AVERY & MACDONALD'S
Neonatology:

Pathophysiology and
Management of
the Newborn

8TH EDITION

Avery & Macdonald's Neonatology

Pathophysiology and Management of the Newborn

8TH EDITION

James P. Boardman, BSc, MSc, MBBS, FRCPCH, PhD
Professor of Neonatal Medicine
The University of Edinburgh
Edinburgh, United Kingdom

Alan M. Groves, MBChB, FRCPCH, MD
Associate Professor
Department of Pediatrics
Dell Medical School
University of Texas at Austin
Austin, Texas

Jayashree Ramasethu, MBBS, DCH, MD, FAAP
Professor of Clinical Pediatrics
Georgetown University Medical Center
Division of Neonatal Perinatal Medicine
MedStar Georgetown University Hospital
Washington, District of Columbia

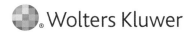

Philadelphia • Baltimore • New York • London
Buenos Aires • Hong Kong • Sydney • Tokyo

Acquisitions Editor: Colleen Dietzler
Development Editor: Thomas Celona
Editorial Coordinator: Julie Kostelnik
Marketing Manager: Kirsten Watrud
Production Project Manager: Bridgett Dougherty
Design Coordinator: Stephen Druding
Manufacturing Coordinator: Beth Welsh
Prepress Vendor: SPi Global

8th Edition

Cataloging-in-Publication Data available on request from the Publisher

ISBN: 978-1-9751-2925-5

shop.lww.com

Dedication

To all the infants, families, and staff who make the NICU environment so extraordinary and in memory of health care workers around the world who lost their lives to the Covid-19 pandemic.

To my parents, Ann and Peter, the most inspiring life-long learners, and to my wife, Kathleen, and children Alexander, Juliet, Luke, and Daniel, who continually teach me about the things in life that have no words.

James P. Boardman

I would personally like to dedicate this book to my family, in particular to my incredible wife Abby, and adorable children Eve and Cormac.

Alan M. Groves

I thank my mother Padma, my husband Prakash and the rest of my family Raji, Viji, Gaurav, and Chandu, my friends, and colleagues at work who are like a second family. This work could not have been accomplished without their steadfast support.

Jayashree Ramasethu

Contributors

Shawn K. Ahlfeld, MD
Assistant Professor
Division of Neonatology and Pulmonary Biology
Department of Pediatrics
University of Cincinnati
Cincinnati Children's Hospital Medical Center
Cincinnati, Ohio

Samia Aleem, MD, MHS
Medical Instructor in Pediatrics
Division of Neonatal–Perinatal Medicine
Department of Pediatrics
Duke University Medical Center
Duke Clinical Research Institute
Durham, North Carolina

Ruben E. Alvaro, MD, FAAP
Medical Director of Neonatology
St. Boniface Hospital
Medical Director
Neonatal Control of Breathing Lab
Department of Pediatrics
Associate Professor of Pediatrics
University of Manitoba
Winnipeg, Manitoba, Canada

Kristian Aquilina, FRCS(SN), MD
Honorary Associate Professor
University College London Great Ormond Street Institute
    of Child Health
Consultant Paediatric Neurosurgeon
Great Ormond Street Hospital
London, United Kingdom

Judy L. Aschner, MD
Professor
Pediatrics
Hackensack Meridian School of Medicine
Nutley, New Jersey

Marvin I. Gottlieb, MD, PhD
Chair of Pediatrics and Physician-in-Chief
Pediatrics
Joseph M. Sanzari Children's Hospital at Hackensack Meridian
University Medical Center
Hackensack, New Jersey

David Askenazi, MD, MSPH, FASN
Professor of Pediatrics
University of Alabama at Birmingham
Medical Director
Pediatric and Infant Center for Acute Nephrology
Children's of Alabama
Birmingham, Alabama

Gerri R. Baer, MD
Supervisory Medical Officer
U.S. Food and Drug Administration, Office of the Commissioner,
    Office of Pediatric Therapeutics
Silver Spring, Maryland

Andrew Berry, AM, MB BS, FRACP
State Director, NETS (NSW)
Senior Lecturer, UNSW
Sydney Children's Hospitals Network
New South Wales, Australia

Elizabeth J. Bhoj, MD, PhD
Assistant Professor of Pediatrics and Human Genetics
Children's Hospital of Philadelphia
University of Pennsylvania
Philadelphia, Pennsylvania

Vinod K. Bhutani, MD, FAAP
Professor of Pediatrics (Neonatology)
Division of Neonatal and Developmental Medicine
Department of Pediatrics
Lucile Packard Children's Hospital at Stanford
Stanford University School of Medicine
Stanford, California

Zulfiqar A. Bhutta, FRS, MBBS, FRCPCH, FAAP, PhD
Distinguished University Professor and Founding Director
Institute for Global Health and Development
The Aga Khan University
South Central Asia, East Africa & United Kingdom
Karachi, Pakistan
Codirector, SickKids Centre for Global Child Health
The Hospital for Sick Children
Toronto, Ontario, Canada

David Blundell, MBChB
Paediatric Cardiology Registrar
Freeman Hospital
Newcastle upon Tyne, United Kingdom

Lauren H. Boal, MD
Instructor in Pediatrics
Harvard Medical School
Assistant in Pediatrics
Division of Pediatric Hematology and Oncology
Department of Pediatrics
Mass General Hospital for Children
Boston, Massachusetts

James P. Boardman, BSc, MSc, MBBS, FRCPCH, PhD
Professor of Neonatal Medicine
The University of Edinburgh
Edinburgh, United Kingdom

Margo Sheck Breilyn, MD
Assistant Professor
Division of Pediatric Genetic Medicine
Albert Einstein College of Medicine
The Children's Hospital at Montefiore
Bronx, New York

Luc P. Brion, MD
Professor of Pediatrics
Division of Neonatal–Perinatal Medicine
Department of Pediatrics
UT Southwestern Medical Center
Parkland Health & Hospital System
Children's Medical Center at Dallas
Clements University Hospital
Texas Health Resources, Presbyterian–Dallas
Dallas, Texas

Jason R. Buckley, MD
Assistant Professor of Pediatrics
Medical Director, Pediatric Cardiac Intensive Care Unit
Division of Cardiology
Department of Pediatrics
Medical University of South Carolina
Charleston, South Carolina

Barbara K. Burton, MD
Professor of Pediatrics
Northwestern University Feinberg School of Medicine
Attending Physician
Division of Genetics, Birth Defects and Metabolism
Ann & Robert H. Lurie Children's Hospital of Chicago
Chicago, Illinois

Susan C. Campisi, PhD
Postdoctoral Research Fellow
Centre for Global Child Health
The Hospital for Sick Children
Toronto, Ontario, Canada

Joseph B. Cantey, MD, MPH
Associate Professor of Pediatrics
Division of Neonatology
Division of Allergy, Immunology, and Infectious Diseases
University of Texas Health San Antonio
University Hospital System
San Antonio, Texas

Bianca Carducci, MSc
Centre for Global Child Health
The Hospital for Sick Children
Toronto, Ontario, Canada

Subarna Chakravorty, MBBS, PhD, FRCP, FRCPath, MRCPCH
Honorary Senior Lecturer
School of Cancer and Pharmaceutical Sciences
King's College London
Consultant Paediatric Haematologist
Paediatrics
King's College Hospital NHS Trust
London, United Kingdom

Ha-young Choi, MD
Assistant Professor of Clinical Pediatrics
Georgetown University Medical Center
Attending Neonatologist
Division of Neonatal Perinatal Medicine
MedStar Georgetown University Hospital
Washington, District of Columbia

Kai-wen Chuang, MD
Assistant Clinical Professor
Department of Urology
University of California, Irvine
Irvine, California
Pediatric Urologist
Children's Hospital of Orange County
Orange, California

Josef M. Cortez, MD
Associate Professor of Pediatrics
Division of Neonatology
College of Medicine Jacksonville
University of Florida
Medical Director, NICU
UF Health Jacksonville
Jacksonville, Florida

John M. Costello, MD, MPH
Professor of Pediatrics
Vice Chair of Clinical Research, Department of Pediatrics
Director of Research, Children's Heart Center
Division of Cardiology
Department of Pediatrics
Medical University of South Carolina
Charleston, South Carolina

Serena J. Counsell, PhD
Professor of Perinatal Imaging & Health
Centre for the Developing Brain
King's College London
Head of Advanced Neuroimaging
Centre for the Developing Brain
King's College London
London, United Kingdom

Ian P. Crocker, PhD
Senior Lecturer
Maternal and Fetal Health Research Centre
School of Medical Sciences
University of Manchester
Manchester, United Kingdom

David S. Crossland, MBChB, MRCPCH
Associate Clinical Lecturer
Congenital Heart Disease Research Group
Population Health Sciences Institute
Newcastle University
Newcastle upon Tyne, United Kingdom
Consultant Paediatric and Adult Congenital Heart Disease
  Cardiologist
Freeman Hospital
Newcastle upon Tyne, United Kingdom

Rose Crowley, BA, MBBS, MRCPCH, MSc
Specialist Registrar in Neonatal Medicine
Neonatal Department
University College London Hospital
London, United Kingdom

Diomel M. de la Cruz, MD
Assistant Professor
Division of Neonatology
Department of Pediatrics
College of Medicine
University of Florida
Gainesville, Florida

Anna L. David, MBChB, PhD, FRCOG
Professor and Consultant in Obstetrics and Maternal Fetal Medicine
Director, Elizabeth Garrett Anderson Institute for Women's Health
University College London
London, United Kingdom
Hon Professor of Fetal Medicine
KU Leuven
Leuven, Belgium
Consultant in Obstetrics and Maternal Fetal Medicine
University College London Hospitals NHS Foundation Trust
London, United Kingdom

Jonathan M. Davis, MD
Vice Chair of Pediatrics
Chief of Newborn Medicine
Tufts Children's Hospital
Professor of Pediatrics
Tufts University School of Medicine
Boston, Massachusetts

Suneetha Desiraju, MD
Instructor, Neonatal–Perinatal Medicine
Sheila S. and Lawrence C. Pakula, MD Fellow
Department of Pediatrics
Johns Hopkins University School of Medicine
Baltimore, Maryland

Miren B. Dhudasia, MBBS, MPH
Research Assistant
Center for Pediatric Clinical Effectiveness
Division of Neonatology
Children's Hospital of Philadelphia
Philadelphia, Pennsylvania

Nicole R. Dobson, MD
Associate Professor of Pediatrics
Uniformed Services University
Program Director
Neonatal–Perinatal Medicine Fellowship
Walter Reed National Military Medical Center
Bethesda, Maryland

George J. Dover, MD
University Distinguished Professor Emeritus
Department of Pediatrics
John's Hopkins Hospital
Johns Hopkins University School of Medicine
Baltimore, Maryland

Leigh E. Dyet, MBBS, MRCPCH, PhD
Honorary Associate Professor
UCL Institute of Women's Health
Consultant in Neonatal Medicine
Neonatal Department
University College London Hospital
London, United Kingdom

Deborah M. Eastwood, FRCS
Consultant Paediatric Orthopaedic Surgeon
Associate Professor
Department of Paediatric Orthopaedics
Great Ormond Street Hospital for Children and the Royal National
    Orthopaedic Hospital
University College London
London, United Kingdom

David Edwards, MA, MBBS, DSc, FRCR, FRCP, FRCPCH, FMedSci
Professor of Paediatrics and Neonatal Medicine
Director, Centre for the Developing Brain
Head of Department of Perinatal Imaging and Health
King's College London
Consultant Neonatologist
Guy's and St Thomas' NHS Trust
Group Leader
MRC Centre for Neurodevelopmental Disorders
NIHR Senior Investigator Emeritus
London, United Kingdom

Afrodite Psaros Einberg, MD, PhD
Senior Consultant
Department of Pediatric Gastroenterology, Hepatology and
    Nutrition
Astrid Lindgren Children's Hospital
Karolinska University Hospital
CLINTEC
Karolinska Institutet
Stockholm, Sweden

Mark I. Evans, MD
Professor of Obstetrics and Gynecology
Icahn School of Medicine at Mt. Sinai
Director, Comprehensive Genetics
President, Fetal Medicine Foundation of America
New York, New York

Shara M. Evans, Msc, MPH
PhD Candidate
Maternal and Child Health
Gillings School of Public Health
University of North Carolina at Chapel Hill
Chapel Hill, North Carolina

Penny M. Feldman, MD
Associate Professor of Pediatrics
Department of Pediatrics
University of Massachusetts Medical School
Pediatric Endocrinologist
UMass Memorial Children's Medical Center
UMass Memorial Health Care
Worcester, Massachusetts

Björn Fischler, MD, PhD
Adjunct Professor of Pediatrics
Senior Consultant
Department of Pediatrics
CLINTEC
Karolinska Institutet and Karolinska University Hospital
Stockholm, Sweden

Dustin D. Flannery, DO, MSCE
Assistant Professor of Pediatrics
Perelman School of Medicine
University of Pennsylvania
Attending Physician
Pennsylvania Hospital
Division of Neonatology
Children's Hospital of Philadelphia
Philadelphia, Pennsylvania

Joseph T. Flynn, MD, MS
Dr. Robert O. Hickman Endowed Chair in Pediatric
    Nephrology
Professor of Pediatrics, University of Washington
Chief, Division of Nephrology
Seattle Children's Hospital
Seattle, Washington

Jonathan M. Gamiao, BS
Research Associate
Department of Pediatrics
School of Medicine
Wayne State University
Detroit, Michigan

Rebekah C. Gardea, BSN
School of Nursing
University of Texas Health San Antonio
University Hospital System
San Antonio, Texas

Bruce D. Gelb, MD
Gogel Family Professor of Child Health and Development
Professor of Pediatrics and Genetics and Genomic Sciences
Director, Mindich Child Health and Development Institute
Icahn School of Medicine at Mount Sinai
New York, New York

Michael K. Georgieff, MD
Martin Lenz Harrison Land Grant Professor
Departments of Pediatrics, Child Psychology and Obstetrics/
    Gynecology
Medical School and College of Education and Human
    Development
University of Minnesota
Minneapolis, Minnesota

Regan E. Giesinger, MD, FRCPC
Clinical Associate Professor
University of Iowa
Director, Neonatal Hemodynamics Program
Director, Neonatal Transport Program
Associate Director, Neonatal–Perinatal Medicine
    Fellowship
Iowa City, IA

Dana Brabbing-Goldstein, MD
Senior Physician
Genetics Institute
Tel Aviv Sourasky Medical Center
Tel Aviv, Israel

Pierre Gressens, MD, PhD
Director
Université de Paris, Inserm UMR 1141
NeuroDiderot
Paris, France
Professor of Foetal and Neonatal Neurology
Centre for the Developing Brain
King's College London
London, United Kingdom
Child Neurologist
Robert Debré Hospital
Paris, France

Alan M. Groves, MBChB, FRCPCH, FAAP, MD
Associate Professor
Department of Pediatrics
Dell Medical School
University of Texas at Austin
Austin, Texas

Sarah Guillon, MD, MRes
Chef de Clinique Assistant
Medical School
University of Paris
Chef de Clinique Assistant
Maternity
Robert Debré Hospital
Paris, France

Kaiane A. Habeshian, MD
Assistant Professor
George Washington School of Medicine
Attending Physician, Pediatric Dermatologist
Dermatology and Pediatrics
Children's National Hospital
Washington, District of Columbia

Annie Harrington, MSN, CPNP-PC
Pediatric Nurse Practitioner
Division of Pediatric Surgery
Department of Surgery
Icahn School of Medicine
Mount Sinai Medical Center
Mount Sinai, New York

J. M. Hawdon, MA, MBBS, MRCP, FRCPCH, PhD
Consultant Neonatologist
Medical Director
Responsible Officer
Royal Free London NHS Foundation Trust
London, United Kingdom

Angela Huertas-Ceballos, MD, MSc, FRCPCH
Consultant Neonatologist
Lead Clinician for the Neurodevelopmental Follow-up Service
University College London Hospitals NHS Foundation Trust
London, United Kingdom

Carl E. Hunt, MD
Research Professor of Pediatrics
Research Director, Neonatology Fellowship Program
F. Edward Hébert School of Medicine–"America's Medical School"
Uniformed Services University
Bethesda, Maryland
Adjunct Professor of Pediatrics
George Washington University
Washington, District of Columbia

Sherwin J. Isenberg, MD
Distinguished Professor Emeritus of Ophthalmology and Pediatrics
Stein Eye Institute
Department of Ophthalmology
UCLA School of Medicine
Los Angeles, California

Amish Jain, MBBS, MRCPCH (UK), PhD (Physiology)
Staff Neonatologist
Mount Sinai Hospital Director
Targeted Neonatal Echocardiography and Hemodynamic Program
Associate Professor
University of Toronto
Clinician-Scientist
Lunenfeld-Tanenbaum Research Institute
Toronto, Ontario, Canada

Caroline Jones, MBBS
Consultant Fetal and Paediatric Cardiologist
Alder Hey Children's NHS Foundation Trust
Liverpool, United Kingdom

Hendrée E. Jones, PhD
Executive Director, UNC Horizons
Professor
Department of Obstetrics and Gynecology
School of Medicine
The University of North Carolina at Chapel Hill
Chapel Hill, North Carolina

Jeremy B. Jones, MBChB, MRCP, FRCR, DipMedEd
Consultant Paediatric Radiologist
Royal Hospital for Children and Young People
Training Programme Director
South East Scotland Radiology Training Programme
Honorary Clinical Senior Lecturer
The University of Edinburgh
Edinburgh, United Kingdom

Karen L. Kamholz, MD, MPH
Associate Professor of Clinical Pediatrics
Georgetown University Medical Center
Program Director, Neonatal–Perinatal Medicine Fellowship
    Program
MedStar Georgetown University Hospital
Washington, District of Columbia

Amanda G. Sandoval Karamian, MD
Pediatric Epilepsy Fellow
Division of Neurology
Children's Hospital of Philadelphia
Philadelphia, Pennsylvania

David W. Kimberlin, MD
Professor and Vice Chair for Clinical and Translational
    Research
Codirector, Division of Pediatric Infectious Diseases
Department of Pediatrics
The University of Alabama at Birmingham
Birmingham, Alabama

Paul S. Kingma, MD, PhD
Adjunct Associate Professor
Division of Neonatology and Pulmonary Biology
Department of Pediatrics
University of Cincinnati
Cincinnati Children's Hospital Medical Center
Cincinnati, Ohio

Joy E. Lawn, MBBS, FRCP (Paeds), MPH, PhD, FMedSci
Professor of Maternal, Reproductive and Child Health
    Epidemiology
Director MARCH Centre (Maternal Adolescent Reproductive &
    Child Health)
London School of Hygiene & Tropical Medicine
London, United Kingdom

Mary M. Lee, MD, FAAP
Executive Vice President and Chief Scientific Officer
Nemours Children's Health
Physician in Chief
Nemours Children's Health
Nemours Children's Hospital
Wilmington, Delaware
Professor of Pediatrics
Sidney Kimmel Medical College
Jefferson University
Philadelphia, Pennsylvania

Shoo K. Lee, OC, DHC, PhD, FRCPC, MBBS
Professor of Paediatrics, Obstetrics & Gynecology, and Public
    Health
University of Toronto
Neonatologist and Director of The Maternal Infant Care Research
    Center (MiCARE)
Mount Sinai Hospital
Toronto, Ontario, Canada

Scott A. Lorch, MD, MSCE
Kristine Sandberg Knisely Professor of Pediatrics
Perelman School of Medicine
University of Pennsylvania
Attending Neonatologist
Associate Chair
Director of Clinical and Epidemiological Research
Division of Neonatology
The Children's Hospital of Philadelphia
Philadelphia, Pennsylvania

Maria Magnusson, MD, PhD
Associated Researcher
Clinical Chemistry and Blood Coagulation Research
MMK
Department of Pediatrics
CLINTEC
Karolinska Institutet
Head of Coagulation Unit
Senior Consultant Pediatric & Adult Coagulation
Department of Hematology
Karolinska University Hospital
Stockholm, Sweden

Krishelle L. Marc-Aurele, MD
Program Director, Neonatal–Perinatal Fellowship Program
Associate Professor
Divisions of Neonatology and Palliative Medicine
Department of Pediatrics
Rady Children's Hospital
University of California San Diego
San Diego, California

Luciana Marcondes, MD, FRACP
Paediatric and Adult Congenital Electrophysiologist
Paediatric and Congenital Cardiac Services
Starship Children's Health
Auckland, New Zealand

Alison Maresh, MD
Assistant Professor
Otolaryngology–Head & Neck Surgery
Weill Cornell Medicine
New York, New York

Gilbert I. Martin, MD
Professor of Pediatrics and Neonatology
Loma Linda Children's Hospital
Loma Linda, California
Director
NICU–Emeritus
Emanate Health
West Covina, California

Nahya Salim Masoud, MD, MMED, PhD
Paediatrician, Research Scientist, and Senior Lecturer
Department of Paediatrics and Child Health
Muhimbili University of Health and Allied Sciences
Dar es Salaam
United Republic of Tanzania

Irene M. McAleer, MD, JD, MBA
Health Science Clinical Professor (ret.)
Department Of Urology
University of California
Irvine, California
Pediatric Urologist
Providence Children's Hospital
El Paso, Texas

Jessica M. McGovern, DO
Assistant Professor of Clinical Pediatrics
Georgetown University Medical Center
Division of Neonatal Perinatal Medicine
MedStar Georgetown University Hospital
Washington, District of Columbia

Katie Mckinnon, MBBS, BA, PGCMedEd, MRCPCH
Clinical Research Fellow, Neonatology
University College London Hospital NHS Foundation Trust
London, United Kingdom

Patrick J. McNamara, MB BCh, BAO, MSc, MRCPCH
Division Chief, Neonatology
Vice Chair Pediatric Acute Care Services
Department of Pediatrics
Stead Family Children's Hospital
Professor of Pediatrics
University of Iowa
Iowa City, Iowa

Eugenio Mercuri, MD
Professor of Pediatric Neurology
Department of Pediatrics
Catholic University
Head of the Pediatric Neurology Unit
Department of Pediatrics
Fondazione Policlinico Gemelli
Rome, Italy

Peter S. Midulla, MD, FACS, FAAP
Surgeon-in-Chief
Kravis Children's Hospital
New York, New York

Neena Modi, MBChB, MD, FRCP, FRCPCH, FFPM, FMedSci
Professor of Neonatal Medicine
Department of Primary Care and Public Health
Imperial College London
Consultant in Neonatal Medicine
Chelsea and Westminster Hospital
London, United Kingdom

Vikash K. Modi, MD
Chief, Pediatric Otolaryngology–Head & Neck Surgery
Associate Professor
Weill Cornell Medical Center
NewYork-Presbyterian Hospital
New York, New York

Gregory P. Moore, MD, FRCPC, MSt (c)
Academic Neonatologist
Department of Pediatrics
CHEO (The Children's Hospital of Eastern Ontario)
Department of Obstetrics, Gynecology and Newborn Care
The Ottawa Hospital
Faculty of Medicine
University of Ottawa
Clinical Investigator
CHEO Research Institute
Clinical Investigator
The Ottawa Hospital Research Institute
Ottawa, Ontario, Canada

Suhas M. Nafday, MD, MRCP (Ire), DCH, FAAP
Professor of Pediatrics
Division of Neonatology
Department of Pediatrics
Albert Einstein College of Medicine
Director, Newborn Services
Children's Hospital at Montefiore–Einstein
Chairman
Neonatal Performance Improvement and Patient Safety at Einstein
Bronx, New York

Amy T. Nathan, MD
Associate Professor
Division of Neonatology and Pulmonary Biology
Department of Pediatrics
University of Cincinnati
Cincinnati Children's Hospital Medical Center
Cincinnati, Ohio

Josef Neu, MD
Professor of Pediatrics
University of Florida
Neonatologist
University of Florida Health Science Center
Gainesville, Florida

Colm P. F. O'Donnell, MB, FRCPI, PhD
Consultant Neonatologist
National Maternity Hospital
Professor
School of Medicine
University College Dublin
Dublin, Ireland

Enrique M. Ostrea Jr, MD
Professor of Pediatrics
Wayne State University
Neonatologist
Hutzel Women's Hospital
Children's Hospital of Michigan
Detroit, Michigan

Marika Pane, MD, PhD
Associate Professor
Child Neurology and Psychiatry
Catholic University
Head of the Neuromuscular Unit
Nemo Center, Department of Pediatrics
Fondazione Policlinico Gemelli, IRCCS
Rome, Italy

Stephen W. Patrick, MD, MPH, MS, FAAP
Director, Vanderbilt Center for Child Health Policy
Associate Professor of Pediatrics and Health Policy
Division of Neonatology
Vanderbilt University Medical Center
Nashville, Tennessee

Stacy L. Pineles, MD, MS
Jerome and Joan Snyder Chair in Ophthalmology
Director, Ophthalmology Residency Program
Pediatric Ophthalmology, Adult Strabismus,
    Neuro-Ophthalmology
Stein Eye Institute
Department of Ophthalmology
UCLA
Los Angeles, California

Swetha G. Pinninti, MD
Assistant Professor of Pediatrics
Division of Pediatric Infectious Diseases
University of Alabama at Birmingham
Birmingham, Alabama

Gloria S. Pryhuber, MD
Professor
Division of Pediatrics and Environmental Medicine
University of Rochester Medical Center
Rochester, New York

Karen M. Puopolo, MD, PhD
Associate Professor of Pediatrics
Perelman School of Medicine
University of Pennsylvania
Chief, Section on Newborn Medicine
Pennsylvania Hospital
Division of Neonatology
Children's Hospital of Philadelphia
Philadelphia, Pennsylvania

Jayashree Ramasethu, MBBS, DCH, MD, FAAP
Professor of Clinical Pediatrics
Georgetown University Medical Center
Division of Neonatal Perinatal Medicine
MedStar Georgetown University Hospital
Washington, District of Columbia

Sara E. Ramel, MD
Associate Professor
Division of Neonatology
Department of Pediatrics
Medical School
University of Minnesota
Minneapolis, Minnesota

Irene Roberts, MBChB, MD(Hons), DRCOG, FRCP, FRCPath, FRCPCH, MD
Emeritus Professor of Paediatric Haematology
Department of Paediatrics
Oxford University
MRC Investigator
Molecular Haematology Unit
Weatherall Institute of Molecular Medicine
John Radcliffe Hospital
Oxford, United Kingdom

Adalina Sacco, MD, MRCOG, MRCP, MBBS
Academic Clinical Lecturer
Institute for Women's Health
University College London
Maternal–Fetal Medicine Subspecialty Trainee
Women's Health
University College London Hospital
London, United Kingdom

Samantha Sadoo, MBBS, BSc, DTMH, MRCPCH
Research Fellow
Centre for Maternal, Adolescent, Reproductive and Child Health
London School of Hygiene and Tropical Medicine
Paediatric Registrar
Neonatal Unit
University College London Hospital
London, United Kingdom

Jeffrey M. Saland, MD, MSCR
Professor and Chief of Pediatric Nephrology and Hypertension
Director, Pediatric Nephrology Fellowship Program
Mount Sinai Kravis Children's Hospital
Icahn School of Medicine at Mount Sinai
New York, New York

Matthew A. Saxonhouse, MD
Associate Professor
Division of Neonatology
Codirector Neonatal Thrombosis Center
Levine Children's Hospital
Atrium Healthcare
Charlotte, North Carolina

Kristin Scheible, MD
Associate Professor
Director, Complex Delivery Team
Division of Neonatology
Department of Pediatrics
University of Rochester Medical Center
Golisano Children's Hospital at Strong
Rochester, New York

Luke W. Schroeder, MD
Assistant Professor of Pediatrics
Division of Cardiology
Department of Pediatrics
Medical University of South Carolina
Charleston, South Carolina

Robert A. Silverman, MD
Clinical Associate Professor
Georgetown University Medical Center
Attending Physician, Pediatric Dermatologist
Departments of Pediatrics and Dermatology
MedStar Georgetown University Hospital
Washington, District of Columbia

Jonathan R. Skinner, MBChB, DCH, MRCP(UK), FRACP, MD
Honorary Professor of Paediatrics, Child and Youth Health
University of Auckland
Auckland, New Zealand
Paediatric Cardiologist/Electrophysiologist
Heart Centre for Children
Sydney Children's Hospitals Network
Sydney, Australia

Judith A. Smith, MHA, ACHE
Principal/Co-Founder
Women and Children's Health Services–Strategic, Operational and Facility Planning
Smith Hager Bajo, Inc.
Scottsdale, Arizona

Martha Sola-Visner, MD
Associate Professor of Pediatrics
Harvard Medical School
Attending Neonatologist
Director of Newborn Medicine Clinical Research
Division of Newborn Medicine
Boston Children's Hospital
Boston, Massachusetts

Ann R. Stark, MD
Professor in Residence of Pediatrics
Department of Neonatology
Beth Israel Deaconess Medical Center
Harvard Medical School
Boston, Massachusetts

Robin H. Steinhorn, MD
Professor and Vice Dean of Children's Services
Department of Pediatrics
University of California, San Diego
Senior Vice President
Rady Children's Hospital
San Diego, California

Cally J. Tann, MSC, DTMH, FRCPCH, PhD
Associate Professor
Neonatal Health & Development
The Centre for Maternal, Adolescent, Reproductive & Child Health
Honorary Principal Scientist
MRC/UVRI & LSHTM Uganda Research Unit
Uganda
Consultant Neonatologist
University College London Hospitals
Department of Infectious Disease Epidemiology
London School of Hygiene & Tropical Medicine
London, United Kingdom

Janice A. Taylor, MD, MEd, FACS, FAAP
Associate Professor, Pediatric Surgery
Department of Surgery
College of Medicine
University of Florida
Gainesville, Florida

Mark W. Thompson, MD
Assistant Professor
Department of Pediatrics
Uniformed Services University of the Health Sciences
Ft. Bragg, NC

Marianne Thoresen, MD, PhD
Professor of Neonatal Neuroscience
University of Bristol
Consultant Neonatologist
St Michael's Hospital
Bristol, United Kingdom
Professor of Physiology
University of Oslo
Oslo, Norway

Mark A. Turner, FRCPCH, PhD, DRCOG, MRCP(UK), FFPM(Hon)
Professor of Neonatology and Research Delivery
Institute of Life Course and Medical Sciences
University of Liverpool
Consultant Neonatologist
Director of Research and Development
Liverpool Women's NHS Foundation Trust
Liverpool Health Partners
Liverpool, United Kingdom

Sabita Uthaya, MBBS, FRCPCH, MD
Clinical Senior Lecturer
Imperial College London
Consultant in Neonatal Medicine
Chelsea and Westminster NHS Foundation Trust
London, United Kingdom

Maria Esterlita T. Villanueva-Uy, MD, MSPH
Research and Clinical Associate Professor
Institute of Child Health and Human Development
National Institutes of Health
University of the Philippines Manila
Attending Neonatologist
Department of Pediatrics
Philippine General Hospital
University of the Philippines Manila
Manila, Philippines

Sally H. Vitali, MD
Assistant Professor of Anaesthesia
Department of Anaesthesia
Harvard Medical School
Senior Associate in Critical Care Medicine
Anesthesiology, Critical Care and Pain Medicine
Boston Children's Hospital
Boston, Massachusetts

Howard J. Weinstein, MD
R. Alan Ezekowitz Professor of Pediatrics
Harvard Medical School
Chief of Pediatric Hematology and Oncology
Department of Pediatrics
Massachusetts General Hospital for Children
Boston, Massachusetts

Dany Weisz, BSc, MD, MSc
Assistant Professor of Paediatrics
University of Toronto
Staff Neonatologist
Department of Newborn and Developmental Paediatrics
Sunnybrook Health Sciences Centre
Director
Neonatal Hemodynamics and Targeted Neonatal Echocardiography Program
Sunnybrook Health Sciences Centre
Toronto, Ontario, Canada

Tara L. Wenger, MD, PhD
Associate Professor of Pediatrics
Division of Genetic Medicine
Department of Pediatrics
Associate Director of Inpatient Genetic Services
Seattle Children's Hospital
Seattle, Washington

Robert D. White, MD
Director, Regional Newborn Program
Beacon Children's Hospital
South Bend, Indiana

Scott W. White, MBBS, PhD, FRANZCOG, CMFM
Senior Lecturer in Maternal Fetal Medicine
Division of Obstetrics and Gynaecology
The University of Western Australia
Consultant in Maternal Fetal Medicine
King Edward Memorial Hospital
Perth, Western Australia

Andrew Whitelaw, MD, FRCPC
Emeritus Professor of Neonatal Medicine
University of Bristol
Bristol, United Kingdom

Jeffrey A. Whitsett, MD
Professor of Pediatrics
Codirector, Perinatal Institute
Chief, Division of Neonatology and Pulmonary Biology
Department of Medicine
University of Cincinnati
Cincinnati Children's Hospital Medical Center
Cincinnati, Ohio

Hilary E. A. Whyte, MB BCh, MSc, FRCPI, FRCPC
Professor
Department of Paediatrics
University of Toronto
Neonatologist
Division of Neonatology
The Hospital for Sick Children
Medical Director, Acute Care Transport Service
Departments of Paediatrics and Critical Care Medicine
The Hospital for Sick Children
Medical Director
SickKids International
Toronto, Ontario, Canada

Dominic J. C. Wilkinson, FRCPCH, DPhil
Consultant Neonatologist
Oxford University Hospital NHS Foundation Trust
Professor of Medical Ethics
Oxford Uehiro Centre for Practical Ethics
University of Oxford
Oxford, United Kingdom

Craig B. Woda, MD, PhD
Pediatric Hospitalist
Assistant in Medicine
Department of Emergency Medicine
Boston Children's Hospital
Boston, Massachusetts
Pediatric Nephrologist
Department of Pediatric Nephrology
Connecticut Children's Medical Center
Hartford, Connecticut
Pediatric Nephrologist
Department of Pediatric Nephrology
University of Massachusetts Medical Center
Worcester, Massachusetts

Ronald J. Wong, MD
Senior Research Scientist
Division of Neonatal and Developmental Medicine
Department of Pediatrics
Stanford University School of Medicine
Stanford, California

Courtney J. Wusthoff, MD, MS
Associate Professor of Neurology & Neurological Sciences
Pediatrics–Neonatal and Developmental Medicine
Stanford University School of Medicine
Neurology Director, Neuro NICU
Lucile Packard Children's Hospital Stanford
Palo Alto, California

Yuval Yaron, MD
Director, Prenatal Genetic Diagnosis Unit
Genetics Institute
Tel Aviv Sourasky Medical Center
Tel Aviv, Israel

Amir M. Zayegh, MBBS, BMedSci, FRACP, MSt, DipMgmt
Consultant Neonatologist
The Royal Women's Hospital Melbourne
Melbourne, Australia

Sinai C. Zyblewski, MD, MSCR
Professor of Pediatrics
Director, Fetal Cardiology
Director, Pediatric Cardiology Fellowship Program
Division of Cardiology
Department of Pediatrics
Medical University of South Carolina
Charleston, South Carolina

Foreword

"Medicine is the only world-wide profession, following everywhere the same methods, actuated by the same ambitions, and pursuing the same ends."

Sir William Osler (1849–1919). Aequanimitas, with other addresses, "Unity, Peace and Concord."

The baton passed to the talented new editors was a heavy one. They have created an eighth edition of *Neonatology* that is valuable in countries with scarcer health care resources, while retaining the utility of the textbook for providers in countries with extensive medical infrastructure. Global health is now an established discipline that recognizes the growing consensus underlying many new medical practices. In lower- and middle-income countries, major funding sources are increasingly investing in the application of care strategies proven in wealthier nations.

The continued emphasis on pathophysiological principles is supported by ongoing positive reader feedback since the publication of the first edition in 1975. To make the new edition more reader-friendly, the flow of subheadings is standardized across chapters and the uniformity of the template for tables and flow charts improved. Redundancy of information across chapters is minimized, in turn enhancing the search/bookmarking program.

The editors have delivered a fine textbook, and the knowledge that the future of *Neonatology* is in such good hands has heightened our serenity in retirement.

Gordon B. Avery, MD, PhD, FAAP
Mhairi G. MacDonald, MBChB, DCH, FRCP(E),
FAAP, FRCPCH

Preface

Neonatal medicine came of age in the second half of the twentieth century. It developed at a rapid pace, building upon principles and methods established by pioneers of medicine and science from earlier eras. Rapid scientific discoveries provided the speciality with intellectual underpinnings that advanced understanding of infant health and illness, and eradicated or diminished diseases. These have had a huge impact on the health and survival of babies around the world.

Our appreciation of chemistry and biochemistry, cellular and molecular biology, physiology and pathophysiology, (epi)genetics and (epi)genomics, immunology, epidemiology, neuroscience, trials methodology, implementation science, and so many other disciplines has mushroomed. This explosion of knowledge and understanding has led to hitherto unimagined therapies that have turned once fatal problems into matters of everyday practice. For example, it has led to vaccines that have eliminated or virtually eliminated diseases that killed or destroyed the lives of millions in the past, and therapies that have saved the lives of hundreds of thousands of children who happen to enter the world too small or too soon. There is still much work to do: we must improve implementation of treatments that we know work in a way that is fair and equitable across societies; mechanistic understanding of many diseases is rudimentary and this hampers the development of preventive and therapeutic strategies; where therapies do exist, we must get better at giving the right treatment at the right time to the right baby; we must place parents and caregivers at the heart of what we do; we must work hard to reduce health disparities within and between countries; and we must strive to shape policy so that the interests of children are promoted amidst ever-increasing demands placed on health care systems. Science and education are at the heart of these goals.

The explosive growth in understanding of infant health and disease and a solid grasp of new technologies and methods that underpin discovery can seem formidable, even overwhelming. As a result, there can arise a tendency to take the scientific foundations of the speciality for granted and to lose sight of the history of the speciality—its triumphs and its (sometimes fatal) failings—and the essential need to understand mechanisms of disease and treatment. This concerns us enormously because it has serious consequences. Diagnosis and prognosis rely increasingly on an ability to mesh careful clinical assessment with pathophysiology, genetics, molecular biology, and advanced imaging; therapeutics is becoming more precise and sophisticated in targeting specific steps and mediators of disease. Changes in the type and amount of data available about a patient and his or her disease require us to understand the nature of disease in greater depth than ever before and to be able to relate this to the individual we are treating. Instead, there is a trend to resort to treatment guidelines for generic groups of patients, often created by others. While treatment guidelines frequently provide the core components of safe, effective care pathways, they may also lead to practitioners taking circuitous routes to diagnoses, reaching imprecise prognoses, and recommending treatments they do not fully understand. We believe that deep understanding of physiology and pathophysiology enhances our ability to understand symptoms and clinical presentations; practice using an individualized approach; have a realistic understanding of effect sizes and side effects of treatments; make the most judicious use of diagnostic and prognostic tools; design research studies with maximum efficiency and impact; and interpret evidence.

This is a textbook of neonatology. In order to help lifelong students of neonatology (all of us), we hope to equip them with the knowledge they need to tackle diseases of the newborn, secure in the knowledge that deep understanding of how pathophysiology drives disease will enable them to be effective practitioners. We have taken deep dives into the principles of disease that have stood the test of time, described advances in technology, and linked both to the practice of neonatal medicine.

Experts from around the world present a thorough but accessible understanding of how diseases occur and how their pathophysiology drives management. This edition of the book differs from its predecessors. Many of the 61 chapters have been rewritten or substantially revised; new author leads of 40 chapters join the outstanding contributors whose continuing efforts have been so valuable. Authors have taken care to recognize that populations and health systems differ around the world, and this impacts the practice of neonatal medicine in different countries. There is timely content about global newborn health, maternal determinants of infant disease, advances in ethical thought about care, neonatal palliative care, family integrated care, early life determinants of life course disease, efficient collection and use of data, and the impact of the Covid-19 pandemic. We have described some of the variations in practice that exist around the world in the hope that we may learn from each other, but this could not be comprehensive for obvious reasons, so where discrepancies or uncertainties exist, we encourage readers to follow the clinical guidance that operates in their own jurisdiction.

We emphasize what is understood, but note the limitations of current knowledge. We hope that enquiring minds will find in this book a door to further exploration and that neonatal practitioners will share the excitement of discovery that we have been privileged to experience in our education and careers so far.

The first edition of this book was published in 1975 as the speciality of neonatal medicine was being born. Subsequent editions retained the founding principles of including information from the bedrock disciplines of anatomy, physiology, and pathology, while keeping pace with scientific and clinical advances and new technologies. For these reasons, each edition has been recognized as *the* authoritative text of the time. We hope that this edition equips all students and practitioners of neonatal medicine with the grounding they need to deliver excellent and effective care in the 2020s.

We are grateful to Julie Kostelnik and Thomas Celona at Wolters Kluwer who worked with enthusiasm, diligence, and organization to help bring the book to fruition; and to Sabari Selvam Venkadachalam, our project manager at SPi Global. Finally, we are indebted to the authors, many of whom made their contributions as Covid-19 upturned their professional, and in some cases, personal lives; they did so with commitment and resolve. We cannot thank them enough.

James P. Boardman, BSc, MSc, MBBS, FRCPCH, PhD
Edinburgh, United Kingdom
Alan M. Groves, MBChB, FRCPCH, MD
Austin, Texas
Jayashree Ramasethu, MBBS, DCH, MD, FAAP
Washington, District of Columbia

Preface to the First Edition

Neonatology means knowledge of the human newborn. The term was coined by Alexander Schaffer, whose book on the subject, *Diseases of the Newborn*, was first published in 1960. This book, together with Clement Smith's *Physiology of the Newborn Infant*, formed cornerstones of the developing field. In the past 15 years, neonatology has grown from the preoccupation of a handful of pioneers to a major subspecialty of pediatrics. Knowledge in this area has so expanded that it now seems important to collect this material into a multiauthor reference work.

Although the perinatal mortality rate has declined over the past 50 years, the best presently attainable survival rates have not been achieved throughout the world, and indeed the United States lags behind 15 other countries, despite its vast resources. New knowledge and improvement in the coordination of services for mother and child are needed to drive down perinatal mortality further. And finally, far greater emphasis must be placed on morbidity, so that surviving infants can lead full and productive lives. One hopes that in the future, the yardstick of success will be the quality of life and not the mere fact of life itself.

In this past decade, neonatology, as a recognized subspecialty of pediatrics, has come into being around the intensive care premature nursery. Needless to say, the problems of prematurity are far from solved. But neonatology is ripe for a broadening out from its prematurity–hyaline membrane disease beginnings. The newborn is heir to so many problems, and his or her physiology is so unique and rapidly changing that all conditions of the newborn should come within the concern of the new and expanding discipline of neonatology. It has long since become standard practice to admit to premature nurseries other high-risk infants such as those of diabetic or toxemic mothers. Here, the criterion is the need for intensive care. However, the neonatologist's specialized knowledge should give him a significant role in the care of other infants in the first 2 to 3 months of life, whether they require intensive care and whether they are readmitted for problems unrelated to prematurity and birth itself. Detailed knowledge of newborn physiology can assist in the management of congenital anomalies; surgical conditions of the neonate; failure to thrive; nutritional problems; genetic, neurologic, and biochemical diseases; and a host of conditions involving delayed maturation. Thus, one can conceive of a subspecialty sharply limited in age to early infancy but broad in its study of the interaction of normal physiology and disease processes.

Neonatology must also grow in its relationship to obstetrics and fetal biology. In the best centers, an active partnership has developed between obstetrics and pediatrics around the management of high-risk pregnancies and newborns. Sometimes training has been cooperative, but in only a few instances have basic scientists concerned with fetal biology been brought into this effort. Important beginnings have been made in studying the fetomaternal unit, such as the endocrine studies of Egon Diczfalusy, the cardiopulmonary studies of Geoffrey Dawes, and the immunologic studies of Arther Silverstein. But fundamental processes such as the controls of fetal growth and the onset of labor are not understood at this time. Centers or institutes bringing together workers of diverse points of view are needed to wrestle with the profound problems of fetal biology. At the clinical level, the interdependence of obstetrics and neonatology is obvious. As an ultimate development, these two specialties may one day be joined as a new entity—perinatology—at least at the level of training and certification. In the meantime, far greater mutual understanding and daily interaction are needed for the optimal care of mothers and their infants.

This book is organized around problems as they occur, as well as by organ systems. It hopes to achieve a balance between presentation of the basic science on which rational management must rest and the advice concerning patient care, which experts in each subarea are qualified to give. Individual chapter authors have approached their subjects in various ways, and no attempt has been made to achieve a completely uniform format. In some instances, there is overlap of subject material, but the somewhat different viewpoints presented, and the desire to spare the reader from hopscotching through the book after cross references, have persuaded me to leave small overlaps undisturbed.

It is appreciated that no volume such as this can have more than a finite useful lifetime. Yet while its currency lasts, I hope it will serve as a practical guide to therapy and an aid in the understanding of pathophysiology for those active in the care of newborns.

Gordon B. Avery, MD, PhD

Contents

PART 1

GENERAL CONSIDERATIONS

1

Newborn Survival in a Global Context

Joy E. Lawn, Samantha Sadoo, Cally J. Tann, and Nahya Salim Masoud

INTRODUCTION

Each year, 5.4 million deaths happen around the time of birth, including 2.5 million newborns within the first 28 days of life, 2.6 million stillbirths, and 0.3 million maternal deaths (1,2). At least 1 million newborns each year survive with long-term disability as a result of complications that occurred around the time of birth (2). Most of these deaths occur in low- and middle-income countries (LMICs) with the highest risk for the poorest families, yet almost all could be prevented.

Remarkable progress has been made for maternal and child health in recent decades. Since 1990, global child deaths under the age of five have been reduced by about two-thirds, and maternal deaths by more than 50% (3). However, progress for neonatal mortality has been much slower and now nearly half of under-five deaths worldwide are in the neonatal period (first 28 days of life) (1). In 2015, the first ever global target for newborn survival was agreed, and many LMICs have made national commitments to this target (4). Some countries are starting to make rapid progress for newborn survival, and many are now investing in hospital care including for preterm newborns. However, stillbirths are reducing more slowly and still have limited global attention.

This chapter provides an overview of the global context including relevant goals and action plans and current status for newborns around the world; and it provides the evidence base for interventions and how to implement these. The final section gives suggestions on what pediatricians, neonatologists, nurses, and all concerned can do to accelerate progress for every newborn around the world.

GLOBAL CONTEXT

Sustainable Development Goals for 2030

The 17 Sustainable Development Goals (SDGs) were adopted by all United Nations (UN) Member States in 2015, with goal 3 being the only one focused on health (**Fig. 1.1**) (4). The first health target (3.1) is focused on ending preventable maternal deaths, reaching a global average maternal mortality ratio of 70/100,000 births, with a number of different thresholds per country, requiring analyses for each country to set targets. Target 3.2 is to end preventable child and newborn deaths. Since 1990 and the global summit for children, there have been several iterations of targets for under-five deaths worldwide. SDG 3.2 gives the current target, which is for all countries to reach a mortality rate of 25 or lower for children under the age of 5 years by 2030 (4).

For the first time ever, there is an explicit global goal for newborn survival: that every country by 2030 reach a neonatal mortality rate (NMR) of 12 deaths or lower per 1,000 live births (**Fig. 1.2**). This target was based on analyses in the Lancet Every Newborn series 2014, with extensive consultation in more than 60 countries, three regional meetings, and many UN-led fora (2,5–8). Despite many appeals by countries, organizations, and individuals, stillbirths were not counted in these SDGs (4).

To advance progress toward these targets, the UN Secretary General launched the "Global Strategy (2016–2030) for Women, Children, and Adolescent health," which was based on three pillars; "Survive," "Thrive," and "Transform" (**Panel 1.1**) (9). Under "Survive," as well as SDG targets for maternal, child, and neonatal mortality, the Strategy does include a stillbirth target: for each country to reduce their stillbirth rate (SBR) to 12 or fewer per 1,000 births by 2030, which was based on analyses in the Lancet Every Newborn 2014, although the stillbirth target was omitted from the SDGs (4–9).

Newborn onto the Global Agenda

Newborn health was neglected on the global health agenda. It was assumed that there would be a "trickle down" effect from improvements in maternal or child health; however, newborn health was often dropped between maternal and child health programs. A number of myths also affected action, including the perception that newborn care was expensive and impossible in resource-poor settings.

In 2005, the Lancet Neonatal Survival Series was published, bringing new data to show where, when, and why newborn deaths occur, and highlighted the potential to reduce global neonatal deaths by two-thirds through high-impact interventions in integrated packages of care (10–13). Importantly, about a third of potential for lives saved was through community-based interventions, since at that point most births in LMICs were at home (11). The series in 2005 also developed an approach for integrated service delivery packages across the continuum of care (antenatal, intrapartum, and postpartum), at community and facility level. In 2014, The Lancet published another series "Every Newborn," providing the basis for the first newborn survival target now included in global goals, and emphasizing the shift beyond survival alone (2,5–8). Following this series, the Every Newborn Action Plan (ENAP) was unanimously passed at the World Health Assembly providing a roadmap to end preventable neonatal mortality and stillbirths, and contribute to reducing maternal mortality (**Panel 1.2**) (14). The ENAP has galvanized commitment and action, with more than 90 countries reporting each year on changes, and more than 78 countries setting a specific target for NMR reduction by 2030.

Stillbirths Are Still Stillborn on the Global Agenda

Stillbirths have been almost invisible on the global health agenda with a notable lack of targets, and progress has been substantially slower than for maternal, neonatal, and under-five child mortality. The Lancet published the first "Stillbirth" series in 2011, highlighting the burden, causes, and cost-effective interventions (15–20). In 2015, there were an estimated 2.6 million third trimester stillbirths globally, with little improvement since 2011, although most stillbirths are preventable (21–25). National SBRs range from less than 5 per 1,000 total births in high-income countries (HICs) to

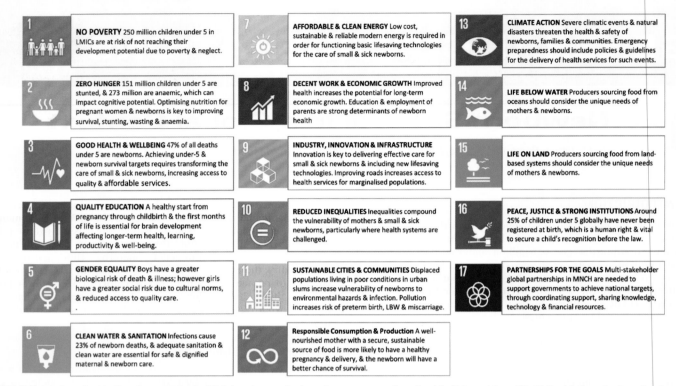

FIGURE 1.1 Sustainable Development Goals (SDGs) noting particular relevance to newborn health. (Adapted from World Health Organization; *Survive and thrive: transforming care for every small and sick newborn*. Geneva: World Health Organization, 2018.)

nearly 50 per 1,000 in some low-income countries (LICs). Ninety-eight percent occur in LMICs with the highest rates and slowest progress seen in sub-Saharan Africa, although stillbirths continue to affect wealthier nations with around 1 in every 300 babies stillborn in HICs (26).

Shockingly, about 1.2 million stillbirths are estimated to occur during labor, the majority associated with a lack of timely, good-quality obstetric care (26). Despite widespread fatalism around stillbirth, less than 10% of stillbirths are due to congenital abnormalities, and some of these are preventable such as neural tube defects (21). Many antepartum conditions associated with stillbirth are addressable through antenatal care, including maternal infections such as malaria and syphilis, noncommunicable diseases such as diabetes and hypertension, maternal under- or

overnutrition, lifestyle factors such as smoking and alcohol use, and placental disorders including preeclampsia. Both maternal age greater than 35 years and adolescent pregnancies increase risk, as does short inter-pregnancy intervals. Fetal factors such as prolonged pregnancy greater than 42 weeks and rhesus disease are also higher risk for stillbirth. Socioeconomic factors such as maternal education and gender-based violence are underlying risks for many stillbirths (21).

Ending preventable stillbirths requires more focus on the political barriers that impede attention, including empowering women. Respectful and supportive care, including bereavement support, is an important yet still neglected aspect of care even in HICs, and may bring more open recognition of the stigma and lead to more action (23).

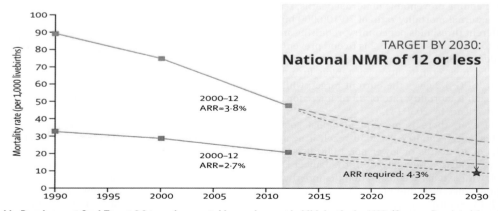

FIGURE 1.2 Sustainable Development Goal Target 3.2 to end preventable newborn and child deaths by 2030. (Source: Reprinted from Lawn JE, Blencowe H, Oza S, et al. Every newborn: progress, priorities, and potential beyond survival. *Lancet* 2014;384(9938):189. Copyright © 2014 Elsevier, with permission.)

PANEL 1.1

The Global Strategy for Women's, Children's, and Adolescents' Health (2016–2030) (9)

The updated 15-year Global Strategy was launched in parallel to that of the SDGs in 2015, by the then UN Secretary General Ban Ki-moon, involving multi-stakeholder groups such as developing country governments, major charities, philanthropists, and the private sector. The Strategy's three overarching objectives are as follows:

1. *Survive*: End preventable deaths
   - Reduce global maternal mortality to <70 per 100,000 live births.
   - Reduce newborn mortality to at least as low as 12 per 1,000 live births in every country.
   - Reduce under-five mortality to at least as low as 25 per 1,000 live births in every country.
   - End epidemics of HIV, tuberculosis, malaria, neglected tropical diseases, and other communicable diseases.
   - Reduce by one-third premature mortality from noncommunicable diseases and promote mental health and well-being.

2. *Thrive*: Ensure health and well-being
   - End malnutrition; address nutritional needs of children, adolescent girls, plus pregnant and lactating women.
   - Ensure universal access to sexual and reproductive health care services (including family planning) and rights.
   - Ensure that all girls and boys have access to good-quality early childhood development.
   - Substantially reduce pollution-related deaths and illnesses.
   - Achieve universal health coverage, including financial risk protection and access to quality essential services, medicines, and vaccines.

3. *Transform*: Expand enabling environments
   - Eradicate extreme poverty.
   - Ensure that all girls and boys complete free, equitable, and good-quality primary and secondary education.
   - Eliminate all harmful practices and all discrimination and violence against women and girls.
   - Achieve universal and equitable access to safe and affordable drinking water and to adequate and equitable sanitation and hygiene.
   - Enhance scientific research, upgrade technologic capabilities, and encourage innovation.
   - Provide legal identity for all, including birth registration.
   - Enhance the global partnership for sustainable development.

PANEL 1.2

The Every Newborn Action Plan (14)

Every newborn is a multipartner initiative providing frameworks for action, guided by the Convention on the Rights of the Child (CRC), the principles of universal health coverage, the WHO Framework on integrated people-centered health services, and the continuum of care. The five strategic objectives set in 2014 were as follows:

1. *Strengthen and invest in care around the time of birth, and in care for small and sick newborns*

   In addition to focusing on improved care during labor, birth, and the first day and week of life, there must be a focus on expanding access to care and improving quality of care for small and sick newborns. Many deaths and complications can be prevented by ensuring access to high-quality essential care for every mother and newborn.

2. *Improve the quality of maternal and newborn care*

   There is substantial variation in the quality of care for women and children. High-quality care, including high-impact, cost-effective interventions, is crucial not only to ensure that newborns survive but also thrive; that they are able to fulfil their potential for health and wellbeing, and that disabilities are minimized.

3. *Reach every woman and newborn to reduce inequities*

   Access to high-quality health care without financial hardship is a human right. Protecting and promoting this right, particularly for the most vulnerable newborns, including those in humanitarian settings, must be a priority. Robust evidence is available on promoting equitable care and ending preventable newborn deaths. Applying this evidence in accordance with the principles of UHC, and using innovative approaches to reach vulnerable groups, can accelerate progress towards equitable coverage of lifesaving care.

4. *Harness the power of parents, families, and communities*

   A family-centered approach, where small and sick newborns are the focus of care, requires parents and families to be actively engaged and empowered during hospitalization, at home postdischarge, and in the community. Education and empowerment of parents, families, and communities to demand quality care, engage meaningfully in that care, and improve follow-up care practices are crucial.

5. *Count and track every small and sick newborn*

   Data and metrics enable managers to monitor progress and take action to improve results. The availability of standardized indicators to monitor expenditures and outcomes is key to promoting accountability. There is a need for accurate, reliable data to facilitate planning efforts and to measure quality, outcomes and the impact of interventions and programs.

The Covid-19 Pandemic

COVID-19 was officially recognized by the World Health Organization (WHO) as a pandemic in March 2020, and has impacted health and well-being in both high-income and low-income countries worldwide. There are major disparities between countries, but everywhere the most vulnerable populations are disproportionately affected, and while the direct effects on women and their babies may be lower than for other demographic groups, the indirect effects are catastrophic (27–30) (Panel 1.3).

DEFINITIONS

In order to monitor trends and progress across countries and regions, standard definitions must be applied; these definitions have been set by the WHO (31). **Neonatal mortality** is defined as the number of deaths of liveborn babies during the first 28 completed days of life (**early**: 0 to 6 days, **late**: 7 to 27 days). The **neonatal mortality rate** (NMR) is the neonatal mortality per 1,000 live births in a given year. **Stillbirths** definition recommended by WHO for international comparison is a baby born with no signs of life at or after 28 weeks' gestation (late fetal deaths), but WHO clearly recommends that all countries also count stillbirths from 22 weeks of gestation (early fetal deaths). Some HICs, including UK, USA, and Australia, have definitions that differ, for example 20 weeks or 23 weeks. The **stillbirth rate (SBR)** is the number of late stillbirths per 1,000 births (both live and stillbirths). **Perinatal mortality** is

variably defined, and the recommendation is not to use this term but rather to report stillbirths and neonatal mortality separately. **Infant mortality** refers to deaths within the first year of life (31).

Preterm birth is defined as a live birth before 37 completed weeks of gestation; moderate-to-late preterm is between 32 and 36 weeks of completed gestation, very preterm between 28 and 31 weeks of gestation, and extremely preterm before 28 weeks of gestation. Deaths are only considered to be due to preterm birth if they are directly attributable, for example, respiratory distress or necrotizing enterocolitis (NEC). **Low birth weight** refers to a weight at birth of less than 2,500 g; very low birth weight is a birth weight of less than 1,500 g, and extremely low birth weight is less than 1,000 g. Infants below the 10th percentile by gestation are classified as small for gestational age (SGA) (31).

UNDERSTANDING NEONATAL MORTALITY AROUND THE WORLD

Progress for Reducing Newborn Deaths?

Progress in NMRs since 1990 have varied substantially, from a reduction of 86% in East Asia to 39% in sub-Saharan Africa (1). However, within sub-Saharan Africa certain countries are making rapid progress, for example Rwanda, which reduced its NMR from

COVID-19 affects newborns in many ways, directly due to infection with the virus itself, and indirectly due to the widespread disruption to health services, families, and the economy.

Direct impact:

The direct effects of SAR-CoV2 infection on mortality and morbidity appear to be low for women of reproductive age, and even lower for newborns. Early data suggest potential rises in preterm birth (some of which may be iatrogenic) and possibly of stillbirth. In the United Kingdom, risks to both women and babies are much higher in people who are Black, Asian or minority ethnic. It is important to identify infection early, reduce transmission, and mitigate risks. After birth, mothers and babies should remain together unless clinically indicated, cohorted, or isolated as necessary. Skin-to-skin contact and breast-feeding should be encouraged as usual; currently there is no evidence of the virus in breast milk, but mothers should be advised to wear masks and observe hand hygiene. Rigorous infection prevention and control is essential, including deep cleaning, PPE for staff, and cohorted waiting rooms. Guidance from WHO, RCPCH, and BAPM provides specifics. Maternal mental health and psychosocial support is even more crucial, given higher anxiety levels. Partners should be allowed to support the mother during labor and visit their babies on the neonatal unit; during the first phase of the pandemic some centers restricted visiting rights, which does not adhere to the principles of right to privacy and family life as per article 8 of the Human Rights Act. It is vital to maintain newborn care that can easily become lost amid competing priorities within health systems reacting to a pandemic.

Indirect impact:

Previous outbreaks such as with the Ebola virus or SARS found that indirect consequences were far greater than the direct effects. Women and their babies are the most vulnerable to major disruptions in health services. Marked reductions have been seen in coverage of care, which may be due to reduced access (movement restrictions and limited public transport) or to reduced provision of care (closures of facilities) or importantly to fear of using health facilities and distrust of the system. Families may access facilities, yet find lower quality of care due to fewer health care providers for newborn care—health worker numbers may be reduced due to sickness, redeployment, or burnout. Essential medicines and supplies may be affected by supply chain disruptions. In some hospitals, oxygen units have been moved from newborn wards to adult wards.

Consequences include the following:
- Deaths: It has been estimated that 45% reduction in coverage of essential health care services for 6 months in 118 LMIC could result in an extra 56,700 maternal deaths and 1,157,000 million newborn and child deaths.
- Other adverse health outcomes, such as disability due to delayed or suboptimal care, are happening in both high- and low-income settings. Reduced primary care services, with gaps in nutrition support and routine immunizations have been predicted to result in many deaths in the years to come.
- Worsened experience of care due to reduced access for partners and visitors, wearing of PPE by caregivers, and less choice for example in personal birth plans.
- Child protection may be threatened due to increased caregiver stress, increasing the risk abuse, including violence or neglect, in the context of disrupted support services.
- Mental health consequences for women and families are only starting to be detailed.

In addition, households and countries are experiencing extensive socioeconomic impact, including a global recession. Families lose income due to the inability to work, along with suffering an increase in prices of essential goods due to the economic recession. Due to increasing poverty and disrupted food and agriculture systems, undernutrition is an important concern. Increasing poverty increases individual health risks and also population health status.

Importantly, there are learnings regarding resilience at individual level, at facility level, or for districts and countries. The pandemic is a test of leadership at all levels. Documenting and rapidly sharing is key to mitigating potentially disastrous effects. Without major commitment and innovation, in "building better" the aspirations of the SDGs may be thrown off course for many countries and the world's poorest families.

References: Data from (1) WHO. COVID-19: operational guidance for maintaining essential health services during an outbreak. Available from: https://www.who.int/publications-detail/covid-19-operational-guidance-for-maintainingessential-health-services-during-an-outbreak. Accessed May 25, 2020; (2) Roberton T, Carter ED, Chou VB, et al. Early estimates of the indirect effects of the COVID-19 pandemic on maternal and child mortality in low-income and middle-income countries: a modelling study. *Lancet Glob Health* 2020; doi: 10.1016/S2214-109X(20)30229-1. (3) Sochas L, Channon AA, Nam S. Counting indirect crisis-related deaths in the context of a low-resilience health system: the case of maternal and neonatal health during the Ebola epidemic in Sierra Leone. *Health Policy Plan* 2017;32(suppl 3):iii32. (4) Rao SPN, Minckas N, Medvedev MM, et al. Small and sick newborn care during the COVID-19 pandemic: global survey and thematic analyses of healthcare providers' voices and experiences. *BMJ Global Health* 2020:e004347. doi: 10.1136/bmjgh-2020-004347 (27-41)

39 to 16 between 2000 and 2017, equating to an average annual rate of reduction (AARR) of 5.1%. Worldwide the most rapid progress has been seen in China (8.9%), Estonia (8.7%), and Belarus (8.2%) (**Panel 1.4**). Most countries have taken decades to reduce their NMRs from 20 to 12 or fewer deaths per 1,000 live births (**Fig. 1.3**). If the same regional AARRs continue as seen between 2000 and 2017, most regions can achieve the target of an NMR of 12 or less per 1,000 live births by 2030; excluding Southern Asia (predicted by 2042) and sub-Saharan Africa (by 2050) (**Panel 1.4**) (32). Countries affected by humanitarian crises have the slowest progress and many are unlikely to meet their targets (1).

Where Do Newborn Deaths Occur?

Almost all neonatal deaths (98%) occur in LMICs, with 75% occurring in Southern Asia and sub-Saharan Africa. Four countries account for almost half of all neonatal deaths in 2019; India (522,000), Nigeria (270,000), Pakistan (248,000), and Democratic Republic of the Congo (97,000). Of the 10 countries with the highest NMRs, 8 are in Africa and most have experienced humanitarian crises (1).

National NMRs vary widely from 0.9 per 1,000 live births, to 44 deaths per 1,000 live births. Some LMICs have made substantial progress, but around 40 countries, mainly in Africa and those with humanitarian crises, need to more than double their current progress in order to achieve the 2030 target (**Fig 1.3**) (1).

When and Why Do Newborn Deaths Occur?

An estimated 36% of all neonatal deaths occurred on the day of birth, and 73% during the first week of life; these proportions are similar across regions and economic settings (33).

The four leading direct causes of newborn deaths are preterm birth complications (35% of all neonatal deaths), intrapartum-related events (primarily through brain insult previously referred to as birth asphyxia) (24%), neonatal infections (15%), and congenital disorders (11%). Newborn deaths now contribute 47% of all child deaths under-five (**Fig. 1.4**) (1). The cause of death profile varies depending on context; in all countries the leading cause of death is direct complications of preterm birth particularly respiratory immaturity (34,35). However, in HICs, the predominant gestational age of those who die is less than 25

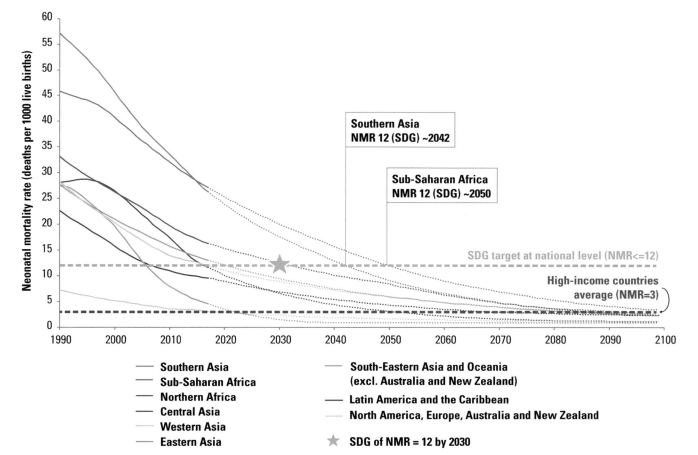

SDG target at national level (NMR<=12)

Note: The projections are calculated at the country level using the AARR 2000–2017 and constrained to not exceed the projected under-5 mortality rate and aggregated to the regional levels. After 2030 countries with populations less than 90 000 inhabitants in 2017 are not included in the regional aggregates.

Source: Analysis update from *The Lancet* Every Newborn (6). Data taken from: United Nations Inter-agency Group for Child Mortality Estimation estimates for NMR ARR 2000–2017 (7).

FIGURE 1.3 Projected time by region to reach SDG national target (NMR = 12) or average for high-income countries (NMR = 3). (Source: Data from Lawn JE, Cousens S, Zupan J. 4 million neonatal deaths: when? Where? Why? *Lancet* 2005;365(9462):891; United Nations inter-agency Group for Child Mortality Estimation estimates for NMR ARR 2000-2017; and Darmstadt GL, Bhutta ZA, Cousens S, et al. Evidence-based, cost-effective interventions: how many newborn babies can we save? *Lancet* 2005;365(9463):977.)

weeks due to availability of high-quality intensive care, whereas in LICs the predominant gestational age is 32 to 37 weeks (34). In the highest burden settings, half of neonatal deaths are due to infections, often acquired at birth or related to hygiene particularly through the umbilical cord (35).

Preterm Birth Complications

There are an estimated 14.8 million preterm births annually, constituting about 11% of all live births (36). Preterm birth rates are increasing in most countries with reliable data, in part due to fertility treatments, increasing maternal age, and early induction

---

PANEL 1.4

National Progress to Reach the Newborn Survival Target by 2030: 10 Fastest Progressors and Regional Fastest Progressors

Average Annual Rate of Reduction in Neonatal Mortality (%), 2000–2017

10 Fastest Progressors Globally		Regional Fastest Progressor		
China	8.9%	Eastern Asia	China	8.9%
Estonia	8.7%	North America, Europe	Estonia	8.7%
Belarus	8.2%	Central Asia	Kazakhstan	8.1%
Kazakhstan	8.1%	Western Asia	Georgia	7.0%
Georgia	7.0%	Sub-Saharan Africa	Rwanda	5.1%
Latvia	7.0%	Northern Africa	Tunisia	5.1%
Turkey	6.9%	Southeastern Asia and Oceana	Cambodia	5.1%
Saudi Arabia	6.4%	Latin America and Caribbean	Nicaragua	4.9%
Azerbaijan	6.2%	Southern Asia	Bangladesh	4.9%
Russian Federation	6.2%	Australia and New Zealand	Australia	3.0%

Source: Chap 2, Lawn et al. in World Health Organization; UNICEF. *Survive and thrive: transforming care for every small and sick newborn*. Geneva: World Health Organization, 2018.

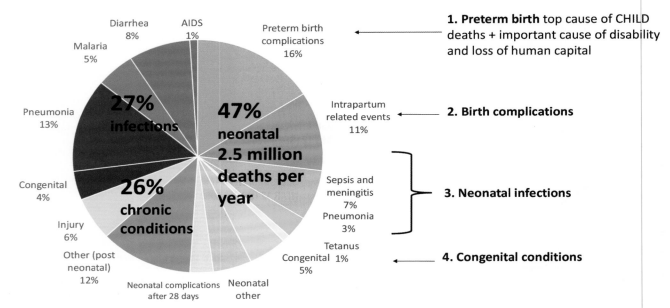

FIGURE 1.4 Global causes of child deaths under 5 years of age in 2018, for 195 countries. (Reprinted from World Health Organization, United Nations Children's Fund. *Survive and thrive: transforming care for every small and sick newborn.* Geneva, Switzerland: World Health Organization, 2019.)

of labor or caesarean section (34,36). Countries with the highest numbers of preterm births include India, China, Brazil, and the USA, demonstrating that preterm birth is a high burden issue across all income settings. Preterm birth rates range from 8.7% in the European region to up to 13.4% in North Africa, with greater variation within individual countries (35). With an estimated 1.01 million deaths per year, preterm birth is now the leading cause of under-5 child mortality worldwide (Fig. 1.4) and an important cause of long-term morbidity including disability and noncommunicable diseases in later life (1). In addition to direct preterm birth complications such as respiratory disease, the risk of death due to other causes, particularly infections, is increased. Preterm birth, particularly moderate preterm (32 to 36 weeks), is a risk factor in over half of all neonatal deaths (35). There is a significant survival gap for preterm babies; a 28-week-gestation newborn has a 95% survival chance in HICs compared to a less than 5% chance in LICs (2). Among the 13 million preterm newborns who survive each year, an estimated 2.7% have moderate-to-severe impairments and 4.4% have mild neurodevelopmental impairments, mostly in middle-income countries (MICs) (2). At 2 years of age, survivors are three times more likely to have language and motor delays, twice as likely to have cognitive delays, and likely to have poorer social–emotional skills compared to those born at term (34,32). Preterm birth accounts for one of the highest numbers of disability-adjusted life years (DALYs) for any single condition, and the majority (97%) are still due to prematurity-related deaths (35).

Intrapartum-Related Events

An estimated 1.15 million newborns suffer neonatal encephalopathy associated with intrapartum-related events each year; 96% are born in LMICs (37). This is descriptive term for a clinical constellation of neurologic dysfunctions in the term infant frequently associated with birth injury; previously referred to as "birth asphyxia". This is the second leading cause of neonatal mortality accounting for an estimated 627,000 neonatal deaths annually, and 1.3 million (half of all third-trimester) stillbirths (38,39). Of the survivors, 233,000 each year are estimated to develop moderate to

severe neurodevelopmental impairment, and 181,000 have mild impairment (37). Accurate estimates are impeded by variable definitions of intrapartum-related events, neonatal encephalopathy and "birth asphyxia," and lack of standardization in measuring neurodevelopmental impairment (40).

Neonatal Infections

There are an estimated 6.7 million newborns in LMICs with possible severe bacterial infections every year, including clinical syndromes of sepsis, meningitis, and pneumonia; approximately 3 million may require intensive care. Neurodevelopmental impairment occurs in 23% of survivors of neonatal meningitis (41). Twenty-three percent of all neonatal deaths are attributed to infection (including diarrhea and tetanus) (1). Group B streptococcal (GBS) disease is the leading global cause of neonatal infections; there are an estimated 320,000 early- and late-onset GBS sepsis cases each year, and 90,000 deaths and 57,000 stillbirths are attributed to GBS disease (42). Additionally, up to 3.5 million preterm births are attributed to maternal GBS colonization/infection worldwide (42,43). It is thought that 3 out of every 10 deaths due to neonatal sepsis are caused by resistant pathogens (44).

Congenital Disorders

Worldwide 11% of neonatal deaths are attributed to congenital anomalies; 9% of all deaths under the age of 5 deaths (1). Ninety-six percent occur in LMICs. Since 1990 the rate of decline has been slower than any other cause of neonatal mortality (45). The four leading conditions are cleft lip and palate, congenital heart anomalies, abdominal malformations, and neural tube defects. As well as mortality, these conditions lead to a significant burden of disability (45).

Risk Factors for Neonatal Mortality

Approximately 80% of neonatal deaths are low birth weight, and two-thirds are preterm. About two-thirds of LBW babies are preterm; the remainder are caused by intrauterine growth restriction and genetic syndromes (2,46). Those at highest risk of mortality and morbidity are in the most marginalized groups, particularly in rural areas, urban slum environments, and humanitarian settings (1). Other socioeconomic factors such as maternal age and educational status also increase the risk. Boys are at higher risk than girls of neonatal death or disability, but in some contexts notably in South Asia, this biologic advantage may be reversed due to social factors (2).

REDUCING NEONATAL MORTALITY AROUND THE WORLD

Context-Specific Approaches According to Phase of Mortality

The United Kingdom and United States of America reached the SDG target for NMR of 12 per 1,000 live births around 1980. The current NMR in many of the lowest income countries is around 25/1,000. The United Kingdom and United States of America took at least 25 years to get from 25 to 12; therefore, to meet the SDG in less than a decade from now, LMICs need to progress faster than this (32). Advances in neonatal care since 1980 have resulted in high-tech approaches and a shift to de-intensivization, enabled for example by wider use of antenatal steroids and use of continuous positive airway pressure (CPAP) for preterms, which are more feasible in LMICs (47). In addition, designing for family-centered care, empowering neonatal nurses, and avoidance of harm (such as retinopathy of prematurity [ROP]) are all themes that can enable faster and safer progress (48).

NMR in the United kingdom and United States of America progressed through three phases (Fig. 1.5). Strategies to reduce newborn deaths depend on the level of mortality and the context, and there are principles that can be applied to countries at the relevant level of mortality now as follows (32):

1. **Public health approaches**
   Between the 1900s and 1940s, high NMRs (40 deaths per 1,000 live births) were reduced by approximately 25% through general improvements in sanitation, socioeconomic and educational status, as well as improved healthy practices such as breast-feeding and clean cord care (47).
   Application now: For very high NMRs (over 30 per 1,000) at least half of deaths may be due to infections, and these contexts may have mainly home births and very limited resources. Many of these countries have humanitarian crises. Approaches that are feasible in these contexts include maternal tetanus immunization, clean birth kits, and breast-feeding. Community health workers (CHWs) or primary care health workers can provide simplified antibiotic treatment for infections, where referral is not possible.

2. **Improved care in pregnancy, at the time of birth and essential newborn care**
   Between the 1940s and 1970s, NMRs were halved. Major changes were the shift of births into hospitals, improved obstetric care (notably more caesarean sections). Immediate newborn care also improved such as clean cord care, breast-feeding, and thermal care. Oxygen and antibiotics both became increasingly available (47).
   Application now: Most of the world's births and neonatal deaths happen in countries with NMRs between 15 and 30 and have the majority of their births in hospitals. Yet there are huge quality gaps with overcrowding, inadequate numbers of health workers, and basic supplies (32). Addressing this quality care gap could save an estimated 2 million lives per year, including women, newborns, and stillbirths (6).

3. **Special and intensive neonatal care**
   Between 1970 and 2005, newborn mortality was further reduced in HICs by 75%, due to high-quality, individualized, advanced neonatal care. Neonatology was established as a specialty. However, the rapid uptake of new technologies without adequate monitoring led to an increase in adverse effects such as visual impairment and lung injury. With advancing hospital care, parents and newborns became more separated, affecting breast-feeding and mother–infant bonding. This was recognized in the 1980s and 1990s after which there began a shift to family-centered care (48,49). Health systems were strengthened with greater financing, regulations, monitoring, human resources, essential technologies and infrastructure, and the use of data to inform quality improvements.
   Application now: Many MICs are transiting toward NMRs of around 15/1,000. It is not possible to reach the SDG target for NMR of 12/1,000 without investing in hospital newborn care, including respiratory support for preterm newborns (47).

Integrating Interventions within the Continuum of Care

The highest impact care packages are care around the time of birth, and care for the small and sick newborn; through universal coverage, an estimated 2.9 million women, stillbirths, and newborns could be saved every year (compared with the 2016 baseline) (Fig. 1.6) (32).

Improving newborn health is part of integrated services for reproductive, maternal, child, and adolescent health. Interventions

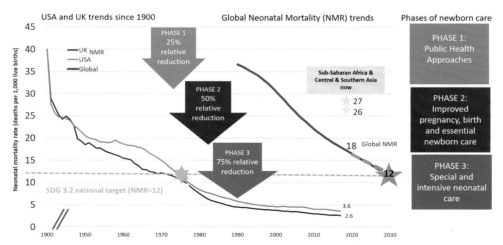

FIGURE 1.5 Learning from historical trends for neonatal mortality rate reduction in the United Kingdom and the United States of America to inform phases of change in LMICs. (Adapted from Lawn JE, Kinney MV, Belizan JM, et al. Born too soon: accelerating actions for prevention and care of 15 million newborns born too soon. *Reprod Health* 2013;10(Suppl 1):S6.)

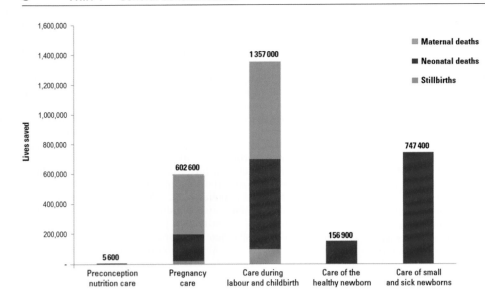

FIGURE 1.6 **Estimated impact of scaling up interventions, on maternal and neonatal deaths and stillbirths by 2030, from a 2016 baseline.** (Adapted from Bhutta ZA, Das JK, Bahl R, et al. Can available interventions end preventable deaths in mothers, newborn babies, and stillbirths, and at what cost? The Lancet 2014;384(9940):347. Copyright © 2014 Elsevier, with permission. From World Health Organization. *Every Newborn: an action plan to end preventable deaths.* Geneva, Switzerland: World Health Organization, 2014.)

are grouped across the "continuum of care"; the life course (from pregnancy and birth, to the postneonatal periods and through childhood and adolescence), the place of care (community, outpatients, and health facilities), and involve both curative and preventive interventions (**Fig. 1.7**) (50).

The focus of care is often either on the woman or on the baby; however, a collaborative approach integrating interventions for both mother and baby by time and place, and by the same health worker, is key. Transformation requires integrated service design, including health care worker teams and funding (50,51).

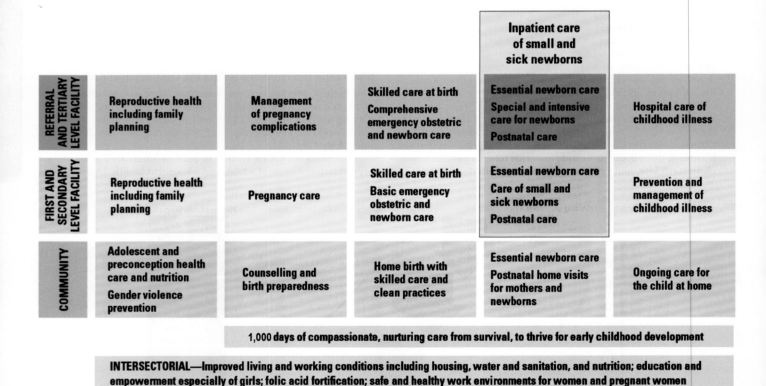

FIGURE 1.7 **Interventions and health service delivery packages across the continuum of care.** (Adapted from Every Newborn Action Plan UNICEF, World Bank Group and United Nations. *Levels & Trends in Child Mortality: Report 2019: Estimates developed by the United Nations Inter-agency group for child mortality estimation.* New York: UNICEF, 2019.)

Prepregnancy Care

Contraception is important to enable girls and women to plan pregnancies, optimize birth spacing (12 to 60 months), and reduce adolescent pregnancies or pregnancy after 35 years; these lower the risk for the mother and risk of preterm birth. However in Africa 22% of women still have an unmet need for family planning (52). Through satisfying the unmet need for family planning a third of maternal deaths a year could be averted, neonatal deaths and stillbirths halved, and human capital including education, improved (6,53). The preconception period is increasingly recognized as important for improving maternal, perinatal, and neonatal and child health outcomes. Interventions include screening for and treating maternal infection (malaria, HIV, tuberculosis, syphilis, and other sexually transmitted infections), addressing maternal smoking and alcohol and substance abuse, avoiding both under- and overnutrition, folic acid supplementation, and optimizing the management of chronic diseases. However, robust evidence is not yet available on packages of care and how to deliver these, especially since a large proportion of pregnancies are unplanned (54).

Pregnancy Care

UN estimates report that 86% women worldwide receive antenatal care at least once during pregnancy, but only 65% receive the previously recommended minimum of four visits (eight visits are now recommended by WHO) (55). Reasons include a lack of transportation, finances, and services, and even when accessed the quality of care may be suboptimal. Women who receive continuity of care from one midwife compared to shared or medical-led care are 24% less likely to experience preterm birth (56). Pregnancy-induced disorders such as preeclampsia, eclampsia, and gestational diabetes should be assessed for and treated promptly (57).

Labor and Birth Care

The day of birth is the highest risk for both mothers and babies, resulting in nearly half of maternal and newborn deaths and stillbirths. Care around the time of birth has the potential to avert a high number of maternal and newborn deaths and stillbirths, providing the highest impact (2). Nearly 80% of births worldwide now occur in facilities, offering an important opportunity to provide safe maternal and newborn care and identify and manage high-risk cases (32). The most important intervention for safe motherhood is to make sure that a skilled birth attendant is present at every birth, linked to high-quality emergency obstetric care (58). Birth preparedness, clean birth kits, and education regarding clean birth practices such as handwashing and the use of sterile cord cutting can reduce maternal and neonatal tetanus and other infections. WHO recommend antenatal corticosteroids for pregnant women at risk of preterm birth at 24 to 34 weeks' gestation where this can be accurately assessed, and there is no clinical evidence of maternal infection, to accelerate lung maturation and reduce the risk of respiratory problems (59). Intrapartum antibiotics for preterm premature rupture of the membranes are recommended to cover an increased risk of infection transmission to the baby (60). Intrapartum prophylaxis is also advised for maternal GBS when known; however, only 30 countries worldwide routinely screen mothers for GBS (41).

Newborn Care

Out of the approximately 140 million newborns born each year, 30 million require hospital care (**Fig. 1.8**) (32). Yet many LMICs have not previously planned and invested in newborn care, and hospital care for small and sick newborns is a major gap worldwide. Newborn deaths, disability, and other long-term effects including of NCDs in later life have a major burden and effect on human capital. Additionally, there are social, economic, and emotional impacts on families (32). Investing in newborn care is highly cost-effective in every health system context (6).

Care for Every Newborn

All babies require basic or "essential" newborn care, including drying and stimulation after birth, and resuscitation for those who do not breathe. Handwashing, sterile cord cutting, and cleansing of the umbilical cord with chlorhexidine can reduce risk of infection (61). All newborns should be kept warm with skin-to-skin care, head covering, and delayed bathing, and early breast-feeding should be initiated (62). Vitamin K should be administered to all babies to prevent hemorrhagic disease of the newborn, along with immunizations as per national protocols. Caregivers should be aware of danger signs and how to seek medical help. Ongoing support for exclusive breast-feeding is crucial (63).

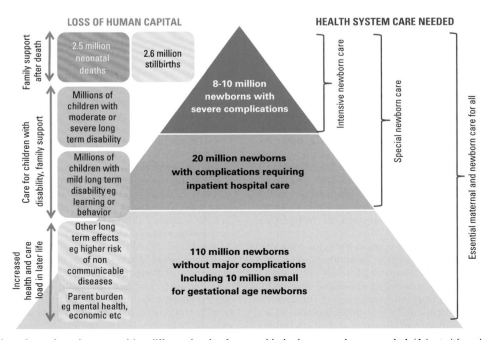

FIGURE 1.8 Estimated numbers of newborns requiring different levels of care, with the impact on human capital. (Adapted from Lawn JE, Davidge R, Paul VK, et al. *Born too soon: care for the preterm baby*. Geneva, Switzerland: World Health Organisation, 2012. Available from: https://www.who.int/pmnch/media/news/2012/201204_borntoosoon-report.pdf)

Level 1	
Immediate and essential newborn care	Immediate newborn Care (delayed cord clamping, drying, skin to skin etc)
	Neonatal resuscitation for those who need it
	Breastfeeding early initiation and support
	Essential newborn care Identification and referal of complications
	Targeted care as needed eg PMTCT of HIV
Level 2	
Special newborn care	Thermal care including KMC for all stable neonates <2 000g
	Assisted feeing and IV fluids
	Safe administration of oxygen
	Detection and management of neonatal sepsis with injection antibiotics
	Detection and management of neonatal jaundice with phototherapy
	Detection and management of neonatal encephalopathy
	Detection and referral/management of congenital abnormalities
Transition	CPAP managment of perform respiratory distress
	Follow up of at risk newborns
	Exchange transfusion
Level 3	
Intensive newborn care	Mechanical/assisted ventilation
	Advanced feeding support (e g parenteral nutrition)
	Investigation and care for congenital aonditions
	Screening and treatment for ROP

FIGURE 1.9 Levels of newborn care with interventions, according to WHO norms and standards. (Adapted from World Health Organization, United Nations Children's Fund. *Survive and thrive: transforming care for every small and sick newborn.* Geneva, Switzerland: World Health Organization, 2019.)

PANEL 1.5

NEST 360: Neonatal Essential Solutions and Technologies

The NEST360 collaborative aims to half neonatal mortality in newborn care units across Africa, implementing a package including a bundle of robust, affordable technologies along with health systems change and infection prevention, driven by data. NEST is being implemented with government leadership in four African countries, providing context-specific solutions to four major gaps that prevent quality newborn care in hospitals:

1. *Technology:* Neonatal units in sub-Saharan Africa often lack lifesaving technologies that have been available in HICs since the 1970s. A bundle of innovative technologies target common newborn conditions such infection, hypothermia, jaundice, and CPAP for respiratory support.

2. *Human resources:* Technology is necessary but not sufficient. Having enough health care providers with skills is crucial, and also device maintenance technicians. Education, both in-service and preservice, is foundational to implement safe, high-quality newborn care and enable local innovators to create new technologies.

3. *Implementation:* Managers of health systems lack data and finances to implement quality programs that meet need. Local data collection tools and analysis to drive change (e.g., hospital quality improvement dashboards) will provide crucial information enabling improvement at the facility level, plus evidence-based planning and investment.

4. *Market shaping:* Manufacturers face challenges of uncertain market size and high costs of distribution in Africa. Donated medical equipment is often inappropriate for the local context; not designed for heat, humidity, and electrical surges; and unable to be maintained locally. Sustainable distribution and maintenance of essential equipment requires new focus on innovative financing options, market shaping to buy in bulk, and more reliable distribution systems.

source: www.nest360.org/

Care for Small and Sick Newborns

An estimated 30 million small and sick newborns will have potentially life-threatening conditions and require special newborn care, including KMC, phototherapy, and antibiotics (32). About 8 to 10 million will need intensive newborn care due to being very small and sick, particularly respiratory support (Fig. 1.9). As the level of care becomes more complex from essential to intensive, there is a need for more advanced specialized staff, infrastructure, equipment, support systems (such as diagnostics and laboratory support), and outpatient follow-up services (63). High-quality essential and special newborn care is the priority, with access to intensive care for the few who may require it. Referral systems are crucial to link families from home and primary care facilities to secondary and tertiary care in case of complications (63).

Practice should be evidence based; international standards and guidance published by WHO for newborn care can be adapted to the local context depending on disease burden and available resources (62). Innovative health care technologies have the potential to enhance access to quality care for all small and sick newborns (**Panel 1.5**) (32). In most LMICs, care of small and sick newborns is mainly delivered by nurses and midwives. The shortage of HCWs worldwide is a barrier to achieving targeted health goals, and "task sharing" has been encouraged, for example training clinical officers to conduct caesarean sections rather than obstetricians (64).

Family-centered care describes an approach to care that promotes a mutually beneficial partnership between families and HCWs to care for newborns in facilities at all levels (48). Developmental care involves a minimal handling approach, responding to baby cues, maximizing comfort, and encouraging the involvement of families on neonatal units (65). Principles include dignity and respect, information sharing, participation, and collaboration. Engaging parents and families strengthens parenting skills and confidence to care for their newborn, reducing stress, enhancing parent–newborn bonding, breast-feeding, long-term neurodevelopmental outcomes, and facilitating earlier discharge (66). Strategies to encourage family-centered care include offering accommodation for parents on or near the ward, encouraging parent involvement in daily cares and feeding, and providing education and peer support (65,66).

Specific interventions to prevent and manage the leading causes of neonatal deaths are as follows.

Preventing Preterm Birth and Caring for Preterm Neonates

Current methods to prevent preterm birth are limited in their impact; these include family planning (particularly avoiding pregnancies under 18 or over 35 years) and treating infections during pregnancy including malaria (56). It has been demonstrated that the provision of antenatal care by the same midwife, rather than shared care or medical-led care, reduces preterm birth by 24% (56). Promising research is under way to improve understanding and strategies to prevent preterm birth.

Major reductions in preterm deaths have primarily been through improving care of preterm neonates, and in high-income settings 22 weeks' gestation neonates are resuscitated and more than half of neonates less than 25 weeks now survive. However, in LMICs many babies who are only moderately preterm die from very preventable conditions (67).

Kangaroo mother care (KMC) is an evidence-based, WHO-recommended intervention for the care of stable LBW, especially preterm newborns. Although originally designed for resource-poor and high-mortality settings, a growing evidence base indicates multiple benefits for newborns and their families in all settings (68). KMC involves early and prolonged skin-to-skin contact between the newborn and caregiver, and has been has been shown to reduce all-cause mortality by up to 50%, reduce sepsis by up to 60%, and improve breast-feeding, weight gain, physiologic stability, parent–infant bonding, and long-term developmental outcomes (68). It also decreases the length of hospital admission, and health care worker workload. Despite the evidence of its cost-effectiveness, KMC is still underutilized in most settings (69). Several trials are examining the impact of KMC on unstable LBW newborns under 2 kg.

The most common pathway to death for preterm neonates is due to respiratory distress syndrome (RDS), which can be managed with oxygen therapy or CPAP to prevent collapse of the airways. Low-cost bubble CPAP is being scaled up in many LMIC, and there are more robust, low-cost devices such as Pumani, which was invented in Malawi and is now available in more than 70 countries (70). Oxygen should be monitored to maintain saturation levels between 91% and 95%; unregulated use can cause Retinopathy of Prematurity (ROP) which is a leading cause of blindness in LMICs and should be screened for to allow for early detection and treatment if needed (71). Additional respiratory support can be provided by surfactant therapy instilled directly into the lungs; however, this costly intervention is not feasible in most LMICs; the same is true for mechanical ventilation (72).

Preterm babies have high nutritional requirements, and feeds should be introduced as soon as possible. However, most babies under 34 weeks' gestation do not have a coordinated sucking and swallowing reflex, and may require intravenous fluids initially, with milk introduced gradually via gastric tubes, potentially followed by a feeding syringe, cup, or spoon. Support can be provided to the mother to express breast milk; exclusive breast milk feeding can reduce the risk of NEC (73).

Preventing and Managing Intrapartum-Related Complications and Neonatal Encephalopathy

Primary prevention with high-quality obstetric care could avert almost 80% of neonatal deaths due to intrapartum-related events; this requires midwives, and basic and comprehensive emergency obstetric care (6). Basic care includes assisted vaginal delivery, parenteral antibiotics, parenteral oxytocics, and parenteral anticonvulsants for preeclampsia or eclampsia. Comprehensive emergency obstetric care additionally includes caesarean section and blood transfusion (74).

Secondary prevention involves neonatal resuscitation. An estimated 5% to 10% of newborns (7 to 14 million per year) require some stimulation immediately after birth to help initiate breathing; approximately 6 million newborns per year require bag and mask ventilation; a much smaller number (<1% of births) may require advanced newborn resuscitation, including intubation, chest compressions, or medications (37). Through the systematic implementation of neonatal resuscitation programs in low-resource settings, an estimated 200,000 intrapartum-related deaths could be averted each year (Panel 1.6) (75–78).

Neonatal encephalopathy is a condition of altered brain functions characterized by a constellation of neurologic symptoms including impaired consciousness, respiration, tone, and seizures and is commonly associated with insult or injury to other organ systems including the kidneys and the liver (79). Supportive care for those with neonatal encephalopathy includes maintaining blood pressure and sugar and electrolyte levels, treating seizures, and providing respiratory support including ventilation, where available (80). Where there is evidence of an intrapartum insult such as poor cord gases or the need for prolonged resuscitation, the term hypoxic–ischemic encephalopathy (HIE) is used to imply causality (80). While the complexity of the aetiology is well recognized, in LMIC the majority are still associated with intrapartum complications (81). Clinical and preclinical studies suggest linkages between perinatal infections, neonatal encephalopathy, and neurodevelopmental impairment (82,83). Evidence from HICs support the use of therapeutic hypothermia for babies with moderate–severe HIE to reduce mortality and risk of abnormal neurodevelopmental outcomes (84,85). However, therapeutic hypothermia is currently not recommended for LICs due to lack of evidence of improved outcomes in these settings, and indeed the potential for harm, especially given much higher prevalence of infections and the challenges of one-to-one nurse ratios plus intensive monitoring (86).

Preventing and Treating Neonatal Infections

An estimated 84% of neonatal deaths due to infections are preventable (6). Neonatal infection can be caused in the antepartum period through transplacental infection, for example congenital syphilis, which is now the leading bacterial cause of congenital infection and stillbirth (87). Intrapartum infection is caused by ascending infection from the maternal genitourinary tract; invasive GBS and *Escherichia coli* are the most common causes. Intrapartum antibiotic prophylaxis should be considered for risk factors such as fever during labor, known GBS colonization in urine or vaginal swab, or a previous baby with invasive GBS disease can reduce the risk of transmission and neonatal infection (60). On average, 18% of pregnant women worldwide are colonized with GBS, but screening is a controversial topic and policies vary. Thirty-five countries including the United States routinely screen and treat all pregnant mothers at 35 to 37 weeks' gestation, and 25 countries utilize a risk factor approach only treating those who have prelabor rupture of membranes or spontaneous preterm labor or who are known to be GBS positive (43). Maternal immunizations such as tetanus and pertussis are important; several GBS vaccines are currently in development and hold great potential but are not yet available (41).

After birth, infections are transferred through the environment; for neonates born in facilities or admitted to the ward there is a risk of health care–associated infections (HAI), which

---

PANEL 1.6

"Helping Babies Breathe" (HBB)

HBB is a neonatal resuscitation program set up by the American Academy of Pediatrics (AAP) and partners for resource-limited settings, which aligns with ILCOR and 2012 WHO Basic Newborn Resuscitation Guidelines. Between 2010 and 2018, this package has been taught to more than 400,000 providers in 25 languages in over 80 countries.

The program teaches the initial steps in neonatal resuscitation for a single provider focusing on "The Golden Minute," when all infants should be dried, kept warm, stimulated, and if not breathing, given bag-and-mask ventilation. HBB is part of the "Helping Babies Survive" program that includes "Essential Care for Every Baby," "Essential Care for Small Babies," "Improving Care of Mothers and Babies: A Guide for Improvement Teams," and a "Helping Mothers Survive" program.

Data from Pediatrics, A.A.o., *Guide for implementation of Helping Babies Breathe® (HBB): strengthening neonatal resuscitation in sustainable programs of essential newborn care.* Itasca, IL: American Academy of Pediatrics, 2011; Singhal N, Lockyer J, Fidler H, et al. Helping Babies Breathe: global neonatal resuscitation program development and formative educational evaluation. *Resuscitation* 2012;83(1):90; and Wall SN, Lee AC, Niermeyer S, et al. Neonatal resuscitation in low-resource settings: what, who, and how to overcome challenges to scale up? *Int J Gynaecol Obstet* 2009;107(Suppl 1):S47, s63.

are more likely to be drug resistant than community-acquired infections (88). Hygiene is key, particularly hand washing. WHO recommend cord washing with chlorhexidine, but only for home births in high-mortality settings (61). Preterm babies are at particular risk due to an immature immune system, reduced maternal antibody transfer during pregnancy, and longer duration of hospital admission.

Prompt diagnosis of signs of infection and treatment with antibiotics is essential; however, signs of newborn infection can be nonspecific and difficult to detect. Neonates with possible infection should be managed in hospital; however, where this is not feasible, the WHO suggest outpatient treatment with simplified regimens (89). Antibiotic choices should be based on up-to-date local, national, and international guidelines; WHO recommends ampicillin and gentamicin as first line. Neonatal tetanus should be managed by cleaning of the umbilicus, intravenous antibiotics, antispasmodic treatment such as diazepam, intravenous magnesium sulfate (for stabilization of the autonomic nervous system), antitetanus immunoglobulin, and tetanus vaccination after recovery. Supportive measures for neonates with sepsis include appropriate fluid resuscitation (90).

Antimicrobial resistance (AMR) is a particular challenge in LMICs where there is a high incidence of infections, limited diagnostics capacity, and unregulated use of second- or third-line antibiotics (44). More rapid detection of outbreaks and systematic surveillance of organisms causing infections are foundational to guide antibiotic stewardship programs. Point-of-care (POC) diagnostics would be transformative in reducing the presumptive use of antibiotics (88).

Preventing Congenital Disorders and Caring for Affected Neonates

Two-thirds of deaths due to congenital conditions are treatable with pediatric surgery and neonatal intensive care (45). Additionally, there are important primary prevention strategies that are feasible at scale, including folic acid fortification (which can prevent more than 50% of neural tube defects such as spina bifida), rubella immunization (congenital rubella syndrome causes heart defects, cataracts and deafness), and genetic counseling. There is a need for stronger national and regional surveillance systems of birth defects in order to guide public health policy and action (45).

Preventing Jaundice and Caring for Jaundiced Neonates

Neonatal jaundice is caused by raised serum bilirubin (SBR) levels, which may be high enough to cause brain injury (kernicterus) leading to death or long-term neurodevelopmental impairment. Jaundice can be due to prematurity, infection, or hemolysis (for example with rhesus disease, G6PD deficiency etc.) (91). Prevention strategies include testing pregnant women for a rhesus-negative blood group and administering an injection of antirhesus immunoglobulin. Screening for G6PD deficiency in areas of high prevalence (>5%) has proved to be cost-effective and is recommended. To improve early detection and treatment, caregivers should receive advice on how to recognize jaundice and seek appropriate help, and predischarge newborn examinations should be carried out. Effective management requires the availability of SBR testing devices and phototherapy equipment (32).

Community Care and Referral Systems

While facility-based care provides the greatest impact, community-based care plays an important role particularly in LMICs and should be well-linked (92). Community-based women's groups have been proven to improve outcomes substantially for mother and baby, through empowering women to make good health-related decisions and improve health seeking behaviors; notably this addresses the first and second delays of the three-delay model (delay in danger sign recognition and delay in care seeking) (93,94). When facility care is not possible, treatment can be provided at community level, including intramuscular antibiotics (89). Transport systems for health emergencies in LMIC are a major gap, and small and sick newborns can die quickly. Where available it is best to stabilize as much as possible prior to transfer, and the baby can be transferred in the KMC position. Communication with the receiving center and appropriate documentation are important for continuity of care (12).

LONG-TERM OUTCOMES AFTER NEONATAL CONDITIONS

Worldwide, approximately 140 million newborns are born each year, and they do not enter the world as equals. Every newborn's risk of death and of disability depends on where it is born, and the care that the newborn and mother receive. An estimated 45 million births still occur at home (**Fig. 1.10**) (95).

For the 30 million babies who experience complications around the time of birth, there may be lifelong consequences on health and development, yet most of these disabilities as well as deaths are preventable. As neonatal intensive care and obstetric care are being scaled up, particularly in MICs, rates of disability are increasing due to increasing survival rates and inadequate quality of care in some instances (64). In the last two decades there has been a growing recognition of the importance of providing developmentally supportive care on neonatal units, and implementing vigilant follow up for at-risk newborns who were born small and sick to identify developmental disability including cerebral palsy, ROP, and auditory and other visual impairments (48).

The first thousand days of life are a critical period for neuroplasticity and an important window of opportunity for interventions that maximize developmental potential (96). An estimated 53 million children under the age of 5 have stunting and/or suboptimal development, 95% of which reside in LMICs (97). The Nurturing Care Framework for Early Childhood Development (ECD) launched in 2018 by WHO, UNICEF, and the World Bank Group indicates that focusing on early childhood development is one of the best investments in national economic growth (98). Nurturing care is crucial for all children, arguably even more so for children with developmental disability as ECD interventions have the potential to limit impairments following newborn brain injury (99).

DATA TO TRACK AND HELP DRIVE CHANGE

Improving the quality and usage of data is crucial to drive monitor and evaluate programs, and tailor strategies to the context (**Panel 1.7**). Half of the world's newborns are not registered at birth, and greater than 95% of neonatal deaths and nearly all stillbirths have no death certificate. Given that greater than 80% of births are in health facilities, there is an opportunity to improve routine facility-based data. Impact indicators such as NMR, preterm birth and LBW rates, and disability rates after neonatal conditions are crucial to monitor progress towards national and global goals. Coverage indicators tracking the proportion of small and sick newborns who receive the care they require are also vital. Maternal and perinatal death surveillance or audit can be a powerful tool for improving quality of care and accountability, if capacity is strengthened to analyze data, and implement solutions (100,101).

High income countries
~12 million births

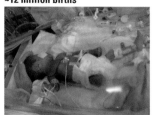

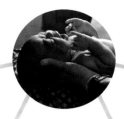

Middle income countries
~39 million births

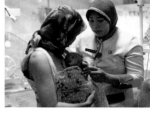

140 million births
per year

2.5 million neonatal deaths

~1.3 million survivors
with major disability

Many more with lost potential
for child development

Low and middle income countries,
especially humanitarian settings
~44 million births at home

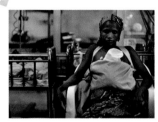

Low and middle income countries
~45 million births in hospitals

FIGURE 1.10 **The four worlds into which 140 million babies are born each year.** (From March of Dimes, PMNCH, Save the Children, WHO; Howson CP, Kinney M, Lawn JE, eds. *Born too soon: the global action report on preterm birth.* Geneva, Switzerland: World Health Organisation, 2012; Reprinted from Lawn JE, Blencowe H, Oza S, et al. Every Newborn: progress, priorities, and potential beyond survival. *Lancet* 2014;384(9938):189. Copyright © 2014 Elsevier, with permission.)

CONCLUSION

Commitment and investment will be needed to achieve the SDG goals, end preventable deaths, and support health and development across the life course. The care of small and sick newborns requires improvement in its access, quality, uptake, and affordability; this can be attained through strategic partnerships and innovative approaches. All of us have a crucial role to play; governments, health care professionals, professional associations, researchers, private sector, parents, and communities.

USEFUL SOURCES FOR MORE INFORMATION

- Lancet Every Newborn series
- Every Newborn Action Plan and annual progress reports
- Survive and Thrive: Transforming care for every small and sick newborn
- Oxford Textbook of Global Health of Women, Newborns, Children, and Adolescents
- Healthy Newborn Network

PANEL 1.7

How Can Health Care Professionals Contribute to Improving Global Newborn Health?

- Evidence-based advocacy through use of data and promoting investment for newborn care in LMICs.
- Empowerment of health professionals in LMICs, including with training such as Helping Babies Breathe, and ETAT+ (Emergency Triage, Assessment and Treatment plus admission of sick newborns and children), and WHO and NEST360 education materials.
- Collaboration through participating in one of the many international organizations that support partnerships with LMICs, aiming to improve quality care that is appropriate to the local context, aligned to the national strategy, and evidence based.
- Implementation and other research, to further address knowledge gaps in LMICs.

REFERENCES

1. UNICEF; World Health Organization; World Bank Group; United Nations. *Levels & Trends in Child Mortality: Report 2019, Estimates developed by the United Nations Inter-agency group for child mortality estimation.* New York: United Nations Children's Fund, 2019.
2. Lawn JE, Blencowe H, Oza S, et al. Every newborn: progress, priorities, and potential beyond survival. *Lancet* 2014;384(9938):189.
3. United Nations DESA. *The Millennium Development Goals Report 2015.* New York: United Nations, 2016.
4. United Nations DESA. *Sustainable Development Goals.* New York: United Nations Department of Economic and Social Affairs, 2015.
5. Darmstadt GL, Kinney MV, Chopra M, et al. Who has been caring for the baby? *Lancet* 2014;384(9938):174.
6. Bhutta ZA, Das JK, Bahl R, et al. Can available interventions end preventable deaths in mothers, newborn babies, and stillbirths, and at what cost? *Lancet* 2014;384(9940):347.
7. Dickson KE, Simen-Kapeu A, Kinney MV, et al. Every newborn: health-systems bottlenecks and strategies to accelerate scale-up in countries. *Lancet* 2014;384(9941):438.
8. Mason E, McDougall L, Lawn JE, et al. From evidence to action to deliver a healthy start for the next generation. *Lancet* 2014;384(9941):455.
9. Every Woman Every Child. *The global strategy for women's, children's and adolescents' health (2016–2030).* New York: United Nations, 2015.
10. Lawn JE, Cousens S, Zupan J. 4 million neonatal deaths: when? Where? Why? *Lancet* 2005;365(9462):891.
11. Darmstadt GL, Bhutta ZA, Cousens S, et al. Evidence-based, cost-effective interventions: how many newborn babies can we save? *Lancet* 2005;365(9463):977.
12. Knippenberg R, Lawn JE, Darmstadt GL, et al. Systematic scaling up of neonatal care in countries. *Lancet* 2005;365(9464):1087.
13. Martines J, Paul VK, Bhutta ZA, et al. Neonatal survival: a call for action. *Lancet* 2005;365(9465):1189.
14. WHO. *Every newborn: an action plan to end preventable deaths.* Geneva: World Health Organisation, 2014.
15. Froen JF, Cacciatore J, McClure EM, et al. Stillbirths: why they matter. *Lancet* 2011;377(9774):1353.
16. Lawn JE, Blencowe H, Pattinson R, et al. Stillbirths: where? When? Why? How to make the data count? *Lancet* 2011;377(9775):1448.
17. Bhutta ZA, Yakoob MY, Lawn JE, et al. Stillbirths: what difference can we make and at what cost? *Lancet* 2011;377(9776):1523.
18. Pattinson R, Kerber K, Buchmann E, et al. Stillbirths: how can health systems deliver for mothers and babies? *Lancet* 2011;377(9777):1610.
19. Flenady V, Middleton P, Smith GC, et al. Stillbirths: the way forward in high-income countries. *Lancet* 2011;377(9778):1703.

20. Goldenberg RL, McClure EM, Bhutta ZA, et al. Stillbirths: the vision for 2020. *Lancet* 2011;377(9779):1798.
21. Lawn JE, Blencowe H, Waiswa P, et al. Stillbirths: rates, risk factors, and acceleration towards 2030. *Lancet* 2016;387(10018):587.
22. Froen JF, Friberg IK, Lawn JE, et al. Stillbirths: progress and unfinished business. *Lancet* 2016;387(10018):574.
23. Heazell AEP, Siassakos D, Blencowe H, et al. Stillbirths: economic and psychosocial consequences. *Lancet* 2016;387(10018):604.
24. Flenady V, Wojcieszek AM, Middleton P, et al. Stillbirths: recall to action in high-income countries. *Lancet* 2016;387(10019):691.
25. de Bernis L, Kinney MV, Stones W, et al. Stillbirths: ending preventable deaths by 2030. *Lancet* 2016;387(10019):703.
26. Blencowe H, Cousens S, Jassir FB, et al. National, regional, and worldwide estimates of stillbirth rates in 2015, with trends from 2000: a systematic analysis. *Lancet Glob Health* 2016;4(2):e98.
27. WHO. COVID-19: operational guidance for maintaining essential health services during an outbreak. Available from: https://www.who.int/publications-detail/covid-19-operationalguidance-for-maintainingessential-health-services-during-an-outbreak. Accessed May 25, 2020.
28. Roberton T, Carter ED, Chou VB, et al. Early estimates of the indirect effects of the COVID-19 pandemic on maternal and child mortality in low-income and middle-income countries: a modelling study. *Lancet Glob Health* 2020; doi: 10.1016/S2214-109X(20)30229-1.
29. Sochas L, Channon AA, Nam S. Counting indirect crisis-related deaths in the context of a low-resilience health system: the case of maternal and neonatal health during the Ebola epidemic in Sierra Leone. *Health Policy Plan* 2017;32(suppl 3):iii32.
30. Rao SPN, Minckas N, Medvedev MM, et al. Small and sick newborn care during the COVID-19 pandemic: global survey and thematic analyses of healthcare providers' voices and experiences. *BMJ Global Health* 2020:e004347. doi: 10.1136/bmjgh-2020-004347.
31. WHO: Recommended definitions, terminology and format for statistical tables related to the perinatal period and use of a new certificate for cause of perinatal deaths. Modifications recommended by FIGO as amended October 14, 1976. *Acta Obstet Gynecol Scand* 1977;56(3):247.
32. World Health Organization; UNICEF. *Survive and thrive: transforming care for every small and sick newborn*. Geneva: World Health Organization, 2018.
33. Oza S, Cousens SN, Lawn JE. Estimation of daily risk of neonatal death, including the day of birth, in 186 countries in 2013: a vital-registration and modelling-based study. *Lancet Glob Health* 2014;2(11):e635.
34. Chawanpaiboon S, Vogel JP, Moller AB, et al. Global, regional, and national estimates of levels of preterm birth in 2014: a systematic review and modelling analysis. *Lancet Glob Health* 2019;7(1):e37.
35. Blencowe H, Cousens S, Chou D, et al. Born too soon: the global epidemiology of 15 million preterm births. *Reprod Health* 2013;10(suppl 1):S.
36. Blencowe H, Cousens S, Oestergaard MZ, et al. National, regional, and worldwide estimates of preterm birth rates in the year 2010 with time trends since 1990 for selected countries: a systematic analysis and implications. *Lancet* 2012;379(9832):2162.
37. Lee AC, Kozuki N, Blencowe H, et al. Intrapartum-related neonatal encephalopathy incidence and impairment at regional and global levels for 2010 with trends from 1990. *Pediatr Res* 2013;74(suppl 1):50.
38. Liu L, Oza S, Hogan D, et al. Global, regional, and national causes of under-5 mortality in 2000–15: an updated systematic analysis with implications for the Sustainable Development Goals. *Lancet (London, England)* 2016;388(10063):3027.
39. Lawn JE, Lee AC, Kinney M, et al. Two million intrapartum-related stillbirths and neonatal deaths: where, why, and what can be done? *Int J Gynaecol Obstet* 2009;107(suppl 1):S5.
40. Boggs D, Milner KM, Chandna J, et al. Rating early child development outcome measurement tools for routine health programme use. *Arch Dis Child* 2019;104(suppl 1):S22.
41. Seale AC, Blencowe H, Zaidi A, et al. Neonatal severe bacterial infection impairment estimates in South Asia, sub-Saharan Africa, and Latin America for 2010. *Pediatr Res* 2013;74(suppl 1):73.
42. Lawn JE, Bianchi-Jassir F, Russell NJ, et al. Group B Streptococcal disease worldwide for pregnant women, stillbirths, and children: why, what, and how to undertake estimates? *Clin Infect Dis* 2017;65(suppl 2):S89.
43. Seale AC, Bianchi-Jassir F, Russell NJ, et al. Estimates of the burden of group B streptococcal disease worldwide for pregnant women, stillbirths, and children. *Clin Infect Dis* 2017;65(suppl 2):S200.
44. Laxminarayan R, Matsoso P, Pant S, et al. Access to effective antimicrobials: a worldwide challenge. *Lancet* 2016;387(10014):168.
45. Higashi H, Barendregt JJ, Kassebaum NJ, et al. The burden of selected congenital anomalies amenable to surgery in low and middle-income regions: cleft lip and palate, congenital heart anomalies and neural tube defects. *Arch Dis Child* 2015;100(3):233.
46. Katz J, Lee AC, Kozuki N, et al. Mortality risk in preterm and small-for-gestational-age infants in low-income and middle-income countries: a pooled country analysis. *Lancet* 2013;382(9890):417.
47. Lawn JE, Kinney MV, Belizan JM, et al. Born too soon: accelerating actions for prevention and care of 15 million newborns born too soon. *Reprod Health* 2013;10(suppl 1):S6.
48. Maree C, Downes F. Trends in family-centered care in neonatal intensive care. *J Perinat Neonatal Nurs* 2016;30(3):265.
49. Gooding JS, Cooper LG, Blaine AI, et al. Family support and family-centered care in the neonatal intensive care unit: origins, advances, impact. *Semin Perinatol* 2011;35(1):20.
50. Kerber KJ, de Graft-Johnson JE, Bhutta ZA, et al. Continuum of care for maternal, newborn, and child health: from slogan to service delivery. *Lancet* 2007;370(9595):1358.
51. Lassi ZS, Majeed A, Rashid S, et al. The interconnections between maternal and newborn health—evidence and implications for policy. *J Matern Fetal Neonatal Med* 2013;26(suppl 1):3.
52. United Nations, Department of Economic and Social Affairs, Population Division (2017). World Family Planning 2017—Highlights (ST/ESA/SER. A/414). Available from: https://www.un.org/development/desa/pd/sites/www.un.org.development.desa.pd/files/files/documents/2020/Jan/un_2017_worldfamilyplanning_highlights.pdf. Accessed January 2021.
53. Singh S, Darroch JE, Ashford LS. *Adding it up: the costs and benefits of investing in sexual and reproductive health*. New York: Guttmacher Institute; 2014.
54. Dean SV, Mason E, Howson CP, et al. Born too soon: care before and between pregnancy to prevent preterm births: from evidence to action. *Reprod Health* 2013;10(suppl 1):S3.
55. WHO. *WHO recommendations on antenatal care for a positive pregnancy experience*. Geneva: World Health Organization, 2016.
56. Chang HH, Larson J, Blencowe H, et al. Preventing preterm births: analysis of trends and potential reductions with interventions in 39 countries with very high human development index. *Lancet* 2013;381(9862):223.
57. Requejo J, Merialdi M, Althabe F, et al. Born too soon: care during pregnancy and childbirth to reduce preterm deliveries and improve health outcomes of the preterm baby. *Reprod Health* 2013;10(suppl 1):S4.
58. PMNCH. *Opportunities for Africa's newborns: practical data, policy and programmatic support for newborn care in Africa*. Cape Town, South Africa: PMNCH, Save the Children, UNFPA, UNICEF, USAID, WHO, 2006.
59. Mwansa-Kambafwile J, Cousens S, Hansen T, et al. Antenatal steroids in preterm labour for the prevention of neonatal deaths due to complications of preterm birth. *Int J Epidemiol* 2010;39(suppl 1):i122.
60. Seale AC, Mwaniki M, Newton CR, et al. Maternal and early onset neonatal bacterial sepsis: burden and strategies for prevention in sub-Saharan Africa. *Lancet Infect Dis* 2009;9(7):428.
61. Blencowe H, Cousens S, Mullany LC, et al. Clean birth and postnatal care practices to reduce neonatal deaths from sepsis and tetanus: a systematic review and Delphi estimation of mortality effect. *BMC Public Health* 2011;11(suppl 3):S11.
62. WHO. *Thermal protection of the newborn: a practical guide*. Geneva: World Health Organization, 1997.
63. Moxon SG, Lawn JE, Dickson KE, et al. Inpatient care of small and sick newborns: a multi-country analysis of health system bottlenecks and potential solutions. *BMC Pregnancy Childbirth* 2015;15(suppl 2):S7.
64. Dickson KE, Kinney MV, Moxon SG, et al. Scaling up quality care for mothers and newborns around the time of birth: an overview of methods and analyses of intervention-specific bottlenecks and solutions. *BMC Pregnancy Childbirth* 2015;15(suppl 2):S1.
65. Davidson JE, Aslakson RA, Long AC, et al. Guidelines for family-centered care in the neonatal, pediatric, and adult ICU. *Crit Care Med* 2017;45(1):103.
66. O'Brien K, Robson K, Bracht M, et al. Effectiveness of Family Integrated Care in neonatal intensive care units on infant and parent outcomes: a multicentre, multinational, cluster-randomised controlled trial. *Lancet Child Adolesc Health* 2018;2(4):245.
67. Lawn JE, Davidge R, Paul VK, et al. Born too soon: care for the preterm baby. *Reprod Health* 2013;10(suppl 1):S5.
68. Conde-Agudelo A, Belizan JM, Diaz-Rossello J. Kangaroo mother care to reduce morbidity and mortality in low birthweight infants. *Cochrane Database Syst Rev* 2011;(3):CD002771.
69. Vesel L, Bergh AM, Kerber KJ, et al. Kangaroo mother care: a multi-country analysis of health system bottlenecks and potential solutions. *BMC Pregnancy Childbirth* 2015;15(suppl 2):S5.
70. Lissauer T, Duke T, Mellor K, et al. Nasal CPAP for neonatal respiratory support in low and middle-income countries. *Arch Dis Child Fetal Neonatal Ed* 2017;102(3):F194.
71. Gilbert C. Retinopathy of prematurity: a global perspective of the epidemics, population of babies at risk and implications for control. *Early Hum Dev* 2008;84(2):77.
72. Vidyasagar D, Velaphi S, Bhat VB. Surfactant replacement therapy in developing countries. *Neonatology* 2011;99(4):355.
73. WHO. *Guidelines on optimal feeding of low birth weight infants in low and middle income countries*. Geneva: World Health Organization, 2011.
74. Hofmeyr GJ, Haws RA, Bergstrom S, et al. Obstetric care in low-resource settings: what, who, and how to overcome challenges to scale up? *Int J Gynaecol Obstet* 2009;107(suppl 1):S21.

75. American Academy of Pediatrics. *Guide for Implementation of Helping Babies Breathe® (HBB): strengthening neonatal resuscitation in sustainable programs of essential newborn care.* IL: American Academy of Pediatrics, 2011.
76. Singhal N, Lockyer J, Fidler H, et al. Helping Babies Breathe: global neonatal resuscitation program development and formative educational evaluation. *Resuscitation* 2012;83(1):90.
77. Wall SN, Lee AC, Niermeyer S, et al. Neonatal resuscitation in low-resource settings: what, who, and how to overcome challenges to scale up? *Int J Gynaecol Obstet* 2009;107(suppl 1):S47.
78. Lee AC, Cousens S, Wall SN, et al. Neonatal resuscitation and immediate newborn assessment and stimulation for the prevention of neonatal deaths: a systematic review, meta-analysis and Delphi estimation of mortality effect. *BMC Public Health* 2011;11(suppl 3):S12.
79. Nelson KB, Leviton A. How much of neonatal encephalopathy is due to birth asphyxia? *Am J Dis Child* 1991;145:1325.
80. Nelson KB. Is it HIE? And why that matters. *Acta Paediatr* 2007;96:1113.
81. Graham EM, Ruis KA, Hartman AL, et al. A systematic review of the role of intrapartum hypoxia-ischemia in the causation of neonatal encephalopathy. *Am J Obstet Gynecol* 2008
82. Hagberg H, Mallard C, Ferriero DM, et al. The role of inflammation in perinatal brain injury. *Nat Rev Neurol* 2015;11(4):192.
83. Fleiss B, Tann CJ, Degos V, et al. Inflammation-induced sensitization of the brain in term infants. *Dev Med Child Neurol* 2015;57(suppl 3):17.
84. Martinello K, Hart AR, Yap S, et al. Management and investigation of neonatal encephalopathy: 2017 update. *Arch Dis Child Fetal Neonatal Ed* 2017;102(4):F346.
85. Jacobs SE, Berg M, Hunt R, et al. Cooling for newborns with hypoxic ischaemic encephalopathy. *Cochrane Database Syst Rev* 2013;(1):CD003311.
86. Pauliah SS, Shankaran S, Wade A, et al. Therapeutic hypothermia for neonatal encephalopathy in low- and middle-income countries: a systematic review and meta-analysis. *PLoS One* 2013;8(3):e58834(3):e58834.
87. McClure EM, Goldenberg RL. Infection and stillbirth. *Semin Fetal Neonatal Med* 2009;14(4):182.
88. Okomo U, Akpalu ENK, Le Doare K, et al. Aetiology of invasive bacterial infection and antimicrobial resistance in neonates in sub-Saharan Africa: a systematic review and meta-analysis in line with the STROBE-NI reporting guidelines. *Lancet Infect Dis* 2019;19(11):1219. doi: 10.1016/S1473-3099(19)30414-1.
89. WHO. *Managing possible serious bacterial infection in young infants when referral is not feasible: guidelines.* Geneva: World Health Organization, 2015.
90. Seale AC, Agarwal R. Improving management of neonatal infections. *Lancet* 2018;392(10142):100.
91. Lissauer T, Fanaroff A, Miall L, et al. *Neonatology at a glance,* 4th ed. Oxford, UK: Wiley Blackwell, 2016.
92. Lassi ZS, Haider BA, Bhutta ZA. Community-based intervention packages for reducing maternal and neonatal morbidity and mortality and improving neonatal outcomes. *Cochrane Database Syst Rev* 2010;(11):CD007754.
93. Manandhar DS, Osrin D, Shrestha BP, et al. Effect of a participatory intervention with women's groups on birth outcomes in Nepal: cluster-randomised controlled trial. *Lancet* 2004;364(9438):970.
94. Prost A, Colbourn T, Seward N, et al. Women's groups practising participatory learning and action to improve maternal and newborn health in low-resource settings: a systematic review and meta-analysis. *Lancet* 2013;381(9879):1736.
95. Lawn JE, Blencowe H, Darmstadt GL, et al. Beyond newborn survival: the world you are born into determines your risk of disability-free survival. *Pediatr Res* 2013;74(suppl 1):1.
96. Wallander JL, McClure E, Biasini F, *et al.* Brain research to ameliorate impaired neurodevelopment—home-based intervention trial (BRAIN-HIT). *BMC Pediatr* 2010;10:27.
97. Olusanya BO, Davis A, Wertlieb D, et al. Developmental disabilities among children younger than 5 years in 195 countries and territories, 1990–2016: a systematic analysis for the Global Burden of Disease Study 2016. *Lancet Glob Health* 2018;6(10):e1100.
98. WHO *Nurturing care for early childhood development: a framework for helping children survive and thrive to transform health and human potential.* Geneva: World Health Organization, 2018.
99. Kohli-Lynch M, Tann CJ, Ellis ME. Early intervention for children at high risk of developmental disability in low- and middle-income countries: a narrative review. *Int J Environ Res Public Health* 2019;16(22):4449. doi: 10.3390/ijerph16224449. PMID: 31766126; PMCID: PMC6888619
100. Moxon, S.G., H. Ruysen, K.J. Kerber, et al. Count every newborn; a measurement improvement roadmap for coverage data. *BMC Pregnancy Childbirth* 2015;15(suppl 2):S8.
101. WHO. *WHO technical consultation on newborn health indicators: every newborn action plan metrics.* Geneva: World Health Organization, 2015.

GENERAL CONSIDERATIONS

2 The Scope and Organization of Perinatal Services: Global Comparisons and Challenges

Judy L. Aschner, Stephen W. Patrick, Ann R. Stark, and Shoo K. Lee

INTRODUCTION

In the past half century, we have witnessed extraordinary advances in perinatal medicine accompanied by dramatic improvements in birth outcomes in high-income countries (HICs). The obstetrical subspecialty of maternal–fetal medicine has improved both maternal and neonatal outcomes for women with high-risk pregnancies due to fetal disorders, maternal chronic diseases, or pregnancy-associated conditions, such as toxemia and gestational diabetes. The emergence of the subspecialty of neonatology and the availability of dedicated neonatal intensive care units with advanced technology designed for newborn infants have improved the survival and outcomes of infants born prematurely or with serious medical or surgical problems. In high-income, high-resource countries, an entire workforce has evolved with expertise in the unique developmental physiology and diseases of the newborn. This convergence of expertise and resources describes most modern-day neonatal intensive care units in the United States, Canada, and HICs in Europe, in Asia, and across the globe. Multidisciplinary care has become the norm, and families are increasingly being integrated into the health care team.

The infrastructure, resources, and workforce realities are quite different in developing countries, particularly in Africa and Southeast Asia but also in low- and middle-income countries (LMICs) of North, Central, and South America. The disparities in maternal and neonatal mortality remain striking, despite recent investments and early signs of improvements in select regions. This chapter will explore the scope and organization of perinatal and neonatal health care with a focus on (a) disparities that persist in many high-resource nations based on race, ethnicity, income, and access to care and (b) the sobering perinatal outcomes statistics in LMICs that remain our collective challenge and are directly or indirectly the result of inequalities in resource allocation, infrastructure, health literacy, and access.

INFANT, NEONATAL, AND PERINATAL MORTALITY

Valid comparisons of infant mortality over time or between different countries or geographic regions require acceptance and application of standard definitions, complete and reliable data collection, and confidence in both the numerator and denominator. The latter two represent challenges when attempting to compare outcomes in countries with vastly different resources, infrastructure for data collection, and cultural expectations and values. Standard definitions for infant and neonatal mortalities, stillbirth, preterm birth (including subcategories), and low birth weight (including subcategories) have been set by the World Health Organization (WHO), see Chapter 1.

Although prematurity and low birth weight are interrelated, they are not synonymous. Only about two-thirds of low–birth-weight infants are preterm. Infants who are below the 10th percentile of the index population's distribution of birth weights by gestation are considered "small for gestational age." In addition to prematurity, causes of low birth weight include fetal growth restriction and genetic syndromes. Low–birth-weight infants (<2.5 kg) at any gestational age are at increased risk of mortality and morbidity. Very-low-birth-weight infants (<1,500 g) are more than 100 times as likely, and low–birth-weight babies are more than 25 times as likely to die in the first year of life compared with infants who weigh 2,500 g or more at birth (1).

Infant Mortality in the United States and Other High-Income Countries

The United States first began to measure and record the infant mortality rate (IMR) in 1915 when the IMR was close to 100 deaths per 1,000 live births. In the past half century, the U.S. IMR has fallen from 32 deaths per 1,000 live births in 1950 to 5.7 deaths per 1,000 live births in 2019 (**Fig. 2.1**) (2). However, steady improvement in U.S. infant survival has slowed in recent years with minimal improvement since 2014 when the IMR was 5.9 per 1,000 live births (2). The progress observed over the past 50 years has been attributed to improved nutrition and sanitation, economic growth, advances in medical care, and improved access to care (3,4).

Despite these positive trends, 22,335 U.S. infants died before their first birthday in 2017 (5). Moreover, the IMR in the United States is higher than in many other developed countries. Out of 36 Organization for Economic Co-operation and Development (OECD) member countries, the United States ranks number 33 in infant mortality (6), with an IMR of 5.7 to 5.8 deaths per 1,000 live infant births. The average rate of infant mortality among the OECD countries is 3.8 deaths per 1,000 live births (**Fig. 2.2**) (6). Over the past 50 years, the decline in the U.S. IMR has not kept pace with that in other OECD countries.

Even accounting for different reporting measures, U.S. infant mortality remains higher than in comparable HICs. Using a minimum threshold of 22 weeks or 500 g, the IMR in the United States was 4.9 infant deaths per 1,000 live births, compared to an average IMR of 2.9 for the comparable countries of United Kingdom, France, Switzerland, Netherlands, Belgium, Austria, Sweden, and Japan (2016 data) (**Fig. 2.3**) (7). For infants born at 24 to 31 weeks of gestation, the IMR in the United States is comparable to the rates in most European nations; however, the United States had among the highest IMR for preterm infants born between 32 and 36 weeks of gestation and the highest rate of infant death at 37 weeks and above (2.2 per 1,000 live births in 2010) among the OECD countries (8).

Since 2005, the decline in IMR among black mothers was steeper than that observed for other racial or ethnic groups. Nonetheless, large disparities by race and ethnicity persist. In 2017, infants of non-Hispanic black women had the highest mortality rate (10.97 infant deaths per 1,000 births), followed by infants of non-Hispanic American Indian or Alaska Native (9.21 infant deaths per 1,000 births), non-Hispanic Native Hawaiian or other Pacific Islander (7.64 infant deaths per 1,000 births), Hispanic (5.10 infant deaths per 1,000 births), non-Hispanic white (4.67 infant deaths per 1,000 births), and non-Hispanic Asian (3.78 infant deaths per 1,000 births) women (**Fig. 2.4**) (9).

In 2017, both the neonatal mortality rate (7.16) and postneonatal mortality rate (death between 29 days and 1 year of age) (3.82) were highest for infants of non-Hispanic black mothers and lowest for non-Hispanic Asian women (2.71 and 1.08, for neonatal and postneonatal mortality rate, respectively) (9). Postneonatal mortality is most often attributed to SIDS, other sleep-related deaths, congenital malformations, and unintentional injuries.

U.S. Infant Mortality Rate 1950-2020

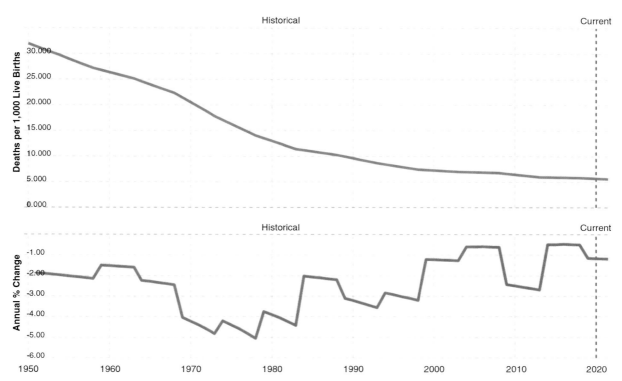

FIGURE 2.1   U.S. infant mortality rate: 1950 to 2020. (Reprinted from https://www.macrotrends.net/countries/USA/united-states/infant-mortality-rate, with permission.)

THE BURDEN OF PRETERM BIRTH: US AND GLOBAL PERSPECTIVES

The preterm birth rate is an important driver of a nation's IMR and a leading cause of childhood disabilities. In 2012, the March of Dimes, the Partnership for Maternal, Newborn and Child Health, Save the Children, and the World Health Organization published "Born Too Soon: The Global Action Report on Preterm Birth" (10). This report provided estimates of preterm birth by country. Approximately 15 million babies, or about 1 in 10 infants, are born preterm annually. Over 1 million of these infants die, making preterm birth complications the leading cause of death among children under 5 years of age. Across 184 countries, the rate of preterm birth ranged from 5% to 18% of all live births (10).

After excluding infants born before 24 weeks of gestation, the United States had the highest preterm birth rate among the 19 countries shown in **Figure 2.5** (11). The percent of preterm births in the United States was about 40% higher than in countries in the United Kingdom and nearly 75% higher than in some Scandinavian countries (11). More recent US data indicate some progress, with the rate of preterm birth falling from a peak of 12.8 in 2006 to 9.6 in 2015, but the rate has steadily risen since then to 10.0 in 2018 (12). There was significant variation in rates of preterm births between states (range Oregon 7.8 to Mississippi 14.2) and among ethnic groups (Pacific Islander 8.7, White 9.0, Hispanic 9.4, American Indian/Alaska Native 11.3, Black 13.6). The reduction in the percent of U.S. babies born prematurely is a strong contributor to the IMR because about two-thirds of all infant deaths occur among those born preterm (13).

Most preterm births happen spontaneously, but in HICs, some preterm births are due to early induction of labor or caesarean birth, for medical and nonmedical reasons. Late preterm births constitute the vast majority of all preterm births. Compared to term infants, these infants have a higher incidence of morbidity, including respiratory distress syndrome, temperature instability, and jaundice and have three times the IMR (1,14,15). Late preterm infants experience longer hospital stays and are more likely to incur higher hospital costs associated with NICU admissions than term infants (16). Even infants born at 37 and 38 weeks of gestation have worse outcomes compared to infants born at 39 and 40 weeks of gestation. Despite a low absolute risk of infant death, singleton infants born at 37 weeks had increased neonatal mortality rates, compared to infants born at 40 weeks (0.66 and 0.34 per 1,000 live births, respectively) (17). Those born electively at 37 and 38 weeks had increased rates of respiratory problems and were more likely to be admitted to a NICU, compared to those born at 39 weeks (18,19).

A public education campaign launched by the March of Dimes, called "Healthy Babies are Worth the Wait," and a similar campaign called "Healthy Start" sponsored by the Department of Health and Human Services discourage scheduled deliveries before 39 weeks. These measures aimed at the public have been accompanied by strong statements by professional organizations including the American College of Gynecologists and the American Academy of Pediatrics to avoid non–medically indicated deliveries before 39 weeks. These recommendations have been reinforced by regional and statewide perinatal quality collaboratives (PQCs) and initiatives championed by individual hospitals and hospital systems.

MAJOR NEONATAL MORBIDITIES

Preterm birth is associated with both short-term (infection, necrotizing enterocolitis, bronchopulmonary dysplasia, intraventricular hemorrhage, and retinopathy of prematurity) and long-term

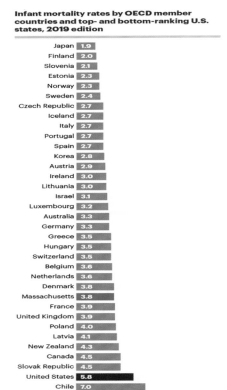

Infant mortality rates by OECD member countries and top- and bottom-ranking U.S. states, 2019 edition

Japan	1.9
Finland	2.0
Slovenia	2.1
Estonia	2.3
Norway	2.3
Sweden	2.4
Czech Republic	2.7
Iceland	2.7
Italy	2.7
Portugal	2.7
Spain	2.7
Korea	2.8
Austria	2.9
Ireland	3.0
Lithuania	3.0
Israel	3.1
Luxembourg	3.2
Australia	3.3
Germany	3.3
Greece	3.5
Hungary	3.5
Switzerland	3.5
Belgium	3.6
Netherlands	3.6
Denmark	3.8
Massachusetts	3.8
France	3.9
United Kingdom	3.9
Poland	4.0
Latvia	4.1
New Zealand	4.3
Canada	4.5
Slovak Republic	4.5
United States	5.8
Chile	7.0
Mississippi	8.6
Turkey	9.2
Mexico	12.1

DEATHS PER 1,000 LIVE BIRTHS

FIGURE 2.2 Infant mortality rate rankings in 2019: United States and other countries in the Organization for Economic Cooperation and Development. (Reprinted from America's Health Rankings® Annual Report 2019 Edition. Available at: www.AmericasHealthRankings.org; https://www.americashealthrankings.org/learn/reports/2019-annual-report/international-comparison.)

complications. Infants born very preterm (<32 weeks' completed gestation) are at greatest risk of death and long-term disability. Many preterm babies face a lifetime of disability, developmental delay, learning disabilities, and neurosensory deficits, with the largest impact occurring in LMICs. Worldwide, it is estimated that over 911,000 preterm survivors (7%) each year suffer long-term neurodevelopmental disabilities, including 345,000 who are moderately or severely affected. For infants born under 28 weeks of gestation, 52% suffer some degree of neurodevelopmental impairment, compared to 24% for infants born at 28 and 31 weeks of gestation and 5% for infants born at 32 and 36 weeks of gestation (10).

MATERNAL RISK FACTORS FOR POOR PREGNANCY OUTCOMES

Common causes of preterm birth include multiple pregnancies, infections, and chronic conditions, such as diabetes and high blood pressure. There is also a genetic influence. However, often no cause is identified. The best predictors of having a preterm birth are multifetal pregnancy or history of previous preterm labor/delivery. The major risk factors for poor pregnancy outcomes in HICs are shown in Table 2.1. Lack of prenatal care may arise from lack of health care facilities, lack of transportation to health care facilities or lack of financial resources to access care, and conditions are often worse in rural areas.

THE NEONATAL WORKFORCE

There are large differences in how countries employ health care resources to look after neonates. Thompson et al. (20) reported that the number of pediatricians varies from 20/10,000 live births in the United Kingdom to 144/10,000 live births in the United States. The reverse is true for family practitioners, with 597 family practitioners/10,000 live births in the United Kingdom, compared to 169 family practitioners/10,000 live births in the United States. These variations reflect differences in how health care professionals are utilized and reimbursed in different countries. In the United States, primary care for infants is often provided by pediatricians, whereas in the United Kingdom, this service is mostly provided by family practitioners. Similarly, neonatologists provide both level II and level III neonatal care in the United States, while they provide mostly level III care in the United Kingdom. Thompson et al. (20) also reported that greater neonatal intensive care resources were not consistently associated with lower birth weight-specific mortality. The United States has high neonatal intensive care capacity, with 6.1 neonatologists per 10 000 live births; Australia, 3.7; Canada, 3.3; and the United Kingdom, 2.7. For intensive care beds, the United States has 3.3 per 10,000 live births; Australia and Canada, 2.6; and the United Kingdom, 0.67. These variations reflect differences in regionalization of care, geography and proximity to health care facilities, and organization of health care services. Despite greater neonatal intensive care resources in the United States, the relative risk (US as reference) of neonatal mortality for infants less than 1,000 g was 0.84 for Australia, 1.12 for Canada, and 0.99 for the United Kingdom; for 1,000 to 2,499 g infants, the relative risk was 0.97 for Australia, 1.26 for Canada, and 0.95 for the United Kingdom.

The capacity of US hospitals to care for preterm or ill newborns is influenced by the availability of qualified physician subspecialists. The American Board of Pediatrics sub-board of Neonatal-Perinatal Medicine conducted its first certifying examination in 1975. Through 2017, 6,880 neonatologists have been certified as diplomates (21), 60% of whom are 50 to 70 years of age, with an average age of 54 years (22). The distribution of diplomates varies widely among states, ranging from 0 in Wyoming to 494 in California (American Board of Pediatrics 2013) (23). The distribution is also not uniform when the number of certified neonatologists is compared to the child population.

The capacity to care for high-risk newborns was expanded with the introduction of neonatal nurse practitioners (NNPs) into the workforce and formalized with certification beginning in the early 1980s. NNPs are registered nurses who have completed a master's degree and advanced clinical training, and they perform many complex activities. A policy statement of the American Academy of Pediatrics Committee of Fetus and Newborn recommended that care provided by NNPs be given in collaboration with or under the supervision of a physician, usually a neonatologist (24). Similar to neonatologists, distribution of NNPs varies regionally and is often not matched to demand. Furthermore, due to factors including declining enrollment in programs, inadequate numbers of preceptors, and plans of currently working NNPs to decrease their work hours, a gap exists between supply and demand (25–27). In some regions of the United States, this gap is being filled by physician assistants and pediatricians working as NICU hospitalists, under the supervision of a neonatologist.

AMERICAN ACADEMY OF PEDIATRICS RECOMMENDED LEVELS OF NEONATAL CARE

The American Academy of Pediatrics Committee on Fetus and Newborn published definitions for Levels of Neonatal Care in 2004 that were subsequently updated in 2012 and reaffirmed in 2015 (28). These updated definitions provide common terms that can be used to compare outcomes, resource use, and health care costs.

Accounting for differential reporting methods, U.S. infant mortality remains higher than in comparable countries

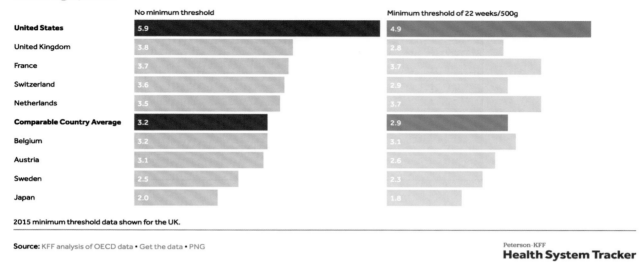

Infant mortality per 1,000 live births, with and without minimum threshold of 22 weeks gestation (or 500 grams birthweight), 2016

	No minimum threshold	Minimum threshold of 22 weeks/500g
United States	5.9	4.9
United Kingdom	3.8	2.8
France	3.7	3.7
Switzerland	3.6	2.9
Netherlands	3.5	3.7
Comparable Country Average	3.2	2.9
Belgium	3.2	3.1
Austria	3.1	2.6
Sweden	2.5	2.3
Japan	2.0	1.8

2015 minimum threshold data shown for the UK.

Source: KFF analysis of OECD data • Get the data • PNG

Peterson-KFF
Health System Tracker

FIGURE 2.3 Infant mortality per 1,000 live births: United States and comparable countries. (Reprinted from Peterson-KFF Health System Tracker. *What do we know about infant mortality in the U.S. and comparable countries?* Available at: https://www.healthsystemtracker.org/chart-collection/infant-mortality-u-s-compare-countries/#item-accounting-for-differential-reporting-methods-u-s-infant-mortality-remains-higher-than-in-comparable-countries, with permission.)

National Vital Statistics Reports, Vol. 68, No. 10, August 1, 2019

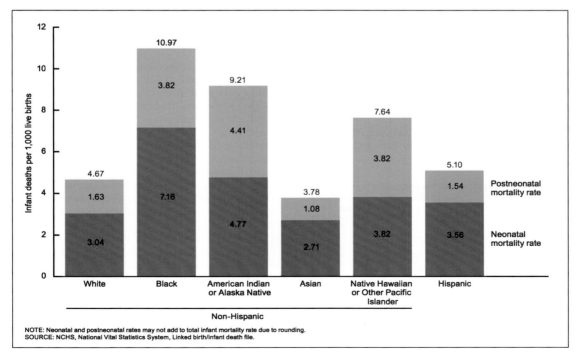

NOTE: Neonatal and postneonatal rates may not add to total infant mortality rate due to rounding.
SOURCE: NCHS, National Vital Statistics System, Linked birth/infant death file.

FIGURE 2.4 Infant, neonatal, and postneonatal mortality rates, by race and Hispanic origin: United States, 2017. (Source: Data from NCHS, National Vital Statistics System, Linked birth/infant death life; Ely DM, Driscoll AK. Infant mortality in the United States, 2017: data from the period linked birth/infant death file. *Natl Vital Stat Rep* 2019;68(10); DHHS publication no. 2019-1120.)

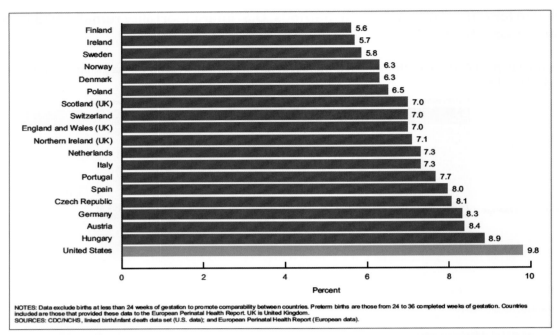

NOTES: Data exclude births at less than 24 weeks of gestation to promote comparability between countries. Preterm births are those from 24 to 36 completed weeks of gestation. Countries included are those that provided these data to the European Perinatal Health Report. UK is United Kingdom.
SOURCES: CDC/NCHS, linked birth/infant death data set (U.S. data); and European Perinatal Health Report (European data).

FIGURE 2.5 Percentage of preterm births: comparison of the United States with selected European countries, 2010. (Source: Data from CDC/NCHS, linked birth/infant death data set (U.S data); and European perinatal Health Report (European data); MacDorman MF, Mathews TJ, Mohangoo AD, et al. International comparisons of infant mortality and related factors: United States and Europe, 2010. *Natl Vital Stat Rep* 2014;63(5).)

Standardized nomenclature is important for public health purposes, for health care professionals who provide neonatal care, and for families making decisions about a delivery hospital. In addition, these national designations can encourage uniform classification by hospitals, state governments and health departments, and other organizations to promote improved perinatal care. The delineation of care levels and recommended capabilities and types of medical providers for each of the four levels of care are shown in Table 2.2 (29). Importantly, all sites that deliver infants should be capable of performing neonatal resuscitation at every delivery, with at least one provider available to be responsible solely for the infant, consistent with the AAP Neonatal Resuscitation Program (30).

Perinatal Regionalization

Perinatal regionalization is an organized system of care in a geographic area in which infants are born at or transferred to hospitals that are able to provide the most appropriate care for each infant's needs. Hospitals within the region are designated by their capability of providing basic or more highly specialized care. The highest level facilities have the most specialized providers and advanced

technology and equipment appropriate to care for the smallest, most critically ill, or most complex infants in order to ensure the best outcomes. The intent of providing risk-appropriate care to the population within a region is to achieve the best outcomes in the most cost-effective manner. This model has been adopted by several health care systems around the world.

Through its leadership of three important publications, the March of Dimes has pioneered the effort for a rational approach to perinatal services that would produce the best results. In 1976, the March of Dimes Committee on Perinatal Health published *Toward Improving the Outcome of Pregnancy* (TIOP I), a coordinated effort of The American College of Obstetricians and Gynecologists, The American Academy of Pediatrics, the American Medical Association, and the American Academy of Family Physicians. TIOP I recommended a regionalized system of care with three levels of neonatal care (I, II, III) defined within the system. High-risk patients would be referred to centers with the appropriate resources and personnel to care for them. At the time, most level III NICUs were at academic centers. TIOP II, published in 1993, adhered to the same principles of regionalization, but changed the definitions of NICUs to Basic, Specialty, and Subspecialty units with expanded criteria. TIOP III, the most recent revision, again promotes the principle of a coordinated continuum of perinatal services in a geographic region to increase survival of high-risk infants (1). Concentrating relatively rare cases at a few locations allows clinical teams to develop expertise and centralize expensive technologies. TIOP III promotes the use of model programs and quality and safety initiatives, including measurement, transparency, and accountability to improve outcomes.

Numerous studies over more than 45 years have documented an increased risk of poor outcome for VLBW infants who are born and receive care outside of a hospital with the highest level NICU (level III), typically associated with a delivery service. A systematic review and meta-analysis of 41 US and international studies published 1976 through 2010 that included more than 113,000 VLBW infants found 62% increased odds of neonatal or

TABLE 2.1	
Risk Factors for Preterm Birth and Poor Pregnancy Outcomes	
Multifetal pregnancy	Low prepregnant weight
History of prior preterm delivery	Folic acid deficiency
Maternal age <17 or >35 years	Obesity
Black race	Infection
Low socioeconomic status	Bleeding
Unmarried	Anemia
Previous fetal or neonatal death	Toxic stress
Three or more spontaneous fetal losses	Lack of social supports
Uterine abnormalities	Tobacco use
Incompetent cervix	Illicit drug use
Genetic predisposition	Alcohol abuse

TABLE 2.2

Definitions, Capabilities, and Provider Types: Neonatal Levels of Care

Level of Care	Capabilities	Provider Types[a]
Level I Well newborn nursery	• Provide neonatal resuscitation at every delivery • Evaluate and provide postnatal care to stable term newborn infants • Stabilize and provide care for infants born 35–37 wk gestation who remain physiologically stable • Stabilize newborn infants who are ill and those born at <35 wk gestation until transfer to a higher level of care	Pediatricians, family physicians, nurse practitioners, and other advanced practice registered nurses
Level II Special care nursery	Level I capabilities plus: • Provide care for infants born ≥32 wk gestation and weighing ≥1,500 g who have physiologic immaturity or who are moderately ill with problems that are expected to resolve rapidly and are not anticipated to need subspecialty services on an urgent basis • Provide care for infants convalescing after intensive care • Provide mechanical ventilation for brief duration (<24 h) or continuous positive airway pressure or both • Stabilize infants born before 32 wk gestation and weighing <1,500 g until transfer to a neonatal intensive care facility	Level I health care providers plus: Pediatric hospitalists, neonatologist, and neonatal nurse practitioners
Level III NICU	Level II capabilities plus: • Provide sustained life support • Provide comprehensive care for infants born <32 wk gestation and weighing <1,500 g and infants born at all gestational ages and birth weights with critical illness • Provide prompt and readily available access to a full range of pediatric medical subspecialists, pediatric surgical specialists, pediatric anesthesiologists, and pediatric ophthalmologists • Provide a full range of respiratory support that may include conventional and/or high-frequency ventilation and inhaled nitric oxide • Perform advanced imaging, with interpretation on an urgent basis, including computed tomography, MRI, and echocardiography	Level II health care providers plus: Pediatric medical subspecialists[b], *pediatric anesthesiologists*,[b] pediatric surgeons, and pediatric ophthalmologists[b]
Level IV Regional NICU	Level III capabilities plus: • Located within an institution with the capability to provide surgical repair of complex congenital or acquired conditions • Maintain a full range of pediatric medical subspecialists, pediatric surgical subspecialists, and pediatric anesthesiologists at the site • Facilitate transport and provide outreach education	Level III health care providers plus: Pediatric surgical subspecialists

[a]Includes all providers with relevant experience, training, and demonstrated competence.

[b]At the site or at a closely related institution by prearranged consultative agreement.

(Reproduced with permission from American Academy of Pediatrics. Committee on Fetus and Newborn. Levels of neonatal care. *Pediatrics* 2012;130(3):587. Copyright © 2012 by the American Academy of Pediatrics.)

predischarge mortality for infants born at hospitals with non–level III compared to those with level III NICUs (31). Studies that identified extremely LBW infants or those born at less than 32 weeks of gestation showed similar results. This differential effect on mortality was sustained regardless of the decade of publication. More recently, a study compared outcomes in a large cohort of infants born 2008 to 2015 at less than 28 weeks of gestation in England, in a system with perinatal regionalization and specialized neonatal transport services (32). Using propensity score matching to minimize confounder variables, they found that death before discharge was not different between infants who were born and stayed in a tertiary center (controls) and those born in a nontertiary center and transferred to a tertiary center within 48 hours. However, the odds of severe brain injury more than doubled in the transferred infants. Infants who remained in nontertiary hospitals had about a 30% increased risk of death but for uncertain reasons, had no increased risk of brain injury. The role of transport itself is uncertain. In a study of more than 60,000 infants transported to a higher level NICU in California, 30.8% had clinical deterioration during transport (33).

Mortality and morbidity in VLBW infants with specific conditions of prematurity are also affected by the level and volume of the birth hospital NICU, as shown in several studies using data from the California Perinatal Quality Care Collaborative. For example, in a study from 2005 to 2011, mortality was greater for VLBW

infants with necrotizing enterocolitis born at centers with low-volume level IIIA and IIIB NICUs than it was for those born at high-volume level IIIB and IIIC NICUs (California definitions) (34). In another study, the rate of bronchopulmonary dysplasia or death before 36 weeks of postmenstrual age was greater in level II than level IV NICUs; the latter typically located in children's hospitals (35). In addition, the rate of death, duration of assisted ventilation, and hospital length of stay in infants with gastroschisis were lowest in those born in the highest level centers (36). However, delivery of preterm or high-risk infants may occur precipitously or emergently at a less equipped facility, and other factors may affect outcome including characteristics of obstetric care (e.g., prenatal steroid use), the experience of nursing staff, nurse-to-patient ratios, or other issues of practice, including approach to resuscitation at the border of viability. Other factors that may play a role in outcomes include regional differences in race or health insurance status.

Studies have shown conflicting results on the effect of volume of patients on outcomes. It seems logical that the experience derived from management of large numbers of patients with similar conditions would be associated with improved outcomes, and this is supported by most studies. For example, in a retrospective population-based cohort study of more than 70,000 VLBW infants without severe congenital anomalies between 1999 and 2009 in California, Missouri, and Pennsylvania, the risk of death or severe intraventricular hemorrhage and death or necrotizing enterocolitis were lowest for infants born in hospitals with a high volume of VLBW deliveries (>50 VLBW infants per year) and a high-level NICU (37). These results were similar to an earlier retrospective study of 48,237 VLBW infants delivered in California 1991 to 2000 in which compared to delivery at a center with a high-volume (>100 VLBW infants per year) high-level NICU, the odds ratio for death increased with both lower volume and lower NICU level (38). In a study of more than 20,000 infants among 165 neonatal units in England contributing data to a National Neonatal Research Database in 2009 to 2011, the odds ratio for neonatal mortality decreased in infants less than 33 weeks of gestation admitted to a high-volume NICU (39). However, the odds ratio for death associated with admission to a tertiary-level NICU was reduced only in infants less than 27 weeks of gestation. By contrast, a study in the Vermont Oxford Network (VON) in 1995 to 2000 showed that volume of admissions explained only 9% of the variation in mortality rate of VLBW infants among participating hospitals (40). Furthermore, although infants with congenital anomalies are typically excluded from investigations of effects of regionalization, studies suggest that delivery and care at a perinatal center with a level III NICU improves neonatal and obstetrical outcomes of infants with prenatally diagnosed anomalies (41–44). More contemporary data will help inform these findings.

In spite of evidence supporting perinatal regionalization and risk-appropriate care for newborns, reimbursement structures, and policy over the past three to four decades have driven changes in delivery site for VLBW infants in the United States, and these have not always supported efficient regionalization of perinatal services. During the years 1987 to 2008, the number of special care beds increased by 89.2%, while the number of births in the United States increased by only 14.6% (1). Similarly, a retrospective study of data from US metropolitan areas during the period 1980 to 1995 showed that while births increased by 18%, hospitals with NICU beds increased by 99% and the number of neonatologists increased by 268%, with a low occupancy rate for NICUs (45). More recently, in California, the proportion of VLBW infants born at and initially managed at hospitals with high volume and providing the highest level of care fell from 42.5% to 26.5% during the period 2005 to 2011 (34). In addition, a cross-sectional study in the United States found that interquartile rates of NICU admission for infants 500 to 1,499 g born in 2013 were 84.5 to 93.2 per 100 births and that admissions were not related to regional bed supply (46). Although federal data are no longer collected by the Maternal Child Health Bureau, as of 2010, only 75 percent of VLBW infants delivered at facilities with a tertiary NICU.

Multiple factors affect the ability to deliver risk appropriate care for VLBW infants. Across the United States, large variation exists in definitions and regulation of neonatal services and many units self-designate their level (48,49). Structural and social factors also impact site of delivery. For example, mothers with a fetus that has a lethal anomaly might benefit from supportive services in their own community. Providers at some nontertiary hospitals may believe that they can adequately manage VLBW infants and that their own capability differs from published data. This may be compounded by competition among hospitals that encourage establishment of NICUs that do not meet all criteria for a tertiary unit. This competition may hamper maternal transport when neonatal transport is available and efficient. Pregnant women may prefer to deliver locally at a community hospital with their known and trusted provider and may not agree to transfer, or rural hospitals may be at significant distance from higher level facilities, making transfer especially burdensome for families. Finally, disparities in adverse birth outcomes disproportionately affect minorities and economically disadvantaged infants (50), and choice of birth hospital may contribute to these disparities (51,52). A comprehensive approach that includes state regulatory requirements for risk appropriate and societal measures to reduce racial and economic inequalities is needed to ensure that high-risk newborns achieve optimal outcomes.

DIFFERENCES IN THE ORGANIZATION AND SCOPE OF NEONATAL CARE IN HIGH-, MIDDLE-, AND LOW-INCOME COUNTRIES

LMICs have fewer resources than HICs and employ them quite differently. The 75 countries with the highest neonatal mortality account for 60% of births and 85% of neonatal deaths in the world. Government health care spending per capita is much lower in LMICs compared to HICs. Consequently, there is higher reliance on traditional birth attendants in low-income countries (20%) compared with middle-income (9%) and high-income (0%) countries. Only 60% of births in low-income countries have skilled attendants at birth. There are fewer doctors, nurses, and midwives in low-income countries (2 doctors/10,000 population, 7 nurses and midwives/10,000 population) compared with middle-income countries (13 doctors/10,000 population, 20 nurses and midwives/10,000 population) and HICs (29 doctors/10,000 population, 57 nurses and midwives/10,000 population). Access to care is therefore a major issue in low-income countries, where only 3% of births have access to neonatal intensive care, compared with 98% in middle-income countries and 100% in HICs. There is also often lack of transport systems for rapidly and safely moving infants to facilities that can provide appropriate care. (10,53)

It is therefore not surprising that different countries have adopted different standards for limits of viability and resuscitation. While many HICs routinely provide active resuscitation for infants at 24 to 25 weeks of gestation and sometimes even as low as 21 weeks of gestation, this is not necessarily the case in low-income countries.

ESTABLISHING INFRASTRUCTURE TO REDUCE MATERNAL AND INFANT MORTALITY IN LOW RESOURCE SETTINGS

The Every Newborn Action Plan (54), the Lancet Every Newborn series (55–58), and the Born Too Soon: The Global Action Report on Preterm Birth (10) proposed actions for policy, programs, and research by all partners, from governments to NGOs to the business community. Much of the learning and principles from these reports have informed the Sustainable Development Goals for 2030 adopted by the United Nations in 2015, as they pertain to women's, children's, and adolescents' health: ending preventable deaths; ensuring health and well-being; and expanding enabling environments (see Panel 1, Chapter 1). Examples of goals within these domains are eradicating extreme poverty; ending malnutrition; achieving universal primary education for girls and boys; promoting gender equality and empowering women; reducing maternal, infant, and childhood mortality; improving maternal health; combating HIV/AIDS, malaria, and other communicable diseases; ensuring environmental sustainability; and developing a global partnership for development. An integrated service delivery package (see Fig. 1.8, Chapter 1) was proposed to provide health care services that cover the spectrum from prepregnancy to birth and childhood.

As noted earlier, one reason for high mortality in resource-limited settings may be the limited numbers of adequately trained health care professionals in community birth facilities (53). Training in basic newborn care and neonatal resuscitation has been proposed as a low-cost intervention to reduce neonatal mortality. In 2010, a simplified, low-cost curriculum for teaching newborn resuscitation in resource-limited areas, Helping Babies Breathe (HBB), was introduced by a consortium led by the American Academy of Pediatrics (59). Using skill-based learning via simulation, peer teaching, and a pictorial action plan that guides care, HBB has been shown to be effective in decreasing neonatal mortality and stillbirths (60,61). The success of HBB led to the design of a simplified educational program, Essential Care for Every Baby (ECEB), based on the principles of HBB, to teach providers knowledge and skills for essential newborn care. The guidelines for essential newborn care include resuscitation at birth, early and exclusive breastfeeding, temperature regulation, hygiene, and prevention of infection (62). A study testing the effectiveness of training birth attendants from rural communities in six countries using a simplified essential newborn care educational program demonstrated that teaching a bundled newborn care curriculum reduces perinatal mortality (63).

Against the backdrop of persistent high maternal and infant mortality in developing countries, the Bill and Melinda Gates Foundation launched their Maternal, Newborn & Child Health program with significant investments to better understand underlying vulnerabilities and promote resilience among women and children (64). Maternal health is closely linked to newborn survival. With improvements in global under-five child mortality, newborns now account for 46% of all childhood deaths. Annually, an estimated 2.5 million newborns die within their first month of life, and an additional 2.6 million are stillborn. Prematurity, complications during delivery, and infection are the main causes. Attended births in a facility have increased, but quality of care remains a challenge, especially when medical complications arise.

The Bill and Melinda Gates Foundation's Maternal, Newborn & Child Health program (64) supports work at the country level and uses national, regional, and global policy and financing levers to develop and implement proven, cost-effective interventions to better target the root causes of poor maternal and newborn health. There is a sense of urgency to reduce newborn mortality to at least as low as 12 per 1,000 live births in every country, which is required to meet the Sustainable Development Goal targets by 2030.

NATIONAL AND REGIONAL QUALITY IMPROVEMENT NETWORKS

In 2000, the National Academy of Medicine (NAM) highlighted that an estimated 98,000 people per year die as a result of medical errors that occur in hospitals (65). *To Err Is Human* and *Crossing the Quality Chasm* served to galvanize national and local efforts to improve the care delivered in U.S. hospitals (65,66). The NAM reports called attention to the problems of medical errors and created a construct to emerge as a safer, more equitable health system by defining ideal health care as: safe, effective, patient-centered, timely, efficient, and equitable (66).

In 2008, Don Berwick, then the President and Chief Executive Officer of the Institute for Healthcare Improvement (IHI), arguing that effective health system change must occur in the continuum of care, introduced the "Triple Aim." The "Triple Aim" includes three interdependent goals of care:

1. Improving the individual experience of care
2. Improving the health of populations
3. Reducing the per capita costs of care for populations

Berwick argued that improvement objectives must include all three laudable goals. For example, reducing per capita costs for populations without taking into account their health could lead to systematic underutilization. Alternatively, reducing per capita costs, while maintaining health, would ensure the sustainability of our health system and potentially create resources to improve our population's overall health (67).

IHI also provided an important framework for patient improvement. A common improvement framework is known as "Plan, Do, Study Act" or a "PDSA cycle." The PDSA cycle provides a scientific method that enables real-time learning. This model allows for testing a potential improvement by planning, trying, observing, and acting on the lessons learned. The cycle creates the structure to test a change on a small scale (e.g., one patient), refine the improvement based upon lessons learned, and then implement the refined change broadly (e.g., unit wide) (67). The PDSA framework is widely used by national, state, and hospital quality improvement efforts.

Improving Neonatal Care

Variations in practice (68) and outcomes (69,70) are well documented in neonatal care. The presence of variation and the unacceptably high rate of care-related preventable complications (e.g., central line–associated bloodstream infections) created the impetus for national, state, and local quality improvement efforts. The most established and well-known improvement organization is the Vermont Oxford Network (VON). VON began in the 1980s as a nonprofit organization "with the goals of improving the quality and safety of medical care for newborn infants and their families through a coordinated program of research, education, and quality improvement" (71). Through the years, VON has grown to include more than 1,300 neonatal intensive care units worldwide. VON's efforts include collaboratives focused on specific topics including infection and chronic lung disease (72), and it serves as a peer network providing feedback on process and outcome indicators. Participating centers collect data for very-low-birth-weight infants and may also gather data for all treated infants. Centers are able to compare their processes and outcomes to other similar units.

VON provides risk-adjusted outcomes for participating centers to compare their unit's performance. Risk adjustment enables the centers to compare outcomes accounting for heterogeneity among neonates (e.g., comorbid conditions). This process enables differences in outcomes to be better attributed to variations in practice (73). Institutions are presented observed or actual outcomes (e.g., mortality) versus what would be predicted to occur based upon their patient case-mix. This feedback enables institutions to identify areas of improvement (71).

State Collaboratives

States throughout the United States have created PQCs to improve care delivered to infants in their states by advancing evidence-based clinical practices and processes. PQCs include a wide array of stakeholders, including hospital leadership, pediatricians and neonatologists, obstetricians and perinatologists, midwives, nurses, state health department staff, and payors. State collaboratives are uniquely positioned to engage local and state stakeholders to improve neonatal care and address issues that may be unique in their local environments. As of 2020, nearly every U.S. state has established or is in the process of developing a perinatal collaborative, many supported by the Centers for Disease Control and Prevention. State-based efforts have been effective in addressing specific problems, such as central line–associated bloodstream infections (74), reducing deliveries before 39 weeks of gestation without medical indication (75), and in some states, data collection efforts enabled comparisons of outcomes in the setting of state-based system change (e.g., de-regionalization) (34). It is clear that the care delivered in U.S. neonatal intensive care units is safer today than it was just a short time ago largely due to quality improvement efforts (76). However, there remains significant opportunity to decrease variable care and improve outcomes for this vulnerable population.

INTERNATIONAL EFFORTS IN QUALITY IMPROVEMENT

Many countries around the world have launched similar national and international efforts aimed at improving quality of care for neonates, and several countries have established national

GENERAL CONSIDERATIONS

networks for benchmarking neonatal outcomes. Canada pioneered the Evidence-based Practice for Improving Quality (EPIQ) initiative aimed at using a more objective and evidence-based process for quality improvement and implemented a national program of quality improvement that resulted in 25% improvement in survival without major morbidity (from 56.6% to 70.9%) as well as reductions in all major morbidities (bronchopulmonary pulmonary dysplasia 44%, necrotizing enterocolitis 39%, nosocomial infections 46%, severe retinopathy of prematurity 41%, severe brain injury 4%) among infants 32 weeks gestational age and under between 2004 and 2017 (77). The EPIQ concept has now been adopted by many hospitals in Asia, Europe, and South America. The International Network for Evaluating Outcomes (iNEO) comprises 11 countries (Australia, Canada, Finland, Israel, Italy, Japan, New Zealand, Spain, Sweden, Switzerland, UK) that pool population based data from their national networks for international comparison of neonatal outcomes for benchmarking and collaborative quality improvement internationally (78,79). Learning from other countries has yielded many benefits and led to the development of several important initiatives such as kangaroo care (80) and family integrated care (81), both of which are aimed at increasing parental involvement in care of their infants and have led to significantly improved short- and long-term infant outcomes. Among 81 LMICs, Chou et al. estimated that improving quality of care by implementing a subset of basic evidence-based antenatal, childbirth, and postnatal care interventions for mothers and newborns can prevent 67,000 maternal deaths, 0.67 million neonatal deaths, and 0.52 million stillbirths annually (82).

HEALTH CARE EXPENDITURES AND THE ECONOMICS OF NEONATAL CARE

U.S. National Health Expenditures

The United States spends more per capita on health care than any other industrialized nation member of the OECD. In 2019, the United States spent an estimated $10,500 per person on health, more than twice the average of $4,000 per person (83). The United States leads other OECD nations in the proportion of Gross Domestic Product (GDP) spent on health—accounting for nearly 17% of the US economy (83). However, when compared to other OECD countries, the US investment in health produces uneven results, lagging behind other OECD countries in many

indicators of health, including infant mortality, and claiming the highest population rate among OECD countries without health coverage (84).

By 2018, aggregate U.S. national health expenditures (NHE) reached $3.6 trillion (85). Businesses, households, and other private venues were responsible for 55% of expenditures, compared to federal and state governments accounting for 45%. The bulk of US health expenditures are attributed to hospital care (33%) and professional services including physicians (26%; Fig. 2.6). In 2018, NHE grew 4.6% from 2017, rising in all facets of health spending (85).

Expenditures for Newborn Care and Prematurity

Estimates of NHE for the provision of care to newborns are difficult to obtain. An analysis of national hospital billing data by the Agency for Healthcare Research and Quality (AHRQ) estimated national hospital costs for 3.8 million births in 2016 to be $18.9 billion. AHRQ estimated that the 93,600 preterm infants diagnosed with "extreme prematurity" or "respiratory distress" born that year accounted for the greatest proportion of expenditures, exceeding $6.5 billion. Overall, newborns accounted for nearly 40% of NHE on children (86). Importantly, such cost estimates likely underestimate actual costs as they include only hospital costs and not professional fees.

The true cost of prematurity beyond the birth hospitalization is more difficult to measure. In the 2007 NAM report, Preterm Birth: Causes, Consequences, and Prevention, estimated annual expenditures related to be $26.2 billion in 2005, which, after adjusting for inflation equals to $34.7 billion in 2020. More than half of annual expenditures are spent on medical care costs for maternal care at delivery and their children's hospitalization in the neonatal period and beyond ($22.3B). Importantly, the NAM also estimated other direct costs of prematurity with early intervention services ($810M), special education ($1.5B), and indirect costs of lost productivity ($7.5B) (Table 2.3). The NAM suggests their estimates are likely conservative as they only include lifetime costs for four conditions (cerebral palsy, mental retardation, vision impairment, and hearing loss) (87).

Paying for Newborn Care

In 2018, private insurance was the payor for 49.1% of births, compared to 43.0% for state Medicaid programs, 4.1% that were uninsured, and 3.8% attributed to sources (e.g., Tricare) (88). From

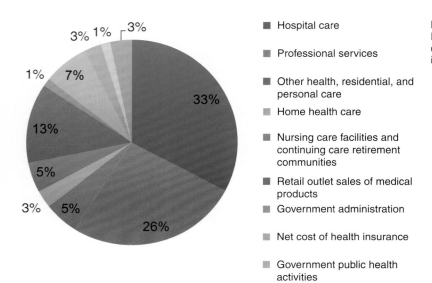

- ■ Hospital care
- ■ Professional services
- ■ Other health, residential, and personal care
- ■ Home health care
- ■ Nursing care facilities and continuing care retirement communities
- ■ Retail outlet sales of medical products
- ■ Government administration
- ■ Net cost of health insurance
- ■ Government public health activities

FIGURE 2.6 National Health Expenditures, 2018. (Adapted from Hartman M, et al. National Health Care spending in 2018: growth driven by accelerations in Medicare and private insurance spending. *Health Aff (Millwood)* 2020;39(1):8.)

TABLE 2.3

Estimates Aggregate and Individual Costs Associated with Prematurity in 2014

	Medical Care Costs			Other Costs				
	Birth to Age 5 Y	6 Y and older (4 DDs)	Total	Early Intervention	Special Education (4 DDs)	Lost Productivity (4 DDs)	Maternal Delivery	Total
Aggregate (millions)	$21,100	$1,300	$22,300	$810	$1,500	$7,500	$2,600	$34,700
Per infant (dollars)	$41,500	$2,500	$44,000	$1,600	$2,900	$14,900	$4,600	$68,400

aData from Estimates from National Academy of Medicine Institute of Medicine Committee on Understanding Premature, B. and O. Assuring Healthy. The National Academies Collection: Reports funded by National Institutes of Health. In: Behrman RE, Butler AS, eds. *Preterm birth: Causes, Consequences, and Prevention*, Washington, DC: National Academies Press (US) National Academy of Sciences, 2007. Adjusted to 2020 US$ using the Consumer Price Index.Statistics, U.S.B.o.L. Consumer Price Index. 2014 [cited July 15, 2014]; Available from http://www.bls.gov/cpi/

2008 to 2018, the proportion of births paid by Medicaid increased from 40.5% to 43.0%, highlighting the importance of this program to maternal child health (88,89). Medicaid is the most common source of payment for births in rural communities (50.0%), among teenaged births (77.5%), and among women with a high school education (65.8%). There is substantial state variation in Medicaid paid births ranging from 62.8% in Louisiana to 25.3% in North Dakota (88).

Today, Medicaid, also known as Title XIX of the Social Security Act, is the single largest purchaser of health care for newborns. The program, which began in 1965, was created to provide coverage for impoverished, women, children, and elderly (90). Since its inception, Medicaid has expanded and, along with the Children's Health Insurance Program, now covers more than 71 million Americans accounting for $592B in annual expenditures. When compared to other populations covered by Medicaid, children account for a relatively small share of total Medicaid expenditures; in total, children account for 51% of Medicaid enrollment and 19% of expenditures (91). The program's important role as a safety net for vulnerable populations has been clear during US economic downturns. The "great recession" from 2007 to 2009 coincided with a rise in unemployment and child poverty but not a rise in the number of uninsured children in the United States. The program's design, as well as additional investment in the program through the American Recovery and Reinvestment Act, ensured that Medicaid insured additional children (92). Whether this will prove true in the severe recession caused by the SARS-CoV-2 pandemic remains to be seen.

Medicaid is jointly financed by federal and state governments and is administered by states. Each state is given federal matching dollars to support their Medicaid program based upon a 3-year running average of their state's per capita income relative to the nation. As such, states vary widely in their contribution to their Medicaid programs (93). For example, in Fiscal Year 2011, Mississippi's federal match is 78% compared to Wyoming at the mandated floor of 50% (91). Therefore, the federal government spends three dollars for every dollar Mississippi spends on Medicaid, compared to one dollar for every dollar Wyoming spends on their program.

Medicaid's role in covering a high proportion of neonates also means that the program has opportunities to manage the quality of care delivered through the use of incentives and penalties, known as pay-for-performance. For example, the Patient Protection and Affordable Care Act mandated that Medicaid not pay for certain hospital-associated infections (HAIs) including central line–associated bloodstream infections (94). While similar programs for adults aimed at preventing HAI in Medicare have not been shown to be effective (95), it is likely that pay-for-performance will continue to play a role in health care financing moving forward.

Another federal-state program that plays a critical role for neonates is the Maternal Child Health Grant, also known as Title V of the Social Security Act. As opposed to Medicaid, which is an entitlement program, Title V is a block grant providing a fixed amount to states of maternal and child health. The program was enacted

in 1935 and provides funding for mothers, infants, and has a specific focus on children with special needs. The program varies in its scope from state-to-state, but each Title V program:

- Focuses exclusively on the entire maternal and child health population
- Encompasses infrastructure, population-based, enabling, and direct services for the maternal and child health population
- Requires a unique partnership arrangement between federal, state, and local entities
- Requires each state to work collaboratively with other organizations to conduct a state-wide, comprehensive Needs Assessment every 5 years
- Based on the findings of the Needs Assessment, requires each state to identify state priorities to comprehensively address the needs of the MCH population and guide the use of the Maternal and Child Health Block Grant funds
- May serve as the payer of last resort for direct services for the maternal and child health population that are not covered by any other program

Patient Protection and Affordable Care Act

In March 2010, the Patient Protection and Affordable Care Act (PPACA) was signed into law. The passage of the PPACA represented the largest change to our health care system since the passage of Medicaid and Medicare in the 1960s. The basic premise of the PPACA is to expand health care coverage through Medicaid expansions to previously ineligible groups (e.g., adults without children), through the creation of federal- and state-based health insurance exchanges and by mandating coverage. Importantly, the PPACA also created standards for coverage that have implications for preterm infants. Prior to the PPACA, annual and lifetime expenditure caps were not an uncommon feature of insurance policies, especially among those purchased on the individual market (i.e., not employer-sponsored). The PPACA eliminated caps for coverage, ensured that no one be denied coverage for preexisting conditions, and ensured coverage for maternity care (96).

COVID-19 AND PERINATAL CARE

At the time of this chapter submission, the world is battling a global pandemic caused by the novel coronavirus SARS-CoV-2. COVID-19, the name of the disease caused by SARS-CoV-2, has been reported on every continent except Antarctica. It can affect persons of all ages, including newborns. Multiple reports document COVID-19 infections among pregnant women (97–104).

Early reports suggested that pregnant women were not at increased risk for severe respiratory illness or death, but had higher rates of preterm birth and cesarean delivery (102). In institutions with universal testing of pregnant women admitted to the hospital, the SARS-CoV-2 screen positive rate is about 15%, with a large proportion of asymptomatic women (103). As confirmed infections continue to rise, there are increasing numbers of pregnant women

GENERAL CONSIDERATIONS

with COVID-19 presenting to hospitals with respiratory symptoms, sometimes severe, similar to reports of women with severe illness during earlier SARS and MERS-CoV outbreaks.

Pediatric data demonstrate that children of all ages are susceptible to SARS-CoV-2. In general, children with COVID-19 tend to have less severe disease and a much lower mortality than older individuals (104–107). While many children infected with SARS-CoV-2 are asymptomatic, severe disease can occur in children (108), especially in those with underlying conditions, and infants under 1 year of age (109). In the United States, children aged less than 1 year accounted for the highest percentage (15% to 62%) of hospitalization among pediatric patients with COVID-19 (110). Among 95 children aged less than 1 year, 59 (62%) were hospitalized, including 5 requiring ICU care (110). Among 345 pediatric cases, 80 (23%) had at least one underlying condition. The most common underlying conditions were chronic lung disease (including asthma), cardiovascular disease, and immunosuppression (110). Just as the pediatric medical community was heaving a collective sigh of relief that the worst of this pandemic generally spared the pediatric age group, a new inflammatory syndrome, currently termed multi-system inflammatory syndrome in children (MIS-C), with presentations resembling atypical Kawasaki disease or toxic shock syndrome, has grabbed the attention of pediatricians and the public health community. Clinical presentation includes persistent fever, variable rash, conjunctivitis, peripheral edema, generalized extremity pain, significant gastrointestinal symptoms and progression to warm, vasoplegic shock, refractory to volume resuscitation, and eventually requiring pressors for hemodynamic support (111). Reported cases are on the rise, and several deaths have been reported. The link to COVID-19 remains unclear, but at this time, the syndrome is thought to be a postviral inflammatory response in children across the full age spectrum from infancy to young adults.

The data for newborns with COVID-19 are still limited. Although there are reports of COVID-19 in newborns, the risk for vertical transmission, however, appears to be low (112–114). Respiratory secretions and saliva are the primary infectious fluids for transmission of SARS-CoV-2, although virus has also been detected in blood and stool. Among tested newborns who were positive for SARS-CoV-2, several had pneumonia by clinical and radiographic criteria; a few had abnormalities in inflammatory markers and transaminase levels (113). At this time, there is insufficient evidence to recommend the optimal mode of delivery for infected mothers or the risk to the newborn of prolonged rupture of membranes. The impact and necessity of mother/newborn separation and the role of breastfeeding in promoting or protecting newborns from infection need further study (115) No study to date has demonstrated the presence of SARS-CoV-2 in breast milk. In the United States, it has been recommended that infected mothers express breast milk (after appropriate breast and hand hygiene) and this milk be fed to the infant by an uninfected caregiver. At the time of writing, different countries are developing different policies with respect to breast feeding: practitioners are advised to follow the guidance that applies to their place and country of work. In addition to the known benefits of breastfeeding, mothers' milk may provide infant protective factors after maternal COVID-19.

In the United States, racial and ethnic disparities in illness severity and outcomes are being reported, with a disproportionately high death rate among black Americans (116). An article under review suggests that Hispanic women are at increased risk for severe disease during pregnancy (117). COVID-19 may further exacerbate racial and ethnic disparities in pregnancy outcomes in the United States and around the globe. In some LMICs, poor sanitation, overcrowded housing, poverty, and limited access to clean water, soap, and sanitizers magnifies the risks of widespread infection. Without access to advanced medical care and testing, the death toll is likely to be extremely high but also difficult to accurately count. The clinical and research communities will need to consider COVID-19 when addressing perinatal services and global comparisons and challenges.

REFERENCES

1. Berns SD, ed. *Toward improving the outcome of pregnancy III: enhancing perinatal health through quality, safety and performance initiatives. Reissued edition*. White Plains, NY: March of Dimes Foundation, 2011.
2. Available from: https://www.macrotrends.net/countries/USA/united-states/infant-mortality-rate
3. Guyer B, Freedman MA, Strobino DM, et al. Annual summary of vital statistics: trends in the health of Americans during the 20th century. *Pediatrics* 2000;106:1307.
4. Centers for Disease Control and Prevention. Advancements in public health, 1900-1999: healthier mothers and babies. *MMWR* 1999;48:849.
5. Murphy SL, Xu JQ, Kochanek KD, Arias E. *Mortality in the United States, 2017*. NCHS Data Brief, no 328. Hyattsville, MD: National Center for Health Statistics, 2018.
6. America's Health Rankings® Annual Report 2019 Edition. Available from: www.AmericasHealthRankings.org; https://www.americashealthrankings.org/learn/reports/2019-annual-report/international-comparison
7. Available from: https://www.healthsystemtracker.org/chart-collection/infant-mortality-u-s-compare-countries/#item-accounting-for-differential-reporting-methods-u-s-infant-mortality-remains-higher-than-in-comparable-countries
8. Horbar LD, Carpenter JH, Badger GJ, et al. Mortality and neonatal morbidity among infants 501-1500 grams from 2000 to 2009. *Pediatrics* 2012;129:1019.
9. Ely DM, Driscoll AK. Infant mortality in the United States, 2017: data from the period linked birth/infant death file. *Natl Vital Stat Rep* 2019;68(10):1.
10. March of Dimes, PMNCH, Save the Children, WHO. In: Howson CP, Kinney MV, Lawn JE, eds. *Born too soon: the global action report on preterm birth*. Geneva, Switzerland: World Health Organization, 2012.
11. MacDorman MF, Mathews TJ, Mohangoo AD, et al. International comparisons of infant mortality and related factors: United States and Europe, 2010. *Natl Vital Stat Rep* 2014;63(5):1.
12. Ref: 2019 March of Dimes Report. Available from: http://https://www.marchofdimes.org/materials/MOD2019_REPORT_CARD_and_POLICY_ACTIONS_BOOKLETv72.pdf
13. Ref: https://www.statista.com/statistics/263738/infant-mortality-in-the-usa/
14. McIntire DD, Leveno KJ. Neonatal mortality and morbidity rates in late preterm births compared with births at term. *Obstet Gynecol* 2008;111:35.
15. Tomashek KM, Shapiro-Mendoza CK, Davidoff MJ, et al. Differences in mortality between late-preterm and term singleton infants in the United States, 1995-2002. *J Pediatr* 2007;151:450, 6 e1.
16. *NICHD Workshop: Optimizing Care and Long-term Outcome of Near-term Pregnancy and Near-term Newborn Infant*. Bethesda, MD. July 18-19, 2005.
17. Zhang X, Kramer MS. Variations in mortality and morbidity by gestational age among infants born at term. *J Pediatr* 2009;154:358, e2 e1.
18. Clark SL, Belfort MA, Byrum SL, et al. Improved outcomes, fewer cesarean deliveries, and reduced litigation: results of a new paradigm in patient safety. *Am J Obstet Gynecol* 2008;199:105 e1.
19. Tita AT, Landon MB, Spong CY, et al. Timing of elective repeat cesarean delivery at term and neonatal outcomes. *N Engl J Med* 2009;360:111.
20. Thompson LA, Goodman DC, Little GA. Is more neonatal intensive care always better? Insights from a cross-national comparison of reproductive care. *Pediatrics* 2002;109(6):1036.
21. Available from: https://www.abp.org/content/pediatric-subspecialists-ever-certified
22. Available from: https://www.abp.org/sites/abp/files/pdf/abp_pediatric_workforce_trends.pdf
23. American Board of Pediatrics. *Workforce Data 2013-2014*. Available from: https://www.abp.org/sites/abp/files/pdf/workforcebook.pdf
24. Wallman C; American Academy of Pediatrics Committee on Fetus and Newborn. Advanced practice in neonatal nursing. *Pediatrics* 2009;123:1606 (reaffirmed January 2014).
25. Freed GL, Dunham KM, Lamarand KE, et al. Neonatal nurse practitioners: distribution, roles and scope of practice. *Pediatrics* 2010;126:856.
26. Cusson RM, Buus-Frank ME, Flanagan VA, et al. A survey of the current neonatal nurse practitioner workforce. *J Perinatol* 2008;12:830.
27. Pressler JL, Kenner CA. The NNP/DNP shortage: transforming neonatal nurse practitioners into DNPs. *J Perinat Neonatal Nurs* 2009;23:272.
28. American Academy of Pediatrics Committee on Fetus and Newborn. Levels of neonatal care. *Pediatrics* 2012;130:587; reaffirmed 2015;136(5):e1418.
29. American Academy of Pediatrics Committee on Fetus and Newborn. Levels of neonatal care. *Pediatrics* 2012;130:587.
30. Weiner GM, Zaichkin J, eds. *Textbook of neonatal resuscitation (NRP)*, 7th ed. American Academy of Pediatrics and American Heart Association, 2016.

31. Lasswell SM, Barfield WD, Rochat RW, et al. Perinatal regionalization for very low-birth-weight and very preterm infants: a meta-analysis. *JAMA* 2010;304:992.

32. Hellenius K, Longford N, Lehtonen L, et al. Association of early postnatal transfer and birth outside a tertiary hospital with mortality and severe brain injury in extremely preterm infants: observational cohort study with propensity score matching. *BMJ* 2019;367:l5678.

33. Pai VV, Kan P, Gould JB, et al. Clinical deterioration during neonatal transport in California. *J Perinatol* 2020;40(3):377. doi: 10.1038/s41372-019-0488.

34. Kastenberg ZJ, Lee HC, Profit J, et al. Effect of deregionalized care on mortality in very-low-birth-weight infants with necrotizing enterocolitis. *JAMA Pediatr* 2015;169(1):26. doi: 10.1001/jamapediatrics.2014.2085.

35. Lapcharoensap W, Gage SC, Kan P, et al. *JAMA Pediatr* 2015;169(2):e143676. doi: 10.1001/jamapediatrics.2014.3676.

36. Apfeld JC, Kastenberg ZJ, Sylvester KG, et al. The effect of level of care on gastroschisis outcomes. *J Pediatr* 2017;190:79.

37. Jensen EA, Lorch SA. Effects of a birth hospital's neonatal intensive care level and annual volume of very-low-birth-weight infant deliveries on morbidity and mortality. *JAMA Pediatr* 2015;169(8):151906.

38. Phibbs CS, Baker LC, Caughey AB, et al. Level and volume of neonatal intensive care and mortality in very-low-birth-weight infants. *N Engl J Med* 2007;356:2165.

39. Watson SI, Arulampalam W, Petrou S, et al. The effects of designation and volume of neonatal care on mortality and morbidity outcomes of very preterm infants in England: retrospective population-based cohort study. *BMJ Open* 2014;4:e004856.

40. Rogowski JA, Horbar JD, Staiger DO, et al. Indirect vs direct hospital quality indicators for very low birth-weight infants. *JAMA* 2004;291:202.

41. Audibert F. Regionalization of perinatal care: did we forget congenital anomalies? *Ultrasound Obstet Gynecol* 2007;29:247.

42. Calisti A, Oriolo L, Giannino G, et al. Delivery in a tertiary center with co-located surgical facilities makes the difference among neonates with prenatally diagnosed major abnormalities. *J Matern Fetal Neonatal Med* 2012;25:1735.

43. Nasr A, Langer JC; Canadian Paediatric Surgery Network. Influence of location of delivery on outcome in neonates with gastroschisis. *J Pediatr Surg* 2012;47:2022.

44. Nasr A, Langer JC; Canadian Paediatric Surgery Network. Influence of location of delivery on outcome in neonates with congenital diaphragmatic hernia. *J Pediatr Surg* 2011;46:814.

45. Howell EM, Richardson D, Ginsburg P, et al. Deregionalization of neonatal intensive care in urban areas. *Am J Public Health* 2002;92:119.

46. Harrison WN, Wasserman JR, Goodman DC. Regional variation in neonatal intensive care admissions and the relationship to bed supply. *J Pediatr* 2018;192:73.

47. Maternal and Child Health Bureau Title V Block Grant. Available from: https://mchdata.hrsa.gov/TVISReports/Charts/PMGMap.aspx?ReportType=NPM&MeasureType=Performance&PMNum=17

48. Blackmon LR, Barfield WD, Stark AR. Hospital neonatal services in the United States: variation in definitions, criteria and regulatory status, 2008. *J Perinatol* 2009;29:788.

49. Kroelinger CD, Okoroh EM, Goodman DA, et al. Designation of neonatal levels of care: a review of state regulatory and monitoring policies. *J Perinatol* 2019. doi: 10.1038/s41372-019-0500-0.

50. Burris HH, Hacker MR. Birth outcome racial disparities: a result of intersecting social and environmental factors. *Semin Perinatol* 2017;6:360.

51. Howell EA, Janevic T, Herbert PL, et al. Differences in morbidity and mortality rates in black, white, and Hispanic very preterm infants among New York City hospitals. *JAMA Pediatr* 2018;172(3):269.

52. Profit J, Gould JB, Bennett M, et al. Racial/ethnic disparity in NICU quality of care delivery. *Pediatrics* 2017;141(3):e20170918.

53. Lawn JE, Wilczynska-Ketende K, Cousens SN. Estimating the causes of 4 million neonatal deaths in the year 2000. *Int J Epidemiol* 2006;35:706. doi: 10.1093/ije/dyl043.

54. WHO. *Every newborn: an action plan to end preventable deaths*, 2014. Available from: http://www.everynewborn.org/Documents/Full-action-plan-EN.pdf. Accessed December 26, 2014.

55. Lawn JE, Blencowe H, Oza S, et al. Every newborn: progress, priorities, and potential beyond survival. *Lancet* 2014;384(9938):132.

56. Bhutta ZA, Das JK, Bahl R, et al. Can available interventions end preventable deaths in mothers, newborn babies, and stillbirths, and at what cost? *Lancet* 2014;384(9940):308.

57. Dickson KE, Simen-Kapeu A, Kinney MV, et al. Every newborn: health-systems bottlenecks and strategies to accelerate scale-up in countries. *Lancet* 2014;384(9941):438.

58. Mason E, McDougall L, Lawn JE, et al. From evidence to action to deliver a healthy start for the next generation. *Lancet* 2014;384(9941):455.

59. Singhal N, Lockyer J, Fidler H, et al. Helping Babies Breathe: global neonatal resuscitation program development and formative educational evaluation. *Resuscitation* 2012;83(1):90.

60. Goudar S, Somannavar M, Clark R, et al. Stillbirth and newborn mortality in India after Helping Babies Breathe training. *Pediatrics* 2013;131(2):e344. doi: 10.1542/peds.2012-2112.

61. Msemo G, Massawe A, Mmbando D, et al. Newborn mortality and fresh stillbirth rates in Tanzania after Helping Babies Breathe training. *Pediatrics* 2013;131(2):e353.

62. World Health Organization. *Pregnancy, childbirth, postpartum and newborn care: a guide for essential practice*, 2nd ed. Geneva, Switzerland: World Health Organization, 2006.

63. Carlo WA, Goudar SS, Jehan I, et al. Newborn-care training and perinatal mortality in developing countries. *N Engl J Med* 2010;362(7):614.

64. Available from: https://www.gatesfoundation.org/what-we-do/global-development/maternal-newborn-and-child-health

65. Institute of Medicine Committee on Quality of Health Care in America. In: Kohn LT, Corrigan JM, Donaldson MS, eds. *To err is human: building a safer health system*. Washington, DC: National Academies Press (US), 2000. Copyright 2000 by the National Academy of Sciences. All rights reserved.

66. Institute of Medicine Committee on Quality of Health Care in America. *Crossing the quality chasm: a new health system for the 21st century*. Washington, DC: National Academies Press (US), 2001. Copyright 2001 by the National Academy of Sciences. All rights reserved.

67. Berwick DM, Nolan TW, Whittington J. The triple aim: care, health, and cost. *Health Aff (Project Hope)* 2008;27(3):759.

68. McCormick MC, Escobar GJ, Zheng Z, et al. Place of birth and variations in management of late preterm ("near-term") infants. *Semin Perinatol* 2006;30(1):44.

69. Sankaran K, Chien LY, Walker R, et al. Variations in mortality rates among Canadian neonatal intensive care units. *CMAJ* 2002;166(2):173.

70. Vohr BR, Wright LL, Dusick AM, et al. Center differences and outcomes of extremely low birth weight infants. *Pediatrics* 2004;113(4):781.

71. Horbar JD, Soll RF, Edwards WH. The Vermont Oxford Network: a community of practice. *Clin Perinatol* 2010;37(1):29.

72. Horbar JD, Rogowski J, Plsek PE, et al. Collaborative quality improvement for neonatal intensive care. NIC/Q Project Investigators of the Vermont Oxford Network. *Pediatrics* 2001;107(1):14.

73. Patrick SW, Schumacher RE, Davis MM. Methods of mortality risk adjustment in the NICU: a 20-year review. *Pediatrics* 2013;131(suppl 1):S68.

74. Fisher D, Cochran KM, Provost LP, et al. Reducing central line-associated bloodstream infections in North Carolina NICUs. *Pediatrics* 2013;132(6):e1664.

75. Donovan EF, Lannon C, Bailit J, et al. A statewide initiative to reduce inappropriate scheduled births at 36(0/7)-38(6/7) weeks' gestation. *Am J Obstet Gynecol* 2010;202(3):243.e241.

76. Horbar JD, Edwards EM, Greenberg LT, et al. Variation in Performance of Neonatal Intensive Care Units in the United States. *JAMA Pediatr* 2017;171(3):e164396.

77. Lee SK, Beltempo M, McMillan DD, et al. Outcomes and care practices for preterm infants <33 weeks' gestation: a quality improvement study. *CMAJ* 2020;192(4):E81. doi: 10.1503/cmaj.190940.

78. Shah PS, Lui K, Reichman B, et al.; International Network for Evaluating Outcomes (iNeo) of Neonates. The International Network for Evaluating Outcomes (iNeo) of neonates: evolution, progress and opportunities. *Transl Pediatr* 2019;8(3):170. doi: 10.21037/tp.2019.07.06.

79. Lui K, Lee SK, Kusuda S, et al.; iNeo Investigators. Trends in neonatal outcomes for very preterm and very low birth weight neonates in 11 countries. *J Pediatr* 2019;215:32. doi: 10.1016/j.jpeds.2019.08.020.

80. Ramanathan K, Paul VK, Deorari AK, et al. Kangaroo Mother Care in very low birth weight infants. *Indian J Pediatr* 2001;68:1019.

81. O'Brien K, Robson K, Bracht M, et al.; SK for the FICare Study Group and FICare Parent Advisory Board. Evaluation of family integrated care: a cluster randomized controlled trial in Canada, Australia, and New Zealand. *Lancet Child Adolesc Health* 2018;2:245. doi: 10.1016/S2352-4642(18)30039-7.

82. Chou VB, Perrson LA. Estimating the global impact of poor quality of care on maternal and neonatal outcomes in 81 low- and middle-income countries: a modeling study. *PLoS Med* 2019;16(12):e1002990.

83. *Health spending*, 2018. Available from: https://data.oecd.org/healthres/health-spending.htm. Accessed March 24, 2020.

84. Lorenzoni L, Belloni A, Sassi F. Health-care expenditure and health policy in the USA versus other high-spending OECD countries. *Lancet* 2014;384(9937):83.

85. Hartman M, et al. National health care spending in 2018: growth driven by accelerations in Medicare and private insurance spending. *Health Aff (Millwood)* 2020;39(1):8.

86. Moore BJ, Freeman WJ, Jiang HJ. Costs of pediatric hospital stays, 2016. In: *HCUP statistical brief*. Rockville, MD: Agency for Healthcare Research and Quality, 2019.

87. Institute of Medicine Committee on Understanding Premature Birth and Assuring Healthy Outcomes. The National Academies Collection. Reports funded by National Institutes of Health. In: Behrman RE, Butler AS, eds. *Preterm birth: causes, consequences, and prevention*. Washington, DC: National Academies Press (US) National Academy of Sciences, 2007.

GENERAL CONSIDERATIONS

88. *Medicaid's role in financing maternity care.* Washington, DC: MACPAC, 2020:1.

89. Kowlessar NM, Jiang HJ, Steiner C. In: A.f.H.R.a. Quality, ed. *Hospital stays for newborns, 2011.* HCUP Statistical Brief #163. Rockville, MD: Agency for Healthcare Research and Quality, 2013.

90. Patrick SW, Freed GL. Intergenerational enrollment and expenditure changes in Medicaid: trends from 1991 to 2005. *BMC Health Serv Res* 2012;12:327.

91. *Medicaid & CHIP,* 2020. Available from: https://www.kff.org/state-category/medicaid-chip/. Accessed March 24, 2020.

92. Patrick SW, Choi H, Davis MM. Increase in federal match associated with significant gains in coverage for children through Medicaid and CHIP. *Health Aff (Millwood)* 2012;31(8):1796.

93. Patrick SW, Davis MM. Reformulating the federal match as a key to the sustainability of Medicaid. *JAMA Pediatr* 2013;167(3):218.

94. Patrick SW, et al. Health care-associated infections among critically ill children in the US, 2007-2012. *Pediatrics* 2014;134(4):705.

95. Lee GM, et al. Effect of nonpayment for preventable infections in U.S. hospitals. *N Engl J Med* 2012;367(15):1428. Summary of the Affordable Care Act. 2013. Available from: http://kff.org/health-reform/fact-sheet/summary-of-the-affordable-care-act/. Accessed December 2, 2014.

96. U.S. Bureau of Labor Statistics. *Consumer price index,* 2014. Available from: http://www.bls.gov/cpi/. Accessed July 15, 2014.

97. Chen L, Li Q, Zheng D, et al. Clinical characteristics of pregnant women with Covid-19 in Wuhan, China. *N Engl J Med* 2020;382(25):e100.

98. Yang H, Sun G, Tang F, et al. Clinical features and outcomes of pregnant women suspected of coronavirus disease 2019. *J Infect* 2020; 81(1):e40.

99. Della Gatta AN, Rizzo R, Pilu G, et al. Coronavirus disease 2019 during pregnancy: a systematic review of reported cases. *Am J Obstet Gynecol* 2020.

100. Yang Z, Wang M, Zhu Z, et al. Coronavirus disease 2019 (COVID-19) and pregnancy: a systematic review. *J Matern Fetal Neonatal Med* 2020:1. doi: 10.1080/14767058.2020.1759541

101. Kasraeian M, Zare M, Vafaei H, et al. COVID-19 pneumonia and pregnancy; a systematic review and meta-analysis. *J Matern Fetal Neonatal Med* 2020:1. doi: 10.1080/14767058.2020.1763952

102. Liu D, Li L, Wu X, et al. Pregnancy and perinatal outcomes of women with coronavirus disease (COVID-19) pneumonia: a preliminary analysis. *AJR Am J Roentgenol* 2020;215(1):127.

103. Sutton D, Fuchs K, D'Alton M, et al. Universal screening for SARS-CoV-2 in women admitted for delivery. *N Engl J Med* 2020;382:2163.

104. Juan J, Gil MM, Rong Z, et al. Effects of coronavirus disease 2019 (COVID-19) on maternal, perinatal and neonatal outcomes: a systematic review. *Ultrasound Obstet Gynecol* 2020.

105. Wu Z, McGoogan JM. Characteristics of and important lessons from the Coronavirus Disease 2019 (COVID-19) outbreak in China: summary of a report of 72314 cases from the Chinese Center for Disease Control and Prevention. *JAMA* 2020.

106. Lu X, Zhang L, Du H, et al. SARS-CoV-2 infection in children. *N Engl J Med* 2020;382:1663.

107. Dong Y, Mo X, Hu Y, et al. Epidemiological characteristics of 2143 pediatric patients with 2019 coronavirus disease in China. *Pediatrics* 2020. doi: 10.1542/peds.2020-0702

108. Shekerdemian LS, Mahmood NR, Wolfe KK, et al. Characteristics and outcomes of children with Coronavirus Disease 2019 (COVID-19) infection admitted to US and Canadian pediatric intensive care units. *JAMA Pediatr* 2020;174(9):86. doi: 10.1001/jamapediatrics.2020.1948.

109. Dong Y, Mo X, Hu Y, et al. Epidemiological characteristics of 2143 pediatric patients with 2019 coronavirus disease in China. *Pediatrics* 2020;145(6):e20200702. doi: 10.1542/peds.2020-0702.

110. Coronavirus disease 2019 in children—United States, February 12–April 2, 2020. *MMWR Morb Mortal Wkly Rep* 2020;69:422. doi: 10.15585/mmwr.mm6914e4external icon.

111. Riphagen S, Gomez X, Gonzalez-Martinez C, et al. Hyperinflammatory shock in children during COVID-19 pandemic. *Lancet* 2020;395(10237):1607. doi: 0.1016/S0140-6736(20)31094-1.

112. Zeng L, Xia S, Yuan W, et al. Neonatal early-onset infection with SARS-CoV-2 in 33 neonates born to mothers with COVID-19 in Wuhan, China. *JAMA Pediatr* 2020;174(7):722.

113. Zhu H, Wang L, Fang C, et al. Clinical analysis of 10 neonates born to mothers with 2019-nCoV pneumonia. *Transl Pediatr* 2020;9:51.

114. Chen H, Guo J, Wang C, et al. Clinical characteristics and intrauterine vertical transmission potential of COVID-19 infection in nine pregnant women: a retrospective review of medical records. *Lancet* 2020;395:809.

115. Puopolo KM, Hudak ML, Kimberlin DW, et al. *INITIALGUIDANCE: management of infants born to mothers with COVID-19.* American Academy of Pediatrics Committee on Fetus and Newborn, Section on Neonatal Perinatal Medicine, and Committee on Infectious Diseases, April 2, 2020. Available from: https://downloads.aap.org/AAP/PDF/COVID%2019%20Initial%20Newborn%20Guidance.pdf

116. Webb Hooper M, Nápoles AM, Pérez-Stable EJ. COVID-19 and racial/ethnic disparities. *JAMA* 2020;323(24):2466. doi: 10.1001/jama.2020.8598.

3 Newborn Intensive Care Unit Design: Scientific and Practical Considerations

Robert D. White, Judith A. Smith, and Gilbert I. Martin

INTRODUCTION

A newborn ICU (NICU) is intended to provide the space and equipment necessary to treat ill newborns safely and effectively. In doing so, it must also facilitate staff efficacy and work quality, encourage parental presence and participation, and provide an optimal physical and sensory environment for high-risk newborns.

In the ideal circumstance there are adequate supplies to accomplish these goals, but in many cases resources, including space, equipment, and staff, are limited. Even then, however, there should be no reduction in the key aspects of cleanliness, parental access, and an optimal physical and sensory environment.

In this chapter, we will outline basic and optimal features of the physical design of a NICU. For those who have the opportunity to undertake new construction, every effort should be made to achieve optimal design. When an existing unit is being renovated, limitations of space and funding may sometimes restrict the extent to which planners can specify these optimal features. When new construction or renovation is not possible, even further limitations will exist, yet efforts to optimize parental presence, cleanliness, and the physical and sensory environment should still be undertaken.

SCIENTIFIC FOUNDATIONS FOR NEWBORN ICU DESIGN CONSIDERATIONS

The evidence supporting recommendations for the optimal NICU design derives from three general lines of inquiry: (a) the optimal sensory environment for the high-risk newborn infant; (b) the optimal environment for adults who spend extended periods of time in the NICU, including both hospital staff and parents; and (c) clinical trials of specific NICU design features, most notably the single-family room.

Optimal Sensory Environment for High-Risk Newborns

There is limited evidence on which to judge the optimal sensory environment for the high-risk newborn infant. Extrapolation from the *in utero* environment presents several difficulties: (a) We have limited information on the sensory input received by the fetus. Sound levels, for example, appear to be fairly high for the fetus but are delivered via a liquid medium rather than through an air medium, so it is difficult to judge what an equivalent sensory experience would be for a high-risk newborn. (b) Certain stimuli cannot be replicated. For example, the fetus receives circadian signals from the mother that include transplacental hormones as well as variation in maternal body temperature and activity. Postnatally, the same stimuli are difficult to replicate. Likewise, the liquid-filled uterus undoubtedly provides a different type of proprioceptive stimulus than any environment currently possible in an incubator. Conversely, the newborn infant receives much more visual stimuli than does a fetus. (c) *In utero*, the fetus is generally in a stable, homeostatic, anabolic condition. After birth, its medical status may be quite tenuous, so certain stimuli that would be appropriate for a more stable infant may not be suitable for one who is critically ill.

In spite of these challenges, there have been a number of efforts to identify the optimal sensory environment of care for high-risk newborns. Comprehensive systems of care, often referred to as "developmental care," have been described and studied; the Newborn Individualized Developmental Care and Assessment Program (NIDCAP) is the most extensively investigated (1,2). Specific forms of stimuli, such as music or parental conversation (3,4), have also been evaluated. The clearest benefit has been described for skin-to-skin (STS) care, also known as kangaroo care. Because it involves extensive human contact with multisensory input, it is likely that STS most closely replicates the *in utero* environment, especially if it is provided by the baby's mother. Benefits of STS has been shown in many trials, some with extended follow-up (5,6).

The optimal sensory environment for the high-risk newborn is likely to have the following characteristics:

1. Minimal noxious stimuli, including noise, bright lights, and unpleasant procedures
2. Generous availability of human contact, ideally provided by a parent in extended, intimate contact
3. Exposure to conversation, soothing music, and circadian lighting (7)

Optimal Environment for Adults in the NICU

There are many stressors for adults in a hospital setting including pervasive auditory alarms, limited access to nature and daylight, and uncomfortable furnishings, especially when used for extended periods of time. Staff and families tend to be willing to make extreme sacrifices for the sake of the patients, but these sacrifices come with a personal cost that could be lessened by appropriate design.

Clinical Trials of Specific NICU Design Features

Single-family room design is the best-studied aspect of NICUs, including a randomized controlled study (8) and several trials using historical controls that have demonstrated multiple benefits (9), including reduced long-term costs (10) and improved outcomes. Single-family rooms may not be optimal in all situations, however (11,12), most notably when parents are largely absent.

BASIC DESIGN PRINCIPLES

Parental Access and Participation

Since parental interaction in general and STS care in particular have been shown to improve both infant outcome and parental well-being, structural and operational aspects of the NICU should be designed to enhance and support parent interaction with their baby. There must be adequate space at the bedside for a parent to comfortably hold the infant for extended periods of time without interfering with ongoing care such as feedings and vital signs, or with the care of infants at adjacent bedsides.

Optimal Sensory Environment for the High-Risk Newborn

The newborn's brain is undergoing extraordinary growth, differentiation, and development during the period of time NICU care may be required. To a large extent, these changes continue in whatever care environment is present. It is likely that human contact is an important component of the sensory environment, providing similar stimuli as might be experienced *in utero*. Noxious stimuli may also be part of the NICU experience, including excessive noise, light, and painful procedures. The environment of care should minimize these noxious stimuli and enhance the likelihood of beneficial stimuli.

- Noxious sounds should be limited whenever possible; undesired sound can be produced by the building (e.g., heating, ventilation, and air conditioning), human activity (e.g., conversation, public address systems, traffic near the bedside), and NICU equipment (e.g., alarms, ventilator operation). Some of this may be modifiable, whereas other components may not be unless new construction is contemplated. Efforts to reduce noise at its origin as well as to increase its absorption (e.g., acoustical ceiling tile and wall treatments, carpet in high-traffic areas) should be ongoing.

- Nurturing stimuli should be provided whenever possible. Parental presence should be encouraged both structurally, by providing adequate space and support at the bedside for parents to stay and interact with their baby, and operationally, with education of their importance to their infant's development and support of their needs. When close parental interaction with the baby is not possible, suitable stimuli should be provided by caregivers, utilizing evidence-based developmental care practices.

Facilitate Staff Efficacy and Work Quality

Hospital-based caregivers are essential to the treatment and sustenance of infants in the NICU. They must be able to practice in an environment conducive to their needs. Many of the considerations previously listed, such as adequate space at the bedside for parents without interfering with provision of medical care, control of noise, and ease of hand washing contribute to provider satisfaction. Staff must also be given appropriate space away from the bedside to collaborate, relax, and learn. Communication is especially important, so systems and spaces must be designed to facilitate this.

▋ NEW CONSTRUCTION

Specific principles for design of a modern, well-resourced NICU are described in the Recommended Standards for Newborn ICU Design (13). Many supporting papers and research are referenced within that document, so comments in this chapter are limited to other considerations necessary to create a NICU that will support excellent care for many years.

The Planning Process

Often, a new NICU is seen as a means of escaping from some increasingly undesirable feature of a current NICU, or an opportunity to incorporate a new, desirable method of delivering care. While both of these considerations are appropriate, they should not obscure the other opportunities offered with new construction. For example, units built prior to 2010 are too noisy according to the Recommended Standards and American Academy of Pediatrics (AAP) guidelines as are most of those built since 2010, yet architectural and operational strategies to achieve more desirable sound levels are well established (14). If noise is not recognized as a major problem in the existing NICU, its control may not be a priority in planning of the new NICU. The opportunity to reduce noise levels is much less difficult and expensive if it is addressed in the planning stage. Access to daylight is of considerable value to both staff and families, but many caregivers have become so used to working without daylight and it is not considered important enough to make this a priority, a decision that cannot be reversed once the planning process is well under way.

In order to avoid these sources of ongoing regret, the team planning a new NICU must be diverse and visionary. Families must be given a prominent voice. A careful literature review is imperative, and site visits to innovative NICUs should be taken. Since the typical NICU is used for 20 to 30 years, trends anticipated to take place over that time frame should be analyzed. In this regard, planners for NICUs in the past have consistently underestimated generational changes. We can suggest some of these generational changes here:

- Increased integration of families into the care process: The exclusion of families from the NICU was not evidence based, and studies and experience have demonstrated the benefits to both baby and parents of encouraging family participation in care. Pioneering units have now concluded that allowing parents almost unlimited access produces improved outcomes with no appreciable downside. It is reasonable to anticipate the continuation of this trend so planning teams should imagine the design and operational implications of its full implementation and assure that their new facility will be prepared to provide this level of support.

- Couplet care: A logical extension of increased parental access and participation is couplet care, in which mothers are admitted to the NICU along with their babies so that both are patients in the same space. Separation of mothers from their babies during this critical stage was not evidence based, and several units have now demonstrated the feasibility and desirability of this design feature.

- Technologic advances: While the previous considerations emphasized the "high-touch" aspect of future neonatal care, there is a considerable "high-tech" aspect to plan for as well. It is likely that in the lifetime of a future NICU, many of our existing devices will disappear and new devices will be introduced. Wired monitors and current-generation respiratory support systems will be replaced by devices that monitor many more parameters continuously and are connected to servo-controlled systems to deliver respiratory, medication, and nutritional support. Compact, readily accessible imaging devices will give us better windows into the infant's body, while artificial intelligence devices will be making decisions on an ongoing basis between medical provider rounds. In some cases, space requirements will be reduced by these changes, but they may be increased in other locations, making flexibility of spaces an important consideration.

- Specialized services and expertise: Just as neonatology became too complex by the 1970s to remain within the purview of a general pediatrician's expertise, no single practitioner today can be fully skilled in every aspect of neonatal care. Optimal care for a high-risk newborn will require specialization of caregivers—and to some extent the NICU structure itself. Some NICUs have created specialized surgical, tiny baby, or neurocritical spaces within their NICU. A similar intent has led to the creation in certain NICUs for dedicated space for the care of infants with neonatal abstinence syndrome (NAS). Other advanced NICUs are launching telemedicine services that offer specialized physician and other professionals' availability to hospital NICUs in rural and poor resource regions. Professional organizations have created medical coding that emphasizes telemedicine and the use of the internet for parental teaching. A careful consideration of demographic and medical trends is essential so that the planned unit can embrace these needs.

- Design economies: NICUs facing pressure to be good stewards of resources seek to achieve design economies without compromising vision. Standardized, acuity-adaptable infant care spaces help achieve design economies while providing operational flexibility and supporting clinical safety. If co-location of cohorts of patients such as surgical or tiny babies is preferred, that approach can be compatible with standardized infant care spaces designed for multiple needs. As specialization increases, standardization and efficiency remain central to NICU design. It is important to clarify that economically designed NICUs often aim for standardized infant patient-care space. Customized design of several unique types of rooms ranging from isolation to couplet care is common.

- Care in other settings: Financial stresses and other considerations will drive some NICUs to explore treating some of their current population in lower-cost, more nurturing settings. It can be argued, for example, that an NICU is the least optimal place to put a baby with NAS, especially as medication becomes a less essential portion of the treatment plan. For another example, many units, especially in Europe where home care is more developed than in the United States, are now discharging infants for the last week or two of their stay when tube feedings are the only factor requiring their continued presence in the NICU. Often, resource-limited countries have taken the lead in demonstrating the benefit of these changes that will likely be driven by more global resource restrictions in the future.

• Healing environments of care: There is abundant literature now on the benefits of sunlight and views of nature to the adult caregivers in hospitals, both staff and parents, who are at high risk for burnout and posttraumatic stress disorder (PTSD). NICUs have often been confined to interior spaces in the hospital because access to nature was considered unimportant (or even detrimental, in the case of sunlight) to a newborn, so rooms on exterior walls were used preferentially for adult patients. It is possible, however, to design a structure that will provide access to nature for all adult inhabitants, both families and staff, in all care settings. These spaces should be available not only for the patient rooms but also for family and staff lounges and other spaces used for respite or collaboration.

Additional Resources for Design and Operation of Newly Built or Renovated NICUs

The most comprehensive descriptions of design features for the NICU are the Recommended Standards for Newborn ICU Design (13) and the European Standards of Care for Newborn Health (15). There is an extensive literature addressing specific aspects of NICU design, including lighting (16), sound control (17), and flooring (18). In addition, several books describe and illustrate examples of optimal design for children, including multiple examples in the NICU (19–22).

▌ SPECIFIC RECOMMENDATIONS

Recommended Standards for Newborn ICU Design are online at https://nicudesign.nd.edu/. These are written for scenarios where substantial resources (funding, space, staff) are available. Even in areas where resources are more limited, though, certain principles are attainable and important. In this section, we have modified the original recommendations to reflect important considerations for NICUs regardless of the location. Whenever possible, efforts should be made to achieve and go beyond the Recommended Standards.

Delivery Room

When an NICU is located within a hospital with a delivery service these services should be adjacent to one another whenever possible. Every delivery room must include an infant resuscitation area with appropriate space, equipment, ventilation, environmental controls, and communication tools as described for an NICU infant space in this chapter.

Unit Configuration

Parental involvement with the care of their infant is important in any setting but especially when other resources are limited. Staff needs are important as well so that they can provide care efficiently without undue stress. The design of the NICU must consider the needs of the parents and staff not only at the bedside but in the support areas as well.

NICU Location within the Hospital

The NICU should be located in an area where traffic from other services will not need to pass through the unit.

Family Entry and Reception Area

The NICU should have a clearly identified entrance and reception area where families and visitors can be greeted. This may also include lockable storage and a hand washing sink.

Signage and Art

Signage and art should help families feel welcome. The language and images should reflect the diversity of the community served and use the language of partnership.

Safety/Infant Security

The NICU should be designed as part of an overall security program to protect the physical safety of infants, families, and staff. This should include limiting entrances and exits to those that can be monitored, yet operated in a family-friendly manner.

Space, Clearance, and Privacy Requirements for the Infant Space

Infant beds should be spaced no closer than 8 feet (2.4 m) with an aisle width of no less than 4 feet (1.2 m), excluding hand washing stations, columns, and aisles. Within this space, there should be sufficient space and furnishing to allow a parent to stay seated at the bedside. The need for visual and acoustic privacy for infants and families should be addressed not only in the design of each bed space but also in the overall unit design—for example, by minimizing traffic flow past each bed.

Private (Single-Family) Rooms

When possible, some single-family rooms should be provided to facilitate privacy and family interaction while reducing sensory overload and nosocomial infections. In addition to providing the optimal environment of care for most infants when their parents are present for most or all of the day, these rooms are also useful for infectious isolation, discharge preparation, and hospice care. Ideally, these rooms would include a kangaroo chair, a recumbent surface suitable for sleeping, wireless monitoring of the infant, and a communication device that allows anyone in the room to call for assistance. The bedside needs for care of the infant, including a hand washing sink, separate work counter, and supply storage should be provided.

Couplet Care Rooms

Couplet care is a new concept in high-resource settings but with a long history in lower resource areas. In its optimal form the couplet care room in an NICU has space and equipment to properly care for both mother and baby. Appropriate space includes direct access to a sink, bath, and toilet facilities for the hospitalized mother. In most cases, separation of a mother from her ill newborn immediately after birth is not necessary for medical reasons. There are logistical and training aspects that must be anticipated, but experience in both high-resource and resource-limited settings has documented the feasibility and success of this concept.

Airborne Infection Isolation Rooms

Each NICU should have or should have access to an airborne infection isolation room, properly equipped with negative air flow capability, a self-closing door, an observation window, and personal protective equipment storage. The quantity of airborne infection isolation rooms should be determined based on an infection control risk assessment conducted by appropriate staff.

Electrical, Gas Supply, and Mechanical Needs

Sufficient electrical and gas outlets should be provided at each bedside and organized in a way to ensure safety, easy access, and maintenance. For most beds, this will require at least eight simultaneously accessible electrical outlets with at least half of these outlets on an emergency power system; at least two each of simultaneously accessible air and oxygen outlets, and at least two vacuum outlets. Higher minimums for electrical, gas supply, and mechanical needs exist for NICUs in some locations, and applicable regulations would apply. This area should also include communication devices, supply storage, and charting space, resulting in an efficient and organized workstation around the infant.

Ambient Temperature and Ventilation

A minimum of six air changes per hour is required, with a minimum of two changes being outside air. The ventilation pattern should be low velocity and filtered and inhibit particulate matter from moving freely in the space, and intake and exhaust vents should be situated to minimize drafts on or near the infant beds. Filters should be located outside the infant care area so they can be changed easily and safely. Ductwork should be designed to minimize noise utilizing less angular construction. Optimal temperature is 72°F to 78°F (22°C to 26°C) with a relative humidity of 30% to 60%, while avoiding condensation on wall and window surfaces.

Hand Washing

The status of ill newborns should not be compromised by hospital-acquired infections. Babies can be protected by the following measures:

- Large, deep hand washing sinks with hands-free faucets and off-set drains should be situated within 20 feet (6 m) of any infant bed, but no closer than 3 feet (1 m) from an infant bed, supply, or counter/work surface unless protected by a splash guard to prevent splatter of contaminated fluid. The sink rim should be thin enough to discourage placement of clean supplies on this potentially contaminated surface. There should be no aerator on the faucet, and the faucet should be offset from the drain. Walls adjacent to sinks should be constructed of nonporous material. Signage above each sink should contain written and pictorial hand washing instructions.
- Containers of liquid hand cleaner should be within easy reach of every infant bed.
- All surfaces in the patient care area should be easily cleanable and durable.
- Separate receptacles should be provided for biohazardous and nonbiohazardous waste.

General Support Space

Distinct spaces are needed for clean and soiled materials, medical equipment, medication management, and unit management services.

- Charting space at each bedside should be provided. An additional separate area or desk for tasks such as compiling more detailed records and telephone communication should be provided in an area acoustically separated from the infant and family areas.
- A clean utility room should be provided for storage of supplies used regularly in the care of newborns. This room should be equipped with easily accessible electrical outlets for recharging of equipment. Storage should also be available at each bedside for frequently used supplies.
- A soiled utility room should be equipped with a hands-free hand washing station, a work counter protected from potential contamination by use of the sink, and negative air pressure with 100% of air exhausted to the outside. It should be situated to allow removal of soiled materials without passing through the infant care area.

Staff Support Space

Space should be provided within the NICU to meet the professional, personal, and administrative needs of the staff. These include, at a minimum, private space for lockers, lounge, toilet facilities, and on-call rooms. Office space should be provided for unit leadership, meetings, and counseling.

Milk Preparation

Space for preparation and storage of human milk, formula, and additives should be provided in a space away from the bedside, equipped with a refrigerator and freezer, a work counter, and a hand washing station. Cleanliness of the floor, walls, and ceiling should be easily maintained.

Lactation Support

Space should be provided for lactation consultation and milk expression either near the bedside or in dedicated lactation space, where separate space is appropriate for cultural, social, or other reasons.

Family Support Space

Space should be provided in or immediately adjacent to the NICU for a family lounge area with educational resources, lockable storage, telephones, and toilet facilities.

Family Transition Room(s)

A family transition room allows families and infants extended private time together prior to discharge and should be considered if space allows. These rooms can also be used for other family support including education and counseling when unoccupied. This room should be situated within an area of controlled public access and may be supplied with electrical, medical gas, and suction outlets depending on the function(s) intended for this area. They should have direct access to sink, bath, and toilet facilities and be equipped with emergency call capability, sleeping facilities for two parents, and sufficient space for the infant's bed and equipment.

Ceiling Finishes

Ceiling materials should have an average noise reduction coefficient (NRC) of 0.85 and a ceiling attenuation class (CAC) minimum of 29. They should be nonfriable and easily cleanable. They should be constructed in a manner to prevent the passage of particles from the cavity above the ceiling plane into the clinical environment. All materials used should be free of volatile organic compounds and other toxic substances whenever possible.

Wall Surfaces

Wall surfaces should be durable, be easy to clean, and use acoustical abatement material whenever possible. They should be free of volatile organic compounds and other toxic substances whenever possible and should be resistant to degradation by ultraviolet light, bleach, hydrogen peroxide, and other exposure elements.

Floor Surfaces

Floor surfaces should be durable, minimize the ability to harbor pathogens, and be easy to clean. They should be designed for impact sound reduction and have a light reflectance value of less than 30%. They should be free of volatile organic compounds and other toxic substances whenever possible and should be resistant to degradation by ultraviolet light, bleach, hydrogen peroxide, and other exposure elements.

Furnishings

All furnishings should be easily cleanable with the fewest possible seams in the integral construction. Exposed surface seams should be sealed. Furnishings should be durable to withstand impact, free of volatile organic compounds and other toxic substances whenever possible, and resistant to degradation by ultraviolet light, bleach, hydrogen peroxide, and other exposure elements. Corners should be rounded, bull-nosed, or coved whenever possible.

Lighting

Ambient lighting levels in the infant care spaces should be adjustable through a range of at least 10 to no more than 600 lux as measured on any plane at each bedside. Both natural and electric light sources should have master controls that allow for immediate darkening of any bed position sufficient for transillumination when necessary. Rheostat controls should be provided so that lighting levels can be adjusted gradually and incrementally. The sources should provide accurate color rendering and avoid unnecessary ultraviolet or infrared radiation through the use of appropriate lamps, lens, and/or filters. Flicker index should not exceed 0.1. No infant should have a direct line of sight to an electric light source or the sun. The lighting design should allow circadian changes in ambient lighting and should provide adequate illumination in staff work areas for their tasks. Control of illumination should be accessible to staff and families, and capable of adjustment across the recommended range of lighting levels.

Procedure Lighting in the Infant Care Areas

Separate procedure lighting should be mounted at each infant bed. This luminaire should be capable of providing no less than 2,000 lux at the plane of the infant bed, and should be framed so that no more than 2% of the light output extends beyond its illumination field. This lighting should be adjustable so that lighting at less than maximal levels can be provided.

Daylighting

At least one source of natural daylight should be visible from all infant care areas, either from the infant care station itself or from an adjacent area. Exterior windows should be glazed with a maximum U value of 0.5, situated at least 2 feet (0.6 m) from any infant bed, equipped with a shading device, and easily cleanable. Care should be taken so that direct sunlight does not strike the infant, IV fluids, or monitor screens.

Access to Nature

Views of nature should be provided in the unit in at least one space that is accessible to all families and at least one space that is accessible to all staff.

Acoustic Environment

Sound levels in infant rooms and adult sleep rooms should not exceed an L_{50} of 45 dB A-weighted, slow response and an L_{10} of 65 dB A-weighted, slow response, as measured three feet from any infant bed or other relevant listener position. Staff and family areas should not exceed an L_{50} of 50 dB A-weighted, slow response, and an L_{10} of 70 dB A-weighted, slow response, as measured 3 feet from any relevant listener position. Achieving these levels will require multiple strategies:

- Building mechanical systems and permanent equipment should conform to Noise Criteria (NC) 30 in infant and adult sleep rooms, and to NC 35 in other spaces within the NICU.
- Speakers and intercoms should have adjustable volume controls.
- Traffic unrelated to patient care should be routed outside patient care areas and adult sleep rooms.
- Speech privacy and freedom from intrusive sounds should be provided by acoustic seals for door, windows, and partitions, and by selecting ceiling, wall, and flooring materials designed for this purpose.

Much of the undesirable noise found in NICUs comes from external sources—heating and ventilation equipment, as well as sources outside the NICU or even the hospital. Some of the noise comes from internal sources, including conversation, monitor alarms, and traffic through the corridors including supply carts

and equipment. All of these sources must be considered and a plan for mitigation developed prior to finalizing construction plans. Addressing noise concerns after construction is complete is rarely satisfactory.

Usability Testing

No design is perfect in the beginning. The design often tries to correct flaws in a previous NICU but may not adequately anticipate or address unintended consequences of these changes, or unknown problems with new concepts or equipment. Latent safety threats are found in every major renovation or new construction; these are much easier to remedy if discovered during the planning process rather than after construction is complete. Before a design is completed or modified, development of scenarios using computer simulations initially and physical mock-ups subsequently encourages staff, families, and planners to explore the proposed new environment and thereby develop a design that will minimize these safety threats.

REFERENCES

1. Westrup B. Newborn Individualized Developmental Care and Assessment Program (NIDCAP)—family-centered developmentally supportive care. *Early Hum Dev* 2007;83:443.
2. Ohlsson A, Jacobs SE. NIDCAP: a systematic review and meta-analyses of randomized trials. *Pediatrics* 2013;131:e881.
3. Filippa M, Lordier L, De Almeida JS, et al. Early vocal contact and music in the NICU: new insights into preventive interventions. *Pediatr Res* 2020;87(2):249.
4. Caskey M, Stephens B, Tucker R, et al. Adult talk in the NICU with preterm infants and developmental outcomes. *Pediatrics* 2014;133:e578.
5. Baley J; Committee on Fetus and Newborn. Skin-to-skin care for term and preterm infants in the Neonatal ICU. *Pediatrics* 2015;136:596.
6. Feldman R, Rosenthal Z, Eidelman AI. Maternal-preterm skin-to-skin contact enhances child physiologic organization and cognitive control across the first 10 years of life. *Biol Psychiatry* 2014;75:56.
7. Morag I, Ohlsson A. Cycled light in the intensive care unit for preterm and low birth weight infants. *Cochrane Database Syst Rev* 2016;(8):CD006982.
8. Ortenstrand A, Westrup B, Brostom EB, et al. The Stockholm Neonatal Family Centered Care Study: effects on length of stay and infant morbidity. *Pediatrics* 2010;125:e278.
9. Kuhn P, Sizun J, Casper, C, et al. Recommendations on the environment for hospitalized newborn infants from the French neonatal society: rationale, methods and first recommendation on neonatal intensive care unit design. *Acta Paediatr* 2018;107:1860.
10. Shepley MM, Smith JA, Sadler BL, et al. The business case for building better neonatal intensive care units. *J Perinatol* 2014;34:811.
11. Pineda RG, Neil J, Dierker D, et al. Alterations in brain structure and neurodevelopmental outcome in preterm infants hospitalized in different neonatal intensive care unit environments. *J Pediatr* 2014;164:52.
12. White R. The next big ideas in NICU design. *J Perinatol* 2016;36:259.
13. Consensus Committee on Recommended Standards for Advanced Neonatal Care. NICU Design Standards. Available from: https://nicudesign.conductor.nd.edu/
14. AAP Committee on Fetus and Newborn and ACOG Committee on Obstetric Practice. *Guidelines for perinatal care.* 8th ed.. American Academy of Pediatrics, Itasca, IL. 2017:82.
15. European standards of care for newborn health—NICU design. Available from: Newborn-health-standards.org/standards/nicu-design/overview/
16. Rea MS, Figueiro MG. The NICU lighted environment. *Newborn Infant Nurs Rev* 2016;16:195.
17. Philbin MK. Planning the acoustic environment of a neonatal intensive care unit. *Clin Perinatol* 2004;31:331.
18. White RD. Flooring choices for newborn ICUs. *J Perinatol* 2007;27 (Suppl 2):S29.
19. Shepley MM. *Design for pediatric and neonatal critical care.* Philadelphia, PA: Routledge, 2014.
20. Komiske BK. *Designing the world's best: children's hospitals.* Melbourne: Images Publishing, 1999.
21. Komiske BK. *Designing the world's best children's hospitals 2: the future of healing environments.* Melbourne: Images Publishing, 2005.
22. Komiske BK. *Designing the world's best children's hospitals 3.* Melbourne: Images Publishing, 2013.

GENERAL CONSIDERATIONS

4 Data Collection Systems for Service Evaluation and Research

Neena Modi

INTRODUCTION

It is an entirely accurate cliché of the modern age that data are being amassed continuously at an incredible rate, to an extent to which we are largely unaware. The controllers of social media platforms have been quick to appreciate the wider uses to which large quantities of data may be put, from selling products and services, to manipulating societies, and influencing the outcomes of elections. But data can also be invaluable in improving health care across the entire research, development, audit, evaluation, and improvement pathway that is necessary to achieve patient benefit. Every patient contact generates data. Traditional paper case notes contain a variety of data, such as objective measurements (e.g., weight, length, head circumference, laboratory results), subjective assessments (e.g., patient affect, mood, symptoms), and clinical inferences (e.g., diagnoses, differential diagnoses, problem lists). Data may be numeric (e.g., kg, cm, SI units), categorical (e.g., Apgar score, Small for Gestational Age), forced choice (e.g., from a menu), or free text (e.g., abdominal distension, poor perfusion, myocardial infarction, heart attack). Data are also generated in the form of images (e.g., x-rays, ultrasound, magnetic resonance, CT, positron emission tomography) from medical or recreational physiologic monitoring systems (e.g., heart and respiratory rate monitors, wearable devices). Data from non–health care sources may also be invaluable in improving patient care. These include, for example, interrogation of meteorologic and air quality data to predict increases in acute asthmatic attacks. This chapter will focus on clinical information; this chapter will describe why clinical data need to be recorded, and how they can be gathered, pooled, stored, and used responsibly to benefit patient care directly and indirectly. This chapter will discuss governance and patient confidentiality, and provide a roadmap for establishing a health data collection. Finally, this chapter will offer a glimpse into future possibilities.

WHY DO HEALTH CARE DATA NEED TO BE RECORDED, COLLECTED, AND SHARED?

Primary Uses

Health care data are needed for primary purposes, to provide a record and convey information about the patient and his or her care. Recording health care data accurately is a fundamental component of good medical care. Imagine caring for a patient without records or without ability to share data. If you had seen the patient before, all you would have is your memory of previous findings and events. If this was first contact, you would have no prior information other than what the patient could tell you, and no way of sharing information to inform future care. If you were able to record data but not share them, each new health care professional encountering the patient would have to obtain information and record data anew.

This is not as farfetched as it may seem. In many health care systems, data may not be recorded or shared. In low-resource settings, staff able to take a comprehensive medical history or document vital signs regularly in traditional paper records, may be limited in number. In low-resource settings, the use of Electronic Patient Records (EPRs), hailed as a powerful advance, is also severely restricted by lack of training, infrastructure, funding, and maintenance support (1,2). However, in high-resource settings, providers of highly commercialized health care systems may be reluctant to share information considered a marketable commodity, rather than an integral component of good patient care. For example, a substantial proportion of the population of the United States is not supported by a provider who integrates their care (3). Even in public sector systems, technical or bureaucratic obstacles may hinder sharing.

Secondary Uses

Health care data can also be used for secondary purposes to benefit patient care, the organization and delivery of health services, and to inform the development of health policy. Examples include bench-marking processes, costs and outcomes, auditing practice against standards, evaluating quality improvement processes, quantifying variation, facilitating the development of medicines and health care products, and a very wide variety of research. To be useful for such secondary purposes, data should ideally be drawn from complete populations in order to avoid drawing biased inferences and conclusions. Once again, this highlights the importance of being able to pool and share data. The distinction between primary and secondary uses of health care data, though superficially logical, may be unhelpful in a modern age as it implies a clear separation between the clinical care provided to a patient and the benefits that flow from research, audit, evaluation, and quality improvement. Today, these wider components of the care pathway are considered as important as the historic duty of immediate care owed by a practitioner toward his or her patient. It follows that there is a strong case to be made for considering the wider purposes of health data at the outset. Figure 4.1 illustrates the basic components of a patient benefit cycle with the delivery of each element facilitated by access to a source of high-quality data.

The Consequences of Not Sharing Health Care Data

The difficulties in sharing data have meant that all too often health care workers providing front-line clinical care, as well as those conducting evaluations, research, and policy development, have opted to collect data specifically for each specific task. This is wasteful of time, expensive, burdensome, and increases the risk of harm as each repetitive recording of data increases the chance that an error may be made. Failure to share information is poor patient care. For example, this can hinder realization that multiple presentations by a child to different health care facilities indicates possible non-accidental injury or that an unconscious patient has a major drug allergy. Can it be acceptable for every health care professional coming into contact with a patient (e.g., triage nurse, casualty doctor, medical registrar, admitting nurse, admitting doctor, and consultant) to ask the same questions repeatedly to that patient and more so, one who is ill, or very young, or frail or confused?

Data were usually captured on paper and then transcribed into computer files, a time-consuming process that also increases the risk of introducing errors. A further problem is that different organizations have different remits and statutory responsibilities and may hold different sections of data. Thus, a department of education may hold information about school performance, a valuable outcome measure for neonatal research studies, yet ancillary clinical information is likely to be in databases held by a department of health. A public health department might have responsibility for identifying disease outbreaks, hot spots, or safety surveillance and again only hold a subset of available data. Among the adverse consequences of constraints on the availability and ability to share so-called "secondary use data" are that much needed research is not conducted, audits and evaluations are limited to only a small number of care processes and outcomes, are frequently not

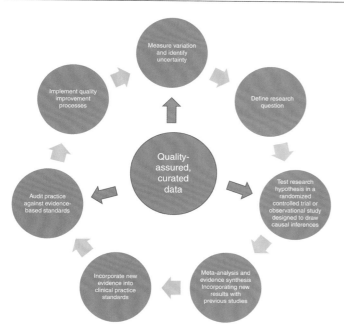

FIGURE 4.1 **The patient benefit cycle.**

generalizable or applicable to the entire relevant population, and health policy is built on incomplete information.

WHAT IS NEEDED TO SHARE HEALTH CARE DATA AND USE IT EFFECTIVELY?

General Requirements

In order to share health care data, they need to be recorded using nomenclature that is comprehensible to all users, for multiple diverse purposes. Data must be reliable, accurate, and readily

retrievable. Records from different sources must be linkable. Data to be pooled must be consistent. They must be held in a secure repository. There must be regulatory processes in place to safeguard patient confidentiality, protect against improper use, and allow access only to legitimate users. There must be information provided to patients and health care professionals, and trust in the processes established and the veracity of the outputs. Research governance processes in many countries, especially for medicines trials, also currently preclude the use of anything other than original source data. The development of data quality assurance processes for clinical data should help make these acceptable for medicines research in the future. A standard EPR system offers opportunity for staff at different locations to enter and access compatible data. However, all too often, hospitals and primary care practices use different systems and are unable to access a common health care record. This also makes it difficult to extract compatible information which can be used for research. **Figure 4.2** summarizes the steps required to create a health care database.

Defining the Dataset

The first step in creating a database to be used for multiple wider purposes is to define a core dataset and reach agreement on the variables to be included. Good general principles are to start with a manageable number of variables, and record only raw, not derived or categorized, variables; for example, do not record birth weight centile or category (i.e., extremely, very or low birth weight) but rather, birth weight, gestational age and sex and calculate birth weight centile, or assign to a category centrally thus ensuring that the same approach and/or definition is applied consistently. Similarly, where case definitions are problematic and lack agreement (e.g., necrotizing enterocolitis, bronchopulmonary dysplasia), record each component (e.g., clinical signs, imaging findings, lab results) separately. This will enable a consistent case definition to be applied, which is essential to ensure like is compared with like, and observer subjectivity and bias are minimized. Research to construct evidence-based case definitions is increasing (4), and

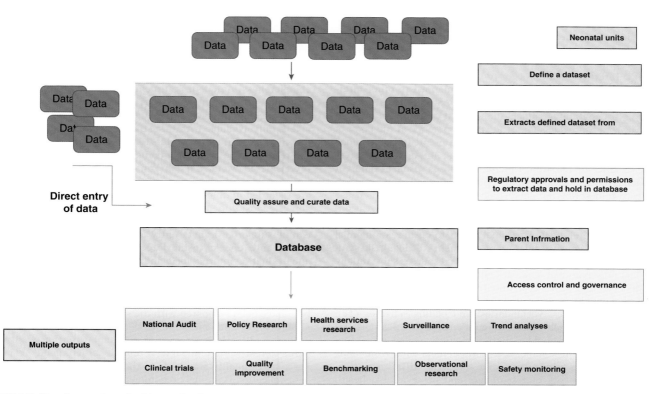

FIGURE 4.2 **Steps for creating a health care database.**

GENERAL CONSIDERATIONS

the need for international consensus and regulatory requirements are likely to drive further developments in this field (5). It is also useful to incorporate core outcomes into the data set. A core outcome set is a group of variables that are considered important to record consistently in all research in a specialty. This is invaluable in enabling high-quality research syntheses and meta-analyses (6). Inconsistent reporting is commonplace and a major cause of research waste (7). The incorporation of core outcomes and the raw variables that make up a case definition will add to the growing utility of neonatal data sets.

Each data variable must be clearly defined in respect of both its clinical meaning and its technical format. These definitions are held in an accompanying meta–data set. Ideally, the data set should be approved in accordance with local requirements and registered as a national asset, for example, the Neonatal Data Set which specifies variables held in the UK National Neonatal Research Database is an approved National Health Service (NHS) Information Standard (8). This means that any supplier of neonatal EPR systems to the NHS in England must show compliance with ability to record Neonatal Data Set variables, and detailed clinical and technical specifications are openly available as a shared resource.

Nomenclature and Technical Data Specifications

If health care data are to be recorded, for primary as well as secondary purposes, it makes sense to do so at the outset in a manner that positively facilitates comparison and sharing. This means not only recording data in a consistent manner, using common definitions, but also using common nomenclature and technical specifications. This sounds obvious, but these seemingly self-evident issues continue to pose major problems. Does information convey a consistent meaning? Do practitioners use the same language? Is the meaning the same when one doctor uses the term chronic lung disease, another bronchopulmonary dysplasia, and another ventilator dependency? If the patient is transferred to another hospital, does the new health care team have ready access to the full records of the first, or only to a summary? Approaches to address these problems are ongoing. SNOMED-CT (Systematized Nomenclature of Medicine Clinical Terms) is an attempt to map medical "concepts" (e.g., heart attack; myocardial infarction) to standard terminologies so that clinical content can be represented consistently. It is a structured clinical vocabulary for use in electronic health records and is owned, developed, and administered by SNOMED International, a not-for-profit organization (9). The terminology is comprehensive, multilingual, mapped to other international standards and is used in more than 80 countries.

Databases containing clinical information can differ in purpose and design. EPR provide support to clinical practice at the point of care, whereas administrative databases are created for insurance reimbursement or other management needs, and disease registers for surveillance or research. Different purposes result in different approaches for the logical structure, physical formats, and terminologies used to describe the data which can be a barrier to their use for secondary uses. The Clinical Data Interchange Standards Consortium (CDISC) is an organization that develops data standards for medical research (10). A cardinal aim is to ensure commercial research sponsors meet regulatory requirements. Utilizing the standards have been shown to decrease research resources substantially (11). The Observational Medical Outcomes Partnership Common Data Model (OMOP-CDM) is an initiative aimed at enabling analysis of disparate data by transforming these into a common format with common terminologies, vocabularies, and coding schemes (12). The Observational Health Data Sciences and Informatics (OHDSI) program is a multistakeholder, multidisciplinary collaborative that aims to maximize the value of real-world clinical data by enabling large-scale analytics using open source solutions. OHDSI has established a global network of researchers and observational health

databases with a central coordinating centre at Columbia University (13) and for Europe, at the Erasmus University Medical Centre in Rotterdam (14). In 2018, a European Health Data and Evidence network project (15) was started under the Innovative Medicines Initiative that will further drive the adoption of OMOP-CDM in Europe.

Retrieving and Pooling Data

If clinical data are to be used for service evaluations and research, they must be retrieved from medical or administrative records, whether these are paper or electronic, pooled, and held in a central repository for use for multiple approved purposes. Extracting data from paper records and entering them into a database has been the mainstay of many neonatal registers around the world but is laborious, expensive, and risks transcription errors. Many databases are created by recording data specifically to populate the database usually using an online system. The UK National Neonatal Research Database (16,17) is an alternative approach where data are extracted from EPR, thus eliminating the burden and expense of duplicate data recording and speeding data availability for secondary uses. When establishing a new database, flexibility in accommodating different ways of bringing in data is advisable. Flexibility within EPR systems is also desirable, with a range of methods for data capture as appropriate, ranging from free text entries to forced choice selections using drop down menus, recording numeric values, and responding to unambiguous questions. Natural Language Processing methods can be used to extract objective information from free text, but the extent to which this can produce high-quality, validated data remains uncertain.

Data Quality

The quality of health care data is rarely checked formally or systematically. Consider for example, when data are entered into an EPR or in old-fashioned paper case notes, what quality checks are made? This is another reason why researchers and others have often been reluctant to use routine sources of health care data for secondary purposes, claiming that only data recorded specifically for a particular need are likely to meet quality standards. If routine data could be shown to meet such standards, the cost and time to complete research studies would likely reduce substantially. It should go without saying that accurate data would also benefit patient care.

Six core data quality dimensions have been defined, namely completeness, uniqueness, timeliness, validity, consistency, and accuracy (18). Completeness can be expressed as the proportion of missing data for each variable. Uniqueness is whether the variable is only available within the database or can be obtained from other sources. Timeliness refers to the delay between the event and the record of the event or its outcome being available. A variable is considered "valid" if it conforms to a predefined syntax (format, type, and range). Consistency is shown by agreement when data are recorded in different ways, times, or places. Accuracy is arguably the most difficult to assess objectively as it requires a knowledge of "truth" or an accepted "gold-standard." However, accuracy can be supported at data entry level for example, by introducing out-of-range checks, using forced choice or drop-down menus, and evaluating internal logic and consistency within an individual record. Involving parents in checking the accuracy of demographic and other data is a promising approach that is also being explored (19). Key data within the UK National Neonatal Research Database have been compared with the same items recorded as part of a multicentre randomized controlled trial and found to have high accuracy (20). However, overall, the application of quality standards to real-world clinical data remains in its infancy. Establishing a set of quality standards at the outset when creating a new data collection is strongly recommended.

Record Linkage

To utilize different types or sources of data, they must be able to be linked or related to each other in some way. This may be through use of personal identifiers (name or a national identity number), a geographical locator (address or postcode), or through probabilistic linkage where a group of nonidentifying data items (e.g., sex, month of birth, year of birth, place of birth) are matched to achieve a high probability that individuals in different datasets can be linked.

Health care records can be linked across different sources at patient level if a single identifier is used nationally or across a health care system, for example the NHS number in the United Kingdom. Linkage using identifiers requires the explicit consent of individuals which can pose major practical difficulties if large numbers of patients or complete populations are involved. There should also be demonstrable assurance that patient confidentiality will be maintained, and the purposes are appropriate and valid. In England, the NHS introduced a national data opt-out in 2018. This enables patients to op-out of the use of their data for research or other purposes beyond their individual care and treatment (21).

The use of a common pseudonym across different data sources can support linkage of deidentified records. Linkage of databases within countries offers opportunity to ascertain long-term outcomes, for example, educational outcomes through linkage of health and educational records. There is also opportunity to explore wider contributors to health, such as the impact of air pollution on long-term respiratory outcomes by linking health and environmental databases. To be successful, linkage requires patient trust in the processes.

Completely anonymized databases can also be linked to enable exploration of between-country variations in care and patient outcomes. The International Network of Evaluations of Outcomes of Neonates (iNeo) is an international quality improvement initiative that has linked data from Australia, Canada, Israel, Japan, New Zealand, Spain, Sweden, Switzerland, and the United Kingdom (22). eNewborn is a platform for benchmarking, quality improvement, and research to date largely confined to European countries (23).

Databases and Repositories

In a systematic review to identify neonatal databases and define their characteristics, 82 were identified worldwide (24). These included 39 regional and 39 national country-specific databases. Five countries accounted for the location of 47 of all identified databases: the United States (n = 24), Canada (n = 11), the United Kingdom (n = 7), and Australia/New Zealand (n = 5). Sixty databases restricted entries to neonatal unit admissions by birth characteristic or insurance cover. Data were captured specifically for 53 databases, were drawn from administrative sources for 21, and were drawn from clinical sources for 8. Of the latter, only two contain information on admissions to neonatal units across defined geographical areas. One of these is the NNRD that captures data from all neonatal units in England, Scotland, and Wales (16,17); the other is the Pediatrix Baby Steps Clinical Data Warehouse that contains data from neonatal units operated by the Pediatrix Medical Group, a private enterprise operating in over 30 U.S. states (25). Both databases also have the largest variety of infant and maternal data fields and record all infants admitted to neonatal units in contrast with some long-standing databases such as the Vermont Oxford Network where only infants meeting specific birth weight or other criteria are included (26). The Pediatrix Clinical Data Warehouse contains clinical information from BabySteps, the company's proprietary EPR, and is used to support quality improvement (27). The NNRD is an award-winning resource, described as an exemplar for the NHS that has resolved many EPR data challenges. It holds defined patient-level information, the Neonatal Data Set an approved NHS Information Standard (ISB1595), extracted from the EPR of all admissions to all neonatal units in

England, Wales, and Scotland. Data undergo multiple rounds of quality assurance. There is objective evidence of accuracy and completeness by, for example, comparison with Case Record Forms from a large randomized controlled trial. To date the NNRD contains data on around a million babies and 10 million days of care, with information on around 100,000 new patients added each year. It is managed on the FAIR principles for data (*Findable, Accessible, Interoperable,* and *Reusable*) (28) as a national resource, used for a wide range of health service evaluations, quality improvement programs, research, and national audit.

Regulatory and Resource Requirements

The regulatory and legal requirements governing the collection of health data, sharing within and between countries, and their uses for secondary purposes differs widely across the world. A detailed discussion of these variations is beyond the scope of this chapter but suffice to say these requirements must be met. It is also important to note that this is a field that is changing rapidly and likely to continue to do so over the coming years. For example, the General Data Protection Regulation is a regulation on data protection, privacy, and data transfer outside the European Union and the European Economic Area that was adopted in law in 2016 and became enforceable in 2018 (29). Although its intent was to give citizens control over their personal data and unify regulations within the European Union, the GDPR has been interpreted differently in different countries, which adds further complexity to an already problematic area.

Resourcing the infrastructural requirements for databases is another potential obstacle that requires to be addressed to realize the full potential of large high-quality patient care databases. Many large-scale collections of health data are now held and managed by for-profit companies. These models raise issues regarding ownership and exploitation of personal data. In public sector health care systems, resources may be funded through grants from governments, research councils, or charities, or operate through cost recovery models applied to supported studies or charges for access.

Access and Visibility

Patients whose data are retained in a database, and the health care staff who record these data, have a right to know how the data will be used and by whom. It is also the case that widest possible legitimate use will benefit patient care and health care services. Therefore, clear processes to enhance the visibility of databases and govern access are essential. Health Data Research UK, established in 2017, a nonprofit company owned by UK Research and Innovation and funded by charities and public bodies (30). Health Data Research UK is uniting the countries health data, standardizing processes for access, and increasing visibility to facilitate the delivery of research and innovation at scale. It is likely that the next decade will see the establishment of registers across the world that list health data resources and provide access and other information in a similar manner to clinical trial registers.

Stakeholder Trust and Involvement

Understanding stakeholder perspectives, and ensuring their trust and involvement in the use of personal health data and clinical information for research and other purposes beyond immediate care are essential. This requires that health care teams as well as patients and the public understand the processes involved of creating clinical databases, the purposes for which they will be used, and have trust and confidence that the data will be used well, patient confidentiality will be assured, and access will be appropriately regulated and managed. This can be accomplished through inclusion of stakeholder representatives in development, oversight and management of databases, and their involvement in conducting research, audit and evaluations using the data, and disseminating

GENERAL CONSIDERATIONS

the outputs. The application of machine learning (ML) and artificial intelligence (AI) to clinical data sets brings added need to ensure that outputs and applications are trustworthy and conform to expected ethical principles for clinical research and that health system managers, policymakers, and analysts are aware of these issues (31,32). In the United Kingdom, neonatal units contributing to the NNRD collectively form the UK Neonatal Collaborative (UKNC). Each neonatal unit has a UKNC lead, the NNRD Steering Board includes UKNC representatives, and the UKNC is acknowledged in all outputs. Every neonatal unit contributes to the NNRD, and data reliability and completeness have grown steadily over the years. Although not a regulatory requirement, the agreement of every contributing clinical team is sought for data from their unit to be included in any research. The NNRD Steering Board includes nurses, health service managers, junior doctors, parents, and representatives from all relevant stakeholder organizations who communicate and engage with their respective constituencies. An annual conference is held, attended by parents, managers, commissioners, and clinicians, and information disseminated about new projects and research studies.

FUTURE DIRECTIONS

Data collections for service evaluations and research in neonatal medicine no less than other clinical specialties have to date largely focused on benchmarking, audit, quality improvement, and observational studies. However, there are also considerable opportunities to be seized to conduct a variety of types of research. Compared with other age groups, the representation of neonates in biomedical research is disproportionately low. Only 2.5% of trials registered in 2019 in the Cochrane Central Register of Controlled Trials involve neonates, and over 90% of infants receive one or more medicines that have been neither developed nor tested in these populations. Novel approaches to generate evidence are therefore urgently needed. New technologies also offer opportunities to involve low-resource settings, which carry the greatest burden of newborn care need, in these big-data opportunities from the outset. For example, there is an increasing range of open-source EPR applications suitable for these underserved areas (1,2), and the use of mobile phone technologies by frontline health care workers offer promising approaches to capturing data for clinical and wider use (33).

As a further example, consider randomized controlled trials. The very high costs of trials are in large part due to data requirements, but it is now possible to conduct large efficient randomized studies using data routinely recorded in clinical databases (34). In situations where randomization is not possible, or would be unethical, impractical, or prohibitively expensive, novel big data approaches can be used for evidence generation. The ability to draw causal inferences from observational data can be maximized using approaches such as propensity score and other matching techniques to create quasi-randomized groups for comparison (35,36). In instrumental variable analyses, the likelihood of a causal relationship between an exposure and an outcome is evaluated by assessing the association between a variable strongly correlated with the exposure (the instrumental variable) but not related at all to the outcome (37,38). In Mendelian randomization, natural, random variation in genes with known functions are used as instrumental variables (39). The outcome of interest is determined in individuals who carry the variant and those who do not. As the genetic variant is typically not associated with confounders, differences in the outcome between those carrying and not carrying the variant can reasonably be attributed to the difference in the risk factor. These approaches, however, all require rich, detailed, high-quality data.

Randomized controlled trials can have important limitations. They only estimate average treatment effects, recruit only a small proportion of eligible patients and take place under strictly defined conditions. Trials are rarely large enough to identify interactions, for example, in relation to sex or age, or the effect on outcomes of complex sets of interacting internal (e.g., race, comorbidities) and time-varying external factors (e.g., medications, nutritional intake). For these reasons, generalizability is often limited, and effectiveness in specific patient subgroups may be uncertain. Uncertainties in clinical practice pose major risks to patient safety and contribute to variation and inequity in outcomes. Technologic advances in ability to store and process very large volumes of data and apply data science techniques, which include AI and ML, have opened up alternative routes to improving patient care, but bring with them new challenges. "Big-data" provides the wherewithal to develop clinical decision support tools, automate image analyses, conduct population surveillance, identify outliers, and predict outbreaks. AI and ML can in theory exploit detailed real-world clinical data to identify personalized care pathways based on individual patient characteristics and deliver responsive, rapid evidence generation. Such research is set to expand rapidly in the coming years.

REFERENCES

1. Syzdykova A, Malta A, Zolfo M, et al. Open-source electronic health record systems for low-resource settings: systematic review. *JMIR Med Inform* 2017;5(4):e44.
2. Alsaffar M, Yellowlees P, Odor A, et al. The state of open source electronic health record projects: a software anthropology study. *JMIR Med Inform* 2017;5(1):e6.
3. Beal AC, Doty MM, Hernandez SE, et al. *Closing the divide: how medical homes promote equity in health care: results from The Commonwealth Fund 2006 Health Quality Survey.* New York: The Commonwealth Fund, 2007. Available from: https://www.commonwealthfund.org/publications/fund-reports/2007/jun/closing-divide-how-medical-homes-promote-equity-health-care. Accessed December 30, 2019.
4. Battersby C, Longford N, Costeloe K, et al.; for UK Neonatal Collaborative Necrotising Enterocolitis Study Group. The development of a gestational age-specific case-definition for neonatal Necrotising Enterocolitis. *JAMA Pediatr* 2017;171:256.
5. Costeloe K, Turner MA, Padula MA, et al. Sharing data to accelerate medicines development and improve neonatal care: data standards and harmonized definitions. *J Pediatr* 2018;203:437.
6. Webbe J, Brunton G, Ali S, et al. Developing, implementing and disseminating a core outcome set for neonatal medicine. *BMJ Paediatr Open* 2017;1(1):e000048.
7. Webbe J, Ali S, Sakonidou S, et al.; COIN Project Steering Committee. Inconsistent outcome reporting in large neonatal trials: a systematic review. *Arch Dis Child Fetal Neonatal Ed* 2020;105(1):69.
8. NHS Digital, Neonatal Data Set. Available from: https://www.datadictionary.nhs.uk/data_dictionary/messages/clinical_data_sets/data_sets/national_neonatal_data_set/national_neonatal_data_set_-_episodic_and_daily_care_fr.asp?shownav=1. Accessed December 31, 2019.
9. SNOMED-CT. Available from: http://www.snomed.org/. Accessed December 24, 2019.
10. Clinical Data Interchange Standards Consortium. Available from: https://www.cdisc.org/. Accessed December 31, 2019.
11. Vadakin A, Kush R. The Case for CDISC Standards 2014. Available from: https://www.cdisc.org/system/files/all/article/PDF/The%20Case%20for%20CDISC%20Standards-FINAL-30SEP.pdf. Accessed December 30, 2019.
12. Observational Medical Outcomes Partnership Common Data Model (OMOP-CDM). Accessed December 31, 2019.
13. www.ohdsi.org. Accessed December 31, 2019.
14. OHDSI Europe. Accessed December 31, 2019.
15. EHDEN. Accessed December 31, 2019.
16. Modi N. Information technology infrastructure, quality improvement and research: the UK National Neonatal Research Database. *Transl Pediatr* 2019;8:193.
17. Modi N, Ashby D, Battersby C, et al. *Developing routinely recorded clinical data from electronic patient records as a national resource to improve neonatal health care: the Medicines for Neonates research programme.* Library Southampton, UK: NIHR Journals, 2019.
18. UK Working Group on Data Quality Dimensions. The six primary dimensions for data quality assessment. October 2013. Available from: https://www.whitepapers.em360tech.com/wp-content/files_mf/1407250286DAMAUKDQDimensionsWhitePaperR37.pdf. Accessed December 30, 2019.

19. Sakonidou S, Andrzejewska I, Kotzamanis S, et al.; BUDS Project Steering Group. Better Use of Data to improve parent Satisfaction (BUDS): protocol for a prospective before-and-after pilot study employing mixed methods to improve parent experience of neonatal care. *BMJ Paediatr Open* 2019;3(1):e000515.

20. Battersby C, Statnikov Y, Santhakumaran S, et al.; the UK Neonatal Collaborative and Medicines for Neonates Investigator Group. The United Kingdom National Neonatal Research Database: a validation study. *PLoS One* 2018;13:e0201815.

21. NHS Digital National Data Opt-Out. Available from: https://digital.nhs.uk/services/national-data-opt-out. Accessed December 31, 2019.

22. International Network for Evaluation of Outcomes of Neonates. Available from: http://ineonetwork.org. Accessed December 31, 2019.

23. Haumont D, NguyenBa C, Modi N. eNewborn: the information technology revolution and challenges for neonatal networks. *Neonatology* 2017; 111(4):388.

24. Statnikov Y, Ibrahim B, Modi N. A systematic review of administrative and clinical databases of infants admitted to neonatal units. *Arch Dis Child Fetal Neonatal Ed* 2017;102(3):F270.

25. Spitzer AR, Ellsbury D, Clark RH. The Pediatrix BabySteps® Data Warehouse: a unique national resource for improving outcomes for neonates. *Indian J Pediatr* 2015;82(1):71.

26. Vermont Oxford Network. Available from: https://public.vtoxford.org/. Accessed December 31, 2019.

27. Spitzer AR, Ellsbury DL, Handler D, et al. The Pediatrix BabySteps Data Warehouse and the Pediatrix QualitySteps improvement project system—tools for "meaningful use" in continuous quality improvement. *Clin Perinatol* 2010;37(1):49.

28. FAIR Principles. Available from: https://www.go-fair.org/fair-principles/. Accessed November 31, 2019.

29. General Data Protection Regulation. Available from: https://gdpr-info.eu/. Accessed December 31, 2019.

30. Health Data Research UK. Available from: https://www.hdruk.ac.uk/about/. Accessed December 31, 2019.

31. Tricco AC, Zarin W, Rios P, et al. Engaging policy-makers, health system managers, and policy analysts in the knowledge synthesis process: a scoping review. *Implement Sci* 2018;13(1):3.

32. Floridi L, Cowls J, Beltrametti M, et al. AI4People: an ethical framework for a good AI society opportunities, risks, principles, and recommendations. *Minds Mach (Dordr)* 2018;28(4):689. https://doi.org/10.1007/s11023-018-9482-5. Accessed December 30, 2019.

33. Agarwal S, Perry HB, Long LA, et al. Evidence on feasibility and effective use of mHealth strategies by frontline health workers in developing countries: systematic review. *Trop Med Int Health* 2015;20:1003.

34. Gale C, Modi N, Jawad S, et al. Study protocol: The WHEAT pilot trial: WithHolding Enteral feeds around packed red cell transfusion to prevent necrotising enterocolitis in preterm neonates: a multi-centre, electronic patient record, randomised controlled point-of-care pilot trial. *BMJ Open* 2019;9(9):e033543.

35. Battersby C, Longford N, Mandalia S, et al.; the UK Neonatal Collaborative Necrotising Enterocolitis (UKNC-NEC) study group. Incidence and enteral feed antecedents of severe neonatal necrotising enterocolitis in England 2012–13: a two-year, population surveillance study. *Lancet Gastroenterol Hepatol* 2017;2:43.

36. Helenius K, Longford N, Lehtonen L, et al.; Neonatal Data Analysis Unit and the United Kingdom Neonatal Collaborative. Association of early postnatal transfer and birth outside a tertiary hospital with mortality and severe brain injury in extremely preterm infants: observational cohort study with propensity score matching. *BMJ* 2019; 367:l5678.

37. Watson SI, Arulampalam W, Petrou S, et al.; on behalf of the Neonatal Data Analysis Unit and the NESCOP Group. The effects of designation and volume of neonatal care on mortality and morbidity outcomes of very preterm infants in England: retrospective, population-based, cohort study. *BMJ Open* 2014;4(7):e004856.

38. Watson SI, Arulampalam W, Petrou S, et al. The effects of a one to one nurse to patient ratio on the mortality rate in neonatal intensive care: a retrospective, longitudinal, population-based study. *Arch Dis Child Fetal Neonatal Ed* 2016;101:F195.

39. Cornish AJ, Tomlinson IP, Houlston RS. Mendelian randomisation: a powerful and inexpensive method for identifying and excluding non-genetic risk factors for colorectal cancer. *Mol Aspects Med* 2019; 69:41.

GENERAL CONSIDERATIONS

5 Quality Assessment and Improvement

Scott A. Lorch

With an increasing number of premature infants surviving to hospital discharge, there has been increasing attention to optimizing the short-term and long-term outcomes of these high-risk patients. One area necessary to achieve this goal is to optimize the quality of care received by patients. Quality of care refers to the ability of a hospital or health care system to provide care for an individual patient that optimally addresses the needs of that patient at a specific time. First described by Donabedian in 1966 (1,2), the original framework proposed that the structure of care of an individual provider influenced the processes of care that provider delivered to a patient, which ultimately determined a patient's outcome (**Fig. 5.1**). These structures, processes, and outcomes of health care may be used to assess the quality of care received by a patient (3,4).

Since Donabedian's seminal publication, there have been numerous quality measures developed for perinatal care, with a growing body of literature on the characteristics of an optimal measure; the use of such measures for individual hospitals performing quality improvement work and for public agencies performing quality assessment work; and the relationship between health care quality and interhospital variations in perinatal outcomes. This chapter will review the fundamental underpinnings of quality measurement in perinatal medicine, highlight the characteristics of an ideal quality measure, and provide examples of how various quality measures are used at the level of the individual hospital and the population as a whole. Understanding this fast-moving field will provide caregivers with the tools to optimize their outcomes while understanding how other stakeholders in health care interpret their quality metrics.

VARIATION IN THE OUTCOMES OF PRETERM NEONATES

In order to understand the need to assess the type of care delivered by an individual health care provider, we first need to examine evidence that mortality and morbidity vary between these providers. The first widespread example of this variation was published in Pediatrics in 1987 (5). Here, Avery and colleagues presented the prevalence of chronic lung disease in infants with birth weight between 700 and 1,500 g at eight major neonatal intensive care units (NICUs) throughout the United States. For infants born between 1982 and 1984, survival rate ranged from 78% to 84% within the eight units. However, one unit had a significantly lower rate of chronic lung disease in survivors. This finding led to extensive research into the different practice patterns at Center number 3, later identified as Columbia University, and their use of continuous positive airway pressure (CPAP) as a primary mode of ventilation for very low birth weight infants.

Evidence of such variation persists into more recent times. The Vermont Oxford Network published data on the rates of mortality and common neonatal morbidity in 756 NICUs in the United States between 2005 and 2014 (6,7). Among the 408,164 infants with a birth weight between 501 and 1,500 g born at units, Horbar and colleagues showed a dramatic improvement in mortality, the rate of late-onset infection, necrotizing enterocolitis (NEC), severe intraventricular hemorrhage (IVH), and severe retinopathy of prematurity (ROP) over this time, while the rate of bronchopulmonary dysplasia (BPD) remained around 30%. Even with a secular improvement in outcomes, there were persistent interhospital variations in the rates of all of these outcomes (**Fig. 5.2**). A similar level of variation is observed in infant mortality across U.S. states, with infant mortality rates ranging from a low of 3.6 per 1,000 live births in New Hampshire to 8.3 per 1,000 live births in Mississippi in 2018 (**Fig. 5.3**) (8).

These differences may exist for a number of reasons, including the overall care provided by individual hospitals within the state; differences in the policies of perinatal care that exist in different states, which guide the perinatal health care system in that state; and differences in patient characteristics within each state. One example of the role of state-level policies is work on the relationship between infant mortality and the presence of certificate of need programs. Such policies limit the ability of hospitals to create, or expand, an NICU unless the hospital demonstrates a community need for the expansion. States without such policies had twice as many NICUs and NICU beds, and a 0.5/1,000 higher infant mortality rate compared to states with such policies (9). However, the development and validation of quality measures for health care systems or states is much less developed than for individual hospitals. Thus, the remainder of this chapter will explore the use of quality measures to explain persistent variations in outcomes between individual hospitals.

TYPES OF QUALITY OF CARE MEASUREMENTS

Most perinatal quality of care metrics come from three potential areas, as defined by the Donabedian theory of health care quality: Structures of care; processes of care; and outcomes of care. These areas can be defined as follows:

1. Structures of care: the setting and types of health care available to providers and patients, including the characteristics of health care providers and the systems of health care delivery. To be a quality measure, these structures of care should be associated with both desired processes of care and improvements in outcomes.
2. Processes of care: the activities of care delivery by health care providers to patients. To be a quality measure, processes of care should be associated with improvements in desired outcomes.
3. Outcomes of care: the result of health care, including "recovery, restoration of function, and survival." To be a quality measure, outcome measures should be associated with processes of care that may be involved with high-quality care.

Each of these topic areas has advantages and disadvantages to its use, as shown in **Table 5.1** (10).

Structure Measures

Structures of care typically focus on the characteristics of the health care delivery team, whether it involves providers, facilities, or the larger health care system. These metrics are frequently used by state policy makers to improve care quality. For example, the most commonly used structural measure today is the level of perinatal care, for either neonatal or obstetrical care. Other examples of these measures include nurse-to-patient ratio and the requirement of specific educational metrics for nurses, the routine availability of auxiliary caregivers such as neonatal pharmacists and social workers, and the availability of specific subspecialty services such as surgery care. Structures-of-care metrics are easy to measure and report to policy makers but are frequently difficult to change quickly. Also, appropriate structure of care measures should be associated with some set of care processes that result in improved outcomes of care

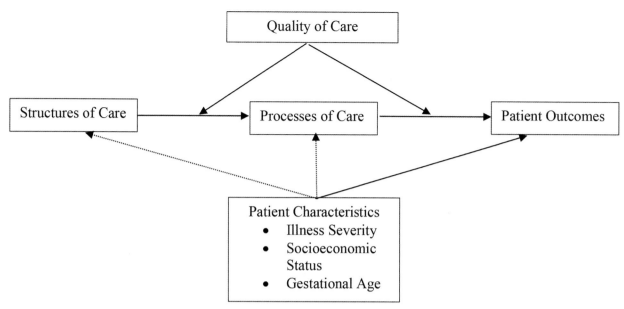

FIGURE 5.1 Modified Donabedian framework for quality of care. Structures of care at a given hospital or for a given health care provider influence the processes of care delivered, which in turn result in a given patient outcome. The quality of care delivery modifies these associations, while patient characteristics impact the ultimate outcomes of the patient, and potentially both the structures and processes of care received.

of value for patients and other stakeholders. However, there are a large number of factors that result in widespread variation in care processes, and even wider variations in outcomes across hospitals with similar structures, as we will see examples of later. For these reasons, many structures-of-care measures are used by stakeholders to limit the number of providers of specific types of care, such as ventilation or the care of infants under 28 weeks of gestation, rather than to measure quality of care.

Process Measures

Processes of care reflect what types of care a health care provider delivered to a patient. Examples include the receipt of antenatal corticosteroids, receipt of recommended screening for ROP by ophthalmology, hand washing prior to examining a patient, and even whether a patient was delivered operatively or vaginally. These measures usually have the greatest face validity

for providers as it assesses what they meant to do (11). However, process of care measures have several significant challenges especially for quality assessment purposes. First, these measures are frequently challenging to assess across multiple providers, or even within the same hospital for a measure that requires direct observation such as hand washing. Also, there should be evidence that a given process of care leads to a desired outcome of care. Demonstrating this association is frequently difficult across different hospitals that care for different types of patients. In addition, if this outcome occurs months or years after the health care encounter, there may be additional factors occurring in the intervening time period that weaken the association between the process and outcome measure. For these reasons, process of care measures are frequently used in quality improvement interventions at the hospital level, with fewer measures used by stakeholders for quality assessment across multiple hospitals.

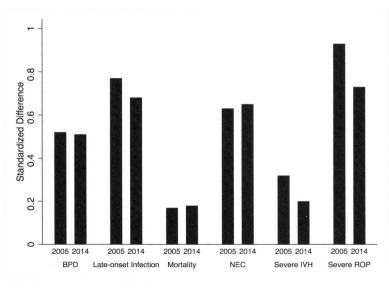

FIGURE 5.2 Standardized difference for various outcome measures between the 10th and 90th percentile hospital in Vermont Oxford Network, 2005 and 2014. Bar graphs show the standardized difference, or the difference between the 10th and 90th percentile hospitals divided by the median value, for five outcome measures in the Vermont Oxford Network hospital network in 2005 and 2014. (Adapted from Horbar JD, Edwards EM, Greenberg LT, et al. Variation in performance of neonatal intensive care units in the United States. *JAMA Pediatr* 2017;171:e164396.)

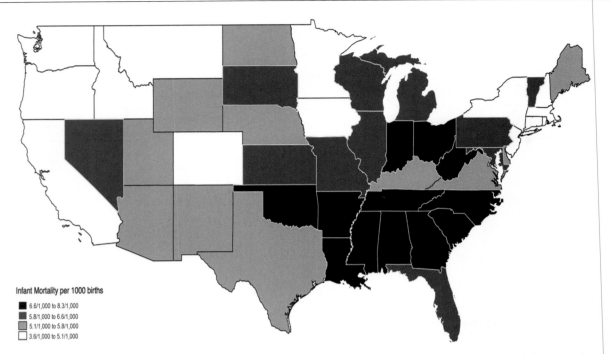

FIGURE 5.3 Variation in infant mortality rates by state, 2018. (Data from wonder.cdc.gov, accessed on https://www.cdc.gov/nchs/pressroom/sosmap/infant_mortality_rates/infant_mortality.htm. Last accessed August 24, 2020.)

Infant Mortality per 1000 births

- 6.6/1,000 to 8.3/1,000
- 5.8/1,000 to 6.6/1,000
- 5.1/1,000 to 5.8/1,000
- 3.6/1,000 to 5.1/1,000

TABLE 5.1

Examples of Types of Quality of Care Measures

Structures of care
- Level of care
- Presence of specific staffing
  - Nurse-to-patient ratio
  - Neonatal pharmacy
  - Social work
- Pediatric subspecialist
- Pediatric surgery and surgery subspecialists
- Availability of neonatal transport

Processes of care
- Receipt of antenatal corticosteroids
- Receipt of intratracheal surfactant
- Adequate hand hygiene
- Appropriate retinal screening for ROP
- Nonindicated early term deliveries
- Maternal smoking cessation
- Deep vein thrombosis prophylaxis
- Hepatitis B vaccine coverage
- Total bilirubin screening

Outcome measures
- Mortality measures
  - Neonatal mortality
  - Infant mortality
- Morbidity measures
  - BPD
  - NEC
  - CLABSI
  - ROP
- Measures of health care use
  - Preventable readmission
  - Emergency department use
- Unexpected complications in term infant measure

Outcome Measures

Outcomes of care measures are primarily the end-products of a health care encounter. Since these measures reflect what ultimately happened to a patient, they are of interest to policy makers and insurers. Examples of such measures in perinatal medicine include mortality, morbidity, and health care use such as hospital readmissions. Many of these measures are easy to measure and identify using vital statistic records or insurance databases. There are, though, challenges in using such measures to assess care quality. As shown in Figure 5.1, there are additional factors that may influence patient outcomes, such as illness severity, gestational age, and sociodemographic factors. As a result, outcome measures typically require *risk adjustment* for use in quality assessment and quality improvement activities. In addition, there may still be unknown or unmeasured patient-level factors that impact the ultimate outcome of patients, such as genetic and epigenetic factors. Without measuring such factors, common risk adjustment methods may not adequately address systematic differences in case mix between health care providers. Also, the time that it takes to measure an outcome may limit use for quality improvement or quality assessment; this is particularly true for long-term neurocognitive outcomes that may require data 3, 7, or even 18 years after the child is born. Thus, while outcome measures are frequently used to assess care quality and used in quality improvement interventions, they require care to ensure that differences in patient case mix and other confounding factors are appropriately accounted for.

WHY ARE THERE SO MANY POTENTIAL QUALITY MEASURES?

While it would be ideal to have a single measure of care quality, there is no true measure of "health care quality." The National Academy of Medicine has identified six domains of health care quality in their publication, *Crossing the Quality Chasm: A New Health System for the 21st Century* (Table 5.2) (12). Similarly, the World Health Organization (WHO) has published standards for improving the quality of maternal and newborn care in health facilities worldwide (13,14). These guidelines identify eight standards of care that mirror the National Academy of Medicine domains (Table 5.2). As we can see, the scope of these domains precludes any one measure to assess all domains or standards. Current measures for neonatal care focus more on effectiveness and safety measures, with little attention to patient-centered and equity areas. Instead, a specific quality measure assesses some part of this overarching construct of "health care quality." A schematic of how a measure may do this is shown in **Figure 5.4** (10,15). This figure reflects a "flashlight" theory of quality measurement. What we are interested in assessing is the black box titled quality. A given measure can be thought of as a flashlight, illuminating some part of the quality box. A measure has two characteristics. First, we can assess how much of the box is illuminated by a given measure. Some measures illuminate a large portion of the box, and may assess multiple domains of health care quality outlined in Table 5.2. Other measures may only illuminate a small portion of the box, and may not even capture one of these domains. Generally, the more domains that are assessed by a given quality measure, the more likely that a change in this measure will influence other potential measures of care. For example, a measure of timeliness may also assess other aspects of a health care provider such as efficiency, but not necessarily safety. We can also take the same approach when examining how different health care providers manage different organ systems: some measures of pulmonary management may also assess the quality of delivery room resuscitation, but have no association with how a provider reduces health care–associated infections.

Second, we can assess how clearly the measure illuminates the box. Some measures provide a clear, bright picture of the box and thus are highly reliable measures. Less reliable measures may provide a blurry picture of the box. Threats to a highly reliable and clear measure include difficulty in defining the measure; a large amount of random variation in the measure, either for different patients with the same baseline risk of developing an adverse outcome, or for different patients over time; rare frequency; and the inability to appropriately adjust for different case mix across facilities.

TABLE 5.2

Domains and Standards of Perinatal Health Care Quality

Domain	Definition
National Academy of Medicine (12)	
Safety	Avoidance of harm to patient with care provided
Effective	Provide care and services to patients based on scientific knowledge about which patients would benefit from specific services
Patient-centered	Provide care that is respectful and responsive to patient values, preferences, and needs
Timely	Provide care without harmful delays
Efficient	Provide care without waste, including equipment, supplies, and ideas
Equitable	Provide care that does not vary in quality because of patient characteristics, geographic location, and socioeconomic status
World Health Organization (14)	
Receipt of evidence-based care and management of complications during labor, childbirth, and early postnatal period	
Use of data to ensure early, appropriate action to improve care of every woman and newborn	
Appropriate referral of women and newborns with conditions that cannot be dealt with effectively with available resources	
Effective communication with women and families	
Respectful care of women and newborns	
Provision of emotional support to every woman and her family that is sensitive to their needs and strengthens the woman's capability	
Competent, motivated staff are available to provide routine care and manage complications	
The health facility has appropriate physical environment for routine maternal and newborn care and to manage complications	

Data from Institute of Medicine. *Crossing the quality chasm: a new health system for the 21st century.* Washington, DC: The National Academies Press, 2001; and World Health Organization. *Standards for improving quality of maternal and newborn care in health facilities.* Geneva, Switzerland: World Health Organization, 2016.

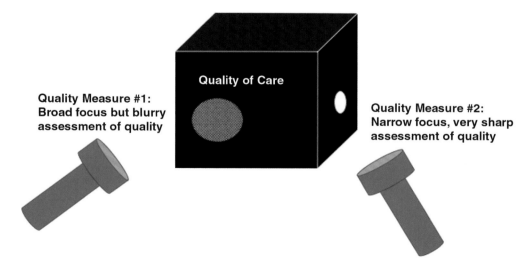

FIGURE 5.4 Flashlight theory of quality. Different measures of quality, whether they are structures, processes, or outcomes of care, assess a different part of the black quality box. No one measure assesses the entire box. Measures may illuminate a larger or smaller portion of the box, depending on how broadly the measure assesses care quality. Measures may also have stronger or weaker assessments of the portion of the box they illuminate, reflecting differences in the reliability of the measure. Quality measure 1 illuminates a large portion of the box, but weakly as reflected by the blurry nature of the light. Quality measure 2 illuminates a smaller portion of this box but provides a clear, reliable assessment of this portion of the box as reflected by the clear nature of the light.

Characteristics of an Ideal Quality of Care Measure

Easy to classify
Easy to measure
High reliability and reproducibility
Face and construct validity
Present in sufficient numbers to minimize loss of statistical power
Adequate risk adjustment

Reprinted from Lorch SA. National quality measures in perinatal medicine. *Clin Perinatol* 2017;44:485. Copyright © 2017 Elsevier. With permission.

CHARACTERISTICS OF AN IDEAL QUALITY MEASURE

Given these challenges, providers and stakeholders rely on multiple quality of care measures to assess the care delivered to patients. An ideal measure would be a bright, reliable measure that assesses a large portion of the quality box for a given health care provider. There are a number of characteristics for an ideal perinatal quality measure (Table 5.3) (10). These characteristics include the following:

1. *Easy to define the measure*: The definition of a measure should be clear to all providers and stakeholders. While this characteristic seems obvious, many potential perinatal measures lack clarity, especially when vital statistics or hospital administrative data are used. For example, most studies of BPD recommend an oxygen titration test at 36 weeks of corrected age to determine whether an infant meets the criteria for BPD (16–18). It is frequently not clear in administrative records whether such tests are performed. In other cases, it may be difficult to ensure that similar patients are included in the eligible cohort across different hospitals. For example, regional and cultural differences in vaccine refusals have hampered the use of immunization adequacy as prevention quality of care measure (19,20).

2. *Easy to measure*: Accurate data about a measure should be readily available and easy to collect for providers and stakeholders. There are a number of potential sources of data for measures (21). These data sources have advantages and disadvantages for the assessment of health care quality, and the use

of a specific data source may depend on what measure is being assessed (Table 5.4). The most familiar data source for providers are data from *prospective cohorts*, such as that used by the Vermont Oxford Network or for statewide perinatal quality collaboratives (PQCs). Prospective data allow for precise measure definitions across all providers participating in the cohort. When combined with routine audits of the data, prospective cohorts offer high data accuracy and data completion. However, these cohorts are frequently expensive and limited to providers that participate in a specific endeavor. Other data sources listed in Table 5.4 include electronic medical records and administrative claims data. While less onerous to collect information, these data have limitations centered on the accuracy of data and the amount of clinical data.

3. *Shows high reliability and reproducibility*: Reliability assesses the ability of a measure to distinguish the performance of one hospital from another, ideally identifying those hospitals with higher performance from lesser performing facilities. It is also known as the ratio of the signal to the noise in the measure, where the variation in outcomes related to provider-level characteristics are the desired signal, and the variation in patient outcomes within a specific hospital is the noise.

   There are numerous measures of reliability. The first level of reliability is whether a measure is consistent for a given patient. This consistency can be over time (test–retest reliability), or between different raters (interrater reliability). The second level of reliability is at the hospital level, where we calculate the percentage of the total variation in a measure that results from variation between providers. Statistical methods are available for the calculation of these statistics when the measure is a continuous or categorical variable. Ideally, a measure will have a reliability above 0.8, although in some cases a reliability above 0.6 is considered acceptable (22).

4. *Shows face and construct validity*: A measure should also show validity, that is, whether a measure actually assesses the aspect of care quality it claims. Validity comes in several forms.
   • *Face validity* measures whether stakeholders and providers believe that a measure assesses some aspect of quality of care based on their general understanding of how the measure is collected. This is the easiest form of validity to obtain, but may be the least helpful if there is little consensus on what

Sources of Data for Quality Measures

Data Source	Advantages	Disadvantages	Examples
Prospective cohort	• Data accuracy • Complete data • Availability of all data fields of interest	• Limited to specific hospitals • Financial and time cost • Time window limited by ability to collect data	Vermont Oxford Network
Electronic medical records	• Data from clinical sources • Available in larger numbers of hospitals	• Requires accurate data entry into medical chart • Onerous abstraction of data from text fields • Financial cost • Variation in data structure and data fields between developers	Kaiser Permanente Health Information System
Linked administrative data (Birth certificates + insurance or billing data)	• Population-based data source, typically states or regions	• Need to link data across multiple data sources • Clinical data limited to fields collected in administrative data or birth certificates • Relies on accurate coding and validation of data	California linked datasets
Administrative claims (Billing data, insurance claims, birth certificates)	• Population-based data, typically national • Low cost	• Limited clinical data • Relies on accurate coding of data • Insurance data from limited group of patients	National birth certificate file Medicaid Analytic eXtract

Modified from Lorch SA, Passarella M, Zeigler A. Challenges to measuring variation in readmission rates of neonatal intensive care patients. *Acad Pediatr* 2014;14:S47. Copyright © 2014 Academic Pediatric Association, with permission.

a measure assesses, or if the general understanding about a measure's assessment of quality is flawed.

- *Construct validity* formally tests how well a measure is associated with care quality, typically by testing various hypotheses about the measure. For example, if we believe that an NICU with a higher level of care should, in general, have better quality than a lower level center, then a higher level NICU should have a superior performance on a specific measure. Other forms of construct validity focus on correlations between different quality measures, with the presumption that these measures assess the same aspect of quality and an NICU should perform equally well on both measures.
- *Criterion validity* assesses how well a measure correlates with a "gold standard" measure that may in many cases be onerous to measure and assess. This test occurs only if such a gold standard quality measure exists in the literature.

5. *Sufficient numbers of events per hospital:* There are unique aspects of assessing care quality in perinatal medicine. One challenge is the relative rarity of many outcomes, especially for a normally small numbers of patients most NICUs care for. The frequency of many outcomes is less than 10%, especially when we study cohorts such as infants born very low birth weight (<1,500 g) or low birth weight (<2,500 g). The prevalence of these outcomes may increase when the cohort is narrowed but decreases the absolute number of patients that we assess the metric upon. Small numbers limit the statistical power to detect significant and meaningful differences between hospitals. An additional issue with small numbers of outcomes is the inability to distinguish random noise in a measurement from a true change in the baseline rate of the outcome. As a result, it can be difficult for hospitals or other stakeholders to assess the impact of specific quality improvement interventions, or to identify poor-performing hospitals when data are less reliable and noisy.

6. *Ability to risk adjust measure:* Risk-adjustment refers to the need to control, or adjust, for the types of patient that a hospital cares for, because the likelihood an infant develops a given outcome depends on characteristics of the child. This is particularly an issue for outcome measures such as mortality and morbidity where such patient characteristics as gestational age, birth weight, and other antepartum and intrapartum complications predispose infants to a higher likelihood to experience adverse outcomes (23–26). In addition, structural measures suffer from selection bias: higher risk infants are more likely to deliver at higher technology, higher level hospitals with the capability to immediately care for those infants (27–29).

There are a variety of methods to perform risk adjustment for a specific quality measure. An in-depth discussion of these methods is beyond the scope of this chapter. Briefly, though, the most common method to risk-adjust quality measures involves the development of a statistical model that assesses the association between a set of risk factors and the outcome to risk adjust. These models estimate an expected rate of a given outcome at a specific hospital based on the characteristics of the patients that receive care at that hospital. By comparing the actual rate of the outcome to this expected rate at a given hospital, and multiplying this observed/expected ratio by the average rate of the outcome in the entire population, we can calculate a hospital-specific risk-adjusted outcome rate.

The challenges to risk adjustment are many, including the need to validate the risk-adjustment model and to update it as changes in clinical practice affect these associations between risk factors and outcomes and the need for measurable variables to account for the most of the patient-level variation in risk (27). Also, many clinicians are skeptical about the ability of a risk-adjustment model to adequately capture the illness severity of patients receiving care in their unit. Since process measures frequently do not require risk adjustment, this is a key reason why process measures are preferred by many clinicians (11).

EXAMPLES OF TYPES OF MEASURES

To see some of the advantages and disadvantages to various types of quality measures we will examine a structural, process, and outcome measure, applying the framework listed above to assess each type of measure.

Structural Measure: Levels of Neonatal Care

Levels of care as a potential structural measure of neonatal quality arise from an extensive literature base starting in the 1980s that found that outcomes of high-risk infants are improved when they are delivered at a hospital with the capability to care for them immediately after birth. This section will provide evidence and challenges for the use of levels of care, and consequently other structural measures of care, as measures of perinatal care quality.

Ease of Use

Structural measures tend to be easy to classify but difficult to measure. Structural measures usually list of characteristics that a facility must have, similar to the recommended list characteristics for a given neonatal level as defined by the American Academy of Pediatrics (30). These guidelines, shown in Table 5.5, show that a level 1 NICU has the capacity to care only for well infants, while a level 4 hospital can manage the sickest infants, including those who require pediatric cardiothoracic surgery, cardiopulmonary bypass, and ECMO. Because these measures are not typically collected with any frequency by state or private groups, these measures require either self-report from the hospital or manual collection of data by investigators or stakeholders. This is particularly an issue for many of the structural measures used by the US News & World Report, which as of 2020 have included such items as the presence of social workers, neonatal pharmacist, and other auxiliary staff services (31).

Levels of care have an additional challenge. Although there are national guidelines to designate levels of neonatal care, most recently published by the American Academy of Pediatrics in 2012, many states have modified these designations to meet local needs (32,33). Such variation is not typically seen in other structural measures noted in Table 5.1.

Reliability and Validity of Measure

Levels of care are an attractive measure of neonatal quality because of the extensive literature base showing an association between delivery at a high-level hospital and improved morbidity and mortality. High-level hospitals in most studies have been defined as a level 3 or level 4 center, with many older studies before 2012 using previous designations where high-level hospitals were classified as having levels 3B and above. This literature base includes data both prior to the diffusion of NICUs into community hospitals, and after deregionalization occurred in the 1990s, as well as in other developed countries such as the Netherlands, Portugal, and Canada. Studies have also shown that outcomes are improved when the mother is transferred to desired hospital versus transporting the infant (29,34). These data were summarized in a meta-analysis of the evidence published through 2010 (35), showing an increased odds of death for very low birth weight infants born at hospitals with a level 1 or level 2 NICU (odds ratio 1.62, 95% CI 1.44 to 1.83). This effect was larger for infants born with a birth weight less than 1,000 g (odds ratio 1.80, 95% CI 1.31 to 2.46).

The reliability of a structures-of-care measure has not been assessed. Studies examining the association between delivery hospital level and outcomes typically reclassify hospitals based on the characteristics of the children that they are caring for, as

TABLE 5.5

Levels of Neonatal Care

Level of Neonatal Care	Characteristics
Level 1: Well baby newborn nursery	• Provide neonatal resuscitation at all deliveries • Evaluate and manage care of stable term newborn infants • Stabilize and provide care to physiologically stable infants born 35–37 wk gestation • Stabilize and transfer infants who are ill, or born <35 wk gestation to a higher level of care
Level 2: Special care nursery	All capabilities of level 1 and • Provide care for infants born ≥32 wk gestation and weighing ≥1,500 g whose illnesses are expected to resolve quickly without need for subspecialty services • Care for infants convalescing after intensive care • Provide brief (<24 h) mechanical ventilation or continuous positive airway pressure • Stabilize and transfer infants born ≤ 32 wk gestation and weighing ≤1,500 g to a higher level of care
Level 3: Neonatal intensive care unit	All capabilities of level 2 and • Provide sustained life support • Provide comprehensive care for infants born at all gestational ages and birth weights with critical illness • Provide prompt and ready access to a full range of pediatric subspecialists, pediatric surgical specialists, pediatric anesthesiologists, and pediatric ophthalmologists • Provide a full range of respiratory support, including conventional and/or high-frequency models and inhaled nitric oxide • Perform advanced imaging
Level 4: Regional neonatal intensive care unit	All capabilities of level 3 and • Can provide surgical repair of complex congenital and acquired conditions, including congenital heart disease • On-site access to a full range of pediatric subspecialists, pediatric surgical specialists, and pediatric anesthesiologists • Facilitate regional transport and outreach education to lower level nurseries

Reproduced with permission from American Academy of Pediatrics Committee on Fetus and Newborn. Levels of neonatal care. *Pediatrics* 2012;130:587. Copyright © 2012 by the American Academy of Pediatrics.

the concordance between reported level of care and the actual care delivered to newborn infants is poor (27–29,34). Such concerns over the self-reported levels of care by hospitals have led the American Academy of Pediatrics to develop a task force to independently assign levels of care to hospitals in states with legislated levels of care policies (36).

Risk Adjustment

Like many of the structures-of-care measures, levels of care require extensive risk adjustment to appropriately account for the fact that the most complicated and highest risk infants tend to be referred to the highest level NICUs for their management (23–29). While older studies accounted for these interhospital differences in case mix using a combination of gestational age, birth weight,

and maternal characteristics, more recent data suggest that population-based data sets that do not include important clinical variables such as maternal vital signs, the severity of maternal coexisting medical conditions, and results from fetal monitoring may fail to adjust for these case mix differences (27). Lorch et al., using an instrumental variables approach to account for this unmeasured selection bias, showed that delivery at a high-level, high-volume center was associated with an 18% to 65% reduction in all hospital mortality for infants with a gestational age between 23 and 37 weeks, and a 23% to 32% reduction in all hospital mortality for infants with a birth weight between 500 and 1,500 g. There was no statistically significant difference in mortality or morbidity between high- and low-level NICUs when traditional risk-adjustment measures were used. Similar reductions in the risk of common morbidities of preterm birth, such as BPD, were also observed when infants were delivered at high-level centers (27).

Other Challenges

The other challenge with using structural measures for assessing care quality is the heterogeneity in the association between improved outcomes and hospitals with a given structural measure strata. As discussed in the introduction, data from the Vermont Oxford Network show wide variations in mortality and common complications of preterm birth between hospitals of similar levels of care (6). One reason may be volume, as several studies have found that outcomes are improved when an infant is referred for delivery at a hospital with a high-volume, high-level NICU compared to a high-level, low-volume NICU (27–29,34,37–42). A volume threshold that improves outcomes remains unknown.

Finally, factors that influence the choice of hospital, such as socioeconomic status, have not been accounted for in studies of levels of care as a measure of quality. Howell et al., using data from New York City between 1996 and 2001, found that 49% of white very low birth weight infants delivered at hospitals in the lowest mortality quartile compared to 29% of black very low birth weight infants (43). Also, women of lower socioeconomic status and minority racial/ethnic status may be less likely to redirect care to hospitals with high-level NICUs when faced with an obstetric unit closure (44). Such results may reduce the reliability and validity of the aforementioned studies.

Summary

As with many structural measures of care, levels of care are a crude assessment of neonatal quality because of the factors that exist in between the structure of care and the ultimate outcome of the infant. While many of these metrics are easy to classify and measure, they typically require prospective collection of data by stakeholders to obtain accurate information. Thus, few structural measures of care are used to assess care delivery other than levels of care legislation in many states. The heterogeneity in outcomes between hospitals of the same level of care, though, suggests that other measures of quality may be superior.

Process Measure: Screening for Retinopathy of Prematurity

This measure arises from evidence that routine ophthalmologic screening reduces the risk of blindness or reduced visual acuity from stage 4 or Stage 5 (ROP) (45). Screening for ROP arose from evidence from 2000 to 2009 that the rates of any visual retinal examination among infants weighing 501 to 1,500 g remained low at 74.5% (46), and that 29% of neonatologists in a survey performed in 2006 agreed that some children in their state develop ROP-related visual impairment that could be prevented by timely screening (47). These data highlight potential areas for improvement in this field. This section will provide evidence and challenges for the use of this measure as a quality metric, highlighting the advantages and barriers to the use of process measures to assess care quality.

Ease of Use

Process measures tend to be difficult to measure and classify depending on how well the measure is defined. Process measures typically cannot be collected using insurance or hospital administrative data. Thus, either the stakeholders or the clinical teams must prospectively collect this information and perform checks of its accuracy, as required by this metric. In addition, process measures require detailed descriptions of what constitutes a successful outcome. For this measure, a successful outcome is the performance of at least one retinal exam for infants born at 22 to 29 weeks of gestation at the postnatal age recommended for ROP screening by the American Academy of Pediatrics. It does not, though, assess whether the infant received retinal examinations at all potential screening times, typically every 1 to 4 weeks depending on the postnatal age of the incident.

Reliability and Validity

Reliability testing for most process measures typically involves interrater reliability, assessing for the consistency of a successful or unsuccessful process measure for a specific patient between multiple raters. Reported reliability for the screening for ROP measure was demonstrated by the stability hospital means on this measure over a 9-year period. Validity for the process measure, as with other process measures, is shown through the association between the lack of a retinal exam with a higher rate of blindness from ROP (45). Such associations between the receipt of the process measure and a clinically relevant outcome can be frequently difficult to achieve, especially for interventions that may occur many months before the outcome of interest typically occurs.

Risk Adjustment

Unlike many structural and outcome measures, process measures are rarely risk adjusted. This is because for most measures, all eligible infants should receive the process measure in a high-quality system.

Summary

As with many process measures, screening for ROP has strong face validity with the advantage that complicated risk adjustment is not required. However, the need to prospectively collect data makes such measures expensive and challenging to implement on a population level.

Outcome Measure: Neonatal Mortality

Neonatal mortality is a frequently proposed measure of quality of care because, in most medical situations, especially in adults, death is an easy-to-measure, easy-to-classify outcome that is associated with care practices. However, in perinatal medicine, neonatal mortality requires extensive risk adjustment and suffers from the small numbers of true outcomes that limit the power to detect clinically meaningful differences between clinical practices. These characteristics are common for outcome measures.

Ease of Use

Outcome measures typically can be easily collected from population-based data, with the caveat that coding misclassification frequently occurs from two areas. First, if centers do not perform the needed tests to detect an outcome, such as a head ultrasound for IVH, or an oxygen tolerance test at 36 weeks of gestation age to accurately diagnose BPD, then misclassification will occur. Second, many outcome measures are assessed or occur at a given postnatal age, such as BPD (measured at 36 weeks of postnatal age) and ROP. Infants who die prior to those postnatal ages may inappropriately lower the rate of these outcomes. For neonatal mortality, additional challenges exist. First, there is no universally accepted minimum gestational age needed to be considered a live birth: some states use a threshold as low as 16 weeks of gestation, while other states use

a threshold as high as 24 weeks (48). Fetal death is also a potential competing measure. Ignoring these deaths may artificially increase the rates of neonatal death at hospitals that successfully resuscitate an infant but ultimately have the infant die, thereby transferring a fetal death that is unmeasured into a neonatal death that is measured (27,29,39,40). Finally, assigning deaths to a specific hospital can be difficult since sicker infants are more likely to be transferred. This transfer of care may bias against hospitals that receive large numbers of transfers. Also, when care is split between centers for substantial periods of time, it is difficult to assign the outcome to a specific hospital. As a result, most research studies assign patients to their birth hospital regardless of where the death occurred, which may overestimate the impact of birth hospital on outcomes. Thus, while many outcome measures appear easy to measure and classify, understanding the nuances of the definitions and any competing measures is important to understanding how well an outcome measure assesses care quality.

Reliability and Validity

For many stakeholders, outcome measures have the strongest face validity because they assess the end result of care on the infant. Mortality has strong face and construct validity. There is ample evidence of variation in mortality rates by the level and volume of care of birth hospitals (27,29,39,40). More recent data from the Vermont Oxford Network show variations in mortality within hospitals of the same level. This fact suggests that mortality may be associated with care received at a specific hospital (6). The reliability of outcome measures is more mixed, especially when there are unclear definitions of the outcome measure. Reliability is typically improved when data are collected prospectively and are validated with multiple raters.

Risk Adjustment and Other Considerations

Because younger and sicker infants are more likely to die, risk adjustment is critical for neonatal mortality measures. Standard risk adjustment models include variables present at delivery, such as gestational age, birth weight, multiple birth, and gender. Although these models have been used in multiple studies, one recent study found that mortality rates between different levels of NICUs were only statistically significant using methods that accounted for unmeasured case-mix differences (27). In addition, mortality is a rare event, occurring overall in six per 1,000 deliveries in the United States. Thus, it is more difficult to detect statistically significant differences in mortality rates between hospitals. Similar challenges are seen with many other so-called common complications of preterm birth that occur in less than 5% to 10% of all preterm infants in developed countries. For other situations, where such outcomes are more prevalent, these measures may have more power to detect such differences.

Summary

While commonly identified as potential quality measures, outcome metrics require validated risk adjustment tools and clear definitions to overcome many of the challenges in their use to assess perinatal quality. Neonatal mortality suffers from the same issues, including concerns about the small numbers of outcomes, the need for risk adjustment, and the need to include some but not all fetal deaths at a given hospital.

USE OF MEASURES

There are many uses for quality measures at both the hospital and population levels. While this chapter is not designed to discuss specific quality improvement methods for an individual hospital, the use of valid and reliable metrics is a crucial part of any successful quality improvement program. We will finish this chapter with an examination of how specific quality measures are used for benchmarking purposes across multiple hospitals, specifically through the Vermont Oxford Network, and in state-level oversight programs through perinatal quality collaboratives (PQCs).

Individual Hospital Quality Improvement and Benchmarking

Quality measures are frequently used by hospitals to benchmark themselves with similar hospitals around the United States. The largest such perinatal group is the Vermont Oxford Network, which includes more than 1,300 hospitals as of 2020 that use data-driven quality improvement programs to improve the health of newborn infants. Benchmarking is a technique where hospitals compare their performance to other hospitals, many or all of whom are similar to the hospital of interest, using similar data collection techniques and data definitions to provide a more accurate comparison of a hospital's performance. Similar techniques are used in public reporting of data, where state agencies publish hospital process or outcome measures so that patients can research potential providers and to choose providers with better outcomes. Such public reporting of data is more common for adult hospitals, where many states publish catheter-associated bloodstream infection rates and other outcome measures (49). A similar program that reports risk-adjusted mortality rates for coronary artery bypass graft has existed for over two decades in New York state (50). Beyond their benchmarking services, the Vermont Oxford network has led several multicenter quality improvement initiatives to improve care in such areas as antibiotic stewardship, the prevention of hospital-acquired bloodstream infections, reduction in the rate of BPD, and the use of human milk to prevent NEC (51,52). Other countries have similar benchmarking organizations for NICUs within their country, including Canada (53) and Australia and New Zealand (54).

There has been recent attention from the WHO at developing metrics for the assessment of care quality at health care facilities in low- and middle-income nations. Simulation models from 81 countries suggest that if high-quality health systems could implement 19 antenatal, childbirth, or postnatal interventions, there would be a 28% decrease in maternal deaths, a 28% decrease in neonatal deaths, and a 22% decrease in stillbirths. The greatest decrease in mortality was seen in key interventions provided at or around childbirth (55). The WHO has thus set up standards for improving maternal and neonatal care that include 8 standards and 31 quality statements (13,14). However, the ability of facilities to obtain these data may be challenging. In a recent study, standardized tools to capture health service delivery data in low- and middle-income countries, such as the Service Provision Assessment and the Service Availability and Readiness Assessment, could only fully generate 4 of the 31 proposed quality statements in the WHO guideline, with 4 to 8 guidelines unable to be assessed at all (56). Similar challenges were faced in a survey of 963 health care facilities in Bangladesh, Ghana, Kenya, Malawi, Nigeria, Pakistan, Sierra Leone, South Africa, Tanzania, and Zimbabwe (57). These challenges to obtaining accurate data for benchmarking and quality improvement programs in low- and middle-income countries, along with limited validation of the meaning of metrics within a specific country or region, remain an important area to overcome.

State-Level Oversight: Perinatal Quality Collaboratives

PQCs are state-based or occasionally multistate-based networks of providers and stakeholders who work to improve the outcomes and health of pregnant women and children. The oldest state PQC is the California Perinatal Quality Care Collaborative founded as an action arm of the California Association of Neonatologists in 1997. As of 2020, 40 States had an operational PQC, with eight states in the process of developing such a program (58,59).

There is an extensive literature showing the impact of State PQCs on improving maternal and neonatal processes and outcomes. Topic areas include the health of opioid-exposed infants experiencing neonatal abstinence syndrome, safe sleep practices, smoking, the reduction of cesarean births in low-risk pregnant women, the reduction of early term deliveries, and reductions in pregnancy complications associated with preeclampsia and maternal hemorrhage (58–64).

Another such statewide program is the Health Resources and Services Administration Maternal and Child Health Bureau Collaborative Improvement and Innovation Network (CoIIN) to reduce infant mortality, implemented in 2012. This collaborative was designed to address persistently high rates of infant mortality in 13 Southern States in public health regions IV and VI. This multistate improvement initiative applied data-driven quality improvement and collaboration innovation at the state levels to address multiple priority areas related to preterm birth and infant mortality. Hirai et al. published the impact of the CoIIN on the change in outcomes between 2011 and 2014, comparing changes in three priority areas (Early elective delivery, smoking cessation, and safe sleep strategies) as well as preterm birth and infant mortality (65). For the three priority areas, participation in the CoIIN in the 13 Southern States was associated with a larger improvement than in other regions in the country. For early elective delivery, there was a 22% reduction in the region IV and VI states, compared to a 14% reduction in all other regions; 11 of the 13 CoIIN states reduced their early elective delivery rates. For smoking cessation, the CoIIN states had a 7% increase in the quit rate during pregnancy compared to 2% in all other regions, while for safe sleep strategies the CoIIN states had a 5% increase in back-only sleep position compared to a 2% increase in all of the regions. However, for preterm birth and infant mortality the reductions in the CoIIN and non-CoIIN states were relatively similar: the CoIIN states had a 4% reduction in births less than 37 weeks' gestation, compared to 2% in the other regions, and the CoIIN states had a 2% reduction in infant mortality compared to a 5% reduction in the other regions. These data show the strength of applying quality measures to a population-based framework that includes both quality improvement measures at the hospital level and data-driven oversight and collaboration between stakeholders and health care providers.

SUMMARY

This brief overview highlights the challenges and opportunities that quality assessment holds to improve the health and outcomes of high-risk newborns and their mothers. The growing evidence that quality measures assess only some part of a given provider's "quality of care" only strengthens the need to understand what a given measure is assessing, how data are collected on a given measure that influences the reliability and validity of said measure, and the underlying threats to use of that measure to assess care quality for both individual hospitals and state and national stakeholders. Current measures for neonatal care focus more on effectiveness and safety measures, with little attention to patient-centered and equity areas. Understanding these metrics and what they reflect about overall quality of care is critical to optimizing hospital and population outcomes of high-risk infants.

REFERENCES

1. Donabedian A. Evaluating the quality of medical care. *Milbank Q* 1966; 44:166.
2. Berwick D, Fox DM. Evaluating the quality of medical care: Donabedian's classic article 50 years later. *Milbank Q* 2016;94:237.
3. Ayanian JZ, Markel H. Donabedian's lasting framework for health care quality. *N Engl J Med* 2016;375:205.
4. Institute of Medicine. *Medicare: a strategy for quality assurance,* Vol. I. Washington, DC: The National Academies Press, 1990.
5. Avery ME, Tooley WH, Keller JB, et al. Is chronic lung disease in low birth weight infants preventable? A survey of eight centers. *Pediatrics* 1987;79:26.
6. Horbar JD, Edwards EM, Greenberg LT, et al. Variation in performance of neonatal intensive care units in the United States. *JAMA Pediatr* 2017;171:e164396.

7. Lorch SA. A Decade of improvement in neonatal intensive care: how do we continue the momentum? *JAMA Pediatr* 2017;171:e164395.

8. Data from wonder.cdc.gov. Available from: https://www.cdc.gov/nchs/pressroom/sosmap/infant_mortality_rates/infant_mortality.htm. Accessed August 24, 2020.

9. Lorch SA, Maheshwari P, Even-Shoshan O. The impact of certificate of need programs on neonatal intensive care units. *J Perinatol* 2012;32:39.

10. Lorch SA. National quality measures in perinatal medicine. *Clin Perinatol* 2017;44:485.

11. Lilford R, Brown CA, Nicholl J. Use of process measures to monitor the quality of clinical practice. *BMJ* 2007;335:648.

12. Institute of Medicine. *Crossing the Quality Chasm: a new health system for the 21st century.* Washington, DC: The National Academies Press, 2001.

13. Tuncalp Ö, Were WM, MacLennan C, et al. Quality of care for pregnant women and newborns—the WHO vision. *BJOG* 2015;122:1045.

14. World Health Organization. *Standards for improving quality of maternal and newborn care in health facilities.* Geneva, Switzerland: World Health Organization, 2016.

15. Lorch SA. Quality measurements in pediatrics: what do they assess? *JAMA Pediatr* 2013;167:89.

16. Jensen EA, Dysart K, Gantz MG, et al. The diagnosis of bronchopulmonary dysplasia in very preterm infants. An evidence-based approach. *Am J Respir Crit Care Med* 2019;200:751.

17. Jobe AH, Bancalari E. Bronchopulmonary dysplasia. *Am J Respir Crit Care Med* 2001;163:1723.

18. Walsh MC, Wilson-Costello D, Zadell A, et al. Safety, reliability, and validity of a physiologic definition of bronchopulmonary dysplasia. *J Perinatol* 2003;23:451.

19. Immunization Action Coalition. *Hepatitis B: what hospitals need to do to protect newborns.* St. Paul, MN: Immunization Action Coalition, 2013. Available from: https://www.immunize.org/protect-newborns/guide/birth-dose.pdf

20. World Health Organization. *Practices to improve coverage of the hepatitis B birth dose vaccine.* Geneva, Switzerland: World Health Organization, 2013.

21. Lorch SA, Passarella M, Zeigler A. Challenges to measuring variation in readmission rates of neonatal intensive care patients. *Acad Pediatr* 2014; 14:S47.

22. Adams JL. *The reliability of provider profiling: a tutorial.* Santa Monica, CA: Rand Corporation, 2009.

23. Richardson DK, Phibbs CS, Gray JE, et al. Birth weight and illness severity: independent predictors of neonatal mortality. *Pediatrics* 1993;91:969.

24. Richardson DK, Gray JE, McCormick MC, et al. Score for neonatal acute physiology: a physiologic severity index for neonatal intensive care. *Pediatrics* 1993;91:617.

25. Richardson DK, Corcoran JD, Escobar GJ, et al. SNAP-II and SNAPPE-II: simplified newborn illness severity and mortality risk scores. *J Pediatr* 2001;138:92.

26. Anonymous. The CRIB (clinical risk index for babies) score: a tool for assessing initial neonatal risk and comparing performance of neonatal intensive care units. The International Neonatal Network. *Lancet* 1993;342:193.

27. Lorch SA, Baiocchi M, Ahlberg CE, et al. The differential impact of delivery hospital on the outcomes of premature infants. *Pediatrics* 2012;130:270.

28. Rogowski A, Horbar JD, Staiger DO, et al. Indirect vs direct hospital quality indicators for very low-birth-weight infants. *JAMA* 2004;291:202.

29. Phibbs CS, Baker LC, Caughey AB, et al. Level and volume of neonatal intensive care and mortality of very-low-birth-weight infants. *N Engl J Med* 2007;356:2165.

30. American Academy of Pediatrics Committee on Fetus and Newborn. Levels of neonatal care. *Pediatrics* 2012;130:587.

31. Olmsted MG, Powell R, Murphy J, et al. *Methodology: U.S. news and world report best children's hospitals 2018-2019.* Available from: https://www.usnews.com/static/documents/health/best-hospitals/BCH_Methodology_2018-19.pdf. Accessed August 21, 2020.

32. Nowakowski L, Barfield WD, Kroelinger CD, et al. Assessment of state measures of risk-appropriate care for very low birth weight infants and recommendations for enhancing regionalized state systems. *Matern Child Health J* 2012;16:217.

33. Blackmon LR, Barfield WD, Stark AR. Hospital neonatal services in the United States: variation in definitions, criteria, and regulatory status. *J Perinatol* 2009;29:788.

34. Phibbs CS, Bronstein JM, Buxton E, et al. The effects of patient volume and level of care at the hospital of birth on neonatal mortality. *JAMA* 1996;276:1054.

35. Lasswell SM, Barfield WD, Rochat RW, et al. Perinatal regionalization for very-low-birth-weight and very preterm infants: a meta-analysis. *JAMA* 2010;304:992.

36. https://www.aap.org/en-us/advocacy-and-policy/aap-health-initiatives/nicuverification/Pages/default.aspx. Accessed August 21, 2020.

37. Marlow N, Bennett C, Draper ES, et al. Perinatal outcomes for extremely preterm babies in relation to place of birth in England: The EPICure 2 study. *Arch Dis Child Fetal Neonatal Ed* 2014;99:F181.

38. Bartels DB, Wypijj D, Wenzlaff P, et al. Hospital volume and neonatal mortality among very low birth weight infants. *Pediatrics* 2006;117:2206.

39. Chung JH, Phibbs CS, Boscardin WJ, et al. Examining the effect of hospital-level factors on mortality of very low birth weight infants using multilevel modeling. *J Perinatol* 2011;31:770.

40. Chung JH, Phibbs CS, Boscardina WJ, et al. The effect of neonatal intensive care level and hospital volume on mortality of very low birth weight infants. *Med Care* 2010;48:635.

41. Cifuentes J, Bronstein J, Phibbs CS, et al. Mortality in low birth weight infants according to level of neonatal care at hospital of birth. *Pediatrics* 2002;109:745.

42. Synnes AR, Macnab YC, Qiui Z, et al. Neonatal intensive care unit characteristics affect the incidence of severe intraventricular hemorrhage. *Med Care* 2006;44:754.

43. Howell EA, Hebert P, Chatterjee S, et al. Black/white differences in very low birth weight neonatal mortality rates among New York City hospitals. *Pediatrics* 2008;121:e407.

44. Lorch SA, Srinivas SK, Ahlberg C, et al. The impact of obstetric unit closures on maternal and infant pregnancy outcomes. *Health Serv Res* 2013; 48:455.

45. American Academy of Pediatrics, American Academy of Ophthalmology, American Association for Pediatric Ophthalmology and Strabismus, American Association of Certified Orthoptists. Screening examination of premature infants for retinopathy of prematurity. *Pediatrics* 2018;142: e20183061.

46. Soll RF, Edwards EM, Badger GJ, et al. Obstetric and neonatal care practices for infants 501 to 1500 g from 2000 to 2009. *Pediatrics* 2013;132(2):222.

47. Kemper AR, Wallace DK. Neonatologists' practices and experiences in arranging retinopathy of prematurity screening services. *Pediatrics* 2007;120:527.

48. MacDorman MF, Kirmeyer S. Fetal and perinatal mortality, United States. *Natl Vital Stat Rep* 2005;57(8):1. Hyattsville, MD: National Center for Health Statistics. Available from: https://www.cdc.gov/nchs/data/misc/itop97.pdf. Accessed August 21, 2020.

49. Reagan J, Hacker C. Laws pertaining to healthcare-associated infections: a review of 3 legal requirements. *Infect Control Hosp Epidemiol* 2012;33:75.

50. https://health.data.ny.gov/Health/30-Day-Risk-Adjusted-Mortality-CABG/9vv6-5ie3. Accessed August 21, 2020.

51. Dukhovny D, Buus-Frank ME, Edwards EM, et al. A collaborative multicenter QI initiative to improve antibiotic stewardship in newborns. *Pediatrics* 2019;144:e20190589.

52. Soll RF, McGuire W. Evidence-based practice: improving the quality of perinatal care. *Neonatology* 2019;116:193.

53. www.canadianneonatalnetwork.org. Accessed August 21, 2020.

54. anznn.net. Accessed August 21, 2020.

55. Chou VB, Walker N, Kanyangarara M. Estimating the global impact of poor quality of care on maternal and neonatal outcomes in 81 low- and middle-income countries: a modeling study. *PLoS Med* 2019;16:e1002990.

56. Sheffel A, Karp C, Creanga AA. Use of Service Provision Assessments and Service Availability and Readiness Assessments for monitoring quality of maternal and newborn health services in low-income and middle-income countries. *BMJ Glob Health* 2018;3:e001011.

57. Madaj B, Smith H, Mathai M, et al. Developing global indicators for quality of maternal and newborn care: a feasibility assessment. *Bull World Health Organ* 2017;95:445.

58. https://www.cdc.gov/reproductivehealth/maternalinfanthealth/pqc.htm. Accessed August 21, 2020.

59. Henderson ZT, Ernst K, Simpson KR, et al. The National Network of State Perinatal Quality Collaboratives: a growing movement to improve maternal and infant health. *Womens Health* 2018;27:221.

60. Walsh MC, Crowley M, Wexelblatt S, et al. Ohio perinatal quality collaborative improves care of neonatal narcotic abstinence syndrome. *Pediatrics* 2018;141:e20170900.

61. Gupta M, Donovan EF, Henderson Z. State-based perinatal quality collaboratives: pursuing improvements in perinatal health outcomes for all mothers and newborns. *Semin Perinatol* 2017;41:195.

62. Kacica MA, Glantz JCJ, Xiong K, et al. A statewide quality improvement initiative to reduce non-medically indicated scheduled deliveries. *Matern Child Health J* 2017;21:932.

63. Kaplan HC, Sherman SN, Cleveland C, et al. Reliable implementation of evidence: a qualitative study of antenatal corticosteroid administration in Ohio hospitals. *BMJ Qual Saf* 2016;25:173.

64. Bailit LJ, Iams J, Silber A, et al. Changes in the indications for scheduled births to reduce nonmedically indicated deliveries occurring before 39 weeks of gestation. *Obstet Gynecol* 2012;120:241.

65. Hirai AH, Sappenfield WM, Ghandour RM, et al. The Collaborative Improvement and Innovation Network (CoIIN) to reduce infant mortality: an outcome evaluation from the US South, 2011 to 2014. *Am J Public Health* 2018;108:815.

GENERAL CONSIDERATIONS

6 Inter-Hospital Transport

Hilary E. A. Whyte and Andrew Berry

BACKGROUND

Regionalization

The need for regionalization in health care was recognized more than 50 years ago in order to achieve optimal patient outcomes in a cost-effective manner. This principle was exemplified by high-risk mothers, newborns, and children, where best outcomes were seen in tertiary perinatal units and children's hospitals (1). Little hope of a good outcome follows transfer of a seriously ill patient, who arrives in a semi-moribund state at the tertiary care center. This "unsatisfactory aspect of neonatal care" was first described in Toronto, in which multiple ambulance providers transported infants who had no appropriate oxygen monitoring or ventilators and were often acidotic and cold on arrival (2). A similar study in Melbourne, Australia, prompted the development of their retrieval service in 1976, to focus on lifesaving resuscitation and stabilization prior to transfer (3–5) requiring specific expertise in this population (6).

Specialization in Transport Teams

Despite the variations seen in patterns of regionalization (7) and variations in transport systems, (8) the need for an interfacility transport service for neonates is rarely disputed. Many countries recommend transfer of high-risk mothers to a tertiary setting (9,10), to avoid "outborn" deliveries with their attendant increase in mortality and morbidity (11,12). Barker described 147 high-risk in utero transfers where only 2 babies delivered during land ambulance transfer (9). The use of fetal fibronectin may enhance the maternal triage process (13), but every mother with a threatened preterm birth should be considered for emergent transport to tertiary care, due to their greatly enhanced outcomes of very low birth weight (VLBW) infants (1). This concurs with older literature reinforcing the much needed incentive to transfer high-risk pregnancies to the nearest tertiary center (14,15). Teams that can respond to both high-risk maternal as well as neonatal populations offer distinct advantages since they diminish the perceived risk of a delivery during transport. When mothers cannot be moved due to emergent or imminent delivery, neonates do better when the specialized neonatal transport teams are present at their delivery (16,17).

Most developed countries have adopted the concept of regionalization with the integration of transport or retrieval programs (18,19), but the importance of that service being specialized to specifically meet the needs of the patient population is still debated. Although no randomized controlled trial has been conducted to demonstrate the superiority of specialized teams (20,21), several studies demonstrated enhanced care and better outcomes by specialized teams, often combining both high-risk neonatal and pediatric patients (22,23). Several prospective "before and after" studies on specialized teams showed a significant decline in adverse events (e.g., 34% to 12.5%) during transport (23–25). In general, the patients transported by specialized teams are sicker and require more interventions (26), and although it may take longer for a specialized team to reach the patient bedside, this is not associated with worse outcomes (27).

Indeed, adverse events are very prevalent when nonspecialized teams are used and generally relate to the severity of illness, duration of transfer, and the lack of experience of the personnel (28,29). In one study of 346 neonatal transports, 36% had an adverse event: 67% due to human error, 21% due to equipment failure, and 9% had ambulance problems (30). There is no evidence that one health care professional group over another has improved outcomes (31). A survey of paramedics in United States reported that 72.5% dealt with pediatric patients and 71.8% were familiar with neonatal equipment (32), but training and maintaining competencies must be addressed (33). Clinical expertise and transport expertise are *both* required to provide safe transport for the critically ill patient, most notably the neonate. Standardization in training and evaluation, equipment, and systems design is required for best practice (33,34).

Levels of Care

The decision to bring intensive care to the newborn is of particular relevance for neonatal interfacility transport; care delivered should never be downgraded during the transport process (35). The aim is to improve clinical stability during the retrieval process (18,19). While the principle of "receiving is retrieving" is generally underscored, most teams transport to the destination hospital, which best meets patient's needs, acuity, and complexity (11). This is of particular note when dealing with extreme prematurity where tertiary perinatal centers offer better outcomes than surgical neonatal intensive care units (NICUs) (36).

Critical patients can only be managed in the short term until the neonatal transport team arrives. The degree of competency in patient care depends on the hospital level of care, in combination with the support provided via telephone or telemedicine connectivity with the tertiary site (37). Thus, situational awareness with knowledge of the specific referring hospital is vitally important when triaging patients for transport. Levels of care have been articulated by several health care systems and share commonalities (38,39) (see Table 5.6). In general terms, the level of obstetrical and neonatal cares should equate. All maternity units must be capable of emergent cesarean section and basic neonatal resuscitation. In level 1 hospitals, care is most frequently provided by nonspecialist physicians or midwives, while level 2 units offer obstetrical and pediatric specialists with some units having neonatologists working as part of the interprofessional neonatal care team. Development of a network of these community-based level 2 NICUs capable of caring for infants requiring short-term respiratory support and/or intravenous nutrition is essential to maintain the capacity at level 3 hospital NICUs. This also reduces health care costs, the need for transport, and keeps babies closer to home, facilitating family-centred care. Improvements in their functional capacity are most frequently overseen and facilitated by the transport service of their tertiary center, which often provide the outreach education necessary for the development of required competencies. Infants who no longer require specialized services should be retrotransferred or repatriated to those community hospitals as soon as appropriate. This helps families and infants' transition to home, engages local physicians who provide on-going care, and reinforces the partnership between all hospitals and providers.

MODEL OF TRANSPORT TEAMS

Team Model—The Professions

The optimal composition of the specialized transport team remains somewhat elusive with all possible models of professionals providing care having been described for both neonatal and pediatric critical care transport (40,41). Most teams consist of two people; a registered nurse (RN), together with a registered respiratory therapist (RRT) or critical care paramedic (CCP) and/or physician (MD), depending on availability of these professional staff and local policies. However, since RRT as a profession do not exist outside of North America and RNs do not have a full scope of advanced practice in many jurisdictions, this may limit the model to an RN/MD team. Nurse practitioners such as in the UK model (42) are increasingly seen where RRTs are unavailable and doctors are in short supply (43). An RN/RN team is less costly (31); however, specially trained emergency medical service (EMS) paramedics are an alternative (44). Regardless of profession, team members must be independent critical thinkers, problem solvers, decisive, flexible, resourceful, and resilient, with good interpersonal and communication skills, capable of the best crisis and crew resource management (45). Karlsen described 26 different compositions of team in the United States, where the RRT/RN model is the most common accounting for 40% of all teams (40).

Studies of teams without physicians in the field have demonstrated acceptable outcomes (46). Indeed, the addition of a physician has not been demonstrated to improve outcomes (16,47,48). Their role ought to focus on triage and medical on-line control (49). Nurse led teams have shorter response times compared to those including physicians (46,50).

McCloskey examined the predictability of the need for a physician before and after transport of critically ill pediatric patients and showed 73% had no decision discrepancy (51). Guidelines published by the American College of Critical Care Medicine have recommended an RN and MD for adult-based retrievals (52).

Ideally, team members should be cross trained where each learns the full scope of practice required for transport, thereby enhancing flexibility in scheduling and stabilization time (45).

Arguably a physician may provide additional benefit with

- Deteriorating clinical condition despite interventions
- Death or withdrawal of ICU support at the community facility
- Long-distance retrieval with risk of deterioration during transport, for example, severe PPHN
- Decision-making for resuscitation at the limits of viability
- Education and training of novice transport team members
- Multiple patients requiring retrieval at the same time, for example, twins/triplets

Team Model—The Location

Neonatal transport teams are usually tertiary hospital-based offering services across a network of hospitals and varying levels of care. This model centralizes the expertise of the transport team members, provides ready access to teaching, and fosters that learning environment. In a survey of 398 different neonatal transport teams in the United States, transporting over 65,000 critically ill neonates per annum, one-third were teams dedicated to transport, while the remainder used unit-based staff. Of the NICU-based teams, 44.3% were fully dedicated (40). Teams may reside at a land or air ambulance base, but these are usually teams with very high annual volumes and/or a high proportion of air transports. Special attention must then be paid to continuing education with contracts with hospitals for teaching and regular evaluation. Dedicated transport teams, rather than trained NICU/PICU staff "on call" for transport, enhance availability and response times (53), with improvements in clinical stability (8,11). Dedicated teams should never be pulled to the bedside on patient assignment when NICU resources are short to ensure their availability. However, dedicated teams must have a sufficient volume of transports to justify their existence. On downtime, dedicated teams can certainly be employed as a resource throughout the hospital; helping the "code team," labor and delivery, NICU, or emergency departments. Teams also decrease adverse events when used on "intramural transports" of neonates for diagnostics or interventions, for example, MRI scans or image-guided therapies (54). They also

provide procedural sedation eliminating an "anesthesia slot." Ideally this is a specific shift assignment.

Increasing the scope of neonatal teams' practice to include pediatric patients in the toddler age range may generate sufficient volumes to justify a dedicated team and maintenance of competencies (45), while ideally a retrieval team for age 0 to 18 meets community needs (11,19,53).

Team Training and Competencies

Although no specific threshold of experience has been tested to predict better outcomes, it seems reasonable to have a minimum of 3 years of prior specialization in neonatal intensive care or related specialty, for example, pediatric or cardiac intensive care. Education and training is essential and varies considerably from days to years depending on the professionals' backgrounds, scope, and sophistication of the team (8). Medical directives may be used and permit the team some autonomy but imply a higher training requirement.

Better nontechnical performance is seen in those with previous ICU or deploy experience (55). Leadership qualities with quick wit, intelligence, and interpersonal skills favor team and crisis resource management creating optimal team dynamics. Health and safety of the team are also of primary importance (56).

Initial Certification

All transport clinician education programs should be built on the principles of adult learning theory, integrating concepts from behaviorism, cognitivism, and constructivism theory (57,58). An outline of the Acute Care Transport Service (ACTS) education program in Toronto, which uses the model of RN/RRT, is shown in **Figure 6.1** with an overview of acquisition of the core competencies in **Table 6.1**. Each recruit spends 1 year on contract as a transport associate (TA) to determine eligibility for further training. If then hired as a clinician, they undergo a 2nd year of intense competency-based assessment as clinician in training (CIT). For both TA and CIT, they undergo a phased approach to meeting their competencies (Fig. 6.1). A small failure rate should be expected in this "high stakes" professional role.

Skills Training

Most transport handbooks provide a comprehensive list of required skills for transport clinicians but do not generally outline a training program (56,59), which should be based on the population being served. Neonatal transfers require more interventions and have more complications compared to other populations (46). In one study of 295 neonatal transfers, 19.8% of the neonates required intubation, compared to 7.5% of infants and 4.9% children; almost half of transport complications in neonates were airway related. Compare this to EMS providers in Oregon with 11,328 annual transports; only 497 (4.4%) were considered emergent, 8.6% were intubated, and 2% with a difficult airway (60).

Training in advanced airway skills is a particular concern with neonatal intubations being the most challenging (61,62). Success rates increase with rapid sequence induction (RSI) on the first attempt (62). Premedication with atropine, followed by fentanyl and succinylcholine, is recommended for neonates (63). Video-assisted devices to facilitate successful intubation have been increasingly used (64). Algorithms to manage the difficult airway are recommended (65). Simulation and task trainers are a necessary adjunct, but high fidelity simulation is not superior (66). Animal models are helpful for teaching intubation, intraosseous needle, or chest tube insertion (67–69). Although no studies relate specific training requirements to outcomes, repetition and training in simple procedures does lead to improvement (70,71). Clinical problems including respiratory failure, hypothermia, hemodynamic instability, and respirator emergencies require specific attention during training schedules (21,72). Campbell and others

Phase 1

• KNOWLEDGE ACQUISITION (0-3 MONTHS)
- Joint Orientation (Neonatal & Pediatric didactic sessions)
- Self-Directed learning modules, Program Materials provided (Binder and access to iShare, Dropbox)
- Resource reading
- Preceptor(s) identified -> first partnership begins
- Clinical placement starts, advanced skills education day(s) & skills OSCE session, clinicial education placements
- Needs assessment completed
- Develop learning plan
- Review Training progress assessment tool, certifications evaluation tool, Competencies

Phase 2

• APPLICATION AND INTEGRATION (3-6 MONTHS)
- Advanced Theory education sessions
- Preceptor/Preceptee clinical experiences on transport
- Participation at Transport Team education days
- Self-directed learning modules, case reviews, high fidelity simulation education day(s), required courses completed
- Ongoing evaluation with Preceptor and Transport Medical Director/delegate
- Written exam (validate knowledge transfer)

Phase 3

• CERTIFICATION (6-12 MONTHS)
- Successful integration of knowledge and skills
- Clinician competencies demonstrated
- OSCEs
- Certification Transport Runs with TSN/Staff Intensivist or delegate; ACTS interprofessional education specialist
- Certification meeting & postcertification CE requirements reviewed

Education Hours

Orientation: integrated over duration of program –didactic, case based learning simulations. Total of 100 hours

Additional hours for course certifications: e.g. neonatal & pediatric sedation & ECG course, infant and child maltreatment course

Additional hours for independent learning activities: e.g. academic rounds, learning packages

Clinical Hours

OR rotation: 24 hours

Labour/Delivery rotation: 36 hours

ED rotation: 72 hours

PICU/CCCU or NICU rotation: 72 hours

PICU/CCCU MD shadow shifts: 36 hours

NICU NNP mentor shifts: 36 hours -> Total: 278 hours (adjusted based on needs assessment)

Transport clinical preceptorship: 9 months (1440 hours)

Evaluation

Clinical evaluation by preceptors during training phases, assessments by educator & medical director/delegate

Call back evaluations: monthly case reviews with physician(s), 2 written exams, advanced procedure/skills OSCEs

High fidelity patient simulation OSCEs (on average 4 simulation cases)

Field certification (on average 6 physician/educator observed transport retrievals)

FIGURE 6.1 Transport clinician in training (CIT) program. (Courtesy of Annette Martens, RN MScN: Acute Care Transport Service [ACTS] Educator.)

TABLE 6.1

Core Requirements for the ACTS Transport Clinician Program

Core clinical certification(s)	1. NRP—Neonatal resuscitation program 2. PALS—Pediatric advanced life support course 3. PTLS—Pediatric trauma life support course 4. BLS—Basic life support 5. Underwater survival training 6. Winter survival training, STABLE Program an asset, ACLS an asset
Equipment certification(s)	1. Neonatal transport incubator configurations → competency-based assessment(s) (CBA) 2. Pediatric transport stretcher configurations → CBA 3. Transport CritiCool whole body cooling and warming system → CBA 4. Inhaled nitric oxide—E tutorial and CBA 5. Transport HAMILTON-T1 ventilator operations—E tutorial and CBA 6. B Braun IV pump operations—E tutorial and CBA 7. Point-of-care testing: i-STAT and glucose meter—E tutorial 8. Capnography I learn module 9. Transport Zoll patient monitor and integrated defibrillator—E tutorial and CBA
Core clinical and technical skills	1. Vascular and arterial access/sampling: peripheral intravenous insertion, umbilical venous and umbilical arterial insertion, intraosseous needle insertion, peripheral arterial line insertion/sampling/puncture, capillary blood sampling, SQ port access 2. O/NGT insertion, urinary catheter insertion, invasive temperature 3. Airway management: positioning, suctioning/patency, oxygen/air administration, nasal cannula low- and high-flow delivery, aerosolized mask and aerogen circuit administration, bag mask ventilation/CPAP, oropharyngeal/nasopharyngeal airway insertion, supraglottic airway insertion, subglottic airway device, intubation, surgical airway assist 4. Noninvasive and invasive ventilation with treatment modalities 5. Needle thoracentesis, chest tube insertion 6. Peritoneal drainage assist 7. Cardioversion, defibrillation, pacing 8. Neonatal therapeutic hypothermia 9. Pediatric therapeutic cooling or rewarming 10. Blood product administration 11. Medication administration 12. C-spine precautions and spinal motion restriction 13. Aero-medical flight physiology, transport safety training: which includes equipment, ground and air transportation, patient and health care professional safety

Courtesy of Acute Care Transport Services (ACTS), The Hospital for Sick Children, Toronto.

make a good case for using simulation scenario-based training for transport teams (73,74).

Team Competencies

One example of competencies adopted by Accreditation Canada is displayed on the Knowledge Exchange Network (KEN) of Children's Health Care Canada (33). They guide education and practice for any interfacility transport team in the following categories:

- **Professional Responsibilities**: Includes membership of their professional college, staying within scope of practice and legislation, ensuring patient privacy and confidentiality, ethical behavior, working as a team player, continuous learning, quality improvement, and research.
- **Communication**: Includes skill in culturally sensitive, verbal, nonverbal, and written communication, focusing on tact, discretion, compassion, and empathy. Some have chosen to use SBAR (Fig. 6.2) as a means of standardized communication and documentation.
- **Health and Safety**: Includes appropriate clothing and footwear to be worn to suit the environment and team identity. Maintaining mental and physical well-being, personal protection against infectious diseases, and infection control should be a focus. Safe lifting and patient movement all fall under this competency.
- **Assessment and Diagnostics**: Includes training in comprehensive history taking, physical assessment, psychiatric assessment, obstetrical assessment, laboratory and radiologic diagnostics, and interpretation.

- **Therapeutics**: Includes courses such as NRP, APLS, STABLE, and procedural sedation. Technical procedures, knowledge of devices and equipment, ventilation strategies, pharmacology, and toxicology are all essential.
- **Integration**: Integration of information into a problem list with differential diagnoses is practiced. Focus on referring and

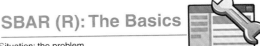

SBAR (R): The Basics

Situation: the problem
What is going on with the patient?

Background: brief, related, to the point
What is the clinical background or context?

Assessment: what you found AND what you think
What do I think the problems?

Recommendation: what you want
What do need to do your job effectively and safely?

Readback: receiver acknowledges information given
Is the summary of the issues/plan consistent with points above?

FIGURE 6.2 SBAR: the basics. (Adapted from Institute for Healthcare Improvement. *SBAR tool: situation-background-assessment-recommendation.* Available from: http://www.ihi.org/resources/Pages/Tools/sbartoolkit.aspx.)

GENERAL CONSIDERATIONS

receiving teams as our clients, as well as the families we serve are fundamental.

- **Transportation**: Mode of transport, that is, ground versus air ambulance is a decision requiring specific expertise. Availability and costs of air ambulance, availability, and proximity of helipads, weather, traffic, size and weight of equipment, number of team, and family members are all considerations. Most frequently, the mode decisions are independently made by pilots unaware of patient condition for optimal decision-making.

Maintaining Competencies

Education is the key to both recruitment and retention, with feedback, self-assessment, mentorship, recognition, and annual retreats as part of this strategy (70–76). Continuing education and skills practice are enhanced by continuous exposure within the hospital milieu (40). Annual written and oral assessments or objective structured assessment of technical skills, plus direct observation of patient care on "ride outs" is encouraged (76). Experience including mistakes or "near misses" provide the basis for learning activities (77).

Physician Trainees

Physicians in training require exposure to prehospital care and/or interfacility transport. However, a U.S.-based survey showed neonatal transport exposure in only 43% pediatric residents, of whom only 23% were evaluated as part of the training; pediatric transport exposure occurred in 55 % with 21% evaluated (78). Exposure to transport medicine must be a focus of their education by our transport teams (79). Even a 1-hour teaching session improves training on the medicolegal aspects of transport (80). Involvement both in "the field" and as medical control is needed for our transport teams to flourish; therefore, a thorough understanding of the challenges and complexities of care in the transport environment is paramount.

Specific training in transport medicine is available for those who wish to make prehospital or interfacility transport a focus of their career. Most subspecialty training programs in neonatology and pediatric emergency medicine will require at least 1 month of transport training in their program. It should be encouraged and offered to trainees during residency as elective time.

STANDARDS FOR SYSTEM, PROCESSES, AND CLINICAL CARE

Standards

There are no mandatory requirements for credentialing or accreditation of teams or their transport systems; participation in accreditation is voluntary (81–83). The Q-Mentum standards for EMS (33), or the National Highway Act (84), do include the neonatal population. Competencies outlined and transportation equipment are open to interpretation (85). Networks established to bench mark their teams' activities can draw inferences on best practices (86,87). The U.S.-based Ground Air Medical qUality Transport (GAMUT) report on 12 core metrics (Table 6.2) with significant overlap with the Canadian Neonatal Transport Network (CNTN) indicators. They include first attempt endotracheal tube intubation (ETI) success rates, unplanned device dislodgement, medicinal administration errors, hypothermia, crew and patient injuries, family accompaniment, and average mobilization times (88,89).

Networks and Quality Improvement Initiative

Transport networks exist in Australasia, Europe, and Canada; one example being the Canadian Neonatal Transport Network (CNTN) where a quality improvement collaborative can compare and contrast efficiency and outcomes of transported patients focusing on

- Improving transport team safety by trending safety/risk events
- Optimizing cost effectiveness
- Guiding content of educational programs for team

TABLE 6.2

AAP Section on Transport Medicine Metrics

1. First attempt intubation success
2. Rate of CPR performed
3. Unintended neonatal hypothermia
4. Use of a standardized patient hand-off
5. Medical equipment failure
6. Verification of endotracheal tube placement
7. Transport-related crew injuries
8. Dislodgement of therapeutic devices
9. Average team mobilization time
10. Transport-related patient injuries
11. Medication administration errors
12. Serious reportable events

* In RED front are indicators also captured in CNTN.

American Academy of Pediatrics Section on Transport Medicine. Key performance indicators (KPIs). Metrics highlighted in red are also captured by the Canadian Neonatal Transport Network (CNTN) as KPIs. Courtesy of Kyong-Soon Lee, MD, FRCPC, Director of CNTN.

- Providing topics for outreach programs
- Clinical or outcomes research in transport, for example, publications on structure and organization (inputs) rather than measurement of performance (outputs)
- Identifying those factors that are modifiable

Failures of communication are found to be responsible for the majority of serious safety events. Transport teams are prone to communication breakdown at every phase of the transport process, especially at time of hand overs (30,90). A structured format or communication tool should be taught and always used to enhance transfer of accurate and complete information (91). Many transport programs have adopted the SBAR tool shown to reduce errors in health care (Figs. 6.2 and 6.3). SBAR use in team call-backs for medical orders enhances efficient and accurate communication (75,91). Communication with families must be handled with utmost sensitivity and tact, focusing on keeping parent and patient together. Factors influencing family presence on transport include land versus air missions (26.6% vs. 6.3%) due to distance and availability of aircraft seats; parents' anxiety should be mitigated through appropriate communication (92).

Key Performance Indicators (KPIs)

The quality of the transport process should be monitored (Table 6.3) (93).

Clinical

Deviations from usual clinical practice, diagnostics, therapeutic interventions, problem solving, and patient- or equipment-related

Vital Communication Approach **Patient & Staff Safety**

Utilize Key phrases understood by all to mean "stop and listen to me – we have a potential problem"

Adapted from the Airline Industry communication method "CUUS"*

I'm Concerned
I'm Uncomfortable
This is Unsafe
I'm Scared

Use these words in order, to escalate your expression of concern if you feel the message hasn't gotten across

 Stop and make sure all are on the same page!!

*Information based on the communication method used by the airline industry, which has supported development of various safety focused communication tools and presentations in healthcare.

FIGURE 6.3 SBAR: important elements.

TABLE 6.3

Checklist to Review for Each Transport Run

Item	Details
System indicators	
Team configuration	Should physician have attended?
Mode of transport	Was most efficient mode (i.e., land vs. air) chosen?
Transport times	• Delay in dispatch or reaction time >15 min • Delay in mobilization time >30 min • Prolonged stabilization time: neonates >120 min, pediatrics >60 min
Clinical indicators	
For all populations	Unintended hypothermia (temperature <36.5 °C or <36.0 °C)
For preterm infants gestational age <32 wk	• Hypocarbia pCO2 <30 • Use of volume boluses • Delay in starting intravenous fluids >1 h
For hypoxic–ischemic encephalopathy	• Age cooling started • Target temperature 34.0 °C reached within 6 h of age • Eligible and not cooled
Complications	
Dislodgment of tubes: endotracheal, PIV, UAC, UVC, PAL, chest tube	
Difficult IV access, inability to establish IV	
Difficult intubation	
Cardiac arrest or need for cardioversion	
Medication error	
Equipment and vehicle	• Supplies not available • Supplies depleted • Equipment incompatible • Equipment failure • Vehicle crash • Arrive at wrong destination
Injury to patient	
Injury to crew	
Clinical deterioration necessitating return to referral	
Clinical deterioration requiring vehicle stoppage	

Courtesy of Kyong-Soon Lee, MD, FRCPC: Associate Medical Director, ACTS, The Hospital for Sick Children, Toronto, Ontario.

From Lee KS. Neonatal transport metrics and quality improvement in a regional transport service. *Transl Pediatr* 2019;8(3):233.

events are highlighted. If they occur prior to arrival of the transport team, feedback to the referring institution team/staff must be undertaken by the medical director or delegate. Challenges with team performance should be addressed in a timely fashion and educational "pearls" shared with the entire transport team.

Process

By review, we identify ways to improve our transport teams' functionality, for example, delays in dispatch or mobilization, delays in access to medical on line control. Sometimes "just do it" will fix it; other times we need more in-depth evaluation, which may lead to project work for the transport team.

System

Challenges outside the control of the transport team such as scope of practice, geographic boundaries, or governance structure require data to bring attention to these matters.

Transport times to measure efficiency and effectiveness include

1. Dispatch time: time of referral call to team dispatch
2. Mobilization time: time of referral call to team departing home base
3. Response time: time of referral call to arrival at patient bedside
4. Stabilization time: time of arrival of team to departure from referring hospital
5. Total transport time: time team dispatched until returned to home base

Transport times in categories 3 and 5 will be influenced by the team location, availability of vehicles, traffic, weather, and distances. Item 4 depends on complexity of neonate and level of care of referral hospital. Triage decisions, dispatch, and mobilization times depend on acuity at time of the first call and reflect team efficiency.

Illness severity scores are required such that teams can compare equivalent populations when bench marking and assessing their efficacy but there is no ideal acuity score as yet. However, the transport risk index of physiologic stability (TRIP) has been validated for newborns during transport. Trends in the TRIP score may be used to assess the patient's response to the stabilization process (94).

Canadian Neonatal Transport Network (CNTN) Database

Sixteen specialized neonatal transport teams in Canada formed their network in 2013. This has provided the opportunity to bench mark across the provincial teams and drives decisions on necessary competencies, such as this example demonstrating the frequency of procedures during neonatal transport (Table 6.4).

TABLE 6.4

Neonatal Procedures Performed by Transport Teams and Success Rates

Procedure	Frequency N (% of Transports)	Success N (% Attempts)
Peripheral intravenous	1,586 (47.3)	1,351 (85.2)
Arterial blood gas	1,410 (42.1)	1,257 (89.1)
Endotracheal intubation	829 (24.8)	790 (95.3)
Venipuncture	569 (17.0)	511 (89.8)
Umbilical venous catheter	293 (8.8)	273 (93.2)
Umbilical arterial catheter	170 (5.1)	121 (71.2)
Peripheral arterial line	99 (3.0)	48 (48.5)
Oral airway	64 (1.9)	60 (93.8)
Chest tube	48 (1.4)	47 (97.9)
Laryngeal mask airway	8 (0.2)	8 (100)

Courtesy of Kyong-Soon Lee, MD, FRCPC, Director of CNTN.

CONSULTATIONS AND REFERRALS

Communication about patients needing a higher level of care has relied on a telephone call from a clinician to a tertiary care physician. More than one consultant may have a contribution to treatment advice, transport organization, or acceptance of the transfer. The risk is that phone calls made in separate "one-to-one" conversations may result in gaps in overall knowledge or contradictory advice. If the critical care transport team is outside of those discussions, there may be further fragmentation of advice.

Since the early 1990s, telephone conference calls became standard practice with the transport team hearing the discussion and able to ask questions. Using a single point of contact (telephone hotline) and a senior transport physician "chairing" the call, specialists are brought into the call as needed with the referring hospital staff. Ideally, the transport service "hosts" this call. If required, a transport plan is executed; the destination hospital can be dealt with after team dispatch. Being able to reach individuals without using intermediaries such as switchboard operators can be achieved by technology, which alerts the individual to the degree of urgency and identifies the source of the call.

What Is Involved in a Transport Call?

The process for call taking to provide advice/consultation and expedite retrieval/transport ideally should be recorded, providing the opportunity for review of the calls for education, quality improvement, quality of care, or medicolegal review (Table 6.5).

Referral

Referring physician or delegate makes initial telephone contact with their designated tertiary center and where possible includes the transport team on that "conference call." The process may differ between regions; however, the following is optimal:

- Dedicated "one number to call" to access immediate consultation from a staff physician with timely dispatch of a specialized transport team, if required. Dispatch on "baby first, bed second" philosophy, regardless of NICU bed availability at that site, brings the "mobile intensive care" to the patient. Bed finding may proceed while patient is stabilized. Air transports of course must have an identified destination to permit pilot assessment of flight path conditions.
- The tertiary center remains responsible for patient care until the alternate destination is determined if required, and a formal hand over between staff physicians occurs.

TABLE 6.5

Steps Involved in Making Referral for Consultation +/− Transport

What Is Involved in a Call?

1. Call received through "one number to call"
2. Staff physician and transport coordinator provide advice/consult; dispatch team if transporting
3. Team mobilizes with dedicated ambulance and paramedic staff
4. Team travels to referral center; air ambulance (fixed wing) required if distance > 250K
5. Team takes report, conducts assessment, and assumes care of patient[a]
6. Team treats, stabilizes, and transport back to receiving center
7. Team transfers patient to ED/PICU/CCCU or NICU and provides SBAR[a] handover

[a]All calls and callbacks for orders are recorded and kept as part of patient record.

Courtesy of Acute Care Transport Service (ACTS), The Hospital for Sick Children, Toronto.

- Ideally, the "dedicated number" facility should track all transferred patients. Trends in referrals and deferrals outside of agreed boundaries are tracked.
- Calls should be taken by a dedicated physician at "consultant level" with expertise in transport medicine. Inclusion of a transport coordinator helps with timely team mobilization.
- A "recorded" telephone conference "bridge line" allows multiple people to participate, enhancing clinical and triage decisions. These recordings become part of the patient chart.
- Communication should always be polite, professional, and complete: the use of a handoff tool such as the SBAR ensures more appropriate advice, along with expectations around response time to the sending facility (91).

Triaging

Simultaneous requests may occur, requiring multiple recorded "bridge lines" and additional personnel identified to handle the referrals. Software platforms exist to optimize this process for dispatch centers often managed by nonclinical staff. Most hospital-based programs provide a clinical triage process.

The urgency of the transport is principally dependent on patient illness severity but also location, competency, and comfort of the referring hospital staff. The ability to respond in a timely fashion is dictated by the number of teams' available, proximity to other teams, and team backup plan. Emergent time sensitive calls take priority. Although no established bench marks exist, patients are usually divided into categories of emergent (transport team mobilization within 10 to 15 minutes and time to definitive care of within 4 hours) or urgent (mobilization within 30 minutes and definitive care within 12 hours). Electives can be transported for specialty consultation at first available opportunity.

When there is more than one critically ill infant/child requiring transport, the following options should be considered:

- Contact a retrieval team from another catchment area to determine their availability. Teams should never operate on the basis of a "may be baby," so they are sometimes operating out of region while their own region is uncovered.
- Consider sending an "on call" transport physician ahead of the next available team, to help with stabilization.
- Create another "ad-hoc" retrieval team, for example, a physician with the transport coordinator or other clinician with transport experience. A backup team on call is an option.
- For stable infants, for example, term infants with imperforate anus or hyperbilirubinemia, the referring hospital may transport the infant. Specialized equipment for securing the infant is still required.

Often the transport staff physician must help support the referring hospital by phone until help arrives. The addition of a "Telemedicine" service or videoconferencing capability at the referring hospital to augment the telephone link is invaluable (95).

Patient Knowledge

While information about patients is often stored in electronic form in hospitals, the capacity of such systems to share information with another hospital is often limited. Solutions are required which permit pertinent clinical information to accompany the patient referral process. The transport service should be able to view static information available on the patient, document their advice, decisions made, and add to the package of information provided by the local hospital. Technologies exist to link and transfer data in this way; even between disparate systems but commercial and administrative boundaries create barriers for such information flow. Such "patient knowledge" should not be proprietary to any particular treating organization or clinician. The information systems should support the underlying analog referral process rather than frustrate it.

Hospital Knowledge

To offer the best advice and support, those offering that advice must be fully immersed in the realities facing the local hospitals. Experienced transport clinicians gain an appreciation of the diversity of local situations, location, and accessibility, through a slow process of acquiring the corporate knowledge of their region. Systems that incorporate this knowledge to make it available for all are enormously helpful. The "local" clinician often does not know enough about processes or systems of their region. A dynamically updated database of all hospitals and clinicians in "the system" is required, and location of airstrips and helipads. Graphical information such as maps, information about logistic options for teams, with times and "normal" referral pathways, plus information on locally available tools for supporting care (e.g., Ventilators, CPAP devices), and treatment options are helpful.

TELEMEDICINE AND ADJUNCTS

Despite impeccable active listening and optimal verbal communication, simply "seeing" the patient helps enormously; "a picture is worth a 1,000 words" (37,95). Various forms of telemedicine, telehealth, or teleconferencing are available with important distinctions between them. *Telehealth* typically supports patients directly with a connection to a remote clinician. Some such systems include clinical examination tools like ophthalmoscopy and otoscopy and imaging devices like ultrasound. *Teleconferencing* is more of a business tool whereby virtual meetings are held. Cameras may be audio activated to highlight the current speaker, for example, Zoom.

Telemedicine in transport may offer enhancements to the abilities and scope of the clinicians since visual as well as auditory contact with base hospital becomes feasible (95). Patel among others demonstrated this enhanced decision-making and decreased transport duration when using video. Triaging calls is also enhanced. A serious concern is the lack of compatibility with Health Information and Privacy Act, but the video is generally not recorded and should desirably be separate from the audio conferencing system anyway. In a survey of potential telemedicine users, 80% believe that these compromises are essential to best practice (96). Videoconferencing systems that are slow to initiate represent a major risk for key participants. Speaking to a hands-free microphone especially if noisy or having questions broadcast into a room may be inappropriate. Audio quality is generally poorer with video conferencing systems. Ideally, a fully duplex landline with a wirelessly connected headset provides the best quality and convenience to the referring clinician. A video camera mounted overhead or at the bedside, with a good view of the patient and environs, should be rapidly accessible by remote viewers who control the camera (pan/zoom/tilt) without any third party. The system should be secure and allow password-protected access to appropriate users. The local hospital staff should not have to operate the technology apart from the "on/off" switch.

The video image should provide high-definition resolution (1920× 1080p or greater), optical zoom (>20×; preferably 40×), accurate color rendition, good performance in low light conditions, and bandwidth to support frame-rates which show smooth clinical movement such as seizure activity or work of breathing. There should be no perception of flicker or individual frames. Technology to support 60 Hz should be a minimum. Some advantage in a two-way video stream may be outweighed by reduction in the quality of the one-way image; further sharing with multiple viewers may add to degradation. Devices fixed in one location are typically three to four times cheaper and less intrusive than mobile alternatives.

Costs of under $2000 USD per unit afford utilization at several bed locations. When these support local care and avoid interhospital transport, telemedicine is a worthwhile cost-saver.

Remote images: Capacity to view images such as x-ray, CT scan, MRI, and ultrasound are often extremely helpful. Images should be of Digital Imaging and Communications in Medicine (DICOM) standard with a capacity to use the tools to modify the image settings and scroll through multiple images. Photographic images can be useful for skin conditions such as vascular anomalies, rashes, and burns with their higher resolution over a still from a video stream, adding diagnostic value.

PREPARING FOR TRANSPORT: REFERRING HOSPITAL AND TRANSPORT TEAM

Referring Hospital

While the transport team is on route, the referring hospital team will continue resuscitation and stabilization as follows:

- Current algorithm for neonatal resuscitation, for example, NRP, in addition to gentle care strategies.
- Securing an Airway, maintaining effective Breathing and achieving Circulatory stability.
- Ensure effective temperature homeostasis.
- Consider Sugar, Temperature, Breathing, Labs, Evaluation, and Emotional family support; STABLE program is often used for training beyond NRP (97).
- Resuscitation and stabilization are coordinated with the transport physician providing advice.
- Definitive treatment (e.g., surfactant, iNO, therapeutic hypothermia) is typically commenced on the arrival of the transport team.
- The designated level of care of the referral NICU (level 1 vs. 2) should determine how much we should expect/request prior to team arrival.

Tertiary Site

The transport team members should review the clinical scenario with tertiary NICU staff prior to departure to outline a management plan. Teams should use a predeparture checklist to ensure all equipment and supplies are intact (Table 6.6).

- Check all equipment, ensure batteries fully charged, gas tanks full (e.g., nitric oxide).
- Team uniform should always be worn including safety footwear with personal protective equipment available when required.
- Consider team nutrition, especially for longer distance retrievals.
- Take money and credit cards for long-distance retrievals; flying time and weather may be unpredictable. Passport or immigration documents are required for cross border transports.
- Plan the roles of each team member on arrival at referring hospital.
- Provide updates using cellular telephones/wireless technology if situation changes.

ONCE THE TRANSPORT TEAM ARRIVES

- Team members introduce themselves to all. Parents are encouraged to be present during the stabilization for maximum communication.
- Assess level of stability on arrival with a quick review of the patient's vital signs. If unstable, an initial brief call back is made to elicit orders for intervention. Use of a tool such as SBAR to explain clinical situation and prioritization of treatment is always preferred (75,91).

GENERAL CONSIDERATIONS

TABLE 6.6

Predeparture Checklist

ACTS—Predeparture Checklist
Neonatal

IV pumps syringe/lg vol—CHECK THAT PUMPS ARE SECURE
Adequate gas supply
Nitric delivery system:
1. Assembled circuit for deck B
2. Second saturation probe
BLUE Neo backpack
GREEN Neo backpack
DRUG KIT: cold, narcotic, and ice packs
Glucometer
iSTAT. Cartridges: G8 × 2/G4 × 2 external simulator
Patient record/binder with parent pack
Warming mattress/hat
Gel rolls < 30 wk < 72h of age
Thermal incubator cover as indicated
Call sheet
Cell phone
Bereavement supplies (transport office)
Individual stethoscopes
Individual black books
Stryker stretcher battery light GREEN
+/– Bili blanket (N1/N2 only provide phototherapy)
+/– Difficult airway kit
+/– CMAC intubation kit
+/– Defibrillator—deck B and C only as required
+/– 2nd SpO₂ probe
+/– EZ IO/vein light
+/– Ice packs

Please ensure black airway bag is attached to transport deck/stretcher

Courtesy of Acute Care Transport Service (ACTS), The Hospital for Sick Children, Toronto.

- A formal medical hand over from the referring physician is obtained, including clarification of medical responsibility, and their ongoing role in patient management if warranted. A shared responsibility for patient care exists, as soon as the tertiary center provides advice from that first telephone call, and continues until the team departure from the referring hospital. In practical terms, it is helpful for the team using their medical directives to assume responsibility for patient care on arrival at the referral center. However, depending on the acuity of the patient, the team and referring staff may work together to provide the patient care.
- The infant is placed on the team's equipment for respiratory support as soon as practical. For those infants requiring intubation, oral intubation is generally preferred using rapid sequence intubation (RSI) (63); there is no advantage to using nasal cannulation. An oro/nasogastric tube will be required to ventilate the stomach.
- Secure or replace inadequate or precarious vascular access. Place umbilical venous (UVC) ± umbilical arterial catheter (UAC) or peripheral arterial line (PAL) for mechanically ventilated patients or those with hemodynamic compromise, where the arterial line can then be transduced.
- Monitor all vital signs using the team's equipment. Formulate management plans and required medical orders beyond

team's medical directives; then call back to medical "on line" control.

- Transport team may administer treatments, that is, surfactant, sedation, analgesia (opiates), muscle relaxation, inotropic agents, and PGE₁ following discussion with tertiary NICU staff. Medical directives exist for a minority of interventions and will change from time to time. Familiarize yourself with which ones are current.
- Obtain electronic or hard copy images of the maternal and newborn records including diagnostics.
- Identify and retrieve the placenta, store fresh in biohazard plastic bag. If stored in formaldehyde, the specimen must be sent separately.
- Transfer patient into the transport incubator as soon as stability is reached in anticipation of departure; ensure the parents/family members see the infant before departure.
- Anticipate potential cardiorespiratory or neurologic deterioration and draw up drugs ready for seizure control, sedation, and/or inotropic support on route.
- Counsel parents regarding problem, diagnosis, and prognosis when pertinent. Provide reading materials about destination hospital, breast-feeding, and pictures of the infant.
- Attempt to get mother's breast milk/colostrum for oral immune therapy.
- Encourage a parent or family member to accompany the team with their infant assuming adequate seating in air/land ambulance (regulations regarding parents or family members accompanying infants in ambulances may vary in different countries).
- Plan a perinatal NICU as receiving site for all infants less than 30 weeks GA as they have greatly enhanced outcomes versus a tertiary surgical NICU (11,12,36).

Family-Centered Care

Transport of a sick newborn infant to another facility has a major impact and puts additional stress on the family, dealing with the medical concerns and being moved to a distant hospital. While it may not be possible to permit a parent to accompany their newborn due to limitations of space, it should be considered in every case (92).

MEDICAL DIRECTIVES AND MEDICAL ON-LINE CONTROL

In 2007, the Federation of Health Regulatory Colleges in Ontario released "An Inter-professional Guide on the Use of Orders, Directives and Delegation for Regulated Health Professionals in Ontario," designed to assist with understanding of guidelines, standards, and regulations developed by the health profession colleges. They outlined which prescriptions can be written pursuant to medical directives. Medical directives are indirect physician orders, used to expedite patient care by competent health professionals. They are used by teams who do not have a physician on the transport team routinely (Table 6.7). A medical directive can

- Apply to a specific patient population who meet specific criteria.
- Is role specific (e.g., NP, RD, RN) and not person specific and users must possess the necessary knowledge, skill, and judgment before implementing.
- The procedure being delegated is in the patient's best interest.
- Enable an implementer to act under specific conditions without a physician.
- Implementers are not ordering a procedure when using a directive; rather they are implementing a physician's order.
- Must have the integrity of a direct order, thus all responsible physicians must approve it.

TABLE 6.7

Medical Directives

Medical Directives, Acute Care Transport Services

Initiating an order to perform a procedure

Initiating an order for airway management, mechanical ventilation, and/or assisted ventilation

Initiating an order for a diagnostic imaging examination

Initiating an order for muscle relaxation for intubation and procedural topical anesthesia and nonpharmacologic analgesia

Initiating an order for emergency drugs for cardiopulmonary resuscitation

Initiating an order for treatment to newborns at delivery

Initiating an order for intravenous therapy

Initiating an order for surfactant and the treatment of respiratory distress syndrome

Initiating an order for volume expanders for hypovolemia and/or hypoperfusion

Initiating an order for investigations; interpreting and/or communicating results from investigations

Initiating an order for antibiotics at risk for/or suspected sepsis

Initiating an order for antipyretic management

Initiating and order for inhalation therapy

Courtesy of Acute Care Transport Services (ACTS), The Hospital for Sick Children, Toronto.

- Is approved only when all affected regulated professionals and relevant administrators participate in their development and thus is written with essential components.

Medical directives are used when assessing or treating patients, when the competent health care provider needs to perform:

- A controlled act or another act that is traditionally held within medicine (e.g., prescribing medications, ordering labs).
- AND the act is not authorized to the health care professionals' scope of practice.

Typically, transport teams have medical directives limited to emergency practice while their mainstay is to have appropriate "on line medical control" as previously outlined.

CLINICAL PRACTICE GUIDELINES, CHECKLISTS, AND SPECIAL CIRCUMSTANCES

The Health Improvement Institute provides a generic definition for a *standard (or protocol)* as "a basis for comparison"; a reference point against which other things can be evaluated; and "they set the measure for all subsequent work." The Institute of Medicine (IOM) defines clinical practice guidelines as "systematically developed statements to assist practitioner and patient decisions about appropriate health care for specific clinical circumstances" (90). Specifically identified common case presentations should trigger establishment of clinical practice guidelines for transport. Standards and guidelines are generally developed using verifiable, systematic literature searches and reviews of existing evidence published in peer-reviewed journals.

High-Risk Preterm Delivery in Community Hospitals

The outcome for very premature infants is improved when delivery occurs at inborn tertiary perinatal centers. In utero transfer of fetus with mothers in threatened preterm labor is preferable as outcomes for transported infants are inferior (9). When in utero transport is not feasible, then the presence of a skilled transport team at the delivery in the community hospitals is beneficial (16).

Dispatch of a transport team to attend a high-risk delivery is an emergency but should never replace the preferred option of transporting the mother to a high-risk perinatal setting. Enhanced predelivery counseling may require dispatch of a physician with the transport team. The transport team provides added value in terms of expertise in NRP and the "golden hour" following delivery (Fig. 6.4).

Prematurity and Respiratory Distress Syndrome (RDS)— Surfactant Replacement Therapy

Management of the premature infant during transport includes supporting the respiratory system. Those 23 to 34 weeks GA will potentially benefit from surfactant replacement therapy to decrease mortality, air leak, and BPD (98). Prophylactic surfactant within 10 to 30 minutes of birth is no longer recommended. Current recommendations include prophylactic CPAP with early rescue therapy with surfactant (natural or synthetic), preferably within 2 hours of delivery (99), and most infants less than 27 weeks will require treatment despite antenatal steroids. If intubated for surfactant treatment, to minimize lung injury, volume-targeted invasive ventilation (PC/AC/VG) is preferred recognizing that lung compliance will dramatically change post-surfactant.

Neonates no longer undergo routine intubation for transport, and CPAP can be delivered effectively with the appropriate ventilator/software, using humidified gases.

Congenital Heart Disease

Many congenital heart diseases (CHDs) are now diagnosed antenatal and preference is for delivery in a tertiary center where duct-dependent lesions can be managed with emergent use of prostaglandin E_1 infusion (PGE1: 0.01 µg/kg/min), pending transfer for surgical intervention.

The distinction between hypoxemia secondary to congenital heart disease versus compromised pulmonary blood flow, for example, tricuspid atresia/pulmonary atresia versus persistent pulmonary hypertension of the newborn (PPHN) may be difficult.

Most recommend commencement of a prostaglandin E_1 infusion when clinical assessment suggests a cardiac lesion, that is, presence of a murmur, cardiomegaly, or failed hyperoxia test. It may also have some utility in PPHN due to pulmonary vasodilation and offloading the right ventricle.

Obstructive left heart lesions should be suspected in all neonates who present with clinical features of circulatory collapse or low cardiac output syndrome, that is, poor perfusion and pulses, hypotension, oliguria, +/– lactic acidosis within the first couple of weeks of life, and a prostaglandin E_1 (PGE1) infusion should be commenced immediately. A dose of 0.05 to 0.1 µg/kg/min of PGE1 is usually recommended while a lower dose (0.01 µg/kg/min) commenced immediately after birth may suffice. Doses in excess of 0.02 µg/kg/min may be associated with apnea, and these patients should be intubated prior to transport if the duration is expected to exceed an hour or more (100).

In profound hypoxemia ($paO_2 < 30$ mm Hg) with low saturations despite prostaglandin infusion, rapid transfer for urgent intervention is mandatory. Transposition of the great arteries (d-TGA) with an intact septum requiring emergent balloon atrial septostomy (BAS) or obstructed total anomalous pulmonary venous drainage (TAPVD), which requires emergency surgery, is most likely. Most other cyanotic and acyanotic lesions will improve with prostaglandins. Care must be taken in single ventricle physiology where pulmonary overcirculation will be detrimental to hemodynamic stability resulting in low cardiac output state. These infants are

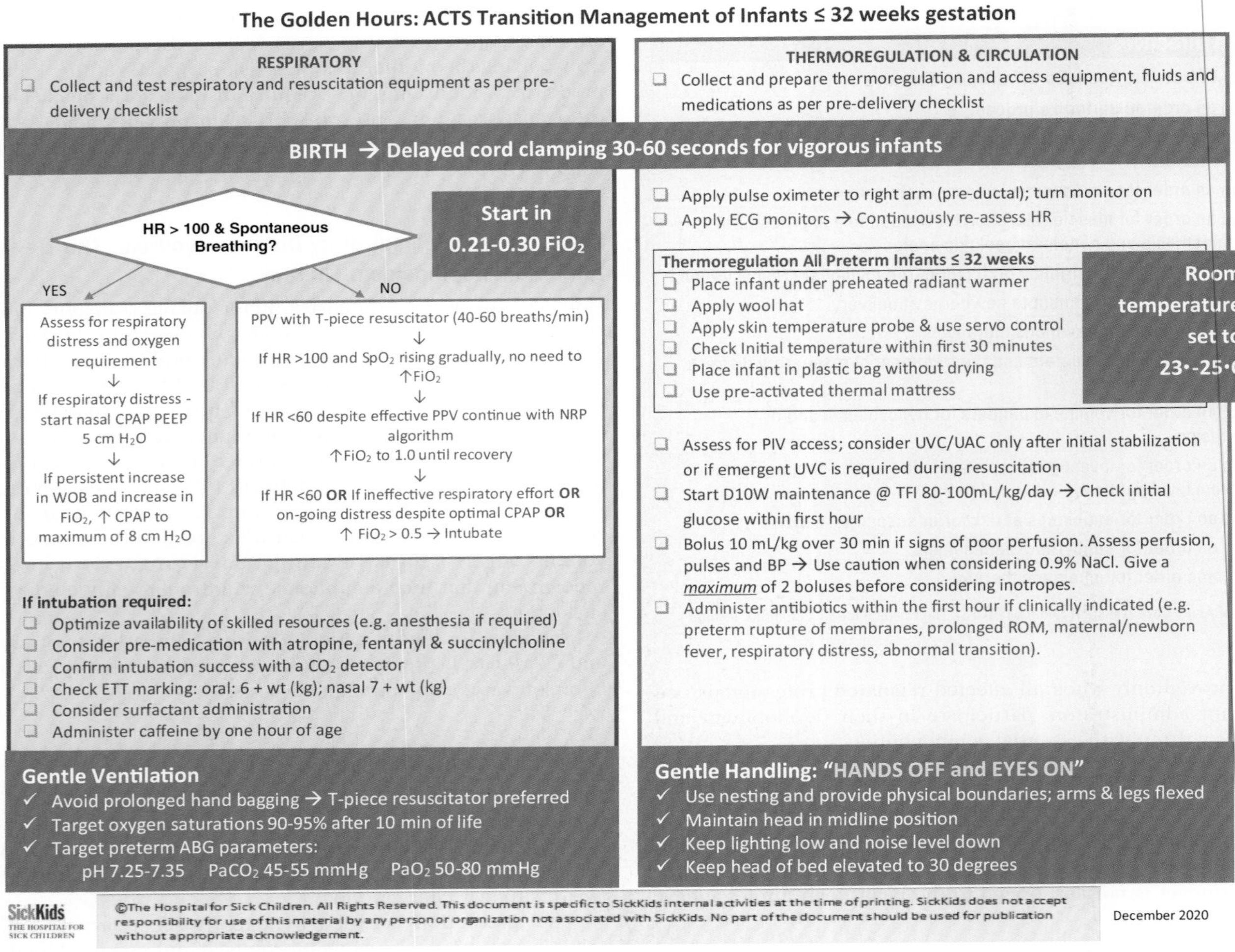
The Golden Hours: ACTS Transition Management of Infants ≤ 32 weeks gestation
RESPIRATORY
Collect and test respiratory and resuscitation equipment as per pre-delivery checklist
THERMOREGULATION & CIRCULATION
Collect and prepare thermoregulation and access equipment, fluids and medications as per pre-delivery checklist
BIRTH → Delayed cord clamping 30-60 seconds for vigorous infants
HR > 100 & Spontaneous Breathing?
Start in 0.21-0.30 FiO2
YES
NO
Assess for respiratory distress and oxygen requirement
If respiratory distress - start nasal CPAP PEEP 5 cm H2O
If persistent increase in WOB and increase in FiO2, ↑ CPAP to maximum of 8 cm H2O
PPV with T-piece resuscitator (40-60 breaths/min)
If HR >100 and SpO2 rising gradually, no need to ↑FiO2
If HR <60 despite effective PPV continue with NRP algorithm
↑FiO2 to 1.0 until recovery
If HR <60 OR If ineffective respiratory effort OR on-going distress despite optimal CPAP OR ↑ FiO2 > 0.5 → Intubate
If intubation required:
Optimize availability of skilled resources (e.g. anesthesia if required)
Consider pre-medication with atropine, fentanyl & succinylcholine
Confirm intubation success with a CO2 detector
Check ETT marking: oral: 6 + wt (kg); nasal 7 + wt (kg)
Consider surfactant administration
Administer caffeine by one hour of age
Apply pulse oximeter to right arm (pre-ductal); turn monitor on
Apply ECG monitors → Continuously re-assess HR
Thermoregulation All Preterm Infants ≤ 32 weeks
Place infant under preheated radiant warmer
Apply wool hat
Apply skin temperature probe & use servo control
Check Initial temperature within first 30 minutes
Place infant in plastic bag without drying
Use pre-activated thermal mattress
Room temperature set to 23•-25•C
Assess for PIV access; consider UVC/UAC only after initial stabilization or if emergent UVC is required during resuscitation
Start D10W maintenance @ TFI 80-100mL/kg/day → Check initial glucose within first hour
Bolus 10 mL/kg over 30 min if signs of poor perfusion. Assess perfusion, pulses and BP → Use caution when considering 0.9% NaCl. Give a maximum of 2 boluses before considering inotropes.
Administer antibiotics within the first hour if clinically indicated (e.g. preterm rupture of membranes, prolonged ROM, maternal/newborn fever, respiratory distress, abnormal transition).
Gentle Ventilation
✓ Avoid prolonged hand bagging → T-piece resuscitator preferred
✓ Target oxygen saturations 90-95% after 10 min of life
✓ Target preterm ABG parameters:
pH 7.25-7.35 PaCO2 45-55 mmHg PaO2 50-80 mmHg
Gentle Handling: "HANDS OFF and EYES ON"
✓ Use nesting and provide physical boundaries; arms & legs flexed
✓ Maintain head in midline position
✓ Keep lighting low and noise level down
✓ Keep head of bed elevated to 30 degrees
SickKids THE HOSPITAL FOR SICK CHILDREN
©The Hospital for Sick Children. All Rights Reserved. This document is specific to SickKids internal activities at the time of printing. SickKids does not accept responsibility for use of this material by any person or organization not associated with SickKids. No part of the document should be used for publication without appropriate acknowledgement.
December 2020

FIGURE 6.4 The golden hours: ACTS transition management of infants ≤32 weeks gestation. (©The Hospital for Sick Children.)

preferentially transported in room air or low FiO_2 to maintain saturations in 75% to 85% range.

Infants with Cardiac Arrhythmias

Bradyarrhythmia

These are most frequently due to hypoxia where respiratory support will usually fix the problem. Congenital heart block or electrolyte disturbance such as hyperkalemia must be ruled out/treated. Commonly, mothers with systemic lupus erythematosus (SLE) may present for the first time during pregnancy because of fetal bradyarrhthymia and emergency C/S has been known to occur as a result of failure to recognize the underlying pathology. Superficial pacing may be required and pads should always be placed front and back on these babies during transport in case of further deterioration pending more definitive action in cardiac pacing.

Tachyarrhythmia

These may also be due to underlying electrolyte disturbances, but central venous lines misplaced in R atrium, for example, high UVC or PICC line may result in tachycardia. Lines must be withdrawn to treat arrhythmia. Commonly supraventricular tachycardia (SVT) due to Wolfe Parkinson White, atrial flutter, or junctional ectopic tachycardia, among others, can result in hemodynamic instability requiring cardioversion. All teams must be versed in the safe use of their defibrillator for cardioversion, although more commonly drug treatment will suffice. Appropriate administration of adenosine using a double plunger technique with IV located as close to SA node as possible (central line or PIV in left antecubital fossa) will result in cardioversion. The patient if resistant should have a continuous infusion of esmolol or other B blocker during transport.

Hydrops Fetalis

These newborns are usually very unstable depending on severity and whether there is cardiac tamponade as a result of pericardial effusion, or pleural effusions and massive ascites. Transport teams should be competent and prepared to initiate and maintain drainage of all these body cavities prior to transport to achieve optimal cardiorespiratory stability. Typically, these infants have an antenatal diagnosis and will be born in a tertiary setting. Milder cases may miss detection.

Persistent Pulmonary Hypertension of the Newborn

The diagnosis of PPHN is frequently challenging outside of the setting in which a confirmatory echocardiogram (ECHO) can be provided. Most transport teams do not have the competency to carry out an ECHO to look for structural anatomy or functional integrity of the heart. However, portable ECHO machines with transmission of the images back to the tertiary center may make this a more common practice in future. This is one use of point of care ultrasound (POCUS) in transport to enhance care especially for decisions on preload versus inotropic support versus afterload reduction (101).

Features that help in making the diagnosis of PPHN include a pre- and postsaturation difference of greater than 10%, lability with handling, presence of a soft tricuspid murmur, and a history consistent with this presentation; seen in infants with a birth asphyxia, meconium aspiration syndrome, prolonged rupture of membranes, intrauterine growth restriction, and cyanotic CHD. Treatment refractory PPHN is often seen in congenital diaphragmatic hernia (CDH), or other pulmonary hypoplasia. Some PPHN infants will require rapid transport for extracorporeal life support (ECLS) (101–103), although most do well with appropriate ventilation, and inhaled nitric oxide (iNO). High-frequency oscillation or jet ventilation is often preferred in the tertiary setting, since few teams can safely offer this option due to availability of suitable ventilators. Vasoactive agents may be required and the "go-to" drugs depend on local preference and the underlying etiology. Many teams will use low-dose epinephrine (0.03 to 0.05 µg/kg/min) if dobutamine (10 µg/kg/min) as inotropic support has failed. Norepinephrine or vasopressin may help if vasoplegia plays a role.

Birth Asphyxia

Transport teams continue to see high numbers of infants with moderate to severe hypoxic ischemic encephalopathy (HIE). Some have multiorgan involvement with cardiac, liver, renal, and adrenal dysfunction, while others present solely with encephalopathy. Randomized controlled trials in HIE showed reduction in combined mortality and morbidity for infants "cooled" within a 6-hour window after birth (104). Transport teams encourage early consultation by referral team prior to initiation of passive cooling, with active cooling provided by transport teams using portable "cooling blankets" or "cool packs" to achieve goal of 33°C to 34°C as soon as possible after birth. Only infants greater than 34 weeks GA with no obvious bleeding/coagulation disturbance or severe PPHN/oxygenation failure should be considered. Due to difficulty with early clinical classification of HIE, 25% of cooled HIE patients will be deemed mild but amplitude integrated EEG (aEEG), also known as cerebral function monitors (CFM), prior to initiation of "cooling" will benefit enrollment decisions. This 2 channel aEEG comes in a portable size but not all countries have health authority approvals to use them. We rely on transport clinician's ability to judge severity of encephalopathy; infants relying on any respiratory support (CPAP or CMV) without a significant oxygen requirement should be considered encephalopathic. Clinical seizures manifest in only half of HIE infants so monitoring aEEG during transport is ideal. All should be considered "*emergency transports*" to ensure timely access to definitive care.

The Surgical Neonate

Many fetuses are diagnosed antenatal and delivered in a high-risk setting. Some surgical emergencies will be missed or present later, which include necrotising enterocolitis, bowel perforation, tracheoesophageal fistula +/− esophageal atresia (TEF/EA), incarcerated hernia, gastroschisis, sacrococcygeal teratoma, and CDH. Others require time-sensitive diagnostic or therapeutic intervention, for example, craniofacial anomalies, meningomyelocele, posterior urethral valves, suspected Hirschsprung disease, etc. If patients present as "life or limb threatened," a no-refusal policy guarantees acceptance at the nearest tertiary surgical center, and deemed emergent. Bilious emesis requires immediate transfer to rule out intestinal volvulus. Noninvasive respiratory support is contraindicated in the majority of infants with concern for bowel obstruction. These infants require the largest bore gastric tube for ventilation and drainage of the stomach on intermittent suction. Unless they are self-ventilating effectively in room air, they require

intubation for respiratory compromise. They will also benefit from transport by a specialized transport team. Some may be escorted by their referring RN, for example, imperforate anus.

Special Populations: The Difficult Airway

Among the newborns requiring an advanced airway for transport are Beckwith-Weidman syndrome, cystic hygroma, Pierre Robin Sequence, Treacher-Collins syndrome, and those where difficulty with intubation was experienced (105); prone position or side lying may be adequate to achieve stability. To optimize intubation success, direct laryngoscopy has been superseded by video-laryngoscopy with improved success on first pass (64). Muscle relaxation is not to be advised in this situation. The introduction of a supraglottic or laryngeal mask airway (LMA) has revolutionized the management of these infants if over 1.5 kg. Airway expertise requires continuous practice through simulation/task trainers, OR shifts, and in some cases human cadaver labs. Neonatal tracheotomy is a skill that should be taught and practiced in the event that other lifesaving maneuvers are not effective (65).

Withdrawal of ICU Support

If neonates have suffered profound hypoxic–ischemic brain injury or have a lethal genetic syndrome, for example, Potters syndrome, or are at limits of viability, the transport team, +/− a physician, will assist in decisions regarding withdrawal of life support, with provision, and support for the bereavement process in the community. Final decisions depend upon the social and medical situation but involve

- Assisting the referring physician in counseling the family around end of life decision-making and withdrawal of life-sustaining technology.
- Parents encouraged to be with and hold their baby when he/she dies.
- Transport teams must be highly sensitive to the needs of the family; cultural, spiritual, religious, and personal views are top priorities. Legacy work includes making foot/hand moulds and prints, photographs, saving locks of hair, etc.
- The role of an autopsy should always be discussed with the family with its potential benefit for genetic counseling.
- If death was not anticipated at onset of labor, and especially if family are questioning the care provided, the regional coroner/medical examiner's (ME) office should be notified prior to requesting consent to postmortem; the coroner/ME may order an autopsy.

TRANSPORT OF INFECTIOUS DISEASE PATIENTS

Screening for infectious disease should be part of every initial transport call, so personal protective equipment (PPE) is "donned" prior to patient contact and isolation or negative pressure room arranged for patient's admission. Agents requiring contact or droplet precaution typically consists of gown and gloves, eye visor or goggles, and procedure mask. This is adequate for patients with respiratory illness who are not on enhanced respiratory support. For aerosol generating medical procedures (AGMPs), increasing risk of transmission and/or if disease specific mortality/morbidity is high, PPE with the addition of N95 respirator mask, appropriately fitted, is recommended. All AGMPs (intubation, ventilation, noninvasive ventilation (NIV) (e.g., CPAP) and/or nebulized medications should include in-line suctioning and use of cuffed ETTs, with closed circuit ventilation preferred, with filters on the expiratory limb of the ventilation circuit, and HMEs rather than humidifiers. Metered dose inhalers and self-inflating bags should be used. A lower threshold for invasive ventilation is preferred especially during air transport given small space and exposure of pilots also. At times of pandemic, limiting the number of staff essential to these procedures is expected. Restrictions on accompanying family members are a must.

AEROMEDICAL PHYSIOLOGY AND AVIATION MEDICINE

Air transport can significantly improve response times and/or can reduce the "out of hospital time" for long-distance transports. The aviation environment differs in many important ways including effects on patients, staff, and equipment. Unless there is a good understanding of this environment, harm may ensue.

Atmosphere

The earth is surrounded by a thin blanket of air; nitrogen (78%), oxygen (21%), and other gases (1%). If the air contains moisture (or humidity), up to 5% may be in a gaseous form, water vapor. The atmosphere comprises several distinct layers with the troposphere closest to the surface ranging up to 60,000 feet at the equator and 20,000 feet at the poles. There is a progressive fall in air and ambient pressure with altitude within the troposphere. The tropopause marks the boundary with the next layer, the stratosphere. The tropopause is the layer in which most aircraft operate, where nearly all the moisture is and where weather phenomena occur.

At sea level, the mean air pressure is 760 mm Hg (29.92 inches of mercury) or 1,012 Hectopascal (hPa) in SI units. In the tropopause, pressure falls in a nearly linear fashion with altitude at a rate of 1 hPa per 30 feet of altitude. The units of altitude are always expressed in feet, agreed by worldwide consensus. Temperature falls with altitude at a rate of around 2 degrees per 1,000 feet.

The two main clinical consequences of reduced air pressure are

1. Available oxygen is reduced, that is, the partial pressure of oxygen falls (along with all other partial pressures) making less oxygen available despite the fraction of oxygen contributing to the total atmospheric pressure remaining constant at 21%.
2. The reduced pressure of ambient air at increasing altitude also has clinical implications.

Aircraft operate at altitudes selected to ensure safety (clear of obstacles), operational efficiency (speed and distance), and minimization of conflict with other aircraft (separation), at least 1,000 feet above the highest obstacle or land mass along the route, within 10 nautical miles on each side. This is known as the "lowest safe altitude" or LSALT, to give pilots this "buffer." Higher altitudes are more efficient for fuel consumption and speed with reduced turbulence and weather. Although rotor and fixed wing aircraft will operate differently, a normally aspirated piston-engine aircraft operates most efficiently between 5,000 and 8,000 feet above sea level. If fitted with a turbocharger, the engine operates over 10,000 feet because the air pressure for combustion is increased. Jet engines compress the ambient air even more permitting flight at much higher levels of 20,000 to 30,000 feet and higher speeds due to thinner air creating less drag. The aerodynamics of the fixed wing aircraft permit flight at higher levels compared to the helicopter rotor system. Forward speed of helicopters is aerodynamically limited to about half that of turboprops and one-third that of jets. They commonly operate at around 5,000 feet as they are not pressurized.

Above 10,000 feet, air pressure is about 60% of that at sea level and consequently the partial pressure of oxygen is about 60% (Table 6.8).

Gas exchange in healthy humans at 96 mm Hg provides sufficient oxygenation to offer arterial oxygen levels (PaO_2) around 60 mm Hg. Any losses from intrapulmonary shunting or VQ mismatch will further reduce PaO_2. Below 10,000 feet is the "physiologic zone"; above this supplementary oxygen would

TABLE 6.8

Effect of Altitude on Barometric Pressure

	Sea Level	10,000 feet
Atmospheric pressure P_{atm}	760 mm Hg	457 mm Hg
Partial pressure of O_2—PO_2	160 mm Hg	96 mm Hg

be required. Usually the cabin is pressurized so the breathable atmosphere is below 10,000 feet; commonly selected cabin pressure altitude (CPA) is 4,000 feet for air ambulances. Requesting a low CPA may incur a slower flight in more turbulent air with reduced range. Commercial airliners routinely pressurize the cabin to around 8,000 feet and will not be able to modify the CPA in the same way.

An aeromedical aircraft must consider many factors before accepting a mission and generally it takes up to 30 minutes to complete preflight assessment. This flight planning task is vital to safety:

1. Can the aircraft carry the required personnel and equipment?
2. Is the flight crew rested and competent for the mission?
3. Is the aircraft able to carry sufficient fuel to reach the destination?
4. Current weather conditions at the start and end of the flight and on route?
5. Can a safe landing be made at the destination?
6. What alternative location is available for the aircraft to safely divert to if required?

Weather must permit the pilot to see to operate the aircraft visually for the take-off and landing. Instruments in the aircraft and/or on the ground at airports assist and permit an aircraft to descend but landing without any visual reference is only available to some passenger jets at a limited number of airports.

Ice can compromise the aircraft flight surfaces, propeller or rotor blades, or engines when operating around 0°C in cloud. Anti-icing equipment exists in most fixed wing aircraft but rarely in helicopters limiting their use in such weather. Weather forecasts include the altitude at which the air is at zero degrees (the "freezing level") and charts show the LSALT for each leg of the flight. It may be possible to operate between the freezing level and the LSALT and avoid both "icing" and being too close to the ground. At higher altitudes, the risk diminishes because the moisture content of the air decreases.

Hypoxia—Dalton's Law

Dalton demonstrated that the total pressure of a gas mixture is the sum of the individual or partial pressures of all the gases in the mixture (106). The total of these "partial" pressures is the atmospheric pressure ($p_{atmos} = p_1 + p_2 + p_3 + \ldots + p_n$). *The reduction in atmospheric pressure with increasing altitude is associated with a corresponding reduction in the partial pressure of oxygen.* This affects patients requiring supplemental oxygen with a fall in SaO_2 and increased oxygen demand with increasing altitude. All fixed wing aircrafts can be pressurized soon after takeoff and kept at that pressure, or one equivalent to 4,000 feet to minimize the effect. At increasing altitude, the reduced PAO_2 progressively diminishes the potential PaO_2. Thus, within the physiologic zone, oxygen saturations in a healthy adult will progressively fall (Table 6.9).

Oxygen deprivation will cause reduced mental and physical functioning and may manifest in slow or inaccurate decision-making or a false sense of well-being. With abrupt failure of pressurization, the symptoms will be more rapid and pronounced. Unconsciousness will occur without supplemental oxygen. The time of "useful consciousness" shortens with altitude to 5 minutes at 22,000 feet and only 30 seconds at 35,000 feet.

TABLE 6.9

Effect of Altitude on Oxygenation

Altitude (feet)	O₂ Sat.	P_AO₂
2,000	96%	87
4,000	94%	78
6,000	90%	70
8,000	88%	60
10,000	85%	50

Quick thinking and action is required to look after yourself so you can look after others, including your patient. The pilot will urgently descend to lower altitudes while you adjust the patient's respiratory support to avoid hypoxia.

Pressure—Boyle Law

The reduction in atmospheric pressure with ascent to altitude is associated with expansion of a collection of gas within a closed space (107).

Consequently, gastrointestinal, sinus, or middle ear gas will expand as altitude increases and may cause pain (or barotrauma). Conversely, on descent, these air spaces may not equilibrate with ambient pressure quickly. Typically, a rate of descent of 500 feet/min or less is well tolerated. Infants may benefit from a pacifier to induce sucking and opening of the eustachian tubes.

A gastric tube should always be inserted to deflate the stomach and reduce air expansion in the gut. With an abnormal collection of air, for example, pneumothorax, pneumoperitoneum, or intracranial air, the climb to altitude will cause the air to expand. Untreated pneumothoraces will enlarge; it is advisable to insert a chest drain prior to "takeoff". Air trapped in the bowel wall may cause pain or perforation; open NG/OG tubes to minimize gastric dilatation. The balloon in urinary catheters or cuffed ETT will expand so water and not air is routinely used to inflate them. Avoiding altitude may mean ground transport, but in most cases, the aircraft, if pressurized, is capable of maintaining a sea level CPA or equivalent to the elevation of the referring hospital.

At increasing altitude, the effect of volume can be summarized in Table 6.10.

Altitude and reduced ambient pressure will not cause an air leak but will cause an expansion of a preexisting air leak.

Although the volumetric effects are smaller, this law also applies to liquids. In tightly constrained spaces such as brain and CSF in the skull, increasing altitude can increase intracranial pressure. In head injuries or an obstructed CSF draining system, this may exacerbate the raised intracranial pressure (108).

Coping with Transport

All transports carry a degree of risk for the patient, crew, and pilots (109,110). Air transports obviously carry a greater mortality risk although ground ambulances are more frequently affected.

Air medical crew should not fly with conditions such as otitis media, GI upset, dental problems, and sinus obstruction with pain

TABLE 6.10

Effect of Altitude on Gas Volume

Altitude (feet)	% Increase in Volume
2,000	10
4,000	20
6,000	30
8,000	40
10,000	50
18,000	100

exacerbation at altitude. Extended periods at significant altitude cause fatigue.

For medical equipment, some gas delivery systems are affected by altitude, for example, flow meter settings will increase with altitude and diminish with descent, and also the pressures set on the ventilator may vary, and may require adjustment. A patient requiring a specific inspired oxygen concentration on the ground should not need an increase in FiO_2 at altitude since the FiO_2 doesn't change with altitude; only the absolute total and partial pressures. However, the reading on the analyzer progressively falls with altitude, as the device is actually measuring only oxygen and assumes an unchanged total atmospheric pressure. In theory, making adjustments to the measured FiO_2 in response to that fall will be enough to compensate for altitude changes.

For mechanical ventilators supplied by both medical oxygen and air, the proportions of each gas to deliver a certain FiO_2 will vary according to altitude. It will be vital to avoid hyperoxia so FiO_2 just sufficient to maintain the targeted PaO_2 or O_2 saturation must be used, which may deplete air supplies. In such circumstances, ask the pilot to fly higher or use a higher CPA than usual levels, which permits a higher FiO_2 setting to be used while still delivering the required PaO_2. Such maneuvers can increase the duration of useful medical air supply by 25% to 40%.

The interior of the aircraft cabin is heated and may have an air conditioner to manage excessive temperature. Air conditioning is less common in helicopters. The cabin air is dry at higher altitudes contributing to team fatigue; increase oral intake of water. Temperature control is important; there may be significant heat loss by conduction, convention, and radiation from the neonate. Incubator temperature may need to be increased to accommodate for increased losses.

Ambient noise levels are high and vibration is common (111–114) and may be associated with hemodynamic instability. Both interfere with the ability to observe, examine, or monitor the patient as well as poor lighting. Be sure to have electronic monitoring of the patient, with equipment settings and alarms visible to be able to rely on visual cues. Monitors provide reliable estimates of vital signs in spite of movement or electromagnetic interference (EMI). Routine use of ear muffs is recommended. Procedures are rare on route, but equipment must be ready in case emergency procedures are necessary, for example, cardiopulmonary arrest, self-extubation.

Newton Laws

Newton's 1st Law of Motion states that *"Every body continues in its state of rest, or of uniform motion in a straight line, unless it is compelled to change that state by forces applied upon it."* Newton's 2nd Law of Motion states *"The change of motion is proportional to the motive force impressed; and is made in the direction of the straight line in which that force is impressed."* (114) Therefore, the baby and all equipment should be secured prior to takeoff. Small objects become missiles when dislodged and are projected at significant speed after acceleration and deceleration of the aircraft. Items of equipment must be secured in a manner which protects everyone in the aircraft from injury. Equipment restraint systems are now designed to secure the item in place when forces of up to 20 times the object's weight are experienced (or "pull testing" at 20G). Air safety regulations require all to be secure in an aircraft when below 1,000 feet above the ground or when the seat belt fastened sign is on (as in turbulence). The ergonomics of the layout of the equipment should permit access to the patient especially the airway, while the staff member is properly restrained.

▌ EQUIPMENT REQUIREMENTS AND SUPPLIES

Medical transport requires vehicles designed to support the needs of teams, their patients, and equipment and supplies required. Ground ambulances are designed to support the carriage of a typical adult patient and are primarily for use in scene response. The intention in this prehospital transport is to get to hospital in the shortest possible time and the facilities in the ambulance reflect this. Helicopter medical transport generally has a similar prehospital role; albeit with higher level of paramedical skills.

For the newborn, the situation is different. The standard task is to transport patients between hospitals as a secondary response with rare exceptions of home births. Use of dedicated specialized vehicles for land transport is the accepted best practice allowing customization of the interior, enhancing team safety and increasing response times (53,83). Often, use of vehicles that are not part of the local ambulance service means "lights and sirens" cannot be operated since this applies only to designated ambulances. Dedicated team vehicles permit the storage of specialized equipment and supplies and electric lifts and/or stretchers needed for safety. Air ambulances are generally not dedicated to neonatal or pediatric transport teams and present a different set of problems focused on compatibility of equipment with the interior design of the aircraft, rotor, and fixed wing.

Selection of Vehicles

Factors influencing this include vehicle availability, patient acuity, geographic location of the referring hospital, climactic conditions, time of day, and day of week. The mode of transport, that is, ground versus air ambulance requires specific expertise. Aside from availability and costs of air ambulances, considerations also include proximity of helipads, traffic, size and weight of equipment, and number of team and family members. While the request for air transport is made by transport team, the decision is most frequently independently made by pilots unaware of patient condition.

Land Ambulance

The majority of retrievals are by road, particular short distance missions less than 150 km. This is also the only option in suboptimal climactic conditions or in cases of extreme respiratory compromise where patient saturation is less than 90% in oxygen FiO_2 1.0 where flying at altitude must to be avoided. It may also be preferable with significant air leak syndromes or bowel obstruction unless the aircraft can be pressurized.

Rotor Wing Aircraft

Helicopters are faster than road and flexible over intermediate distances (150 to 250 km). They may land at both the referring and receiving hospitals assuming availability of helipads but availability, space and flight restrictions, and weather conditions are considerations. Rotor may also be preferred for shorter transport times in extreme traffic congestion. They cannot be pressurized and usually fly between 2,000 and 5,000 feet above sea level, which may be deleterious to the patient's condition.

Fixed Wing Aircraft

Propeller and jet airplanes are the only option for long-haul retrievals and ideally for greater than 250 km. They are more spacious and can be pressurized to sea level if requested. They usually fly with pressure adjusted between 4,000 and 8,000 feet above sea level. Limitations include availability, weather, and the need to travel to and from the landing strip.

Equipment

Neonates should be transported in suitable neonatal incubator "decks" customized to fit securely and certified for both land or air ambulances (e.g., **Fig. 6.5**). This "life-support" equipment should be capable of providing full intensive care support. Equipment is thoroughly cleaned using infection control protocols between transports. All equipment and supplies are checked at the beginning of every shift using appropriate checklists and restocked as

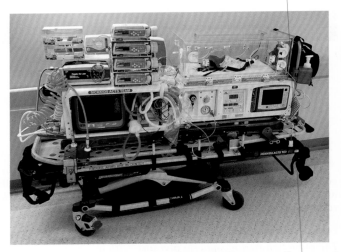

FIGURE 6.5 Specialized equipment for neonatal transport. (Courtesy of Acute Care Transport Service (ACTS), The Hospital for Sick Children, Toronto.)

necessary ready for the next transport (Table 6.6). Typically, the equipment list for such "level 3" transport contains

- Incubator; with active heating, effective thermal insulation, and good ergonomic design
- Appropriate and certified patient restraint system
- Infusion pumps capable of a range of accurate infusion rates. Pumps should include electronic systems to guide dosing based on a library of specific drugs
- Mechanical ventilator capable of multiple modes of ventilation; invasive and all noninvasive methods using oxygen concentrations from 0.21 to 1.0
- Physiologic monitor for vital signs, ECG, capnography, at least 2 of invasive pressure readings, and temperature channels
- Point of care testing for blood work

Increasingly, equipment includes

- Defibrillator (separate or built in to monitor)
- Heated humidification for gases
- Data storage/electronic record
- Real-time data and video streaming

Specialty treatments may be on the standard "deck" or easily added options:

- Inhaled nitric oxide (iNO)
- High-frequency ventilation (HFV)
- Cooling blanket
- Phototherapy
- Amplitude-integrated EEG (aEEG)
- Point of care ultrasound (POCUS) for vascular access, abdominal scan, functional/diagnostic imaging of the head, heart, and lungs
- ECMO—extracorporeal membrane oxygenation

A "level 2" neonatal transport or retrotransfer/repatriation of a patient might operate with a simple life-support system, capable of physiologic monitoring +/− ventilation.

The mission profile of the transport service and its clinical approach to various disease conditions will determine what is considered "default" technology and what is considered "discretionary." Whereas in a hospital, many assumptions can be made about the patient care environment, these cannot be assumed in transport. During transport, there is the ever present concern that equipment batteries may become exhausted, vehicle power may fail, and gas supplies might run low—especially if anticipated travel times become unexpectedly extended.

To mitigate these risks, a power and gas continuity strategy is required for all essential components of care. Electrically powered equipment; monitors, pumps, and ventilators have batteries expected to last for several hours. This equipment is always connected to mains power and re-charged between missions. Reliance on the various sources of external power such as ambulances helps to conserve battery power, which should be a temporary support "between" sources of mains power, for example, ward to ambulance. Batteries then do not require quite as much capacity. The goal is to have security of power and gas such that teams do not have to worry.

Patient Safety

The patient being transported is vulnerable to the transport environment. Their physical safety in a moving vehicle must be considered. National and international bodies prescribe standards for occupant safety, which should provide a framework for achieving the content or at least the spirit of those standards (81–83).

Local road vehicle and aviation regulations for passenger safety, including restraint and protection in case of an accident, must be addressed. A harness designed for the patient size and to meet the "crashworthiness" standard must be used. Hearing protection should be offered. Vibration exposure sometimes exceeds the acceptable threshold for adults in the workplace, which currently remains the only existing standard. Overlap of the natural frequency of the incubator system with that of the ambulance causes accentuation of vibration (resonance). Likely, a lower frequency peak originates from resonance of vehicle suspension and higher frequency peak (7 to 14 Hz) from the engine and transmission (115).

Staff Safety

All staff occupants of the vehicle must be equally safe. Equipment carried is a potential hazard unless secured in accordance with engineering certifications. An extra infusion pump lying loose on the mattress might become a projectile with potential to harm. Even something weighing 500 g, in an abrupt deceleration from 40 km/h, increases the mass 20 fold, to become a 10 kg missile. All devices need to be secured in an approved manner or incorporated into the "certified" life-support system.

Aircraft Safety

All equipment carried in aircraft must not present a hazard to its operation. Apart from physical restraint, equipment devices must not emit EMI, which could jeopardize the aircraft's navigation or communications system. These risks could transmit through air (radiation) or via cables (conduction). Moreover, in the case that a device became faulty, it cannot place the aircraft at risk; consider faults in batteries, leaks from gas bottles containing hazardous materials, for example, nitric oxide or oxygen. These are potential fire hazards with increased risk in a small aircraft. The flight may be conducted to "save a life" but does not relieve the obligation of transport service and aircraft operator to properly address and mitigate the risks to each other. We also must examine whether the proper functioning of the medical equipment is adversely affected by the aircraft systems. That is called "electromagnetic compatibility" or EMC.

Historically, medical equipment often radiated significant energy but improved shielding, filtering, and "earthing" has reduced this problem for EMI and EMC. However, the use of a device in any particular aircraft type will have to be verified by in flight testing and will need certification as meeting the relevant EMC and EMI standards in the country of operation.

The ergonomics of the relationship between patient, life-support equipment, and team also needs careful design. Aircraft designers spent the first 100 years of aviation on the pilot in the cockpit, but the same attention for critical care transport is needed.

Interoperability

In transport medicine, we need life-support equipment to operate in different vehicles even within a single mission. Equipment should move from one land vehicle type to the next and then to aircraft seamlessly and without interruption in the process such that the team focus is the patient. But it is often at these vehicle changes that adverse incidents occur or errors are made. Certification of all equipment should meet aviation and ground specifications. The challenge is to ensure that the internal configuration of the aircraft selected for air medical transport meet the needs of neonatal transport providers. This is best achieved through a collaborative process to design a standardized "transport system" efficient and ergonomic interoperability, which includes all the elements considered vital to patient care and their local aircraft provider. Ideally, the specification for neonatal transport considers

- Carrying capacity—life-support system(s)
- Range of operation of ambulance/aircraft
- Power: Ground 12vDC rated at 30A. Air 28vDC rated at 25A
- Mains power 120vAC or 230vAC (*see below)
- Oxygen (and medical air for some services) with appropriate capacity
- Suction
- Seating capacity min. 3 to 5 persons (team + paramedic +/– trainee, +/– parent)
- Refrigerator/freezer—drugs/human milk
- Parent accommodation (seated/stretcher)
- Loading/unloading in a nonlift environment
- Communication technology
- Approval for carriage/use of therapeutic agents such as iNO

*To replicate wall socket capacity requires an invertor with 15A (120vAC) or 10A (230vAC) capacity. Ambulances often have smaller invertors, which will not support draw of "transport deck," especially heated humidification and high-flow devices. Alternatively, some ambulances are fitted with an AC generator.

▌MEDICOLEGAL AND LIABILITY ISSUES

This aspect of transport medicine is not well articulated in literature, in large part due to the fact that legalities will vary across countries and states (83). Those involved in interfacility transport should become familiar with local State laws and court decisions, which may impact liability in their jurisdiction(s) served.

While the usual medicolegal considerations for patient care underpin all else, there is an added disadvantage or higher risk in the setting of transport medicine. High acuity vulnerable patients are cared for in suboptimal settings or facilities where local demography, geography, climate, and resources can delay retrieval and impact the outcome. Every health care professional has a legal duty to exercise that degree of knowledge, skill, and judgment that is expected of a comparably trained practitioner of the same class, acting in similar circumstances. It is the obligation of each licensed and/or certified professional to know and understand the standard to which he or she will be held and should not be pressured into functioning beyond their intended role for which they are prepared, trained, and legally authorized. Medical malpractice insurance is a must for all physicians with those in emergency medicine, obstetrics, neurosurgery, and orthopedics carrying the highest premiums.

Regulation around "on-line" medical control may differ between jurisdictions. Any one of the referring physician, the accepting physician, the transport system's medical director, the subspecialty consultant, or some combination of the above may be responsible for the patient being transferred. It may benefit from a contract, a memorandum of understanding, or other legal document between the agencies or jurisdictions to provide clarification. It needs to be clearly defined in advance and not decided while the transport is taking place. Advance knowledge of the protocol by all stakeholders is helpful in proactively addressing potential situations concerning medical oversight and responsibility.

A commonly held view is that the responsibility for patient care is shared by the sending and receiving physician or their delegate as soon as phone or telemedicine consultation occurs. The responsibility to provide advice to our referral base is mandatory regardless of bed capacity at that tertiary center. We remain responsible for advice until we have executed a "staff to staff" hand over to another center, which agrees to accept the patient and their care.

At time of arrival of the transport team, a "graded responsibility" for the patient and their stabilization occurs until the team departure from the hospital. In some cases, the transport teams will accept *full responsibility* for patient care at the point of arrival at the sending facility but clear documentation in patient record is required and the team must then operate independent of the referring hospital staff. During the transport of the patient, or "out of hospital" time, the responsibility lies solely with the transport team under their medical "on line control" and using their medical directives where appropriate.

The transport service is responsible for ensuring that policies, procedures, and protocols are in place, which cover the care provided by the transport team. These documents should be consistent with laws, regulations, and administrative rules for their jurisdiction(s). Thus, quality assurance/quality management, which uses patient and referring facility/physician satisfaction surveys, chart/case reviews, and peer reviews, are required to identify problems or areas for improvement that could serve as models for other services.

Regulations, which protect patient medical records and other identifiable health information, are outlined by the Health Insurance Portability and Accountability Act (HIPPA) of 1996 (117,118). These have implications for all transport services where medical records or information are being transferred from one facility to another. The use and disclosure of protected health information along with measures to ensure the secure transmission and storage of medical records and other individually identifiable or demographic information are covered by these standards.

REFERENCES

1. Lasswell SM, Barfield WD, Rochat RW, et al. Perinatal regionalization for very low-birth-weight and very preterm infants: a meta-analysis. *JAMA* 2010;304(9):992.
2. Chance G, O'Brien M, Swyer P. Transportation of sick neonates, 1972: an unsatisfactory aspect of medical care. *Can Med Assoc J* 1973;109(9):847.
3. Roy RN, Kitchen WH. NETS: a new system for neonatal transport. *Med J Aust* 1977;2(26–27):855.
4. Chance GW, Matthew JD, Gash J, et al. Neonatal transport: a controlled study of skilled assistance. *J Pediatr* 1978;93(4):662.
5. Gunn T, Outerbridge EW. Effectiveness of neonatal transport. *Can Med Assoc J* 1978;118(6):646.
6. Hood JL, Cross A, Hulka B, et al. Effectiveness of the neonatal transport team. *Crit Care Med* 1983;11(6):419.
7. Zeitlin J, Papiernik E, Breart G; EUROPET Group. Regionalization of perinatal care in Europe. *Semin Neonatol* 2004;9(2):99.
8. Eliason S, Whyte HE, Dow K, et al.; Canadian Neonatal Network. Variations in transport outcomes of very low birth weight infants among Canadian NICUs. *Am J Perinatol* 2013;30(5):377.
9. Barker CL, Costello C, Clark PT. Obstetric air medical retrievals in the Australian outback. *Air Med J* 2013;32(6):329.
10. Kelly LE, Shah PS, Hakansson S, et al.; for International Network for Evaluating Outcomes of Neonates (iNEO). Perinatal health services organization for preterm births: a multinational comparison. *J Perinatol* 2013;37(7):762.
11. Lui K, Abdel-Latif ME, Allgood CL, et al.; New South Wales and Australian Capital Territory Neonatal Intensive Care Unit Study. Improved outcomes of extremely premature outborn infants: effects of strategic changes in perinatal and retrieval services. *Pediatrics* 2006;118(5):2076.
12. Hossain S, Shah PS, Ye XY, et al.; Canadian Neonatal, Australian and New Zealand Neonatal Networks. Outborns or inborns: where are the differences? A comparison study of very preterm neonatal intensive care unit infants cared for in Australia and New Zealand and in Canada. *Neonatology* 2016;109(1):76.
13. Bergella V, Saccone G. Fetal Fibronectin testing for reducing the risk of preterm birth. *Cochrane Database Syst Rev* 2019;7(7):CD006843.
14. Deutchman ME, Sills D, Connor PD. Perinatal outcomes: a comparison between family physicians and obstetricians. *J Am Board Fam Pract* 1995;(6): 440.
15. Cifuentes J, Bronstein J, Phibbs CS, et al. Mortality in low birth weight infants according to level of neonatal care at hospital of birth. *Pediatrics* 2002;109(5):745.
16. McNamara PJ, Mak W, Whyte HE. Dedicated neonatal retrieval teams improve delivery room resuscitation of outborn premature infants. *J Perinatol* 2005;25(5):309.
17. McEvoy CG, Descloux E, Barazzoni MS, et al. Evaluation of Neonatal Transport in Western Switzerland: a model of perinatal regionalization. *Clin Med Insights Pediatr* 2017;11:1179556517709021.
18. Leslie AJ, Stephenson TJ. Audit of neonatal intensive care transport closing the loop. *Acta Paediatr* 1997;86(11):1253.
19. Fenton AC, Leslie A, Skeoch CH. Optimising neonatal transfer. *Arch Dis Child Fetal Neonatal Ed* 2004;89(3):F215.
20. Belway D, Henderson W, Keenan SP, et al. Do specialist transport personnel improve hospital outcome in critically ill patients transferred to higher centers? A systematic review. *J Crit Care* 2006;21(1):8; discussion 17-18.
21. Chang AS, Berry A, Jones LJ, et al. Specialist teams for neonatal transport to neonatal intensive care units for prevention of morbidity and mortality. *Cochrane Database Syst Rev* 2005;(10):CD007485.
22. Edge WE, Kanter RK, Weigle CG, et al. Reduction of morbidity in interhospital transport by specialized pediatric staff. *Crit Care Med* 1994;22(7):1186.
23. Vos GD, Nissen AC, Nieman FH, et al. Comparison of interhospital pediatric intensive care transport accompanied by a referring specialist or a specialist retrieval team. *Intensive Care Med* 2004;30(2):302.
24. Orr RA, Felmet KA, Han Y, et al. Paediatric specialised teams are associated with improved outcomes. *Pediatrics* 2009;124(1):40.
25. Wiegersma JS, Droogh JM, Zijlstra JG, et al. Quality of interhospital transport of the critically ill: impact of a Mobile Intensive Care Unit with a specialized retrieval team. *Crit Care* 2011;15(1):R75.
26. Meyer MT, Mikhailov TA, Kuhn EM, et al. Pediatric specialty transport teams are not associated with decreased 48-hour pediatric intensive care unit mortality: a propensity analysis of the VPS, LLC database. *Air Med J* 2016;35(2):73.
27. Patel SC, Murphy S, Penfel S, et al. Impact of interfacility transport method and specialty teams on outcomes of paediatric trauma patients. *Pediatr Emerg Care* 2018;34(7):467.
28. Wallen E, Venkataraman ST, Grosso MJ, et al. Intrahospital transport of critically ill pediatric patients. *Crit Care Med* 1995;23(9):1588.
29. van den Berg J, Olsson L, Svensson A, et al. Adverse events during air and ground neonatal transport: 13 years' experience from a neonatal transport team in Northern Sweden. *J Matern Fetal Neonatal Med* 1995;28(10):1231.
30. Lim MT, Ratnavel N. A prospective review of adverse events during interhospital transfers of neonates by a dedicated neonatal transfer service. *Pediatr Crit Care Med* 2008;9(3):289.
31. Lee SK, Zupancic JA, Sale J, et al. Cost-effectiveness and choice of infant transport systems. *Med Care* 2002;40(8):705.
32. Raynovich W, Hums J, Stuhlmiller DF, et al. Critical care transportation by paramedics: a cross-sectional survey. *Air Med J* 2013;32(5):280.
33. International accreditation program 2019—Q-mentum standards. Available from: http://accreditation.ca
34. Commission on Accreditation of Medical Transport Systems. Accreditation Standards. Available from: http://camts.org/Resource-Materials.html
35. Social Security Act: Section 1867 [42 U.S.C. 1395dd]. April 5, 2013. Available from: https://www.ssa.gov/OP_Home/ssact/title18/1867.htm.
36. Shah P, Shah V, Zhenguo Q, et al.; the Canadian Neonatal Network. Improved outcomes of outborn preterm infants if admitted to perinatal centers versus free standing childrens hospitals. *J Pediatr* 2005;146(5):626.
37. Fang J, Campbell M, Schuning V. A retrospective study on the impact of telemedicine on the quality of newborn resuscitation. *Pediatrics* 2018;142:159. doi: 10.1542/peds.142.1_MeetingAbstract.159.
38. Standardised maternal and newborn levels of care definitions. 2013. Available from: https://www.pcmch.on.ca
39. Maternal/fetal and neonatal services: tiers in brief to support system planning. 2020. Available from: www.perinatalservicesbc.ca

40. Karlsen K, Trautman AM, Price-Douglas W, et al. National survey of neonatal transport teams in the United States. *Pediatrics* 2011;128(4):685.

41. Tanem J, Triscari D, Chan M, et al. Workforce survey of pediatric interfacility transport systems in the United States. *Pediatr Emerg Care* 2016;32(6):364.

42. Leslie A, Stephenson T. Neonatal transfers by advanced neonatal nurse practitioners and paediatric registrars. *Arch Dis Child Fetal Neonatal Ed* 2003;88(6):F509.

43. Davies J, Bickell D, Tibby SM. Attitudes of paediatric intensive care nurses to development of a nurse practitioner role for critical care transport. *J Adv Nurs* 2011;67(2):317.

44. von Vopelius-Feldt J, Benger JR. Prehospital anaesthesia by a physician and paramedic critical care team in Southwest England. *Eur J Emerg Med* 2003;20(6):382.

45. Whyte HE, Jefferies AL; Canadian Paediatric Society Fetus and Newborn Committee. The interfacility transport of critically ill newborns. *Paediatr Child Health* 2015;20(5):265.

46. King BR. King TM, Foster RL, et al. Pediatric and neonatal transport teams with and without a physician: a comparison of outcomes and interventions. *Pediatr Emerg Care* 2007;23(2):77.

47. Beyer AJ III, Land G, Zaritsky, A. Nonphysician transport of intubated pediatric patients: a system evaluation. *Crit Care Med* 1992;20(7):961.

48. Rashid A, Bhuta T, Berry A. A regionalised transport service, the way ahead? *Arch Dis Child* 1999;80(5):488.

49. Thomas SH, Williams KA, Claypool DW; 2002 Air Medical Services Task Force of the National Association of EMS Physicians. Medical director for air medical transport programs. *Prehosp Emerg Care* 2002;6(4):455.

50. Fox C, Newell F, Stewart M. Evaluation of a neonatal nurse practitioner model of neonatal emergency retrieval. *J Paediatr Child Health* 2016;52:19.

51. McCloskey KA, Johnston C. Critical care interhospital transports: predictability of the need for a pediatrician. *Pediatr Emerg Care* 1990;6(2):89.

52. Warren J, Fromm RE Jr, Orr RA, et al. Guidelines for the inter- and intrahospital transport of critically ill patients. *Crit Care Med* 2004;32(1):256.

53. De Vries S, Wallis LA, Maritz D. A retrospective evaluation of the impact of a dedicated obstetric and neonatal transport service on transport times within an urban setting. *Int J Emerg Med* 2001;4(1):28.

54. Laffan EE, McNamara PJ, Amaral J, et al. A six–year review of interventional procedures in very low–birth weight infants (<1.5 kg): Complications lessons learned and current practice. *Pediatr Radiol* 2009;39(8):781.

55. Jernigan PL, Wallace MC, Novak CS, et al. Measuring intangibles: defining predictors of non-technical skills in critical care air transport team trainees. *Mil Med* 2016;181(10):1357.

56. Canadian Association of Paediatric Health Centres. Competencies profile—Interfacility critical care transport of maternal, neonatal, and paediatric patients. Available from: https://www.caphc.org/neonatalpaediatric-transport-systems/. 2011.

57. Merriam S, Bierma LL. *Adult learning: linking theory and practice.* John Wiley and Sons Inc., 2014.

58. Benner P. *From Novice to expert: excellence and power in clinical nursing practice.* Menlo Park, CA: Addison-Wesley, 1984.

59. Droogh JM, Smit M, Absalom AR, et al. Transferring the critically ill patient: are we there yet? *Crit Care* 2015;19:62.

60. Hansen M, Meckler G, Lambert W, et al. Patient safety events in out-of-hospital paediatric airway management: a medical record review by the CSI-EMS. *BMJ Open* 2016;6(11):e012259.

61. Lockey DJ, Healey B, Crewdson K, et al. Advanced airway management is necessary in prehospital trauma patients. *Br J Anaesth* 2015;114(4):657.

62. Smith KA, Gothard MD, Schwartz HP, et al. Risk factors for failed tracheal intubation in pediatric and neonatal critical care specialty transport. *Prehosp Emerg Care* 2015;19(1):17.

63. Barrington KJ; Canadian Paediatric Society, Fetus and Newborn Committee. Premedication for Endotracheal Intubation in the Newborn Infant. *Paediatr Child Health* 2011;16(3):159.

64. Wallace MC, Britton ST, Meek R, et al. Comparison of five video-assisted intubation devices by novice and expert laryngoscopists for use in the aeromedical evacuation environment. *Mil Med Res* 2017;4:20.

65. Practice guidelines for management of the difficult airway. A report by the American Society of Anesthesiologists Task Force on Management of the Difficult Airway. *Anesthesiology* 1993;78(3):597.

66. Finan E, Bismilla Z, Whyte HE, et al. High-fidelity simulator technology may not be superior to traditional low-fidelity equipment for neonatal resuscitation training. *J Perinatol* 2012;32(4):287.

67. Powell DA, Gonzales C, Gunnels RD. Use of the ferret as a model for pediatric endotracheal intubation training. *Lab Anim Sci* 2001;41(1):86.

68. Hourihane JO, Crawshaw PA, Hall MA. Neonatal chest drain insertion—an animal model. *Arch Dis Child Fetal Neonatal Ed* 1995;72(2):F123.

69. Anastakis DJ, Regehr G, Reznick RK, et al. Assessment of technical skills transfer from the bench training model to the human model. *Am J Surg* 1991;177(2):167.

70. Britt RC, Novosel TJ, Britt LD, et al. The impact of central line simulation before the ICU experience. *Am J Surg* 2009;197(4):533.

71. Hunt EA, Duval-Arnould JM, Nelson-McMillan KL, et al. Pediatric resident resuscitation skills improve after "rapid cycle deliberate practice" training. *Resuscitation* 2014;85(7):945.

72. Singh JM, Gunz AC, Dhanani S, et al. Frequency, composition, and predictors of in-transit critical events during pediatric critical care transport. *Pediatr Crit Care Med* 2016;17(10):984.

73. Cheng A, Donoghue A, Gilfoyle E, et al. Simulation-based crisis resource management training for pediatric critical care medicine: a review for instructors. *Pediatr Crit Care Med* 2012;13(2):197.

74. Campbell DM, Dadiz R. Simulation in neonatal transport medicine. *Semin Perinatol* 2016;40(7):430.

75. Wilson D, Kochar A, Whyte-Lewis A, et al. Evaluation of situation, background, assessment, recommendation tool during neonatal and pediatric interfacility transport. *Air Med J* 2017;36(4):182.

76. Whyte HE, Narvey M. Team models in interfacility and maintaining competencies. *Curr Treat Options Pediatr* 2017;3(4):327.

77. Knowles M. *The adult learner: a neglected species*, 3rd ed. Houston, TX: Gulf Publishing, 1984.

78. Kline-Krammes S, Wheeler DS, Schwartz HP, et al. Missed opportunities during pediatric residency training: report of a 10-year follow-up survey in critical care transport medicine. *Pediatr Emerg Care* 2012;28(1):1.

79. Mickells GE, Goodman DM, Rozenfeld RA. Education of pediatric subspecialty fellows in transport medicine: a national survey. *BMC Pediatr* 2017;17(1):13.

80. Becker TK, Skiba JF, Sozener CB. An educational measure to significantly increase critical knowledge regarding interfacility patient transfers. *Prehosp Disaster Med* 2015;30(3):244.

81. Standards—CAMTS. 2015. Available from: www.camts.org

82. Accreditation Canada. 2013. Available from: https://accreditation.ca

83. College of Intensive Care Medicine of Australia and New Zealand. Available from: www.cicm.org.au

84. National Highway Traffic Safety Administration. Guide for interfacility patient transfer. Available from: www.nhtsa.gov/people/injury/ems/interfacility/images/interfacility.pdf

85. Kempley ST, Ratnavel N, Fellows T. Vehicles and equipment for land-based neonatal transport. *Early Hum Dev* 2009;85(8):491.

86. Bigham MT, Schwartz HP, Ohio C; Neonatal/Pediatric Transport Quality. Quality metrics in neonatal and pediatric critical care transport: a consensus statement. *Pediatr Crit Care Med* 2013;14(5):518.

87. Gunz AC, Dhanani S, Whyte H, et al. Identifying significant and relevant events during pediatric transport: a modified Delphi study. *Pediatr Crit Care Med* 2014;15(7):653.

88. Schwartz HP, Bigham MT, Schoettker PJ, et al.; American Academy of Pediatrics Section on Transport Medicine. Quality metrics in neonatal and pediatric critical care transport: A National Delphi Project. *Pediatr Crit Care Med* 2015;16(8):711.

89. Romito J, Alexander SN. Chapter 8: Section on transport medicine. In: Insoft RM, Schwartz HP. *Guidelines for air & ground transport of neonatal and pediatric patients manual*, 4th ed. American Academy of Paediatrics, 2015.

90. To Err is Human: Building a Safer Health System. Summary. Available from: www.nationalacademies.org

91. Weingart C, Herstich T, Baker P, et al. Making good better: implementing a standardized handoff in pediatric transport. *Air Med J* 2013;32(1):40.

92. Joyce CN, Libertin R, Bigham MT. Family-centered care in pediatric critical care transport. *Air Med J* 2015;34(1):32.

93. Lee KS. Neonatal transport metrics and quality improvement in a regional transport service. *Transl Pediatr* 2019;8(3):233.

94. Lee SK, Zupancic JA, Pendray M, et al.; Canadian Neonatal Network. Transport risk index of physiologic stability: a practical system for assessing infant transport care. *J Pediatr* 2001;139(2):220.

95. Spooner SA, Gotlieb EM; Committee on Clinical Information Technology; Committee on Medical Liability. Telemedicine: pediatric applications. *Pediatrics* 2004;(6):e639.

96. Patel S, Hertzog JH, Penfil S, et al. A prospective pilot study of the use of telemedicine during pediatric transport: a high-quality, low-cost alternative to conventional telemedicine systems. *Pediatr Emerg Care* 2015;31(9):611.

97. Karlsen AK, Scott AP, Kendall AB. The S.T.A.B.L.E Program: the evidence behind the 2012 update. *J Perinat Neonatal Nurs* 2012;26(2):147-157. Available from: https.//stable program.org

98. Polin RA, Carlo WA; Committee on fetus and newborn, American Academy of Pediatrics. Surfactant replacement therapy for preterm and term neonates with respiratory distress. *Pediatrics* 2014;133(1):156.

99. Bahadue FL, Soll R. Early vs. late surfactant therapy for RDS. *Cochrane Database Syst Rev* 2010;11(11):CD001456.

100. Carmo KA, Barr P, West M, et al. Transporting newborn infants with suspected duct dependent congenital heart disease on low-dose prostaglandin E1 without routine mechanical ventilation. *Arch Dis Child Fetal Neonatal Ed* 2007;92(2):F117.

101. Carmo KA, Lutz T, Berry A, et al. Feasibility and Utility of portable ultrasound during retrieval of sick preterm infants. *Acta Paediatr* 2016;105(12):e549.

102. Broman L. Interhospital transport on extracorporeal membrane oxygenation of neonates—perspective for the future. *Front Pediatr* 2019;7:329. doi: 10.3389/fped.2019.00329.

103. *Guidelines for ECMO Transport Extracorporeal Life Support Organization (ELSO)*. Ann Arbor, MI: 2019. Available from: https://www.elso.org/portals/o/files

104. Shankaran S. Therapeutic hypothermia for neonatal encephalopathy. *Curr Treat Options Neurol* 2012;14(6):608.

105. Weiss E, Tsarouhas N. Transport of the neonate with a difficult / critical airway disorders of the neonatal airway. *Pediatrics* 2018; 142(5):327.

106. Dalton J. Essay IV. On the expansion of elastic fluids by heat. *Mem Lit Philos Soc Manch* 1802;5 pt. 2:595.

107. Jewell W. *The golden cabinet of true treasure*. L[owens] for Iohn Crosley, 1612. Ann Anbor, MI: text creation partnership, 2011. Available from: http:name.umdl.umich.edu/A04486.0001.001

108. Henry W. Experiments on the quantity of gases absorbed by water, at different temperatures, and under different pressures. *Philos Trans R Soc Lond* 1803;93 29

109. Becker LR, Zaloshnja E, Levick N, et al. Relative risk of injury and death in ambulances and other emergency vehicles. *Accid Anal Prev* 2003;35(6):941.

110. Bouchut JC, Van Lancker E, Chritin V, et al. Physical stressors during neonatal transport: Helicopter compared with ground ambulance. *Air Med J* 2011;30(3):134.

111. Hankins D. Air versus ground transport studies. *Air Med J* 2010;29(3):102.

112. Karlsson BM, Lindkvist M, Lindkvist M, et al. Sound and vibration: effects on infants' heart rate and heart rate variability during neonatal transport. *Acta Paediatr* 2012;101(2):148.

113. Gajendragadkar G, Boyd JA, Potter DW, et al. Mechanical vibration in neonatal transport: a randomized study of different mattresses. *J Perinatol* 2000;20(5):307.

114. Blaxter L, Yeo M, McNally D, et al. Neonatal head and torso vibration exposure during inter-hospital transfer. *Proc Inst Mech Eng H* 2017;231(2):99.

115. Bellieni CV, Pinto I, Stacchini N, et al. Vibration risk during neonatal transport. *Minerva Pediatr* 2004;56(2):207.

116. Newton I. *Philosophiae Naturalis Principia Mathematica*. Facsimile of the Third Edition (1726) with Variant Readings. Volumes 1 and 2. Harvard University Press, 1972.

117. Health Insurance Portability and Accountability Act. 1996, Public Law 104-191, Section 264, 110 Stat 1996. Available from: https://hipaa.com

118. Personal Health Information Protection Act 2004, SO 2004, C3, Sec A. Available from: www.ontario.ca

7 Perinatal Medical Ethics, Decision-Making, and Legal Principles

Dominic J. C. Wilkinson, Gregory P. Moore, and Amir M. Zayegh

ETHICAL AND LEGAL PRINCIPLES

Neonatology is full of ethical questions (Table 7.1). The approach to these questions is necessarily different from the approach in other chapters of this book. While scientific evidence can be relevant, answers to ethical questions require values and judgment.

There are various different approaches to answering ethical questions. One approach is to apply a particular ethical theory or framework (e.g., consequentialism or the "four principles" approach (1)) to a problem. There is then a need to decide which ethical theory to apply (and which version of the theory). In this chapter, we are applying a practical, reason-based approach to clinical ethics (2), which can be applied without drawing directly on specific theory. To address ethical dilemmas, one needs to clarify the central ethical question in a particular case, identify the possible actions that could be taken, and evaluate or weigh up the arguments and reasons in favor of different courses of action.

There are some overarching ethical principles that apply in perinatal care and on which there is general agreement internationally. The law often reflects these principles. (We will discuss general legal principles in this chapter; however, we recommend that readers seek advice specific to their local jurisdiction for any legal questions.)

The Best Interests of the Child

Since newborn infants cannot express their wishes or make decisions, there is a need for others to make decisions for them. There is wide agreement that this should be on the basis of their "best interests" (i.e., what course of action would be best for them overall) (3,4). The United Nations convention on the rights of the child states that the child's best interests should be a "primary consideration" when decisions are made about them (5). Law often incorporates this principle. Yet, while acting in the infant's best interests is a laudable goal, it can be extremely challenging to determine what this means in practice. There can be different reasonable views about what would be best. Also, there can be legitimate questions about whether or to what extent the interests of others (e.g., parents, siblings, other neonatal patients, society, etc.) can be taken into account. See Withdrawing Intensive Care (below) for further discussion of best interests in relation to decisions to forego life-prolonging treatment.

Autonomy of Parents

The second, widely accepted, ethical principle relating to newborn care is that parents' view should be sought about treatment decisions. Physicians usually must seek parental consent prior to administering treatments or performing procedures that involve anything more than minimal risk (Table 7.2) (7). There are several reasons to give weight to parents' interests and views in decision-making (8,9). Most societies think that it is good for parents to have significant latitude in deciding how to bring up their child. After the child himself or herself, they are the ones likely to be most affected by those decisions.

Parental freedom to make decisions for and about their children closely resembles the principle of respect for individual autonomy. However, parents' freedom to decide about treatment for their children is necessarily more constrained than their freedom to decide about their own health (7). If respecting parents' wishes would conflict with the best interests of the child, the interests of the child should usually take precedence (Fig. 7.1). In

Continuing Intensive Care (below), we discuss in more detail the challenge of disagreement between parents and health professionals about treatment.

Sanctity of Life

Ethical and legal frameworks relating to newborns (as for older patients) often emphasize the importance of preserving life. This is a valuable principle for health professionals in perinatal care (as in the rest of medicine). Most ethical frameworks, though, also accept that there are limits to this principle. For example, continued life sustaining treatment may be regarded as futile or potentially inappropriate (see Continuing Intensive Care). In the setting of limited resources, providing life-prolonging treatment to one infant may conflict with the ability of professionals to provide treatment for other infants (10). The sanctity of life principle may also be interpreted as prohibiting certain actions (e.g., those that deliberately hasten death) (11). See Withdrawing Intensive Care for discussion of some differences in interpretation of this principle.

Permissibility of Withdrawing or Withholding Life-Prolonging Treatment

Sometimes it may not be in the best interests of the newborn to prolong life, and parents may not wish for the provision of such life-prolonging treatment. Most ethical and many religious frameworks accept that it is not obligatory to prolong life in such circumstances (3,12,13). Clinicians and parents may make decisions not to commence treatment (e.g., withholding resuscitation) or may decide to stop treatment already started (e.g., withdrawing mechanical ventilation). Many ethicists and professional guidelines consider that such decisions are ethically equivalent—if it would be ethical to withhold treatment, it would also be ethical to withdraw the same treatment (if already started, and assuming that all other factors are unchanged) (3,14,15). On the other hand, some ethicists and some religious approaches consider withdrawing treatment a more ethically controversial decision. Parents and health professionals often find withdrawing treatment psychologically more difficult (14).

In contrast, some argue that it may be preferable to withdraw treatment than to withhold it, as that can allow gathering of more evidence of the patient's prognosis or response to treatment (16).

COMMENCING INTENSIVE CARE

Antenatal Consultation

Neonatologists frequently have antenatal consultations with pregnant women/couples when concerning fetal abnormalities have been detected, a maternal condition may adversely affect the fetus, or preterm birth is anticipated. There are different purposes for these consultations, though many will involve more than one purpose. In some settings, the aim is simply to provide information and answer questions about the likely neonatal course and treatment (e.g., surgery) that would be required. In other settings, the consultations inform decisions about management during pregnancy that will ultimately be made by the pregnant woman and her obstetric care providers (e.g., about the timing or mode of delivery, maternal or fetal interventions, or termination of pregnancy). Finally, the consultations may involve discussion and counseling that focuses on determining the plan for neonatal management at delivery, including whether to attempt resuscitation and stabilization of the neonate using all intensive care measures or to

TABLE 7.1
Ethical Questions in Neonatal Care

When?	Which newborn infants should receive treatment? E.g., Which extremely premature infants should be resuscitated?
	When is it ethical to withhold or withdraw life-sustaining treatment?
	When is it ethical to perform a randomized controlled trial?
What?	What decisions are permitted? E.g., Is withdrawing treatment different from withholding treatment? Is it permissible to withhold artificial nutrition and hydration? Is it ethical to hasten dying in newborn infants?
How? Who?	How should decisions about treatment for newborn infants be made?
	Who should have the final say? (What should you do if there is disagreement?)

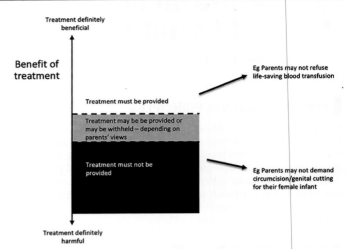

FIGURE 7.1 The role of parents in decisions about medical treatment for a child. If treatment would be harmful for a newborn, it should not be provided, even if parents demand it. If not-receiving treatment would be harmful, treatment must be provided, even if parents refuse consent.

commence a perinatal palliative care plan that includes withholding some (or all) life-sustaining intensive care measures. A final purpose for all such consultations is to develop a trusting relationship between the neonatologist and pregnant woman, as this will optimize any decision-making during the prenatal and postnatal period (17).

One major challenge during antenatal consultations is prognostic uncertainty (18,19). There may be little data on fetal or neonatal outcomes for the specific condition that has been detected. Where there are data, it may be of questionable relevance because it includes a spectrum of severity or comorbidities. There is often the potential for selection bias in published cohorts, since more severely affected fetuses may die due to termination of pregnancy or *in utero* demise. Alternatively, the institution of perinatal palliative care for some fetuses or neonates may result in overly negative outcomes due to self-fulfilling prophecies (20,21). Neonatologists should understand such limitations of published literature and ensure any data use is

TABLE 7.2
Parental Consent in Neonatal Care

Urgency of treatment

Emergency treatment: Treatment usually provided in the best interests of the infant. Providing information/seeking consent at the time not possible. Parents updated afterward (or during, if they are present)

Semiurgent treatment: Parents should be updated and informed prior to treatment

Routine/nonurgent treatment: Usual to inform parents prior to procedures (for some low-risk procedures, consent may be implied, and parents updated when feasible)

Types of consent

Explicit written consent: Usually required for procedures that involve significant risk, or where documentation of consent process is essential, e.g., surgical procedures, research studies

Explicit verbal consent: Usually required for more invasive procedures that are routinely provided as part of neonatal care (but where risk is not so great as to require written informed consent), e.g., lumbar puncture, blood transfusion

Implicit consent: Especially for routine, low risk, minimally invasive procedures/investigations. Where parents have indicated their agreement to admission for neonatal care, consent is often inferred for such treatments, e.g., insertion of nasogastric tube, measurement of blood glucose or other routine blood tests, x-ray

Adapted with permission from British Association of Perinatal Medicine. *Enhancing shared decision-making in neonatal care: a framework for practice.* 2019. Available from: https://hubble-live-assets.s3.amazonaws.com/bapm/attachment/file/180/Shared_Making_in_Neonatal_Care.pdf

ethically sound by explaining to women the extent of any uncertainty and avoiding framing bias (e.g., stating both the survival rate and mortality rate).

Where antenatal consultations may inform obstetric decision-making, disagreement can occur as the ethical perspectives and priorities of neonatologists (particularly focused on fetal and neonatal well-being) may differ from those of obstetricians (focused on maternal and fetal well-being) (22). Collaborative discussions between the health care providers involved in a given case will support families as they consider the various options during decision-making. On occasion, families may ask neonatologists, "What would you do?" Neonatologists should carefully explore the reasons for this question before potentially answering it directly (23). There are strong ethical norms that counseling relating to termination of pregnancy should be nondirective (i.e., that counselors should be neutral and avoid influencing decisions to either continue or terminate a pregnancy) (24).

Perinatal Palliative Care

"Perinatal palliative care" refers to holistic, multidisciplinary compassionate care for pregnant women and their families following antenatal diagnosis of a fetal life-limiting condition (25). The care continues beyond the expected delivery of their neonate, providing integrated ongoing support through the pregnancy, delivery, postnatal period, and (where appropriate) bereavement. Table 7.3 lists some situations where it may be considered ethical to manage the baby with a palliative care plan that includes withholding some or all life-sustaining intensive care measures at delivery or postnatally. (See Withdrawing Intensive Care for discussion of the ethical basis for withholding or withdrawing intensive care.)

As part of perinatal palliative care, antenatal consultation with the neonatologist helps understand and clarify the parents' values and priorities, and plan the management for the delivery and early postnatal period. In confirmed life-limiting conditions, decision-making is sometimes more straightforward but counseling and planning still needs care and compassion (26). In potentially life-limiting conditions (Table 7.3), where the diagnosis and/or prognosis are not clear, decision-making is even more challenging. Parallel planning can be crucial in such situations; this enables clinicians to explore care in the event of death *in utero*, death shortly after birth with the withholding of life-sustaining intensive care measures, or survival with potential ongoing palliative care (27). In some situations, there may be a provisional plan to initiate

TABLE 7.3

Situations When Perinatal Palliative Care May Be Considered

Confirmed life-limiting conditions:

Very high chance of death *in utero*, in the newborn period or in early infancy. Diagnosis and prognosis are clear. Examples include (but are not limited to):

- Anencephaly
- Bilateral renal agenesis
- Severe skeletal dysplasia
- Severe osteogenesis imperfecta
- Hydranencephaly
- Holoprosencephaly
- Trisomy 13, 18 (see text)

Potentially life-limiting conditions:

Significant chance of death *in utero*, in the newborn period, or early infancy. Diagnosis and/or prognosis are not always clear. Examples include (but are not limited to):

- Severe multicystic dysplastic kidneys and oligohydramnios
- Severe hydrocephalus
- Severe congenital cardiac conditions that may not be amenable to surgery, or only with severe morbidity
- Severe fetal cardiomyopathy
- Hydrops fetalis

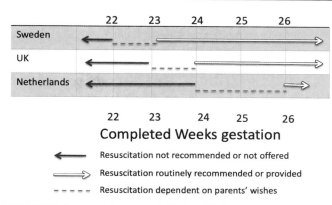

FIGURE 7.2 Gestational age thresholds for initiating intensive care in three Northern European countries. (From British Association of Perinatal Medicine. Enhancing shared decision-making in neonatal care: a framework for practice. 2019. Available from: https://www.bapm.org/resources/158-enhancing-shared-decision-making-in-neonatal-care. Accessed November 13 2020. Ref. (6).

Countries and institutions vary in their thresholds (Fig. 7.2) (37,38). There are common prenatal factors other than gestation that affect an infant's prognosis (e.g., birth weight, sex, multiple pregnancy, use of antenatal steroids, days within week of gestation) (39,40). The result is that infants with the same gestation can have very different prognoses; some infants with a lower gestation can have a better prognosis than other infants with a higher gestation. Guidelines appear to endorse a different ethical standard for decisions than would be permitted in older children (41), perhaps due to a devaluing of preterm infants (42).

The most ethically relevant factor for decisions about the initial care plan is an infant's prognosis. Where possible, clinicians should individualize counseling, using locally relevant outcome data to estimate the outlook for a particular infant. Decisions should not be based on gestational age alone (43). Consideration should be given to initiating intensive care if there is uncertainty regarding the decision as the prognosis of the individual infant may become clearer postnatally (Table 7.4) (44).

There is limited evidence about how best to counsel women facing extremely preterm delivery. A recent systematic review summarizes literature reporting on parents' views of such antenatal consultations (45). One main finding was that parents want the consultations—including the degree of involvement in the decision—individualized based on their needs and situation. First-hand accounts, from those who have experienced such decisions, suggest that prospective parents benefit from empathic efforts to understand their circumstances and priorities and that they do not always value or find helpful statistics or extensive information about the potential complications of prematurity (46). The use of decision aids, including written information, may improve recall

all necessary intensive care measures for stabilization and assess the baby's condition after birth. Time with the baby, further investigations (e.g., metabolic studies, echocardiogram/ultrasound), or assessment of response to treatment may be helpful to support the medical team and family's continued decision-making. Depending on the clinical situation, following confirmation of prognosis and decisions made, intensive care may continue or management may shift to palliative care.

One situation where perinatal palliative care may be considered appropriate is following antenatal diagnosis of trisomy 13 or 18. These conditions used to be regarded as "lethal" anomalies; however, this terminology has been criticized (28). It is now clear that a small proportion of infants survive for more than 1 year, without requiring major medical interventions (29). Survival rates may be higher in infants who receive interventions (including cardiac surgery) (30), and it is more common now for families to request life-prolonging treatment (31). There are challenging ethical questions about how to manage such requests (32). Neonatologists should provide families with balanced information about treatment options and outcomes and engage with them in a process of shared decision-making about treatment (33).

Initiating Intensive Care for Extremely Preterm Infants

Decisions about provision of intensive care or palliative care may arise where extremely preterm birth is anticipated (particularly birth at 22 through 25 weeks of gestation).

Extremely preterm infants have a high mortality rate compared to term infants, even with attempted intensive care. Furthermore, intensive care treatment can be burdensome, prolonged, expensive and, if successful in terms of survival, associated with one or more long-term complications. In many parts of the world, local or national guidelines suggest that below a certain gestation (the "Lower Threshold"), prognosis is so poor that resuscitation should not be offered, while past another point (the "Upper Threshold") resuscitation should be mandatory given the better prognosis (34). One perceived advantage of such guidelines is that they may reduce arbitrary variation in practice between centers or between clinicians.

Yet, there are also problems with this approach, even if guidelines are of adequate quality (35) and implemented properly (36).

TABLE 7.4

Questions to Facilitate an Ethical Approach to Decision-Making Regarding the Initial Care Plan for an Extremely Preterm Infant

Is there a local or national guidance relevant to the decision?

What is the estimated prognosis for this individual infant (is it anticipated to be better or worse than average for infants of this gestation)?

What are parents' values and priorities? (Some parents prioritize survival, others are concerned about the possibility of long-term neurodisability; some value an attempt at intensive care, others want their infant to experience minimal to no suffering)

In the face of uncertainty about outcome (or parents' priorities), is it best to consider providing intensive care initially? If yes, consider changing to palliative care with withdrawal of life-sustaining intensive care measures later if the prognosis subsequently appears poor and parents agree

GENERAL CONSIDERATIONS

and support decision-making (47,48). **Figure 7.3** illustrates some practical guidance for antenatal consultation.

WITHDRAWING INTENSIVE CARE

In many neonatal units, the majority of deaths in neonatal intensive care follow decisions to withhold or discontinue active treatment (49–51). It can be challenging, however, to determine when the outlook for an infant is sufficiently poor that it is ethical to allow them to die. For example, such questions sometimes arise in the care of term newborn infants with severe hypoxic–ischemic encephalopathy, or extremely preterm infants who have developed complications or are not responding to intensive care.

As noted above, it is ethically permissible to forego life-prolonging treatment if that would not be in the child's best interests. There are a number of distinct situations where life-prolonging treatment may not be in a child's best interests (**Table 7.5**). In practice, a combination of these may apply.

Quality of Life

In published studies of end of life decisions in neonatal intensive care units, up to 1/3 of such decisions took place in infants who were stable (51,52). In such cases, assessments of quality of life appear to be playing an important role in the justification for the decision (Table 7.5).

Quality of life decisions in perinatal care are controversial (53). One challenge relates to uncertainty and difficulty in predicting future quality of life. As with antenatal counseling, it may be

TABLE 7.5

Situations in Which It May Be Ethical to Withdraw or Withhold Life-Prolonging Treatment

Reduced Quantity of Life	Reduced Quality of Life
Brain death: An infant has been diagnosed as meeting neurologic criteria for death	Burdensome treatment: Medical treatment that is keeping an infant alive is burdensome and unpleasant and is doing more harm than good overall. E.g., long-term ventilation in severe neuromuscular disorder
Imminent death: An infant is deteriorating despite maximal treatment and is expected to die within minutes or hours even if active medical treatment continues. E.g., infant with sustained severe hypoxia on maximum ventilator settings, or extremely preterm infant not responding to attempted stabilization in delivery room	Burdensome illness: An infant's illness causes them to suffer substantially, and this suffering cannot be adequately relieved by medical treatment. E.g., severe epidermolysis bullosa
Inevitable death: An infant has a life-limiting condition that is likely or certain to lead to death in infancy or early childhood even if active medical treatment continues. E.g., severe metabolic disorder	Lack of benefit: An infant is not necessarily suffering from their illness or from treatment; however, the severity of their condition means that they appear to gain little benefit from life. E.g., profound cognitive impairment/minimally conscious state

Adapted from Larcher V, Craig F, Bhogal K, et al. Making decisions to limit treatment in life-limiting and life-threatening conditions in children: a framework for practice. *Arch Dis Child* 2015;100(Suppl 2):s1. doi: 10.1136/archdischild-2014-306666.

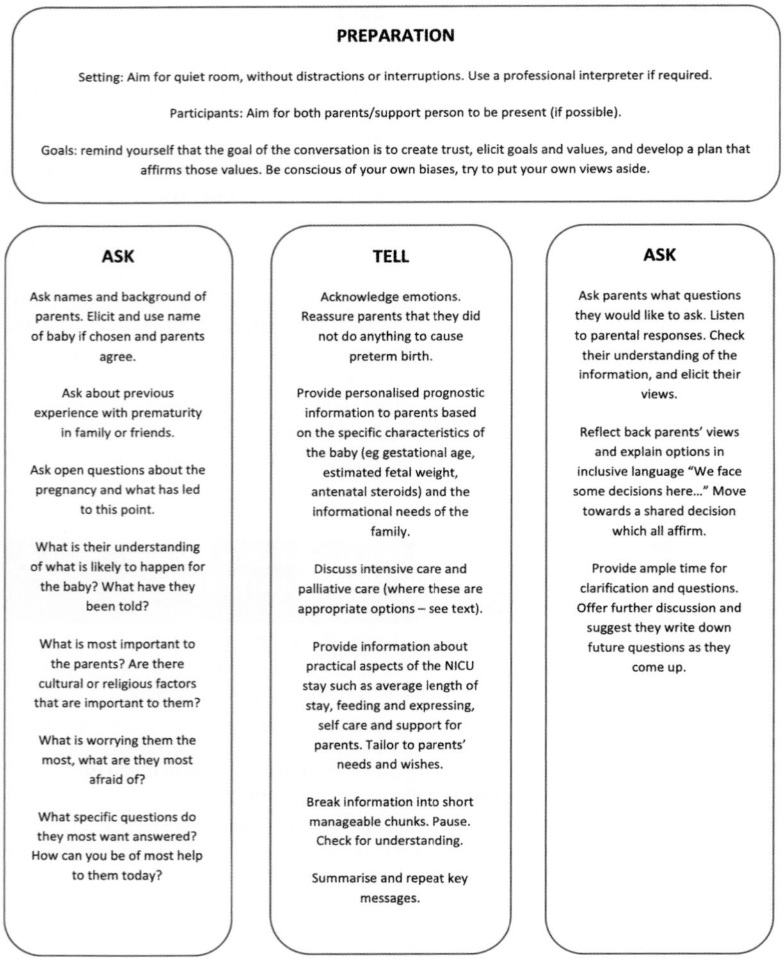

FIGURE 7.3 A practical guide to antenatal consultations prior to extremely preterm delivery.

PREPARATION

Setting: Aim for quiet room, without distractions or interruptions. Use a professional interpreter if required.

Participants: Aim for both parents/support person to be present (if possible).

Goals: remind yourself that the goal of the conversation is to create trust, elicit goals and values, and develop a plan that affirms those values. Be conscious of your own biases, try to put your own views aside.

ASK

Ask names and background of parents. Elicit and use name of baby if chosen and parents agree.

Ask about previous experience with prematurity in family or friends.

Ask open questions about the pregnancy and what has led to this point.

What is their understanding of what is likely to happen for the baby? What have they been told?

What is most important to the parents? Are there cultural or religious factors that are important to them?

What is worrying them the most, what are they most afraid of?

What specific questions do they most want answered? How can you be of most help to them today?

TELL

Acknowledge emotions. Reassure parents that they did not do anything to cause preterm birth.

Provide personalised prognostic information to parents based on the specific characteristics of the baby (eg gestational age, estimated fetal weight, antenatal steroids) and the informational needs of the family.

Discuss intensive care and palliative care (where these are appropriate options – see text).

Provide information about practical aspects of the NICU stay such as average length of stay, feeding and expressing, self care and support for parents. Tailor to parents' needs and wishes.

Break information into short manageable chunks. Pause. Check for understanding.

Summarise and repeat key messages.

ASK

Ask parents what questions they would like to ask. Listen to parental responses. Check their understanding of the information, and elicit their views.

Reflect back parents' views and explain options in inclusive language "We face some decisions here..." Move towards a shared decision which all affirm.

Provide ample time for clarification and questions. Offer further discussion and suggest they write down future questions as they come up.

difficult to find studies that are relevant and reliable regarding the outcome (54,55), particularly for infants with rare life-limiting conditions (56). There may be a range of severity of possible outcomes. Where there is outcome data (57,58), there is often little specific information on the quality of life of surviving children.

Furthermore, there is some evidence suggesting that as a group, health care professionals evaluate the quality of life of disabled children more negatively than parents, or than the children/young people themselves (59). Other literature has pointed to a "disability paradox": individuals with disabilities that would be judged (by others) to be very severe, nevertheless report positive levels of well-being and quality of life (60).

It is not surprising that there can sometimes be disagreements between professionals and between professionals and families about decisions to withdraw intensive care treatment on the basis of predicted quality of life (61). Such decisions should be taken following careful consideration, be based on the best available information and evidence, and fully involve parents (62).

Analgesia and Sedation

Symptom control is an important part of end of life care. Judicious use of analgesics such as opioids is widely accepted as ethically permissible (63). This is sometimes justified by drawing on the ethical "doctrine of double effect" (64,65). According to this principle, actions taken with good intention (e.g., to relieve symptoms) are ethically permitted even if they sometimes have unintended side effects (e.g., respiratory depression). In fact, recent evidence suggests that this doctrine may often be unnecessary in palliative care. There is some evidence in adults (and a little in infants) that such agents, titrated to the patient's symptoms, do not hasten death (66–68). Yet, sometimes health professionals give higher doses of analgesia/sedation, with the aim to hasten death (69). That would not be sanctioned by the doctrine of double effect and is not legal in many jurisdictions (70).

Withdrawal of Artificial Nutrition and Hydration

Where infants have predicted poor prognosis, but are not dependent on respiratory support, questions sometimes arise about provision of other potentially life-prolonging treatment. For example, profoundly neurologically compromised infants may not be able to safely coordinate sucking and swallowing and hence be permanently dependent on feeding via external tubes (oro/nasogastric/gastrostomy). In such infants, artificial feeding is a life-prolonging intervention and may be judged not to be in the best interests of some infants.

Professional guidance (3,71) has accepted that artificial feeding, like all other medical treatments, should be evaluated on its merits; in some circumstances, the burdens may outweigh the benefits and hence it may be withheld or withdrawn (72). Where this occurs, however, the dying phase may be drawn out, and both family members and clinical staff may find the process extremely difficult (73). There is a need to forewarn parents and to draw on the expertise of specialized palliative care teams in supporting the infant, parents, and staff.

Active Ending of Life

Where the end of life phase for an infant may be protracted and distressing, some ethicists have argued that it would be preferable to hasten death rather than withdrawing or withholding life-prolonging treatment (74). Few jurisdictions permit active ending of life in newborn infants. In the Netherlands, it is lawful if specific criteria have been met (75). Two distinct practices have been described. In infants who have been extubated as part of palliative care and who are "gasping," neonatologists have sometimes administered neuromuscular blockers to alleviate parental distress and shorten the dying phase (76). This has been described in 13% to 24% of dying infants in Dutch intensive care units (66,77) though may be less common in recent years (78). A separate process (the Groningen Protocol) has been described for infants who are not dependent on respiratory support, are not actively dying, but are perceived to be suffering unbearably without hope of this suffering being relieved. In such situations (with parental consent, and following the assessment of an independent physician) neonatologists in The Netherlands have ended the life of infants (e.g., in an infant with severe epidermolysis bullosa) (78,79). Cases must be reported to an expert panel, and the prosecutor subsequently makes a decision whether or not to prosecute. These legal provisions appear have been used only rarely in The Netherlands (78,79).

Organ Donation

While organ donation after death has been a relatively common option in adult or pediatric intensive care, until recently it has rarely occurred in newborns. Some newborn infants, though, may be eligible to donate organs (e.g., en bloc kidneys, hepatocyte/liver, or even heart) (80).

This can occur following diagnosis of brain death. It is rare for newborn infants to meet neurologic criteria for death, partly because open sutures and fontanelles limit acute increases in intracranial pressure and prevent coning. Nevertheless, recent guidance accepts that newborn infants at or close to term may be diagnosed with brain death on the basis of the same criteria as in older children/adults (81,82).

Infants may also be able to donate solid organs after diagnosis of death by circulatory criteria (i.e., irreversible cessation of circulation) (83). This can occur in infants who have respiratory support withdrawn and who develop asystole within a short period (e.g., up to 1 hour) after extubation (84). There are often practical limits on organ donation relating to the size of infants, which mean that organ donation is usually restricted to term or near-term infants.

Widely accepted ethical principles governing organ donation in infants include that donation is only possible after death, decisions to withdraw treatment should be separated from decisions about donation, and parental consent is necessary for donation to occur (85).

CONTINUING INTENSIVE CARE

Potentially Inappropriate Treatment

One of the most frequent sources of ethical discomfort in neonatal intensive care arises when parents wish life-prolonging treatment to continue, but health professionals believe that it would be better to discontinue this treatment and allow the infant to die.

Sometimes health professionals express the view that further life-prolonging treatment would be futile. The concept of medical futility arose as an attempt to resolve or to avoid disputes like this (86). It reflects a perceived need by doctors to set limits on patient or family autonomy and a way to justify a decision not to provide life-sustaining treatment (87).

What does it mean for treatment to be "futile"? There are multiple different ways that futility has been interpreted. All of these have been criticized (88,89). A distinction has been made between a higher medical concept of futility and the stricter physiologic definition often used in law (61). The former describes treatments as futile when they have no hope of curing the patient's illness or alleviating their suffering. The latter describes a treatment as futile when it will be ineffective and provide no benefit to the patient (89).

The most frequent criticism is that despite its air of objectivity, a determination that treatment is futile is subjective and based on the values of the doctor or medical team (89). For example, treatment is sometimes judged futile because the chance of recovery is very small (e.g., 0.5%) ("quantitative futility") (90). Yet some parents would regard this chance as worth taking if there were a possibility of recovery or long-term survival and the alternative were death. At other times, treatment may be judged *qualitatively* futile, because the infant's current and predicted future quality of life is so poor (90). As the above discussion in Withdrawing Intensive Care makes clear, the nature of quality of life judgments makes it hard to define or determine with confidence a level of quality of life that would justify unilaterally withholding treatment.

Recent guidelines have encouraged a shift from referring to "futile" treatment, to denoting treatment as "potentially inappropriate" (91). This language reflects both the uncertainty and value-based nature of such determinations.

There are two distinct ethical reasons for professionals not to provide treatment that parents strongly desire. First, such treatment may be judged to be contrary to the infant's best interests. Professionals may judge that continued treatment would harm the infant. The second, and more controversial, justification is that providing treatment would be harmful to other patients (92). In a setting of limited resources (e.g., intensive care beds), providing treatment to a patient with an extremely low chance of benefit would mean denying treatment to other patients with a significantly greater chance of benefit (93,94). Sometimes both of these reasons may be present (95). The ethical approach to addressing requests for potentially inappropriate treatment is different, depending on which of these reasons applies (61).

Moral Distress

With the increasing ability to prolong life with intensive care support, medical and nursing staff in the neonatal intensive care unit encounter an increasing number of ethically confronting situations where they believe that continuing intensive care may not be in the infant's best interests (96). Moral distress is defined as a situation where an individual makes a clear moral judgment but is unable to act according to it, due to institutional, societal, or contextual barriers (97). Moral dilemmas, in contrast, occur when multiple ethical judgments are competing, with uncertainty about the correct action to take (98). Moral distress is important as it has been linked with a compromise of personal integrity, dissatisfaction within the workplace, burnout of staff, and a negative impact on patient care (99,100). While it is mostly described in relation to nursing staff, intensive care physicians may have similar rates of moral distress (96).

In a pluralistic society and given the challenge of determining when continued treatment is potentially inappropriate, some moral distress may be inevitable. Moral distress may also be productive in promoting thoughtfulness and deliberation in ethically difficult or uncertain cases, and in questioning current practice as medical technologies advance (101).

Given its negative effects on some intensive care staff and intensive care unit morale, measures to reduce moral distress in neonatal care are being explored (102). While evidence to guide recommendations is limited, improving the ethical environment of intensive care units appears to be important. Multidisciplinary meetings facilitated by a senior clinician or ethicist can encourage members of staff to voice their views and to feel empowered to advocate for the patient (103). It is also useful to help staff to differentiate distress felt due to the nature of the patient's condition from distress due to the presence of conflicting moral views. Clinical education to improve staff awareness of the outcomes of patients and ethical education on the range of reasonable ethical views have also been suggested, although conflicting data exist as to whether this reduces or increases moral distress given the uncertainty and subjectivity involved in these difficult situations (104,105).

Resolving Disagreement

Protracted cases of disagreement between parents and health care teams can be damaging for families, professionals, and infants (106). Table 7.6 lists some of the landmark court cases in the United States and united Kingdom arising from conflict between health professionals and parents. It is important, where possible, to identify and aim to resolve disagreement at an early stage, as conflicts can become entrenched over time (120). A structured resolution approach to resolving disagreements may be helpful (Fig. 7.4). The aim is to separate fact-based from value-based disagreements, to obtain additional information or perspectives to help both sides to understand each other, and to apply a fair due process to resolve disputes (Fig. 7.5) (121). If health professionals and parents are unable to reach agreement, the court may have a role to play in arbitrating and reaching a decision in the best interests of the infant.

OTHER ETHICAL ISSUES

Ethical issues in perinatal care go beyond questions of life and death. As in the rest of pediatrics and medicine, there can be a wide range of ethical questions, such as those relating to confidentiality, capacity (e.g., where parents' decision-making abilities may be compromised), resource allocation, or genetic testing. For the most part, the ethical approach to these questions for newborn infants will be identical to the approach taken elsewhere in pediatrics. One ethical issue that differs in some respects is neonatal research ethics.

Research Ethics

There are many questions in neonatology for which there is little scientific evidence, or the evidence is conflicting. There have been, unfortunately, a number of prominent examples in the history of neonatology where treatments have been provided with good intention but have later been shown to be harmful (122–124). This gives rise to a strong ethical reason to conduct research in the neonatal intensive care unit and to rigorously evaluate existing and novel therapies (125,126).

One potentially challenging area is to determine when it would be ethical to conduct a trial. Because infants are unable to consent to participation, research is typically only permitted if the risk to the infant is deemed to be very low (127). How should doctors or researchers assess if the risk is low enough? There may be opposing risks in trials of new therapies: a risk of missing out on the benefit of the new treatment (if randomized to standard care and the new treatment is effective) or a risk of harm from the new treatment (if it is harmful overall). Treatment provided as standard care frequently varies in and between neonatal units. Trials comparing these different ways of treating infants may or may not be perceived as risky. In a large international trial (the SUPPORT Oxygen trial), preterm infants were randomized to have their oxygen saturation level targeted within one of two commonly used ranges: a higher or a lower range. At the time, neonatal units varied in the range they routinely used. The trial found a significantly lower mortality rate in infants with the high target. Some experts strongly criticized the researchers for potentially placing infants at risk through the trial (128,129). Others argued that this risk was not predictable at the time of commencing the trial; infants enrolled in the trial were not placed at higher risk by being involved in the research (130,131).

One principle, commonly cited in research ethics, is that a controlled trial may proceed if there is equipoise. This means clinicians are generally unsure which treatment would be superior such that they have equal reason to give either (132,133). Yet, equipoise can be hard to obtain for many therapies that need evaluation. There can be more reason in favor of one treatment than the other (but it is not conclusive, or the reasoning remains arguable), or, some professionals may strongly favor a new treatment, while others

TABLE 7.6

Landmark Legal Cases of Conflict in the NICU

Year of Clinical Case/Birth of Neonate	Case or Child Name	Clinical Situation	Outcome
1971	"Johns Hopkins Case" (107)	Trisomy 21 with duodenal atresia. Parents refused permission for corrective surgery.	Parental wishes prioritized above all else; infant died after withholding of hydration and nutrition.
1974	*Maine Medical Center v. Houle* (108)	Multiple anomalies including trachea-esophageal fistula. Parents and treating doctor decided to forego treatment. Other physicians objected.	Right to life (of neonate) prioritized above all else. Infant died following surgical repair.
1976	Andrew Stinson (109,110)	24 weeks gestation, 800 g preterm infant. Developed multiple complications. Parents did not wish for intensive treatment, however, doctors refused to withdraw treatment.	Patient eventually died following accidental extubation. Parents published book describing their experience.
1982	Baby Doe (111–114)	Trisomy 21 with esophageal atresia and trachea-esophageal fistula. Parents declined consent for surgery.	Parental wishes prioritized by the courts; patient died without surgery at 6 days of life. Federal legislation ("Baby Doe Regulations") after this case prioritized right to life above parental wishes or disability/quality of life considerations.
1992	Baby K (115,116)	Anencephaly. Parents wishing for intensive care to continue, while health professionals were opposed.	Medical stabilization at mother's request was required since it wasn't considered futile (i.e. neonate would live and could be extubated and continue to live); after repeated stabilizations, died at 2.5 years of age.
2000	Jodie and Mary (117)	Conjoined twins, joined at the abdomen. If they remained conjoined, both predicted to die. If separated, one would die. Parents refused consent for separation. Doctors wished to proceed with surgery.	Court approved surgery separating twins. One twin survived.
2004	Sun Hudson (118,119)	Thanatophoric dysplasia Type 1 on mechanical ventilation.	Final court decision approved withdrawal of life-sustaining therapy against parents' wishes; patient died when ventilator was removed at 5 months of age.
2016	Charlie Gard (61)	Infantile onset encephalomyopathic mitochondrial DNA depletion syndrome. Parents wished for continuing intensive care and transfer to United States for experimental treatment. Health professionals opposed to this.	Final court decision supported withdrawal of life-sustaining therapy without experimental treatment. Infant died after withdrawal of life-sustaining treatment.

strongly favor the alternative. This is particularly challenging for therapies for which evidence is emerging gradually. When is the evidence enough? Equipoise can be particularly difficult to achieve for potentially life-saving interventions for infants who are extremely unwell. One example was the controversy over trials of extra-corporeal membrane oxygenation (ECMO) in the 1990s (134,135). Physicians in the United Kingdom were uncertain about the overall benefits compared to harms of ECMO and commenced the UK Collaborative ECMO trial in 1993. In contrast, U.S. neonatologists at that time were already convinced of the benefits of ECMO and

believed that the available evidence was sufficient to make such trials unethical (136). The UK trial was completed and found a significantly lower mortality in infants randomized to ECMO: it led to the establishment of a national ECMO service for newborns (137).

An alternative way of understanding "equipoise" is the concept of "clinical equipoise" (133). This refers to a situation where there is uncertainty across a community of professionals; individual doctors may be certain, but there are opposing views on the benefit of treatment. (There appeared to be clinical equipoise at the time of the ECMO trials and the SUPPORT trial.)

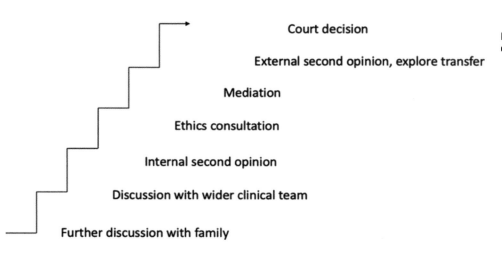

Court decision

External second opinion, explore transfer

Mediation

Ethics consultation

Internal second opinion

Discussion with wider clinical team

Further discussion with family

FIGURE 7.4 A stepwise approach to resolve disagreements.

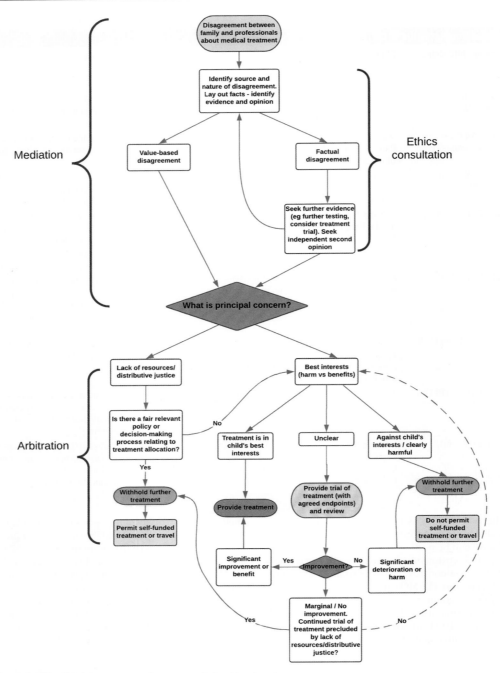

FIGURE 7.5 Mediation and arbitration in response to disagreement about treatment.

The second challenging area for ethics in neonatal research relates to consent (138). As noted above in Ethical and Legal Principles, parental consent is necessary prior to many interventions. It is particularly important for interventions that health care professionals consider optional. Yet, obtaining consent for neonatal research can be challenging. For interventions that are required very soon after birth, it may be difficult or impossible to obtain consent in time. Two options are to: (a) say that research cannot take place in such circumstances or (b) only perform it where consent has taken place antenatally. The first option would result in an inability to study potentially life-saving interventions. The second option may introduce selection bias since antenatal consent is only possible in a subgroup of cases. Because of these challenges, neither option is ideal. Another ethically acceptable option for some trials of newborn

resuscitation is to *waive* the requirement for informed consent prior to participation (139). In that situation, parents are usually informed about the research subsequently and given the option of withdrawing their child (and their child's data) from the study. There is some evidence that parents who have been involved in such studies have found the process of waiving or deferring consent acceptable (140).

REFERENCES

1. Beauchamp TL, Childress JF. *Principles of biomedical ethics*, 7th ed. New York/Oxford: Oxford University Press, 2012.
2. Wilkinson D, Herring J, Savulescu J. *Medical ethics and law: a core curriculum for the 21st century*. Edinburgh: Elsevier, 2019.
3. Larcher V, Craig F, Bhogal K, et al. Making decisions to limit treatment in life-limiting and life-threatening conditions in children: a framework

for practice. *Arch Dis Child* 2015;100(Suppl 2):s1. doi: 10.1136/archdis-child-2014-306666

4. Kopelman LM. The best-interests standard as threshold, ideal, and standard of reasonableness. *J Med Philos* 1997;22(3):271.

5. United Nations Human Rights. Convention on the Rights of the Child. 2002. Available from: http://www.ohchr.org/EN/ProfessionalInterest/Pages/CRC.aspx

6. British Association of Perinatal Medicine. Enhancing shared decision-making in neonatal care: a framework for practice (Draft). 2019. Available from: https://www.bapm.org/resources/draft-framework-enhancing-shared-decision-making-neonatal-care?tQSafariFixApplied=true. Accessed October 9, 2019.

7. Katz AL, Webb SA. Informed consent in decision-making in pediatric practice. *Pediatrics* 2016;138(2):e20161485. doi: 10.1542/peds.2016-1485

8. Navin MC, Wasserman JA. Reasons to amplify the role of parental permission in pediatric treatment. *Am J Bioeth* 2017;17(11):6. doi: 10.1080/15265161.2017.1378752

9. Wilkinson D. How much weight should we give to parental interests in decisions about life support for newborn infants? *Monash Bioeth Rev* 2010;29(2):13.1. doi: 10.2104/mber1013

10. Wilkinson D, Petrou S, Savulescu J. Rationing potentially inappropriate treatment in newborn intensive care in developed countries. *Semin Fetal Neonatal Med* 2018;23(1):52. doi: 10.1016/j.siny.2017.10.004

11. Koch T. Does the "sanctity of human life" doctrine sanctify humanness, or life? *Camb Q Healthc Ethics* 1999;8(4):557.

12. Weise KL, Okun AL, Carter BS, et al. Guidance on forgoing life-sustaining medical treatment. *Pediatrics* 2017;140(3):e20171905. doi: 10.1542/peds.2017-1905

13. Bülow H-H, Sprung CL, Reinhart K, et al. The world's major religions' points of view on end-of-life decisions in the intensive care unit. *Intensive Care Med* 2008;34(3):423. doi: 10.1007/s00134-007-0973-8

14. Wilkinson D, Butcherine E, Savulescu J. Withdrawal aversion and the equivalence test. *Am J Bioeth* 2019;19(3):21. doi: https://doi.org/10.1080/15265161.2019.1574465

15. Sulmasy LS, Bledsoe TA; for the ACP Ethics, Professionalism and Human Rights Committee. American College of Physicians Ethics Manual: Seventh Edition ACP Ethics Manual. *Ann Intern Med* 2019;170(2_Supplement):S1. doi: 10.7326/m18-2160

16. Vincent JL. Withdrawing may be preferable to withholding. *Critical Care (London, England)* 2005;9(3):226.

17. von Hauff P, Long K, Taylor B, et al. Antenatal consultation for parents whose child may require admission to neonatal intensive care: a focus group study for media design. *BMC Pregnancy Childbirth* 2016;16(1):103.

18. Wilkinson D. *Death or disability? The Carmentis Machine and treatment decisions for critically ill children.* Oxford: OUP, 2013.

19. Rysavy MA. Prognosis as an intervention. *Clin Perinatol* 2018;45(2):231.

20. Mercurio MR. Physicians' refusal to resuscitate at borderline gestational age. *J Perinatol* 2005;25(11):685. doi: 10.1038/sj.jp.7211395

21. Wilkinson D. The self-fulfilling prophecy in intensive care. *Theor Med Bioeth* 2009;30(6):401. doi: 10.1007/s11017-009-9120-6

22. Brown SD, Donelan K, Martins Y, et al. Does professional orientation predict ethical sensitivities? Attitudes of paediatric and obstetric specialists toward fetuses, pregnant women and pregnancy termination. *J Med Ethics* 2014;40(2):117.

23. Tucker EB, Torke A, Helft P, et al. Doctor, what would you do? An answer for patients requesting advice about value-laden decisions. *Pediatrics* 2015;136(4):740.

24. Elwyn G, Gray J, Clarke A. Shared decision making and non-directiveness in genetic counselling. *J Med Genet* 2000;37(2):135.

25. Carter B. Pediatric palliative care in infants and neonates. *Children* 2018;5(2):21.

26. Sidgwick P, Harrop E, Kelly B, et al. Fifteen-minute consultation: perinatal palliative care. *Arch Dis Child Educ Pract* 2017;102(3):114.

27. Marty CM, Carter BS. Ethics and palliative care in the perinatal world. *Semin Fetal Neonatal Med* 2018;23(1):35.

28. Wilkinson D, de Crespigny L, Xafis V. Ethical language and decision-making for prenatally diagnosed lethal malformations. *Semin Fetal Neonatal Med* 2014;19(5):306. doi: http://dx.doi.org/10.1016/j.siny.2014.08.007

29. Cereda A, Carey JC. The trisomy 18 syndrome. *Orphanet J Rare Dis* 2012;7(1):81.

30. Lorenz JM, Hardart GE. Evolving medical and surgical management of infants with trisomy 18. *Curr Opin Pediatr* 2014;26(2):169. doi: 10.1097/MOP.0000000000000076

31. Haug S, Goldstein M, Cummins D, et al. Using patient-centered care after a prenatal diagnosis of trisomy 18 or trisomy 13: a review. *JAMA Pediatr* 2017;171(4):382. doi: 10.1001/jamapediatrics.2016.4798

32. Kukora S, Firn J, Laventhal N, et al. Infant with trisomy 18 and hypoplastic left heart syndrome. *Pediatrics* 2019;143(5):e20183779.

33. Andrews SE, Downey AG, Showalter DS, et al. Shared decision making and the pathways approach in the prenatal and postnatal management of the trisomy 13 and trisomy 18 syndromes. *Am J Med Genet C Semin Med Genet* 2016;172(3):257.

34. Wilkinson D. The grey zone in neonatal treatment decisions. In: McDougall R, Delany C, Gillam L, eds. *Parents, ethics and healthcare decision-making.* Melbourne: Federation Press, 2016.

35. Binepal N, Lemyre B, Dunn S, et al. Systematic review and quality appraisal of international guidelines on perinatal care of extremely premature infants. *Curr Pediatr Rev* 2015;11(2):126.

36. Moore G, Reszel J, Daboval T, et al. Qualitative evaluation of a guideline supporting shared decision making for extreme preterm birth. *J Matern Fetal Neonatal Med* 2020;33(6):973.

37. Guillen U, Weiss EM, Munson D, et al. Guidelines for the management of extremely premature deliveries: a systematic review. *Pediatrics* 2015;136(2):343. doi: 10.1542/peds.2015-0542

38. Rysavy MA, Li L, Bell EF, et al. Between-hospital variation in treatment and outcomes in extremely preterm infants. *N Engl J Med* 2015;372(19):1801. doi: 10.1056/NEJMoa1410689

39. Tyson JE, Parikh NA, Langer J, et al. Intensive care for extreme prematurity—moving beyond gestational age. *N Engl J Med* 2008;358(16):1672. doi: 10.1056/NEJMoa073059

40. Nguyen TP, Amon E, Al-Hosni M, et al. "Early" versus "late" 23-week infant outcomes. *Am J Obstet Gynecol* 2012;207(3):226.e1.

41. Janvier A, Barrington KJ, Aziz K, et al. Ethics ain't easy: do we need simple rules for complicated ethical decisions? *Acta Paediatr* 2008;97(4):402. doi: 10.1111/j.1651-2227.2008.00752.x

42. Janvier A, Leblanc I, Barrington KJ. Nobody likes premies: the relative value of patients' lives. *J Perinatol* 2008;28:821. doi: 10.1038/jp.2008.103

43. Wilkinson DJ. Gestational ageism. *Arch Pediatr Adolesc Med* 2012;166(6):567. doi: 10.1001/archpediatrics.2011.1262

44. Andrews B, Myers P, Lagatta J, et al. A comparison of prenatal and postnatal models to predict outcomes at the border of viability. *J Pediatr* 2016;173:96.

45. Kharrat A, Moore GP, Beckett S, et al. Antenatal consultations at extreme prematurity: a systematic review of parent communication needs. *J Pediatr* 2018;196:109.

46. Staub K, Baardsnes J, Hebert N, et al. Our child is not just a gestational age. A first-hand account of what parents want and need to know before premature birth. *Acta Paediatr* 2014;103(10):1035. doi: 10.1111/apa.12716

47. Guillen U, Suh S, Munson D, et al. Development and pretesting of a decision-aid to use when counseling parents facing imminent extreme premature delivery. *J Pediatr* 2012;160(3):382. doi: S0022-3476(11)00900-0 [pii] 10.1016/j.jpeds.2011.08.070

48. Moore GP, Lemyre B, Daboval T, et al. Field testing of decision coaching with a decision aid for parents facing extreme prematurity. *J Perinatol* 2017;37(6):728. doi: 10.1038/jp.2017.29

49. Hellmann J, Knighton R, Lee SK, et al. Neonatal deaths: prospective exploration of the causes and process of end-of-life decisions. *Arch Dis Child Fetal Neonatal Ed* 2016;101(2):F102. doi: 10.1136/archdischild-2015-308425

50. Aladangady N, Shaw C, Gallagher K, et al. Short-term outcome of treatment limitation discussions for newborn infants, a multicentre prospective observational cohort study. *Arch Dis Child Fetal Neonatal Ed* 2017;102(2):F104. doi: 10.1136/archdischild-2016-310723

51. Verhagen A, Janvier A, Leuthner S, et al. Categorizing neonatal deaths: a cross-cultural study in the United States, Canada, and The Netherlands. *J Pediatr* 2010;156(1):33. doi: 10.1016/j.jpeds.2009.07.019

52. Lam V, Kain N, Joynt C, et al. A descriptive report of end-of-life care practices occurring in two neonatal intensive care units. *Palliat Med* 2016;30(10):971. doi: 10.1177/0269216316634246

53. Camosy C. *Too expensive to treat? Finitude, tragedy and the neonatal ICU.* Grand Rapids, MI: Eerdmans, 2010.

54. Wilkinson D. Magnetic resonance imaging and withdrawal of life support from newborn infants with hypoxic-ischemic encephalopathy. *Pediatrics* 2010;126(2):e451. doi: 10.1542/peds.2009-3067

55. Rysavy MA, Tyson JE. The problem and promise of prognosis research. *JAMA Pediatr* 2016;170(5):411. doi: 10.1001/jamapediatrics.2015.4871

56. Kukora S, Gollehon N, Weiner G, et al. Prognostic accuracy of antenatal neonatology consultation. *J Perinatol* 2017;37(1):27. doi: 10.1038/jp.2016.171

57. James J, Munson D, DeMauro SB, et al. Outcomes of preterm infants following discussions about withdrawal or withholding of life support. *J Pediatr* 2017;190:118. doi: 10.1016/j.jpeds.2017.05.056

58. Brecht M, Wilkinson DJ. The outcome of treatment limitation discussions in newborns with brain injury. *Arch Dis Child Fetal Neonatal Ed* 2015;100(2):F155. doi: 10.1136/archdischild-2014-307399

59. Saigal S, Stoskopf B, Pinelli J, et al. Self-perceived health-related quality of life of former extremely low birth weight infants at young adulthood. *Pediatrics* 2006;118(3):1140. doi: 10.1542/peds.2006-0119

60. Albrecht GL, Devlieger PJ. The disability paradox: high quality of life against all odds. *Soc Sci Med* 1999;48(8):977.

61. Wilkinson D, Savulescu J. *Ethics, conflict and medical treatment for children: from disagreement to dissensus.* London: Elsevier, 2018.

62. Janvier A, Barrington K, Farlow B. Communication with parents concerning withholding or withdrawing of life-sustaining interventions in neonatology. *Semin Perinatol* 2014;38(1):38. doi: 10.1053/j.semperi.2013.07.007

GENERAL CONSIDERATIONS

63. Mancuso T, Burns J. Ethical concerns in the management of pain in the neonate. *Paediatr Anaesth* 2009;19(10):953. doi: 10.1111/j.1460-9592.2009.03144.x

64. Frey R. The doctrine of double effect. In: Frey R, Wellman C, eds. *A companion to applied ethics.* Malden, MA: Blackwell Publishing, 2005:464.

65. McIntyre A. The double life of double effect. *Theor Med Bioeth* 2004;25(1):61.

66. Janvier A, Meadow W, Leuthner SR, et al. Whom are we comforting? An analysis of comfort medications delivered to dying neonates. *J Pediatr* 2011;159(2):206. doi: 10.1016/j.jpeds.2011.01.022

67. Thorns A, Sykes N. Opioid use in last week of life and implications for end-of-life decision-making. *Lancet* 2000;356(9227):398. doi: 10.1016/S0140-6736(00)02534-4

68. Maltoni M, Pittureri C, Scarpi E, et al. Palliative sedation therapy does not hasten death: results from a prospective multicenter study. *Ann Oncol* 2009;20(7):1163. doi: 10.1093/annonc/mdp048

69. Provoost V, Cools F, Bilsen J, et al. The use of drugs with a life-shortening effect in end-of-life care in neonates and infants. *Intensive Care Med* 2006;32(1):133. doi: 10.1007/s00134-005-2863-2

70. Meisel A, Snyder L, Quill T. Seven legal barriers to end-of-life care: myths, realities, and grains of truth. *JAMA* 2000;284(19):2495.

71. Diekema DS, Botkin JR. Clinical report—forgoing medically provided nutrition and hydration in children. *Pediatrics* 2009;124(2):813.

72. Carter BS, Leuthner SR. The ethics of withholding/withdrawing nutrition in the newborn. *Semin Perinatol* 2003;27(6):480.

73. Hellmann J, Williams C, Ives-Baine L, et al. Withdrawal of artificial nutrition and hydration in the neonatal intensive care unit: parental perspectives. *Arch Dis Child Fetal Neonatal Ed* 2013;98(1):F21. doi: 10.1136/fetalneonatal-2012-301658

74. Kuhse H. Death by non-feeding: not in the baby's best interests. *J Med Humanit Bioeth* 1986;7(2):79.

75. Verhagen E, Sauer PJ. The Groningen protocol—euthanasia in severely ill newborns. *N Engl J Med* 2005;352(10):959. doi: 10.1056/NEJMp058026

76. Willems DL, Verhagen AA, van Wijlick E, et al. Infants' best interests in end-of-life care for newborns. *Pediatrics* 2014;134(4):e1163. doi: 10.1542/peds.2014-0780

77. Koper JF, Bos AF, Janvier A, et al. Dutch neonatologists have adopted a more interventionist approach to neonatal care. *Acta Paediatr* 2015;104(9):888. doi: 10.1111/apa.13050

78. ten Cate K, van de Vathorst S, Onwuteaka-Philipsen BD, et al. End-of-life decisions for children under 1 year of age in the Netherlands: decreased frequency of administration of drugs to deliberately hasten death. *J Med Ethics* 2015;41(10):795. doi: 10.1136/medethics-2014-102562

79. Eduard Verhagen AA. Neonatal euthanasia: lessons from the Groningen Protocol. *Semin Fetal Neonatal Med* 2014;19(5):296. doi: 10.1016/j.siny.2014.08.002

80. Charles E, Scales A, Brierley J. The potential for neonatal organ donation in a children's hospital. *Arch Dis Child Fetal Neonatal Ed* 2014;99(3):F225. doi: 10.1136/archdischild-2013-304803

81. Royal College of Paediatrics and Child Health. The diagnosis of death by neurological criteria (DNC) in infants less than two months old. 2015 [updated April 2015]. Available from: http://www.rcpch.ac.uk/improving-child-health/clinical-guidelines-and-standards/published-rcpch/death-neurological-criteria

82. Nakagawa TA, Ashwal S, Mathur M, et al. Guidelines for the determination of brain death in infants and children: an update of the 1987 Task Force recommendations. *Am Acad Pediatrics* 2011;128(3):e720.

83. Workman JK, Myrick CW, Meyers RL, et al. Pediatric organ donation and transplantation. *Pediatrics* 2013;131(6):e1723.

84. Stiers J, Aguayo C, Siatta A, et al. Potential and actual neonatal organ and tissue donation after circulatory determination of death. *JAMA Pediatr* 2015;169(7):639.

85. Weiss MJ, Sherry W, Hornby L. Pediatric donation after circulatory determination of death (pDCD): a narrative review. *Paediatr Respir Rev* 2019;29:3.

86. Wilkinson D. Medical futility. The International Encyclopedia of Ethics. 2017.

87. Pope TM. Legal briefing: medical futility and assisted suicide. *J Clin Ethics* 2009;20(3):274.

88. Brody BA, Halevy A. Is futility a futile concept? *J Med Philos* 1995;20(2):123.

89. Truog RD, Brett AS, Frader J. The problem with futility. *N Engl J Med* 1992;326(23):1560.

90. Schneiderman LJ, Jecker NS, Jonsen AR. Medical futility: its meaning and ethical implications. *Ann Intern Med* 1990;112(12):949.

91. Bosslet GT, Pope TM, Rubenfeld GD, et al. An Official ATS/AACN/ACCP/ESICM/SCCM Policy Statement: responding to requests for potentially inappropriate treatments in intensive care units. *Am J Respir Crit Care Med* 2015;191(11):1318. doi: 10.1164/rccm.201505-0924ST

92. Niederman M, Berger J. The delivery of futile care is harmful to other patients. *Crit Care Med* 2010;38(10 (Suppl)):S518.

93. Orentlicher D. Rationing health care: its a matter of the health care system's structure. *Ann Health Law* 2010;19:449.

94. McDermid RC, Bagshaw SM. Prolonging life and delaying death: the role of physicians in the context of limited intensive care resources. *Philos Ethics Humanit Med* 2009;4:3.

95. Wilkinson D. Beyond resources: denying parental requests for futile treatment. *Lancet* 2017;389(10082):1866. doi: 10.1016/S0140-6736(17)31205-9

96. Trotochaud K, Coleman JR, Krawiecki N, et al. Moral distress in pediatric healthcare providers. *J Pediatr Nurs* 2015;30(6):908. doi: 10.1016/j.pedn.2015.03.001

97. Jameton A. *Nursing practice: the ethical issues.* Englewood Cliffs/London: Prentice-Hall, 1984.

98. Prentice T, Janvier A, Gillam L, et al. Moral distress within neonatal and paediatric intensive care units: a systematic review. *Arch Dis Child* 2016;101(8):701. doi: 10.1136/archdischild-2015-309410

99. Carse A. Moral distress and moral disempowerment. *Narrat Inq Bioeth* 2013;3(2):147.

100. Cavaliere TA, Daly B, Dowling D, et al. Moral distress in neonatal intensive care unit RNs. *Adv Neonatal Care* 2010;10(3):145.

101. Lantos JD. Moral distress and ethical confrontation: problem or progress? *J Perinatol* 2007;27:201. doi: 10.1038/sj.jp.7211679

102. Prentice TM, Gillam L, Davis PG, et al. The use and misuse of moral distress in neonatology. *Semin Fetal Neonatal Med* 2018;23(1):39. doi: 10.1016/j.siny.2017.09.007

103. Sauerland J, Marotta K, Peinemann MA, et al. Assessing and addressing moral distress and ethical climate Part II: neonatal and pediatric perspectives. *Dimens Crit Care Nurs* 2015;34(1):33. doi: 10.1097/DCC.0000000000000083

104. Janvier A, Nadeau S, Deschenes M, et al. Moral distress in the neonatal intensive care unit: caregiver's experience. *J Perinatol* 2007;27(4):203.

105. Penticuff JH, Walden M. Influence of practice environment and nurse characteristics on perinatal nurses' responses to ethical dilemmas. *Nurs Res* 2000;49(2):64.

106. Meller S, Barclay S. Mediation: an approach to intractable disputes between parents and paediatricians. *Arch Dis Child* 2011;96(7):619. doi: 10.1136/adc.2010.191833

107. Gustafson JM. Mongolism, parental desires, and the right to life. *Perspect Biol Med* 1973;16(4):529. doi: 10.1353/pbm.1973.0049

108. McCormick RA. To save or let die. The dilemma of modern medicine. *JAMA* 1974;229(2):172.

109. Stinson R, Stinson P. On the death of a baby. *J Med Ethics* 1981;7(1):5. doi: 10.1136/jme.7.1.5

110. Stinson R, Stinson P. *The long dying of baby Andrew.* Boston, MA: Little, Brown, 1983.

111. Angell M. Handicapped children: Baby Doe and Uncle Sam. *N Engl J Med* 1983;309(11):659. doi: 10.1056/nejm198309153091109

112. Harrison H. Parents and handicapped infants. *N Engl J Med* 1983;309(11):664. doi: 10.1056/nejm198309153091113

113. Pless JE. The story of Baby Doe. *N Engl J Med* 1983;309(11):664. doi: 10.1056/nejm198309153091111

114. Weir RF. The government and selective nontreatment of handicapped infants. *N Engl J Med* 1983;309(11):661. doi: 10.1056/nejm198309153091110

115. Annas GJ. Asking the courts to set the standard of emergency care—the case of Baby K. *N Engl J Med* 1994;330(21):1542. doi: 10.1056/nejm199405263302120

116. Flannery EJ. One advocate's viewpoint: conflicts and tensions in the Baby K case. *J Law Med Ethics* 1995;23(1):7; discussion 13.

117. Annas GJ. Conjoined twins—the limits of law at the limits of life. *N Engl J Med* 2001;344(14):1104. doi: 10.1056/nejm200104053441419

118. Lightfoot L. The ethical health lawyer. Incompetent decisionmakers and withdrawal of life-sustaining treatment: a case study. *J Law Med Ethics* 2005;33(4):851.

119. Paris JJ, Billinngs JA, Cummings B, et al. Howe v. MGH and Hudson v. Texas Children's Hospital: two approaches to resolving family-physician disputes in end-of-life care. *J Perinatol* 2006;26(12):726. doi: 10.1038/sj.jp.7211591

120. Forbat L, Teuten B, Barclay S. Conflict escalation in paediatric services: findings from a qualitative study. *Arch Dis Child* 2015;100(8):769. doi: 10.1136/archdischild-2014-307780

121. Wilkinson D, Barclay S, Savulescu J. Disagreement, mediation, arbitration: resolving disputes about medical treatment. *Lancet* 2018;391(10137):2302.

122. Robertson A. Reflections on errors in neonatology III. The "experienced" years, 1970 to 2000. *J Perinatol* 2003;23(3):240. doi: 10.1038/sj.jp.7210873

123. Robertson AF. Reflections on errors in neonatology: II. The "Heroic" years, 1950 to 1970. *J Perinatol* 2003;23(2):154. doi: 10.1038/sj.jp.7210843

124. Robertson AF. Reflections on errors in neonatology: I. The "Hands-Off" years, 1920 to 1950. *J Perinatol* 2003;23(1):48. doi: 10.1038/sj.jp.7210842

125. Modi N. Ethical and legal issues in neonatal research. *Semin Neonatol* 1998;3(4):303. doi: https://doi.org/10.1016/S1084-2756(98)80085-7

126. Modi N, McIntosh N. The effect of the neonatal Continuous Negative Extrathoracic Pressure (CNEP) trial enquiries on research in the UK. *Arch Dis Child* 2011;96(6):500. doi: 10.1136/adc.2010.188243

127. Binik A. On the minimal risk threshold in research with children. *Am J Bioeth* 2014;14(9):3. doi: 10.1080/15265161.2014.935879

128. Drazen JM, Solomon CG, Greene MF. Informed consent and SUPPORT. *N Engl J Med* 2013;368(20):1929. doi: 10.1056/NEJMe1304996

129. Macklin R, Shepherd L, Dreger A, et al. The OHRP and SUPPORT—another view. *N Engl J Med* 2013;369(2):e3. doi: 10.1056/NEJMc1308015#SA1

130. Lantos JD. Learning the right lessons from the SUPPORT study controversy. *Arch Dis Child Fetal Neonatal Ed* 2014;99(1):F4. doi: 10.1136/archdischild-2013-304916

131. Lantos JD. Neonatal research ethics after SUPPORT. *Semin Fetal Neonatal Med* 2018;23(1):68. doi: 10.1016/j.siny.2017.10.003

132. Miller FG, Brody H. A critique of clinical equipoise. Therapeutic misconception in the ethics of clinical trials. *Hastings Cent Rep* 2003;33(3):19.

133. Weijer C, Shapiro SH, Cranley Glass K. For and against: clinical equipoise and not the uncertainty principle is the moral underpinning of the randomised controlled trial. *BMJ* 2000;321(7263):756.

134. Lantos JD. Was the UK collaborative ECMO trial ethical? *Paediatr Perinatal Epidemiol* 1997;11(3):264.

135. Mike V, Krauss A, Ross G. Neonatal extracorporeal membrane oxygenation (ECMO): clinical trials and the ethics of evidence. *J Med Ethics* 1993;19(4):212. doi: 10.1136/jme.19.4.212

136. Lantos JD, Frader J. Extracorporeal membrane oxygenation and the ethics of clinical research in pediatrics. *N Engl J Med* 1990;323(6):409. doi: 10.1056/NEJM199008093230610

137. Swanevelder JLC, Firmin RK. Extracorporeal circulatory/life support: an update. *J Card Crit Care* 2017;01(02):65. doi: 10.1055/s-0038-1626674

138. Wilman E, Megone C, Oliver S, et al. The ethical issues regarding consent to clinical trials with pre-term or sick neonates: a systematic review (framework synthesis) of the empirical research. *Trials* 2015;16(1):502. doi: 10.1186/s13063-015-0957-x

139. Schreiner MS, Feltman D, Wiswell T, et al. When is waiver of consent appropriate in a neonatal clinical trial? *Pediatrics* 2014;134(5):1006. doi: 10.1542/peds.2014-0207

140. Rich WD, Katheria AC. Waiver of consent in a trial intervention occurring at birth—how do parents feel? *Front Pediatr* 2017;5:56. doi: 10.3389/fped.2017.00056

GENERAL CONSIDERATIONS

8 Care of the Family, Palliative Care, Brain Death, and Organ Donation

Krishelle L. Marc-Aurele

Family-centered and palliative care approaches broaden treatment goals to include a patient's family and quality of life. Both take a more holistic view of illness in the context of a baby's life. Both are necessary to provide compassionate healing in the intensive care unit. When the limits of intensive care are reached, palliative care offers ways to address distressing symptoms and plan for end of life. For some families, organ donation is a way to create a legacy and give the gift of life to others. Organ donation may occur after brain death criteria are met or sometimes after circulatory death.

CARE OF THE FAMILY

In the 1960s when the first neonatal intensive care units (NICUs) were established, parents were not considered to be integral to the care of sick newborns (1). The focus was on medicalization of the baby's care, using incubators and feeding tubes. Over time however, studies on mother–infant bonding demonstrated a positive impact on infant well-being, and newborn care moved away from excluding parents toward more family-centered care. In 2003, the American Academy of Pediatrics published *Family Pediatrics: Report of the Task Force on the Family*, stating, "It is essential that pediatricians realize that the family is their patient—not just the child" (2). This section will review applicable neonatal recommendations in the 2017 *Guidelines for Family-Centered Care in the Neonatal, Pediatric, and Adult ICU* as well as the pertinent research supporting these recommendations.

Family is broadly defined. The following serves as an example of such a definition: "We all come from families. Families are big, small, extended, nuclear, multigenerational, with one parent, two parents, and grandparents. We live under one roof or many. A family can be as temporary as a few weeks, as permanent as forever. We become part of a family by birth, adoption, or marriage or from a desire for mutual support. As family members, we nurture, protect, and influence one another. Families are dynamic and are cultures unto themselves, with different values and unique ways of realizing dreams. Together, our families become the source of our rich cultural heritage and spiritual diversity. Each family has strengths and qualities that flow from individual members and from the family as a unit. Our families create neighborhoods, communities, states, and nations" (New Mexico's Memorial Task Force on Children and Families and the Coalition for Children, 1990) (3).

What Do the Guidelines for Family-Centered Care Recommend for Neonates?

In 2017, an international multidisciplinary team published *Guidelines for Family-Centered Care in the Neonatal, Pediatric, and Adult ICU* (4). The team defined family-centered care as "an approach to health care that is respectful of and responsive to individual families' needs and values." For ICU patients of all ages, they recommended that families be offered the option to be present at the bedside, participate in interdisciplinary team rounds, and with an assigned staff member for support, be present during resuscitations.

For babies in the ICU, these recommendations are based on several studies including a 2010 randomized control trial conducted in an Iranian NICU that compared standard of care to a more family-centered approach. At the time of the study, the standard of care for the majority of Iranian hospitals was to restrict parents from being at the bedside for long periods of time and from

participating in their babies' care (5). For this study, the group randomized to family-centered care received specific education on aspects of neonatal care and were then responsible for being in the NICU to assist in the care for their newborn. Parents in the control group were only allowed to be present at admission. For the family-centered care group, parent satisfaction was significantly higher and highest related to the ability to be present in the NICU. The study also showed that babies with parents in the family-centered care group had significantly lower average length of NICU stay: 6 days shorter (5).

A study in Stockholm similarly showed decreased lengths of hospital stay with increased parent participation and unrestricted entry to the NICU (6). With regard to resuscitation, interviewed parents have shared their desire to be by their child's side and expressed feelings of guilt if they were not present. Some parents report that being present despite knowing their child might die is an inherent parental need that supersedes any possible trauma of witnessing a resuscitation (7). Overall, allowing parents more time, access, and involvement at the bedside in the NICU has been shown to increase parent satisfaction and help parents feel less stressed (8,9).

Some of the recommendations from the *Guidelines for Family-Centered Care in the Neonatal, Pediatric, and Adult ICU* were specific to the neonatal population. A summary of recommendations for family-centered care in the NICU are listed in Table 8.1. One explicit recommendation emphasizes the importance of teaching families of critically ill babies how to assist with care for their infant in order to improve parental confidence and psychological health (4). This is supported by a survey of families from eight American NICUs, which showed significant correlation with direct involvement in the care for their baby and increased parental comfort and confidence (11). Additionally, several studies including randomized trials have shown that helping parents to recognize infant behavioral cues and to meet their infants' needs results in significantly lower parental stress (14–16). Mothers randomized to a Creating Opportunities for Parent Empowerment program reported improved mental health outcomes (17). In the intervention group, parents were given education regarding infant behavior and development as well as parenting activities to complete during the first weeks of admission and at discharge. When compared to those in the control group, the mothers in the intervention group had fewer maternal state anxiety and depressive symptoms. In addition, babies with parents randomized to the intervention had a nearly 4-day shorter average length of NICU hospitalization. One hypothesis is that family-centered care in the NICU helps parents feel more prepared to take their baby home.

Other NICU specific recommendations are to provide psychological support for parents, including peer-to-peer support and multimodal cognitive behavioral therapy by a psychologist (11). In fact, Hynan et al. recommend that all NICUs with 20 or more beds have at least one doctoral-level psychologist embedded in the NICU staff and proportionately more NICU mental health professionals if the NICU is larger (18). Although having a child in the NICU can be transformative, it can also be stressful or lead to depression and anxiety (19,20). The explicit recommendation for psychological support for NICU parents stems from several studies. Compared with a group of mothers in the control group, mothers who received telephone support by trained mothers with experience of having a very premature infant in the NICU reported less

GENERAL CONSIDERATIONS

TABLE 8.1

Recommendations for Family-Centered Care

Unrestricted parent presence (10)

Daily interdisciplinary team bedside rounds for parent participation

Invitation for parents to be present during resuscitation and other medical procedures

Education and support for parental caregiving, including kangaroo care, breast-feeding (11)

Hospital design:

    Single-patient rooms

    Family sleeping areas, preferably in the patient room (3)

    Kitchen, laundry, and lounge for family (3)

    Bathroom with shower for parents

Family education programs about the environment and care plan

Involvement of grandparents and siblings

Peer-to-peer support for families, including breast-feeding and lactation support (12)

Proactive palliative care consultation (4)

Psychological support, including cognitive–behavioral therapy by a psychologist (12)

Social work support in family meetings

Spiritual support by hospital chaplain or spiritual advisor (13)

Continued education for staff on family-centered care

stress and less depression (21). Having trained breast-feeding peer counselors on staff has increased mothers' confidence with providing breast milk, promoted feelings of empowerment, and helped mothers develop their maternal identity (22). Furthermore, cognitive behavioral therapy in a randomized controlled trial and specific care by a psychologist have been associated with reduced maternal anxiety, depression, and symptoms of trauma (23,24).

Despite its recognition as an important component of patient care, family-centered care is still a growing practice in neonatology. In 2016, a group in New Delhi, India, advocated for family-centered care as a low-cost intervention to improve neonatal quality of care in resource-limited settings and a potential strategy to compensate for restricted staffing in low and middle income countries (25). Their randomized controlled study using an audiovisual training module was found to be feasible and approved for introduction within the national public health services. A survey of NICUs from 2004 to 2005 in eight European countries showed that 90% to 100% of all NICUs in Sweden, Denmark, the Netherlands, Belgium, and the United Kingdom allowed unrestricted parent access to their baby but that NICUs in France, Italy, and Spain had not universally adopted the family-centered practice (10). Interviews with neonatologists and senior nurses from five European countries in 2014 identified several barriers to enabling physical parent–infant closeness in neonatal units (26). Barriers included limited parental leave and rights, design of the neonatal unit, institutional culture, as well as lack of adequate staffing.

What Is the Difference between Family-Centered Care and Family-Integrated Care?

Family-centered care is delivered by the medical team while family-integrated care (FICare) is delivered by the family. The FICare model was developed specifically for the Canadian NICU environment, based on the principle that families should be empowered to provide as much of their baby's care in the neonatal unit as they are able (27). In a clustered randomized controlled trial, the primary caregiver parent committed to at least 6 hours per day to be in the NICU. Enrolled parents were expected to be present at daily medical rounds using the chart they completed every day on feedings, output, and activity as well as a parent diary of special

events, attend small group parent education sessions, and track their skill development in a parent checklist. All medical providers in the NICU attended a 2-day training program in FICare at the Mount Sinai Hospital in Toronto. After 21 days into the program, the FICare intervention improved neonatal weight gain, decreased parent stress and anxiety scores, and increased exclusive breast milk feeding rates at discharge (28). FICare promotes parents as necessary members of the neonatal team and, some may argue, is a step ahead of family-centered care (29).

What Is the Neonatologist's Role in Family-Centered Care?

As the leader of the medical team, the neonatologist's role is to make explicit the expectation to collaborate with families and to modify systems of care to improve families' experiences (3). This includes conducting interdisciplinary team rounds at the bedside so that parents can participate as well as seeking out parental observations and preferences for the care plan. It also includes raising awareness of how medical jargon prevents families from fully engaging in bedside discussions and using plain language to talk about their babies' care. Additionally, it means modeling and educating all trainees and staff members how to provide family-centered care.

PALLIATIVE CARE

Before ventilators, surfactant, and modern day NICUs were available, medical care for sick infants was essentially palliative care. When it was difficult to prevent death, the goal was to keep babies warm, fed, and protected (30). Over time, neonatal mortality fell and physicians began to question, "Because we can, should we?" (31). Palliative care for infants thus began with a focus on end-of-life care but has grown in depth and breadth over the last several decades. This chapter will explore the growth and three main aims of palliative care in the NICU: (a) To relieve symptoms, (b) To facilitate informed decision-making, and (c) To improve the quality and enjoyment of life.

Why Do We Need Palliative Care in the NICU?

Palliative care is essential to neonatal care not just because nearly half of all children who die do so during infancy, but also because many life-limiting conditions are diagnosed in the NICU (32). Specialized training in communication and symptom management is necessary to provide excellent care for babies and their families. Additionally, NICU staff members need support in caring for babies with life-limiting conditions and their families (33). Unfortunately, surveys of residents, fellows, and nurses, have identified an unmet need for neonatal and pediatric palliative care education (34,35). In the absence of a formal palliative care curriculum, pediatric residents have reported minimal competence and comfort in nearly all areas of pediatric palliative care (36,37). When asked, residents felt they would benefit from additional training that would be important for the primary care physician and not just for subspecialists.

What Is Palliative Care in the NICU?

Neonatal palliative care developed in tandem with the recognition that some babies were dying in the NICU after withdrawing or withholding life-sustaining treatment (31). In the beginning, palliative care for babies primarily focused on end-of-life care (38). Palliative care studies about dying infants emphasize providing adequate pain management with compassionate extubation and at the end of life (39,40). In 2001, Caitlin and Carter published, *Creation of a Neonatal End of Life Palliative Care Protocol*, which included consensus-based recommendations on how to institute a palliative care program, categories of newborns who have needed comfort care, communication strategies, and symptom management

TABLE 8.2

Sample Perinatal Hospice Birth Plan

Plan of Care for Mom (Name)

1. Please call the baby by the name, ___ Baby's name ___. This is very comforting to hear.
2. We [want/do not want] fetal monitoring. We understand that [she/he] may not survive the labor.
3. I am [hoping for a natural vaginal delivery/anticipating a cesarean section].
4. I would like the following people to support me during the labor process: _____ I would like [some of them/all of them] to be present during the birth.
5. I will bring music to play [during labor or after our baby is born]. Please remind me to play it.
6. This time is special and intimate and we wish to share it with our family. We would appreciate it if only the necessary and essential hospital personnel were present.
7. Please counsel me on my pain management options. I want to be consulted during the birthing process re: an epidural or other pain medications. I would like the medication to be given to me in the smallest dose that would be effective to provide maximum pain relief and comfort while still allowing me to remain alert.
8. After the delivery, I wish to be in a private room with less exposure to pending births or any newborns with their mothers as this would be painful for me to bear.
9. Upon discharge, please give me information on both maintaining a milk supply and information that I may need later, including milk suppression and physical comfort measures.

Plan of Care for Baby (___ Baby's name ___)

1. After the delivery, we ask that ___ Partner's name ___ be allowed to cut the umbilical cord.
2. When the baby is born, we would like the NICU team to be present to assess ___ Baby's name ___ and tell us how [she/he] is doing. We would like all information to be shared so that we can fully understand what might happen next.
3. We understand that ___ Baby's name ___ may quickly show signs that [she/he] cannot breathe on [her/his] own. We do not want a breathing tube to be placed.
4. Following delivery, we wish to hold our baby immediately and ask that vital signs, weighing of baby, medications, and labs be postponed if possible.
5. Instead of going to the NICU after birth, we would like to be together with ___ Baby's name ___ in our labor and delivery or postpartum room.
6. We request that oral/nasal suctioning only be used for comfort and any further treatment be discussed with us prior to performing them on our baby.
7. We would like our baby to be given pain or other medications for comfort only.
8. We request that a ceremony—blessing—be performed upon birth by _____.
9. Please help us bathe and dress ___ Baby's name ___. We would like to make as many memories as possible during our time together.
10. We understand that our baby may be born with more or fewer problems than anticipated. If this is the case, we ask that [her/his] doctor discuss with us how best to care for our baby and plan for the future.
11. If our baby survives delivery and cannot suck or breast-feed, we wish to provide oral comfort with drops of breast milk.
12. We wish to hold our baby if [she/he] is dying or has died. We wish to keep our baby in the room with us as long as possible and to spend time with [her/him] after [she/he] has died.
13. We would like to keep the following items as keepsakes: cord clamp, lock of hair, ID band, tape measure, crib card, weight card, hat/blanket/clothes, fetal monitor tape, bulb syringe, footprints/handprints, thermometer, photographs. We would like Now I Lay Me Down To Sleep to be contacted to take photographs. Volunteer photographers can be contacted at https://volunteers.nowilaymedowntosleep.org/find-photographers.
14. Please allow my partner, ___ Partner's name ___, to stay with me overnight in the room.

Used with permission by Krishelle Marc-Aurele, MD.

at the end of life (41). Available studies evaluating the effect of palliative care in the NICU focus mainly on babies who have died (42–45).

The initial palliative care movement included helping families during pregnancy plan for neonatal comfort care, a practice called perinatal hospice (46). When pregnancy termination for a life-threatening fetal diagnosis is not acceptable because of their faith or values, receiving support to continue with the pregnancy is important for families. Perinatal hospice provides additional support to enable parents to find hope, to aid them with decision-making, and to provide prebereavement counseling (47). Frequently, a palliative team helps a family create a birth plan to maximize memory-making opportunities with their infant (Table 8.2). A major barrier to providing adequate perinatal hospice is late referral to services (33).

Over time, neonatal palliative care has evolved from comfort care, also known as end-of-life care, to include patients with potentially life-limiting but not necessarily life-threatening conditions. As a field, palliative care for infants has grown tremendously over the last 60 years (Fig. 8.1). Demonstrating this upstream approach, Petteys et al. published their hospital-based policy triggers for

NICU palliative consultation upon admission, including gestational age 28 weeks or less at birth, known or suspected congenital or chromosomal anomalies, and need for coordination of multidisciplinary support (48). In broadening the scope of palliative care to include babies with goals for life prolongation but increased risk for morbidity, Petteys et al. greatly improved parental satisfaction.

Who Is Eligible for Palliative Care?

Palliative care is for babies in the NICU with uncertain prognoses and high mortality or morbidity regardless of whether the goals are for life prolongation or comfort care. In fact, many babies with a good prognosis can benefit from a palliative care approach (Fig. 8.2). Some categories of infants who meet criteria for palliative care are (49)

- Infants with extreme prematurity
- Infants with genetic anomalies associated with life-limiting prognoses (e.g., infants with mitochondrial disorders or trisomy 13 or 18)
- Infants with congenital malformations that may threaten vital functions (e.g., infants with renal agenesis, or anencephaly)

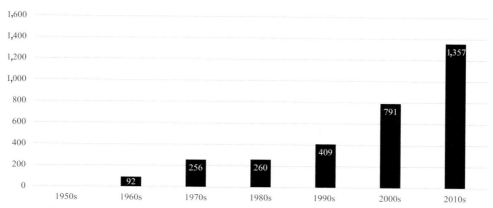

FIGURE 8.1 Pubmed citations for "Palliative care" and "Infants birth to 23 months": 1953–2019. (Data from PubMed. 2020. National Center for Biotechnology Information. Available from: https://pubmed.ncbi.nlm.nih.gov.)

The 2013 Pediatric *Palliative Care and Hospice Care Commitments, Guidelines, and Recommendations* outline three main aims of pediatric palliative care: (a) To relieve symptoms, (b) To facilitate informed decision-making, and (c) To improve the quality and enjoyment of life (50). There is significant overlap in the goals for palliative and neonatal intensive care. However, the philosophy of palliative medicine remains unique. The word "palliaire" means to cloak or conceal. This is in contrast with neonatal intensive care, which hopes to prevent and cure. While the neonatal team aims to reduce mortality, chronic lung disease, and retinopathy of prematurity, the palliative team focuses on reducing symptoms that negatively impact a baby's quality of life as well as helping families to adapt and function during illness. The palliative team is not trying to reduce disease but to improve life with disease.

What Is the Palliative Care Approach to Relieve Symptoms?

Symptoms that can negatively impact one's quality of life can stem from physical, psychological, existential, or spiritual issues. The most common physical symptoms that can affect a baby's quality of life include feeding intolerance specifically nausea, vomiting, constipation, and diarrhea, disordered sleep, seizures, shortness of breath, and pain. Treating most of these symptoms, specifically the manifestations of feeding intolerance, disordered sleep, and seizures, is part of routine daily NICU care. Feeding tolerance often takes the center stage of neonatal rounds, and every

effort is made to reduce vomiting, constipation, and diarrhea. Neonatal nurses treat disordered sleep with regular sleep schedules and cycled lighting in the NICU. Pharmacologic treatment for infant sleep disturbance is rare and limited to melatonin if at all (51,52). Babies are carefully monitored and treated for seizures in the NICU. Lastly, if the goals are for life prolongation, the neonatal team treats shortness of breath with noninvasive ventilation, diuretics, and bronchodilators. If the goal is to compassionately extubate or provide comfort care, then many neonatologists feel comfortable giving morphine or benzodiazepines to relieve shortness of breath.

In 2016, the American Academy of Pediatrics Committee on Fetus and Newborn Care and Section on Anesthesiology and Pain Medicine updated a policy stating, "The prevention of pain in neonates should be the goal of all pediatricians and health care professionals who work with neonates" (53). The policy emphasized that every neonatal facility should implement, "(a) a pain-prevention program that includes strategies for minimizing the number of painful procedures performed and (b) a pain assessment and management plan that includes routine assessment of pain" using both pharmacologic and nonpharmacologic therapies. However, treating neonatal pain can be complicated. When the goals of care are to prolong life, neonatologists must balance treating pain, minimizing respiratory depression, and avoiding long-term sequelae of opiates. Pharmacologic treatment of neonatal pain only becomes simpler when the goals are to prioritize symptom management over life prolongation. To help with this balance, many NICU teams have adopted care plans to treat procedural or surgical pain in a stepwise and judicious manner starting with nonpharmacologic strategies, and then oral sucrose or glucose, acetaminophen, and nonsteroidal anti-inflammatories, before moving to opiates and dexmedetomidine (54–56). To treat pain, some therapies are less commonly used in babies. Gabapentin, ketamine, and propofol, although infrequently used by neonatologists, are valuable especially for very painful conditions like epidermolysis bullosa (57). In these unique and more challenging situations, a palliative specialist may provide additional experience and training to support adequate pain control. Additionally, a palliative approach to pain might incorporate integrative modalities like massage, healing touch, music therapy, acupressure, or acupuncture, which may not be as routine in the NICU.

Identifying and treating symptoms from mental health issues in both child and parent is a necessary part of palliative care and is increasingly recognized as integral to excellent general pediatric care (58). Caring for the mental health of NICU parents who are at risk for experiencing depression, posttraumatic stress disorder, grief, and anxiety is part of family-centered care. Although

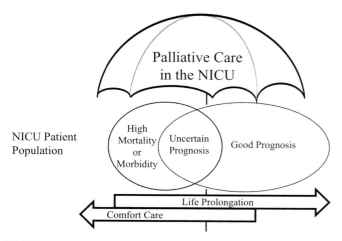

FIGURE 8.2 Palliative care in the NICU. An umbrella term or philosophy that can benefit most babies in the NICU. (Courtesy of Krishelle Marc-Aurele, MD.)

GENERAL CONSIDERATIONS

screening for depression is not possible in babies, older infants can manifest anxiety. At times, it can be difficult to separate pain from anxiety. Persistent crying or irritability in an older infant that does not improve with an adequate dose of an opiate may actually be anxiety. Providing medication for pain prior to repeated painful procedures can be effective in reducing anticipatory anxiety for older babies. Because a Cochrane Review raised concerns about the safety of routine intravenous midazolam and few data exist on the safety of other benzodiazepines in babies, this class of medication is more commonly reserved for end-of-life care (59).

Additionally, palliative care aims to relieve symptoms from existential or spiritual distress mainly through the expertise of a chaplain on the team. In the setting of any serious illness, whether acutely life-threatening, life-limiting, or chronic, families often look to their faith for comfort or meaning. They may feel hopeless, lonely, or regret. They may have questions about why suffering happens or about dying in the context of their spirituality. Frequently these spiritual concerns need to be addressed before families can make decisions about treatment and are the key to understanding their beliefs and values particularly important to advanced care planning.

One validated tool for nurses, doctors, and social workers to identify spiritual concerns and needs is the FICA Spiritual History Tool (60). The letter "F" stands for questions about Faith, Belief, and Meaning. Questions for "I," or Importance and Influence, include the following: What importance does your faith or belief have in your life? The letter "C" stands for questions about Community support. Finally, "A" stands for Addressing Spirituality or Faith in Care. The FICA tool recommends asking, "How can health care providers best support your spirituality? How would you like health care providers to use this information about your spirituality in the care they provide?" Although this tool gives the team the opportunity to identify spiritual and religious beliefs that might affect health care decision-making, it is important to remember that patients and families facing serious illness should also be referred to spiritual providers who are trained to address spiritual distress.

What Is the Palliative Care Approach to Facilitate Informed Decision-Making?

In addition to providing expertise in symptom management, palliative teams hone specific communication skills to facilitate informed decision-making. While neonatologists have experience in giving unexpected and often unwanted news, palliative specialists have additional training in use of silence, ways to express empathy, and strategies to disclose tough information. In the same way that an intensivist practices and refines a procedural skill, palliative practitioners examine and seek feedback on how and what they say or do not say both in role-play and actual family meetings. Palliative physicians learn additional skills from the palliative social worker, chaplain, and nurse because they do consultations as a team and debrief afterward.

What Are Palliative Care Approaches to Giving Unexpected News?

It's important to remember that what a parent might interpret as "bad news" can be anything a parent does not want to hear (61). The information may be "good news" to a physician because "All tests for meningitis are negative" but in fact, is actually "bad news" for a parent who is hoping for an explanation after an extended workup. Instead, experts recommend reporting news as unexpected or serious to avoid framing information with our own biases. Carroll et al. recommends being mindful that words we use as medical professionals "will be part of the family's story forever ... and consider how the family will retell this moment for years to come" (62).

The "Ask–Tell–Ask" strategy is useful when disclosing unexpected or serious information (63). First, *ask* permission to give

unexpected news. Parents may want to wait until they can be together for support or may want to block out more time in their schedule to receive serious news. At the beginning of the meeting, *ask* what parents understand in order to assess their knowledge and customize what you will tell them. Using open-ended questions and asking parents to "Tell me more" demonstrates your interest in listening to what parents have to say and gives permission for them to elaborate. Then *tell* no more than three short digestible pieces of information. After saying something difficult, stop talking. Most people will have a strong emotional response to unexpected or serious news and will not be able to process additional information. Support families with silence at least 15 seconds and wait for them to speak. After they have returned to the conversation, *ask* parents to restate what they heard in their own words to check for understanding. *Ask* for questions and concerns.

During the meeting, watch for and acknowledge emotions with empathy statements using the NURSE mnemonic (Naming, Understanding, Respecting, Supporting, Exploring) (64). *Naming* refers to stating an observation of a parent's emotions (i.e., "It sounds like you are frustrated"), being careful to suggest and not tell parents what they are feeling (i.e., "I wonder if you are feeling overwhelmed"). *Understanding* is the action of summarizing what you heard parents say (i.e., "My understanding of what you said is that you are afraid we are missing something in trying to find the diagnosis. Did I get that right?"). Back et al. recommend against "giving premature reassurance at this point, even though the temptation to do this is strong" and instead recommend verifying concerns that parents have (63). *Respecting* can be nonverbal by nodding, leaning in, or showing concern in body language. However, verbally acknowledging your respect for parents is a powerful way to show empathy (i.e., "You are loving and brave parents. I can see that you are just trying to make sure your child gets the best care."). *Supporting* is to express a willingness to help (i.e., "We'll do this together" or "How can we help you?"). Lastly, *exploring* is to inquire more about an emotion or concern a parent has already mentioned (i.e., "You said that you lay awake at night worrying. Can you tell me more about that?").

To complement the NURSE mnemonic, "I wish" statements are helpful in responding to feelings of disappointment. Saying "I wish things were different" acknowledges what parents have lost and validates their hopes and dreams. It's normal to feel responsible for causing and therefore want to "fix" strong emotions expressed by parents. Some doctors, overwhelmed by feelings of guilt and helplessness, offer treatment options that are not indicated because bearing witness to parents' distress is so difficult. Instead, saying something like "I wish I had a treatment that could reverse the injury to his brain," will both give a clear and consistent message and also express that as a physician on their side, you had similar hopes.

What Are Palliative Care Approaches to Negotiating Goals of Care?

If reasonable parents in a given situation could disagree on whether to focus on prolonging their child's life or whether to focus instead on their child's comfort and quality of life, then having a goals-based discussion is required to achieve shared decision-making. In general, goals of care conversations are best done at a separate time from when serious or unexpected news are given. Most families require time and space to process difficult information and its associated emotions. After that, families typically need even more time before they are ready to make changes to the plan of care. Ideally, conversations about the goals of care begin early in the course of a child's illness to allow families to adapt as the illness changes. Sometimes stated goals of care can be overlapping (e.g., to improve function and maximize quality of life) or conflicting (e.g., to pro-long life and maximize quality of life). If goals of care seem to be in opposition, then determine which goal has the highest priority.

It's important to recognize that parents often want to hear hope from doctors and express hope as a survival strategy during goals of care conversations. As they cope with their child's illness, their hope will adjust. Janvier et al. explain, "When parents decide to have a child, they hope for a healthy pregnancy and a strong child ... when their baby is sick ... they hope their child will not have disabilities. They may hope their child simply survives, or that they can at least take their child home" (65). Doctors, on the other hand, are afraid of providing false hope to families. It is possible, however, to convey hope to parents in a way that is honest (i.e., "I'm worried that your baby will die, but I hope that I'm wrong"). Avoid saying, "There's nothing more we can do" because even when preventing death is no longer feasible, maximizing comfort or working to get a child home is "something we *can* do." Palliative care specialists frequently say, "Let's hope for the best but also plan for the worst."

One guide to navigate goals of care discussions is VITALtalk's REMAP tool (Reframe, Expect Emotion, Map, Align, and Plan) (66). After assessing for parental understanding, *reframe* the conversation with a question such as "With this new information, may we talk about next steps?" *Expect Emotion* is a reminder to watch for and acknowledge emotions using the previously described NURSE mnemonic or supportive silence. The importance of silence cannot be overemphasized. If physicians continue to talk when parents are in shock or expressing strong emotions, then they eliminate the opportunity for families to process the information and their feelings. Remember to wait in silence as much as possible. *Map* out the future by eliciting goals for their child (i.e., "When you think about the future, what are you worried about and what is most important for your child?"). Then *align* with the family's values by repeating back to parents what was said to be important (i.e., "What I heard you say is that what's most important is..."). Lastly, *plan* treatments that match values. Offer to give a recommendation and do so only if permission is granted.

How Can Palliative Care Improve Quality and Enjoyment of Life for a Child and Family?

Early referral to palliative care may reduce a child's symptom burden and prepare family members for what to expect during their child's illness. The palliative team will encourage families to plan for the future and anticipated decisions ahead, but also to enjoy the present by making memories. Memory making in the NICU can include performing a ceremony, whether a blessing, anointing, or the act of putting on heirloom baby clothes. It can be done with a portrait session by Now I Lay Me Down To Sleep, a worldwide nonprofit organization of volunteer photographers who offer professionally retouched family photos at no cost (67). Creating keepsakes like handprints and foot molds or bathing their infant with music playing in the background can be important moments for families to reflect upon as they grieve.

In promoting shared decision-making with families to plan for their child's future medical care and discuss preferences for end of life, palliative teams can improve communication with the medical team and reduce a family's decisional burden. Having these conversations has the potential to reduce parental anxiety and distress about what to expect during illness and or dying. Palliative care can help families adapt and function during illness.

Who Provides Neonatal Palliative Care?

Neonatal palliative care requires a combination of both consultative and primary palliative care teams to work together and provide support to one another (68). In 2006, the American Board of Medical Specialties granted Hospice and Palliative Medicine its formal subspecialty status, and hospital-based palliative consultation services

grew in numbers. However, it became clear that the demand for palliative care exceeded the supply of palliative medicine subspecialists. In 2002, von Gunten coined the phrase *primary palliative care*, referring to the basic skills and competencies required of all physicians and health care professionals to provide palliative care (69). In the NICU, primary palliative care would ideally be provided by all members of the primary team (i.e., neonatologists, neonatal nurses, and all neonatal professionals including respiratory therapists, pharmacists, occupational, speech, and physical therapists, lactation consultants, social workers, chaplains, and neonatal trainees of all disciplines). The NICU team would manage an infant's pain and other symptoms, a family's depression and anxiety, and initiate discussions about prognosis and goals of care. For more complex or refractory situations that exceed the skills or available time of the primary team, palliative subspecialist consultation can provide additional support and expertise. A palliative subspecialist could offer recommendations for advanced symptom management, like starting gabapentin or ketamine for intractable pain, as well as take the time to further explore situations with perceived conflict about goals of care. For the most difficult cases, the palliative consultant could serve as an ongoing educational and continuity provider to support the relationship between primary providers and families. This mixed model allows babies and families to receive palliative care concurrently and avoids having to "switch to palliative care." The combination of primary and subspecialty consultation palliative care is necessary to meet the needs of seriously ill babies and their families.

What Is the Difference between Palliative and Hospice Care?

Palliative care can be provided at any time in a person's life whether the goals are for life prolongation or comfort care, while hospice care is generally considered to be end-of-life care with comfort-focused goals. Hospices can serve families in their home to support goals to allow a baby to have a natural death outside of hospital settings. Many babies need ongoing medical treatment of pain, seizures, spasticity, etc. in order to make life at home comfortable, and many families need anticipatory guidance. The hospice team typically includes a palliative physician, nurse, social worker, and chaplain that each periodically visits with patients and families to provide symptom management, bereavement counseling, and emotional support through the dying process. As of 2011, hospice care is still developing internationally with 42% of the world's countries still without any hospice-palliative services (70).

BRAIN DEATH

The Uniform Determination of Death Act (UDDA) was originally created in 1980 to provide a legal basis for determining death in all situations. It defined death by circulatory as well as neurologic criteria (i.e., brain death) but only in children older than 5 years of age. In 1987, the American Academy of Pediatrics *Clinical Report—Guidelines for the Determination of Brain Death in Infants and Children* outlined brain death criteria for newborns greater than 38 weeks of gestational age and at least 7 days of life, as well as for infants and young children (71). This section will review the 2011 American Academy of Pediatrics update to the 1987 Task Force recommendations and the controversies surrounding brain death in pediatrics.

WHAT ARE THE CRITERIA TO DETERMINE BRAIN DEATH FOR ADULTS?

The UDDA was originally created in 1980 by a National Conference of Commissioners on Uniform State Laws in cooperation with the American Bar Association, the American Medical Association, and the President's Commission for the Study of Ethical Problems in Medicine and Biomedical and Behavioral Research (72). The goal was to provide a legal basis for determining death in all situations. The UDDA defined death, stating that "an individual who has sustained either (a) irreversible cessation of circulatory and respiratory functions, or (b) irreversible cessation of all functions of the entire brain, including the brainstem, is dead. A determination of death must be made in accordance with accepted medical standards" (73).

The latest update to the criteria for determination of brain death in adults, or persons 18 years of age and older, was published by the American Academy of Neurology in 2010 (74). After meeting certain clinical prerequisites, one neurologic examination is sufficient to pronounce brain death for adults in most states. The publication discusses various ancillary tests that are currently used but not necessary nor suitable as a substitute for the clinical diagnosis of brain death.

What Are the Criteria to Determine Brain Death for Neonates?

The American Academy of Pediatrics *Clinical Report—Guidelines for the Determination of Brain Death in Infants and Children* was initially published in 1987, revised in 2011, and reaffirmed in 2019 with no changes (75). Although the 2011 recommendations expanded the guidelines to include infants and newborns, or children younger than 1 year of age, they do not apply to newborns less than 37 weeks of gestational age. Similarly, the 2014 Royal College of Paediatrics and Child Health guidelines exclude infants less than 37 weeks of gestation age (76). At this time, no guideline to determine brain death exists for the premature infant. In the United States and the United Kingdom, determining brain death in pediatric patients, as in adults, is a clinical diagnosis and ancillary studies are not required nor substitutive.

Although the Canadian Neurocritical Care Group agrees that brain death can be established by clinical criteria alone, the Canadian guidelines recommend a radionuclide brain flow study to test for cerebral perfusion in newborns greater than 38 weeks of gestation and young infants, aged 7 days to 2 months, as well as two electroencephalograms for infants 2 months to 1 year of age (77). Other countries recommend or require ancillary studies to determine brain death in infants (78–80). Confirmatory tests check for either loss of electrical activity of the brain or absence of cerebral blood flow. Unfortunately, false-negative and false-positive results for both electroencephalography and tests for cerebral blood flow have been published for infants who otherwise met neurologic criteria for death (76). For this reason, there is no international consensus regarding the application and interpretation of ancillary tests for brain death determination.

As in adults, the pediatric guidelines require certain clinical prerequisites and the exclusion of reversible conditions. For example, infants undergoing therapeutic hypothermia cannot be examined until normothermic, and hypotension as well as metabolic derangements must be corrected before neurologic examination for brain death. Additionally, analgesics, sedatives, and neuromuscular blockades should be discontinued for a reasonable amount of time based on the elimination half-life of the medication. The American, Canadian, and British guidelines recommend deferring examination for at least 24 hours after any cardiopulmonary resuscitation or sustained severe brain injury (75–77).

In contrast to the criteria used for adults, pediatric guidelines recommend two neurologic examinations performed by different attending physicians, including apnea testing with each exam, separated by an observation period. There is variability among different national guidelines regarding the recommended observation period (77,79). In the United States for newborns (born at gestational age 37 weeks or greater) at birth to 30 days of age, the recommended observation period between neurologic exams is 24 hours, and for infants greater than 30 days of age and children up to 18 years of age, the observational period is 12 hours (75). One exam is to determine whether the child has met the clinical criteria and the second is to confirm that he/she has fulfilled the criteria for brain death.

TABLE 8.3

Neurologic Examination to Assess for Brain Death

1. Coma	Complete loss of consciousness, vocalization, and volitional activity
2. Loss of all brainstem reflexes	Midposition or fully dilated pupils that do not respond to light
	Absence of movement of bulbar musculature including facial and oropharyngeal muscles
	Absent gag, cough, sucking, and rooting reflex
	Absent corneal reflexes
	Absent oculovestibular reflexes
3. Apnea	Complete absence of documented respiratory effort (if feasible) by formal apnea testing demonstrating a $PaCO_2 \geq 60$ mm Hg and ≥ 20 mm Hg increase above baseline
4. Flaccid tone and absence of spontaneous or induced movements	Excluding spinal cord events such as reflex withdrawal or spinal myoclonus

Data from Nakagawa TA, Ashwal S, Mathur M, et al. Guidelines for the determination of brain death in infants and children: an update of the 1987 task force recommendations. *Pediatrics* 2011;128(3):e720.

The working group for the British guidelines could not find a rationale to specify a precise interval between clinical examinations and recommended only that the interval between examinations "need not be prolonged" (76). Table 8.3 details the elements of the neurologic exam to assess for brain death. The neurologic exam must demonstrate a child's flaccid tone as well as complete loss of consciousness, vocalization, volitional activity, all brainstem reflexes, and spontaneous or induced movements. Spinal cord reflexes do not count as spontaneous movements. The apnea test must demonstrate complete absence of documented respiratory effort with a $PaCO_2 \geq 60$ mm Hg and ≥ 20 mm Hg above the baseline. The guidelines state, "Once death has occurred, continuation of medical therapies, including ventilator support, is no longer an option unless organ donation is planned" (75).

What Are the Controversies Surrounding Brain Death in Pediatrics?

Although the medical, ethical, and legal community in the United States accepts the absence of either neurologic or circulatory function as death, brain death can be a difficult concept to understand when a child's heart rate, blood pressure, and oxygen saturations remain normal due to advanced life-sustaining technology. One such example is the case of JM, a 13-year-old girl who was declared brain dead after complications from a tonsillectomy (81). JM's mother said, "She's warm and soft. She's not cold and stiff like death. She smells good and when I rub her feet she pulls away... She is not dead. She needs time to get better...[she] is dead only if her heart stops" (82). Her family cited religious objections to the UDDA and asked that she be moved to New Jersey where religious beliefs must be considered in determining death. New Jersey is the only state that requires the circulatory definition of death and provides health insurance coverage when there is religious exemption to the neurologic definition of death (83). After 4 years, doctors removed JM's life support when she was having internal bleeding due to liver failure. Cases like JM demonstrate what challenges medical teams face to prepare families for how brain death will look different from the societal view of circulatory death.

What Are Recommendations for Clinicians Regarding Declaring Pediatric Brain Death?

The words "brain death" suggest that only one part of a person has died: an incomplete death (84). Experts recommend avoiding the phrase "brain dead" to prevent confusion or false hope (82). Instead, they advise physicians tell parents that their child has met the definition of death by neurologic criteria and that their child is dead, thus eliminating the choice to remove life-sustaining technology. According to the UDDA, there is no decision to be made and so offering a choice creates additional misunderstanding. Furthermore, strict adherence to published guidelines and the medical, ethical, and legal criteria for determining brain death is more likely to maintain public trust (85).

ORGAN DONATION

Each year since 1988, an average of 269 U.S. infants receive organ transplants, but only 107 deceased U.S. infants donate organs based on Organ Procurement and Transplantation Network (OPTN) data. In 2020, almost 110 American infants remain on the transplant waitlist. The limited infant donor pool results in a gap in supply and demand for organ transplantation. In this section, we will review the current status of infant and neonatal organ donation in the United States.

What Is the Current Status of Infant Organ Donation?

Most infants, younger than 1 year of age, who need a transplant are on the waitlist for a liver or heart, based on OPTN data as of February 20, 2020. The most common conditions that ultimately lead to liver and cardiac transplantation during infancy are biliary atresia and congenital heart disease, respectively. Unfortunately, nearly 25% of American infants listed for heart transplant die waiting for a heart, with the majority of children who die weighing less than 15 kg (86). Infants have the highest waiting-list mortality for transplant regardless of age or solid organ type (87). This reflects a very small donor pool for infant and neonatal organs.

Why Is the Infant and Neonatal Organ Donor Pool So Small?

Currently less than 2% of all organ and tissue donations ($N \sim 3,400$) are from donors under 1 year of age based on OPTN data as of February 20, 2020. Traditionally, organ donation occurs after the determination of brain death and organs are procured from donors whose hearts are still beating. Underrepresentation of infant organ donors may be related to lack of awareness that brain death determination can apply to newborns and infants or variation in practice to evaluate for brain death (87). Alternatively, inexperience with neonatal organ transplantation along with no or late referral for organ donation may play a bigger role (88).

What Are Ways to Reduce High Waiting-List Mortalities for Infants Awaiting Transplantation?

Living donor and split-liver transplantation avoid the need for infant donor organs. The most common type of living donation is directly from either a biologic relative or an unrelated person who has a connection with the transplant candidate. Typically, living persons donate liver or kidney transplants to neonates. Split-liver transplantation, or dividing an adult donor liver into two, provides double the grafts: one for a child and the other for an adult (89).

Another strategy involves recovery of organs after planned withdrawal of life-sustaining medical treatment, also known as non-heart-beating organ donation or controlled donation after circulatory death (DCD). Most organs obtained from pediatric DCD have been livers and kidneys (90). Although the number of organs from pediatric DCD has increased, more education and awareness about DCD is needed. Labrecque et al. reviewed deaths in three Boston NICUs over a 3-year period and found about 16% of deaths met criteria for potential DCD donation (90). Based on the time interval from withdrawal of life-sustaining treatment to circulatory death, about half of the potential donors could have been candidates for liver and kidney DCD and half were potential cardiac DCD candidates. Identified DCD candidates in this study were most likely to have been diagnosed with either hypoxic ischemic encephalopathy or chronic lung disease. Similarly, in the United Kingdom, where neonatal organ donation is rare, Charles et al. reviewed 6 years of deaths at the Great Ormond Street Hospital and found that 36% of infants ($N = 30$) younger than 2 months of age might have been potential DCD donors. The study also identified 13% of infants ($N = 11$) who could have been potential donors after brain death, if determination of neonatal brain death in the United Kingdom were not prohibited (91). In 2013, the American Academy of Pediatrics released the *Ethical Controversies in Organ Donation after Circulatory Death* policy statement (92). It states that DCD is an ethically acceptable option and recommends decoupling the decision-making and even the medical teams involved in the withdrawal of life-sustaining treatment and organ donation. The committee advises waiting 2 to 5 minutes after fulfillment of circulatory death before organ procurement and that physicians should help institutions develop policies to manage inherent conflicts of interest in the DCD process.

Approaches to reduce the neonatal cardiac waiting-list mortality includes transplanting ABO-incompatible hearts as well as employing investigational cardiac assist devices (87,93). In 2001, a group from the Hospital for Sick Children in Toronto published outcomes for 10 infants who received ABO-incompatible cardiac transplants (94). Normally, solid organ transplantation is contraindicated between donors and recipients with incompatible blood groups because of the risk of acute rejection. But newborns have underdeveloped antibody, isohemagglutinin, and complement production and so their immature immune system gives them an advantage in terms of graft acceptance (95).

Currently, there is only one FDA-approved long-term mechanical cardiac assist device for neonates and infants: the Berlin Heart EXCOR (96). In a review of 97 children weighing less than 10 kg who were supported with the Berlin Heart EXCOR ventricular assist device, 57% either underwent transplantation ($N = 53$) or were weaned from the device ($N = 2$) (97). For children weighing less than 10 kg, the median age for ventricular assist device implantation was 6.2 months and median duration of support was 26 days. Currently, pediatric cardiac assist devices are primarily used as a bridge to transplant and not considered "destination therapies," or permanent treatment options.

Can Patients with Anencephaly Donate Organs?

Because infants with anencephaly have intact brainstem reflexes while their heart is still beating, they cannot meet the criteria for brain death determination (98). The 2005 Canadian Paediatric Society statement on *Use of Anencephalic Newborns as Organ Donors* recommends no alteration of the infant brain death criteria to include infants with anencephaly and in fact, recommends against organ donation from infants with anencephaly. The Canadian Paediatric Society Fetus and Newborn Committee argued that infants with anencephaly will not satisfy brain death criteria and DCD is unlikely to result in suitable organs due to ischemic damage sustained from anticipated apnea before circulatory death (99). Since that published statement, organ DCD has been shown to be feasible for infants with anencephaly (100). Although there is no guarantee that organs will be recovered or transplanted successfully, the choice to donate after circulatory death provides an opportunity for parents of babies with anencephaly to experience a sense of meaning in the setting of their loss (101).

CONCLUSIONS

Effective family-centered care recognizes that patients' healing relies on the involvement of their families. Integrating family in the everyday care for their infant not only reduces parental stress and improves short-term outcomes for infants but may also reduce

GENERAL CONSIDERATIONS

NICU lengths of stay. NICUs should focus on adopting policies and guidelines as standards of care to support parents as primary providers in the ICU environment.

Palliative care is essential for the infant and family with life-limiting and uncertain prognoses. It includes management of symptoms that commonly affect quality of life as well as specific communication skills for giving serious news and goals of care conversations. Like all good care, palliative care relies on all members of the NICU team and support from subspecialty consultation. It is a team effort.

In 2011, the AAP published guidelines for the determination of brain death for infants born at 37 weeks' gestation and older. Although the determination of brain death has been ethically, medically, and legally adopted, the concept of brain death can be difficult for families to accept.

The gap between supply and demand for infant organ transplantation, mostly for heart and liver organs, remains high. Education alongside optimization of the infant donor pool is important to decreasing the high transplant waiting-list mortality.

ACKNOWLEDGEMENT

Data from the Organ Procurement and Transplantation Network was supported by the Health Resources and Services Administration contract 234-2005-37011C. The content of this chapter is the responsibility of the authors alone and does not necessarily reflect the views or policies of the Department of Health and Human Services, nor does mention of trade names, commercial products, or organizations imply endorsement by the U.S. Government.

REFERENCES

1. Maree C, Downes F. Trends in family-centered care in neonatal intensive care. *J Perinat Neonatal Nurs* 2016;30(3):265.
2. Schor EL; American Academy of Pediatrics Task Force on the Family. Family pediatrics: report of the Task Force on the Family. *Pediatrics* 2003;111(6 Pt 2):1541.
3. Committee on Hospital Care and Institute for Patient- and Family-Centered Care. Patient- and family-centered care and the pediatrician's role. *Pediatrics* 2012;129(2):394.
4. Davidson JE, Aslakson RA, Long AC, et al. Guidelines for family-centered care in the neonatal, pediatric, and adult ICU. *Crit Care Med* 2017;45(1):103.
5. Bastani F, Abadi TA, Haghani H. Effect of family-centered care on improving parental satisfaction and reducing readmission among premature infants: a randomized controlled trial. *J Clin Diagn Res* 2015;9(1):SC04.
6. Ortenstrand A, Westrup B, Broström EB, et al. The Stockholm Neonatal family centered care study: effects on length of stay and infant morbidity. *Pediatrics* 2010;125(2):e278.
7. Maxton FJ. Parental presence during resuscitation in the PICU: the parents' experience. *J Clin Nurs* 2008;17(23):3168.
8. De Bernardo G, Svelto M, Giordano M, et al. Supporting parents in taking care of their infants admitted to a neonatal intensive care unit: a prospective cohort pilot study. *Ital J Pediatr* 2017;43(1):36.
9. Voos KC, Ross G, Ward MJ. et al. Effects of implementing family-centered rounds (FCRs) in a neonatal intensive care unit (NICU). *J Matern Fetal Neonatal Med* 2011;24(11):1403.
10. Greisen G, Mirante N, Haumont D, et al. Parents, siblings and grandparents in the neonatal intensive care unit. A survey of policies in eight European countries. *Acta Paediatr* 2009;98(11):1744.
11. Cooper LG, Gooding JS, Gallagher J, et al. Impact of a family-centered care initiative on NICU care, staff and families. *J Perinatol* 2007;27(S2):S32.
12. Roué J-M, Kuhn P, Lopez Maestro M, et al. Eight principles for patient-centred and family-centred care for newborns in the neonatal intensive care unit. *Arch Dis Child Fetal Neonatal Ed* 2017;102(4):F364.
13. Feudtner C, Haney J, Dimmers MA. Spiritual care needs of hospitalized children and their families: a national survey of pastoral care providers' perceptions. *Pediatrics* 2003;111(1):e67.
14. Matricardi S, Agostino R, Fedeli C, et al. Mothers are not fathers: differences between parents in the reduction of stress levels after a parental intervention in a NICU. *Acta Paediatr* 2013;102(1):8.
15. Landsem IP, Handegård BH, Tunby J, et al. Early intervention program reduces stress in parents of preterms during childhood, a randomized controlled trial. *Trials* 2014;15:387.
16. Balbino FS, Balieiro MMFG, Mandetta MA. Measurement of family-centered care perception and parental stress in a neonatal unit. *Rev Lat Am Enfermagem* 2016;24:e2753.
17. Melnyk BM, Feinstein NF, Alpert-Gillis L, et al. Reducing premature infants' length of stay and improving parents' mental health outcomes with the creating opportunities for parent empowerment (COPE) neonatal intensive care unit program: a randomized, controlled trial. *Pediatrics* 2006;118(5):e1414.
18. Hynan MT, Steinberg Z, Baker L, et al. Recommendations for mental health professionals in the NICU. *J Perinatol* 2015;35(suppl 1):S14.
19. Janvier A, Lantos J, Aschner J, et al. Stronger and more vulnerable: a balanced view of the impacts of the NICU experience on parents. *Pediatrics* 2016;138(3):e20160655.
20. Al Maghaireh DF, Abdullah KL, Chan CM, et al. Systematic review of qualitative studies exploring parental experiences in the neonatal intensive care unit. *J Clin Nurs* 2016;25(19–20):2745.
21. Preyde M, Ardal F. Effectiveness of a parent "buddy" program for mothers of very preterm infants in a neonatal intensive care unit. *CMAJ* 2003;168(8):969.
22. Rossman B, Greene MM, Meier PP. The role of peer support in the development of maternal identity for "NICU moms". *J Obstet Gynecol Neonatal Nurs* 2015;44(1):3.
23. Shaw RJ, St John N, Lilo E, et al. Prevention of traumatic stress in mothers of preterms: 6-month outcomes. *Pediatrics* 2014;134(2):e481.
24. Jotzo M, Poets CF. Helping parents cope with the trauma of premature birth: an evaluation of a trauma-preventive psychological intervention. *Pediatrics* 2005;115(4):915.
25. Maria A, Dasgupta R. Family-centered care for sick newborns: a thumbnail view. *Indian J Community Med* 2016;41(1):11.
26. Dykes F, Thomson G, Gardner C, et al. Perceptions of European medical staff on the facilitators and barriers to physical closeness between parents and infants in neonatal units. *Acta Paediatr* 2016;105(9):1039.
27. O'Brien K, Bracht M, Robson K, et al. Evaluation of the family integrated care model of neonatal intensive care: a cluster randomized controlled trial in Canada and Australia. *BMC Pediatr* 2015;15:210.
28. O'Brien K, Robson K, Bracht M, et al. Effectiveness of family integrated care in neonatal intensive care units on infant and parent outcomes: a multicentre, multinational, cluster-randomised controlled trial. *Lancet Child Adolesc Health* 2018;2(4):245.
29. Banerjee J, Aloysius A, Platonos K, et al. Family centred care and family delivered care—what are we talking about? *J Neonatal Nurs* 2018;24(1):8.
30. Hartline J. *Historical perspectives* [Internet]. AAP.org. [Cited June 1, 2019]. Available from: http://www.aap.org/en-us/about-the-aap/Committees-Councils-Sections/Neonatal-Perinatal-Medicine/TECAN/Pages/Historical-Perspectives.aspx
31. Duff RS, Campbell AG. Moral and ethical dilemmas in the special-care nursery. *N Engl J Med* 1973;289(17):890.
32. Field MJ, Behrman RE; Institute of Medicine, Committee on Palliative and End-of-Life Care for Children and Their Families. *When children die: improving palliative and end-of-life care for children and their families.* Washington, DC: The National Academies Press, 2003.
33. Marc-Aurele KL, Nelesen R. A Five-year review of referrals for perinatal palliative care. *J Palliat Med* 2013;16(10):1232.
34. Michelson KN, Ryan AD, Jovanovic B, et al. Pediatric residents' and fellows' perspectives on palliative care education. *J Palliat Med* 2009;12(5):451.
35. Davies B, Sehring SA, Partridge JC, et al. Barriers to palliative care for children: perceptions of pediatric health care providers. *Pediatrics* 2008;121(2):282.
36. Baker JN, Torkildson C, Baillargeon JG, et al. National survey of pediatric residency program directors and residents regarding education in palliative medicine and end-of-life care. *J Palliat Med* 2007;10(2):420.
37. Kolarik RC. Pediatric resident education in palliative care: a needs assessment. *Pediatrics* 2006;117(6):1949.
38. Whitfield JM, Siegel RE, Glicken AD, et al. The application of hospice concepts to neonatal care. *Am J Dis Child* 1982;136(5):421.
39. Carter BS, Howenstein M, Gilmer MJ, et al. Circumstances surrounding the deaths of hospitalized children: opportunities for pediatric palliative care. *Pediatrics* 2004;114(3):e361.
40. Janvier A, Meadow W, Leuthner SR, et al. Whom are we comforting? An analysis of comfort medications delivered to dying neonates. *J Pediatr* 2011;159(2):206.
41. Catlin A, Carter BS. Creation of a neonatal end-of-life palliative-care protocol. *J Clin Ethics* 2001;12(3):316.
42. Gilmour D, Davies MW, Herbert AR. Adequacy of palliative care in a single tertiary neonatal unit. *J Paediatr Child Health* 2017;53(2):136.
43. Samsel C, Lechner BE. End-of-life care in a regional level IV neonatal intensive care unit after implementation of a palliative care initiative. *J Perinatol* 2015;35(3):223.
44. Younge N, Smith PB, Goldberg RN, et al. Impact of a palliative care program on end-of-life care in a neonatal intensive care unit. *J Perinatol* 2015;35(3):218.

45. Pierucci RL, Kirby RS, Leuthner SR. End-of-life care for neonates and infants: the experience and effects of a palliative care consultation service. *Pediatrics* 2001;108(3):653.

46. Hoeldtke NJ, Calhoun BC. Perinatal hospice. *Am J Obstet Gynecol* 2001;185(3):525.

47. Rocha Catania T, Stein Bernardes L, Guerra Benute GR, et al. When one knows a fetus is expected to die: palliative care in the context of prenatal diagnosis of fetal malformations. *J Palliat Med* 2017;20(9):1020.

48. Petteys AR, Goebel JR, Wallace JD, et al. Palliative care in neonatal intensive care, effects on parent stress and satisfaction: a feasibility study. *Am J Hosp Palliat Care* 2015;32(8):869.

49. Carter BS. Pediatric palliative care in infants and neonates. *Children* 2018;5(2):21.

50. Section on Hospice and Palliative Medicine and Committee on Hospital Care. Pediatric palliative care and hospice care commitments, guidelines, and recommendations. *Pediatrics* 2013;132(5):966.

51. Mindell JA. Pharmacologic management of insomnia in children and adolescents: consensus statement. *Pediatrics* 2006;117(6):e1223.

52. Aversa S, Marseglia L, Arco A, et al. 1640 efficacy and safety of melatonin in neonates. *Arch Dis Child* 2012;97(suppl 2):A464.

53. Committee on Fetus and Newborn and Section on Anesthesiology and Pain Medicine. Prevention and management of procedural pain in the neonate: an update. *Pediatrics* 2016;137(2):e20154271.

54. Deindl P, Unterasinger L, Kappler G, et al. Successful implementation of a neonatal pain and sedation protocol at 2 NICUs. *Pediatrics* 2013;132(1):e211.

55. Aukes D, Roofthooft DW, Simons SH, et al. Pain management in neonatal intensive care: evaluation of the compliance with guidelines. *Clin J Pain* 2015;31(9):830.

56. Hall RW, Anand KJS. Pain management in newborns. *Clin Perinatol* 2014;41(4):895.

57. Carter BS, Brunkhorst J. Neonatal pain management. *Semin Perinatol* 2017;41(2):111.

58. *Roadmap to resilience, emotional, and mental health* [Internet]. The American Board of Pediatrics, 2018. Available from: https://www.abp.org/foundation/roadmap. Accessed April 13, 2019.

59. Ng E, Taddio A, Ohlsson A. Intravenous midazolam infusion for sedation of infants in the neonatal intensive care unit. *Cochrane Database Syst Rev* 2017;1(1):CD002052.

60. Borneman T, Ferrell B, Puchalski CM. Evaluation of the FICA tool for spiritual assessment. *J Pain Symptom Manage* 2010;40(2):163.

61. Feudtner C. Hospice & palliative medicine: breaking bad news [Internet]. In: *Contemporary pediatrics*. 2015. Available from: https://www.contemporarypediatrics.com/contemporary-pediatrics/news/hospice-palliative-medicine-breaking-bad-news. Accessed August 28, 2019.

62. Carroll C, Carroll C, Goloff N, et al. When bad news isn't necessarily bad: recognizing provider bias when sharing unexpected news. *Pediatrics* 2018;142(1):e20180503.

63. Back AL, Arnold RM, Baile WF, et al. Approaching difficult communication tasks in oncology. *CA Cancer J Clin* 2005;55(3):164.

64. Smith RC. *Patient-centered interviewing: an evidence-based method.* Philadelphia, PA: Lippincott Williams & Wilkins, 2002.

65. Janvier A, Barrington K, Farlow B. Communication with parents concerning withholding or withdrawing of life-sustaining interventions in neonatology. *Semin Perinatol* 2014;38(1):38.

66. Transitions/Goals of Care: Using the REMAP tool [Internet]. VitalTalk. Available from: https://www.vitaltalk.org/guides/transitionsgoals-of-care/. Accessed August 28, 2019.

67. Now I Lay Me Down To Sleep [Internet]. Available from: https://www.nowilaymedowntosleep.org/. Accessed August 29, 2019.

68. Marc-Aurele KL, English NK. Primary palliative care in neonatal intensive care. *Semin Perinatol* 2017;41(2):133.

69. von Gunten CF. Secondary and tertiary palliative care in US hospitals. *JAMA* 2002;287(7):875.

70. Connor SR, Bermedo MCS. *Global atlas of palliative care at the end of life*. London, England: Worldwide Palliative Care Alliance, World Health Organization, 2014.

71. Report of Special Task Force. Guidelines for the determination of brain death in children. American Academy of Pediatrics Task Force on Brain Death in Children. *Pediatrics* 1987;80(2):298.

72. McCabe J. The new determination of death act. *Am Bar Assoc J* 1981;67(11):1476.

73. National Conference of Commissioners on Uniform State Laws. *Uniform determination of death act* [Internet]. Available from: https://www.law.upenn.edu_bll_archives_ulc_fnact99_1980s_udda80.htm

74. Wijdicks EFM, Varelas PN, Gronseth GS. Evidence-based guideline update: determining brain death in adults. *Neurology* 2010;74:1911.

75. Nakagawa TA, Ashwal S, Mathur M, et al.; Society of Critical Care Medicine, Section on Critical Care and Section on Neurology of American Academy of Pediatrics, Child Neurology Society. Clinical report—guidelines for the determination of brain death in infants and children: an update of the 1987 task force recommendations. *Pediatrics* 2011;128(3):e720.

76. Marikar D. The diagnosis of death by neurological criteria in infants less than 2 months old: RCPCH guideline 2015. *Arch Dis Child Educ Pract Ed* 2016;101(4):186.

77. Guidelines for the diagnosis of brain death. Canadian Neurocritical Care Group. *Can J Neurol Sci* 1999;26(1):64.

78. Toida C, Muguruma T. Pediatric brain death in a Japanese pediatric hospital. *Acute Med Surg* 2016;3(1):10.

79. Al-Bar MA, Chamsi-Pasha H. Brain death. In: *Contemporary bioethics*. Cham: Springer International Publishing, 2015:227.

80. Brain Injury Evaluation Quality Control Centre of National Health and Family Planning Commission. Criteria and practical guidance for determination of brain death in children (BQCC version) *Chin Med J (Engl)* 2014;127:4140.

81. Brierley J. UK court accepts neurological determination of death. *Lancet* 2015;385(9984):2254.

82. Paris JJ, Cummings BM, Moore MP. "Brain death," "dead," and parental denial. *Camb Q Healthc Ethics* 2014;23(04):371.

83. Son RG, Setta SM. Frequency of use of the religious exemption in New Jersey cases of determination of brain death. *BMC Med Ethics* 2018;19(1):76.

84. De Georgia MA. History of brain death as death: 1968 to the present. *J Crit Care* 2014;29(4):673.

85. Volakli EA, Mantzafleri PE, Kalamitsou S, et al. Brain death in children. In: *Intensive Care*. IntechOpen, 2017:115. Available from: https://www.intechopen.com/books/intensive-care/brain-death-in-children

86. Almond CSD, Thiagarajan RR, Piercey GE, et al. Waiting list mortality among children listed for heart transplantation in the United States. *Circulation* 2009;119(5):717.

87. Mah D, Singh TP, Thiagarajan RR, et al. Incidence and risk factors for mortality in infants awaiting heart transplantation in the USA. *J Heart Lung Transplant* 2009;28(12):1292.

88. Lechner BE. Of tragedies and miracles—neonatal organ donation. *N Engl J Med* 2018;379(22):2089.

89. Emre S, Umman V. Split liver transplantation: an overview. *Transplant Proc* 2011;43(3):884.

90. Labrecque M, Parad R, Gupta M, et al. Donation after cardiac death: the potential contribution of an infant organ donor population. *J Pediatr* 2011;158(1):31.

91. Charles E, Scales A, Brierley J. The potential for neonatal organ donation in a children's hospital. *Arch Dis Child Fetal Neonatal Ed* 2014;99(3):F225.

92. Committee on Bioethics. Ethical controversies in organ donation after circulatory death. *Pediatrics* 2013;131(5):1021.

93. Boucek MM, Mashburn C, Dunn SM, et al. Pediatric heart transplantation after declaration of cardiocirculatory death. *N Engl J Med* 2008;359(7):709.

94. West LJ, Pollock-Barziv SM, Dipchand AI, et al. ABO-incompatible heart transplantation in infants. *N Engl J Med* 2001;344(11):793.

95. Urschel S, West LJ. ABO-incompatible heart transplantation. *Curr Opin Pediatr* 2016;28(5):613.

96. Mascio C. *Mechanical circulatory support in congenital heart disease: expert analysis*. American College of Cardiology, 2018. Available from: https://www.acc.org/latest-in-cardiology/articles/2018/03/28/12/51/mechanical-circulatory-support-in-congenital-heart-disease

97. Conway J, St Louis J, Morales DLS, et al. Delineating survival outcomes in children <10 kg bridged to transplant or recovery with the Berlin Heart EXCOR Ventricular Assist Device. *JACC Heart Fail* 2015;3(1):70.

98. Powers RJ, Schultz D, Jackson S. Anencephalic organ donation after cardiac death: a case report on practicalities and ethics. *J Perinatol* 2015;35(10):785.

99. CPS Fetus and Newborn Committee. Use of anencephalic newborns as organ donors. *Paediatr Child Health* 2005;10(6):335.

100. Williams L, Kennedy K, Boss RD. The decision to donate: helping families make meaning during neonatal loss. In response to: anencephalic organ donation after cardiac death: practicalities and ethics—a case report. *J Perinatol* 2015;35(10):777.

101. *Neonatal donation* [Internet]. IIAM. Available from: https://www.iiam.org/neonatal-donation/. Accessed February 4, 2019.

Discharge Planning, Follow-Up Care, and Outcome Evaluation

Angela Huertas-Ceballos and Katie Mckinnon

INTRODUCTION

The goal of perinatal care is to improve survival, minimize the occurrence and severity of long-term adverse neurodevelopmental outcomes, and enhance health-related quality of life. Advances in neonatal intensive care have led to a dramatic reduction in infant mortality rates, and as survival improves, it is essential to understand the long-term outcome of survivors. Without this information, possible negative effects of medical interventions may not be identified, life course effects of complications during the perinatal period will not be fully appreciated, and patient outcomes are unlikely to continue improving.

Neurodevelopmental surveillance for the high-risk infant begins antenatally when parents are identified and counseled, or after a complex birth. It then follows the child throughout admission to the neonatal unit where they are exposed to multiple interventions, aiming first for survival, but also brain protection and promotion of growth and general health.

Discharge planning, follow-up care, and outcome evaluation are key elements of the ongoing assessment and management of children at risk of developmental problems. Medical and environmental risk factors identified before, during, and after birth are taken into account, as these all increase the child's vulnerabilities for adverse outcome. Active early intervention, provided from the start of medical care and throughout admission, all the way to discharge and then into infancy and childhood, may provide opportunities to influence growth and developmental trajectories, and improve outcomes (1).

More widely, a state-of-the-art neurodevelopmental surveillance program for high-risk populations of neonates can provide essential outcome data for informing neonatal care quality improvement initiatives, and for planning future service provision for children according to their needs.

Measurement of outcomes in high-risk neonates requires valid and standardized instruments, and currently, there are a wide variety of tests and questionnaires available. No test is the "gold standard," and sometimes, a combination of several tests may give the most accurate outcome for a particular group. It is important, therefore, that the researcher and clinician are familiar with the population under surveillance and aims of testing in order to make the right selection.

Surveillance of neonatal unit graduates with formal testing is also useful to answer research questions and evaluate various aspects of neonatal care. This is important given the variations in care in neonatal practices across the globe, and the variations in morbidity and mortality rates within and between countries (2). In low- and middle-income countries, where the population of neonates at high risk is much wider and is more vulnerable, outcome data can also be used to assess factors affecting the basic provision of health, nutrition, and socioeconomic status, so that improvement initiatives and funding can be targeted (3).

DISCHARGE PLANNING

Discharge planning is a proactive process that begins at the time of admission to the neonatal unit, when the needs of the patient and family are identified, and culminates in a plan of care that can be shared with community services.

Preparations for home are an important step in a child's progress through the neonatal unit, particularly after a prolonged or complex stay. Firstly, medical status is key, but other important factors to consider include family readiness, home care provision, and pressure to reduce length of stay (4).

Good discharge planning can reduce the risk of future hospital admissions (5) and allow ongoing or anticipated problems to be managed through care plans. As survival of preterm and unwell infants rises, they are frequently discharged with chronic or unresolved medical problems, needing more care and follow-up and involvement of other specialities and services than previously (4). The primary concern is to ensure infants are not at undue increased risk of morbidity and mortality by untimely discharge home.

A list of routine predischarge tests should be developed locally and reviewed before discharge. Guidelines may vary from institution to institution, and the tests performed should be individualized based on the patient's history and clinical course. An example of the tests that are recommended and the assessment of readiness from all stakeholders in this process are described in Table 9.1.

As well as focusing on the logistics and practical aspects of discharge, planning must also include emotional and psychological support for families. Practical elements, including knowledge and training of parents, will vary depending on the child's requirements but could include NG (nasogastric) tube feed training, home oxygen arrangements, understanding medication regimens, immunization schedules, and other national screening programs (hearing, metabolic). An assessment of parental requirements is also important as social and family support, housing, and finances may impact their ability to care for their child.

Ongoing involvement of families throughout admission to the neonatal unit helps with support and education about their child's development. Programs like Family-Integrated Care (FIC), such as outlined in the Bliss Baby Charter (6), and other initiatives informing preparation for discharge (5,7) (Fig. 9.1) help to involve families early, enhance communication, improve parental experience, and promote emotional and technical readiness for discharge (8).

WHO TO FOLLOW-UP AND WHY

Normal Development and Defining Disability

In order to deliver a comprehensive service for the identification of children that may need referrals or intervention, it is important to concentrate initially on what normal development is. Understanding normal growth and developmental trajectories is as important as acquiring the skills and training on tests to measure these because the definition of normality may differ slightly depending on the population. For example, preterm infants grow, move, and behave differently compared to term infants, but they may still be within a range of normality for their condition of prematurity.

Development of the child starts at conception but continues into early adulthood (Fig. 9.2). In preterm neonates, or those with complex medical problems, a significant stretch of development occurs in the neonatal unit. Postural challenges, abnormal sensory triggers, sedation, and isolation in the extrauterine environment of the NICU may impact how a premature infant grows and develops, and even with nurturing therapies such as NIDCAP (newborn individualized developmental care and assessment program) (11), preterm

term infants at 5 years of age. The lower the gestation, the wider the gap. The etiology of low IQ is complicated because IQ is the product of the social environment, genetic factors, cultural background, and nutritional background and is probably not just the effect of prematurity. It is also well known that environment has a much bigger impact on IQ as the child grows.

At school age, reading and mathematics in preterm infants were significantly below their classmates, and the deficits are not fully explained by low IQ. Specific deficits in executive function seem to be underlying, and these effects are also present, to a lesser extent, in the late preterm population (26,41).

Other studies have reported significant deficits in basic cognitive processes including short-term memory, processing speed, visual-perceptual skills, sensorimotor integration, and attention in extreme preterm infants when compared to term born controls (42). Such deficits have been observed from school entry all the way through adolescence. Meta-analyses have demonstrated impairment in executive functions (cognitive processes that allow individuals to respond flexibly to the environment and to engage in purposeful, goal-directed behavior) especially in those born less than 26 weeks (43). Such processes include inhibition, planning, shifting or cognitive flexibility, working memory, or verbal fluency (27).

Adult Outcomes
EP children with CP and neurosensory disabilities can have increasing limitations as they mature to adulthood, and those without CP or diagnosed neurosensory disabilities can also experience difficulties. They do not appear to outgrow their cognitive problems, and deficits are still present to a similar magnitude as in earlier assessments, including significantly poorer performance in tests of IQ and executive functions, and increased rates of intellectual disabilities and lower educational attainment compared with adults born at term (44).

The increased risk of psychiatric disorders in adulthood for the ex-preterm population (ASD, ADHD, and mood disorders) may be a progression of signs and symptoms seen earlier in life, such as behavioral problems and attention deficits, developing into diagnosable conditions in adulthood (45). There is evidence of reduced social interactions and reduced risk-taking behaviors in adolescents, higher introversion, and autistic trends. Fewer are married or cohabiting, and reproductive rates are lower than term controls (46).

There is also some evidence that adult emotional outcomes in those born preterm may be influenced by bullying experiences in school; these effects account for a large proportion of the impact on emotional development, suggesting school interventions could be beneficial (47). The risk of psychiatric disorders in adults born preterm is three times the risk for term-born controls.

However, the majority of ex-preterm adults lead independent and self-supporting lives (48,49), with evidence that although there are difficulties in developing relationships, the quality of those relationships is similar to term/normal birth weight controls (46). There remain similar rates of employment, and self-perceived quality of life is similar to controls, with quality of life measures higher than predicted by health professionals (50).

The Term Baby
Various factors can make the term baby more susceptible to neurodevelopmental or medical complications (Table 9.4).

Term infants who are growth restricted, even with apparently normal placental function, have also been reported to have lower developmental scores at 2 years (51). NE (neonatal encephalopathy) is a significant cause of neurodisability. Despite the age of therapeutic hypothermia, the burden of disability in neonates with NE remains a problem. (149)

Hearing loss related to medication and other noxious agents has improved significantly as ototoxic medication is carefully monitored. However, there remain a number of risk factors, including low birth weight, neonatal unit stay greater than 5 days, ECMO (extracorporeal membrane oxygenation), mechanical ventilation, hyperbilirubinemia, craniofacial abnormalities, CNS infections, congenital infections, and some syndromes (52).

The neurodevelopmental outcome in PAIS (perinatal arterial ischemic stroke) is primarily dependent on the location of the territory affected—the MCA (middle cerebral artery) territory is most commonly affected in PAIS and also most likely to cause impairment in at least one domain (53). As such, imaging and other neurologic investigations are key to early predictions of outcome (54) which is important for tailoring interventions.

Congenital abnormalities include both structural and functional abnormalities and are individually rare, but cumulatively frequent (55). Children with CP are more likely to have congenital anomalies than the general population, and many congenital anomalies require follow-up for neurodevelopmental and medical outcomes. The types and incidence of these outcomes is very dependent on the specific type of congenital anomaly. For certain conditions such as complex congenital heart disease and diaphragmatic hernias, however, they are well known to be associated with a range of long-term morbidities including neurodevelopmental difficulties in a range of domains, and surveillance programs should be in place for these groups of infants (56,57).

Intervention-Associated Outcomes and the NICU Environment
Exchanging the womb for the neonatal unit environment at a time of rapid brain growth is likely to compromise preterm infants' early development, which can result in long-term physical and mental health problems and developmental disabilities.

Postnatal high-dose dexamethasone steroid therapy, for example, may confer respiratory benefits to infants who are ventilator dependent, but the treatment is associated with abnormal growth, and abnormal neurodevelopmental and cardiac outcomes (58).

Prolonged empirical antibiotic exposure after very preterm birth maybe prescribed for "suspicion of sepsis" but is also associated with increased odds of morbidity (severe neurologic injury, ROP, NEC, BPD, or hospital-acquired infection) and mortality (59).

Painful procedures such as heel lances, venipuncture, and insertion of tubes are essential in the management of the infant in the neonatal unit, but there is growing evidence that pain is associated with altered somatosensory function and modulation (60). Pain relief with opiates is considered paramount in some neonatal units; it is however a controversial intervention. Some studies show no effect of opiate exposure on neurodevelopment (61), but others have shown a reduction in cerebellar growth proportionate to opiate exposure, with consequential effects on motor and cognitive outcomes (62).

NIDCAP aims to prevent the iatrogenic sequelae of intensive care and to maintain the intimate connection between parent and infant, one expression of which is kangaroo mother care. Studies have shown improvements in brain development, functional competence, health, and quality of life (11,63).

Prevention of pain is mandatory for surgical conditions at any age. However, the choice and type of analgesia and anesthesia should be considered carefully because uncertainties have been raised about the safety of anesthetic agents during critical periods of brain development (64,65).

Some interventions may have protective effects on neurodevelopment. For example, caffeine is given for management of apnea of prematurity (66), but there is evidence that it may also be associated with improved neurodevelopmental outcomes when given early (67), although some animal studies have suggested that different doses can have positive or negative effects on the developing brain (68). Antenatal magnesium sulfate is an intervention that is well established as having a positive impact on development, with a number needed to treat to avoid CP in one baby of 63 (69). A more

TABLE 9.4

Risks and Associated Outcomes in Term Infants

Category	Risk	Associated Outcomes
Maternal	Diabetes, hypertension, infection, thyroid disease	Developmental delays
	Socioeconomic status	Speech delay
Antenatal	Placental malfunction (hypoxia, anemia)	Cognitive impairment
	Isoimmunization, kernicterus	Motor impairment
	Infection (CMV, other)	Hearing loss
	Paradoxical emboli (stroke)	Delayed/impaired visual maturation
		Impaired speech
Perinatal	Cord obstruction (hypoxia)	Cognitive and motor impairment
	Trauma (anemia, hypoxia)	Seizures
Neurologic	Grey/white matter damage	Cognitive impairment
	Encephalopathy (including hypoxic, infectious, viral, metabolic, bilirubin)	Motor impairment
	Trauma	Seizures
	Stroke	Early mortality
	Congenital neurologic conditions	
Respiratory	CDH	Prolonged assisted ventilation
	Lung sequestration (needing surgery)	Pulmonary hypertension
	Pulmonary hypertension	Feeding difficulties
	ECMO	Cognitive problems
Cardiac	Complex congenital heart disease	Pulmonary hypertension
		Impaired quality of life (multiple admissions, surgical procedures)
		Neurodevelopmental delay
		Feeding problems
Gastrointestinal	Surgical problems	Feeding issues
	Gastroschisis, exomphalos	Short bowel
	Extrophies	Growth failure
		Behavioral problems secondary to feeding issues
		Impaired quality of life (surgical procedures)
Sensory	HIE	Delayed/impaired visual maturation
	Infection (acute, congenital)	Hearing loss
	Ototoxic medication (e.g., aminoglycosides)	Abnormal pain responses
	Painful procedures	
	Analgesia, anesthetics	

CDH, congenital diaphragmatic hernia; CMV, cytomegalovirus; CP, cerebral palsy; ECMO, extracorporeal membrane oxygenation; HIE, hypoxic ischemic encephalopathy.

recent meta-analysis suggested that a single bolus dose could be sufficient, with reduction of CP by 30% (70).

ECMO maybe a life-saving therapy for infants with severe lung or heart conditions, but poor neurodevelopmental outcomes have been associated with this intervention. For example, in children with complex cardiac conditions, infants who received ECMO had moderate delay at 2-year Bayley III assessment, compared to those who did not (71).

With regard to growth and nutrition interventions, we must mention the Barker hypothesis or the "fetal origins of adult diseases," which relates to interventions in the fetus or immediate neonatal period that have a long-lasting impact in child or adulthood. ELBW and EP in particular have been shown to have effects on early mortality, nutrition, and cardiometabolic syndrome, as well as diabetes and hypertension (72).

Breast milk is beneficial for the high-risk population (72,73). In EP infants, it provides nutrients that are well tolerated and achieves growth in a steady way. There is evidence from observational studies that it is brain protective and that growth outcomes are better than with formula. Breastfeeding is recommended for at least 6 months, and there is evidence of improved neurodevelopmental outcomes on breastfed infants (74).

Social and Environmental Factors

It is well known that sociodemographic factors such as socioeconomic status, social support, ethnicity, and maternal physical and mental health are important determinants of outcome in high-risk infants. These should be addressed during discharge planning, and as surveillance progresses, there should be provision for parental support and prompt intervention when adverse social factors are identified (75).

Special mention to electronic devices should be acknowledged—given the high risk of adverse sensory outcomes in this population, the advice from national pediatric institutions in various countries is to promote extended sensory input and avoid any screens below the age of 3 years (76), although the potential role of technology in promoting child development is a fervent area of research.

Neurologic Investigations

In the rapidly moving landscape of research in neonatology, neurologic investigations as surrogate outcomes are increasing in demand. In clinical care, these are a fundamental part of the neurodevelopmental surveillance program.

Cranial ultrasound continues to be a useful tool in the hands of experienced neonatologists or radiologists. Sequentially done, it reliably identifies intraventricular hemorrhage, post-hemorrhagic ventricular dilatation, and severe white matter lesions but is less reliable for detecting mild and moderate injury when compared to MRI (77). The neurologic examination can add useful context to cranial ultrasound or MRI for predicting neurosensory impairment at 1 year (78).

Brain MRI is used consistently in prediction of outcome in NE, as well as other lesions and pathologies (79). In the preterm population, conventional MRI imaging is useful for prediction of outcome, although it is dependent on experienced interpretation (80), and routine MRI in preterm infants increases costs with only modest benefits for predicting outcome in comparison to ultrasound (81) (see chapter 50).

MRI can also be used for specific biomarkers. In particular, conventional T1 and T2 weighted structural scans, and lactate/N-acetylaspartate (NAA) (N-acetylaspartate), from proton magnetic resonance spectroscopy, are useful in prediction of motor outcomes at 1 year in infants with NE (82) and at 2 years, even after undergoing therapeutic hypothermia (83). Other imaging modalities and biomarkers are promising as surrogates for long-term outcomes in research on neonatal interventions.

In low resource settings, cranial ultrasound scanning may be the only imaging technique available. In Ugandan infants with NE, these have been used to categorize patterns of pathology and correlate well with outcome (84,85).

HOW TO FOLLOW-UP

General Medical Care

The program starts by identifying those aspects of an infant's life that require monitoring. These include growth and nutrition, neurodevelopment, immunizations, lung and airway, surgical conditions, environmental factors, seizures, and intercurrent illnesses that may impact on the infants' normal growth. Table 9.5 outlines

areas that the pediatrician may consider evaluating at every consultation and is presented for preterm and for term infants.

Growth and Nutrition
Growth Velocity
There are various charts for measuring growth velocity of neonates in and beyond the neonatal unit, with the most commonly used from INTERGROWTH-21st and WHO (86–88). There are also local standards for various countries, such as the CDC (Centers for Disease Control and Prevention) charts for the United States (89).

Growth trajectories provide important information about infant well-being. The infant's weight, length, and HC (head circumference) must be plotted using appropriate charts and compared with the standardized centiles expected for that particular infant. Preterm infants should have measurements plotted according to corrected age (age adjusted for prematurity) until 2 years of age.

Much work on growth has previously been based on predictions of intrauterine growth, and there is now a drive for more physiologic measures (90). Adequate nutrition, caloric intake, and healthy appearance with normal biochemistry labs all together seem to be more appropriate measures of good nutrition (91).

It is important to remember that caloric requirements for healthy ex-preterm infants are usually higher than for healthy term infants especially during the rapid catch-up growth.

Causes for impaired growth are usually increased expenditure in BPD, increased losses due to malabsorption after NEC or significant gastro-oesophageal reflux disease, and decreased intake caused by fatigue, hypoxia, swallow problems, sensory issues, and chromosomal abnormalities (92,93).

Head Circumference
During the first 2 years, the head of the preterm infant grows faster than other anthropometric measures. The head often has suture diastasis, a distinctive turricephalic shape, and the anterior fontanelle may remain open for several months. If the HC crosses two centile lines, or is enlarging at twice the normal rate over two weeks, hydrocephalus should be considered and investigated. A term infant with history of hypoxia or significant encephalopathy may present with their HC dropping centiles, which may be consistent with brain atrophy or microcephaly. In this case, it may be associated with visual and developmental impairment (94).

Nutritional Requirements
Caloric intake requirements have been calculated for term and preterm infants and are presented in extensive publications and textbooks. ESPGHAN (the European Society of Paediatric Gastroenterology, Hepatology and Nutrition) have provided helpful guidance (95), with advice of a requirement of 110 to 135 kcal/kg/d, plus specific advice about constituent nutrient requirements. After discharge, calories are usually provided in the form of breast milk or formula (96). There is controversy on whether supplementation with fortifiers should be used or whether high-calorie formulas should be alternated with breast milk (97).

Sometimes, like in the case of complex cardiac conditions, reduction of energy expenditure maybe achieved through NG or percutaneous gastric tubes; a multidisciplinary approach is recommended for infants who require special nutritional support post discharge.

Feeding Problems
If not recognized, feeding problems may lead to significantly impaired nutritional intake and negatively affect the parent–infant relationship, as well as long-term neurodevelopmental outcomes (98). The assessment of a child with feeding problems includes a detailed history of feeding behaviors and nutritional intake, a physical examination with assessment of motor reflexes, and observation of feeding behaviors. If the infant desaturates during feeding, then supplemental oxygen should be increased. Also evaluate the

TABLE 9.5
Medical Considerations for Preterm and Term Infants

Category	Preterm	Term
Growth and nutrition	Growth charts (HC, height, weight)	Growth charts (HC, height, weight)
	Growth velocity	Feeding issues
	Caloric supplements	NGT, PEG
	Feeding issues	
Immunizations	Schedule as per routine immunizations	Schedule as per routine immunizations
	Specific recommendations for BPD	Specific recommendations for seizures
Home oxygen, diuretics	For BPD	For complex cardiac disease, pulmonary hypertension, ECMO
Tracheostomy, ENT	Severe BPD	For congenital conditions
	Postintubation laryngeal cysts	Laryngomalacia
	Post-PDA ligation	
Seizures	High risk if brain injury	NE
		Congenital/genetic conditions
Sensory	ROP, vision impairment	Delayed visual maturation
	Hearing loss	Glue ear
Blood investigations	Metabolic bone disease	Hypercalcemia/ hypercalciuria (therapeutic hypothermia)

BPD, bronchopulmonary dysplasia; ECMO, extracorporeal membrane oxygenation; ENT, ear/nose/throat; HC, head circumference; NE, neonatal encephalopathy; NGT, nasogastric tube; PDA, patent ductus arteriosus; PEG, percutaneous endoscopic gastrostomy; ROP, retinopathy of prematurity.

teat and hole size, as well as milk volume (breast or bottle), as these can also cause fatigue and overwhelming (99). For infants with prolonged feeding tube dependence, specialized tube weaning programs may be required, such as the Graz model, which has shown good results (100).

Gastroesophageal reflux should be addressed by positioning. There is enough evidence that antireflux medication may be more harmful than beneficial and decision on its use should be carefully assessed (101,102).

Management of feeding problems usually requires psychological support for mothers and family, as well as a multidisciplinary team consisting of a speech and language therapist, occupational therapist, dietitian, and other as required.

Immunizations

It is important for premature infants to continue their immunization regimen at appropriate chronologic age, not correcting for gestational age at birth. The benefits of vaccination outweigh risks, so the schedule should not be delayed or withheld. Efforts to minimize side effects include that ensuring prophylactic paracetamol is given as recommended for term infants, and in those with concerns about apnea, bradycardia, or desaturations, consider administration in a hospital setting with adequate respiratory monitoring (103). Starting immunizations prior to discharge improves vaccine coverage (104).

Immunization schedules differ in some details between countries but are broadly similar. The U.S. guidelines provide an easy to follow reference (105), but practitioners should follow the immunization schedule that exists in their own country. Some diagnoses require special consideration; for example, in some countries, palivizumab prophylaxis for respiratory syncytial virus is recommended for infants with chronic lung disease (106).

Home Oxygen

The ATS (American Thoracic Society) has published guidelines on home oxygen therapy for children (107). The publication defines hypoxemia and the indications for oxygen at home with the description of the various conditions. In the United Kingdom, the BTS (British Thoracic Association) last updated their guidance in 2009 (108). Most management for BPD is empirical, individualized, and based on observations.

There is agreement in both guidelines that target oxygen saturations are 95% to 98%; because outside this range, there is some evidence of impaired neurodevelopmental outcome, increased risk of pulmonary hypertension, poor growth, and poor sleep. In addition to intermittent monitoring of oxygen saturations, a good physical assessment is important, including growth, signs of respiratory distress, presence of apneas, wheezing, and cough.

Empirical strategies for weaning off oxygen and diuretics vary, but the speed of reduction of oxygen should be inversely related to the severity of the disease with approximately 0.1 L/min per month during the day and then during the night, with saturations maintained. By consensus, the ATS recommended room air challenges be considered for clinically stable children under 1 year of age receiving less than 0.1 L/min and children up to preschool age receiving 0.1 to 0.25 L/min. A flow rate less than 0.25 to 0.5 L/min could be considered for school-age and older children (107). It is not pertinent to wean or discontinue oxygen use on the basis of FiO₂ alone.

Post-discharge diuretics for the management of BPD remains controversial. If in use, doses should be adjusted with weight and electrolytes monitored. Empirical use of bronchodilators and inhaled steroids is sometimes required for the management of wheeze and cough episodes during the first 5 years of life.

Infants with BPD and RHH (right heart hypertrophy) represent a particularly high-risk group and should be managed jointly with pediatric cardiology and respiratory physicians.

Ear, Nose, and Throat and Tracheostomy

Clinical guidelines on tracheostomy management have been published (109). In general, few children require tracheostomy before discharge and if they do, home readiness should be assessed for the amount of equipment and visitors they will require. The majority of children are weaned off tracheostomy by the age of three, and the remainder by the age of five.

Dysphonia in ex-premature infants is not infrequent and can be caused by vocal cord palsy after duct ligation and vocal cord cysts or subglottic stenosis after intubation (110). Children present with hoarse voice, history of apneas, snoring, and mouth breathing. A laryngoscopy should be considered, including assessment of laryngomalacia, with surgical management if required.

Seizures

0.1% of term newborn infants present with seizures (111). Seizures during the newborn period maybe subtle or overt and may occur once or repetitively. Seizures are present in approximately 29% to 35% of infants with moderate or severe hypoxic-ischemic encephalopathy (HIE) (112), 10% of preterm infants with intraventricular hemorrhage (IVH), and 17% of preterm infants with periventricular leukomalacia (PVL) (113,114). By the time the child is ready for discharge, a plan for anticonvulsive medication should be in place if required, as well as follow-up and parental education. New seizures developing during the follow-up period deserve further investigation. See Chapter 51.

Sensory
Visual Impairment

The incidence of ROP increases as gestational age and birth weight decrease. In the outpatient setting, the most important aspect of ongoing care is an understanding of the urgency of the first follow-up appointment with ophthalmology especially if the state of the retina is uncertain, or if the infant has received treatment.

Premature infants without ROP are at increased risk of other ophthalmologic problems, such as loss of visual acuity, errors of refraction, and strabismus. Children with complex problems including partial blindness, severe myopia, and nystagmus should be evaluated by a vision therapist and referred for vision therapy both of which can help with the rehabilitation of the infant.

Term babies may present with delayed visual maturation—a diagnosis of exclusion in otherwise normal children (115). In HIE, it is important to review imaging for evidence of problems in the visual pathway (116). Once imaging and other tests have excluded other causes, reassurance of improvement within the first year of life may be appropriate.

Hearing Impairment

Screening for auditory brainstem responses and/or otoacoustic emissions should be offered to all infants in the newborn period. Countries in resource rich settings often have screening programs, and practitioners should adhere to these for the setting in which they work. The goal is early detection of hearing impairment for early intervention, because this can restore hearing and is associated with improved language skills, school performance, and behavior.

Children at risk of hearing impairment should be offered alternatives to verbal communication, such as sign language, alternative methods of gesturing, language boards, or computer-assisted communication devices, as early as possible. Candidates for hearing aids or cochlear implants should be promptly referred to specialists.

Renal and Bone

The premature infant is at high risk of metabolic bone disease, particularly if there has not been fortification and/or supplementation with vitamin D, calcium, or phosphate during their neonatal unit stay. Follow-up, therefore, should include investigations for bone and kidney, and supplementation as necessary.

Term infants exposed to hypothermia should be carefully examined during follow-up for subcutaneous fat necrosis, which will be noticeable after 3 months of life (117). This is associated with hypercalcemia, hypercalciuria, and nephrocalcinosis, and early referral to endocrinology and nephrology may be required.

Necrotizing Enterocolitis

The most common complications of NEC are strictures, adhesions, and short bowel syndrome. Short bowel is a challenging condition in terms of growth and nutrition. It often needs long-term parenteral nutrition at home and prognosis is guarded. See Chapter 36.

Hydrocephalus

It is important to differentiate hydrocephalus from normal catch up head growth. If hydrocephalus is suspected, it should be evaluated with cranial imaging. Any suspicion of increased intracranial pressure should be referred to a neurosurgeon for assessment, without delay. Any implanted device for cerebrospinal fluid (CSF) drainage requires monitoring for evidence of obstruction or infection, and urgent referral to neurosurgical colleagues is required if these complications are suspected. See Chapter 53.

Apnea and Bradycardia

Apnea is defined as cessation of breathing for 20 seconds or longer, or a shorter respiratory pause associated with bradycardia, cyanosis, pallor, and/or marked hypotonia. In preterm infants, the incidence of apneas is inversely proportional to gestational age and the severity of ongoing problems. CNS immaturity is the most common cause, but it is important to rule out medical problems such as anemia, sepsis, meningitis, other infections, seizures, upper airway obstruction, hypoxia, bronchospasm, or reflux.

Although controversial, persisting apneas that have been investigated may need monitoring at home. The AAP recommendation is only to use monitoring until 43 weeks corrected age or cessation of episodes, and for infants who require prolonged ventilatory support. Monitoring does not prevent sudden infant death syndrome (SIDS), and families should be aware of the recommendations of supine sleep, safe sleep, and elimination of tobacco smoke (118).

Neurodevelopment Surveillance

Background and Definition

Surveillance is the sequential measurement of outcomes in a high-risk population during a specific period of time, with the goal of early identification of problems enabling prompt intervention. Surveillance starts from antenatal care, continues through NICU admission, discharge, and all the way until adulthood.

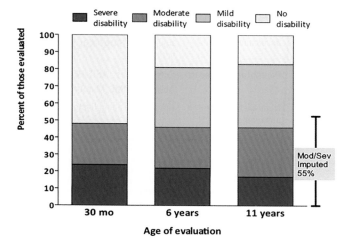

FIGURE 9.5 Outcomes of extreme prematurity (22 to 25 weeks' gestation) changing by age of evaluation. (Source: Courtesy of Dr. N. Marlow, EPICure data.)

In the last 20 years, the landscape of follow-up services has changed significantly, and in addition to local developments, national and worldwide initiatives have been published and implemented. The United States (119) and the World Bank have recommended guidelines and toolkits for measuring childhood development in low- and middle-income countries (3). The United Kingdom has recommendations in NICE (National Institute of Clinical Excellence) guidance (120,121), and Europe-wide standards have been produced by EFCNI (European Foundation for the Care of Newborn Infants) (122).

Increasingly, the recommendation is for comprehensive clinical services aimed at supporting families, measuring outcomes, implementing early intervention, and auditing provision of care. There is still, however, a large variation in service provision. Chisholm described the situation in the United Kingdom (123), where areas of close monitoring contrasted with areas of no standardized provision, and there were variations in composition of MDT involvement in assessments and provision of early intervention services. Similar to the United Kingdom but in much larger magnitude is the great variability in follow-up care and service provision across Europe (124) and in low- and middle-income countries (125).

Surveillance can be used to support research activity and for clinical care and service design (119). Research in neurodevelopment is used to answer a specific question or to test a hypothesis. Here, surveillance may be incorporated into a range of study designs that investigate the impact of obstetric or neonatal factors on outcome; these include randomized controlled trials, systematic reviews, and cohort studies. Clinical care surveillance is used for monitoring, informing, diagnosing, referring, managing, and supporting children and their families, and for informing quality improvement initiatives.

Duration of Surveillance

The minimum agreed length of follow-up for high-risk neonates is 2 years (126), although as evidence grows about the adverse life course outcomes of certain groups of neonates, this is likely to change: indeed, recent UK guidance suggests follow-up until 4 years for those born less than 28 weeks (120).

There is variation in outcome depending on when assessments are performed (Fig. 9.5); 2-year outcomes are insufficient to pick up all developmental concerns, and longer follow-up is required to detect disabilities that manifest later in childhood.

It is generally accepted that correcting for gestational age is important to the age of 2 years, but there remains controversy on how long this should continue for, and it has been suggested that failure to adjust at school level entry could impact educational attainment (127). A final consideration is that age correction may be appropriate for some domains of the Bayley Scales of Infant Development but not others, even before the age of 2 years; further work is required to determine optimal use of chronologic versus corrected age in clinical and research practice (128).

Developmental Tests

Once the high-risk population is defined, and the setting and outcomes have been decided, the selection of a tool for measuring the outcome must be made. Ideally, a test should be standardized, valid, appropriate, easy to administer, low cost (particularly if screening or low-income setting), biologically plausible, and acceptable. In deciding the most suitable child development assessment tools for a population, a number of psychometric properties of the should be considered (Table 9.6).

Although not ideal, developmental tests are useful and popular as an objective measurement of an infant's skills by an independent assessor. The areas for assessment generally include cognition, language, motor, social-emotional, behavioral, adaptation, psychiatric, preacademics, learning ability, memory, executive function, quality of life, and adult outcomes, depending on the population.

TABLE 9.6
Basic Psychometric Properties Used to Evaluate CDATs

Relevance/Importance		Comment	
Reliability	Internal consistency	Evaluates the similarity of test items assessed in one domain. One measure is split-half reliability, which compares the scores on two halves of a test in a single domain.	High internal consistency suggests that some items are too similar, so no additional information is gained from assessing them. Low internal consistency suggests that the items may not be assessing the same domain.
	Interobserver	Evaluates variability between different assessors on the same subject.	There may be systematic errors, specific to a particular group of assessors, and this parameter may not be generalizable when the tool is used by a different group of assessors.
	Intraobserver	Evaluates variability within a single assessor on a single subject.	Commonly evaluated by the same assessor scoring video recordings of their own assessments. This is not essential unless there is low interobserver reliability.
Validity	Test–retest	Evaluates variability within the subject (influenced by random factors such as familiarity with items and mood).	Difficult to interpret in early childhood when changes in development occur over a short time. Usually the repeat assessment should be carried out within 2 weeks of the first test.
	Content	Experts in the field make consensus agreement on whether the individual item and the range of items adequately sample and represent the domain of interest.	Subjective measure that cannot be used in isolation to evaluate validity.
	Criterion	Ideally assessed by comparison to an established "gold standard" test assessing the same construct.	Usually "gold standard" tests are not available, so the comparison is typically against another recognized test regularly used in the same population and thought to measure the same domain.
	Discriminatory/convergent	Evaluates expected positive and negative correlations between scores in different domains or between different tests of the same or differing underlying construct.	Scores from two independent tests (e.g., one using report method, the other a direct test) of one domain should correlate where neither test is considered a "gold-standard." To ensure the test is not overlapping with constructs not of interest, the scores evaluating different constructs should poorly correlate, e.g., test scores on "fine motor" should correlate poorly with "social emotional."
	Construct	Statistical evaluation to see whether values of observed data fit a theoretical model of the constructs (confirmatory) or to explore a possible model of the "underlying traits" being measured.	Large numbers of assessments are required to evaluate this.

CDAT, Child Development Assessment Tools.

From Sabanathan S, Wills B, Gladstone M. Child development assessment tools in low-income and middle-income countries: how can we use them more appropriately? *Arch Dis Child* 2nd ed. 2015;100(5):482. Available from: http://creativecommons.org/licenses/by/4.0/

Assessment tools should be selected based on psychometric properties (Table 9.6), local capabilities, and the purpose of testing (129). Table 9.7 presents a basic categorization of some of the most commonly used developmental assessments available. Sometimes a combination of tests is necessary for answering a specific question.

The World Bank has created the Early Childhood Development Measurement Inventory, an extensive list of tests, describing their characteristics, indications, and cost (3). A more descriptive review by WHO is also available (75), and an analysis of the routine use of various early child development assessment tools and outcomes in global health settings has been recently published (130,131). Recent innovations in testing include the Parent Report of Children's Abilities, Revised (PARCA-R), which has good reliability and validity, is cost effective, and is recommended by NICE guidance (132); and Quantitative Checklist for Autism in Toddlers (Q-CHAT)—modified from the M-CHAT and used in comparison with Bayley assessments (133,134).

Timing of Testing

Any time is good for testing as long as the selected test is designed to measure that particular time in the child's development. Each assessment should provide an opportunity for early intervention therapy according to the child's developmental progress. After the second year, surveillance should be continued by family and local services on a yearly basis until school age. At school, age-specific tools for teachers and parents are added to the surveillance.

TABLE 9.7
Taxonomy of Child Development Measures

Measure	System/Type	Test
Physiology measures	ANS	HR, RR, stress (e.g., cortisol)
	Brain structure	Structural MRI
	Brain function	fMRI, fNIRS, ERP
Behavior measures	Direct child assessment	Screening test: RNDA, GMCD
		Ability test: MDAT, KDI, BSID, NEPSY, WISC, KABC
	Parent/teacher report	Screening test: ASQ, PEDS, TQQ
		Ability test: DMC, MacArthur-Bates CDI
	Naturalistic/structured observational	IEA's Child Coding System

ANS, autonomic nervous system; ASQ, ages and stages questionnaires; CDI, communicative development inventories; DMC, developmental milestones checklist; ERP, event-related potentials; fMRI, functional magnetic resonance imaging; fNIRS, functional near-infrared spectroscopy; GMCD, guide for monitoring child development; HR, heart rate; IEA, International association for the evaluation of educational achievement; KABC, Kaufman assessment battery for children; KDI, Kilifi developmental inventory; BSID, Bayley Scales of Infant Development; MDAT, Malawi developmental assessment tool; MRI, magnetic resonance imaging; NEPSY, developmental neuropsychologic assessment; PEDS, parents' evaluation of developmental status; TQQ, ten questions questionnaire; WISC, Wechsler intelligence scale for children; RNDA, rapid neurodevelopmental assessment; RR, respiratory rate.

From Fernald L, Prado E, Kariger P, et al. A toolkit for measuring early childhood development in low and middle-income countries. 2017. Washington, DC: World Bank. Copyright © World Bank. Available from: https://openknowledge.worldbank.org/handle/10986/29000 License: CC BY 3.0 IGO.

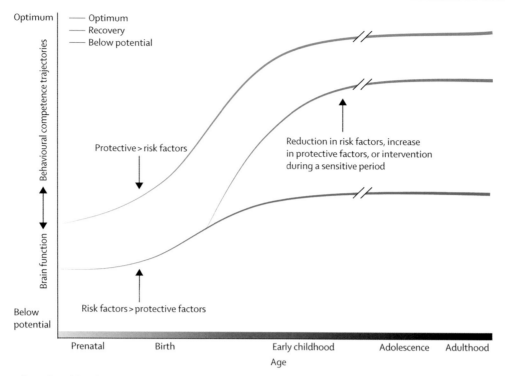

FIGURE 9.6 Differing trajectories of development, with impacts of risks and protective factors. (Reprinted from Walker SP, Wachs TD, Grantham-McGregor S, et al. Inequality in early childhood: risk and protective factors for early child development. *Lancet* 2011;378(9799):1325. Copyright © 2011 Elsevier, with permission.)

Finally, there are several tests on cognition and dexterity available for young adults, plus other measures of quality of life, adaptability to environment, and inclusion into society (119).

The NICE guideline suggests assessments for those with a developmental problem, or those at risk of a developmental problem, should include at least assessments at term/discharge, 3 to 5 months, 12 months, and 24 months of age and be organized by the neonatal team in liaison with the community services available (120).

Assessment Settings and Outcome Assessors

Tests in the form of questionnaires, surveys, or photos/videos can be used by parents at home, teachers in school, nurses in the neonatal unit environment, or therapists and allied health professions in their own environments. As children grow, they can also be their own assessors, especially on measures of quality of life, attainment, and fulfillment (50).

Most tests are done in formal settings, generally in children's clinics with appropriately trained staff, but special consideration is made when these settings are not available or appropriate, and in these circumstances, the home environment may be more suitable.

Ideally a multidisciplinary team should be available for resolution of concerns, as well as for the provision of anticipatory guidance and early intervention. This is dependent on availability but could include neonatologists or pediatricians with neonatal/child development interest, outreach nurses, occupational therapists, physiotherapists, speech/language therapists, dietitians, community nurse or health visitor, and educational/clinical psychologist (120).

Developmental Trajectories

Repeated measurements over time are required for understanding developmental trajectories of individuals and populations and for measuring the impact of interventions (Fig. 9.6). A number of useful insights have come from studying trajectories.

Durrant et al. (Fig. 9.7) report data from greater than 2,000 EP infants in the North Central London Region collected over 15 years

and followed to 2 years. They used the SITAR (superimposition by translation and rotation) model (136) to standardize Bayley III scores to this high-risk population and map domain curves over time.

Important insights have come from longitudinal follow-up of the EPICure cohort from birth to adulthood. Examples are the recent reports showing that the impact of prematurity on cognition remains constant from early childhood to adulthood (Fig. 9.8) (44) and that attention, social and emotional problems in EP individuals persist into early adulthood (45). The Bayley III trajectories also show variation by skill (Fig. 9.9).

The Neurology Examination

The neurology examination is an essential part of any neuro-developmental assessment. Sequential neurology assessments in infants initially described by Amiel-Tison have been widely published and used as outcome measures for diagnosing motor problems and prompting interventions for motor development (137).

The Hammersmith Newborn and Infant Neurology examinations are validated tools for use in children from birth to 2 years of age. They are comprehensive, giving a score that is predictive of motor outcomes, and can be used for clinical trajectories (138).

The Prechtl GM video assessment is currently the most reliable examination as a predictor of motor outcome in high-risk infants either preterm or term. The fidgety movements are seen at around 12 weeks of age, and their absence is highly specific and sensitive for prediction of CP. The generated optimality score is useful for research, and work is ongoing for validating this tool for nonmotor prognoses. GM assessment has been added to neurodevelopmental surveillance in Europe and the United Kingdom (20,139).

Other neurology examinations have been described elsewhere. Regardless of the test, for clinical purposes, a sequence of at least three examinations is needed for a reliable trajectory.

The HC trajectory should always be included in the neurology examination.

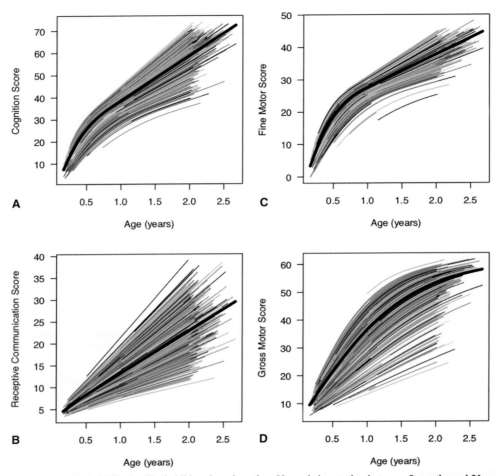

FIGURE 9.7 Developmental trajectories with Bayley III of children born less than 30 weeks' gestation between 3 months and 24 months: (A) cognition, (B) receptive communication, (C) fine motor, (D) gross motor, with mean curve in *black*. (Used with permission from Durrant C, Wong H, Cole TJ, et al. Developmental trajectories of children born at less than 30 weeks gestation on the Bayley-III scales. Neonatal Society Autumn Meeting; 2018:3. Courtesy of Dr. Angela Huertas.)

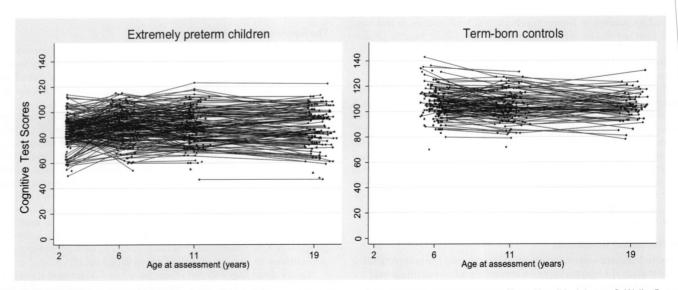

FIGURE 9.8 Cognitive trajectories of extremely preterm children and their term controls, from 2.5 years to 19 years. (From Linsell L, Johnson S, Wolke D, et al. Cognitive trajectories from infancy to early adulthood following birth before 26 weeks of gestation: a prospective, population-based cohort study. *Arch Dis Child* 2nd ed. 2018;103(4):363. Available from: https://creativecommons.org/licenses/by/4.0/)

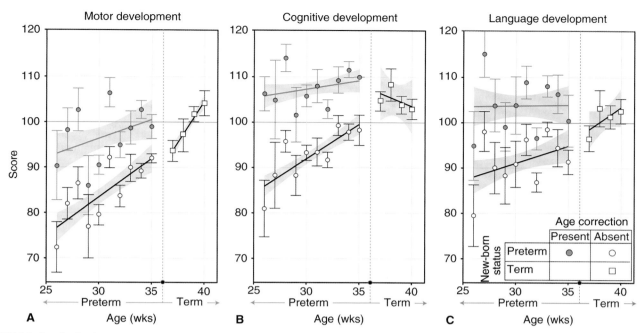

FIGURE 9.9 Standardized average uncorrected and corrected age scores (±standard error of the mean) as a function of gestational age (in weeks) for the (A) motor, (B) cognitive, and (C) language developmental domains. The newborn status (preterm 26 to 35 weeks vs. term 37 to 40 weeks) and the age correction (present, absent) are coded by color and shape, respectively. The *lines* indicate the multiple regression model, and the *shaded area* corresponds to ±1 standard error of the regression. (From Morsan V, Fantoni C, Tallandini MA. Age correction in cognitive, linguistic, and motor domains for infants born preterm: an analysis of the Bayley Scales of Infant and Toddler Development, Third Edition developmental patterns. *Dev Med Child Neurol* 2018;60(8):820. Copyright © 2018 Mac Keith Press. Reprinted by permission of John Wiley & Sons, Inc.)

EARLY INTERVENTION

General Principles of Early Intervention

Early Intervention (EI) programs have the potential to influence growth and developmental trajectories. It has been hypothesized that the earlier the intervention, the greatest likelihood of beneficial effect (135).

EI programs aim to promote health and well-being, protect neurodevelopment, and prevent deterioration in developmental domains. Early cognitive, communication, growth, and development are influenced by many factors, and social and emotional development are directly influenced by caregiver relationships. Therefore, these programs should integrate the environment, community, parents, families, communication strategies, information on sensory awareness, and motor development. A comprehensive review by Hutchon describes the principles by which we should manage these settings and families (1).

Important clinical interventions happen before, during, and after delivery, after discharge, and at different points during preschool, school, and adult life. EI beyond discharge have shown some initial benefits, although the evidence for sustained impact on long-term outcomes is not robust across all developmental domains. However, there is extensive literature advocating EI as good practice guidance.

Before Delivery

Prevention of Preterm Birth and Antenatal Counseling

Antenatal medical interventions and involvement of parents and family in antenatal counseling and decisions are key early interventions to improve neurodevelopmental outcomes in high-risk infant.

In the Neonatal Unit

Family Care

FIC is a widely recognized form of neonatal care where parents are the primary caregivers, and neonatal staff provide support and education. Alongside state-of-the-art clinical skills, evidence-based

management protocols, and highly skilled professionals, FIC has been suggested to improve neurodevelopmental outcomes (140).

Initiatives using developmentally supportive care environments include NIDCAP, developmental care, family nurture interventions, kangaroo mother care, and early intervention strategies that extend beyond discharge (141,142).

Support for families goes beyond clinical care for their infants. In term and EP/ELBW infants, feeding problems and maternal interactions with their child are interrelated, with increasing feeding problems over time (143).

Communication and Language Problems

Children born preterm were found to have specific deficits in social communication and symbolic skills. They spend the first part of their lives exposed to a range of atypical sensory stimuli. After discharge, they experience higher rates of oromotor impairments, which have been hypothesized to link to language deficits. Further investigations into the impact of early environment on language outcomes, and effective language interventions, are critical in facilitating improved outcomes (35).

After Discharge

Early interventions in the post-discharge period currently rely on early assessments and identification of those at risk, with targeting of therapy services and other support to those most vulnerable. An example of early intervention is the EI SMART framework, addressing sensorimotor development, attention and regulation, relationships, and therapist support (1). These must be personalized based on the individual, with their diagnoses and problems, as well as the environment and local capabilities.

ECONOMICS AND FINANCIAL ASPECTS OF MEDICAL AND NEURODEVELOPMENTAL SURVEILLANCE

Manghan et al. estimated the economic consequences of preterm birth from birth to adult life stratified by gestational age and compared them to term birth in the United Kingdom. They concluded that despite concerns about ongoing costs after discharge from perinatal services, the largest contribution to the economic impact of preterm birth are hospital inpatient costs after birth, which are responsible for 92.0% of the incremental costs per preterm survivor (144).

A systematic review of the economic consequences of preterm birth for health services, the economy, families and carers, and more broadly for society has been published. Initial hospitalization costs varied from $576,972 per infant born at 24 weeks to $930 per infant born at term, and from $169,132 per surviving infant born at less than 1,500 g to $1,200 per infant born at greater than 2,500 g (U.S., 2015 prices). Average duration of initial hospitalization varied between 116 days per surviving infant born at 24 weeks' gestation to 2.4 days per infant born at term. A consistent inverse association was observed between gestational age and economic costs regardless of period of follow-up and age at assessment (145).

In terms of specific diagnoses, Petrou et al. presented estimated costs and health-related quality of life outcomes associated with childhood psychiatric disorders during the 11th year of life of the EPICure cohort. Compared to the term-born control population, the preterm population had an average annual cost difference of over £2,000. This exceeds that identified for several other childhood conditions, including childhood asthma and juvenile idiopathic arthritis, and compares with annual cost burdens reported elsewhere of £890 (1996–1997 prices) for childhood depression, and U.S. $1,100 to 1,800 (1996 prices) for ADHD (146).

The World Bank reviewed evidence for interventions in low- and middle-income countries in a variety of domains that would benefit child development—these included nutrition, health, water, sanitation, education, social protection, physical environment, and nurturing care. Early childhood interventions are important economic investments, with higher returns in terms of human capital than those in later life (147). The WHO made clear that informal support services are insufficient for children at risk, and governmental policy, funding, and service provision is necessary to ensure that those who require additional support can access it (148).

CONCLUSION

The main purpose of perinatal care is to raise healthy babies who are able to reach their full potentials in life. Maternal conditions, problems during pregnancy, and complications at delivery predispose the newborn to short and long-term problems with general health and development. Added risks include medical and pharmaceutical interventions, environmental exposures, and associated altered parent interactions. These cumulative vulnerabilities mean follow-up is needed for the optimization of ongoing growth and development.

Follow-up care for these high-risk infants begins antenatally when parents are counselled, or at birth for those whose antenatal risks are not known or not present, and families are to be encouraged to participate in their children's growth and developmental progress throughout admission.

Measurements of outcomes throughout admission provide useful trajectories on growth, HC, nutrition, sensory systems, behavior, and neurobehavioral profiles, which help build the foundation for developmental trajectories after discharge into infancy and childhood.

Interventions including promotion of maternal health, prevention of preterm birth, delivery in the right place, evidence-based clinical guidelines, available breast milk, continuous parental support, provision for developmental care and skin-to-skin, and preparation for discharge from the point of admission are just some of the many interventions that may redirect trajectories in future development of children at risk.

Research has helped us understand that EI in the early years may provide a cost-effective window of opportunity to promote better outcomes (135), although further research is required to identify which interventions should be used. It has also shown that developmental trajectories are influenced by socio-environmental factors, including the families and communities in which they live (3).

Funding for research and innovation should aim to reduce the burden of prematurity, improve technology in obstetric management, facilitate delivery at the right place with the right expertise, improve neonatal unit environments, promote bonding and attachment with families, and support communities responsible for delivering the interventions.

Demand for assessments that are standardized valid, objective, and generalizable to inform research and services has significantly increased, and there is now a wide variety of tests, questionnaires, checklists, and surveys available to measure outcomes in at-risk children. However, the essential questions on quality of life are not always addressed.

The needs of this high-risk group of infants must be recognized globally in line with other health and welfare priorities, to ensure that they are identified as a vulnerable population. The development of basic surveillance programs, with the potential for creating early intervention strategies for supporting infants and their families, should be added to the political agenda, as well as to the social, health, and educational agendas.

Global initiatives in low- and middle-income countries, aiming to promote the rights of children to grow, develop, and live a happy life, are now concentrating on improving basic risk factors related to their environment, such as the provision of safe water, adequate nutrition, and basic education. Further funding has been devoted to improving access to health services in an attempt at reaching not only the high-risk population of children but also the community where they live. Good antenatal and neonatal care globally, with supportive surveillance, may allow high-risk infants to live active and fulfilling lives.

REFERENCES

1. Hutchon B, Gibbs D, Harniess P, et al. Early intervention programmes for infants at high risk of atypical neurodevelopmental outcome. *Dev Med Child Neurol* 2019;(11):CD005495.
2. Edstedt Bonamy AK, Zeitlin J, Piedvache A, et al. Wide variation in severe neonatal morbidity among very preterm infants in European regions. *Arch Dis Child Fetal Neonatal Ed* 2018;104(1):F36.
3. Fernald L, Prado E, Kariger P, et al. *A toolkit for measuring early childhood development in low and middle-income countries*. Washington, DC: World Bank, 2017.
4. Committee on Fetus and Newborn. Hospital discharge of the high-risk neonate. *Pediatrics* 2008;122(5):1119.
5. Ingram JC, Powell JE, Blair PS, et al. Does family-centred neonatal discharge planning reduce healthcare usage? A before and after study in South West England. *BMJ Open* 2016;6(3):e010752.
6. Bliss. *Bliss Family Friendly Accreditation Scheme*. 2015 Jan 14:1.
7. Berman L, Raval MV, Ottosen M, et al. Parent perspectives on readiness for discharge home after neonatal intensive care unit admission. *J Pediatr* 2019;205:98.
8. Gupta M, Pursley DM, Smith VC. Preparing for discharge from the neonatal intensive care unit. *Pediatrics* 2019;143(6):e20182915.
9. Grantham-McGregor S, Cheung YB, Cueto S, et al. Developmental potential in the first 5 years for children in developing countries. *Lancet* 2007;369(9555):60.
10. Thompson RA, Nelson CA. Developmental science and the media. *Early brain development. Am Psychol* 2001;56(1):5.
11. Als H. *Newborn Individualized Developmental Care and Assessment Program (NIDCAP)*. Boston, MA: NIDCAP Federation International, 2011.
12. World Health Organization. *International Classification of Functioning, Disability and Health—Children & Youth Version*. Geneva: World Health Organization, 2008:1.
13. BAPM RCPCH Working Group. *Classification of health status at 2 years as a perinatal outcome*. London: British Association of Perinatal Medicine, 2008.
14. Overman AE, Liu M, Kurachek SC, et al. Tracheostomy for infants requiring prolonged mechanical ventilation: 10 years' experience. *Pediatrics* 2013;131(5):e1491.

15. Cristea AI, Carroll AE, Davis SD, et al. Outcomes of children with severe bronchopulmonary dysplasia who were ventilator dependent at home. *Pediatrics* 2013;132(3):e727.

16. Tsang AKL. The special needs of preterm children—an oral health perspective. *Dent Clin North Am* 2016;60(3):737.

17. Huang P, Zhou J, Yin Y, et al. Effects of breast-feeding compared with formula-feeding on preterm infant body composition: a systematic review and meta-analysis. *Br J Nutr* 2016;116(1):132.

18. Koyama S, Ichikawa G, Kojima M, et al. Adiposity rebound and the development of metabolic syndrome. *Pediatrics* 2014;133(1):e114.

19. Rochow N, Raja P, Liu K, et al. Physiological adjustment to postnatal growth trajectories in healthy preterm infants. *Pediatr Res* 2016;79(6):870.

20. Ferrari F, Frassoldati R, Berardi A, et al. The ontogeny of fidgety movements from 4 to 20 weeks post-term age in healthy full-term infants. *Early Hum Dev* 2016;103(C):219.

21. National Guideline Alliance (UK). *Cerebral palsy in under 25s: assessment and management.* London: National Institute for Health and Care Excellence (UK), 2017.

22. Alexander B, Kelly CE, Adamson C, et al. Changes in neonatal regional brain volume associated with preterm birth and perinatal factors. *NeuroImage* 2019;185:654.

23. Marlow N. Outcome following extremely preterm birth. *Curr Paediatr* 2004;14(4):275.

24. Boyle EM, Johnson S, Manktelow B, et al. Neonatal outcomes and delivery of care for infants born late preterm or moderately preterm: a prospective population-based study. *Arch Dis Child Fetal Neonatal Ed* 2015;100(6):F479.

25. Petrini JR, Dias T, McCormick MC, et al. Increased risk of adverse neurological development for late preterm infants. *J Pediatr* 2009;154(2):169.

26. Chan E, Quigley MA. School performance at age 7 years in late preterm and early term birth: a cohort study. *Arch Dis Child Fetal Neonatal Ed* 2014;99(6):F451.

27. Aarnoudse-Moens CSH, Weisglas-Kuperus N, van Goudoever JB, et al. Meta-analysis of neurobehavioral outcomes in very preterm and/or very low birth weight children. *Pediatrics* 2009;124(2):717.

28. Costeloe KL, Hennessy EM, Haider S, et al. Short term outcomes after extreme preterm birth in England: comparison of two birth cohorts in 1995 and 2006 (the EPICure studies). *BMJ* 2012;345(dec04 3):e7976.

29. Patel RM, Rysavy MA, Bell EF, et al. Survival of infants born at periviable gestational ages. *Clin Perinatol* 2017;44(2):287.

30. Adams-Chapman I, Heyne RJ, DeMauro SB, et al. Neurodevelopmental impairment among extremely preterm infants in the neonatal research network. *Pediatrics* 2018;141(5):e20173091.

31. Johnson S, Marlow N. Growing up after extremely preterm birth: lifespan mental health outcomes. *Semin Fetal Neonatal Med* 2014;19(2):97.

32. Moore T, Johnson S, Hennessy E, et al. Screening for autism in extremely preterm infants: problems in interpretation. *Dev Med Child Neurol* 2012;54(6):514.

33. Kuban KCK, O'Shea TM, Allred EN, et al. Positive screening on the Modified Checklist for Autism in Toddlers (M-CHAT) in extremely low gestational age newborns. *J Pediatr* 2009;154(4):535.

34. Johnson S, Marlow N. Preterm birth and childhood psychiatric disorders. *Pediatr Res* 2011;69(5 Pt 2):11R.

35. Sanchez K, Spittle AJ, Cheong JL, et al. Language in 2-year-old children born preterm and term: a cohort study. *Arch Dis Child* 2019;104(7):647.

36. Fierson WM; American Academy of Pediatrics Section on Ophthalmology, American Academy of Ophthalmology, American Association for Pediatric Ophthalmology, American Association of Certified Orthoptists. Screening examination of premature infants for retinopathy of prematurity. *Pediatrics* 2018;142(6):e20183061.

37. MacKay DF, Smith GCS, Dobbie R, et al. Gestational age at delivery and special educational need: retrospective cohort study of 407,503 school-children. Lau TK, editor. *PLoS Med* 2010;7(6):e1000289.

38. Keunen K, Benders MJ, Leemans A, et al. White matter maturation in the neonatal brain is predictive of school age cognitive capacities in children born very preterm. *Dev Med Child Neurol* 2017;59(9):939.

39. Moore GP, Lemyre B, Barrowman N, et al. Neurodevelopmental outcomes at 4 to 8 years of children born at 22 to 25 weeks' gestational age. *JAMA Pediatr* 2013;167(10):967.

40. Kerr-Wilson CO, Mackay DF, Smith GCS, et al. Meta-analysis of the association between preterm delivery and intelligence. *J Public Health* 2012;34(2):209.

41. Simms V, Cragg L, Gilmore C, et al. Mathematics difficulties in children born very preterm: current research and future directions. *Arch Dis Child Fetal Neonatal Ed* 2013;98(5):F457.

42. Anderson PJ. Neuropsychological outcomes of children born very preterm. *Semin Fetal Neonatal Med* 2014;19(2):90.

43. Johnson S, Marlow N. Early and long-term outcome of infants born extremely preterm. *Arch Dis Child* 2016;102(1):97.

44. Linsell L, Johnson S, Wolke D, et al. Cognitive trajectories from infancy to early adulthood following birth before 26 weeks of gestation: a prospective, population-based cohort study. *Arch Dis Child* 2018;103(4):363.

45. Linsell L, Johnson S, Wolke D, et al. Trajectories of behavior, attention, social and emotional problems from childhood to early adulthood following extremely preterm birth: a prospective cohort study. *Eur Child Adolesc Psychiatry* 2018;28(4):531.

46. Mendonça M, Bilgin A, Wolke D. Association of Preterm Birth and Low Birth Weight With Romantic Partnership, Sexual Intercourse, and Parenthood in Adulthood: a systematic review and meta-analysis. *JAMA Netw Open* 2019;2(7):e196961.

47. Wolke D, Baumann N, Strauss V, et al. Bullying of preterm children and emotional problems at school age: cross-culturally invariant effects. *J Pediatr* 2015;166(6):1417.

48. Saigal S. Functional outcomes of very premature infants into adulthood. *Semin Fetal Neonatal Med* 2014;19(2):125.

49. Hack M. Young adult outcomes of very-low-birth-weight children. *Semin Fetal Neonatal Med* 2006;11(2):127.

50. Saigal S. Quality of life of former premature infants during adolescence and beyond. *Early Hum Dev* 2013;89(4):209.

51. Savchev S, Sanz-Cortes M, Cruz-Martinez R, et al. Neurodevelopmental outcome of full-term small-for-gestational-age infants with normal placental function. *Ultrasound Obstet Gynecol* 2013;42(2):201.

52. McGrath AP, Vohr BR. Hearing loss in the newborn infant: early hearing detection and intervention. *Neoreviews* 2017;18(10):e587.

53. Wagenaar N, Martinez-Biarge M, van der Aa NE, et al. Neurodevelopment after perinatal arterial ischemic stroke. *Pediatrics* 2018;142(3):e20174164.

54. De Vis JB, Alderliesten T, Hendrikse J, et al. Magnetic resonance imaging based noninvasive measurements of brain hemodynamics in neonates: a review. *Pediatr Res* 2016;80(5):641.

55. World Health Organization. *Congenital anomalies.* Geneva: World Health Organization, 2016:1.

56. Peetsold MG, Heij HA, Kneepkens CMF, et al. The long-term follow-up of patients with a congenital diaphragmatic hernia: a broad spectrum of morbidity. *Pediatr Surg Int* 2008;25(1):1.

57. Nattel SN, Adrianzen L, Kessler EC, et al. Congenital heart disease and neurodevelopment: clinical manifestations, genetics, mechanisms, and implications. *Can J Cardiol* 2017;33(12):1543.

58. Scott SM, Rose SR. Use of glucocorticoids for the fetus and preterm infant. *Clin Perinatol* 2018;45(1):93.

59. Ting JY, Roberts A, Sherlock R, et al. Duration of initial empirical antibiotic therapy and outcomes in very low birth weight infants. *Pediatrics* 2019;143(3):e20182286.

60. Walker SM. Long-term effects of neonatal pain. *Semin Fetal Neonatal Med* 2019;24(4):101005.

61. Giordano V, Deindl P, Fuiko R, et al. Effect of increased opiate exposure on three years neurodevelopmental outcome in extremely preterm infants. *Early Hum Dev* 2018;123:1.

62. Zwicker JG, Miller SP, Grunau RE, et al. Smaller cerebellar growth and poorer neurodevelopmental outcomes in very preterm infants exposed to neonatal morphine. *J Pediatr* 2016;172:81.

63. Akbari E, Binnoon-Erez N, Rodrigues M, et al. Kangaroo mother care and infant biopsychosocial outcomes in the first year—a meta-analysis. *Early Hum Dev* 2018;122:22.

64. Charlton AJ, Davies JM, Rimmer S. Anaesthesia and brain damage in the newborn. *Anaesthesia* 1989;44(8):641.

65. Davidson AJ, Disma N, de Graaff JC, et al. Neurodevelopmental outcome at 2 years of age after general anaesthesia and awake-regional anaesthesia in infancy (GAS): an international multicentre, randomised controlled trial. *Lancet* 2016;387(10015):239.

66. Kua KP, Lee SWH. Systematic review and meta-analysis of clinical outcomes of early caffeine therapy in preterm neonates. *Br J Clin Pharmacol* 2016;83(1):180.

67. Lodha A, Entz R, Synnes A, et al. Early caffeine administration and neurodevelopmental outcomes in preterm infants. *Pediatrics* 2019;143(1):e20181348.

68. Atik A, Harding R, De Matteo R, et al. Caffeine for apnea of prematurity: Effects on the developing brain. *Neurotoxicology* 2017;58:94.

69. Doyle LW, Crowther CA, Middleton P, et al. Magnesium sulphate for women at risk of preterm birth for neuroprotection of the fetus. Cochrane Pregnancy and Childbirth Group, editor. *Cochrane Database Syst Rev* 2009;290(20):2669.

70. Crowther CA, Middleton PF, Voysey M, et al. Assessing the neuroprotective benefits for babies of antenatal magnesium sulphate: an individual participant data meta-analysis. Myers JE, editor. *PLoS Med* 2017;14(10):e1002398.

71. Sadhwani A, Cheng H, Stopp C, et al. Early neurodevelopmental outcomes in children supported with ECMO for cardiac indications. *Pediatr Cardiol* 2019;40(5):1072.

72. Markopoulou P, Papanikolaou E, Analytis A, et al. Preterm birth as a risk factor for metabolic syndrome and cardiovascular disease in adult life: a systematic review and meta-analysis. *J Pediatr* 2019;210:69.

GENERAL CONSIDERATIONS

73. ESPGHAN Committee on Nutrition; Agostoni C, Braegger C, Decsi T, et al. Breast-feeding: a commentary by the ESPGHAN Committee on Nutrition. *J Pediatr Gastroenterol Nutr* 2009;49:112.

74. Bar S, Milanaik R, Adesman A. Long-term neurodevelopmental benefits of breastfeeding. *Curr Opin Pediatr* 2016;28(4):559.

75. World Health Organization. *Developmental difficulties in early childhood.* Geneva: World Health Organization, 2012.

76. Canadian Paediatric Society, Digital Health Task Force, Ottawa, Ontario, Ponti M, Bélanger S, Grimes R, et al. Screen time and young children: promoting health and development in a digital world. *Paediatr Child Health* 2017;22(8):461.

77. Leijser LM, de Bruïne FT, van der Grond J, et al. Is sequential cranial ultrasound reliable for detection of white matter injury in very preterm infants? *Neuroradiology* 2010;52(5):397.

78. Setänen S, Lahti K, Lehtonen L, et al. Neurological examination combined with brain MRI or cranial US improves prediction of neurological outcome in preterm infants. *Early Hum Dev* 2014;90(12):851.

79. Sánchez Fernández I, Morales-Quezada JL, Law S, et al. Prognostic value of brain magnetic resonance imaging in neonatal hypoxic-ischemic encephalopathy: a meta-analysis. *J Child Neurol* 2017;32(13):1065.

80. Anderson PJ, Cheong JLY, Thompson DK. The predictive validity of neonatal MRI for neurodevelopmental outcome in very preterm children. *Semin Perinatol* 2015;39(2):147.

81. Edwards AD, Redshaw ME, Kennea N, et al. Effect of MRI on preterm infants and their families: a randomised trial with nested diagnostic and economic evaluation. *Arch Dis Child Fetal Neonatal Ed* 2017;103(1):F15.

82. Kendall GS, Melbourne A, Johnson S, et al. White matter NAA/Cho and Cho/Cr ratios at MR spectroscopy are predictive of motor outcome in preterm infants. *Radiology* 2014;271(1):230.

83. Mitra S, Kendall GS, Bainbridge A, et al. Proton magnetic resonance spectroscopy lactate/N-acetylaspartate within 2 weeks of birth accurately predicts 2-year motor, cognitive and language outcomes in neonatal encephalopathy after therapeutic hypothermia. *Arch Dis Child Fetal Neonatal Ed* 2019;104(4):F424.

84. Tann CJ, Webb EL, Lassman R, et al. Early childhood outcomes after neonatal encephalopathy in uganda: a cohort study. *EClinicalMedicine* 2018;6(C):26.

85. Tann CJ, Nakakeeto M, Hagmann C, et al. Early cranial ultrasound findings among infants with neonatal encephalopathy in Uganda: an observational study. *Pediatr Res* 2016;80(2):190.

86. Villar J; Giuliani F, Bhutta ZA, et al. Postnatal growth standards for preterm infants; the Preterm Postnatal Follow-up Study of the INTERGROWTH-21(st) Project. *Lancet Glob Health* 2015;3(11):e681.

87. World Health Organization. *WHO Child Growth Standards and the Identification of Severe Acute Malnutrition in Infants and Children: A Joint Statement by the World Health Organization and the United Nations Children's Fund.* Geneva: World Health Organization, 2009.

88. Cole TJ, Statnikov Y, Santhakumaran S, et al.; on behalf of the Neonatal Data Analysis Unit and the Preterm Growth Investigator Group. Birth weight and longitudinal growth in infants born below 32 weeks' gestation: a UK population study. *Arch Dis Child Fetal Neonatal Ed* 2013; 99(1):F34.

89. Ogden CL, Kuczmarski RJ, Flegal KM, et al. Centers for Disease Control and Prevention 2000 Growth Charts for the United States: improvements to the 1977 National Center for Health Statistics Version. *Pediatrics* 2002;109(1):45.

90. Villar J, Giuliani F, Figueras-Aloy J, et al. Growth of preterm infants at the time of global obesity. *Arch Dis Child* 2019;104(8):725.

91. Schwarzenberg SJ, Georgieff MK; Committee on Nutrition. Advocacy for improving nutrition in the first 1000 days to support childhood development and adult health. *Pediatrics* 2018;141(2):e20173716.

92. Hack M. Catch-up growth during childhood among very-low-birth-weight children. *Arch Pediatr Adolesc Med* 1996;150(11):1122.

93. Saigal S, Stoskopf BL, Streiner DL, et al. Physical growth and current health status of infants who were of extremely low birth weight and controls at adolescence. *Pediatrics* 2001;108(2):407.

94. Silver HK, Deamer WC. Graphs of the head circumference of the normal infant. *J Pediatr* 1948;33(2):167.

95. Agostoni C, Buonocore G, Carnielli VP, et al. Enteral nutrient supply for preterm infants: commentary from the European Society of Paediatric Gastroenterology, Hepatology and Nutrition Committee on Nutrition. *J Pediatr Gastroenterol Nutr* 2010;50(1):85.

96. Peters T, Pompeii-Wolfe C. Nutrition considerations after NICU discharge. *Pediatr Ann* 2018;47(4):e154.

97. Young L, Embleton ND, McCormick FM, et al. Multinutrient fortification of human breast milk for preterm infants following hospital discharge. Cochrane Neonatal Group, editor. *Cochrane Database Syst Rev* 2013;49(4):456.

98. Patra K, Greene MM. Impact of feeding difficulties in the NICU on neurodevelopmental outcomes at 8 and 20 months corrected age in extremely low gestational age infants. *J Perinatol* 2019;39(9):1241.

99. Orton JL, Olsen JE, Ong K, et al. NICU graduates: the role of the allied health team in follow-up. *Pediatr Ann* 2018;47(4):e165.

100. Marinschek S, Pahsini K, Scheer PJ, et al. Long-term outcomes of an interdisciplinary tube weaning program. *J Pediatr Gastroenterol Nutr* 2019;68(4):591.

101. Rosen R, Vandenplas Y, Singendonk M, et al. Pediatric gastroesophageal reflux clinical practice guidelines. *J Pediatr Gastroenterol Nutr* 2018;66(3):516.

102. Tighe M, Afzal NA, Bevan A, et al. Pharmacological treatment of children with gastro-oesophageal reflux. Cochrane Upper GI and Pancreatic Diseases Group, editor. *Cochrane Database Syst Rev* 2014;49(9):852.

103. Public Health England. *Immunisation against infectious disease.* London: Public Health England, 2017:1–5.

104. Denizot S, Fleury J, Caillaux G, et al. Hospital initiation of a vaccinal schedule improves the long-term vaccinal coverage of ex-preterm children. *Vaccine* 2011;29(3):382.

105. Centers for Disease Control and Prevention. *Recommended Childhood and Adolescent Immunization Schedules:* Atlanta: CDC, 2019. *AAP books.* 2019;879.

106. American Academy of Pediatrics Committee on Infectious Diseases, American Academy of Pediatrics Bronchiolitis Guidelines Committee. Updated guidance for palivizumab prophylaxis among infants and young children at increased risk of hospitalization for respiratory syncytial virus infection. *Pediatrics* 2014;134:415.

107. Hayes D Jr, Wilson KC, Krivchenia K, et al. Home oxygen therapy for children. An Official American Thoracic Society Clinical Practice Guideline. *Am J Respir Crit Care Med* 2019;199(3):e5.

108. Balfour-Lynn IM, Field DJ, Gringras P, et al. BTS guidelines for home oxygen in children. *Thorax* 2009;64(Suppl 2):ii1.

109. Ross E, Stephenson K. Fifteen-minute consultation: emergency management of tracheostomy problems in children. *Arch Dis Child Educ Pract Ed* 2019;104(4):189.

110. Reynolds V, Meldrum S, Simmer K, et al. Dysphonia in very preterm children: a review of the evidence. *Neonatology* 2014;106(1):69.

111. Glass HC, Pham TN, Danielsen B, et al. Antenatal and intrapartum risk factors for seizures in term newborns: a population-based study, California 1998–2002. *J Pediatr* 2009;154(1):24.

112. Simbruner G, Mittal RA, Rohlmann F, et al.; neo.nEURO.network Trial Participants. Systemic hypothermia after neonatal encephalopathy: outcomes of neo.nEURO.network RCT. *Pediatrics* 2010;126(4):e771.

113. Strober JB, Bienkowski RS, Maytal J. The incidence of acute and remote seizures in children with intraventricular hemorrhage. *Clin Pediatr* 1997;36(11):643.

114. Kohelet D, Shochat R, Lusky A, et al. Risk factors for seizures in very low birthweight infants with periventricular leukomalacia. *J Child Neurol* 2006;21(11):965.

115. Azmeh R, Lueder GT. Delayed visual maturation in otherwise normal infants. *Graefes Arch Clin Exp Ophthalmol* 2012;251(3):941.

116. Mercuri E, Atkinson J, Braddick O, et al. The aetiology of delayed visual maturation: Short review and personal findings in relation to magnetic resonance imaging. *Eur J Paediatr Neurol* 1997;1(1):31.

117. Adams L, Basu TN, Orrin E. Subcutaneous fat necrosis in a newborn. *BMJ* 2018;363:k4062.

118. Task Force on Sudden Infant Death Syndrome. SIDS and other sleep-related infant deaths: updated 2016 recommendations for a safe infant sleeping environment. *Pediatrics* 2016;138(5):e20162938.

119. Vohr B, Wright LL, Hack M. Follow-up care of high-risk infants. *Pediatrics* 2011;114(Supplement 5):1377.

120. National Guideline Alliance (UK). *Developmental follow-up of children and young people born preterm.* London: National Institute for Health and Care Excellence (UK), 2017.

121. Mckinnon K, Huertas-Ceballos A. Developmental follow-up of children and young people born preterm, NICE guideline 2017. *Arch Dis Child Educ Pract Ed* 2019;104(4):221.

122. EFCNI. *European Standards of Care for Newborn Health: follow-up and continuing care.* Munich: EFCNI, 2018. 101 p.

123. Chisholm P, Arasu A, Huertas-Ceballos A. Neurodevelopmental follow-up for high-risk neonates: current practice in Great Britain. *Arch Dis Child Fetal Neonatal Ed* 2017;102(6):F558.1.

124. Seppänen AV, Elizabeth D, Barros H, et al. 3rd Congress of Joint European Neonatal Societies (jENS 2019). *Pediatr Res* 2019;86(Suppl 1):1.

125. Yousafzai AK, Lynch P, Gladstone M. Moving beyond prevalence studies: screening and interventions for children with disabilities in low-income and middle-income countries. *Arch Dis Child* 2014;99(9):840.

126. Neonatal NADOH. *Toolkit for high quality neonatal services.* London: Department of Health, 2009.

127. Odd D, Evans D, Emond A. Preterm birth, age at school entry and long term educational achievement. Schooling CM, editor. *PLoS ONE* 2016;11(5):e0155157.

128. Morsan V, Fantoni C, Tallandini MA. Age correction in cognitive, linguistic, and motor domains for infants born preterm: an analysis of the

Bayley Scales of Infant and Toddler Development, Third Edition developmental patterns. *Dev Med Child Neurol* 2018;60(8):820.

129. Sabanathan S, Wills B, Gladstone M. Child development assessment tools in low-income and middle-income countries: how can we use them more appropriately? *Arch Dis Child.* 2015;100(5):482.

130. Boggs D, Milner KM, Chandna J, et al. Rating early child development outcome measurement tools for routine health programme use. *Arch Dis Child* 2019;104(Suppl 1):S22.

131. Woodward LJ, Huppi PS. Neurodevelopmental follow-up. In: Volpe JJ, ed. *Volpe's neurology of the newborn.* 6th ed. Philadelphia, PA: Elsevier, 2018:255.

132. Johnson S, Bountziouka V, Brocklehurst P, et al. Standardisation of the Parent Report of Children's Abilities–Revised (PARCA-R): a norm-referenced assessment of cognitive and language development at age 2 years. *Lancet Child Adolesc Health* 2019;3(10):705.

133. Allison C, Baron-Cohen S, Wheelwright S, et al. The Q-CHAT (Quantitative CHecklist for Autism in Toddlers): a normally distributed quantitative measure of autistic traits at 18–24 months of age: preliminary report. *J Autism Dev Disord* 2008;38(8):1414.

134. Wong HS, Huertas-Ceballos A, Cowan FM, et al. Evaluation of early childhood social-communication difficulties in children born preterm using the quantitative checklist for autism in toddlers. *J Pediatr* 2014;164(1):26.

135. Walker SP, Wachs TD, Grantham-McGregor S, et al. Inequality in early childhood: risk and protective factors for early child development. *Lancet* 2011;378(9799):1325.

136. Durrant C, Wong H, Cole TJ, et al. Developmental trajectories of children born at less than 30 weeks gestation on the Bayley-III scales. Neonatal Society Autumn Meeting; 2018. 3 p.

137. Amiel-Tison C. Update of the Amiel-Tison neurologic assessment for the term neonate or at 40 weeks corrected age. *Pediatr Neurol* 2002;27(3):196.

138. Haataja L, Mercuri E, Regev R, et al. Optimality score for the neurologic examination of the infant at 12 and 18 months of age. *J Pediatr* 1999;135(2 I):153.

139. Einspieler C, Prechtl HFR. Prechtl's assessment of general movements: a diagnostic tool for the functional assessment of the young nervous system. *Ment Retard Dev Disabil Res Rev* 2005;11(1):61.

140. Young A, McKechnie L, Harrison CM. Family integrated care: what's all the fuss about? *Arch Dis Child Fetal Neonatal Ed* 2019;104(2):F118.

141. Bann CM, Wallander JL, Do B, et al. Home-based early intervention and the influence of family resources on cognitive development. *Pediatrics* 2016;137(4):e20153766.

142. van Wassenaer-Leemhuis AG, Jeukens-Visser M, van Hus JWP, et al. Rethinking preventive post-discharge intervention programmes for very preterm infants and their parents. *Dev Med Child Neurol* 2016;58:67.

143. Bilgin A, Wolke D. Associations between feeding problems and maternal sensitivity across infancy: differences in very preterm and full-term infants. *J Dev Behav Pediatr* 2017;38(7):538.

144. Mangham LJ, Petrou S, Doyle LW, et al. The cost of preterm birth throughout childhood in England and Wales. *Pediatrics* 2009;123(2):e312.

145. Petrou S, Yiu HH, Kwon J. Economic consequences of preterm birth: a systematic review of the recent literature (2009–2017). *Arch Dis Child* 2019;104(5):456.

146. Petrou S, Johnson S, Wolke D, et al. Economic costs and preference-based health-related quality of life outcomes associated with childhood psychiatric disorders. *Br J Psychiatry* 2018;197(5):395.

147. Denboba AD, Sayre RK, Wodon QT, et al. *Stepping up early childhood development.* Washington, DC: World Bank; 2014.

148. World Health Organization, UNICEF. *Early childhood development and disability.* Geneva: World Health Organization, 2012. 40 p.

149. Shankaran S, Pappas A, McDonald SA, et al. Childhood outcomes after hypothermia for neonatal encephalopathy. *N Engl J Med* 2012;366(22):2085.

GENERAL CONSIDERATIONS

PART 2

The Fetal Patient

10 Prenatal Diagnosis and Management in the Molecular Age—Indications, Procedures, and Laboratory Techniques

Mark I. Evans, Dana Brabbing-Goldstein, Shara M. Evans, and Yuval Yaron

INTRODUCTION

In the beginning of the 20th century, the leading cause of infant mortality (approximately 150/1,000) was infectious diseases. With the development of antibiotics and increasingly sophisticated medical and surgical therapies, the primary causes of child mortality have shifted to genetic and congenital disorders (1). Particularly for syndromic conditions, the pediatrician is commonly the first medical provider to raise the issue of future pregnancies and the possibilities for prenatal diagnosis.

Over the course of the past four decades, there have been revolutionary changes in our approach to prenatal diagnosis and screening (2). In the 1960s and 70s, we evolved from merely wishing patients "Good luck" to asking "How old are you?" Maternal age was, and still is, a cheap screening test for aneuploidy, but there has been an explosion of techniques that have dramatically enhanced the statistical performance of screening tests to identify high-risk patients. Screening for elevated maternal serum alpha-fetoprotein (MSAFP) for neural tube defects (NTDs) began in the 1970s, and low MSAFP's were discovered to be associated with Down syndrome (DS) and trisomy 18 in the 1980s (3). Nuchal translucency (NT) and several other ultrasound (US) markers then emerged, which increased the efficacy of both ultrasound screening and detection of anomalies. Biochemical and now molecular markers have moved to the forefront of screening and diagnostic testing. These have both revolutionized our abilities and challenged some of the basic tenets of the past decades (2).

We have seen a pendulum swinging back and forth between the primacy of screening and testing as new technologies have been developed (Fig. 10.1). Overall, prenatal diagnosis has moved along two parallel paths that sometimes converge (i.e., imaging and tissue diagnoses). See also Chapter 57. In many instances, clinicians are experts in one diagnostic modality or the other; there are a very limited number who are true experts in both. As a result, there is often huge variability in approach to counseling, screening, and diagnosis depending upon by whom and where a patient is seen. We can, oversimplistically, divide overall approaches into "basic," "selective," and "comprehensive."

As they internalize reproductive risks, both physicians and patients have to decide how much effort and expense they are willing to exert to evaluate those risks, and what they would do with the results (Fig. 10.2). As with all advances in medicine, science and culture within any society, there is a gradual acceptance and incorporation of new technologies that proceeds at highly different paces in different locales. The Internet has exploded the dissemination process; sophisticated patients even from remote areas can now access information on what is available if they are willing to travel to get it. At tertiary/"quaternary" centers such as ours, a significant proportion of patients travel considerable distances for services that are not available at home (4,5).

Thousands of papers and hundreds of textbooks have been written over the past decades about the subjects addressed in this chapter, but only a miniscule percentage of the available literature can be cited here. We will provide a summary of key points, but no short chapter can possibly do justice to the enormous technical advances in multiple disciplines that have contributed to our abilities to screen, diagnose, and treat fetal conditions.

Prenatal diagnosis can reduce morbidity and mortality by guiding delivery plans and early treatment for fetuses with some genetic abnormalities such as early enzymatic treatment in cases of inborn error of metabolism (6). Furthermore, diagnosing a lethal genetic condition before birth allows parents time to make reproductive choices about the pregnancy management by offering additional and accurate prognostic information for the parents. This includes termination or palliative care after delivery (6) and reproductive options in subsequent pregnancies, such as prenatal diagnosis and preimplantation genetic testing (PGT). Providing women and partners detailed genetic counseling with a careful and detailed explanation of the risks and benefits of each approach results in outcomes that are best aligned with women's preferences.

GENETIC COUNSELING

As the complexity of genetic information has increased massively in scope and amount, the need to explain it has skyrocketed in parallel. The best analogy is to that of computers, for which "Moore's law" predicted that capabilities would double every 18 to 24 months, and cost would decrease by 50%. At least the first half of the equation has applied in genetics. The situation has been made even more challenging because currently advances in clinical medicine are often beholden to technologic advances in disciplines that are outside the "culture" of medicine (7). For example, many of the noninvasive screening techniques rely upon the ingenuity and intellectual capabilities of electrical engineers backed by venture capitalists who do not necessarily adhere to the ethos of putting patient care above all else. They have pushed to introduce tests into practice without sufficient testing, medical peer review, and user/patient education. Numerous direct-to-consumer genetic companies have emerged that provide frequently alarming information, often without context or easy access to proper counseling. Well-publicized charges of fraud against high-profile operations (e.g., Theranos) have also created a culture of suspicion about the reliability of new technologies that have been introduced into practice with venture capital backing as opposed to traditional academic approaches (8). Likewise, shopping mall

SWINGING PENDULUM

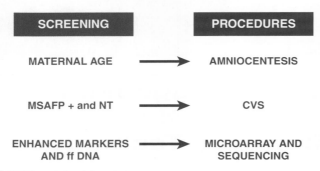

FIGURE 10.1 Pendulum slide.

ultrasound "boutiques" have emerged to supply "baby pictures" (9). In these instances, patients often believe they have received complete services when in fact important questions about their specific situation have neither been asked nor answered (8).

Genetic counseling is the foundation of educating patients as to the risks of reproduction, opportunities to investigate those risks, and options for dealing with the information obtained. There is no one standard for what genetic counseling is in practice. Numerous studies have documented that the education of most obstetricians in genetics is suboptimal; thus, relatively few physicians caring for pregnant women are in a position to have a substantive discussion

about complex genetic issues (10). There are approximately 200 obstetrician–gynecologists in the United States who are also formally trained and board certified in Clinical Genetics, so that the approximately 2,000 maternal–fetal medicine subspecialists perform a disproportionate proportion of genetic evaluations. However, while they usually have considerably more knowledge than do general obstetricians, perinatologists are commonly very time challenged and may not maintain a "state-of-the-art" understanding of the rapid changes in screening and testing technology options nor do they have the time for in-depth, unrushed discussions with patients.

Genetic counseling as a profession emerged over the past few decades. Genetic Counselors are Masters-trained individuals who have both an in-depth knowledge of genetic fundamentals and an understanding of screening principles and testing options. Their credo includes respect for one of the key tenets of genetics, that is, nondirective presentation of information. In many clinical settings, the counselors have far more understanding of genetic issues than do the attending physicians, which can raise quality of patient care issues if overall care is not regarded as a team effort. The authors believe that it is optimum to have a coordinated team approach to patient care. What too frequently occurs is that a "vending machine" selection of possible testing options is offered to the patient without adequate guidance. Only when there is an abnormal result does the primary medical provider call for help to explain to an often panicked patient what the results actually mean. When possible, we believe that dedicated centers providing the continuum of genetic counseling, diagnosis, and treatment

Evolving Approach to Screening, Diagnosis, and Prenatal Management

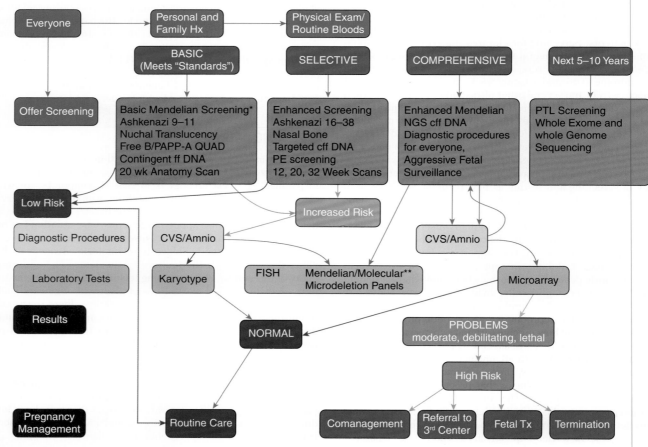

FIGURE 10.2 Flow chart for prenatal genetic evaluation and management.

are optimal. Alternatively, in this digital age, it should be possible to create a hierarchy of services from networked providers that approximates the kind of care that would be available in a comprehensive center.

Throughout this chapter, the importance of skilled genetic counseling will be reinforced. Whatever technologies are available now or in the future, their application will vary across and within cultures. Physicians should be aware of this and accommodate the patient's preference whenever it is possible to do so.

INDICATIONS

Prenatal Screening

Mendelian Disorders

To the pediatrician, screening for mendelian disorders has been central to care for decades (11). The routine use of newborn heel stick blood sample screening is nearly universal in the United States and many high-income countries and continues to rapidly expand in both utilization and quantity of tests available (12). In the 1970s, prenatal screening for mendelian disorders in the United States was simplistic, being based primarily on ethnicity. Since then there has been an explosion of testing possibilities, and a serious disconnect has developed between the individual risk for a specific disorder and the availability of screening tests. For example, the panel offered to persons of Ashkenazi Jewish descent increased from 1 to 3 available tests in the 1970s to over 35 current "routine" test offerings in some labs (13). More tests are

always under development. For many of the diseases tested, however, the incidence in the Jewish population is actually no higher than in other ethnic groups, and the incidence of some is less than 1/100,000. We frequently see new patients who state that they have already been screened for "everything" and who are very upset to learn that there is no such thing.

Multiple companies now offer screening for dozens of disorders across all ethnic groups (14). Although there were some serious problems in the implementation of these screens, including confusion regarding the actual risks of a disease for individual couples, the emerging consensus among tertiary physicians is that this "expanded carrier screening" is considerably more cost-effective than targeted panels. Furthermore, several studies have shown that at least 1/100 couples are found, unexpectedly, to be at risk for a serious mendelian disorder, and 1/300 fetuses are diagnosed as affected (14). Overall, the incidence of affected children is higher for these than for DS until women reach about age 35. In over half of couples found to be unexpectedly at risk, the disorder at risk is not one that one would have guessed from their ethnic background (14).

Public policy always has to catch up with technologic reality (15). In the early 2000s, there was minimal acceptance of screening for rare disorders such as Usher syndrome. National organizations such as the American College of Obstetrics and Gynecology (ACOG) elected not to endorse universal screening for disorders such as Fragile X and spinal muscular atrophy (SMA) whose incidences are far higher (Table 10.1). It was the considerable advances in technologic capabilities that changed the cost/benefit

TABLE 10.1

Expanded Mendelian Disorder Panel

Conditions Tested	Gene	Exons	Variants	Detection Rate
11-Beta-hydroxylase-deficient congenital adrenal hyperplasia	CYP11B1. Autosomal recessive. Sequencing with copy number analysis	NM_000497:1-9		Ashkenazi Jewish 94%
6-Pyruvoyl-tetrahydropterin synthase deficiency	PTS. Autosomal recessive. Sequencing with copy number analysis	NM_000317:1-6		Ashkenazi Jewish >99%
ABCC8-related familial hyperinsulinism	ABCC8. Autosomal recessive. Sequencing with copy number analysis	NM_000352:1-39		Ashkenazi Jewish >99%
Adenosine deaminase deficiency	ADA. Autosomal recessive. Sequencing with copy number analysis	NM_000022:1-12		Ashkenazi Jewish >99%
Alpha-thalassemia	HBA1, HBA2. Autosomal recessive. Analysis of homologous regions		**(13):** -(alpha)20.5, --BRIT, --MEDI, --MEDII, --SEA, --THAI or --FIL, -alpha3.7, -alpha4.2, HBA1+HBA2 deletion, Hb Constant Spring, anti3.7, anti4.2, del HS-40	Unknown due to rarity of disease
Alpha-mannosidosis	MAN2B1. Autosomal recessive. Sequencing with copy number analysis	NM_000528:1-23		Ashkenazi Jewish >99%
Alpha-sarcoglycanopathy	SGCA. Autosomal recessive. Sequencing with copy number analysis	NM_000023:1-9		Ashkenazi Jewish >99%
Alström syndrome	ALMS1. Autosomal recessive. Sequencing with copy number analysis	NM_015120:1-23		Ashkenazi Jewish >99%
AMT-related glycine encephalopathy	AMT. Autosomal recessive. Sequencing with copy number analysis	NM_000481:1-9		Ashkenazi Jewish >99%
Andermann syndrome	SLC12A6. Autosomal recessive. Sequencing with copy number analysis	NM_133647:1-25		Ashkenazi Jewish >99%
Argininemia	ARG1. Autosomal recessive. Sequencing with copy number analysis	NM_000045:1-8		Ashkenazi Jewish 97%
Argininosuccinic aciduria	ASL. Autosomal recessive. Sequencing with copy number analysis	NM_001024943:1-16		Ashkenazi Jewish >99%
Aspartylglucosaminuria	AGA. Autosomal recessive. Sequencing with copy number analysis	NM_000027:1-9		Ashkenazi Jewish >99%

THE FETAL PATIENT

(Continued)

TABLE 10.1

Expanded Mendelian Disorder Panel (*Continued*)

Conditions Tested	Gene	Exons	Variants	Detection Rate
Ataxia with vitamin E deficiency	TTPA. Autosomal recessive. Sequencing with copy number analysis	NM_000370:1-5		Ashkenazi Jewish >99%
Ataxia–telangiectasia	ATM. Autosomal recessive. Sequencing with copy number analysis	NM_000051:2-63		Ashkenazi Jewish >99%
ATP7A-related disorders	ATP7A. X-linked recessive. Sequencing with copy number analysis	NM_000052:2-23		Ashkenazi Jewish 92%
Autoimmune polyglandular syndrome type 1	AIRE. Autosomal recessive. Sequencing with copy number analysis	NM_000383:1-14		Ashkenazi Jewish >99%
Autosomal recessive osteopetrosis type 1	TCIRG1. Autosomal recessive. Sequencing with copy number analysis	NM_006019:2-20		Ashkenazi Jewish >99%
Autosomal recessive polycystic kidney disease, PKHD1-related	PKHD1. Autosomal recessive. Sequencing with copy number analysis	NM_138694:2-67		Ashkenazi Jewish >99%
Autosomal recessive spastic ataxia of Charlevoix-Saguenay	SACS. Autosomal recessive. Sequencing with copy number analysis	NM_014363:2-10		Ashkenazi Jewish 99%
Bardet-Biedl syndrome, BBS1-related	BBS1. Autosomal recessive. Sequencing with copy number analysis	NM_024649:1-17		Ashkenazi Jewish >99%
Bardet-Biedl syndrome, BBS10-related	BBS10. Autosomal recessive. Sequencing with copy number analysis	NM_024685:1-2		Ashkenazi Jewish >99%
Bardet-Biedl syndrome, BBS12-related	BBS12. Autosomal recessive. Sequencing with copy number analysis	NM_152618:2		Ashkenazi Jewish >99%
Bardet-Biedl syndrome, BBS2-related	BBS2. Autosomal recessive. Sequencing with copy number analysis	NM_031885:1-17		Ashkenazi Jewish >99%
BCS1L-related disorders	BCS1L. Autosomal recessive. Sequencing with copy number analysis	NM_004328:3-9		Ashkenazi Jewish >99%
Beta-sarcoglycanopathy	SGCB. Autosomal Recessive. Sequencing with copy number analysis	NM_000232:1-6		Ashkenazi Jewish >99%
Biotinidase deficiency	BTD. Autosomal recessive. Sequencing with copy number analysis	NM_000060:1-4		Ashkenazi Jewish >99%
Bloom syndrome	BLM. Autosomal recessive. Sequencing with copy number analysis	NM_000057:2-22		Ashkenazi Jewish >99%
Calpainopathy	CAPN3. Autosomal recessive. Sequencing with copy number analysis	NM_000070:1-24		Ashkenazi Jewish >99%
Canavan disease	ASPA. Autosomal recessive. Sequencing with copy number analysis	NM_000049:1-6		Ashkenazi Jewish 98%
Carbamoyl phosphate synthetase I deficiency	CPS1. Autosomal Recessive. Sequencing with copy number analysis	NM_001875:1-38		Ashkenazi Jewish >99%
Carnitine palmitoyltransferase IA deficiency	CPT1A. Autosomal recessive. Sequencing with copy number analysis	NM_001876:2-19		Ashkenazi Jewish >99%
Carnitine palmitoyltransferase II deficiency	CPT2. Autosomal recessive. Sequencing with copy number analysis	NM_000098:1-5		Ashkenazi Jewish >99%
Cartilage-hair hypoplasia	RMRP. Autosomal recessive. Sequencing with copy number analysis	NR_003051:1		Ashkenazi Jewish >99%
Cerebrotendinous xanthomatosis	CYP27A1. Autosomal recessive. Sequencing with copy number analysis	NM_000784:1-9		Ashkenazi Jewish >99%
Citrullinemia type 1	ASS1. Autosomal recessive. Sequencing with copy number analysis	NM_000050:3-16		Ashkenazi Jewish >99%
CLN3-related neuronal ceroid lipofuscinosis	CLN3. Autosomal recessive. Sequencing with copy number analysis	NM_001042432:2-16		Ashkenazi Jewish >99%
CLN5-related neuronal ceroid lipofuscinosis	CLN5. Autosomal recessive. Sequencing with copy number analysis	NM_006493:1-4		Ashkenazi Jewish >99%
CLN6-related neuronal ceroid lipofuscinosis	CLN6. Autosomal recessive. Sequencing with copy number analysis	NM_017882:1-7		Ashkenazi Jewish >99%
CLN8-related neuronal ceroid lipofuscinosis	CLN8. Autosomal recessive. Sequencing with copy number analysis	NM_018941:2-3		Ashkenazi Jewish >99%
Cohen syndrome	VPS13B. Autosomal recessive. Sequencing with copy number analysis	NM_017890:2-62		Ashkenazi Jewish 97%
COL4A3-related Alport syndrome	COL4A3. Autosomal recessive. Sequencing with copy number analysis	NM_000091:1-52		Ashkenazi Jewish 97%
COL4A4-related Alport syndrome	COL4A4. Autosomal Recessive. Sequencing with copy number analysis	NM_000092:2-48		Ashkenazi Jewish 98%

TABLE 10.1

Expanded Mendelian Disorder Panel (*Continued*)

Conditions Tested	Gene	Exons	Variants	Detection Rate
Combined pituitary hormone deficiency, PROP1-related	PROP1. Autosomal recessive. Sequencing with copy number analysis	NM_006261:1-3		Ashkenazi Jewish >99%
Congenital adrenal hyperplasia, CYP21A2-related	CYP21A2. Autosomal recessive. Analysis of homologous regions		**(13):** CYP21A2 deletion, CYP21A2 duplication, CYP21A2 triplication, G111Vfs*21, I173N, L308Ffs*6, P31L, Q319*, Q319*+CYP21A2dup, R357W, V281L, [I237N;V238E;M240K], c.293-13C>G	Ashkenazi Jewish >99%
Congenital disorder of glycosylation Type Ia	PMM2. Autosomal recessive. Sequencing with copy number analysis	NM_000303:1-8		Ashkenazi Jewish >99%
Congenital disorder of glycosylation Type Ic	ALG6. Autosomal recessive. Sequencing with copy number analysis	NM_013339:2-15		Ashkenazi Jewish >99%
Congenital disorder of glycosylation, MPI-related	MPI. Autosomal recessive. Sequencing with copy number analysis	NM_002435:1-8		Ashkenazi Jewish >99%
Costeff optic atrophy syndrome	OPA3. Autosomal recessive. Sequencing with copy number analysis	NM_025136:1-2		Ashkenazi Jewish >99%
Cystic fibrosis	CFTR. Autosomal recessive. Sequencing with copy number analysis	NM_000492:1-27. IVS8-5T allele analysis is only reported in the presence of the R117H mutation		Ashkenazi Jewish >99%
Cystinosis	CTNS. Autosomal recessive. Sequencing with copy number analysis	NM_004937:3-12		Ashkenazi Jewish >99%
D-bifunctional protein deficiency	HSD17B4. Autosomal recessive. Sequencing with copy number analysis	NM_000414:1-24		Ashkenazi Jewish 98%
Delta-sarcoglycanopathy	SGCD. Autosomal recessive. Sequencing with copy number analysis	NM_000337:2-9		Ashkenazi Jewish 99%
Dihydrolipoamide dehydrogenase deficiency	DLD. Autosomal recessive. Sequencing with copy number analysis	NM_000108:1-14		Ashkenazi Jewish >99%
Dysferlinopathy	DYSF. Autosomal recessive. Sequencing with copy number analysis	NM_003494:1-55		Ashkenazi Jewish 98%
Dystrophinopathy (including Duchenne/Becker muscular dystrophy)	DMD. Autosomal recessive. X-linked Recessive. Sequencing with copy number analysis	NM_004006:1-79		Ashkenazi Jewish >99%
ERCC6-related disorders	ERCC6. Autosomal recessive. Sequencing with copy number analysis	NM_000124:2-21		Ashkenazi Jewish 99%
ERCC8-related disorders	ERCC8. Autosomal recessive. Sequencing with copy number analysis	NM_000082:1-12		Ashkenazi Jewish 95%
EVC-related Ellis-van Creveld syndrome	EVC. Autosomal recessive. Sequencing with copy number analysis	NM_153717:1-21		Ashkenazi Jewish 96%
EVC2-related Ellis-van Creveld syndrome	EVC2. Autosomal recessive. Sequencing with copy number analysis	NM_147127:1-22		Ashkenazi Jewish >99%
Fabry disease	GLA. X-linked recessive. Sequencing with copy number analysis	NM_000169:1-7		Ashkenazi Jewish 98%
Familial dysautonomia	IKBKAP. Autosomal Recessive. Sequencing with copy number analysis	NM_003640:2-37		Ashkenazi Jewish >99%
Familial mediterranean fever	MEFV. Autosomal recessive. Sequencing with copy number analysis	NM_000243:1-10		Ashkenazi Jewish >99%
Fanconi anemia complementation group A	FANCA. Autosomal recessive. Sequencing with copy number analysis	NM_000135:1-43		Ashkenazi Jewish 92%
Fanconi anemia, FANCC-related	FANCC. Autosomal recessive. Sequencing with copy number analysis	NM_000136:2-15		Ashkenazi Jewish >99%
FKRP-related disorders	FKRP. Autosomal recessive. Sequencing with copy number analysis	NM_024301:4		Ashkenazi Jewish >99%
FKTN-related disorders	FKTN. Autosomal recessive. Sequencing with copy number analysis	NM_001079802:3-11		Ashkenazi Jewish >99%
Fragile X syndrome	FMR1. X-linked dominant. Triplet repeat detection		**(1):** FMR1 CGG repeat number	Ashkenazi Jewish >99%

THE FETAL PATIENT

TABLE 10.1

Expanded Mendelian Disorder Panel (*Continued*)

Conditions Tested	Gene	Exons	Variants	Detection Rate
Galactokinase deficiency	GALK1. Autosomal recessive. Sequencing with copy number analysis	NM_000154:1-8		Ashkenazi Jewish >99%
Galactosemia	GALT. Autosomal recessive. Sequencing with copy number analysis	NM_000155:1-11		Ashkenazi Jewish >99%
Gamma-sarcoglycanopathy	SGCG. Autosomal recessive. Sequencing with copy number analysis	NM_000231:2-8		Ashkenazi Jewish 88%
Gaucher disease	GBA. Autosomal recessive. Analysis of homologous regions		**(10):** D409V, D448H, IVS2+1G>A, L444P, N370S, R463C, R463H, R496H, V394L, p.L29Afs*18	Ashkenazi Jewish 95%
GJB2-related DFNB1 nonsyndromic hearing loss and deafness	GJB2. Autosomal recessive. Sequencing with copy number analysis	NM_004004:1-2		Ashkenazi Jewish >99%
GLB1-related disorders	GLB1. Autosomal recessive. Sequencing with copy number analysis	NM_000404:1-16		Ashkenazi Jewish >99%
GLDC-related glycine encephalopathy	GLDC. Autosomal recessive. Sequencing with copy number analysis	NM_000170:1-25		Ashkenazi Jewish 94%
Glutaric acidemia, GCDH-related	GCDH. Autosomal recessive. Sequencing with copy number analysis	NM_000159:2-12		Ashkenazi Jewish >99%
Glycogen storage disease type Ia	G6PC. Autosomal recessive. Sequencing with copy number analysis	NM_000151:1-5		Ashkenazi Jewish >99%
Glycogen storage disease type Ib	SLC37A4. Autosomal recessive. Sequencing with copy number analysis	NM_001164277:3-11		Ashkenazi Jewish >99%
Glycogen storage disease type III	AGL. Autosomal recessive. Sequencing with copy number analysis	NM_000642:2-34		Ashkenazi Jewish >99%
GNE myopathy	GNE. Autosomal recessive. Sequencing with copy number analysis	NM_001128227:1-12		Ashkenazi Jewish >99%
GNPTAB-related disorders	GNPTAB. Autosomal recessive. Sequencing with copy number analysis	NM_024312:1-21		Ashkenazi Jewish >99%
HADHA-related disorders	HADHA. Autosomal recessive. Sequencing with copy number analysis	NM_000182:1-20		Ashkenazi Jewish >99%
Hb beta chain–related hemoglobinopathy (including beta thalassemia and sickle cell disease)	HBB. Autosomal recessive. Sequencing with copy number analysis	NM_000518:1-3		Ashkenazi Jewish >99%
Hereditary fructose intolerance	ALDOB. Autosomal recessive. Sequencing with copy number analysis	NM_000035:2-9		Ashkenazi Jewish >99%
Herlitz junctional epidermolysis bullosa, LAMB3-related	LAMB3. Autosomal recessive. Sequencing with copy number analysis	NM_000228:2-23		Ashkenazi Jewish >99%
Hexosaminidase A deficiency (including Tay-Sachs disease)	HEXA. Autosomal recessive. Sequencing with copy number analysis	NM_000520:1-14		Ashkenazi Jewish >99%
HMG-CoA Lyase deficiency	HMGCL. Autosomal recessive. Sequencing with copy number analysis	NM_000191:1-9		Ashkenazi Jewish 98%
Holocarboxylase synthetase deficiency	HLCS. Autosomal recessive. Sequencing with copy number analysis	NM_000411:4-12		Ashkenazi Jewish >99%
Homocystinuria, CBS-related	CBS. Autosomal recessive. Sequencing with copy number analysis	NM_000071:3-17		Ashkenazi Jewish >99%
Hydrolethalus syndrome	HYLS1. Autosomal recessive. Sequencing with copy number analysis	NM_145014:4		Ashkenazi Jewish >99%
Hypophosphatasia	ALPL. Autosomal recessive. Sequencing with copy number analysis	NM_000478:2-12		Ashkenazi Jewish >99%
Isovaleric acidemia	IVD. Autosomal recessive. Sequencing with copy number analysis	NM_002225:1-12		Ashkenazi Jewish >99%
Joubert syndrome 2	TMEM216. Autosomal recessive. Sequencing with copy number analysis	NM_001173990:1-5		Ashkenazi Jewish >99%
Junctional epidermolysis bullosa, LAMA3-related	LAMA3. Autosomal recessive. Sequencing with copy number analysis	NM_000227:1-38		Ashkenazi Jewish >99%
Junctional epidermolysis bullosa, LAMC2-related	LAMC2. Autosomal recessive. Sequencing with copy number analysis	NM_005562:1-23		Ashkenazi Jewish >99%
KCNJ11-related familial hyperinsulinism	KCNJ11. Autosomal recessive. Sequencing with copy number analysis	NM_000525:1		Ashkenazi Jewish >99%

TABLE 10.1

Expanded Mendelian Disorder Panel (*Continued*)

Conditions Tested	Gene	Exons	Variants	Detection Rate
Krabbe disease	GALC. Autosomal recessive. Sequencing with copy number analysis	NM_000153:1-17		Ashkenazi Jewish >99%
LAMA2-related muscular dystrophy	LAMA2. Autosomal recessive. Sequencing with copy number analysis	NM_000426:1-65		Ashkenazi Jewish >99%
Leigh syndrome, French-Canadian type	LRPPRC. Autosomal recessive. Sequencing with copy number analysis	NM_133259:1-38		Ashkenazi Jewish >99%
Lipoid congenital adrenal hyperplasia	STAR. Autosomal recessive. Sequencing with copy number analysis	NM_000349:1-7		Ashkenazi Jewish >99%
Lysosomal acid lipase deficiency	LIPA. Autosomal recessive. Sequencing with copy number analysis	NM_000235:2-10		Ashkenazi Jewish >99%
Maple syrup urine disease type Ia	BCKDHA. Autosomal recessive. Sequencing with copy number analysis	NM_000709:1-9		Ashkenazi Jewish >99%
Maple syrup urine disease type Ib	BCKDHB. Autosomal recessive. Sequencing with copy number analysis	NM_183050:1-10		Ashkenazi Jewish >99%
Maple syrup urine disease type II	DBT. Autosomal recessive. Sequencing with copy number analysis	NM_001918:1-11		Ashkenazi Jewish 96%
Medium chain Acyl-CoA dehydrogenase deficiency	ACADM. Autosomal recessive. Sequencing with copy number analysis	NM_000016:1-12		Ashkenazi Jewish >99%
Megalencephalic leukoencephalopathy with subcortical cysts	MLC1. Autosomal recessive. Sequencing with copy number analysis	NM_015166:2-12		Ashkenazi Jewish >99%
Metachromatic leukodystrophy	ARSA. Autosomal recessive. Sequencing with copy number analysis	NM_000487:1-8		Ashkenazi Jewish >99%
Methylmalonic acidemia, cblA type	MMAA. Autosomal recessive. Sequencing with copy number analysis	NM_172250:2-7		Ashkenazi Jewish >99%
Methylmalonic acidemia, cblB type	MMAB. Autosomal recessive. Sequencing with copy number analysis	NM_052845:1-9		Ashkenazi Jewish >99%
Methylmalonic aciduria and homocystinuria, cblC type	MMACHC. Autosomal recessive. Sequencing with copy number analysis	NM_015506:1-4		Ashkenazi Jewish >99%
MKS1-related disorders	MKS1. Autosomal recessive. Sequencing with copy number analysis	NM_017777:1-18		Ashkenazi Jewish >99%
Mucolipidosis III gamma	GNPTG. Autosomal recessive. Sequencing with copy number analysis	NM_032520:1-11		Ashkenazi Jewish >99%
Mucolipidosis IV	MCOLN1. Autosomal recessive. Sequencing with copy number analysis	NM_020533:1-14		Ashkenazi Jewish >99%
Mucopolysaccharidosis type I	IDUA. Autosomal recessive. Sequencing with copy number analysis	NM_000203:1-14		Ashkenazi Jewish >99%
Mucopolysaccharidosis type II	IDS. X-linked recessive. Sequencing with copy number analysis	NM_000202:1-9		Ashkenazi Jewish 88%
Mucopolysaccharidosis type IIIA	SGSH. Autosomal recessive. Sequencing with copy number analysis	NM_000199:1-8		Ashkenazi Jewish >99%
Mucopolysaccharidosis type IIIB	NAGLU. Autosomal recessive. Sequencing with copy number analysis	NM_000263:1-6		Ashkenazi Jewish >99%
Mucopolysaccharidosis type IIIC	HGSNAT. Autosomal recessive. Sequencing with copy number analysis	NM_152419:1-18		Ashkenazi Jewish >99%
MUT-related methylmalonic acidemia	MUT. Autosomal recessive. Sequencing with copy number analysis	NM_000255:2-13		Ashkenazi Jewish >99%
MYO7A-related disorders	MYO7A. Autosomal recessive. Sequencing with copy number analysis	NM_000260:2-49		Ashkenazi Jewish >99%
NEB-related nemaline myopathy	NEB. Autosomal recessive. Sequencing with copy number analysis	NM_001271208:3-80,117-183		Ashkenazi Jewish >99%
Nephrotic syndrome, NPHS1-related	NPHS1. Autosomal recessive. Sequencing with copy number analysis	NM_004646:1-29		Ashkenazi Jewish >99%
Nephrotic syndrome, NPHS2-related	NPHS2. Autosomal recessive. Sequencing with copy number analysis	NM_014625:1-8		Ashkenazi Jewish >99%
Niemann-Pick disease type C1	NPC1. Autosomal recessive. Sequencing with copy number analysis	NM_000271:1-25		Ashkenazi Jewish >99%
Niemann-Pick disease type C2	NPC2. Autosomal recessive. Sequencing with copy number analysis	NM_006432:1-5		Ashkenazi Jewish >99%
Niemann-Pick disease, SMPD1-related	SMPD1. Autosomal recessive. Sequencing with copy number analysis	NM_000543:1-6		Ashkenazi Jewish >99%

THE FETAL PATIENT

(Continued)

TABLE 10.1

Expanded Mendelian Disorder Panel (*Continued*)

Conditions Tested	Gene	Exons	Variants	Detection Rate
Nijmegen breakage syndrome	NBN. Autosomal recessive. Sequencing with copy number analysis	NM_002485:1-16		Ashkenazi Jewish >99%
Ornithine transcarbamylase deficiency	OTC. X-linked recessive. Sequencing with copy number analysis	NM_000531:1-10		Ashkenazi Jewish 97%
PCCA-related propionic acidemia	PCCA. Autosomal recessive. Sequencing with copy number analysis	NM_000282:1-24		Ashkenazi Jewish 95%
PCCB-related propionic acidemia	PCCB. Autosomal recessive. Sequencing with copy number analysis	NM_000532:1-15		Ashkenazi Jewish >99%
PCDH15-related disorders	PCDH15. Autosomal recessive. Sequencing with copy number analysis	NM_033056:2-33		Ashkenazi Jewish 93%
Pendred syndrome	SLC26A4. Autosomal recessive. Sequencing with copy number analysis	NM_000441:2-21		Ashkenazi Jewish >99%
Peroxisome biogenesis disorder type 1	PEX1. Autosomal recessive. Sequencing with copy number analysis	NM_000466:1-24		Ashkenazi Jewish >99%
Peroxisome biogenesis disorder type 3	PEX12. Autosomal recessive. Sequencing with copy number analysis	NM_000286:1-3		Ashkenazi Jewish >99%
Peroxisome biogenesis disorder type 4	PEX6. Autosomal recessive. Sequencing with copy number analysis	NM_000287:1-17		Ashkenazi Jewish 97%
Peroxisome biogenesis disorder type 5	PEX2. Autosomal recessive. Sequencing with copy number analysis	NM_000318:4		Ashkenazi Jewish >99%
Peroxisome biogenesis disorder type 6	PEX10. Autosomal recessive. Sequencing with copy number analysis	NM_153818:1-6		Ashkenazi Jewish >99%
Phenylalanine hydroxylase deficiency	PAH. Autosomal recessive. Sequencing with copy number analysis	NM_000277:1-13		Ashkenazi Jewish >99%
POMGNT-related disorders	POMGNT1. Autosomal recessive. Sequencing with copy number analysis	NM_017739:2-22		Ashkenazi Jewish 96%
Pompe disease	GAA. Autosomal recessive. Sequencing with copy number analysis	NM_000152:2-20		Ashkenazi Jewish >99%
PPT1-related neuronal ceroid lipofuscinosis	PPT1. Autosomal recessive. Sequencing with copy number analysis	NM_000310:1-9		Ashkenazi Jewish >99%
Primary carnitine deficiency	SLC22A5. Autosomal recessive. Sequencing with copy number analysis	NM_003060:1-10		Ashkenazi Jewish >99%
Primary hyperoxaluria type 1	AGXT. Autosomal recessive. Sequencing with copy number analysis	NM_000030:1-11		Ashkenazi Jewish >99%
Primary hyperoxaluria type 2	GRHPR. Autosomal recessive. Sequencing with copy number analysis	NM_012203:1-9		Ashkenazi Jewish >99%
Primary hyperoxaluria type 3	HOGA1. Autosomal recessive. Sequencing with copy number analysis	NM_138413:1-7		Ashkenazi Jewish >99%
Pycnodysostosis	CTSK. Autosomal recessive. Sequencing with copy number analysis	NM_000396:2-8		Ashkenazi Jewish >99%
Pyruvate carboxylase deficiency	PC. Autosomal recessive. Sequencing with copy number analysis	NM_000920:3-22		Ashkenazi Jewish >99%
Rhizomelic chondrodysplasia punctata type 1	PEX7. Autosomal recessive. Sequencing with copy number analysis	NM_000288:1-10		Ashkenazi Jewish >99%
RTEL1-related disorders	RTEL1. Autosomal recessive. Sequencing with copy number analysis	NM_032957:2-35		Ashkenazi Jewish >99%
Salla disease	SLC17A5. Autosomal recessive. Sequencing with copy number analysis	NM_012434:1-11		Ashkenazi Jewish 98%
Sandhoff disease	HEXB. Autosomal recessive. Sequencing with copy number analysis	NM_000521:1-14		Ashkenazi Jewish 99%
Short-chain acyl-CoA dehydrogenase deficiency	ACADS. Autosomal recessive. Sequencing with copy number analysis	NM_000017:1-10		Ashkenazi Jewish >99%
Sjögren-Larsson syndrome	ALDH3A2. Autosomal recessive. Sequencing with copy number analysis	NM_000382:1-10		Ashkenazi Jewish 96%
SLC26A2-related disorders	SLC26A2. Autosomal recessive. Sequencing with copy number analysis	NM_000112:2-3		Ashkenazi Jewish >99%
Smith-Lemli-Opitz syndrome	DHCR7. Autosomal recessive. Sequencing with copy number analysis	NM_001360:3-9		Ashkenazi Jewish >99%
Spastic paraplegia type 15	ZFYVE26. Autosomal recessive. Sequencing with copy number analysis	NM_015346:2-42		Ashkenazi Jewish >99%

TABLE 10.1

Expanded Mendelian Disorder Panel (*Continued*)

Conditions Tested	Gene	Exons	Variants	Detection Rate
Spinal muscular atrophy	SMN1. Autosomal recessive. Spinal muscular atrophy		**(1):** SMN1 copy number	Ashkenazi Jewish 94%
Spondylothoracic dysostosis	MESP2. Autosomal recessive. Sequencing with copy number analysis	NM_001039958:1-2		Ashkenazi Jewish >99%
TGM1-related autosomal recessive congenital ichthyosis	TGM1. Autosomal recessive. Sequencing with copy number analysis	NM_000359:2-15		Ashkenazi Jewish >99%
TPP1-related neuronal ceroid lipofuscinosis	TPP1. Autosomal recessive. Sequencing with copy number analysis	NM_000391:1-13		Ashkenazi Jewish >99%
Tyrosine hydroxylase deficiency	TH. Autosomal recessive. Sequencing with copy number analysis	NM_199292:1-14		Ashkenazi Jewish >99%
Tyrosinemia type I	FAH. Autosomal recessive. Sequencing with copy number analysis	NM_000137:1-14		Ashkenazi Jewish >99%
Tyrosinemia type II	TAT. Autosomal recessive. Sequencing with copy number analysis	NM_000353:2-12		Ashkenazi Jewish >99%
USH1C-related disorders	USH1C. Autosomal recessive. Sequencing with copy number analysis	NM_005709:1-21		Ashkenazi Jewish >99%
USH2A-related disorders	USH2A. Autosomal recessive. Sequencing with copy number analysis	NM_206933:2-72		Ashkenazi Jewish 94%
Usher syndrome type 3	CLRN1. Autosomal recessive. Sequencing with copy number analysis	NM_174878:1-3		Ashkenazi Jewish >99%
Very-long-chain Acyl-CoA dehydrogenase deficiency	ACADVL. Autosomal recessive. Sequencing with copy number analysis	NM_000018:1-20		Ashkenazi Jewish >99%
Wilson disease	ATP7B. Autosomal recessive. Sequencing with copy number analysis	NM_000053:1-21		Ashkenazi Jewish >99%
X-linked adrenoleukodystrophy	ABCD1. X-linked recessive. Sequencing with copy number analysis	NM_000033:1-6		Ashkenazi Jewish 77%
X-linked Alport syndrome	COL4A5. X-linked recessive. Sequencing with copy number analysis	NM_000495:1-51		Ashkenazi Jewish 95%
X-linked congenital adrenal hypoplasia	NR0B1. X-linked recessive. Sequencing with copy number analysis	NM_000475:1-2		Ashkenazi Jewish 99%
X-linked juvenile retinoschisis	RS1. X-linked recessive. Sequencing with copy number analysis	NM_000330:1-6		Ashkenazi Jewish 98%
X-linked myotubular myopathy	MTM1. X-linked recessive. Sequencing with copy number analysis	NM_000252:2-15		Ashkenazi Jewish 98%
X-linked severe combined immunodeficiency	IL2RG. X-linked recessive. Sequencing with copy number analysis	NM_000206:1-8		Ashkenazi Jewish >99%
Xeroderma pigmentosum group A	XPA. Autosomal recessive. Sequencing with copy number analysis	NM_000380:1-6		Ashkenazi Jewish >99%
Xeroderma pigmentosum group C	XPC. Autosomal recessive. Sequencing with copy number analysis	NM_004628:1-16		Ashkenazi Jewish 97%

analyses of how much it is "worth doing." Unfortunately, it is commonly only after litigation of something "missed" that the standards change to demand the offering of services previously thought to be either experimental or to have a very high cost-to-yield ratio.

One thing is clear, however, that there has been a shift in how and when we see patients. Thirty years ago, most of the time we were doing prenatal diagnosis for a mendelian disorder, it was because they already have a child at home who is affected. Now, we are much more likely to know that couples are at risk before they have such a child. As such, they have much more control over their destiny than before.

Chromosomal Disorders

In 1970, only about 5% of births were to women over 35 years of age, rising to 10% by 1990. In the United States today, the number of births to women over 35 years of age has reached almost 15%, and in selected areas such as Manhattan, it is approximately 20% (16). In 1970, the typical 40-year-old pregnant woman had been

married for 20 years and was having her fourth child. Today, a 40-year-old is more likely to be a professional woman having her first child. Not surprisingly, acceptance and tolerance of genetic risk and indeed approach to the conditions themselves differs between societies, between women, and over time in both societies and individuals.

Much of the change in attitude has come from improvements in our ability to accurately detect genetic health status of the fetus. Although Down syndrome (DS) represents only a small proportion of the serious genetic disorders observed worldwide, it continues to be at the forefront of patient concern as that is the name "they know" (17) (Table 10.2).

The efficacy of DS screening has evolved dramatically over 50 years with evolving protocols. The unifying theme of all these advances has been progressive improvement of sensitivity with lower false-positive rates. Methodologies have included three different categories of techniques (biochemical, ultrasound, and now molecular markers).

THE FETAL PATIENT

TABLE 10.2

Worldwide Birth Defects	
Congenital heart defects	1,040,835
Neural tube defects	323,904
Hemoglobin disorders	307,897
Down syndrome	217,293
G6-PD	177,032

Reprinted with permission from March of Dimes Birth Defects Foundation, 2006.

Available second trimester biochemical testing increased from single screening using low MSAFP in the early 1990s to double screening with MSAFP and human chorionic gonadotropin (hCG), triple screening by adding testing for unconjugated estriol (uE3), and currently quadruple testing by adding Inhibin A. In the mid to late 90s came the beginning of the shift of focus to the first trimester, and the best markers have proven to be pregnancy-associated plasma protein-A (PAPP-A) and human chorionic gonadotropin (β hCG), with the free β component being far more efficacious than total hCG (18). The next generation now include alpha-fetal protein (AFP), placental growth factor (PlGF), and others as some programs simultaneously screen for various aneuploidies, preeclampsia, and potentially preterm labor (19) (Table 10.3).

Over the years, a change in the pattern of clinically recognized indications for chromosomal prenatal diagnosis has been observed. Overall, the most common indication for genetic counseling and prenatal diagnosis is still the risk for nondysjunctional aneuploidy stemming from "advanced maternal age," the risk threshold of which is still defined as being 35 years of age or older at delivery or having a risk equivalent to that. Other "classic" indications to evaluate fetal karyotype include a previous affected offspring, a balanced structural rearrangement of parental chromosomes, abnormal ultrasound, or abnormal screening tests (20).

In the 1980s and 1990s, increased use of biochemical serum screening and of ultrasonographic screening for fetal chromosome anomalies identified more young patients at risk. Previously, young pregnant women were considered to be at low risk for fetal aneuploidy based merely on age. Positive screening results allowed them to consider having diagnostic prenatal testing. Various combinations of double, triple, or quadruple serum screening (multiplied by the a priori risk of their maternal age) selected a subgroup of patients among whom about 65% of chromosomally abnormal conceptions were identified. Using a risk cutoff for fetal aneuploidy equal to that of age 35 years, some 5% of "young" pregnant patients would have a positive screening test. About 1 in 50 amniocenteses performed for this indication revealed a chromosomally abnormal conceptus (21,22). Today, in the second trimester, sonographic markers for fetal chromosome anomalies are observed in 3% to 5% of pregnancies (21) and are another

indication for fetal karyotyping (23,24). In the 1990s, Benacerraf et al. developed a scoring system in which a score of "2," regardless of maternal age, was high enough to warrant diagnostic studies (karyotype by amniocentesis). Unfortunately, the quality of ultrasound assessment is much more variable than laboratory markers so that automatically combining ultrasound results from multiple centers lowers the detection rate of ultrasound, per se, and combined methodology algorithms (25).

There are also many soft US markers that have sometimes been associated with increased risk, but whose statistics are not adequate to become incorporated into routine use. Unfortunately, a lack of understanding of what such soft markers can and, more importantly, cannot indicate has led to a number of baseless malpractice actions claiming that patients had a "clear indication" for amniocentesis when there have been no appropriate studies demonstrating actual increased risk associated with the particular US finding (26). Merely because a given finding has a somewhat higher statistical occurrence in association with a given outcome, it does not automatically mean that it is reasonable or cost-effective to alter the patient care plan. Deleterious outcomes can be either having a child with a genetic disorder or having a complication from performing diagnostic procedures on incorrectly labeled high-risk patients.

A very important conceptual advance in the prenatal diagnosis of DS over the past 2 to 3 decades was the understanding that the US visualization of fetal NT, when performed correctly, was a very powerful marker of DS (27). The technology assessment literature is replete with failures to expand the use of successfully piloted techniques into routine clinical practice as the technology emerges (28). Organizations such as the Fetal Medicine Foundation (FMF) in London and later the Nuchal Translucency Quality Review program of the Society for Maternal-Fetal Medicine (SMFM) began quality assessment programs and credentialing (29). These programs were designed to minimize the likelihood of poor-quality ultrasound measurements impacting the accuracy of the algorithm for risk assessment and, thus, lowering the sensitivity and specificity of the US test (30,31). Credentialed training improved the outcomes of US testing to some degree, but sadly most providers have declined to participate in such quality assurance programs.

For about 15 years (roughly 1998 to 2013), the mainstay of screening was "combined" first trimester screening, which includes free beta hCG, PAPP-A, and the US screening for NT. Experience with well over a million patients has shown that when the biochemical parameters are measured appropriately and the US is performed and interpreted with proper quality control and assessment measures, combined screening can identify about 85% of DS pregnancies (18).

Pregnancies with increased NT measurements and normal karyotypes represent a distinct risk group. Over 100 genetic conditions have been found in such cases—the most common of which are cardiac anomalies and Noonan syndrome (32). We believe that

TABLE 10.3

Down Syndrome Screening Protocols over Past 50 Years				
Method	**Components**	**Time Frame**	**Sensitivity**	**FPR***
Maternal age	Birthday	1960s to present	35%	15%
Low MSAFP + age	AFP	1980s	50%	~5%
Double	AFP/hCG	1990s	55%	~5%
Triple	AFP/hCG/estriol	1990s	60%	~5%
Quad	AFP/hCG/estriol/inhibin	1990s/2000s	65%	~5%
NT	US measurements	1990s to present	60%	~5%
Combined	Free β hCG/PAPP-A/NT	2000s to present	85%	~5%
Sequential	Combined + quad	2000s to present	85%–90%	~5%
Free fetal DNA	Sequencing/targeted	Since 2011	98%	0.2%–1%

FPR, false-positive rate.

all patients with NT measurements over 3 mm (some say 3.5 mm) should be offered a fetal echocardiogram to search for cardiac anomalies, even if the 20-week anatomy scan is normal. It is also likely that with increased utilization of chromosomal microarray (CMA) analysis, some cases with increased NT will be shown to have previously unrecognized deletions or duplications (33).

Noninvasive Prenatal Screening

The "holy grail" of prenatal screening was for decades the concept that fetal cells could be obtained from a maternal blood sample and, thus, avoid the need and risk of an invasive diagnostic procedure for aneuploidy (34). Ectopic trophoblastic tissue in pregnant women has been documented since the late 1890s, when such tissues were found in the lungs of women who died of eclampsia. In the 1990s, the focus was on methods to separate out the rare fetal cells (perhaps 1/10,000,000) in the circulation. Numerous papers and a large NIH-sponsored trial (NIFTY) explored various separation strategies (fluorescent-activated and magnetic-activated cell sorting), but ultimately the technologies were not substantive enough to permit fetal cells in maternal blood to emerge as a viable screening approach (34).

In 1997, Lo and Wainscoat patented and then published a method for taking paternal DNA, amplifying it, and using it for the diagnosis of fetal gender (35). Over the years, there have been a number of approaches attempted, for example, using digital polymerase chain reaction (PCR) of DNA and RNA, and methylation differences. These approaches attempted, with inadequate success, to reliably investigate free fetal DNA (ffDNA) (36). Since 2011, the main approach has been using next-generation sequencing (NGS), also called massive parallel sequencing (MPS), in which DNA amplification is performed millions of times simultaneously using probes of approximately 36 base pairs, which provides enough specificity to accurately identify from which chromosome the excess fragments derive. Overall, the genome is interrogated over a 100 times, so that there is enough power to reliably determine the relative concentrations of DNA fragments for a given chromosomal region compared to the expected concentrations (37–39). For example, chromosome 21 normally encompasses approximately 1.32% of the genome DNA. If one were to observe approximately 2%, then it could readily be concluded that there was a trisomy for chromosome 21. Obviously, however, it is realistically not possible to obtain a noninvasive specimen that is exclusively fetal. Thus, the number of chromosome probes from the fetus is figuratively drowned in maternal DNA, such that the actual percentage increase is about 0.1%. However, by counting the genome over 100 times using the multiple parallel shotgun sequencing (MPSS) approach, the reliability is significantly improved.

Furthermore, as with any parameter, there is always a bell-shaped curve of counts that is amenable to being treated as a parametric measurement. As such, the algorithm looks at the standard deviation (SD) of the counts and considers values beyond 3+SD as being abnormal. With MPSS, this is done for all chromosomes. For the targeted probe or targeted sequencing protocols, only the chromosomes of interest are interrogated (39). Of those cases "at risk," diagnostic procedures such as amniocentesis or chorionic villous sampling (CVS) are then offered for confirmation; these techniques can produce both false positives and false negatives. Ultrasound imaging may or may not be consistent with the abnormality. It is important to recognize that, despite a literature reporting sensitivities approaching 99% for DS, a 99% sensitivity is NOT a 99% positive predictive value (40).

It is also well-appreciated statistical dogma that while sensitivity and specificity do not vary with prevalence, the predictive values do (41). Thus, while in a 40-year-old with a DS+ NIPS screen the likelihood of actually having a fetus with DS may be greater than 70%, in younger women the likelihood is much lower. For example, if there is a 99% sensitivity and a 99% specificity

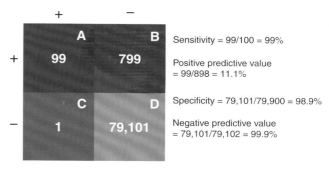

99–99 Screening

	+	−
+	**A** 99	**B** 799
−	**C** 1	**D** 79,101

Sensitivity = 99/100 = 99%

Positive predictive value = 99/898 = 11.1%

Specificity = 79,101/79,900 = 98.9%

Negative predictive value = 79,101/79,102 = 99.9%

FIGURE 10.3 Reality of screening. Example of a screening test with 99% sensitivity and 99% specificity. With a rare condition (in this case an incidence of 1:800), even a "great test" will have a low positive predictive value (here 11%). Patients and physicians all too often confuse the sensitivity with PPV.

(1% false positives) in a younger woman with a baseline risk of 1:800, the actual positive predictive value can be as low as 11%. That would be comparable to a 3-mm NT measurement on US. After several years of concern after NT measurements were introduced, it is now reasonably well understood that this finding is only an indicator of odds, and not a definitive answer (**Fig. 10.3**). Nevertheless, it is still critical for both physicians and patients to understand that the same limitations apply to cell ffDNA (NIPS) and act accordingly.

Public health policy debates over the role of NIPS screening methods are already very harsh, as the costs for these methods approach the total reimbursements from Medicaid in many jurisdictions for 9 months' worth of care, including labor and delivery (42). Blunt cost assessments, including the savings from pregnancies with serious problems that are terminated, will be necessary to determine a true financial cost/benefit ratio (43). Ultimately, these authors believe that all patients should be offered diagnostic testing (discussed below). For those who choose screening, it is still debatable based upon improving detection and lower costs as to what is the best protocol. Once again recommendations on screening versus testing vary significantly in different regions. Rates of diagnostic testing in the United Kingdom, for example, are only around 5% (RCOG Consensus). As we have previously written, *"In a diverse society, however, there will never be a uniform acceptance of any stance on this subject. The concept of taking a procedure risk for diagnostic capabilities has been at the center of genetic counseling and prenatal diagnosis for 50 years. The issues for NIPS… are no different than many that have come previously—just the names of the conditions that can be discovered and what resources are used and risks taken to find them"* (44).

PRENATAL DIAGNOSTIC PROCEDURES

Overview

Diagnostic (invasive) procedures for prenatal diagnosis of fetal disease are available throughout gestation from conception. Assisted reproduction technologies (ART) enable diagnosis (or exclusion) of several disorders on the 4- to 8-cell embryo before implantation.

Prenatal diagnosis requires direct assessment of fetal tissue. Since the late 1960s, this has been possible by the aspiration of amniotic fluid (AF). Beginning in the 1980s, chorionic villi have been obtained either transcervically or transabdominally. Other tissues, such as skin, muscle, liver, and fetal blood have been obtained occasionally (and now rarely) for those diagnoses that cannot be accomplished by sampling AF or villi. We think of these procedures as a continuum of approaches, rather than distinct entities that are independent of one another (43) (Table 10.4).

TABLE 10.4

Screening and Testing Options in 2020

Choices	Method	Sensitivity	False-Positive Rate	No Answer	Detection	Subchromosomal
Screening	First TM combined (free β, PAPP-A, NT)	84%	~5%	<1%	Trisomies 21, 18,13,	No
	First TM combined (total, PAPP-A, NT)	80%	~5%	<1%	Trisomies 21, 18,13,	No
	Second TM quad	65%	~5%	<1%	Trisomies 21, 18,13	No
	NIPS	98%	0.5%–1%	1%–7%	Trisomies 21, 18,13, sex	Limited
			Loss rate			
Testing	CVS	~100%	1/800	~0.2%	Full karyotype	Microarray—yes
	Amniocentesis	~100%	1/800	~0.2%	Full karyotype	Microarray—yes

TM, trimester; free β, free β sub-unit of hCG; total, combined sub-units of hCG; quad, quadruple screening (AFP, hCG, estriol, inhibin); NIPS, noninvasive prenatal screening.

Invasive procedures for diagnosis of fetal genetic disorders that have relied upon techniques for culturing and karyotyping of AF fibroblasts were developed (45) in the late 1960s to early 1970s. The first diagnosis of a fetal chromosome anomaly by amniocentesis (46) was followed shortly by the diagnosis of an enzyme deficiency in AF cells (43). Collaborative studies then established the safety and accuracy of mid-trimester amniocentesis, which became a routine part of prenatal care in high-risk patients and the gold standard against which other procedures for prenatal diagnosis are compared (47).

A major disadvantage of amniocentesis, however, is that results are usually not available until late in the second trimester, generally 17 to 20 weeks of gestation, by which time the pregnancy is very visible, the mother has felt the baby moving, the bonding process is accelerated, and consideration of termination is even more emotionally and physically onerous than earlier in gestation (48). Improvements in ultrasonography machinery and increasing expertise in US-guided procedures enabled physicians in the 1980s to attempt prenatal diagnosis in the first trimester, introducing CVS and then early amniocentesis. These technical developments were backed and reinforced by increasing preference on the part of patients for first trimester prenatal diagnosis, with second trimester terminations having higher complication rates, being more emotionally onerous, and having a higher health care cost (49). In the 80s, CVS was usually performed between 9 and 10 weeks, but currently, it is more commonly done between 11.5 and 13 weeks of gestation so that an NT measurement can be done simultaneously on the same US.

The accuracy and safety of CVS are quite comparable to those of mid-trimester amniocentesis (50–53), and the concerns that the procedure might cause fetal limb reduction defects (LRDs) at the gestational age at which CVS is generally performed have been shown to be unwarranted (54). Recent data suggest that CVS is as safe or may even be safer than mid-trimester amniocentesis (55,56). An alternative to CVS was offered by early amniocentesis performed between 10 and 14 weeks of gestation, but this technique was abandoned because, despite initial enthusiasm for the method based upon its alleged comparative safety compared with CVS (55) early amniocentesis was quickly associated with AF leakage that lead to talipes (56).

Amniocentesis

It has long been appreciated that prenatal diagnostic procedures should be performed by an obstetrician trained and experienced in the procedure, and that it should be preceded by genetic counseling (57,58), in which the family pedigree and genetic risk are evaluated, and the advantages, limitations, and risks of relevant procedures are explained.

A detailed US examination should assess gestational age, AF volume, and fetal and placental location and include an anatomic examination for fetal malformations (57). The mother's blood type and antibody status should be known prior to amniocentesis.

Rh-negative women with negative antibody screening with a father of the baby that is known to be Rh positive or unknown should receive Rh immunoprophylaxis after the procedure (58). Historically, it was believed that in Rh-negative patients, the selected needle path should avoid, if reasonably possible, the placenta. However, we do not hesitate to go through the placenta to reach a pocket of AF if it is the best approach.

After sterile preparation of the skin, we reach the amniotic cavity transabdominally mostly with a 20-gauge, 3.5-inch long, spinal needle. Longer needles are sometimes needed. The needle, held in one hand with the finger on top of the stylet, should be inserted smoothly, in a single, rapid motion, into the AF pocket. We prefer to use the 20-gauge needle at 15 weeks and beyond, because the procedure can be performed significantly faster than with the 22-gauge needle. Although it is, in practicality, impossible to prove, we believe that an important consideration in the safety of fetal procedures is speed. The larger needle allows a procedure duration of less than 1 minute. Real-time ultrasonographic guidance during amniocentesis has been routine since the 1980s, since it reduces the frequency of multiple needle insertions, bloody taps, trauma, tenting, and failure to obtain AF, but we still believe that "feel" is an important component of safety and efficacy (59,60).

When the needle tip, seen on ultrasound as a bright spot, is placed satisfactorily into the AF pocket, the stylet is removed, and a 3- to 5-mL syringe is attached. The first 2 to 3 mL of fluid are aspirated and discarded, in order to minimize the risk of contamination with maternal cells drawn from the path of the needle. Typically, 20 mL of AF are then drawn into the syringe, transferred to sterile tubes, and transported at room temperature to the laboratory for processing (if a procedure is performed prior to 15 weeks of gestational age, 1 cc per week of gestation is withdrawn). If multiple studies, such as microarray or other DNA tests, are being performed up to 30 cc can be obtained if the fetus is over 16 to 17 weeks' gestation and even more at 20+ weeks (61).

Patients are released after ultrasound documentation of fetal viability. Following amniocentesis, we recommend to defer sexual activity, baths, and strenuous exercise for 2 or 3 days. We do not believe that bed rest or severe limitations of routine activity make any difference. Patients are also instructed to report immediately signs of infection, heavy vaginal bleeding, leakage of AF, and regular uterine contractions.

Multiple Gestations

With infertility treatments, multiple births in the United States have tripled to about 3% of births and represent an even higher percentage of patients presenting for prenatal diagnosis (16). One-third of naturally occurring multiple gestations are monozygotic, and approximately overall 20% of twins are monozygotic with infertility therapies. Thus, in most cases separate sampling of AF from both sacs is required to assess correctly the karyotype of each fetus. In general, the chance that at least one dizygotic twin has an abnormal karyotype is essentially twice the age-related risk

(61). However, the risks of procedures in multiples do not appear to be increased significantly, probably because such procedures are disproportionately performed by subspecialists (perinatologists and geneticists) who generally have more experience and expertise (62). When the anatomic relationship of the sacs and the chorioamniotic membrane between them is clearly discernible, it is generally straightforward to sample both sacs, with continuous ultrasound guidance.

Historically, injection of a dye into the first sac after aspiration of AF was considered a helpful marker (63,64). We have long ago abandoned this. Our technique is, after obtaining the specimen from a sac, to use the aspiration syringe to fill it to 5 cc of AF and then, without disconnecting it, immediately eject it back into the cavity. The fluid injected creates contrast that demarcates the different sacs (**Fig. 10.4**).

Abnormally elevated AF AFP in the absence of an obvious cause, such as spina bifida, observable on ultrasound indicates the need to test for acetylcholinesterase (AChE). The combination of an abnormally elevated AF AFP and a positive AChE is associated in most cases with fetal malformations or with fetal death. Transfer of these materials across the membranes may confuse clinical interpretation of AF AFP, and AChE results in twin pregnancies. Discordant AF AFP results are more common in dizygotic twins, perhaps due to the dichorionic diamniotic membrane between the sacs. AChE diffuses readily across the membranes and cannot be used to determine which twin is abnormal (65).

"Early" Amniocentesis

Improved ultrasound technology, increasing experience with ultrasound-guided needle manipulation and patient preference for more private, earlier genetic diagnosis have motivated a shift from second trimester amniocentesis toward earlier procedures, mostly CVS. When CVS was being developed in the 1980s, and the United States Federal Drug Administration severely limited the number of centers who could obtain the investigational device exemption for the catheter, many centers began to offer "early" amniocenteses (EA), which has never been rigorously defined and has been described for procedures from as early as 10 weeks up to 15 6/7 weeks. When the possibility that CVS could cause LRDs was first reported in the early 1990s (54,66), there was further interest in early amniocentesis as an alternative (67). However, a number of reports documented an increased incidence of talipes with EA. Approximately 15% of procedures resulted in tenting of

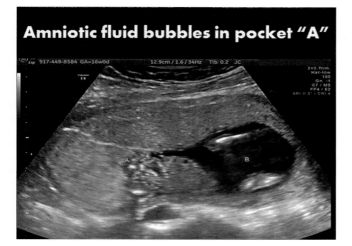

FIGURE 10.4 Amniotic fluid bubbles. After obtaining specimen from sac "A" 5 cc of extra fluid is drawn into the syringe and immediately injected back into the sac stirring up debris in sac producing "bubbles," which clearly outline one sac from the other (sac B).

membranes with transient oligohydramnios, and in about 15% of those cases, talipes was present in the newborn. Overall, the 1.5% total risk of talipes was too high to be considered a reasonable risk; thus, EA was abandoned (68,69).

Safety and Complications of Amniocentesis

Multiple studies over the past four decades have investigated the risks of amniocentesis (51,70–72). As with all prenatal procedures, there is a constellation of factors developing concurrently that render definitive assessment of risk difficult. Most importantly, there is a well-understood background rate of fetal loss that diminishes with advancing gestational ages, and there is a dramatic correlation between maternal age and the risk of spontaneous loss. If the data are limited to those fetuses known to be euploid, the correlation persists, but it is less dramatic.

The only randomized trial of amniocentesis versus no amniocentesis in low-risk patients was done in the mid 1980s by Tabor et al. in Copenhagen. They found nearly a 1% increase in pregnancy loss following amniocentesis (70). However, true risk is today significantly lower. Uncertainty over risks of amniocentesis are produced by different definitions of which losses are associated (days after the procedure, up to 24 weeks, or anytime in pregnancy), assumptions about the baseline risk of loss, and variability between centers. There continues to be considerable variability in quoted fetal loss rates following amniocentesis. In the United Kingdom, rates of up to 1% are still regularly cited (73). The Society of Obstetrics and Gynecology of Canada states that multiple factors are involved and that overall risk is between 0.6% and 1.0% (74).

More recent studies suggest a much lower complication rate, with the general consensus in experienced hands being that fetal loss after amniocentesis may be as low as 0.1% to 0.2% above background rates (71,72). One often quoted study from the FASTER trial suggested that the risk was as low as 1/1,600, but this too-low estimate resulted from an error in statistical analysis (75–77).

Three large-scale studies have now concluded that amniocentesis is far safer than previously thought, and that CVS and amniocentesis are of comparable risks (51–53). More recent data from Denmark suggest that the procedure risks of CVS and amniocentesis are the same and that the incidence of late-term complications is actually lower in the CVS group than in those who have amniocentesis (52). Finally, Akolekar in England confirmed the above and the very minimal risks of procedures in competent hands (53).

Maternal complications such as sepsis and death are also very rare, but never zero.

Trauma to the fetus during amniocentesis has been reported, including central nervous system injury and amniotic band syndrome (78). However, fetal injury caused by the amniocentesis needle was never very common and should now be virtually nonexistent with ultrasound-guided procedures performed by experienced physicians.

Chorionic Villous Sampling

Since the introduction of amniocentesis into high-risk obstetrics in the 1970s, there has been a constant desire to move prenatal diagnoses to as early in gestation as possible (2). In the mid-1980s, the combination of increasingly sophisticated ultrasound imaging and laboratory cytogenetic advances made first trimester sampling of chorionic villi possible.

Indications

With the possible exception of those patients whose primary risk is for an NTD, virtually any patient seen in the first trimester who would be considered a candidate for amniocentesis is also a candidate for CVS (49). CVS has the advantage of earlier diagnosis, increased privacy, and allowing earlier intervention when chosen by patients. Developments in screening, both combined and NIPS, mean that the majority of DS pregnancies, for example, can be identified in the first trimester. We believe that it is not acceptable to routinely identify high risk in the first trimester and then force the patient to wait a month for an amniocentesis when a CVS could provide the answer much sooner and with privacy for the parents.

In the 1980s, we generally scheduled CVS patients to be seen at about 9 to 10 weeks after their last menstrual period (LMP). Now, 12 weeks is the most common time because:

1. NT screening cannot be reliably performed (for determination that the results are in the normal range) until nearly 12 weeks gestation.
2. The concerns about LRDs, despite being proven to be unfounded, still create patient concern, and some physicians are concerned about liability exposure.
3. If an abnormality is found at 12 to 13 weeks, it is still early enough for the patient to choose to terminate by the safer, easier, quicker, and cheaper suction method that can be used in the first trimester. Second trimester termination techniques are more expensive, have higher complication rates, and are without privacy because the pregnant status of the patient has usually become obvious by this time (49).

Multiple Gestations

As there has been a significant drop in the use of CVS and amniocentesis on singletons, many physicians do not have the training even on singletons and so should not even begin to think about performing procedures on multiples. We routinely perform CVS on multiple gestations because we believe strongly that CVS has significant advantages over amniocentesis. When patients choose fetal reduction (FR), either because of a diagnosed fetal abnormality or because of the increased risks of abnormality associated with multiples, *per se*, FR has better outcome statistics in the late first trimester than either very early (6 to 7 weeks) or later in the second trimester. For the past 25 years, we almost always performed CVS, analyze the specimens with fluorescent *in situ* hybridization (FISH) analysis overnight, and then performed the FR the next afternoon (79). The development of microarrays has added to the choices and management schema (discussed below).

Placental and fetal locations must be meticulously noted in order to avoid sampling one twin twice and the other not at all (**Fig. 10.5**). Nevertheless, there is always the small risk of cross-contamination of samples. Operators must be facile with both the transabdominal (TA) and the transcervical (TC) approaches,

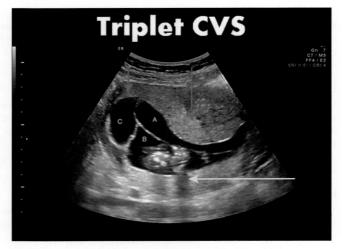

FIGURE 10.5 CVS multiples. *Yellow arrow* shows posterior placental *"B,"* which is reached transcervically. *Red arrows* show path of transabdominal CVS needles to anterior placentas *A* and *C*. Placenta *C* looks small only because picture shows only a small portion of it.

to maximize the ability to obtain specimens and to minimize the chance of cross contamination. Furthermore, the operators must make sure they are not getting the specimens from the placenta of a "vanishing twin," which may occur in up to 3% of pregnancies, and which is disproportionately likely to show chromosomal abnormalities (79,80).

CVS Technique

After counseling, ultrasound confirms fetal viability. In our experience, about 2% of patients are discovered to have a blighted ovum or an embryonic/fetal demise (81,82). Fetal size discordances should also be noted. Of significant concern is the smaller-than-expected fetus, even in the first trimester. We have found that such fetuses are at increased risk for aneuploidy (83), and such cases merit CVS to hasten diagnosis.

In general, placental location determines whether the approach will be TC or TA. For most cases, this decision will be straightforward. If the placenta is low-lying, posterior, or previa, a TC approach is appropriate (80). CVS is relatively easy to perform in these cases and may be attempted by trainees under supervision. As placental position moves upward or lateral, or if the uterus is retroverted, or there are fibroids, for example, TC CVS is more technically challenging. The placenta can often be maneuvered into a more horizontal (TC) or vertical (TA) configuration by judicious manipulation of bladder volume and using the speculum handle to alter the angle of the cervical canal. If the placenta is anterior and fundal, an abdominal approach is often indicated. Large subchorionic hematomas and fibroids should be avoided if possible and sometimes dictate the approach. Overall, the TC approach requires more experience than does TA. In our experience, either TA or TC is clearly indicated in about 20% of cases each; in the remaining 60%, either approach can be used (80). Acceptability of screening methods varies across and within cultures. Physicians should be aware of this and accommodate the patient's preference, when it is possible to do so.

In multiple gestations, sampling using both approaches is the routine, and the operator's ability to do both well is essential.

Other factors must be considered before attempting CVS. For patients with a history of genital herpes simplex or a recent group B streptococcus (GBS) infection, the small or theoretical risk of introducing an infection into the fetal–placental tissues should be discussed with the patient. While routine culturing is not warranted, transabdominal CVS TA-CVS or amniocentesis is usually offered when a significant risk of active GBS is appreciated (84).

Transabdominal CVS also has been applied successfully in the second and third trimesters for prenatal diagnosis, with results comparable to amniocentesis and probably associated with a smaller risk of pregnancy loss than cordocentesis. The major advantage of late CVS is the possibility of obtaining rapid results in situations where such information is needed for decisions about mode and timing of delivery, pregnancy termination, or fetal therapy. Such situations include the ultrasonographic diagnosis of fetal anomalies late in the second trimester, close to the legal limit in gestational age after which termination of pregnancy is no longer legally possible in many locations. Late CVS also offers a distinct advantage over cordocentesis in cases complicated by oligohydramnios. Prenatal availability of fetal FISH and karyotype in pregnancies complicated by severe intrauterine growth restriction (IUGR) or fetal anomalies may influence the mode of delivery; the management of intrapartum fetal distress, which is a common phenomenon in fetuses with chromosome anomalies; or the decision for surgical intervention within the first few hours after birth (80).

Safety of CVS

For first trimester diagnosis, either TA-CVS or TC-CVS is the preferred method of choice, while EA carries a significant risk for both fetal loss and fetal malformations and has been abandoned. Skill in both TC and TA methods is necessary to provide the most complete, practical, and safe approach to first trimester diagnosis.

In the early 90s, it was suggested that CVS may be associated with specific fetal malformations, particularly LRDs (54,66). Today, based on the published data, it is clear that there is no increased risk for LRDs or any other birth defect when CVS is performed at greater than 70 days of gestation (from LMP). There is a minimal risk between 8 and 9 weeks, but there is about a 1% risk of limb reduction defections if the procedure is performed between 24 and 42 days postfertilization (6 to 7 weeks LMP) (80).

Accuracy of CVS Cytogenetic Results

A major concern with all prenatal diagnostic procedures is the possibility of discordance between the prenatal cytogenetic diagnosis and the actual fetal karyotype. With CVS, these discrepancies can occur from either maternal tissue contamination or from true biologic differences between the extraembryonic tissue (i.e., placenta) and the fetus. It was demonstrated in the 1980s that genetic evaluation of chorionic villi provides a high level of accuracy, particularly in regard to the diagnosis of common trisomies (85,86). Clinical errors or misinterpretations are rare, and the need for repeat testing continues to decrease as more knowledge about the characteristics of chorionic villi was obtained. Today, approximately 0.5% of CVS cases have an ambiguous finding that requires further confirmation by amniocentesis (87). Overall, CVS is associated with a low rate of maternal cell contamination or chromosomal abnormalities confined to the placenta, as will be described below (88).

Confined Placental Mosaicism

Mosaicism occurs in about 0.5% to 2% of all CVS samples (86–88), and it is confirmed in the fetus in 10% to 40% of these cases. Grati has shown that the likelihood of a mosaicism being clinically important varies significantly by the specific chromosome involved such that it can be included in counseling (89). In contrast, AF cell mosaicism is observed in only 0.1% to 0.3% of cultures, but when found, it is confirmed in the fetus in approximately 70% of cases (86–88). Fetoplacental discrepancies are known to occur because the chorionic villi consist of a combination of extraembryonic tissue of different sources that become separated and distinct from those of the embryo in early developmental stages. Specifically, at the 32- to 64-celled blastocyst, only 3 to 4 blastomeres differentiate into the inner cell mass (ICM), which forms the embryo, mesenchymal core of the chorionic villi, the amnion, yolk sac, and chorion, whereas the rest of the cells become the precursors of the extraembryonic tissues (86–90).

A chromosomal aberration that does not involve the fetal cell lineage will produce a confined placental mosaicism (CPM), in which the trophoblast and perhaps the extraembryonic mesoderm may demonstrate aneuploid cells, but the fetus is euploid.

Another adverse outcome that may be associated with CPM is that of uniparental disomy (UPD). In UPD, both chromosomes of a given pair are inherited from a single parent, rather than one from each. UPD results when the original trisomic embryo is "rescued" by the loss of the one extra chromosome. Because trisomic embryos have two chromosomes from one parent and one from the other, there is a theoretical 1 in 3 chance that the two remaining chromosomes originate from the same parent, leading to UPD. This may have clinical consequences if the chromosome involved harbors imprinted genes whose expression vary according to the parent of origin or if the two remaining chromosomes carry a mutant recessive gene, creating a homozygous state. In general, UPD has been reported for almost every chromosomal pair, although clinical consequences have been observed mainly in cases involving specific chromosomes (i.e., chromosomes 2, 6, 7, 10, 11, 14, 15, 16, 20) (91).

When discordances between CVS and AF cell karyotypes were first appreciated in the 1980s, they were interpreted as a "problem" of CVS. We now realize that, in fact, they represent an opportunity to identify real issues such as UPD that can have significant clinical impact that otherwise would not be detectable.

Tissue Biopsies

On rare occasion fetal liver and muscle biopsy are still needed when molecular analyses of amniocytes or chorionic villi are insufficient for diagnosis. Improved molecular approaches have dramatically decreased the need for these over the past decade. Biopsies are indicated only in the absence of other alternatives, because the risk for pregnancy loss associated with these invasive procedures is higher than CVS or amniocentesis. For example, in the late 1980s, we developed fetal muscle biopsy for rare cases of Duchenne muscular dystrophy (DMD), when molecular analysis of trophoblasts, amniocytes, or fetal leukocytes was nondiagnostic, and family studies were uninformative. We have performed dozens of *in utero* fetal muscle biopsies in the middle of the second trimester to assess dystrophin levels in myoblasts by *in situ* hybridization (92,93). Absence of dystrophin suggests an affected fetus. The technique uses a kidney biopsy needle in which the full trocar is placed into the fetal gluteal muscle, the trocar extended, and then the trigger pulled creating a core biopsy (**Fig. 10.6**). Muscle specimens are flash frozen with dry ice for storage and shipping.

Fetal liver biopsy can be performed for certain rare enzyme deficiencies. For example, in one type of glycogenosis, glucose-6-phosphatase is decreased; this enzyme is expressed only in fetal liver and kidney. In the absence of direct DNA techniques, the only option available for prenatal diagnosis is fetal liver biopsy in which glucose-6-phosphatase activity can be measured. Fetal liver biopsy also is applicable in rare cases of ornithine transcarbamylase deficiency for which family studies are uninformative, and known deletions cannot be detected (94,95). Over time most of these procedures will continue to diminish, and prenatal diagnosis of virtually all DNA-derived genetic disorders will be performed by molecular analysis, including some mitochondrial disorders that may be amenable to prenatal diagnosis.

Fetal skin biopsies were originally developed to diagnose dermatologic disorders such as epidermolysis bullosa lethalis. More recently, we have found skin biopsy to be a better alternative for settling discordances between CVS and amniocentesis results than cordocentesis (95). Some trisomies such as 12 and 20 are not detected in fetal blood, and chromosome 8 is variable (96).

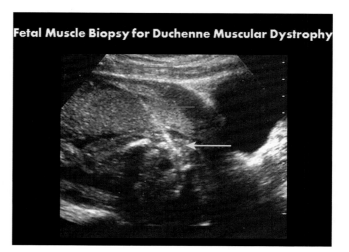

FIGURE 10.6 Fetal muscle biopsies. *Yellow arrow* shows core biopsy needle in fetal gluteal muscle. *Red arrows* show path of the needle through the placenta.

The technique is the same as for fetal muscle biopsy except that the trocar is extended before penetration of the skin, so that the biopsy includes the skin.

Cordocentesis

Cordocentesis has been performed since the 1980s for multiple indications. As with tissue biopsies, its use rose and then fell dramatically. Fifty years ago, Freda and Adamsons originally attempted to access the vascular system of the fetus for treatment of Rh isoimmunization by hysterotomy and fetal exposure (97). This method soon was abandoned because of the unacceptably high risk for the mother and fetus.

Daffos introduced ultrasonography-guided percutaneous umbilical blood sampling (PUBS) in 1983 for the diagnosis of fetal infections (98). The procedure gained rapid and wide acceptance. However, with the development of better molecular tests, the use of cordocentesis has dramatically decreased over the past decade. The risk of fetal loss is relatively small, usually about 1% or less in very experienced hands (98). Different guidance techniques (i.e., fixed-needle guides vs. freehand), needles of lengths varying from 8 to 15 cm, gauges varying from 20 to 27 g, and differing patient preparation protocols are used by various centers. Nicolaides and colleagues have shown that an outpatient setting in a standard ultrasonography room, without need for maternal fasting, sedation, tocolytics, antibiotics, or fetal paralysis for the procedure works very well (99).

In alloimmune thrombocytopenia, cordocentesis allows the determination of fetal platelet phenotype and count. A low fetal platelet count in this situation can be treated by weekly infusion of platelets until delivery or other approaches (see Chapter 44) (100).

In Rh isoimmunization, fetal blood sampling was performed for immediate confirmation of fetal antigenic status, obviating the need for further intervention in the Rh-negative fetus. Today, we accomplish the same by noninvasive prenatal screening (NIPS). If the fetus is Rh positive, cordocentesis enables a more accurate assessment of fetal anemia and an immediate rise in fetal erythrocyte count on correction by intravascular transfusion. From case–control studies, it appears that at all gestational ages studied and at all levels of disease severity, intravascular correction of fetal anemia is more efficient and less risky to the mother and fetus than the intraperitoneal approach (101).

The diagnosis of fetal infection is based commonly on the demonstration of the agent-specific immunoglobulin (IgM) in fetal blood, because the large molecule does not cross the placenta. Fetal blood sampling should be scheduled to allow enough time from initial exposure to infection for IgM to appear after immunocompetence develops in the fetus. For first trimester exposures, the best time for cordocentesis is probably after 20 weeks' gestation. In a few specific cases, *in utero* treatment also is available. Thus, after toxoplasmosis infection in the mother, and demonstration of IgM specific for toxoplasmosis in fetal blood, antibiotic treatment with spiramycin reduced significantly the risk of congenital toxoplasmosis, as well as the risk of late sequelae (102). Cordocentesis has also been used for repeated blood transfusions *in utero* to hydropic fetuses with hemolytic anemia caused by parvovirus B19 infection (102).

Severe, early-onset IUGR commonly is associated with fetal chromosome anomalies. Cordocentesis allows for rapid fetal karyotyping, which can be available within 48 to 72 hours. Routine use of cordocentesis sampling for chromosomal analysis has dramatically fallen and currently is usually reserved for settling discrepancies between CVS and amniocentesis specimens, although we generally prefer skin biopsies.

Testing versus Screening

Since the early development of prenatal diagnosis in the late 1960s, there has been a pendulum constantly swinging back and forth between the primacy of screening versus testing. Diagnostic

procedures have progressively gotten safer as centers of excellence developed with specialized, experienced operators and with better ultrasound to visualize those procedures. At the same time, screening procedures have also improved with increasing rounds of improved sensitivity and specificity as generations of technology have progressed (Table 10.3).

Over the past several years, cell ffDNA for NIPS has emerged as the most popular method for screening for common aneuploidies and sex identification. Literally millions of cases have been performed, and the utilization of diagnostic testing (mostly amniocentesis) has decreased significantly as have other methods of screening such as the combined screen.

In our own program for the past 35 years, about 80% of patients following genetic counseling decide to proceed with a diagnostic procedure. That has not changed. What has changed is that the proportion of patients coming for consultations has dramatically decreased (103,104).

NIPS and CMA (see below) are both disruptive technologies that have had major impact upon the practice of obstetrics and gynecology and reproductive genetics. The introduction of NIPS has been primarily industry driven. Large-scale studies were done mostly only after widespread clinical introduction and extensive marketing such that the costs of the studies were mostly paid for by patient revenues (105). CMA followed the more traditional paradigm of academic studies, grant funding, and large-scale multicenter investigations before introduction; it has not had the mass sales force efforts of NIPS. The noninvasive nature of NIPS allows the primary provider to initiate screening without referral to subspecialists. We believe this practice generally does a disservice to patients who may desire a complete diagnostic evaluation but who often are not told that there is more available than what they are being offered (104,105). In particular, the accessibility of NIPS may come at the expense of full genetic counseling, which is a vital component of the antenatal genetic assessment.

Our data are consistent with a general concept we have presented for several years that the focus of prenatal diagnosis needs to move beyond DS to consider all sources of neurologic and structural impairment (103,104). With the advent of screening for preeclampsia, further progress is also being added to maternal health disorder screening (106). For the majority of pregnant women, the incidence of abnormal copy number variants (CNVs) is actually greater than the standard aneuploidies. For younger women, the detection of abnormal CNVs can be 10 times the expected yield of aneuploidies (49,106). Eventually, with deeper NGS and whole exome sequencing, noninvasive methods may approximate the diagnostic capabilities of diagnostic procedures and microarray (105–108). Until that time, however, literally tens of thousands of CNVs are not being detected because of reliance upon the screening practices of NIPS today (104,109).

From a public health perspective, including public policy, cost/benefit analysis, and maximizing patient autonomy, moving toward the direction of much higher diagnostic capabilities at the risk of complications including pregnancy loss should be considered very compelling.

Once again, this is an area with massive variability in acceptance, and tolerance of genetic risk differs across and between cultures. There will never be a uniform acceptance of any stance on this subject. The concept of accepting a procedure risk for diagnostic capabilities has been at the center of genetic counseling and prenatal diagnosis for 50 years (20). The issues for NIPS versus microarray are in parallel with many that have come previously—just the names of the conditions that can be discovered and what resources are used and risks taken to find them have evolved.

We have recently estimated that the cost of care of abnormal CNVs such as beta thalassemia major, Prader-Willi syndrome, and Marfan syndrome in the US health care system could be $500,000

TABLE 10.5

USA Societal Comparisons

	Cases per Year	Cost Lifetime per Case	Total Costs
Down syndrome births	6,000	$1,000,000	$6 Billion
Cerebral palsy	8,000	$1,000,000	$8 Billion
HIV cases	40,000	$400,000	$16 Billion
Auto fatalities	38,000		
Gunshot deaths	34,000		
Missed CNV's	34,000	$500,000	$17 Billion

or more (43). If we compare these numbers against estimated costs for several other medical conditions, it becomes apparent that abnormal CNVs, for which we are doing very little as a public health measure, are costing the medical "system" far more than many issues for which we devote tremendous efforts to detect and parents often choose to prevent (43,103,104). In toto, abnormal CNVs represent about three times the cost of DS and cerebral palsy (103). The incidences of auto fatalities, gunshot deaths, and HIV are comparable to abnormal CNVs, and the costs of HIV are roughly comparable (Table 10.5) (110–112). Far more public health efforts are being directed at these other situations such that the tremendous expense for NIPS for DS represents a very inefficient use of health care expenditures.

We believe that it is time to take a step back and view prenatal screening and diagnosis from the wider perspective of its impact upon society in more than just the strict statistical performance metrics. Because the yield of diagnosed abnormalities is essentially twice that of karyotypes in dysmorphic children, CMA have essentially replaced karyotypes in pediatric genetics (113). The NICHD trial and many others now show that in fetuses with normal ultrasounds and karyotype, the detection of CNV's of well-documented pathology is about 1.5% (114,115). For the past 40 years, high risk has been defined as age 35, so now "everyone's risk" is over 35, which is why we offer diagnostic procedures to essentially all pregnant women regardless of their age (104).

Once again there is a huge range of practice across and within cultures, with decisions being as much ethics as science driven.

For NIPS, never before have we seen one technology substantially replace another (diagnostic tests) when it is both simultaneously less efficacious and ultimately more expensive (103,104). The shift from diagnostics to screening is not new, however. Over two decades, ultrasound reliance has also decreased diagnostic testing, but has resulted in more anomalies being missed (116).

NIPS has high performance for DS but much less for other conditions (103). Although originally proposed for only the high-risk population, its use had migrated to being used mostly on low-risk, routine patients. By definition, all screening tests have poorer performance for lower incidence conditions and are less cost beneficial. Our own work and others have suggested that the cost of finding additional DS cases over combined screening may be about $3 million per case (103). In the United States, Aetna Insurance Company began coverage for NIPS for "routine" pregnancies in 2015 but in 2017 reversed their decision. We believe this was a reasonable decision. The cost/benefits of routine NIPS versus combined screening (β hCG, PAPP-A, and NT) will evolve as the costs of NIPS inevitably lower with new technology and higher volumes.

The "goalposts" of what can be diagnosed by microarray analysis have also improved considerably. About 1% of all children develop neurologic developmental delays (ND), and over 1% develop autism (117). CMA studies suggest that as much as 40% of ND and 20% of autism can be identified (103–105). The 2012 NICHD data showed that, at the most conservative, 0.5% of patients with no other findings had well-documented, pathologic CNVs (114), and 1.7% had a CNV that was either well documented or likely to be pathologic. We believe 1.5% is a reasonable, conservative number. Modeling variable detection, costs, and patient choices allows us to develop both high- and low-cost estimates under differing scenarios.

Laboratory Analyses

In previous editions of this book, our discussion of the use of laboratory techniques included the basics of the techniques. In the current edition, the book has been reorganized placing the fundamentals of laboratory tests in Chapter 56. Here, we focus on the use of these techniques as a fundamental component of prenatal diagnosis and screening.

Standard Cytogenetic Techniques

Described in Chapter 56

Molecular Cytogenestic Techniques

In addition to the standard cytogenetic techniques, several methods have originated from the interface between cytogenetics and molecular biology, commonly referred to as "molecular cytogenetics." In general, these techniques use fluorescently labeled DNA probes that bind to a specific chromosomal region and thus allow assessment of the presence and number of specific genomic loci within a cell.

Fluorescent *in situ* Hybridization

FISH was first introduced in the early 1990s. FISH functions as a bridge between conventional cytogenetics and molecular DNA testing, enables sensitive and relatively fast evaluation of the number and location of large pieces of chromosomes by direct visualization of specific regions under the microscope (118). It is based on the fact that single-stranded DNA probes can anneal to complementary DNA strands to form a double-stranded helix under proper conditions, a process called hybridization (119). The probe is composed of a specific DNA segment that incorporates modified nucleotides tagged by fluorescence markers (120). It is also possible to use multiple FISH probes, each with a different fluorochrome in a single hybridization procedure. FISH can be used when there is a high index of clinical suspicion for a condition associated with a deletion or duplication of a specific gene(s). Hence, the most critical element in FISH is the selection of the specific probe that will help to answer the clinical question.

FISH probes produce a fluorescent signal on whichever chromosome they hybridize to, that is, if a signal is present, DNA complementary to the probe is present. Thus, a paired chromosomal region produces two dots. Cells, monosomic for the chromosomal region (i.e., a chromosomal deletion), show only a single dot per nucleus, while trisomic cells show three dots. It is important to remember that a technical failure of hybridization may also result in absence of signal, providing a false-positive result. Reducing false-positive rates may be accomplished by analyzing numerous cells.

One of the major advantages of FISH over the standard banding methods is its ability to recognize subtle chromosomal changes such as deletions or duplications, which result in an alteration of normal gene dosage (121). Specific commercial FISH probes are available to recognize specific microdeletions, for example, DiGeorge/velocardiofacial syndrome that most often results from a 3 Mb deletion on chromosomal region 22q11.2. Unlike standard cytogenetic techniques, which require dividing cells in metaphase, FISH may be applied to interphase nuclei of nondividing cells (121) obviating the need for cell culture, which usually requires 10 to 14 days. Use of FISH significantly shortens the procedure time for analysis of chromosomal numeric aberrations in prenatal diagnosis and preimplantation genetic diagnosis (PGD) (120).

The fundamental limitation of using FISH in the clinical setting is that in most cases the clinician must have a prior knowledge of or high index of suspicion for the specific chromosome aberration in question.

Chromosomal Microarray

The fundamental limitation of FISH, obligating clinical suspicion and targeted probe selection for a specific chromosome location, made it clear that a genome-wide molecular cytogenetic approach for detecting copy number imbalances at a higher resolution is needed. In the past few years, advances in molecular cytogenetic techniques enabled the detection of small genomic alterations (e.g., deletions and duplications) generally termed "submicroscopic alterations" (i.e., under the 5- to 10-Mb resolution for conventional karyotyping), on a genome-wide scale. Some of these microdeletions or microduplications are associated with well-described clinical syndromes and others may have significant clinical implications. These conditions result from changes in the amount of genetic material along the chromosome, and thus are termed CNVs. These include deletions and duplications in the range of thousands to millions of base pairs.

CNVs can be either benign or pathogenic, depending on their location and genetic content. It is well documented that such alterations are an important cause of unexplained developmental delay/intellectual disability (DD/ID), autism spectrum disorders (ASDs), and multiple congenital anomalies (MCA) (**Fig. 10.7**). For patients with these conditions, CNVs account for 10% to 20% of cases, despite normal results on conventional cytogenetic studies (114).

CMA analysis enables the simultaneous analysis of the entire genome to identify deletions and duplications 100 to 1,000 times smaller than those identified by karyotype, without the need to preselect the target. In general, the technique is based on the hybridization properties of DNA. One such approach is comparative genomic hybridization (CGH). This involves patient DNA, labeled with a green dye and a control DNA labeled with a red dye, mixed in equal proportions and hybridized to an array of unique genomic DNA sequences spotted individually on a surface. Spots corresponding to sequences that are present in equal amounts in the patient and in the control will give a yellow signal. If the patient has a deletion in a specific region, all spots corresponding to the sequences will disproportionately hybridize more of the control DNA and thus have a red color. Conversely, if the patient has a duplication in a specific region, all spots corresponding to the sequences will hybridize more of the patient's DNA and thus have a green color. In the earliest version of CGH, both sets of DNA were hybridized to normal metaphase chromosomes on a slide and analyzed under a fluorescence microscope. Currently, a higher resolution, array CGH is used (also termed "DNA chips"), in which test and control DNA are hybridized with a microarray that contains probes corresponding to specific regions of the genome. A variety of different probes are in clinical usage, including large ones derived from bacterial artificial chromosomes (BAC array), small ones consisting of oligonucleotide sequences (oligo-array), and even smaller single nucleotide polymorphisms (SNP arrays).

Earlier array CGHs contained hundreds to thousands of BAC probes, which were about 1 Mb apart, enabling detection of CNVs greater than 1 Mb in size. Newer technology was based on hundreds of thousands of smaller and denser oligonucleotide probes, providing resolution to 50 to 100 kb, allowing detection of duplications and deletions that may affect only a single gene. The major advantage of SNP arrays over other platforms, and of particular relevance to prenatal diagnosis, is the additional data

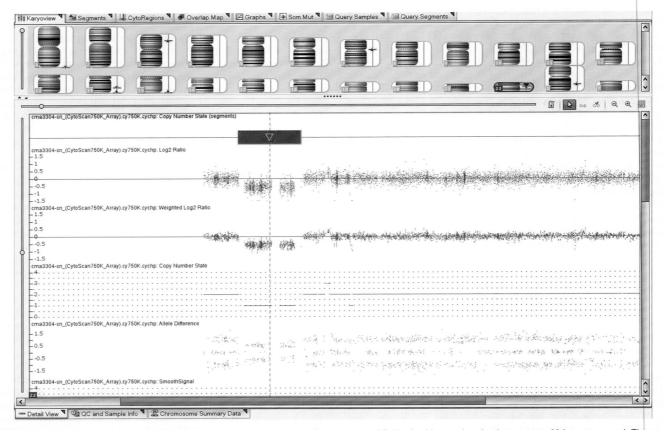

FIGURE 10.7 Microarray in tetralogy of Fallot. CMA analysis in a fetus with tetralogy of Fallot. In this panel, only chromosome 22 is represented. The graphs show a segment of chromosome 22, which falls below the baseline compatible with 2 copies (area below the *red horizontal bar*). This represents a 22q11.2 deletion characteristic of velocardiofacial syndrome/DiGeorge syndrome (VCF/DGS).

gained by the SNP probes: triploidy, diploid–triploid mosaicism, maternal cell contamination, and loss of heterozygosity (LOH). The presence of LOH could be either due to common ancestry of the parents (consanguinity) or due to uniparental isodisomy (122). Therefore, there is increasing use of SNP arrays for chromosomal evaluation in the prenatal setting. Currently there are array designs that incorporate high-quality nonpolymorphic copy number probes along with sufficient SNP probes to identify CNVs as well as LOH and UPD.

Performing such a genome-wide analysis is not flawless. It has long been known that there are significant CNVs in the human genome that have no apparent phenotypic effects (2). Given the large degree of cytogenetically visible polymorphism in the human karyotype, it is not surprising that there would be even more variation within normal individuals at a submicroscopic level. When used as a clinical diagnostic tool, it is not desirable to detect a large number of CNVs that are either benign or represent "variants of uncertain clinical significance" (VUS). For this reason, clinical array designs disperse their probes on those regions of the genome containing single-copy sequence and most known coding sequences and functional genes, attempting to maximize the yield of pathogenic CNVs but minimize the detection of benign CNVs found in the normal population.

Nonetheless, CMA has been fruitful in the elucidation of numerous novel syndromes manifesting as congenital anomalies or altered neurocognitive development, including ASDs (123–125). CMA analysis provides additional clinically relevant information in 1.7% (1:60) of pregnancies with standard indications for prenatal diagnosis (such as advanced maternal age and positive aneuploidy screening result). In cases of an anomaly diagnosed on ultrasonography, additional clinically relevant information from CMA is gained in 6.0% to 6.5% of cases (114,115). The overall incidence of VUSs is 1.1% to 1.5% for all indications (6,126). A meta-analysis of 10,314 fetuses from 8 large studies showed that CNVs associated with early-onset syndromic disorders occurred in 1:270 (0.37%) pregnancies, late-onset diseases were detected in 1:909 (0.11%) pregnancies, and susceptibility CNV was observed in 1:333 (0.3%) cases (127).

Pediatricians have largely abandoned karyotype as the primary cytogenetic in analysis in favor of CMA. Some authorities (including the authors of this chapter) believe that CMA should replace standard cytogenetic analysis in prenatal diagnosis. Obviously, the detection rate is increased, but there is a trade-off. Balanced chromosomal rearrangements (translocations and inversions) are not detected with CMA because there is no gain or loss of genetic material. Thus, de novo, apparently balanced rearrangement identified by standard karyotyping will be missed; these may be associated with some risk of congenital abnormalities (106), such as by interruption of genes at the breakpoints.

Several studies have found that, at a minimum, there is a 0.5% baseline risk for the identification of a significant microdeletion or microduplication, even in women with an uneventful prenatal examination (114,115). By adding the individual risk for pathogenic CNVs to the individual risk for cytogenetically visible chromosome aberrations, Srebniak and colleagues showed that overall a pregnant women has a risk higher than 1:180 for a clinically significant cytogenetic aberration, and that pregnant women younger than 36 years of age have a higher risk for pathogenic CNVs than for DS (127). Variants of uncertain origin (VUS) prenatally can also create challenges in counseling expectant parents. However, with new knowledge and greater sharing of results in public databases, the number of genomic regions definitively associated with disease has increased and the incidence of variants of uncertain significance has decreased over time (128). Ultimately, we believe that the true incidence of finding significant abnormalities on CMA that cannot be detected by traditional karyotype or ultrasound is at least 1%, which is a far higher threshold than the 0.5% seen

with maternal age 35. As such, our practice routinely now offers all patients—regardless of maternal age—a diagnostic test (preferably CVS in the first trimester) with CMA analysis.

Other genetic experts have taken a different stance, highlighting the economic and ethical consequences of universal diagnostic testing along with the societal impact of abandoning the presumption of a normal infant in otherwise uncomplicated pregnancies (129).

Whole Exome Sequencing and Whole Genome Sequencing

Fetal malformations are detected in approximately 3% of all pregnancies. As previously discussed, prenatal CMA analysis has become the first-tier diagnostic test in the evaluation of structural anomalies during pregnancy (130) with an added yield of 3% to 6% over standard cytogenetic analysis. Yet, a substantial proportion of the cases remain undiagnosed because fetal malformations may be the result of many monogenic disorders and genetic syndromes. This is even more likely in the presence of multiorgan involvement. It is of note that even apparently innocuous anomalies are associated with intellectual disability that cannot be ruled solely by imaging. Many of these syndromes are caused by pathogenic sequence variants in developmental genes. These intragenic variants, such as missense, nonsense, or small insertions/deletions (indels) of a few base pairs are not recognizable by CMA that has a resolution of only tens of thousands of base pairs.

To complicate matters even further, only a minority of these genetic conditions present with recognizable fetal phenotypes, enabling targeted gene sequencing (e.g., fetal cardiac rhabdomyomas in tuberous sclerosis). During the last few years, genome-wide sequencing strategies, such as whole-exome sequencing (WES), has greatly increased the detection rate over CMA in cases with neurodevelopmental disorders and malformations to about 25% to 30% (131,132) (Fig. 10.8).

In recent years, prenatal WES has become more frequent in the diagnosis of fetuses with multiple malformations and recurrent fetal phenotypes undetected by standard genetic testing including chromosomal microarrays. Several small studies have investigated the utility of WES in the clinical setting. Best et al. summarized 31 studies of series of 5 or more fetuses. Varying diagnostic rates, between 6.2% and 80%, were demonstrated (6,126,133). The highly variable results are explained by highly different inclusion criteria, with greatest yield in highly selected cases. In our center we have focused on recurrent brain abnormalities (133). In the largest cohort published thus far, including 610 fetuses with structural anomalies and 1,202 matched parental samples, a diagnostic genetic variant was identified in 52 fetuses (8.5%) with highest yield (15.4%) in fetuses with more than one structural anomaly and lowest yield (3.2%) in fetuses with isolated increased NT (126). Petrovski et al. sampled 234 WES trios in fetuses with malformations and their parents. They identified diagnostic genetic variants in 24 (10%) families (134). Both studies include unselected fetuses with structural anomalies and normal CMA results. The diagnostic yield of WES varies according to the anatomic system involved, with highest detection rates in cases of central nervous system anomalies and skeletal and lymphatic malformations and the lowest detection rate among cases with cardiac malformations (134). The highest rate of positive results was in the presence of multiple anomalies (134).

Unique characteristics of the prenatal setting brings new challenges: Firstly, prenatal diagnosis in an ongoing pregnancy requires rapid turnaround time. However, as has been shown in the postnatal setting where WES and WGS have been successfully adopted for very rapid emergency genetic diagnoses on pediatric and neonatal intensive care units (135), turnaround times may no longer be a true limitation for prenatal WES. Secondly, the most efficient process for examining the exome in prenatal diagnosis involves

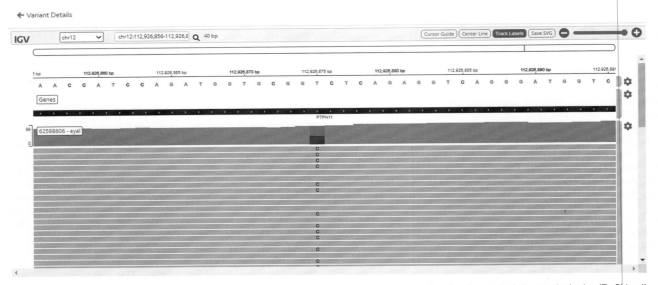

FIGURE 10.8 Whole exome sequencing (WES) results in a fetus with increased nuchal translucency. Results show a single base substitution (T>C) leading to a missense mutation in the PTNP11 gene. Pathogenic variants in PTPN11 are causative of Noonan syndrome in 50% of the cases. Noonan syndrome is characterized by characteristic facies, short stature, congenital heart defect, and developmental delay of variable degree. Increased nuchal translucency can be the presenting sign in the prenatal period.

sequencing the fetus as well as the biologic parents (trio). WES of trios could reveal nonpaternity, consanguinity, and incidental findings in parents that are medically actionable (130). Thirdly, difficulties in fetal phenotyping make prenatal genotype–phenotype correlation more challenging than in the postnatal setting. Developmental delay, hearing loss, and subtle dysmorphic features cannot be determined using fetal ultrasound. This may accidentally cause excluding appropriate candidate genes. Lastly, interpreting variants of uncertain significance is extremely difficult in the prenatal setting, where the phenotype may be incomplete, particularly in the absence of fetal variant database equivalent to postnatal databases.

Genome-wide testing will undoubtedly become more prevalent in the coming years. This will be made available with increasing sequencing power and decreasing cost, as well as improvement in bioinformatics. Furthermore, it is not difficult to envision the use of whole genome sequencing (WGS) as the first-tier approach that will provide sequencing as well as structural variants, eliminating the stepwise approach currently used.

Preimplantation Genetic Testing

PGT was previously known as PGD. PGT is a term used to describe the testing of human embryos in a laboratory for genetic disorders by means of obtaining a cellular biopsy sample from a developing human oocyte or embryo, acquired via a cycle of *in vitro* fertilization (IVF), evaluating the genetic composition of this sample. It uses this information to determine which embryos will be optimal for subsequent uterine transfer (**Fig. 10.9**). There are three types of PGT: PGT for aneuploidies (PGT-A), PGT for monogenic/single gene defects (PGT-M), and PGT for chromosomal structural rearrangements (PGT-SR) (136).

For couples at risk of transmitting a genetic disease or a chromosomal aberration to their offspring, PGT and transfer of unaffected embryos offers an alternative to prenatal diagnosis by CVS or amniocentesis, followed by termination of pregnancy of an affected fetus. Molecular PGT was initially employed for embryo sexing in couples at risk for X-linked diseases. The technique used PCR to amplify Y-chromosome specific sequences, and only female embryos were transferred (137). During the last two decades, the range of genetic abnormalities that can be detected by PGT has

increased exponentially, and the only prerequisite for PGT is that the disease-causing mutation is known. Even if the mutation is not specified, molecular analysis can often be made employing linked polymorphic markers-based haplotype analysis of family members.

Initially, PGT was employed for early-onset severe conditions (such as cystic fibrosis, fragile X, etc.). However, PGT can also be used to prevent late-onset conditions such as in carriers of cancer predisposition genes (e.g., familial adenomatous polyposis [FAP]) and other late-onset conditions. This latter use raises many ethical and practical questions. Moreover, it is possible to perform combined PGT and HLA typing. This may prove beneficial in cases where the parents already have a child affected with a genetic disease amenable to bone marrow transplantation (BMT) (such as thalassemia or Fanconi anemia). Using this approach, double-PGT ensures that subsequent offspring are not only disease free but also suitable bone marrow donors, "saver siblings," for the affected child, again raising significant ethical issues (138).

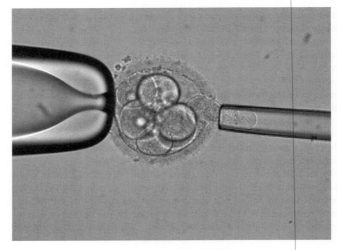

FIGURE 10.9 Embryo biopsy. Embryo held in place by low suction on left while single cell is aspirated into catheter on right.

Because PGT requires the analysis of DNA from single cells, PCR has been the primary method used for the analysis. Technical difficulties due to the minute amount of genetic material and the inherent pitfalls of the PCR, such as amplification failure, allele dropout (ADO), and foreign DNA contamination (e.g., paternal genome) continue to limit the use of PGT. Intracytoplasmic sperm injection (ICSI), using a single sperm that is injected into the oocyte, eliminates the possibility of paternal DNA contamination. Another source of contamination may arise from maternal cumulus cells adherent to the oocytes. Allelic dropout might occur when the initial input quantity of DNA is too low, resulting in the failure to amplify one or more alleles in the sample.

In an embryo carrying an autosomal dominant mutation, ADO might conceal the presence of the disease by amplifying only the unaffected allele, and thus a false-negative result could give rise to a pregnancy with an affected fetus. To analyze the embryo's genetic material, PGT begins with an IVF followed by the growth of the embryo to the 6- to 8-cell stage. At this point, a single cell is removed from the embryo to supply the DNA for the diagnostic test (i.e., embryo biopsy). The removal does not impair further development of the embryo.

PCR, first introduced in the mid-1980s, makes single cell molecular analysis possible. The technique enriches a DNA sample for one specific oligonucleotide fragment, across several orders of magnitude, generating thousands to millions of copies of a PCR product or amplicon. Finally, the precise composition of the amplified fragment (i.e., the amplicon) may be studied by direct sequencing. More advanced molecular methods for PGT may include multiplex PCR (simultaneous amplification of more than one fragment in the same PCR reaction) (138) and even whole genome amplification (WGA). All the PCR techniques amplify the DNA of a single cell to a detectable level. In disorders caused by large-scale deletions such as DMD, the actual PCR amplification reaction is sufficient for making a diagnosis since it is based on the lack of amplification of the corresponding deleted portion of the gene. When a gene mutation is in question, the amplified fragment harboring the mutation is indistinguishable from the normal one using the standard visualization methods such as gel electrophoresis. In such cases, further analysis of the amplified fragment is required for mutation detection.

Array CGH is another potentially important method for aneuploidy diagnosis and screening in the setting of PGT-A, to a greater extent than standard FISH and allowing a larger number of abnormalities to be detected (113–115). Recently, the method of NGS has been introduced into the clinic for aneuploidy screening (139,140). The NGS approach has the advantage of simultaneous assessment of aneuploidy, translocations, single-gene disorders, small copy number variations, and low-level mosaicism. NGS was suggested to be superior over other molecular methods (e.g., aCGH) in detection of mosaicism, which might have a positive impact on the clinical outcomes by decreasing the incidence of miscarriage (140,141). Nonetheless, this may pose a potential risk of overdiagnosing euploid embryos as mosaic, and a high rate of false-positive results (142).

In 1995, the first reports of the "next step" of PGT, the "preimplantation genetic testing for aneuploidy" (PGT-A), started to appear. The objective of PGT-A was to transfer embryos that had been screened for aneuploidies. The underlying rationale for this screening was no longer prevention of a genetic disease, but an expected increase in live birth rates after IVF, because embryos containing aneuploidies were thought not to implant or develop to term and hence to contribute to low live birth rates in specific groups of patients (137,138). The beneficial effect of PGT-A was expected to be greatest in women of advanced maternal age (over 35), women with a history of recurrent miscarriage, women with a history of repeated implantation failure (i.e., several failed IVF cycles), and women with a partner with low sperm quality (severe

male factor), mainly since high percentages of aneuploidies have been found in the embryos of these women. More recently, PGT-A has been offered to younger women (under 35 years of age). Unfortunately, current literature clearly shows no evidence of a beneficial effect of PGT-A as currently conducted on live birth rates after IVF. Trials from multiple independent established groups showed the same negative results, and therefore, it seems justified to conclude that there is no beneficial effect of PGS in terms of increased live birth rates (141,142).

There are currently three sources of cellular material that can be used for PGT: polar bodies from oocytes and zygotes, blastomeres from cleavage-stage embryos (day 3 embryos), and trophectoderm cells from blastocysts. Historically, cleavage-stage (blastomere) biopsy has been the most popular; however, higher abnormality levels, mosaicism, and potential for embryo damage have led to it being superseded by blastocyst (trophectoderm) biopsy, which provides more cells for analysis but generally requires embryo freezing and transfer later than the current cycle (143).

The next question is whether embryo biopsy could have any harmful effects. Prospective follow-up trials have shown that neither birth weight nor major malformation rates were statistically different from those of ICSI children. Perinatal death rates among PGT singleton and ICSI singleton children were also similar, but significantly more perinatal deaths were seen in post-PGT multiple pregnancies compared with ICSI multiple pregnancies (115).

MANAGEMENT OF ABNORMALITIES

Barriers to Access to Care

One cannot treat something until it has been diagnosed. Despite this, there is perhaps no aspect of medicine that engenders more vigorous societal disputes than prenatal diagnosis. Of course, prenatal diagnosis is tightly linked to the entire abortion debate which in the United States, at least, has manifested itself in multiple waves of legal restrictions to patient's rights to have a termination (144). In 2019, more than 400 policies restricting abortion were introduced in the United States (144). There have been multiple court challenges to existing and newly enacted laws from both sides, and the situation is likely to become more intense in the next several years.

Termination

One of the traditional arguments against prenatal diagnosis has been that it is merely a "search and destroy" mission. Many years of experience and data show that, because of the availability of prenatal diagnosis, far more pregnancies have resulted in live births than have been terminated. The following four points summarize our experience (2):

1. Even in the highest risk programs, we are able to give good news to perhaps as many as 95% of patients.
2. When we do find an anomaly, not everyone chooses to terminate. We have published our own data showing about a 50/50 split between those couples with problems choosing to continue versus choosing to terminate (145). Not surprisingly, there has been a direct correlation between the severity of the problem and likelihood of choosing to terminate. Likelihood of choosing to terminate obviously also varies significantly between and within countries (146–148).
3. There are many couples who already have a child with a serious condition—whom they love very much and would not "trade" under any circumstances. They would like another child, but the family unit cannot "afford" (comprehensively including administratively, financially, physically, and emotionally) to have another child with special needs. They request prenatal diagnosis to ensure that the next child does not have the same problem.

4. Congenital abnormalities such as spina bifida can be diagnosed relatively early in pregnancy but by the time of delivery have inflicted considerable phenotypic damage to the baby. In some cases, repairs can be attempted *in utero* that can prevent many of the manifestations of the problem.

When, for whatever reason, patients do make the decision that they do not wish to continue a pregnancy, there are both procedural and legal considerations. Overall, from the perspective of maternal health, termination is considerably safer than having a baby (149,150). It also needs to be recognized that the political and religious controversies will never be completely resolved, and termination and women's rights will always be a source of considerable conflict in our society (150).

The approach varies by gestational age. In the first trimester, the usual method is a suction dilatation and curettage, which has been demonstrated over 50 years to be a very safe and effective procedure. Medical abortion using mifepristone and misoprostol are 95.5% effective through 63 days (8 weeks) of pregnancy (151). This time frame is almost always too early to have had prenatal diagnosis by any method other than PGT or ultrasound showing a severe abnormality (151).

Unfortunately, despite the availability of CVS and first trimester screening, most chromosomal and structural abnormalities are not found until the second trimester (2,22,23,104). When patients choose to terminate, the second trimester choices are either dilatation and extraction (D&E) or prostaglandin induction of labor. Both procedures, when done by experienced physicians, are very safe but not as low risk as first trimester options. Prostaglandin inductions have the advantage of allowing for a complete autopsy in syndromic cases, but they take longer and can be of more emotional distress to patients and their families than D&E procedures for which the patient can have heavy sedation or general anesthesia (152).

All too often, patients do not have screening or diagnosis until "something" is found, often serendipitously, and late in pregnancy. Additionally, fetal abnormalities may not be recognized by providers, or they may be unclear. In many such cases, physicians delay diagnosis in favor of awaiting further development (153). Delays in diagnosis or in decision making about whether to whether to continue or terminate can result in patients approaching or exceeding the legal limit to have a termination in their home locale (154,155). This problem is exacerbated in the United States, as increasingly restrictive legislation limits the legal gestational age

of abortions, increasingly with either very strict definitions of fetal anomaly exceptions or no exceptions at all (156).

There are still a few US centers at which late terminations are legal. These centers have often been the target of picketing and legal and illegal attacks upon them and the providers, and several abortion providers have been assassinated. In 2013, the attorney general of Kansas, who filed hundreds of motions and cases against Dr. George Tiller before his murder in 2009, was ultimately disbarred for repeated abuse of power (156). That has not been the general experience, however.

The experience of several centers has shown that, paradoxically, when the upper gestational age limit of terminations is lowered, the utilization of abortion goes up, and vice versa. With uncertainties in individual cases, patients may have the luxury of waiting a few weeks to see if the problem gets better or worse, whereas if forced to make an immediate decision, they may be more likely to terminate (149).

Fetal Reduction and Selective Termination

Assisted reproductive technologies have helped literally millions of women to have their own children. There have been more than 8 million IVF births since Louise Brown in 1978. A price to pay for that success, however, has been the generation of multiple pregnancies (157). High-profile media stories such as the McCoy septuplets of the 1990s were mostly positive about the miracles of having "that many" and did not focus on the long-term risks of those children having disabilities or dying. A major change occurred in 2009 when the "octomom" story of a woman having octuplets (in addition to the 6 she already had at home) raised considerable public concern (158). Partly as a consequence, the incidence of all multiples has been reduced, with higher orders such as sextuplets returning to levels seen in the late 1980s, but the incidence of twins and triplets is still several multiples above expected rates without IVF (**Fig. 10.10**) (158).

More than 30 years ago, we and others began publishing on the use of FR to reduce the risks of loss and prematurity from multiples mostly resulting from infertility treatments (159). Our experience has been that FR significantly reduces both loss and prematurity (158). Starting with triplets or quadruplets reduced down to twins or a singleton results in pregnancy outcomes similar to starting with the finishing numbers. With quintuplets or more, there are vast improvements in outcomes, but the results do not

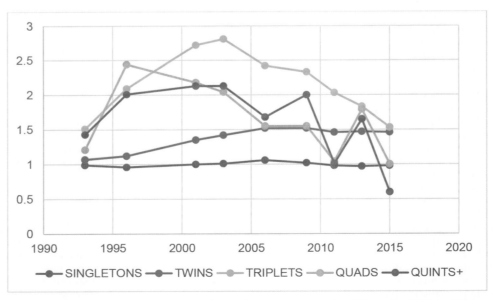

FIGURE 10.10 Incidence of multiples. Births of higher-order multiples (quads+) has in 2015 returned to 1989 baseline (1989 data). Twins and triplets still elevated.

quite reach the point of never having been a high order multiple. Over the years, with better control of infertility therapies, average starting numbers have decreased, and couples are now commonly reducing twins to a singleton (160).

We have found that over the past two decades, performing CVS with FISH analysis for chromosomes 21, 18, and 13 and sex chromosomes improves the chances of healthy children (79). Our data suggest that performing CVS and FR on 2 consecutive days minimizes the chance of mistaking which fetus is which and permits couples to only have to travel to our center once. While FISH cannot diagnose everything the karyotype does, we modeled the residual risk of a problem to be about 1/400 and recently have published our data showing 1/350 (79). We have also seen many couples with risks for mendelian disorders for whom we can do CVS on all fetuses, run the analyses, and prioritize reduction of the affected fetuses.

In recent years, the availability of microarray analysis has created an alternative, that is, waiting for the microarray result before FR. We find that most of our patients who are traveling considerable distances (e.g., by airplane) still choose to have CVS/FR on 2 consecutive days. For patient who are "local," many of them will wait before FR—particularly when reducing to a singleton. For triplets or more, we sometimes use a hybrid approach: reduce down to twins based upon the FISH and then wait for the microarray before reducing to a singleton (79,103,104).

In earlier years, although we determined gender as part of the genetic evaluation, we would not consider it during fetal selection because there appeared to be a tendency in the 1980s to favor males. In the last 20 years, we have found couples of all ethnic backgrounds being interested in gender, and that there now appears to be an equal desirability of both sexes (161). For couples reducing to twins, the most common request is for one of each.

A separate category includes patients with both natural and infertility treatment twin pregnancies, in whom an abnormality is detected in one of the fetuses. We distinguish between FR, which are procedures mostly performed in the first trimester and done for fetal number, and selective terminations (ST), which are mostly second trimester and are done for a diagnosed fetal abnormality. Several individual center and collaborative reports over the last 30 years have shown that the earlier the procedure is performed (but after 11 weeks), the better the perinatal outcome, thus leading us to the conclusion that for all multiples, offering CVS for diagnosis is better than waiting for amniocentesis.

Regardless of when the diagnosis is made, as long as it is legal in the jurisdiction, ST can be performed. In dichorionic twins, intracardiac KCl is the most effective method. Our older data suggested that after 16 weeks, the loss rate of the survivor was increased, but our experience now shows even after 20 weeks, the outcomes of the normal twin are generally improved by reduction of the abnormal twin (162).

The situation is much more complex for the monochorionic twin pair for whom the incidence of structural fetal anomalies is actually considerably higher than for fraternal twins (163). Unfortunate experiences from the 1970s and 1980s showed that if KCl terminations were performed (because the monozygosity was not appreciated), loss rates approached 50% with as much as 75% neurologic impairment in the survivor (164). Even with spontaneous death of one twin, certainly in the late second and third trimester, there is a risk of impairment to the survivor of approximately 12%, which results from bleeding into the placenta as opposing intravascular pressure from the other fetus ceases at death. There is considerable debate as to optimal management of the abnormal twin, varying from performing immediate cesarean section, at term, intrauterine transfusion of the surviving twin, or expectant management. It is usually not possible to determine prospectively the risk of damage to the remaining twin (164).

In the1990s, we developed the concept of umbilical cord ligation to perform ST and minimize the risk to the survivor (165).

Several approaches have been utilized, including umbilical cord ligation, cauterization, radio frequency ablation of the hepatic artery, and embolization. All have survival statistics of approximately 90%, but they also have a 6% to 10% risk of a damaged survivor (166).

Fetal Therapy

In the 1960s, the first attempts at fetal treatment were performed by Liley in New Zealand. He attempted to treat hemolytic anemia, mostly due to RH isoimmunization, by performing intraperitoneal transfusions under x-ray guidance (167). Fetal interventions have been categorized into percutaneous, open fetal surgical, medical, and stem cell groups.

Percutaneous

An exciting potential in the early 1980s was to treat fetal hydrocephalus. The hope was to prevent damage from ongoing CNS compression. The reality was that fetuses with multisystem and syndromic conditions who might have (perhaps mercifully) died, were left alive but impaired (168). Not surprisingly, trisomy 18 fetuses were not going to have a normal neurodevelopmental prognosis merely because their hydrocephalus was reduced. Only after the painful recognition that hydrocephalus was generally a multisystem disorder and that diagnostic capabilities were still limited was the procedure abandoned.

Fetal bladder enlargement, termed lower urinary tract obstruction (LUTO), has been treated by percutaneous bladder shunting since the early 1980s (169). Most often LUTO represents an isolated defect so that, in theory, with resolution of LUTO, every other aspect of development could revert to normal. The general consensus was that there had to be demonstration of adequate renal function at the time of the procedure, because poor to zero renal function in utero has dire multiorgan consequences that neonatal transplants are not likely to overcome. Initially, criteria for intervention included oligohydramnios, but later they were liberalized because, by the time oligohydramnios was significant, considerable irreversible renal parenchymal damage had already been done (169).

As the results of long-term studies have become available, it has been recognized that, despite resolution of AF volume for the remainder of the pregnancy, the incidence of later renal impairments and failure are much higher than hoped. These data have called into question the ability to correct fetal renal function once abnormalities have become recognizable (170).

Another, rarely used, percutaneous therapy has been the treatment of fetal goiter caused by the treatment of maternal hyperthyroidism with medications such as propylthiouracil (PTU) and propranolol, which cross the placenta and cause fetal hyperthyroidism (**Fig. 10.11**). There have not been a sufficient number of treated cases, to date, on which to base a generalizable conclusion regarding the effectiveness of this procedure (171).

Over the past 20 years, the most utilized in utero percutaneous therapy has been laser treatment of monochorionic twin placentas in pregnancies that have developed twin-to-twin transfusion syndrome (TTTS) (172,173). The procedure, first developed in the 1990s, based upon a crude concept of creating separate halves of the placenta, has evolved into discrete lasering of communicating vessels to preserve a more physiologic environment. There is a large literature on the methods to diagnose, classify, and treat these cases, with statistics generated for outcomes based on the severity of the problem. It is now abundantly clear that TTTS is better treated by laser than by amnioreduction (173). Multiple studies have reported widely variable outcomes, in part depending upon the relative severity of the condition (Quintero staging) and the experience of the center (174). See also Chapter 13. Unfortunately, residual neurologic impairment in survivors has been reported to be as high as 10%, and there are no real biomarkers other than prematurity, which merely provides odds adjustments (166,173).

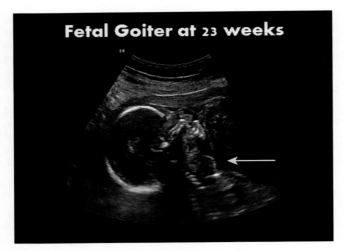

FIGURE 10.11 Fetal goiter. *Yellow arrow* shows fetal goiter. Intra-amniotic thyroxine injections slowed progression of goiter growth.

Open

The classic model is open fetal surgery for congenital diaphragmatic hernia (CDH). Over a decade of work, evolving from animal experimentation to determine the pathophysiology, therapeutics, and surgical techniques led to the first successful case, reported by Harrison et al. in 1989 (175,176). It was originally anticipated that open fetal surgery could increase survival in CDH from the 35% resulting from traditional methods of treatment, including ECMO, to about 70%. However, with standardization and improvement of the treatment of the "control" group with ECMO, at the same tertiary centers that were performing fetal surgery, the differences in survival essentially disappeared, removing the justification for open fetal surgery for CDH (177).

As has been seen in many situations, the development of a technology turns out to have considerable benefit for purposes not considered when originally developed. For example, fetal surgery results in improved survival in severe cases of congenital cystadenomatoid malformations (CCAMs) of the lung, (now called congenital pulmonary airway malformation [CPAM]). Even that approach has receded as now many of the cases can be treated by either shunting or steroid administration. Likewise, sacrococcygeal teratomas can produce high-output cardiac failure, and interruption of the blood supply to the tumor *in utero* has been achieved (178).

The major emphasis for fetal surgery in the past 15 years has been the treatment of meningomyelocele. The several centers combined for the "MOMs" trial demonstrated that, for couples committed to continuing with pregnancies affected by spina bifida, motor function was better in those babies operated on *in utero* than in those that waited for postpartum treatment. Overall, however, neurologic function is less than expected in unaffected children, and there are frequently significant long-term impairments with or without fetal surgery (179,180).

Much, but not all of fetal surgery, has moved from open to laparoscopic approaches that have the advantage of smaller incisions—particularly on the uterus. The shift has reduced the recovery of mothers and the likelihood of preterm labor and rupture of membranes. The disadvantage is a more complex surgical methodology with some limitations on the extensiveness of procedures. Centers tend to be devotees of one approach or the other rather than an even mixture (181,182).

A major side benefit of the enormous efforts extended to develop fetal surgery has been the development of the "EXIT" procedure (*ex utero* intrapartum treatment), which is used when there are concerns about establishing an airway at birth (183). In such cases, an extended cesarean delivery is performed. A tradi-

tional cesarean section is modified by meticulous maintenance of hemostasis at surgery and the use of heavy-dose tocolytic anesthetics to keep the uterus from contracting. It is not unusual for the overall surgical time to be extended by an hour to perform the fetal manipulations. The benefit is, while the fetus/baby is still hooked up to the world's best heart lung machine (the placenta), pediatric surgeons/ENT/or neonatologists can establish the airway and do whatever surgery is required without the problem of maintaining oxygenation after the cord is cut.

Medical

Fetal surgery has been the focus of media attention for 30 years. However, numerically, medical therapies have been far more prevalent and, in the case of NTD prevention, are universal in many countries. With major public health implications around the globe, the single most effective fetal therapy has been supplementation of breads and grains with folic acid. Supplementation has cut the incidence of NTDs by over half (184,185). We have recently shown that the 4-mg increased dose for prevention of recurrences is too high as the body cannot absorb much more than 1 mg/d (186). This conclusion de facto increases the proportion of high-risk patients who are actually being adequately treated for prevention of recurrence.

The classic medical fetal therapy has been the prevention of masculinization of females with 21 hydroxylase deficiency using prenatally administered dexamethasone, beginning in the first trimester. This therapy blocks the conversion of excess 17-hydroxyprogesterone to androstenedione and testosterone (187). Since we first published results of this therapy 35 years ago, hundreds of fetuses have been successfully treated, although some now argue that therapy is not appropriate because it leads to unnecessary treatment in some fetuses that are then exposed to the potential complications of steroid therapy (188,189). Other biochemical alterations have been treated *in utero*, including use of B12 therapy in methylmalonic aciduria and biotin in multiple carboxylase deficiency, but resulting improvement in overall patient outcomes has been difficult to prove (190).

Genetic/Stem Cell

Anatomic abnormalities are most directly treated by surgery. For metabolic abnormalities, the approach can be either to supplement or replace the end product by medical therapy. A more elegant approach is to enable the fetus to have the capability of making its own missing product. Ultimately gene therapy might be feasible, but for the past 20 years a limited number of stem cell transplants have been employed. We achieved the first successful treatment of a fetus diagnosed with X-linked severe combined immunodeficiency disorder (SCID) in the mid 1990s, by obtaining bone marrow from the father, "cleaning" it (mostly T-cell depletion), and then transplanting it intraperitoneally × 3, beginning at 15 weeks (191). In this case, and subsequently others, low to medium levels of engraftment have been demonstrated with amelioration of disease. In general, treatment of immunodeficiencies has had more beneficial results than treatment of other metabolic disorders. It now appears that fetal immunocompetency against grafts is developed much earlier than previously recognized, but the results of a decade's work now suggest that the source of the immune response is maternal rather than fetal (192,193).

▌CONCLUSION

Advances in the understanding of genetic and congenital disorders, major improvement in prenatal diagnostic capabilities both clinically and in the laboratory, and the opportunity to treat a selected number of disorders *in utero* have radically altered the concepts of prenatal care. As a consequence, a much higher proportion of problems is now detected *in utero*, and there are significantly fewer surprises at delivery. Maternal (*in utero*) rather than neonatal patient transport to tertiary/quaternary centers has clearly improved care, combined with an ability to plan for the optimal place and mode of delivery well in advance and for the appropriate care team and equipment to be present at the time of delivery. There has been a dramatic decrease in *in utero* and perinatal mortality, which has sometimes been replaced with increased perinatal morbidity. We can anticipate an ever-increasing overall acuity of illness in the NICU, as fetal therapies effectively treat minor to moderate abnormalities but also save those who previously would have died but now survive but have significant problems.

As with all new technologies, there is a phase of development in which a small number of investigators pioneer a new approach. It is followed by a phase of diffusion during which new centers emerge, numbers increase but complications skyrocket. Fetal therapy is no exception to this rule. Many new centers, typically started by trainees from more established ones, have sprung up. As many of the procedures have transitioned from experimental to highly specialized clinical care, competition for cases has become significant. Fetal therapy programs are seen as high-profile, high-prestige programs with considerable "pull through" business for the medical center.

The International Fetal Medicine and Surgery Society has written guidelines for emerging centers to try to minimize the downside of expansion of capacity with newer providers with less experience (194). History has suggested that it takes about a decade for quaternary procedures to take their place in the routine armamentarium of high-risk care with regional capabilities. There is no reason to believe fetal therapy will be an exception.

REFERENCES

1. Wegman ME. Infant mortality in the 20th century, dramatic but uneven progress. *J Nutr* 2001;131:401s.
2. Evans MI, Johnson MP, Yaron Y, et al., eds. *Prenatal diagnosis: genetics, reproductive risks, testing, and management.* New York, NY: McGraw Hill Publishing Co., 2006.
3. Gastel B, Haddow JE, Fletcher JC, et al., eds. *Maternal Serum alpha-fetoprotein: issues in the prenatal screening and diagnosis of neural tube defects. NCHCT conference proceedings.* Washington, DC: US Gov't Printing Office, 1980.
4. Cohen AH, Hanft RS, eds. *Technology in American Health Care: Policy directions for effective evaluation and management.* Ann Arbor, MI: University of Michigan Press, 2004.
5. Evans MI, Hanft RS. The introduction of new technologies. *ACOG Clin Rev* 1997;2:1.
6. Best S, Wou K, et al. Promises, pitfalls and practicalities of prenatal whole exome sequencing. *Prenat Diagn* 2018;38(1):10.
7. Weizman T, Berger AC. *Generating evidence for genomic diagnostic test development: workshop summary.* Washington, DC: Institute of Medicine, 2011.
8. https://techcrunch.com/2019/06/28/theranos-founder-elizabeth-holmes-to-stand-trial-in-2020/
9. Committee Opinion. *Direct to consumer marketing of genetic testing. Ethics committee.* Washington, DC: American College of Obstetricians and Gynecologists, 2008.
10. Ready K, Hague IS, Srinivasan BS, et al. Knowledge and attitudes regarding expanded genetic carrier screening among women's health care providers. *Fertil Steril* 2012;97:407.
11. National Newborn Screening and Global Resource Center. History and overview of newborn screening. Available from: http://genes-r-us.uthscsa.edu/resources/newborn/overview.htm
12. President's Council on Bioethics. The Changing moral focus of newborn screening: an ethical analysis by the president's council on bioethics. Available from: http://bioethics.georgetown.edu/pcbe/reports/newborn_screening/index.html. Accessed September 20, 2019.
13. Ashkenazi Jewish Carrier Screening. Available from: https://www.webmd.com/a-to-z-guides/ashkenazi-jewish-genetic-panel#1. Accessed August 28, 2019.
14. Haque IS, Lazarin GA, Kang H, et al. Modeled fetal risk of genetic diseases identified by expanded carrier screening. *JAMA* 2016;316:734.
15. National Human Genome Research Institute. Regulation of genetic tests. Available from: http://www.genome.gov/10002335
16. Martin JA, Hamilton BE, Osterman MJK, et al. *Births: final data for 2012. National vital statistics report: 62 #9.* December 2013.
17. Christianson A, Howson CP, Modell B. *Global Report on birth defects.* White Plains, NY: March of Dimes Birth Defects Foundation, 2006.
18. Evans MI, Hallahan TW, Krantz D, et al. Meta-analysis of first trimester Down Syndrome screening studies: free beta hCG significantly outperforms intact hCG in a multi-marker protocol. *Am J Obstet Gynecol* 2007;196:198.
19. Hassan S, Romero R, Vidyadhari D, et al. Vaginal progesterone reduces the rate of pre-term birth in women with a sonographic short cervix: a multicenter, randomized, double-blind, placebo-controlled trial. *Ultrasound Obstet Gynecol* 2011;38:18.
20. Shane Michaels H, Nazareth S, Tambini L. Genetic counseling. In: Evans MI, Johnson MP, Yaron Y, et al., eds. *Prenatal diagnosis: genetics, reproductive risks, testing, and management.* New York, NY: McGraw Hill Publishing Co., 2006:71.
21. Drugan A, Reichler A, Bronshtein M, et al. Abnormal biochemical serum screening versus second trimester ultrasound-detected minor anomalies as predictors of aneuploidy in low-risk patients. *Fetal Diagn Ther* 1996;11(5):301.
22. Drugan A, Johnson MP, Evans MI. Ultrasound screening for fetal chromosome anomalies. *Am J Med Genet* 2000;90:98.
23. Benacerraf BR, Nadel A, Bromley B. Identification of second trimester fetuses with autosomal trisomy by use of a sonographic scoring index. *Radiology* 1994;193:135.
24. Wiwantikit V. Adjusted classification for ultrasound scoring index for antenatal detection of fetal trisomy. *Indian J Hum Genet* 2012;18:226.
25. Evans MI, Cuckle HS. Performance Adjusted Risks (PAR): a method to improve the quality of algorithm performance while allowing all to play. *Prenat Diagn* 2011;31:797.
26. Lau TK, Evans MI. Second trimester sonographic soft markers: what can we learn from the experience of first trimester nuchal translucency screening? *Ultrasound Obstet Gynecol* 2008;32:123.
27. Wright D, Syngelaki A, Bradbury D, et al. First trimester screening for Trisomies 21, 18, and 13 by ultrasound and biochemical testing. *Fetal Diagn Ther* 2014;35:118.
28. Haddow JE, Palomaki GE, Knight GJ, et al. Screening of maternal serum for fetal Down's Syndrome in the first trimester. *N Engl J Med* 1998;338:955.
29. D'Alton ME. Nuchal translucency quality monitoring: the transition from research to clinical care. *Obstet Gynecol* 2010;116:806.
30. Evans MI, Krantz DA, Hallahan TW, et al. Undermeasurement of nuchal translucencies: implications for screening. *Obstet Gynecol* 2010;116:815.
31. Evans MI, Krantz D, Hallahan T, et al. Impact of NT credentialing by FMF, NTQR, or both upon screening distribution and performance. *Ultrasound Obstet Gynecol* 2012;39:181.
32. Souka AP, Von Kaisenberg CS, Hyett JA, et al. Increased nuchal translucency with normal karyotype. *Am J Obstet Gynecol* 2005;192:1005.
33. Wapner RJ, Martin CL, Levy B, et al. Chromosomal microarray versus karyotyping for prenatal diagnosis. *N Engl J Med* 2012;367:2175.
34. Bianchi DW, Simpson JL, Jackson LG, et al. Fetal gender and aneuploidy detection using fetal cells in maternal blood: analysis of NIFTY I data. *Prenat Diagn* 2002;22:609.
35. Lo YM, Corbetta N, Chamberlain PF, et al. Presence of fetal DNA in maternal plasma and serum. *Lancet* 1997;350:485.
36. Lo YMD. Noninvasive prenatal detection of fetal chromosomal aneuploidies by maternal plasma nucleic acid analysis: a review of the current state of the art. *BJOG* 2009;116:152.
37. Ehrich M, Deciu C, Zwiefelhofer T, et al. Noninvasive detection of fetal trisomy 21 by sequencing of DNA in maternal blood: a study in a clinical setting. *Am J Obstet Gynecol* 2011;204:205.e1-11.
38. Sparks AB, Wang ET, Struble CA, et al. Selective analysis of cell free DNA in maternal blood for evaluation of fetal trisomy. *Prenat Diagn* 2012;32:3.
39. Bianchi DW, Wilkins-Haug L. Integration of noninvasive DNA testing for aneuploidy into prenatal care: what has happened since the rubber met the road? *Clin Chem* 2014;60:78.
40. Chitty LS, Bianchi DW. Noninvasive prenatal testing: the paradigm is shifting rapidly. *Prenat Diagn* 2013;33:511.
41. Galen RS, Gambino SR. *Beyond normality: the predictive value and efficacy of medical diagnoses.* Baltimore, MD: John Wiley and Sons, 1975.
42. Krantz DA, Hallahan TW, Carmichael JB, et al. Utilization of a 1/1000 cutoff in combined screening for Down Syndrome in younger women AMA patients provides cost advantages compared with NIPS. *Am J Obstet Gynecol* 2014;210:S111.
43. Evans MI, Evans SM, Bennett TA, et al. The price of abandoning diagnostic testing for cell free fetal DNA Screening. *Prenat Diagn* 2018;38:243.
44. Evans MI, Andriole S, Curtis J, et al. The epidemic of abnormal copy number variant cases missed because of reliance upon noninvasive prenatal screening. *Prenat Diagn* 2018;38(10):730.
45. Steel MW, Breg WR. Chromosome analysis of human amniotic fluid cells. *Lancet* 1966;1:383.

46. Jacobson JB, Barter RH. Intrauterine diagnosis and management of genetic defects. *Am J Obstet Gynecol* 1967;99:795.
47. National Institute of Child Health and Human Development Amniocentesis Registry. *The safety and accuracy of midtrimester amniocentesis. DHEW publication no (NIH) 788dtr.* Washington, DC: United States Department of Health, Education and Welfare, 1978.
48. Fletcher JC, Evans MI. Maternal bonding in early fetal ultrasound examinations. *N Engl J Med* 1983;308:392.
49. Evans MI, Drugan A, Koppitch FC, et al. Genetic diagnosis in the first trimester: the norm for the 90s. *Am J Obstet Gynecol* 1989;160:1332–1336.
50. Rhoads GG, Jackson LG, Schlesselman SE, et al. The safety and efficacy of chorionic villus sampling for early prenatal diagnosis of cytogenetic abnormalities. *N Engl J Med* 1989;320:609.
51. Mujezinovic F, Alfirevic Z. Procedure related complications of amniocentesis and chorionic villus sampling: a systematic review. *Obstet Gynecol* 2007;110:687.
52. Wulff CB, Gerds TA, Rode L, et al. Risk of fetal loss associated with invasive testing following combined first trimester screening for Down Syndrome: a national cohort of 147,987 singleton pregnancies. *Ultrasound Obstet Gynecol* 2016;47:48.
53. Akolekar R, Beta J, Picciarelli G, et al. Procedure-related risk of miscarriage following amniocentesis and chorionic villus sampling: a systematic review and meta-analysis. *Ultrasound Obstet Gynecol* 2015;45:16.
54. Firth HV, Boyd PA, Chamberlain P, et al. Severe limb abnormalities after chorionic villus sampling at 56–66 days' gestation. *Lancet* 1991;337:762.
55. Hanson FW, Happ RL, Tennant FR, et al. Ultrasonography-guided early amniocentesis in singleton pregnancies. *Am J Obstet Gynecol* 1990;162:1376.
56. Wilson RD. Early amniocentesis: a clinical review. *Prenat Diagn* 1995;15:1259.
57. NHS fetal Anomaly Screening Program. Available from: www.fetalanomaly.screening.nhs.uk. Accessed August 28, 2019.
58. Cohn GM, Gould M, Miller RC, et al. The importance of genetic counseling before amniocentesis. *J Perinatol* 1996;16:352.
59. Evans MI, Hume RF, Johnson MP, et al. Integration of genetics and ultrasonography in prenatal diagnosis: just looking is not enough. *Am J Obstet Gynecol* 1996;174:1925.
60. Benaceraff BR, Frigoletto FD. Amniocentesis under continuous ultrasound guidance: a series of 232 cases. *Obstet Gynecol* 1983;62:760.
61. Drugan A, Evans MI. Amniocentesis. In: Evans MI, Johnson MP, Yaron Y, et al., eds. *Prenatal diagnosis: genetics, reproductive risks, testing, and management.* New York, NY: McGraw Hill Publishing Co., 2006:415.
62. Cuckle HS. Epidemiology of aneuploidy. In: Evans MI, Johnson MP, Yaron Y, et al., eds. *Prenatal diagnosis: genetics, reproductive risks, testing, and management.* New York, NY: McGraw Hill Publishing Co., 2006.
63. Yukobowich E, Anteby EY, Cohen SM, et al. Risk of fetal loss in twin pregnancies undergoing second trimester amniocentesis. *Obstet Gynecol* 2001;98:876.
64. Van der Pol JS, Wolf H, Boer K, et al. Jejunal atresia related to the use of methylene blue in genetic amniocentesis in twins. *Br J Obstet Gynaecol* 1992;99:141.
65. Drugan A, Sokol RJ, Syner FN, et al. Clinical implications of amniotic fluid AFP in twin pregnancies. *J Reprod Med* 1989;34:977.
66. Firth HV, Boyd PA, Chamberlain PF, et al. Analysis of limb reduction defects in babies exposed to chorionic villus sampling. *Lancet* 1994;343(8905):1069.
67. Elejalde BR, deElejalde MM, Acuna JA, et al. Prospective study of amniocentesis performed between weeks 9 and 16 of gestation: its feasibility, risks, complications and use in early genetic prenatal diagnosis. *Am J Med Genet* 1964;35:188.
68. Hanson FW, Tennant F, Hune S, et al. Early amniocentesis: outcome, risks and technical problems at less than 12.8 weeks. *Am J Obstet Gynecol* 1992;166:1707.
69. Johnson JM, Wilson RD, Winsor EJ, et al. The early amniocentesis study: a randomized clinical trial of early amniocentesis versus midtrimester amniocentesis. *Fetal Diagn Ther* 1996;11:85.
70. Tabor A, Phillip J, Masden M, et al. Randomized controlled trial of genetic amniocentesis in 4606 low risk women. *Lancet* 1986;1:1287.
71. Odibo AO, Gray DL, Dicke JM, et al. Revisiting the fetal loss rate after second trimester genetic amniocentesis: a single center's 16 year experience. *Obstet Gynecol* 2008;111:589.
72. Blessed WB, Lacoste H, Welch RA. Obstetrician-gynecologists performing genetic amniocentesis may be misleading themselves and their patients. *Am J Obstet Gynecol* 2001;184:1340.
73. Royal College of Obstetricians and Gynaecologists (RCOG). *Amniocentesis and Chorionic Villus Sampling. Green Top Guideline No.8.* London, England: RCOG Press, 2010.
74. Wilson RD, Langlois S, Johnson JA; SOGC Genetics Committee; CCMG Prenatal Diagnosis Committee. Mid-trimester amniocentesis fetal loss rate. *J Obstet Gynaecol Can* 2007;29:586.
75. Eddleman KA, Malone FD, Sullivan L, et al. Pregnancy loss rates after midtrimester amniocentesis. *Obstet Gynecol* 2006;108:1067.
76. Wapner RJ, Evans MI, Platt LD. Pregnancy loss rates after amniocentesis. *Obstet Gynecol* 2007;109:780.
77. Nicolaides KH. Pregnancy loss rates after amniocentesis. *Obstet Gynecol* 2007;109:781.
78. Squier M, Chamberlain P, Zaiwalla Z, et al. Five cases of brain injury following amniocentesis in mid-term pregnancy. *Dev Med Child Neurol* 2000;42(8):554.
79. Rosner M, Pergament E, Andriole S, et al. Detection of genetic abnormalities using CVS and FISH prior to fetal reduction in sonographically normal appearing fetuses. *Prenat Diagn* 2013;33:940.
80. Evans MI, Rozner N, Yaron Y, et al., eds. *Prenatal diagnosis: genetics, reproductive risks, testing, and management.* New York, NY: McGraw Hill Publishing Co., 2006:433.
81. Rudnicki M, Vejerslev LO, Junge J. The vanishing twin: morphologic and cytogenetic evaluation of an ultrasonographic phenomenon. *Gynecol Obstet Invest* 1991;31:141.
82. Johnson MP, Drugan A, Koppitch FC, et al. Postmortem CVS is a better method for cytogenetic evaluation of early fetal loss than culture of abortus material. *Am J Obstet Gynecol* 1990;163:1505.
83. Drugan A, Johnson MP, Isada NB, et al. The smaller than expected first trimester fetus is at increased risk for chromosome anomalies. *Am J Obstet Gynecol* 1992;167:1525.
84. Silverman NS, Sullivan MW, Jungkind DL, et al. Incidence of bacteremia associated with chorionic villus sampling. *Obstet Gynecol* 1994;84(6):1021.
85. Rhoads GG, Jackson LG, Schlesselman SE, et al. The safety and efficacy of chorionic villus sampling for early prenatal diagnosis of cytogenetic abnormalities. *N Engl J Med* 1989;320:609.
86. Ledbetter DH, Martin AO, Verlinsky Y, et al. Cytogenetic results of chorionic villus sampling: high success rate and diagnostic accuracy in the United States collaborative study. *Am J Obstet Gynecol* 1990;162:495.
87. Brun JL, Mangione R, Gangbo F, et al. Feasibility, accuracy and safety of chorionic villus sampling: a report of 10741 cases. *Prenat Diagn* 2003;23(4):295.
88. Ledbetter DH, Zachary JL, Simpson MS, et al. Cytogenetic results from the US collaborative study on CVS. *Prenat Diagn* 1992;12(5):317.
89. Grati FR. Chromosomal mosaicism in human feto-placental development: implications for prenatal diagnosis. *J Clin Med* 2014;3:809.
90. Ledbetter DH, Zachary JM, Simpson JL, et al. Cytogenetic results from the U.S. collaborative study on CVS. *Prenat Diagn* 1992;12:317.
91. Kotzot D. Abnormal phenotypes in uniparental disomy (UPD): fundamental aspects and a critical review with bibliography of UPD other than 15. *Am J Med Genet* 1999;265.
92. Evans MI, Greb A, Kazazian Jr HH, et al. In utero fetal muscle biopsy for the diagnosis of Duchenne muscular dystrophy. *Am J Obstet Gynecol* 1991;165:728.
93. Evans MI, Krivchenia EL, Johnson MP, et al. *In utero* fetal muscle biopsy alters diagnosis and carrier risks in Duchenne and Becker muscular dystrophy. *Fetal Diagn Ther* 1995;10(2):71.
94. Holzgreve W, Golbus MS. Prenatal diagnosis of ornithine transcarbamylase deficiency utilizing fetal liver biopsy. *Am J Hum Genet* 1984;36:320.
95. Evans MI, Holzgreve W, Krivchenia, et al. Tissue biopsies. In: Evans MI, Johnson MP, Yaron Y, et al., eds. *Prenatal diagnosis: genetics, reproductive risks, testing, and management.* New York, NY: McGraw Hill Publishing Co., 2006:449.
96. Hsu LYF, Kaffe S, Perlis TE. A revisit of trisomy 20 mosaicism—an overview of 103 cases. *Prenat Diagn* 1991;11:7.
97. Freda VJ, Adamson KJ. Exchange transfusion in utero. *Am J Obstet Gynecol* 1964;89:817.
98. Daffos F, Cappella-Pavlovsky M, Forestier F. Fetal blood sampling via the umbilical cord using a needle guided by ultrasound: report of 66 cases. *Prenat Diagn* 1983;3:271.
99. Nicolaides KH, Soothill PW, Rodeck CH, et al. Ultrasound guided sampling of umbilical cord and placental blood to access fetal well being. *Lancet* 1986;1:1065.
100. Berkowitz RL, Bussel JB, McFarland JG. Alloimmune thrombocytopenia: state of the art 2006. *Am J Obstet Gynecol* 2006;195:907.
101. Harman CR, Bowman JM, Manning FA, et al. Intrauterine transfusion: intraperitoneal versus intravascular approach: a case control comparison. *Am J Obstet Gynecol* 1990;162:1053.
102. Gilbert R, Petersen E. *Toxoplasmosis and pregnancy.* 2018. Available from: https://www.uptodate.com/contents/toxoplasmosis-and-pregnancy. Accessed October 1, 2019.
103. Evans MI, Anriole S, Curtis J, et al. The epidemic of abnormal copy number variants missed because of reliance upon noninvasive prenatal screening. *Prenat Diagn* 2018;38:730.
104. Evans MI, Wapner RJ, Berkowitz RL. Non invasive prenatal screening or advanced diagnostic testing: caveat emptor. *Am J Obstet Gynecol* 2016;215:298.

105. Evans MI, Vermeesh JR. Current controversies in prenatal diagnosis 3: industry drives innovation in research and clinical application of genetic prenatal diagnosis and screening. *Prenat Diagn* 2016;36:1172.
106. Williams J, Rad S, Beauchamp S, et al. Utilization of noninvasive prenatal testing: impact upon referrals for diagnostic testing. *Am J Obstet Gynecol* 2015;213:102.e1-6.
107. Best S, Wou K, Vora N, et al. Promises, pitfalls and practicalities of prenatal whole exome sequencing. *Prenat Diagn* 2018;38:10.
108. Gregg AR, Skotko BG, Benkendorf JL, et al. Noninvasive prenatal screening for fetal aneuploidy, 2016 update: a position statement of the American College of Medical Genetics and Genomics. *Genet Med* 2016;18:1056.
109. Angelis A, Tordrup D, Kanavos P. Socio-economic burden of rare diseases: a systematic review of cost of illness evidence. *Health Policy* 2015;119:964.
110. http://www.iihs.org/iihs/topics/t/general-statistics/fatalityfacts/state-by-state-overview. October 1, 2019.
111. http://time.com/5011599/gun-deaths-rate-america-cdc-data/. October 1, 2019.
112. https://www.cdc.gov/hiv/statistics/overview/ataglance.html. October 1, 2019.
113. Coulter ME, Miller DT, Harris DJ, et al. Chromosomal microarray testing influences medical management. *Genet Med* 2011;13:770.
114. Wapner RJ, Martin CL, Levy B, et al. Chromosomal Microarray versus karyotyping for prenatal diagnosis. *N Engl J Med* 2012;367:2175.
115. Shaffer LM, Dabell MP, Fisher AJ, et al. Experience with microarray-based comparative genomic hybridization for prenatal diagnosis in over 5000 pregnancies. *Prenat Diagn* 2012;32:976.
116. Henry GP, Britt DW, Evans MI. Screening advances and diagnostic choice: the problem of residual risk. *Fetal Diagn Ther* 2008;23:308.
117. Rosenfeld JA, Patel A. Chromosomal microarrays: understanding genetics of neurodevelopmental disorders and congenital anomalies. *J Pediatr Genet* 2017;6:42.
118. van Ommen GJ, Breuning MH, Raap AK. FISH in genome research and molecular diagnostics. *Curr Opin Genet Dev* 1995;5(3):304.
119. Trask BJ. Fluorescence in situ hybridization: applications in cytogenetics and gene mapping. *Trends Genet* 1991;7(5):149.
120. Pinkel D, Straume T, Grey JW. Cytogenetic analysis using quantitative, high-sensitivity, fluorescence hybridization. *Proc Natl Acad Sci U S A* 1986;83:2934.
121. Sullivan BA, Leana-Cox J, Schwartz S. Clarification of subtle reciprocal rearrangements using fluorescent *in situ* hybridization. *Am J Med Genet* 1993;47:223.
122. Karampetsou M, Morrogh D, Chitty L. Microarray technology for the diagnosis of fetal chromosome aberrations: which platform should we use? *J Clin Med* 2014;20:663.
123. Miller DT, Adam MP, Aradhya S, et al. Consensus statement: chromosomal microarray is a first-tier clinical diagnostic test for individuals with developmental disabilities or congenital anomalies. *Am J Hum Genet* 2010;86:749.
124. Sagoo GS, Butterworth AS, Sanderson S, et al. Array CGH in patients with learning disability (mental retardation) and congenital anomalies: updated systematic review and meta-analysis of 19 studies and 13,926 subjects. *Genet Med* 2009;11(3):139.
125. Manning M, Hudgins L. Array-based technology and recommendations for utilization in medical genetics practice for detection of chromosomal abnormalities. *Genet Med* 2010;12(11):742.
126. Lord J, McMullan DJ, et al. Prenatal exome sequencing analysis in fetal structural anomalies detected by ultrasonography (PAGE): a cohort study. *Lancet* 2019;393(10173):747.
127. Srebniak MI, Joosten M, Knapen MFCM, et al. Frequency of submicroscopic chromosomal aberrations in pregnancies without increased risk for structural chromosomal aberrations: systematic review and meta-analysis. *Ultrasound Obstet Gynecol* 2018;51:445.
128. Levy B, Wapner RJ. Prenatal diagnosis by chromosomal microarray analysis. *Fertil Steril* 2018;109:201.
129. Hui, L, Norton M. What is the real "price" of more prenatal screening and fewer diagnostic procedures? Costs and trade-offs in the genomic era. *Prenat Diagn* 2018;38:246.
130. Committee opinion No. 682: microarray and next-generation sequencing technology: the use of advanced genetic diagnostic tools in obstetrics and gynecology. Committee on Genetics. *Obstet Gynecol* 2016;128:e262.
131. Yang Y, Muzny DM, Reid JG, et al. Clinical whole-exome sequencing for the diagnosis of Mendelian disorders. *N Engl J Med* 2013;369:1502.
132. Deciphering Developmental Disorders Study. Large-scale discovery of novel genetic causes of developmental disorders. *Nature* 2015;519:223.
133. Reches A, Hiersch L, et al. Whole-exome sequencing in fetuses with central nervous system abnormalities. *J Perinatol* 2018;38(10):1301.
134. Petrovski S, Aggarwal V, et al. Whole-exome sequencing in the evaluation of fetal structural anomalies: a prospective cohort study. *Lancet* 2019;393:758.
135. Willig LK, Petrikin JE, Smith LD, et al. Whole-genome sequencing for identification of Mendelian disorders in critically ill infants: a retrospective analysis of diagnostic and clinical findings. *Lancet Respir Med* 2015;3:377.
136. Zegers-Hochschild F, Adamson GD, et al. The International Glossary on Infertility and Fertility Care, 2017. *Hum Reprod* 2017;32:1786.
137. Handyside AH, Robinson MD, Simpson RJ, et al. Isothermal whole genome amplification from single and small numbers of cells: a new era for preimplantation genetic diagnosis of inherited disease. *Mol Hum Reprod* 2004;10:767.
138. Eggerding FA. A one-step coupled amplification and oligonucleotide ligation procedure for multiplex genetic typing. *PCR Methods Appl* 1995;4, 337.
139. Zheng H, Jin H, Liu L, et al. Application of next-generation sequencing for 24 chromosome aneuploidy screening of human preimplantation embryos. *Mol Cytogenet* 2015;8:38. doi: 10.1186/s13039-015-0143-6
140. Maxwell SM, Colls P, Hodes-Wertz B, et al. Why do euploid embryos miscarry? A case control study comparing the rate of aneuploidy within presumed euploid embryos that resulted in miscarriage or live birth using next-generation sequencing. *Fertil Steril* 2016;106:1414.
141. Lai HH, Chuang TH, Wong LK, et al. Identification of mosaic and segmental aneuploidies by next-generation sequencing in preimplantation genetic screening can improve clinical outcomes compared to array-comparative genomic hybridization. *Mol Cytogenet* 2017;10:14. doi: 10.1186/s13039-017-0315-7
142. Gleisher N, Vidali A, Braverman J, et al. Accuracy of preimplantation genetic screening (PGS) is compromised by degree of mosaicism of human embryos. *Reprod Biol Endocrinol* 2016;14:54. doi: 10.1186/s12958-016-0193-6
143. Griffin DK, Ogur C. Chromosomal analysis in IVF: just how useful is it? *Reproduction* 2018;156:F29. doi: 10.1530/REP-17-0683
144. Nash E. *Unprecedented wave of abortion bans is an urgent call for action.* Guttmacher Institute, 2019.
145. Pryde PG, Odgers AE, Isada NB, et al. Determinants of parental decision to abort (DTA) or continue for non-aneuploid ultrasound detected abnormalities. *Obstet Gynecol* 1992;80:52.
146. Natoli JL, Ackerman DL, McDermott S, et al. Prenatal diagnosis of Down Syndrome: a systematic review of termination rates (1995-2011). *Prenat Diagn* 2012;32:142.
147. Deng C, Yi L, Mu Y, et al. Recent trends in the birth prevalence of Down Syndrome in China: impact of prenatal diagnosis and subsequent terminations. *Prenat Diagn* 2015;35:311.
148. *Abortion Statistics, England and Wales 2018.* UK Dept of Health and Social Care, 2019. Available from: https://assets.publishing.service.gov.uk/government/uploads/system/uploads/attachment_data/file/808556/Abortion_Statistics__England_and_Wales_2018__1_.pdf
149. *Abortion resources.* Guttmacher Institute, January 2014. Available from: http://www.guttmacher.org/sections/abortion.php
150. Raymond ED, Grimes DA. The comparative safety of legal induced abortion and childbirth in the United States. *Obstet Gynecol* 2012;119:215.
151. Gatter M, Cleland K, Nucatola DL. Efficacy and safety of medical abortion using mifepristone and buccal misoprostol through 63 days. *Contraception* 2015;91:269.
152. Chasen ST, Kalish RB, Gupta M, et al. Dilatation and evacuation at >or =20 weeks: comparison of operative techniques. *Am J Obstet Gynecol* 2004;190:1180.
153. Dommergues M, Benachi A, Benifla J, et al. The reasons for termination of pregnancy in the third trimester. *Br J Obstet Gynaecol* 1999;106:297.
154. Cartwright AF, Karunaratne M, Barr-Walker J, et al. Identifying national availability of abortion care and distance from major US cities: systematic online search. *J Med Internet Res* 2018;20:e156.
155. Hern WM. Fetal diagnostic indications for second and third trimester outpatient pregnancy termination. *Prenat Diagn* 2014;34:438.
156. *Phil Kline is indefinitely suspended from practicing law.* Kansas City Star. October 18, 2013. Available from: http://www.kansascity.com/2013/10/18/4560734/kline-indefinitely-suspended-from.html
157. *An overview of abortion laws.* Guttmacher Institute. October 1, 2019. Available from: https://www.guttmacher.org/state-policy/explore/overview-abortion-laws
158. Evans MI, Andriole SA, Britt DW. Fetal reduction—25 years' experience. *Fetal Diagn Ther* 2014;35:69.
159. Evans MI, Dommergues M, Wapner RJ, et al. Efficacy of transabdominal multifetal pregnancy reduction: collaborative experience among the world's largest centers. *Obstet Gynecol* 1993;82:61.
160. Evans MI, Kaufman M, Urban AJ, et al. Fetal reduction from twins to a singleton: a reasonable consideration. *Obstet Gynecol* 2004;104:232.
161. Evans MI, Rosner M, Andriole S, et al. Evolution of gender preferences in multiple pregnancies. *Prenat Diagn* 2013;33:935.

THE FETAL PATIENT

162. Evans MI, Goldberg J, Horenstein J, et al. Selective termination (ST) for structural (STR), chromosomal (CHR), and Mendelian (MEN) anomalies: international experience. *Am J Obstet Gynecol* 1999;181(4):893.

163. Hack KE, Derks JB, Elias SG, et al. Increased perinatal mortality and morbidity in monochorionic versus dichorionic twin pregnancies: clinical implications of a large Dutch cohort study. *BJOG* 2008;115:58.

164. Evans MI, Lau TK. Making decisions when no good options exist: delivery of the survivor after intrauterine death of the co-twin in monochorionic twin pregnancies. *Fetal Diagn Ther* 2010;28:191.

165. Quintero RA, Reich H, Puder KS, et al. Brief report: umbilical cord ligation of an acardiac twin by fetoscopy at 19 weeks of gestation. *N Engl J Med* 1994;330:469.

166. Gebb J, Rosner M, Dar P, et al. Long term neurologic outcomes after fetal interventions: meta-analysis. *Am J Obstet Gynecol* 2014;210:S115.

167. Liley AW. Intrauterine transfusion of foetus in haemolytic disease. *Br Med J* 1963;2 1107.

168. Manning FA, Harrison MR, Rodeck C. Catheter shunts for fetal hydronephrosis and hydrocephalus. Report of the international fetal surgery registry. *N Engl J Med* 1986;315:336.

169. Evans MI, Sacks AL, Johnson MP, et al. Sequential invasive assessment of fetal renal function, and the in utero treatment of fetal obstructive uropathies. *Obstet Gynecol* 1991;77:545.

170. Wu S, Johnson MP. Fetal lower urinary tract obstruction. *Clin Perinatol* 2009;36:377.

171. Munoz J, Kessler AA, Felig P, et al. Sequential amniotic fluid thyroid hormone changes correlate with goiter shrinkage following in utero thyroxine therapy. *Fetal Diagn Ther* 2016;39:222.

172. Senat MV, Deprest J, Boulvain M, et al. Endoscopic laser surgery versus serial amnioreduction for severe twin to twin transfusion syndrome. *N Engl J Med* 2004;351:136.

173. Papanna R. *Twin-twin transfusion syndrome: management and outcome.* Up to date.com. Available from: https://www.uptodate.com/contents/twin-twin-transfusion-syndrome-management-and-outcome/print

174. Quintero RA, Morales WJ, Allen MH, et al. Staging of twin-twin transfusion syndrome. *J Perinatol* 1999;19:550.

175. Harrison MR, Longaker MT, Adzick NS, et al. Successful repair in utero of a fetal diaphragmatic hernia after removal of herniated viscera from the left thorax. *N Engl J Med* 1990;322:1582.

176. Harrison MR, Evans MI, Adzick NS, et al., eds. *The unborn patient: the art and science of fetal therapy*, 3rd ed. Philadelphia, PA: W.B. Saunders Publishing Company, 2001.

177. Hedrick HL. Management of prenatally diagnosed congenital diaphragmatic hernia. *Semin Pediatr Surg* 2013;22:37.

178. Egloff A, Bulas DI. Prenatal diagnosis and management of congenital pulmonary airway malformation. Available from: https://www.uptodate.com/contents/prenatal-diagnosis-and-management-of-congenital-pulmonary-airway-malformation

179. Bruner JP, Tulipan N, Paschall RL, et al. Intrauterine repair of myelomeningocele, "hindbrain restoration" and the incidence of shunt-dependent hydrocephalus. *JAMA* 1999;282:1826.

180. Adzick NS, Thom EA, Spong CV, et al. A randomized trial of prenatal versus postnatal repair of myelomeningocele. *N Engl J Med* 2011;364:993.

181. Joyeux L, Engels AC, Russo FM, et al. Fetoscopic versus open repair for spina bifida aperta: a systematic review of outcomes. *Fetal Diagn Ther* 2016;39:161.

182. Committee on Obstetric Practice, Society for Maternal–Fetal Medicine. Committee Opinion No. 720: Maternal-Fetal Surgery for Myelomeningocele. *Obstet Gynecol* 2017;130:e164.

183. Moldenhauer JS. Ex utero intrapartum therapy. *Semin Pediatr Surg* 2013;22:44.

184. Czeizel AE, Dudas I. Prevention of the first occurrence of neural-tube defects by periconceptional vitamin supplementation. *N Engl J Med* 1992;327:1832.

185. Evans MI, Llurba E, Landsberger EJ, et al. Impact of folic acid supplementation in the United States: markedly diminished high maternal serum AFPs. *Obstet Gynecol* 2004;103:474.

186. Dolin CD, Deierlein AL, Evans MI. Folic acid supplementation to prevent recurrent neural tube defects: 4 mg is too much. *Fetal Diagn Ther* 2018;44:161.

187. Evans MI, Chrousos GP, Mann DL, et al. Pharmacologic suppression of the fetal adrenal gland in utero: attempted prevention of abnormal external genital masculinization in suspected congenital adrenal hyperplasia. *JAMA* 1985;253:1015.

188. New M, Abraham M, Yuen T, et al. An update on prenatal diagnosis and treatment of congenital adrenal hyperplasia. *Semin Reprod Med* 2012;30:396.

189. Heland S. Preventing female virilisation in congenital adrenal hyperplasia: The controversial role of antenatal dexamethasone. *Aust N Z J Obstet Gynaecol* 2016;56:225.

190. Evans MI, Duquette DA, Rinaldo P, et al. Modulation of B12 dosage and response in fetal treatment of methylmalonic aciduria (MMA); Titration of treatment dose to serum and urine MMA. *Fetal Diagn Ther* 1997;12:21.

191. Flake AW, Puck JM, Almieda-Porada G, et al. Successful in utero correction of X-linked recessive severe combined immuno-deficiency (X-SCID): fetal intraperitoneal transplantation of CD34 enriched paternal bone marrow cells (EPPBMC). *N Engl J Med* 1996;335:871.

192. Pearson EG, Flake AW. Stem cell and genetic therapies for the fetus. *Semin Pediatr Surg* 2013;22:56.

193. Riley JS, McClain LE, Stratigis JD, et al. Pre-existing maternal antibodies cause rapid prenatal rejection of allotransplants in mouse model of in utero hematopoietic cell transplantation. *J Immunol* 2018;201:1549.

194. Moon-Grady AJ, Baschat A, Cass D, et al. Fetal Treatment 2017: the evolution of fetal therapy centers—a joint opinion from the International Fetal Medicine and Surgical Society (IFMSS) and the North American Fetal Therapy Network (NAFNet). *Fetal Diagn Ther* 2017;42:241.

11 Multiple Gestation

Scott W. White

INTRODUCTION

Multiple pregnancy occurs in 1% to 2% of pregnancies and has increased in incidence in line with the median age of pregnant mothers and the rate of assisted reproductive technologies (ARTs) (1). The bulk of multiple pregnancies are twins, with higher order multiples making up only 2% of multiple pregnancies (2). Although multiple pregnancies are relatively uncommon, they disproportionately contribute to maternal and perinatal morbidity as well as long-term disability in children, with most of the offspring morbidity related to preterm birth and to complications of monochorionic placentation. Recent advances in ultrasound surveillance of monochorionic pregnancies and treatment of their complications, together with advances in neonatal intensive care of preterm infants, have reduced the morbidity in offspring of multiple pregnancies.

PHYSIOLOGY

Twins may arise from a single embryo (monozygotic) or two separate embryos (dizygotic), with the latter making up two-thirds of spontaneously conceived twins. Dizygotic twins are always dichorionic and diamniotic whereas the chorionicity and amnionicity of monozygotic twins are determined by the gestation at which the single zygote cleaves. Early cleavage prior to day 3, as occurs in one-third of cases, will result in dichorionic diamniotic twins (Fig. 11.1). Most common, in two-thirds of cases, is cleavage between day 3 and 8, where a shared placenta is formed (monochorionic) but each twin remains in its own amniotic sac (diamniotic). More rarely, late cleavage results in monochorionic monoamniotic twins (days 8 to 13) or conjoined twins (beyond day 13).

Chorionicity and amnionicity are the most important determinants of perinatal outcomes in multiple pregnancies. Monochorionic placentae universally contain vascular anastomoses between twins allowing the sharing of blood across the placenta from each twin to the other. This has implications for the unique complications of monochorionicity including twin–twin transfusion syndrome (TTTS) and twin anemia–polycythemia sequence (TAPS), among others. Because of these unique complications obstetric management varies significantly between monochorionic and dichorionic pregnancies, and the accurate ascertainment of chorionicity early in pregnancy is vital. It is also of relevance to prenatal diagnosis of aneuploidy and other genetic conditions, influencing screening test performance characteristics as well as the methods of prenatal diagnostic testing.

Chorionicity and amnionicity can be reliably determined by first trimester ultrasound. Monochorionic diamniotic twins have a single placenta into which the thin intertwin membrane inserts to form a "T sign" with no placental tissue extending into the membrane attachment. Monochorionic monoamniotic twins have a single placenta with no dividing membrane between the twins and in almost all cases have identifiable entanglement of the umbilical cords of the two fetuses. Dichorionic twins may have obviously separate placentae or fused placentae with a thicker intertwin membrane with placental tissue extending between the leaves of the membrane as it inserts into the placental surface to form a "lambda" or "twin peak sign." Beyond the first trimester, ultrasound determination of chorionicity can be more difficult as the features of dichorionicity may become less apparent with advancing gestation. Fetal phenotypic sex discordance reliably signifies dizygosity and therefore dichorionicity, except in the very rare circumstance of sex chromosome heterokaryotypic monozygotic twins.

EPIDEMIOLOGY

Monozygotic twinning occurs relatively uniformly across populations, with clinically apparent monozygotic pregnancies occurring in 3 to 4 per 1,000 pregnancies. This rate likely underestimates the true frequency of early zygotic cleavage as up to 30% of such pregnancies will result in early demise of one or both fetuses (3). Monozygotic twinning in spontaneously conceived pregnancies is unaffected by age, ethnicity, maternal physical factors, fertility, or environmental conditions. In artificially conceived pregnancies, the rate is significantly higher, in particular with techniques such as blastocyst transfer and artificial hatching that, although increasing the rate of pregnancy overall, may interfere with the function of the zona pellucida and promote zygotic cleavage in 1% to 3% of such conceptions (4–6).

By contrast, dizygotic twinning occurs with varying frequency in different populations. Ethnicity is a major determinant of the rate of such twinning with a lower rate in East Asia (6 per 1,000 live births in Japan) and a higher rate in Africa (50 per 1,000 live births in Nigeria) (7,8). Further, the rate of dizygotic twinning is influenced by maternal characteristics such as matrilineal family history, age, obesity, height, parity, as well as coital frequency, seasonality, and the use of ovulation-inducing medication.

IMPACT OF ASSISTED REPRODUCTIVE TECHNOLOGY

ARTs, including ovulation induction and *in vitro* fertilization (IVF), are now commonplace with over 250,000 babies born annually worldwide through such techniques (9). One of the consequences of the rise of ART has been an increase in the incidence of multiple pregnancy. The rate of multiple pregnancy following ART varies considerably geographically related to local practices surrounding multiple embryo transfers at IVF and ultrasound monitoring during controlled ovarian hyperstimulation. For example, in the United States in 2000, 44% of ART-conceived births were twins, 9% were triplets, and 0.6% were quadruplets or greater (10). By contrast, in Sweden, twins are born from 6% of IVF transfers and triplets from 0.1% (9). This principally reflects the number of embryos transferred, with 70% of transfers in Sweden being single embryo, compared to 10% in the United States (9).

ANTENATAL COMPLICATIONS

Aneuploidy

Aneuploidy should occur equally commonly in multiple conceptions as in singleton conceptions. For monozygotic multiple pregnancies, the overall pregnancy aneuploidy rate should be equal to that of singletons whilst for dizygotic multiple pregnancies it should be double that given the two separate fertilization events. The observational evidence, however, shows that aneuploidy occurs less commonly in clinically apparent multiple pregnancies than in singleton pregnancies. This is likely to be related to a synergistic risk of early miscarriage of aneuploidy and multiple

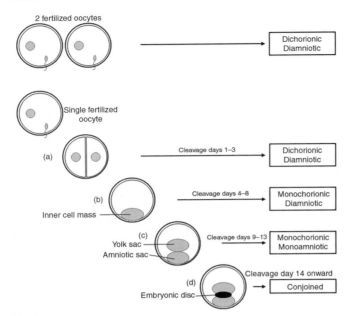

FIGURE 11.1 The timing of cleavage determines the chorionicity and amnionicity of monozygotic twins. (*a*) Cleavage between days 1 and 3, prior to the development of the inner cell mass; (*b*) Cleavage between days 4 and 8 after development of the inner cell masses but before the development of the amniotic sac; (*c*) Cleavage between days 9 and 13 before the development of the embryonic disc; (*d*) Cleavage after day 13 and the development of the embryonic disc.

pregnancy such that a greater proportion of aneuploid multiple pregnancies miscarry leaving a smaller proportion to become clinically recognized pregnancies (11,12).

Contemporary screening for aneuploidy in twins may be performed by combined ultrasound and biochemistry or with cell-free DNA-based approaches. An advantage of ultrasound-based approaches is the capacity to generate a fetus-specific probability based on each twin's nuchal translucency. In dichorionic twins, this provides around 70% sensitivity for trisomy 21 at a 5% screen positive rate (13). In monochorionic twins, a single probability is given for both fetuses who are (with rare exceptions) concordant in their chromosome complement. The sensitivity and screen positive rate are influenced by the choice of nuchal translucency measurement between the maximum of the twins, the minimum, or the mean (14). Nuchal translucency–based aneuploidy screening is also confounded in monochorionic twins as discordance in nuchal translucency is seen in impending TTTS (15). Cell-free DNA-based aneuploidy screening techniques are now well established for twin pregnancies, with sensitivity of 99% and false positive rate of less than 1% for trisomy 21, performance similar to that in singleton pregnancies (16). A downside to this technique is its inability to provide an assessment for the twins individually. Cell-free DNA-based screening has not yet been robustly validated for higher order multiple pregnancies where there is potential for significantly poorer test performance due to interference of multiple fetal cf-DNA profiles in the same maternal sample.

Fetal Anomalies

Structural fetal anomalies are three times more common among monozygotic twins than dizygotic twins and five times more common than in singletons (17). Despite being genetically very highly concordant, structural anomalies in monozygotic multiple pregnancies are discordant between fetuses in 85% of cases, reflecting the many postzygotic influences upon anatomical development (18). In a series of 312 monochorionic twins with major structural

anomalies, 90% involved a single system and 10% multiple systems (19). Of the single system anomalies, neurologic (39%) and cardiac (30%) malformations were most common, followed by musculoskeletal (13%) and urinary (11%). The presence of a structurally anomalous fetus also potentially affects the normal co-twin, with an increased risk of preterm birth either related to interventions performed upon the anomalous twin or as a complication of the anomaly itself (18). The prenatal detection of structural anomalies may be lower in multiple pregnancies due to the adverse effect upon ultrasound imaging.

Selective Reduction

Selective reduction of multiple pregnancies is the targeted termination of one of more fetuses in the setting of discordant fetal anomalies, as therapy for complications of monochorionicity, to reduce the complications associated with higher order multiple pregnancy, or at parental request. The method of selective fetal reduction varies according to chorionicity and amnionicity, operator experience and available equipment, and gestational age and may include intracardiac or intrafunic potassium chloride or lidocaine, radiofrequency ablation, interstitial or umbilical cord laser ablation, bipolar cord ligation, and cord transection. In monochorionic pregnancies, the presence of vascular anastomoses between fetuses sharing a placenta precludes drug administration and requires immediate cord occlusion to prevent acute intertwin transfusions and embolization.

Selective reduction of multiple pregnancies carries a risk of procedure-related loss of the entire pregnancy, which is higher at earlier gestations. This risk of earlier gestation procedures must be balanced against the greater reduction in complications of higher order multiple pregnancy by earlier reduction. In general, where selective reduction is being carried out to avoid complications of higher order multiple pregnancy or for parental choice, procedures prior to 16 weeks' gestation provide optimal reduction in late complications while carrying a 10% to 15% risk of complete pregnancy loss. Occasionally, late selective fetal reductions may be performed in the setting of discordant fetal anomalies in order to minimize procedure-related complications for the healthy twin although this approach comes with a risk that selective reduction may become technically impossible at the later gestation or that preterm birth may occur prior to the procedure being carried out.

With comprehensive prenatal and neonatal care, the long-term morbidity of trichorionic triplet pregnancies is now relatively low, with a median gestation of birth around 32 weeks and the risk of extreme prematurity being around 10% (20). When performed in the first trimester, selective reduction of triplets to twins significantly reduces the rate of extreme preterm birth to similar to that of dichorionic twins. This benefit is accompanied by a similar-magnitude risk of entire pregnancy loss. The decision in such cases therefore is effectively a trade-off between extreme preterm birth and procedure-related loss, with the decision ultimately being individualized to the perceptions of these competing risks by the parents. The contemporary outcomes of dichorionic twin pregnancies are generally favorable such that selective reduction of nonanomalous twins to a singleton would be considered not to be medically indicated. The high rates of extreme preterm birth and maternal complications in quadruplets and above warrant consideration of selective reduction to twins in order to optimize maternal and fetal outcomes.

PRETERM BIRTH

Preterm birth is an enduring challenge in multiple pregnancies with birth prior to 37 weeks' gestation occurring in 63% of dichorionic twins, 78% of monochorionic twins (21), 78% of triplets (22), and 97% of higher order (23) multiple pregnancies (**Fig. 11.2**). Preterm birth accounts for half of complications of multiple pregnancies,

LIVE BIRTHS

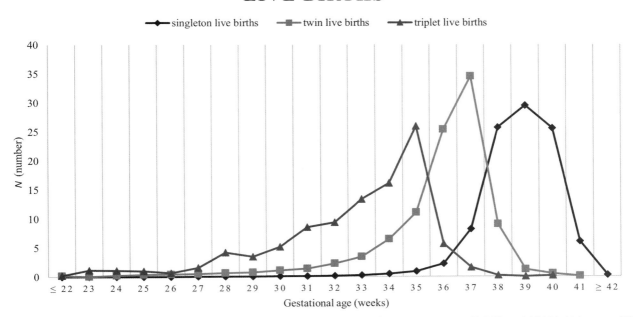

FIGURE 11.2 Overall distributions of singleton, twin, and triplet births by gestational age. (From Ko HS, Wie JH, Choi SK, et al. Multiple births rates of Korea and fetal/neonatal/infant mortality in multiple gestation. *PLoS One* 2018;13(8):e0202318. Copyright © 2018 Ko et al. Available from: https://creativecommons.org/licenses/by/4.0/)

and these infants represent a disproportionately large subset of those admitted to neonatal nurseries (24).

The mechanisms of preterm birth are different in multiple compared with singleton pregnancies. Uterine overdistension is a contributory mechanism leading directly to the onset of preterm labor, but cervical dysfunction, ascending infection, decidual hemorrhage, and placental dysfunction are also negatively impacted by multiple pregnancy. Other maternal complications such as hypertensive disease, gestational diabetes, obstetric cholestasis, and peripartum cardiomyopathy are more common in multiple pregnancy, leading to increased rates of medically indicated preterm delivery. Obstetric concerns about the risk of late pregnancy complications and difficulty in ultrasound-based fetal surveillance lead commonly to iatrogenic preterm birth, particularly in monochorionic twins and higher order multiples.

Identification of women with multiple pregnancies at particular risk of preterm birth may take into account maternal factors such as personal and family history of preterm birth and other comorbidities, which may predict pregnancy complications in general. The two most studied screening approaches are ultrasound-assessed cervical length and fetal fibronectin (25). Mid-pregnancy cervical length is proportional to gestation of onset of labor, with an exponential increase in the rate of preterm birth at shorter cervical lengths (26). In asymptomatic women with cervical length less than 25 mm, the risk of extreme preterm birth prior to 28 weeks is 25% (27). Fetal fibronectin is a biomarker for preterm labor quantifiable from a vaginal swab. It is clinically most useful in women with symptoms of preterm labor where the positive and negative predictive values are higher, particularly in multiple pregnancy, but is of less use in predicting preterm birth in asymptomatic women (28).

Several interventions aiming to reduce preterm birth in multiple pregnancies and its complications have been evaluated as follows.

Vaginal progesterone in unselected twin pregnancies appears to be of no benefit in reducing either preterm birth or its consequent neonatal and childhood morbidity. An individual participant data (IPD) meta-analysis of over 3,600 twin pregnancies comparing

vaginal progesterone versus placebo demonstrated no significant difference between groups in the rate of preterm birth before 32 weeks (RR 0.91, 95% CI 0.68 to 1.2) nor in the rate of composite neonatal morbidity (RR 0.97, 95% CI 0.77 to 1.2) (29). Included in this meta-analysis, the STOPPIT randomized controlled trial of 500 women went on to assess childhood outcomes at 3 and 6 years of age and found no significant benefit or harm in those randomized to vaginal progesterone versus placebo (30,31).

Vaginal progesterone has more of a role in women with twin pregnancies and a sonographically short cervix in the mid-trimester. An IPD meta-analysis (32) found that women with cervical length less than 25 mm who were prescribed vaginal progesterone had significantly reduced rates of preterm birth before 30 weeks and 35 weeks (RRs ranging from 0.47 to 0.83), neonatal mortality (RR 0.53, 95% CI 0.35 to 0.81), and neonatal morbidity. Reassuringly, there was no evidence of adverse childhood neurodevelopmental outcomes in those individuals exposed to progesterone suggesting that this is a safe intervention with substantial immediate benefits.

Cervical cerclage in multiple pregnancies appears to be less effective than in singletons. Two systematic reviews of cervical cerclage in twin pregnancies found no evidence of benefit in preterm birth reduction when performed for either history- or ultrasound-based indications (33,34). Of concern was that both reviews found a possible increase in harm from the intervention with an increase in the risk of perinatal death. There may be a more limited role for cervical cerclage in those women with a very short cervix (<15 mm) in whom a subgroup analysis showed a 58% reduction in preterm birth after cervical cerclage compared to no treatment (OR 0.42, 95% CI 0.24 to 0.81). Further evidence from larger trials is required to better dictate management in such cases.

The Arabin cervical pessary is a silicon ring that is placed around the cervix in mid-pregnancy aiming to reduce spontaneous preterm labor. In unselected twin populations, pessary use does not appear to reduce the rate of preterm birth, associated perinatal morbidity, or childhood neurodevelopmental outcomes (35,36). The use of cervical pessary in women with twins and a short cervix may be beneficial, although this is based on subgroup analyses and small trials and may only be effective at very early gestations (35,37). The use of cervical pessary in high-risk twin pregnancies requires further evaluation in larger clinical trials.

Bed rest has been proposed to reduce the rate of preterm birth in multiple pregnancies by alleviating pressure in the uterus and upon the cervix. In their Cochrane review, however, da Silva Lopes et al. found no difference in the rate of preterm birth or related adverse perinatal outcomes between those randomized to bed rest be it strict or partial, inpatient or outpatient, compared to those without physical activity limitation (38). This is in keeping with other research suggesting a lack of benefit, or even potential harm, from bed rest in women at increased risk of preterm birth (39–42). Currently, there is insufficient evidence to recommend a policy of strict physical activity modification in women carrying multiple pregnancies.

Various tocolytic agents are used in the setting of threatened preterm labor including calcium channel blockers, betamimetics, nonsteroidal anti-inflammatories, oxytocin receptor antagonists, magnesium sulfate, and progestogens. Overall, the literature suggests a likely benefit of short-term tocolytic therapy in symptomatic women to allow time for administration of antenatal corticosteroids (ACSs) and *in utero* transfer to an appropriately equipped perinatal center. Women with multiple pregnancies are insufficiently captured in the published literature to demonstrate efficacy, but it is reasonable to extrapolate the benefit in singletons to multiples. The use of maintenance tocolysis after acute treatment of symptomatic women or in asymptomatic women is not supported by evidence.

ACSs have been well established to reduce neonatal morbidity and mortality. In twins specifically, the recent EPIPAGE-2 cohort study (43) demonstrated benefit from ACS administration prior to birth from 24 to 31 weeks, with reductions in grade III-IV intraventricular hemorrhage or periventricular leukomalacia (OR 0.27, 95% CI 0.13 to 0.60) and in-hospital mortality (OR 0.31, 95% CI 0.14 to 0.69) but no difference in severe bronchopulmonary dysplasia (OR 1.02, 95% CI 0.35 to 2.93), with particular benefit seen in those receiving ACS within 7 days prior to birth. There was no additional benefit from a repeat course of ACS compared with a single completed course. Similarly, Vaz et al. also demonstrated benefit of ACS from 25 to 34 weeks, with reductions in respiratory distress syndrome (OR 0.17, 95% CI 0.05 to 0.59) and requirement for mechanical ventilation (OR 0.19, 95% CI 0.05 to 0.64) (44).

Maternal magnesium sulfate administration prior to preterm birth is associated with a reduction in cerebral palsy in surviving offspring and is now recommended by national societies and the World Health Organization. Overall, cerebral palsy is reduced by 32% in the offspring of women receiving magnesium sulfate compared to placebo (OR 0.68, 95% CI 0.54 to 0.87) (45). There is a lack of specific evidence for this intervention in twins and higher order multiples, but it is reasonable in the absence of such evidence to extrapolate the known benefit to singletons in recommending the use of magnesium sulfate also in multiple pregnancies.

COMPLICATIONS OF MONOCHORIONIC PLACENTATION

Monochorionicity, after gestation at birth, is the most significant predictor of perinatal outcome in multiple pregnancies. In all monochorionic placentae there are vascular anastomoses through which sharing of blood between twins occurs. Although in most situations this is of no overt consequence, unbalanced sharing may lead to TTTS or TAPS and acute massive transplacental hemorrhage may lead to death or hypovolemic injury after co-twin demise. Further, monochorionic placentae may provide disproportionate villous area to the fetuses leading to selective fetal growth restriction (sFGR). Monochorionic pregnancies are notoriously difficult to predict, with changes in clinical status often occurring

rapidly and without prior sonographic abnormalities, and as such these pregnancies require frequent monitoring by experienced clinicians.

Twin–Twin Transfusion Syndrome

TTTS occurs in 10% to 15% of monochorionic twin pregnancies (46) and is the result of hemodynamically significant imbalance in transplacental blood sharing between twins. Placental vascular anastomoses may be described by the vessels involved as arterioarterial (AA) where an artery from each twin meets, venovenous (VV) where a vein from each twin meets, or arteriovenous (AV) where an artery from one twin meets a vein from the other. Unbalanced AV anastomoses are thought to lead to TTTS where the "donor" twin supplies more blood across the placenta to the "recipient" twin than it receives. The donor twin becomes anemic and oliguric whilst the recipient twin becomes polycythemic and polyuric. Either twin may become hydropic, due to chronic anemia in the donor twin or to chronic volume overload–related cardiac failure in the recipient.

TTTS most commonly becomes apparent between 16 and 24 weeks although there may be signs prior to this such as discordant nuchal translucency measurements in the first trimester, and late-onset cases also occur, which are often acute and severe. Untreated TTTS has a very high rate of perinatal mortality for both twins related to progressive cardiac dysfunction and extreme prematurity.

The clinical hallmark of TTTS is amniotic fluid volume discordance between twins with oligohydramnios in the donor and polyhydramnios in the recipient. Quintero et al. described an ultrasound-based description of five stages based on amniotic fluid volume discordance (stage 1), absence of a visible urine-filled bladder in the donor twin (stage 2), critically abnormal Doppler studies (stage 3), hydrops (stage 4), or fetal death (stage 5) (47). Although this provides a useful tool to describe the ultrasound findings, it is less useful in predicting the progression of disease and the outcome following treatment, and fetuses may progress from one stage to another without ever showing features of an intermediate stage.

Untreated severe TTTS has an extremely high perinatal mortality rate of around 90% (48). Early treatments for TTTS aimed to correct amniotic fluid volume discordance by serial amnioreduction or septostomy (deliberate puncture of the intertwin membrane to allow amniotic fluid to equilibrate across the defect). Although these treatments may reduce the risk of preterm birth by preventing the uterine overdistension of polyhydramnios, they do not address the underlying pathophysiology and are ineffective in a significant proportion of cases. Subsequently, fetoscopic laser ablation of placental surface anastomoses was developed, which was shown to be superior to amnioreduction and has now been universally adopted as the gold standard treatment. In the Eurofetus trial of fetoscopic laser ablation versus amnioreduction (49), the former was associated with a reduced risk of death of both twins before 28 days of age (RR 0.63, 95% CI 0.25 to 0.93) and a reduced risk of periventricular leukomalacia (6% vs. 14%, p = 0.02) and neurologic complications overall (48% vs. 69%, p = 0.003) at 6 months of age. A neurodevelopmental advantage remained evident at 4 years of age in those randomized to laser ablation (50).

The outcomes of pregnancies complicated by TTTS treated by fetoscopic laser ablation are dependent on the Quintero stage at treatment as well as the experience of the unit in which treatment is performed, with higher-volume units having superior outcomes to smaller units (51). Typical perinatal outcomes for stage 2 to 3 disease are around 70% survival of both twins, 90% survival of at least one twin, and 10% death of both twins (48). The median gestation at birth after laser therapy is around 34 weeks (51). Longer-term follow-up studies demonstrate a significant impact of severe TTTS requiring treatment upon neurodevelopment, with cerebral palsy in 6% and neurodevelopmental impairment more generally in 10% of survivors, both mediated in part by preterm birth (52). Long-term cardiac outcomes appear to be favorable in TTTS survivors who show comparable outcomes to singletons in childhood follow-up studies despite demonstrable cardiac dysfunction prenatally (53). Chronic renal disease appears to be relatively common after TTTS, with 31% developing some form of chronic impairment during childhood of whom half required long term renal replacement therapy (54). There are also likely to be long-term health consequences of TTTS where it is complicated fetal growth restriction and preterm birth, in line with the developmental origins of health and disease.

Twin Anemia–Polycythemia Sequence

TAPS is the result of chronic transplacental transfusion from one monochorionic twin to the other where the volume is insufficient to cause hemodynamic consequences such as in TTTS. In contrast to TTTS, TAPS tends to occur late in pregnancy. It may occur spontaneously in around 5% of monochorionic diamniotic pregnancies or following fetoscopic laser ablation for TTTS in around 3% of cases treated by the Solomon technique (55–58). The perinatal outcomes are better for TAPS than for TTTS, with survival in 85% of fetuses (59). There are, however, significant risks of longer-term adverse neurodevelopmental outcomes, particularly for donor twins. Overall, neurodevelopmental impairment is observed in 30% of surviving twins and is more common in donors compared to recipients (44% vs. 18%). Severe impairment occurs in 9% and again is more common in donors than recipients (18% vs. 3%). Cognitive scores and parental concern for neurodevelopment are worse in recipients than donors. Independent predictors of neurodevelopmental outcome include gestational age at birth and severe anemia at birth.

Selective Fetal Growth Restriction

Selective fetal growth restriction is defined variably but most commonly prenatally as 25% discordance in ultrasound-estimated fetal weight between twins with the smaller twin being below the 10th centile (60). Although growth discordance is common in severe TTTS, sFGR is that which occurs in the absence of other features of TTTS. As monochorionic twins have identical genetic growth potential and grow within the same intrauterine environment, the growth of each twin is determined by the proportion of function each receives from the shared placenta. Abnormalities of placental cord insertion are commonly observed in sFGR, with the smaller twin often having a velamentous cord insertion compared to the central insertion of the larger twin, providing evidence of unequal vascular distributions within the placenta.

sFGR occurs in around 10% to 15% of monochorionic twin pregnancies (61) and is associated with poorer perinatal and longer-term outcomes compared with concordantly grown monochorionic twins (62–64). sFGR may be classified according to Gratacos type, which describes the pattern of umbilical arterial flow in the smaller twin (65). Gratacos type 1 sFGR (**Fig. 11.3A**) is that where the smaller twin has persistent forward end-diastolic flow in the umbilical artery. Type 2 sFGR is that where the smaller twin has persistent absent end-diastolic flow in the umbilical artery (**Fig. 11.3B**) and indicates more severe placental dysfunction. Type 3 sFGR is that where the umbilical arterial flow cycles between forward, absent, and reversed end-diastolic flow (**Fig. 11.3C**), relating to oscillatory flow in large arterioarterial anastomoses between twins (66).

Type 3 sFGR is the most challenging for obstetric management as the fetoplacental Doppler studies are altered by intertwin anastomotic hemodynamics and are therefore less reliable indicators of fetal status (61). Furthermore, the clear presence of significant calibre anastomoses suggests vulnerability of the larger twin to large volume hemodynamically compromising shifts should the smaller twin suffer *in utero* demise, which may occur in as many as two-thirds of cases of type 3 sFGR (67,68). Even in cases where both twins survive, the larger twin is at increased risk of neurologic complications as described by abnormal neonatal neuroimaging (67), most likely related to recurrent acute intertwin transfusions during periods of fetal bradycardia of the smaller twin. For these reasons, type 3 sFGR is generally associated with an earlier gestation at iatrogenic delivery than type 1 sFGR (69).

Perhaps the only benefit of monochorionicity is the observation that type 2 sFGR is often much more slowly progressive than equivalent Doppler abnormalities in a singleton fetus such that deferral of delivery to a later gestation may often be safely achieved.

Twin Reversed Arterial Perfusion Sequence

Twin reversed arterial perfusion (TRAP) sequence occurs in monochorionic pregnancies in the setting of early fetal demise of one twin where there is ongoing perfusion of the demised twin's body by the surviving twin through an AA placental anastomosis. Blood flows from the umbilical artery of the live "pump" twin via the anastomosis and in a retrograde direction through an umbilical artery of the "acardiac" twin. This retrograde flow generally

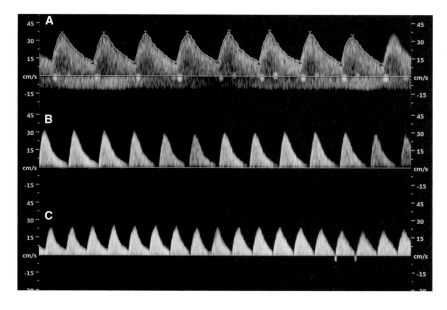

FIGURE 11.3 Umbilical artery Doppler waveforms in selective fetal growth restriction. A: Type 1: persistent forward diastolic flow. **B:** Type 2: persistent absent end-diastolic flow. **C:** Type 3: cyclical forward, absent, and reversed end-diastolic flow.

THE FETAL PATIENT

perfuses only the lower half of the demised twin's body and, depending only the volume of flow, permits growth of the abdomen, pelvis, and legs to a certain extent. The additional cardiac burden upon the pump twin confers a risk of cardiac failure and *in utero* demise.

The natural history of TRAP sequence is a high rate of fetal loss around 35% to 50%, frequently in the early second trimester of pregnancy (70,71). Although some cases may be safely managed expectantly, the prognostic factors that differentiate these cases are not well defined (70,72). It is likely that small acardiac masses without significant blood flow and no signs of cardiac decompensation in the pump twin are reasonably managed without intervention but with close surveillance for deterioration (73). Larger acardiac masses, those with more significant blood flow, and those with signs of pump twin cardiac dysfunction or hydrops do better with intervention. Intervention for TRAP sequence requires immediate occlusion of flow between the fetuses, which may be achieved with a variety of techniques including radiofrequency ablation, interstitial laser ablation, laser or bipolar cord occlusion, or high-intensity focused ultrasound, with ablative techniques apparently superior to cord occlusion (72). Early intervention is technically feasible but may be associated with a higher fetal loss rate (74), with most centers preferring to treat stable cases between 12 and 16 weeks' gestation.

Monoamniotic Twins

Monoamniotic twins occur in approximately less than 5% of monochorionic pregnancies (75). These pregnancies are at increased risk of complications, both due to the usual increase seen in monochorionic pregnancies and also due to unique complications of monoamnionicity, principally related to umbilical cord entanglement that is present to some extent in essentially all monoamniotic pairs. Monoamnionicity results from late division of the embryo and is diagnosed in the first trimester of pregnancy by the lack of an intertwin membrane and by demonstration of umbilical cord entanglement.

Umbilical cord entanglement with acute occlusion is the presumed mechanism for the observed increase in sudden unexpected fetal death in monoamniotic twins compared to monochorionic diamniotic twins, reported in as many as 70% of cases (76,77). There are also significant increases in miscarriage, fetal malformations, and preterm birth compared to monochorionic twins in general (78). Interestingly, and probably related to a greater presence of protective AA anastomoses, TTTS is less common in monoamniotic twins than in diamniotic twins (79). When it does occur, however, fetoscopic treatment is more difficult due to cord entanglement and close cord insertion proximity and perinatal outcomes may be less favorable than those of treated diamniotic pregnancies (80).

The prenatal management of monoamniotic twins focuses on surveillance for complications of monochorionicity and the avoidance of late stillbirth presumed related to cord entanglement. Various monitoring strategies have been employed with the aim of detecting acute cord compromise allowing emergency delivery in order to prevent otherwise unpredictable fetal deaths. Such strategies range from frequent ultrasound assessment to intensive fetal heart rate monitoring (multiple times per day or even continuous cardiotocography) in either an inpatient or outpatient setting. The evidence to guide such practice is limited. There may be some benefit to inpatient versus outpatient monitoring with a systematic review demonstrating fewer stillbirths in those managed mainly as inpatients (3% vs. 7%), although this may reflect variation in other features of clinical management and likely also comes at a cost of increased very early iatrogenic preterm birth (81). A subsequent well-designed prospective cohort study showed no such benefit of inpatient management (82). It is likely more important which monitoring strategy is employed, rather than where it is physically carried out, and there is currently insufficient evidence to support one protocol over others (83). Given the paucity of evidence, variation in clinical practice is still broad.

The timing of elective delivery of monoamniotic twins is similarly focused on avoiding unpredictable stillbirth while minimizing complications of prematurity. The risk of stillbirth in late monoamniotic twin pregnancies is difficult to accurately quantify as early iatrogenic delivery has been commonplace for some time and data are therefore lacking. It is probable that most fetal losses occur prior to 30 weeks and that the risk at later gestations may be lower than previously believed (81). By contrast, however, the rate of nonrespiratory complications of prematurity, particularly those of major individual long-term significance, falls rapidly in the third trimester such that at some point the risk of a major complication of prematurity becomes lower than that of unpredictable antepartum fetal demise, estimated to be 32+4 weeks (84). This has led to recommendations such as that of the Royal College of Obstetricians and Gynaecologists that uncomplicated monoamniotic twins should be delivered between 32 and 34 weeks (85). As there is a significant risk of acute cord entanglement during labor and delivery, it is recommended that monoamniotic twins are delivered by cesarean section.

Conjoined Twins

Conjoined twinning is a rare complication in monozygotic twins resulting from very late embryonic cleavage in around 1 in 1,000 monochorionic pregnancies (86). Perinatal death is common in such twins, with around half being stillborn and another one-third dying within the first 24 hours of life (87,88).

Conjoined twins are categorized anatomically according to the aspect and site of union (88). Dorsal union includes craniopagus, pygopagus, and rachipagus where the twins are joined at the skull, coccyx, and spine, respectively. Lateral union results in parapagus, where twins are joined laterally at the abdomen and pelvis. Further classification of parapagus involves description of further sites of union or separation such as dithoracic (separate heads and thoraces), dicephalic (separate heads but fused thoraces), and diprosopus (fused heads and thoraces). Depending on the degree of fusion, parapagus twins may have two or three legs and between two and four arms. Ventral unions are further defined by the site and extent of fusion. Ischiopagus twins are joined at the pelvis (either face-to-face or end-to-end). Thoracopagus and omphalopagus twins are joined from the chest wall to the umbilicus, with the former involving shared cardiac structures and the latter not. Cephalopagus twins are joined at the face as well as the chest and abdomen.

Advances in prenatal and postnatal imaging modalities and anesthetic and surgical techniques has allowed the evolution of the surgical separation of conjoined twins. Decisions surrounding termination of pregnancy, maintaining conjoined anatomy, and attempting separation are complex and require multidisciplinary input from a broad range of specialists in order to guide families' decisions. Inherent to all of these decisions will be individual and personal considerations of ethics and morals as well as perceptions of quality of life. In some cases, due to shared vital organs, separation with the aim of survival of both twins is clearly not feasible, whereas in others with less significant organ sharing, separation may be considered relatively straightforward. The literature now contains case series and reviews of hundreds of cases of successful separation procedures demonstrating that such treatment is feasible in appropriately selected cases. Given the rarity and complexity of such cases, separation should only be considered in experienced surgical units well equipped to deal with complex major surgery in multiple anatomical regions and the substantial physiologic insults that may accompany such treatment.

Single Fetal Demise in Monochorionic Twins

Monochorionic twins are at increased of unanticipated *in utero* death, either due to the known complications of monochorionicity such as TTTS and sFGR or even in the absence of an apparent cause (89). Given the ubiquity of intraplacental intertwin anastomoses among these twins, circulatory events in one twin lead to vulnerability in the other. In the event of fetal demise, the cardiac output and blood pressure dramatically fall in the deceased twin, creating a large pressure differential between the twins that can result in exsanguination of the surviving twin across the placental anastomoses into the body of the deceased twin. The resultant hypovolemia and hypotension may lead to critical organ hypoperfusion in the survivor, which may be lethal or sublethal. Sublethal hypoperfusion may result in ischemic injuries, particularly to the fetal brain, with long-term functional outcomes.

In their review and meta-analysis, Hillman et al. assessed the outcomes of 343 monochorionic twin pregnancies complicated by single fetal demise (90). Of the originally surviving twin, death occurred in 15% compared with 3% in dichorionic twin pregnancies after single fetal demise. Preterm birth occurred in 68% of surviving monochorionic co-twins. Abnormal postnatal neuroimaging and neurodevelopmental delay (defined variably between studies but generally "severe," "cerebral palsy," or "paralysis") were present in 34% and 26% of survivors, respectively. The authors noted significant heterogeneity in outcomes between the included studies. They hypothesized that this may have been due to altered risk of adverse outcomes according to the gestation at fetal demise, but the data were conflicting. The risk of co-twin death may be higher at later gestations, but that of adverse neurodevelopmental outcomes appears to be lower at later gestations.

A more recent series of 50 cases of single fetal demise was described by van Klink et al. (91). In this series, perinatal mortality of the co-twin was 16%, although only one of these was spontaneous fetal death and the remainder were due to termination of pregnancy for demonstrated abnormal prenatal neuroimaging or neonatal death, all of which were ascribed to neurologic injury. Cerebral injury was demonstrated either pre- or postnatally in 26% of twins overall, and in 10% of those children surviving one postnatal year. This study showed that deaths associated with TTTS were particularly likely to result in neurologic injury in the surviving co-twin, as were those at a later gestational age, and those where birth was at an earlier gestational age.

MATERNAL ANTENATAL COMPLICATIONS

Most of the common maternal complications of pregnancy are more frequent in multiple compared to singleton pregnancies. Gestational diabetes is roughly three times as common in women carrying twins than singletons, and four times as common in those carrying triplets (92). This reflects mainly the endocrine effects of a larger placental mass in multiple pregnancies, such as greater production of human placental lactogen. Although gestational diabetes is associated with increased adverse maternal and neonatal outcomes in singletons including hypertensive disorders of pregnancy, preterm birth, growth restriction and macrosomia, respiratory morbidity, neonatal nursery admission, hypoglycemia, and jaundice (93), these risks may be less significant in twins. Several studies demonstrate amelioration of these additional risks in twin pregnancies complicated by gestational diabetes, and it may be that the presence of glucose intolerance in pregnancy, if identified and treated, contributes little to the additional burden attributable to multiple pregnancy itself (94–97).

Hypertensive disorders of pregnancy are two to three times more common among women carrying twins than singletons, and up to 10 times more common in those with triplets (98,99). Gestational hypertension (the new development of hypertension in pregnancy without other features of preeclampsia) appears equally common in monochorionic and dichorionic pregnancies, occurring in 5% to 6% of each (100). Preeclampsia overall is more common in dichorionic than monochorionic twins (13% vs. 4%) (100) although this likely reflects a longer duration of pregnancy (and a longer time in which to develop preeclampsia) in dichorionic twins, as the rate of preterm preeclampsia is equally common among these groups (98).

Antepartum hemorrhage and its associated morbidity is increased in multiple pregnancies. Placenta previa is around 50% more common in dichorionic twins than in singletons (101). The rate is not significantly higher in monochorionic twins than in singletons. Although most second trimester low-lying placentas, even in twins, will resolve by the third trimester and not result in antepartum hemorrhage, the greater incidence of preterm labor and the greater uterine distension in twins compared to singletons render women with twins more vulnerable to early placental shearing in the setting of placenta previa and therefore to antepartum hemorrhage. Placental abruption is twice as common in twins as it is with singleton pregnancies (12% vs. 6%) (102). The epidemiologic risk factors for abruption is different in singleton and multiple pregnancies, and it is likely that there are different underlying pathophysiologic mechanisms in each group.

Some rare complications of pregnancy appear to have a predilection for women carrying twins or higher order multiples. Obstetric cholestasis (or intrahepatic cholestasis of pregnancy) is around five times more common in twins than in singleton pregnancies (6.7% vs. 1.3%) and is more severe, with higher levels of maternal serum bile salts and greater risks of preterm birth, perinatal death, and meconium staining of amniotic fluid (103,104). Peripartum cardiomyopathy is a serious complication of around 1 in 3,500 live births and is more common in women carrying multiple pregnancies (105). As it generally occurs at late gestations, it is not usually associated with significant neonatal morbidity unless there is fetal compromise in the setting of maternal decompensation in undiagnosed or untreated disease (106).

MODE OF BIRTH

First-born twins are at lower risk of neonatal morbidity (3.0% vs. 4.6%, OR 0.55, 95% CI 0.39 to 0.70) and mortality (0.3% vs. 0.6%, OR 0.55, 95% CI 0.38 to 0.81) than their second-born co-twins (107). It was often thought that this is due to acute intrapartum compromise in the case of intrapartum placental abruption or difficult delivery of the second twin raising the question of whether twins, in particular the second-born twin, may have improved outcomes with planned cesarean section. However, Rossi et al., in their 2011 systematic review (107) refuted that suggestion, finding that planned cesarean section was associated with a higher rate of neonatal morbidity for the first twin and a similar rate of morbidity for the second twin compared to planned vaginal birth. Further, after stratification for presentation and mode of birth, neonatal mortality was lower for both twins following vaginal birth than cesarean section for both vertex and nonvertex presentation of the second twin. Similar results were found by Steins Bisschop et al. in their subsequent review (108).

On the basis of such observational data, the Twin Birth Study (109) was undertaken in order to determine whether planned vaginal birth or planned cesarean section was associated with improved maternal, neonatal, and long-term neurodevelopmental outcomes. This study was a randomized controlled trial of twin pregnancies delivering at 32 to 38 weeks' gestation with the first twin in cephalic presentation and included 2,804 women and their 5,607 fetuses. Delivery by cesarean section ultimately occurred in 91% and 44% of women randomized to planned cesarean section and planned vaginal birth, respectively. The composite primary outcome of perinatal death or serious neonatal morbidity was no different between study groups. Maternal composite mortality and severe morbidity were also similar between groups. Planned subgroup analyses according to parity, stratified gestational age, maternal age, chorionicity, presentation of the second twin, and national perinatal mortality rate of the trial center showed no differences in outcomes between groups according to any of these factors. The primary neonatal outcome was more common for the second-born twin, but this was independent of the study group allocation.

Follow-up studies to this randomized trial assessed other outcomes for both the mothers and the offspring. At 3 months postpartum, there were no significant differences in maternal outcomes of depression, quality of life, incontinence, or breast-feeding between trial groups (110). At 2 years postpartum, problematic maternal urinary incontinence was less common in women randomized to planned cesarean section than planned vaginal birth (8% vs. 12%, OR 0.63, 95% CI 0.47 to 0.83) (111). When present, urinary incontinence had no greater impact on quality of life in either study group. At 2 years of age, neurodevelopmental assessment was performed in 83% of offspring using the Ages and Stages Questionnaire and validation of abnormal scores by clinical neurodevelopmental assessment (112). There were no significant differences in death or neurodevelopmental delay according to planned mode of birth. Overall, planned cesarean birth for term or late preterm twins provides a modest reduction in problematic maternal urinary incontinence at 2 years postpartum but is not associated with any differences in other maternal, neonatal, or neurodevelopmental outcomes.

Epidemiologic data show that, despite a lack of apparent major benefit from planned cesarean section for uncomplicated twin pregnancies, the rate of cesarean section in such pregnancies continues to rise. Recent Australian data demonstrate that the proportion of twins born by cesarean section rose from 24% to 71% between 1983 and 2015, with twins as the sole indication for cesarean section rising from 1.8% to 21% over this time (113). Similar increases have been observed in Europe and in North America (114–116). In the Australian study there was significant regional variation in cesarean section rates, suggesting that this reflects more clinician practice than changing clinical criteria. The authors, among others, suggest that this reduction in twin vaginal births combined with an increased number of clinicians among whom these births are divided may have important ramifications for acquisition and maintenance of skill in the management of vaginal twin delivery that may alter the risk of vaginal birth (115,117,118). There is clear evidence that adverse outcomes for the second twin are increased in the setting of cesarean section for the second twin after vaginal birth for the first twin, which is likely to be more common in cases managed by less experienced obstetricians (107).

MATERIAL PERIPARTUM MORBIDITY

Severe maternal morbidity is increased among women carrying multiple pregnancies compared to singletons (119). Complications such as intensive care unit admission (OR 4.3, 95% CI 3.5 to 5.8), eclampsia (OR 4.8, 95% CI 3.1 to 7.5), and major obstetric hemorrhage (OR 5.2, 95% CI 4.4 to 6.2) are all significantly increased, as is maternal mortality (OR 4.5, 95% CI 1.6 to 12.5). Factors associated with increased maternal morbidity in twins include maternal age greater than 40 years, nulliparity, conception with IVF, and induction of labor or prelabor cesarean section. Perhaps unsurprisingly, postnatal depression and stress are significantly more common in mothers of twins and higher order multiples than singletons (120).

NEONATAL OUTCOMES

Overall neonatal outcomes are poorer for the offspring of multiple pregnancies than for their singleton counterparts. In the main this relates to an increase in complications of these pregnancies,

principally preterm birth, fetal growth restriction, and unique complications of monochorionicity. Reassuringly, for most outcomes, twins do not appear to face additional burden of morbidity independent of that related to obstetric complications.

Mortality

Fetal, neonatal, and infant mortality are all greater in twins and triplets compared to singletons. Relative risks for these outcomes are around 3, 9, and 6, respectively, in twins and 10, 37, and 20, respectively, in triplets (121).

Prematurity

Preterm birth is significantly more common in twins and higher-order multiples compared to singletons and, therefore, multiple pregnancy increases the risk of complications of prematurity overall. However, the outcomes of preterm twins are generally similar to those of gestation-matched singletons. Gnanendran et al. (122) undertook neurodevelopmental assessments on 1,473 ex-preterm children at 2 to 3 years of corrected age and found no significant differences between multiples and singletons. This is consistent with other studies of neurodevelopment of ex-preterm twins (123–125). Chorionicity is an important determinant of offspring outcomes, with preterm monochorionic twins having higher rates of neurodevelopmental impairment than dichorionic twins (126).

Late Prematurity

Neonatal outcomes are poorer in late preterm twins compared to term twins, with increased requirement for NICU admission, mechanical ventilation, and respiratory distress syndrome (127). Respiratory morbidity rates are similar or slighter lower in late preterm twins compared to singletons (128,129). Length of hospital stay is slightly greater in twins than similar-aged singletons (13.5 vs. 12.6 days, $p = 0.011$). Neonatal jaundice is less common in twins (29% vs. 50%, $p < 0.001$) and the mean duration of phototherapy is shorter (1.45 vs. 1.99 days, $p < 0.001$) (130). Other neonatal morbidity is not significantly different between late preterm twins and singletons (131). Monochorionic twins are at greater risk of neonatal morbidity after late preterm birth than dichorionic twins (127).

Growth Restriction

Small for gestational age and fetal growth restriction are more common in twin pregnancies than in singletons. Multiple pregnancy does not appear to compound the adverse neonatal outcomes seen in growth-restricted infants, with similar rates of length of hospital stay, assisted ventilation, complications of prematurity, congenital anomalies, and neonatal death when compared to singletons matched for gestational age, degree of growth restriction, and sex (132,133).

Neurodevelopmental Outcomes

The evidence surrounding a direct contribution of multiple pregnancy to neurodevelopmental outcomes has been conflicting. Although twins and triplets are clearly at increased risk of abnormal neurodevelopment, most of that risk relates to complications of multiple pregnancy, particularly preterm birth (133). Cerebral palsy is 5 to 6 times more common in twins than in singletons overall (134–137). However, when analyses are stratified by gestational age, a difference between twins and singletons is only apparent at term gestations or birth weight greater than 2,500 g, where the risk for cerebral palsy is as much as six-fold higher in twins than in singletons (136). The observation that cerebral palsy is greater for twins than in singletons in the absence of apparent pregnancy complications suggests that there may be an inherent contribution of developmental outcome inherent to the process of twinning (138).

In twins, the independent risk factors for abnormal neuro-motor outcomes include death of a co-twin (139), chorionicity (140,141), discordant growth where the risk is increased similarly for both twins of a discordant pair compared to normally grown twins (142), and TTTS and other specific complications of mono-chorionicity (143–145). ARTs appear not to independently impact neurologic outcomes in multiple pregnancies independent of other confounding factors (146).

Nutrition

Women breast-feeding multiple infants face several additional challenges to those with singletons, and this contributes to lower rates of prenatal intention to breast-feed, breast-feeding initiation, exclusive breast-feeding, and continuation of breast-feeding at hospital discharge, and higher rates of formula and donor breast milk use (147,148). Given the high rate of preterm birth in multiple pregnancies and the specific benefits of breast-feeding for preterm infants, these mothers are important targets of strategies to improve breast-feeding outcomes. There is evidence that prenatal and postnatal clinician-led education and support can improve outcomes such as the rates of breast-feeding initiation and exclusive breast-feeding at 6 months (149–151). There is no evidence to guide specific breast-feeding education and support interventions for women with multiple pregnancies (147). Given the unique challenges that these women face, specific tools are likely to be beneficial, and development of such tools should be a priority.

▎CONCLUSION

Multiple pregnancies are associated with an increase in adverse outcomes for the mother and the offspring across the fetal–neonatal–childhood course. The neonatal outcomes principally reflect the increased incidence of preterm birth among all multiple pregnancies in addition to specific complications in monochorionic pregnancies. In some outcomes, such as congenital anomalies, there may also be contributions to adverse outcomes as a result of multiple pregnancy itself. Although the rate of multiple pregnancy has increased with the use of artificial reproductive technologies, this has more recently slowed, particularly for higher order multiples, with more judicious use of multiple embryo transfers after IVF. Advances in neonatal care in recent decades, particularly in the management of prematurity, has reduced the morbidity of multiple pregnancy such that most offspring of multiple pregnancies will now have favorable long-term outcomes. Optimizing the outcomes of such pregnancies requires input from a broad multidisciplinary team with experience in the management of multiple pregnancy and its prenatal and neonatal complications.

REFERENCES

1. Office for National Statistics. *Birth Statistics 2008*. FM1 No 37. London, England, 2010.
2. Australian Institute of Health and Welfare. Australia's mothers and babies 2017—in brief. In: *Perinatal Statistics Series*. Canberra, Australia, 2019..
3. Dickey RP, et al. Spontaneous reduction of multiple pregnancy: incidence and effect on outcome. *Am J Obstet Gynecol* 2002;186(1):77.
4. Chang HJ, et al. Impact of blastocyst transfer on offspring sex ratio and the monozygotic twinning rate: a systematic review and meta-analysis. *Fertil Steril* 2009;91(6):2381.
5. Ikemoto Y, et al. Prevalence and risk factors of zygotic splitting after 937 848 single embryo transfer cycles. *Hum Reprod* 2018;33(11):1984.
6. Hattori H, et al. The risk of secondary sex ratio imbalance and increased monozygotic twinning after blastocyst transfer: data from the Japan Environment and Children's Study. *Reprod Biol Endocrinol* 2019;17(1):27.
7. Imaizumi Y. Twinning rates in Japan, 1951-1990. *Acta Genet Med Gemellol (Roma)* 1992;41(2-3):165.
8. Nylander PP. The factors that influence twinning rates. *Acta Genet Med Gemellol (Roma)* 1981;30(3):189.
9. Mansour R, et al. International Committee for Monitoring Assisted Reproductive Technologies world report: Assisted Reproductive Technology 2006. *Hum Reprod* 2014;29(7):1536.
10. Reynolds MA, et al. Trends in multiple births conceived using assisted reproductive technology, United States, 1997-2000. *Pediatrics* 2003;111(5 Pt 2):1159.
11. Boyle B, et al. Prevalence and risk of Down syndrome in monozygotic and dizygotic multiple pregnancies in Europe: implications for prenatal screening. *BJOG* 2014;121(7):809; discussion 820.
12. Sparks TN, et al. Observed rate of Down Syndrome in twin pregnancies. *Obstet Gynecol* 2016;128(5):1127.
13. Malone FD, et al. First-trimester or second-trimester screening, or both, for Down's syndrome. *N Engl J Med* 2005;353(19):2001.
14. Vandecruys H, et al. Screening for trisomy 21 in monochorionic twins by measurement of fetal nuchal translucency thickness. *Ultrasound Obstet Gynecol* 2005;25(6):551.
15. Sebire NJ, et al. Increased nuchal translucency thickness at 10-14 weeks of gestation as a predictor of severe twin-to-twin transfusion syndrome. *Ultrasound Obstet Gynecol* 1997;10(2):86.
16. Liao H, Liu S, Wang H. Performance of non-invasive prenatal screening for fetal aneuploidy in twin pregnancies: a meta-analysis. *Prenat Diagn* 2017;37(9):874.
17. Nobili E, Paramasivam G, Kumar S. Outcome following selective fetal reduction in monochorionic and dichorionic twin pregnancies discordant for structural, chromosomal and genetic disorders. *Aust N Z J Obstet Gynaecol* 2013;53(2):114.
18. Mahalingam S, Dighe M. Imaging concerns unique to twin pregnancy. *Curr Probl Diagn Radiol* 2014;43(6):317.
19. Rustico MA, et al. Major discordant structural anomalies in monochorionic twins: spectrum and outcomes. *Twin Res Hum Genet* 2018;21(6):546.
20. Zipori Y, et al. Multifetal reduction of triplets to twins compared with non-reduced twins: a meta-analysis. *Reprod Biomed Online* 2017;35(1):87.
21. Kosinska-Kaczynska K, et al. Perinatal outcome according to chorionicity in twins—a Polish multicenter study. *Ginekol Pol* 2016;87(5):384.
22. Razavi AS, et al. Preterm delivery in triplet pregnancies. *J Matern Fetal Neonatal Med* 2017;30(21):2596.
23. Chibber R, et al. Maternal and neonatal outcome in triplet, quadruplet and quintuplet gestations following ART: a 11-year study. *Arch Gynecol Obstet* 2013;288(4):759.
24. National Perinatal Information System Quality Analytical Services, March of Dimes. *Special care nursery admissions*. White Plains, NY: March of Dimes Perinatal Data Center, 2011.
25. Murray SR, et al. Spontaneous preterm birth prevention in multiple pregnancy. *Obstet Gynaecol* 2018;20(1):57.
26. Kindinger LM, et al. The effect of gestational age and cervical length measurements in the prediction of spontaneous preterm birth in twin pregnancies: an individual patient level meta-analysis. *BJOG* 2016;123(6):877.
27. Conde-Agudelo A, et al. Transvaginal sonographic cervical length for the prediction of spontaneous preterm birth in twin pregnancies: a systematic review and metaanalysis. *Am J Obstet Gynecol* 2010;203(2):128.e1-12.
28. Conde-Agudelo A, Romero R. Cervicovaginal fetal fibronectin for the prediction of spontaneous preterm birth in multiple pregnancies: a systematic review and meta-analysis. *J Matern Fetal Neonatal Med* 2010;23(12):1365.
29. Schuit E, et al. Effectiveness of progestogens to improve perinatal outcome in twin pregnancies: an individual participant data meta-analysis. *BJOG* 2015;122(1):27.
30. McNamara HC, et al. STOPPIT baby follow-up study: the effect of prophylactic progesterone in twin pregnancy on childhood outcome. *PLoS One* 2015;10(4):e0122341.
31. Norman JE, et al. Progesterone for the prevention of preterm birth in twin pregnancy (STOPPIT): a randomised, double-blind, placebo-controlled study and meta-analysis. *Lancet* 2009;373(9680):2034.
32. Romero R, et al. Vaginal progesterone decreases preterm birth and neonatal morbidity and mortality in women with a twin gestation and a short cervix: an updated meta-analysis of individual patient data. *Ultrasound Obstet Gynecol* 2017;49(3):303.
33. Roman A, et al. Efficacy of ultrasound-indicated cerclage in twin pregnancies. *Am J Obstet Gynecol* 2015;212(6):788.e1-6.
34. Saccone G, et al. Cerclage for short cervix in twin pregnancies: systematic review and meta-analysis of randomized trials using individual patient-level data. *Acta Obstet Gynecol Scand* 2015;94(4):352.
35. Liem S, et al. Cervical pessaries for prevention of preterm birth in women with a multiple pregnancy (ProTWIN): a multicentre, open-label randomised controlled trial. *Lancet* 2013;382(9901):1341.
36. Simons NE, et al. Child outcomes after placement of a cervical pessary in women with a multiple pregnancy: a 4-year follow-up of the ProTWIN trial. *Acta Obstet Gynecol Scand* 2019;98(10):1292.
37. Xiong YQ, et al. Cervical pessary for preventing preterm birth in singletons and twin pregnancies: an update systematic review and meta-analysis. *J Matern Fetal Neonatal Med* 2020:1.
38. da Silva Lopes K, et al. Bed rest with and without hospitalisation in multiple pregnancy for improving perinatal outcomes. *Cochrane Database Syst Rev* 2017;(3):CD012031.

THE FETAL PATIENT

39. Sosa CG, et al. Bed rest in singleton pregnancies for preventing preterm birth. *Cochrane Database Syst Rev* 2015;(3):CD003581.

40. Saccone G, et al. Effects of exercise during pregnancy in women with short cervix: secondary analysis from the Italian Pessary Trial in singletons. *Eur J Obstet Gynecol Reprod Biol* 2018;229:132.

41. Zemet R, et al. Quantitative assessment of physical activity in pregnant women with sonographic short cervix and the risk for preterm delivery: a prospective pilot study. *PLoS One* 2018;13(6):e0198949.

42. Levin HI, et al. Activity restriction and risk of preterm delivery. *J Matern Fetal Neonatal Med* 2018;31(16):2136.

43. Palas D, et al. Efficacy of antenatal corticosteroids in preterm twins: the EPIPAGE-2 cohort study. *BJOG* 2018;125(9):1164.

44. Vaz A, et al. Effect of antenatal corticosteroids on morbidity and mortality of preterm singletons and twins. *J Matern Fetal Neonatal Med* 2018;31(6):754.

45. Shepherd E, et al. Antenatal and intrapartum interventions for preventing cerebral palsy: an overview of Cochrane systematic reviews. *Cochrane Database Syst Rev* 2017;(8):CD012077.

46. Benoit RM, Baschat AA. Twin-to-twin transfusion syndrome: prenatal diagnosis and treatment. *Am J Perinatol* 2014;31(7):583.

47. Quintero RA, et al. Staging of twin-twin transfusion syndrome. *J Perinatol* 1999;19(8 Pt 1):550.

48. Hecher K, et al. Long-term outcomes for monochorionic twins after laser therapy in twin-to-twin transfusion syndrome. *Lancet Child Adolesc Health* 2018;2(7):525.

49. Senat MV, et al. Endoscopic laser surgery versus serial amnioreduction for severe twin-to-twin transfusion syndrome. *N Engl J Med* 2004;351(2):136.

50. Salomon LJ, et al. Long-term developmental follow-up of infants who participated in a randomized clinical trial of amniocentesis vs laser photocoagulation for the treatment of twin-to-twin transfusion syndrome. *Am J Obstet Gynecol* 2010;203(5):444.e1-7.

51. Bamberg C, Hecher K. Update on twin-to-twin transfusion syndrome. *Best Pract Res Clin Obstet Gynaecol* 2019;58:55.

52. van Klink JM, et al. Long-term neurodevelopmental outcome in survivors of twin-to-twin transfusion syndrome. *Twin Res Hum Genet* 2016;19(3):255.

53. Halvorsen CP, et al. Childhood cardiac outcome after intrauterine laser treatment of twin-twin transfusion syndrome is favourable. *Acta Paediatr* 2015;104(3):252.

54. Melhem NZ, Ledermann S, Rees L. Chronic kidney disease following twin-to-twin transfusion syndrome-long-term outcomes. *Pediatr Nephrol* 2019;34(5):883.

55. Ruano R, et al. Fetoscopic laser ablation of placental anastomoses in twin-twin transfusion syndrome using 'Solomon technique'. *Ultrasound Obstet Gynecol* 2013;42(4):434.

56. Slaghekke F, et al. Fetoscopic laser coagulation of the vascular equator versus selective coagulation for twin-to-twin transfusion syndrome: an open-label randomised controlled trial. *Lancet* 2014;383(9935):2144.

57. Ashwal E, et al. Twin anemia-polycythemia sequence: perinatal management and outcome. *Fetal Diagn Ther* 2016;40(1):28.

58. Baschat AA, et al. Outcome after fetoscopic selective laser ablation of placental anastomoses vs equatorial laser dichorionization for the treatment of twin-to-twin transfusion syndrome. *Am J Obstet Gynecol* 2013;209(3):234.e1-8.

59. Tollenaar LSA, et al. High risk of long-term neurodevelopmental impairment in donor twins with spontaneous twin anemia-polycythemia sequence. *Ultrasound Obstet Gynecol* 2020;55(1):39.

60. Khalil A, et al. ISUOG Practice Guidelines: role of ultrasound in twin pregnancy. *Ultrasound Obstet Gynecol* 2016;47(2):247.

61. Bennasar M, et al. Selective intrauterine growth restriction in monochorionic diamniotic twin pregnancies. *Semin Fetal Neonatal Med* 2017;22(6):376.

62. Algeri P, et al. Selective IUGR in dichorionic twins: what can Doppler assessment and growth discordancy say about neonatal outcomes? *J Perinat Med* 2018;46(9):1028.

63. Groene SG, et al. The impact of selective fetal growth restriction or birth weight discordance on long-term neurodevelopment in monochorionic twins: a systematic literature review. *J Clin Med* 2019;8(7):944.

64. Victoria A, Mora G, Arias F. Perinatal outcome, placental pathology, and severity of discordance in monochorionic and dichorionic twins. *Obstet Gynecol* 2001;97(2):310.

65. Gratacos E, et al. A classification system for selective intrauterine growth restriction in monochorionic pregnancies according to umbilical artery Doppler flow in the smaller twin. *Ultrasound Obstet Gynecol* 2007;30(1):28.

66. Gratacos E, et al. Incidence and characteristics of umbilical artery intermittent absent and/or reversed end-diastolic flow in complicated and uncomplicated monochorionic twin pregnancies. *Ultrasound Obstet Gynecol* 2004;23(5):456.

67. Gratacos E, et al. Prevalence of neurological damage in monochorionic twins with selective intrauterine growth restriction and intermittent absent or reversed end-diastolic umbilical artery flow. *Ultrasound Obstet Gynecol* 2004;24(2):159.

68. Pasquini L, et al. Application of umbilical artery classification in complicated monochorionic twins. *Twin Res Hum Genet* 2015;18(5):601.

69. Buca D, et al. Outcome of monochorionic twin pregnancy with selective intrauterine growth restriction according to umbilical artery Doppler flow pattern of smaller twin: systematic review and meta-analysis. *Ultrasound Obstet Gynecol* 2017;50(5):559.

70. Mone F, Devaseelan P, Ong S. Intervention versus a conservative approach in the management of TRAP sequence: a systematic review. *J Perinat Med* 2016;44(6):619.

71. Pagani G, et al. Intrafetal laser treatment for twin reversed arterial perfusion sequence: cohort study and meta-analysis. *Ultrasound Obstet Gynecol* 2013;42(1):6.

72. Wong AE, Sepulveda W. Acardiac anomaly: current issues in prenatal assessment and treatment. *Prenat Diagn* 2005;25(9):796.

73. Zhang ZT, et al. Treatment of twin reversed arterial perfusion sequence with radiofrequency ablation and expectant management: a single center study in China. *Eur J Obstet Gynecol Reprod Biol* 2018;225:9.

74. Roethlisberger M, et al. First-trimester intervention in twin reversed arterial perfusion sequence: does size matter? *Ultrasound Obstet Gynecol* 2017;50(1):40.

75. Litwinska E, et al. Outcome of twin pregnancy with two live fetuses at 11-13 weeks' gestation. *Ultrasound Obstet Gynecol* 2020;55(1):32.

76. Post A, Heyborne K. Managing monoamniotic twin pregnancies. *Clin Obstet Gynecol* 2015;58(3):643.

77. Ezra Y, et al. Intensive management and early delivery reduce antenatal mortality in monoamniotic twin pregnancies. *Acta Obstet Gynecol Scand* 2005;84(5):432.

78. Madsen TE, et al. Temporal trends of sex differences in transient ischemic attack incidence within a population. *J Stroke Cerebrovasc Dis* 2019;28(9):2468.

79. Baxi LV, Walsh CA. Monoamniotic twins in contemporary practice: a single-center study of perinatal outcomes. *J Matern Fetal Neonatal Med* 2010;23(6):506.

80. Murgano D, et al. Outcome of twin-to-twin transfusion syndrome in monochorionic monoamniotic twin pregnancy: systematic review and meta-analysis. *Ultrasound Obstet Gynecol* 2020;55(3):310.

81. D'Antonio F, et al. Perinatal mortality, timing of delivery and prenatal management of monoamniotic twin pregnancy: systematic review and meta-analysis. *Ultrasound Obstet Gynecol* 2019;53(2):166.

82. Monomono Working Group. Inpatient vs outpatient management and timing of delivery of uncomplicated monochorionic monoamniotic twin pregnancy: the MONOMONO study. *Ultrasound Obstet Gynecol* 2019;53(2):175.

83. Mieghem TV, Shub A. Management of monoamniotic twins: the question is not 'where?', but 'how?'. *Ultrasound Obstet Gynecol* 2019;53(2):151.

84. Van Mieghem T, et al. Prenatal management of monoamniotic twin pregnancies. *Obstet Gynecol* 2014;124(3):498.

85. Kilby MD, Bricker L; Royal College of Obstetricians and Gynaecologists. Management of monochorionic twin pregnancy. *BJOG* 2016;124:e1.

86. Syngelaki A, et al. Diagnosis of fetal defects in twin pregnancies at routine 11-13-week ultrasound examination. *Ultrasound Obstet Gynecol* 2020;55(4):474.

87. Mian A, et al. Conjoined twins: from conception to separation, a review. *Clin Anat* 2017;30(3):385.

88. Kaufman MH. The embryology of conjoined twins. *Childs Nerv Syst* 2004;20(8-9):508.

89. Sebire NJ, et al. The hidden mortality of monochorionic twin pregnancies. *Br J Obstet Gynaecol* 1997;104(10):1203.

90. Hillman SC, Morris RK, Kilby MD. Co-twin prognosis after single fetal death: a systematic review and meta-analysis. *Obstet Gynecol* 2011;118(4):928.

91. van Klink JM, et al. Single fetal demise in monochorionic pregnancies: incidence and patterns of cerebral injury. *Ultrasound Obstet Gynecol* 2015;45(3):294.

92. Weissman A, Drugan A. Glucose tolerance in singleton, twin and triplet pregnancies. *J Perinat Med* 2016;44(8):893.

93. Crowther CA, et al. Effect of treatment of gestational diabetes mellitus on pregnancy outcomes. *N Engl J Med* 2005;352(24):2477.

94. Sheehan ACM, et al. Does gestational diabetes cause additional risk in twin pregnancy? *Twin Res Hum Genet* 2019;22(1):62.

95. McGrath RT, et al. Outcomes of twin pregnancies complicated by gestational diabetes: a meta-analysis of observational studies. *J Perinatol* 2017;37(4):360.

96. Hiersch L, et al. Gestational diabetes mellitus is associated with adverse outcomes in twin pregnancies. *Am J Obstet Gynecol* 2019;220(1):102.e1.

97. Foeller ME, et al. Neonatal outcomes in twin pregnancies complicated by gestational diabetes compared with non-diabetic twins. *J Perinatol* 2015;35(12):1043.

98. Francisco C, et al. Hidden high rate of pre-eclampsia in twin compared with singleton pregnancy. *Ultrasound Obstet Gynecol* 2017;50(1):88.

99. Morency AM, et al. Obstetrical and neonatal outcomes of triplet births—spontaneous versus assisted reproductive technology conception. *J Matern Fetal Neonatal Med* 2016;29(6):938.

100. Bartnik P, et al. Twin chorionicity and the risk of hypertensive disorders: gestational hypertension and pre-eclampsia. *Twin Res Hum Genet* 2016;19(4):377.

101. Weis MA, et al. Natural history of placenta previa in twins. *Obstet Gynecol* 2012;120(4):753.

102. Ananth CV, et al. Placental abruption among singleton and twin births in the United States: risk factor profiles. *Am J Epidemiol* 2001;153(8):771.

103. Liu X, et al. Perinatal outcomes with intrahepatic cholestasis of pregnancy in twin pregnancies. *J Matern Fetal Neonatal Med* 2016;29(13):2176.

104. Batsry L, et al. Perinatal outcomes of intrahepatic cholestasis of pregnancy in twin versus singleton pregnancies: is plurality associated with adverse outcomes? *Arch Gynecol Obstet* 2019;300(4):881.

105. Pearson GD, et al. Peripartum cardiomyopathy: National Heart, Lung, and Blood Institute and Office of Rare Diseases (National Institutes of Health) workshop recommendations and review. *JAMA* 2000;283(9):1183.

106. Abboud J, et al. Peripartum cardiomyopathy: a comprehensive review. *Int J Cardiol* 2007;118(3):295.

107. Rossi AC, Mullin PM, Chmait RH. Neonatal outcomes of twins according to birth order, presentation and mode of delivery: a systematic review and meta-analysis. *BJOG* 2011;118(5):523.

108. Steins Bisschop CN, et al. Mode of delivery in non-cephalic presenting twins: a systematic review. *Arch Gynecol Obstet* 2012;286(1):237.

109. Barrett JF, et al. A randomized trial of planned cesarean or vaginal delivery for twin pregnancy. *N Engl J Med* 2013;369(14):1295.

110. Hutton EK, et al. Maternal outcomes at 3 months after planned caesarean section versus planned vaginal birth for twin pregnancies in the Twin Birth Study: a randomised controlled trial. *BJOG* 2015;122(12):1653.

111. Hutton EK, et al. Urinary stress incontinence and other maternal outcomes 2 years after caesarean or vaginal birth for twin pregnancy: a multicentre randomised trial. *BJOG* 2018;125(13):1682.

112. Asztalos EV, et al. Twin Birth Study: 2-year neurodevelopmental follow-up of the randomized trial of planned cesarean or planned vaginal delivery for twin pregnancy. *Am J Obstet Gynecol* 2016;214(3):371.e1.

113. Liu YA, et al. Changes in the modes of twin birth in Victoria, 1983-2015. *Med J Aust* 2020;212(2):82.

114. Antsaklis A, Malamas FM, Sindos M. Trends in twin pregnancies and mode of delivery during the last 30 years: inconsistency between guidelines and clinical practice. *J Perinat Med* 2013;41(4):355.

115. Zhang JW, et al. In which groups of pregnant women can the caesarean delivery rate likely be reduced safely in the USA? A multicentre cross-sectional study. *BMJ Open* 2018;8(8):e021670.

116. Smith GC, et al. Mode of delivery and the risk of delivery-related perinatal death among twins at term: a retrospective cohort study of 8073 births. *BJOG* 2005;112(8):1139.

117. Reitter A, et al. Mode of birth in twins: data and reflections. *J Obstet Gynaecol* 2018;38(4):502.

118. de Castro H, et al. Trial of labour in twin pregnancies: a retrospective cohort study. *BJOG* 2016;123(6):940.

119. Witteveen T, et al. Severe acute maternal morbidity in multiple pregnancies: a nationwide cohort study. *Am J Obstet Gynecol* 2016;214(5):641.e1.

120. van den Akker O, Postavaru GI, Purewal S. Maternal psychosocial consequences of twins and multiple births following assisted and natural conception: a meta-analysis. *Reprod Biomed Online* 2016;33(1):1.

121. Ko HS, et al. Multiple birth rates of Korea and fetal/neonatal/infant mortality in multiple gestation. *PLoS One* 2018;13(8):e0202318.

122. Gnanendran L, et al. Neurodevelopmental outcomes of preterm singletons, twins and higher-order gestations: a population-based cohort study. *Arch Dis Child Fetal Neonatal Ed* 2015;100(2):F106.

123. Ylijoki M, et al. Neurodevelopmental outcome of preterm twins at 5 years of age. *Pediatr Res* 2020;87(6):1072.

124. Christensen R, et al. Longitudinal neurodevelopmental outcomes in preterm twins. *Pediatr Res* 2020. doi: 10.1038/s41390-020-0840-7

125. Babatunde OA, et al. Neurodevelopmental outcomes of twins compared with singleton children: a systematic review. *Twin Res Hum Genet* 2018;21(2):136.

126. Ichinomiya K, et al. Comparison of neurodevelopmental outcomes between monochorionic and dichorionic twins with birth weight ≤1500 g in Japan: a register-based cohort study. *J Perinatol* 2018;38(10):1407.

127. Sung JH, et al. Neonatal outcomes of twin pregnancies delivered at late-preterm versus term gestation based on chorionicity and indication for delivery. *J Perinat Med* 2016;44(8):903.

128. Salem SY, et al. Neonatal outcomes of low-risk, late-preterm twins compared with late-preterm singletons. *Obstet Gynecol* 2017;130(3):582.

129. Simchen MJ, et al. Neonatal morbidities and need for intervention in twins and singletons born at 34-35 weeks of gestation. *J Perinat Med* 2016;44(8):887.

130. Zdanowicz JA, et al. Do late preterm twins face an increased neonatal morbidity compared with singletons? *Swiss Med Wkly* 2018;148:w14581.

131. Ribicic R, et al. Perinatal outcome of singleton versus twin late preterm infants: do twins mature faster than singletons? *J Matern Fetal Neonatal Med* 2016;29(9):1520.

132. Baker ER, et al. A comparison of neonatal outcomes of age-matched, growth-restricted twins and growth-restricted singletons. *Am J Perinatol* 1997;14(8):499.

133. Briana DD, Malamitsi-Puchner A. Twins and neurodevelopmental outcomes: the effect of IVF, fetal growth restriction, and preterm birth. *J Matern Fetal Neonatal Med* 2019;32(13):2256.

134. Grether JK, Nelson KB, Cummins SK. Twinning and cerebral palsy: experience in four northern California counties, births 1983 through 1985. *Pediatrics* 1993;92(6):854.

135. Petterson B, et al. Twins, triplets, and cerebral palsy in births in Western Australia in the 1980s. *BMJ* 1993;307(6914):1239.

136. Williams K, Hennessy E, Alberman E. Cerebral palsy: effects of twinning, birthweight, and gestational age. *Arch Dis Child Fetal Neonatal Ed* 1996;75(3):F178.

137. Glinianaia SV, et al. Intrauterine growth and cerebral palsy in twins: a European multicenter study. *Twin Res Hum Genet* 2006;9(3):460.

138. Luu TM, Vohr B. Twinning on the brain: the effect on neurodevelopmental outcomes. *Am J Med Genet C Semin Med Genet* 2009;151C(2):142.

139. Pharoah PO, Cooke T. Cerebral palsy and multiple births. *Arch Dis Child Fetal Neonatal Ed* 1996;75(3):F174.

140. Adegbite AL, et al. Neuromorbidity in preterm twins in relation to chorionicity and discordant birth weight. *Am J Obstet Gynecol* 2004;190(1):156.

141. Hack KE, et al. Increased perinatal mortality and morbidity in monochorionic versus dichorionic twin pregnancies: clinical implications of a large Dutch cohort study. *BJOG* 2008;115(1):58.

142. Scher AI, et al. The risk of mortality or cerebral palsy in twins: a collaborative population-based study. *Pediatr Res* 2002;52(5):671.

143. Dickinson JE, et al. The long term neurologic outcome of children from pregnancies complicated by twin-to-twin transfusion syndrome. *BJOG* 2005;112(1):63.

144. Cincotta RB, et al. Long term outcome of twin-twin transfusion syndrome. *Arch Dis Child Fetal Neonatal Ed* 2000;83(3):F171.

145. Crombleholme TM, et al. A prospective, randomized, multicenter trial of amnioreduction vs selective fetoscopic laser photocoagulation for the treatment of severe twin-twin transfusion syndrome. *Am J Obstet Gynecol* 2007;197(4):396.e1-9.

146. Middelburg KJ, et al. Neuromotor, cognitive, language and behavioural outcome in children born following IVF or ICSI-a systematic review. *Hum Reprod Update* 2008;14(3):219.

147. Whitford HM, et al. Breastfeeding education and support for women with twins or higher order multiples. *Cochrane Database Syst Rev* 2017;(2):CD012003.

148. Kim BY. Factors that influence early breastfeeding of singletons and twins in Korea: a retrospective study. *Int Breastfeed J* 2016;12:4.

149. McFadden A, et al. Support for healthy breastfeeding mothers with healthy term babies. *Cochrane Database Syst Rev* 2017;(2):CD001141.

150. Kim SK, et al. Interventions promoting exclusive breastfeeding up to six months after birth: a systematic review and meta-analysis of randomized controlled trials. *Int J Nurs Stud* 2018;80:94.

151. Jacobsen N. Antenatal breastfeeding education and support: summary and analysis of 2 Cochrane Publications. *J Perinat Neonatal Nurs* 2018;32(2):144.

THE FETAL PATIENT

12 Placental Physiology, the *In Utero* Environment, and Antenatal Determinants of Disease

Ian P. Crocker

PLACENTAL DEVELOPMENT AND ANATOMY

Successful pregnancy is established through the interaction of the human blastocyst with the maternal uterine wall, usually within the mid-secretory (receptive) phase of the menstrual cycle, about 1 week after ovulation. It is facilitated by preimplantation events within the implanting blastocyst and uterine endometrium. Within the blastocyst, at around the 32 to 64 cell stage, two distinct embryonic cell types emerge: the outer trophoblast cells, termed trophectoderm, which eventually become the placenta, and the inner cell mass, which originates the fetus and fetal membranes. For the blastocyst, disintegration of the zona pellucida at around 6 days postfertilization, so called "hatching," is followed by trophoblast adherence to the endometrium ("apposition"), epithelial cell displacement, and trophoblast migration (see **Fig. 12.1**); aided by protease secretion and temporal decidualization of the uterine stroma, in response to maternal progesterone and androgen. Once resident, the epithelium seals around the embryo and trophoblast begin to infiltrate the newly differentiated endometrial decidua.

By day 8 of pregnancy, the trophoblast cells form an outer multinucleated syncytiotrophoblast that erodes the maternal tissues. This primary syncytiotrophoblast, distinct from its later namesake, expands through fusion with underlying mononuclear cytotrophoblast, until spaces termed lacunae emerge and combine. Encroaching interactions with uterine capillaries allows maternal blood to occupy this lacunar network, but any uteroplacental circulation at this stage remains stagnant, with the developing placenta reliant solely on carbohydrate and lipid-rich secretions from endometrial glands (1). With continued morphogenesis, inner cytotrophoblast cells coalesce into finger-like projections, termed villi, which permeate the surrounding syncytium. Within these primary villi, the extra-embryonic mesoderm establishes a core of connective tissue, which by the end of the 3rd week of pregnancy becomes vascularized through *de novo* blood vessel formation (vasculogenesis) and angiogenesis; development from preexisting blood vessels. Although nucleated fetal red cells are evident within primal vessels at this time, likely through hematopoiesis, a true fetoplacental circulation isn't established until gestational week 5.

Within the developing placenta, arbitration generates secondary then tertiary villi with various specialisms. Those that grow out toward the maternal decidua basalis form a protective cytotrophoblastic shell to plug maternal spiral arteries and provide anchoring points for stability. While those that pervade the lacunae, the branching chorionic villi, will eventually afford the exchange surface of the placenta, increasing the surface area for nutrient and waste exchange until delivery. For anchoring villi, two specialized invasive extravillous cytotrophoblast cells (EVTs) emerge from proliferative columns, penetrating and colonizing the decidual stroma, proximal myometrium (interstitial EVT), and maternal spiral arterioles directly (endovascular EVT) (**Fig. 12.2**). Their coordinated goal is to remodel the spiral arteries, removing and replacing the vascular endothelium and muscoelastic tissues, to generate dilated sinusoids of high flow, low pulsatility and resistance with which to (a) protect the immature placenta from the ensuing maternal blood and (b) meet the ever-growing demands of the fetus.

At around 10 weeks gestation, the aforementioned trophoblastic plugs disintegrate allowing oxygenated maternal blood access to the placental intervillous space for the first time. This histiotrophic to hemotrophic shift establishes a true hemochorial system

of notable fetal evolutionary advantage, including an unprecedented capacity for *in utero* brain development. The accompanying threefold rise in intraplacental oxygen elicits further placental remodeling, stimulating villus atrophy and regression around the superficial chorionic sac, creating the smooth chorion laeve, which ultimately combines with amnion and decidua parietalis as the fetal membrane, to encapsulate the fetus and amniotic fluid. Although mandatory, this exaggerated oxygenation may also confer a major oxidative challenge to the early placenta; maladaptation of which may hold gross anatomical consequences, such as eccentric, marginal or velamentous umbilical cord insertion, and/or pathophysiologic implications, including sparse villus vascular development and perturbed placenta transport (2). Intraplacental fluctuations in oxygen delivery are also proposed consequences of deficits in uterine spiral artery conversion; in which defective invasion by EVT, and retained vasomotive activity, likely impacts the metabolic and angiogenic capacity of the placenta, as defined in fetal growth restriction (FGR) and early-onset preeclampsia. It is also speculated that exaggerated blood delivery and its turbulent and inconsistent nature, as a result of these inadequate transformations, begets villus maldevelopment, with eventual sonographic appearance of intraplacental "lakes"; echogenic cystic lesions of thrombotic material deemed prognostic for adverse pregnancy outcomes (3).

Placental Adaptations to Blood Flow

Continued chorionic villous development is orchestrated by the uteroplacental milieu, under the influence of numerous maternal and fetal factors. Of note are the growth factors, vascular endothelial growth factor (VEGF), placental growth factor (PGF) and fibroblast growth factor 2 (bFGF), epidermal growth factor (EGF), and angiopoitin-1 and -2 (Ang-1 and Ang-2), which coordinate vasculogenesis and angiogenesis, and are themselves regulated by variations in oxygen partial pressure. These factors not only induce the differentiation of hematopoietic and hemangioblastic cells but also yield the first placental macrophages, the so-called Hofbauer cells, as a further source of VEGF (4). Placental secreted VEGF is detected in maternal plasma as early as 6 weeks gestation, peaking at the end of the first trimester (5). Responsible for vascular endothelial proliferation and vessel tube formation, resultant branching angiogenesis predominates throughout the first and second trimesters, decreasing vascular resistance and increasing the fetoplacental surface for exchange. From the third trimester, VEGF declines with concomitant increases in PLGF, shifting angiogenesis to a nonbranching phenotype, as typified by elongation and coiling of the capillary loops within the terminal villi, and achieving the well-branched and multilooped vascular network of the maturing placenta.

Under normal circumstances, the maternal supply and fetal extraction of oxygen are carefully balanced. However, with two independent circulations (maternal and fetal), intraplacental oxygen may theoretically vary from hypoxia to normoxia and even to hyperoxia, depending on environmental and clinical factors (i.e., high altitude pregnancies, maternal anemia) and/or degree of placental pathology. Under hypoxic conditions, terminal villi may become frequent and pronounced, presumably to encourage oxygen uptake (6). Alternatively, under hyperoxia, where fetal oxygen extraction is impaired, reduced endothelial proliferation offers explanation for observed reductions in terminal villi and longer

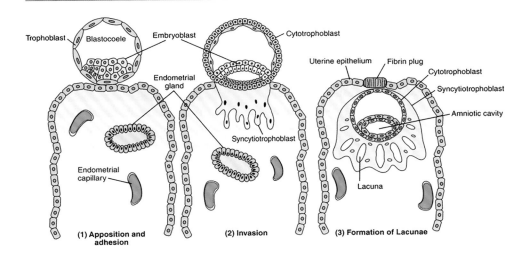

FIGURE 12.1 Implantation of the human blastocyst and rudimentary formation of the human placenta. After fertilization, the blastocyst differentiates into the inner cell mass (embryo) and trophoblast shell (placenta). Following attachment, implantation within the decidualized endometrium is accompanied by syncytiotrophoblast invasion and further differentiation. By day 9, lacunae appear in the syncytiotrophoblast and interact with the maternal endometrial sinusoids. At this stage, the primary yolk sac is the main source of embryo nutrition. (Reprinted with permission from Rhoades RA, Bell DR. *Medical physiology*. 5th ed. Philadelphia, PA: Wolters Kluwer, 2017, Figure 38.2.)

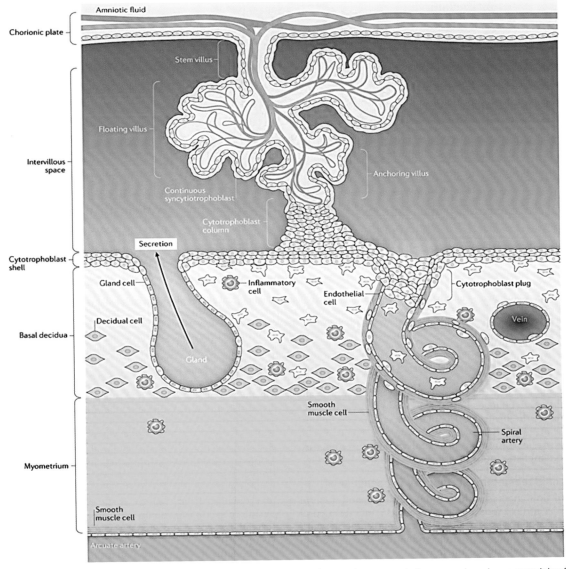

FIGURE 12.2 The placental villus and uterine spiral artery remodeling. The villous placenta is composed of a mesenchymal core containing fetal vessels and capillaries emerging from the stem villi and chorionic plate. The villi are surrounded by outer multinucleated syncytiotrophoblast and inner cytrophoblast cells. Some villi remaining floating for nutrient exchange, others anchor the placenta to the decidual bed, containing component stromal cells, inflammatory cells, spiral arteries, and secretory glands. Initialing the spiral arteries remain plugged by cytotrophoblast and undergo upstream remodeling (by invasive extravillous trophoblast, EVT) for conversion to dilated high flow and low resistance vessels for optimal maternal blood delivery. (Reprinted by permission from Nature: Aplin JD, Myers JE, Timms K, et al. Tracking placental development in health and disease. *Nat Rev Endocrinol* 2020;16:479. Copyright © 2020 Springer Nature.)

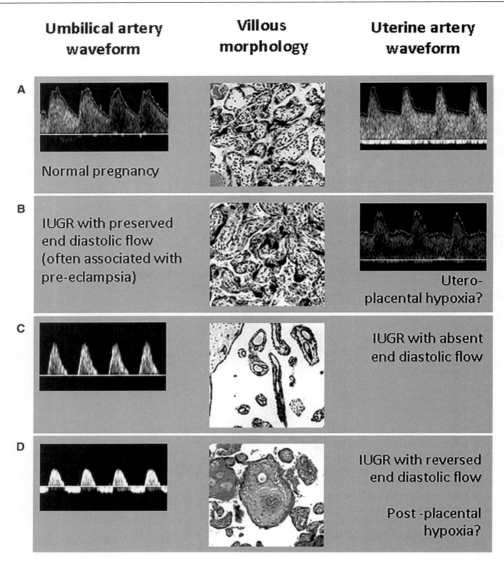

Umbilical artery waveform   **Villous morphology**   **Uterine artery waveform**

A — Normal pregnancy

B — IUGR with preserved end diastolic flow (often associated with pre-eclampsia) — Utero-placental hypoxia?

C — IUGR with absent end diastolic flow

D — IUGR with reversed end diastolic flow — Post-placental hypoxia?

FIGURE 12.3 Relationship between umbilical and uterine artery Doppler flow velocities and villous placental morphology. A: Normal umbilical flow and uterine waveforms corresponding to highly branched villi. **B:** Intrauterine growth restriction (IUGR = FGR) with abnormal uterine waveforms with prediastolic notch, suggestive of increased resistance and uteroplacental hypoxia/oxidative stress. With compensatory villous branching and restricted intervillous space. **C:** IUGR with umbilical artery Doppler with absent end-diastolic component, corresponding to increased placental resistance and postplacental hypoxia associated with unbranched and filiform villi. **D:** IUGR with reversed end-diastolic umbilical flow, common with severe fetal growth restriction and fetal hypoxia–associated histology showing fibrin-type fibrinoid deposition and stem vessel constriction. (From Kay H, Nelson DM, Wang Y. *The placenta: from development to disease.* John Wiley & Sons, 2011. Copyright © 2011 Blackwell Publishing Ltd. Reprinted by permission of John Wiley & Sons, Inc.)

slender intermediate villi, with limited capillary loops and terminal branches (6). Such changes in histology and villus maturation may be reflected in the upstream Doppler assessments of umbilical blood flow (7). Nevertheless, apportioning flow resistance in the cord purely to aberrations in placental vascular architecture remains an oversimplistic interpretation.

Determinants of Placental Blood Flow and Consequences

Umbilical blood flow increases throughout gestation and at term represents over a fifth of fetal cardiac output. In the absence of autonomic innervation, vascular tone in the placental network is dependent solely on autocrine and circulating vasoactive factors, most notably flow-induced nitric oxide (NO) (8). Although estimates of umbilical flow are afforded by Doppler ultrasound, through a resistance and pulsatile index (RI and PI), true quantification and downstream determinants remain elusive. Within the fetoplacental circulation, low resistance is a prerequisite for fetal health as reflected by sustained diastolic flow. However, an absence or reversal of this end-diastolic component is indicative of

vascular compromise; correlating strongly with FGR, raised perinatal risk and encroaching fetal demise (Fig. 12.3). Nevertheless, even in the face of fetal adversity, placental blood flow is usually well preserved. Perhaps remarkably, computer modeling predicts 50% obliteration of small placental arteries is necessary before Doppler resistance is attenuated, illustrating the organs considerable reserve capacity (9). Moreover, akin to ventilation flow matching in the human lung, it has been purported that flow is diverted away from areas of "insufficiency," such as that imparted by infarcts, microthrombi and vascular stagnation, and directed instead toward regions of more sustained oxygen and nutrient provision (10).

The fetus itself may also adapt to placental insufficiency; this time through dilation of its cerebral circulation. This preferential flow of blood to the brain at the expense of other organs, the "brain sparing effect," is indicated by raised umbilical artery PI to middle cerebral artery (MCA) PI ratio (commonly termed U/C). Although fetal cerebral redistribution represents an effort to preserve brain development in the face of chronic hypoxemia, prolonged "sparing" may lead to attenuations within the cerebral vasculature. In experimental animals, induced placental insufficiency alters brain structure in the offspring, reducing brain weight and causing ventriculomegaly and volumetric reductions in basal ganglia and hippocampus (11). In humans, attenuations in cerebral hemodynamics before birth may persist postnatally but usually normalize within days of delivery (12). Notwithstanding, studies of term and preterm infants in brain-sparing pregnancies consistently report prolonged cognitive and behavioral deficits in affected children and an exaggerated risk of stroke in later life (12).

While persistent redistribution of fetal blood serves to maintain necessary flow to the brain, sustained reductions in oxygen and nutrients to peripheral organs may also trigger life-long adverse effects. Prolonged brain sparing can instil asymmetric intrauterine growth, where the fetus is not just small, but thinner for its length, with a relatively normal sized head but shorter body. Sonographically, this is defined by the head to abdominal circumference ratio (HC/AC) and is more prevalent in cases of severe preeclampsia, fetal distress, and lower Apgar scores than their symmetrically grown counterparts (13). Although it's unclear how these *in utero* adaptions permanently affect the cardiovascular, metabolic, and endocrine functions of the baby in childhood and more notably adulthood, resounding evidence supports this case, with the Baker hypothesis and the notion of developmental origins of human disease (DOHad), stipulating a greater risk of adult coronary heart disease, hypertension, type-2 diabetes mellitus, insulin resistance, and hyperlipidemia in affected babies (14). Equally, given the prognostic value of both asymmetric growth and cerebral redistribution, it is understandable that each remains an important consideration for obstetric invention, either induction of labor or cesarean section. Although there are reports of severely compromised fetuses returning their MCA-PI to normal, this reversal is more frequently a preterminal signal to expedite delivery, than one of fetal recovery with which to delay it.

Uterine Blood Flow and Its Consequences

The rise in uterine artery (UtA) blood flow in pregnancy is arguably the greatest physiologic challenge in the human body, as a trade-off for bipedalism, brain expansion, and evolutionary advantage. Throughout pregnancy, uterine blood flow is enriched through dilation of uterine arteries, a progressive increase in maternal blood volume and reductions in blood viscosity, reaching around 500 to 750 mL/min at term and 10% to 15% of maternal cardiac output. In general, these hemodynamic adaptations, specifically those in the uterus, follow a continuum established in the menstrual cycle and are critical in early pregnancy, as epitomized in IVF embryo transfer, where transvaginal Doppler pulsatility, as a measure of UtA blood velocity, strongly aligns with uterine receptivity and pregnancy success (15).

During pregnancy, maternal UtAs are readily monitored by Doppler ultrasound and pulse-wave velocimetry. Resistance falls with advancing gestation, a finding attributed to downstream spiral artery transformations (as described above), but more likely through distal myometrial dilations, as evidenced through consistent waveforms for extra-uterine placentas, and unwavering indexes even as the placental is being delivered (16). Notwithstanding, raised resistance (pulsatility index) and waveform notching are still attributed to inadequate uterine transformations in both preeclampsia (PE) and FGR (Fig. 12.3). As such, UtA Doppler assessments have found prominence as best predicators of early-onset PE, often now supplemented with additional clinical factors of moderate predictive value, that is body mass index (BMI), serum PGF, placental protein 13 (PP13), and others (17). Although a long held belief that the placenta is underperfused and oxygen deplete in such circumstances, little evidence supports this notion. Instead, an alternative prediction is one of placental oxidative and metabolic stress, likely generated by ischemia–reperfusion and aberrant rheology of maternal blood entering the placental intervillous space. Such circumstances are considered stimulatory for liberated antiangiogenic factors, including soluble fms-like tyrosine kinase-1 (sFlt-1), with direct and indirect maternal vascular consequences (18). Although systemic in preeclampsia, such vascular dysfunction may also exacerbate acute decidual vasculopathy, further perpetuating a pathogenic loop.

Placental Transport Functions

The mature hemochorial placenta has a tree-like topography, with large stem vessels emanating from cord and chorionic plate, to support more bulbous intermediate villi from which terminal villi emerge, that is the dominate sites of placenta transfer and maternal–fetal exchange. These smaller terminal villi are characterized by a high degree of vascularization and microvilli to significantly increase surface area. The fetal capillaries of the terminal villi expand into sinusoids opposing an increasingly thin layer of syncytiotrophoblast, the so called "vasculosyncytial membrane." There are three mechanisms by which solutes are transferred across this membrane; diffusion, transporter-mediated transcellular transfer, and endocytosis/exocytosis. In line with Flick law, placental diffusion is directly proportional to the exchange surface area and inversely proportional to thickness of the barrier, which in this case decreases with gestation. The concentration of solutes and electrical hydrostatic gradients provide a driving force for transfer, dependent on maternal side concentrations and fetal metabolism. A panoply of transport proteins is also present within the maternal facing syncytiotrophoblast microvillus membrane (MVM) and fetal facing basal membrane (BM), conferring facilitated diffusion and carrier-mediated transfer for glucose and essential/nonessential amino acids. Lipids, on uptake by lipoproteins and scavenger receptors, are hydrolyzed and transferred within the placenta as nonesterified fatty acids, although the precise mechanism remains unclear. Along with documented alterations in maternal and fetal blood flow in conditions such as FGR and preeclampsia, there are equally reported changes in the structural variables of the exchange barriers in these placentas and a growing wealth of literature describing changes in transporter expression and activities, which may contribute to "placental insufficiency" (19).

Placental Endocrine Functions

As well as a major source of steroid and protein hormones, the placenta is also responsible for modulating fetal exposure to hormones produced by the mother, with aberrations impacting upon fetal growth/development and neonatal health. The principle hormones and growth factors in play across gestation are progesterone and estrogen, leptin, glucocorticoids, insulin-like growth factor (IGF), PGH, human chorionic gonadotropin (hCG), and the thyroid hormones. Of these, maternal thyroxine, triiodothyronine, and leptin cross the human placenta and benefit the fetal CNS, while liberated progesterone and estrogen are also neuroprotective (20,21). hCG, IGF, and PGH feedback following placental secretion to influence placental growth, indirectly assisting fetal well-being. Glucocorticoids are required for normal fetal development, but an excess may hold developmental consequences and restrict placental function. As such, the fetus is protected from maternal glucocorticoids by placental 11β-hydroxysteroid dehydrogenase type 2 (11β-HSD2), which metabolizes the majority of cortisol to inactive cortisone. Restrictions in hormones and growth factors are frequently associated with FGR, while homozygous mutations in 11β-HSD2 gene invariably result in birthweight reductions (22). Although knowledge of these reproductive factors is in many ways rudimentary, the placenta clearly plays a pivotal role as gatekeeper and orchestrator of *in utero* fetal health, shielding the fetus and improving resilience to maternal and environmental stressors.

Placental and Reproductive Immunology

Immune responses are crucial for reproductive processes, be that ovulation, menstruation, fetal acceptance, or parturition. For humans, the idea of the fetus as a semiallograft (the "paradox of pregnancy") was first purposed by Medawar in 1953, who surmised that fetal survival hinged upon maternal immune suppression (23). In essence, Medawar made three bold claims: (a) there is an anatomical separation between mother and fetus; (b) there is a lack of fetal antigen expression; and (c) there is functional suppression of maternal lymphocytes. Over the years, these ideas have been confirmed and refuted in equal measure, but what is now clear is that direct contact between fetus and maternal (immune) cells is offered by trophoblasts within the placenta and fetal membranes, but these trophoblasts lack major histocompatibility complex antigens, which would otherwise stimulate fetal rejection. Moreover, although maternal lymphocyte function in pregnancy is by no means suppressed (in fact quite the opposite), it is undoubtedly modified, as a pre-requisite for embryo implantation, uterine modifications, fetal tolerance, and eventual parturition.

In dealing directly with the placenta as an immunologic barrier, trophoblast cells offer direct contact with maternal tissues and resident or recruited leucocytes. In this regard, four different trophoblasts can be considered. Firstly, the villous cytotrophoblast, which remain in the villi as a pool of dividing progenitors. Secondly, the syncytiotrophoblast, the multinucleated layer that envelops the villi, bathed directly in maternal blood. Thirdly, extravillous cytrophoblast, which migrate into the decidua and myometrium, locating and transforming uterine spiral arteries for optimal uteroplacenta blood flow. Fourthly, and certainly the least considered, is the primary syncytiotrophoblast, which is the rudimentary invasive syncytium, liberated from the attached blastocyst at implantation. Lamentably, very little is known about the impact of this primary syncytium on maternal immunity. However, given its position as first contact between blastocyst and maternal immune system, with likely role in orchestrating all fetal/placental acceptance, this void in knowledge perhaps singlehandedly underpins the roadblock in truly understanding the "paradox of pregnancy." Nevertheless, the immunogenic features of the remaining trophoblast are considered below, alongside their related pathologies and fetal and neonatal sequelae.

There is broad expectation that maternal peripheral immunity must adapt to pregnancy but remain active against local and systemic infections. Peripheral leukocytes are elevated in early pregnancy and a shift in the ratio of type 1 to type 2 T lymphocytes and their cytokines is considered important to dampen the inflammatory response, much akin to a parasitic infection (24). This Th2-type prevalence may be instigated by pregnancy hormones (estrogen and progesterone) and/or trophoblast-derived cytokines/proteins, such as indoleamine dioxygenase (IDO), with importance exemplified in situations of pregnancy loss, where type-2 cytokines are reportedly diminished (25,26). In addition to these peripheral adaptations, placental trophoblasts evade immune detection through their limited expression of low-immunogenic nonclassical antigens (MHC Ia) and the immunomodulatory properties of expressed HLA-G (27). Together, these protective mechanisms limit paternal antigen sensitization and maternal anti-HLA antibody production; both known determinants of preterm delivery and chronic chorioamnionitis.

Within the uterus, following fertilization and embryo implantation, uterine natural killer cells (uNKs) are the dominant leucocyte population (>50%) but exhibit attenuated cytotoxicity toward invasive (extravillous) trophoblast. Here, again HLA-G plays a central role, suppressing uNK recognition and cytotoxic T-cell proliferation, with trophoblast themselves inducing apoptosis in resident leucocytes that become inadvertently activated. After uNKs, macrophages are the second most abundant decidual leukocytes and persist throughout pregnancy, maintaining their capacity for

antigen presentation but also prompting differentiation of tolerogenic regulatory T cells (Tregs). These cells, above others, have the primary role of suppressing antigen-specific maternal immunity, even expanding in response to semen and seminal fluid, and accelerating their capabilities in subsequent pregnancies, suggesting a "memory"-like recognition of paternal antigens.

With protection of the trophoblast assured, a responsive maternal immune system remains essential to control bacterial, viral, and protozoal infections, which can beget infertility, miscarriages, stillbirth, and neonatal morbidities, associated with aberrant fetal growth and prematurity. In reality, the villus syncytiotrophoblast is a highly effective barrier against pathogens, but small breaches occur through hemodynamic/hypoxic injury and stress. The resident Hofbauer cells (villous macrophages) remove pathogens and detritus, and where the syncytiotrophoblast is breached maternal macrophages and complement deposit placental fibrinoid to keep the fetal and maternal circulations divided. The intact syncytial surface has immunoglobulin Fc receptors to facilitate transfer of passive humoral immunity to the fetus and toll-like receptors TLR4 to further recognize bacterial products and signal (through antimicrobial peptides) local immune activity. Shed material from the syncytiotrophoblast, including DNA, microRNA, and even whole trophoblast and fetal hematopoietic cells, can traffic into maternal blood and persist for decades as chimeric elements in a woman's organs and tissues (28). Whether this material assists in healthy physiology or contributes to adult pathology is hotly debated, but its presence is speculated to convey remittance in rheumatoid arthritis during pregnancy, and subsequent development of autoimmune diseases, such as systemic lupus erythematous (SLE) and antiphospholipid syndrome (APS), which paradoxically impact future pregnancy success (29).

As discussed, some placental pathologies show direct involvement of immune cells, either maternal or fetal, even in the absence of overt infection. Although the reasons remain unclear, all are associated (to a greater or lesser extent) with increased obstetric complications. However, in most situations, the assumptions of maternal immune rejection of the fetus are unfounded. For example, placentas with villitis of unknown etiology (VUE) exhibit infiltration of maternal CD8+ T cells and activation of Hofbauer cells, but this is likely an exaggeration of normal placental physiology. More rare, but arguably more in line with graft vs host rejection, is chronic histiocytic intervillositis (CHI) and massive perivillous fibrin deposition (MPVFD); two serious placental conditions, often resulting in stillbirth and FGR; both of which are solely defined from placental examination after delivery; with clear-cut signs of maternal immune rejection, that is maternal macrophage, complement, and fibrin involvement (30). Highly recurrent in subsequent pregnancies (70% to 100%), sensitization from a previous pregnancy is likely in CHI/MPVFD, akin to rhesus disease. Moreover, with links to neonatal alloimmune thrombocytopenia and prevalence in women with autoimmune disease, placental and paternal antigen recognition, with or without HLA incompatibility, is a strong possibility. Further neonatal complications can arise with autoimmunity and maternal transfer of antibodies across the placenta. In neonatal lupus (NL), transplacental migration of maternal anti-Ro and/or anti-La autoantibodies frequently results in fetal cardiac disease, including congenital heart block and cardiomyopathy (31).

The Placenta and Parturition

Arguably, all maternal immunologic steps following implantation have the singular aim of limiting inflammation in the placenta and fetal membranes, as a means of suppressing the untimely initiation of labor. Although parturition in humans remains ill-defined, inflammatory components are heavily recognized, alongside the substantiated roles of myometrial stretch, hormones (i.e., functional progesterone withdrawal) and prostaglandins (PGE_2 and $PGF_{2\alpha}$). It is recently argued that human labor requires an inflammatory event, triggered from a number of concurrent "clocks," within the fetus, fetal membranes, placenta, uterus, and maternal system (32). With the harmonic maturation of these clocks defining parturition, the premature fruition or exaggerated triggering of any single clock (regardless of others) may prove enough to elicit mistimed labor onset. Spontaneous human labor is marked by leukocyte infiltration and elevations in proinflammatory cytokines within the uterus, cervix, and fetal membranes, prior to and during labor, which propagate uterine excitability and cervical ripening. Similarly, this proinflammatory upsurge is evident in preterm labor, following intrauterine hemorrhage, infection, preterm rupture of membrane (PROM), and overdistention of the intrauterine cavity (i.e., through multiple gestations and polyhydramnios). The specific role of placenta and fetal membranes is arguably to convey maturation signals from fetus to uterus, be that fetal brain maturation (indicated by the HPA axis) or fetal lung maturation (proffered by appearance of surfactant in the amnion). The placenta and membranes, however, cannot be mere bystanders, as evidenced from fetectomy in apes, where pregnancy continues and labor onset is restricted to term, even in the absence of the fetus (33). The mechanisms of this placental-determined labor are unclear, but a cellular age-driven process linked with telomere shortening is postulated, along with emergence of so-called alarmins (HMGB1, uric acid, cffDNA) and sterile inflammation, triggered through excess cell decline or stress-induced injury (34).

Placental Pathologies

Placental examination after delivery can have immediate or nuanced implications for new-born care, highlighting the need for abrupt intervention or assigning risk of more chronic developmental issues and disease. Immediate histiopathic diagnosis is possible for hematogenic infections from the mother (i.e., sepsis or viremia) or from congenital infections, usually from polymicrobial bacteria "ascending" from the cervicovagina, causing acute chorioamnionitis (ACA) or funisitis. Of all the placental pathologies, ACA is the most frequent, defined by neutrophil infiltration of the placental membranes. Adverse maternal outcomes from ACA include postpartum infections and sepsis, while adverse infant outcomes include stillbirth, premature birth, neonatal sepsis, chronic lung disease, and brain injury, leading to cerebral palsy and neurodevelopmental impairments (35). Twelve percent of primary cesarean births at term involve ACA, with failure to progress following rupture of membranes the most common indication. Less frequent are the histiopathic umbilical cord infections (funisitis) involving the umbilical vein (phlebitis) and/or one or more arteries (arteritis) and sometimes extending into the Wharton jelly. In all scenarios, infectious agents can prompt the release of proinflammatory cytokines/chemokines, leading to the untimely release of prostaglandin, cervical ripening and labor in the woman, or fetal inflammatory response syndrome (FIRS) and sepsis in the newborn, with damaging cerebral white matter implications (36). With thrombogenic foci within placental vessels also possible, the placenta can be considered a potential source of thromboemboli, following neonatal diagnosis of visceral infarcts or embolic strokes (37).

Alternative transplacental routes for congenital infections are less common, as the syncytiotrophoblast offers substantial protection from transmission of infectious agents and toxins. Viral particles can transfer passively across the villus, while others are actively transported; the most common being cytomegalovirus (CMV), with parvovirus, herpes simplex virus, hepatitis B and C, rubella, and coxsackie virus also included. Although overt histopathology for these infections may be present, evidence is often more subtle. Bacterial infections are equally difficult to determine, particularly given the recent (controversial) recognition of a commensal placental microbiota (38). However, certain histologic changes,

such as lymphoplasmacytic and granulomatous villitis, can be tell-tale signs of infectious etiologies (i.e., syphilis, CMV). The accumulation of mononuclear cells within villous stroma, that is villitis, is always a common readout, alongside fibrin deposition and avascularization, but direct placental damage is often unclear, regardless of the infection or consequences for the fetus/neonate. Blood disorders on both sides of the placenta, fetal, or maternal (i.e., sickle cell disease, dyserythropoietic anemia, thalassemia, etc.) may also impact upon placental histology. However, here again these features are never definitive.

FGR is related to a decrease in placental weight and reduction in placenta functional units, termed cotyledons. These placentas are often greater in thickness and predisposed to eccentric umbilical cord insertions. Sonographic examination may be unrevealing, but areas of hypoechogenicity and appearance of a "jelly-like" placenta may be observed in severe case, histologically confirmed after delivery as ischemic thrombotic lesions, attributed to decidual vasculopathy and aberrant spiral artery remodeling (39). Other histologic lesions are also common in FGR, including chronic villitis and localized hemorrhagic endovaculitis (vasculopathy of the placenta capillaries), but their appearance is not specific. Overlaps with preeclampsia are also clear, specifically in early-onset syndrome (<32 weeks gestation) confounded by FGR. Additional placental features in preeclampsia are infarcts and placental abruption, impaired villus growth and Tenny-Parker changes, increased aggregates and budding of the syncytiotrophoblast, as proposed adaptions to altered maternal blood flow. Other placental pathologies associated with poor pregnancy outcomes include villus edema, expanded spaces within the villi that restrict placental transport and capillary flow, and mesenchymal dysplasia (PMD), a placentomegaly with "grapelike" vesicles, resembling a molar pregnancy on ultrasound. Serve villous edema (placental hydrops) is a nonimmune hydrops, arising from fetal and maternal factors, such as cardiac anomalies, fetal anemia or hemorrhage, congenital abnormalities, chromosomal disorders, and tumors (neuro- and hepatoblastoma, and Beckwidth-Weidemann syndrome). PMD is a benign condition of cystic spaces associated with polyhydramnios and fetal hydrops, maternal diabetes, and even FGR. Although some pathologies of the placenta may be localized and others more gross, it should be remembered that the human placenta has significant multiplicity and reserve capacity, and as such the accumulation of uteroplacental lesions may be necessary before any clinically apparent disruption is observed.

Noninvasive Placental Monitoring

Prior to delivery, ultrasound provides the main tool for noninvasive elevations of the placenta, utilizing uterine and umbilical velocimetry as functional proxies. Together with improved measures of placental volume and vascularization (as afforded by more recent advances), this modality now offers potential beyond the routine documentation of the placenta's location and gross anomalies (i.e., previa and accreta). Although the normal placenta, viewed by ultrasound, is relatively homogenous, areas of echogenicity appear as gestation progresses, and these can become excessive in pregnancies affected by FGR, maternal hypertension, diabetes, and smoking. Improvements in 3D scanning and power Doppler now provide more precise estimates of placental volume (i.e., placental quotient; placenta volume:fetal crown-rump length) and vascular measures within the fetoplacenta, uterus, and chorionic villus itself (e.g., vascularization flow index, VFI) (40). Although many of these parameters remain experimental, some are finding increased use as clinical tools. Magnetic resonance imaging (MRI) has been part of clinical practice for many years and most commonly performed to aid diagnosis of abnormal placentation (i.e., accreta, increta, and percreta). With its capability to image the whole placenta at any gestation, MRI holds unique advantages over ultrasound, but its expense and limited access make its use challenging. The ability of MRI to measure placental function is becoming realized over conventional relaxometry, with multicontrast models and dynamic contrast-enhanced (DCE) MRI, beginning to reveal quantitative placental pharmacokinetics and fetal blood oxygen saturation (41). As an obstetric tool, MRI may never be incorporated into routine antenatal care, but in combination with other techniques, it may well contribute to the future monitoring of high-risk pregnancies and aid in complex decision-making around placental issues, such as monochorionic twins.

SUMMARY

When intrauterine growth trajectory is disturbed, the fetus becomes vulnerable to perinatal and neonatal complications. A reduction in oxygen to the placenta is long held to impact fetal development, particularly the brain, but a more effective standpoint is a fetus that has outstripped its placental capacity. In reducing its growth and metabolic needs to balance placental provision, organs, vessels, and signaling pathways within the fetus are transiently or permanently modified, predisposing the neonate, child, and adult to clinical complications and morbidities. Evidence implies that placenta-derived cytokines and thrombi (as a consequence of inflammation) exacerbate this prospect, either alone or in concert with relative hypoxemia, to generate excitotoxicity and neurologic impairments. Linking placental pathology to neonatal sequelae would seem essential in this regard, helping predict those prone to intrapartum events and also offering tailored therapeutic advantages. While antenatal ultrasound remains the mainstay of fetal surveillance, its measures of placental function *in utero* are arguably inadequate. Improvements may be proffered by MRI, with its more precise measures of size, perfusion, oxygenation, and metabolism, facilitating risk stratification in cases of fetal compromise and preterm birth. However, its role in routine antenatal care requires further evaluation.

REFERENCES

1. Spencer TE. Biological roles of uterine glands in pregnancy. *Semin Reprod Med* 2014;32:346.
2. Jauniaux E, Hempstock J, Greenwold N, et al. Trophoblastic oxidative stress in relation to temporal and regional differences in maternal placental blood flow in normal and abnormal early pregnancies. *Am J Pathol* 2003;162:115.
3. Burton GJ, Woods AW, Jauniaux E, et al. Rheological and physiological consequences of conversion of the maternal spiral arteries for uteroplacental blood flow during human pregnancy. *Placenta* 2009;30:473.
4. Seval Y, Korgun ET, Demir R. Hofbauer cells in early human placenta: possible implications in vasculogenesis and angiogenesis. *Placenta* 2007;28:841.
5. Regnault TRH, de Vrijer B, Galan HL, et al. The relationship between transplacental O$_2$ diffusion and placental expression of PlGF, VEGF and their receptors in a placental insufficiency model of fetal growth restriction. *J Physiol* 2003;15:641.
6. Kingdom J, Huppertz B, Seaward G, et al. Development of the placental villous tree and its consequences for fetal growth. *Eur J Obstet Gynecol Reprod Biol* 2000;92:35.
7. Galan HL, Ferrazzi E, Hobbins JC. Intrauterine growth restriction (IUGR): biometric and Doppler assessment. *Prenat Diagn* 2002;22:331.
8. Poston L. The control of blood flow to the placenta. *Exp Physiol* 1997;82:377.
9. Thompson S, Trudinger BJ. Doppler waveform pulsatility index and resistance, pressure and flow in the umbilical placental circulation: an investigation using a mathematical model. *Ultrasound Med Biol* 1990;16:449.
10. Nye GA, Ingram E, Johnstone ED, et al. Human placental oxygenation in late gestation: experimental and theoretical approaches. *J Physiol* 2018;596:5523.
11. Rehn AE, Van Den Buuse M, Copolov D, et al. An animal model of chronic placental insufficiency: relevance to neurodevelopmental disorders including schizophrenia. *Neuroscience* 2004;129:381.
12. Cohen E, Baerts W, van Bel F. Brain-sparing in intrauterine growth restriction: considerations for the neonatologist. *Neonatology* 2015;108:269.
13. Sharma D, Shastri S, Sharma P. Intrauterine growth restriction: antenatal and postnatal aspects. *Clin Med Insights Pediatr* 2016;10:67.
14. Joung KE, Lee J, Kim HJ. Long-term metabolic consequences of intrauterine growth restriction. *Curr Pediatr Rep* 2020;8:45.
15. Steer CV, Tan SL, Dillion D, et al. Vaginal color Doppler assessment of uterine artery impedance correlates with immunohistochemical markers of endometrial receptivity required for the implantation of an embryo. *Fertil Steril* 1995;63:101.
16. Schaaps JP, Tsatsaris V, Goffin F, et al. Shunting the intervillous space: new concepts in human uteroplacental vascularization. *Am J Obstet Gynecol* 2005;192:323.
17. Allen RE, Rogozinska E, Cleverly K, et al. Abnormal blood biomarkers in early pregnancy are associated with preeclampsia: a meta-analysis. *Eur J Obstet Gynecol Reprod Biol* 2014;182:194.
18. Roberts JM, Rajakumar A. Preeclampsia and soluble fms-like tyrosine kinase 1. *J Clin Endocrinol Metab* 2009;94:2252.
19. Gaccioli F, Susanne Lager S. Placental nutrient transport and intrauterine growth restriction. *Front Physiol* 2016;7:40.
20. Bouret SG. Neurodevelopmental actions of leptin. *Brain Res* 2010;1350:2.
21. Williams GR. Neurodevelopmental and neurophysiological actions of thyroid hormone. *J Neuroendocrinol* 2008;20:784.
22. Seckl JR, Holmes MC. Mechanisms of disease: glucocorticoids, their placental metabolism and fetal 'programming' of adult pathophysiology. *Nat Clin Pract Endocrinol Metabol* 2007;3:479.
23. Medawar PD. Some immunological and endocrinological problems raised by the evolution of viviparity in vertebrates. Symposia of the Society for Experimental Biology, vol. 7, 1952:320.
24. Saito S, Nakashima A, Shima T, et al. Th1/Th2/Th17 and regulatory T-cell paradigm in pregnancy. *Am J Reprod Immunol* 2010;63:601.
25. Veenstra van Nieuwenhoven AL, Heineman MJ, Faas MM. The immunology of successful pregnancy. *Hum Reprod Update* 2003;4:347.
26. Kudo Y, Boyd CA, Sargent IL, et al. Tryptophan degradation by human placental indoleamine 2,3-dioxygenase regulates lymphocyte proliferation. *J Physiol* 2001;535:207.
27. Hunt JS, Petroff MG, Morales P, et al. HLA-G in reproduction: studies on the maternal-fetal interface. *Hum Immunol* 2000;61:1113.
28. Khosrotehrani K, Bianchi DW. Multi-lineage potential of fetal cells in maternal tissue: a legacy in reverse. *J Cell Sci* 2005;118:1559.
29. Mardera W, Littlejohn EA, Somer EC. Pregnancy and autoimmune connective tissue diseases. *Best Pract Res Clin Rheumatol* 2016;30:63.
30. Romero R, Whitten A, Korzeniewski SJ, et al. Maternal floor infarction/massive perivillous fibrin deposition: a manifestation of maternal antifetal rejection? *Am J Reprod Immunol* 2013;70:285.
31. Fischer-Betz R, Specker C. Pregnancy in systemic lupus erythematosus and antiphospholipid syndrome. *Best Pract Res Clin Rheumatol* 2017;31:397.
32. Menon R, Bonney EA, Condon J, et al. Novel concepts on pregnancy clocks and alarms: redundancy and synergy in human parturition. *Hum Reprod Update* 2016;22:535.
33. Albrecht ED, Pepe GJ. The placenta remains functional following fetectomy in baboons. *Endocrinology* 1985;116:843.
34. Girard S, Heazell AEP, Derricott H, et al. Circulating cytokines and alarmins associated with placental inflammation in high-risk pregnancies. *Am J Reprod Immunol* 2014;72:422.
35. Kim CJ, Romero R, Chaemsaithong P, et al. Acute chorioamnionitis and funisitis: definition, pathologic features, and clinical significance. *Am J Obstet Gynecol* 2015;213:S29.
36. Kuypers E, Ophelders D, Jellema RK, et al. White matter injury following fetal inflammatory response syndrome induced by chorioamnionitis and fetal sepsis: lessons from experimental ovine models. *Early Hum Dev* 2012;88:931.
37. Kraus FT, Acheen VI. Fetal thrombotic vasculopathy in the placenta: cerebral thrombi and infarcts, coagulopathies, and cerebral palsy. *Hum Pathol* 1999;30:759.
38. Perez-Muñoz ME, Arrieta MC, Ramer-Tait AE, et al. A critical assessment of the "sterile womb" and "in utero colonization" hypotheses: implications for research on the pioneer infant microbiome. *Microbiome* 2017;5:48.
39. Raio L, Ghezzi F, Cromi A, et al. The thick heterogeneous (jellylike) placenta: a strong predictor of adverse pregnancy outcome. *Prenat Diagn* 2004;24:182.
40. Tuuli MG, Houser M, Odibo L, et al. Validation of placental vascular sonobiopsy for obtaining representative placental vascular indices by three-dimensional power Doppler ultrasonography. *Placenta* 2010;31:192.
41. Turk AE, Stout JN, Ha C, et al. Placental MRI: developing accurate quantitative measures of oxygenation. *Top Magn Reson Imaging* 2019;28:285.

13 The Impact of Maternal Illness and Therapy on the Fetus and Neonate

Adalina Sacco, Sarah Guillon, and Anna L. David

Chronic and acute maternal illness can have implications for the developing fetus and newborn, some of which may be lifelong. The topic is broad, and this chapter focuses on several important areas pertaining to the effect of maternal illness on the developing fetus and the newborn (**Fig. 13.1**). For several conditions in this chapter, practice varies between countries and readers are advised to work within their country's guidance.

PRETERM BIRTH

Preterm birth (PTB) is defined as a birth prior to 37 weeks' gestation, and can be either spontaneous or iatrogenic based on concerns about the mother or fetus requiring delivery. The frequency of PTB varies between countries from 5% and up to 12, or even 18% depending on the particular populations studied. Preterm is divided in moderate to late preterm (32 to 36 weeks), very preterm (28 to 31 weeks), and extremely preterm (<28 weeks) as defined by the World Health Organization (WHO).

The causes of PTB are multifactorial and differ between spontaneous and iatrogenic births. Spontaneous PTB may be associated with ascending vaginal infection, multiple pregnancies, polyhydramnios, maternal infections such as pyelonephritis and bacterial vaginosis, uterine anomalies, placental abruption, or cervical weakness. Often, a cause is not found. In women who are high risk for PTB, screening in pregnancy is performed by transvaginal ultrasound assessment of the cervical length, with or without tests of vaginal fibronectin. PTB may also be iatrogenic either for fetal concerns (e.g., fetal growth restriction) or maternal concerns (e.g., preeclampsia). If spontaneous PTB occurs, then investigations for maternal infection and placental histology are recommended. If a placental abruption has occurred, then a maternal thrombophilia screen would be advised. In situations of recurrent PTB, an ultrasound scan outside of pregnancy should be performed to identify any uterine anomalies.

Several interventions are used to lower the risk of PTB in high-risk women. Cervical cerclage has been shown to reduce the incidence of spontaneous PTB in women at high risk of PTB who are identified with a short cervix (1). The evidence for use of vaginal progesterone is as yet unclear, but there appears to be no evidence of harm in neonates at 2 years of age (2). When active preterm labor occurs (i.e., uterine contractions and cervical shortening) prolongation of the pregnancy is difficult. There are, however, some interventions aimed at reducing neonatal mortality and morbidity. If possible, transfer of the mother to a center with sufficient neonatal resources improves outcomes (3). Maternal antenatal corticosteroid administration prior to 34 weeks' gestation has been shown to decrease the risk of perinatal death, respiratory distress syndrome, intraventricular hemorrhage, necrotizing enterocolitis, need for mechanical ventilation, and infections in the first 48 hours of life (4). Maternal magnesium sulfate is also given if preterm labor occurs, usually prior to 32 weeks' gestation as this reduces the risk of neurodevelopmental disorders for preterm infants, particularly cerebral palsy (5). Tocolytics such as oxytocin receptor antagonists or calcium channel blockers (e.g., nifedipine) are not associated with a reduction of neonatal morbidity and mortality but can be used to delay birth long enough to permit the administration of corticosteroids and/or maternal transfer (6). Antibiotics are recommended in threatened preterm delivery if a maternal infection (e.g., urinary tract) is identified, and for all women with preterm rupture of membranes or in spontaneous

preterm labor as prophylaxis against group B streptococcus infection (7). In all infants, but particularly those born prematurely, delayed cord clamping is recommended to improve neonatal outcomes including a decreased need for transfusion and an improved transitional circulation (8).

PTB can have a lasting impact on the neonate and child, and prematurity complications are responsible of 15% of infant deaths below 5 years of age. Prematurity is also associated with long-term morbidities such as chronic lung disease, neurodevelopmental issues, visual impairment, prolonged hospital stay, and gastrointestinal and renal dysfunction (9).

HYPERTENSIVE DISORDERS OF PREGNANCY

Chronic Hypertension

Chronic hypertension (HTN) is the presence of HTN in the woman prior to pregnancy; this may be undiagnosed and present in pregnancy for the first time, usually prior to 20 weeks' gestation. Chronic HTN affects between 1% and 5% of pregnancies (10). Outside pregnancy, in the United Kingdom it is defined by a blood pressure (BP) above 140/90 mm Hg on ambulatory blood pressure monitoring (ABPM) (11) and in the United States by a BP above 135/85 on ABPM (12). The prevalence of chronic HTN in pregnancy is rising, most likely due to demographic changes such as an increase in maternal age at childbirth, maternal obesity, and metabolic syndrome.

Low-dose aspirin, taken at night, and initiated by 16 weeks of gestation is recommended for all women with chronic HTN to reduce the risk of severe preeclampsia (11). The exact dose of aspirin advised varies between countries and institutions, usually between 75 and 100 mg once a day. HTN in pregnancy is treated with a limited number of antihypertensives, most commonly labetalol, nifedipine, and methyldopa. Angiotensin-converting enzyme (ACE) inhibitors can be teratogenic if used in the first trimester of pregnancy and can lead to oligohydramnios and fetal renal failure if used later in the pregnancy. Diuretics are also not recommended for use in pregnancy. It has been suggested that target BP during pregnancy should be 135/85 mm Hg or less, guided by the Control of Hypertension in Pregnancy Study (CHIPS) trial, which showed tighter control reduced the rate of severe maternal HTN (13).

Chronic HTN is associated with poor perinatal outcomes. Women have 2.7 times increased risk of PTB and birth weight less than 2,500 g, 3.2 times increased risk of neonatal admission, 4.2 times increased risk of perinatal death, and 2.4 times risk of stillbirth (14,15).

Preeclampsia

Preeclampsia (PET) is a common pregnancy complication involving the development of HTN and proteinuria, with or without other organ involvement. The rate of PET in the United Kingdom is 2.8% but varies in different populations (16). PET is a multisystemic syndrome including a genetical predisposition, an up-regulation of the placental angiogenic factors leading to an angiogenic state and environmental factors. It is usually divided in early onset (<34 weeks of gestation) and late onset.

Low-dose aspirin as above is recommended for all women at high risk of PET. Antihypertensive treatment of PET is the same as treatment of chronic HTN (above).

Early-onset preeclampsia, defined as PET before 34 weeks of gestation, confers a high risk of maternal and/or fetal morbidity.

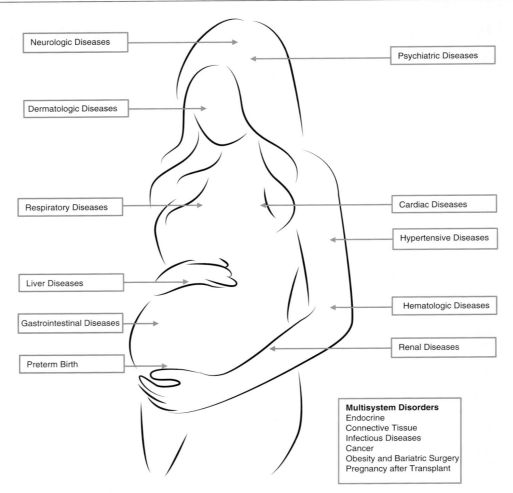

FIGURE 13.1 Maternal illnesses and the effect of therapy that can impact on the developing fetus and neonate.

Fetal mortality can be high in cases of severe early-onset preeclampsia, with only 57% survival prior to 27 weeks' gestation (17). The fetal morbidity is also increased compared to late-onset PET, with a higher rate of fetal growth restriction, oligohydramnios, stillbirth, and lower Apgar score at birth (18–20). Maternal complications occur in more than 50% of the cases due to hemolysis, elevated liver enzymes, and low platelet count (HELLP) syndrome, lung edema, eclampsia (seizures), and placental abruption (21).

Late-onset preeclampsia is accountable for 80% to 90% of cases of preeclampsia. Maternal and fetal outcomes are more favorable in the case of late-onset compared to early-onset disease (22), although prematurity and late fetal growth restriction can still occur. It is a source of debate whether late-onset and early-onset PET are on a spectrum or represent different disease processes.

ENDOCRINE DISEASE

Diabetes

Preexisting type 1 or 2 diabetes mellitus affects 0.4% to 1.2% of all pregnancies (23,24) (NICE Diabetes). The prevalence of type 2 diabetes in pregnancy is increasing particularly in certain populations, likely due to higher rates of maternal obesity, sedentary lifestyles, and older maternal age.

The diagnosis of type 1 or 2 diabetes is usually made prior to pregnancy, although type 2 diabetes can sometimes be detected

for the first time in pregnancy—this is usually early onset and persists postnatally. In pregnancy, metformin is typically the only oral hypoglycemic medication used and patients taking other oral hypoglycemics are recommended to discontinue these. Rapid-acting insulin analogs, either alone or in combination with long-acting insulin, are typically used when needed. Women who are already stable on an insulin regimen, including insulin pumps, are usually continued on these with increased frequency of monitoring to try to achieve a low HbA1C. In the United Kingdom, delivery of women with preexisting diabetes is recommended between 37+0 and 38+6 weeks' gestation.

Gestational diabetes mellitus (GDM) is the onset of diabetes during pregnancy. It is estimated that up to 5% of pregnancies are affected by diabetes, of which the majority (87.5%) is GDM, depending on which criteria are used for diagnosis (25). Some countries recommend routine screening for all, whereas others recommend that only women with risk factors for gestational diabetes, such as body mass index (BMI) >30 kg/m², previous baby weighing ≥4.5 kg, previous GDM, first-degree relative with diabetes, or high-risk ethnic origin should be offered a glucose-tolerance test in pregnancy. Treatment of GDM is similar to preexisting diabetes in pregnancy, with close monitoring, dietary modification, metformin, and escalating to subcutaneous injection of rapid-acting insulin forming the basis of treatment. In the United Kingdom, delivery of women with uncomplicated GDM is recommended no later than 40+6 weeks' gestation; in practice, this is generally interpreted as diet-controlled GDM, and women on treatment are offered delivery around 38 to 39 weeks' gestation.

Poor glycemic control during organogenesis (if diabetes is pre-existing) increases the risk of congenital abnormalities such as cardiac and neural tube defects (26). Women of reproductive age with preexisting insulin should plan conception by achieving low stable HbA1C levels, which can reduce the risk of structural defects. The incidence of miscarriage, stillbirth, macrosomia, and birth trauma are all increased with poor glycemic control (27). Babies born to mothers with insulin-treated diabetes are at risk of neonatal hypoglycemia due to the high levels of insulin and the absence of glucose supply from the mother. Other increased risks for babies born to diabetic mothers include respiratory distress syndrome, transient metabolic disorders (e.g., hypocalcemia, hypomagnesemia), polycythemia, hyperbilirubinemia and transient hypertrophic cardiomyopathy. Some recent studies have shown possible long-term effects such as an increased risk of autism (28) and lower cognitive development (29).

Thyroid Disease
Hypothyroidism

Hypothyroidism is defined by elevated concentrations of thyroid-stimulating hormone (TSH) and low concentrations of free thyroxine (T3/T4) and occurs in 0.2% to 0.6% of pregnancies. Treatment is based on administration of levothyroxine. Causes of hypothyroidism include autoimmune (Hashimoto disease), drugs, postviral, iatrogenic (e.g., following treatment for hyperthyroidism), and iodine deficiency. Subclinical hypothyroidism occurs when there is a mildly raised TSH with normal T3/T4, and occurs in 5% to 37% of pregnancies.

Overt hypothyroidism if untreated is known to be linked to adverse perinatal outcomes. It is associated with infertility, miscarriage and fetal loss. It is also linked to preterm labor, fetal growth restriction, pregnancy-induced HTN, and reduced childhood IQ (30,31). If adequate treatment is given, maternal and fetal outcomes are usually good. The effects of subclinical hypothyroidism are a source of debate and are often extrapolated from overt hypothyroidism. Treatment for subclinical hypothyroidism during pregnancy does not improve cognitive outcomes for children at the age of 5 years (32).

Hyperthyroidism

Hyperthyroidism is defined by reduced levels of TSH with high levels of T3/T4. In women of reproductive age, the prevalence is approximately 0.5% (33). The commonest cause is autoimmune (Graves' disease); rarer causes include a toxic multinodular goiter, functional adenoma, or TSH-secreting tumor. Graves' disease is associated with thyrotropin receptor antibodies (TRAb). Treatment is with antithyroid drugs such as carbamazepine and propylthiouracil (PTU).

Untreated hyperthyroidism is associated with subfertility, miscarriage, fetal growth restriction, and PTB (34). Maternal TRAb antibodies cross the placenta and in 1% of pregnancies cause fetal goiter and thyrotoxicosis. In the non-pregnant population, carbimazole is the commonest treatment used. However, this has been associated with birth defects in 2% to 4% of pregnancies, such as aplasia cutis (a skin defect on the scalp) and abdominal wall, digestive, urinary, cardiac, and respiratory defects. For this reason, pregnant women are often treated with PTU instead. PTU also is associated with birth defects in 2% to 3% of pregnancies although these tend to be milder than with carbimazole. PTU has a higher rate of maternal liver damage than carbimazole, and the practice of changing women with hyperthyroidism from carbimazole to PTU is debatable. Neonates at risk of hyperthyroidism should have cord blood sent for TRAb antibodies and thyroid function checked, and plans should be made for clinical and biochemical follow-up

as neonatal thyrotoxicosis may not present at birth and can be life threatening.

Parathyroid, Pituitary, and Adrenal Disease
Parathyroid

Parathyroid disease is rare during pregnancy. Hyperparathyroidism is defined by high levels of parathyroid hormone (PTH) with hypercalcemia, although this may not be evident in pregnancy due to increased calcium demands. Its prevalence is around 0.03% in pregnant women (35). Hyperparathyroidism may be caused by hyperplasia or parathyroid adenomas, and treatment is usually surgical, which can be performed in pregnancy (ideally second trimester) if needed. Adverse pregnancy outcomes are associated with severe hypercalcemia (>3.5 mmol/L) and include miscarriage, stillbirth, preeclampsia, and preterm labor. The neonate has a risk of tetany or seizures due to hypocalcemia caused by suppression of fetal PTH (36).

Pituitary

Hyperprolactinemia (high levels of circulating prolactin) is most commonly caused by pituitary adenomas, which may be micro (<1 cm) or macro (>1 cm) (37). Other causes include stalk lesions, medication, and kidney disease. Mild rises in prolactin are seen in normal pregnancy and following exercise or sexual intercourse. Prolactinomas may cause subfertility, headache, and visual field defects. Treatment is with dopamine-receptor agonists such as bromocriptine or cabergoline, which are usually discontinued after pregnancy is confirmed. As the pituitary enlarges during pregnancy, it is possible to observe expansion of a prolactinoma. This could lead rarely to a disturbance of the visual field and pituitary apoplexy (38). Prolactinomas are not associated with adverse pregnancy outcomes.

Acromegaly is usually caused by growth hormone–secreting pituitary adenomas. They are rare in pregnant women but may expand during pregnancy. Management is surgical, with medication (e.g., somatostatin analogs) second line. In pregnancy there is an increased risk of gestational diabetes, HTN, and fetal macrosomia but no direct adverse effects on the fetus.

Adrenal

Cushing syndrome is defined by an increased circulating cortisol level and low adrenocorticotropic hormone (ACTH). The cause may be pituitary (Cushing disease) or due to adrenal tumors. Outside pregnancy, Cushing disease is commonest, but in pregnancy, adrenal adenomas (44%) and carcinomas (12%) are the commonest cause. Surgical management is first line. In pregnancy there is an increased risk of HTN, diabetes, PTB, stillbirth, and perinatal death. At birth the neonate may have suppressed cortisol due to the high maternal levels and may present with vomiting, lethargy, or collapse (39).

Addison's disease occurs when there are low levels of circulating cortisol, raised ACTH, and a low cortisol response to a stimulation test. The commonest cause is autoimmune due to adrenal antibodies. Management is with replacement of glucocorticoids and mineralocorticoids, which will need to be increased during illness and labor. Although adrenal antibodies cross the placenta, there is usually no effect on the neonate (39).

CONNECTIVE TISSUE DISEASES

Connective tissue diseases can cover different organs and systems leading to various symptoms with variable effects in pregnancy.

Systemic Lupus Erythematosus

These conditions commonly affect women of reproductive age. Systemic lupus erythematosus (SLE) prevalence in the United

Kingdom is 0.12% and affects six times more women than men (40). Continuation of hydroxychloroquine during pregnancy is usually required to control the disease and lower the need for corticosteroid therapy. Maternal complications of SLE in pregnancy include HTN, preeclampsia, nephritis, and eclampsia. Those complications are particularly seen when lupus nephritis and antiphospholipid antibodies are present (41). On the fetal side, SLE increases the risk of miscarriage, fetal growth restriction and PTB. Anti-Ro/La antibodies can cross the placenta and are associated with neonatal lupus syndromes such as the cutaneous form of neonatal lupus and congenital heart block (42). Congenital heart block can occur antenatally and can be a dangerous condition with associated morbidity and mortality. On the contrary, cutaneous neonatal lupus is impressive by the visible aspect of the rash but usually leads to no adverse events and no scarring.

Antiphospholipid Syndrome

Antiphospholipid syndrome (APS) affects up to 5% of women of childbearing age. This condition is diagnosed by a combination of clinical and biologic features. Patients are at high risk of thromboses and pregnancy loss. The most common complications during pregnancy are miscarriage, fetal growth restriction, preeclampsia, PTB, placental abruption and stillbirth (43,44). The antibody β2 glycoprotein-I is associated with the higher risks of complications compared to anticardiolipin antibodies and lupus anticoagulant antibodies alone. This risk also increases if the pregnant woman has more than one antibody. The chance of a liveborn neonate is only 30% when the women are triple positive (45).

Rheumatoid Arthritis

Rheumatoid arthritis (RA) is an autoimmune disease resulting in a chronic inflammatory state of the joints. The prevalence is around 0.3% in pregnant women (46). Treatment during pregnancy consists of analgesia, corticosteroids, disease-modifying drugs such as azathioprine and hydroxychloroquine, and biologics such as TNF-alpha antagonists. There is growing evidence that biologics are safe to use in pregnancy (47). RA can be associated with adverse pregnancy outcomes such as fetal growth restriction and PTB. If anti-Ro antibodies are present then there is a risk of neonatal lupus and heart block, as above.

Ehlers-Danlos Syndrome (EDS)

This is a group of disorders with symptoms ranging from joint hypermobility syndrome to vascular effects. Vascular type IV is more threatening during pregnancy than others and is associated with risks of uterine rupture, PTB, postpartum hemorrhage, and maternal mortality (48).

▌CARDIAC DISEASES

Overall cardiac diseases affect 1% to 4% of pregnancies (49). However, they are a leading cause of indirect maternal death in developed countries (50).

Acquired Heart Disease

Ischemic heart disease, including myocardial infarction, is becoming more frequent in pregnancy. Diagnosis of acute coronary syndromes (ACS) involves history, electrocardiogram (ECG) changes, and a rise in cardiac enzymes, particularly troponin. Management is with percutaneous coronary intervention or antiplatelet and thrombolytic medication.

Valve disease is uncommon in pregnancy; mitral stenosis or regurgitation may be seen following rheumatic fever in women from countries of high prevalence. The main risks are atrial fibrillation and heart failure. Metallic heart valves pose a particular issue in pregnancy whereby full anticoagulation is crucial to avoid valve thrombosis. Warfarin is the best treatment option for this but is teratogenic and associated with increased stillbirth and miscarriage (51). The other option is high dose low molecular weight heparin (LMWH), which is safe for the fetus but is associated with a higher risk of a thromboembolic event for the mother (52).

Peripartum cardiomyopathy is a dilated cardiomyopathy that occurs during pregnancy or postpartum. A full recovery is only made in approximately half of patients, and there is a risk of relapse in future pregnancies leading to the need for iatrogenic PTB if it recurs.

Congenital Heart Disease

Pregnancy in women with congenital heart disease (CHD) is becoming more common. Amongst these patients, structural defects such as patent ductus arteriosus (PDA), septal defects, aortic coarctation, and tetralogy of Fallot are most frequently seen. Management depends upon the individual lesion, with PDA and septal defects usually being well tolerated. Babies of mothers with congenital heart defects are also at 3% to 5% risk to have CHD themselves, and women should have detailed fetal echocardiography in the mid-trimester anomaly scan (53).

▌RESPIRATORY DISEASES

Asthma

Asthma is an inflammatory disease characterized by recurrent attacks of wheezing and breathlessness. It is the most common pulmonary disease seen in pregnancy, occurring in 8% to 13% of pregnancies worldwide (54). Treatment includes inhaled short- or long-acting beta agonists, inhaled corticosteroids, and oral corticosteroids. Asthma medications are safe in pregnancy, and for most women asthma has no effect on the pregnancy. Severe uncontrolled asthma may increase the risk of congenital malformations, fetal growth restriction, and PTB (55). Babies are at an increased risk of transient tachypnea of the newborn and low birth weight.

Obstructive Sleep Apnea

Obstructive sleep apnea (OSA) is defined by more than five episodes per hour of apnea or hypopnea during sleep. The prevalence of OSA during pregnancy is around 7 per 10,000 in the United States (56). It is associated with preeclampsia, gestational diabetes, maternal mortality, pulmonary embolism (PE), and cardiomyopathy. Neonates are more likely to be growth restricted, which is likely due to the high rate of hypertensive complications (57).

Tuberculosis

Tuberculosis (TB) is a major issue in low- and middle-income countries and affects nine million people worldwide. Treatment of TB during pregnancy, as in non-pregnant patients, includes the use of isoniazid, rifampicin, pyrazinamide, and ethambutol in combination. These medications are considered safe in pregnancy. Fetal growth restriction may occur in mothers with pulmonary TB in pregnancy. Congenital TB is rare.

Cystic Fibrosis

Women with cystic fibrosis (CF) frequently reach childbearing age, and pregnancy in these patients is becoming more common. Management is multidisciplinary with particular attention paid to lung infections, nutrition, and pancreatic failure. Pregnancy complications include fetal growth restriction and PTB. CF is inherited in an autosomal recessive manner, so partner testing and/or prenatal testing may be performed to diagnose fetal CF.

▌HEMATOLOGIC DISEASES

Anemia

Anemia is very common during pregnancy. Due to physiologic hemodilution, anemia is defined as a hemoglobin concentration below 10.5 g/dL during pregnancy. The commonest cause is iron or folate deficiency. Maternal anemia may increase the risk of low birth weight, PTB, and perinatal and neonatal mortality in low- and middle-income countries (58).

Thromboembolic Disease

Venous thromboembolism is the commonest direct cause of maternal death in the United Kingdom (59). Changes in the balance of coagulation system during pregnancy leads to a propensity toward thrombosis both antenatally and postpartum. Risk factors include increasing age and parity, obesity, medical comorbidities, and inherited or acquired thrombophilias. Treatment during pregnancy is with LMWH. Adverse pregnancy outcomes are rare except in the case of massive PE.

Thrombocytopenia

Thrombocytopenia during pregnancy is common and affects around 5% to 10% of pregnancies. The commonest cause is gestational thrombocytopenia, which is responsible for up to three-quarters of thrombocytopenia. Only 3% of the cases of thrombocytopenia during pregnancy are due to idiopathic thrombocytopenic purpura (ITP). This immune condition is characterized by a low platelet count and the presence of platelet autoantibodies. The autoantibodies cross the placenta and can affect the fetus. Overall the outcomes of pregnancies with ITP are good (60), but neonates are at increased risk of fetal thrombocytopenia and hemorrhage complications (61). For this reason, in known or suspected cases of ITP, instrumental vaginal delivery and fetal blood sampling are avoided.

Hemoglobinopathies

Sickle cell disease (SCD) is defined by the presence of hemoglobin S in the blood. It is relatively common in Sub-Saharan Africa, the Middle East, and India and occurs in less than 1 in 10,000 people in North America (62). It is commonly treated by hydroxyurea and blood exchange. This condition is associated with a higher risk of adverse maternal and perinatal outcomes, which is highest risk for HbSS phenotypes (63). There is an increased risk of miscarriage, severe preeclampsia, fetal growth restriction, PTB, and perinatal mortality (64).

Thalassemias are inherited disorders of alpha- or beta-globin genes. Women with alpha- or beta-thalassemia trait may become anemic during pregnancy. Alpha-thalassemia major is commonly lethal due to overwhelming hydrops and anemia, unless fetal blood transfusion is provided. Women with beta-thalassemia major are usually transfusion dependent and experience complications of iron overload.

Both SCD and thalassemias are recessively inherited, so partner and/or invasive testing can be considered for diagnosis of the fetus.

RENAL DISEASE

Chronic kidney disease (CKD) is classified according to estimated glomerular filtration rate (GFR). In pregnancy, creatinine levels are used instead of eGFR, which increases naturally in pregnancy. CKD occurs in 0.3% to 3% of women of reproductive age (65). Management of CKD in pregnancy depends on the underlying cause, and involves surveillance for complications. Most women with mild renal impairment do not experience any change in their renal function during pregnancy. In severe CKD, there is a risk of irreversible worsening of their renal function. Women with severe CKD are at risk of adverse pregnancy outcomes such as preeclampsia, fetal growth restriction, and PTB (66).

LIVER DISEASES

Intrahepatic Cholestasis of Pregnancy

Intrahepatic cholestasis of pregnancy (ICP), formerly known as obstetric cholestasis, is relatively common during pregnancy with a prevalence between 0.2% to 2% and occurs mostly during the third trimester (67). The main symptom is pruritus. The diagnosis is made by an elevation of maternal serum of bile acids after excluding other causes. Treatment is commonly with ursodeoxycholic acid, although a recent study has shown that this does not reduce adverse perinatal outcomes nor itching severity (68). Neonatal complications are related to the absolute level of bile acids. In women with high levels of bile acids, there is an increased risk of stillbirth, PTB, low Apgar scores, and neonatal unit admission (69).

Acute Fatty Liver of Pregnancy

Acute fatty liver of pregnancy (AFLP) is an uncommon and extremely serious condition that affects approximately 1 in 10,000 pregnancies. It occurs mainly in the third trimester, more commonly in multiple pregnancies, with clinical features of nausea, HTN, abdominal pain, and jaundice (70). It leads to liver and renal dysfunction, hypoglycemia, coagulopathy, and encephalopathy. It is associated with a perinatal mortality rate of approximately 11%.

GASTROINTESTINAL DISEASES

Inflammatory Bowel Disease (IBD)

Crohn disease (CD) and ulcerative colitis (UC) are chronic inflammatory diseases of the bowel and are relatively frequent in women of childbearing age. Diagnosis is typically made following biopsies of gastrointestinal (GI) tract mucosa taken during endoscopy studies. Treatment involves disease-modifying agents, corticosteroids, immunosuppressants, biologics, and surgery. In quiescent or well-controlled inflammatory bowel disease (IBD), pregnancy outcomes are usually good. In active or severe disease there is a risk of infertility, miscarriage, fetal growth restriction, and PTB. Cesarean section is usually not required unless there is perianal CD (71).

Celiac Disease

Celiac disease is an autoimmune disorder of gluten intolerance. The prevalence of this disease is around 1% in Europe and in the United States. Active celiac disease in pregnancy is associated with an increased risk of miscarriage, fetal growth restriction, PTB, and stillbirth. Treatment with a gluten-free diet reduces these risks (72).

Gallbladder Disease

Pregnancy affects gallbladder contractility and biliary stone formation, with gallstones reported to occur in 1% to 3% of all pregnant women (73). Acute cholecystitis affects 0.1% of pregnant women. The clinical presentation is similar to that of the non-pregnant patient (right upper quadrant pain, fever, tachycardia, leukocytosis, and inflammation of the gallbladder wall). Imaging with transabdominal ultrasound is the most useful modality to confirm the diagnosis. Magnetic or endoscopic retrograde cholangiopancreatography can be performed in pregnancy, as can surgical cholecystectomy if required due to sepsis or complications.

The Acute Abdomen in Pregnancy

Acute abdominal pain with signs of peritonism can occur in pregnancy for a number of non-obstetric reasons, as in non-pregnant women. These include acute appendicitis, acute pancreatitis, torted or ruptured ovarian cysts, infection such as pyelonephritis, cholecystitis, or calculi in the urinary or biliary tracts. These diseases should be kept in mind alongside obstetric causes when assessing pregnant women with abdominal pain. Acute appendicitis in pregnancy should be treated surgically as it can become severe and complications such as perforation and abscess can occur. Fetal loss occurs in approximately 1.5% of cases of simple appendicitis in pregnancy, rising to 36% if perforation occurs (74).

NEUROLOGIC DISEASE

Epilepsy

Epilepsy affects 0.5% to 1% of women and is the commonest neurologic disorder in pregnancy. Treatment involves the use of antiepileptic drugs (AEDs), and the majority of women have stable seizure control in pregnancy. Optimization of medication and seizure control prior to pregnancy is important. Studies have not shown any increase in miscarriage or fetal hypoxic brain injury in women with epilepsy, although fetal bradycardias during seizures have been documented. There is an increased risk of congenital malformations in pregnancies affected by epilepsy; this risk is increased by certain AEDs and polytherapy. High-dose folic acid supplementation (5 mg/day) should ideally be taken women with epilepsy prior to conception. Anomalies commonly seen include neural tube defects, cardiac anomalies, orofacial clefts, and limb reduction defects. Sodium valproate is associated with double the risk of other AEDs and should not be used in women of reproductive age unless other treatments are ineffective or not tolerated (75). Children born to mothers with epilepsy have an increased risk of developing the condition themselves.

Multiple Sclerosis

Multiple sclerosis (MS) is an inflammatory disease that affects the white matter of the spinal cord and brain. It affects up to 0.1% of women of reproductive age. Relapses in pregnancy are often treated with corticosteroids; outside of pregnancy beta-interferon and other disease-modifying agents are used, and there is increasing evidence for their safety in pregnancy. MS has not been shown to increase adverse pregnancy outcomes for the neonate.

Migraine

Headaches and migraines are common in pregnancy and may increase in frequency throughout gestation. Management typically involves simple analgesia; if migraines are severe or occurring frequently then prophylaxis with aspirin or beta-blockers may be used. Treatment of acute migraine with triptans in pregnancy is not common but has not been shown to have any adverse effects. Migraine increases the risk of preeclampsia; it is unclear if other adverse fetal outcomes are associated separate to this (76).

INFECTIONS IN PREGNANCY

Maternal Infections
Human Immunodeficiency Virus

Human immunodeficiency virus (HIV) affects 1.5 per 1,000 people in the United Kingdom, with higher rates in low and middle income countries, particularly in sub-Saharan Africa. Management is with antiretroviral therapy (ART), which should be continued in pregnancy. HIV is associated with an increased rate of miscarriage, fetal growth restriction, and PTB. Mother-to-child transmission (MTCT) can occur during pregnancy, delivery, and breast-feeding. This is reduced significantly by ART therapy, cesarean birth, and formula feeding, although in women with very low viral loads vaginal birth does not increase the risk of MTCT (77). The availability of elective cesarean birth and safe formula feeding varies between countries and, depending upon socioeconomic and cultural factors, may not be possible or appropriate.

Malaria

Malaria may affect pregnant women living in countries with high incidence or in women who travel to such countries. It has a high morbidity and mortality rate in pregnancy, and prompt treatment with antimalarial medication should be undertaken. Adverse effects on the fetus or neonate include miscarriage, fetal growth restriction, stillbirth, PTB, and anemia (78).

Hepatitis

Viral hepatitis is a common cause of hepatic dysfunction in pregnancy. Hepatitis A and E viruses are spread by the fecal-oral route and are most commonly seen following travel. Hepatitis A is usually self-limiting and without serious consequences; hepatitis E is the same outside of pregnancy but in pregnant women hepatitis E can cause maternal liver failure, encephalopathy, and death.

Hepatitis B and C are transmitted via blood products; hepatitis D is also transmitted via blood products and only affects people already infected with hepatitis B. Hepatitis B and C are typically screened for in pregnancy; they are not known to cause congenital malformations, but vertical transmission can occur in 3% to 5% of cases. Hepatitis B vaccination and immunoglobulin can be administered to the neonate to reduce this risk.

Other causes of hepatitis include the herpes simplex virus, Epstein-Barr virus, and cytomegalovirus (CMV). Acute hepatitis can also occur due to nonimmune etiology, such as autoimmune hepatitis and alcohol use.

Upper Respiratory Tract Infections

The common "cold" is not associated with adverse perinatal outcomes. Influenza during pregnancy, particularly in the third trimester and early in the postpartum period, can be associated with more severe effects than in the nonpregnant population, and the seasonal influenza vaccination is recommended for all pregnant women.

On current data, there is no definitive evidence of maternal fetal transmission of SARS-CoV-2 to the fetus and it is as yet unclear if maternal infection increases adverse outcomes such as preterm birth or stillbirth.

Pneumonia

Severe pneumoniae could occur during the pregnancy. The diagnosis is often delayed leading to severe maternal morbidity (79). It seems to increase the risk of preeclampsia in the rest of the pregnancy.

Lower Urinary Tract Infections

Urinary tract infections (UTIs) occur in approximately 8% of pregnancies and have been associated with low birth weight and prematurity (80). Recurrent UTIs can be managed with antibiotic prophylaxis as in nonpregnant women. UTIs in pregnancy are more likely to develop into ascending infection (pyelonephritis) than in nonpregnant women.

Pyelonephritis

Pyelonephritis occurs in approximately 2% of pregnancies and can cause serious maternal morbidity, septicemia, and shock. Treatment involves hospitalization and antimicrobial therapy. Miscarriage or preterm labor can occur during an acute episode.

Fetal Infections
Cytomegalovirus

CMV usually causes a subclinical maternal infection but can have severe fetal effects. Fetal transmission is more common with primary infections, with infection rates of 30% to 40%, although only half of these will be symptomatic at birth. Fetal abnormalities may include ventriculomegaly, hepatosplenomegaly, intracranial calcifications, and fetal growth restriction. Other abnormalities that may occur in childhood include sensorineural hearing loss, chorioretinitis, hepatitis, and psychomotor retardation. Congenital CMV should be confirmed at birth and, if positive, postnatal treatment with valganciclovir or ganciclovir should be considered as there is evidence that this can reduce hearing loss and improve neurodevelopmental outcomes (81).

Toxoplasmosis

Primary toxoplasmosis infection during pregnancy is usually mild or undetected in women but can have significant effects on a developing fetus. Later gestational age at the time of exposure is associated with higher chance of transmission, though infection earlier in pregnancy is associated with more severe fetal or neonatal effects (81). Fetal complications may include ventriculomegaly, intracranial calcifications, microcephaly, ascites, and fetal growth restriction. Clinical findings often are not seen at birth; however, 55% to 85% of infants infected will develop symptoms such as chorioretinitis, hearing loss, and psychomotor retardation and 4% will die within the first year of life. Post-exposure treatment with spiramycin or pyrimethamine–sulfonamide does not eliminate the risk of congenital infection.

Varicella–Zoster Virus

Over 90% of women in Western Europe have previously been exposed to varicella–zoster virus (VZV), and primary chickenpox in pregnancy is rare (82). If it occurs, the maternal infection can be severe including pneumonia, hepatitis, and encephalitis. Varicella immunoglobulin should be offered to pregnant women with a history of VZV exposure up to 10 days after the contact but is not effective if a rash has already developed. Oral acyclovir is used if pregnant women present within 24 hours of rash onset. Fetal varicella syndrome can occur with primary maternal infection until approximately 28 weeks' gestation. Clinical findings include skin scarring in a dermatomal distribution, eye defects (microphthalmia, chorioretinitis, or cataracts), limb hypoplasia, and neurologic abnormalities (microcephaly, cortical atrophy, mental retardation, or dysfunction of bowel and bladder sphincters). If primary maternal VZV develops around delivery or immediately postpartum, there is a 20% risk of neonatal varicella infection.

Parvovirus

Parvovirus B19 causes a flu-like illness that may be unnoticed. Primary infection in pregnancy is not associated with congenital defects but can cause severe fetal anemia. The virus infects fetal erythroid progenitor cells, which can lead to miscarriage, high output cardiac failure and nonimmune hydrops fetalis (NIHF). *In utero* red cell transfusion or delivery may be indicated.

Rubella

Primary maternal rubella infection in pregnancy may be symptomatic in approximately half of women. Fetal infection is commonest in the first trimester and is not reported to occur after 20 weeks' gestation. Congenital rubella infection can involve ocular defects (cataracts, microphthalmia), heart defects (PDA, septal defects), sensorineural hearing loss, microcephaly, and mental retardation.

Zika Virus

Primary infection with Zika virus during pregnancy causes a mild, often unnoticed, maternal infection. Congenital Zika virus syndrome is more likely to occur with maternal infections early in gestation. Clinical abnormalities include cranial abnormalities (microcephaly, ventriculomegaly, cranial calcifications, cerebellar atrophy, vermian agenesis, Blake's pouch cyst), microphthalmia, oligohydramnios, and fetal growth restriction (83).

SKIN DISEASE

Eczema and Psoriasis

These preexisting conditions may improve or flare during pregnancy and generally do not have any adverse pregnancy outcomes. Most treatment, particularly topical, is safe in treatment, although methotrexate is teratogenic and should be avoided.

Polymorphic Eruption of Pregnancy

This occurs in 0.5% of pregnancies, usually in the third trimester, and has a specific distribution of pruritic papules on the abdomen (within striae but with umbilical sparing), upper thighs, and upper arms. Treatment is with emollients and steroid cream, and there are no known adverse fetal effects.

Pemphigoid Gestationis

Pemphigoid gestationis is an autoimmune bullous disorder that occurs in 1 in 2,000 to 1 in 60,000 pregnancies (84). Urticarial papules and plaques typically develop on the abdomen and mostly within the umbilical region (as opposed to polymorphic eruption of pregnancy [PEP]). Tense blisters may occur. Treatment is with topical or systemic corticosteroids. Fetal effects can occur, with an increased risk of low birth weight, PTB, and stillbirth.

PSYCHIATRIC DISORDERS

Eating Disorders

Eating disorders affecting up to 7.2% of pregnant women (85). Binge-eating and self-induced vomiting among women with preexisting eating disorders decrease during the pregnancy (86). Anorexia and bulimia are associated with an increased risk of fetal growth restriction. Anorexia is also associated with an increased risk of postpartum hemorrhage due to vitamin K deficiency.

Addiction

It is reported that of the 600,000 pregnancies recorded in the United Kingdom each year, 30,000 involve substance abusers (87). Fetal alcohol syndrome is estimated to affect 0.2 to 0.9 in 1,000 births in the United States. Clinical features include short height, low body weight, small head size, poor coordination, low intelligence and behavioral problems. Tobacco use in pregnancy increases the risk of PTB, low birth weight, and sudden infant death syndrome (SIDS). Opioid addiction can increase the risk of PTB, stillbirth, and neonatal abstinence syndrome (NAS). NAS is a group of withdrawal symptoms that most commonly occurs in newborns after exposure to opioids during pregnancy (See Chapters 14 and 54).

Depression and Anxiety

Depression and anxiety are the most common mental health problems during pregnancy, affecting approximately 12% of women in pregnancy and 15% to 20% of women in the first year after childbirth (88). During pregnancy and the postnatal period, anxiety disorders (e.g., panic disorder, generalized anxiety disorder, obsessive–compulsive disorder, and posttraumatic stress disorder) can occur on their own or can coexist with depression. These conditions can affect infant bonding and the ability to provide appropriate care to the infant and child.

Psychosis

Psychosis can be exacerbated during pregnancy and the postnatal period. Postpartum psychosis affects between 1 and 2 in 1,000 women, with preexisting bipolar disorder being a particular risk factor (88). Symptoms can include hallucinations, delusions, mania, and confusion. For the neonate, there is a risk of neglect or, rarely, physical harm.

OBESITY

Obesity, defined as a BMI ≥ 30 kg/m^2 is increasing in women of reproductive age in many countries. In the United Kingdom for the first time over half (50.4%) of women giving birth in 2016–2017 were recorded as overweight or obese at the time of booking (59). Pregnant women who are obese are at greater risk of a variety of pregnancy-related complications compared with women of normal BMI, including preeclampsia and gestational diabetes. For the fetus and child, maternal obesity is associated with an increased risk of a range of structural anomalies including neural tube defects, cardiovascular abnormalities, cleft lip

THE FETAL PATIENT

and palate, hydrocephaly, and limb reduction defects (89). The increased rate of these abnormalities is not fully explained by the increased rate of gestational diabetes. Ultrasound scanning and screening (e.g., noninvasive prenatal testing) are both adversely affected by increased maternal weight, which may lead to abnormalities not being detected. Women with obesity have an increased risk of stillbirth, induction of labor, and emergency cesarean section.

Bariatric surgery has become an increasingly common method for morbidly obese individuals to achieve sustainable weight loss, with 40% of procedures performed in women of reproductive age. Women who have undergone bariatric surgery have a reduced rate of gestational diabetes and preeclampsia in subsequent pregnancies, but an increased rate of maternal anemia, fetal growth restriction, and PTB (89). It is recommended that women wait 12 to 18 months following bariatric surgery before becoming pregnant as conception before then is during the time of rapid weight loss and is associated with very poor fetal outcomes.

SOCIOECONOMIC DEPRIVATION

Both between countries and within countries, socioeconomic deprivation is associated with worse outcomes for both mother and baby. Maternal mortality and morbidity, miscarriage, PTB, and low birth weight are all associated with increasing socioeconomic deprivation. Potential mechanisms for this are multiple and complex, and include interactions with ethnicity, obesity, health-related behaviors such as smoking, illicit drug taking and access to screening programs, domestic violence, and access to services (e.g., contraception, abortion, preconceptual counseling and antenatal care). The London Measure of Unplanned Pregnancy (LMUP), an international and psychometrically validated six-part questionnaire assesses pregnancy planning/intention. In high- and low-income populations, it has been found to identify women with a higher risk of adverse pregnancy outcomes such as preterm birth and low birth weight (90).

CANCER IN PREGNANCY

Cancer affects 1 of every 1,000 pregnancies, and the rate is predicted to rise given as the age of childbearing increases (91). The most common cancers during pregnancy are cervical, breast, melanoma, acute leukemias and lymphomas, and colorectal carcinoma. Stage for stage, carcinoma identified during pregnancy may be more advanced comparing non-pregnant and pregnant women, likely reflecting a delay in diagnosis due to physiologic changes of pregnancy rather than more aggressive disease during pregnancy. Pregnancy termination has not been found to alter cancer progression. Metastasis to the fetus or placenta has been reported in fewer than 70 cases, mostly cancers of the breast, cervix, melanoma, thyroid, and leukemia and lymphoma (92).

Decisions regarding management of malignancies during pregnancy are compounded by the timing in gestation as well as assessing risks to both mother and fetus. Treatment strategies should be coordinated through a multidisciplinary team involving the obstetrician, maternal–fetal medicine specialist, medical oncologist and/or radiation oncologist, neonatologist, surgeon, and psychologist. Cytotoxic chemotherapy should be avoided in the first trimester, although its use in the second and third trimesters is considered relatively safe. Concerns include risks of stillbirth, fetal growth restriction, and premature birth (91). Radiation should be delayed until the postpartum period. Most authorities recommend delivery after 32 to 34 weeks when there is a high likelihood of fetal maturity and survival. Adequate maternal and neonatal follow-up are critical.

Radiation exposure to the pelvis can result in damage to the uterus, and in subsequent pregnancies some reports suggest higher risks of miscarriage, fetal growth restriction, PTB, stillbirth, and placenta accreta (93).

PREGNANCY AFTER TRANSPLANTATION

The first successful pregnancy following organ transplantation occurred in 1958 in a woman who received a kidney from her identical twin sister (94). Since then, thousands of successful pregnancies have been completed after organ transplants (kidney, heart, lung, liver, intestine, pancreas, bone marrow, and combinations of organs); the most data exist for pregnancies following kidney transplants. Great success has been achieved in this field, although pregnancy can present unique challenges after transplantation. There may be medical concerns due to the underlying condition leading to the transplant—for example, for women with kidney transplants, specific issues include HTN, elevated creatinine levels, or proteinuria. Other concerns are for teratogenicity from immunosuppressive medications, graft failure/rejection, and overall risks of pregnancy complications.

In the United States, updated data regarding pregnancy outcomes among transplant recipients, especially regarding use of newer immunosuppressive agents, are collected by the National Transplantation Pregnancy Registry that was established in 1991 (95). Birth defects are reported in 5% to 40% of infants born to patients after transplant compared to the background rate of 1% to 2%; this is primarily thought to be related to medication exposure during organogenesis. Most experts advise waiting 1 to 2 years after transplant before conceiving. Graft failure or host rejection occurs infrequently during gestation, although it may occur unpredictably, and graft function does not seem to be affected by pregnancy if it was stable prior to conception (94). PTB and lower birth weight infants are commonly seen in pregnancies among transplant patients. Total body irradiation and bone marrow transplant is associated with an increased risk of PTB and fetal growth restriction, particularly in women who had a transplant as a child.

CONCLUSIONS

When considering pregnancy on the background of maternal illness there are some key concepts. Firstly, all women of reproductive age with medical conditions should have fertility and reproductive choices discussed and be offered specific advice about their own conditions and risk to enable them to plan pregnancies at an optimal time for themselves. Women desiring pregnancy should be encouraged to optimize their condition before they conceive through careful consideration of their lifestyle and diet, and by switching to the optimal medications if indicated. They should take folic acid periconceptually, at an increased dose if indicated. Secondly, once pregnant, multidisciplinary team management including obstetricians, relevant specialists, and neonatologists is usually indicated so that recommendations about pregnancy management may be made reflecting an appropriate breadth of expertise, in order to comprehensively balance risks and benefits for the women and her fetus. Finally, women should have a dating scan in the first trimester to confirm accurate gestational age and should be prescribed low-dose aspirin by 16 weeks of gestation if there are risks of fetal growth restriction or preeclampsia associated with their condition. Fetal growth and well-being should be monitored, if necessary with serial fetal growth scans usually every 4 weeks. Routine antenatal care such as testing for maternal blood group antibodies at 28 weeks, vaccination against whooping cough and influenza, and screening for diabetes should follow on as usual. Planning the optimal gestational age and route of delivery is important taking into consideration the pregnant woman's choices.

REFERENCES

1. Alfirevic Z, Stampalija T, Medley N. Cervical stitch (cerclage) for preventing preterm birth in singleton pregnancy. *Cochrane Database Syst Rev* 2017;6:CD008991.

2. Norman JE, Marlow N, Messow C-M, et al. Vaginal progesterone prophylaxis for preterm birth (the OPPTIMUM study): a multicentre, randomised, double-blind trial. *Lancet* 2016;387(10033):2106.

3. Costeloe KL, Hennessy EM, Haider S, et al. Short term outcomes after extreme preterm birth in England: comparison of two birth cohorts in 1995 and 2006 the EPICure studies). *BMJ* 2012;345:e7976.

4. Roberts D, Brown J, Medley N, et al. Antenatal corticosteroids for accelerating fetal lung maturation for women at risk of preterm birth. *Cochrane Database Syst Rev* 2017;(3):CD004454.

5. Doyle LW, Crowther CA, Middleton P, et al. Antenatal magnesium sulfate and neurologic outcome in preterm infants: a systematic review. *Obstetr Gynecol* 2009;113(6):1327.

6. Sentilhes L, Sénat M-V, Ancel P-Y, et al. Prevention of spontaneous preterm birth: guidelines for clinical practice from the French College of Gynaecologists and Obstetricians (CNGOF). *Eur J Obstet Gynecol Reprod Biol* 2017;210:217.

7. Hughes RG, Brocklehurst P, Steer PJ, et al.; on behalf of the Royal College of Obstetricians and Gynaecologists. Prevention of early-onset neonatal group B streptococcal disease. Green-top Guideline No 36. *BJOG* 2017;124:e280.

8. Delayed umbilical cord clamping after birth. ACOG Committee Opinion Number 684. January 2017. Available from: https://www.acog.org/clinical/clinical-guidance/committee-opinion/articles/2020/12/delayed-umbilical-cord-clamping-after-birth

9. Liu L, Johnson HL, Cousens S, et al. Global, regional, and national causes of child mortality: an updated systematic analysis for 2010 with time trends since 2000. *Lancet* 2012;379(9832):2151.

10. Bateman BT, Bansil P, Hernandez-Diaz S, et al. Prevalence, trends, and outcomes of chronic hypertension: a nationwide sample of delivery admissions. *Am J Obstet Gynecol* 2012;206(2):134.e1.

11. NICE. Hypertension in adults: diagnosis and management. 2019 October 1. Available from: https://www.nice.org.uk/guidance/ng136

12. American College of Cardiology. Guideline for high blood pressure in adults. 2017. Available from: https://www.acc.org/latest-in-cardiology/ten-points-to-remember/2017/11/09/11/41/2017-guideline-for-high-blood-pressure-in-adults#:~:text=For%20adults%20with%20confirmed%20hypertension,Hg%20is%20recommended%20as%20reasonable

13. Magee LA, von Dadelszen P, Rey E, et al. Less-tight versus tight control of hypertension in pregnancy. *N Engl J Med* 2015;372(5):407.

14. Bramham K, Parnell B, Nelson-Piercy C, et al. Chronic hypertension and pregnancy outcomes: systematic review and meta-analysis. *BMJ* 2014;348:g2301.

15. Panaitescu AM, Syngelaki A, Prodan N, et al. Chronic hypertension and adverse pregnancy outcome: a cohort study. *Ultrasound Obstet Gynecol* 2017;50(2):228.

16. Tan MY, Wright D, Syngelaki A, et al. Comparison of diagnostic accuracy of early screening for pre-eclampsia by NICE guidelines and a method combining maternal factors and biomarkers: results of SPREE. *Ultrasound Obstet Gynecol* 2018;51(6):743.

17. Bombrys AE, Barton JR, Nowacki EA, et al. Expectant management of severe preeclampsia at less than 27 weeks' gestation: maternal and perinatal outcomes according to gestational age by weeks at onset of expectant management. *Am J Obstet Gynecol* 2008;199(3):247.e1.

18. Madazli R, Yuksel MA, Imamoglu M, et al. Comparison of clinical and perinatal outcomes in early- and late-onset preeclampsia. *Arch Gynecol Obstet* 2014;290(1):53.

19. Stubert J, Ullmann S, Dieterich M, et al. Clinical differences between early- and late-onset severe preeclampsia and analysis of predictors for perinatal outcome. *J Perinat Med* 2014;42(5):617.

20. van Esch JJA, van Heijst AF, de Haan AFJ, et al. Early-onset preeclampsia is associated with perinatal mortality and severe neonatal morbidity. *J Matern Fetal Neonatal Med* 2017;30(23):2789.

21. van Oostwaard MF, van Eerden L, de Laat MW, et al. Maternal and neonatal outcomes in women with severe early onset pre-eclampsia before 26 weeks of gestation, a case series. *BJOG* 2017;124(9):1013.

22. Ni Y, Cheng W. Comparison of indications of pregnancy termination and prognosis of mothers and neonates in early- and late-onset preeclampsia. *Hypertens Pregnancy* 2016;35(3):315.

23. NICE guidelines. Diabetes in pregnancy: management from preconception to the postnatal period. 2015 August. Available from: https://www.nice.org.uk/guidance/ng3

24. Admon LK, Winkelman TNA, Moniz MH, et al. Disparities in chronic conditions among women hospitalized for delivery in the United States, 2005–2014. *Obstet Gynecol* 2017;130(6):1319.

25. Management of diabetes from preconception to the postnatal period: summary of NICE guidance. *BMJ* 2008;336(7646):714.

26. Agha MM, Glazier RH, Moineddin R, et al. Congenital abnormalities in newborns of women with pregestational diabetes: a time-trend analysis, 1994 to 2009. *Birth Defects Res Part A Clin Mol Teratol* 2016;106(10):831.

27. Sacks DA, Hadden DR, Maresh M, et al. Frequency of gestational diabetes mellitus at collaborating centers based on IADPSG Consensus Panel–Recommended

Criteria: The Hyperglycemia and Adverse Pregnancy Outcome (HAPO) Study. *Diabetes Care* 2012;35(3):526.

28. Xiang AH, Wang X, Martinez MP, et al. Maternal type 1 diabetes and risk of autism in offspring. *JAMA* 2018;320(1):89.

29. Adane AA, Mishra GD, Tooth LR. Diabetes in pregnancy and childhood cognitive development: a systematic review. *Pediatrics* 2016;137(5):e20154234.

30. Cleary-Goldman J, Malone FD, Lambert-Messerlian G, et al. Maternal thyroid hypofunction and pregnancy outcome. *Obstet Gynecol* 2008;112(1):85.

31. Sahu MT, Das V, Mittal S, et al. Overt and subclinical thyroid dysfunction among Indian pregnant women and its effect on maternal and fetal outcome. *Arch Gynecol Obstet* 2010;281(2):215.

32. Casey BM, Thom EA, Peaceman AM, et al. Treatment of subclinical hypothyroidism or hypothyroxinemia in pregnancy. *N Engl J Med* 2017;376(9):815.

33. Cooper DS, Laurberg P. Hyperthyroidism in pregnancy. *Lancet Diabetes Endocrinol* 2013;1(3):238.

34. Luewan S, Chakkabut P, Tongsong T. Outcomes of pregnancy complicated with hyperthyroidism: a cohort study. *Arch Gynecol Obstet* 2011;283(2):243.

35. Hirsch D, Kopel V, Nadler V, et al. Pregnancy outcomes in women with primary hyperparathyroidism. *J Clin Endocrinol Metab* 2015;100(5):2115.

36. Nelson-Piercy C. *Handbook of obstetrics medicine*, 5th ed. Boca Raton, FL: CRC Press, 2015. Available from: https://www.taylorfrancis.com/books/9780429330766

37. Molitch ME. Endocrinology in pregnancy: management of the pregnant patient with a prolactinoma. *Eur J Endocrinol* 2015;172(5):R205.

38. Lambert K, Rees K, Seed PT, et al. Macroprolactinomas and nonfunctioning pituitary adenomas and pregnancy outcomes. *Obstet Gynecol* 2017;129(1):185.

39. Kamoun M, Mnif MF, Charfi N, et al. Adrenal diseases during pregnancy: pathophysiology, diagnosis and management strategies. *Am J Med Sci* 2014;347(1):64.

40. Rees F, Doherty M, Grainge M, et al. The incidence and prevalence of systemic lupus erythematosus in the UK, 1999–2012. *Ann Rheum Dis* 2016;75(1):136.

41. Smyth A, Oliveira GHM, Lahr BD, et al. A systematic review and meta-analysis of pregnancy outcomes in patients with systemic lupus erythematosus and lupus nephritis. *Clin J Am Soc Nephrol* 2010;5(11):2060.

42. Zuppa AA, Riccardi F, Frezza S, et al. Neonatal lupus: follow-up in infants with anti-SSA/Ro antibodies and review of the literature. *Autoimmun Rev* 2017;16(4):427.

43. Cervera R, Serrano R, Pons-Estel GJ, et al. Morbidity and mortality in the antiphospholipid syndrome during a 10-year period: a multicentre prospective study of 1000 patients. *Ann Rheum Dis* 2015;74(6):1011.

44. Alijotas-Reig J, Esteve-Valverde E, Ferrer-Oliveras R, et al. The European Registry on Obstetric Antiphospholipid Syndrome (EUROAPS): a survey of 1000 consecutive cases. *Autoimmun Rev* 2019;18(4):406.

45. Saccone G, Berghella V, Maruotti GM, et al. Antiphospholipid antibody profile based obstetric outcomes of primary antiphospholipid syndrome: the PREGNANTS study. *Am J Obstet Gynecol* 2017;216(5):525.e1.

46. Tsuda S, Sameshima A, Sekine M, et al. Pre-conception status, obstetric outcome and use of medications during pregnancy of systemic lupus erythematosus (SLE), rheumatoid arthritis (RA) and inflammatory bowel disease (IBD) in Japan: multi-center retrospective descriptive study. *Mod Rheumatol* 2020;30(5):852.

47. Komaki F, Komaki Y, Micic D, et al. Outcome of pregnancy and neonatal complications with anti-tumor necrosis factor-α use in females with immune mediated diseases; a systematic review and meta-analysis. *J Autoimmun* 2017;76:38.

48. Murray ML, Pepin M, Peterson S, et al. Pregnancy-related deaths and complications in women with vascular Ehlers-Danlos syndrome. *Genet Med* 2014;16(12):874.

49. Regitz-Zagrosek V. 'Ten Commandments' of the 2018 ESC Guidelines for the management of cardiovascular diseases during pregnancy. *Eur Heart J* 2018;39(35):3269.

50. Knight M, Nair M, Tuffnell D, et al., eds; on behalf of MBRRACE-UK. *Saving lives, improving mothers' care—lessons learned to inform maternity care from the UK and Ireland confidential enquiries into maternal deaths and morbidity 2013–15.* Oxford: National Perinatal Epidemiology Unit, University of Oxford, 2017.

51. Soma-Pillay P, Nene Z, Mathivha TM, et al. The effect of warfarin dosage on maternal and fetal outcomes in pregnant women with prosthetic heart valves. *Obstet Med* 2011;4(1):24.

52. McLintock C, McCowan LME, North RA. Maternal complications and pregnancy outcome in women with mechanical prosthetic heart valves treated with enoxaparin. *BJOG* 2009;116(12):1585.

53. Gill HK, Splitt M, Sharland GK, et al. Patterns of recurrence of congenital heart disease: an analysis of 6,640 consecutive pregnancies evaluated by detailed fetal echocardiography. *J Am Coll Cardiol* 2003;42(5):923.

54. Hansen C, Joski P, Freiman H, et al. Medication exposure in pregnancy risk evaluation program: the prevalence of asthma medication use during pregnancy. *Matern Child Health J* 2013;17(9):1611.

55. Blais L, Kettani F-Z, Forget A, et al. Asthma exacerbations during the first trimester of pregnancy and congenital malformations: revisiting the association in a large representative cohort. *Thorax* 2015;70(7):647.

56. Louis JM, Mogos MF, Salemi JL, et al. Obstructive sleep apnea and severe maternal-infant morbidity/mortality in the United States, 1998–2009. *Sleep* 2014;37(5):843.

57. Bourjeily G, Danilack VA, Bublitz MH, et al. Obstructive sleep apnea in pregnancy is associated with adverse maternal outcomes: a national cohort. *Sleep Med* 2017;38:50.

58. Rahman MM, Abe SK, Rahman MS, et al. Maternal anemia and risk of adverse birth and health outcomes in low- and middle-income countries: systematic review and meta-analysis. *Am J Clin Nutr* 2016;103(2):495.

59. HQIP. National Maternity and Perinatal Audit (NMPA) clinical report 2019. 2019 September 12. Available from: https://www.hqip.org.uk/resource/national-maternity-and-perinatal-audit-nmpa-clinical-report-2019/#.X8TpaxP7TzI

60. Subbaiah M, Kumar S, Roy KK, et al. Pregnancy outcome in patients with idiopathic thrombocytopenic purpura. *Arch Gynecol Obstet* 2014;289(2):269.

61. Melekoğlu NA, Bay A, Aktekin EH, et al. Neonatal outcomes of pregnancy with immune thrombocytopenia. *Indian J Hematol Blood Transfus* 2017;33(2):211.

62. Hassell KL. Population estimates of sickle cell disease in the U.S. *Am J Prev Med* 2010;38(4 Suppl):S512.

63. Oteng-Ntim E, Meeks D, Seed PT, et al. Adverse maternal and perinatal outcomes in pregnant women with sickle cell disease: systematic review and meta-analysis. *Blood* 2015;125(21):3316.

64. Kuo K, Caughey AB. Contemporary outcomes of sickle cell disease in pregnancy. *Am J Obstet Gynecol* 2016;215(4):505.e1.

65. Zhang L, Wang F, Wang L, et al. Prevalence of chronic kidney disease in China: a cross-sectional survey. *Lancet* 2012;379(9818):815.

66. Zhang J-J, Ma X-X, Hao L, et al. A systematic review and meta-analysis of outcomes of pregnancy in CKD and CKD outcomes in pregnancy. *Clin J Am Soc Nephrol* 2015;10(11):1964.

67. Williamson C, Geenes V. Intrahepatic cholestasis of pregnancy. *Obstet Gynecol* 2014;124(1):120.

68. Chappell LC, Bell JL, Smith A, et al. Ursodeoxycholic acid versus placebo in women with intrahepatic cholestasis of pregnancy (PITCHES): a randomised controlled trial. *Lancet* 2019;394(10201):849.

69. Geenes V, Chappell LC, Seed PT, et al. Association of severe intrahepatic cholestasis of pregnancy with adverse pregnancy outcomes: a prospective population-based case–control study. *Hepatology* 2014;59(4):1482.

70. Liu J, Ghaziani TT, Wolf JL. Acute fatty liver disease of pregnancy: updates in pathogenesis, diagnosis, and management. *Am J Gastroenterol* 2017;112(6):838.

71. Alstead EM, Nelson-Piercy C. Inflammatory bowel disease in pregnancy. *Gut* 2003;52(2):159.

72. Saccone G, Berghella V, Sarno L, et al. Celiac disease and obstetric complications: a systematic review and metaanalysis. *Am J Obstet Gynecol* 2016;214(2):225.

73. Jelin EB, Smink DS, Vernon AH, et al. Management of biliary tract disease during pregnancy: a decision analysis. *Surg Endosc* 2008;22(1):54.

74. Weston P, Moroz P. Appendicitis in pregnancy: how to manage and whether to deliver. *Obstet Gynaecol* 2015;17(2):105.

75. Shakespeare J, Sisodiya SM. Guidance document on valproate use in women and girls of childbearing years. 28. Available from https://www.rcog.org.uk/globalassets/documents/guidelines/valproate-guidance-march-2019.pdf

76. Goadsby PJ, Goldberg J, Silberstein SD. Migraine in pregnancy. *BMJ* 2008;336(7659):1502.

77. British HIV Association. BHIVA guidelines for the treatment of HIV-1-positive adults with antiretroviral therapy. 2018 (2019 third interim update). 2018. Available from: https://www.bhiva.org/pregnancy-guidelines

78. GUIDELINE, RCOG Green-Top. *The diagnosis and treatment of malaria in pregnancy*. Royal College of Obstetricians and Gynaecologist, 2010:2.

79. Sobhy S, Babiker Z, Zamora J, et al. Maternal and perinatal mortality and morbidity associated with tuberculosis during pregnancy and the postpartum period: a systematic review and meta-analysis. *BJOG* 2017;124(5):727.

80. McCormick T, Ashe RG, Kearney PM. Urinary tract infection in pregnancy. *Obstetr Gynaecol* 2008;10(3):156.

81. Effectiveness of prenatal treatment for congenital toxoplasmosis: a meta-analysis of individual patients' data. *Lancet* 2007;369(9556):115.

82. Royal College of Obstetricians and Gynaecologists. Chickenpox in pregnancy (Green-top Guideline No. 13). 2015. Available from: https://www.rcog.org.uk/en/guidelines-research-services/guidelines/gtg13/

83. Royal College of Obstetricians and Gynaecologists. Zika virus infection and pregnancy. 2016. Available from: https://www.rcog.org.uk/en/guidelines-research-services/guidelines/zika-virus-infection-and-pregnancy/

84. Jones SV, Ambros-Rudolph C, Nelson-Piercy C. Skin disease in pregnancy. *BMJ* 2014;348:g3489.

85. Easter A, Bye A, Taborelli E, et al. Recognising the symptoms: how common are eating disorders in pregnancy? *Eur Eat Disord Rev* 2013;21(4):340.

86. Nunes MA, Pinheiro AP, Hoffmann JF, et al. Eating disorders symptoms in pregnancy and postpartum: a prospective study in a disadvantaged population in Brazil. *Int J Eat Disord* 2014;47(4):426.

87. NICE. *Pregnancy and complex social factors. A model for service provision for pregnant women with complex social factors*. National Institute for Health and Clinical Excellence, 2010;1. Available from: https://www.nice.org.uk/guidance/cg110

88. Howard LM, Megnin-Viggars O, Symington I, et al. Antenatal and postnatal mental health: summary of updated NICE guidance. *BMJ* 2014;349:g7394.

89. Royal College of Obstetricians and Gynaecologists. Care of women with obesity in pregnancy (Green-top Guideline No. 72). Available from: https://www.rcog.org.uk/en/guidelines-research-services/guidelines/gtg72/

90. Barrett G, Smith SC, Wellings K. Conceptualisation, development, and evaluation of a measure of unplanned pregnancy. *J Epidemiol Commun Health* 2004;58(5):426.

91. Pentheroudakis G, Orecchia R, Hoekstra HJ, et al. Cancer, fertility and pregnancy: ESMO Clinical Practice Guidelines for diagnosis, treatment and follow-up. *Ann Oncol* 2010;21(suppl_5):v266.

92. Dildy GA, Moise KJ, Carpenter RJ, et al. Maternal malignancy metastatic to the products of conception: a review. *Obstet Gynecol Surv* 1989;44(7):535.

93. Chiarelli AM, Marrett LD, Darlington GA. Pregnancy outcomes in females after treatment for childhood cancer. *Epidemiology* 2000;11(2):161.

94. Mastrobattista JM, Gomez-Lobo V. Pregnancy after solid organ transplantation. *Obstetr Gynecol* 2008;112(4):919.

95. Armenti VT, Constantinescu S, Moritz MJ, et al. Pregnancy after transplantation. *Transplant Rev* 2008;22(4):223.

The Impact of Prenatal Exposure to Nonnarcotic Drugs: Maternal, Fetal, Neonatal, and Long-Term Outcomes

Enrique M. Ostrea Jr., Josef M. Cortez, Maria Esterlita Villanueva-Uy, and Jonathan M. Gamiao

Drug abuse has reached epidemic proportions in the past two decades, with increases in the number of drug users and the types of drugs used. Equally alarming is an increase in the proportion of drug users among women of childbearing age, because the effects of drugs on the pregnancy and fetus can be far-reaching. Existing information in the literature on maternal, neonatal, and long-term complications of drug use during pregnancy will be presented. There are instances when the data discussed are conflicting; this may be explained by confounding factors such as polydrug drug use, socioeconomic status, environmental factors, parental education, and maternal psychopathology, which are not adequately controlled for in many studies. This chapter is confined to the discussion of nonnarcotic drugs of abuse in pregnant women (Table 14.1).

EPIDEMIOLOGY

In 2017, an estimated 271 million people worldwide aged 15 to 64 had used drugs at least once in the previous year, equivalent to 5.5% of the global population (1). In the United States, 7.2 million women aged greater than 18 years reported substance use disorder (2). Among pregnant women, substance use was lower in 2018 than in 2017: 5.4% of pregnant women used illicit drugs in 2018 versus 8.5% in 2017. This trend was also observed for tobacco and alcohol use during pregnancy: 11.6% (2018) versus 14.7% (2017) and 9.9% (2018) versus 11.5% (2017), respectively (2).

Substance exposure during pregnancy may cause congenital anomalies and/or fetal growth restriction, increase the risk of preterm birth, produce signs of withdrawal or toxicity in the neonate, or impair normal neurodevelopment (3–9). The antenatal, intrapartum, neonatal, and long-term complications associated with maternal drug misuse during pregnancy are shown in Table 14.2.

COCAINE

In 2018, about 2 million American women used cocaine and the majority are 18 to 25 years old (2). The rate of cocaine use during pregnancy is harder to estimate than other illicit substances largely due to variability in methods of detection, and partly due to social and legal consequences of its use. Maternal interviews can be unreliable; for example, in one multicenter study involving 8,527 neonates, meconium analysis was positive for cocaine exposure in 38% of cases in which the mother denied usage (10). In another study, cocaine use during pregnancy was detected by standardized maternal interview in 50.8%, meconium analysis in 67.8%, and hair analysis in 78% of cases (11).

Cocaine is an alkaloid extracted from the leaves of *Erythroxylon coca* bush. Its chemical name is methylbenzoylecgonine, and it is a naturally occurring local anesthetic. Cocaine is metabolized by plasma and hepatic esterases into three major water-soluble metabolites, ecgonine methyl ester, benzoylecgonine, and ecgonine, although other minor metabolites are also present. The half-life of cocaine in adults depends on the route of administration: on average, it is 0.6 hours after intravenous administration, 0.9 hours after oral use, and 1.3 hours after intranasal use. Cocaine metabolites can be found in the urine 72 hours after administration. In infants, metabolites can be found for up to 2 weeks after administration (12).

Pathophysiology

The pathophysiologic effects of cocaine on fetal development may be considered according to two major pathways: neurochemical and vasoconstrictive (12). The neurochemical effects result from three neurotransmitters: norepinephrine, dopamine, and serotonin. Cocaine inhibits reuptake of norepinephrine and dopamine, which accumulate at the synaptic cleft, leading to prolonged stimulation of their corresponding receptors. Therefore, the effects of norepinephrine stimulation (e.g., tachycardia, hypertension, arrhythmia, diaphoresis, tremors) and dopamine stimulation (e.g., increased alertness, euphoria or enhanced feeling of well-being, sexual excitement, heightened energy) are experienced. Cocaine also decreases the uptake of tryptophan, which affects serotonin biosynthesis (12). A diminished serotonin level is associated with diminished need for sleep, because serotonin regulates the sleep–wake cycle. Cocaine may also alter fetal programming by altering gene expression, increasing exposure to catecholamines and influencing fetal neuroendocrine pathways, which can lead to infant behavioral dysregulation, poor behavioral control and emotion regulation during childhood, and possibly a susceptibility to substance use in adolescence (13).

The mechanism of cocaine addiction is likely mediated by its effects on the dopaminergic system (5,9). The immediate response to cocaine is an increased extracellular concentration of dopamine, and in the brain, the nucleus accumbens appears to be involved in the initial rewarding effects of cocaine. Chronic cocaine exposure may affect other regions of the brain such as the caudate–putamen, which may result in prolonged addiction to the drug.

Adverse Effects of Cocaine in Pregnant Women, Obstetric Effects, and Placental Transfer

Maternal use of cocaine has been associated with a number of obstetric complications: increased rate of preterm labor, preterm premature rupture of membranes, precipitous labor, placental abruption, meconium-stained amniotic fluid, abnormal fetal heart tracings, and fetal death (5). Acute cocaine toxicity in pregnancy has been associated with acute thrombocytopenia, hypertension, blurred vision, headache, abdominal pain, seizures, myocardial infraction, and stroke (14,15).

Cocaine-induced vasoconstriction, mediated by adrenergic stimulation, may play a role in the development of obstetric complications. In pregnant animal models, the following hemodynamic changes occur following cocaine administration: (a) maternal blood pressure increases within 5 minutes after cocaine infusion, (b) uterine vascular resistance increases, (c) uterine blood flow decreases, (d) fetal heart rate and blood pressure increase, and (e) fetal partial pressure of oxygen and oxygen content decrease as a result of reduced uterine blood flow (16). Pregnancy can potentiate the toxic effects of cocaine, because progesterone can increase the adrenergic sensitivity of the receptors or delay cocaine metabolism. Further, cocaine enhances umbilical artery vasoconstrictor action of catecholamines and serotonin, presumably by increasing sensitivity of α-adrenergic receptors of arterial smooth muscle.

Effects of Cocaine Exposure on the Fetus and Neonate

Cocaine is highly lipid soluble and has a low molecular weight, thus it readily crosses the placenta. The fetal concentration of

TABLE 14.1
Nonnarcotic Drugs of Abuse in Pregnant Women

A. Stimulant/antidepressant

Cocaine

Alcohol (ethanol)

Nicotine

Amphetamines and congeners

Phencyclidine (PCP)

Marijuana

Selective serotonin reuptake inhibitors—venlafaxine, sertraline, paroxetine

B. Nonnarcotic hypnosedative

Benzodiazepines

Diazepam, chlordiazepoxide, clorazepate, flurazepam, halazepam, prazepam, clonazepam, lorazepam, quazepam, estazolam, alprazolam, oxazepam, temazepam, midazolam, triazolam

Barbiturates

Others

Baclofen

Valproate

cocaine is only a fraction of the mother's, because the placenta retains large amounts of cocaine, which offers some protection against cocaine toxicity.

The cocaine-exposed fetus is at risk for a number of complications (5). Cocaine decreases placental perfusion, which leads to poor gas exchange and impaired fetal oxygenation. Fetal hypoxemia can lead to fetal distress, meconium staining of the amniotic fluid, and low Apgar score. Meconium staining was reported in 23% of the births in cocaine-using women—approximately twice the incidence among nondrug users. There is also an increased incidence of premature birth. Many reports associate cocaine use during pregnancy with fetal growth restriction/small for gestational age, low birth weight, and small head circumference (5). However, caution should be taken in interpreting these reports—concomitant exposure to other substances such as nicotine, alcohol, opiates, and lead are confounders that contribute to impaired growth *in utero* (3). The risk of growth restriction is increased with severity of drug use. Somatic growth deceleration is evident after 32 weeks of gestation. The dose-related, negative effect of cocaine on head circumference may reflect a specific central nervous system insult that interferes with prenatal brain growth (17). A summary of the organ dysfunctions associated with cocaine use during

TABLE 14.2
Complications Associated with Maternal Abuse of Drugs during Pregnancy

Drugs	Antenatal	Intrapartum	Neonatal	Long Term
Narcotics	Stillbirth	Fetal distress	Prematurity	Persistence of withdrawal
	Spontaneous abortion	Low Apgar score	Low birth weight	Child neglect and abuse
	Fetal asphyxia	Neonatal depression	Increased mortality	Sudden infant death syndrome (SIDS)
	Maternal infection	Meconium-stained fluid	Small-for-gestational-age (SGA)	Psychomotor delay
	Premature rupture of membranes (PROM)		Aspiration pneumonia	Strabismus/nystagmus
			Meconium aspiration	Behavior problems, for example, hyperactivity, aggression, inattention, impulsiveness, short attention span
			Persistent pulmonary hypertension (PPHN)	
			Transient tachypnea	
			Hyaline membrane disease	Language problems
			Altered sleep pattern	Preschool—problems in perception, short-term memory and organization
			Thrombocytosis	
			Jaundice	
			Abstinence syndrome	
			Abnormal Brazelton Neonatal Assessment Scale (BNAS)	
Nonnarcotic hypnosedatives	Spontaneous abortion		Abstinence syndrome	
	Malformation		Floppy baby syndrome	
	IUGR		Neonatal depression (high dose)	
			Omphalocele-exstrophy (diazepam)	
			Spina bifida complex (overdose)	
			Delayed feeding, poor suck	
			Depressed respiration	
			Hyperphagia	
Cocaine	Stillbirth	Abruptio placenta	Prematurity	Strabismus/nystagmus
	Spontaneous abortion	Premature labor	Low birth weight	Problem in expressive and receptive language
	Increased uterine vascular resistance	PROM	Small for gestation	Low verbal comprehension
	Maternal infection	Shortened duration of labor	Small head circumference	Poor recognition, memory and information processing
	Placental infarcts	Meconium-stained fluid	Multiorgan dysfunction	
	Intrauterine growth retardation (IUGR)		Abnormal EEG	Low Fagan score
	Abnormal fetal breathing		Abnormal auditory brain stem responses (ABR)	Low Bayley score
			Transient hypertonia	Poor cognitive functions
			Subependymal cysts	Decreased visual attention
			Cerebral infarction	
			Moebius syndrome	
			Heart rate/rhythm abnormalities	

Long-Term Effects of Prenatal Alcohol Use

Variations in long-term growth retardation have been observed with alcohol use in pregnancy (64). Growth retardation at 8 months of age and significant effects on height and head circumference in children at 6 years of age have been reported. Some catch up growth after 8 months of age has been observed whether the children were exposed to alcohol in the first and second trimesters or throughout gestation. However, head circumference remained smaller among children who were exposed throughout pregnancy (65). Some children who had prenatal alcohol exposure continued to be smaller in weight, length, and head circumference at 3 years of age even after controlling for nutrition, postnatal environment, exposure to alcohol during lactation, and other significant covariates (64).

Behavioral and Cognitive Effects

A review of literature showed that the impact of prenatal alcohol exposure on early neurodevelopmental outcomes is poorly understood—whether the teratogenic effects of alcohol during early gestation, or the effects of alcohol on later brain development are detrimental to specific functional domains is unclear (66). One systematic review of longitudinal studies reported that prenatal alcohol exposure influenced delays in receptive and expressive communication up to 36 months (67). Furthermore, prenatal alcohol exposure predicted neurobehavioral changes up to 22 years of age as measured by the adult self-report on various domains such as internalizing, externalizing, attention, and critical items scales (68). Alcohol use throughout pregnancy was associated with a higher rate of behavioral problems although there is a complex association between dose, pattern, and timing of prenatal alcohol exposure and childhood behavior (69). More research is needed to better understand the mechanisms by which prenatal alcohol exposure affects neurobehavior and dysmorphisms (70).

Fetal Alcohol Spectrum Disorders (FASD): Definitions, Prevalence, and Risk Factors

FASD encompasses the range of adverse effects associated with alcohol use in pregnancy, including the fetal alcohol syndrome (FAS), ARBDs, and alcohol-related neurodevelopmental disorders (ARND) (71). FAS refers to a clinical diagnosis involving specific physical, behavioral, and cognitive abnormalities following prenatal alcohol exposure (71,72). ARBD refers to physical findings related to congenital structural dysplasias and malformations affecting organ systems including minor anomalies but with normal neurodevelopment (71). ARBD may account for 5% of all congenital anomalies (68). Table 14.4 shows the various dysmorphic

TABLE 14.4

Fetal and Neonatal Dysmorphogenesis Secondary to Prenatal Exposure to Alcohol

Central nervous system	
Neurobehavioral	Intellectual impairment (i.e., mild to moderate mental retardation),[a] low IQ (65–70), hypotonia,[b] developmental delay, poor coordination, cognitive and sensory deficits, attention deficits, hyperactivity and irritability in infancy, hyperactivity in childhood, language disabilities and sleep–wake cycle disturbances, electroencephalogram hypersynchrony, delayed or deficient myelination, corpus callosum hypoplasia, echolalia, cerebral palsy
Craniofacial	
Head	Microcephaly,[a] Dandy-Walker malformation, anencephaly, porencephaly, meningomyelocele, spasmus nutans
Eyes	Ocular retinal tortuosity, ptosis, strabismus, epicanthal folds, myopia, retinal coloboma, astigmatism, steep corneal curvature, anterior chamber anomalies, sensorineural hearing loss
Ears	Poorly formed conchae and posterior rotation of the ear and eustachian tube
Nose	Short, upturned[b] hypoplastic philtrum[a]
Mouth	Dental malalignments, small teeth with faulty enamel, retrognathia in infancy[a] or relative prognathia in adolescence, cleft lip or cleft palate, malocclusions, prominent palatine ridges, thinned upper vermillion,[a] poor suck reflex
Maxilla	Hypoplastic[b]
Cardiovascular	
Heart	All cardiac defects (57%), particularly ventricular septal defect, atrial septal defects, murmurs, tetralogy of Fallot, double-outlet right ventricle, dextrocardia, patent ductus arteriosus, and great vessel anomalies
Pulmonary	
Chest	Pectus excavatum, bifid xiphoid
Lungs	Pulmonary atresia, atelectasis, upper respiratory infections
Gastrointestinal	
Abdomen	Inguinal and abdominal hernias, diastasis recti, gastroschisis, hepatic fibrosis, childhood cirrhosis, extrahepatic biliary atresia, hyperbilirubinemia in childhood
Urogenital	
Renal	Hydronephrosis; small rotated kidneys; aplastic, dysplastic, or hypoplastic kidneys; horseshoe kidneys; ureteral duplications; megaloureter, cystic diverticula; vesicovaginal fistula, pyelonephritis
Dermatologic	
Dermatoglyphic	Aberrant fingerprint and palmar creases, hemangiomas in one-half of the cases, disproportionately diminished adipose tissue,[b] abnormal whorls on scalp, hirsutism in infancy, nail hypoplasia, poor proprioception
Orthopedic	
Skeletal	Polydactyly, radioulnar synostosis, talipes equinovarus, dislocated hip, scoliosis, Klippel-Feil syndrome, limited joint movement, lumbosacral lipoma, shortened fifth digit, syndactyly, camptodactyly, clinodactyly, flexion contractures
Endocrinology	
Congenital	DiGeorge syndrome

[a]Feature seen in 80% of patients.
[b]Feature seen in more than 50% of patients.

THE FETAL PATIENT

features that may be observed in the fetus and infant after prenatal alcohol exposure.

In a 2017 meta-analysis, the global prevalence of alcohol use in pregnancy is 9.8% (6). Further, the authors reported that the prevalence of FAS in the general population was 14.6 per 10,000, or 1 in every 67 women who consumed alcohol while pregnant (6). There are regional differences in the prevalence of FASD: the WHO European region had the highest prevalence (19.8 per 1,000), and the WHO Eastern Mediterranean region had the lowest prevalence (0.1 per 1,000) likely due to cultural variations in alcohol consumption (73).

The Collaborative Initiative on Fetal Alcohol Spectrum Disorders (CI-FASD) defined three specific criteria for the diagnosis of FASD; infants must exhibit an abnormality from each category (72,74):

1. Prenatal or postnatal growth retardation, that is, weight, length, or head circumference less than 10th percentile when corrected for gestational age
2. CNS involvement, which includes signs of neurologic abnormalities (e.g., irritability in infancy, hyperactivity during childhood), developmental delay, hypotonia or intellectual impairment (e.g., mental retardation)
3. Characteristic facial dysmorphology (at least two of the three must be present)
   - Microcephaly (head circumference <3rd percentile)
   - Microphthalmia or short palpebral fissures
   - Poorly developed philtrum, thin upper lip, that is, vermillion border, and flattening of the maxilla

Physical findings of smooth philtrum, thin upper lip, and short palpebral fissure are very common in FAS. Presence of some, but not all, of these features is defined as ARBDs, or fetal alcohol effects. Current criteria for diagnosis of FAS depend on recognition of subtle physical anomalies, growth retardation, and nonspecific developmental aberrations, which may change with time and varying degrees of severity. Underdiagnosis of FAS usually occurs when complete patterns of abnormalities cannot be substantiated or when there is clinician concern of stigmatizing the mother and child.

Maternal risk factors for FAS relate to quantity, frequency, and timing of alcohol consumption during pregnancy; maternal age; body size; nutritional status; socioeconomic status; mental health; genetic predisposition; and gravidity and parity (75). Some biologic factors increase the risk of FAS when they are associated with heavy drinking, for example, advanced maternal age. In a study of maternal nutritional status, infants with FAS had nutritional deficiencies in both macronutrients (i.e., proteins and total energy) and micronutrients (various vitamins and minerals such as vitamins C, D, thiamine, pantothenic acid, selenium) (76).

Follow-Up of Infants with Fetal Alcohol Syndrome

Postnatal growth restriction and delayed motor performance are hallmarks of prenatal alcohol exposure, especially of FAS (77). However, variations in long-term growth retardation have been observed with alcohol use in pregnancy (64). Growth restriction at 8 months of age, and significant effects on height and head circumference in children at 6 years of age have been reported. Some catch up growth after 8 months of age have been observed depending on whether the children were exposed to alcohol in the first and second trimester or throughout gestation, while head circumference remained smaller among children who were exposed throughout pregnancy (65). Some children with prenatal alcohol exposure continued to be smaller in weight, length, and head circumference at 3 years of age even after controlling for nutrition, current environment, exposure to alcohol during lactation, and other significant covariates (64). Long-term study of children with FAS showed that the characteristic craniofacial malformations of

FAS diminished with time but the microcephaly and, to a lesser degree, short stature, and underweight persisted in boys.

Neurodevelopmental delays can persist into childhood (78), with long-term effects including attention and memory deficits, and poor adaptability and organization (66,78). Significant adaptive behavioral deficits in adolescents and adults with FAS and FAE, particularly in areas of socialization and communicative skills, are also reported. Behavioral problems include general spatial memory deficit, distorted spatial arrangement, verbal and learning deficits, stereotyped behaviors, irritability, hyperactivity, attention deficits, tremulousness, and hyperdistractibility. Hyperkinetic disorders, emotional disorders, and sleep disorders are reported to persist over time. Speech may be delayed or impaired, which may arise partly as a result of hearing impairments. Slow growth of the head circumference can indicate poor brain growth in children with moderate to severe FAS. MRI reveals reduced growth in the cerebellar vermis, cerebral vault, basal ganglia, and diencephalon, and basal ganglia changes may relate to behavioral abnormalities (79).

Ophthalmic abnormalities are also found in children with FAS. These consist primarily of fundus anomalies and optic nerve hypoplasia, which are attributed to competition of ethanol with retinol at ADH-binding sites (80). Other eye findings include strabismus, blepharoptosis, epicanthus, cataract, glaucoma, persistent hyperplastic primary vision, and increased tortuosity of retinal vessels with reduced vascular branching.

Four types of hearing disorders are associated with FAS: (a) developmental delay in auditory maturation, (b) sensorineural hearing loss, (c) intermittent conductive hearing loss as a result of recurrent serous otitis media, and (d) central hearing loss (81). Seventy-seven percent of children with FAS have conductive hearing loss secondary to recurrent, serous otitis media. Twenty-seven percent have sensorineural hearing loss, and central hearing dysfunction is common. In turn, patients may have associated speech pathology, expressive language defects, and receptive language defects. Craniofacial abnormalities may also increase susceptibility to peripheral hearing disorders.

NICOTINE AND SMOKING DURING PREGNANCY

Nicotine is the primary stimulant in tobacco smoke. It is absorbed readily from the lungs, almost with the same efficiency as intravenous administration, and is distributed rapidly throughout the body.

Cigarette smoke contains about 4,000 chemical compounds. Most are found in the gas phase of cigarette smoke and include carbon monoxide, carbon dioxide, nitrogen oxide, ammonia, hydrogen cyanide, and other compounds. A smaller number of undesirable compounds are in the particulate phase of cigarette smoke (nicotine and tar). Tar consists primarily of polycyclic aromatic hydrocarbons (e.g., nitrosamines, aromatic amines, polycyclic hydrocarbons) and numerous other compounds, including metallic ions and radioactive compounds.

At present, fewer Americans are smoking tobacco. Among pregnant women in the United States, 11.6% used tobacco in 2018, which was down from 14.7% in 2017 (2). Women who continue to smoke during pregnancy tend to have lower socioeconomic status and are more likely to have a partner who smokes.

Absorption and Metabolism

Nicotine is distributed rapidly throughout the body and reaches the brain within 8 seconds after consumption. Peak concentrations of nicotine in plasma after a cigarette is smoked are typically between 25 and 50 ng/mL. After a single cigarette, concentrations decline rapidly over 5 to 10 minutes, primarily reflecting distribution. After long-term smoking, the elimination half-life of nicotine is approximately 2 hours.

Nicotine is metabolized mainly in the liver into two main metabolites, cotinine and nicotine-1′-N-oxide. Cotinine has few or no cardiovascular effects and is cleared more slowly than nicotine, with a half-life of about 19 hours. Cotinine concentrations in plasma, breast milk, and infant urine all reflect the smoking habits of mothers during pregnancy (82). Cotinine can be measured in meconium, and the highest concentrations are found in infants whose mothers are heavy smokers (>2 packs per day). Interestingly, equivalent amounts of cotinine were found in meconium of infants whose mothers were passive smokers and mothers who smoked 1 pack per day, which indicates the significant exposure to nicotine in the mother and her fetus from passive smoking (83).

Nicotine crosses the placenta and is excreted in the milk of lactating women (82). There is a close correlation between nicotine concentration in the mother's plasma and her breast milk after smoking. Cotinine is also detected in amniotic fluid and placenta (82).

During pregnancy, nicotine and cotinine clearances are increased by 60% and 140%, respectively, compared with postpartum clearance due to the induction of the CYP2A6 enzyme by increased estrogen and progesterone (84).

Outcomes of Maternal Smoking during Pregnancy

Maternal smoking, both active and passive, is associated with pregnancy complications including placenta previa, premature rupture of membranes, placental abruption; poor neonatal outcomes including preterm birth, growth restriction, SIDS, preterm-related deaths; and poor long-term childhood outcomes (85,86). Maternal smoking is associated with decidual necrosis and reduced intervillous blood flow, which can lead to problems of ectopic pregnancy, placental calcification, placenta previa, and placental abruption (87). Passive tobacco exposure is associated with increased risk for spontaneous abortion to almost twice that observed in nonexposed mothers. There was no differential effect of passive or active exposure between normal or abnormal karyotypes of the abortuses (88). Maternal smoking alters the balance between cytotrophoblast proliferation and differentiation. Similar to hypoxic conditions, there is an up-regulation of molecules such as von Hippel-Lindau tumor suppressor protein, hypoxia-inducible transcription factors, and VEGFs, all of which control the cellular response to oxygen tension. Passive exposure to tobacco smoke also has the same ill effects on the placenta (89). Maternal smoking is associated with thickening of the trophoblastic basement membrane, increase in collagen content of the villous mesenchyme, and decrease in vascularization, likely affecting placental excretory and nutritive functions, possibly contributing to growth restriction (87).

Prematurity

Maternal smoking, both passive and active, is a risk factor for preterm birth (85). Mechanisms for smoking affecting preterm birth have been attributed to nicotine-induced vasoconstriction, fetal hypoxia, disruption of calcium signaling, altered steroid hormone production, disruption of prostaglandin synthesis, and aberrant responses to oxytocin (90). The impact of smoking on preterm birth and other adverse long-term outcomes may be mediated by epigenetic mechanisms (90). Smoking cessation during pregnancy leads to a reduction in prematurity, stillbirths, LBW, and SGA (91).

Fetal and Neonatal Deaths

Among first-born infants, one study reported a 25% greater risk of fetal or neonatal death for less than one-pack-per-day smokers and a 56% greater risk for more than one-pack-per-day smokers, compared to nonsmokers (92). Among pregnant adolescents, smokers were 50% more likely to experience intrapartum fetal death compared with nonsmokers; highest risk was found among those who smoked 10 to 19 cigarettes per day (93).

Postmortem examinations of fetuses and neonates who died following exposure to tobacco smoke reveal histologic and immunohistochemical changes including increased epithelial dark cells and cystic stromal cells, decreased capillary formation, and increased expression of substance P and apoptosis. Furthermore, there is accumulation of iron in the brainstem and cerebellum suggestive of methemoglobinemia, a biomarker of oxidative stress due to nicotine exposure (94,95). Ependymal damage as shown by pseudostratified cytoarchitecture with numerous apoptotic and reactive astrocytes were seen among sudden death victims implicating the entry of nicotine in the cerebral spinal fluid of the fetus (95).

Effects on Fetus and Neonate

Nicotine is a neuroteratogen. It targets specific neurotransmitter receptors in the fetal brain, leading to decreased cell numbers and altered synaptic activity. The adverse effects of nicotine involve multiple neurotransmitter pathways that alter immediate developmental events and programming of synaptic competence. These defects may eventually lead to disabilities in learning and cognition, which appear later in childhood or adolescence (96). Alterations in development of the autonomic nervous system may also lead to increased susceptibility to hypoxic–ischemic brain injury, stillbirth, and SIDS (94).

Smoking in pregnancy is associated with fetal growth restriction, likely from the toxic effects of nicotine and other metabolites to the placenta (3,85–87). Maternal smoking was associated with reduced second trimester head size, femur length, reduced third trimester head size, femur length, and estimated fetal weight (86). Nicotine down-regulates insulin growth factor 1 (IGF-1) and delays chondrogenesis leading to decreased length in offsprings of smokers (97).

Reports of birth defects associated with maternal smoking include cardiovascular/heart disease, musculoskeletal disorders (limb reduction defects, missing/extra digits, clubfoot), craniosynostosis, ocular disease, orofacial clefts, gastrointestinal defects (gastroschisis, anal atresia), herniae, and undescended testes (98).

Neurobehavioral Effects and Long-Term Outcomes

Nicotine exposure has been implicated in problems with newborn behavior and child development (96). For example, prenatal tobacco exposure is associated with altered stress reactivity at ages 2 to 6 years leading to peer isolation, hyperactivity, conduct, and emotional problems at ages 7 to 11 (99).

Prenatal tobacco smoke exposure increases the risk of attention-deficit hyperactivity disorder (ADHD) (100) and is associated with both maternal and paternal smoking (101). Other neurobehavioral problems in the ADHD spectrum include greater impulsivity and externalizing symptoms, more conduct and oppositional defiant disorders, lower verbal IQ, and cognitive dysfunction, although this association may be due to unmeasured confounding (102).

Long-term follow-up evaluation of children's cognitive and developmental functions indicate that, when sociodemographic factors were controlled, children exposed to cigarette smoke *in utero* performed less well in cognitive, psychomotor, and language tests. After adjusting for confounders, prenatal tobacco exposure in the first and second trimesters was associated with abnormal language function by the Bayley Scales of Infant development at 2 years of age; specifically, cotinine concentrations greater than 1.5 ng/mL adversely affected child cognition at 2 years of age (103). Thus, smoking during pregnancy has a negative impact on the child's psychomotor development within the first 2 years of life, which underscores the need to reduce smoking.

Children of smoking mothers have a phenotype that is associated with maternal undernutrition, likely due to the effects of *in utero* hypoxia: they are born smaller than children of nonsmokers but are at increased risk of being overweight or obese and of developing the metabolic syndrome in later life (104,105). Both *in utero* exposure to tobacco and ongoing childhood exposure to smoking in the first years of life are important contributors to childhood obesity up to 6 years of age (105). Altered DNA methylation has been documented in smoking mothers' offspring, and it has been suggested that these epigenetic alterations may link prenatal smoke exposure with the metabolic syndrome and obesity (90).

Sudden Infant Death Syndrome

Maternal smoking before and during pregnancy is a risk factor for SIDS (106,107). It is proposed that nicotine affects catecholamine metabolism in the brain causing attenuated responses to hypoxia, which impacts respiratory and cardiovascular control mechanisms. On post-mortem examination of SIDS victims, the choroid plexus of the fourth ventricle which contains important structures for autonomic vital functions, showed more histologic and immunohistologic alterations, increased iron deposition, ependymal damage, and gliosis (94,95). Furthermore, there were differences in expression of nicotinic acetylcholine receptors in the brain stem (responsible for respiration and arousal) between SIDS victims exposed to tobacco smoke versus those who were not exposed. Animal studies have shown loss or suppression of acute hypoxic sensitivity in adrenal chromaffin cells and impairment of central chemoreceptor function, leading to longer and irregular respiratory cycles (108).

Nicotine and Electronic Cigarettes (Vaping)

Electronic cigarettes (ECs) are devices that produce an aerosol that contains nicotine, commonly referred to as vapor, that the user inhales (109). The vapor contains considerable amounts of other toxicants, including volatile organic compounds, and carbonyls, which are formed when e-liquids are heated to high temperatures. Carbonyls include formaldehyde, acetaldehyde, acetone, and butanol. Propylene glycol–based e-liquids generate higher levels of carbonyls than other fluids and higher levels of carcinogenic formaldehyde compared with the range seen in tobacco smoke. Thus, e-cigarettes present a potential harm to users and nonusers through second-hand or third-hand exposure, especially in vulnerable populations such as children, elderly, pregnant females, and those with cardiovascular disease.

The effects of ECs on the pregnant woman, her fetus, and infant are thought to be due to nicotine, and users should recognize that nicotine varies significantly between brands (109). The effects of other EC toxicants are still unknown.

AMPHETAMINES AND CONGENERS

Amphetamines are a group of chemically related sympathomimetic amines with CNS stimulant and peripheral α- and β-adrenergic actions. Amphetamines bind to presynaptic membrane transporters responsible for the reuptake of norepinephrine, dopamine, and serotonin, resulting in efflux of these monoamines from the cytoplasmic pool into the extracellular space (110). Amphetamine causes the intracellular vesicular release of catecholamines within the nerve terminal causing redistribution of monoamines from the storage vesicles into the cytoplasmic pool. There is strong abuse potential because of their neuropsychiatric effects, which include a decreased sense of fatigue, wakefulness, alertness, mood elevation, self-confidence, and often euphoria and elation. They have been to treat obesity, narcolepsy, hyperkinesis, ADHD, and depression.

Epidemiology

A major public health concern is the abuse of amphetamines, particularly methamphetamines. In 2017, there were 29 million people worldwide who were past-year users of amphetamines and prescription stimulants (1). In the United States, the number of fatalities attributed to the use of psychostimulants including methamphetamine has risen from 1,300 to greater than 10,000 from 2007 to 2017. Among American women of child-bearing age (15 to 44 years), approximately 208,000 reported methamphetamine use and 3.3% were pregnant (2).

Amphetamine and Methamphetamine

Methamphetamine is the methylated derivative of amphetamine and is prepared through the reduction of ephedrine or pseudoephedrine, which are common ingredients in cough medications. The ease of its synthesis, its availability and affordability, and a state of prolonged high have made it an increasingly popular drug of abuse. High doses may cause aggressive behavior, arrhythmias, severe anxiety, seizures, shock, strokes, abdominal cramps, insomnia, and death. Chronic use can produce paranoid psychosis.

In a study of pregnant methamphetamine users, intake decreased over the three trimesters (84.3% vs. 56% vs. 42.4%), but a significant proportion of women remained with high methamphetamine use and polysubstance exposure (111). In general, pregnant users are likely to be less than 24 years of age, may use multiple drugs, are at increased risk of domestic violence, are more likely to be homeless, and have higher incidence of comorbid psychiatric illnesses (112).

Pregnancy and Neonatal Perinatal Outcome

Methamphetamine use among pregnant women is associated with fetal death, growth restriction, and preterm birth (9,113). However, other covariates such as polysubstance use, malnutrition, under-reporting of drug use, and other social stressors accompanying general drug use need to be considered when reporting such outcomes (112,113).

The Infant Development Environment and Lifestyle (IDEAL) study was a multicenter, longitudinal prospective study designed to determine outcomes following prenatal exposure to methamphetamine from birth up to 7 years of age. Within the first 5 days of life, infants demonstrated neurobehavioral patterns of decreased arousal, increased stress, and poor movement quality suggestive of neurotoxic effects of methamphetamine (7). Other clinical manifestations included diaphoresis, episodes of agitation alternating with lassitude, meiosis, and vomiting. Infants exposed to both cocaine and methamphetamine were described as having abnormal sleep patterns, tremors, poor feeding, hypertonia, sneezing, a high-pitched cry, frantic fist sucking, tachypnea, loose stools, fever, yawning, hyperreflexia, and excoriation (7). An abstinence syndrome after exposure to cocaine and amphetamine has not been clearly defined, and these signs may likely be due to drug effects rather than withdrawal (4,7). Prenatal methamphetamine exposure was associated with fetal growth restriction even after adjusting for covariates such as other substances (marijuana, cigarettes, and alcohol), low socioeconomic status, male sex, and inadequate prenatal care (113). It is inferred that amphetamines decrease the delivery of nutrition to the fetus due to vasoconstriction (112).

In a large population-based study involving the United States and five Nordic countries, authors reported a small increase in risk of cardiac malformations associated with intrauterine exposure to methylphenidate, a different kind of stimulant, but there were no congenital malformations associated with amphetamine exposure (114).

Methamphetamine is likely to be neurotoxic to the fetus (115). The effects of methamphetamine on the fetal brain is gestational age dependent, with earlier exposure producing long-lasting effects on serotonergic systems. Neuroimaging studies of intrauterine exposure to methamphetamine revealed smaller subcortical volumes and increased neurocognitive deficits, and alterations in cellular metabolism in the basal ganglia (116).

Long-Term Effects

The IDEAL study showed that despite absence of true abstinence syndrome with intrauterine methamphetamine exposure, heavy drug exposure was associated with increased stress responses in the neonatal period (7). As older children, they were at higher risk for impaired executive function, possibly arising from poor inhibitory control. Early cognitive outcomes of methamphetamine exposure included lower scores on global IQ, and adverse effects on working memory, attention, executive function, and inhibitory control. Nevertheless, stable home environments mitigated many of these adverse outcomes, and children without socioeconomic deprivation were at lower risk for internalizing and externalizing behavior (7).

Methylenedioxymethamphetamine (MDMA), Gamma Hydroxybutyrate (GHB), Ketamine

The illicit use of club drugs such as MDMA, GHB, and ketamine have increased during the past decade, and there is growing concern about their potential toxicity and effects on pregnancy because they are used by a significant number of women of child-bearing age. However, only sparse data are available regarding the effects of these drugs on pregnancy and the fetus.

The use of MDMA, better known as "ecstasy" or Molly, has become a public health concern (117). Among American women of childbearing age, about 251,000 reported MDMA use in 2016, and approximately 0.4% reported using MDMA while pregnant (2). In animal studies, the effect of MDMA on the developing brain manifests as locomotor deficits and impaired spatial learning, likely associated with decreased serotonin in the hippocampus (117). The Drugs and Infancy Study (DAISY) was a prospective, longitudinal study from 2003 to 2008 that followed a cohort of infants who had prenatal exposure to MDMA from birth to 24 months of age (118). There were persistent neurotoxic effects of heavy prenatal MDMA exposure on motor development through the first and second years of life. MDMA may also have a teratogenic effect on the developing fetus, mostly as cardiovascular and musculoskeletal anomalies (119).

Ketamine

Ketamine is a non-competitive antagonist of *N*-methyl-D-aspartate (NMDA) receptor that is used as general anesthetic but has become a popular recreational drug among partygoers in the last 25 years because of its euphoric and hallucinogenic effects (120). There is growing concern about detrimental effects on brain development after maternal administration of ketamine, but research in humans is limited to date, and animal studies have been inconclusive (120). In rabbits, 2 hours of maternal administration of ketamine and laparotomy was associated with slower motor development among pups, but this effect was negligible by 7 weeks of age (121). Rat pups who had ketamine exposure *in utero* had increased neuronal apoptosis and impaired synaptic protein expression in the prefrontal cortex (122). Among rhesus monkeys, there were altered behaviors relating to maternal separation, recognition memory, and contact with novel objects reported at 3 to 4 months of age (123). Collectively, these all point to ketamine's neurotoxic effects on the developing fetal brain. Researchers from Taiwan reported a female infant with ketamine exposure who was born small-for-gestational age and had generalized hypotonia, poor reflexes, and moderate cerebral dysfunction on electroencephalogram (124). Hypotonia eventually resolved after 3 weeks.

█ MARIJUANA OR CANNABIS

In 2018, marijuana was the most commonly used drug in the United States with an estimated 26 million past-month users aged greater than 18 years (2). Among pregnant women, marijuana is the most commonly used drug and is likely to increase with its legalization in many states. In the United States, demographic and social characteristics associated with marijuana use before and during pregnancy include (a) use by a partner, (b) single status, (c) childhood trauma, and (d) prior delinquent behavior, but its use was not associated with maternal age, ethnicity, psychopathology, and perceived stress (125). Marijuana use in pregnancy is associated with concurrent exposure to tobacco and alcohol, as well as other illicit drugs (125). These demographics and patterns are dynamic and could change with the intensified push to legalize marijuana, and its promotion as an antiemetic in some social media. However, both the American Academy of Pediatrics and American College of Obstetrics and Gynecology are unified in stating that there are concerns about marijuana crossing the placenta, affecting the fetus, and being associated with adverse pregnancy outcomes and long-term neurodevelopmental consequences (126–128).

Marijuana or cannabis comes from the plant *Cannabis sativa*. Cannabis contains more than 400 chemicals, of which 61 are unique to cannabis and are referred to collectively as cannabinoids. The primary psychoactive component is δ-9-tetrahydrocannabinol (THC). Other cannabinoids, however, such as cannabidiol and cannabinol, also have biologic activity and potentially can affect the fetus.

Placental Transfer

THC readily crosses the placenta and enters the fetus, but a major metabolite, 11-nor-9-carboxy-THC does not cross as rapidly (129). In rats, the placenta contained 10 times more radiolabeled THC than fetal serum. Fetal THC serum concentrations in animal models were well below maternal serum concentrations. In humans, however, the concentrations of THC in maternal and fetal sera are similar (129). Prolonged fetal exposure is likely when maternal marijuana lasts up to 30 days.

Effects on Pregnancy, Fetus, and Neonate

Many of the reported effects of marijuana on pregnancy outcomes are equivocal partly due to under-reporting and partly due to methodologic variation in the studies. For example, some studies rely on self-reporting of marijuana exposure, while others rely on biologic specimens (e.g., meconium, urine). Another confounding variable is the concomitant use of smoking and other drugs among marijuana users (125), and some studies do not adjust for these confounders, while some report composite outcomes. A meta-analysis that adjusted for tobacco use reported that marijuana use during pregnancy was not associated with growth restriction, prematurity, or increased NICU admission (130). However, another report showed an association between marijuana use during pregnancy and adverse outcomes including growth restriction, prematurity, NICU admission, neonatal infection, and neonatal death (131). In another large cohort of pregnant women, marijuana exposure alone was not associated with any significant perinatal adverse outcomes after adjustment for confounders, but concomitant smoking increased the risk (132). Stillbirth has been associated with marijuana use during pregnancy but results are equivocal, likely due to methodologic challenges of adjustment for confounders (131,132). There are reports of congenital anomalies following marijuana exposure *in utero* in animal studies, but these have largely not been validated in human cohorts (127).

Subtle neonatal behavioral changes associated with marijuana use during pregnancy include increased startles and tremors with some similarities to the withdrawal symptoms associated with narcotic exposure (Chapter 54), although neonatal abstinence syndrome has not been associated with prenatal marijuana exposure (4).

Long-Term Neurodevelopmental Outcome

The effects of marijuana on the central nervous system are mediated by cannabinoid-1 receptors (CB1Rs), and the endogenous endocannabinoid system is present as early as day 16 of gestation

THE FETAL PATIENT

mostly in the mesocorticolimbic brain structures. With advancing gestation, there is increasing expression of these receptors suggesting a key role by endocannabinoids in human brain development that may affect neuronal survival, proliferation, migration, and differentiation (133). Exogenous marijuana in pregnancy could interfere with normal brain growth and neurodevelopment: neuroimaging provides evidence of regional increases in cortical thickness in children with prenatal exposure (134).

Epidemiologic data support the association of prenatal marijuana exposure with adverse long-term neurodevelopmental outcomes (135–138). During infancy, third trimester marijuana use was associated with decreased mental development index on the Bayley Scales of Infant Development. At age 3 years, prenatal marijuana exposure was associated with lower scores on short-term memory functioning and verbal reasoning on the Stanford-Binet Intelligence Scale among African-Americans, but this relationship was attenuated among Caucasians (135). At age 6 years, children of heavy users during the first trimester had decreased verbal reasoning skills (136). By 10 years, children with prenatal marijuana exposure had more hyperactivity, impulsivity, and decreased attention (137). In high school, children who were exposed had lower reading, math, and spelling scores (138).

Associations between prenatal exposure and neuropsychologic impairments include depressive symptoms at 10 years, impaired executive functioning and aggressive behavior in young adulthood (139), and increased externalizing behaviors (impulsivity, hyperactivity, and delinquency) in adolescence (140).

▌ PHENCYCLIDINE

Phencyclidine (PCP) was first introduced in 1957 as a dissociative anesthetic. Despite its wide margin of safety in humans, its clinical use was discontinued after reports of adverse effects that included agitation, confusion, delirium, and persistent hallucinations. Other untoward effects include feelings of paranoia, impending death, outbursts of bizarre, agitated, or violent behavior, and psychosis mimicking schizophrenia. It remains popular as a drug of abuse because of its sedative and hallucinogenic effects, synthesis from readily available precursors, low cost, and various routes of administration. Most users smoke PCP; others sniff or snort the powder, drink the liquid form mixed with lemonade or alcohol, or inject it intravenously.

Placental Transfer and Metabolism

Placental transfer of PCP has been studied in animals. In piglets, serum concentrations of PCP were 10 times higher than in the sow; in fetal rabbits, similarly high serum concentrations were found that reached a peak 2 hours after parenteral drug administration to the doe. There was almost a 10-fold higher concentration of PCP in fetal tissue than in maternal blood and PCP appeared in the pup's brain as early as 15 minutes after subcutaneous injection to the dam. PCP has also been detected in amniotic fluid and umbilical cord blood at high concentrations (141,142).

PCP appears rapidly in breast milk, appearing within 15 minutes of maternal administration. By 3 hours, the ratio of concentration in milk to plasma is approximately 10:1 (143).

PCP is lipophilic and is stored in body fat and the CNS for prolonged periods, with slow release into the bloodstream. The major routes of elimination involve metabolism of PCP in the liver and excretion in the urine and feces. The half-life of the drug is about 3 days, although it has been found in the urine as long as 8 days after last use. The half-life of PCP in the fetus is approximately twice that in the mother (141).

Mode of Action

PCP has strong, centrally mediated effects in animals and humans and influences many different neuronal systems. It inhibits uptake and increases release of monoamines in the brain, interacts with cholinergic and serotonergic systems, and antagonizes neuronal stimulation caused by the excitatory amino acid, N-methyl aspartate. PCP is an N-methyl-D-aspartate receptor (NMDAR) blocker, which induces neuronal apoptosis during early brain development, and in later years causes schizophrenia-like behavior (144). In brain culture studies of 2.5-day old rat pups, the apoptotic effects of PCP were prevented by the brain-derived neurotrophic factor (BDNF) in a dose-dependent fashion. Inhibition by BDNF was through parallel activation of phosphatidylinositol-3 kinase (PI3K)/Akt and extracellular signal-regulated kinase (ERK) pathways, which both have trophic functions during early brain development (145). PCP may produce a general enhancement of neurotransmitter release by blocking voltage-sensitive potassium channels and thus might act at several different loci.

Epidemiology

Between 2011 and 2017, global demand of PCP accounted for 44% of the total quantity of hallucinogens (1). Among pregnant women, the prevalence of PCP use has not been firmly established, although its use is thought to be downward trending in the United States. Although the number of new users of hallucinogens continues to rise, this is largely attributable to other drugs such as MDMA (1).

Neonatal Outcomes

Studies reporting neonatal outcomes of prenatal PCP exposure are equivocal. In one study, there were no significant differences in birth weight, length, and head circumference in PCP-exposed newborns compared to matched controls (146). However in contrast, Tabor et al. reported growth restriction, neonatal withdrawal/intoxication, and longer hospital stay among PCP-exposed newborns (147).

Although PCP has not been reported to be teratogenic and is not associated with congenital malformations in humans, animal studies have shown either neurodegenerative or anti-apoptotic changes in various regions of the brain, leading to decreased motor coordination and hyperactivity in newborn pups (148). PCP has also been shown to produce widespread apoptotic neurodegeneration throughout the developing brain when administered to immature rodents during periods of synaptogenesis. PCP also affects NMDA pathways, eventually resulting in decreased brain mass, possibly accounting for neurobehavioral disturbances later on (149).

Neurobehavioral Effects

PCP-exposed newborns showed abnormal neurobehavioral findings: irritability, tremors, hypertonicity, poor attention, bizarre eye movements, staring spells, hypertonic ankle reflexes, and depressed grasp and rooting reflexes (150). A most characteristic feature in infants is a sudden change in level of consciousness, with lethargy alternating with irritability. The behavioral outcome of these newborns has been attributed to PCP intoxication, rather than withdrawal (147).

Long-Term Outcome

In animal models, the NMDAR is antagonized by PCP through the impairment of neuronal progenitors (148,151). In mice, PCP-exposed pups exhibit deficits in cognitive memory and sensorimotor gating up to adulthood. Prenatal inhibition of NMDA receptor function was associated with abnormalities in presynaptic glutamate transmission and altered neuregulin 1 (Nrg1)/erbB4 expression, plausibly contributing to schizophrenia pathology (149,152). There are not many reports on neurodevelopmental outcomes of PCP-exposed infants, but an earlier study stated that the Bayley psychomotor and mental developmental indices of PCP-exposed infants at 3 months and 1 year of age were not statistically different from those of controls (153).

ANTIDEPRESSANTS (SELECTIVE SEROTONIN REUPTAKE INHIBITORS, SSRIs)

Since the introduction of SSRIs in 1988, this class of drug has become a leading treatment for depression and other mood/behavioral disorders. The use of SSRIs during pregnancy has also become more common. Based on meta-analysis of 40 cohort studies in 15 countries, the international pooled prevalence estimate was 3.0% with the highest prevalence in North America (5.5%) followed by Europe and Australasia at 1.6% and 1.3%, respectively (154). Sertraline (1.10%) was the most commonly used SSRI followed by citalopram (0.77%) and fluoxetine (0.76%).

The existence of a withdrawal syndrome with antidepressants, both the classic tricyclic antidepressants (TCA) and the newer SSRIs, is well documented in adults. Withdrawal or "discontinuation" syndrome have been described in newborn infants following third trimester fluoxetine, paroxetine, sertraline, and venlafaxine exposure (155,156). The withdrawal signs include acrocyanosis, tachypnea, tachycardia, respiratory distress, temperature instability, irritability, sweating, and convulsions. Onset of signs typically occur within the first 4 days and last for 2 to 21 days. The withdrawal syndrome associated with maternal SSRI use could be attributed to the cholinergic receptor, or dependence on the serotonin system. Nearly two-thirds of reported cases of suspected SSRI-induced neonatal withdrawal are associated with paroxetine, a more potent inhibitor of norepinephrine reuptake than sertraline or citalopram. Paroxetine also has a distinctive effect on muscarinic receptors compared with fluoxetine and other SSRIs. These aspects of paroxetine's mechanism are more suggestive of a cholinergic withdrawal syndrome, also described in adults (156).

A systematic review reported pregnancy and neonatal outcomes following antidepressant use in pregnancy (157). There was no association between antidepressant medication exposure and spontaneous abortion, but there were associations with preterm birth, lower birth weight, and 1- and 5-minute Apgar scores. In addition, there was a higher risk of preterm birth among women with depression who received SSRI during pregnancy than women with depression who did not receive SSRI (158). Prenatal exposure to SSRI is associated with neonatal persistent pulmonary hypertension (PPHN). In a systematic review of women and their offspring exposed to SSRI during pregnancy, the risk of PPHN was higher than controls, especially if exposure occurred at later than 20 weeks' gestation (159). Sertraline has the lowest risk for PPHN among the SSRIs. Although there was a risk for PPHN among those exposed to SSRIs, the absolute risk remained low, and the benefits of SSRI for pregnant mothers outweigh the risk of PPHN (160).

It has been suggested that children of mothers who took fluoxetine during the first trimester have a slightly increased risk for cardiovascular malformations, septal defects, and nonseptal defects (161), although some have questioned the association (162).

Intelligence does not seem to be affected by prenatal exposure to SSRIs. The Danish National Birth Cohort showed no difference in IQ at 5 years of age between those exposed to SSRI/anxiolytics and those who were not exposed (163). Similarly in a prospective study of children with prenatal exposure to SSRI, children with prenatal exposure to maternal depression without SSRI, and unexposed children, maternal report of executive function, nonverbal intelligence at 5 years, and neuropsychologic tests at 7 years did not show any differences among the three groups. It was exposure to maternal depression without SSRI that was related to emotional control problems at 4 years old (164). Antidepressant dose and duration during pregnancy did not affect the intelligence and behavior of the children. Instead, severity of maternal depression during pregnancy and at testing predicted the child's behavior (165).

Several meta-analyses have shown an increased risk for autistic spectrum disorder (ASD) and attention deficit hyperactivity disorder (ADHD) ranging from 1.45 to 1.96 times odds among children

with prenatal exposure to SSRIs. However, there were concerns about heterogeneity of studies as well as influence of other potential confounding factors, such as underlying maternal psychopathology. Furthermore, sibling matched analysis and preexisting maternal affective disorders yielded no significant differences on the incidence of ASD/ADHD (166–168).

Serotonin has a critical role in embryonic and fetal brain development, with roles in neuronal maturation, migration, synaptogenesis, and differentiation of neural crest cells, which are involved in facial and cardiac development. It is also important in epigenetic processes such as stress responsivity at the hypothalamic–pituitary axis (169). It is still unclear whether epigenetic changes occur with maternal use of SSRIs during pregnancy. In a review of six studies, three showed an increase in DNA methylation in CpG sites using cord blood of infants exposed to SSRIs prenatally, while the remaining three showed an association between epigenetic changes in the umbilical cord blood and maternal mood, but not antidepressant medication use (170).

Alteration in serotonin signaling either by exposure to SSRIs or genetic factors affects early brain development and may result in neurobehavioral deficits. SSRIs readily cross the placenta and the fetal blood brain barrier, and thus increase brain serotonin. Altered serotonin signaling may lead to increased sensitivity to negative social context in some individuals and could serve as a buffer or plasticity factor, which increases resilience of the individual. Other factors such as the primary maternal mood disorder, and postnatal and childhood social experience, may play a role in determining childhood susceptibility (171). These factors may interact with each other in a complex manner, which may explain why robust evidence to show that prenatal SSRI exposure affects neurodevelopmental outcome is lacking, in spite of large systematic reviews. The challenge is to understand the interplay of these factors and to be able to identify those who are at risk for later neurobehavioral compromise.

Overall, successful treatment of depression during pregnancy is very important. It should be individualized, and optimal treatment should be decided between the woman and her physician.

NONNARCOTIC HYPNOSEDATIVES

Abuse of nonnarcotic hypnosedatives during pregnancy can have complications on the fetus and neonate, including withdrawal. The manifestations of nonnarcotic withdrawal in the neonate are similar to those of narcotic withdrawal (4). However, in a few instances (e.g., with barbiturate withdrawal or ethchlorvynol withdrawal), hyperphagia has been described as a prominent feature.

The manifestations of the nonnarcotic abstinence syndrome are more frequently intense and life-threatening compared to narcotic withdrawal, and seizures are more frequent. Most of the withdrawal from narcotics is seen within the first 3 days of postnatal life, as a result of the short half-life of narcotics. In contrast, withdrawal from the nonnarcotics, for example, phenobarbital, diazepam, or chlordiazepoxide, may occur 7 to 21 days after birth, due to slow clearance of the drug in the infant (172). Not infrequently, withdrawal from nonnarcotic substances observed in the NICU is iatrogenic, resulting from the use of hypnosedative agents among critically ill neonates and infants, especially those who received regular doses for ≥72 hours (173).

BENZODIAZEPINES

Benzodiazepines are commonly used for the treatment of generalized anxiety disorder, panic disorder, seizures, perioperative sedation, and skeletal muscle relaxation. Because of the effect of benzodiazepines on the brain's reward pathway, benzodiazepine use disorder (BUD) may occur by misuse of medication and is associated with physical dependence and withdrawal (174). Among pregnant women, benzodiazepines are frequently prescribed to reduce anxiety (175). According to the 2019 World Drug Report by the United Nations, nonmedical use of benzodiazepines is ranked in the top 3 of commonly used substances in 40 countries and is higher in women (1). Not uncommonly, benzodiazepines are used in various combinations with opioids, alcohol, and other drugs.

Pregnant women may be susceptible to BUD because of a heightened prevalence of anxiety during pregnancy (175). The calming effect of benzodiazepines results from their action on gamma-aminobutyric acid type A (GABA-A) receptors, which allows greater affinity for GABA, the main inhibitory neurotransmitter in the central nervous system. Several pathways are induced when GABA attaches to GABA-A receptors causing postsynaptic hyperpolarization and decreased action potential, the end results being relaxation, sedation, hypnosis, amnesia, and cessation of seizures if present. At higher doses, symptoms of euphoria, confusion, mood swings, and visual distortion can be felt (176).

During pregnancy, benzodiazepines cross the placenta easily, resulting in significant drug concentrations in fetal serum and tissues. Placental transfer of diazepam can occur from the 6th week of gestation and accumulate in fetal tissues during organogenesis, providing substantial theoretical justification for abnormal development (177). However, recent evidence from meta-analyses and larger cohorts shows that congenital malformations are not associated with prenatal benzodiazepine exposure (178,179).

Preterm birth, low birth weight, smaller head circumference, increased cesarean delivery, higher rates of NICU admission, and increased use of ventilator in the NICU have been described in infants prenatally exposed to benzodiazepines (180).

Chronic and high doses of benzodiazepine exposure are associated with neonatal abstinence syndrome (4). When used concomitantly with opioids, the risk of NAS is increased and may be of greater severity and associated with longer hospitalization (4,172). When high doses of benzodiazepines are administered late in pregnancy, neonates are may be born with poor muscle tone, poor feeding, drowsiness, and delayed feeding, although these effects are self-limiting (174).

In a large cohort of children from the Norwegian Mother and Child Cohort Study at age 1.5 to 3 years, benzodiazepine exposure *in utero* was reported to be associated with child internalizing problems consisting of anxiousness, emotional reactivity, and somatic complaints (181). These manifestations may be predictive of later psychopathology in children and adolescents. In another study, children at age 6 who had prenatal exposure to benzodiazepines were more likely to score higher on tests for oppositional-defiant behavior disorder and aggression (182). However, when the study was adjusted for maternal anxiety without benzodiazepine exposure, aggressive behavior was no longer observed.

BARBITURATES

Barbiturates are classified as ultrashort, intermediate, and long acting. The intermediate-acting barbiturates are most frequently abused, for example, secobarbital, pentobarbital, amobarbital, and butabarbital. The abuse of the long-acting barbiturates (e.g., phenobarbital) is not as common as the shorter-acting forms. Phenobarbital, however, is more frequently involved in withdrawal syndrome in the newborn because it is used frequently by the mother for insomnia, for the relief of anxiety, as an anticonvulsant, or for sedation during toxemia of pregnancy.

Barbiturates cross the placenta readily and establish high concentrations in maternal and cord blood, as well as in fetal brain, liver, and adrenal glands (183). A withdrawal syndrome is described following prenatal barbiturate exposure consisting of irritability, severe tremors, hyperacusis, excessive crying, vasomotor instability, diarrhea, restlessness, increased tone, hyperphagia, vomiting, disturbed sleep, and the onset is on the first day of life or as late as 10 to 14 days of age (4). There is no pattern in the anomalies observed with prenatal barbiturate exposure (184). A slightly higher incidence of learning problems was observed among offsprings with prenatal phenobarbital, compared to controls (185).

OTHER DRUGS ASSOCIATED WITH NEONATAL WITHDRAWAL

Baclofen

Baclofen reduces spasticity among patients with neurologic disorders. Due to its pain-relieving qualities, the medication eventually became the subject of abuse on its own. In pregnancy, prenatal exposure to baclofen was associated with neonatal withdrawal in a small number of case reports (186,187). A term infant born to a mother on baclofen pump had withdrawal signs of feeding difficulty, hypertonicity, tremors, hyperactive Moro reflex, diarrhea, and sneezing occurring between 12 and 48 hours of life and resolving after oral administration of baclofen (186). Another case of baclofen-induced neonatal withdrawal was reported in a preterm infant whose mother was also on baclofen pump during pregnancy (187).

Valproate

Valproate is an effective drug for generalized or focal epilepsy. Neonatal hypoglycemia and withdrawal manifestations have been reported with maternal use of valproate for epilepsy. Valproate readily crosses the blood–brain barrier and is a potent teratogen. Its use during pregnancy can lead to fetal valproate syndrome, which is characterized by facial dysmorphism, congenital anomalies (neural tube defects and cardiac defects), and neurodevelopmental delay. Lower doses may decrease but not mitigate the risk of anomaly (188). In a 17-year longitudinal study, prevalence of major congenital malformations was highest among infants exposed prenatally to valproate (10.3%) compared with other antiepileptic drugs (189).

Prenatal exposure to valproic acid increases the risk for autism. Prenatal valproate is widely used in animal models to induce autism in offspring and to evaluate new therapies for ASD (190). Valproate-exposed non-human primates showed disruption of normal gene expression during embryonic development, and features of autism such as impaired social interaction, pronounced stereotypies, and disrupted visual attention to social stimulus (191).

There is also a higher risk for attention deficit/hyperactivity disorder (ADHD) among children with prenatal exposure to valproate. In a 14-year Danish study, 8.4% of children prenatally exposed to valproate had ADHD compared to 3.2% of the unexposed children (192). Also, 6- to 8-year-old children exposed to valproate prenatally had memory dysfunction as shown by lower than expected scores in list learning, story recall, and figure recall tasks (193). Current guidelines and FDA regulations strongly discourage the use of valproate among women of childbearing age due to teratogenic risks (194). Valproate should only be started in girls and women when other options have been fully explored (188). A number of women of child-bearing age who take VPA make an informed choice to continue it after thorough consideration of risks, either because pregnancy is unlikely or because other treatments have failed (194).

METHODS TO DETECT DRUG EXPOSURE IN THE MOTHER AND INFANT

Identifying prenatal exposure to illicit substances is not easy. Mothers may not disclose drug use for fear of consequences and stigmatization. Even with disclosure, information on the type and extent of drug use may be inaccurate (10). Methods to detect substance abuse in a pregnant woman or intrauterine drug exposure in a neonate ideally should address not only the types of drug abused but also the amount, frequency, and duration of drug exposure. Two general methods are used to achieve this: maternal interview and laboratory tests.

Maternal Interview

Maternal interview has the greatest potential for providing comprehensive information on the type, amount, frequency, and duration of drug use. Routine interview forms an integral part of the obstetric history, which is obtained either prenatally or when a woman is admitted in labor. The accuracy of the data obtained by this method depends on the attention devoted to the interview. Cursory interview often results in underreporting of drug use, whereas the incidence increases threefold to fivefold if a more organized protocol is used (195). Maternal fear of the consequences of disclosure, underestimation of drug use, physical discomfort experienced by the woman, particularly if in labor, all affect the accuracy of self-report. Under these circumstances, the reporting of drug use by the mother can be as low as one-fourth of the true incidence (11).

Laboratory Diagnosis of Neonatal Drug Exposure

Most of the laboratory tests for drug detection are used for screening purposes. Confirmation with use of another unrelated method is needed if test results are to withstand challenge. Various analytical procedures are used for drug detection and include thin-layer chromatography, immunoassays, high-performance liquid chromatography (HPLC), gas chromatography for screening, and gas chromatography–mass spectrometry (GCMS) for confirmation. A review of the use and limitations of these procedures is published (196).

Specimens for Drug Testing

Urine. The testing of biologic fluids for drugs is by far the most common method to detect illicit drugs in a pregnant woman, or prenatal drug exposure in a neonate. However, there are several limitations to this method. Identification of drugs in biologic fluids will differentiate only those who have been exposed to drugs versus those who were not. The test cannot provide reliable information on the frequency, duration, or the time of last drug use. Among biologic fluids, urine has been most often tested owing to several advantages: urine collection is easy; drug metabolites in urine are usually found in higher concentrations than in serum due to the concentrating ability of the kidneys; large volumes of urine can be collected; urine is easier to analyze than blood because it usually is devoid of protein and other cellular constituents; metabolites in urine are usually stable especially if frozen; and urine is amenable to most of the drug-testing methods.

However, there are several drawbacks to urine testing. Foremost is the high rate of false-negative results. In the mother, unless collection is closely watched, urine can easily be substituted with a clean specimen or adulterated by dilution or addition of salt, which may interfere with the testing methods, particularly with the immunoassays. Drug in urine reflects recent use, so negative results may occur if the woman has abstained for some time before testing. In the infant, the incidence of false-negative urine tests also is high, ranging from 32% to 63% because the infant's urine has to be collected as close to birth as possible (197). The later after birth that urine is collected, the higher is the likelihood of a false-negative test. Recent abstention by the mother from the use of drugs may also result in a negative urine test in the infant (197).

Meconium. The concept behind meconium drug testing was based on studies in pregnant rhesus monkeys that were given morphine throughout gestation. A high concentration of morphine and its metabolites were found in the gastrointestines or "meconium" of their fetuses (10). Drugs accumulate in meconium secondary to fetal swallowing of drugs in amniotic fluid or from the excretion of drug metabolites in the bile from the liver. Studies in pregnant rats

showed that the concentration of morphine and cocaine in meconium were related to the dose, timing, and duration of drug administration to the dam (198).

Meconium drug testing can be used to detect a variety of licit and illicit drugs (10). Included among the drugs of abuse are opiates, cocaine, cannabinoids, amphetamines, nonnarcotic hypnosedatives, nicotine, and alcohol (fatty acid ethyl esters). Meconium analysis has been adapted to various analytical methods which include radioimmunoassay technique (EMIT), fluorescence polarization immunoassay (FPIA), HPLC, and GCMS (196).

There are several advantages to using meconium to detect prenatal drug exposure in the infant: ease and noninvasiveness of meconium collection which is particularly useful in anonymous drug prevalence studies; high sensitivity and specificity of the test; a wide window for detecting intrauterine drug exposure to as early as the 12th to 16th week of gestation; ability to test meconium even in samples obtained beyond 24 hours after birth; and positive correlation between concentration of drugs in meconium and the amount of drug use by the mother during gestation. The main disadvantage of meconium drug testing is that meconium is a stool specimen that requires preparative procedures before analysis.

Hair. Hair analysis is based on the principle that illicit substances and their metabolic products are incorporated from the serum into the hair follicle and grow into the cuticle and hair shaft (199). The drug, once deposited in the hair shaft, remains for an indefinite period. As the hair grows at the rate of 1 to 2 cm month, deposited drugs follow the growth of the hair shaft. The section of the hair closest to the scalp represents the most recent exposure. Sectional analysis of hair can be performed to provide information on the timing and duration of drug use. Information on the chronicity of drug use makes hair analysis advantageous compared with urine or other body fluid testing. Furthermore, quantitative detection of drugs in hair has been correlated with the amount of drug use in the past.

Hair has been analyzed to detect opiates, cocaine, PCP, methamphetamine, antidepressants, and nicotine (199). However, there are some significant drawbacks to hair analysis for drugs. Patients who are not chronic drug users may not be detected by hair analysis, because drug deposition in hair relies on serum levels during hair growth. Use of hair dye, bleach, and other cosmetic agents by the woman may alter the presence and amount of drug in hair. Some ethnic groups weave hair from other individuals into their own hair, and this may interfere with the appropriate collection of hair sample. Obtaining hair samples is invasive and some patients may refuse hair testing. Hair can also be passively exposed to drugs that can be smoked (e.g., cocaine, marijuana). In newborn infants, the amount of hair collected may not be enough for testing.

Others. Other types of specimens have been tested for drugs, for example, sweat, nail clippings, gastric juice, and saliva. The use of these specimens for drug detection is uncommon.

▌TREATMENT

Initial management of the infant exposed to substances *in utero* is directed toward the serious antenatal and neonatal complications that are associated with maternal drug use such as asphyxia, fetal distress, prematurity, and meconium aspiration. Thereafter, the infant is tested for illicit drug exposure, sexually transmitted infections, assessed/treated for drug withdrawal, and referred to social and child protection services.

Supportive Treatment of Drug Withdrawal

The care of drug withdrawal in the neonate primarily is supportive. Appropriate measures include swaddling to decrease sensory stimulation, close attention to nutrition and feeding, as well as observation of sleeping habits, temperature stability, weight loss, diarrhea,

THE FETAL PATIENT

and change in clinical status. Daily caloric intake should provide up to 150 to 250 cal/kg/day for proper growth in neonates exhibiting withdrawal.

Assessment of the Severity of Neonatal Withdrawal

The assessment of withdrawal from narcotics is discussed in Chapter 54. There are no studies available that specifically assess the severity of neonatal withdrawal from nonnarcotics drugs and current methods to assess neonatal narcotic withdrawal are used.

Pharmacologic Treatment of Drug Withdrawal

The decision to use pharmacologic agents to treat neonatal non-narcotic withdrawal is based on the assessment of its severity. The use of pharmacologic agents for withdrawal from narcotic drugs, as compared to supportive care alone, is discussed in detail in Chapter 54.

Compared to narcotic withdrawal, there are no adequate studies to determine the most appropriate pharmacologic agents to treat non-narcotic neonatal withdrawal. As a rule, drug selection should match the class of agent that the infant is withdrawing from. For hypnosedatives, phenobarbital or benzodiazepines are used. There is cross reaction between the different drugs in the alcohol/hypnosedative group, and each drug is effective in treating withdrawal from any drug in the group. Thus, barbiturates or benzodiazepines can be used to treat withdrawal from nonbarbiturates, including alcohol, or vice versa. Phenobarbital is given at a dose of 3 to 6 mg/kg/d in divided doses every 6 to 12 hours, and the dose is titrated based on the infant's response. The aim of treatment with drugs is to render the infant comfortable, without altering conscious state.

During the treatment of withdrawal, attention should also focus on the nutrition and fluid and electrolyte balance of the infant, particularly if vomiting, diarrhea, hyperpyrexia, and hyperhidrosis are present. Intravenous fluids may be required to correct deficits or prevent the occurrence of imbalances.

COMPLICATIONS OF NEONATAL DRUG WITHDRAWAL

The complications of neonatal drug withdrawal are related to its severity. Biochemical aberrations in serum electrolytes, pH, and dehydration may occur secondary to vomiting and diarrhea. Weight loss may be profound not only due to excess fluid losses, but to poor oral intake and hyperactivity. Aspiration pneumonia may occur secondary to vomiting and incoordinate sucking and swallowing. Respiratory alkalosis can occur because of tachypnea. Convulsions may be present and are observed more frequently in withdrawal from non-narcotic drugs.

Other Supportive Measures

Mothers with substance use disorder may have serious impediments to a successful parenting role. Similarly, neurobehavioral abnormalities and the effects of withdrawal can prevent gratifying infant feedback, which is important in bonding. Thus, the mother and child should have early and repeated contacts and support. Social services and appropriate child welfare authorities should be engaged to ensure that appropriate family supports and community resources are in place. The infant's disposition is influenced by the child welfare policies of the local community. Considerations are given as to whether the mother is in drug recovery, what drugs she is using, if she is enrolled in drug treatment, if she has resources, and whether the extent of her family or support network is sufficient. The staff personnel should frequently inform the mother of her infant's condition and reassure her that with adequate control of the withdrawal, the infant will begin to feed better and respond more positively to her over time.

If plans have been made to place the infant in a foster home, the infant will need human contact in the interim and should receive stimulation through regular handling and cuddling by staff.

BREASTFEEDING

Most drugs taken by a lactating mother will cross into her breast milk. The concentration of illicit drug/s in breast milk depends on the type, amount, and timing of drug intake by the mother. There also is the danger of transmission of the human immunodeficiency virus (HIV) through the breast milk; thus, breastfeeding may not be recommended in a mother who is HIV positive.

For the infant whose mother has continued to use illicit substances throughout pregnancy, breastfeeding may be unsafe (200). For some mothers, breastfeeding can be instituted with support and close monitoring, adequate weight gain of the infant, and discussions about the risks to the infant from exposure to illicit substances through breast milk. Guidelines about breastfeeding of infants born to drug using mothers vary, and clinicians are advised to follow breastfeeding guidelines that apply in their area of practice.

Cocaine and its metabolites are detectable in breast milk and the concentration varies, depending on whether the mother uses cocaine frequently, or recreationally. Newborn infants are extremely sensitive to cocaine because they cannot metabolize cocaine well. The Academy of Breastfeeding Medicine suggests that women who have used cocaine generally should not breastfeed unless they have a negative maternal urine toxicology at delivery, have been abstinent for at least 90 days, are in a substance abuse treatment program and plan to continue it in the postpartum period, have the approval of their substance abuse counselor, have been engaged and compliant in their prenatal care, and have no other contraindications to breastfeeding (201).

Alcohol is distributed in breast milk, but the amount ingested by the infant is only a small fraction of the amount consumed by the mother. Short-term alcohol consumption by lactating women had an immediate effect on the odor of their milk and the feeding behavior of their infant (200). The infants suck more frequently during the first minute after their mothers had consumed alcohol, but consume significantly less milk.

SOCIAL AND PROTECTIVE SERVICE REFERRAL AND FOLLOW-UP

All infants of drug-dependent mothers should have a social service referral to assess the adequacy of parenting and care of the infant at home. Discharge of the infant to the mother's care, with the help of a support person, is the primary objective, unless serious conditions dictate otherwise. Discharge of the infant to a person other than the mother (foster parent) or an agency should be attempted only when it is apparent that the infant will be neglected, poorly cared for, or abused. Mothers hesitate to admit to the use of drugs during pregnancy because of fear that their infants will be taken away from them. They should be assured otherwise; in fact, they should be encouraged to be responsible for the primary care of their infants. The social worker and physician also should advise the mother regarding the availability of medical and social services in the community, including substance abuse counseling and family planning.

As part of child protection laws operative in many countries, infants born to drug-dependent mothers are considered as potentially abused and are required by law to be reported to a child protection agency. The agency will often require a positive drug screen in the infant before safeguarding actions are taken. Referral to a child protection agency is helpful when the intent is to ensure the protection and adequacy of care of the infant at home.

However, when the objective is to initiate punitive measures against the mother, referral to the child protection agency can be counter-productive.

The infant of a drug using mother is at risk of many long-term problems and ongoing exposure to drugs in the household. Follow-up of these infants should be planned not only to assess their medical and physical well-being but also to ascertain that further risks to drug exposure and neglect are prevented.

REFERENCES

1. World Drug Report 2019. United Nations Office on Drugs and Crime. June 2019. Available from: https://wdr.unodc.org/wdr2019/. Accessed April 8, 2020.
2. McCance-Katz EF. The National survey on drug use and health: 2018. In: McCance-Katz EF, ed. *NSDUH*. Rockville, MD: Substance Abuse and Mental Health Services Administration, August 2019. http://www.samhsa.gov/data/report/dr-elinore-f-mccance-katz-webcast-slides-national-survey-drug-use-and-health-2018. Accessed March 27, 2020.
3. Soto E, Bahado-Singh R. Fetal abnormal growth associated with substance abuse. *Clin Obstet Gynecol* 2013;56(1):142. doi: 10.1097/GRF.0b013e31827e6b60
4. Hudak ML, Tan RC; Committee on Drugs; Committee on Fetus and Newborn; American Academy of Pediatrics. Neonatal drug withdrawal. *Pediatrics* 2012;129(2):e540. doi: 10.1542/peds.2011-3212
5. Cain MA, Bornick P, Whiteman V. The maternal, fetal, and neonatal effects of cocaine exposure in pregnancy. *Clin Obstet Gynecol* 2013;56(1):124. doi: 10.1097/GRF.0b013e31827ae167
6. Popova S, Lange S, Probst C, et al. Estimation of national, regional, and global prevalence of alcohol use during pregnancy and fetal alcohol syndrome: a systematic review and meta-analysis. *Lancet Glob Health* 2017;5(3):e290. doi: 10.1016/S2214-109X(17)30021-9
7. Smith LM, Diaz S, LaGasse LL, et al. Developmental and behavioral consequences of prenatal methamphetamine exposure: a review of the Infant Development, Environment, and Lifestyle (IDEAL) study. *Neurotoxicol Teratol* 2015;51:35. doi: 10.1016/j.ntt.2015.07.006
8. Dejong K, Olyaei A, Lo JO. Alcohol use in pregnancy. *Clin Obstet Gynecol* 2019;62(1):142. doi: 10.1097/GRF.0000000000000414
9. Smid MC, Metz TD, Gordon AJ. Stimulant use in pregnancy: an under-recognized epidemic among pregnant women. *Clin Obstet Gynecol* 2019;62(1):168. doi: 10.1097/GRF.0000000000000418
10. Ostrea EM Jr, Brady M, Gause S, et al. Drug screening of newborns by meconium analysis: a large-scale, prospective, epidemiologic study. *Pediatrics* 1992;89(1):107.
11. Ostrea EM Jr, Knapp DK, Tannenbaum L, et al. Estimates of illicit drug use during pregnancy by maternal interview, hair analysis, and meconium analysis. *J Pediatr* 2001;139(3):344. doi: 10.1067/mpd.2001.111429
12. Benowitz NL. Clinical pharmacology and toxicology of cocaine. *Pharmacol Toxicol* 1993;72(1):3. doi: 10.1111/j.1600-0773.1993.tb01331.x
13. Lester BM, Padbury JF. Third pathophysiology of prenatal cocaine exposure. *Dev Neurosci* 2009;31(1–2):23. doi: 10.1159/000207491
14. Towers CV, Pircon RA, Nageotte MP, et al. Cocaine intoxication presenting as preeclampsia and eclampsia. *Obstet Gynecol* 1993;81(4):545.
15. Castleman J, Veal L, Ganapathy R. Peripartum cocaine use and postpartum myocardial infarction. *Heart* 2012;98(21):1609. doi: 10.1136/heartjnl-2012-302758
16. Moore TR, Sorg J, Miller L, et al. Hemodynamic effects of intravenous cocaine on the pregnant ewe and fetus. *Am J Obstet Gynecol* 1986;155(4):883. doi: 10.1016/s0002-9378(86)80044-8
17. Bateman DA, Chiriboga CA. Dose-response effect of cocaine on newborn head circumference. *Pediatrics* 2000;106(3):E33. doi: 10.1542/peds.106.3.e33
18. van de Bor M, Walther FJ, Sims ME. Increased cerebral blood flow velocity in infants of mothers who abuse cocaine. *Pediatrics* 1990;85(5):733.
19. Konkol RJ, Tikofsky RS, Wells R, et al. Normal high-resolution cerebral 99mTc-HMPAO SPECT scans in symptomatic neonates exposed to cocaine. *J Child Neurol* 1994;9(3):278. doi: 10.1177/088307389400900311
20. John V, Dai H, Talati A, et al. Autonomic alterations in cocaine-exposed neonates following orthostatic stress. *Pediatr Res* 2007;61(2):251. doi: 10.1203/01.pdr.0000252436.62151.67
21. Lipshultz SE, Frassica JJ, Orav EJ. Cardiovascular abnormalities in infants prenatally exposed to cocaine. *J Pediatr* 1991;118(1):44. doi: 10.1016/s0022-3476(05)81842-6
22. Mehta SK, Finkelhor RS, Anderson RL, et al. Transient myocardial ischemia in infants prenatally exposed to cocaine. *J Pediatr* 1993;122(6):945. doi: 10.1016/s0022-3476(09)90025-7

23. Frassica JJ, Orav EJ, Walsh EP, et al. Arrhythmias in children prenatally exposed to cocaine. *Arch Pediatr Adolesc Med* 1994;148(11):1163. doi: 10.1001/archpedi.1994.02170110049008
24. Conradt E, Sheinkopf SJ, Lester BM, et al.; Maternal Lifestyle Study. Prenatal substance exposure: neurobiologic organization at 1 month. *J Pediatr* 2013;163(4):989. doi: 10.1016/j.jpeds.2013.04.033
25. McCann EM, Lewis K. Control of breathing in babies of narcotic- and cocaine-abusing mothers. *Early Hum Dev* 1991;27(3):175. doi: 10.1016/0378-3782(91)90193-7
26. Wennberg RP, Yin J, Miller M, et al. Fetal cocaine exposure and neonatal bilirubinemia. *J Pediatr* 1994;125(4):613. doi: 10.1016/s0022-3476(94)70020-6
27. Downing GJ, Horner SR, Kilbride HW. Characteristics of perinatal cocaine-exposed infants with necrotizing enterocolitis. *Am J Dis Child* 1991;145(1):26. doi: 10.1001/archpedi.1991.02160010028005
28. Silva-Araujo A, Tavares MA, Patacao MH, et al. Retinal hemorrhages associated with in utero exposure to cocaine. Experimental and clinical findings. *Retina* 1996;16(5):411. doi: 10.1097/00006982-199616050-00008
29. Lester BM, Corwin MJ, Sepkoski C, et al. Neurobehavioral syndromes in cocaine-exposed newborn infants. *Child Dev* 1991;62(4):694. doi: 10.1111/j.1467-8624.1991.tb01563.x
30. Richardson GA, Conroy ML, Day NL. Prenatal cocaine exposure: effects on the development of school-age children. *Neurotoxicol Teratol* 1996;18(6):627. doi: 10.1016/s0892-0362(96)00121-3
31. Bada HS, Bann CM, Bauer CR, et al. Preadolescent behavior problems after prenatal cocaine exposure: relationship between teacher and caretaker ratings (Maternal Lifestyle Study). *Neurotoxicol Teratol* 2011;33(1):78. doi: 10.1016/j.ntt.2010.06.005
32. Warner TD, Behnke M, Eyler FD, et al. Diffusion tensor imaging of frontal white matter and executive functioning in cocaine-exposed children. *Pediatrics* 2006;118(5):2014. doi: 10.1542/peds.2006-0003
33. LaGasse LL, Gaskins RB, Bada HS, et al. Prenatal cocaine exposure and childhood obesity at nine years. *Neurotoxicol Teratol* 2011;33(2):188. doi: 10.1016/j.ntt.2010.11.002
34. Bandstra ES, Morrow CE, Accornero VH, et al. Estimated effects of in utero cocaine exposure on language development through early adolescence. *Neurotoxicol Teratol* 2011;33(1):25. doi: 10.1016/j.ntt.2010.07.001
35. Buckingham-Howes S, Berger SS, Scaletti LA, et al. Systematic review of prenatal cocaine exposure and adolescent development. *Pediatrics* 2013;131(6):e1917. doi: 10.1542/peds.2012-0945
36. Singer LT, Minnes S, Short E, et al. Cognitive outcomes of preschool children with prenatal cocaine exposure. *JAMA* 2004;291(20):2448. doi: 10.1001/jama.291.20.2448
37. Tronick EZ, Messinger DS, Weinberg MK, et al. Cocaine exposure is associated with subtle compromises of infants' and mothers' social-emotional behavior and dyadic features of their interaction in the face-to-face still-face paradigm. *Dev Psychol* 2005;41(5):711. doi: 10.1037/0012-1649.41.5.711
38. Fisher PA, Lester BM, DeGarmo DS, et al. The combined effects of prenatal drug exposure and early adversity on neurobehavioral disinhibition in childhood and adolescence. *Dev Psychopathol* 2011;23(3):777. doi: 10.1017/S0954579411000290
39. Bada HS, Das A, Bauer CR, et al. Impact of prenatal cocaine exposure on child behavior problems through school age. *Pediatrics* 2007;119(2):e348. doi: 10.1542/peds.2006-1404
40. Behnke M, Eyler FD, Warner TD, et al. Outcome from a prospective, longitudinal study of prenatal cocaine use: preschool development at 3 years of age. *J Pediatr Psychol* 2006;31(1):41. doi: 10.1093/jpepsy/jsj027
41. Liu J, Lester BM, Neyzi N, et al. Regional brain morphometry and impulsivity in adolescents following prenatal exposure to cocaine and tobacco. *JAMA Pediatr* 2013;167(4):348. doi: 10.1001/jamapediatrics.2013.550
42. Delaney-Black V, Chiodo LM, Hannigan JH, et al. Prenatal and postnatal cocaine exposure predict teen cocaine use. *Neurotoxicol Teratol* 2011;33(1):110. doi: 10.1016/j.ntt.2010.06.011
43. Warner TD, Behnke M, Eyler FD, et al. Early adolescent cocaine use as determined by hair analysis in a prenatal cocaine exposure cohort. *Neurotoxicol Teratol* 2011;33(1):88. doi: 10.1016/j.ntt.2010.07.003
44. Strathearn L, Mayes LC. Cocaine addiction in mothers: potential effects on maternal care and infant development. *Ann N Y Acad Sci* 2010;1187:172. doi: 10.1111/j.1749-6632.2009.05142.x
45. Fares I, McCulloch KM, Raju TN. Intrauterine cocaine exposure and the risk for sudden infant death syndrome: a meta-analysis. *J Perinatol* 1997;17(3):179.
46. Burd L, Blair J, Dropps K. Prenatal alcohol exposure, blood alcohol concentrations and alcohol elimination rates for the mother, fetus and newborn. *J Perinatol* 2012;32(9):652. doi: 10.1038/jp.2012.57
47. Hard ML, Einarson TR, Koren G. The role of acetaldehyde in pregnancy outcome after prenatal alcohol exposure. *Ther Drug Monit* 2001;23(4):427. doi: 10.1097/00007691-200108000-00018

THE FETAL PATIENT

48. Sundermann AC, Zhao S, Young CL, et al. Alcohol use in pregnancy and miscarriage: a systematic review and meta-analysis. *Alcohol Clin Exp Res* 2019;43(8):1606. doi: 10.1111/acer.14124

49. Kaufman MH. The teratogenic effects of alcohol following exposure during pregnancy, and its influence on the chromosome constitution of the pre-ovulatory egg. *Alcohol Alcohol* 1997;32(2):113. doi: 10.1093/oxfordjournals.alcalc.a008245

50. Randall CL, Taylor J, Walker DW. Ethanol-induced malformations in mice. *Alcohol Clin Exp Res* 1977;1(3):219. doi: 10.1111/j.1530-0277.1977.tb05876.x

51. Day NL, Richardson GA. Prenatal alcohol exposure: a continuum of effects. *Semin Perinatol* 1991;15(4):271.

52. Savoy-Moore RT, Dombrowski MP, Cheng A, et al. Low dose alcohol contracts the human umbilical artery in vitro. *Alcohol Clin Exp Res* 1989;13(1):40. doi: 10.1111/j.1530-0277.1989.tb00281.x

53. McLeod W, Brien J, Loomis C, et al. Effect of maternal ethanol ingestion on fetal breathing movements, gross body movements, and heart rate at 37 to 40 weeks' gestational age. *Am J Obstet Gynecol* 1983;145(2):251. doi: 10.1016/0002-9378(83)90501-x

54. Hoff SF. Synaptogenesis in the hippocampal dentate gyrus: effects of in utero ethanol exposure. *Brain Res Bull* 1988;21(1):47. doi: 10.1016/0361-9230(88)90119-0

55. Patra J, Bakker R, Irving H, et al. Dose-response relationship between alcohol consumption before and during pregnancy and the risks of low birth-weight, preterm birth and small for gestational age (SGA)—a systematic review and meta-analyses. *BJOG* 2011;118(12):1411. doi: 10.1111/j.1471-0528.2011.03050.x

56. de la Monte SM, Kril JJ. Human alcohol-related neuropathology. *Acta Neuropathol* 2014;127:71. doi: 10.1007/s00401-013-1233-3

57. Donald KA, Fouche JP, Roos A, et al. Alcohol exposure in utero is associated with decreased gray matter volume in neonates. *Metab Brain Dis* 2016;31(1):81. doi: 10.1007/s11011-015-9771-0

58. Fried PA, Makin JE. Neonatal behavioural correlates of prenatal exposure to marihuana, cigarettes and alcohol in a low risk population. *Neurotoxicol Teratol* 1987;9(1):1. doi: 10.1016/0892-0362(87)90062-6

59. Richardson S, de Vincenzi I, Pujol H, et al. Alcohol consumption in a case-control study of breast cancer in southern France. *Int J Cancer* 1989;44(1):84. doi: 10.1002/ijc.2910440116

60. Rosett HL, Snyder P, Sander LW, et al. Effects of maternal drinking on neonate state regulation. *Dev Med Child Neurol* 1979;21(4):464. doi: 10.1111/j.1469-8749.1979.tb01650.x

61. Inkelis SM, Thomas JD. Sleep in infants and children with prenatal alcohol exposure. *Alcohol Clin Exp Res* 2018. doi: 10.1111/acer.13803

62. Anderson PO. Alcohol use during breastfeeding. *Breastfeed Med* 2018;13(5):315. doi: 10.1089/bfm.2018.0053

63. May PA, Hasken JM, Blankenship J, et al. Breastfeeding and maternal alcohol use: prevalence and effects on child outcomes and fetal alcohol spectrum disorders. *Reprod Toxicol* 2016;63:13. doi: 10.1016/j.reprotox.2016.05.002

64. Carter RC, Jacobson JL, Sokol RJ, et al. Fetal alcohol-related growth restriction from birth through young adulthood and moderating effects of maternal prepregnancy weight. *Alcohol Clin Exp Res* 2013;37(3):452. doi: 10.1111/j.1530-0277.2012.01940.x

65. Sampson PD, Bookstein FL, Barr HM, et al. Prenatal alcohol exposure, birthweight, and measures of child size from birth to age 14 years. *Am J Public Health* 1994;84(9):1421. doi: 10.2105/ajph.84.9.1421

66. Subramoney S, Eastman E, Adnams C, et al. The early developmental outcomes of prenatal alcohol exposure: a review. *Front Neurol* 2018;9:1108. doi: 10.3389/fneur.2018.01108

67. Hendricks G, Malcolm-Smith S, Adnams C, et al. Effects of prenatal alcohol exposure on language, speech and communication outcomes: a review longitudinal studies. *Acta Neuropsychiatr* 2019;31(2):74. doi: 10.1017/neu.2018.28

68. Day NL, Helsel A, Sonon K, et al. The association between prenatal alcohol exposure and behavior at 22 years of age. *Alcohol Clin Exp Res* 2013;37(7):1171. doi: 10.1111/acer.12073

69. O'Leary CM, Nassar N, Zubrick SR, et al. Evidence of a complex association between dose, pattern and timing of prenatal alcohol exposure and child behaviour problems. *Addiction* 2010;105(1):74. doi: 10.1111/j.1360-0443.2009.02756.x

70. Mattson SN, Foroud T, Sowell ER, et al.; CIFASD. Collaborative initiative on fetal alcohol spectrum disorders: methodology of clinical projects. *Alcohol* 2010;44(7–8):635. doi: 10.1016/j.alcohol.2009.08.005

71. Williams JF, Smith VC; Committee On Substance Abuse. Fetal alcohol spectrum disorders. *Pediatrics* 2015;136(5):e1395. doi: 10.1542/peds.2015-3113

72. Hoyme HE, Kalberg WO, Elliott AJ, et al. Updated clinical guidelines for diagnosing fetal alcohol spectrum disorders. *Pediatrics* 2016;138(2):e20154256. doi: 10.1542/peds.2015-4256

73. Lange S, Probst C, Gmel G, et al. Global prevalence of fetal alcohol spectrum disorder among children and youth: a systematic review and meta-analysis. *JAMA Pediatr* 2017;171(10):948. doi: 10.1001/jamapediatrics.2017.1919

74. Arenson AD, Bakhireva LN, Chambers CD, et al. Implementation of a shared data repository and common data dictionary for fetal alcohol spectrum disorders research. *Alcohol* 2010;44(7–8):643. doi: 10.1016/j.alcohol.2009.08.007

75. Roozen S, Peters GY, Kok G, et al. Systematic literature review on which maternal alcohol behaviours are related to fetal alcohol spectrum disorders (FASD). *BMJ Open* 2018;8(12):e022578. doi: 10.1136/bmjopen-2018-022578

76. May PA, Hamrick KJ, Corbin KD, et al. Maternal nutritional status as a contributing factor for the risk of fetal alcohol spectrum disorders. *Reprod Toxicol* 2016;59:101. doi: 10.1016/j.reprotox.2015.11.006

77. Feldman HS, Jones KL, Lindsay S, et al. Prenatal alcohol exposure patterns and alcohol-related birth defects and growth deficiencies: a prospective study. *Alcohol Clin Exp Res* 2012;36(4):670. doi: 10.1111/j.1530-0277.2011.01664.x

78. Mamluk L, Jones T, Ijaz S, et al. Evidence of detrimental effects of prenatal alcohol exposure on offspring birthweight and neurodevelopment from a systematic review of quasi-experimental studies. *Int J Epidemiol* 2020:dyz272. doi: 10.1093/ije/dyz272

79. Boronat S, Sanchez-Montanez A, Gomez-Barros N, et al. Correlation between morphological MRI findings and specific diagnostic categories in fetal alcohol spectrum disorders. *Eur J Med Genet* 2017;60(1):65. doi: 10.1016/j.ejmg.2016.09.003

80. Stromland K, Hellstrom A. Fetal alcohol syndrome—an ophthalmological and socioeducational prospective study. *Pediatrics* 1996;97(6 Pt 1):845.

81. Church MW, Kaltenbach JA. Hearing, speech, language, and vestibular disorders in the fetal alcohol syndrome: a literature review. *Alcohol Clin Exp Res* 1997;21(3):495. doi: 10.1111/j.1530-0277.1997.tb03796.x

82. Llaquet H, Pichini S, Joya X, et al. Biological matrices for the evaluation of exposure to environmental tobacco smoke during prenatal life and childhood. *Anal Bioanal Chem* 2010;396(1):379. doi: 10.1007/s00216-009-2831-8

83. Ostrea EM Jr, Knapp DK, Romero A, et al. Meconium analysis to assess fetal exposure to nicotine by active and passive maternal smoking. *J Pediatr* 1994;124(3):471. doi: 10.1016/s0022-3476(94)70378-7

84. Benowitz NL, Hukkanen J, Jacob P III. Nicotine chemistry, metabolism, kinetics and biomarkers. *Handb Exp Pharmacol* 2009(192):29. doi: 10.1007/978-3-540-69248-5_2

85. Crume T. Tobacco use during pregnancy. *Clin Obstet Gynecol* 2019;62(1):128. doi: 10.1097/GRF.0000000000000413

86. Abraham M, Alramadhan S, Iniguez C, et al. A systematic review of maternal smoking during pregnancy and fetal measurements with meta-analysis. *PLoS One* 2017;12(2):e0170946. doi: 10.1371/journal.pone.0170946

87. Jauniaux E, Burton GJ. Morphological and biological effects of maternal exposure to tobacco smoke on the feto-placental unit. *Early Hum Dev* 2007;83(11):699. doi: 10.1016/j.earlhumdev.2007.07.016

88. George L, Granath F, Johansson AL, et al. Environmental tobacco smoke and risk of spontaneous abortion. *Epidemiology* 2006;17(5):500. doi: 10.1097/01.ede.0000229984.53726.33

89. Genbacev O, McMaster MT, Zdravkovic T, et al. Disruption of oxygen-regulated responses underlies pathological changes in the placentas of women who smoke or who are passively exposed to smoke during pregnancy. *Reprod Toxicol* 2003;17(5):509. doi: 10.1016/s0890-6238(03)00094-7

90. Rogers JM. Smoking and pregnancy: epigenetics and developmental origins of the metabolic syndrome. *Birth Defects Res* 2019;111(17):1259. doi: 10.1002/bdr2.1550

91. Berard A, Zhao JP, Sheehy O. Success of smoking cessation interventions during pregnancy. *Am J Obstet Gynecol* 2016;215(5):611.e1. doi: 10.1016/j.ajog.2016.06.059

92. Cnattingius S, Haglund B, Meirik O. Cigarette smoking as risk factor for late fetal and early neonatal death. *BMJ* 1988;297(6643):258. doi: 10.1136/bmj.297.6643.258

93. Aliyu MH, Salihu HM, Alio AP, et al. Prenatal smoking among adolescents and risk of fetal demise before and during labor. *J Pediatr Adolesc Gynecol* 2010;23(3):129. doi: 10.1016/j.jpag.2009.10.008

94. Lavezzi AM, Mehboob R, Matturri L. Developmental alterations of the spinal trigeminal nucleus disclosed by substance P immunohistochemistry in fetal and infant sudden unexplained deaths. *Neuropathology* 2011;31(4):405. doi: 10.1111/j.1440-1789.2010.01190.x

95. Lavezzi AM, Mohorovic L, Alfonsi G, et al. Brain iron accumulation in unexplained fetal and infant death victims with smoker mothers—the possible involvement of maternal methemoglobinemia. *BMC Pediatr* 2011;11:62. doi: 10.1186/1471-2431-11-62

96. Ernst M, Moolchan ET, Robinson ML. Behavioral and neural consequences of prenatal exposure to nicotine. *J Am Acad Child Adolesc Psychiatry* 2001;40(6):630. doi: 10.1097/00004583-200106000-00007

97. Deng Y, Cao H, Cu F, et al. Nicotine-induced retardation of chondrogenesis through down-regulation of IGF-1 signaling pathway to inhibit matrix synthesis of growth plate chondrocytes in fetal rats. *Toxicol Appl Pharmacol* 2013;269(1):25. doi: 10.1016/j.taap.2013.02.008

98. Hackshaw A, Rodeck C, Boniface S. Maternal smoking in pregnancy and birth defects: a systematic review based on 173 687 malformed cases and 11.7 million controls. *Hum Reprod Update* 2011;17(5):589. doi: 10.1093/humupd/dmr022

99. Park A, O'Malley SS, King SL, et al. Mediating role of stress reactivity in the effects of prenatal tobacco exposure on childhood mental health outcomes. *Nicotine Tob Res* 2014;16(2):174. doi: 10.1093/ntr/ntt131

100. Huang L, Wang Y, Zhang L, et al. Maternal smoking and attention-deficit/hyperactivity disorder in offspring: a meta-analysis. *Pediatrics* 2018;141(1):e20172465. doi: 10.1542/peds.2017-2465

101. Langley K, Heron J, Smith GD, et al. Maternal and paternal smoking during pregnancy and risk of ADHD symptoms in offspring: testing for intrauterine effects. *Am J Epidemiol* 2012;176(3):261. doi: 10.1093/aje/kwr510

102. Gustavson K, Ystrom E, Stoltenberg C, et al. Smoking in pregnancy and child ADHD. *Pediatrics* 2017;139(2):e20162509. doi: 10.1542/peds.2016-2509

103. Polanska K, Krol A, Merecz-Kot D, et al. Environmental tobacco smoke exposure during pregnancy and child neurodevelopment. *Int J Environ Res Public Health* 2017;14(7):796. doi: 10.3390/ijerph14070796

104. Behl M, Rao D, Aagaard K, et al. Evaluation of the association between maternal smoking, childhood obesity, and metabolic disorders: a national toxicology program workshop review. *Environ Health Perspect* 2013;121(2):170. doi: 10.1289/ehp.1205404

105. Raum E, Kupper-Nybelen J, Lamerz A, et al. Tobacco smoke exposure before, during, and after pregnancy and risk of overweight at age 6. *Obesity (Silver Spring)* 2011;19(12):2411. doi: 10.1038/oby.2011.129

106. Anderson TM, Lavista Ferres JM, Ren SY, et al. Maternal smoking before and during pregnancy and the risk of sudden unexpected infant death. *Pediatrics* 2019;143(4):e20183325. doi: 10.1542/peds.2018-3325

107. Lavista Ferres JM, Anderson TM, Johnston R, et al. Distinct populations of sudden unexpected infant death based on age. *Pediatrics* 2020;145(1):e20191637. doi: 10.1542/peds.2019-1637

108. Eugenin J, Otarola M, Bravo E, et al. Prenatal to early postnatal nicotine exposure impairs central chemoreception and modifies breathing pattern in mouse neonates: a probable link to sudden infant death syndrome. *J Neurosci* 2008;28(51):13907. doi: 10.1523/JNEUROSCI.4441-08.2008

109. Rehan HS, Maini J, Hungin APS. Vaping versus smoking: a quest for efficacy and safety of e-cigarette. *Curr Drug Saf* 2018;13(2):92. doi: 10.2174/1574886313666180227110556

110. Sandtner W, Schmid D, Schicker K, et al. A quantitative model of amphetamine action on the 5-HT transporter. *Br J Pharmacol* 2014;171(4):1007. doi: 10.1111/bph.12520

111. Della Grotta S, LaGasse LL, Arria AM, et al. Patterns of methamphetamine use during pregnancy: results from the Infant Development, Environment, and Lifestyle (IDEAL) Study. *Matern Child Health J* 2010;14(4):519. doi: 10.1007/s10995-009-0491-0

112. Oei JL, Kingsbury A, Dhawan A, et al. Amphetamines, the pregnant woman and her children: a review. *J Perinatol* 2012;32(10):737. doi: 10.1038/jp.2012.59

113. Smith LM, LaGasse LL, Derauf C, et al. The infant development, environment, and lifestyle study: effects of prenatal methamphetamine exposure, polydrug exposure, and poverty on intrauterine growth. *Pediatrics* 2006;118(3):1149. doi: 10.1542/peds.2005-2564

114. Huybrechts KF, Broms G, Christensen LB, et al. Association between methylphenidate and amphetamine use in pregnancy and risk of congenital malformations: a Cohort Study From the International Pregnancy Safety Study Consortium. *JAMA Psychiat* 2018;75(2):167. doi: 10.1001/jamapsychiatry.2017.3644

115. Won L, Bubula N, Heller A. Fetal exposure to methamphetamine in utero stimulates development of serotonergic neurons in three-dimensional reaggregate tissue culture. *Synapse* 2002;43(2):139. doi: 10.1002/syn.10026

116. Chang L, Smith LM, LoPresti C, et al. Smaller subcortical volumes and cognitive deficits in children with prenatal methamphetamine exposure. *Psychiatry Res* 2004;132(2):95. doi: 10.1016/j.pscychresns.2004.06.004

117. Barenys M, Reverte I, Masjosthusmann S, et al. Developmental neurotoxicity of MDMA. A systematic literature review summarized in a putative adverse outcome pathway. *Neurotoxicology* 2020;78:209. doi: 10.1016/j.neuro.2019.12.007

118. Singer LT, Moore DG, Min MO, et al. Motor delays in MDMA (ecstasy) exposed infants persist to 2 years. *Neurotoxicol Teratol* 2016;54:22. doi: 10.1016/j.ntt.2016.01.003

119. McElhatton PR, Bateman DN, Evans C, et al. Congenital anomalies after prenatal ecstasy exposure. *Lancet* 1999;354(9188):1441. doi: 10.1016/s0140-6736(99)02423-x

120. Olutoye OA, Baker BW, Belfort MA, et al. Food and Drug Administration warning on anesthesia and brain development: implications for obstetric and fetal surgery. *Am J Obstet Gynecol* 2018;218(1):98. doi: 10.1016/j.ajog.2017.08.107

121. Van der Veeken L, Van der Merwe J, Devroe S, et al. Maternal surgery during pregnancy has a transient adverse effect on the developing fetal rabbit brain. *Am J Obstet Gynecol* 2019;221(4):355.e1. doi: 10.1016/j.ajog.2019.07.029

122. Zhao T, Li C, Wei W, et al. Prenatal ketamine exposure causes abnormal development of prefrontal cortex in rat. *Sci Rep* 2016;6:26865. doi: 10.1038/srep26865

123. Capitanio JP, Del Rosso LA, Calonder LA, et al. Behavioral effects of prenatal ketamine exposure in rhesus macaques are dependent on MAOA genotype. *Exp Clin Psychopharmacol* 2012;20(3):173. doi: 10.1037/a0026773

124. Su PH, Chang YZ, Chen JY. Infant with in utero ketamine exposure: quantitative measurement of residual dosage in hair. *Pediatr Neonatol* 2010;51(5):279. doi: 10.1016/S1875-9572(10)60054-X

125. Ko JY, Farr SL, Tong VT, et al. Prevalence and patterns of marijuana use among pregnant and nonpregnant women of reproductive age. *Am J Obstet Gynecol* 2015;213(2):201.e1. doi: 10.1016/j.ajog.2015.03.021

126. Ryan SA, Ammerman SD, O'Connor ME; Committee on Substance Use And Prevention; Section on Breastfeeding. Marijuana use during pregnancy and breastfeeding: implications for neonatal and childhood outcomes. *Pediatrics* 2018;142(3):e20181889. doi: 10.1542/peds.2018-1889

127. Volkow ND, Compton WM, Wargo EM. The risks of marijuana use during pregnancy. *JAMA* 2017;317(2):129. doi: 10.1001/jama.2016.18612

128. Committee on Obstetric Practice. Committee Opinion No. 722: Marijuana use during pregnancy and lactation. *Obstet Gynecol* 2017;130(4):e205. doi: 10.1097/AOG.0000000000002354

129. Ganapathy VV, Prasad PD, Ganapathy ME, et al. Drugs of abuse and placental transport. *Adv Drug Deliv Rev* 1999;38(1):99. doi: 10.1016/s0169-409x(99)00009-5

130. Conner SN, Bedell V, Lipsey K, et al. Maternal marijuana use and adverse neonatal outcomes: a systematic review and meta-analysis. *Obstet Gynecol* 2016;128(4):713. doi: 10.1097/AOG.0000000000001649

131. Metz TD, Allshouse AA, Hogue CJ, et al. Maternal marijuana use, adverse pregnancy outcomes, and neonatal morbidity. *Am J Obstet Gynecol* 2017;217(4):478.e1. doi: 10.1016/j.ajog.2017.05.050

132. Chabarria KC, Racusin DA, Antony KM, et al. Marijuana use and its effects in pregnancy. *Am J Obstet Gynecol* 2016;215(4):506.e1. doi: 10.1016/j.ajog.2016.05.044

133. Wu CS, Jew CP, Lu HC. Lasting impacts of prenatal cannabis exposure and the role of endogenous cannabinoids in the developing brain. *Future Neurol* 2011;6(4):459. doi: 10.2217/fnl.11.27

134. El Marroun H, Tiemeier H, Franken IH, et al. Prenatal cannabis and tobacco exposure in relation to brain morphology: a prospective neuroimaging study in young children. *Biol Psychiatry* 2016;79(12):971. doi: 10.1016/j.biopsych.2015.08.024

135. Day NL, Richardson GA, Goldschmidt L, et al. Effect of prenatal marijuana exposure on the cognitive development of offspring at age three. *Neurotoxicol Teratol* 1994;16(2):169. doi: 10.1016/0892-0362(94)90114-7

136. Goldschmidt L, Richardson GA, Willford J, et al. Prenatal marijuana exposure and intelligence test performance at age 6. *J Am Acad Child Adolesc Psychiatry* 2008;47(3):254. doi: 10.1097/CHI.0b013e318160b3f0

137. Goldschmidt L, Day NL, Richardson GA. Effects of prenatal marijuana exposure on child behavior problems at age 10. *Neurotoxicol Teratol* 2000;22(3):325. doi: 10.1016/s0892-0362(00)00066-0

138. Goldschmidt L, Richardson GA, Willford JA, et al. School achievement in 14-year-old youths prenatally exposed to marijuana. *Neurotoxicol Teratol* 2012;34(1):161. doi: 10.1016/j.ntt.2011.08.009

139. Smith AM, Mioduszewski O, Hatchard T, et al. Prenatal marijuana exposure impacts executive functioning into young adulthood: an fMRI study. *Neurotoxicol Teratol* 2016;58:53. doi: 10.1016/j.ntt.2016.05.010

140. Porath AJ, Fried PA. Effects of prenatal cigarette and marijuana exposure on drug use among offspring. *Neurotoxicol Teratol* 2005;27(2):267. doi: 10.1016/j.ntt.2004.12.003

141. McCarron MM. Phencyclidine intoxication. *NIDA Res Monogr* 1986;64:209.

142. Ali SF, Ahmad G, Slikker W Jr, et al. Effects of gestational exposure to phencyclidine: distribution and neurochemical alterations in maternal and fetal brain. *Neurotoxicology* 1989;10(3):383.

143. Nicholas JM, Lipshitz J, Schreiber EC. Phencyclidine: its transfer across the placenta as well as into breast milk. *Am J Obstet Gynecol* 1982;143(2):143. doi: 10.1016/0002-9378(82)90643-3

144. Morris BJ, Cochran SM, Pratt JA. PCP: from pharmacology to modelling schizophrenia. *Curr Opin Pharmacol* 2005;5(1):101. doi: 10.1016/j.coph.2004.08.008

145. Xia Y, Wang CZ, Liu J, et al. Brain-derived neurotrophic factor prevents phencyclidine-induced apoptosis in developing brain by parallel activation of both the ERK and PI-3K/Akt pathways. *Neuropharmacology* 2010;58(2):330. doi: 10.1016/j.neuropharm.2009.10.009

THE FETAL PATIENT

146. Chasnoff IJ, Burns WJ, Hatcher RP, et al. Phencyclidine: effects on the fetus and neonate. *Dev Pharmacol Ther* 1983;6(6):404. doi: 10.1159/000457343

147. Tabor BL, Smith-Wallace T, Yonekura ML. Perinatal outcome associated with PCP versus cocaine use. *Am J Drug Alcohol Abuse* 1990;16(3–4):337. doi: 10.3109/00952999009001595

148. Jebelli AK, Doan N, Ellison G. Prenatal phencyclidine induces heightened neurodegeneration in rats in some brain regions, especially during 2nd trimester, but possible anti-apoptotic effects in others. *Pharmacol Toxicol* 2002;90(1):20. doi: 10.1034/j.1600-0773.2002.900105.x

149. Lu L, Mamiya T, Lu P, et al. Prenatal exposure to phencyclidine produces abnormal behaviour and NMDA receptor expression in postpubertal mice. *Int J Neuropsychopharmacol* 2010;13(7):877. doi: 10.1017/S1461145709990757

150. Strauss AA, Modaniou HD, Bosu SK. Neonatal manifestations of maternal phencyclidine (PCP) abuse. *Pediatrics* 1981;68(4):550.

151. Toriumi K, Mouri A, Narusawa S, et al. Prenatal NMDA receptor antagonism impaired proliferation of neuronal progenitor, leading to fewer glutamatergic neurons in the prefrontal cortex. *Neuropsychopharmacology* 2012;37(6):1387. doi: 10.1038/npp.2011.324

152. du Bois TM, Newell KA, Huang XF. Perinatal phencyclidine treatment alters neuregulin 1/erbB4 expression and activation in later life. *Eur Neuropsychopharmacol* 2012;22(5):356. doi: 10.1016/j.euroneuro.2011.09.002

153. Howard J, Kropenske V, Tyler R. The long-term effects on neurodevelopment in infants exposed prenatally to PCP. *NIDA Res Monogr* 1986;64:237.

154. Molenaar NM, Bais B, Lambregtse-van den Berg MP, et al. The international prevalence of antidepressant use before, during, and after pregnancy: a systematic review and meta-analysis of timing, type of prescriptions and geographical variability. *J Affect Disord* 2020;264:82. doi: 10.1016/j.jad.2019.12.014

155. Sanz EJ, De-las-Cuevas C, Kiuru A, et al. Selective serotonin reuptake inhibitors in pregnant women and neonatal withdrawal syndrome: a database analysis. *Lancet* 2005;365(9458):482. doi: 10.1016/S0140-6736(05)17865-9

156. Costei AM, Kozer E, Ho T, et al. Perinatal outcome following third trimester exposure to paroxetine. *Arch Pediatr Adolesc Med* 2002;156(11):1129. doi: 10.1001/archpedi.156.11.1129

157. Ross LE, Grigoriadis S, Mamisashvili L, et al. Selected pregnancy and delivery outcomes after exposure to antidepressant medication: a systematic review and meta-analysis. *JAMA Psychiat* 2013;70(4):436. doi: 10.1001/jamapsychiatry.2013.684

158. Eke AC, Saccone G, Berghella V. Selective serotonin reuptake inhibitor (SSRI) use during pregnancy and risk of preterm birth: a systematic review and meta-analysis. *BJOG* 2016;123(12):1900. doi: 10.1111/1471-0528.14144

159. Masarwa R, Bar-Oz B, Gorelik E, et al. Prenatal exposure to selective serotonin reuptake inhibitors and serotonin norepinephrine reuptake inhibitors and risk for persistent pulmonary hypertension of the newborn: a systematic review, meta-analysis, and network meta-analysis. *Am J Obstet Gynecol* 2019;220(1):57.e1. doi: 10.1016/j.ajog.2018.08.030

160. Grigoriadis S, Vonderporten EH, Mamisashvili L, et al. Prenatal exposure to antidepressants and persistent pulmonary hypertension of the newborn: systematic review and meta-analysis. *BMJ* 2014;348:f6932. doi: 10.1136/bmj.f6932

161. Gao SY, Wu QJ, Zhang TN, et al. Fluoxetine and congenital malformations: a systematic review and meta-analysis of cohort studies. *Br J Clin Pharmacol* 2017;83(10):2134. doi: 10.1111/bcp.13321

162. Koren G, Nordeng HM. Selective serotonin reuptake inhibitors and malformations: case closed? *Semin Fetal Neonatal Med* 2013;18(1):19. doi: 10.1016/j.siny.2012.10.004

163. Eriksen HL, Kesmodel US, Pedersen LH, et al. No association between prenatal exposure to psychotropics and intelligence at age five. *Acta Obstet Gynecol Scand* 2015;94(5):501. doi: 10.1111/aogs.12611

164. El Marroun H, White TJ, Fernandez G, et al. Prenatal exposure to selective serotonin reuptake inhibitors and non-verbal cognitive functioning in childhood. *J Psychopharmacol* 2017;31(3):346. doi: 10.1177/0269881116665335

165. Nulman I, Koren G, Rovet J, et al. Neurodevelopment of children following prenatal exposure to venlafaxine, selective serotonin reuptake inhibitors, or untreated maternal depression. *Am J Psychiatry* 2012;169(11):1165. doi: 10.1176/appi.ajp.2012.11111721

166. Kim JY, Son MJ, Son CY, et al. Environmental risk factors and biomarkers for autism spectrum disorder: an umbrella review of the evidence. *Lancet Psychiatry* 2019;6(7):590. doi: 10.1016/S2215-0366(19)30181-6

167. Uguz F. Maternal antidepressant use during pregnancy and the risk of attention-deficit/hyperactivity disorder in children: a systematic review of the current literature. *J Clin Psychopharmacol* 2018;38(3):254. doi: 10.1097/JCP.0000000000000868

168. Kaplan YC, Keskin-Arslan E, Acar S, et al. Prenatal selective serotonin reuptake inhibitor use and the risk of autism spectrum disorder in children: a systematic review and meta-analysis. *Reprod Toxicol* 2016;66:31. doi: 10.1016/j.reprotox.2016.09.013

169. Ornoy A, Koren G. SSRIs and SNRIs (SRI) in pregnancy: effects on the course of pregnancy and the offspring: how far are we from having all the answers? *Int J Mol Sci* 2019;20(10):2370. doi: 10.3390/ijms20102370

170. Viuff AC, Pedersen LH, Kyng K, et al. Antidepressant medication during pregnancy and epigenetic changes in umbilical cord blood: a systematic review. *Clin Epigenetics* 2016;8(1):94. doi: 10.1186/s13148-016-0262-x

171. Oberlander TF. Fetal serotonin signaling: setting pathways for early childhood development and behavior. *J Adolesc Health* 2012;51(2 suppl):S9. doi: 10.1016/j.jadohealth.2012.04.009

172. Huybrechts KF, Bateman BT, Desai RJ, et al. Risk of neonatal drug withdrawal after intrauterine co-exposure to opioids and psychotropic medications: cohort study. *BMJ* 2017;358:j3326. doi: 10.1136/bmj.j3326

173. Duceppe MA, Perreault MM, Frenette AJ, et al. Frequency, risk factors and symptomatology of iatrogenic withdrawal from opioids and benzodiazepines in critically Ill neonates, children and adults: a systematic review of clinical studies. *J Clin Pharm Ther* 2019;44(2):148. doi: 10.1111/jcpt.12787

174. Shyken JM, Babbar S, Babbar S, et al. Benzodiazepines in pregnancy. *Clin Obstet Gynecol* 2019;62(1):156. doi: 10.1097/GRF.0000000000000417

175. Dennis CL, Falah-Hassani K, Shiri R. Prevalence of antenatal and postnatal anxiety: systematic review and meta-analysis. *Br J Psychiatry* 2017;210(5):315. doi: 10.1192/bjp.bp.116.187179

176. Mohler H, Fritschy JM, Rudolph U. A new benzodiazepine pharmacology. *J Pharmacol Exp Ther* 2002;300(1):2. doi: 10.1124/jpet.300.1.2

177. Jauniaux E, Jurkovic D, Lees C, et al. In-vivo study of diazepam transfer across the first trimester human placenta. *Hum Reprod* 1996;11(4):889. doi: 10.1093/oxfordjournals.humrep.a019272

178. Okun ML, Ebert R, Saini B. A review of sleep-promoting medications used in pregnancy. *Am J Obstet Gynecol* 2015;212(4):428. doi: 10.1016/j.ajog.2014.10.1106

179. Enato E, Moretti M, Koren G. The fetal safety of benzodiazepines: an updated meta-analysis. *J Obstet Gynaecol Can* 2011;33(1):46. doi: 10.1016/S1701-2163(16)34772-7

180. Yonkers KA, Gilstad-Hayden K, Forray A, et al. Association of panic disorder, generalized anxiety disorder, and benzodiazepine treatment during pregnancy with risk of adverse birth outcomes. *JAMA Psychiat* 2017;74(11):1145. doi: 10.1001/jamapsychiatry.2017.2733

181. Brandlistuen RE, Ystrom E, Hernandez-Diaz S, et al. Association of prenatal exposure to benzodiazepine and child internalizing problems: a sibling-controlled study. *PLoS One* 2017;12(7):e0181042.

182. Radojcic MR, El Marroun H, Miljkovic B, et al. Prenatal exposure to anxiolytic and hypnotic medication in relation to behavioral problems in childhood: a population-based cohort study. *Neurotoxicol Teratol* 2017;61:58. doi: 10.1016/j.ntt.2017.02.005

183. Ploman L, Persson BH. On the transfer of barbiturates to the human foetus and their accumulation in some of its vital organs. *J Obstet Gynaecol Br Emp* 1957;64(5):706. doi: 10.1111/j.1471-0528.1957.tb08460.x

184. Barroso FV, Araujo Junior E, Guazelli CA, et al. Perinatal outcomes from the use of antiepileptic drugs during pregnancy: a case-control study. *J Matern Fetal Neonatal Med* 2015;28(12):1445. doi: 10.3109/14767058.2014.955004

185. Shankaran S, Papile LA, Wright LL, et al. Neurodevelopmental outcome of premature infants after antenatal phenobarbital exposure. *Am J Obstet Gynecol* 2002;187(1):171. doi: 10.1067/mob.2002.122445

186. Freeman EH, Delaney RM. Neonatal Baclofen withdrawal: a case report of an infant presenting with severe feeding difficulties. *J Pediatr Nurs* 2016;31(3):346. doi: 10.1016/j.pedn.2015.12.004

187. Duncan SD, Devlin LA. Use of baclofen for withdrawal in a preterm infant. *J Perinatol* 2013;33(4):327. doi: 10.1038/jp.2012.107

188. Sen A, Nashef L. New regulations to cut valproate-exposed pregnancies. *Lancet* 2018;392(10146):458. doi: 10.1016/S0140-6736(18)31672-6

189. Tomson T, Battino D, Bonizzoni E, et al. Comparative risk of major congenital malformations with eight different antiepileptic drugs: a prospective cohort study of the EURAP registry. *Lancet Neurol* 2018;17(6):530. doi: 10.1016/S1474-4422(18)30107-8

190. Roullet FI, Lai JK, Foster JA. In utero exposure to valproic acid and autism—a current review of clinical and animal studies. *Neurotoxicol Teratol* 2013;36:47. doi: 10.1016/j.ntt.2013.01.004

191. Zhao H, Wang Q, Yan T, et al. Maternal valproic acid exposure leads to neurogenesis defects and autism-like behaviors in non-human primates. *Transl Psychiatry* 2019;9(1):267. doi: 10.1038/s41398-019-0608-1

192. Christensen J, Pedersen L, Sun Y, et al. Association of prenatal exposure to valproate and other antiepileptic drugs with risk for attention-deficit/hyperactivity disorder in offspring. *JAMA Netw Open* 2019;2(1):e186606. doi: 10.1001/jamanetworkopen.2018.6606

193. Barton S, Nadebaum C, Anderson VA, et al. Memory dysfunction in school-aged children exposed prenatally to antiepileptic drugs. *Neuropsychology* 2018;32(7):784. doi: 10.1037/neu0000465

194. Bosak M, Slowik A, Turaj W. Why do some women with epilepsy use valproic acid despite current guidelines? A single-center cohort study. *Epilepsy Behav* 2019;98(Pt A):1. doi: 10.1016/j.yebeh.2019.06.031

195. Khavari KA, Farber PD. A profile instrument for the quantification and assessment of alcohol consumption. The Khavari Alcohol Test. *J Stud Alcohol* 1978;39(9):1525. doi: 10.15288/jsa.1978.39.1525

196. Ostrea EM Jr. Detection of prenatal drug exposure in the pregnant woman and her newborn infant. *NIDA Res Monogr* 1992;117:61.

197. Osterloh JD, Lee BL. Urine drug screening in mothers and newborns. *Am J Dis Child* 1989;143(7):791. doi: 10.1001/archpedi.1989.02150190041017

198. Silvestre MA, Lucena JE, Roxas R Jr, et al. Effects of timing, dosage, and duration of morphine intake during pregnancy on the amount of morphine in meconium in a rat model. *Biol Neonate* 1997;72(2):112. doi: 10.1159/000244473

199. Garcia-Bournissen F, Rokach B, Karaskov T, et al. Cocaine detection in maternal and neonatal hair: implications to fetal toxicology. *Ther Drug Monit* 2007;29(1):71. doi: 10.1097/ftd.0b013e3180310ddd

200. Ostrea EM Jr, Mantaring JB III, Silvestre MA. Drugs that affect the fetus and newborn infant via the placenta or breast milk. *Pediatr Clin North Am* 2004;51(3):539, vii. doi: 10.1016/j.pcl.2004.01.001

201. Reece-Stremtan S, Marinelli KA. ABM clinical protocol #21: guidelines for breastfeeding and substance use or substance use disorder, revised 2015. *Breastfeed Med* 2015;10(3):135. doi: 10.1089/bfm.2015.9992

THE FETAL PATIENT

PART 3

Care Around Birth

15 Transition and Stabilization

Ruben E. Alvaro

INTRODUCTION

Respiratory physiologists and physicians have long been interested in the respiratory and cardiovascular events that occur at birth. However, apart from occasional references to the pulmonary circulation, the fetal circulation only received serious consideration in the middle of the 20th century, when it was recognized that dramatic changes in blood flow through the lungs occurred after birth.

The first detailed description of circulation in the mammalian fetus was provided by Harvey in 1628 (1). Although he correctly described blood flow from the inferior vena cava through the foramen ovale, he thought that the blood had to enter the pulmonary veins before returning to the left atrium. He was also perplexed by how the fetus survives *in utero* without the aid of respiration. The answer to the last question came in 1799 when Scheel noted light red blood in the umbilical vein and dark red blood in the umbilical artery in the fetal sheep as well as darkening of that color when the pregnant ewe was asphyxiated (2). However, it was Zweifel in 1876 who categorically stated that the placenta was the lung of the fetus, describing the presence of oxyhemoglobin in the umbilical blood before any breathing had occurred (3).

The conventional belief during the 19th century was that the fetal pulmonary blood flow progressively increased over gestation and that it was relatively higher in the fetus than after birth (4,5). It was not until the first part of the 20th century that the right ventricular pressure was demonstrated to fall and pulmonary blood flow to increase after the establishment of breathing (6,7). It was only 50 years ago that Dawes et al. demonstrated by direct measurements in fetal lambs that pulmonary blood flow increased when the lungs were ventilated with air (8). Over these past 50 years, the developmental changes in the pulmonary circulation and in its responses to stresses of hypoxia, and increases in pulmonary arterial pressure and blood flow, have become subjects of intense investigation (9).

The transition from the placenta to the lungs at birth is accomplished by three main cardiopulmonary processes: (a) onset of breathing, resulting in lung expansion with concomitant decrease in pulmonary vascular resistance (PVR) and increase pulmonary blood flow; (b) increase in blood oxygen content that further decreases PVR; and (c) loss of the placental circulation with resultant increase in systemic vascular resistance leading to the closure of the fetal cardiovascular shunts and transition from fetal to neonatal circulation. Thus, to establish the lungs as the site of gas exchange after birth, significant changes in the cardiac and pulmonary circulation as well as the initiation of pulmonary ventilation must occur. Other essential adaptations to extrauterine life are changes in endocrine function, substrate metabolism, and thermogenesis. Many abnormal maternal, placental, and fetal conditions may interfere with this physiologic transition and compromise the newborn infant.

The establishment of effective pulmonary ventilation at birth requires that the lungs develop to a stage where the alveoli can be inflated to provide adequate gas exchange. It also requires the lowering of the PVR to allow for the increase in pulmonary blood flow to accommodate the entire cardiac output. The successful transition also requires that the lung liquid volume be removed from the alveolar spaces and that surfactant material be secreted into the acinus to allow for satisfactory physical expansion of the lungs after the initial postnatal breaths. Adequate neurologic drive to generate and maintain spontaneous continuous breathing is essential to maintain ventilation postnatally.

In this chapter, I review some of the most important cardiorespiratory adjustments that occur at the time of delivery allowing the fetus to achieve a successful extrauterine transition.

PULMONARY ADAPTATION

Fetal Lung Fluid

During fetal life, the internal volume of the lungs is maintained by the secretion of liquid into the pulmonary lumen. This liquid expansion of potential air spaces is essential for the growth and the development of normal lung structure before birth, which in turn may influence lung function after birth (10).

The fluid in the fetal lung was for many years assumed to be aspirated amniotic fluid as a result of fetal breathing movements (FBMs) (11). In 1941, Potter and Bohlender observed alveolar fluid in two human fetuses with malformations of the respiratory tract which blocked the entrance of amniotic fluid, thus establishing that the lung fluid was secreted, not inhaled (12). Experiments performed in other species confirmed that fetal pulmonary fluid was indeed generated within the lungs (13–15).

We know now that the fetal lung fluid is neither a mere ultrafiltrate of plasma nor aspirated amniotic fluid. Compared to plasma, this lung fluid is rich in chloride and potassium, is significantly lower in bicarbonate, and has similar sodium concentration. It is also quite different from amniotic fluid having much higher osmolality, Na+ and Cl− concentrations, and significantly lower K+, protein, and urea concentration (table) (10,16–18). This distinctive composition of the lung liquid changes very little during gestation (17,19). The high Cl− and the low protein content characteristics of the lung fluid result from active Cl− secretion and tight junctions between epithelial cells, respectively.

It is not known exactly when this secretory activity begins, but already during the glandular stage of lung development at about 3 months of gestation, the lung epithelium actively secretes fluid (20,21). In fetal lambs, the volume of lung liquid increases from about 5 mL/kg of body weight at midgestation (18) to about 30 to 50 mL/kg at term (18,22–25). The secretion rate increases from about 2 mL/kg body weight at midgestation (18) to about 5 mL/kg at term (25,26). The lung liquid secretion decreases with increased luminal hydrostatic pressure induced by a prolonged obstruction of the fetal trachea and increases when luminal pressure falls below amniotic fluid pressure and when FBMs are abolished (24).

This liquid secreted by the fetal lungs flows intermittently up the trachea with FBMs. Some of this fluid is swallowed and the remainder contributes directly to the formation of amniotic fluid production accounting for approximately 25% to 50% of the amniotic fluid turnover in the sheep fetus, with the rest being formed by the fetal urine (10). The mechanism by which amniotic fluid is not aspirated into the lungs was demonstrated by Brown et al. in 1983, when they showed that the larynx acts as a one-way valve allowing only liquid outflow under normal circumstances (27). The continuous secretion of liquid by the lungs confronted with a flow impediment produced by the larynx and the amniotic fluid pressure creates a small but important positive intrapulmonary pressure, which is essential for normal growth and for the structural and biochemical maturation of the developing lung (10,27,28). Thus, in fetal sheep, unimpeded leakage of tracheal liquid decreases lung size by arresting pulmonary tissue growth, whereas prolonged obstruction of tracheal outflow leads to lung hyperplasia (28,29). Nardo et al. have shown that lung hypoplasia in fetal sheep can be considerably improved by short-term obstruction at the tracheal level (30). On the other hand, pulmonary hypoplasia in humans can be observed in pathologic conditions such as diaphragmatic hernia, pleural effusion, or severe oligohydramnios (Potter syndrome) as a result of the compression of the fetal lungs and the decrease in their internal volume (31,32).

Congenital high airway obstruction syndrome (CHAOS) is a clinical condition caused by complete or near-complete obstruction of the fetal airway that results in elevated intratracheal pressure, distension of the tracheobronchial tree, and lung hyperplasia. The enlarged lungs may cause cardiac and caval compression leading to *in utero* heart failure manifested by ascites, hydrops fetalis, and placentomegaly (33,34).

The production of fetal lung liquid depends on a system of active ion transport across the alveolar type II cells of the pulmonary epithelium (10,35,36). Olver and Strang demonstrated that lung liquid secretion is coupled with active transport of Cl− toward the pulmonary lumen, generating an electrical potential difference of −5 mV (lumen negative) (37). This chloride secretion generates an osmotic gradient that causes liquid to flow from the microcirculation through the interstitium into the potential air spaces. This chloride secretion occurs through chloride channels in the apical membrane (alveolar side) and depends largely on chloride influx at a bumetanide-sensitive Na+ −K+ −2Cl− (NKCC) cotransporter system in the basolateral membrane (interstitial side) (38). Thus, Cl− enters the cell on a cotransporter linked with K+ and Na+ down the electrochemical potential gradient for Na+ generated by Na+ −K+ −ATPase in the basolateral membrane of the cell. Consequently, Cl− concentration increases inside the cell, above its equilibrium potential, which provides an electrochemical gradient for Cl− exit across the luminal membrane of the epithelial cell through Cl− permeant ion channels (Fig. 15.1) (10). Addition of the loop diuretic bumetanide or furosemide (specific NKCC inhibitors) into the fetal lung liquid decreases fluid secretion by decreasing Cl− entry into the epithelial cell through the basolateral membrane.

Clearance of Lung Fluid

Pulmonary fluid, essential to fetal lung and airway development, must be rapidly removed at birth in order to allow adequate postnatal gas exchange (39–41). Thus, the transition from intra to extrauterine life requires the effective clearance of lung liquid to support air breathing and the conversion of the pulmonary epithelium in the distal air spaces from fluid secretion to fluid absorption. Disruption of this process has been implicated in several disease states, including transient tachypnea of the newborn (TTN) and hyaline membrane disease (HMD) (40,42–44). Preterm delivery and Cesarean section without prior labor result in excessive retention of lung fluid and may contribute to respiratory compromise in the newborn infant (43,45–49).

Although a complete understanding is still lacking, it is now clear that the mechanisms by which fetal lungs are able to clear themselves of fluid at birth are multidimensional and can occur via a number of processes before, during, and after birth (50).

Lung Fluid Clearance before Birth

It is well known now that net alveolar fluid clearance occurs at a rapid rate late in gestation and that this clearance is driven by elevations of endogenous epinephrine. The critical link between β-adrenergic stimulation and lung fluid clearance was made in 1978 by Walters and Olver who found that intravenously infused epinephrine caused rapid absorption of lung fluid in near-term fetal lambs and that this response could be inhibited by prior treatment with propranolol (51). The intravenous epinephrine caused an immediate and reversible increase in luminal electronegativity by stimulating the active transport of Na+ out of the lung lumen (52). In the absence of adrenergic stimulation, the amiloride-sensitive Na+ channels remain closed (secretory state). Thus, the opened or closed state of the Na+ channels determines whether the fetal lungs, at any particular time, are secretory or reabsorptive (10). Cell culture, animal, and human studies have shown that activation of sodium channels (ENaCs) by increased circulating levels of adrenaline and vasopressin are important mechanisms of lung liquid reabsorption during labor (10,27,40,52–55).

The movement of sodium across the pulmonary epithelium from the alveolar lumen to the interstitium with subsequent absorption into the vasculature can be considered a two-step process. In the first step, sodium passively enters the apical membrane of the alveolar type II cell, through amiloride-sensitive Na+ channels (ENaC). In the second step, sodium is actively pumped out of the cell into the interstitium through the basolateral membrane by the ouabain inhibitable Na+ −K+ −ATPase. Thus, Na+ −K+ −ATPase pump inhibition with ouabain consistently reduces liquid clearance in various species (56–61). To equilibrate the osmotic pressure, generated by the movement of Na+, water diffuses from the alveolar to the interstitial space either through specific water channels (aquaporins) or through the paracellular junctions (Fig. 15.2) (40,62,63).

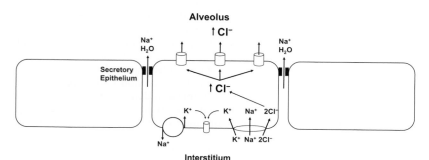

Alveolus

FIGURE 15.1 Lung liquid secretion. Schematic drawing of lung liquid secretion in fetal life. Type II cells secrete chloride (Cl−) by a process that involves Na/K/2Cl cotransporter and the Na-K-ATPase (Na+ pump) activity on the basolateral membrane. This energy-dependent process increases the concentration of Cl− within the cell exceeding its electrochemical equilibrium, which leads to opening of the apical Cl− channels and flow of this anion into the lung lumen. Na+ and water will follow Cl− through a paracellular route.

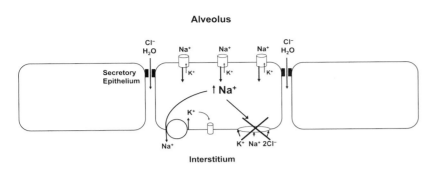

Alveolus

FIGURE 15.2 Lung liquid absorption. Schematic drawing of lung liquid absorption in the fetal lung near birth. To offset Cl– secretion, Na channels on the apical membrane of epithelial cells are activated establishing conduit for the osmotically active Na+ ion. Na enters the cell by the gradient generated by the Na/K/ATPase activity on the basolateral membrane. The net movement of Na+ to the basolateral direction induces a parallel movement of Cl– and fluid through the paracellular route.

Lung Fluid Clearance during Birth

There are two different mechanisms mostly responsible for airway liquid clearance during birth, and their relative contribution will likely depend on the mode and timing of delivery. Firstly, small increases in transpulmonary pressure across the highly compliant fetal respiratory system with uterine contractions during labor can cause an increase in airway pressure and liquid loss via the trachea. Secondly, the stress response elicited by the passage of the fetal head through the cervix and vagina results in a large increase in fetal adrenaline concentrations. As explained above, this catecholamine surge stimulates sodium reabsorption via activation of ENaCs (64). Thus, the mode and time of delivery could influence how much of the fetal lung fluid is reabsorbed by these mechanisms.

Lung Fluid Clearance after Birth

Although the switch from Cl– secretion to sodium absorption is one of the critical mechanism for lung fluid clearance at the time of delivery, other mechanical factors play an important role in clearing the residual liquid present in potential air spaces at birth. Studies in rabbit pups using time-lapsed phase contrast x-ray imaging have demonstrated that transpulmonary hydrostatic pressures generated during inspiration play a major role in airway liquid clearance and functional residual capacity (FRC) development at birth (65,66). These studies have shown that FRC accumulates with each breath and the FRC volume increase equals the volume of liquid leaving the airways resulting in a "step-like" increase in FRC with each breath (**Fig. 15.3**) (65,66). The same research group observed that the FRC development was not dependent on

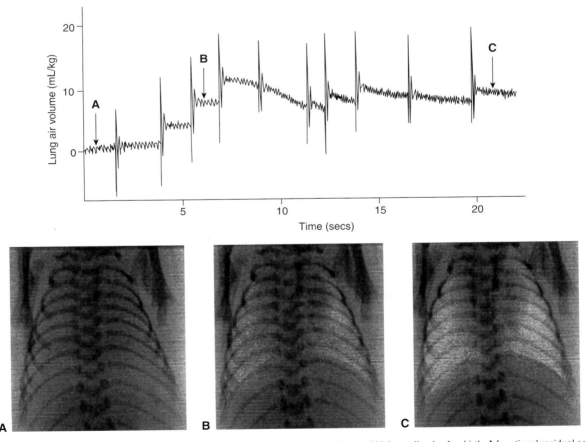

FIGURE 15.3 Top: A plethysmograph recording of a spontaneously breathing near term, newborn rabbit immediately after birth. A functional residual capacity (FRC) was recruited following each spontaneous breath (large increase in gas volume), resulting in a FRC of 10 mL/kg after only 4 breaths. The rapid periodic fluctuation in volume between breaths (when the lung is at FRC) is the heartbeat. **Bottom:** Phase contrast x-ray images (**A–C**) were recorded at each time point on the plethysmograph trace. In image (**A**), as no air was present in the lungs they were not visible, but as the different regions of the lung aerated they become visible (images **B and C**). The degree of aeration in the images directly corresponds with the amount of air in the lungs as measured by plethysmography. (Adapted from Hooper SB, Siew ML, Kitchen MJ, et al. Establishing functional residual capacity in the nonbreathing infant. *Semin Fetal Neonatal Med* 2013;18:336. Copyright © 2013 Elsevier, with permission.)

CARE AROUND BIRTH

ENaC activity and that increased airway pressures can compensate for the absence of ENaC activity and facilitate liquid clearance. Thus, lung inflation from either a spontaneous breath or a positive pressure inflation increases airway pressure above the pressure of the surrounding interstitial tissue producing a pressure gradient for liquid to move out of the airways, into the interstitium around distensible perivascular spaces of large pulmonary blood vessels and airways. These perivascular cuffs progressively diminish in size as the fluid is removed by small pulmonary blood vessels and lymphatics. Bland et al. have shown that the pulmonary circulation absorbs most of the residual liquid present in potential air spaces at birth and that elevated left atrial pressure or reduction of plasma protein concentration slows the rate of liquid clearance in mature animals (67–69).

RESPIRATORY ADAPTATION

Fetal Breathing

The discovery of fetal breathing in the late 1960s immediately stimulated interest in the factors that control breathing *in utero* (70–72). Besides conditioning respiratory muscles, FBMs contribute to normal lung differentiation and growth and likely to the development of neural circuits involved in respiratory control (73). Shortly after its discovery, the Oxford group showed that, although fetal breathing was influenced by fetal behavior, occurring essentially in rapid eye movements (REMs) sleep, it was clearly regulated by other chemical factors, such as carbon dioxide and oxygen concentration (74). Subsequent work confirmed and expanded these findings by recording the electrical activity of the diaphragm and clearly demonstrating the central origin of the respiratory output *in utero* (75–79). Using ultrasound technology, breathing movements were also identified in the human fetus, being present about 40% of the time during late pregnancy, a figure similar to that in sheep (70,80–82).

The discovery of fetal breathing not only stimulated the development of the area of fetal assessment but also brought a new dimension to the events occurring at birth. What has been traditionally called "the initiation of breathing at birth" must now be called "the establishment of continuous breathing at birth." Breathing begins long before birth. The question is not what determines the appearance of breathing at birth, but what makes it continuous. From another angle, what makes fetal breathing episodic in late gestation and present only during low voltage electrocortical activity? The answer to this question remains unknown.

Fetal breathing in sheep is mostly continuous in early gestation (90 to 115 days) but becomes episodic in late gestation, primarily occurring during periods of low-voltage electrocortical activity (71,72,79,83,84). During high-voltage electrocortical activity, there is no established breathing present, but occasional breaths may surface after episodic, generalized, tonic muscular discharges associated with body movements (**Fig. 15.4**) (79). During low-voltage electrocortical activity, breathing is irregular, the diaphragmatic EMG being characterized by an abrupt beginning and end. The physiologic mechanism responsible for the occurrence of fetal breathing only during low-voltage electrocortical activity is unknown.

Many studies have clearly shown that the fetal breathing apparatus is capable of responding well to chemical stimuli and other agents known to modify breathing postnatally. Thus, it became clear that the fetus responds to an increase in $PaCO_2$ with an increase in breathing (74,80,85–89). The increased breathing activity is prolonged into the transitional high-voltage ECoG but does not continue into the established high-voltage ECoG (**Fig. 15.5**). There is much evidence suggesting that the actions of CO_2 are central.

Administration of low oxygen to the fetus by having the ewe breathe hypoxic mixtures abolished fetal breathing; this was associated with a decrease in body movements and in the amplitude of the ECoG (74,90,91). Transection of the brain at the upper level of the pons prevents the inhibitory action of hypoxia and induces continuous breathing. Conversely, increase in arterial PO_2 to levels above 200 Torr through the administration of 100% O_2 to the fetus via an endotracheal tube stimulated breathing and induced continuous breathing in 35% of the experiments in fetal sheep (92). These findings suggest that low partial tension of O_2 in the fetus at rest may be a normal mechanism inhibiting breathing *in utero*.

Establishment of Continuous Breathing at Birth

The traditional view has been that labor and delivery produce a transient fetal asphyxia, which stimulates the peripheral chemoreceptors to induce the first breath. Breathing would then be maintained through the input of other stimuli, such as cold or touch (93,94). More recent observations have questioned this general view. **First**, the denervation of the carotid and aortic chemoreceptors does not alter fetal breathing or the initiation of continuous breathing at birth (95,96). **Second**, continuous breathing can be established *in utero*, with manifestations of arousal, by raising fetal PO_2 and occluding the umbilical cord (**Fig. 15.6**) (92). These observations during administration of high O_2 or cord occlusion suggest that the fetus can be made to resemble a neonate *in utero* without the transient hypoxemia to stimulate the peripheral chemoreceptors and without any of the sensory stimuli, such as cold, for example, once thought to be important for the establishment of continuous breathing at birth.

It has been debated whether the key factors in inducing the changes in fetal breathing at birth are intrinsic to the fetal brain or are in the placenta. Because placental separation at birth is

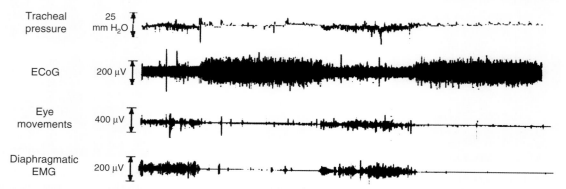

FIGURE 15.4 Fetal breathing in a fetal lamb at 134 days of gestation. The deflections in tracheal pressure and diaphragmatic activity occur during periods of rapid-eye-movement (REM) in low-voltage electrocortical activity only. In high-voltage electrocortical activity (quiet sleep), breathing is absent. (Republished with permission of CSIRO, from Rigatto H. Regulation of fetal breathing. *Reprod Fertil Dev* 1996;8:23; permission conveyed through Copyright Clearance Center, Inc.)

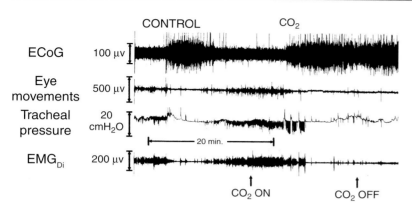

FIGURE 15.5 Fetal breathing during control and during CO_2 rebreathing. Note the increase in tracheal pressure and diaphragmatic activity during CO_2 rebreathing. Fetal breathing was prolonged into the transitional low- to high-voltage ECoG, but stopped in established high-voltage ECoG. (Republished with permission of CSIRO, from Rigatto H. Regulation of fetal breathing. *Reprod Fertil Dev* 1996;8:23; permission conveyed through Copyright Clearance Center, Inc.)

associated with the onset of continuous breathing, we together with others have hypothesized that placental factors might be responsible for the inhibition of fetal breathing (97–102). This line of thinking is based on the assumption that the release of a factor by the placenta into the fetal circulation prevents fetal breathing from being continuous, with inhibition during high-voltage ECoG, and present only during periods of reticular activation as it occurs during low-voltage ECoG. In the absence of this factor from the placenta at birth, after cord clamping, the state-related inhibition observed during high-voltage ECoG is insufficient to disrupt continuous breathing. Teleologically, it is interesting that nature may have delegated to the placenta the important role of providing the fetus with gas exchange and nutrients, and it is conceivable that it may also have endowed the placenta with some form

of chemoreceptor activity regulating fetal breathing and behavior by the secretion of chemical substances into the fetal circulation.

More evidence for a placental role has been present since Dawes and Harned and Ferreiro (93,94) showed that only after clamping the umbilical cord does the newborn lamb start breathing and behaving like a neonate. Subsequently, Adamson et al. induced breathing in the fetus with umbilical cord occlusion and supply of O_2 via an endotracheal catheter (99). Upon release of the cord, breathing ceased immediately, before any change in blood gases or pH, suggesting that a factor from the placenta might be involved. In our laboratory, we were able to induce continuous breathing and wakefulness in fetal sheep by occluding the umbilical cord, as long as we provided a gas exchange area for the fetus via an endotracheal tube (98,101–104). These experiments suggest the origin

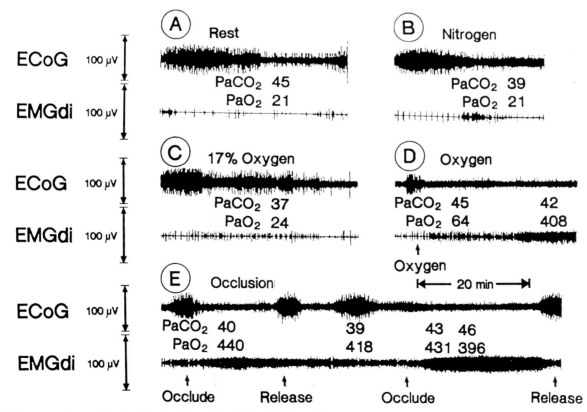

FIGURE 15.6 Representative tracing showing the effect of fetal FiO₂ on fetal breathing and electrocortical activity. A: Control cycle showing little breathing in fetus in early labor at 143 days of gestation. **B:** Lung distension (mean airway pressure 30 cm H_2O) and inspired N_2 does not affect baseline tracing. **C:** 17% O_2 also does not alter breathing. **D:** 100% O_2 induces continuous breathing. **E:** Occlusion on two occasions induces more forceful breathing than that observed with O_2 alone. Note that continuous breathing was elicited despite preventing the rise of $PaCO_2$ by ventilating the fetus with high-frequency ventilation (15 Hz, stroke = 7 cm H_2O). (Republished with permission of CSIRO, from Rigatto H. Regulation of fetal breathing. *Reprod Fertil Dev* 1996;8:23; permission conveyed through Copyright Clearance Center, Inc.)

CARE AROUND BIRTH

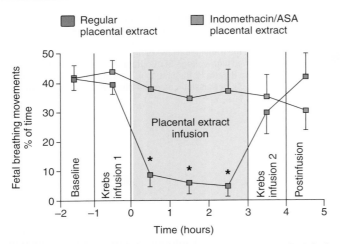

FIGURE 15.7 Incidence of fetal breathing movements during the infusion of placental extracts. The regular placental extracts (*solid circles*) induced a profound inhibition of fetal breathing that progressively recovered upon discontinuation of the infusions. This effect disappeared when the extracts were treated with indomethacin/ASA (open circle). Values are mean ± SE. *$p < 0.05$.

in the placenta of a compound which inhibits fetal breathing and fetal activity.

In trying to prove the hypothesis that a factor is released by the placenta, we injected the fetal sheep with a placental extract (juice of cotyledons acutely dissected, sliced, and immersed in Krebs solution) after continuous breathing was induced by cord occlusion (98). In all experiments, the placental extract decreased or abolished breathing. The infusion of the placental extract into the fetal circulation also inhibited spontaneous fetal breathing present during low voltage electrocortical activity without inducing significant changes in blood gas tensions, pH, heart rate, and blood pressure (105). We have recently demonstrated that this factor in the placental extract is likely a prostaglandin, since treatment of the extract with Indomethacin/ASA, which significantly reduced the concentration of prostaglandins, eliminated the activity of the extract (**Fig. 15.7**) (106).

Indirect evidence that placental prostaglandins, especially PGE₂, are the mediators responsible for the inhibition of breathing in fetal life have been demonstrated by Kitterman et al. (107) and Wallen et al. (108) who have shown that infusion of PGE₂ into the circulation of the fetal sheep induced a prompt and complete cessation of breathing movements. In addition, the incidence of FBM was inversely correlated with both the PGE₂ dose and the mean PGE₂ concentration. Conversely, intravenous infusion of prostaglandin synthetase inhibitors, such as indomethacin or meclofenamate, induces continuous breathing for many hours in the fetus (107,109,110). Thus, the rate of placental prostaglandin production plays a significant role in setting the level of fetal breathing activity by producing a sleep-related inhibition in the fetal brainstem.

It is unlikely, however, that prostaglandins are involved in the inhibition of fetal breathing observed during hypoxia, since this inhibition persists after the administration of prostaglandin inhibitors. Several studies have shown that adenosine is the likely mediator of the respiratory depression observed during hypoxia since intravascular administration of adenosine inhibits fetal breathing and eye movements (111) and the infusion of adenosine receptor antagonists blunts this inhibition (111,112). Also, brain disruptions that eliminate hypoxic inhibition of breathing also abolish the depressant effects of adenosine (113). Koos et al. have recently shown that hypoxia inhibits fetal breathing

through activation of central adenosine receptors, specially the A(2A) subtype (114).

Mechanics of the First Postnatal Breaths

There have been many explanations and controversies on how air enters the lung at birth. Several authors have reported that the first inspiration in vaginally delivered human infants does not require diaphragmatic contraction (115,116). Pfister et al. have found large negative intrapulmonary pressure in fetal sheep during labor, which implied that the lung volume was less than FRC (117). The elastic recoil of the chest wall, once it is delivered from the birth canal, would cause passive inflow of air without diaphragmatic contraction. However, using cineradiography, recording of breathing patterns, and more recently phase-contrast x-ray imaging of the lung, several authors have shown that the entry of air into the lung at birth is dependent on the generation of a transpulmonary pressure created mainly from contraction of the diaphragm (66,116,118,119). This first inspiration of air is also associated with dilation of the intrathoracic trachea and the movement of air into the posterior portions of the lung (119).

Although lung fluid is partially reabsorbed during labor and delivery, a significant amount of fluid is still present in the lungs at the time the newborn infant is ready to take the first postnatal breath. In spontaneously breathing infants, a transpulmonary pressure of about 60 cm H_2O is required to make this fluid flow through the airways with the first inspiration (120). Vyas et al. observed that infants can generate very high inspiratory pressures and positive expiratory pressures during the first breath to achieve those inspired volumes (121). However, according to the Laplace equation for a cylinder state ($P = t/r$), a much higher pressure gradient between the mouth opening and the alveolus would be needed to overcome the high surface tension forces if the airways were not partially distended with fluid because of the small radius of curvature (122). Thus, the normal fluid content of the lung at birth facilitates the first breath by lowering the opening pressure and ensuring a more homogeneous filling of the lung with air. A significant reduction in the volume of fetal pulmonary fluid, as seen sometimes in post-term deliveries, may not be beneficial at birth (123). First, greater pressures would be required to inflate the air sacs in fluid-free lungs, and secondly, the distribution of inspired air during the first breath may not be as uniform. Faridy has shown that the highest opening pressure was seen in fluid-free lungs and the lowest in lungs containing fluid of about 25% of maximum lung volume (122).

The transpulmonary pressure needed to aerate the lungs at birth also depends on the compliance of the alveolar tissue and the surface forces at air-fluid interface. During labor and birth, a massive release of surfactant in pulmonary fluid facilitates lung opening by lowering the opening pressure through the decrease in surface forces and the improvement of lung compliance (122–125). Thus, as seen in Figure 15.9, the first postnatal breath (I) begins with no air volume in the lungs and no transpulmonary pressure gradient. As the chest wall expands, the transpulmonary pressure increases until it overcomes the surface tension of small airways and alveoli. At this point, actively inspired air begins to enter the lungs and according to the Laplace equation, as the radius increases, the distending pressure required to open up those units decreases.

Although the first inspiratory effort is extremely important for lung opening, the creation of FRC at the end of the first expiratory effort is essential for the normal pulmonary adaptation at birth. It is obvious that if all the air that entered the lung were to leave the lung, every breath would necessarily resemble the first breath (126). Several mechanisms are required to maintain FRC after birth. It has been well described that the first postnatal breath tends to be the deepest and the slowest of the early pattern of breathing primarily due to a short deep inspiration followed by a prolonged expiratory time (127). These initial breaths are actively exhaled by the high negative transpulmonary pressures. These expiratory breaths are also associated with interruptions in the expiratory flow (braking of the expiration) that help maintaining FRC. There are two mechanisms for stopping or slowing expiratory flow. The first one is the diaphragmatic post-inspiratory activity that slows the rate of lung deflation by counteracting its passive recoil. The second one is the closure or narrowing of the pharyngeal/laryngeal region, as indicated by the radiographic studies of Bosma et al. (118) Te Pas et al. have recently found that this expiratory braking is achieved most commonly by crying (128). Siew et al. have recently shown that although transpulmonary hydrostatic pressure gradient generated during inspiration may be able to clear liquid from the airway, FRC tends to decrease between breaths in both spontaneously breathing and mechanically ventilated term and preterm newborn rabbits (65,128,129). This decreasing FRC likely represents the reentry of liquid into the airways from the interstitial tissue compartment when transpulmonary hydrostatic pressure gradients are low, as during expiration (66). The resulting positive pressure in the airway generated by the expiratory braking mechanisms would not only facilitate liquid absorption but also improve air retention at the end of expiration as well as increase lung compliance.

Surfactant also plays an important role in maintaining FRC. The near-zero surface tension and the bubble formation produced by surfactant allows for retention of large volumes of air at the end of the first expiration. When surfactant is deficient, the consequences are a tendency to airlessness with each expiration and the application of high inspiratory pressures to maintain respiration. This leads to the marked retractions so commonly associated with atelectasis and HMD as seen in preterm infants with surfactant deficiency.

CIRCULATORY ADAPTATION

Fetal Circulation

A combination of preferential flow and streaming through structural shunts in the liver (ductus venosus) and heart (foramen ovale and ductus arteriosus), allows the highest oxygen content blood coming from the placenta to be delivered to the heart, brain, and upper torso (Fig. 15.8). This relative parallel flow contrasts with the flow in series and without shunts of the adult circulation. Thus, the volume of blood in the fetal heart ventricles is not equal. In fact, the right ventricle ejects approximately two-thirds of total fetal cardiac output (300 mL/kg/min), whereas the left ventricle ejects only a little more than one-third (150 mL/kg/min) (130).

Placenta blood is delivered to the fetus through the umbilical vein. Approximately 50% of this umbilical blood flow passes through the ductus venosus directly into the inferior vena cava and mixes with the systemic venous drainage from the lower body. The other 50% of the umbilical blood flow joins the hepatic–portal venous system and passes through the hepatic vasculature (131). Preferential streaming allows the well-oxygenated blood derived from the ductus venosus to travel through the dorsal and leftward wall of the inferior vena cava (132). A tissue flap called the eustachian valve, located at the junction of the inferior vena cava and right atrium, serves to direct the highly oxygenated blood from the ductus venosus across the foramen ovale into the left atrium and then the left ventricle and ascending aorta (132–134). The less oxygenated anterior stream (mainly blood from the lower body and the hepatic circulation) joins the oxygen poor blood from the superior vena cava (which drains the head and upper body) and the coronary sinus (which delivers venous return from the myocardium) at the right atrium, directing the blood through the tricuspid valve into the right ventricle (Fig. 15.8).

Since the placenta is responsible for gas exchange *in utero*, very little blood flow is sent to the lungs. The pulmonary circulation is a high-resistance, low-flow circuit that receives less than 10% of the ventricular output. Instead of entering the pulmonary arteries, most of the right ventricular blood is diverted away from the lungs through the widely patent ductus arteriosus to the descending aorta, reaching the placenta for oxygenation through the umbilical arteries.

The well-oxygenated blood coming across the foramen ovale joins the small amount of blood returning from the lungs via the pulmonary veins in the left atrium and traverses the mitral valve into the left ventricle. This blood is then ejected across the aortic valve into the ascending aorta bringing well-oxygenated blood to the myocardium, brain, head, and upper torso (Fig. 15.8).

Regulation of Fetal Pulmonary Vascular Resistance

There is a close association between pulmonary arterial development and airway development. As gestation progresses, synchronization of airway and vessel branching occurs, suggesting they may be regulated by common mediators or exchange messenger molecules (135,136). The embryonic endothelial channels later acquire a smooth muscle layer, and thus, the ability to regulate vascular tone and blood flow.

During early gestation, pulmonary blood flow is limited by the paucity of pulmonary vessels. However, although the number of small blood vessels per unit of lung volume increases 10-fold during the last trimester, pulmonary blood flow remains low due to a high PVR (Fig. 15.9). In addition to the mechanical compression of pulmonary vessels by the fluid-filled, atelectatic lungs and the lack of rhythmic distension, this high-resistance low-flow state, is probably maintained in part by vasoconstriction since the fetal pulmonary vascular bed responds readily to vasodilators.

The discovery that the effects of some vasodilators agents, such as acetylcholine, bradykinin, and histamine were dependent on release of an endothelium-derived relaxing factor (EDRF), later shown to be nitric oxide (NO) (137,138), led to the exploration of its possible role in the perinatal decrease in PVR. NO, an inorganic, gaseous free radical discovered in the late 1980s, is produced by the endothelial cells from the terminal nitrogen of L-arginine by nitric oxide synthase (NOS). NOS can be stimulated by pharmacologic agents such as acetylcholine or bradykinin and by birth, shear stress, and oxygen. NO activates soluble guanylate cyclase (cGMP), which produces smooth muscle relaxation by activation of protein kinase C (Fig. 15.10) (139). Hydrolysis of cGMP is accomplished by phosphodiesterases, which control the intensity and duration of cGMP signal transduction (140). In fetal life, NO production is also stimulated by activation of ATP-dependent K+ channels. A maturational increase in NO-mediated relaxation has been documented during the late fetal and early postnatal period, which parallels the dramatic fall in PVR at birth (141–145). In fetal lambs, inhibiting NO synthesis increases resting PVR and inhibits the ventilation-induced fall in PVR. Increase in oxygen tension increases both basal and stimulated NO release, and inhibition of NO blocks virtually the entire increase in fetal pulmonary blood flow caused by hyperbaric oxygenation without ventilation (146–148). Shear stress resulting from increased pulmonary blood flow and rhythmic distension of the lung without changing oxygen tension also induces endothelial NOS gene expression and contribute to pulmonary vasodilatation at birth (149,150).

Endothelin-1 (ET-1), a 21-amino acid peptide also produced by vascular endothelial cells, has potent vasoactive activities (151).

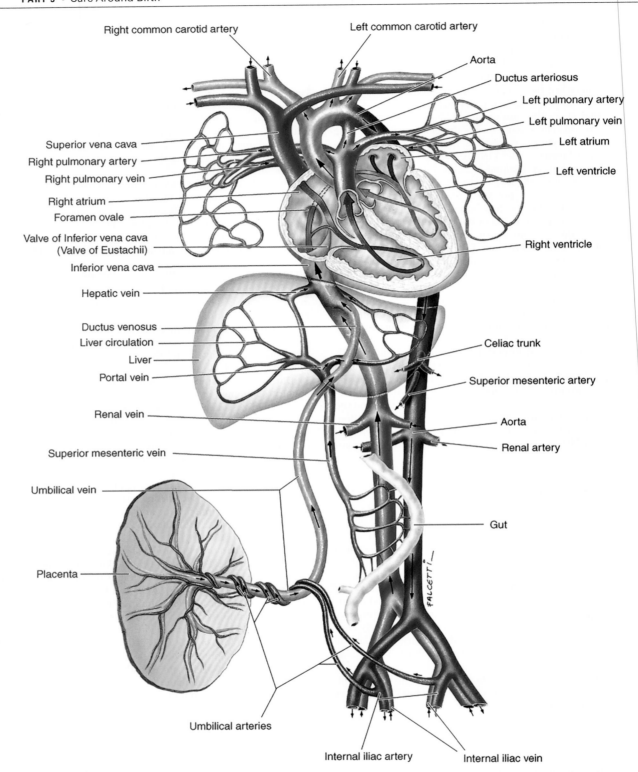

FIGURE 15.8 Fetal blood circulation. (Reprinted with permission from Kawamura D, Nolan T. Abdomen and superficial structures, 4th ed. Philadelphia, PA: Wolters Kluwer, 2017, Figure 5.1.)

Although endothelin-1 appears to play an important and active role in mediating PVR, *in vivo* studies indicate that the effects of exogenous endothelin are complex and depend on the site, developmental age, and tone of the vascular bed (152–154). Thus, exogenous ET-1 predominantly vasodilates the fetal and newborn pulmonary circulations by acting on the ET$_B$ receptors located on the endothelial cells but causes vasoconstriction in the adult pulmonary circulation by acting on the ET$_m$ receptors located in the smooth muscle cells (155,156). Increasing data also suggest that endogenous NO and ET-1 participate in the regulation of each other through an autocrine feedback loop. Thus, ET-1 stimulates the release of NO, and NO inhibits the ET-1 system (157,158).

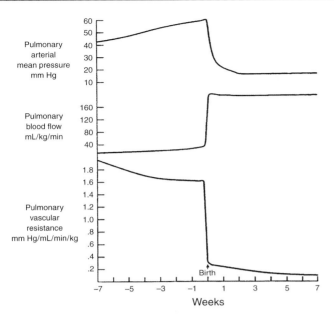

FIGURE 15.9 Representative changes in the pulmonary hemodynamics during transition from the late-term fetal circulation to the neonatal circulation. Pulmonary vascular resistance (PVR) decreases progressively during later gestation due to lung growth and increased cross-sectional area for flow. PVR decreases dramatically at birth due to the vasodilating effect of lung aeration. PVR continues to fall more gradually over the first 6 to 8 weeks of life. Pulmonary blood flow remains at relatively low levels during fetal growth, then increases abruptly with lung expansion and the rapid fall in PVR. Mean pulmonary artery pressure falls rapidly immediately after birth because the pulmonary vasodilation causes PVR to fall more than pulmonary blood flow increases. (Adapted with permission of McGraw-Hill, from Rudolph AM. Fetal circulation and cardiovascular adjustment after birth. In Rudolph AM, Hoffman JIE, Rudolph CD, eds. *Rudolph's pediatrics*. 19th ed. Norwalk, CT: Appleton & Lange, 1991:1309, permission conveyed through Copyright Clearance Center, Inc.)

The low oxygen tension in fetal life is a physiologic stimulus for the pulmonary vasculature to be constricted. This hypoxic pulmonary vasoconstriction develops over the period of gestation when the cross-sectional area of the vascular bed is increasing rapidly. Increasing oxygen tension before 100 days of gestation does not decrease PVR, but by 135 days, it decreases resistance markedly and increases pulmonary blood flow to normal newborn levels. Its mechanism of action may be in part through regulation of activity and gene expression of voltage-gated K+ channels (159), NOS, and/or endothelin (160,161).

Unlike the mature pulmonary circulation, the fetal pulmonary vasculature appears to regulate flow through a myogenic response. The fetal pulmonary vasculature exhibits a time-limited vasodilation in response to dilating stimuli, including shear stress, oxygen, and many pharmacologic vasodilators, with return to the constricted resting state despite continued exposure to the vasodilating stimulus. This unique mechanism limits pulmonary blood flow and preserves placental perfusion and gas exchange.

Transition to Extrauterine Circulation

At birth, a number of complex events must take place so that the fetal circulation that depends on the placenta for gas exchange and intracardiac and extracardiac shunts to deliver oxygenated blood to the heart and brain switch to the neonatal circulation in which the gas exchange is transferred to the lungs and the fetal shunts are eliminated. A rapid and sustained decrease in PVR during the first breaths facilitate this adaptation. Although this normal pulmonary vascular transition occurs spontaneously and quickly in

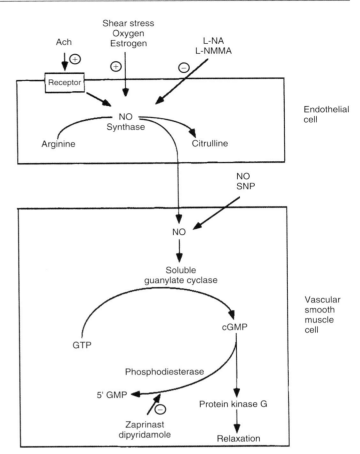

FIGURE 15.10 The proposed mechanism of synthesis and action of nitric oxide. Nitric oxide is produced in the endothelium from the terminal guanido nitrogen of L-arginine by NO synthase. NO synthase can be stimulated by pharmacologic agents such as acetylcholine or bradykinin, and by birth, shear stress, and oxygen. Endothelial production of NO can be blocked by arginine analogues that have modifications of the guanido nitrogen of the molecule. Nitric oxide activates soluble guanylate cyclase, increases cGMP concentrations in vascular smooth muscle, and initiates the cascade resulting in smooth muscle relaxation. The magnitude and duration of the effect of cGMP is controlled by its inactivation by specific phosphodiesterases. (Reproduced from Lakshminrusimha S, Steinhorn R. Pulmonary Vascular biology during neonatal transition. *Clin Perinatol* 1999;26(3):601. Copyright © 1999 Elsevier, with permission.)

most neonates, failure of the pulmonary circulation to undergo this change results in persistent pulmonary hypertension of the newborn (PPHN). This condition, which carries significant morbidity and mortality, develops when the PVR fails to decrease adequately during the transition to extrauterine life. Altered intrauterine environment producing structural changes in the pulmonary circulation or hypoxemia, acidosis and/or hypercarbia secondary to meconium aspiration, surfactant deficiency, or pneumonia at birth abnormally constrict the transitional pulmonary circulation. In this condition, right to left shunts at the atrial and ductus arteriosus levels continue secondary to the high PVR, producing significant hypoxemia which in turn causes increase pulmonary vasoconstriction. Thus, two major hemodynamic events must occur at delivery to allow for a normal transition from fetal to neonatal circulation.

Pulmonary Vasodilatation

At birth, pulmonary arterial blood flow increases 8- to 10-fold, and PVR decreases by 50% within the first 24 hours, as the lung assumes the function of gas exchange (**Fig. 15.11**) (162–166). This decrease in PVR is brought about by active vasodilation, which is

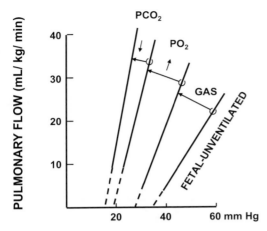

PULMONARY ARTERIAL-LEFT ATRIAL PRESSURE

FIGURE 15.11 Pulmonary vascular conductance increases with the onset of ventilation. Separate curves depict the contributions of gaseous inflation, increased PO_2, and decreased PCO_2. (Adapted from Strang LB. The lungs at birth. *Arch Dis Child* 1965;40:575.)

regulated by a complex and incompletely understood interaction between metabolic, hormonal, and mechanical factors, triggered by a number of birth-related stimuli. Three main factors contribute to the increase in pulmonary blood flow during this transition: 1. ventilation of the lungs, 2. increased oxygenation, and 3. hemodynamic forces, such as increased shear stress. The effects of these factors on pulmonary circulation at birth appears to be mediated primarily by the release of NO from the vascular endothelium, which results in smooth muscle relaxation via activation of the intracellular cGMP-dependent protein kinase (167). The initial partial increase in pulmonary vasodilation may be independent of oxygenation and may be caused by physical expansion of the lungs and the production of prostaglandins (166). The next component is maximal pulmonary vasodilation associated with oxygenation, which may be mainly caused by NO synthesis. The increased shear forces related to the rise in pulmonary blood flow may stimulate endothelial cells to produce NO, which helps maintain pulmonary vasodilation (**Fig. 15.11**).

1. **Ventilation of the lungs:** It has long been known that the initiation of rhythmic breathing causes vasodilation, even in the absence of increase in oxygen tension (**Fig. 15.11**) (8,163). However, physical expansion of the lungs alone produces only partial increase in pulmonary blood flow and a decrease in PVR. A small proportion of this relates to the mechanical distension of the lungs and the establishment of an air–liquid interface, as alveolar fluid is replaced by gas, which increases vessel radius by exerting a negative dilating pressure on the small pulmonary arteries, and veins (168,169). Ventilation of the lung also releases vasoactive substances such as PGI_2 from vessel walls, which increases pulmonary blood flow and decreases PVR (170). Cyclooxygenase inhibition, which blocks PGI_2 production, prevents the normal decrease in PVR with lung expansion, but not the changes that occur with oxygenation (170–173). Other prostaglandins like PGD2 and histamine released by the mast cells during lung expansion may also contribute to the initial postnatal pulmonary vasodilation. (174) Nitric Oxide Synthase (NOS) and calcium sensitive K+ channel (K_{ca}) inhibition also blunt ventilation-induced pulmonary vasodilatation (175,176).

2. **Increased oxygenation:** Oxygen is a potent stimulus for pulmonary vasodilation. Even in the absence of ventilation, increased oxygen tension reduces PVR. Ventilation plus increased oxygen tension produces complete pulmonary vasodilation and both are particularly crucial in the normal transition to postnatal

circulation and pulmonary gas exchange (**Fig. 15.11**) (163). Although the mechanisms of oxygen-induced pulmonary vasodilation are not completely understood, several factors appear to contribute to this response. Many studies have shown that the effect of oxygen on perinatal pulmonary circulation appears to be mediated primarily by the effects of NO on K+ channels in arterial smooth muscle cells either directly or through a cGMP-sensitive kinase (177–179). Thus, the sudden increase in oxygen tension that occurs at birth appears to enhance NO synthesis, and NOS inhibition blunts the oxygen-induced decrease in PVR. Although it is assumed that oxygen may act directly on endothelial cells to increase NO production, it is possible that it stimulates release of another agent, such as bradykinin, calcitonin gene-related peptide, or adrenomedullin, which in turn stimulates NO production (180,181).

Oxygen could also increase plasma and red blood cell adenosine triphosphate (ATP), which releases NO from endothelial cells and is a potent fetal pulmonary vasodilator (182). It is known that the release of NO from cultured human vascular endothelial cells is stimulated by ATP and that the inhibition of NOS by N-nitro-L-arginine attenuates the vasodilation caused by ATP and its metabolites in the fetal circulation. Konduri et al. have recently suggested that increase in oxidative phosphorylation and release of ATP can also mediate the endothelium-dependent pulmonary vasodilation that occurs in response to oxygen exposure (183).

Other studies have shown that NO release and pulmonary vasorelaxation can also be mediated by endothelial α2-adrenoreceptors activation (184–186). Magnenant et al. have recently suggested that α2-adrenoreceptors are involved in the control of basal pulmonary vascular tone and in the pulmonary vasodilator effect of norepinephrine during fetal life through activation of the NO-dependent pulmonary vasodilation (187).

Recent studies have also supported the hypothesis that hypoxia causes ET_A-mediated inhibition of a K+ channels, which leads to vessel depolarization and calcium influx, resulting in vasoconstriction (188–191). Goirand et al. have recently shown that ET_A receptor blockade opposes hypoxic pulmonary vasoconstriction in the rat isolated perfused lung through the suppression of the inhibition of K+ channels by endogenous ET-1 (192). Thus, the increase in oxygen, together with the perinatal decrease in ETA receptor message, probably contributes also to decreased hypoxic pulmonary vasoconstriction observed at birth.

3. **Increased shear stress:** Partial or complete compression of the ductus arteriosus *in utero* increases pulmonary blood flow and causes a progressive fall in PVR in response to flow- or shear stress-induced pulmonary vasodilation (193,194). The initial increase in pulmonary blood flow that occurs with lung expansion and oxygenation at birth raise shear stress in the pulmonary vascular endothelium causing further pulmonary vasodilation (166). This blood flow-dependent pulmonary vasodilation is mainly caused by NO, which is produced by an increase in shear stress of vascular endothelium (194–196). Stepwise elevations in flow increased exhaled NO, and nonselective inhibition of NOS completely blocks the shear stress–induced pulmonary vasodilation (194,196). This NO shear stress–induced vasodilation is mediated by activation of both voltage- and Ca2+-dependent K+ channels (195–198). Ralevic et al. have shown that vascular endothelial cells also release ATP when they are exposed to shear stress (199). Inhibition of receptors for ATP attenuates the pulmonary vasodilation that occurs in response to stepwise increases in flow (200).

Loss of the Placental Circulation and Closure of the Fetal Shunts

At birth, the umbilical circulation is abolished as the vascular smooth muscle of the umbilical cord go into spasm in response to the abrupt longitudinal stretching and the increased oxygenation (201). The removal of the low-resistance bed of the placenta produces much of the increase in systemic vascular resistance at birth. As the pulmonary blood flow in fetal life is very low, most of the left ventricular preload *in utero* comes from the placenta through the ductus venosus, inferior vena cava, and through the foramen ovale to directly enter the left atrium. At birth, immediate cord clamping before lung aeration produces a marked reduction in cardiac output due to a reduction in preload to the left ventricle. The cardiac output remains reduced until the pulmonary blood flow increases in response to lung aeration becoming the primary source of preload for the left ventricle. This marked reduction in cardiac output caused by immediate cord clamping can be avoided by aerating the lung and increasing pulmonary blood flow before the umbilical cord is clamped (202).

Without umbilical venous flow, the ductus venosus receives little blood flow and a passive, as well as active constriction begins. Complete closure of the ductus venosus usually occurs by the end of the first week of life. The reasons for closure of the foramen ovale after birth are twofold. First, the occlusion of the umbilical cord decreases the volume of blood flowing up the inferior vena cava decreasing the right-left atrial pressure difference. Secondly, the increase in pulmonary venous return to the left atrium in response to the marked increase in pulmonary blood flow increases left atrial pressure. The reverse pressure difference across the foramen ovale pushes the foramen ovale flap against the atrial septum closing the shunt. The foramen ovale remains patent, with no flow through it for weeks or months. The closure of the third fetal shunt, the ductus arteriosus, depends predominantly on the net balance between vasodilators, mainly oxygen and prostaglandins and other vasoactive substances (203,204). Increased oxygen tension is known to be a potent stimulant of ductal smooth muscle constriction after birth (204). Prostaglandins, mainly PGE2, are major mediators of ductal relaxation pre- and postnatally. The rapid fall in circulating prostaglandins at birth, caused by increased lung metabolism (from increased pulmonary blood flow) and the loss of placental prostaglandins, facilitates the constrictive effects of oxygen on the ductal tissue. Although functional closure of the ductus arteriosus occurs in the first 72 hours of life (205), permanent or anatomical closure takes several days per weeks and is achieved by endothelial destruction, subintimal proliferation, and connective tissue formation (206). When the ductus arteriosus fails to close or reopens in the first days of life, as frequently observed in small preterm infants, a significant left to right shunt may occur. The incidence of reopening is inversely related to birth weight. The closure of the patent ductus arteriosus effectively separates the pulmonary and systemic circulations and establishes the normal postnatal circulatory pattern.

CONCLUSION

The transition from fetal to neonatal life represents one of the most dynamic and difficult periods in human life cycle. Dramatic neurohormonal, metabolic, and cardiorespiratory adjustments must occur over hours to days around the time of delivery to insure the smooth and successful transition to extrauterine life. These changes are invoked by a variety of processes including perinatal surges in hormones, labor, delivery, gaseous ventilation and oxygenation of the lungs, cord occlusion, and decrease in environmental temperature. Intensive research over the last century has significantly improved our understanding of the normal development of the cardiorespiratory system that allows the fetus to rapidly and efficiently adapt to air breathing at birth. This transitional period is characterized by removal of the lung liquid volume from the alveolar spaces and by the secretion of surfactant material into the acinus for satisfactory physical expansion of the lungs after the initial postnatal breaths. To maintain adequate ventilation and oxygenation, the newborn infant must also switch from intermittent

fetal breathing to continuous breathing at birth, a process that is still not completely understood. The switch from placental to pulmonary gas exchange also requires the elimination of the fetal shunts and a rapid and sustained decrease in PVR to allow a significant increase in pulmonary blood flow. Thus, the circulation changes from one characterized by a relatively low combined ventricular output, right ventricular dominance, and pulmonary vasoconstriction, to a circulation in series with a high cardiac output equally divided between the two ventricles, and a greatly dilated pulmonary vascular bed. Many factors can disrupt this physiologic process causing significant morbidity and mortality.

REFERENCES

1. Harvey W. In: Barnes WR, ed. *Exercitatio anatomica de motu cordis et sanguinis in animalibus.* London, England, 1628:1847.
2. Scheel P. Comentatio de Liquoris amnii aspiras arteriae foetuum humanorum natura et usu. *HFNIAE.* 1799:86.
3. Zweifel P. Die Respiration des Fötus. *Arch Gynakol* 1876;9:291.
4. Bichat X. *Anatomie générale, àppliqueé à la physiologie et à la médecine.* Paris, France: Brosson, Gabon, 1801.
5. Kilian HF. *Ueber den Kreislauf des Blutes im Kinde, welches noch nicht geathmet hat.* Karlsruhe, Germany: Muller, 1826.
6. Hamilton WF, Woodbury RA, Woods EB. The relation between systemic and pulmonary blood pressures in the fetus. *Am J Physiol* 1937;119:206.
7. Barclay AE, Barcroft J, Barron DH, et al. A radiographic demonstration of the circulation through the heart in the adult and in the foetus, and the identification of the ductus arteriosus. *Br J Radiol* 1939;12:505.
8. Dawes GS, Mott JC, Widdicombe JG, et al. Changes in the lungs of the newborn lamb. *J Physiol (Lond)* 1953;121:141.
9. Rudolph AM. Fetal and neonatal pulmonary circulation. *Annu Rev Physiol* 1979;41:383.
10. Strang LB. Fetal lung liquid: secretion and reabsorption. *Physiol Rev* 1991;71:991.
11. Preyer W. *Specielle Physiologic des Embryo.* Leipzig, Germany: Greeben Verlag (L.Fernau), 1885:149.
12. Potter EL, Bohlender GP. Intrauterine respiration in relation to development of the fetal lung. *Am J Obstet Gynecol* 1941;42:14.
13. Jost A, Policard A. Contribution experimental a l'etude du development prenatal du poumon chez le lapin. *Arch Anat Microsc Morphol Exp* 1948;37:323.
14. Reynolds SRM. A source of amniotic fluid in the lamb nasopharyngeal and buccal cavities. *Nature* 1953;175:307.
15. Dawes GS, Mott JC, Widdicombe JG. The foetal circulation in the lamb. *J Physiol* 1954;126(3):563.
16. Adams, FH, Moss AJ, Fagan L. The tracheal fluid in the fetal lamb. *Biol Neonate* 1963;5:151.
17. Adamson TM, Boyd RDH, Platt HS, et al. Composition of alveolar liquid in the fetal lamb. *J Physiol (Lond)* 1969;204:159.
18. Olver RE, Schneeberger EE, Walters DV. Epithelial solute permeability, ion transport and tight junction morphology in the developing lung of the fetal lamb. *J Physiol* 1981;315:395.
19. Mescher EJ, Platzker ACG, Ballard PL, et al. Ontogeny of tracheal fluid, pulmonary surfactant, and plasma corticoids in the fetal lamb. *J Appl Physiol* 1975;39:1017.
20. Burri PH. Fetal and postnatal development of the lung. *Annu Rev Physiol* 1984;46:617.
21. Adamson IYR. Development of lung structure. In: Crystal RG, West JB, Barnes PJ, et al., eds. *The Lung: Scientific Foundations.* New York, NY: Raven Press, 1991:663.
22. Humphrey's PW, Normand ICS, Reynolds EOR, et al. Pulmonary lymph flow and the uptake of liquid from the lungs of the lamb at the start of breathing. *J Physiol (Lond)* 1967;193:1.
23. Normand ICS, Olver RE, Reynolds OR, et al. Permeability of lung capillaries and alveoli to non-electrolytes in the fetal lamb. *J Physiol (Lond)* 1971;219:303.
24. Harding R, Hooper S. Regulation of lung expansion and lung growth before birth. *J Appl Physiol* 1996;81:209.
25. Hooper SB, Harding R. Fetal lung liquid; a major determinant of the growth and functional development of the fetal lung. *Clin Exp Pharmacol Physiol* 1995;22:235.
26. Adamson TM, Brodecky V, Lambert TF, et al. Lung liquid production and composition in the 'in utero' foetal lamb. *Aust J Exp Biol Med Sci* 1975;53:65.
27. Brown MJ, Olver RE, Ramsden CA, et al. Effects of adrenaline and of spontaneous labour on the secretion and absorption of lung liquid in the fetal lamb. *J Physiol* 1983;344:137.

28. Alcorn D, Adamson TM, Lambert TF, et al. Morphological effects of chronic tracheal ligation and drainage in the fetal lamb lung. *J Anat* 1977;123:649.

29. Fewell JE, Johnson P. Upper airway dynamics during breathing and during apnea in fetal lambs. *J Physiol (Lond)* 1983;339:495.

30. Nardo I, Hopper SB, Harding R. Lung hypoplasia can be reversed by short-term obstruction of the trachea in fetal sheep. *Pediatr Res* 1995;38:690.

31. Scurry JP, Adamson TM, Cussen LJ. Fetal lung growth in laryngeal atresia and tracheal agenesis. *Aust Paediatr J* 1989;25:47.

32. Souza P, O'Brodovich H, Post M. Lung fluid restriction affects growth, but not airway branching of embryonic rat lung. *Int J Dev Biol* 1995;39:629.

33. Crombleholme TM, Albanese CT. The fetus with airway obstruction. In: Harrison MR, Evans MI, Adzick NS, et al., eds. *The unborn patient: The art and science of fetal therapy*, 3rd ed. Philadelphia, PA: Saunders, 2001;357.

34. Lim F, Crombleholme M, Hedrick HL, et al. Congenital high airway obstruction syndrome: natural history and management. *J Pediatr Surg* 2003;38:940.

35. Matalon S. Mechanisms and regulation of ion transport in adult mammalian alveolar type II pneumocytes. *Am J Physiol* 1991;261:C727.

36. Saumon G, Basset G. Electrolyte and fluid transport across the mature alveolar epithelium. *J Appl Physiol* 1993;74:1.

37. Olver RE, Strang LB. Ion fluxes across the pulmonary epithelium and the secretion of the lung liquor in the fetal lamb. *J Physiol (Lond)* 1974;241:327.

38. Frizzell RA, Field M, Schultz SG. Sodium-coupled chloride transport by epithelial tissues. *Am J Physiol* 1979;236:F1.

39. Bland RD, Nielson DW. Developmental changes in lung epithelial ion transport and liquid movement. *Annu Rev Physiol* 1992;54:373.

40. O'Brodovich HM. Immature epithelial Na+ channel expression is one of the pathogenetic mechanisms leading to human neonatal respiratory distress syndrome. *Proc Assoc Am Physicians* 1996;108:345.

41. Adams FH, Yanagisawa M, Kuzela D, et al. The disappearance of fetal lung fluid following birth. *J Pediatr* 1971;78:837.

42. O'Brodovich HM, Hannam V. Exogenous surfactant rapidly increases PaO$_2$ in mature rabbits with lungs that contain large amounts of saline. *Am Rev Respir Dis* 1993;147:1087.

43. Egan EA, Dillon WP, Zorn S. Fetal lung liquid absorption and alveolar epithelial solute permeability in surfactant deficient, breathing fetal lambs. *Pediatr Res* 1984;18:566.

44. Barker PM, Gowen CW, Lawson EE, et al. Decreased sodium ion absorption across nasal epithelium of very premature infants with respiratory distress syndrome. *J Pediatr* 1997;130:373.

45. Aherne W, Dawkins MJR. The removal of fluid from the pulmonary airways after birth in the rabbit, and the effect on this of prematurity and pre-natal hypoxia. *Biol Neonate* 1964;7:214.

46. Bland RD, et al. Lung fluid balance in lambs before and after premature birth. *J Clin Invest* 1989;84:568.

47. Bland RD, McMillan DD, Bressack MA, et al. Clearance of liquid from lungs of newborn rabbits. *J Appl Physiol* 1980;49:171.

48. Sundell HW, et al. Lung water and vascular permeability-surface area in newborn lambs delivered by cesarean section compared with the 3–5 day old lamb and adult sheep. *J Dev Physiol* 1980;2:191.

49. Sundell HW, et al. Lung water and vascular permeability-surface area in premature newborn lambs with hyaline membrane disease. *Circ Res* 1987;60;923.

50. Hooper SB, et al. Establishing functional residual capacity in the non-breathing infant. *Semin Fetal Neonatal Med* 2013;18:336.

51. Walters DV, Olver RE. The role of catecholamines in lung liquid absorption at birth. *Pediatr Res* 1978;12:239.

52. Olver RE, Ramsden CA, Strang LB, et al. The role of amiloride-blockable sodium transport in adrenaline-induced lung liquor reabsorption in the fetal lamb. *J Physiol (Lond)* 1986;376:321.

53. Walters DV, Ramsden CA, Olver RE. Dibutyryl cAMP induces a gestation-dependant absorption of fetal lung liquid. *J Appl Physiol* 1990;68:2054.

54. Chapman DL, Carlton DP, Cummings JJ, et al. Intrapulmonary terbutaline and aminophylline decrease lung liquid in fetal lambs. *Pediatr Res* 1991;29:357.

55. Hooper SB, Wallace MJ, Harding R. Amiloride blocks the inhibition of fetal lung liquid secretion caused by AVP but not by asphyxia. *J Appl Physiol* 1993;74:111.

56. Basset G, Crone C, Saumon G. Significance of active ion transport in transalveolar water absorption: a study on isolated rat lung. *J Physiol* 1987;384:311.

57. Sakuma T, Okaniwa G, Nakada T, et al. Alveolar fluid clearance in the resected human lung. *Am J Respir Crit Care Med* 1994;150:305.

58. Sakuma T, Pittet JF, Jayr C, et al. Alveolar liquid and protein clearance in the absence of blood flow or ventilation in sheep. *J Appl Physiol* 1993;74:176.

59. Jayr C, Garat C, Meignan M. et al. Alveolar liquid and protein clearance in anesthetized ventilated rats. *J Appl Physiol* 1994;76:2636.

60. Icard P, Saumon G. Alveolar sodium and liquid transport in mice. *Am J Physiol Lung Cell Mol Physiol* 1999;277:L1232.

61. Matthay MA, Folkesson HG, Clerici C. Lung epithelial fluid transport and the resolution of pulmonary edema. *Physiol Rev* 2002;82:569.

62. Walters DV. Fetal lung liquid: secretion and absorption. In: Hanson MA, Spencer JAD, Rodeck CH, et al., eds. *Fetus and neonate: physiology and clinical application. Vol 2: breathing*. Cambridge, England: Cambridge University Press, 1994;43.

63. Umenishi F, Carter EP, Yang B, et al. Sharp increase in rat lung water channel expression in the perinatal period. *Am J Respir Cell Mol Biol* 1996;15:673.

64. Hooper SB, Polgrase GR, Roehr CC. Cardiopulmonary changes with aeration of the newborn lung. *Paediatr Respir Rev* 2015;16:147.

65. Siew ML, et al. Inspiration regulates the rate and temporal pattern of lung liquid clearance and lung aeration at birth. *J Appl Physiol* 2009;106:1888.

66. Hooper SB. Imaging lung aeration and lung liquid clearance at birth. *FASEB J* 2007;21:3329.

67. Bland RD, et al. Lung fluid balance in lambs before and after birth. *J Appl Physiol* 1982;53:992.

68. Raj JU, Bland RD. Lung luminal liquid clearance in newborn lambs. Effect of pulmonary microvascular pressure elevation. *Am Rev Respir Dis* 1986;134:305.

69. Cummings JJ, et al. Hypoproteinemia slows lung liquid clearance in young lambs. *J Appl Physiol* 1993;74:153.

70. Dawes GS, Fox HE, Leduc BM, et al. Respiratory movements and paradoxical sleep in the fetal lamb. *J Physiol* 1970;210:47P.

71. Merlet C, Hoerter J, Devilleneuve C, et al. Mise en evidence de mouvements respiratoires chez le foetus d'agneau au cours du dernier mois de la gestation. *C R Acad Hebd Seances Acad Sci D* 1970;270:2462.

72. Dawes GS, Fox HE, Leduc MB, et al. Respiratory movements and rapid eye movement sleep in the fetal lamb. *J Physiol* 1972;220:119.

73. Koos BJ, Rajaee A. Fetal breathing movements and changes at birth. In: Zhang L, Ducsay CA, eds. *Advances in fetal and neonatal physiology, advances in experimental medicine and biology*. New York, NY: Springer Science + Business Media, 2014;89–101.

74. Boddy K, Dawes GS, Fisher R, et al. Fetal respiratory movements, electrocortical and cardiovascular responses to hypoxaemia and hypercapnia in sheep. *J Physiol (Lond)* 1974;243:599.

75. Maloney JE, Adamson TM, Brodecky V, et al. Modification of respiratory center output in the unanesthetized fetal sheep "in utero". *J Appl Physiol* 1975;39:552.

76. Maloney JE, Bowes G, Wilkinson M. "Fetal breathing" and the development of patterns of respiration before birth. *Sleep* 1980;3:299.

77. Ioffe S, Jansen AH, Russell BJ, et al. Respiratory response to somatic stimulation in fetal lambs during sleep and wakefulness. *Pflugers Arch* 1980;388:143.

78. Ioffe S, Jansen AH, Russell BJ, et al. Sleep, wakefulness and themonosynaptic reflex in fetal and newborn lambs. *Pflugers Arch* 1980;388:149.

79. Rigatto H, Moore M, Cates D. Fetal breathing and behavior measured through a double wall Plexiglas window in sheep. *J Appl Physiol (1985)* 1986;61:160.

80. Boddy K, Dawes GS. Fetal breathing. *Br Med Bull* 1975;31:3.

81. Patrick J, Campbell K, Carmichael L, et al. A definition of human fetal apnea and the distribution of fetal apneic intervals during the last ten weeks of pregnancy. *Am J Obstet Gynecol* 1980;136:471.

82. Patrick J, Campbell K, Carmichael L, et al. Patterns of human fetal breathing during the last 10 weeks of pregnancy. *Obstet Gynecol* 1980;56:24.

83. Dawes GS. Breathing before birth in animals and man. *N Engl J Med* 1974;290:557.

84. Kitterman JA, Liggins GC, Clements JA, et al. Stimulation of breathing movements in fetal sheep by inhibitors of prostaglandin synthesis. *J Dev Physiol* 1979;1:453.

85. Dawes GS, Gardner WN, Johnston BM, et al. Effects of hypercapnia on tracheal pressure, diaphragm and intercostal electromyograms in unanesthetized fetal lambs. *J Physiol (Lond)* 1982;326:461.

86. Jansen AH, Ioffe S, Russell BJ, et al. Influence of sleep state on the response to hypercapnia in fetal lambs. *Respir Physiol* 1982;48:125.

87. Moss IR, Scarpelli EM. Generation and regulation of breathing in utero: fetal CO$_2$ response test. *J Appl Physiol Respir Environ Exerc Physiol* 1979;47:527.

88. Rigatto H. A new window on the chronic fetal sheep model. In: Nathanielsz PW, ed. *Animal models in fetal medicine*. Ithaca, NY: Perinatology Press, 1984;57.

89. Rigatto H, Hasan SU, Jansen A, et al. The effect of total peripheral chemodenervation on fetal breathing and on the establishment of breathing at birth in sheep. In: Jones CT, ed. *Fetal and neonatal development*. Ithaca, NY: Perinatology Press, 1988;613.

90. Clewlow F, Dawes GS, Johnston BM, et al. Changes in breathing, electrocortical and muscle activity in unanesthetized fetal lambs with age. *J Physiol (Lond)* 1983;341:463.

91. Koos BJ, Sameshima H, Power GG. Fetal breathing, sleep state, and cardiovascular responses to graded hypoxia in sheep. *J Appl Physiol* 1987;62:1033.

92. Baier RJ, Hasan SU, Cates DB, et al. Effects of various concentrations of O2 and umbilical cord occlusion on fetal breathing and behavior. *J Appl Physiol* 1990;68:1597.

93. Dawes GS. The establishment of pulmonary respiration. In: Dawes GD, ed. *Foetal and neonatal physiology.* Chicago, IL: Year Book Medical Publishers, 1968:125.

94. Harned H, Ferreiro J. Initiation of breathing by cold stimulation: effects of change in ambient temperature on respiratory activity of the full-term fetal lambs. *J Pediatr* 1973;88:663.

95. Jansen AH, Ioffe S, Russell BJ, et al. Effect of carotid chemoreceptor denervation on breathing in utero and after birth. *J Appl Physiol Respir Environ Exerc Physiol* 1981;51:630.

96. Rigatto H, Lee D, Davi M, et al. Effect of increased arterial CO_2 on fetal breathing and behavior in sheep. *J Appl Physiol* 1988;64:982.

97. Alvaro R, Weintraub Z, Alvarez J, et al. The effects of 21 or 30% O_2 plus umbilical cord occlusion on fetal breathing and behavior. *J Dev Physiol* 1992;18:237.

98. Alvaro R, deAlmeida V, Al-Alaiyan S, et al. A placental extract inhibits breathing induced by umbilical cord occlusion in fetal sheep. *J Dev Physiol* 1993;19:23.

99. Adamson SL, Richardson BS, Homan J. Initiation of pulmonary gas exchange by fetal sheep in utero. *J Appl Physiol* 1987;62:989.

100. Adamson SL, Kuiper IM, Olson DM. Umbilical cord occlusion stimulates breathing independent of blood gases and pH. *J Appl Physiol* 1991;70:1796.

101. Thorburn GD. The placenta and the control of fetal breathing movements. *Reprod Fertil Dev* 1995;7:577.

102. Alvarez JE, Baier RJ, Fajardo CA, et al. The effect of 10% O_2 on the continuous breathing induced by O_2 or O_2 plus cord occlusion in the fetal sheep. *J Dev Physiol* 1992;17:227.

103. Baier, RJ, Fajardo CA, Alvarez J, et al. The effects of gestational age and labour on the breathing and behavior response to oxygen and umbilical cord occlusion in the fetal sheep. *J Dev Physiol* 1992;18:93.

104. Baier, RJ, Hasan SU, Cates DB, et al. Hyperoxemia profoundly alters breathing pattern and arouses the fetal sheep. *J Dev Physiol* 1992;18:143.

105. Alvaro RE, Robertson M, Lemke R, et al. Effects of a prolonged infusion of a placental extract on breathing and electrocortical activity in the fetal sheep. *Pediatr Res* 1997;41:300A.

106. Alvaro RE, Hasan SU, Chemtob S, et al. Prostaglandins are responsible for the inhibition of breathing observed with a placental extract in fetal sheep. *Respir Physiol Neurobiol* 2004;144(1):35–44.

107. Kitterman J, Liggins GC, Fewell JE, et al. Inhibition of breathing movements in fetal sheep by prostaglandins. *J Appl Physiol Respir Environ Exerc Physiol* 1983;54:687.

108. Wallen LD, Mural DT, Clyman RI, et al. Regulation of breathing movements in fetal sheep by prostaglandin E2. *J Appl Physiol* 1986;60:526.

109. Koos BJ. Central stimulation of breathing movements in fetal lambs by prostaglandin synthetase inhibitors. *J Physiol (Lond)* 1985;362:455.

110. Kitterman J. Arachidonic acid metabolites and control of breathing in the fetus and newborn. *Semin Perinatol* 1987;11:43.

111. Koos BJ, Maeda T. Fetal breathing, sleep state and cardiovascular response to adenosine in sheep. *J Appl Physiol* 1990;68:489.

112. Bissonette JM, Hohimer AR, Knopps SJ. The effect of centrally administered adenosine on fetal breathing movements. *Respir Physiol* 1991;84:273.

113. Koos BJ, Maeda T, Jan C. Adenosine A1 and A2A receptors modulate sleep state and breathing in fetal sheep. *J Appl Physiol* 2001;91:343.

114. Koos BJ, Phil D, Takatsugu M, et al. Adenosine A2A receptors mediate hypoxic inhibition of fetal breathing in sheep. *Am J Obstet Gynecol* 2002;186:663.

115. Karlberg P. The adaptive changes in the immediate postnatal period, with particular reference to respiration. *J Pediatr* 1960;56:585.

116. Karlberg P, Cherry RB, Escardo FE, et al. Respiratory studies in newborn infants. II Pulmonary ventilation and mechanics of breathing in the first minutes of life, including the onset of respiration. *Acta Paediatr* 1962;51:121.

117. Pfister RE, Ramsden CA, Neil HL, et al. Volume and secretion rate of lung liquid in the final days of gestation and labour in the fetal sheep. *J Physiol* 2001;535(3):889.

118. Bosma JF, Lind J, Gentz N. Motions of the pharynx associated with initial aeration of the lungs of the newborn infant. *Acta Paediatr Suppl* 1959;48:117.

119. Fawcitt J, Lind J, Wegelius C. The first breath: a preliminary communication describing some methods of investigation of the first breath of a baby and the results obtained from them. *Acta Paediatr Suppl* 1960;49:5.

120. Agostoni E, Talietti A, Agostoni AF, et al. Mechanical aspects of the first breath. *J Appl Physiol* 1958;13:344.

121. Vyas H, Field D, Milner AD, et al. Determinants of the first inspiratory volume and functional residual capacity at birth. *Pediatr Pulmonol* 1986;2:189.

122. Faridy EE. Air opening pressure in fluid filled lungs. *Respir Physiol* 1987;68:279.

123. Faridy EE. Fetal lung development in surgically induced prolonged gestation. *Respir Physiol* 1981;45:153.

124. Faridy EE. Air opening pressure in fetal lungs. *Respir Physiol* 1987;68:293.

125. Lowson EE, Brown ER, Torday DL, et al. The effect of epinephrine on tracheal fluid flow and surfactant efflux in fetal sheep. *Am Rev Respir Dis* 1978;118:1023.

126. Avery ME, Mead J. Surface properties in relation to atelectasis and hyaline membrane disease. *Am J Dis Child* 1959;97:517.

127. Mortola JP, Fisher JT, Smith JB, et al. Onset of respiration in infants delivered by cesarean section. *J Appl Physiol* 1982;52(3):716.

128. Te Pas AB, et al. Breathing patterns in preterm and term infants immediately after birth. *Pediatr Res* 2009;65:352.

129. Siew ML, et al. Positive end-expiratory pressure enhances development of a functional residual capacity in preterm rabbits ventilated from birth. *J Appl Physiol* 2009;106:1487.

130. Heymann MA, Creasy RK, Rudolph AM. Quantitation of blood flow patterns in the foetal lamb in utero. In: *Proceedings of the Sir Joseph Barcroft Centenary Symposium: Foetal and Neonatal Physiology.* Cambridge, UK: Cambridge University Press, 1973.

131. Edelstone DI, Rudolph AM, Heymann MA. Liver and ductus venosus blood flows in fetal lambs in utero. *Circ Res* 1978;42:426.

132. Edelstone DI, Rudolph AM. Preferential streaming of ductus venosus blood to the brain and heart in fetal lambs. *Am J Physiol* 1979;237:1172.

133. Berhman RE, Lees MH, Peterson EN, et al. Distribution of the circulation in the normal and asphyxiated fetal primate. *Am J Obstet Gynecol* 1970;108:957.

134. Reuss ML, Rudolph AM, Heymann MA. Selective distribution of microspheres injected into the umbilical veins and inferior venae cavae of fetal sheep. *Am J Obstet Gynecol* 1981;141:427.

135. Hislop A, Reid L. Intrapulmonary arterial development during fetal life: branching pattern and structure. *J Anat* 1972;113:35.

136. Hislop A, Reid L. Formation of the pulmonary vasculature. In: Wa H, ed. *Development of the Lung.* New York, NY: Marcel Dekker, 1977:37.

137. Furchgott RF, Zawadzki JV. The obligatory role of endothelial cell in the relaxation of arterial smooth muscle by acetylcholine. *Nature* 1980;288:373.

138. Ignarro LJ, Byrns RE, Buga GM, et al. Endothelium-derived relaxing factor from pulmonary artery and vein possesses pharmacologic and chemical properties identical to those of nitric oxide radical. *Circ Res* 1987;61:866.

139. Warner T, Mitchell J, Sheng H, et al. Effects of cyclic GMP on smooth muscle relaxation. In: Murad F, ed. *Advances in pharmacology,* vol 26. San Diego, CA: Academic Press, 1984:171.

140. Thompson W. Cyclic nucleotide phosphodiesterases: pharmacology, biochemistry and function. *Pharmacol Ther* 1991;51:13.

141. Perreault T, De Marte JM. Maturational changes in endothelium-derived relaxation in newborn piglet pulmonary circulation. *Am J Physiol* 1993;264:H302.

142. Steinhorn RH, Morin FC III, Gugino SF, et al. Developmental differences in endothelium-dependent responses in isolated ovine pulmonary arteries and veins. *Am J Physiol* 1993;264:H2162.

143. Shaul PW, Farrar MA, Magness RR. Pulmonary endothelial nitric oxide production is developmentally regulated in the fetus and newborn. *Am J Physiol* 1993;265:H1056.

144. North AJ, Star RA, Brannon TS, et al. Nitric oxide synthase type I and type III gene expression are developmentally regulated in rat lung. *Am J Physiol* 1994;266:L635.

145. Bloch KD, Filippov G, Sanchez LS, et al. Pulmonary soluble guanylate cyclase, a nitric oxide receptor, is increased during the perinatal period. *Am J Physiol* 1997;272:L400.

146. Moore P, Velvis H, Fineman JR, et al. EDRF inhibition attenuates the increase in pulmonary blood flow due to O_2 ventilation in fetal lambs. *J Appl Physiol* 1992;73:2151.

147. McQueston JA, Cornfield DN, McMurtry IF, et al. Effects of oxygen and exogenous L-arginine on EDRF activity in fetal pulmonary circulation. *Am J Physiol* 1993;264:H865.

148. Tiktinsky MH, Morin FC III. Increasing oxygen tension dilates fetal pulmonary circulation via endothelium-derived relaxing factor. *Am J Physiol Heart Circ Physiol* 1993;265:H376.

149. Abman SH, Chatfield BA, Hall SL, et al. Role of endothelium-derived relaxing factor during transition of pulmonary circulation at birth. *Am J Physiol* 1990;259:H1921.

150. Cornfield DN, Reeve HL, Tolarova S, et al. Oxygen causes fetal pulmonary vasodilation through activation of a calcium-dependent potassium channel. *Proc Natl Acad Sci U S A* 1996;93:8089.

151. Yangisawa M, Kurihara H, Kimura S, et al. A novel potent vasoconstrictor peptide produced by vascular endothelial cells. *Nature* 1998;332:411.

152. Chatfield BA, McMurtry IF, Hall SL, et al. Hemodynamic effects of endothelin-1 on ovine fetal pulmonary circulation. *Am J Physiol* 1991;261:R182.

CARE AROUND BIRTH

153. Hislop AA, Zhao YD, Springall DR, et al. Postnatal changes in endothelin-1 binding in porcine pulmonary vessels and airways. *Am J Respir Cell Mol Biol* 1995;12:557.

154. Wong J, Vanderford PA, Fineman JR, et al. Developmental effects of endothelin-1 on the pulmonary circulation in sheep. *Pediatr Res* 1994;36:394.

155. Arai H. Hori S, Aramori I, et al. Cloning and expression of a cDNA encoding an endothelin receptor. *Nature* 1990;348:730.

156. Sakurai T, Yanagisawa M, Takuwa Y, et al. Cloning of a cDNA encoding a non-isopeptide-selective subtype of the endothelin receptor. *Nature* 1990;348:732.

157. Boulanger C, Luscher TF. Release of endothelin from the porcine aorta. Inhibition by endothelium-derived nitric oxide. *J Clin Invest* 1990;85:587.

158. Luscher, TF, Yang Z, Tschudi M, et al. Interaction between endothelin-1 and endothelium-derived relaxing factor in human arteries and veins. *Circ Res* 1990;66:1088.

159. Gosch JR. Oxygen dilation in fetal pulmonary arterioles: role of K+ channels. *J Surg Res* 2001;97:159.

160. Weir EK, Archer SL. The mechanism of acute hypoxic pulmonary vasoconstriction: the tale of two channels. *FASEB J* 1995;9:183.

161. Sham JS, Crenshaw EB Jr, Deng LH, et al. Effects of hypoxia in porcine pulmonary arterial myocytes: roles of K(V) channel and endothelin-1. *Am J Physiol* 2000;279:L262.

162. Dawes GS, Mott JC. Vascular tone of the foetal lung. *J Physiol (Lond)* 1962;164:465.

163. Cassin S, Dawes GS, Ross BB. Pulmonary blood flow and vascular resistance in immature foetal lambs. *J Physiol (Lond)* 1964;171:80.

164. Emmanouilides GC, Moss AJ, Duffie ER, et al. Pulmonary arterial pressure changes in human newborn infants from birth to 3 days of age. *J Pediatr* 1964;65:327.

165. Heymann MA, Soifer SJ. Control of fetal and neonatal pulmonary circulation. In: Weir EK, Reeves JT, eds. *Pulmonary vascular physiology and pathophysiology*. New York, NY: Marcel Dekker, 1989:33.

166. Heymann MA. Control of the pulmonary circulation in the fetus and during the transitional period to air breathing. *Eur J Obstet Gynecol Reprod Biol* 1999;84:127.

167. Raj U, Shimoda L. Oxygen-dependent signaling in pulmonary vascular smooth muscle. *Am J Physiol Lung Cell Mol Physiol* 2002;283:L671.

168. Enhorning G, Adams FH, Norman A. Effect of lung expansion on the fetal lamb circulation. *Acta Paediatr Scand* 1996;55:441.

169. Gilbert RD, Hessler JR, Eitzman DV, et al. Site of pulmonary vascular resistance in fetal goats. *J Appl Physiol* 1972;32:47.

170. Leffler C, Hessler J, Green R. Mechanism of stimulation of pulmonary prostacyclin synthesis at birth. *Prostaglandins* 1984;28:877.

171. Leffler CW, Hessler JR, Green RS. The onset of breathing stimulates pulmonary vascular prostacyclin synthesis. *Pediatr Res* 1984;18:938.

172. Leffler C, Tyler T, Cassin S. Effect of indomethacin on pulmonary vascular response to ventilation of fetal goats. *Am J Physiol* 1978;234:H346.

173. Leffler CW, Hessler JR, Terragno NA. Ventilation-induced release of prostaglandin-like material from fetal lungs. *Am J Physiol* 1980;238:H282.

174. Soifer SJ, Morin FC III, Kaslow DC, et al. The developmental effects of prostaglandin D2 on the pulmonary and systemic circulations in the newborn lamb. *J Dev Physiol* 1983;5:237.

175. Cornfield DN, Resnik ER, Herron JM, et al. Pulmonary vascular K+ channel expression and vasoreactivity in a model of congenital heart disease. *Am J Physiol Lung Cell Mol Physiol* 2002;283:L1210.

176. Tristani-Firouzi M, Martin E, Tolarova S, et al. Ventilation-induced pulmonary vasodilation at birth is modulated by potassium channel activity. *Am J Physiol* 1996;271:H2353.

177. Bolotina VM, Najibi S, Palacino JJ, et al. Nitric oxide directly activates calcium-dependent potassium channels in vascular smooth muscle. *Nature* 1994;368:850.

178. Robertson BE, Schubert R, Hescheler J, et al. cGMP dependent protein kinase activates Ca-activated K channels in cerebral artery smooth muscle cells. *Am J Physiol* 1993;265:C299.

179. Saqueton CB, Miller RB, Porter VA, et al. NO causes perinatal pulmonary vasodiltion through K+ −channels activation and intracellular Ca2+ release. *Am J Physiol* 1999;276:L925.

180. De Vroomen M, Takahashi Y, Roman C, et al. Calcitonin gene-related peptide increases pulmonary blood flow in fetal sheep. *Am J Physiol* 1998;274:H277.

181. Godecke A, Decking U, Ding Z, et al. Coronary hemodynamics in endothelial NO synthase knockout mice. *Circ Res* 1998;82:186.

182. Konduri G, Woodard L. Selective pulmonary vasodilation by low-dose infusion of adenosine triphosphate in newborn lambs. *J Pediatr* 1991;199:94.

183. Konduri GG, Mattei J. Role of oxidative phosphorylation and ATP release in mediating birth-related pulmonary vasodilation in fetal lambs. *Am J Physiol Heart Circ Physiol* 2002;283:H1600.

184. Pepke-Zaba J, Higenbottam TW, Dinh-Xuan AT, et al. Alpha-adrenergic stimulation of porcine pulmonary arteries. *Eur J Pharmacol* 1993;235:169.

185. MacLean MR, McCulloch KM, McGrath JC. Influences of the endothelium and hypoxia on α2-adrenoceptor-mediated responses in the rabbit isolated pulmonary artery. *Br J Pharmacol* 1993;108;155.

186. Miller VM. Vanhoutte PM. Endothelial α2-adrenoceptors in canine pulmonary and systemic blood vessels. *Eur J Pharmacol* 1985;118:123.

187. Magnenant E, Jaillard S, Deruelle P, et al. Role of the alpha2-adrenoceptors on the pulmonary circulation in the ovine fetus. *Pediatr Res* 2003;54:1.

188. Shimoda LA, Sylvester JT, Sham JS. Inhibition of voltage-aged K+ current in rat intrapulmonary arterial myocytes by endothelin-1. *Am J Physiol* 1998;274:L842.

189. Barman SA. Pulmonary vasoreactivity to endothelin-1 at elevated vascular tone is modulated by potassium channels. *J Appl Physiol* 1996;80:91.

190. Li H, Elton TS, Chen YF, et al. Increased endothelin receptor gene expression in hypoxic rat lung. *Am J Physiol* 1994;266:L553.

191. Peng W, Michael JR, Hoidal JR, et al. ET-1 modulates Kca-channel activity and arterial tension in normoxic and hypoxic human pulmonary vasculature. *Am J Physiol* 1998;275:L729.

192. Goirand F, Bardou M, Guerard P, et al. ETA, mixed ETA/ETB receptor antagonists, and protein kinase C inhibitor prevent acute hypoxic pulmonary vasoconstriction: influence of potassium channels. *J Cardiovasc Pharmacol* 2003;41:117.

193. Adman SH, Accurso FJ. Acute effects of partial compression of ductus arteriosus on fetal pulmonary circulation. *Am J Physiol* 1989;257:H626.

194. Rairigh RL, Storme L, Parker TA, et al. Inducible NO synthase inhibition attenuates shear stress-induced pulmonary vasodilation in the ovine fetus. *Am J Physiol* 1999;276:L513.

195. Cornfield DN, Chatfield BA, McQueston JA, et al. Effects of birth-related stimuli on L-arginine-dependent pulmonary vasodilation in ovine fetus. *Am J Physiol* 1992;262:H1474.

196. Ogasa T, Nakano H, Ide H, et al. Flow-mediated release of nitric oxide in isolated, perfused rabbit lungs. *J Appl Physiol* 2001;91(1):363.

197. Storme L, Rairigh RL, Parker TA, et al. K+−channel blockade inhibits shear stress-induced pulmonary vasodilation in the ovine fetus. *Am J Physiol* 1999;276:L220.

198. Cooke JP, Rossitch E Jr, Andon NA, et al. Flow activates an endothelial potassium channel to release an endogenous nitrovasodilator. *J Clin Invest* 1991;88:1663.

199. Ralevic V, Milner P, Kirkpatrick KA, et al. Flow-induced release of adenosine 5'-triphosphate from endothelial cells of the rat mesenteric arterial bed. *Experientia* 1992;48:31.

200. Hassessian H. Bodin P, Burnstock G. Blockade by glibenclamide of the flow-evoked endothelial release of ATP that contributes to vasodilation in the pulmonary vascular bed of the rat. *Br J Pharmacol* 1993;109:466.

201. Nelson N. Physiology of transition. In: Avery GB, Fletcher MA, MacDonald MG, eds. *Neonatology: Pathophysiology and management of the newborn*, 4th ed. Philadelphia, PA: J.B. Lippincott Company, 1994:223.

202. Bhatt S, Polglase GR, Wallace EM, et al. Ventilation before umbilical cord clamping improves the physiological transition at birth. *Front Pediatr* 2014;2:113.

203. Starling MB, Elliott RB. The effects of prostaglandins, prostaglandin inhibitors, and oxygen on the closure of the ductus arteriosus, pulmonary arteries and umbilical vessels in vitro. *Prostaglandins* 1974;8(3):187.

204. Sharpe GL, Larsson KS. Studies on closure of the ductus arteriosus. X. In vivo effect of prostaglandin. *Prostaglandins* 1975;9(5):703.

205. Lim MK, Hanretty K, Houston AB. Intermittent ductal patency in healthy newborn infants: Demonstration by colour Doppler flow mapping. *Arch Dis Child* 1992;67:1218.

206. Hammerman C. Patent ductus arteriosus: clinical relevance of prostaglandins and prostaglandin inhibitors in PDA pathophysiology and treatment. *Clin Perinatol* 1995;22(2):457.

16 Delivery Room Management

Colm P.F. O'Donnell and Alan M. Groves

INTRODUCTION

Context

Delivery rooms (DRs)—that is, labor wards and operating theatres—are not the natural habitat of the neonatologist. We are summoned there when the regular inhabitants are worried, so our presence indicates tension in the room. To enable everyone to do their best for the family, it is important that all of the staff understand the roles and responsibilities of everyone on the team.

Getting to know the layout of the DRs and what equipment is available is absolutely essential for the neonatal care team, and all staff should ensure they do this prior to being called to a delivery. It is good practice to develop a process/algorithm for checking and preparing your equipment when you are called to a delivery so that any potential shortages are identified and corrected. It is very easy to open the valve on an air or oxygen tank in the calm before a delivery: very hard in the middle of a full resuscitation.

All delivery centers should have an agreed list of when and how you will be called when there are concerns about a baby. And do not forget that the key resource at a delivery is the people. Introduce yourself to the nurses, midwives, obstetricians, and anesthesiologists before you are called there urgently. Cultivating relationships with your DR colleagues will help make sure they go the extra mile to optimize conditions for the baby, whether by turning up the heat, giving antenatal steroids, or calling for more help. If problems arise at a delivery, do not try to resolve them in the heat of the moment; concentrate on helping the baby to the best of your ability. Come back later to address any problems in a clear-headed fashion in calmer circumstances. Many centers now have a semiformal debrief after resuscitations to help improve personnel and systems issues.

While distinctions in treatment approaches are sometimes made for "resource-limited" settings, resources are limited everywhere—it is just a matter of where the limit is set. In all settings, the most important resource is the people who attend the delivery. In a tight spot in the DR, experienced and calm staff are invaluable. Though people believe that the relationship between any two variables in life is mostly linear (i.e., if some is good, more must be better ad infinitum), it is usually quadratic (i.e., neither too little nor too much, moderation in all things [including moderation!]). It is not good when no one attends the delivery of a baby who needs help. However, there can be too many people at a delivery—it can become unclear who is in charge and people can distract one another. Staff attending deliveries should have a defined role. If they do not, they should stand back and observe unless specifically invited to participate by someone involved.

Every neonatal nurse and doctor who goes to the DR wants to do something to help and to do their best. Their presence at deliveries can be upsetting for families and for other staff. This can encourage panic. DO NOT PANIC. In life, nothing goes better when you panic. Watch the baby closely and intelligently. Fortunately, most newborn babies breathe spontaneously. And many DR interventions—stimulation, suction, applying a face mask, giving positive pressure ventilation (PPV)—may cause a spontaneously breathing newborn to stop breathing. If you need to intervene to help a baby, take a deep breath and hurry slowly. It is more important to do things well and in as timely a fashion as possible, rather than to do them quickly and poorly.

Evidence-Based Clinical Practice

It is important to distinguish between association and cause and effect. Just because a baby received an intervention after birth and survived, it does not necessarily mean that the baby survived because of the intervention. The baby may have survived despite it. Neonatology is littered with examples of plausible treatments that were applied in good faith that later proved useless or, more worryingly, harmful. Our practice, in particular the treatments that we use, should be supported by scientific proof that quantify the benefits and harms that they bring. Do not be intimidated by the clunky term "evidence-based clinical practice"—the important concepts are easily understood.

To see whether a therapy is useful, useless, or harmful, it needs to be evaluated in the context of a randomized controlled trial (RCT). Such studies give the most reliable and unbiased judgment of what the real effects of treatments are. In a true RCT, a treatment is given to half of an adequately large group of patients and compared to the other half—the control group—who are given standard care. End points (outcomes) that are clearly defined at the beginning are measured for all participants. Ideally, neither the clinicians who are caring for the babies nor the people who are measuring the results (outcome assessors) should know whether they received treatment or standard care (they should be blinded or masked). In systematic reviews of treatments, RCTs are sought, and if suitable studies are identified, their findings may be combined in a meta-analysis in an attempt to better understand their effects.

For many years, it seemed that heightened emotion and fraught circumstances in the DR precluded coherent scientific study. That is not the case. Over recent years, there has been a lot of DR research that has increased our knowledge. Of course, not all aspects are optimal—in practice, adequate blinding of the care team can be very difficult to achieve. However, if precise repeatable endpoints are chosen, the absence of blinding need not be an insurmountable problem. High-quality evidence has now been produced for optimizing DR temperature, timing of umbilical cord clamping, approach to suctioning of meconium-stained fluid, use of supplemental oxygen, choice of positive pressure delivery device, and many more interventions.

However, much more needs to be done. We owe it to babies to refine our care. It is difficult to study every aspect of DR care in the context of an RCT, particularly for events that are infrequent and unanticipated (e.g., giving chest compressions or epinephrine). However, it is wise to maintain a healthy degree of skepticism about therapies that are not supported by evidence from RCTs.

Historical Perspective

The reanimation of apparently lifeless newborns is described in ancient religious scriptures. Claims for efficacy for many different, and some quite bizarre, interventions—for example, violent swinging (Fig. 16.1), electrocution, alternate immersion in hot and cold water, insufflations of tobacco smoke into the baby's rectum, and rubbing brandy and garlic to the baby's chest—were made over the years (1). Pioneered in Europe in the 1700s, the purpose of hospital maternity care was to prevent maternal death that was then rampant. Neonatal survival was not the priority—if babies survived, well and good; if they survived intact, that was a bonus. Falling maternal mortality in the early 20th century allowed some focus to shift to babies. In the late 1950s, anesthesiologist Virginia Apgar introduced a score that was pivotal in drawing

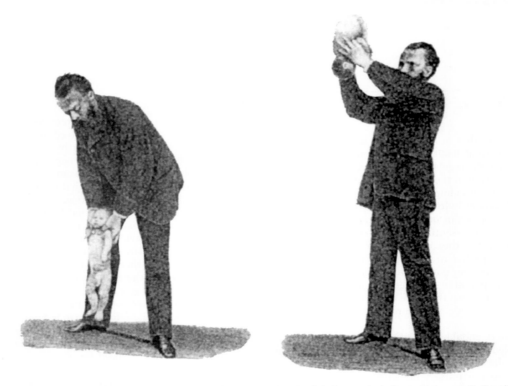

FIGURE 16.1 Illustration (reputedly of Dr Bernhard Schultze himself) demonstrating the Schultze method of neonatal resuscitation. (From Schultze BS. *Der Scheintod Neugeborener.* Jenna: Mauke's Verlag, 1871.)

attention to newborns in the DR (2). Caregivers were forced to assess their condition in a structured fashion at 1 minute of life, drawing attention in a manner that had been lacking up to that point ("9 months' observation of the mother surely warrants 1 minute's observation of the baby") (3). A pattern of treatment of newborn babies evolved, based largely on animal experiments performed by the group of Geoffrey Dawes (4). Term rhesus monkeys were subjected to acute profound asphyxia by ligating the umbilical cord and placing a saline-filled bag (we have been unable to confirm/refute the rumor that condoms were used) over the head to prevent spontaneous breathing. The monkeys initially tried to breathe, then stopped, became progressively more acidemic and bradycardic, and slid inexorably toward death unless they were resuscitated with endotracheal PPV.

The relevance of these experiments to perinatal events in humans can of course be questioned. Physiology often differs between species, and human fetuses and newborns are rarely if ever subjected to the all-or-nothing asphyxia insult used by Dawes et al. However, the data obtained did at least inform initial advances in DR practice in the 1980s and 1990s and continue to remind clinicians of the importance of adequately inflating the chest of a newborn in secondary apnea and of closely monitoring heart rate (HR) as the first sign of effective resuscitation.

In the 1980s, practice in the DR that was largely based on the consensus opinion of experts was formalized into organized courses (5,6). In 1999, the International Liaison Committee on Resuscitation (ILCOR) issued its first recommendations on techniques that should be used to support newborns (7). The Neonatal Task Force of ILCOR is an international collaboration of neonatal health care professionals that review the literature, achieve a consensus on the science, and make treatment recommendations accordingly. Initially, this was done at 5-yearly intervals and has more recently evolved to a more continuous evidence evaluation process. ILCOR recommendations underpin the resuscitation guidelines that apply around the world (8).

Epidemiology and International Perspective

The majority of newborn babies who die are born in low- and middle-income countries. All of the greatest challenges newborns face—asphyxia, prematurity, sepsis, and congenital anomalies—occur more frequently in these settings (9) (see Chapter 1). Frequently, access to antenatal care is limited in these countries, and there is an additional and substantial "hidden" mortality of late antenatal and intrapartum stillbirth. In high-income countries, prematurity occurs more frequently (c. 5 to 18/100 births) than birth asphyxia, early-onset neonatal sepsis (both c. 1/1,000 births), or congenital anomalies. In high-income countries, antenatal care is usually more readily available and consistent so more information is available (e.g., more accurate dating and identification of anomalies from antenatal ultrasound examinations), which allows for better planning in advance of deliveries.

PRINCIPLES OF DELIVERY ROOM MANAGEMENT

Despite variations in available resources, the newborn babies themselves are pretty much the same everywhere. All are naked and wet and at risk of getting cold. All have fluid-filled lungs with relatively little circulating blood that must rapidly become aerated and better perfused. Fortunately, most babies breathe independently; however, some do not or do so ineffectively. For these babies, encouraging them to breathe spontaneously and supporting their breathing is the priority. The principles of DR care of the newborn are the same everywhere—attend the delivery; support the baby's temperature; assess their condition; support their breathing if it is not effective; assess their response; adjust their breathing support; and support their circulation if that is not working. It is worth restating—even for babies who receive circulatory support, the priority is ALWAYS to support breathing. The availability of technology does not preclude the use of more simple methods and is not the be all and end all. Also, the elements are not equally important. All babies need help to regulate their temperature; some babies need help to establish breathing; a minority are intubated for breathing support; and a vanishingly small number get circulatory support. Again, assisting babies to breathe independently is the key to DR care.

Team

All people attending births—birth attendants, midwives, and doctors—should have knowledge of basic life support measures, that is, how to keep a baby warm, stimulate the baby gently, and give mask PPV. There should be at least one person at the delivery specifically for the baby if problems—for example, suspected asphyxia, prematurity, congenital anomalies—are anticipated. Someone should attend for the baby when cesarean delivery is performed under maternal general (as opposed to regional) anesthesia, even if no other problems are anticipated. General anesthetic agents rapidly diffuse into the fetal circulation and can cause apnea of uncertain duration, during which the baby may need breathing support. If it is likely that the baby may need help beyond stimulation and brief mask ventilation, two (or more) people should attend. Likewise, more help will be needed for multiple births. Local resources will dictate the size and composition of the team. If there is a reasonable chance that a baby might need to be intubated (e.g., known congenital diaphragmatic hernia, extreme prematurity), someone with advanced airway skills should attend. When you arrive, check that the equipment you need is present and working. Introduce yourself to the clinicians, and to the family if possible and appropriate to do so. When more than one person attends the delivery, identify a leader and assign roles (e.g., who will collect the baby, listen to the HR, apply the pulse oximeter, and give breathing support).

Equipment

See Table 16.1 for a list of suggested equipment for the DR. Equipment is analogous to cars—many different models with different features are available at varying prices, but they mostly do the same thing. In addition to cost, other local considerations (e.g., the availability of supplies of reliable power, compressed gases, and clean water) will influence the choice of equipment. It may be helpful to have largely one type of any piece of equipment at

TABLE 16.1

Equipment Required for Delivery Room Resuscitation

Resuscitation cot

Resuscitation cot—a firm surface/table top with on overhead radiant heat source

Assessment—clock or stopwatch, stethoscope, pulse oximeter, ECG[a]

Thermoregulation—overhead radiant heat source, clean towels, hat, polyethylene bag, exothermic mattress[a]

Breathing support

Breathing support device—one of self-inflating bag, flow-inflating bag, and T-piece

Compressed gases—air, oxygen, and a blender; heater/humidifier[a]

Airway support—face mask; laryngoscope blades (size and endotracheal tubes of varying sizes; exhaled carbon dioxide detector[a]; supraglottic airway device (e.g., laryngeal mask airway)[a]

Suction device—wall-mounted suction with catheters of varying size

Circulation

Umbilical venous catheter (single lumen 3.5F and 5F) with syringes, three-way stopcock, and 0.9% saline to flush

Adrenaline/Epinephrine 1:10,000 or 0.1 mg/mL

Access to O Rhesus-negative blood for emergency transfusion

[a]Optional.

an institution; uniformity and familiarity may make it easier for people to perform, particularly in stressful situations. It is essential that the equipment works as intended; it should be checked regularly by someone who uses it in their clinical practice. It is also essential that the people who are expected to use the equipment know how to; they need to practice with it regularly.

CLAMPING THE UMBILICAL CORD

Umbilical cords have been divided hundreds of thousands of times each day for hundreds of thousands of years. One might expect, then, that the time at which it occurs would not be contentious. Traditionally, there was little urgency about clamping the umbilical cord, which was usually done once it was no longer pulsating. More modern obstetric management and the active management of labor advocated clamping the cord and giving uterotonics immediately after delivery of the baby in an attempt to effect speedy delivery of the placenta and reduce postpartum bleeding. As intervention for newborns increased, pressure mounted to hand the babies over to the pediatricians without delay. As a default, cords were clamped within seconds of birth, with "delayed" (an adjective that rarely has positive connotations, especially for pediatricians) describing clamping that occurred 30 seconds or more later.

At birth, approximately one-third of the baby's blood volume is in the placenta. Animal studies suggest that the benefit of clamping the cord is not simply one of net transfusion of blood into the newborn (10). After delivery, blood continues to flow in both umbilical vein and arteries, both toward and away from the baby. As the lung aerates, pulmonary vascular resistance falls and pulmonary blood flow markedly increases. When the cord is not clamped, blood flow from the umbilical vein maintains cardiac preload and a smooth circulatory transition. If the cord is clamped before the lung aerates, cardiac preload drops leading to fluctuations and instability in cardiac output that takes time to recover. Animal studies convincingly demonstrate that ensuring lung aeration prior to cord clamping significantly improves both pulmonary and systemic blood flow (11).

Randomized studies in term infants demonstrated that delaying cord clamping increases their hemoglobin level and iron stores without increasing the rate of maternal postpartum hemorrhage (12). This cost-free intervention should be the standard of care everywhere, particularly in countries where iron deficiency anemia is prevalent and associated with adverse childhood outcomes (e.g., lower IQ). The question of when to clamp the cord for preterm infants is more vexed. They are at higher risk of anemia than term infants; however, they are also more likely to have apnea and become hypothermic after birth, which may make neonatologists reluctant to wait. Meta-analysis of small randomized studies suggested that delayed cord clamping might reduce intraventricular hemorrhage in preterm infants (13). In a large randomized study, 26% of babies who were assigned to have their cord clamped ≥60 seconds had it clamped beforehand, mostly due to clinician concern (14). This study found no difference in the rate of survival without major morbidity at 36 weeks corrected. However, a meta-analysis that included this study demonstrated lower in-hospital mortality for preterm infants with delayed cord clamping (15). A study that compared immediate clamping with planned clamping ≥120 seconds in preterm infants (16) suggested improved survival free of disability to 2 years of corrected age with delayed clamping (17). The mechanism by which delayed cord clamping may lead to improved outcomes has not yet been fully described. Animal studies show significant benefits on systemic perfusion, and these findings have been replicated in some human studies (18). However, other large RCTs have shown no impact of timing of cord clamping on measures of systemic blood flow or hypotension (19). Some association with improved autoregulation of cerebral blood flow has been suggested as a mechanism for reduction in IVH (20). On a simpler level, during the transition from placental oxygenation to pulmonary oxygenation of the blood, it seems entirely logical that having the former in place while the latter is established creates a more stable transition.

Neonatologists' eagerness to get their hands on the baby in case resuscitation is needed generated interest in the practice of cord milking or stripping, where immediately after birth, blood is repetitively squeezed through the length of the umbilical cord toward the baby, before the cord is clamped and divided, usually within a minute of birth. A randomized trial that compared cord milking to planned cord clamping at 1 minute in preterm infants showed little difference in the time to arrive at the resuscitation cot but was stopped early because of an increased rate of intraventricular hemorrhage in babies less than 28 weeks (21). The effects of the timing of cord clamping on infants born in need of resuscitation or with congenital anomalies are unclear.

It is an attractive notion that in any given situation (e.g., time at which the cord should be clamped), there is one number suitable for everyone. However, as with sizes of shoes, hats, or gloves, it is unlikely to be the case. It is likely that the "ideal" time for cord clamping varies, and it is unlikely to be within seconds of birth. From the current state of knowledge, it is prudent to wait to see if the baby breathes, and if they do, to clamp the cord at a minute or later. Ongoing studies are focusing on the timing of cord clamping relative to the onset of lung aeration and other metrics of cardio-respiratory stability (22) and if it is desirable and how to provide warmth and breathing support to newborns before clamping. With increased desire to be able to provide breathing support to babies who are still attached to the cord, mobile resuscitation cots that can be brought into close proximity with the mother have been developed and are the subject of study (16,23).

POSITIONING

Newborn infants are placed on their back (supine) after birth. This contrasts with the belief that infants with respiratory distress, preterm infants in particular, breathe more effectively, when placed prone. One small randomized study reported that preterm infants had similar oxygen saturations at 5 minutes whether they were placed on their left side or supine (24). While either appears reasonable, infants are generally placed supine. Infants with suspected upper airway obstruction due the Pierre-Robin sequence are an exception, where turning them on their side or prone may relieve a degree of obstruction.

THERMOREGULATION

Maintaining a newborn's temperature is of critical and often underrated importance. The "gold standard" is core temperature, temperature of blood in the hypothalamus. As it is impractical to measure this in humans, rectal or esophageal temperature is considered to be the gold standard in clinical practice. This was originally measured with mercury-in-glass (MIG) thermometers, which are no longer in routine clinical use given concerns about the safety of mercury. Today, a baby's temperature is usually measured with digital thermometer at the rectum or axilla. Though they are thought of as interchangeable, they do not correlate particularly well. In the past, temperature was rarely measured in the DR; it was usually first measured on admission to the neonatal unit.

Normal temperature for a newborn is defined as a core temperature of 36.5°C to 37.5°C (25). In contrast to many parameters that are measured in the first hours of life, abnormal temperature has been repeatedly shown for more than 60 years and in many settings to have strong association with mortality (26). The colder you are, the more likely you are to die. The strength of this association and its repeated identification make it profoundly unlikely to be due to chance. While it is likely that it is partially just an association (babies who are likely to die get cold), it is also likely at least partially causative (being cold is very bad for babies and makes them more likely to die). Hyperthermia is rarer and less well understood. Associations between hyperthermia at birth and chorioamnionitis may explain some of the reported increased rate of adverse neurologic outcome in babies; however, cause and effect cannot be excluded. And since it is unlikely that being hot would be good for you, it is prudent to avoid overheating.

Newly born babies are warmer (c. 37°C) than the room in which they are born (usually 22°C), so they will lose heat to the environment. Increasing the room temperature lessens the gradient and should reduce heat loss. Newborns are naked and wet and lose heat by evaporation, radiation, convection, and conduction (Fig. 16.2). All are a problem in the DR to a greater or lesser extent and measures should be taken to lessen the effect of each.

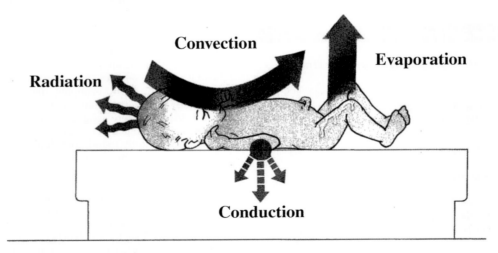

Four ways a newborn may lose heat to the environment

FIGURE 16.2 The routes by which newly born infants lose heat. (From World Health Organisation. *Thermal control of the newborn: a practical guide.* Geneva, Switzerland: World Health Organisation, 1993. WHO/FSE/MSMS 93.2.)

Also, babies do not generate heat well themselves, so they need an external heat source.

The traditional approach to prevent heat loss was to dry the baby, remove the wet linen, and place the baby under a radiant heat source (5). As newborn babies have large heads from which they can lose a lot of heat, placing a hat on the head is also recommended. Randomized studies demonstrate that wrapping babies in (readily available and cheap) food-grade polyethylene bags while leaving their heads exposed, without necessarily first drying them, reduces admission hypothermia in preterm infants (27–30) and in term infants in a resource-poor setting (31). Polyethylene bags reduce evaporative and convective heat loss while still allowing radiant heat to reach the baby. The external heat sources used are generally radiant heat source placed above the resuscitation cot. However, adult humans are also a good heat source and placing babies skin-to-skin is effective (32,33). Other heat sources used include exothermic mattresses; these are filled with a gel that crystallizes and produces heat when a metal disk contained within the gel is snapped (34).

The measures that are appropriate for your setting depend firstly on how much of a problem you have with hypothermia and hyperthermia; and secondly on your resources (e.g., availability of a stable power supply). Firstly, to know whether you've got an issue, you need to measure temperature consistently (i.e., rectally on admission to the neonatal unit with a digital thermometer in all babies) and accurately. Take simple (and cheap) measures to reduce heat loss. Increase the DR temperature to reduce the temperature gradient. Avoid placing babies on cold surfaces (conduction), near large windows (radiation), or near open doors and windows (convection). Put a hat on their head (radiation) and put them in a polyethylene bag (evaporation and convection). Combining methods of preventing heat loss and providing heat can reduce hypothermia but may also increase hyperthermia (27,34). Again, to determine what is appropriate for your setting, you need to measure the babies' temperatures to determine how prevalent hypothermia and hyperthermia where you work. We are quite focused on admission temperature and quite ignorant of what really happens to a baby's temperature in the interval between birth and admission. A growing number of neonatal intensive care units (NICUs) are employing continuous core temperature measurement and servocontrolling of temperature from birth as part of a thermoregulation quality improvement bundle (35).

ASSESSMENT

Clinical
When examining babies clinically, most information is derived from observation; palpation, percussion, and auscultation are much less important. All babies are assessed clinically at birth (even subconsciously), whether or not other technology is used.

Tone and Activity
When you first see a newborn in the DR, observe whether the newborn has tone or whether he or she is limp like a rag doll. This is easily discerned if you are handed the baby. If (like the majority) the baby has got tone, take a deep breath, keep calm, and keep going. If a baby with tone is crying, he/she is also breathing, and in all likelihood, the HR is good. If the baby is active and moving, things are fine. On the other hand, if the baby is limp, be very concerned. The likelihood is that the baby is not breathing effectively, and the HR may be slow.

Breathing
Babies who are crying are breathing. If they are not crying, they may still be breathing. Watch closely for abdominal movement and chest excursion. It can be tricky to assess, particularly in

preterm infants. Chest excursion can be subtle and difficult to see in the crash-bang-clatter of the DR. Breathing should be sufficient to maintain the baby's HR greater than 100 beats per minute (bpm).

Heart Rate
HR is the single most important indicator of the need for and response to resuscitation in the DR. In general, a baby's breathing should be sufficient to maintain HR greater than 100 bpm. If it is less than 100 bpm, it usually means that the baby needs help to improve his/her breathing. Ideally, we should be able to measure the HR easily, quickly, accurately, continuously, and cheaply. HR may be assessed clinically by listening to the heart with a stethoscope or by feeling for pulsations in the umbilical cord. This is usually done by counting the number of beats/pulsations in 6 seconds and multiplying by 10 to give a value in bpm. Auscultation is more reliable than palpation (36,37). While auscultation is not continuous and is less accurate than other methods, its lack of precision is offset by the ease and speed with which it can be obtained with reasonable accuracy (38). HR can also be counted with pulse oximetry (PO) and electrocardiogram (ECG) in the DR. Both count the HR continuously and more accurately than auscultation. ECG displays HR marginally more quickly than PO (38–40). However, having the HR earlier does not appear to influence intervention in the DR (39,40). ECG is more prone to interruption and technical difficulties than PO (41) and does not replace the need for PO in the DR, which is recommended for guiding oxygen supplementation. Pulseless electrical activity—ECG complexes identified in the absence of detectable cardiac output—has been reported (42,43); if it is suspected, clinical assessment is recommended to rule it out.

Color
Babies may be one of three colors at birth. The vast majority of babies are cyanosed. This is normal; fetal oxygen saturation (c. 40% to 60%) is substantially lower than that in postnatal life (>90%). A small number of babies are pale lemon yellow color. This is very unusual and implies poor perfusion and acidosis. In the context of a limp baby, it is a matter for grave concern and calls for immediate intervention. Even more rarely, a newborn baby may be a ghostly milky-white color. Such babies may have exsanguinated, which may happen in the context of an overt antepartum hemorrhage (e.g., vasa previa) or may be unheralded (e.g., fetomaternal hemorrhage). Again, limp ghostly white babies demand immediate intervention and may not respond without transfusion, sometimes of uncrossmatched O-negative blood.

Color perception is affected by many factors including the ambient light in which the baby is observed, the skin color and ethnicity of the baby, and the ability of individual clinicians to perceive color. Color is an unreliable guide to oxygen saturations (SpO$_2$) (43). However, rather than judging the color, you are looking for an improvement in color—babies should become "pinker"—as time passes.

Pulse Oximetry
PO can be used to assess the SpO$_2$ and HR of babies in the minutes after birth. Data are obtained quickest (within a minute or so) when the sensor is placed preductally (i.e., on the right upper limb) and then attached to the monitor. Centile charts are available derived from the progression of SpO$_2$ in babies who were not resuscitated serve as a guide (**Fig. 16.3**) (44). A large proportion of babies were delivered by cesarean section, and all had their umbilical cords clamped immediately after birth. While this may affect the values somewhat, a few things are clear; the range of SpO$_2$ is wide; the values are substantially lower than that seen in babies who have transitioned to air breathing; and they increase steadily over 10 minutes.

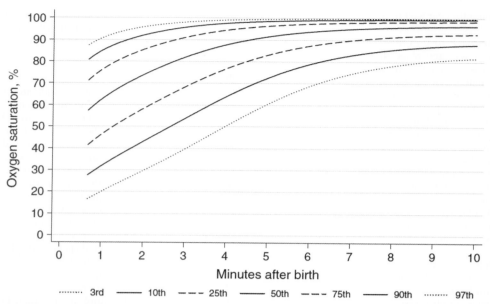

FIGURE 16.3 Dawson centiles. (Reproduced with permission from Dawson JA, Kamlin COF, Vento M, et al. Defining the reference range for oxygen saturations for infants after birth. *Pediatrics* 2010;125:e1340. Ref. (44). Copyright © 2010 by the American Academy of Pediatrics.)

Electrocardiogram

See HR above. In adult and child resuscitation, ECG is used in to look for arrhythmias that may be corrected with cardioversion (a "shockable rhythm"). In babies, it is used for counting the HR. The attraction of ECG appears to be the speed of acquisition of HR—it gives a number quicker than PO. It does not appear to be quicker than auscultation, though it is more accurate. It has more technical difficulties and comes at a cost (equipment, human resources, and potential distraction) and does not replace oximetry.

Assessment Summary

When assessing a baby in the DR, observe (and feel) their tone and activity, listen for crying, and watch for breathing. If a baby is not vigorous and crying, listen to the precordium for the heartbeat, confirm that it is present and count it over 6 seconds to get an estimate of the HR. If you are concerned that the baby is not breathing well and may have a slow HR, get a colleague to place a PO sensor on the right upper limb (see below); you should have a HR reading within a minute. Use ECG leads if you wish.

▌AIRWAY

Most babies are born with a patent airway. Their heads are large and may lead to inadvertent flexion of the neck. It is recommended to keep their heads in a neutral or slightly extended ("sniffing") position, as holding their flexion or extension can compromise their airway.

Suction

Suctioning the airway was extrapolated from adult medicine, where regurgitation of stomach contents and airway obstruction in unconscious patients is a real risk. Newborn babies have empty stomachs and so are at low risk of aspiration. It is normal for clear lung fluid to come out of a baby's mouth after birth. Suctioning can cause local trauma and provoke apnea and bradycardia through vagal stimulation. As routine suctioning does not offer any advantage over no suctioning (45), it shouldn't be done.

Meconium is contained in the fetal bowel, and babies become more likely to pass it before birth the closer they get to term and, particularly, the further they get beyond term. While it is a well-recognized sign of fetal distress, the vast majority of babies who pass meconium before birth are well. However, it may be aspirated and cause a nasty meconium aspiration syndrome (a combination of physical obstruction of smaller airways causing atelectasis and hyperinflation, parenchymal inflammation provoking persistent pulmonary hypertension, and resulting ventilation/perfusion mismatch—see Chapter 28). From the 1970s, it was recommended that babies born through meconium-stained amniotic fluid (MSAF) were to have their nose and mouth suctioned before complete delivery ("intrapartum suctioning") and be immediately intubated after birth for endotracheal suction. However, as no benefit was demonstrated in large randomized trials of intrapartum suction (46) or of endotracheal suction of vigorous babies (47), neither is now recommended. The rates of MAS fell markedly in developed countries from the 1980s; this is more likely due to reduction in postterm births courtesy of more accurate pregnancy dating with the introduction of obstetric ultrasound.

On rare occasions, the airway may be blocked by a clot or thick mucus, so suction must be available to remove them. It must also be available to remove secretions that may obscure the view at laryngoscopy during intubation attempts (see below). While bulb syringe suction devices that automatically reexpand after compression are available, they are not suitable for removing secretions at laryngoscopy. Wall-mounted or portable suction devices with catheters of various sizes (e.g., 6 to 8 Fr) are preferable.

Airway Adjuncts

Oropharyngeal (Guedel) airways have been recommended to relieve obstruction during mask ventilation of unconscious adults. Though models small enough for babies exist, they may increase rather than decrease the degree of airway obstruction during mask ventilation (48), and they are not widely used. They do however continue to be advocated for in the UK Newborn Life Support course and may be of value in the presence of micrognathia or other upper airway obstruction.

Nasal/nasopharyngeal airways are discussed below.

▌BREATHING

The majority of babies—including the majority of extremely preterm infants (49,50)—breathe spontaneously at birth. For the minority of babies who do not, stimulation may help and has long been practiced and recommended. Despite this, we know relatively little about stimulation. Very vigorous stimulation, such as the old practice of holding babies upside down by their ankles and slapping their bottoms, can injure babies and is not recommended. Babies more often have their backs rubbed, the soles of their feet stimulated, or their abdomen or chest rubbed (51,52). In a small randomized study, premature babies who were repeatedly stimulated every 10 seconds over the first 4 minutes of life had higher average SpO$_2$ than babies who were stimulated two to three times (53). Babies who do not breathe following stimulation should be given breathing support with a ventilation device.

Ventilation Devices

These are used to give positive pressure inflations (PPV) to infants who are determined to be apneic. The majority of devices used in the DR are one of three types of manually operated devices—a self-inflating bag, a flow-inflating bag, or a T-piece. There are subtle but important differences between these devices, in particular whether they provide positive end-expiratory pressure (PEEP). Devices that deliver PEEP may also be used to give continuous positive airway pressure (CPAP) to spontaneously breathing infants. It is important that you are familiar with the equipment that you use and to check it regularly.

Self-inflating bags come in varying sizes (for newborns typically approximately 240 mL) and are made of material that automatically reexpands after compression (e.g., silicone). The peak inflating pressure (PIP) delivered during inflation is determined by the force of the squeeze and limited by a pressure relief ("pop-off") valve. It does not need a gas source to function, but oxygen can be attached to give supplementary oxygen. Self-inflating bags do not reliably deliver PEEP, and they cannot be used to give CPAP. Flow-inflating (or anesthetic) bags require a compressed gas source to function. The PIP delivered is determined by the force of the squeeze and may not be limited. A manometer is usually placed in the circuit to monitor the PIP. PEEP can be delivered by controlling the rate of escape of gas from the bag, usually with a valve, and so CPAP can be delivered. T-pieces have increased in popularity over recent years. They require a compressed gas source to function. The PIP is usually set and predetermined. PEEP is delivered, so T-pieces can be used to give CPAP.

Each device has its pros and cons. Self-inflating bags do not depend on compressed gas and are simpler and more intuitive to use than flow-inflating bags or T-pieces; however, they do not reliably deliver PEEP (even with a PEEP valve attached) and cannot be used to give CPAP. The PIP delivered with flow-inflating bags can be varied quickly, and PEEP can be delivered; however, they require more practice and skill to use, and very high PIP and/or PEEP may be unintentionally delivered. T-pieces are relatively easy to use and deliver PEEP and CPAP; however, many versions require multiple steps to be taken to adjust the PIP, acting as a disincentive to providing higher pressures that are sometimes required to recruit lung tissue. In addition, the PEEP is very sensitive to changes in flow rate, giving scope for inadvertent high PEEP and reduced tidal volumes from reduced delta pressure (the difference between PEEP and PIP). There is relatively little information from human studies as to which device may be most effective. One small study found no difference in the SpO$_2$ at 5 minutes of preterm infants who received PPV with a self-inflating bag or T-piece (54). One large study that compared self-inflating bags and T-pieces did not show a difference in the proportion of babies who had HR greater than 100 bpm at 2 minutes of age, though fewer babies treated with the T-piece were intubated (55). The choice of device may be dictated by local concerns and resources. For example, the T-piece is used at my hospital because there is ready access to compressed gas and it allows for CPAP to be given, which is useful as many of the babies who receive breathing support are

born preterm. Whichever device is chosen the key requirement is that the operator is familiar with how to use it, and how to troubleshoot it if things aren't going to plan.

Interfaces

Whichever ventilation device is chosen, it must be used in conjunction with an interface. Various interfaces may be attached to ventilation devices and applied to babies—face masks, nasal interfaces, endotracheal tubes (ETTs), or supraglottic airways.

Face Masks

Mask ventilation is considered the cornerstone of neonatal resuscitation. Masks are usually made silicone or another pliable material. They may be round or more anatomically shaped and may or may not have a cushioned rim. They are intended to encircle the nose and mouth but not overlap the eyes and chin; the size that is appropriate therefore varies with the size of the baby.

Mannequin studies demonstrate that there is substantial leak from commercially available masks (56); that leak is increased if the mask is held by the rim as opposed to the stem (57); that a second operator holding the mask may reduce leak (58); and that substantial force may be applied to the mannequin's head during mask PPV (59). Studies in babies confirm that there are large leaks from commercially available masks (60) and that leaks seen in premature babies are not necessarily reduced with smaller masks (61). It is not clear the extent to which leak matters. The role of mask ventilation is not to provide long-term tidal ventilation of the lungs as when intubated. Rather a short-term period of lung inflation should be enough to oxygenate the blood returning to the heart in the pulmonary veins, with the increase in oxygenation then stimulating spontaneous respiration. Leak presumably matters if/when it interferes with the ability of PPV to stimulate breathing. This is tricky to determine, because the act of applying a face mask may cause apnea in a spontaneously breathing baby; and it is difficult to measure spontaneous breathing in the presence of large leaks.

Nasal interfaces are commonly used to support the breathing of preterm infants in the neonatal unit. ETTs of an appropriate internal diameter (ID) (see ETT below)—which are shortened to around 5 cm and inserted into the nose at right angles to the baby's face and into the nasopharynx—may be useful in relieving airway obstruction in babies with Pierre-Robin sequence. When used to support breathing in preterm infants, they have similar efficacy to face masks at preventing intubation in the DR (62) and by 24 hours (63). Commercially made nasopharyngeal tubes are also manufactured for the same purpose.

Endotracheal Tubes

ETTs are plastic tubes that are inserted through the vocal cords into the trachea for the purpose of providing PPV. A major challenge for all newborn babies, especially premature babies, is establishing and maintaining aeration of the lungs. When the baby is intubated and the larynx is bypassed, gas will continue to leave the lung until the pressure inside the lung equilibrates with atmospheric pressure, unless a continuous pressure is applied to keep gas in there. When a baby is intubated, PEEP should be used if and whenever possible. A ventilator, a T-piece or a flow-inflating bag that provides PEEP should be used in preference to a self-inflating bag for providing ET PPV whenever possible.

The ETTs used for newborns are generally straight, uniform diameter tubes (as opposed to "shouldered" Coles ETTs) that are uncuffed. The ETTs used in adults and children generally have an inflatable cuff to reduce or abolish leak. These are not generally used in newborns due to reports of tracheal injury. The size of the ID of the ETT used varies with the size of the baby (e.g., 2.5 mm ID for babies <1,000 g, 3.0 for 1,000 to 2,500 g, 3.5 for >3,000 g). They have markings at 1-cm intervals from the tip. They may be inserted by the oral route or, less commonly, by the nasal route.

They are inserted under laryngoscopy, which is usually direct (i.e., operator views the larynx by looking directly into the mouth) but may be indirect (i.e., operator views the larynx on a screen that displaying the image captured by a video camera at the tip of the laryngoscope). The laryngoscope blades used to intubate babies are generally straight and come in varying sizes, again determined by the size of the baby being intubated (e.g., 00 for infants <1 kg, 0 for 1 to 2.5 kg, 1 for >2.5 kg).

Intubation is an important skill for neonatologists to learn. Like any physical skill—riding a bike or playing guitar or football—performance improves with repetition. It has become trickier to learn how to intubate babies in recent years, as doctors have had dwindling opportunities to learn; unsurprisingly, proficiency has deteriorated. When attempting intubation, some basic information should be borne in mind. It is an invasive, unpleasant, and painful procedure. Babies should be given analgesia and sedation beforehand, and probably muscle relaxants as they increase the rate of success. In general, babies should only be intubated without prior medication when they are in extremis. Intubation is a two-person procedure—while you get a view of the larynx, you need someone else to observe the baby and to hand you the ETT and suction catheter if needed.

The skill in intubation is all in getting a view of the larynx. If you can't see the larynx and the vocal cords, you won't intubate the baby. To maximize your chances of intubating successfully, optimize ergonomics—make sure the baby is on a firm flat surface that is at an adequate (above your waist) height, that his/her body is in a straight line, and that his/her head is in a neutral position. Make sure that your laryngoscope blade is long enough—a 00 blade will not do for a term baby—and that the light is good. Hold the laryngoscope in your left hand, irrespective of your hand dominance. Hold the handle at the bottom with your thumb running vertically up along (not encircling) it. Start in the midline—find the groove in the middle of the tongue and advance the blade along it, looking for the epiglottis. Once you find it, "grab" it with the tip of the blade or advance the tip of the blade into the vallecula behind it and lift the laryngoscope blade upward (i.e., give a "thumbs up"). Do not pull the laryngoscope handle backward like a lever. You shouldn't need to use a lot of force to view the larynx, particularly in premature babies. The purpose of the laryngoscope is to use it to lift the tongue and jaw out of the way; how heavy can the tongue and jaw of a 750 g baby be? You may need a suction catheter to clear secretions that obscure your view. Once you identify the larynx, do not look away. Wait for the vocal cords to open. When they do, insert an ETT of appropriate size through them and advance it a little (not a lot—people tend to insert it too far). Many people use stylets or introducers (plastic-coated wires) inserted through the ETT to keep it straight. While they may be useful for smaller diameter ETTs that are more pliable, particularly when exposed to radiant heat, they did not increase the success rate of pediatric trainees (64). Confirm that the baby has been correctly intubated by prompt increase in HR in bradycardic babies, "misting" (condensation) in the ETT during exhalation and exhaled carbon dioxide (CO_2) as detected with a colorimetric detector or CO_2 monitor. Once you are happy it is in the trachea, secure it. If you can only hear breath sounds on one side of the chest, it suggests that the ETT may be inserted too far and needs to be withdrawn a little. The depth at which you secure an oral ETT may be estimated various ways; the most commonly used method—add 6 to the baby's weight in kg (e.g., 7 cm for a 1-kg baby)—appears as good or bad as other methods (65–67), though very small (23 week/500 g) infants need even shorter (5.5 to 6.0 cm) tubes.

Supraglottic Airways

Supraglottic airways (e.g., laryngeal mask airway) were developed for short-term breathing support of unconscious adults (e.g., for brief periods of anesthesia). Their main attraction is that they are easier to insert than ETTs. Their use has been reported in babies for the resuscitation of newborns, in the setting of upper airway anomalies and for giving surfactant. Different models are available—some have an inflatable cuff, some do not, and a mannequin study suggests there is wide variation in their performance (68). Currently, models are not available for babies who weigh less than 1.5 kg. This limits their use as a large proportion of babies who receive invasive respiratory support, and certainly who receive exogenous surfactant, are very low birth weight babies. Their use has been reported and shows promise in low- and middle-income countries, where they were found to be more effective than face masks in a small trial of term and near-term babies (69).

Gases

Air versus Oxygen

When supporting the breathing of a newborn, clinicians must decide which gas to use—21% oxygen, 100% oxygen, or some intermediate concentration. At birth, all babies are cyanosed (and have lower SpO_2) compared to babies who have transitioned. Traditionally, it was recommended to give babies 100% oxygen during PPV to reverse this "hypoxia." This explains why the only gas available in the resuscitation area in many old DRs was 100% oxygen. However, concerns about the potential for pure oxygen to cause oxidative damage in newborns prompted studies where term and near-term infants who received PPV at birth were randomly assigned to receive air (21% oxygen) or 100% oxygen. In these studies, infants received either 21% or 100% oxygen, not intermediate concentrations; and when clinicians determined that infants assigned to 21% oxygen were not responding, they switched over to 100% oxygen. Meta-analysis of these trials demonstrated a higher risk of death for babies who were started in 100% oxygen (70).

The current (2020) ILCOR guidance for resuscitation of the term newborn recommends commencing with 21% oxygen and only increasing up the inspired oxygen concentration if the infant is not responding.

The situation for preterm infants is less clear. Preterm infants are at higher risk of having respiratory distress and needing supplemental oxygen to keep their SpO_2 in the normal range; however, they have less well-developed antioxidant defenses and are at higher risk of oxidant damage than term infants. Increasingly, the approach for preterm infants has been to adjust (titrate) the concentration of oxygen aiming for target SpO_2 values that were reported for babies who do not require support after birth. This approach requires a pulse oximeter and an air/oxygen blender. Randomized studies compared strategies of starting in lower (typically ≤30%) versus higher (typically ≥60%) oxygen. They found that most preterm infants received oxygen supplementation to achieve target SpO_2. A suggestion from one study (71) that mortality might be increased in extremely preterm infants randomized to start in air was not borne out in meta-analysis (72). Administration of 100% oxygen has been associated with prolonged increase in inflammatory markers (tumor necrosis factor, interleukin-8) and with increased duration of respiratory support and incidence of BPD in preterm infants (73). However, larger studies are required to reliably determine the effects of each strategy.

The current (2020) ILCOR guidance for resuscitation of the preterm newborn recommends commencing with 21% to 30% oxygen and increasing the inspired oxygen concentration if the infant is not responding and using oxygen saturation targeting.

Heating and Humidification

The gases that babies receive in the NICUs are conditioned (i.e., heated and humidified). Humidifiers are not routinely used in the DR, so the gases used in respiratory circuits there are dry and colder. A randomized study demonstrated that heating and humidifying the gases reduced the prevalence of hypothermia on admission among preterm infants without showing effects on other respiratory outcomes (74).

The equipment you need will depend on the approach you wish to take; or perhaps, the equipment you have available will determine the approach you can take. Term babies who receive PPV should start in 21% oxygen. This may be given with a self-inflating bag without supplemental oxygen to start (you can attach it later if the baby does not respond). If you use a device that requires compressed gas (T-piece or flow-inflating bag), 21% oxygen (medical air) should be available. For preterm infants, the ideal initial oxygen concentration is not known; it is likely less than 100%, but many seem to need more than 30% oxygen. It is desirable to be able to vary the amount of oxygen you are using for preterm infants. An air/oxygen blender will allow you to easily adjust the concentration of oxygen. If you wish to titrate oxygen, you should use a pulse oximeter. Conditioned gases are not necessary but may be used.

Techniques
Continuous Positive Airway Pressure
Spontaneously breathing preterm infants are often given CPAP in the DR, whether or not they show signs of respiratory distress. The amount of pressure that is used is measured in cmH$_2$O. It is not clear what level of pressure should be used, though levels used in the NICU are usually in the region of 5 to 10 cmH$_2$O. This may be delivered with a face mask or nasal interfaces.

Positive Pressure Ventilation
If infants are not breathing and/or are bradycardic, PPV is required. Recommendations seem to be based on levels that were commonly used during pressure-limited ET ventilation of preterm infants in the NICU (e.g., PIP 25 cmH$_2$O). However, it is difficult to extrapolate this to mask ventilation (where leak from the interface may be much larger), particularly in the immediate postnatal period where the lung is still largely fluid-filled and noncompliant. It is recommended that inflations are given for around half a second at a frequency of about 40 to 60 per minute. Efficacy of PPV is best assessed by both visualizing chest expansion with each breath and by ensuring an increase in HR if the infant was bradycardic.

Sustained Inflations
Observational studies in animals and humans suggested that giving a sustained inflation—that is, applying a PIP for 10–15 to 20 seconds rather than 0.5 seconds—may achieve more rapid and even aeration of the lung. In preterm infants, sustained inflations showed benefit in some studies, not in others and uncertain effects overall (75). However, a large study in extremely preterm infants was stopped early due to concerns about increased mortality among the most immature infants randomly assigned to receive sustained inflation (76).

High-Flow Nasal Cannula Therapy
Heated and humidified oxygen-enriched gas given at flow rates ≥1 L/min is frequently used to support the breathing of preterm infants in the NICU. Randomized studies have demonstrated it to be noninferior to nasal CPAP for preterm infants who were extubated (77) and inferior to nasal CPAP as primary treatment for respiratory distress in very moderately preterm infants in the NICU (78). While its use to support preterm infants in the DR has been reported (79), it needs further evaluation and is not currently recommended.

CIRCULATION
The context for resuscitation in newborns is very different to that seen in adults. In adults, the lungs are aerated, and the heart usually stops beating due to arrhythmia. The priority is to maintain circulation while trying to determine whether there is an arrhythmia that may be corrected with cardioversion (a "shockable rhythm"). In newborns, the lungs are not aerated and the heart slows and stops in response to acidemia and hypoxia. Even hearts with serious structural anomalies beat normally after birth when acid–base and oxygenation are normal. A bradycardic or stopped heart will not recover unless the hypoxia and acidemia improve. The quickest way of fixing both is to breathe. PPV is the cornerstone of effective resuscitation in the newborn. The resuscitation team should take whatever steps are necessary to ensure effective PPV (repositioning the airway, increasing pressure, giving prolonged breaths, using airway adjuncts) such that the chest is clearly moving with each breath. Chest compressions should not be given before the chest has been clearly seen to move with PPV.

Newborns are rarely given circulatory support in the DR (80). That makes it difficult to study in a systematic and coherent fashion in humans. Most of the studies on which practice is based are animal studies. Some of animal models used for these studies are a few days old and so with aerated lungs and their circulation has transitioned, making extrapolation of findings difficult in some cases.

Chest Compressions
The main purpose of chest compressions in neonatal resuscitation is to perfuse the heart itself with oxygenated blood, rather than to maintain systemic circulation. Give chest compressions to babies whose HR remains less than 60 bpm despite PPV that has been optimized (ideally, ventilation with adequate PIP and PEEP through a correctly placed ETT). Place both of your thumbs on the sternum and press to a depth of 1/3 to 1/2 of the diameter of the chest about 100 times a minute. Do not squeeze the chest with your whole hand—your thumbs should be working, not your fingers—as this may impair chest excursion and ventilation. Two (index and middle) fingers may also be used to deliver chest compressions; however, thumbs are stronger and are less prone to fatigue (81). To perfuse the coronary arteries, you need an end-diastolic blood pressure. Animal studies suggest that in cardiac arrest, adrenaline helps to raise the end-diastolic blood pressure, improving coronary artery perfusion and chances of return of spontaneous circulation (see below).

Intravenous (IV) Access
On the rare occasions when there is serious circulatory compromise, IV access may be required. Serious circulatory compromise means that peripheral perfusion is poor. In such circumstances, it will be nigh on impossible to insert a peripheral IV cannula. Moreover, cannulae of the caliber typically used to give drugs to newborns in the NICU (e.g., 24F yellow) are not sufficiently large for volume resuscitation. If the baby needs IV access, insert a catheter into the umbilical vein. Attach a three-way stopcock to a sterile 3.5F or 5F catheter and flush it through with normal saline. Tie a tourniquet firmly around the base of the cord. Wear sterile gloves and in as sterile a fashion as possible, clean the cord with an antiseptic solution, cut it low, clean the cut surface, identify the umbilical vein (usually thin-walled, oval shaped and largest of the three vessels that are visible), insert the catheter to a depth 5 to 10 cm, aspirate to check for blood return, and secure it. This provides access directly into the central circulation, ideally the inferior vena cava. If umbilical venous catheterization proves impossible, an intraosseous needle may be inserted into the midtibia as a last resort.

Adrenaline (Epinephrine)
Based on case reports, it used to be recommended that adrenaline be given as a bolus down the ETT; however, negligible plasma levels of adrenaline were found following ET administration in animal studies. If at all possible, give adrenaline as an IV bolus (dose

CARE AROUND BIRTH

0.02 mg/kg or 0.2 mL/kg) centrally through the umbilical vein and follow it with a 3 mL flush of normal saline. This maximizes the chances it will reach the heart and exert effects on the coronary circulation. While adrenaline can be given via the ETT (dose 0.1 mg/kg or 1 mL/kg), it shouldn't be given at the cost of delay in giving IV adrenaline.

Volume Expansion

Volume is rarely given in DR resuscitation (80). Usually babies appear pale and poorly perfused at birth as a result of acidosis, rather than volume depletion. Assisting breathing is the priority and usually improves matters. An important exception is the baby who has exsanguinated.

Acute exsanguination may be heralded by an antepartum hemorrhage (e.g., ruptured vasa previa) or may be unanticipated in the case of fetomaternal hemorrhage. Depending on how recent and how severe the blood loss is, these babies may be conscious, ghostly pale, tachypneic, and tachycardic. As their condition deteriorates, they may remain bradycardic despite PPV through a correctly placed ETT. These babies are unlikely to improve without volume expansion with normal saline or, more likely, blood. Acute exsanguination is a clinical diagnosis. It is not usually possible to get a full blood count or an estimation of hemoglobin/hematocrit from a blood gas in a timely fashion. Even if results are available, the exsanguination may be so sudden as for there not to be sufficient time for it to be reflected by a drop in the value. You should have access to a unit of O Rhesus-negative blood for emergency unmatched transfusion. It should be given through a catheter placed in the umbilical vein. I personally suggest starting with an aliquot of 10 mL/kg (i.e., 30 to 40 mL for a term baby) that you push in manually over a short time (2 to 3 minutes) and titrate to response in HR, color, and perfusion.

SPECIFIC CONSIDERATIONS

Meconium

See SUCTION above. Routine intrapartum suctioning of meconium is not recommended, nor is routine ET suctioning of vigorous infants born through MSAF. It is less certain whether nonvigorous infant born through MSAF should be routinely intubated. While local practice may be influenced by the availability of advanced airway skills, the resuscitation of bradycardic infants should not delayed specifically to suction meconium, that is, if there is not someone immediately available to intubate, begin PPV as you would in any other infant. Blowing some liquid meconium into the lungs will likely have minimal effect on the severity of any ensuing meconium aspiration syndrome, which is generally thought to require deep, gasping respirations for prolonged periods rather than a one-off aspiration. If you suspect that the airway is truly blocked by particulate meconium (the chest is not moving with PPV and there is no response in HR), then suction is required. Subsequent management of meconium aspiration syndrome is covered in Chapter 28.

Congenital Anomalies

The widespread use of midtrimester antenatal ultrasound now identifies many anomalies that once first became apparent in the DR; this allows for better planning. While antenatal ultrasound has been a great advance, it does not identify every anomaly and is better at detecting some lesions (e.g., diaphragmatic hernias) than others (e.g., congenital heart lesions).

Diaphragmatic Hernia

Diaphragmatic hernia is a developmental abnormality that may occur in isolation or in association with other abnormalities. The diaphragm does not form properly to seal the thorax off from the abdomen, resulting in protrusion of organs that should be in the abdomen into the thorax. The lungs are physically smaller, and the alveoli and blood vessels in these physically smaller lungs are also abnormally formed. Historically, the condition was suspected in newborns presenting with profound respiratory distress, a scaphoid abdomen, and absence of breath sounds on one side. The majority of these lesions may now be diagnosed on antenatal ultrasound. The prognosis varies. Some babies have severe respiratory dysfunction and may not survive long, despite intensive care. Others are less severely affected and on rare occasions a baby presents weeks or months after birth with mild tachypnea.

When a fetus is known to have a diaphragmatic hernia antenatally and active (not palliative) care is planned, the family should be referred to a hospital with neonatal intensive care facilities. Experienced staff should attend the delivery as the majority of infants are intubated shortly after birth; this can be tricky as these babies are generally born at or near term and have not received medications. Avoid mask ventilation so as not to inflate the bowel and cause extrinsic lung compression and insert a wide bore nasogastric tube to deflate the bowel. Many babies have serious pulmonary hypertension and need a few days to stabilize before surgical repair is performed. This is followed by another period of intensive care and often by issues in getting enteral feeds established—see Chapter 30 for further details.

Abdominal Wall Defects

Gastroschisis describes a condition where bowel protrudes through a small defect in the anterior abdominal wall and is not covered by a membrane. This condition is increasing in prevalence in high-income countries and is usually isolated. While babies are often growth restricted, they usually aren't especially sick immediately at birth. The bowel, however, is at risk of compromised blood supply and massive fluid loss. Before delivery, place a length of clear polyethylene food-grade wrap on the resuscitation cot. After birth, place the baby supine on the wrap. The bowel should be handled minimally and carefully with sterile gloves. Place the bowel centrally on the abdomen and cover it with the polyethylene wrap. This should reduce fluid loss but still allow for observation, so you can ensure that the bowel remains perfused and does not appear dusky. Bring the baby to the neonatal unit for IV access and urgent referral for surgical treatment (see Chapter 36).

Exomphalos (omphalocele), a condition more frequently associated with other anomalies, describes herniation of the abdominal contents into the base of the umbilical cord. The bowel is covered by a membrane and does not need to be routinely covered; however, great care should be taken not to puncture the membrane and should be covered if it is breached. Babies are usually well in the DR, unless the lesion is massive and makes breathing difficult (particularly if it is so large that the sternum is involved) (see Chapter 36).

Congenital Heart Lesions

Most babies with very abnormal cardiac anatomy (e.g., hypoplastic left heart syndrome, complete AVSD) are not sick in the DR; they become progressively sicker as the days or weeks progress. The exceptions are babies who have transposition of the great vessels with an intact ventricular septum. If this diagnosis is suspected antenatally, it is critical that the baby be delivered at a tertiary center where they can be stabilized for urgent assessment and intervention by a pediatric cardiologist. These babies cannot oxygenate and so remain cyanotic and very quickly become profoundly acidemic. This is not appreciably affected by the standard treatments that we apply (e.g., ventilation, inotropic support). While their breathing and circulation should be supported as far as possible, this should not be done at the expense of urgent cardiac assessment and intervention (e.g., balloon atrial septostomy).

Upper Airway Obstruction

Antenatal ultrasound may identify a fetus as having upper airway obstruction due to a combination of a small chin (micrognathia) and cleft palate (Pierre Robin sequence), or occasionally due to a lesion like a cystic hygroma or teratoma. Further antenatal imaging may help (e.g., magnetic resonance imaging) to define the extent of the lesion or identify other lesions (e.g., brain lesions) that may inform the decision whether to proceed with intensive care and/or surgery or to plan for palliative care from birth. Turning the babies with Pierre-Robin sequence prone (onto their front) encourages the jaw to fall forward and may help relieve the airway obstruction that occurs when the tongue slips backward (glossoptosis). Nasal/nasopharyngeal airways (ETT of appropriate ID shortened to about 5 cm or a distance equivalent to the distance from the nose to tragus of the ear) may also help to further relieve obstruction.

The EXIT—*ex utero* intrapartum therapy—procedure describes a multidisciplinary team approach to the delivery of such babies. Anesthesiologists give the mother deep general anesthesia and tocolytics before obstetricians partially deliver the baby through an incision in the uterus. Critically, the cord is not divided and the baby remains on the placental circulation. This gives airway specialists (neonatologists, pediatric anesthesiologists, and otolaryngologists) a limited period of time to attempt to secure an airway, either by directly intubating the baby or by performing a tracheostomy should that prove impossible. It is a resource-intensive intervention that potentially has significant morbidity for the mother. It is not undertaken lightly and not if there is not a reasonable prospect of a good outcome for the baby.

Hypothermia for Neonatal Encephalopathy

Therapeutic hypothermia—reducing core body temperature to 33.5°C for 72 hours—increases the rate of survival free of serious impairment among term infants who are diagnosed with neonatal encephalopathy (see Chapter 49) (82). Many of these babies are in poor condition and are resuscitated at birth. In the randomized human studies, babies had to have cooling initiated within 6 hours of birth. This was based on animal data that showed that the sooner after the brain injury that animals were cooled, the greater the neuroprotective effect and that there was little effect after 6 hours (83). The babies included in trials of cooling were not cooled in the DR and reached their target temperature many hours later. It is not clear what should be done in the DR. Some clinicians advocate turning off radiant heat sources when it becomes clear that therapeutic hypothermia will be required. However, most would currently argue that while keeping babies warm may not be the priority, babies should be kept normothermic until a definite decision to cool is made. Overheating may add to the severity of the neurologic insult and should be avoided.

Surfactant

Preterm infants lack endogenous surfactant; this increases their difficulties in establishing and maintaining lung aeration. Their risk of respiratory distress syndrome (RDS) increases the more prematurely they are born. Exogenous surfactant replacement therapy was a massive leap forward for preterm infants who were intubated for RDS—it increased their survival and reduced the incidence of pneumothorax and intraventricular hemorrhage (84). Early administration of "rescue" surfactant proved preferable to later (85), and practice evolved to where preterm infants were routinely intubated in the DR for "prophylactic" surfactant before a diagnosis of RDS could be established (86). Concerns about the adverse short- and long-term effects of ET ventilation renewed interest in noninvasive respiratory support and studies subsequently demonstrated that starting babies on CPAP and reserving intubation and "rescue" surfactant for those who deteriorate is superior to routine intubation of all infants for "prophylactic" surfactant (86). However, half or more of those who start on CPAP are ultimately intubated for "rescue" surfactant. This led to approaches that aim to minimize the period of intubation with an ETT by immediate

extubation after surfactant is given (87) or by substituting a thin catheter for an ETT for the purpose of surfactant administration (88). The decision clinicians face is when to intervene to give "rescue" surfactant. Some practitioners choose to give it in the DR, while others choose to do so in the NICU at varying thresholds of oxygen requirement (e.g., 25%, 30%, or 40% oxygen). This means that there is a spectrum where "early rescue" blurs into "prophylaxis." Other methods of administration—for example, giving prophylactic oropharyngeal surfactant immediately after birth aiming to have babies aspirate it—are being investigated. A discussion of the relative merits of these approaches is beyond the scope of this chapter; see Chapter 28.

Hydrops Fetalis

This condition is characterized by fluid collections in at least two fetal compartments (e.g., pleural effusions, ascites, skin edema) and is readily diagnosed on antenatal ultrasound. It is now an unusual presentation in high-income countries. Before the widespread introduction of anti-Rhesus D immune globulin, Rhesus isoimmunization (see Chapter 42) was responsible for the majority of cases. Today cases are caused by variety of conditions (e.g., chromosomal abnormalities, cardiac arrhythmias, viral infections). Overall, the prognosis is poor, but highly dependent on the underlying cause. On occasion, breathing and ventilation in the DR may be very difficult due to the presence of large pleural effusions. The standard approach to resuscitation for all babies should be followed. If after intubating the baby and giving PPV with high PIP, ventilation is still compromised, it may be worth draining a pleural effusion. Get a wide bore adult (e.g., 18G green) IV cannula from your friendly anesthesiologist and attach a syringe. Identify the fifth intercostal space (approximately in a vertical plane beneath the nipple when baby is supine), clean it with an antiseptic swab, and insert the needle at right angles to the chest in the midaxillary line. Stop when you feel a change in resistance—that means you have traversed the (usually thickened) chest wall and entered the pleural cavity. You should be able to aspirate clear straw-colored fluid. Advance the plastic catheter and remove the trocar (it is not a good idea to have a sharp object in a body cavity when you cannot see what it might be sticking into). Aspirate the fluid with a syringe or leave it to drain spontaneously into a container. If the baby does not improve, you may consider also draining the effusion on the other side. Even more rarely, if you believe that tense ascites is "splinting" the diaphragm and interfering with lung aeration, you may consider emergency paracentesis—that is, draining fluid from the abdomen. This should only be attempted as a last resort. The same steps are largely the same; pick a spot in the mid flank but first feel for organomegaly before inserting the needle. Remember, a hydropic baby often has an enlarged liver and spleen and may well be coagulopathic. It is relatively easy to stick a large bore needle into an enlarged viscus and cause serious bleeding that is unlikely to help matters.

▌ STOPPING RESUSCITATION EFFORTS

When should unsuccessful resuscitation attempts stop? This is a fraught and difficult question. I believe clinicians should stop when the chances of survival without devastating brain injury are so low that continued resuscitation is futile. In practical terms, this is difficult to determine. Traditionally, it was thought reasonable to stop resuscitation if there was no response after 10 minutes. Reports followed of babies who had no detected HR at 10 minutes who survived in reasonable condition (89). In long-term outcome of the National Institute of Child Health and Human Development Neonatal Research Network cooling study, 20% of term infants with an Apgar of 0 at 10 minutes survived without disability (90). These data include infants who did and did not undergo therapeutic hypothermia.

It is attractive but naïve to think that there is a "correct" time that is appropriate in all cases. These babies are unusual, and the circumstances in which they arise are individual. Many factors should be taken into account. Consider the "pre-event probability" that the baby would survive without severe multiple impairments. The family's wishes are of paramount importance. When serious anomalies have been diagnosed antenatally (e.g., major brain anomaly) and/or the possible need for extensive resuscitation can be anticipated (e.g., delivery of an extremely preterm infant following prolonged preterm rupture of the membranes), the family's views on to what extent resuscitation is appropriate should be sought. A plan should be agreed between clinicians and family before delivery; this is much preferable to a vague understanding that "we will see how they go when they are born." Babies are sometimes born in poor condition unexpectedly, precluding meaningful discussion with the family. In such circumstances, the decisions fall more squarely on the shoulders of clinicians who are called urgently to a situation they know little or nothing about. They must consider other factors. Does the baby have dysmorphic features that suggest a particular diagnosis (e.g., Patau syndrome)? Does a term baby have skin maceration that suggests he/she has been dead for some time before birth? Has this baby received a brief period of mask ventilation by a junior midwife or has he/she received extensive resuscitation by an experienced clinician? It is unusual for babies to be "unresuscitatable" in the DR; many babies who do not have a detectable heart beat for many minutes after birth ultimately respond. Babies who respond can then be admitted to the NICU where they can be further assessed and a discussion about withdrawal of intensive care can occur if and as appropriate. In such situations, many clinicians worry that a baby may now survive with severe multiple impairments and a consequent poor quality of life who may not have otherwise survived, and agonize over whether continuing resuscitation was the correct thing to do.

Several issues arise, principally the certainty with which we can determine that severe brain injury is inevitable, armed only with limited information available within minutes. Many babies who are extensively resuscitated in the DR and are profoundly brain injured will die despite intensive care. Many more die quickly when breathing support is withdrawn. Admitting these babies to the NICU gives more time for the family to adjust to the situation in which they find themselves.

Some babies do not respond despite extensive resuscitation in the DR. Not only is stopping resuscitation appropriate, it is inevitable. This decision should be made, if at all possible, with the most senior responsible clinician present in the DR. My approach (not necessarily the correct one, it is just mine) for an apparently normally formed term baby is to plan to continue resuscitation for 10 minutes after we are certain that the ETT was correctly sited; for us, that is usually after we have intubated or visualized the tube passing through the cords ourselves. In that time, I ensure that the baby gets PPV with sufficiently high pressures through the ETT, good-quality chest compressions, and adrenaline through a UVC. Some clinicians may also want to satisfy themselves that a pneumothorax is not present. While on rare occasions, a pneumothorax may compromise the ventilation of babies in the DR (e.g., babies with pulmonary hypoplasia), in reality, it is not a cause for a normally formed term baby to be "unresuscitatable." A chest x-ray will not be available in a timely fashion. Be reassured by audible breath sounds bilaterally (and perhaps transilluminate the thorax with a cold light source if it is readily available); I personally think thoracocentesis is unnecessary. If there is no detectable HR at that point, I ask colleagues to continue PPV and chest compressions while I explain to the family that their baby has not responded and that we need to stop. In practice, this interval between birth and stopping is highly variable, but usually longer than 10 minutes.

TRAINING

Organized courses in neonatal resuscitation evolved on the back of recognition of increased mortality of babies born at relatively small hospitals where clinicians were thought to lack experience in resuscitation techniques (1). These courses have largely consisted of didactic teaching and practice of technical skills such as mask ventilation, chest compressions, and endotracheal intubation on mannequins. The dissemination of these courses has been phenomenal, with millions of health care providers having attended courses. Basic life support courses have been demonstrated to reduce mortality in infants in low- and middle-income countries (91). Neonatal resuscitation training in developed countries has evolved now to include more elaborate techniques. High-fidelity simulation has seen the introduction of more sophisticated and life-like mannequins and training venues. Using a respiratory function monitor has been shown to reduce leak during mask PPV in mannequins (92). However, it is difficult to quantify the effect of advanced training techniques including simulation on infant outcomes.

Health care providers who attend births should attend a neonatal resuscitation course. They should know the principles and techniques of basic life support of newborns and be familiar with the equipment used at their workplace. They should practice together to understand the teamwork that is essential.

FUTURE DIRECTIONS

Evolution in health care must be underpinned by careful study and research. In the DR care of newborns, animal studies are vitally important for understanding physiology, the effects of different interventions, and identifying and refining potentially beneficial interventions. However, interventions should ideally be tested in RCTs in human infants.

RCTs in the DR present several challenges. A major one is the choice of appropriate outcomes for clinical trials. Clinicians correctly question whether many short-term outcomes measured in the DR—for example, SpO_2 at 5 minutes, intubation—are meaningful. It is attractive to think that a new intervention will make a "life-or-death" difference. In reality, however, DR death is rare in high-income countries. And I think it is implausible that the most common causes of DR death—extreme prematurity, profound asphyxia, congenital anomaly, or perinatal infection—would be influenced to such a degree by any new intervention (e.g., training technique, interface, ventilation device, monitoring device, or dose of adrenaline) that it would be measurable by a change in the rate of DR death in a clinical trial. The "gold standard" for trials enrolling newborn infants is considered survival free of serious impairment on detailed examination at 2 years corrected age or later. A multitude of factors are likely to influence the outcome of a 25-week infant in the 3 months they spend in hospital (if they survive). Without even considering the influences in the 2 years that follow, I think it is fanciful to believe that a 30-second to 5-minute intervention will have a measurable impact on outcome at 2 years. We must continue to struggle to find a balance between identifying measurable short-term outcomes that are clinically meaningful and long-term outcomes that are likely to be influenced by the intervention being studied.

Another major challenge is the consent procedures used to enroll babies in clinical studies. People correctly debate the ethics of enrolling babies in research, when they are unable to give consent for themselves and their parent(s) find themselves in exceptional and stressful circumstances (93). Similar ethical issues are of course faced by research in emergency settings in adults (94). Less often discussed it the ethics of not doing research in babies. Preventing or making it difficult to perform research in babies implicitly says that we can accept a lower standard of proof that treatments are effective and safe for babies than that required for adults. Studying rare events is difficult, even more so when they arise unpredictably and as an emergency, as is often the case in the DR. It is difficult or impossible to follow the normal consent procedure where verbal and written information are given to a potential participant or their next-of-kin, who has time to consider the material, mull it over it for hours or days, ask questions of the researchers, and get back with a decision. Alternative consent mechanisms—including deferred consent and waivers—are sometimes necessary to do studies that enroll representative populations of babies so that we can continue to refine and improve the care they receive in the DR (95). Studies that are carefully designed by researchers in partnership with families and Institutional Review Boards/Ethics Committees are required.

REFERENCES

1. O'Donnell CPF, Gibson AT, Davis PG. Pinching, electrocution, ravens' beaks and positive pressure ventilation: a brief history of neonatal resuscitation. *Arch Dis Child Fetal Neonatal Ed* 2006;91:F369.
2. Apgar V. A proposal for a new method of evaluation of the newborn infant. *Curr Res Anesth Analg* 1953;32:260.
3. Apgar V. The newborn (Apgar) scoring system. Reflections and advice. *Pediatr Clin North Am* 1966;13:645.
4. Dawes GS. *Foetal and neonatal physiology: a comparative study of the changes at birth.* Chicago, IL: Year Book Medical Publishers, Inc., 1968.
5. Kattwinkel J, ed. *Textbook of neonatal resuscitation.* Elk Grove, IL: American Heart Academy/American Academy of Pediatrics, 1987.
6. Richmond S, ed. *Resuscitation at birth: newborn life support provider manual.* London, UK: Resuscitation Council, 2001.
7. Kattwinkel J, Niermeyer S, Nadkarni V, et al. Resuscitation of the newly born infant: an advisory statement from the Pediatric Working Group of the International Liaison Committee on Resuscitation. *Resuscitation* 1999;40:71.
8. Perlman JM, Wyllie J, Kattwinkel J, et al. Part 7: Neonatal resuscitation: international consensus on cardiopulmonary resuscitation and emergency cardiovascular care science with treatment recommendations. *Pediatrics* 2015;136:S120.
9. The Million Death Study Collaborators. Causes of neonatal and child mortality in India: a nationally representative mortality survey. *Lancet* 2010;376:1853.
10. Kluckow M, Hooper SB. Using physiology to guide time to cord clamping. *Semin Fetal Neonatal Med* 2015;20:225.
11. Bhatt S, Alison BJ, Wallace EM, et al. Delaying cord clamping until ventilation onset improves cardiovascular function at birth in preterm lambs. *J Physiol* 2013;591(8):2113.
12. McDonald SJ, Middleton P, Dowswell T, et al. Effect of timing of umbilical cord clamping of term infants on maternal and neonatal outcomes. *Cochrane Database Syst Rev* 2013;(7):CD004074.
13. Rabe H, Diaz-Rossello JL, Duley L, et al. Effect of timing of umbilical cord clamping and other strategies to influence placental transfusion at preterm birth on maternal and infant outcomes. *Cochrane Database Syst Rev* 2012;8:CD003248.
14. Tarnow-Mordi W, Morris J, Kirby A, et al. Delayed versus immediate cord clamping in preterm infants. *N Engl J Med* 2017;377:2445.
15. Fogarty M, Osborn DA, Askie L, et al. Delayed vs. early umbilical cord clamping for preterm infants: a systematic review and meta-analysis. *Am J Obstet Gynecol* 2018;281:1.
16. Duley L, Dorling J, Pushpa-Rajah A. Randomised trial of cord clamping and initial stabilisation at very preterm birth. *Arch Dis Child Fetal Neonatal Ed* 2018;103:F6.
17. Armstrong-Buisseret L, Powers K, Dorling J, et al. Randomised trial of cord clamping at very preterm birth: outcomes at 2 years. *Arch Dis Child Fetal Neonatal Ed* 2020;105(3):292. doi: 10.1136/archdischild-2019-316912
18. Meyer MP, Mildenhall L. Delayed cord clamping and blood flow in the superior vena cava in preterm infants: an observational study. *Arch Dis Child Fetal Neonatal Ed* 2012;97(6):F484.
19. Popat H, Robledo KP, Sebastian L, et al. Effect of delayed cord clamping on systemic blood flow: a randomized controlled trial. *J Pediatr* 2016;178:81.
20. Vesoulis ZA, Liao SM, Mathur AM. Delayed cord clamping is associated with improved dynamic cerebral autoregulation and decreased incidence of intraventricular hemorrhage in preterm infants. *J Appl Physiol (1985)* 2019;127(1):103.
21. Katheria A, Reister F, Essers J, et al. Association of umbilical cord milking vs delayed umbilical cord clamping with death or severe intraventricular hemorrhage among preterm infants. *JAMA* 2019;322:1877.
22. Knol R, Brouwer E, van den Akker T, et al. Physiological-based cord clamping in very preterm infants—randomised controlled trial on effectiveness of stabilisation. *Resuscitation* 2020;147:26.
23. Brouwer E, Knol R, Vermooij ASL, et al. Physiological-based cord clamping in preterm infants using a new purpose-built resuscitation table: a feasibility study. *Arch Dis Child Fetal Neonatal Ed* 2019;104:F396.
24. Stenke E, Kieran EA, McCarthy LK, et al. A randomized trial of placing preterm infants on their back or left side after birth. *Arch Dis Child Fetal Neonatal Ed* 2016;101(5):F397.
25. World Health Organisation. *Thermal protection of the newborn: a practical guide.* Geneva, Switzerland, 1997.
26. Laptook AR, Bell EF, Shankaran S, et al. Admission temperature and associated mortality and morbidity among moderately and extremely preterm infants. *J Pediatr* 2018;192:53.
27. McCall EM, Alderdice F, Halliday HL, et al. Interventions to prevent hypothermia at birth in preterm and/or low birth weight infants. *Cochrane Database Syst Rev* 2018:CD004210. doi: 10.1002/14651858.CD004210.pub5
28. Vohra S, Frent G, Campbell V, et al. Effect of occlusive polyethylene skin wrapping on heat loss in very low birth weight infants at delivery: a randomized trial. *J Pediatr* 1999;134:547.
29. Vohra S, Roberts RS, Zhang B, et al. Heat loss prevention (HeLP) in the delivery room: a randomized controlled trial of polyethylene occlusive skin wrapping in very preterm infants. *J Pediatr* 2004;145:750.
30. Reilly MC, Vohra S, Rac VE, et al. Randomized trial of occlusive wrap for heat loss prevention in preterm infants. *J Pediatr* 2015;166:262.
31. Leadford AE, Warren JB, Manasyan A, et al. Plastic bags for prevention of hypothermia in preterm and low birth weight infants. *Pediatrics* 2013;132:e128.
32. Belsches TC, Tilly AE, Miller TR, et al. Randomized trial of plastic bags to prevent term neonatal hypothermia in a resource-poor setting. *Pediatrics* 2013;132:e656.
33. Bergman NJ, Linley LL, Fawcus SR. Randomized controlled trial of skin-to-skin contact from birth versus conventional incubator for physiological stabilization in 1200 to 2199 gram newborns. *Acta Paediatr* 2004;93:770.
34. McCarthy LK, Molloy EJ, Twomey AR, et al. A randomized trial of exothermic mattresses for preterm infants in polyethylene bags. *Pediatrics* 2013;132:e135.
35. Bhatt DR, Reddy N, Ruiz R, et al. Perinatal quality improvement bundle to decrease hypothermia in extremely low birthweight infants with birth weight less than 1000 g: single-center experience over 6 years. *J Investig Med* 2020;68(7):1256.
36. Kamlin COF, O'Donnell CPF, Everest NJ, et al. Accuracy of clinical assessment of infant heart rate in the delivery room. *Resuscitation* 2006;71:319.
37. Cavallin F, Cori MS, Negash S, et al. Heart rate determination in infants at risk for resuscitation in a low-resource setting: a randomized controlled trial. *J Pediatr* 2020;221:88.
38. Murphy MC, McCarthy LK, O'Donnell CPF. Comparison of infant heart rate assessment by auscultation, ECG and oximetry in the delivery room. *Arch Dis Child Fetal Neonatal Ed* 2018:F490.
39. Katheria A, Arnell K, Brown M, et al. A pilot randomized trial of EKG for neonatal resuscitation. *PLoS One* 2017;12(11):e0187730. doi: 10.1371/journal.pone.0187730
40. Mizumoto H, Tomotaki S, Shibata H, et al. Electrocardiogram shows reliable heart rate much earlier than pulse oximetry during neonatal resuscitation. *Pediatr Int* 2012;54:205.
41. Murphy MC, De Angelis L, McCarthy LK, et al. Randomised study comparing heart rate measurement in newly born infants using a monitor incorporating electrocardiogram and a pulse oximeter versus pulse oximeter alone. *Arch Dis Child Fetal Neonatal Ed* 2019;104:F447.
42. Luong D, Cheung PY, Barrington KJ, et al. Cardiac arrest with pulseless electrical activity rhythm in newborn infants: a case series. *Arch Dis Child Fetal Neonatal Ed* 2019;104:F572.
43. O'Donnell CPF, Kamlin COF, Davis PG, et al. Clinical assessment of infant colour at delivery. *Arch Dis Child Fetal Neonatal Ed* 2007;92:F465.
44. Dawson JA, Kamlin COF, Vento M, et al. Defining the reference range for oxygen saturation for infants after birth. *Pediatrics* 2010;125:e1340.
45. Foster JP, Dawson JA, Davis PG, et al. Routine oro/nasopharyngeal suction versus no suction at birth. *Cochrane Database Syst Rev* 2017;4:CD010332. doi: 10.1002/14651858.CD010332.pub2
46. Vain NE, Szyld EG, Prudent LP, et al. Oropharyngeal and nasopharyngeal suction of meconium-stained neonates before delivery of their shoulders: multicenter, randomized, controlled trial. *Lancet* 2004;364:597.
47. Wiswell TE, Gannon CM, Jacob J, et al. Delivery room management of the apparently vigorous meconium-stained neonate: results of the multicenter, international collaborative trial. *Pediatrics* 2000;105:1.
48. Kamlin COF, Schmölzer GE, Dawson JA, et al. A randomized trial of oropharyngeal airways to assist stabilization of preterm infants in the delivery room. *Resuscitation* 2019;144:104.
49. O'Donnell CPF, Kamlin COF, Davis PG, et al. Crying and breathing by extremely preterm infants immediately after birth. *J Pediatr* 2010;156:846.

50. Murphy MC, McCarthy LK, O'Donnell CPF. Crying and breathing by newborn preterm infants after early or delayed cord clamping. *Arch Dis Child Fetal Neonatal Ed* 2020;105(3):331. doi: 10.1136/archdis-child-2018-316592

51. Pietravalle A, Cavllin F, Opocher A, et al. Neonatal tactile stimulation at birth in a low-resource setting. *BMC Pediatr* 2018;18:306.

52. Van Henten TMA, Dekker J, Te Pas AB, et al. Tactile stimulation in the delivery room: do we practice what we preach? *Arch Dis Child Fetal Neonatal Ed* 2019;104:F661.

53. Dekker J, Hooper SB, Martherus T, et al. Repetitive versus standard tactile stimulation of preterm infants at birth – a randomized controlled trial. *Resuscitation* 2018;127:37.

54. Dawson JA, Schmolzer GM, Kamlin COF, et al. Oxygenation with T-piece versus self-inflating bag for ventilation of extremely preterm infants at birth: a randomized trial. *J Pediatr* 2011;158:912.

55. Szyld E, Aguilar A, Musante GA, et al. Comparison of devices for newborn ventilation in the delivery room. *J Pediatr* 2014;165:243.

56. O'Donnell CPF, Davis PG, Lau R, et al. Neonatal resuscitation 2: an evaluation of manual ventilation devices and face masks. *Arch Dis Child Fetal Neonatal Ed* 2005;90:F392.

57. Wood FE, Morley CJ, Dawson JA, et al. Improved techniques reduce face mask leak during simulated neonatal resuscitation: study 2. *Arch Dis Child Fetal Neonatal Ed* 2008;93:F230.

58. Tracy MB, Klimek J, Coughtrey H, et al. Mask leak in one-person mask ventilation compared to two-person in newborn infant manikin study. *Arch Dis Child Fetal Neonatal Ed* 2011;96:F195.

59. van Vonderen JJ, Kleijn TA, Schilleman K, et al. Compressive force applied to a manikin's head during mask ventilation. *Arch Dis Child Fetal Neonatal Ed* 2012;97:F254.

60. Schmölzer GM, Dawson JA, Kamlin COF, et al. Airway obstruction and gas leak during mask ventilation of preterm infants in the delivery room. *Arch Dis Child Fetal Neonatal Ed* 2011;96:F254.

61. O Currain E, O'Shea JE, McGrory L, et al. Smaller face masks for positive pressure ventilation in preterm infants: a randomised trial. *Resuscitation* 2019;134:94.

62. McCarthy LK, Twomey AR, Molloy EJ, et al. A randomized trial of nasal prong or face mask for respiratory support for preterm newborns. *Pediatrics* 2013;132:e389.

63. Kamlin COF, Schilleman K, Dawson JA, et al. Mask versus nasal tube for stabilization of preterm infants at birth: a randomized controlled trial. *Pediatrics* 2013;132:e381.

64. Kamlin COF, O'Connell LA, Morley CJ, et al. A randomized trial of stylets for intubating newborn infants. *Pediatrics* 2013;131:e198.

65. Flinn A, Travers C, Laffan EE, et al. A randomized trial of estimating neonatal endotracheal tube insertion depth using weight or gestation. *Neonatology* 2015;107:167.

66. Gill I, Stafford A, Murphy MC, et al. Randomised trial of estimating oral endotracheal tube insertion depth in newborns using weight or vocal cord guide. *Arch Dis Child Fetal Neonatal Ed* 2018;103:F312.

67. Murphy MC, Donoghue VB, O'Donnell CPF. Randomised trial of estimating oral endotracheal tube insertion depth in newborns using suprasternal palpation of the tip or weight. *Arch Dis Child Fetal Neonatal Ed* 2020;105:196.

68. Tracy MB, Priyadarshi A, Goel D, et al. How do different brands of size 1 laryngeal mask airway compare with face mask ventilation in a dedicated laryngeal mask airway teaching manikin? *Arch Dis Child Fetal Neonatal Ed* 2018;103:271.

69. Pejovic NJ, Trevisanuto D, Lubulwa C, et al. Neonatal resuscitation using a laryngeal mask airway: a randomised trial in Uganda. *Arch Dis Child* 2018;103:255.

70. Welsford M, Nishiyama C, Shortt C, et al. Room air for initiating term newborn resuscitation: a systematic review with meta-analysis. *Pediatrics* 2019;143:pii: e20181825. doi: 10.1542/peds.2018-1825

71. Oei JL, Saugstad OD, Lui K, et al. Targeted oxygen in the resuscitation of preterm infants, a randomized clinical trial. *Pediatrics* 2017;139:e20161452.

72. Welsford M, Nishiyama C, Shortt C, et al. Initial oxygen use for preterm newborn resuscitation: a systematic review with meta-analysis. *Pediatrics* 2019;143(1). pii: e20181828. doi: 10.1542/peds.2018-1828

73. Vento M, Moro M, Escrig R, et al. Preterm resuscitation with low oxygen causes less oxidative stress, inflammation, and chronic lung disease. *Pediatrics* 2009;124(3):e439.

74. McGrory L, Owen LS, Thio M, et al. A randomized trial of conditioned or unconditioned gases for stabilization of preterm infants at birth. *J Pediatr* 2018;193:47.

75. Bruschettini M, O'Donnell CPF, Davis PG, et al. Sustained versus standard inflations during neonatal resuscitation to prevent mortality and improve respiratory outcomes. *Cochrane Database Syst Rev* 2017:CD004953. doi: 10.1002/14651858.CD004953.pub

76. Kirpalani H, Ratcliffe SJ, Keszler M, et al. Effects of sustained inflation vs intermittent positive pressure ventilation on bronchopulmonary dysplasia or death among extremely preterm infants: the SAIL randomized clinical trial. *JAMA* 2019;321:1165.

77. Manley BJ, Owen LS, Doyle LW, et al. High-flow nasal cannulae after extubation in very preterm infants. *N Engl J Med* 2013;369:1423.

78. Roberts CT, Owen LS, Manley BJ, et al. Nasal high-flow therapy for primary respiratory support in preterm infants. *N Engl J Med* 2016;375:1142.

79. Reynolds P, Leontiadi S, Lawson T, et al. Stabilisation of premature infants in the delivery room with nasal high flow. *Arch Dis Child Fetal Neonatal Ed* 2016;101:F284.

80. Wyckoff MH, Perlman JM, Laptook AR. Use of volume expansion in delivery room resuscitation of term and near-term infants. *Pediatrics* 2005;115:950.

81. Christman C, Hemway RJ, Wykcoff MH, et al. The two-thumb is superior to the two-finger method for administering chest compressions in a manikin model of neonatal resuscitation. *Arch Dis Child Fetal Neonatal Ed* 2011;96:F99.

82. Jacobs SE, Berg M, Hunt RW, et al. Cooling for newborns with hypoxic ischaemic encephalopathy. *Cochrane Database Syst Rev* 2013;(1):CD003311. doi: 10.1002/14651858.CD003311.pub3

83. Roelfsema V, Bennet L, George S, et al. Window of opportunity of cerebral hypothermia for postischemic white matter injury in the near-term fetal sheep. *J Cereb Blood Flow Metab* 2004;24:877.

84. Seger N, Soll R. Animal derived surfactant extract for treatment of respiratory distress syndrome. *Cochrane Database Syst Rev* 2009;(2):CD007836. doi: 10.1002/14651858.CD007836

85. Bahadue FL, Soll R. Early versus delayed selective surfactant treatment for neonatal respiratory distress syndrome. *Cochrane Database Syst Rev* 2012;11:CD001456. doi: 10.1002/14651858.CD001456.pub2

86. Soll RF, Morley CJ. Prophylactic versus selective use of surfactant in preventing morbidity and mortality in preterm infants. *Cochrane Database Syst Rev* 2012;(3):CD000510.

87. Blennow M, Bohlin K. Surfactant and non-invasive ventilation. *Neonatology* 2015;107:330.

88. More K, Sakhuja P, Shah PS. Minimally invasive surfactant administration in preterm infants: a meta-narrative review. *JAMA Pediatr* 2014;168:901.

89. Kasdorf E, Laptook A, Azzopardi D, et al. Improving infant outcome with a 10 min Apgar of 0. *Arch Dis Child Fetal Neonatal Ed* 2015;100(2):F102.

90. Natarajan G, Shankaran S, Laptook AR, et al.; Extended Hypothermia Subcommittee of the Eunice Kennedy Shriver National Institute of Child Health and Human Development Neonatal Research Network. Apgar scores at 10 min and outcomes at 6-7 years following hypoxic-ischaemic encephalopathy. *Arch Dis Child Fetal Neonatal Ed* 2013;98(6):F473.

91. Dempsey EM, Pammi M, Ryan AC, et al. Standardised formal resuscitation training programmes for reducing mortality and morbidity in newborn infants. *Cochrane Database Syst Rev* 2015;(9):CD009106. doi: 10.1002/14651858.CD009106.pub2

92. O Currain E, Thio M, Dawson JA, et al. Respiratory monitors to teach newborn facemask ventilation: a randomised trial. *Arch Dis Child Fetal Neonatal Ed* 2019;104:582.

93. Megone C, Wilman E, Oliver S, et al. The ethical issues regarding consent to clinical trials with pre-term or sick neonates: a systematic review (framework synthesis) of the analytical (theoretical/philosophical) research. *Trials* 2016;17(1):443.

94. Morrison CA, Horwitz IB, Carrick MM. Ethical and legal issues in emergency research: barriers to conducting prospective randomized trials in an emergency setting. *J Surg Res* 2009;157(1):115.

95. Rich WD, Katheria AC. Waived consent in perinatal/neonatal research-when is it appropriate? *Front Pediatr* 2019;7:493.

17 Physical Assessment and Classification

Leigh E. Dyet and Rose Crowley

INTRODUCTION

The essential skill that is fundamental to any examination of the newborn infant is observation. So much can be gained by observing the infant's color, activity, movements, and behavior. This in no way detracts from the importance of a complete systematic examination, but it guides the examiner toward pathology and to taking a methodical approach in assessing it and making an accurate diagnosis.

The approach to clinical examination of a young infant needs to be flexible. During a quiet moment, the opportunity needs to be taken to listen to the heart sounds or auscultate the chest. Similarly, during an awake, active period, simple observation may yield a plethora of information regarding the neurologic status of the infant. Inspection, palpation, percussion, and auscultation are important tools for clinical examination, and the neonatal examination is no exception.

Physical assessment in neonates serves to determine anatomic normality, but it may be challenging to determine which findings are transient, which are variations of normal, and which are markers of major malformations or syndromes. For example, in extremely premature infants with Down syndrome, the typical features may be difficult to identify at birth but with further growth and maturation they become clearly detectable.

There is considerable overlap between normal processes associated with physiologic changes occurring during the postnatal transition period and those of pathologic states. Once the examiner has determined that findings represent a disease process, it is necessary to decide just how ill the infant is or is likely to become. To that end, a number of acuity of illness scores have been developed that range from the very simple to complex systems that include physiologic monitoring and laboratory values (1–3). The primary advantage of such scoring systems is in forcing a systematic and quantitative assessment that can be compared among observers and over time. The first neonatal examination occurs immediately after birth in the assigning of Apgar scores at 1 and 5 minutes of age and every 5 minutes thereafter until the total is above 7. Scoring is based on assigning values of 0, 1, or 2 for observations of color, heart rate, respiratory effort, tone, and muscle activity. At this time, priority should be given to determination of sex and identification of any major abnormalities. If there are no initial concerns, a more thorough examination should be completed within the first 24 hours, after initial transition, and a formal newborn and infant physical examination (NIPE) should be completed before 72 hours of age (4). This assessment particularly includes the following:

- Eyes to rule out cataracts
- Hips for instability
- Heart sounds and presence of a murmur to identify congenital heart disease
- Descent of testes in boys

Any review in the newborn period should always consider skin and sclera color for hyperbilirubinemia and this should be measured formally if there is any evidence of jaundice, as subjective assessment of its severity is very inaccurate (5).

The following is a discussion of the steps for assessing the newborn infant and interpreting some of the findings.

NEWBORN HISTORY

Unless an infant is critically ill, the newborn examination should be preceded by a review of the maternal history to identify details that may raise the index of suspicion for certain conditions. Some of these are outlined below.

Important elements of the maternal history include the following:

- Age, gravidity, parity, premature births/outcomes, prior fetal losses, and fertility issues
- Illnesses before/during pregnancy, family history, consanguinity, extent of prenatal care
- Drug, alcohol, and tobacco use; medications used whether prescription or not
- Prenatal testing and screening, especially for hepatitis, human immunodeficiency virus (HIV), syphilis, and group B streptococcus; and any concerns raised about fetal development or well-being from ultrasound scans
- Labor: duration, assessments of fetal health, medications administered, mode of delivery
- Social information, educational level, employment or vocation, and ethnic or racial background

EXAMINATION OF THE PLACENTA AND CORD

Examination of the cord and the placenta is an important part of the newborn assessment, especially in an infant who is acutely unwell. This is covered in more detail in Chapter 12.

The umbilical cord is assessed for appearance, length and diameter, number of vessels, and insertion site. The cord is a uniform ivory, ranging in length from 30 to 100 cm; a shorter cord suggests decreased fetal movement and a reason for fetal distress, failed descent, or avulsion. Deep green staining of the cord is a sign of prior fetal distress reflecting the passage of meconium at least several hours prior to delivery. Superficial staining reflects very recent passage of meconium. Longer cords are more likely to result in fetal entanglement or prolapse. At term, the cord diameter is an average of 1.5 cm and is relatively uniform throughout its length, without strictures. If the base of the umbilical cord itself is especially broad or remains fluctuant after vascular pulsations have stopped, there may be a herniation of abdominal contents into the cord representing an exomphalos.

At birth, the presence of two arteries and a single vein should be identified. Single umbilical arteries occur in approximately 1% of pregnancies, with nearly 10% of identified cases having another congenital malformation. A thin cord with a paucity of Wharton jelly is present in neonates with intrauterine growth restriction (IUGR) and may be compressed more easily by fetal parts. The cord should be examined over its entire length for the presence of true or false knots (**Fig. 17.1A and B**). Umbilical cord blood sampling is essential if there are concerns about intrapartum hypoxia–ischemia, hemolytic disease of the newborn, or fetal anemia from another cause.

Several features of the placenta can be readily assessed on gross examination at the time of delivery. There should be a uniform thickness and density throughout. Depressions and adherent clots

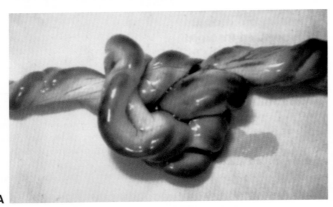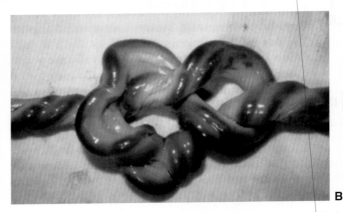

FIGURE 17.1   A and B: True and false knots in the umbilical cord. (Reprinted with permission from Fletcher MA. *Physical diagnosis in the neonatology.* Philadelphia, PA: Lippincott-Raven Publishers, 1998:74.)

or changes in firmness on the maternal surface suggest abruption or infarction. The normal placenta has only a slight odor of fresh blood.

The color of the fetal surface changes with gestational age (GA), but pallor or plethora suggests abnormalities in fetal blood volume or hemoglobin level. Elevated bilirubin in the amniotic fluid stains the placenta bright yellow. Both old blood and meconium will discolor the fetal surface greenish-brown. If either meconium passage or bleeding occurred more than 1 day prior to delivery, it can be difficult to differentiate the two by gross examination.

The fetal surface should be examined for cloudiness of fetal membranes, which suggests an inflammatory reaction but not necessarily due to infection. Nodules on the fetal surface of the amnion (amnion nodosum) indicate prolonged, extreme oligohydramnios. The nodules are usually only a few millimeters in diameter and are slightly raised round or oval plaques that have a shiny surface and leave a depression when picked off (Fig. 17.2). Fetal pulmonary hypoplasia is highly probable in this setting and is a key finding in renal agenesis.

In multiple gestations with a single placenta, the dividing membranes should be assessed; however, it can be very difficult to differentiate monochorionic from dichorionic twins even with careful examination. See Chapter 11 for assessment of multiple gestation.

There are a number of clinical situations in which gross and microscopic examination by a pathologist may offer additional important diagnostic information. There are a number of textbooks that provide a thorough discussion of the abnormalities that can be found (6).

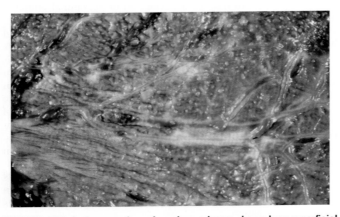

FIGURE 17.2   A close-up view of amnion nodosum shows how superficial and variably sized the nodules are. Any infant born with this finding would have marked compression facies and probably severe pulmonary hypoplasia. Renal agenesis is the most common reason for severe oligohydramnios. (Reprinted with permission from Fletcher MA. *Physical diagnosis in the neonatology.* Philadelphia, PA: Lippincott-Raven Publishers, 1998:83.)

GESTATIONAL AGE ASSESSMENT

Determination of GA and birth weight is required both for determining normalcy and for accurate reporting of health statistics. First-trimester ultrasonography has improved the accuracy of pregnancy dating, and studies have been published showing increased accuracy of estimating GA at a later stage in pregnancy (7); however, if there has been little prenatal care, physical assessment remains the primary method for estimating GA.

GA is noted in completed weeks after the onset of the last menstrual period (LMP). Accurate determination is critical for discussing outcomes for a given infant based on the appropriate comparative group. GA should never be *rounded up*, so an infant born at 24 weeks and 6 days is classified as 24, not 25 weeks of GA. Postdates is an obstetric term meaning a pregnancy that has continued to any time after the expected date of delivery but is not necessarily postterm, defined as 42 weeks' gestation and beyond.

Assessment Techniques

There have been a number of standardized examinations used to estimate GA (7–10) with the Ballard score (11) probably being the most frequently used. As the GA of preterm infants surviving has gradually fallen any method for its estimation now has to include infants born at extreme prematurity and extremely low birth weight (ELBW). The New Ballard Score (NBS) (12) included larger numbers of infants born between 20 and 26 weeks in the study cohort (Fig. 17.3). However, subsequent studies have found that the NBS overestimates the GA of infants born at less than 28 weeks (13) and SGA infants (14). For this reason, maternal LMP and early ultrasound remain the gold standard for determining GA, especially at the edge of viability when plans for care may be informed by best estimates of GA (see also Chapters 7 and 16). In their absence, the NBS remains the best method available to estimate GA, accepting that it may be influenced by additional factors such as:

* Maternal medications or drugs
* Position *in utero*
* Sleep state
* Significant hypertonia or hypotonia

Finally, examination as soon as possible after initial stabilization or by 12 hours of postnatal life increases the accuracy of assessment in gestations shorter than 28 weeks (12).

Neuromuscular Maturity

Tone increases in a caudocephalad direction to a pattern of full flexion at term. To properly assess tone, the infant must be in an unrestrained resting state.

The square window is assessed by flexing the wrist and measuring the minimal angle between the palm and flexor surface

Neuromuscular Maturity

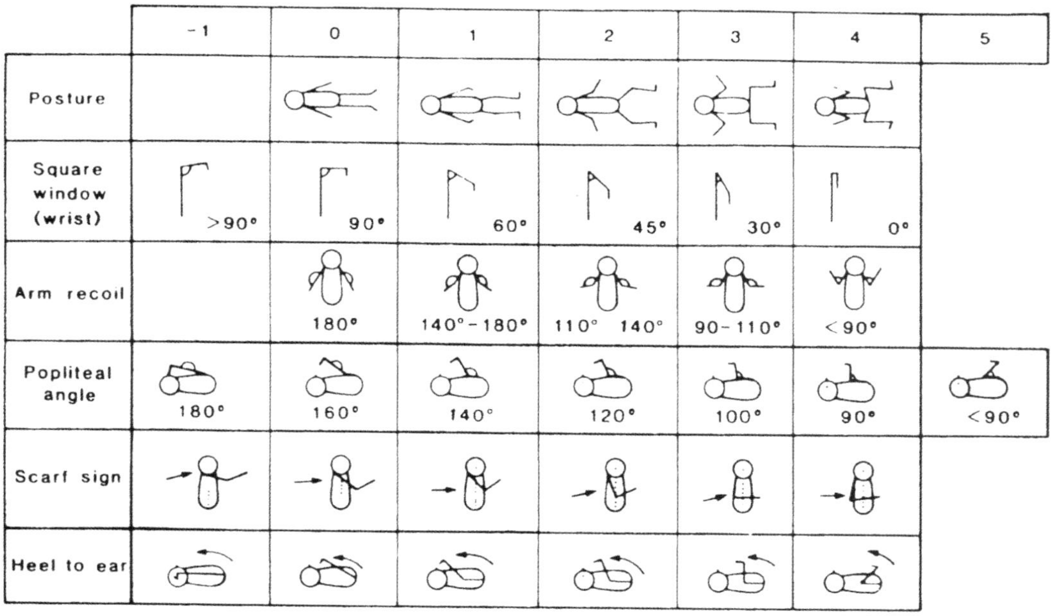

	−1	0	1	2	3	4	5
Posture							
Square window (wrist)	>90°	90°	60°	45°	30°	0°	
Arm recoil		180°	140°−180°	110° 140°	90−110°	<90°	
Popliteal angle	180°	160°	140°	120°	100°	90°	<90°
Scarf sign							
Heel to ear							

Physical Maturity

Skin	sticky friable transparent	gelatinous red, translucent	smooth pink, visible veins	superficial peeling &/or rash. few veins	cracking pale areas rare veins	parchment deep cracking no vessels	leathery cracked wrinkled
Lanugo	none	sparse	abundant	thinning	bald areas	mostly bald	
Plantar surface	heel−toe 40−50 mm: −1 <40 mm: −2	>50 mm no crease	faint red marks	anterior transverse crease only	creases anterior 2/3	creases over entire sole	
Breast	imperceptible	barely perceptible	flat areola no bud	stippled areola 1−2 mm bud	raised areola 3—4 mm bud	full areola 5−10 mm bud	
Eye/ear	lids fused loosely:−1 tightly:−2	lids open pinna flat stays folded	slightly curved pinna; soft; slow recoil	well−curved pinna; soft but ready recoil	formed & firm instant recoil	thick cartilage ear stiff	
Genitals, male	scrotum flat, smooth	scrotum empty faint rugae	testes in upper canal rare rugae	testes descending few rugae	testes down good rugae	testes pendulous deep rugae	
Genitals, female	clitoris prominent labia flat	prominent clitoris small labia minora	prominent clitoris enlarging minora	majora & minora equally prominent	majora large minora small	majora covers clitoris & minora	

Maturity Rating

Score	Weeks
−10	20
−5	22
0	24
5	26
10	28
15	30
20	32
25	34
30	36
35	38
40	40
45	42
50	44

CARE AROUND BIRTH

FIGURE 17.3 Assessment of maturity by the expanded Ballard score. (Reprinted from Donovan EF, Tyson JE, Ehrenkranz RA, et al. Inaccuracy of Ballard scores before 28 weeks' gestation. *J Pediatr* 1998;135:147. Copyright © 1999 Elsevier, with permission.)

of the forearm. With advancing GA, this angle decreases, and it is worthwhile noting that this progression proceeds at a slower rate *ex utero* than if the fetus had continued to develop undisturbed.

The scarf sign, indicative of shoulder and superior axial tone, is assessed by moving the arm across the chest to encircle the neck as a scarf and observing the position of the elbow in relation to the midline. Factors that may lead to increased GA score by limiting mobility include marked obesity, chest wall edema, and shoulder girdle hypertonicity, while conditions causing generalized hypotonia have the opposite effect.

Arm recoil is assessed by placing the infant supine with the arm fully flexed at the elbow. After holding this position for a few seconds, the forearm is fully extended and then released. The degree to which the arm returns to a flexed state is noted. Similar to the scarf sign, conditions affecting muscle tone can have significant impact on this score.

To determine the popliteal angle, the hips are flexed, and the thighs brought up *alongside* the abdomen. While keeping the pelvis flat, the knee is then extended as far as possible to estimate the popliteal angle. Frank breech positioning *in utero* may yield a greater angle than expected for a particular GA.

In contrast to the above test, in the heel-to-ear maneuver, the legs are held together *over* the abdomen and pressed as far as possible toward the ears without lifting the pelvis from the table. The angle made by an arc from the back of the heel to the table decreases with maturity.

Physical Maturity

Skin varies from nearly transparent in the premature infant to opaque with cracking in the postmature newborn.

Lanugo is the fine light-colored hair that is evenly distributed over the body, which first appears at 19 to 20 weeks of GA and becomes maximally apparent at 27 to 28 weeks. After this time, lanugo begins shedding from areas of greatest contact. It is distinct from dark body hair seen in infants of medium to dark complexion.

Assessment of the plantar surface of the foot includes measuring the foot because its length reliably corresponds to early GA (15). With normal muscle activity and uterine compression, creases develop in the sole, progressing from the toes toward the heel. Neuromotor impairments affecting the lower extremities may lead to decreased and/or deep vertical sole creasing, while the opposite can be seen in the presence of oligohydramnios.

The breast develops with an increase in color, stippling of the areola, and increase in the volume of the breast tissue. Volume may be affected by the nutritional state of the fetus and is less consistent with advancing GA than is areolar development, which is, therefore, a better measure of maturity.

With advancing GA, the number of ear folds and firmness of the ear cartilage increases. Extrinsic pressure may impair this process and yield a lower score than expected for a particular GA. Unfusing of the eyelids may begin as early as 22 weeks, with complete unfusing by 28 weeks at the latest (12).

The progression of the testes into the scrotum is a reliable marker of GA. The testes are high in the scrotum at 36 weeks and fully descended by 40 weeks. The presence of a mature scrotal sac (pendulous, rugose) indicates that testicular descent has occurred even if the sac is empty at the time of birth, as may occur due to an *in utero* vascular compromise late in gestation.

Much like the breast volume, the labia majora may appear underdeveloped in the setting of poor *in utero* nutrition. The clitoris, however, approaches term size well before 38 weeks and thus appears disproportionately large in premature females (16). The appearance of a pigmented vertical line, the linea nigra, originating above the pubis, directed toward the umbilicus suggests a GA of at least 36 weeks.

▌ GROWTH

Measurement Techniques

Weight classification coupled with GA helps to determine levels of risk for neonatal and long-term morbidity and mortality. Weights are classified as low birth weight (LBW) if less than 2,500 g; very LBW if less than 1,500 g, and ELBW if less than 1,000 g.

Crown–heel length is most subject to variability and may require repeat measurements if not congruent with weight or head circumference. Proper positioning involves full extension of the supine infant with the top of the head and bottom of the feet both at 90-degree angles to the horizontal. Anomalies of the lower extremities make accurate measurement of crown–heel length impossible; however, the crown–rump measurement may still be feasible. Crown–rump length is measured with the infant supine and the hips flexed 90 degrees. Infants with congenital restricted stature syndromes, for example, achondroplasia, may be classified as those with a short trunk, short legs, or both. These subtypes can be readily differentiated by the crown–rump to total length ratio. From 27 to 41 weeks of gestation, the value is fairly consistent at 0.665 ± 0.027 (17). Proportional reductions in length of the

upper and lower body yield a normal ratio. The ratio is increased if the legs are shortened to a greater degree and decreased if the trunk is foreshortened. Standards for separate lengths of the upper and lower limbs as well as circumferential measurement standards have recently been published (18).

The occipital–frontal head circumference (OFC) is the largest dimension around the head obtained with a tape measure placed snugly above the ears. Head circumference undergoes a marked increase during the last trimester, averaging 25 cm at 28 weeks and 35 cm at term (19). The average head circumference is 0.5 cm greater in male, compared with female, neonates (20). Due to greater reliability of repeated measurements, paper rather than reusable cloth tape measures should be used (21). Molding seen after prolonged breech positioning can lead to an OFC measurement that is as much as 2 cm higher than it will be after molding resolves.

If the OFC differs from length by more than one quartile, the cause should be sought because head size in part reflects brain growth. The most frequent reason for a head percentile to exceed that of length is familial and typically demonstrates a pattern of following a persistently higher but consistent growth curve through childhood. By contrast, pathologic macrocephaly tends to cross to higher percentile curves as it progresses. A decreased rate of head growth, manifested by a flat curve or by dropping to a lower percentile, may indicate poor brain growth, atrophy, or premature suture fusion (craniosynostosis [CS]).

Interpretation of Growth Parameters

Interpretation of growth parameters requires plotting the measurements on percentile charts based on data from a similar population. If birth weight falls between the 10th and 90th percentiles for a given GA, the infant is appropriate for gestational age (AGA); if less than the 10th percentile, the infant is small for gestational age (SGA); and if above the 90th percentile, the infant is large for gestational age (LGA). Some literature cites the 3rd and 97th percentiles as outer limits, but for most clinical purposes, this broader range may under select some at-risk infants, particularly in the lower weight range. AGA infants born at term are at lowest risk for problems associated with neonatal mortality and morbidity.

Infants are considered symmetric if the three parameters of weight, length, and head circumference fall within 25 percentile points of each other. The infant is asymmetric if the parameters are on different curves more than 25 percentile points apart, usually with the weight on a curve lower than those of the head circumference or length. If an infant has either a slowing of intrauterine growth rate documented by serial fetal sonography or a presumed slowing by very low weight for length measurements, he or she is classified as having fetal growth restriction (FGR). All infants who fall below the 10th percentile for weight are SGA; this may or may not result from FGR (19). Infants above the 10th percentile are AGA but may have FGR, such as the infant who demonstrates a deceleration in growth from the 50th to the 20th percentile during the last trimester due to maternal hypertension. A full-term newborn who has suffered FGR and is SGA secondary to neonatal thyrotoxicosis is shown in **Figure 17.4**. Newborns with this condition are also at increased risk of premature fusion of the cranial sutures.

Infants who are SGA, FGR, or LGA are at risk for perinatal and long-term problems.

Problems encountered by LGA infants include the following:

- Iatrogenic prematurity due to overestimation of GA based upon size *in utero*
- Increased requirement for delivery by cesarean section
- Pulmonary hypertension
- Shoulder dystocia
- Birth injuries (brachial plexus, fractures, cephalohematoma)
- Ecchymoses with increased risk of hyperbilirubinemia from RBC degradation

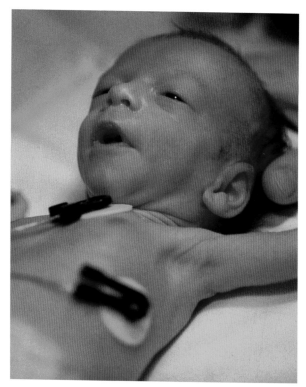

FIGURE 17.4 A full-term SGA newborn with thyrotoxicosis. Premature fusion of the cranial sutures was not detected at birth but presented in early infancy.

- Increased risk of cyanotic heart disease particularly transposition of the great vessels
- The complications associated with poorly controlled maternal diabetes or maternal obesity, including hypoglycemia
- Local fat necrosis associated with instrumented delivery
- Polycythemia with hyperviscosity syndrome
- Seizures
- Renal vein thrombosis
- Increased total blood volume
- Poor feeding

Problems encountered by SGA/FGR infants include the following:

- Prematurity
- Perinatal asphyxia
- Impaired thermoregulation
- Hypoglycemia
- Hypocalcemia
- Polycythemia
- Impaired immune function
- Pulmonary hypertension
- Meconium aspiration
- Necrotizing enterocolitis

EXAMINATION

Examination Conditions

A routine neonatal examination, normally 5 to 10 minutes in duration, should take place in a quiet, warm environment. Lighting should be such that skin markings and color are visible and may require dimming in order to encourage eye opening. If an infant is ill, the examination should focus on those findings that are important for determining the course of management, with a comprehensive exam being deferred until the clinical condition is more stable.

Performing the examination in the presence of one or both parents offers an opportunity to explain any relevant findings and answer any questions they may have.

General Assessment

The specifics of neonatal examination are discussed in the following sections. Some systems that are discussed in more detail in other chapters are given less emphasis in this chapter than they would merit in an actual examination.

Inspection

Inspection begins from a sufficient distance to visualize the infant as a whole. An immediate assessment of wellness can come from simply noting the state, color, respiratory effort, posture, and spontaneous activity. Even simple observations of spontaneous movement patterns can suggest future neurologic deficits or well-being (22).

State

Important indicators of infant well-being are the states or levels of arousal that the infant achieves throughout the examination, and the day, as described by the parents or nursing staff. One categorization of states listed here was originally defined by Prechtl and Beintema (23); modifications have been made but are not clinically important for general assessments (24–29):

- Deep sleep
- Light sleep
- Awake, light peripheral movements
- Awake, large movements, not crying
- Awake, crying

During examination, a healthy infant should demonstrate several levels of arousal. Examination conditions are optimal during light sleep and quiet awake; this is often found approximately two-thirds of the way between feeds when the baby has not just fed and is not yet hungry. It is therefore important to know the feeding history. Portions of the examination requiring a cooperative infant, such as auscultation, are best done during sleep and quiet awake states, while components of the examination that require manipulation of the infant are better left until the end.

Newborns spend nearly two-thirds of each day in sleep (30). Each 24-hour period involves cycling between periods of active sleep (AS) and quiet sleep (QS) with stress shifting the balance toward AS (30). These periods are also known as rapid eye movement (REM) and non-REM sleep, respectively. During AS, infants demonstrate phasic limb movements, eye movements, and irregular respirations. Breathing is typically rapid and shallow, interspersed with periods of more regular respiration (31). In comparison, QS is characterized by regular respirations and the absence of eye and limb movements. As GA increases, the proportion of time spent in QS increases (32).

Unstimulated crying is normally limited in the first 24 hours and should resolve with gentle touch or talking. Excessive crying that requires more than routine consoling, particularly if there are no intervals of quiet alert state, indicates abnormal irritability, but other causes include an appropriate response to pain or to a cold environment (33,34).

Color

Color assessment includes judging perfusion and skin color for the presence of cyanosis, jaundice, pallor, plethora, or any unusual pigmentation (Fig. 17.5). It is important to distinguish cyanosis from the effects of a tight nuchal cord as this may cause facial duskiness and petechiae (35). These can be distinguished by checking the color of the lips and tongue and not relying on the color of the skin.

Respiratory Effort

The examiner can observe the respiratory rate, depth of excursions, use of accessory muscles with retractions or nasal flare, any sounds

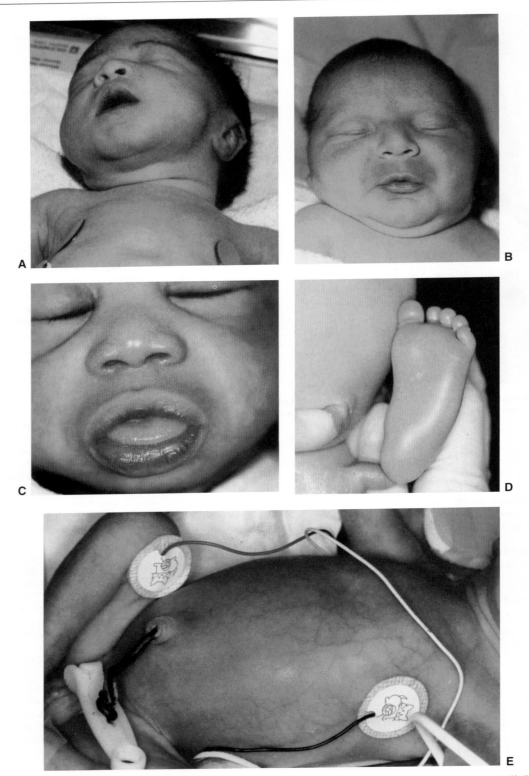

FIGURE 17.5 Cyanosis. A: Generalized cyanosis due to total anomalous pulmonary venous return with an oxygen saturation level of 80%. **B:** Perioral cyanosis. The mucous membranes and area over the chest remain *pink* in the presence of mild cyanosis above the lips. Petechiae make the forehead area appear *blue*. **C:** Lips appear *blue* from normal pigment deposition in vermilion border, but the mucous membranes are *pink*. **D:** Acrocyanosis in the first half hour of life in a 32-week infant. **E:** Cyanosis localized to the abdominal wall. The *blue* color is caused by meconium peritonitis after an intrauterine bowel perforation. If peritoneal meconium is of long enough standing, an abdominal x-ray would show calcifications.

during the respiratory cycle (e.g., grunting or wheezing), and crying pattern. Understanding the infant's pattern of respiratory effort can suggest a specific illness and direct the examination. As the severity of a condition increases, these distinctions may be lost.

Posture

Normal resting posture for GA is determined first (Fig. 17.3). While observing neck position, the examiner looks for symmetry between the sides and compares the upper and lower extremities. If there is lateral asymmetry and the head is turned to one side, there may be an asymmetric tonic neck reflex with the extremities on the mental side in extension and those on the occipital side in flexion. In this case, the head should be turned to the opposite side to verify that the asymmetry reverses. The most common cause of a fixed position of the neck is congenital torticollis, due to unilateral shortening of the sternocleidomastoid muscle (36).

Spontaneous Activity

During light sleep and awake states, the infant should stretch, move all extremities equally, open and close hands, root and start sucking when something touches his or her face, and yawn with facial expression. If the infant lies quietly and moves only in response to stimulation, then this is a more concerning situation.

Premature infants spend more time sleeping but should have spontaneous activity and resting postures appropriate for their GA. It is critical that this inspection is done prior to handling as premature infants may stress quickly and activity levels decline in response.

Vital Signs

Temperature

It is unusual for neonates to develop fever except in response to increased environmental temperature. If an infant's skin temperature is above 38°C and remains elevated after the environmental temperature is lowered, then evaluation for infectious or neurologic causes is indicated. Hypothermia or temperature instability can also be a sign of sepsis in neonates and also requires additional evaluation (37).

In a warm environment, over bundling may cause temperature elevation into the febrile range (38). In the absence of neuromuscular impairment, the infant's postural response to hyperthermia is arm and leg extension, decreased spontaneous activity, and increased sleep duration in order to maximally dissipate heat (39). Conversely, hypothermic infants assume a flexed posture to conserve heat.

Term infants in the first day of life perspire in response to overheating but not as efficiently as a child or adult (40). Infants less than 36 weeks, in comparison, are incapable of perspiring on the first day but do so by 2 weeks of age (41). Furthermore, the minimal temperature required to induce sweating is higher in preterm than in term infants. Perspiration first appears on the forehead, with recruitment of other sites proceeding in a caudal direction. Visible sweating at rest or on feeding in an afebrile infant is abnormal and may indicate distress, typically from cardiac disease.

Respiratory Rate and Heart Rate

The respiratory rate is obtained by observing the movement of the upper abdomen for a full minute. As soon as an infant is touched, the respiratory rate and depth change. The normal respiratory rate is 30 to 60 per minute in a term infant, but during the first day of life, intermittent tachypnea may be noted in some otherwise normal infants. These infants are able to feed well despite these episodes.

The heart rate is 110 to 160 beats per minute (bpm) in healthy term infants, but it may vary significantly during deep sleep or active awake states. Preterm infants have resting heart rates at the higher end of the normal range. Tachycardia, with a rate persistently greater than 160 bpm, may be a sign of many conditions, including central nervous system (CNS) irritability, congestive heart failure, sepsis, anemia, fever, or hyperthyroidism. Conversely, low resting heart rates may be observed following mild perinatal asphyxia.

Blood Pressure

Measuring blood pressure is not routine in most normal newborn nurseries but is used for infants requiring special care and for screening for coarctation of the aorta. There are wide variations of normal blood pressure at different GAs (42–44), and any values consistent with hypertension require three repeated measurements to confirm the abnormality (45).

The range of normal blood pressure in neonates depends on the method used for assessment and GA. Blood pressure is best obtained with the infant in a quiet state, using a cuff with a length covering at least 80% of the arm circumference (45). Noninvasive measurements tend to be higher in more preterm infants and lower in larger infants than those registered by direct intravascular methods (46,47). If the arm blood pressure is elevated or if there is any suspicion antenatally or postnatally of coarctation of the aorta, then the blood pressure should be measured in all four limbs.

Overall Facial Appearance

Overall inspection of the face includes looking for the symmetry, size, shape, and relations of all parts of the face and how the infant holds or uses them. Closer analysis of a seemingly unusual facial appearance can help determine if the constellation represents malformation, deformation, a syndrome, or merely familial appearance. Key features to note when assessing for possible dysmorphic facies include:

- Eyes: size and angle of palpebral fissures, presence of epicanthic folds and hypo- or hypertelorism (abnormally narrowly or widely spaced eyes). Typically, the distance between the medial canthi is approximately equal to the length of the palpebral fissures.
- Nose and jaw: appropriate size and positioning when the face is viewed from the front and in profile
- Philtrum: its size and whether it is abnormally smooth or deeply grooved
- Mouth: tongue size relative to oral cavity
- Ears: position and rotation. When viewed from the front, the top of the helix of the ear should not be below a line passing through the medial canthi. When viewed from the side, low set ears are usually posteriorly rotated (more than 15 degrees posteriorly rotated relative to the plane of the face).

Asymmetry of the face may be noted at rest or when the infant is crying. It is important to differentiate facial nerve palsy (Fig. 17.6) from asymmetric crying facies. Facial nerve palsy involves paucity of movement of the entire affected side of the face and impaired eye closure, together with flattening of the nasolabial fold. It may result from pressure on the facial nerve during forceps delivery or unassisted vaginal delivery and typically improves over the first few weeks of life. Eye protection and lubrication is needed until full eye closure is achieved. Asymmetric crying facies involves normal eye closure and a normal facial appearance at rest with presence of the nasolabial fold. On crying, one side of the mouth does not move down due to absent depressor anguli oris function. It may be an isolated finding, but the baby should be carefully examined for other congenital malformations, particularly cardiovascular abnormalities.

Birthmarks over the face requiring further investigation and treatment may also be noted at this stage. A port-wine stain in the trigeminal nerve distribution may be associated with intracerebral vascular malformation (Sturge Weber syndrome), retinal

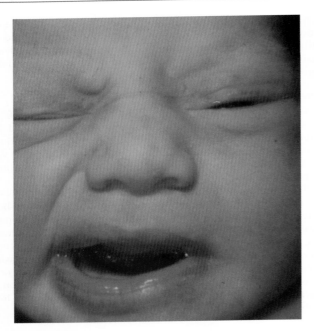

FIGURE 17.6 Facial palsy.

hemangiomas, or glaucoma so requires neuroimaging and ophthalmology review. Capillary hemangiomas over the face may require treatment if they are likely to impede vision as they grow or are affecting the lips, while there is an association between hemangiomas over the jaw or anterior neck and airway hemangiomas.

Head and Neck

Inspection of the head includes assessment of the shape and size relative to the rest of the body, facial structure and character, and distribution of the hair.

Head circumference was discussed previously. Even when the OFC is normal, it is important to note whether the size of the head seems appropriate for the size of the face. The shape of the cranial vault reflects interaction of internal forces (i.e., brain anatomy, volume, intracranial pressure) against external forces (i.e., intrauterine and extrauterine molding, suture mobility). Normal intrauterine molding for a vertex presentation leads to a narrowed biparietal diameter and a maximal occipitomental dimension. After breech presentation, there may be marked accentuation of the occipitofrontal dimension with parietal flattening, an occipital shelf, and apparent frontal prominence. This normal breech shape requires differentiation from the abnormal occipital prominence found in posterior fossa masses (e.g., Dandy-Walker malformation), frontal prominence due to increased cranial volume, or the boat-shaped scaphocephaly from synostosis of the sagittal suture.

Unusual head shapes are found in approximately 10% of newborns, with the most common abnormality being posterior or lateral plagiocephaly (i.e., flattening) (48). Associated risk factors are primiparity, assisted delivery, prolonged labor, and twin pregnancies (48). Plagiocephaly and torticollis often coexist, and the range of motion of the neck should be assessed: the infant's head should turn as far as the shoulder in both directions and farther if it is premature. Fronto-occipital plagiocephaly may be manifested by a unilateral epicanthal fold (49), in addition to occipital flattening with ipsilateral frontal prominence and asymmetrical ear position when viewed from the top of the head.

Inspection of the Hair and Scalp

The hair should be inspected for color, texture, distribution, and directional patterns. Reddish or blond hair in a dark-skinned infant may indicate albinism. Polioses are random patches of white hair, which can be inconsequential or may be part of Waardenburg syndrome (white forelocks associated with other pigment defects and hearing loss (50)). Hirsute infants may have hair extending down the forehead but the eyebrows should not be fused. A posterior hairline that extends well below the neck creases may indicate a short or webbed neck. The texture of hair at term is relatively fine and is increasingly sparse and fine with decreasing GA. There is generally a single parietal hair whorl, and multiple or unusually positioned whorls can suggest associated brain or genetic abnormalities. Unruly hair with multiple directions of growth, particularly with unusual facies, microcephaly, or SGA, may be seen in Down syndrome or Cornelia de Lange syndrome or reflect poor brain growth of early fetal onset (51).

Superficial ecchymoses and abrasions of the scalp are common after vaginal deliveries, especially after extraction by forceps or vacuum. Incision sites for fetal scalp electrodes or blood sampling should be small and inconsequential, although some are deep enough to require closure. They should be differentiated from aplasia cutis congenita, a defect consisting of an area of skin absence. Cutis aplasia especially if in the midline and surrounded by a long thick whorl of hair (the "hair collar sign") or overlain by a port-wine stain (52) can be associated with defects in the underlying skull or brain. In these situations, neuroimaging is indicated. Telangiectatic or staining lesions appear over the scalp, neck, and face, ranging from the superficial and transient flammeus nevus or stork bite to the more intense, permanent port-wine stain.

Scalp rugae with a normal scalp hair pattern are an unusual finding indicating that the skull beneath the rugae has collapsed during fetal development; they predict a very poor neurologic outcome.

Palpation of the Head

Palpation detects motility and firmness of adjacent bones, size of the sutures, bony or dermal defects, and fluid accumulation within the scalp (caput succedaneum, cephalohematoma, or subgaleal hemorrhage). There are six bony plates to the cranial vault; one frontal, two parietal, two temporal, and one occipital. Normally at birth, these bones are separated by six suture lines: metopic, sagittal, and paired coronal and lambdoid (**Fig. 17.7**). Mild overlap of sutures may be seen with molding, but the bony plates should feel mobile. Sutures that are fused feel more like a mountain range, with equal buildup on both sides, and do not shift with pressure. Primary CS is usually apparent at birth or within the first few months of life and may affect one or multiple sutures (**Fig. 17.8**), most commonly the sagittal suture (53). Secondary CS is most commonly caused by a primary failure of brain growth resulting in premature closure of the sutures and is associated with adverse neurodevelopment, but thyrotoxicosis is another cause and should be excluded (54). Normal molding resolves within a few weeks, while deformation from CS worsens over time.

Any suture, particularly the metopic, may be normally widened in the absence of increased intracranial pressure; the exception is a wide lambdoid suture, which indicates increased intracranial pressure. Palpation of the bones adjacent to the sagittal suture may reveal a sensation similar to that felt when gently pressing on an aluminum can or ping pong ball. These softer areas, indicating craniotabes, occur most often in premature infants. In term infants, they can be normal in situations where the fetal head was compressed against the maternal bony pelvis for several weeks (physiologic) or can be a sign of rickets secondary to vitamin D deficiency (55).

The fontanelles vary in size between and within race and by GA (56–58), but the anterior fontanelle of a term infant is typically 1 to 4 cm in length (59). Regardless of size, a pulsatile bulging fontanelle is a strong indicator of increased intracranial pressure. The posterior fontanelle is typically less than 1 cm in diameter at birth. Infants with a closed posterior fontanelle have smaller anterior

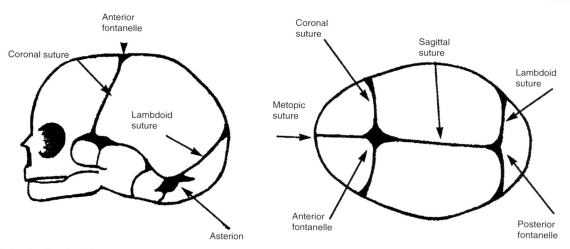

FIGURE 17.7 Lateral and sagittal views of the cranial sutures. (Reprinted with permission from Fletcher MA. *Physical diagnosis in the neonatology.* Philadelphia, PA: Lippincott-Raven Publishers, 1998:175.)

fontanelles, and those with smaller anterior fontanelles also have smaller head circumferences (60). Although aberrantly large fontanelles are seen in genetic syndromes, metabolic or endocrine diseases and vitamin D deficiency, they are not pathognomonic. A third fontanelle between the anterior and posterior ones can be a normal variant but is more common in Down syndrome (61). The anterior fontanelle closes at a median age of 13 months, and by 24 months of age, it is closed in 96% of infants, with no significant differences related to gender, growth parameters, or bone age (57).

There are several other findings on head palpation that are unique to the neonatal period. The most frequent, caput succedaneum, presents at birth with pitting edema and initially is most prominent over the presenting area. Caput succedaneum represents fluid accumulation within and under the scalp. Although a caput initially may be limited to overlying a single bone, it will shift to dependent regions and cross sutures.

Cephalohematoma is less common and rarely is present immediately upon delivery. Any nonfluctuant swelling that is palpable in the delivery suite is more likely to be a caput. Typically, a cephalohematoma develops after delivery and expands during the first few hours as blood accumulates between the surface of a calvarial bone and its pericranial membrane. The cephalohematoma is rounded, discrete, and fluctuant, with boundaries limited by suture lines. Because of periosteal reflection at the margins, there is often a

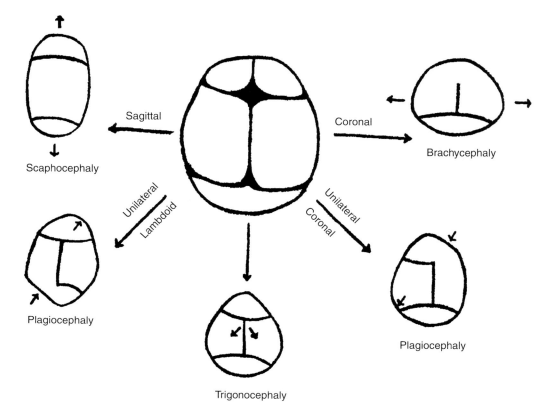

FIGURE 17.8 The various forms of craniosynostosis displaying lack of growth perpendicular to the prematurely fused suture line. (Modified with permission from Fletcher MA. *Physical diagnosis in the neonatology.* Philadelphia, PA: Lippincott-Raven Publishers, 1998:186.)

CARE AROUND BIRTH

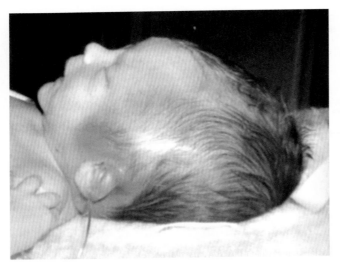

FIGURE 17.9 Large subgaleal hematoma. There is discoloration and swelling that extends across suture lines onto the neck, even onto the ear, causing protuberance of the pinna. There may be some degree of crepitation to palpation, particularly at the margins. The area containing blood can advance well down the forehead and neck because there is little inhibition, and there can be major blood extravasation. (Reprinted with permission from Fletcher MA. *Physical diagnosis in the neonatology.* Philadelphia, PA: Lippincott-Raven Publishers, 1998:185.)

false sensation of underlying bony depression. The blood contained in a cephalohematoma may take several weeks to resorb and may prolong neonatal jaundice. In the longer term, they can calcify and result in hard, bony swellings.

The least frequent but most serious scalp injury is a subgaleal hematoma (**Fig. 17.9**), a fluctuant swelling with less pitting and more discoloration than found in caput succedaneum and often a visible fluid thrill. Because there is little anatomic restriction to accumulation of fluid under the aponeurosis, large amounts may redistribute to the nape of the neck and deplete total body blood volume in a massive subgaleal hemorrhage (62). Serial measurements of OFC and close monitoring of vital signs including BP and hematocrit should be performed in the first 24 hours in all cases of suspected subgaleal hemorrhage, in order to anticipate the need for volume replacement. Cephalohematomas and subgaleal hematomas occur most often after vacuum or difficult forceps extractions but may develop spontaneously even in cesarean or unassisted vaginal deliveries (63).

A thorough examination of the head includes auscultating for bruits over the temporal arteries and anterior fontanelle, particularly in conditions involving high-output cardiac failure such as vein of Galen malformations (64) or arteriovenous malformations.

The neck should be extended to look for branchial cleft cysts or sinuses anywhere from the ear along the anterior border of the sternocleidomastoid. The normal thyroid is rarely palpable, but midline enlargements may represent a goiter or other congenital mass, such as cystic hygroma, lymphangioma, or cervical teratoma. Any mass may produce feeding difficulties, torticollis, and respiratory distress if airway compression is present. A firm mass in the belly of the sternocleidomastoid is a fibroma (sometimes called a sternomastoid tumor (65)), which may cause torticollis. If present, the head is tilted to the involved side with the chin pointing away from the involved muscle.

Eyes

Examining the eyes of a neonate requires patience and a cooperative infant. Trying to pry the eyes open will usually make the examination more difficult due to crying, while positioning the infant in an upright position and rocking gently back and forth or

stimulating sucking may encourage spontaneous eye opening. The emphasis of the neonatal eye examination is on the structure and appearance of the eye and its surroundings rather than assessment of visual acuity or extraocular muscles.

The eyebrows are examined for symmetry and normal separation. Synophrys (fusion of the eyebrows) may be observed in several syndromes such as Cornelia de Lange (see Chapter 57). With opening of the eyelids, failure of one side to elevate may indicate a congenital ptosis. A miotic pupil on the ipsilateral side suggests the presence of congenital Horner syndrome. Disorders of the ectoderm may present with absent eyelashes.

Subconjunctival hemorrhages are very common following vaginal delivery and are due to increased intravascular pressure. It is common for a small amount of mucoid discharge to crust the eyelashes during sleep, due to congenital obstruction of the nasolacrimal duct that occurs in 20% of newborns, 95% of whom are symptomatic in the first month of life (66). This resolves spontaneously within the first year of life in the majority of infants but can take longer (67). Supporting signs include the following:

- Large tear meniscus at the lower lid
- Tearing without stimulation
- Dried mucoid residue after a nap
- Discharge during waking

However, purulent discharge or associated redness or swelling of the lid indicates infection. Maternal history of chlamydia or gonorrhea should be sought; gonococcal infection typically presents within the first few days while chlamydial conjunctivitis typically presents between 5 days and 2 weeks. Rarely, the lacrimal drainage system is obstructed at both ends, resulting in a dacryocystocele (tense, cystic swelling below the medial canthus, often blue-grey in color).

Each eye is compared for relative size, shape, and position in the socket (sunken or protruding) and whether pupils constrict to light. Standard measurements for the eyes are available (68). Eyes that appear too large may be one sign of congenital glaucoma, together with photophobia, excessive tearing, and corneal clouding (see Chapter 58). A dimly lit room with a moderately bright light should be used to elicit the pupillary reaction to light. Too bright a light and reflexive eye closure will occur. The pupil diameter decreases toward term as its response to light increases, with the normal mean +/− SD of pupillary diameter in a term infant being 3.8 to ±0.8 mm and no more than 1 mm difference between left and right (69). Iris color is poorly defined at birth. The iris should form a continuous circle without interruptions (colobomas) or unusual stretching or banding. In some infants less than 28 weeks of gestation, corneal cloudiness or haze permits only a limited inspection of the iris and pupils (70).

The red reflex is best visualized using a direct ophthalmoscope with the widest beam of light possible. It is held 20 to 30 cm from the infant such that both eyes are within the field of light. An abnormal red reflex indicates an ocular abnormality anywhere from the cornea to the retina and warrants an urgent ophthalmologic assessment to determine its exact location. Failure to visualize the red reflex may be secondary to pathology requiring urgent treatment such as a cataract or to benign conditions such as corneal edema. Corneal edema is often present in the first 2 days after birth particularly in infants with darkly pigmented eyes.

Ears

Each ear is examined for shape, size, position, presence of a canal, and any extraneous tags or pits. Any abnormality should prompt closer inspection of the ear canal to verify patency. Pre-auricular skin tags or pits are common but should prompt hearing testing if this is not universally provided. Ear length measurements at different GAs are available (71) but may be approximated as the vertical distance from the arch of the brow to the level at which the nasal columella meets the upper lip. Posteriorly rotated or low-set ears occur when cephalad migration and anterior rotation fail to complete. Molding or deformation from the birth process may give a false impression of abnormal ear position but will resolve after a few days. The position at term should be similar on both sides, with the helix above a line extended between the medial canthi. Using the lateral canthus as a marker may give the false impression that the ears are low set in individuals with upslanting palpebral fissures.

A behavioral reaction to a standardized sound excludes only gross bilateral deficits, but it should be elicited in all neonates. Universal hearing screening at birth is now standard in many institutions worldwide. Common risks for hearing deficit include severe hyperbilirubinemia, congenital infections, or obvious anomalies of the external auditory structures.

Nose

The nose is assessed for shape, size, patency, presence of swelling over the nasolacrimal duct, size of the philtrum, and definition of the nasolabial folds. Deviation from the midline commonly results from facial compression and molding during delivery, but rarely the nasal cartilage can be dislocated causing septal deviation. Since the latter is best treated by septal relocation during the first week of life (72), it is important to identify it. When the tip of the nose is depressed, a dislocated septum appears increasingly angled within the nares but a normal septum merely compresses. After release, a dislocated septum does not return to upright nor can it be passively molded into a normal shape (Fig. 17.10). Passing a small catheter through each naris to the stomach may be required to confirm patency in situations where choanal atresia (anatomical obstruction of the posterior choanae) is suspected. Since neonates are obligate nasal breathers, bilateral choanal atresia presents with acute respiratory distress and cyanosis characteristically relieved by crying and worsened by attempted feeding (73). Unilateral choanal atresia rarely causes symptoms in infancy but may be found incidentally during attempted passage of a nasogastric tube.

Mouth and Throat

The shape of the mouth is a marker of fetal position and neuromotor activity. A cleft of the hard palate may leave insufficient resistance to tongue movement *in utero* and culminate in underdevelopment of the mandible. If the hard palate is intact but the tongue inactive, the hard palate may have a high arch or have prominent lateral palatine ridges. Significant oral asymmetry causes difficulty in breastfeeding on one side compared to the other.

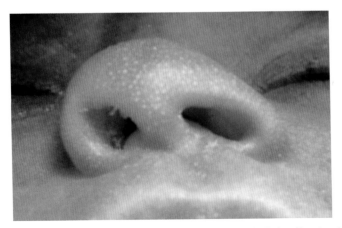

FIGURE 17.10 At rest it is difficult to distinguish a true deviation. (Reprinted with permission from Fletcher MA. *Physical diagnosis in the neonatology.* Philadelphia, PA: Lippincott-Raven Publishers, 1998:211.)

The tongue, buccal surface, palate, uvula, and back of the mouth should be visualized. The gums and hard palate must also be assessed by palpating with a gloved finger while the strength of the suck and gag reflexes also are assessed. A bifid uvula may indicate presence of a submucous cleft palate.

Symmetry of mouth opening should be observed with the infant at rest and crying. Causes of asymmetric opening include the following:

• Head tilting *in utero* for an extended period
• Facial nerve paresis (Fig. 17.6) with ipsilateral flattening of the nasolabial fold
• Absence of the depressor anguli oris muscle (no flattening of the nasolabial fold).

The more common oral findings have counterparts in neonatal dermatology and are benign (Table 17.1). One to six pairs of small benign midline cysts known as "Epstein pearls" may be present at the junction of the hard and soft palates. Other benign cysts (Bohn nodules) may be found along the maxillary or mandibular alveolar ridges or on the buccal surfaces, resolving by 3 months of age. Epstein pearls are always found in the midline except when there is a submucous cleft, in which case they appear as paired cysts along either side of the median raphe (74).

Natal teeth, often in pairs, may be found most commonly along the mandibular alveolar ridge. These teeth are present in 1:2,000 to 3,500 live births and are often removed due to concerns about aspiration or tongue ulceration (Riga-Fede disease) (75). Removal is not always indicated as the majority are part of the normal complement of teeth but should be considered if they are fully erupted and poorly fixed to the alveolus. The Hebling classification (Fig. 17.11) of natal teeth can be used to identify which teeth should be retained, in particular Hebling classification 3 or 4.

• Hebling 1—Shell-shaped crown poorly fixed to the alveolus by gingival tissue, with absence of a root
• Hebling 2—Solid crown poorly fixed to the alveolus by gingival tissues, with little or no root
• Hebling 3—Eruption of the incisal margin of the crown through the gingival tissue
• Hebling 4—Edema of gingival tissue with an unerupted but palpable tooth

A prominent tight frenulum (ankyloglossia or "tongue tie") has been cited as causing poor latch and maternal nipple pain during breastfeeding (Fig. 17.12). Frenuloplasty may be considered for the infant with severe persistent feeding problems or nipple pain unresponsive to usual therapeutic interventions (76). It is a functional diagnosis and frenuloplasty is not routinely required if the baby is feeding well.

Other abnormalities involving the tongue include one that is too large, preventing mouth closure, and tongue protrusion because of low oral–facial tone or small oral cavity. Causes of macroglossia include Down syndrome, Beckwith-Wiedemann syndrome, mucopolysaccharidoses, and congenital hypothyroidism (77).

Skin and Lymph Nodes

The skin should be assessed for the following:

• General color
• Presence of any extra markings or rashes
• Texture
• Turgor
• Edema or areas of induration
• Thickness of underlying fat
• Maturity

Icterus typically progresses in a cephalocaudal pattern and is best appreciated in natural light or by gently blanching the skin to remove blood from the dermal capillaries. The spread of jaundice

TABLE 17.1

Neonatal Oral Findings

Finding	White (%)	Nonwhite (%)	Comments
Palatal cysts (e.g., Bohn nodules, Epstein pearls)	73–85	65–79	Yellow-white elevated cysts 1 mm in diameter; nests of epithelial cells in the midpalatal raphe at the fusion points of the soft and hard palates
Alveolar or gingival cysts	54	40	Appear similar to palatal cysts
Alveolar lymphangioma	0	4	Blue-domed, fluid-filled cysts in posterior regions; no more than one per quadrant; may cause discomfort during feeding if cysts are large
Alveolar eruption of cysts with or without teeth	<0.1	<0.1	Clear, fluid-filled cysts; mandibular central incisor; rates range from 1:2,500 in Hong Kong to 1:3,392 in Canada
Leukoedema	11	43	Filmy, white hue of mucosa, nonblanching; of no significance compared with thrush
Median alveolar notch	16	26	Reduces when teeth erupt or persists as notch between central incisors
Ankyloglossia	~2	~2	Male-to-female ratio of 3:1; lingual frenum prevents protrusion of the tongue, extends to papillated surface of the tongue, or causes fissure in the tip
Commissural lip pits	1	3	Blind-ended pits at corners of the mouth; autosomally dominant; associated with preauricular pits; medial pits more syndromic
Thrush			Adherent white plaques on tongue and buccal and palatal surfaces; will scrape off; caused by *Candida* sp.
Bifid uvula	<1	<1	Associated with submucous cleft palate
Ranula	<<1	<<1	Cyst of sublingual salivary gland
Epulis	<<1	<<1	Large, pedunculated cyst of incisor region

Reprinted with permission from Fletcher MA. *Physical diagnosis in neonatology.* Philadelphia, PA: Lippincott-Raven Publishers, 1998.

cannot reliably be used to estimate serum bilirubin levels and visibly jaundiced infants should have either a blood or transcutaneous bilirubin measurement (78). The distribution and types of pigmentation should also be noted. Areas of hypo- or hyperpigmentation such as café au lait spots and swirling patterns are important to document as they may be associated with neurologic disorders.

A common, benign finding is the presence of a line of demarcation with pallor above and deep erythema in the dependent area below (harlequin color change). Another frequent skin pattern is marbling of the extremities from vasoconstriction (cutis marmorata) occurring when the infant undergoes hypothermic stress.

Common rashes are covered more extensively in Chapter 61 but include erythema toxicum and transient neonatal pustular melanosis. Erythema toxicum is characterized by widespread erythematous macules and papules that vary in size and come and go over several days. Neonatal pustular melanosis consists of small pustules with a friable surface that rupture to leave a hyperpigmented macule, often with surrounding scale. Unlike staphylococcal infection, there is no surrounding erythema and the infant is systemically well.

Many infants are noted at birth to have one or more birthmarks. Common findings include the following:

- Blue spots: blue-gray macules that resemble bruising and occur commonly over the back and buttocks, particularly in darker skinned babies
- Café au lait spots: hyperpigmented macules. If more than six develop prior to the age of five, the child will need evaluation for neurofibromatosis.
- Melanocytic nevi: round or oval-shaped hyperpigmented patches with a rough surface. Giant congenital melanocytic nevi (>20 cm) are associated with an increased risk of melanoma.

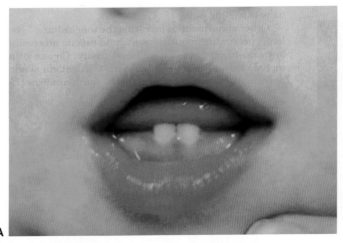 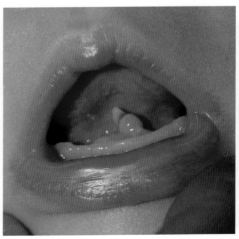

FIGURE 17.11 **A: Hebling classification 3, neonatal tooth not indicated for extraction. B:** Hebling classification 2, neonatal tooth; this tooth was extracted. (Reprinted with permission from Chung J, Morgan SH. Management of natal and neonatal teeth. In: MacDonald MG, ed. *Atlas of procedures in neonatology*, 5th ed. Philadelphia, PA: Lippincott Williams & Wilkins, 2012:390.)

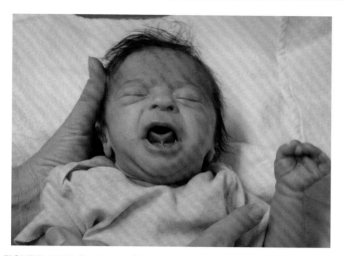

FIGURE 17.12 Newborn with significant ankyloglossia. Note the heart-shaped tongue, inability to raise tongue tip toward the roof of the mouth. (Reprinted with permission from Marinelli K. Lingual frenotomy. In: MacDonald MG, ed. *Atlas of procedures in neonatology*, 5th ed. Philadelphia, PA: Lippincott Williams & Wilkins, 2012:397.)

- Infantile hemangiomas: superficial capillary or "strawberry" hemangiomas usually develop within a few weeks of birth and proliferate rapidly in the first few months of life as raised, bright red lesions. If they have a deeper cavernous component, they may have a bluish tinge.
- Port-wine stains: deep purple macules caused by capillary malformations
- Stork marks: red or pink macules that commonly occur over the eyelids, head, or back of neck

Lymph nodes are palpable in more than one-third of all neonates, most commonly in the inguinal region and independent of perinatal history. These nodes, from 3 to 12 mm in diameter, tend to persist (79).

The most frequent, abnormal congenital lymphatic masses are cystic hygroma or cystic lymphangiomas, which are soft, compressible, and often poorly defined masses in almost any part of the body but commonly in the head, neck, abdomen, and axilla. Ultrasonography can help to determine the constitution of the mass.

Chest and Abdomen
Size and Symmetry
The thorax is normally symmetric, with compliant ribs that may be impacted by external and internal forces. For example, compression from the infant's own arm or a twin's body part may lead to marked asymmetry in thoracic shape and pattern on inspiration. By encouraging the infant to assume the fetal position, the cause of a chest deformation may become apparent.

The abdomen should be mildly protuberant, with a greater fullness above the umbilicus than below. In congenital diaphragmatic hernia, there is herniation of abdominal contents into the thorax that may result in a scaphoid abdomen. Bowel obstruction or hepatomegaly can cause greater distension above the umbilicus, while obstruction of the bladder can lead to increased fullness below this point. Diastasis recti, a separation between the rectus abdominus muscles, is a normal finding during the newborn exam.

Retractions
Mild subcostal and intercostal retractions are common even in healthy neonates because of their compliant chest walls. Suprasternal retractions, indicating proximal airway resistance, are normally less pronounced; supraclavicular retractions are never normal. Due to the compliant chest wall, the presence of

TABLE 17.2

Patterns of Neonatal Respiratory Effort[a]

Conditions	Pattern Observed
Distal airway or lung parenchyma	Intercostal retractions, sternal retractions, flaring, tachypnea, grunts, increased work in breathing
Upper airway obstruction	Suprasternal retraction, subcostal retractions
Cardiac pattern	Tachypnea without effort; infant is quiet but not somnolent
Neurodepression	Poor effort compared with physiologic need, apnea
Metabolic acidosis of sepsis	Tachypnea, apnea, lethargy, whining, minimal retractions

[a]Early in disease process before patterns merge with multiple system involvement.

parenchymal disease may result in paradoxical chest wall movement, with collapse of the chest wall on inspiration leading to a "seesaw" movement.

Because the diaphragm is the primary muscle of breathing with little contribution from accessory muscles, quiet breathing is abdominal, with only mild but equal subcostal retractions. In a spontaneously breathing infant without abdominal abnormalities, any lateral deviation of the umbilicus with inspiration suggests a diaphragmatic paresis with the deviation toward the nonfunctioning side; the "belly dancer sign" (80). Different patterns of neonatal respiratory effort are summarized in Table 17.2.

Auscultation of Breath Sounds
Breath sounds should be symmetric and are typically more bronchial than vesicular because of better transmission of large airway sounds across a small chest. Decreased breath sounds on one side may indicate a fluid collection, air leak, or herniation of abdominal contents across the diaphragm. Changes in the pitch of bronchial sounds from one side to the other or between regions of the lung most likely represent main stem or conducting bronchial narrowing. Coarse crackles at the start of inspiration usually signal proximal airway secretions, while those at the end of inspiration are heard when areas of microatelectasis open. The extrathoracic level of obstruction in inspiratory stridor may be determined by auscultating at various points over the upper airway.

A sound of crushing Styrofoam (polystyrene) or walking on dry snow is characteristic of pulmonary interstitial emphysema.

Clavicles
Asymptomatic clavicular fracture is the most common form of birth trauma, usually noted as an incidental finding on a chest x-ray. These fractures most commonly occur in pregnancies complicated by macrosomia, shoulder dystocia, or operative vaginal delivery and have been found in at least 1.7% to 2.9% of term deliveries and more frequently on the right side (81). Examination may reveal asymmetric bone contour, swelling from hematoma, and crepitations, together with brachial plexus injury or pseudoparesis. There is poor movement in the affected arm and an asymmetric Moro reflex. The infant may not be willing to breastfeed on one side because of discomfort with positioning or may cry with passive movement. Finally, the clavicles may be hypoplastic or absent as in cleidocraniodysostosis. If they are absent, the shoulders may be passively positioned to almost touch in the anterior midline.

Nipples
The breasts of term infants vary in diameter from 0.5 cm to several centimeters. They may be asymmetrical, but they should not be hot, red, or tender. Larger breasts, influenced by maternal hormones, may secrete a thin, milky substance ("witches' milk") for a few days

or weeks. The inter nipple distance varies with GA and body weight but the ratio of the inter-nipple distance to the chest circumference should be less than 0.28 (82). Supernumerary nipples may be seen in the milk line below and lateral to the true breast, more commonly in dark-skinned infants. They are usually rudimentary and may only be distinguishable because of a small mark or dimple.

Umbilicus

The umbilicus normally is positioned approximately halfway between the xiphoid and the pubis. A caudally placed cord insertion occurs in conditions of caudal regression or underdeveloped lower body segment. If there is only a single umbilical artery present, the baby should be examined carefully for any other abnormalities, particularly dysmorphic features, abdominal masses, and cardiovascular abnormalities. Periumbilical erythema or induration at the base of the cord indicates omphalitis, which requires prompt antibiotic treatment. The average cord separation time is 6.61 days (83). Delayed cord separation is seen in preterm infants, following antibiotic administration and with urachal abnormalities, but it can also be associated with leucocyte adhesion deficiency, which is a rare form of immunodeficiency (84). After the cord falls off, intermittent bleeding may indicate a granuloma. Continued leakage of fluid requires investigation to rule out a patent urachus or a vitellointestinal duct.

Palpation of the Abdomen

The infant tolerates palpation of the abdomen best when the organs are brought to the examining hand rather than the fingertips pushing into the abdomen and probing for the organs. Standing at the right side of the infant, with the left hand lifting the legs to flex the hips and knees and raise the pelvis slightly off the mattress to relax the abdominal muscles, the examiner can keep the right hand flat and use the fingerpads rather than fingertips to palpate the abdominal organs. Palpation should start below the umbilicus on both sides and proceed toward the diaphragm. The liver is normally palpable up to 3.5 cm below the costal margin in the midclavicular line, with a thin, soft edge and smooth hepatic surface (85). A false impression of hepatomegaly may be given by lung hyperinflation, in which case assessing the liver span by percussing the upper and lower margins may be more accurate. Brushing a fingernail lightly over the liver (or any solid abdominal mass) while auscultating outlines the margins and provides an alternative method for assessing span as the pitch of the scratching sound rises when it is over the solid mass of the liver. The normal liver span is approximately 6 cm by 35 weeks gestation but may be reduced by 1 cm in those who are SGA (86). In the first 24 to 48 hours after birth, the liver often decreases markedly in size, probably reflecting redistribution of circulating blood volume.

Although difficult to palpate in some infants, the examination of the spleen begins in the right lower quadrant, gently palpating with the right hand in a direction cephalad and to the left side of the abdomen until the fingers come to rest under the left subcostal margin. Successful palpation may be achieved by placing the left hand under the left posterior subcostal margin and applying gentle anterior pressure to bring the spleen forward. If this maneuver is not successful, then positioning the infant in the right lateral decubitus position may displace the spleen in an anteromedial direction, allowing for easier palpation.

The kidneys are palpable if the abdomen is soft, and they are moderately firm and rounded. It is often easier to palpate the right kidney, as it is displaced more caudally than the left by the liver. A fullness in the lower abdomen may be a distended bladder in an infant with infrequent voiding.

An infant reveals abdominal tenderness by a grimace, cry, drawing up of the legs, or tachycardia on light palpation. True guarding is unusual. The presence of localized edema or discoloration of the abdominal wall below the umbilicus is an important indicator of intraperitoneal disease (**Fig. 17.5E**). Unusual

exceptions are ecchymosis caused by leaking of an umbilical vessel or urine edema from a patent urachus leaking into the subcutaneous space above the peritoneum. Transillumination can reveal fluid or gas-filled masses, including distended stomach or bowel, hydronephrotic kidneys or a distended bladder. A transillumination pattern that shifts with patient rotation suggests free air.

Auscultation of the abdomen includes listening for pitch and activity of bowel sounds and for bruits. Infants normally have relatively inactive bowel sounds on their first day of life or if they are extremely premature and not enterally fed for several days or weeks. Even in infants with clinical ileus, bowel sounds tend to persist to some extent; however, a true absence of bowel sounds is always significant. Detecting changes in the pattern of bowel sounds is more helpful than the findings of a single examination. Auscultation may reveal the presence of a bruit over the liver, indicating an arteriovenous fistula, or over the kidneys in the presence of renal artery stenosis.

Cardiovascular System

The role for most clinicians in the newborn examination is not to determine precisely what the cardiac anatomy is, but to rule out cardiac disease. In a symptomatic infant, it is to determine whether there is a cardiac etiology for abnormal physical signs. The timing of presenting signs may offer clues to the cardiovascular condition. For example, the infant who presents with cyanosis as a concern on the first day of life may have a ductal-dependent lesion with a left-to-right shunt (e.g., pulmonary atresia), while the infant with cardiogenic shock at a week of age has a dependence on a right-to-left ductal shunt (e.g., hypoplastic left heart syndrome) until proven otherwise.

The physician must determine the urgency of the condition by asking some basic questions:

- Is this a cardiac disease that could be fatal if not immediately diagnosed and treated (e.g., ductal-dependent lesions)?
- Is its presence potentially aggravating or relieving other conditions (e.g., patent ductus arteriosus [PDA] in the presence of lung disease or pulmonary hypertension)?
- Is this something that requires following the patient because future intervention may be needed (e.g., mild pulmonic stenosis)?

Palpation of the chest may be informative in several ways. In the presence of heart failure, the point of maximal impulse (PMI) may be displaced downward and laterally from its usual location in the fourth or fifth intercostal space in the midclavicular line. A similarly displaced, enhanced maximal impulse, with or without a parasternal heave, is indicative of significant right or biventricular enlargement. Thrills may be present with significant murmurs.

Unless there is significant tachycardia, auscultation of the chest will reveal two heart sounds, with an occasional splitting of the second heart sound due to changes in pulmonary blood flow with normal respiration. In addition to examining the heart sounds, it is important to palpate the strength of the peripheral pulses, taking special note of the intensity of the femoral pulse relative to the brachial pulse. It is very difficult to appreciate a radial–femoral delay, but decreased strength of the distal pulse can be appreciated and when present requires urgent echocardiographic investigation to rule out coarctation of the aorta. Conversely, bounding peripheral pulses are indicative of a *runoff* situation, such as a PDA or, less commonly, an arteriovenous malformation with resultant low diastolic blood pressure.

Although murmurs persisting after the first 12 hours are likely to reflect structural abnormalities, not all will be hemodynamically significant. The decision to perform an echocardiographic examination depends on a number of factors including the ability to re-examine the patient over time, the family history, and the other pertinent findings on clinical examination. In one study (87) of infants referred for an echocardiogram between 1 and 5 days of life purely because of a cardiac murmur, 86% had identifiable cardiac lesions. Ventricular septal defects (37%) were the single most common lesion followed by a PDA (23%). Pulmonary stenosis was the diagnosis in 4% and aortic stenosis in 3%. Unforeseen complex structural heart disease was identified in 5% of infants. A normal heart with an innocent murmur was found in 13% who had no identifiable structural heart disease. Very commonly, a systolic murmur from a closing PDA will be present in the first 24 to 48 hours of life and is diagnosed by the typical disappearance on repeated examinations. Of note, infants with the most serious forms of congenital heart disease may have no murmur, because the defect/s across which blood is flowing may be so large that the blood flow disruption required to produce a murmur does not occur.

At birth, a line of demarcation may be observed, with the head, right arm, and right side of the chest pink and the rest of the infant pale or cyanotic until there is functional closure of the ductus arteriosus. The disappearance of this demarcation with vigorous crying indicates an appropriate drop in pulmonary vascular resistance and transductal shunting. Another reassuring milestone in cardiac transition, often noticed at the first bath, which is a brief but bright red flush over the entire body and extremities. This blush is not seen in infants with cyanotic cardiac disease. Specific points to be considered in the cardiac examination are outlined in Table 17.3.

Genitourinary System

In the delivery room, one of the first documented observations of the neonate is assignment of sex. Genital abnormalities are relatively uncommon but cause significant stress to parents, so it is important to urgently distinguish variations of normal from disorders of sex development using appropriate investigations if necessary.

In the male infant, the penile length should be at least 2.5 cm, but it is related to body and foot length (88). The presence of chordee prevents complete stretching, but a twisted median raphe is of no significance. In some infants, the shaft may appear retracted and covered by suprapubic fat, but this can usually be accommodated to allow accurate clinical assessment. Any significant glandular hypospadias generally is accompanied by incomplete foreskin and, therefore, is readily apparent on simple inspection. The normal newborn male readily provides an opportunity to observe the origin, direction, and force of his urine stream.

The presence of both testes deep in the scrotal sac indicates term gestation. If a testicle is not felt within the sac or canal, use a finger to sweep from the anterior iliac crest along the canal while palpating the scrotum. The volume of the testes should be estimated. Table 17.4 summarizes the normal values for testicular volume. If the scrotum or a testis is distended but soft and nontender, transillumination may reveal a hydrocele. Deep discoloration suggests hematoma or torsion and the need for immediate surgical

TABLE 17.3		
Neonatal Cardiac Examination		
Finding	**Key Location**	**Points to Consider**
Color	Over entire surface except presenting part; inside oral mucous membranes	Peripheral cyanosis may include the area around the mouth but not inside mucous membranes
		Prominent venous–capillary plexus around the mouth and eyes simulates cyanosis
		Acrocyanosis of extremities reverses with warming
		Mild cyanosis may appear as pallor or mottling
		Infant with PDA runoff looks washed out, particularly in the feet
Respiratory pattern	Lateral view of the chest and abdomen Alae nasi	Most often have respiratory rate within normal range
		May be cyanotic but tachypneic without distress (e.g., retractions, labored breathing) unless there is pulmonary edema or severe acidosis
Heart rate rhythm	PMI	Resting rate 120–130 bpm (range 100–150); higher 2nd to 4th wk and in premature infants
		Most premature beats are transient and benign
Precordial bulge	Thorax compared side to side and to the abdomen	Thoracic asymmetry indicates bulge with AVM, tricuspid regurgitation (i.e., Ebstein anomaly), tetralogy with absent PV, intrauterine arrhythmia, or cardiomyopathy
		Most commonly, asymmetry indicates pneumothorax, diaphragmatic hernia, atelectasis, or lobar emphysema
PMI	Left parasternal area	Visible until 4–6 h of life during transition; beyond 12 h, associated with volume overload lesions (e.g., AP shunt, transposition, or outflow obstruction)
		Normally more visible in premature infants but increases with PDA
		Abnormal to have PMI beyond 1–2 cm left of LSB at <1 wk of age
		Right sided indicates dextrocardia vs. shift due to intrathoracic pressures
		Absence of increased impulse with cyanosis indicates pulmonary atresia, tetralogy, and/or tricuspid atresia
		Increase with cyanosis indicates transposition
		Thrill: gross insufficiency of AV valve, severe pulmonary stenosis, absent PV
BP	Right arm and leg	Pressure in lower extremities is equal to or minimally higher than pressure in upper extremities in the first week
		Pressures are preserved by ductal flow in the presence of severe left-sided obstructive disease
		Norms vary by gestational and chronologic age and method
Pulses	Right and left brachial and simultaneous femoral and right brachial	Look for equality of intensity and timing, synchronicity, slope of impulse curve, no delay in peak between preductal and postductal pulses
		Easily seen axillary pulses suggest runoff or wide pulse pressure
Pulse pressure	Systolic minus diastolic BP	25–30 cm of H_2O in term; 15–25 cm of H_2O in preterm
		Narrow indicates myocardial failure, vasoconstriction, and/or vascular collapse
		Widened indicates AV malformation, truncus arteriosus, AP window, and/or PDA; may not be widened until pulmonary vascular resistance has dropped
S_1	Upper LSB	Usually single and relatively accentuated; audible split indicates Ebstein anomaly or slow heart rate; decreased with CHF, prolonged AV conduction
	Lower LSB	Increased accentuation with increased flow across AV valve indicates PDA, MI, VSD, TAPVR, AVM, and/or tetralogy

(Continued)

TABLE 17.3

Neonatal Cardiac Examination (Continued)

Finding	Key Location	Points to Consider
S_2	Upper LSB	Two components should be heard by 6–12 h of age
		Single sound indicates aortic atresia, pulmonary atresia, truncus arteriosus, and/or transposition of great arteries
		Wide split indicates pulmonary stenosis, Ebstein anomaly, TAPVR, tetralogy, and/or occasionally left-to-right atrial shunts
		Loud sounds indicate systemic or pulmonary hypertension
S_3 and S_4	Base or apex	S_3 indicates increased atrioventricular valve flow, PDA, and/or CHF
		S_4 indicates severe myocardial disease with diminished LV compliance
Click	Lower LSB	Benign first several hours; abnormal after transition
		Dilation of great vessel indicates truncus arteriosus, tetralogy of Fallot, left- or right-sided ventricular outflow obstructions
Murmur	Precordium, back, under both axillae	Many serious cardiac malformations do not have their classic murmurs in early neonatal period but will have some combination of signs suggesting pathology; absence of murmur does not preclude presence of serious malformation (e.g., transposition, TAPVR)
		At least 60% of infants have murmurs during the first 48 h of life; PDA, peripheral pulmonary stenosis, and/or tricuspid regurgitation may be indicated
		Quiet is necessary to auscultate murmurs; may need to disconnect the infant from the ventilator for a few beats
		Persistent murmurs first heard right after birth indicate ventricular outflow obstruction; most often pulmonic stenosis
Venous pulse	Jugular vein, liver	Jugular a and v waves in sleeping infant
		In the presence of cyanosis, pulsating liver suggests RA or RV obstruction
Abdomen	Liver (left and right)	Span >5.5 cm at term; late sign of CHF, presence of left-sided or central liver suggests likely cardiac anomaly
Edema	Presacrum, eyelids, legs, and feet	Causes are more often noncardiac except when associated with abnormalities of renal blood flow (e.g., left-sided obstruction of severe hydrops associated with myocardiopathy, such as severe anemia)
	Chest: hydrops	

AP, aortopulmonary; AV, atrioventricular; AVM, arteriovenous malformation; BP, blood pressure; bpm, beats per minute; CHF, congestive heart failure; LA, left atrium; LSB, left sternal border; LV, left ventricle; MI, mitral insufficiency; PDA, patent ductus arteriosus; PMI, point of maximal impulse; PV, pulmonary valve; RA, right atrium; RV, right ventricle; S_1, first heart sound; S_2, second heart sound; S_3, third heart sound; S_4, fourth heart sound; TAPVR, total anomalous pulmonary venous return; VSD, ventricular septal defect.
Data from Goldbloom RB, ed. *Pediatric clinical skills*, 2nd ed. New York, NY: Churchill Livingstone, 1997; and Smith DW, Takashima H. Ear muscles and ear form. *Birth Defects Orig Artic Ser* 1980;16:299.

evaluation. Superficial scrotal cyanosis may represent benign ecchymosis after breech presentation. Only in rare instances of deep scrotal discoloration will a salvageable testicle be found because; most commonly, a remote vascular insult has occurred, and the testicle has been resorbed before birth ("vanishing testicle"). The nubbin of tissue that remains does not need to be excised as it rarely contains any testicular tissue that might have malignant potential (89).

The female genitalia should be inspected for size and location of the labia, clitoris, meatus, vaginal opening, and the relations of the posterior fourchette to the anus (Table 17.4). Virtually all female newborns have redundant hymenal tissue, which tends to be annular with a smooth or fimbriated edge and a central or ventrally displaced opening. Tags of tissue may extend from 1 to 15 mm beyond the rim of the hymen, occur in at least 13% of female neonates, but disappear within a few weeks. A complete review of hymenal variations in newborns is available (90). An imperforate hymen can present with a hydrometrocolpos, a build-up of mucoid or bloody secretions causing a mass protruding from the vagina, which usually resolves with spontaneous rupture or regression but can enlarge significantly and cause urinary obstruction or discomfort.

Assessment for virilization in the female is difficult because there are varying degrees of clitoral hypertrophy and labioscrotal fusion. With full clitoral size realized by 27 weeks of gestation but with little deposition of fat in the labia, there is particular confusion about clitoral hypertrophy in premature infants. By term, the labia majora should completely cover the labia minora. Masculinization causes posterior fusion of the labioscrotal folds independent of clitoral hypertrophy. The distance of the anus from the posterior fourchette varies by GA and body size, but its relation relative to other genital landmarks is more constant (Table 17.4). Measurements are made with the hips flexed and the infant relaxed so that the perineum does not bulge. It is important in both sexes to identify a normally positioned anus. Anterior displacement of the anus, while not problematic in the early months of life, frequently causes significant constipation after the stools become more formed.

TABLE 17.4

Newborn Genitalia

	Parameter	Normal Range	Abnormal Range
Penis	Length	3.5 ± 1 cm	<2.5 cm
	Width	0.9–1.2 cm	
Testis	Volume	1–2 cm	
Anus			
Location, male	Anus to scrotum/coccyx to scrotum	0.58 ± 0.06 cm	<0.46 cm
Location, female	Anus to fourchette/coccyx to fourchette	0.44 ± 0.05 cm	<0.34 cm
Size	Diameter	7 mm + (1.3 × weight in kg)	
Masculinization (i.e., labioscrotal fusion)	Anus to fourchette/anus to clitoris	<0.5 cm	>0.5 cm

From Flatau E, Josefsberg Z, Resner SH, et al. Penile size in the newborn infant. *J Pediatr* 1975;87:663; Reisner SH, Sivan Y, Nitzan M, et al. Determination of anterior displacement of the anus in newborn infants and children. *Pediatrics* 1984;73:216.

Musculoskeletal System

Examination of the spine includes observation for abnormal curving and cutaneous manifestations of underlying deformities. Long tufts of hair, an overlying hemangioma, lipoma, or pigmented nevus potentially indicate a spina bifida occulta or tethered cord, unless well below the origin of the cauda equine. Pilonidal sinus is suspected when the bottom of a sacral pit cannot be visualized or there is moisture in an otherwise dry area.

A sacrococcygeal teratoma tends to be a fixed mass just lateral to midline, and spinal dysraphism presents as a midline mass, most frequently without full skin coverage.

One assesses the extremities for symmetry, size and length, range of active and passive motion, and obvious deformity. The length of the upper extremities should allow the fingers to reach to the upper thighs on extension. The muscles are not well defined but should not feel atrophic or fibrotic.

Examination of the hand consists of observing its activity and appearance, including the nails, joints, and palmar creases. Shortening of the fifth finger mid phalanx leads to incurving termed clinodactyly, which typically is greater than 10 to 15 degrees. The thumb should reach just beyond the base of the index finger. Extra digits that are postaxial or on the ulnar side are most often equivalent to skin tags and of no significance. They may be familial and are most often seen in families of non-Caucasian background. Extra digits on the preaxial or radial side are associated with hematologic and cardiac abnormalities and warrant further evaluation regardless of racial background.

The hips require ongoing assessment after discharge because dislocations may not be detectable on every examination (see Chapter 60). If the femur freely dislocates, it may appear to jerk spontaneously when the infant voluntarily extends or flexes the hip. The legs should be symmetric in length on extension and with the knees flexed as the feet rest on the bed. If they are unequal, suggesting hip dislocation of the shorter leg (i.e., Galeazzi sign), the next maneuver is to attempt reduction on the shorter side while stabilizing the pelvis (i.e., Ortolani maneuver). With the hip and knee flexed, the thigh is grasped with the third finger over the greater trochanter and the thumb near the lesser trochanter. The other hand stabilizes the pelvis. As the thigh is abducted, gentle pressure applied to the greater trochanter reduces the dislocated femoral head into the acetabulum with a clunking sensation. The commonly felt benign clicks are distinct from the pathologic clunks, which often are seen as well as felt when the femoral head jerks into place. If the legs are of equal length or if they rest in full abduction, the first maneuver is to attempt to dislocate the head of the femur (i.e., Barlow maneuver). With the hip and knee flexed, the thigh is grasped and adducted to 15 degrees beyond midline while applying downward pressure. If the hip dislocates on the maneuver, the Ortolani maneuver should then reduce it. If the hip rides to the edge but not out of the acetabulum during the Barlow maneuver, it is subluxable. Even if dislocation is undetectable, there may be telescoping, with free movement of the femur up and down, indicating some degree of instability. The Ortolani maneuver may be falsely negative if a teratologic hip dysplasia cannot be reduced. Unless both hips are involved, discrepancy in leg length and inability to abduct fully to the affected side should be present.

Nervous System

A structured approach to the examination of the nervous system helps to identify neurologic abnormalities to aid diagnosis; to differentiate between CNS, peripheral nervous system, neuromuscular and systemic disorders; to monitor progress with consecutive examinations; and to provide information for prognosis.

A detailed history of the pregnancy and also any past pregnancies including stillbirths, congenital anomalies, or genetic or syndromic conditions is important, but also the family history may help to put any examination into context. As part of this, meeting the parents and potentially assessing their neurology as well can provide clues to a diagnosis, for example, myopathic facies and grip myotonia.

In order to interpret the examination correctly, certain information about the infant needs to be available, in particular the GA, the postnatal age, the timing of the last feed, administration of any sedating medication including antiepileptics and also, if the underlying diagnosis is known, the point in the natural history of this process, for example, in HIE, the findings of the neurologic examination change as the injury evolves.

There are a number of different neurologic examinations that can be used to provide a systematic and thorough assessment (91–95). It is less important which examination is used, but essential that a neurologic examination is performed when appropriate and then repeated if necessary, as an insult evolves. The examination used as an outline within this chapter is that developed by Drs Lilly and Victor Dubowitz (91), which has been shown to be quick, repeatable, reliable, and predictive of long-term neurologic outcome (96).

Ideally, a neurologic examination is best performed in the quiet, alert behavioral state. This is found approximately two-thirds of the way between feeds, when the infant is not sated and sleepy and not too hungry. If the infant is not in an appropriate behavioral state, the examiner will need to delay the examination if they want to ensure an accurate assessment of the infants' neurology. The examination needs to be carried out in a room without bright lights and the room and the examiners hands should be warm.

Observation

Observation is one of the key tools in a neurologic examination. The assessment of the quantity and quality of movements, asymmetries, behavioral state, eye movements, and response to sound do not require any handling. However, more subtle differences in tone or use require more specific evaluation. During observation of an infant, questions to consider are as follows:

- Is the infant awake and alert? (**Fig. 17.13A**)
- Is the infant excessively irritable? If crying, is the character of the cry unusual?
- Are there external signs of congenital anomaly?
- Are there signs of injury, for example, bruising or swelling?
- What is the infant's spontaneous posture? A term infant will usually have flexed limbs (**Fig. 17.13B**). Are there any contractures?
- Are there spontaneous movements of the limbs? Are there tremors or rhythmic movements? Are there antigravity movements? Is there any asymmetry to the movement?
- Are eye movements in all directions and coordinated? Is there nystagmus?
- Does the infant arouse to sound? (**Fig. 17.13C**) Does the baby startle to noise?
- Is there an abnormal breathing pattern?
- Are there any patches of abnormal pigmentation of the skin?

Level of Consciousness

An abnormal level of consciousness is one of the most common neurologic findings. Assessing alertness is achieved by performing arousal maneuvers such as shaking a rattle, ringing a bell, tactile stimulation, shining a light in the eyes, or if necessary, a slightly more noxious stimulus such as a sternal rub. Altered levels of alertness are common in conditions causing cortical dysfunction and range from mild stupor to coma.

Examination of the Head

The head circumference should be measured and plotted on an appropriate chart in order to identify microcephaly or macrocephaly. The average OFC at 40 weeks gestation is 35 cm (33 to 37 cm being approximately the 10th to 90th centiles). Microcephaly is identified if the OFC is more than two standard deviations (SDs) below the mean, so less than 3rd centile and is often associated with genetic, metabolic or infectious etiologies. Macrocephaly is defined as two SDs above the mean (>97th centile) and can be related to an increase in any of the components of the cranium including brain tissue, CSF or bone. Both situations can also be familial if other causes have been excluded. Measuring the parent's heads and plotting their size on an appropriate adult growth chart is an important part in the investigation of an abnormal head size.

The shape of the head should also be considered, and the bones of the skull carefully examined to identify CS or plagiocephaly.

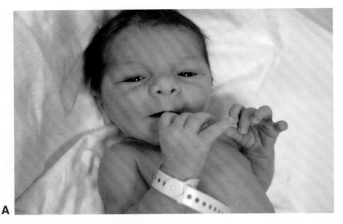
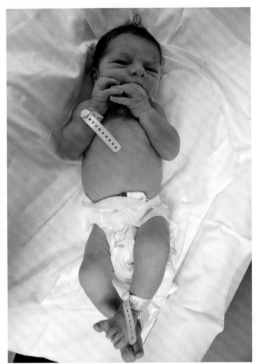
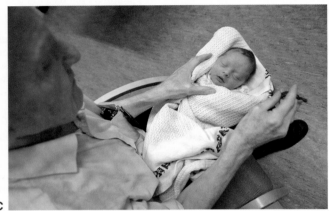

FIGURE 17.13 Observation in the neurologic examination of a term infant. A: This term infant is awake alert and looking around. **B:** This term infant shows a normal posture with arms flexed, hands open (not fisted), and legs semiflexed. **C:** Shaking a bell beside the head to around the infant from sleep and check response to sound. (Photos courtesy of Dr. Andrew Whitelaw and Dr. Damjan Osredkar.)

The tension in the anterior fontanelle increases during crying, but a continually tense or bulging fontanelle, even when the infant is held upright suggests raised intracranial pressure. This may be associated with "sunsetting" of the eyes, where the iris dips downward and allows the white sclera to be visible superiorly. Auscultation over the fontanelle may identify a bruit in cases with a Vein of Galen or arteriovenous malformation.

Any swelling or trauma to the head should also be assessed as outlined in the section earlier in this chapter.

Spine

The spine should be assessed as part of any neurologic examination. A neural tube defect such as a myelomeningocele is an obvious abnormality, but it is also important to identify any smaller pits, dimples or abnormalities in the midline that might overly a spina bifida occulta.

Reaction to Visual Stimulus

Shining a light in front of a newborn infant will normally induce blinking. If the eyes remain open, pupillary constriction can be observed. If the eyes remain closed, holding the infant vertically and away from bright lights may open the eyes. A healthy, alert term infant is able to fix on an object and track it as it moves across a horizontal plane (Fig. 17.14A and B). The most commonly used targets are a red object, a black and white contrasting target or a human face and they should be held approximately 20 cm from the infant's face. Term infants can also track vertically and in some they will be able to follow a target in a full arc. The visual development of preterm infants by term equivalent age is often more advanced than their term born peers and they can

follow a target in an arc more reliably (97). Assessment of fixing and following may need to be repeated if the infant is not initially in the optimal state; it also reveals abnormal eye movements such as nystagmus. Nystagmus is a normal finding in the term infant when they follow a target to the extremes of lateral gaze.

Reaction to Sound

If the infant appears to be asleep, it is useful to begin the examination by shaking a rattle or a bell about 15 cm from each ear. Usually, this will stimulate movement of the limbs or face. The stimulus is about 80 dB and will therefore provide evidence that the infant has some level of hearing. If the sound is repeated a number of times, the infant will eventually stop responding. This "habituation" is a normal response. Awake, healthy term infants will "still" to sound and will orient toward the source of sound by movement of their eyes. They may turn their head toward sound, although it is a slower response that that seen in older infants (98).

Movement Pattern—Quality and Quantity

Infants display patterns of spontaneous muscular activity referred to as general movements. Around term these movements are writhing in nature, they involve the whole body in a variable sequence of arm, leg, neck, and trunk movements and vary in intensity, force, and speed (99). Infants who have fewer movements that are less variable are described as having poor repertoire. This pattern is often seen in infants born preterm but is not specifically predictive of future neurodevelopmental outcome (100). More concerning abnormal movements are described as "cramped synchronised" and are characterized by repetitive rigid

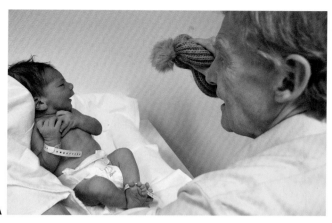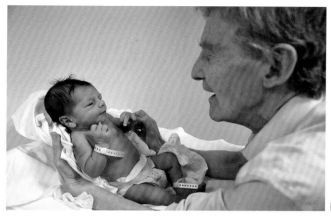

FIGURE 17.14 Visual assessment of the term infant. A: The infant is visually following a red object moving horizontally. **B:** The infant is visually following a face moving horizontally. (Photos courtesy of Dr. Andrew Whitelaw and Dr. Damjan Osredkar.)

movements of the limbs and trunk where the muscles appear to contract and relax almost simultaneously. These movements are often seen in infants with neurologic abnormalities such as HIE or PVL. They have been closely linked to the later development of cerebral palsy (101).

Severely reduced antigravity movements are a reliable marker of neuromuscular disorders (102). This suggests muscle weakness and is often associated with joint contractures. Closer inspection can also sometimes identify skin dimpling and poor dermatoglyphic patterns that are indicators of poor fetal movements.

Jitteriness, characterized by rhythmic tremors of equal amplitude around a fixed axis in an extremity or the jaw, may occur in 41% to 44% of healthy newborns in the first hours of life and thus deserves special comment (103). It occurs more often if the infant is awake, after a startle, or after crying. Accompanying symptoms of CNS irritation, hypertonicity, and low-threshold startle may also be present. Jitteriness is distinguishable from clonic seizure activity because of its more rapid rate and its cessation either in response to gentle pressure or by stimulating sucking; it is most often a physiologic activity. Jitteriness that fails to cease during sucking is atypical and may be a sign of hypoglycemia,

hypocalcemia, or drug withdrawal (103). Jitteriness may persist for many months, but in the absence of other abnormal neurologic signs, it may be considered a benign phenomenon (104).

Neck and Truncal Tone

Neck and truncal tone is examined by assessing head control and "head lag." Head control is assessed in a sitting position by encircling the infant's chest with the examiner's hands and allowing the head to gently fall backward or forward to assess the infant's ability to raise the head back to the vertical. They should be allowed 30 seconds to see whether they attempt this action. A healthy term infant will try to lift the head to the vertical, but may not manage or maintain this (Fig. 17.15A and B). A preterm infant will not achieve this.

Head lag is assessed with the infant in the supine position, with one hand gently supporting the head and the other holding the wrists and pulling the infant gently toward a sitting position. A healthy term infant's response to this would be to flex the head forward to be in line with the trunk. Preterm infants and those with hypotonia cannot achieve this. It is important to differentiate "head lag" due to general hypotonia from neck extensor

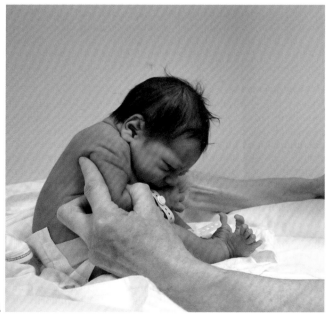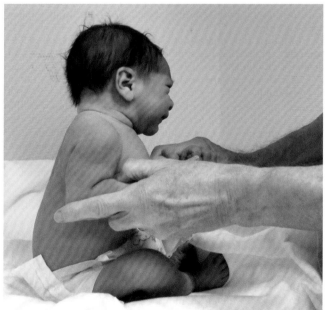

FIGURE 17.15 Assessment of head control. A: From sitting, the infant is gently flexed forward. Initially, the head flexes onto the chest. **B:** The infant tries to extend the head in line with the trunk. (Photos courtesy of Dr. Andrew Whitelaw and Dr. Damjan Osredkar.)

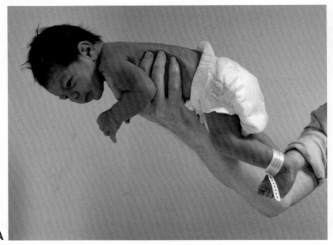
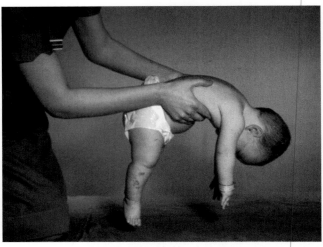

A   **B**

FIGURE 17.16 Ventral suspension. A: A healthy infant holds the head in line with the trunk without head lag. **B:** In ventral suspension, this "floppy infant" has dangling head and limbs. (Photos courtesy of Dr. Andrew Whitelaw and Dr. Damjan Osredkar.)

hypertonia, in which neck flexion is present, but is overcome by tense neck extension.

The response to ventral suspension should also be assessed looking at the position of the head and the limbs as well as the degree of curvature of the back. A healthy term infant will normally hold the head in line with the trunk (**Fig. 17.16A**). A hypotonic infant lets the head flop down (**Fig. 17.16B**), while neck extensor hypertonia will keep the head above the line of the trunk.

A normal truncal tone pattern should see flexor tone being slightly greater than extensor tone. Increased extensor tone can be a transient phenomenon but is also a common sign in neurologic abnormality.

Limb Tone

Limb tone should be assessed with the head in the midline position. The term newborn infant lies with the limbs symmetrically flexed when in the supine position. Tone develops in a caudal direction with tone in the legs developing before the arms and often being slightly greater. This can be reduced by a breech position *in utero* and can be increased in the normal crying infant. In preterm infants, limb tone is reduced and they lie in a more extended posture.

Passive tone can be assessed by arm and leg traction and recoil. To examine arm traction the supine infant is held by the wrist and the arm is gently pulled in a vertical direction. The degree of resistance to extension and the angle of flexion at the elbow is noted when the shoulder lifts from the surface. Leg traction is performed using the same maneuver, but holding the ankle. Resistance to the maneuver and the angle of flexion at the knee are noted when the buttock becomes elevated. Assessment of limb recoil and measurement of the popliteal angel bilaterally are also used to assess passive limb tone and have been outlined in the earlier section on neuromuscular maturity. Any evidence of asymmetry should be noted.

Primitive Reflexes

Abnormalities of the sucking reflex are nonspecific as they may indicate a baby who has a reduced level of consciousness or a baby who has a neuromuscular disorder, so its assessment has to take into context the rest of the examination. A feeding history will provide important information about sucking, or the reaction to a gloved finger can be used. The rooting reflex is elicited with a gentle stroke to the side of the mouth.

The Moro reflex is assessed by holding the infant supine with arms crossed, at a slight angle to the horizontal and then allowing the upper trunk and head to drop gently backward toward

the horizontal. The complete Moro response is full abduction and extension of the arms followed by full adduction and flexion (**Fig. 17.17A–C**). In the normal premature infant, the abduction and extension will occur, but the subsequent adduction and flexion against gravity may be limited. Asymmetry of the Moro reflex can be an important sign of brachial plexus injury (**Fig. 17.17D**). If there is full flexion of the biceps and the whole shoulder can be lifted (deltoid), as in the Moro reflex, this rules out the commonest brachial plexus injury, Erb palsy. Asymmetric movement may also be due to pain from a fracture or bone/joint infection. Asymmetric movement is not usually a feature of unilateral cerebral infarction (unlike adult stroke).

The stepping response is present after 32 weeks' GA. It is assessed by holding the infant vertically and placing the feet on a flat surface. The response is for the infant to lift and then place the foot down again, as if stepping.

There is a palmar and plantar grasp reflex, the palmar being elicited by placing a finger across the palm of the hand with the normal response of fingers curling around it and the plantar by pressing a thumb onto the ball of the foot and the toes curling down and around the thumb. The palmar reflex disappears by around 3 months of age when voluntary grasping begins to develop.

The asymmetric tonic neck reflex is elicited by turning the infants head to one side. The arm on the side the infant is looking toward will extend and the other arm will flex in a "fencing" posture.

Tendon Reflexes

Deep tendon reflexes in newborn infants can be difficult to obtain and to interpret. Reflexes can be absent, present, exaggerated, or asymmetrical and need to be interpreted in the context of other examination findings. In the presence of an otherwise normal neurologic examination reflexes that are difficult to demonstrate are unlikely to be significant. Reflexes should be demonstrated by the examiner placing a finger over the tendon to be tested and tapping it lightly with a tendon hammer or with two fingers. Clonus at the ankle is an indication of abnormality if maintained for more than three beats.

Common Birth-Related Nerve Injuries

A neonate with facial asymmetry while crying and who has a flattened or absent nasolabial fold has a facial palsy (**Fig. 17.6**). These are most often acquired during forceps delivery and have an incidence of 1.8 per 1,000 deliveries (105). The majority recover within the first few months of life (106). In rare cases, there can be a developmental abnormality with aplasia or hypoplasia of the facial nerve (107).

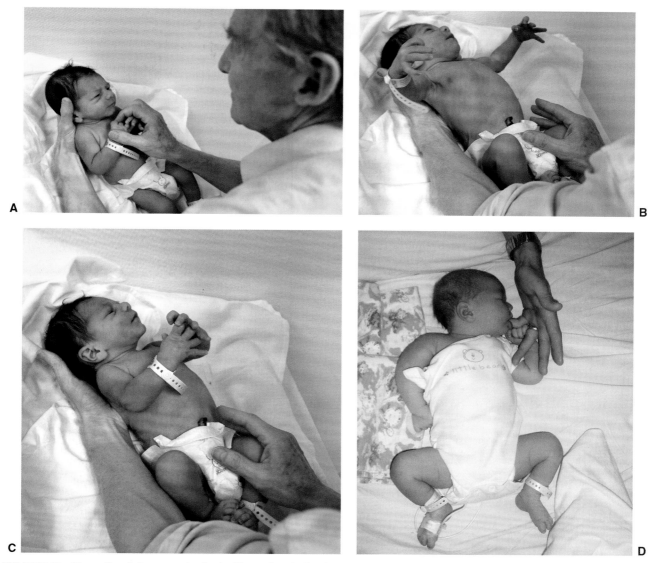

FIGURE 17.17 The Moro reflex. A: In preparation for the Moro reflex, the head and the hands are in the midline. **B:** The Moro reflex. The head is allowed to fall backward. The arms abduct and extend. **C:** The Moro reflex. After abduction, the arms then flex and adduct and the hands return to the midline. **D:** Right-sided brachial plexus injury (Erb palsy). The biceps, deltoid, and supinator are flaccid. (Photos courtesy of Dr. Andrew Whitelaw and Dr. Damjan Osredkar.)

The most common peripheral nerve injury associated with vaginal delivery is a brachial plexus injury. Traction on the arm may damage roots C5 and C6, leaving the infant with a prone adducted arm (Fig. 17.17D). Operative repair may be considered if function is not recovered by 3 months of age (105), but earlier referral for specialist assessment is recommended (108). Bilateral injuries may be confused with spinal cord involvement; however, examination will reveal that the lower extremities have retained their tone and movement. Lesions above the C5 level may impair the function of the diaphragm and have associated cardiovascular instability that may also falsely implicate spinal cord injury (105).

The basics of the neonatal neurologic examination include assessment of conscious state, quality, and quantity of spontaneous movements, truncal and limb tone, sensory functions of vision and hearing, and primitive and deep tendon reflexes. The neurologic examination in the preterm infant differs from that in a term infant, and these differences are outlined in Table 17.5. There are certain physical signs, if definitely present, that should alert the neonatologist to neurologic abnormality (Table 17.6).

TABLE 17.5

Neurologic Examination in the Preterm Infant Differs from that in the Full-Term Infant

- Posture is more extended
- Muscle tone is reduced in the neck/trunk and in the limbs
- Muscle strength is reduced
- Sucking and swallowing reflexes are often inadequate for nutrition until 34 wk, and coordination of sucking, swallowing, and breathing may not be present before 32 wk.
- Breathing is more periodic with lower gestational age
- The Moro reflex consists only of abduction and extension before 32 wk, and below 28 wk may be limited to opening of the hands
- Reaction to sound is present down to 24–26 wk of gestation, and some orientation may be found at 28 wk
- Blinking to light is present at 25–26 wk, but pupil constriction may not be present below 29 wk of gestation. Visual fixing and following are usually present from 32 to 36 wk.

CARE AROUND BIRTH

TABLE 17.6
Warning Signs in Neonatal Neurology

- Persistent hypotonia in a term infant
- Persistently increased muscle tone. This may be seen in infants with moderate encephalopathy after birth asphyxia, traumatic subarachnoid hemorrhage, and meningitis
- Asymmetric reflexes or movements
- Persistent absence of visual following on repeated examinations under optimal conditions. The eyes must be examined for microphthalmia, cataract, retinoblastoma, nystagmus, etc.
- Persistent inability to become awake, alert, and responsive
- Persistent inability to suck and swallow

SUMMARY

Examination of the newborn is an art that requires expertise and practice. Its findings can, when considered in the context of a thorough maternal and antenatal history, enhance greatly the physician's ability to diagnose problems, decide on appropriate investigations, and on many occasions, to reassure parents. Exciting developments in the area of newborn assessment are likely to involve new technologies including, for example, the use of Apps to estimate accurately GA from postnatal images, in settings where antenatal ultrasound is unavailable.

REFERENCES

1. Richardson DK, Corcoran JD, Escobar GJ, et al. SNAP-II and SNAPPE-II: simplified newborn illness severity and mortality risk scores. J Pediatr 2001;138:92.
2. Mendler MR, Mendler I, Hassan MA, et al. Predictive value of Thompson-Score for long-term neurological and cognitive outcome in term newborns with perinatal asphyxia and hypoxic-ischemic encephalopathy undergoing controlled hypothermia treatment. Neonatology 2018;114:341.
3. The International Neonatal Network. The CRIB (clinical risk index for babies) score: a tool for assessing initial neonatal risk and comparing performance of neonatal intensive care units. Lancet 1993;342:193.
4. Public Health England. Newborn and infant physical examination (NIPE) screening programme handbook. Available from: https://www.gov.uk/government/publications/newborn-and-infant-physical-examination-programme-handbook/newborn-and-infant-physical-examination-screening-programme-handbook
5. Rennie J, Burman-Roy S, Murphy MS; Guideline Development Group. Neonatal jaundice: summary of NICE guidance. BMJ 2010;19:c2409.
6. Khong TY Mooney E, Nikkels PGJ, et al. Pathology of the placenta. A practical guide. Switzerland: Springer International Publishing, 2019.
7. Papageorghiou AT, Kemp B, Stones W, et al. Ultrasound-based gestational-age estimation in late pregnancy. Ultrasound Obstet Gynecol 2016;48:719.
8. Saint-Anne-Dargassies S. Neurological development in the full-term and premature neonate, 1st ed. Amsterdam, The Netherlands: Elsevier, 1977.
9. Amiel-Tison C. Neurological evaluation of the maturity of newborn infants. Arch Dis Child 1968;43:89.
10. Dubowitz LM, Dubowitz V, Goldberg C. Clinical assessment of gestational age in the newborn infant. J Pediatr 1970;77:1.
11. Ballard JL, Novak KK, Driver M. A simplified score for assessment of fetal maturation of newly born infants. J Pediatr 1979;95:769.
12. Ballard JL, Khoury JC, Wedig K, et al. New Ballard score, expanded to include extremely premature infants. J Pediatr 1991;119:417.
13. Donovan EF, Tyson JE, Ehrenkranz RA, et al. Inaccuracy of Ballard scores before 28 weeks' gestation. J Pediatr 1998;135:147.
14. Singhal R, Jain S, Chawla D, et al. Accuracy of New Ballard Score in small-for-gestational age neonates. J Trop Pediatr 2017;63:489.
15. Hall JG, Froster-Iskenius UG, Allanson JE. Handbook of normal physical measurements. Oxford, UK: Oxford University Press, 1989.
16. Oberfield SE, Mondok A, Shahrivar F, et al. Clitoral size in full-term infants. Am J Perinatol 1989;6:453.
17. Merlob P, Sivan Y, Reisner SH. Ratio of crown-rump distance to total length in preterm and term infants. J Med Genet 1986;23:338.
18. Abdel-Rahman SM, Paul IM, Delmore P, et al. An anthropometric survey of US pre-term and full-term neonates. Ann Hum Biol 2017;44:678.
19. Beune IM, Bloomfield FH, Ganzevoort W, et al. Consensus based definition of growth restriction in the newborn. J Pediatr 2018;196:71.
20. Amiel-Tison C, Gosselin J, Infante-Rivard C. Head growth and cranial assessment at neurological examination in infancy. Dev Med Child Neurol 2002;44:643.
21. Raymond GV, Holmes LB. Head circumference standards in neonates. J Child Neurol 1994;9:63.
22. Sutter K, Engstrom JL, Johnson TS. Reliability of head circumference measurements in preterm infants. Pediatr Nurs 1997;23:485.
23. Prechtl HF, Einspieler C, Cioni G, et al. An early marker for neurological deficits after perinatal brain lesions. Lancet 1997;349:1361.
24. Prechtl H, Beintema D. The neurologic examination of the full-term newborn infant. Clinics in developmental medicine, Vol. 12. London, UK: SIMP Heinemann, 1964.
25. Brazelton TB. Neonatal behavioral assessment scale. Clinics in developmental medicine, Vol. 88, 2nd ed. Philadelphia, PA: JB Lippincott, 1984.
26. Lester BM, Boukydis CF, McGrath M, et al. Behavioral and psychophysiologic assessment of the preterm infant. Clin Perinatol 1990;17:155.
27. Thoman EB. Sleeping and waking states in infants: a functional perspective. Neurosci Biobehav Rev 1990;14:93.
28. Haddad GG, Jeng HJ, Lai TL, et al. Determination of sleep state in infants using respiratory variability. Pediatr Res 1987;21:556.
29. Sadeh A, Dark I, Vohr BR. Newborns' sleep-wake patterns: the role of maternal delivery and infant factors. Early Hum Dev 1996;44:113.
30. Hathorn MK. The rate and depth of breathing in new-born infants in different sleep states. J Physiol 1974;243:101.
31. Stern E, Parmelee AH, Akiyama Y, et al. Sleep cycle characteristics in infants. Pediatrics 1969;43:65.
32. Poole SR. The infant with acute, unexplained, excessive crying. Pediatrics 1991;88:450.
33. Heine RG, Jaquiery A, Lubitz L, et al. Role of gastro-oesophageal reflux in infant irritability. Arch Dis Child 1995;73:121.
34. Als H, Lester BM, Tronick EC, et al. Manual for the assessment of preterm infants' behavior (APIB). In: Fitzgerald HE, Lester BM, Yogman MW, eds. Theory and research in behavioral pediatrics, Vol. 1. New York, NY: Plenum Press, 1982:65.
35. Peesay M. Nuchal cord and its implications. Matern Health Neonatol Perinatol 2017;3:28.
36. Sargent B, Kaplan SL, Coulter C, et al. Congenital muscular torticollis: bridging the gap between research and clinical practice. Pediatrics 2019;144:e20190582.
37. Hofer N, Müller W, Resch B. Neonates presenting with temperature symptoms: role in the diagnosis of early onset sepsis. Pediatr Int 2012;54:486.
38. Grover G, Berkowitz CD, Lewis RJ, et al. The effects of bundling on infant temperature. Pediatrics 1994;94:669.
39. Harpin VA, Chellappah G, Rutter N. Responses of the newborn infant to overheating. Biol Neonate 1983;44:65.
40. Rutter N, Hull D. Response of term babies to a warm environment. Arch Dis Child 1979;54:178.
41. Harpin VA, Rutter N. Sweating in preterm babies. J Pediatr 1982;100:614.
42. Kent AL, Kecskes Z, Shadbolt B, et al. Normative blood pressure data in the early neonatal period. Pediatr Nephrol 2007;22:1335.
43. Park MK, Lee DH. Normative arm and calf blood pressure values in the newborn. Pediatrics 1989;83:240.
44. Hegyi T, Carbone MT, Anwar M, et al. Blood pressure ranges in premature infants. I. The first hours of life. J Pediatr 1994;124:627.
45. Dionne JM, Flynn JT. Management of severe hypertension in the newborn. Arch Dis Child 2017;102:1176.
46. Dasnadi S, Aliaga S, Laughon M, et al. Factors influencing the accuracy of noninvasive blood pressure measurements in NICU infants. Am J Perinatol 2015;32:639.
47. Dannevig I, Dale HC, Liestøl K, et al. Blood pressure in the neonate: three non-invasive oscillometric pressure monitors compared with invasively measured blood pressure. Acta Paediatr 2005;94:191.
48. Peitsch WK, Keefer CH, LaBrie RA, et al. Incidence of cranial asymmetry in healthy newborns. Pediatrics 2002;110:e72.
49. Jones MD. Unilateral epicanthal fold: diagnostic significance. J Pediatr 1986;108:702.
50. Sleiman R, Kurban M, Succaria F, et al. Poliosis circumscripta: overview and underlying causes. J Am Acad Dermatol 2013;69:625.
51. Smith DW, Greely MJ. Unruly scalp hair in infancy: its nature and relevance to problems of brain morphogenesis. Pediatrics 1978;61:783.
52. Patel DP, Castelo-Soccio L, Yan AC. Aplasia cutis congenita: evaluation of signs suggesting extracutaneous involvement. Pediatr Dermatol 2018;35:e59.
53. Cornelissen M, Ottelander B, Rizopoulos D, et al. Increase in prevalence of craniosynostosis. J Craniomaxillofac Surg 2016;44:1273.
54. Carmichael S, Clarke C, Cunningham M. Craniosynostosis; the potential contribution of thyroid-related mechanisms. Curr Epidemiol Rep 2015;2:1.
55. Paterson CR, Ayoub D. Congenital rickets due to vitamin D deficiency in the mothers. Clin Nutr 2015;34:793.
56. Faix RG. Fontanelle size in black and white term newborn infants. J Pediatr 1982;100:304.

57. Duc G, Largo RH. Anterior fontanel: size and closure in term and preterm infants. *Pediatrics* 1986;78:904.

58. Adeyemo AA, Omotade OO. Variations in fontanelle size with gestational age. *Early Hum Dev* 1999;54:207.

59. Boran P, Oguz F, Furman A, et al. Evaluation of fontanel size variation and closure time in children followed up from birth to 24 months. *J Neurosurg Pediatr* 2018;22:323.

60. Kataria S, Frutiger AD, Lanford B, et al. Anterior fontanelle closure in healthy term infants. *Infant Behav Dev* 1988;11:229.

61. Chemke J, Robinson A. The third fontanelle. *J Pediatr* 1969;75:617.

62. Benaron D. Subgaleal hematoma causing hypovolemic shock during delivery after failed vacuum extraction: a case report. *J Perinatol* 1993;13:228.

63. Levin G, Mankuta D, Eventov-Friedman S, et al. Neonatal subgaleal hemorrhage unrelated to assisted vaginal delivery: clinical course and outcomes. *Arch Gynecol Obstet* 2020;301:93.

64. Spada C, Pietrella E, Caramaschi E, et al. Heart failure caused by VGAM: a lesson for diagnosis and treatment from a case and literature review. *J Matern Fetal Neonatal Med* 2019;18:1.

65. Skelton E, Howlett D. Fibromatosis colli: the sternocleidomastoid pseudotumour of infancy. *J Paediatr Child Health* 2014;50:833.

66. Ogawa GS, Gonnering RS. Congenital nasolacrimal duct obstruction. *J Pediatr* 1991;119:12.

67. Sathiamoorthi S, Frank RD, Mohney BG. Spontaneous resolution and timing of intervention in congenital nasolacrimal duct obstruction. *JAMA Ophthalmol* 2018;136:1281.

68. Sivan Y, Merlob P, Reisner H. Eye measurements in preterm and term newborn infants. *J Craniofac Genet Dev Biol* 1982;2:239.

69. Roarty JD, Keltner JL. Normal pupil size and anisocoria in newborn infants. *Arch Ophthalmol* 1990;108:94.

70. Lai Y, Chen H, Yang S, et al. The characteristics of premature infants with transient corneal haze. *PLoS One* 2018;13:e0195300.

71. Sivan Y, Merlob P, Reisner SH. Assessment of ear length and low set ears in newborn infants. *J Med Genet* 1983;20:213.

72. MacDonald MG. Relocation of a dislocated nasal septum. In: MacDonald MF, Ramasethu J, Rais-Bahrami K, eds. *Chapter 56 in Atlas of procedures in neonatology*, 5th ed. Philadelphia, PA: Wolters Kluwer/Lippincott Williams & Wilkins, 2013.

73. Kwong M. Current updates on choanal atreasia. *Front Pediatr* 2015;3:52.

74. Richard BM, Qiu CX, Ferguson MW. Neonatal palatal cysts and their morphology in cleft lip and palate. *Br J Plast Surg* 2000;53:555.

75. Ritwick P, Musselman RJ. Management of natal and neonatal teeth. In: MacDonald MG, Ramasethu J, Rais-Bahrami K, eds. *Chapter 55 in Atlas of procedures in neonatology*, 5th ed. Philadelphia, PA: Wolters Kluwer/Lippincott Williams & Wilkins, 2013.

76. Power RF, Murphy JF. Tongue-tie and frenotomy in infants with breastfeeding difficulties: achieving a balance. *Arch Dis Child* 2015;100:489.

77. Núñez-Martínez PM, García-Delgado C, Morán-Barroso VF, et al. Congenital macroglossia: clinical features and therapeutic strategies in paediatric patients. *Bol Med Hosp Infant Mex* 2016;73:212.

78. Keren R, Tremont K, Luan X, et al. Visual assessment of jaundice in term and late preterm infants. *Arch Dis Child Fetal Neonatal Ed* 2009;94:F317.

79. Bamji M, Stone RK, Kaul A, et al. Palpable lymph nodes in healthy newborns and infants. *Pediatrics* 1986;78:573.

80. Nichols MM. Shifting umbilicus in neonatal phrenic palsy (the belly dancer's sign). *Clin Pediatr* 1976;15:342.

81. Joseph PR, Rosenfeld W. Clavicular fractures in neonates. *Am J Dis Child* 1990;144:165.

82. Hassan A, Karna P, Dolanski EA. Intermamillary indices in premature infants. *Am J Perinatol* 1988;5:54.

83. López-Medina MD, López-Araque AB, Linares-Abad M, et al. Umbilical cord separation time, predictors and healing complications in newborns with dry care. *PLoS One* 2020;15:e0227209.

84. Wolach B, Gavrieli R, Wolach O, et al. Leucocyte adhesion deficiency—a multicenter national experience. *Eur J Clin Invest* 2019;49:e13047.

85. Wolf A, Lavine JE. Hepatomegaly in neonates and children. *Pediatr Rev* 2000;21:303.

86. Reiff MI, Osborn LM. Clinical estimation of liver size in newborn infants. *Pediatrics* 1983;71:43.

87. Rein AJ, Omokhodion SI, Nir A. Significance of a cardiac murmur as the sole clinical sign in the newborn. *Clin Pediatr* 2000;39:511.

88. Bhakhri BK, Meena SS, Rawat M, et al. Neonatal stretched penile length: relationship with gestational maturity and anthropometric parameters at birth. *Paediatr Int Child Health* 2015;35:53.

89. Woodford E, Eliezer D, Deshpande A, et al. Is excision of testicular nubbin necessary in vanishing testis syndrome? *J Pediatr Surg* 2018;53:2495.

90. Berenson A, Heger A, Andrews S. Appearance of the hymen in newborns. *Pediatrics* 1991;87:458.

91. Dubowitz LM, Dubowitz V, Palmer P, et al. A new approach to the neurological assessment of the preterm and full-term newborn infant. *Brain Dev* 1980;2:3.

92. Dubowitz L, Mercuri E, Dubowitz V. An optimality score for the neurologic examination of the term newborn. *J Pediatr* 1998;133:406.

93. Amiel-Tison C. A method for neurologic evaluation within the first year of life. *Curr Probl Pediatr* 1976;7:1.

94. Sheridan-Pereira M, Ellison PH, Helgeson V. The construction of a scored neonatal neurological examination for assessment of neurological integrity in full-term infants. *J Dev Behav Pediatr* 1991;12:25.

95. Campbell SK, Kolobe TH, Osten ET, et al. Construct validity of the test of infant motor performance. *Phys Ther* 1995;75:585.

96. Novak I, Morgan C, Adde L, et al. Early, accurate diagnosis and early intervention in cerebral palsy: advances in diagnosis and treatment. *JAMA Pediatr* 2017;171:897.

97. Ricci D, Cesarini L, Romeo DM, et al. Visual function at 35 and 40 weeks' postmenstrual age in low-risk preterm infants. *Pediatrics* 2008; 122:e1193.

98. Muir DW, Clifton RK, Clarkson MG. The development of a human auditory localization response: a U shaped function. *Can J Psychol* 1989;43:199.

99. Einspieler C, Prechtl HF, Ferrari F. The qualitative assessment of general movements in the preterm, term and young infants—review of the methodology. *Early Hum Dev* 1997;50:47.

100. Nakajima Y, Einspieler C, Marschik PB, et al. Does a detailed assessment of poor repertoire general movements help to identify those infants who will develop normally? *Early Hum Dev* 2006;82:53.

101. Ferrari F, Cioni G, Einspieler C, et al. Cramped synchronized general movements in preterm infants as an early marker for cerebral palsy. *Arch Pediatr Adolesc Med* 2002;156:460.

102. Vasta I, Kinali M, Messina S, et al. Can clinical signs identify newborns with neuromuscular disorders? *J Pediatr* 2005;146:73.

103. Kramer U, Nevo Y, Harel S. Jittery babies: a short-term follow-up. *Brain Dev* 1994;16:112.

104. Shuper A, Zelzelej J, Weitz R, et al. Jitteriness beyond the neonatal period: a benign pattern of movement in infancy. *J Child Neurol* 1991;6:243.

105. Medlock MD, Hanigan WC. Neurologic birth trauma. Intracranial, spinal cord, and brachial plexus injury. *Clin Perinatol* 1997;24:845.

106. Duval M, Daniel SJ. Facial nerve palsy in neonates secondary to forceps use. *Arch Otolaryngol Head Neck Surg* 2009;135:634.

107. Decraene L, Boudewyns A, Venstermans C, et al. Developmental unilateral facial palsy in a newborn: six cases and literature review. *Eur J Pediatr* 2020;179:367.

108. Coroneos CJ, Woineskos SH, Christakis MK, et al. Obstetrical brachial plexus injury (OBPI): Canada's national clinical practice guideline. *BMJ Open* 2017;7:e014141.

CARE AROUND BIRTH

18 Care of the Normal Newborn

Karen L. Kamholz and Jessica M. McGovern

ONGOING CARE OF THE NEWBORN FOLLOWING DELIVERY

The first few days after delivery are a time of transition and adjustment for newborns and their parents. Infants establish feeding practices and start to regulate their glucose levels and body temperature in the extrauterine environment. They receive prophylactic treatments and begin their routine immunization schedule. Screening tests are performed to evaluate for heart disease, hearing loss, jaundice, and an expanding array of inherited disorders. Within just a couple of days, most normal newborns then transition to home with further care provided in the outpatient setting. This chapter will focus on the care of the normal newborn following the immediate postpartum period delivery and through initial hospital discharge. Table 18.1 provides a summary of care, screening tests, and interventions of normal newborn infants in the first few days after birth in health care facilities in the United States.

Early Assessments and Hospital Care

Newborns should have frequent assessments following delivery with temperature, color, heart rate, respiratory rate, tone, and level of activity and alertness assessed every 30 minutes for the first 2 hours of life. A more complete evaluation by hospital staff should be completed around 1 hour of life and not later than 2 hours of life including full physical examination, review of the prenatal and perinatal history, assessment of growth parameters, and evaluation of need for infectious workup (1,2). The covering pediatrician or other licensed health care provider should be alerted to any concerns promptly and should examine the baby by 24 hours of life if not clinically indicated sooner (1). Well newborns should room in with their mothers as this facilitates infant bonding, empowers mothers to become more comfortable providing infant care, supports cue-based feeding and more frequent breast-feeding, and has been associated with lower rates of jaundice in the newborn (1–3). Skin-to-skin care, with the unclothed infant placed in direct contact with its mother or another family member, should be encouraged in the postpartum period. For safety, the newborn is positioned with the head turned to the side and the neck neutral without flexion or extension. The mouth and nose remain uncovered and the face visible. Having infants skin-to-skin with the mother or another family member has been associated with a decreased incidence of hypothermia and hypoglycemia, a more organized breast-feeding pattern with increased rates of exclusive breast-feeding, less crying and decreased pain responses with procedures, less maternal stress and depression, and a reduction in postpartum hemorrhage (3).

It is important to maintain safety standards while infants are skin-to-skin or rooming in with the mother to prevent unsafe sleeping practices or patient falls, especially given maternal pain, fatigue, and limited mobility in the postpartum period. Providing anticipatory guidance, frequent assessments, good lighting, and appropriate staffing to allow for timely responses to patient calls is important in postpartum care. When a mother needs to rest, the newborn should be placed with another person or in a bassinet to sleep. Safe hospital practices are especially important because they are likely to influence parents' behaviors following discharge (3).

Temperature Regulation

The normal temperature of a newborn is 36.5°C to 37.5°C. Due to a high surface to volume ratio, a large head, thin skin, and little subcutaneous fat, infants have a limited ability to protect themselves from heat loss and require thermal protection, especially in the delivery room and in the first few days of life (4,5). In fact, the heat loss from an unclothed newborn in a 23°C environment is equivalent to the heat loss from an unclothed adult in a 0°C environment (4).

There are four mechanisms by which newborns lose heat: evaporation, conduction, radiation, and convection. Evaporation is the loss of heat from wet skin to the surrounding air and is most problematic in the delivery room and after bathing (5). Promptly drying the infant and removing any wet linens or clothing decreases evaporative heat losses (4). Conduction is the loss of heat when a baby is placed in contact with a cold surface. Prewarming equipment and using warm towels will decrease heat losses due to conduction. Radiation is the loss of heat from an infant's skin to distant cold objects. Positioning newborns away from cold walls and windows helps to prevent radiation heat loss (5). Finally, convection is the loss of heat from the baby's skin to the surrounding air. Keeping infants clothed and away from drafts and ventilation systems helps to reduce convective heat losses (1,5). Newborns should be dressed in 1 to 2 additional layers compared to adults (6). Caps can decrease heat loss in term infants by about 25% (7). Attention to keeping an infant skin-to-skin or covered during transport helps to minimize convective heat losses during these transitions (5).

Maintaining a normal body temperature requires energy and oxygen consumption. A neutral thermal environment is the setting in which an infant can maintain normothermia with the least amount of metabolic demand and varies with infants' gestational age (GA), weight, and postnatal age (4,5). The neutral thermal zone range is narrower for newborns than it is for adults because infants are less efficient at thermogenesis, the metabolic reactions that produce heat (5,8).

Hypothermia results when heat loss exceeds an infant's ability to produce heat (5). Mild hypothermia, also known as cold stress, occurs when an infant's temperature is 35.0°C to 36.4°C. Moderate hypothermia (32.0°C to 34.9°C) and severe hypothermia (<32.0°C) are more significant as they correlate with an increase in morbidity and mortality (4,5,8). Moderate hypothermia is associated with lethargy, poor feeding, hypoglycemia, and hypoxia. With severe hypothermia, infants develop metabolic acidosis, sclerema, respiratory distress or depression, hemorrhage, and impaired cardiac function (4,8).

Newborns respond to cold stress by releasing norepinephrine, which causes changes in behavior including irritability and increased movement to produce more heat (5). Additionally, the release of norepinephrine causes peripheral and pulmonary vasoconstriction to conserve heat losses (8). Finally, in term and late preterm (LPT) infants, the release of norepinephrine signals a process known as nonshivering thermogenesis in which heat is produced through the metabolism of brown fat, a highly innervated and vascularized adipose tissue located in the interscapular region, and around major blood vessels and organs in infants (5,8). Brown adipose tissue has abundant expression of adrenergic receptors to bind norepinephrine, facilitating heat production from the oxidation of free fatty acids and increased transcription of the cAMP-dependent glucose transporter 1 (GLUT1) to increase the uptake and subsequent metabolism of glucose (5,9). It is important to

TABLE 18.1

Summary of General Care, Interventions, and Screening Tests for Well Newborns

Age	Care	Screening	Interventions
Birth to 24 hours of life	Temperature regulation Feeding Umbilical cord care Skin care Bathing (preferably after 6–24 h) Voiding/stooling	Hypoglycemia Jaundice screening if indicated	Vitamin K Erythromycin ophthalmic ointment Hepatitis B vaccine
24–48 hours of life	Temperature control Feeding Weight change Voiding/stooling Discharge examination Discharge counseling and teaching	Jaundice screening Critical congenital heart disease screen Newborn metabolic screen Hearing screen	Male circumcision (if desired) Car seat testing (for infants <37 wk or with risk factors)

note that even with a temperature measuring in the normal range, attention to oxygen consumption, respiratory rate, and heart rate remains important because the infant could be in a state of compensated thermal stress (5,8).

As noted above, in the days following delivery infants should be kept dry, clothed, have a head covering, and be kept away from drafts to help protect against excess heat loss (5,10). Bathing should be delayed at least 6 to 24 hours and until the newborn's temperature is stable. The delivery and postdelivery rooms should have independently adjustable environmental temperature controls, and skin-to-skin care should be encouraged (4,6,8). Term newborns who are progressing well should have their temperature taken at least once daily until discharge (4). Infants born at less than 37 weeks of GA or less than 2,500 g have an increased risk of heat loss and a decreased ability to generate heat (10). These infants, if they are well enough to room in with their mothers, should have their temperature checked at least twice daily until discharge. When under a heat source, a baby's temperature should be checked more frequently (4).

The World Health Organization (WHO) recommends following axillary temperatures in newborns as a safe, easy, hygienic, and reliable approximation of core body temperature. A clean thermometer should be held high in the axilla with the arm adducted until the temperature reading has stabilized. When hypothermia is suspected, a rectal temperature provides a more accurate measure of core body temperature. The thermometer should be inserted into the rectum not more than 2 cm and should be held in position until the temperature reading has stabilized. The infant should not be left unattended during this time, and the thermometer should be cleaned thoroughly after use. The standard thermometer should read down to 35°C. When monitoring the temperature of an infant who is rewarming, the thermometer should read down to 25°C (4).

Caregivers should pay attention to cold feet, decreased activity, poor feeding, and weak cry as possible signs of hypothermia (4,8). For newborns who have become cold, caregivers should take corrective measures, and the temperature should be checked hourly until normal. Blood glucose should also be monitored in cases of hypothermia as low glucose is a common problem in these infants (4). Hypothermia can be an important sign of infection or illness, so infants should be further assessed if they become hypothermic without a definitive environmental cause, or if they fail to rewarm despite appropriate measures (1,4).

Infants who are in a hot and humid environment, are placed too close to a heat source, or are dressed or wrapped in too many layers can develop hyperthermia. Hyperthermia is associated with restlessness, red extremities, an increased metabolic rate with tachypnea and tachycardia, and water loss increasing the risk of dehydration (4). In these cases, the infant should be unwrapped, the air temperature decreased, and the infant fed or given fluids as needed for dehydration. Hyperthermia is occasionally a sign of

infection. Central nervous system abnormalities, like brain injury, can also be associated with temperature instability (8). Health care providers should consider further diagnostic workup as indicated.

Feeding, Weight Loss, Voiding, and Stooling

Careful assessments of feeding, weight loss, voiding, and stooling are essential to both identifying potential problems as well as creating a foundation for successful transition to home. Breast milk provides the best nutrition for infants. Breastfeeding has been associated with decreased neonatal mortality rates as well as decreased morbidities, including lower rates of diarrheal illness, sepsis, and respiratory infections (2). Successful breastfeeding often requires a great deal of support during the initial hospitalization with continuing support after hospital discharge. The WHO and several pediatric professional organizations including the American Academy of Pediatrics (AAP) recommend exclusive breastfeeding for the first 6 months after birth. After this time, breastfeeding should be continued along with gradual introduction of age-appropriate solids until the infant is at least 1 year old. Breastfeeding can be continued past 1 year of life if mutually desired by the mother and her infant. Clinicians should review the mother's medications and health conditions as there are rare contraindications to breastfeeding, such as maternal use of certain medications, active maternal substance abuse, and maternal HIV-positive status (11,12). In resource poor countries, exclusive breastfeeding up to 6 months of age is recommended for infants born to HIV positive mothers, when no alternatives are available. For infants who cannot breastfeed, caregivers should provide an iron-fortified cow's milk–based formula, unless a medical need for an alternative has been identified (13). Caregivers should start a vitamin D supplement of 340 to 400 IU (8.5 to 10 µg) daily within the first few days of life in all breastfeeding infants and in formula-fed infants until they are consuming more than 500 to 1,000 mL of formula per day (14,15).

Infants should begin breastfeeding ideally within 1 hour after birth and room in with mothers to promote frequent on-demand breastfeeding. An initial assessment of mother's delivery history, surgical breast history, and presence of flat or inverted nipples could predict difficulty establishing breastfeeding. Lactation support should be offered, and breastfeeding adequacy, including mother's milk production and infant's latch, should be documented. In addition, evaluation of the infant's voiding, stooling, and weight loss should take place. Supplementation of breastfeeding with formula or banked breast milk may be required in certain clinical situations that will benefit the infant such as persistent hypoglycemia, hyperbilirubinemia, dehydration, and excessive weight loss of 10% or greater (13). Weight loss greater than 10% is not uncommon. Studies show that 5% of vaginally delivered and nearly 10% of cesarean delivered newborns lose 10% or more of their birth weight by 48 hours of life. Assessing weights at least daily during the birth hospitalization and timely postdischarge follow-up may help to

CARE AROUND BIRTH

identify newborns at risk for excessive weight loss (16). While pediatric texts suggest that infants should regain birth weight by 10 to 14 days of life, Paul et al. found that 14% of infants born by vaginal delivery and 24% of infants born by cesarean section are not back to birth weight by 14 days of life. Furthermore, after reaching their weight nadir, infants gained 35 to 40 g/d on average (17).

Most infants will void in the first 12 hours of life. Failure to void by 24 hours of life warrants further investigation with special attention paid to feeding history, hydration status, and signs of genitourinary abnormalities. Ninety-nine percent of full-term healthy infants pass meconium within the first 48 hours of life. If an infant does not pass meconium by this time, the infant should be evaluated for signs of intestinal obstruction (1).

Bathing

Babies are born with a protective layer of vernix caseosa coating the skin. The vernix is composed of sloughed skin and lanugo hair and has a high lipid content. It acts as a moisturizer, lowers the pH of the skin surface, decreases transepidermal water losses, and has antioxidant and antimicrobial properties (18,19). Babies should be wiped lightly with a dry towel after birth to prevent evaporative heat losses, but the vernix should be retained. Placing an infant skin to skin following delivery helps to promote colonization with normal skin flora (19).

Infants born to mothers with hepatitis B, hepatitis C, HIV, active herpes simplex virus, or other similar infectious concerns should have a bath once temperature stability is achieved as this could minimize the transmission of the infection to the baby (1). In addition, the skin should be cleaned carefully prior to the administration of intramuscular (IM) injections. When culturally acceptable and when the transmission of infection is not a concern, delaying the infant's first bath promotes maternal bonding and can increase breastfeeding success (1,19). While each newborn unit should develop their own newborn bathing guidelines, the WHO recommends that a newborn's first bath be delayed until at least 6 hours of life, and preferably until after 24 hours of life (2). Bathing before an infant's temperature has stabilized is not recommended as it can result in hypothermia and respiratory distress (18).

Bathing can be done with water alone or with a mild, synthetic, nonmedicated cleanser that is neutral to mildly acidic and soap free. Caregivers should take measures to prevent heat loss including using warm water (37°C to 37.5°C), maintaining adequate room temperature (21°C to 24°C), keeping the bath time to no more than 10 minutes, and patting the infant dry with a towel and applying a cap after bathing to prevent evaporative heat loss (1,18). Protocols for first washing and drying the face and head before unwrapping the infant to bathe the body could also improve thermal control (20). Tub (or immersion) bathing is preferred to sponge bathing based on studies reporting less infant distress and better temperature regulation with comparable effect on the skin including transepidermal water loss (19–22). Furthermore, there is no difference in cord healing or infection risk with immersion bathing (18,20,21). Newborns require bathing only two or three times a week. Bathing too frequently can disrupt the infant's bacterial skin flora and can cause excessive drying, which can compromise the skin's barrier function (19).

Skin Care

Attention to skin care in the diaper area helps to prevent diaper dermatitis. Diapers should be changed as needed to keep the area clean and dry (18). The skin should be cleaned gently using water and a soft cloth and patted dry. Alternatively, caregivers can use disposable wipes with a pH buffer provided they are free of irritants such as alcohol, fragrance, or detergent (18,19). Zinc oxide or petrolatum-based ointments are used in the diaper area for both prevention and treatment of diaper dermatitis (19).

Bland emollients can be applied more diffusely to infants' skin. These moisturizers can support the skin's barrier function by trapping water and hydrating the stratum corneum (19). Studies

have suggested that daily use of an emollient beginning within the first few weeks of life and continuing through about 6 to 9 months of age can decrease the incidence of atopic dermatitis by about 30% to 50% in infants with a family history of this condition (19,23,24). Any preservative left on an infant's skin has the potential to be absorbed, so any lotions or oils used in this population should be allergen-free, safety tested, and should maintain a pH around 5.5 at the skin surface (18,22). Sunscreen is not recommended for infants less than 6 months of age, though it may be used sparingly on uncovered skin if sun exposure is unavoidable (19).

Umbilical Cord Care

The WHO and the AAP recommend that an infant's umbilical cord be kept clean and dry (2,25). The environment of the umbilical cord is one in which bacteria can flourish including Gram-positive cocci, like *Staphylococcus*, Group A and B *Streptococcus*, and gram-negative rods, like *Escherichia coli*, *Klebsiella*, and *Pseudomonas*. Furthermore, infection of the umbilical stump, known as omphalitis, can serve as an entry point with direct access to the blood stream. In rare cases, omphalitis progresses to more serious infections including periumbilical cellulitis, thrombophlebitis, peritonitis, intra-abdominal abscess, systemic sepsis, or necrotizing fasciitis. Mortality rates for omphalitis have been reported as high as 13%, so medical personnel should instruct caregivers to be alert for signs of evolving omphalitis including redness, warmth, tenderness, swelling, and purulent discharge around the umbilical stump (25). Omphalitis is rare in high-income countries with rates estimated at 0.7 to 1 per 1,000 babies (25,26).

Attention to hygiene is important in all aspects of cord care. Conditions should be clean at delivery and the umbilical cord should be clamped or tied off and then cut with a sterile blade or scissor, preferably using sterile gloves. Caregivers should keep the umbilical cord stump dry and exposed to air or covered loosely with a cloth. Regional customs to apply unhygienic substances, such as cow dung to the cord are discouraged. If soiled, the cord should be cleaned with soap and sterile water (25). Median time to cord separation for a cord that is kept clean and dry is 6 to 7 days (27). For births occurring in a health care facility, including those in low- and middle-income countries, routine treatment of the umbilical cord stump with an antiseptic such as chlorhexidine, as compared to dry cord care, has not been shown to decrease morbidity or mortality (2,26,28,29). Furthermore, treatment can delay cord separation and lead to measurable levels of chlorhexidine in the bloodstream (2,25). In contrast, when a baby is born at home in a region with a neonatal mortality rate in excess of 3%, the WHO does recommend that caregivers apply 7.1% chlorhexidine digluconate aqueous solution or gel, delivering 4% chlorhexidine, to the cord daily for the first week of life (2).

ROUTINE TREATMENTS AND PROPHYLAXIS IN THE NEWBORN

Neonatal Conjunctivitis and Ophthalmia Neonatorum

Conjunctivitis in the newborn can be infectious (bacterial or viral) in nature or due to noninfectious causes (chemical). The incidence of ophthalmia neonatorum, or conjunctivitis occurring within the first 28 days of life, is 1% to 2% in the United States, but as high as 33% in developing countries (30). The most worrisome pathogen causing conjunctivitis in the neonatal period is *Neisseria gonorrhoeae*, with possible long-term complications including corneal scarring, ocular perforation, and blindness (31).

In the United States, the rate of gonococcal ophthalmia neonatorum is estimated at 0.4 per 100,000 live births although, due to limitations in reporting, this may be an underestimate. In mothers with active gonococcal infections at the time of delivery, transmission to the newborn is 30% to 50% in the absence of ocular prophylaxis. Symptoms typically manifest 2 to 5 days after delivery with severe and permanent complications developing in as little as 24 hours (31).

Historically silver nitrate, tetracycline, or gentamicin ophthalmic ointments were applied after birth to prevent gonococcal ophthalmia neonatorum; however, due to a high incidence of chemical conjunctivitis, these agents are no longer routinely used. The only drug currently approved for ophthalmia neonatorum prophylaxis in the United States is erythromycin 0.5% ophthalmic ointment. A single application of a 1-cm ribbon to each lower conjunctival sac is recommended shortly after birth (1,31). Although some countries such as Canada, Norway, Denmark, Sweden, and the United Kingdom have moved away from universal prophylaxis, instead adopting a more aggressive prenatal screening and prevention strategy, several medical professional societies in the United States as well as the WHO continue to recommend universal topical prophylaxis (32,33). A single IV or IM dose of ceftriaxone 25 to 50 mg/kg (not to exceed 125 mg) treats gonococcal ophthalmia neonatorum. This dosing also serves as prophylaxis for disseminated disease in high-risk infants, although caution should be taken with ceftriaxone use in infants with hyperbilirubinemia. Providers should consider consultation with an infectious disease specialist or ophthalmologist if there is concern for active infection (1).

Topical application of 2.5% povidone-iodine solution is also effective in preventing gonococcal ophthalmia neonatorum, and its use outside of North America is increasing. It is an inexpensive antiseptic that can be prepared locally, making it suitable for use in low income countries, with no coinciding risk of drug resistance. However, povidone–iodine does temporarily stain the skin and sclera and has a slightly higher rate of chemical conjunctivitis compared to erythromycin (34,35).

Chlamydia trachomatis, with an incidence of 1.6 to 2.3 per 100,000 live births, is the most common cause of ophthalmia neonatorum in the United States (36). Symptoms tend to be milder and later in onset than gonococcal ophthalmia, presenting 5 to 12 days after delivery. Infants born to mothers with chlamydial infection should be monitored closely and treated for any signs of conjunctivitis since erythromycin ointment is not effective prophylaxis for chlamydial ophthalmia neonatorum (1,32).

Vitamin K Prophylaxis

Vitamin K is a fat-soluble vitamin necessary for the proper function of coagulation factors II, VII, IX, and X. There are two naturally occurring forms: K_1, or phylloquinone, is found in foods such as green vegetables and dairy products and K_2, or menaquinone, is synthesized by intestinal flora. Due to poor placental transfer of vitamin K, newborn levels are approximately 30% to 60% of adult levels. Adult levels are not attained for about 6 months due to naturally low levels in breast milk and low acquisition of vitamin K-producing gut flora. As a result, infants in their first 6 months of life are at risk for hemorrhagic complications known as vitamin K deficiency bleeding (VKDB), formerly called hemorrhagic disease of the newborn (37,38) (see Chapter 44).

VKDB is categorized into three distinct clinical groups: early, classic, and late. Early VKDB occurs in the first 24 hours of life and is related to medications taken by the mother, most notably antiepileptics, cephalosporin antibiotics, rifampin, and isoniazid, or to significant maternal vitamin K deficiency. Classic VKDB, occurring between day 2 and 7 of life, is related to the low placental transfer of vitamin K. It manifests as bleeding in the gastrointestinal tract, umbilicus, nose, skin, or following circumcision with an incidence as high as 1.7%. Late VKDB arises between 7 days and 6 months of life with the highest incidence between 2 and 12 weeks. It is associated with poor intake, secondary to low levels of vitamin K in breast milk, but is also observed in infants with primary malabsorption and hepatobiliary disorders. Data from Europe and Asia suggest rates of late VKDB between 4.4 and 7.2 per 100,000 live births. Complications of VKDB can be serious including intracranial hemorrhage

resulting in life-long neurologic morbidities or death. Mortality is estimated between 20% and 50% in various studies (39–41).

Experiments with both oral and IM administration of vitamin K to prevent VKDB began in the 1940s (37). By 1961, the AAP began recommending the administration of 1 mg of IM vitamin K to newborns following delivery as prophylaxis against classic and late VKDB. The dose is decreased to 0.5 mg in infants weighing 1,500 g or less at birth (42). Infants not receiving vitamin K prophylaxis after delivery are 81 times more likely to develop bleeding complications (41). Studies published in 1990 and 1992 by Golding et al. suggested an association between IM vitamin K administration, but not oral vitamin K prophylaxis, and increased rates of childhood cancer (43,44). Since then, several studies enrolling thousands of children with and without cancer have failed to support a link between prophylactic vitamin K administration and childhood cancer, regardless of the route of administration (37). Several countries have adopted guidelines for oral vitamin K administration. These regimens vary from a single oral dose at birth, to three doses over the first 2 months of life, to daily dosing for 4 months. The Canadian Pediatric Society recommends oral dosing of 2 mg of vitamin K with the first feeding plus repeat doses at 2 to 4 weeks and 6 to 8 weeks of age. Although some oral regimens have shown benefit compared to no prophylaxis, data supporting IM vitamin K administration to prevent classic and late VKDB outweigh that of oral vitamin K. Given this, the AAP continues to recommend only IM vitamin K prophylaxis. Parents who decline IM vitamin K should be counseled on the risks of VKDB, the effectiveness of IM vitamin K, the limited evidence of effectiveness of oral dosing regimens, and the lack of evidence to support a correlation between IM vitamin K administration and childhood cancer (40).

Hepatitis B Vaccine

Hepatitis B is a highly infectious virus that causes acute and chronic liver disease. It is contracted by contact with infected blood or body fluids and occasionally by transplacental transmission (1). The WHO estimates that 257 million people worldwide are living with hepatitis B virus (HBV) with the highest prevalence in the Western Pacific and African regions, where greater than 6% of the adult population is infected (45). While less than 1% of adults in the United States are believed to be infected with HBV, the rates of maternal infection have increased annually since 1998. This is in part due to women immigrating to the United States from endemic areas but also to increased intravenous drug abuse and the opioid epidemic. There is a higher risk of developing chronic infection when HBV is acquired in infancy or childhood, making the three-dose HBV vaccination series in childhood important to addressing the global health burden (46).

Prior to the development of the HBV vaccine in 1981, an estimated 40% of infants born to HBV-positive mothers, and 85% of infants born to mothers with the hepatitis B e antigen, contracted the virus. Eighty to ninety percent of these infants developed chronic infections. The American Committee on Immunization Practices first began recommending universal HBV vaccination in 1991 (47). Current guidelines for prevention of HBV include screening all pregnant women at the first prenatal visit and again at time of delivery if they have new or continuing risk factors (46). For medically stable infants weighing 2 kg or more at birth whose mothers test negative for HBV, the single-antigen HBV vaccine should be administered within 24 hours of birth. This dose is crucial as it protects infants in situations in which lab results are incorrectly transcribed or falsely negative and in the event of household exposure risks after discharge. Infants weighing less than 2 kg at birth have decreased immunogenicity that improves over the first month of life (48). Given this, the vaccine should be administered to these infants on day of life 30 or on the day of hospital discharge, whichever comes first (49).

When mothers test HBV positive, all infants regardless of birth weight should receive both the HBV vaccine and hepatitis B immune globulin (HBIG) within 12 hours of birth but administered at different injection sites (49). HBIG delivers HBV surface antigen antibodies to the newborn providing protection for up to 6 months. The birth dose of HBV vaccine is counted as a part of the three-dose vaccine series for infants greater than 2 kg at birth but not for those weighing less than 2 kg at birth (48). The HBV vaccine alone is 75% to 95% effective in preventing perinatal HBV transmission when administered within 24 hours of birth. Treatment with HBIG in conjunction with the complete HBV vaccine series given over the first 6 months of life has decreased perinatal infection rates to 0.7% to 1.1% in the United States.

All infants whose mothers' HBV status is unknown at time of delivery should receive the HBV vaccine within 12 hours of birth. For infants weighing less than 2 kg, HBIG should also be given within the first 12 hours unless the maternal HBV status can be confirmed as negative. For infants weighing 2 kg or greater, HBIG can be delayed as long as 7 days while the HBV status of the mother is confirmed (49). After completing a three or four dose HBV vaccine series, infants born to mothers who are HBV positive or unknown should undergo postvaccination serologic testing (48).

HBV-positive mothers may breastfeed provided the infant received appropriate HBV prophylaxis after birth. There is insufficient evidence to recommend for or against breast-feeding by mothers who are HBV or hepatitis C virus positive when they have cracked or bleeding nipples. In these cases, it may be of benefit to discontinue nursing and provide appropriate lactation support to maintain supply until the mother's nipples have healed (50).

ROUTINE NEWBORN TESTING

Screening for Hypoglycemia

Healthy newborns experience a physiologic decrease in blood glucose concentration after birth. This decline occurs over the first few hours after the umbilical cord is clamped and the continuous supply of glucose from the placenta stops. Consequent hormone release in response to the physiologic decrease in glucose, including an increase in glucagon and epinephrine, stimulates glycogenolysis resulting in increased blood glucose levels. Gluconeogenesis and fatty acid oxidation as mechanisms to increase glucose levels are less established in the neonate (51) (see Chapter 41). While most healthy term newborns undergo this process without difficulty, some infants are at increased risk for more severe or prolonged hypoglycemia. These infants require routine screening (52).

The AAP recommends regular glucose screening over the first 24 hours of life for all infants who are late preterm (LPT) (34 0/7 to 36 6/7 weeks GA), small for GA, large for GA, and infants of diabetic mothers (52). The Pediatric Endocrine Society (PES) recommends expanding screening criteria to include infants who experience perinatal stress such as a hypoxic/ischemic event or hypothermia, postterm delivery, have a family history of hypoglycemia, or congenital syndrome or abnormal physical features that may be associated with hypoglycemia (53). Additionally, both the AAP and PES recommend screening any infant that shows signs of possible symptomatic hypoglycemia including sweating, temperature instability, irritability, tremulousness, apnea, hypotonia, or seizure. Most institutions use a point-of-care device that rapidly results whole blood glucose concentrations. Because there can be up to a 15% difference between point-of-care and laboratory results, it is essential to send a confirmatory plasma sample if the point-of-care value is concerning (54).

As there is no clear consensus in the literature regarding specific glucose values or duration of hypoglycemia that is associated with neurologic injury, variation in acceptable levels exists within the United States and worldwide. In Canada and New Zealand, hypoglycemia is defined as a glucose less than 47 mg/dL (2.6 mmol/L) in the first 48 to 72 hours (55). According to AAP guidelines, the goal prefeed glucose level is at least 40 mg/dL (2.2 mmol/L) in the first 4 hours of life and at least 45 mg/dL

(2.5 mmol/L) from 4 to 24 hours of age. The PES recommends blood glucose values greater than 50 mg/dL (2.8 mmol/L) for the first 48 hours and greater than 60 mg/dL (3.3 mmol/L) after that time. Any symptomatic infant, regardless of risk factors, should be screened at the time symptoms are noted (53,53).

Newborn Metabolic Screening

Screening newborns for metabolic disorders was first introduced in the early 1960s when Guthrie and Susi performed a study on 400,000 newborns in 29 states testing an inexpensive and reliable method of identifying phenylketonuria (56). As states adopted universal screening programs, additional disorders such as congenital hypothyroidism, congenital adrenal hyperplasia and galactosemia were added based on criteria published by Wilson and Jungner (57). These principles stress that included conditions should be important health problems with a latent or early symptomatic stage and an acceptable treatment available (58,59).

With the advent of tandem mass spectrometry in the 1990s, it became possible to test for many metabolites, and therefore many diseases, using a single drop of blood (57). The result was an increase in the average number of metabolic conditions being screened from around 7 in 1995 to 27 in 2006. In 2005, the American College of Medical Genetics (ACMG) recommended new minimal criteria for inclusion of a new disorder in newborn screening: identifiable at 24 to 48 hours after birth when it would not ordinarily be detected clinically, an available test with appropriate sensitivity and specificity, and demonstrated benefit of early detection and intervention with an efficacious treatment. Per these standards, ACMG released practice guidelines recommending that all states screen for 29 specific "primary" disorders. An additional 25 optional "secondary" disorders meeting the inclusion criteria were also identified. As of 2018, this list had expanded to 35 primary disorders and 26 secondary disorders. The ACMG list remains a recommendation only, with states independently deciding which conditions to include on their screens. Currently, all states are screening for the original 29 recommended disorders with an overall range of 31 to 71 conditions tested per state. The newborn metabolic screen is obtained from a heel stick and collected on filter paper between 24 and 48 hours of life, allowing for timely results while minimizing false-positive or false-negative outcomes (59–61) (**Fig. 18.1**).

With expanded newborn screening comes challenges. Many of the conditions assessed are rare with incidence rates of 1 in 100,000 or fewer. False-positive rates can be significant, mandating the expense of further testing and causing additional parental concern. Furthermore, primary care physicians faced with positive screening results may have limited knowledge of the condition and may be unable to counsel parents adequately. To meet this need, the ACMG has developed a web-based resource called action (ACT) sheets. For each disorder tested, ACT sheets provide clinicians and families with a focused summary of the condition, additional diagnostic evaluations to be performed, and reporting requirements (62).

Critical Congenital Heart Disease (CHHD) Screening

Significant congenital heart disease (CHD) affects about 8 per 1,000 live births; 2 per 1,000 newborn infants will have critical congenital heart disease (CCHD), defined as lesions requiring intervention within the first month of life. These conditions, including hypoplastic left heart syndrome, pulmonary atresia, Tetralogy of Fallot, total anomalous pulmonary venous return, transposition of the great arteries, truncus arteriosus, tricuspid atresia, interrupted aortic arch, and critical coarctation, may cause hypoxia upon closure of the ductus arteriosus, resulting in significant morbidity and mortality. Most of these infants will appear well at birth. Only about half of cases are detected by prenatal testing, and without pulse oximetry screening, up to 30% of infants with CCHD could be discharged from the nursery undiagnosed (63). Although these infants may be asymptomatic, their oxygen saturation is usually

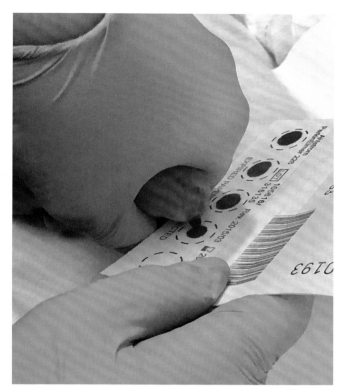

FIGURE 18.1 Newborn metabolic screen sampling. (Reprinted from Ramasethu J, Seo S. *MacDonald's atlas of procedures in neonatology*, 6th ed. Philadelphia, PA: Wolters Kluwer, 2019.)

sufficiently lower than normal to allow detection by pulse oximetry screening. Pulse oximetry is a quick, painless, and cost-effective procedure with an estimated 33% decrease in CCHD-related mortality attributed to the widespread adoption of universal screening (64).

CCHD screening involves obtaining the oxygen saturation in a newborn's right hand and one foot using a motion-tolerant, validated sensor. Details of screening algorithms vary among nations and regions, although all are similar. The United States Department of Health and Human Services and the AAP have recommended universal screening since 2011. Per this guideline, an infant must have an oxygen saturation of at least 95% in either extremity with not more than a three-point difference in saturation between the two measurements to pass. Any saturation of 89% or less is a failed test requiring further evaluation. If the oxygen saturation is between 90% and 94% for measurements in both extremities, or if there is a 3% or greater absolute difference between the two measurements, the test may be repeated up to twice. After three attempts, the test is failed and the infant requires further evaluation (65). Some have suggested modifying this algorithm to evaluate infants after just two failed screening attempts (66). Sweden has similar guidelines to the AAP guideline above, except that any saturation of 90% is considered a failed test (67). In the United Kingdom, there is currently no national recommendation for CCHD screening, but an oxygen saturation of <95% in either extremity, or a difference between the limbs of more than 2% on two repeated occasions, is considered a failed test (68). A European consensus statement published in 2017 recommended CCHD screening be performed in all European countries using either the Swedish or United Kingdom algorithms (69). Any failed screening prompts follow-up echocardiography, preferably with consultation by a pediatric cardiologist (65,69).

The optimal timing for CCHD testing varies among the different guidelines. To decrease the frequency of false-positive results, the United States recommends testing well newborns on day of life 2 after at least 24 hours of life, except in cases of earlier discharge home. The European consensus statement recommends testing after 6 hours of life but before 24 hours on the expectation that 50% of newborns with CCHD could become symptomatic at less than 24 hours of life. With any of the standard algorithms, false-positive rates tend to be low, ranging from 0.04% to 0.8% (63,66,68). There are fewer false positives when the infant is alert during testing (65). Evaluation following false-positive tests often reveals other significant conditions causing hypoxia including pulmonary hypertension, infection, or other non–duct-dependent heart lesions. Studies have consistently found that 30% to 45% of infants with false-positive CCHD screens have an etiology identified other than CCHD, many requiring additional ICU-level care (66,67).

CCHD screening costs about $5 to $10 USD per infant and takes about 10 minutes including testing, paperwork, and counseling time (65,70). Pulse oximetry is not a perfect test, especially for detecting lesions such as aortic arch obstructions (66,67). Sensitivity is about 75% overall, or 58% to 66% among those cases not detected antenatally (63,67,68). Careful physical examination remains an important component in the detection of CHD. Findings such as poor perfusion, decreased lower extremity pulses, murmur, or tachypnea warrant further investigation. Together, pulse oximetry screening plus a good physical examination can increase CCHD detection rates in the newborn to 90% to 96% (67,69).

Newborn Hearing Screen

The WHO reports that 466 million people worldwide suffer from disabling hearing loss, 34 million of whom are children. The prevalence of congenital or early-onset permanent hearing loss varies by country and has been reported as 0.5 to 5 per 1,000 live births with the highest numbers reported in South Asia and sub-Saharan Africa. Recent data from Nigeria suggest a prevalence as high as 28 per 1,000 live births for all degrees of sensorineural hearing impairment. Globally, about 60% of childhood hearing loss is related to preventable causes including congenital infections, ear infections, prematurity, and lack of access to maternal and child health care among others (71). It is imperative to diagnose and treat hearing loss early because children with hearing impairment can have increased difficulty with both verbal and nonverbal communication, lower educational attainment, and are more likely to have behavioral problems and poorer psychosocial well-being (72).

Universal newborn hearing screening (UNHS) was officially recommended in the United States in 1993 and current guidelines have been in place since 2008, endorsed by both the AAP and United States Preventative Services Task Force. Hearing loss affects 0.1% to 0.3% of newborns annually in the United States with only 50% of these infants having an identifiable risk factor for hearing loss. This makes UNHS critical to maximize early detection. It is recommended that all infants undergo hearing screening by 1 month of age. Infants who do not pass this screen are referred for medical evaluation and audiologic testing by 3 months of age and are enrolled in intervention services by 6 months of age. These UNHS guidelines have resulted in more rapid diagnosis and treatment of hearing loss and improved receptive vocabulary (72,73).

Screening is performed with a one- or two-step protocol using otoacoustic emissions (OAE) or auditory brainstem response (ABR) testing. OAE testing evaluates cochlear function by placing small microphones in the external auditory canal to detect sound produced by the cochlea, either spontaneously or evoked with stimuli (**Fig. 18.2**), while the ABR uses scalp electrodes to evaluate the entire auditory pathway (**Fig. 18.3**). Many institutions use a two-step screening process with an initial OAE screen followed by an ABR screen in newborns who fail OAE testing (71). Although the OAE screen is easier to perform, results can be impacted by debris in the external ear canal. The ABR test is more time consuming but is the only way to evaluate for auditory neuropathy (74). This two-step screening approach has a 92% sensitivity and nearly 99% specificity in detecting hearing loss. It is estimated,

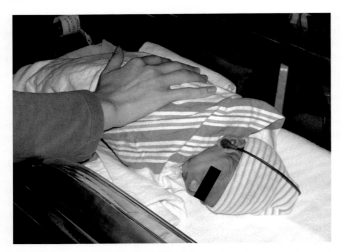

FIGURE 18.2 Infant undergoing OAE screening. (Reprinted from Ramasethu J, Seo S. *MacDonald's atlas of procedures in neonatology*, 6th ed. Philadelphia, PA: Wolters Kluwer, 2019.)

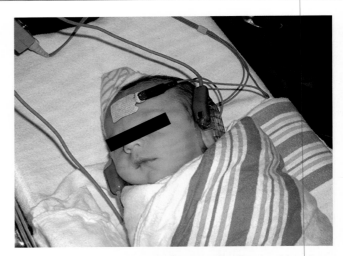

FIGURE 18.3 Infant undergoing AABR screening. (Reprinted from Ramasethu J, Seo S. *MacDonald's atlas of procedures in neonatology*, 6th ed. Philadelphia, PA: Wolters Kluwer, 2019.)

however, that 22% to 33% of infants who fail the OAE screen but pass the ABR screen are later diagnosed with some degree of hearing loss (72,74,75).

Screening for Jaundice

Approximately 60% of full-term and 80% of preterm newborns worldwide develop jaundice due to hyperbilirubinemia (76) (see Chapter 45). In rare cases, significant elevations in bilirubin can lead to acute bilirubin encephalopathy which can result in kernicterus, or life-long neurologic sequelae of bilirubin toxicity. Therefore, it is important to assess all newborn infants for the risk of developing significant hyperbilirubinemia. This assessment should consist of both clinical risk factors and bilirubin measurement. Factors that increase the risk of jaundice include decreased GA (<38 weeks), presence of significant bruising or cephalohematoma, ABO incompatibility, positive direct antiglobulin test (DAT), formerly known as the Direct Coombs test, hemolytic disease, East Asian race, exclusive breast-feeding, and previous sibling with jaundice (77,78). Clinical jaundice present at less than 24 hours of life requires evaluation (79). Because visual estimation alone is unreliable and may lead to errors, every infant should have a transcutaneous (TcB) or total serum (TSB) bilirubin performed prior to hospital discharge (77,78).

TcB measurements should be obtained on the infant's forehead or sternum (**Figs 18.4 and 18.5**). TcB values above 15 mg/dL may not be accurate, possibly underestimating the serum bilirubin level. The AAP recommends obtaining a confirmatory TSB if the TcB value is 70% of the serum bilirubin threshold for phototherapy. All TcB and TSB levels should be plotted on standard nomograms based on the hour of life that the test was performed to determine the risk of hyperbilirubinemia and need for phototherapy (77,79).

Infant Car Seats and Car Seat Challenge Testing

Infants should be discharged home in an appropriate car seat for their size, rear-facing, in the back seat of the vehicle, with well-fitted harness straps and secure attachment of the car seat to the vehicle at the correct angle. When used properly, car seats can decrease infant deaths in passenger motor vehicle accidents by 71% (80). The rear-facing position provides the best support for the head, neck, torso, and pelvis in a head-on collision, distributing forces over the child's full body and decreasing the risk of injury. Since 2018, the AAP has recommended that infants stay rear-facing as long as possible until they reach the height and weight allowed by the manufacturer of the car seat (81). The safest place for any child is in the backseat of the vehicle. Infants should never be in the front seat of

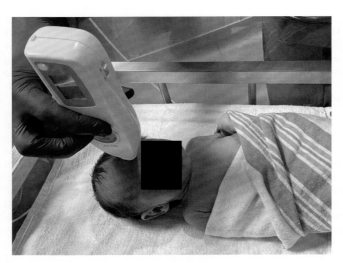

FIGURE 18.4 Transcutaneous bilirubin measurement on the forehead.

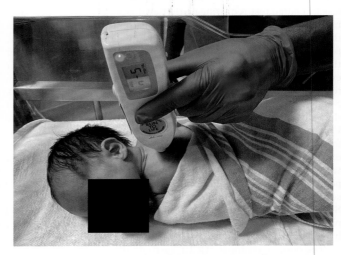

FIGURE 18.5 Transcutaneous bilirubin measurement on the sternum.

a vehicle that has an air bag as air bag deployment itself can itself cause injury. Products should be used with a car seat only if they are approved by the car seat's manufacturer, and infants should never be left unattended in a car (80).

Hospitals should educate parents about proper car seat use prior to discharge, including correct positioning of the infant in the car seat. Improper use of the car seat can decrease its effectiveness. Families should also be counseled that car seats are to be used only for travel and that the infant should be removed from the car seat when travel is complete. Infants can develop worsening gastroesophageal reflux and increased cardiorespiratory events in a car seat as well as plagiocephaly with prolonged use. Furthermore, 8,000 infants per year in the United States are evaluated in emergency departments for car seat related injuries not related to motor vehicle accidents. Most involve infants falling out of a car seat or falling in a car seat that was placed on a counter, ledge, or other height (81).

Preterm infants have immature physiology and are at increased risk of apnea, bradycardia, and/or desaturation when slightly upright position in a car seat. The AAP recommends that an infant car seat challenge be performed prior to discharge for all premature infants (<37 weeks GA) as well as for other at-risk infants like those who have hypotonia, micrognathia, or are recovering from congenital heart surgery (80). For this testing, a newborn's heart rate and oxygen level are monitored while the infant is positioned correctly in its own car seat at the proper incline for at least 90 to 120 minutes (or longer for infants with additional travel time to home). Infants who are unable to tolerate the upright position of a car seat might require discharge in a car bed. Similarly, these infants could be at risk in other upright equipment such as infant swings, bouncer chairs, or infant carriers (80). The car seat challenge is also a test of cardiorespiratory maturity in LPT infants. Providers have found underlying morbidities or diagnoses in some infants who fail the car seat challenge. In one study of LPT infants who failed their car test challenge more than once, 40% actually required home oxygen for safe discharge (82).

Most countries in North America and Europe have similar regulations for placing infants in the back seat of the vehicle in a rear-facing car seat, but not all experts agree on the utility of car seat tolerance screening for premature infants. A 2006 Cochrane review concluded that "additional studies are needed to determine if the car seat test accurately predicts the risk of clinically significant adverse events in preterm infants traveling in car seats." (83) In 2016, after reviewing the available medical literature, the Canadian Paediatric Society withdrew their recommendation for predischarge car seat challenge testing for premature infants (84). Car seat challenge testing is not uniformly practiced in the United Kingdom, but experts have recommended that providers should advise parents on correct use the car seat at hospital discharge (85).

▌NEWBORN MALE CIRCUMCISION

Circumcision is the removal of the foreskin (or prepuce) from the penis. It has been performed since ancient times and often has religious or cultural significance, especially in Muslim and Jewish populations. It is the most common surgical procedure in pediatric patients with about 1.4 million circumcisions performed annually in the United States alone. Ninety-three percent of all circumcisions in the United States are performed in the newborn period, which is also when the procedure has the lowest risk of complications and the greatest accumulated benefit (86,87).

Circumcisions should be performed only in stable, healthy patients by trained medical or nonmedical professionals under sterile conditions. Operative methods used for circumcisions include the Gomco clamp, the Plastibell device, and the Mogen clamp. These devices carry similar complication and revision rates, so the method used is left to practitioner preference (13,86). Adequate analgesia should be provided during the procedure. Dorsal penile nerve blocks or ring blocks provide the

most safe and effective pain control. Topical analgesics, including 4% lidocaine or lidocaine–prilocaine creams, are somewhat less effective in controlling pain and should not be used in premature or low birth weight infants as they can cause skin irritation such as erythema, blistering, and swelling in these populations. Nonpharmacologic measures like positioning, swaddling, sucrose, and pacifiers can be helpful adjuncts, but alone they are inadequate for proper pain management during circumcision (1,86). Use of general anesthesia in conjunction with a local anesthetic is suggested for circumcisions performed after the newborn period (86).

Adverse event rates with newborn circumcision are low with estimates of about 0.2% for minor adverse events and 0.005% for severe adverse events (13,86,87). The most frequent complication is bleeding, which is typically mild. Other complications include infection or the removal of an imperfect amount of tissue. About 0.2% of circumcisions have later correctional procedures, most cosmesis related for incomplete removal of foreskin or for the development of adhesions or skin bridges (87,88). Successful treatment of adhesions with clobetasol, a topical steroid, has also been described (88). Rare complications of circumcision include meatal stenosis, stricture, sepsis, urinary retention, scarring, urethral cutaneous fistula, suture sinus tract, epithelial inclusion cyst, partial or complete amputation, and degloving (86–88). Three deaths related to circumcision have been reported over a period of 35 years for a rate of 0.08 per million newborn male circumcisions. Complication rates are several fold higher when circumcision is performed outside of the newborn period or in infants with minor genitourinary anomalies (87).

The health benefits to circumcision include a reduced incidence of urinary tract infections (UTIs) and decreased transmission of sexually transmitted diseases. UTIs are most prevalent in boys in their first year of life and are more common in male infants diagnosed with hydronephrosis. Newborn circumcision decreases the risk of UTI three- to tenfold (86,89). Circumcision also decreases the transmission of several sexually transmitted diseases. There is an estimated 40% to 60% protective effect of circumcision against heterosexual acquisition of HIV in men in areas with a high prevalence of the disease. The WHO has stated that "urgent consideration must be given to the need to provide increased access to safe, affordable male circumcision services on a large scale, embedded within a comprehensive package of proven HIV prevention measures." (90) Male circumcision is associated with a 28% to 34% reduction in HSV2 acquisition and a 30% to 40% reduction in HPV acquisition. There is also a protective effect of male circumcision on male to female transmission of the higher risk forms of HPV. While circumcision does not decrease the risk of chlamydia or gonorrhea infection, evidence suggests that it protects men from acquiring syphilis. Circumcised males also have a lower risk of penile cancer. Circumcision has no adverse effect on sexual function or sensitivity (86).

There are several contraindications to circumcision during the newborn hospitalization. Circumcision should not be performed in infants with a family history of a bleeding disorder and might need to be delayed in premature or low birth weight infants for small penile size at the time of hospital discharge. Infants with congenital penile malformations including epispadias, hypospadias, chordee, penoscrotal fusion or foreshortened penile ventral skin, penile torsion of more than 60 degrees, buried penis, or micropenis (<1.9 cm stretched penile length) should be referred to a urologist prior to circumcision given the significantly increased rate of circumcision revision procedures in males with minor genitourinary anomalies. Providers should perform a careful examination as minor penile anomalies are quite common. For example, from 2002 to 2012, hypospadias was reported in almost 1 of every 150 male births in the United States (91).

There is wide geographic variability in the frequency with which circumcisions are performed, and recommendations for or against this procedure are quite divergent. The 2012 AAP policy statement on circumcision concluded that "the health benefits of circumcision outweigh the risks." The AAP noted that while there is not enough benefit to recommend routine circumcision, parents should receive unbiased information early in pregnancy to assist them in making an informed decision and health insurance companies should cover the cost of the procedure (92). Conversely, the British and Royal Dutch Medical Associations discourage nontherapeutic male circumcisions, while the Danish Medical Association proposes that the procedure should only be performed with the informed consent of the person himself (93). Overall, the WHO estimates that 30% of males in the world older than age 15 have been circumcised. Two-third of these are Muslim; less than 1% are Jewish; and 13% are non-Muslim, non-Jewish men in the United States, where the circumcision rate is about 55% to 60% (86,90).

The AAP recommends that whether or not a newborn is circumcised, parents should be taught to wash the genital area gently when bathing the infant. Following a circumcision, the area should be kept clean. Petroleum jelly should be applied either to the glans of the penis or to the diaper for 4 to 7 days following the circumcision to prevent adhesion and subsequent irritation or bleeding. The foreskin of an uncircumcised male should not be forcibly retracted. Any adhesions present usually resolve by 2 to 4 months of age (1).

INITIAL HOSPITAL DISCHARGE AND FOLLOW-UP CARE

The WHO recommends at least a 24-hour stay in a care facility following an uncomplicated vaginal delivery, while federal law in the United States mandates that insurance companies cover hospitalizations of at least 48 hours for vaginal deliveries and 96 hours for cesarean sections (2,94). Actual lengths of stay after delivery vary significantly, with one study that compared 92 low- and middle-income countries finding average lengths of stay ranging from 0.5 to 6.2 days for vaginal deliveries and 2.5 to 9.3 days for cesarean sections (95). Ideally, the newborn and mother should be discharged together when both are medically stable, risks of evolving problems have been addressed, the family is able to provide care, and adequate follow-up is in place (13,94).

The AAP recommends that a physician or licensed health provider perform a complete physical examination within 24 hours prior to the newborn's hospital discharge. Infants are deemed to be medically stable for discharge when normal vital signs have been documented for at least 12 hours prior including temperature between 36.5°C and 37.4°C, respiratory rates less than 60, and heart rates between 100 and 190 while awake with good perfusion. (Heart rates dipping as low as 70 while sleeping in an otherwise stable newborn are acceptable.) The infant should have regular urine output, no excess bleeding from a circumcision site for 2 hours, spontaneous stooling, and at least two successful breast-feeding sessions. There should not be concerns for sepsis, and jaundice should be assessed with a follow-up plan in place as needed. Providers are advised to review all relevant lab work including the mother's HBV, HIV, and syphilis results and baby's blood type and Coombs testing. The infant should have received the first HBV vaccine, and the mother should be given the tetanus, diphtheria, acellular pertussis (Tdap), and influenza vaccines if needed. Clinicians should confirm that screening tests are completed including the newborn metabolic screen, CCHD screen, and hearing screen with follow-up arranged as needed. Education should be provided on signs of newborn illness, breastfeeding and its benefits, normal urine and stooling patterns, umbilical cord care, skin care, and circumcision care, newborn temperature measurement, jaundice, safe sleep, hand hygiene, and protection from tobacco exposure. Mothers should also receive instruction on proper swaddling with attention to keeping the infant's hips abducted rather than held in

extension. A car seat should be available for transportation home and parents should be educated about proper car seat use. Providers should ensure that any postdischarge follow-up required for either the mother or the newborn is arranged.

Clinicians should screen for high-risk home environments including presence of drug or alcohol abuse, domestic violence or child abuse, mental illness, homelessness, adolescent parents, lack of social supports, or barriers to good follow-up care. High-risk families might require additional supports to ensure safe discharge (94). Infants with chronic opioid exposure in utero should remain hospitalized to monitor for signs of withdrawal. The recommended time of observation ranges from 3 days for immediate-release opioid exposure to 5 to 7 days for exposure to sustained-release opioids like methadone.

The AAP recommends that infants discharged less than 48 hours after delivery should see their outpatient provider within 48 to 72 hours of discharge, while infants discharged later than 48 hours should follow-up within 3 to 5 days (96). The goal of this visit is to assess the newborn's weight, feeding history, voiding and stooling patterns, hydration status, jaundice, and overall health. Providers should review the infant's prenatal, perinatal, and postpartum history and identify any new problems. They should also provide routine anticipatory guidance and screen for postpartum depression, which can affect about 13% of mothers (97). In addition, the WHO recommends that breastfeeding counseling be incorporated into each postnatal contact (2).

Readmission after initial hospital discharge is not uncommon. In the United States, about 1% to 2% of healthy newborns are readmitted in the first 30 days after initial hospital discharge, most commonly due to feeding problems or jaundice. Appropriate and timely newborn outpatient follow-up has been associated with decreased early newborn readmission rates (96). In addition, a WHO review found an 18% decrease in neonatal mortality in low- and middle-income countries when community health workers performed additional home visits on days 1 and 3 of life and referred any newborns with concerning findings to a health facility (2). Parents should also be taught to recognize danger signs for which they should seek immediate care including rapid breathing or chest indrawing, lethargy, poor feeding, seizure, temperature instability, or jaundice of the palms and soles (2).

Safe Sleep and Tobacco Exposure

Sudden infant death syndrome (SIDS) is the sudden, unexplained death of an infant less than 1 year of age, most often occurring during sleep. Because of this, some people will refer to SIDS as "crib death." Sudden unexpected death in infancy (SUDI), or sudden unexpected infant death (SUID), includes deaths ascribed to SIDS in addition to sudden infant deaths that, after investigation, can be attributed to causes such as suffocation, asphyxia, entrapment, infection, ingestion, metabolic or cardiac disease, or trauma. There are about 3,500 sleep-related infant deaths annually in the United States including SIDS and accidental suffocation or strangulation (98). The majority of cases occur in the first 4 months of life (99).

The number of sleep-related infants' deaths declined about 40% in the United States in the 1990s following the AAPs Back to Sleep campaign (100). In 2016, the AAP published updated safe sleep guidelines. Their recommendations included having infants sleep in the supine position on a firm, infant-approved sleep surface without additional bedding or other soft objects nearby. They noted that breast-feeding, remaining up-to-date with vaccines, pacifier use with sleep, and having regular prenatal care are protective and should be encouraged. Use of tobacco, alcohol, or illicit drugs by caregivers increases an infant's risk of sleep-related death and should be avoided. Overheating and head covering should also be avoided (98).

The AAP guidelines point out that supine sleeping does not increase the risk of reflux, choking, or aspiration, even in infants with a history of gastroesophageal reflux, and that having the infant sleep at an incline could cause the infant to slide into an unsafe position. The sleep surface should be firm enough to maintain its shape. Home cardiorespiratory monitors should not be used routinely as they do not decrease the risk of SIDS. Sitting devices are not recommended for routine sleep. Furthermore, placing infants to sleep on couches or armchairs has been found to be extremely dangerous given the risk of suffocation or entrapment, so providers should counsel parents against this (98).

New to the 2016 AAP guidelines is the recommendation to have the infant's bed placed in the parents' room for at least 6 months, which facilitates feeding and monitoring and may decrease SIDS by as much as 50%. Conversely, bed-sharing, including the use of in-bed sleepers, is not recommended (98). Germany and Canada similarly advise against bed-sharing given the risks of suffocation or entrapment. On the other hand, the Academy of Breastfeeding Medicine argues that in absence of additional hazards such as the infant being placed prone, near soft bedding, on a sofa, or next to an adult who is a smoker or is impaired by alcohol or drugs, there is not a significant risk to bed-sharing. They highlight that since bed-sharing may be culturally valued, and since many breast-feeding women end up bed-sharing either intentionally or unintentionally, providers should discuss how to do this safely. The United Kingdom and Australia also suggest that providers have an open, judgment-free conversation with parents about bed-sharing, reviewing the hazards that would increase the risks of this practice. If parents choose to bed-share or "breast sleep," they should use a bed with a firm surface that is kept away from walls and furniture to avoid entrapment. The parent should sleep on his or her side curled around the infant for protection (101).

In the United States, experts estimate that 8% of infant deaths and 17% of SIDS cases are caused by tobacco smoke exposure. Tobacco smoke exposure increases the risk of stillbirth, preterm birth, low birth weight, congenital malformations, and sudden infant death. Children who are regularly in contact with tobacco smoke have higher risks of ear infections, wheezing, pneumonia, decreased lung function, and cancer. More than half of children in the United States are regularly exposed to tobacco smoke. Given this, the AAP recommends that pediatricians screen caregivers for tobacco dependence during well visits while providing counseling and facilitating treatment as needed (102,103).

▌LATE PRETERM INFANTS

Infants born between 34 0/7 and 36 6/7 weeks GA, known as late preterm (LPT) infants account for about 7% of births annually in the United States and about 70% of all preterm births (104). In an effort to emphasize the vulnerability of this population, an expert panel from a 2005 National Institute of Child Health and Human Development (NICHD) workshop recommended that providers use the name "late preterm" to describe these infants instead of "near-term." (105) Although LPT newborns can appear similar to full-term infants, and although they often receive care in the normal nursery alongside their term counterparts, these babies have immature physiology and metabolism resulting in amplified risks and special needs (106) (see Chapter 25).

LPT infants frequently require admission to a NICU, ranging from 88% of babies born at 34 weeks' GA to 25% of infants born at 36 weeks' GA. LPT infants are two to three times more likely to require an emergency room visit or readmission after hospital discharge (97). In one study, LPT infants had a readmission rate of 4.4% in the first 2 weeks after hospital discharge compared to 2.2% of term infants (107). The most common reasons for early readmission are jaundice, concern for infection, dehydration, and feeding difficulty. Risk factors included LPT infants who were first-born children, were breast-fed, were never admitted to the NICU, and those born to moms with a complicated delivery or postpartum course, on public insurance, or of Pacific Island descent (106,107).

Rehospitalization rates for LPT infants remain higher than their term counterparts between 2 weeks and 6 months of life with rates of 6.8% to 9.1% in LPT babies compared to 3.1% to 5.6% in term infants (107). Others have found a 15% rate of rehospitalization in the first year of life among LPT infants. In addition, mothers of LPT infants are less likely to initiate breast-feeding or to continue breast-feeding for more than 10 weeks, they are more likely to be smoking 10 or more weeks after delivery, and they are less likely to position their infants' supine for sleep, further increasing the risks of this population (108).

Parental education and close provider follow-up have the potential to mitigate some of these risks. Early discharge is discouraged as the AAP notes that LPT infants are unlikely to achieve all the criteria for newborn hospital discharge prior to 48 hours of life. The AAP also recommends that these infants be followed in the outpatient setting within 24 to 48 hours of hospital discharge (1,108). Arranging for a postdischarge follow-up appointment, either at home or in an outpatient clinic, within 72 hours of hospital discharge has been associated with decreased rates of hospital readmission for LPT newborns (106). Additional instruction and support for mothers of LPT infants including increased assistance with breast-feeding as well as extra education on topics such as jaundice, hydration status, back-to-sleep, and tobacco exposure risks could further help support this vulnerable population (106,108). Finally, attention to the long-term developmental follow-up needs of these infants is warranted.

REFERENCES

1. Kilpatrick SJ, Papile L, Macones GA, eds. *Guidelines for perinatal care*, 8th ed. Elk Grove Village, IL/Washington, DC: American Academy of Pediatrics/the American College of Obstetricians and Gynecologists, 2017.
2. World Health Organization. *WHO recommendations on postnatal care of the mother and newborn*. Geneva, Switzerland: World Health Organization, 2014.
3. Feldman-Winter L, Goldsmith JP; Committee on Fetus and Newborn; Task Force on Sudden Infant Death Syndrome. Safe sleep and skin-to-skin care in the neonatal period for healthy term newborns. *Pediatrics* 2016;138(3):e20161889.
4. World Health Organization, Maternal and Newborn Health/Safe Motherhood. *Thermal protection of the newborn: a practical guide*. Geneva, Switzerland: World Health Organization, 1997.
5. Ringer, SA. Core concepts: thermoregulation in the newborn part I: basic mechanisms. *NeoReviews* 2013;14(4):e161.
6. World Health Organization. *WHO recommendations on newborn health: guidelines approved by the WHO Guidelines Review Committee*. Geneva, Switzerland: World Health Organization, 2017.
7. Stothers JK. Head insulation and heat loss in the newborn. *Arch Dis Child* 1981;56(7):530.
8. Ringer, SA. Core concepts: thermoregulation in the newborn, Part II: prevention of aberrant body temperature. *NeoReviews* 2013;14(5):e221.
9. Chondronikola M. The role of brown adipose tissue and the thermogenic adipocytes in glucose metabolism: recent advances and open questions. *Curr Opin Clin Nutr Metab Care* 2020;23(4):282.
10. World Health Organization Dept. of Reproductive Health and Research, United Nations Population Fund, UNICEF. *WHO Managing newborn problems: a guide for doctors, nurses, and midwives*. Geneva, Switzerland: World Health Organization, 2003.
11. American Academy of Pediatrics Section on Breastfeeding. Breastfeeding and the use of human milk. *Pediatrics* 2012;129(3):e827.
12. World Health Organization, UNICEF. *Global strategy for infant and young child feeding*. Geneva, Switzerland: World Health Organization, 2003.
13. Barkemeyer BM. Discharge Planning. *Pediatr Clin North Am* 2015;62(2):545.
14. Wagner CL, Greer FR; American Academy of Pediatrics Section on Breastfeeding; American Academy of Pediatrics Committee on Nutrition. Prevention of rickets and vitamin D deficiency in infants, children, and adolescents. *Pediatrics* 2008;122(5):1142.
15. United Kingdom Scientific Advisory Committee on Nutrition: Working Group on Vitamin D. *Vitamin D and health*. Report available on the Scientific Advisory Committee on Nutrition (SACN) website. Available from: https://assets.publishing.service.gov.uk/government/uploads/system/uploads/attachment_data/file/537616/SACN_Vitamin_D_and_Health_report.pdf. Updated July 2016. Accessed on July 18, 2020.

16. Flaherman VJ, Schaefer EW, Kuzniewicz MW, et al. Early weight loss nomograms for exclusively breastfed newborns. *Pediatrics* 2015;135(1):e16.
17. Paul IM, Schaefer EW, Miller JR, et al. Weight change nomograms for the first month after birth. *Pediatrics* 2016;138(6):e20162625.
18. Blume-Peytavi U, Lavender T, Jenerowicz D, et al. Recommendations from a European roundtable meeting on best practice healthy infant skin care. *Pediatr Dermatol* 2016;33(3):311.
19. Johnson E, Hunt R. Infant skin care: updates and recommendations. *Curr Opin Pediatr* 2019;31(4):476.
20. Bryanton J, Walsh D, Barrett M, et al. Tub bathing versus traditional sponge bathing for the newborn. *J Obstet Gynecol Neonatal Nurs* 2004;33(6):704.
21. Loring C, Gregory K, Gargan B, et al. Tub bathing improves thermoregulation of the late preterm infant. *J Obstet Gynecol Neonatal Nurs* 2012;41(2):171.
22. Renesme L, Allen A, Audeoud F, et al. Recommendation for hygiene and topical in neonatology from the French Neonatal Society. *Eur J Pediatr* 2019;178(10):1545.
23. Horimukai K, Morita K, Narita M, et al. Application of moisturizer to neonates prevents development of atopic dermatitis. *J Allergy Clin Immunol* 2014;134(4):824.
24. Simpson EL, Chalmers JR, Hanifin JM, et al. Emollient enhancement of the skin barrier from birth offers effective atopic dermatitis prevention. *J Allergy Clin Immunol* 2014;134(4):818.
25. Stewart D, Benitz W; Committee on Fetus and Newborn. Umbilical cord care in the newborn infant. *Pediatrics* 2016;138(3):e20162149.
26. Gras-Le Guen C, Caille A, Launay E, et al. Dry care versus antiseptics for umbilical cord care: a cluster randomized trial. *Pediatrics* 2017;139(1):e20161857.
27. Lo´pez-MedinaI MD, Lo´pez-AraqueI AB, Linares-Abad M, et al. Umbilical cord separation time, predictors and healing complications in newborns with dry care. PLoS One 2020;15(1):e0227209.
28. Semrau KEA, Herlihy J, Grogan C, et al. Effectiveness of 4% chlorhexidine cord care on neonatal mortality in Southern Province, Zambia (ZamCAT): a cluster-randomised controlled trial. *Lancet Glob Health* 2016;4(11):e827.
29. Sazawal S, Dhingra U, Ali SM, et al. Efficacy of chlorhexidine application to umbilical cord on neonatal mortality in Pemba, Tanzania: a community-based randomised controlled trial. *Lancet Glob Health* 2016;4(11):e837.
30. Thanathanee O, O'Brien TP. Conjunctivitis: systematic approach to diagnosis and therapy. *Curr Infect Dis Rep* 2011;13(2):141.
31. Curry SJ, Krist AH, Owens DK, et al. Ocular prophylaxis for gonococcal ophthalmia neonatorum: US Preventive Services Task Force reaffirmation recommendation statement. *JAMA* 2019;321:394.
32. Moore DL, MacDonald NE; Canadian Paediatric Society, Infectious Diseases and Immunization Committee. Preventing ophthalmia neonatorum. *Can J Infect Dis Med Microbiol* 2015;26(3):122.
33. World Health Organization. *WHO guidelines for the treatment of Neisseria gonorrhoeae*. Geneva, Switzerland: World Health Organization, 2016.
34. Wilson CB, Nizet V, Maldonado Y, et al., eds. *Remington and Klein's infectious diseases of the fetus and newborn infant*, 8th ed. Philadelphia, PA: Elsevier Saunders Health Sciences, 2015.
35. Darling E, McDonald H. A meta-analysis of the efficacy of ocular prophylactic agents used for the prevention of gonococcal and chlamydial ophthalmia neonatorum. *J Midwifery Womens Health* 2010;55(4):319.
36. Centers for Disease Control and Prevention. *Sexually transmitted disease surveillance 2017*. Atlanta: U.S. Department of Health and Human Services, 2018.
37. Majid A, Blackwell M, Broadbent RS, et al. Newborn vitamin K prophylaxis: a historical perspective to understand modern barriers to uptake. *Hosp Pediatr* 2019;9(1):55.
38. Puckett RM, Offringa M. Prophylactic vitamin K for vitamin K deficiency bleeding in neonates. *Cochrane Database Syst Rev* 2000;(4):CD002776.
39. Burke C. Vitamin K deficiency bleeding: overview and considerations. *J Pediatr Health Care* 2013;27(3):215.
40. Ng G, Lowey, AD. Position statement: guidelines for vitamin K prophylaxis in newborns: a joint statement of the Canadian Paediatric Society and the College of Family Physicians of Canada. *Can Fam Physician* 2018;64(10):736.
41. American Academy of Pediatrics Committee on Fetus and Newborn. Controversies concerning vitamin K and the newborn. *Pediatrics* 2003; 112(1 Pt 1):191.
42. American Academy of Pediatrics. Vitamin K compounds and the water-soluble analogues: use in therapy and prophylaxis in pediatrics. *Pediatrics* 1961;28:501.
43. Golding J, Paterson M, Kinlen LJ, et al. Factors associated with childhood cancer in a national cohort study. *Br J Cancer* 1990;62:304.
44. Golding J, Greenwood R, Birmingham K, et al. Childhood cancer, intramuscular vitamin K, and pethidine given during labour. *BMJ* 1992;305:341.
45. World Health Organization. *Global hepatitis report, 2017*. Geneva, Switzerland: World Health Organization, 2017.
46. US Preventive Services Task Force; Owens DK, Davidson KW, et al. Screening for hepatitis B virus infection in pregnant women US Preventive Services Task Force Reaffirmation Recommendation Statement. *JAMA* 2019;322(4):349.
47. Henderson JT, Webber EM, Bean SI. Screening for hepatitis B infection in pregnant women: updated evidence report and systematic review for the US Preventive Services Task Force. *JAMA* 2019;322(4):360.
48. Schillie S, Vellozzi C, Reingold A, Harris A, et al. Prevention of hepatitis B virus infection in the United States: recommendations of the Advisory Committee on Immunization Practices. *MMWR Recomm Rep* 2018;67(1):1.
49. American Academy of Pediatrics Committee on Infectious Diseases and Committee on Fetus and Newborn. Elimination of perinatal hepatitis B: providing the first vaccine dose within 24 hours of birth. *Pediatrics* 2017;140(3):e20171870.
50. Centers for Disease Control and Prevention (CDC). *Hepatitis B or C infections*. CDC. Available from: https://www.cdc.gov/breastfeeding/breast-feeding-special-circumstances/maternal-or-infant-illnesses/hepatitis.html. Updated January 24, 2018. Accessed January 18, 2020.
51. Tas E, Garibaldi L, Muzumdar R. Glucose homeostasis in newborns: an endocrinology perspective. *NeoReviews* 2020;21(1):e14.
52. Committee on Fetus and Newborn; Adamkin DH. Postnatal glucose homeostasis in late-preterm and term infants. *Pediatrics* 2011;127:575.
53. Thornton PS, Stanley CA, De Leon DD, et al. Recommendations from the Pediatric Endocrine Society for evaluation and management of persistent hypoglycemia in neonates, infants, and children. *J Pediatr* 2015;167:238.
54. Thompson-Branch A, Havranek T. Neonatal hypoglycemia. *Pediatr Rev* 2017;38:147.
55. Narvey MR, Marks SD. The screening and management of newborns at risk for low blood glucose. *Paediatr Child Health* 2019;24:536.
56. Guthrie R, Susi A. A simple phenylalanine method for detecting phenylketonuria in large populations of newborn infants. *Pediatrics* 1963;32:338.
57. Tarini, B. The current revolution in newborn screening: new technology, old controversies. *Arch Pediatr Adolesc Med* 2007;161:767.
58. Wilson JMG, Jungner G. *Public health papers no. 34: principles and practice of screening for disease*. Geneva, Switzerland: World Health Organization, 1966.
59. El-Hattab AW, Almannai M, Sutton VR. Newborn screening: history, current status, and future directions. *Pediatr Clin North Am* 2018;65:389.
60. Forman J, Coyle F, Levy-Fisch J, et al. Screening criteria: the need to deal with new developments and ethical issues in newborn metabolic screening. *J Community Genet* 2012;4:59.
61. Fabie N, Pappas K, Feldman G. The Current State of Newborn Screening in the United States. *Pediatr Clin North Am* 2019;66(2):369.
62. American Academy of Pediatrics Newborn Screening Authoring Committee. Newborn screening expands: recommendations for pediatricians and medical homes—implications for the system. *Pediatrics* 2008;121(1):192.
63. Plana MN, Zamora J, Suresh G, et al. Pulse oximetry screening for critical congenital heart defects. *Cochrane Database Syst Rev* 2018;3:CD011912.
64. Abouk R, Grosse SD, Ailes EC, et al. Association of US State implementation of newborn screening policies for critical congenital heart disease with early infant cardiac deaths. *JAMA* 2017;318(21):2111.
65. Kemper AR, Mahle WT, Martin GR, et al. Strategies for implementing screening for critical congenital heart disease. *Pediatrics* 2011;128(5):e1259.
66. Diller CL, Kelleman MS, Kupke KG, et al. A modified algorithm for critical congenital heart disease screening using pulse oximetry. *Pediatrics* 2018;141(5):e20174065.
67. de-Wahl Granelli A, Wennergren M, Sandberg K, et al. Impact of pulse oximetry screening on the detection of duct dependent congenital heart disease: a Swedish prospective screening study in 39,821 newborns. *BMJ* 2009;338:a3037.
68. Ewer AK, Middleton LJ, Furmston AT, et al. Pulse oximetry screening for congenital heart defects in newborn infants (PulseOx): a test accuracy study. *Lancet* 2011;378(9793):785.
69. Manzoni P, Martin GR, Sanchez Luna M, et al. Pulse oximetry screening for critical congenital heart defects: a European consensus statement. *Lancet Child Adolesc Health* 2017;1(2):88.
70. Grosse SD, Peterson C, Abouk R, et al. Cost and cost-effectiveness assessments of newborn screening for critical congenital heart disease using pulse oximetry: a review. *Int J Neonatal Screen* 2017;3(4):34.
71. World Health Organization. *Childhood hearing loss: strategies for prevention and care*. Geneva, Switzerland: World Health Organization, 2016.
72. American Academy of Pediatrics, Joint Committee on Infant Hearing. Year 2007 position statement: principles and guidelines for early hearing detection and intervention programs. *Pediatrics* 2007;120(4):898.
73. Wake M, Ching TYC, Wirth K, et al. Population outcomes of three approaches to detection of congenital hearing loss. *Pediatrics* 2016;137(1):1.
74. Dedhia K, Graham E, Park A. Hearing loss and failed newborn hearing screen. *Clin Perinatol* 2018;45:629.
75. Levit Y, Himmelfarb M, Dollberg S. Sensitivity of the automated auditory brainstem response in neonatal hearing screening. *Pediatrics* 2015;136(3):641.

76. Olusanya BO, Kaplan M, Hansen TWR. Neonatal hyperbilirubinaemia: a global perspective. *Lancet Child Adolesc Health* 2018;2(8):610.

77. Maisels MJ, Bhutani VK, Bogen D, et al. Hyperbilirubinemia in the newborn infant ≥35 weeks' gestation: an update with clarifications. *Pediatrics* 2009;124(4):1193.

78. Bhutani VK, Stark AR, Lazzeroni LC, et al. Predischarge screening for severe neonatal hyperbilirubinemia identifies infants who need phototherapy. *J Pediatr* 2012;162(3):477.

79. American Academy of Pediatrics Subcommittee on Hyperbilirubinemia. Management of hyperbilirubinemia in the newborn infant 35 or more weeks of gestation. *Pediatrics* 2004;114(1):297.

80. Bull MJ, Engle WA; the Committee on Injury, Violence, and Poison Prevention and the Committee on Fetus and Newborn. Safe transportation of preterm and low birth weight infants at hospital discharge. *Pediatrics* 2009;123(5):1424.

81. Durbin DR, Hoffman BD; Council on Injury, Violence, and Poison Prevention. Child passenger safety. *Pediatrics* 2018;142(5):e20182460.

82. Magnarelli A, Shah Solanki N, Davis NL. Car seat tolerance screening for late-preterm infants. *Pediatrics* 2020;145(1):e20191703.

83. Pilley E, McGuire W. Pre-discharge "car seat challenge" for preventing morbidity and mortality in preterm infants. *Cochrane Database Syst Rev* 2006;(1):CD005386.

84. Narvey MR; the Canadian Paediatric Society, Fetus and Newborn Committee. Assessment of cardiorespiratory stability using the infant car seat challenge before discharge in preterm infants (<37 weeks' gestational age). *Paediatr Child Health* 2016;21(3):155.

85. Pilley E, McGuire W. The car seat: a challenge too far for preterm infants? *Arch Dis Child Fetal Neonatal Ed* 2005;90:F452.

86. American Academy of Pediatrics Task Force on Circumcision. Male circumcision: technical report. *Pediatrics* 2012;130(3):e756.

87. Beheraoui CE, Zhang X, Cooper CS, et al. Rates of adverse events associated with male circumcision in U.S. medical settings, 2001 to 2010. *JAMA Pediatr* 2014;168(7):625.

88. Chan PS, Penna FJ, Holmes AV. Gomco Versus Mogen? No effect on circumcision revision rates. *Hosp Pediatr* 2018;8(10):611.

89. Ellison JS, Dy GW, Fu BC, et al. Neonatal circumcision and urinary tract infections in infants with hydronephrosis. *Pediatrics* 2018;142(1):e20173703.

90. World Health Organization Department of Reproductive Health and Research and Joint United Nations Programme on HIV/AIDS (UNAIDS). *Male circumcision: global trends and determinants of prevalence, safety and acceptability.* Geneva, Switzerland: World Health Organization and Joint United Nations Programme on HIV/AIDS, 2007.

91. Mai CT, Isenburg J, Langlois PH, et al. Population-based birth defects data in the United States, 2008 to 2012: presentation of state-specific data and descriptive brief on variability of prevalence. *Birth Defects Res A Clin Mol Teratol* 2015;103(11):972.

92. American Academy of Pediatrics Task Force on Circumcision. Circumcision policy statement. *Pediatrics* 2012;130(3):585.

93. British Medical Association. *Non-therapeutic male circumcision (NTMC) of children—practical guidance for doctors.* London, United Kingdom: British Medical Association, BMA House, 2019.

94. Benitz WE; Committee on Fetus and Newborn, American Academy of Pediatrics. Hospital stay for healthy term newborn infants. *Pediatrics* 2015;135(5):948.

95. Campbell OM, Cegolon L, Macleod D, et al. Length of stay after childbirth in 92 countries and associated factors in 30 low- and middle-income countries: compilation of reported data and a cross-sectional analysis from nationally representative surveys. *PLoS Med* 2016;13(3):e1001972.

96. Shakib J, Buchi K, Smith E, et al. Timing of initial well-child visit and readmissions of newborns. *Pediatrics* 2015;135(3):469.

97. Vohr B. Long-term outcomes of moderately preterm, late preterm, and early term infants. *Clin Perinatol* 2013;40(4):739.

98. American Academy of Pediatrics Task Force on Sudden Infant Death Syndrome. SIDS and other sleep-related infant deaths: updated 2016 recommendations for a safe infant sleeping environment. *Pediatrics* 2016;138(5):e20162938.

99. Lavista Ferres JM, Anderson TM, Johnston R, et al. Distinct populations of sudden unexpected infant death based on age. *Pediatrics* 2020;145(1):e20191637.

100. Behnam-Terneus M, Clemente M. SIDS, BRUE, and safe sleep guidelines. *Pediatr Rev* 2019;40(9):443.

101. Blair PS, Ball HL, McKenna JJ, et al. Bedsharing and breastfeeding: the academy of breastfeeding medicine protocol #6, Revision 2019. *Breastfeed Med* 2020;15(1):5.

102. Farber HJ, Nelson KE, Groner JA, et al. Public policy to protect children from tobacco, nicotine, and tobacco smoke. *Pediatrics* 2015;136(5):998.

103. Farber HJ, Walley SC, Groner JA, Clinical practice policy to protect children from tobacco, nicotine, and tobacco smoke. *Pediatrics* 2015;136(5):1008.

104. Stewart DL, Barfield WD; Committee on Fetus and Newborn. Updates on an at-risk population: late-preterm and early-term infants. *Pediatrics* 2019;144(5):e20192760.

105. Raju TNKR. The "Late preterm" birth-ten years later. *Pediatrics* 2017;139(3):e20163331.

106. Engle WA, Tomashek KM, Wallman C, et al. "Late-preterm" infants: a population at risk. *Pediatrics* 2007;120(6):1390.

107. Escobar GJ, Clark RH, Greene JD. Short-term outcomes of infants born at 35 and 36 weeks gestation: we need to ask more questions. *Semin Perinatol* 2006;30(1):28.

108. Hwang SS, Barfield WD, Smith RA, et al. Discharge timing, outpatient follow-up, and home care of late-preterm and early-term infants. *Pediatrics* 2013;132(1):101.

CARE AROUND BIRTH

PART 4

The Newborn Infant

19 Fluid and Electrolyte Management

Sabita Uthaya

INTRODUCTION

This chapter will discuss the physiological mechanisms that govern water and electrolyte balance and provide the reader with an understanding of the principles of fluid and electrolyte therapy as well as an approach to the management of common clinical problems encountered in the neonate.

BODY COMPOSITION OF THE NEWBORN INFANT AND POSTNATAL CHANGES IN BODY WATER DISTRIBUTION

At birth, the newborn baby is composed predominantly of water. Total body water (TBW) is divided into two main compartments, intracellular water (ICW) and extracellular water (ECW). The ECW is further divided into the interstitial water and plasma volume. Plasma volume is the intravascular component of the ECW (Fig 19.1).

Body fluid compartments change throughout development from fetal to adult life (1). With increasing gestational age during fetal life, TBW as a proportion of weight decreases from approximately 86% at 24 weeks to 78% at term (2–4) (Fig. 19.2).

Alongside the changes in TBW, changes in relative proportions of ICW and ECW occur. ECW decreases from 59% of body weight at 24 weeks of gestation to 44% at term, while ICW increases from 27% to 34% of body weight (Table 19.1) (1,2,4). Therefore, infants born preterm have higher TBW and ECW compared to term born infants, as do those born small for gestational age (5). After birth TBW continues to decrease as a result of contraction of the ECW (6). In the main, the contraction of ECW is in the interstitial component of ECW. This is triggered by release of atrial natriuretic peptide (ANP) secondary to reduction in pulmonary vascular resistance and increased atrial stretch from increased left atrial venous return (7). ANP stimulates diuresis and natriuresis, and levels peak at 48 to 72 hours at the peak of maximal postnatal diuresis (8–10). The contraction of ECW accounts for the early postnatal weight loss, which is delayed in babies with respiratory distress syndrome (RDS) who have delayed cardiopulmonary adaptation (11). Delayed contraction of ECW compartment and increased weight gain in the initial postnatal period is associated with an increased risk of developing chronic lung disease (12). It should be noted, however, that studies of associations between delayed ECW contraction and severity of RDS and chronic lung disease that have led clinicians to adopt restrictive fluid and sodium intakes in the first couple of days after birth were conducted before antenatal steroids and postnatal surfactant, both of which reduce the incidence and severity of RDS, became standard of care. In the current era of improved antenatal and postnatal care, there should be no reason to overly restrict intakes of fluid and sodium as ECW contraction will occur as it does in healthy term infants.

ICW increases in proportion to body weight after birth and exceeds ECW by 3 months of age (Fig. 19.2).

Electrolytes

Each body water compartment has a different electrolyte composition (Fig. 19.3) (13).

Sodium is the main cation in plasma with potassium, calcium, and magnesium making up the remainder of the cation fraction. The main anion is chloride, with protein and bicarbonate constituting the rest of the anions. Interstitial fluid has a similar solute composition to plasma but for the content of protein, which is higher in plasma. Potassium and magnesium are the main cations in ICW with phosphate (organic and inorganic), bicarbonate, protein, and sulfate making up the rest. In the newborn infant body fluid, electrolyte composition is determined by the gestational age. Preterm infants have higher ECW content and correspondingly higher sodium and chloride per kilogram of body weight (3,4) (Table 19.1). Conversely, potassium content per kilogram of body weight is lower than at term owing to the lower ICW. In fetal life, fluid and electrolyte balance is dependent on maternal homeostasis and management of the mother in labor. At birth, fluid and electrolyte status is therefore reflective of maternal status and not that of the fetus (14,15).

INSENSIBLE WATER LOSS

Insensible water loss (IWL) is water lost by the process of evaporation from the skin and respiratory tract as well as that from stool. The respiratory tract accounts for 30% of IWL with the remaining 70% lost through skin (16–18). Stool water loss is minimal in the days after birth. IWL is dependent on surface area as well as the maturity of skin at birth. Preterm babies have greater surface area to body weight ratio, and this is reflected in higher IWL compared to term infants. Additionally, preterm babies have increased transepidermal water loss because of a thin epidermis and lack of the stratum corneum layer of the skin that contains keratin and prevents water loss by evaporation. Before 30 weeks of gestation the epidermis is thin, with a poorly formed stratum corneum. Skin matures by 34 weeks of gestation. Maturation of the skin is also influenced by postnatal age, such that 2 weeks following birth, the skin of an extremely preterm infant resembles that of a term infant (19). Transepidermal water loss falls exponentially with increasing gestational age and postnatal age (20–23) (Fig. 19.4).

Various factors affect IWL in newborn infants including ambient humidity, humidity of inspired gases, skin integrity, environmental temperature, radiant heat sources including phototherapy, body temperature, congenital skin defects (gastroschisis, omphalocele, neural tube defects, etc.), activity of the infant, and crying (Table 19.2). Measures to reduce IWL by reducing radiant, convective, and conductive heat loss are most effective in extremely preterm infants who are also the most vulnerable to excessive IWL. At similar skin temperature of an infant, a radiant warmer increases IWL by 50% compared to an infant nursed in an incubator because the humidity under a radiant warmer is lower than that in an incubator (24). Use of incubators with

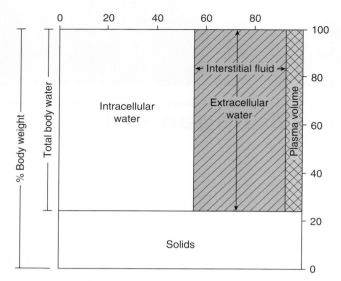

FIGURE 19.1 Distribution of body water in a term newborn infant.

high ambient humidity reduces IWL, decreases maximal weight loss, and lowers the incidence of hypernatremia (25). In settings without access to incubators with humidification systems, use of a plastic blanket under a radiant warmer or in an incubator reduces IWL by 30% to 70% by reducing convective heat loss (26–28). Plastic chambers and heat shields also reduce IWL (27,29). Avoiding the use of tapes, using adhesive removers, and use of skin barriers before the application of items with adhesives can reduce skin breakdown. Humidifying inspired gases in babies receiving mechanical ventilation reduces the respiratory IWL by 30% (17). Humidification should also be used when delivering noninvasive ventilation with low-flow oxygen, high-flow therapy, and continuous positive airway pressure (30). The use of semipermeable membranes (31) and topical ointments (32,33) have been shown to reduce IWL, but these are not widely used because of concerns around increasing the risk of bacterial infection (34).

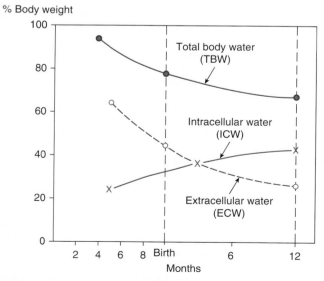

FIGURE 19.2 Changes in body water during gestation and infancy. (From Friis-Hansen B. Changes in body water compartments during growth. *Acta Paediatr Suppl* 1957;46:207. Reprinted by permission of John Wiley & Sons, Inc.)

TABLE 19.1

Changes in Body Water and Electrolyte Composition during Intrauterine and Early Postnatal Life

Component	Gestational Age (wk)					1–4 wk after term birth
	24	28	32	36	40	
Total body water (%)	86	84	82	80	78	74
Extracellular water (%)	59	56	52	48	44	41
Intracellular water (%)	27	28	30	32	34	33
Sodium (mEq/kg)	99	91	85	80	77	73
Potassium (mEq/kg)	40	41	40	41	41	42
Chloride (mEq/kg)	70	67	62	56	51	48

Regulation of Fluid and Electrolyte Balance

The most rapid period of nephrogenesis is between 20 and 30 weeks of gestational age and is complete by term (Fig. 19.5).

This process continues if a baby is born preterm. However, ongoing nephrogenesis may be impacted by the postnatal extrauterine environment, and nephrons that are lost are not replaced. Glomerular filtration rate (GFR) is low in the fetus and at birth. GFR increases with increasing gestational age and postnatal age (35). Creatinine clearance, which is reflective of GFR, has been estimated in the human fetus and shows increase with increasing gestational age (36). Tubular function also increases with gestational age and postnatal age (36). Fractional sodium excretion, the best index of renal tubular sodium reabsorption, which is the fraction of filtered sodium that is excreted in the final urine, is high in the fetus and rapidly declines in the first 2 weeks after birth (37). In healthy term infants it is less than 1% (Fig. 19.6).

The preterm newborn, however, has a limited ability to conserve and excrete sodium. Therefore, sodium depletion and retention can occur. The inability to conserve sodium is due to lower absorption in the proximal tubule of the nephron in the preterm neonate coupled with reduced absorption in the distal tubule, secondary to a blunted aldosterone responsiveness in the distal tubule. Increased expression and activity of the basolateral sodium–potassium ATPase and luminal membrane sodium–hydrogen exchanger within the proximal tubule in the postnatal period result in sodium conservation (38). Glucocorticoids increase the activity of sodium–potassium ATPase and transporter proteins.

Nonrenal regulation of water and electrolyte balance is mediated by hormones produced in the pituitary, adrenal cortex, and heart. Antidiuretic hormone (ADH) or arginine vasopressin (AVP) is produced in the posterior pituitary gland and is functional in the term and preterm infants although there is no linear correlation between urine osmolality and urinary ADH levels (39–41). Preterm infants during water deprivation are able to concentrate urine but not to the same extent as adults (42,43). Newborn infants, both premature and term, can maximally dilute their urine and are able to excrete a fluid load, though not as rapidly as adults (44,45).

OBJECTIVES OF FLUID AND ELECTROLYTE MANAGEMENT

The objectives of fluid and electrolyte management are

1. maintenance of the normal balance of fluid, electrolytes, and normoglycemia
2. supporting the transition of the fetus to extrauterine life
3. avoidance of deficits or excess of either fluid or electrolytes during transition or during periods of illness
4. correction of deficits or excess that may occur either during transition or during periods of acute or chronic illness
5. optimisation of nutritional intake

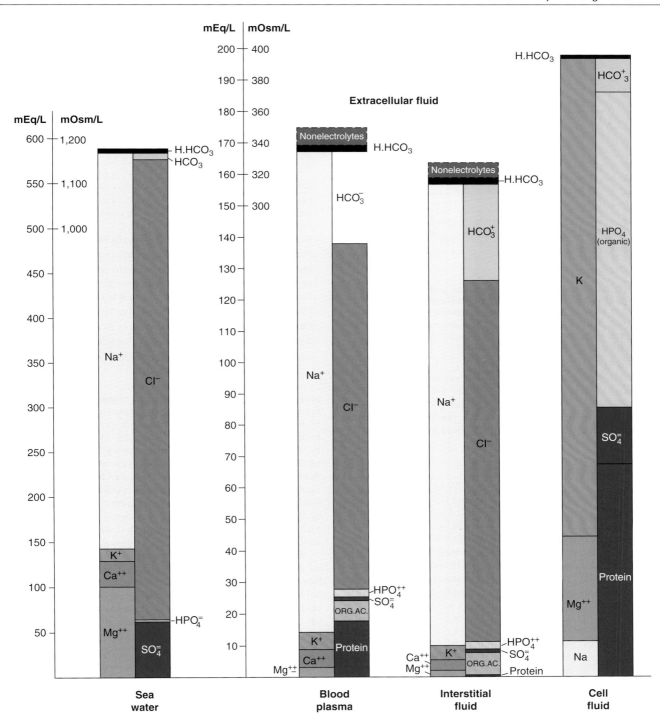

FIGURE 19.3 Ion distribution in seawater, blood plasma, interstitial fluid, and intracellular compartment.

PRINCIPLES OF FLUID AND ELECTROLYTE MANAGEMENT

The principles that underpin management of fluid and electrolyte balance in the newborn are as follows:

1. Management of fluid and electrolyte balance in the immediate postnatal period is different to that in the latter phase of growth and development. Once postnatal adaptation has occurred and extracellular fluid contraction has taken place, delivery of nutrition to allow growth should take precedence.

2. Calculation of fluid and electrolyte intake in the early postnatal period should take into account the baby's IWL based on gestational and postnatal age, the environment, receipt of maternal antenatal steroids, ongoing losses, metabolic stability, and nutritional requirements of the baby.

3. Once postnatal adaptation has taken place, ongoing maintenance intakes should take into account ongoing normal and abnormal losses, nutritional requirements, and monitoring of fluid and electrolyte balance.

4. Although intake of sodium should be avoided in the immediate postnatal period until ECF contraction occurs, preterm

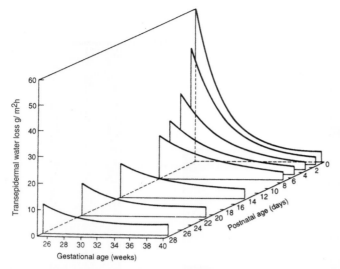

FIGURE 19.4 Insensible water loss in relation to gestational age at birth at different postnatal ages in appropriate for gestational age infants. (From Hammarlund K, Sedin G, Strömberg B. Transepidermal water loss in newborn infants. VIII. Relation to gestational age and post-natal age in appropriate and small for gestational age infants. *Acta Paediatr Scand* 1983;72(5):721. Reprinted by permission of John Wiley & Sons, Inc.)

TABLE 19.2	
Factors Affecting Insensible Water Loss in Newborn Infants	
Factor	**Effect on IWL**
Level of maturity	Inversely proportional to birth weight and gestational age (Fig. 19.4)
Respiratory distress	Respiratory IWL increases with rising minute ventilation when dry air is being breathed
Environmental temperature above neutral thermal zone	Increased in proportion to increment in temperature
Elevated body temperature	Increased by up to 300%
Skin breakdown or injury	Increased by uncertain magnitude
Congenital skin defect (e.g., gastroschisis, omphalocele, neural tube defect)	Increased by uncertain magnitude until surgically corrected
Radiant warmer	Increased by about 50%
Phototherapy	Increased by about 50%
Motor activity and crying	Increased by up to 70%
High ambient or inspired humidity	Reduced by 30% when ambient vapor pressure is increased by 200%
Plastic heat shield	Reduced by 30%–70%
Plastic blanket or chamber	Reduced by 30%–70%
Semipermeable membrane	Reduced by 50%
Topical agents	Reduced by 50%

infants receiving amino acids in parenteral nutrition need adequate early intake of phosphate, usually provided as sodium glycerophosphate, to prevent the increasingly recognized complications of severe hypercalcemia, hypophosphatemia, and hypokalemia that is akin to the "refeeding syndrome" if adequate phosphate is not provided (46).

Fluid and Electrolyte Requirements

Using the principles above, it should be possible to estimate the fluid and electrolyte requirements of both term and preterm babies. IWL, urine output, fecal water, and water retained in new tissue laid down during growth are the four components to be considered in determining daily water requirement. This is offset by water produced as a result of oxidation of macronutrients, which is in the region of 10 mL/kg/d. Fecal water loss is around 5 to 10 mL/kg/d (47). Water retained for growth is around 10 mL/kg/d, assuming a weight gain of 10 to 20 g/kg/d of which 60% to 70% is water (4). Fecal water loss is minimal in the first few days after birth as is water retained in new tissue. In the first postnatal days, the goal of fluid management is to allow isotonic contraction of ECW without compromising nutritional intake unless the clinical condition of the baby requires fluid management to trump that of nutrition. In a term baby the IWL is approximately 20 mL/kg/d (16). In order to excrete a renal solute load of 15 to 30 mOsm/L/d at a urine concentration that can be achieved by the newborn kidney (e.g., 300 mOsm/L or 0.3 mOsm/mL, which is in the middle of the range of urine osmolality), a urine output of 50 to 100 mL/kg/d would be required (volume of urine in mL/kg/d = urine concentration in mOsm/mL/renal solute load in mOsm/kg/d). The renal solute load in the first few days after birth is around 15 mOsm/L; therefore, assuming minimal growth and fecal losses, the requirement of water in a term infant is 20 + 50 = 70 mL/kg/d. Preterm infants in the early postnatal period require higher fluid intakes because of a higher IWL and lower renal solute load. Babies of gestational age less than 27 weeks will require a starting fluid intake of around 150 mL/kg/d assuming an ambient humidity of 50%. Lower volumes may be considered if ambient humidity is higher (20). Table 19.3 shows suggested starting volumes of intravenous intake in babies depending on gestational age.

Sodium supplementation should be minimized until postnatal adaptation has taken place, which is when a postnatal weight loss of around 6% of birth weight has been achieved (48). Preterm babies receiving amino acids in parenteral nutrition should receive phosphate to prevent electrolyte disturbances as described above (46). This is usually provided as sodium glycerophosphate and so some sodium supplementation is inevitable. In order to provide 1 mmol/kg/d of phosphate as sodium glycerophosphate, 2 mmol/kg/d of sodium will be administered.

After postnatal ECW contraction has taken place, the goals of fluid and electrolyte management are to provide adequate nutrition for growth taking into account the renal solute load. With parenteral nutrition, this would equate to approximately a minimum volume of

TABLE 19.3					
Estimated Starting Intravenous Intake, at Ambient Humidity of 50%[a]					
Gestational Age (wk)	**Birth Weight (kg)**	**Approximate IWL (mL/kg/d)**	**Allowance for Urine Output (mL/kg/d)**	**Estimated Intake Range (mL/kg/d)**	**Suggested Starting Volume (mL/kg/d)**
<27	<1.0	120	30–60	150–180	150
27–30	1.0–1.5	40	30–60	70–100	90
31–36	1.5–2.5	15	30–60	45–75	60
>36	>2.5	10	30–60	40–70	60

[a]Lower intake if ambient humidity is higher.

Reprinted from Rennie J. *Rennie and Roberton's textbook of neonatology*, 5th ed. Philadelphia, PA: Churchill Livingstone, 2012:334. Copyright © 2012 Elsevier, with permission. Table 18.3.

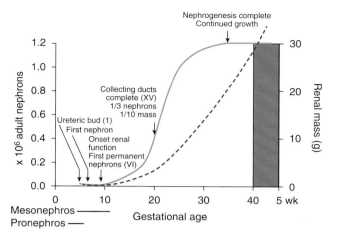

FIGURE 19.5 Development of the human kidney through 40 weeks of gestational age. (Reprinted from Harrison MR, Golbus MS, Filly RA, et al. Management of the fetus with congenital hydronephrosis. *J Pediatr Surg* 1982;17:728. Copyright © 1982 Elsevier, with permission.)

120 mL/kg/d and enteral intake of either breast milk or formula milk of between 150 and 200 mL/kg/d depending on the gestational age of the baby. Although clinicians have traditionally favored "restricting" fluid intake in the early postnatal period, studies have shown that the preterm infant is capable of tolerating a range of water intakes that is not dependent on GFR and healthy preterm infants can tolerate up to 200 mL/kg/d from day 3 after birth (49). Once postnatal adaptation has taken place, a preterm infant requires approximately 4 mmol/kg/d of sodium whereas a term baby's requirement is around

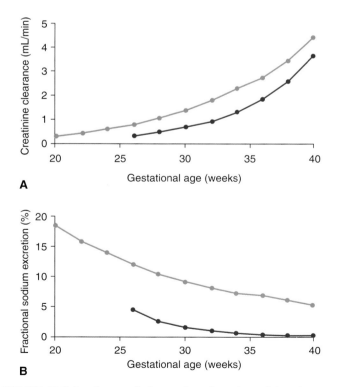

FIGURE 19.6 Developmental changes in estimated creatinine clearance (A) and calculated fractional excretion of sodium (B) between 20 and 40 weeks of gestation in the human fetus and neonate. (From Haycock GB. Development of glomerular filtration and tubular sodium reabsorption in the human fetus and newborn. *Br J Urol* 1998;81(suppl 2):33. Reprinted by permission of John Wiley & Sons, Inc.)

2 to 3 mmol/kg/d. Sodium is a permissive factor for growth, but serum sodium cannot be relied upon to guide supplementation as growth failure precedes a fall in serum sodium.

Monitoring Fluid and Electrolyte Balance

Monitoring fluid and electrolyte balance involves clinical assessment, laboratory tests, and record of intakes and outputs. Clinical assessment should include changes in body weight, cardiovascular sufficiency (heart rate, blood pressure, toe–core gap, capillary refill time), and clinical examination (presence of dehydration or edema). Laboratory tests include measurement of serum electrolytes, urea, creatinine, bone profile, acid–base balance, and blood glucose. Babies in intensive care should be weighed daily and urine output measured continuously either with a catheter *in situ* or by weighing of nappies. Review of urine output should take place more frequently (2-hourly) in acutely unwell babies. Failure to recognize a low urine output can result in prerenal failure progressing to renal failure and cardiovascular compromise. In extremely preterm babies, aim for a urine output of 0.5 mL/kg/h on the first postnatal day. Subsequently aim for an output of 2 to 3 mL/kg/h and intervene should the urine output drop below 1 mL/kg/h. Serum electrolytes and creatinine should be checked daily, with more frequent monitoring if abnormal.

Fluid and Electrolyte Disturbances
Hypernatremia

Hypernatremia (serum sodium >145 mmol/L) could be a result of decreased fluid intake, increased fluid loss, or excessive sodium intake. The most common cause of hypernatremia in the newborn infant is dehydration or relative deficit of water in relation to sodium. In the preterm infant this is due to excessive IWL and in the term infant due to inadequate breast milk intake. Establishing the cause of hypernatremia involves an assessment of the weight of the baby. If a baby has lost weight, it would suggest a loss of water alone as in the situations of excessive IWL and dehydration. If a baby has hypernatremia with an accompanying weight gain in excess of that expected, it would suggest an excess of both sodium and water.

Hypernatremia in the preterm infant due to excessive IWL is often exacerbated by hyperglycemia and attendant high urine output from osmotic diuresis. Managing hypernatremia in this scenario involves increasing fluid intake without increasing sodium intake concurrently and also managing hyperglycemia by reducing glucose intake and insulin therapy as required.

The incidence of hypernatremia in healthy breast-fed term infants has variously been reported to be 2.5 per 10,000 live births in a population-wide study in the United Kingdom (50) to 277 per 10,000 referrals of breast-fed neonates referred to a single neonatal unit in Italy (51).

Hypernatremia can cause significant morbidity and if very severe result in death (52). Neurologic sequelae include seizures, intraventricular hemorrhage, thromboses, and infarction (52). Hypernatremia is accompanied by weight loss in excess of 10% of birth weight. Babies may be lethargic and may not have a sunken fontanelle as would be expected in the presence of dehydration because of cerebral edema that occurs as a result of changes in the osmolarity of brain cells in response to extracellular hyperosmolarity (53). Correction of hypernatremia that has developed over a period of days should be corrected slowly to avoid the risk of cerebral edema, which can occur as a result of compensatory retention of organic osmolytes in brain cells in response to chronic extracellular hyperosmolarity. Rapid drop in serum sodium will result in water entering brain cells resulting in worsening of cell swelling and cerebral edema. Mild hypernatremic dehydration may be managed with enteral feeds. Initial management may require fluid resuscitation with normal saline, 20 mL/kg over 30 minutes if the baby has signs of shock. Correction with rehydration should occur slowly over 2 to 3 days initially with 0.9% saline in 5% to 10% dextrose and changing to 0.45% saline in 5% to 10% dextrose after 24 hours (52). Total fluid volume is calculated as the sum of maintenance fluid and the volume of deficit. Fluid deficit is calculated from the percentage weight loss. For example, a 3-kg baby who has lost 10% of birth weight will have a fluid deficit of 300 mL. Serum electrolytes should be measured 6 hourly, and aim for a reduction of serum sodium of 0.5 mmol/L/h.

In hypernatremic dehydration, output is decreased and the urine becomes concentrated. Polyuria in the presence of hypernatremia would indicate a loss of urine concentrating ability pointing to a diagnosis of diabetes insipidus. In this situation, the urine osmolality will be low in the presence of a simultaneous high plasma osmolality.

Hyponatremia

Establishing the cause of hyponatremia (serum sodium <130 mmol/L), as in the case of hypernatremia, also requires an assessment of the weight of a baby. Hyponatremia with weight loss or suboptimal weight gain indicates a deficit of sodium. Hyponatremia with weight gain suggests an excess of water. Hyponatremia present at birth is reflective of maternal sodium levels. This occurs when the mother has consumed large volumes of water in labor, received sodium-free fluid infusions or secondary to syntocinon infusion to augment labor or in cases of preeclampsia. Hyponatremia in the newborn results from water excess (dilutional) or sodium depletion. Water excess can result from an excess of fluid administration or an impairment in excretion of water. Extracellular fluid may be increased or decreased or may remain the same. Sodium depletion occurs from either insufficient intake or excessive loss. Examples of situations of impaired excretion of water include acute kidney injury, appropriate and inappropriate section of ADH, and in response to treatment with nonselective cyclooxygenase (COX) inhibitors such as ibuprofen and indomethacin.

Sodium depletion from insufficient intake of sodium may occur during transition from parenteral nutrition to enteral feeds especially if intake is predominantly donor-expressed breast milk and supplementation in parenteral nutrition is delayed or inadequate. Excess loss of sodium may be renal (use of diuretics), gastrointestinal (increased nasogastric or stoma losses), or endocrine (congenital adrenal hyperplasia or hypoaldosteronism).

In the case of sodium depletion, management involves administration of sodium, either enterally if the infant is on milk feeds (at least 45 mL/kg/d) (54) or parenterally. Parenteral sodium supplementation may be given either as an additional infusion of 0.9% saline (an infusion of 20 mL/kg/d will give an additional 3 mmol/kg/d of sodium) or in the case of more severe hyponatremia (serum sodium <120 mmol/L) as an infusion of 30% sodium chloride added to 5% or 10% dextrose infusion of, for example, 20 mL/kg/d. Serum sodium should not rise faster than 1 mmol/L/h. Preterm infants should commence sodium supplements of at least 4 mmol/kg/d once postnatal contraction of the ECF has taken place.

Perinatal Asphyxia

Perinatal asphyxia can lead to an inappropriate secretion of ADH from brain injury and renal failure from hypoxic injury to the kidneys. Both scenarios require restriction of fluid intake. Fluid intake should be restricted to IWL and urine output. This is in the region of 30 mL/kg/d. Once urine output is restored, fluid requirement can be liberalized to maintenance intakes. If there is evidence of renal impairment with either oliguria or anuria, potassium should not be administered unless serum levels are below normal. Oliguria may be followed by polyuria before urine output returns to normal levels. This phase may require replacement of excess loss of fluid and sodium. Monitoring of urine output, serum electrolytes, urea and creatinine, and weight are essential.

Management of Neonatal Surgical Patients

Fluid and electrolyte balance and acid–base status should be optimized before surgery to minimize risks of anesthesia and surgery. Certain operations, for example laparotomies, result in increased IWL. IWL can be minimized by using plastic sheets to cover other than the field of interest. Intraoperative fluids should be commenced just prior to the infant's transfer to theater. The choice of fluid is either dextrose 5% or 10% with 0.9% saline (55). Maintenance fluid should be reduced to anticipated IWL and allowance for urine output. For babies less than 32 weeks of postmenstrual age (PMA), this is around 100 mL/kg/d and for those above 32 weeks of PMA 60 mL/kg/d. Intra- and postoperatively administer a bolus of 0.9% saline at 10 to 20 mL/kg if there is evidence of cardiovascular compromise. Postoperatively continue infusion rate at a similar rate to that intraoperatively for at least 12 hours unless urine output is low despite volume expansion, in which case further restriction may be required. Once the infant has a urine output greater than 1.5 mL/kg/h, change to fluids with maintenance potassium and in line with nutritional requirements of the infant. Gastrointestinal losses of greater than 10 mL/kg/d should be replaced mL for mL with intravenous 0.9% saline and potassium chloride of 20 mmol/L or 10 mmol potassium chloride in a 500 mL bag of 0.9% saline. Using a perioperative fluid regimen of 0.9% saline in 5% or 10% dextrose at lower than usual maintenance intake reduces the risk of intra- or postoperative hypovolemia and consequent increased secretion of ADH, oliguria, and hyponatremia. ADH secretion occurs in response to both hyperosmolarity and hypovolemia. The response to hypovolemia and hypotension mediated by baroreceptors in the left atrium, carotid artery, and aortic arch takes precedence over that of maintaining osmolarity. There is a concomitant increase in plasma renin activity, which supports the non-osmotic cardiovascular mediated ADH activity (56). Hypovolemia precedes hypotension and may go unrecognized. Hypovolemia also does not correlate well with hypotension (57). Postoperative hyponatremia is a result of appropriate secretion of ADH where the secretion of ADH is appropriate to the volume status of the baby (57,58). ADH exerts its effect by causing increased reabsorption of water in the distal tubules and collecting ducts of the kidney. The combination of increased intravascular volume and increased peripheral resistance restores blood pressure. The increased reabsorption of water results in reduced osmolarity, hyponatremia, and oliguria. This is worsened with the administration of salt-poor fluid. Management with fluid restriction and treatment with 0.9% saline reduces ADH secretion and restores osmolality and reverses hyponatremia.

SYNDROME OF INAPPROPRIATE ANTIDIURETIC HORMONE

Syndrome of inappropriate antidiuretic hormone (SIADH) is rare in the neonate. ADH secretion occurs in the absence of osmolar and nonosmolar triggers (59). It is distinguished from appropriate ADH secretion by presence of hyponatremia, urinary sodium loss, and hyperosmolar urine with normal blood pressure and renal function. Urine osmolality is less than maximally dilute (60). SIADH may be present in the situation of acute brain injury and central nervous system infections. Treatment involves fluid restriction and treating the underlying cause.

Bronchopulmonary Dysplasia

Babies with bronchopulmonary dysplasia (BPD) have several factors that contribute to perturbation in fluid and electrolyte balance. Diuretic treatment may result in sodium depletion and hyponatremia. In addition, a study has found that some infants with chronic BPD have elevated vasopressin levels (61). The authors concluded that excessive stimulation of vasopressin secretion may explain some of the pulmonary and nonpulmonary signs and symptoms in infants with BPD.

REFERENCES

1. Friis-Hansen B. Changes in body water compartments during growth. *Acta Paediatr Suppl* 1957;46(suppl 110):1.
2. Friis-Hansen B. Body water compartments in children: changes during growth and related changes in body composition. *Pediatrics* 1961;28:169.
3. Romahn A, Burmeister W. Body composition during the first two years of life: analysis with the potassium 40 method (author's transl). *Klin Padiatr* 1977;189(5):321.
4. Ziegler EE, O'Donnell AM, Nelson SE, et al. Body composition of the reference fetus. *Growth* 1976;40(4):329.
5. Hartnoll G, Betremieux P, Modi N. Body water content of extremely preterm infants at birth. *Arch Dis Child Fetal Neonatal Ed* 2000;83(1):F56.
6. Shaffer SG, Bradt SK, Hall RT. Postnatal changes in total body water and extracellular volume in the preterm infant with respiratory distress syndrome. *J Pediatr* 1986;109(3):509.
7. Modi N, Betremieux P, Midgley J, et al. Postnatal weight loss and contraction of the extracellular compartment is triggered by atrial natriuretic peptide. *Early Hum Dev* 2000;59(3):201.
8. Liechty EA, Johnson MD, Myerberg DZ, et al. Daily sequential changes in plasma atrial natriuretic factor concentrations in mechanically ventilated low-birth-weight infants. Effect of surfactant replacement. *Biol Neonate* 1989;55(4–5):244.
9. Rozycki HJ, Baumgart S. Atrial natriuretic factor and postnatal diuresis in respiratory distress syndrome. *Arch Dis Child* 1991;66(1 Spec No):43.
10. Shaffer SG, Geer PG, Goetz KL. Elevated atrial natriuretic factor in neonates with respiratory distress syndrome. *J Pediatr* 1986;109(6):1028.
11. Modi N, Hutton JL. The influence of postnatal respiratory adaptation on sodium handling in preterm neonates. *Early Hum Dev* 1990;21(1):11.
12. Van Marter LJ, Leviton A, Allred EN, et al. Hydration during the first days of life and the risk of bronchopulmonary dysplasia in low birth weight infants. *J Pediatr* 1990;116(6):942.
13. Macallum AB. The paleochemistry of the body fluids and tissues. *Physiol Rev* 1926;6:316.
14. Battaglia F, Prystowsky H, Smisson C, et al. Fetal blood studies. XIII. The effect of the administration of fluids intravenously to mothers upon the concentrations of water and electrolytes in plasma of human fetuses. *Pediatrics* 1960;25:2.
15. Zimmer EZ, Goldstein I, Feldman E, et al. Maternal and newborn levels of glucose, sodium and osmolality after preloading with three intravenous solutions during elective cesarean sections. *Eur J Obstet Gynecol Reprod Biol* 1986;23(1–2):61.
16. Hey EN, Katz G. Evaporative water loss in the new-born baby. *J Physiol* 1969;200(3):605.
17. Sosulski R, Polin RA, Baumgart S. Respiratory water loss and heat balance in intubated infants receiving humidified air. *J Pediatr* 1983;103(2):307.
18. Sulyok E, Jequier E, Prod'hom LS. Respiratory contribution to the thermal balance of the newborn infant under various ambient conditions. *Pediatrics* 1973;51(4):641.
19. Evans NJ, Rutter N. Development of the epidermis in the newborn. *Biol Neonate* 1986;49(2):74.
20. Hammarlund K, Sedin G. Transepidermal water loss in newborn infants. III. Relation to gestational age. *Acta Paediatr Scand* 1979;68(6):795.
21. Hammarlund K, Sedin G, Stromberg B. Transepidermal water loss in newborn infants. VII. Relation to post-natal age in very pre-term and full-term appropriate for gestational age infants. *Acta Paediatr Scand* 1982;71(3):369.
22. Hammarlund K, Sedin G, Stromberg B. Transepidermal water loss in newborn infants. VIII. Relation to gestational age and post-natal age in appropriate and small for gestational age infants. *Acta Paediatr Scand* 1983;72(5):721.
23. Sedin G, Hammarlund K, Nilsson GE, et al. Measurements of transepidermal water loss in newborn infants. *Clin Perinatol* 1985;12(1):79.
24. Bell EF, Weinstein MR, Oh W. Heat balance in premature infants: comparative effects of convectively heated incubator and radiant warmer, with and without plastic heat shield. *J Pediatr* 1980;96(3 Pt 1):460.
25. Kim SM, Lee EY, Chen J, et al. Improved care and growth outcomes by using hybrid humidified incubators in very preterm infants. *Pediatrics* 2010;125(1):e137.
26. Baumgart S, Fox WW, Polin RA. Physiologic implications of two different heat shields for infants under radiant warmers. *J Pediatr* 1982;100(5):787.
27. Baumgart S, Engle WD, Fox WW, et al. Effect of heat shielding on convective and evaporative heat losses and on radiant heat transfer in the premature infant. *J Pediatr* 1981;99(6):948.
28. Marks KH, Friedman Z, Maisels MJ. A simple device for reducing insensible water loss in low-birth-weight infants. *Pediatrics* 1977;60(2):223.
29. Fitch CW, Korones SB. Heat shield reduces water loss. *Arch Dis Child* 1984;59(9):886.
30. Roberts CT, Kortekaas R, Dawson JA, et al. The effects of non-invasive respiratory support on oropharyngeal temperature and humidity: a neonatal manikin study. *Arch Dis Child Fetal Neonatal Ed* 2016;101(3):F248.
31. Mancini AJ, Sookdeo-Drost S, Madison KC, et al. Semipermeable dressings improve epidermal barrier function in premature infants. *Pediatr Res* 1994;36(3):306.
32. Nopper AJ, Horii KA, Sookdeo-Drost S, et al. Topical ointment therapy benefits premature infants. *J Pediatr* 1996;128(5 Pt 1):660.
33. Wananukul S, Praisuwanna P. Clear topical ointment decreases transepidermal water loss in jaundiced preterm infants receiving phototherapy. *J Med Assoc Thai* 2002;85(1):102.
34. Conner JM, Soll RF, Edwards WH. Topical ointment for preventing infection in preterm infants. *Cochrane Database Syst Rev* 2004;(1):CD001150.
35. Leake RD, Trygstad CW, Oh W. Inulin clearance in the newborn infant: relationship to gestational and postnatal age. *Pediatr Res* 1976;10(8):759.
36. Haycock GB. Development of glomerular filtration and tubular sodium reabsorption in the human fetus and newborn. *Br J Urol* 1998;81(suppl 2):33.
37. Al-Dahhan J, Haycock GB, Chantler C, et al. Sodium homeostasis in term and preterm neonates. I. Renal aspects. *Arch Dis Child* 1983;58(5):335.
38. Baum M, Quigley R. Ontogeny of renal sodium transport. *Semin Perinatol* 2004;28(2):91.
39. Wiriyathian S, Rosenfeld CR, Arant BS Jr, et al. Urinary arginine vasopressin: pattern of excretion in the neonatal period. *Pediatr Res* 1986;20(2):103.
40. Marchini G, Stock S. Thirst and vasopressin secretion counteract dehydration in newborn infants. *J Pediatr* 1997;130(5):736.
41. Rees L, Brook CG, Shaw JC, et al. Hyponatraemia in the first week of life in preterm infants. Part I. Arginine vasopressin secretion. *Arch Dis Child* 1984;59(5):414.
42. Hansen JD, Smith CA. Effects of withholding fluid in the immediate postnatal period. *Pediatrics* 1953;12(2):99.
43. Calcagno PL, Rubin MI, Weintraub DH. Studies on the renal concentrating and diluting mechanisms in the premature infant. *J Clin Invest* 1954;33(1):91.
44. Aperia A, Herin P, Lundin S, et al. Regulation of renal water excretion in newborn full-term infants. *Acta Paediatr Scand* 1984;73(6):717.
45. Mc CR, Naylor NJ, Widdowson EM. The response of infants to a large dose of water. *Arch Dis Child* 1954;29(144):104.
46. Bonsante F, Iacobelli S, Latorre G, et al. Initial amino acid intake influences phosphorus and calcium homeostasis in preterm infants—it is time to change the composition of the early parenteral nutrition. *PLoS One* 2013;8(8):e72580.
47. Lemoh JN, Brooke OG. Frequency and weight of normal stools in infancy. *Arch Dis Child* 1979;54(9):719.
48. Hartnoll G, Betremieux P, Modi N. Randomised controlled trial of postnatal sodium supplementation in infants of 25–30 weeks gestational age: effects on cardiopulmonary adaptation. *Arch Dis Child Fetal Neonatal Ed* 2001;85(1):F29.
49. Coulthard MG, Hey EN. Effect of varying water intake on renal function in healthy preterm babies. *Arch Dis Child* 1985;60(7):614.
50. Oddie S, Richmond S, Coulthard M. Hypernatraemic dehydration and breast feeding: a population study. *Arch Dis Child* 2001;85(4):318.
51. Manganaro R, Mami C, Marrone T, et al. Incidence of dehydration and hypernatremia in exclusively breast-fed infants. *J Pediatr* 2001;139(5):673.
52. Laing IA, Wong CM. Hypernatraemia in the first few days: is the incidence rising? *Arch Dis Child Fetal Neonatal Ed* 2002;87(3):F158.
53. Strange K. Maintenance of cell volume in the central nervous system. *Pediatr Nephrol* 1993;7(5):689.
54. Srinivasan L, Bokiniec R, King C, et al. Increased osmolality of breast milk with therapeutic additives. *Arch Dis Child Fetal Neonatal Ed* 2004;89(6):F514.
55. Judd BA, Haycock GB, Dalton N, et al. Hyponatraemia in premature babies and following surgery in older children. *Acta Paediatr Scand* 1987;76(3):385.
56. Gerigk M, Gnehm HE, Rascher W. Arginine vasopressin and renin in acutely ill children: implication for fluid therapy. *Acta Paediatr* 1996;85(5):550.
57. Barr PA, Bailey PE, Sumners J, et al. Relation between arterial blood pressure and blood volume and effect of infused albumin in sick preterm infants. *Pediatrics* 1977;60(3):282.
58. Bauer K, Linderkamp O, Versmold HT. Systolic blood pressure and blood volume in preterm infants. *Arch Dis Child* 1993;69(5 Spec No):521.
59. Al-Dahhan J, Haycock GB, Chantler C, et al. Sodium homeostasis in term and preterm neonates. II. Gastrointestinal aspects. *Arch Dis Child* 1983;58(5):343.
60. Bartter FC, Schwartz WB. The syndrome of inappropriate secretion of antidiuretic hormone. *Am J Med* 1967;42(5):790.
61. Hazinski TA, Blalock WA, Engelhardt B. Control of water balance in infants with bronchopulmonary dysplasia: role of endogenous vasopressin. *Pediatr Res* 1988;23(1):86.

Nutrition

Sara E. Ramel and Michael K. Georgieff

INTRODUCTION

The provision of nutrition to term and preterm newborn infants remains one of the most important aspects of neonatal care. With increasing survival rates among sick newborns, the nourishment of full-term and preterm infants has assumed an increasingly greater role in the neonatal intensive care unit (NICU) in the past 30 years, particularly since the link between nutritional management and relevant long-term health outcomes, such as neurodevelopment (1), cardiovascular health (2), bone health (3), immune health, and cancer risk (4) in preterm infants has become more obvious. Great strides have been made in understanding neonatal nutritional physiology and pathophysiology in these years, allowing physicians to more precisely assess the nutritional requirements and delivery approaches to preterm and term, ill and well infants in their care (5,6). Two consensus panels made up of stakeholders in neonatal nutrition including the American Academy of Pediatrics (AAP), the National Institute on Child Health and Development (NICHD), the Academy of Nutrition and Dietetics (AND), and the United States Department of Agriculture (USDA) recently published the results of their proceedings discussing the evidence base and need for research in four areas of neonatal nutrition: (a) nutritional requirements; (b) nutrient delivery; (c) special circumstances; and (d) assessment of nutritional status (5,6). Knowledge of newborn infants' nutritional requirements and capacity to assimilate nutrients are prerequisites to informed decision-making about nutritional therapy in the nursery. Additionally, it is important to consider how illness alters those requirements and capacities. Ultimately, assessment of the efficacy of nutritional therapy depends on the tools available for assessment of neonatal nutritional status.

The goal of nutritional therapy in the term neonate is to ensure a successful growth transition from the fetal to the postnatal period. In the preterm infant, the stated goal for the past 43 years (7) has been to continue the quantity and quality of intrauterine growth in the extrauterine environment until 40 weeks postconception and to foster catch-up growth and nutrient accretion in the postdischarge period. Until lately, the goal for the growing preterm infant has been to match the third-trimester intrauterine rates of weight gain, linear growth, and brain growth. Even when these rates are successfully attained, the body composition of the preterm infant raised in an extrauterine environment remains remarkably different than that of the same postconceptional age fetus who has remained in utero (7,8). Current efforts are aimed at understanding the metabolic processes that determine the body composition of the preterm infant (9). The preterm infant is at risk for being well below the standard gestational growth curves at the time of hospital discharge because of nutrient deficits that have accrued during the prolonged period of neonatal illness (10). The effect of illness on neonatal metabolism and nutritional requirements is being recognized (11). Pathologic conditions such as bronchopulmonary dysplasia (BPD), congestive heart failure (CHF), acute respiratory distress, intrauterine growth restriction, and sepsis (and their treatments) have negative effects on neonatal energy and protein and mineral and vitamin requirements. These conditions may also affect the digestive and absorptive capacities of the neonate.

In this chapter, the nutritional requirements, methods of nutritional delivery, effect of illness on nutritional status, and nutritional assessment of term and preterm infants are reviewed.

NUTRIENT REQUIREMENTS FOR TERM AND PRETERM INFANTS

Estimation of nutrient requirements is an inexact process, particularly when the goal is unclear (5). To date, the goal has been to achieve the same growth rates and body composition as the "reference" infant. For term infants, the "gold standard" remains the healthy breastfed infant, whose ideal growth was clarified by the World Health Organization (WHO) with the release of standard growth charts (12). Human milk composition varies greatly among mothers, and the length of time that it remains sufficient for all the nutrient needs of the infant is not uniform. Breastfed infants may have lower iron stores after 4 months of age and may also be at greater risk for vitamin D deficiency (13).

Determining the ideal growth goals for the infant born before term is more problematic than in the term infant. The ideal growth rate and body composition of the "healthy" preterm infant remains unknown and is likely to be different from his or her gestationally age-matched fetal counterpart. Further studies collecting long-term outcome data are needed to better define optimal growth patterns for this vulnerable population. Until recently, the daily and weekly accretion rates of various nutrients in the preterm infant have been modeled on in utero accretion rates of these nutrients in gestationally age-matched fetuses. The "reference fetus" described by Ziegler has served as the benchmark by which neonatal nutritionists judge fetal growth and body composition (7). Like the infant and child, healthy fetuses from uncomplicated pregnancies have remarkably similar intrauterine growth trajectories (14). Whether these curves can therefore be utilized as postnatal standard growth curves for infants born preterm remains debatable. The goal rates of weight gain, linear growth, and head growth between the ages of 24 and 36 weeks' gestation can also be estimated from the standard growth curves generated from infants born prematurely at each of those gestational ages (15). However, it must be recognized that the data used to generate these plots are by definition cross-sectional and thus need smoothing to create the resemblance of a curve. Additionally, since premature birth is an abnormal event and up to 30% of VLBW infants are small for dates (often as a result of the pregnancy failing over time), the reliability of using newborn data to assess the growth velocity of healthy fetuses is suspect. Nevertheless, these methods of assessment are used extensively as guideposts for neonatal growth of the preterm infant. On average, these curves predict that the preterm infant should gain 15 to 18 g/kg body weight each day, grow 1 cm/wk linearly, and demonstrate 1 cm/wk of head growth. However, greater weight gain velocity (20 to 30 g/kg/d) may be necessary for preterm infants to achieve normal birth weight z-scores by term after a period of early growth restriction and to optimize neurodevelopment (16). Finally, while g/kg/d is the most common method of growth velocity assessment, there are other methods that are being advocated which include tracking g/d and z-score change over time (17). Thus, the nutrient requirements of term and preterm infants can be calculated based on fetal accretion reference calculations, individual nutrient balance studies, serum nutrient biomarker values, or a combination of these. Which of these methods, if any, best correlates with relevant long-term outcomes (1–5) remains a subject of intense research.

Energy Requirements

Energy requirements must take into account the amount and caloric density of the solution ingested, the route of administration (enteral vs. parenteral), the amount lost in stool or urine, and the energy requirements in the body (e.g., basal metabolic rate, cost of growth, energy cost of food processing by the body). Many of these parameters are now measurable, and reasonable estimates of energy requirements to maintain optimal weight gain and linear growth velocities can be made for both term and preterm infants.

Energy is predominantly derived from carbohydrates and fat in the diet, which provide 4 and 9 kcal/g, respectively. The infant fed human milk receives calories predominantly from fat, whereas the formula-fed infant receives calories more evenly distributed between fat and carbohydrate (18). The calories derived from these sources are used first to maintain the total energy need of the infant, which consists of the basal metabolic rate, the thermic effect of feeding, and physical activity. Energy intake beyond this baseline is stored and recorded as weight gain. Protein is not normally utilized as an energy source, unless the total energy intake is less than the total energy expenditure of the infant. In those cases, certain amino acids can be deaminated and shunted into the gluconeogenic pathways to provide approximately 4 kcal/g of protein (19). This emphasis on maintaining glucose delivery is a consequence of the high metabolic rate of the neonatal brain, which relies primarily on glucose as its energy substrate.

Energy requirements can be affected by numerous factors, including the route of delivery and the disease state. Energy requirements are approximately 10% lower when infants are fed parenterally as opposed to enterally because no energy is excreted in the stool. Diseases that increase energy needs include congestive heart failure (CHF) (20), chronic lung disease (21), acute respiratory disease (11), and sepsis (22). Diseases that decrease energy needs include hypoxic–ischemic encephalopathy and degenerative neurologic conditions in which there is paucity of physical movement. Therapies can also alter energy requirements. Catecholamine infusions and caffeine can increase energy expenditure (23), while mechanical ventilation, extracorporeal membrane oxygenation (ECMO), and total body cooling can reduce it.

Term Infants

Healthy breastfed term infants show adequate growth on as little as 85 to 100 kcal/kg body weight per day during the first 4 months of life (24). Formula-fed infants have higher energy requirements (100 to 110 kcal/kg), most likely as a result of a lower efficiency of digestion and absorption of fat (25).

Preterm Infants

Preterm infants have higher energy requirements than term infants because of a higher resting energy expenditure and greater stool losses as a result of immature absorptive capacities. Whereas the resting energy expenditure of the term infant is 45 to 50 kcal/kg/d, the preterm infant less than 34 weeks' gestation consumes 50 to 60 kcal/kg/d (26). Stool losses vary between 10% and 40% of intake, depending on the diet. For example, a diet in which the fats are predominantly long-chain triglycerides will promote more stool losses because of the low levels of lipase and the small bile salt pools in the premature infant. Replacement of up to 50% of the lactose with glucose polymers and between 10% and 40% of the fat with medium chain triglyceride (MCT) appears to reduce malabsorption to approximately 10% (27). The preterm infant will need an additional 50 to 60 kcal/kg/d beyond the daily energy expenditure and the loss of energy in the stool to maintain weight gain along the intrauterine growth curve (15 to 18 g/kg of body weight daily). Thus, barring any excess needs from diseases that increase oxygen consumption or from malabsorption, the preterm infant will gain weight parallel to the growth curve on approximately 120 kcal/kg/d. Assuming that 2.5 kcal are needed to achieve 1 g of weight

gain, the upward adjustment to a greater weight gain velocity of 20 to 30 g/kg/d would require feeding an additional 10 to 15 kcal/kg body weight per day to the preterm infant. Thus, it is likely that energy intake on the order of 130 to 135 kcal/kg/d is a more reasonable target for the premature infant than the previous recommended intake of 120 kcal/kg/d, especially given that most infants will have fallen away from the curve during their initial period of illness and will have accrued deficits that need to be made up in addition to standard expected weight gain (10). Many are hesitant to increase caloric intake due to concerns of increased adiposity and long-term metabolic risk; however, to date, this has not been verified in the literature. Increasing caloric intake (as high as 150 kcal/kg/d) increases fat-free mass (FFM) gains and linear growth without increasing fat mass (28). More research is needed to further evaluate the optimal weight gain velocity, taking into account both long-term metabolic and neurodevelopmental outcomes. Additionally, all growth parameters (weight, length, head circumference, body composition) must be taken into account when evaluating the energy requirements of preterm infants.

Energy Sources

Carbohydrates

Newborn infants are highly dependent on a source of glucose for normal brain metabolism (29). The primary source of glucose in the term infant is lactose in human milk and cow's milk formulas. Soy-based formulas provide glucose from the metabolism of dietary sucrose or glucose polymers. Preterm infants also receive glucose, initially as dextrose in parenteral solutions, but subsequently enterally from lactose and glucose polymers. Galactose is also important to the newborn, as it is needed for glycogen storage. The newborn infant typically utilizes between 4 and 8 mg/kg/min of glucose (29). This figure is commonly used as the glucose infusion rate for parenteral nutrition. Because of their low glycogen stores and poorer gluconeogenic capacities, preterm infants are more prone to hypoglycemia than term infants. Higher rates of glucose delivery (up to 15 mg/kg/min) may be required in growth-restricted infants and in infants of diabetic mothers to maintain normal glucose concentrations.

Intravenous dextrose infusion rates up to 12.5 mg/kg/min are commonly used in preterm infants to supply energy to promote weight gain. Beyond this rate, a cost/benefit analysis must be made. Although faster rates of weight gain can be achieved on higher glucose infusion rates (especially if the serum glucose is controlled with exogenous insulin infusion) (30), a higher metabolic rate and a shift in the respiratory quotient may occur. Thus, a higher oxygen consumption rate coupled with proportionately more carbon dioxide generated by the cells may significantly affect serum carbon dioxide and ventilatory requirements. Some concern has been voiced that increased carbohydrate-based caloric intake will lead to increased adiposity. This is not however supported by the literature; in contrast, there is some early evidence that increased calories in the first week of life may improve FFM gains throughout hospitalization (31). There are also concerns regarding the long-term effects of early hyperglycemia, with worsened growth and neurodevelopmental outcomes in those infants with more days of hyperglycemia (32); however, the etiology of these changes remains uncertain, as it may be due to caloric restriction used as a strategy to manage the hyperglycemia. Therefore, the risks and benefits of aggressive support with high (>12.5) glucose infusion rates must be carefully considered.

Fats

Lipids are a major energy source for neonates. Certain fatty acids, such as linoleic (omega-6, 18:2) and linolenic (omega-3, 18:3), are essential in the diet, and their absence will produce deficiency syndromes. Essential fatty acid concentrations decline rapidly within 1 week of discontinuing lipid intake. Infants receiving parenteral nutrition or on a fat-restricted enteral diet require at least 0.5 mg/kg/d of an intravenous fat blend containing these fatty acids at least three times per week to prevent severe essential fatty acid deficiency. The AAP has recommended that at least 3% of total energy intake in infants should be in the form of linoleic acid (33).

Daily fat intake varies greatly based on the method of delivery (enteral vs. parenteral) and the dietary source (human milk vs. formula). Enterally fed term infants consume approximately 5 to 6 g/kg/d of fat, whereas parenterally fed infants rarely receive greater than 3.5 g/kg/d. Infants receiving human milk (especially human milk expressed by mothers who have delivered preterm) may receive up to 7 g/kg/d.

Infants fed human milk receive a unique blend of fats that cannot be precisely replicated in infant formulas. Cow's milk fat is generally not well tolerated by newborn infants, requiring formula manufacturers to use vegetable oils as substitutes. The spectrum of fatty acids found in infant formula are distinctly different from human milk fats.

The role of omega fatty acids such as docosahexaenoic acid (DHA) and arachidonic acid (AA) in the infant diet continues to be a subject of intense research. These fatty acids are products of an elongation pathway from linoleic acid and are important in cell membrane structure, in cell-signaling cascades and in myelination (34). The synthetic pathways are usually immature in preterm infants and for some undetermined period of time after birth in term infants (35). Levels of DHA and AA decline immediately after birth (35). Sources of these fatty acids include the placenta and human milk. In contrast, cow's milk fat and vegetable oil do not contain these compounds. Because the preterm infant may be less capable of synthesizing the compounds and would have received them *in utero*, the European Society for Pediatric Gastroenterology and Nutrition has recommended that a source of these fatty acids be added to preterm infant formula (36). Evidence of their efficacy includes studies that demonstrate better visual acuity, more mature electroretinograms, and short-term gains in general neurodevelopment in supplemented infants (37). Studies of the longer-term growth and developmental outcomes of infants who have been supplemented with these fatty acids suggest continued positive effects on the visual system at 1 year of age (37). It remains unclear whether potential early neurodevelopmental gains are sustained beyond the first year. Cochrane reviews assessing whether supplementation of long-chain polyunsaturated fatty acid (LC-PUFA) in infant formula improves neurodevelopment in term (38) and preterm (39) infants have been performed multiple times over the past 12 years. The most recent, which included 15 high-quality trials in term infants and 17 high-quality trials in preterm infants, concluded that the studies do not support a positive long-term neurodevelopmental effect following supplementation via infant formula in the neonatal period (38,39). On the other hand, no adverse effects were noted. An important consideration in the addition of any one compound to an infant's diet is whether the component exerts its nutritional effect individually or in consort with other compounds. Based on their "generally recognized as safe" (GRAS) status, DHA and AA have been added to term, preterm hospital, and preterm discharge formulas by the major formula manufacturers.

The lack of a consistent neurodevelopmental effect may be as a result of suboptimal dosing of the compounds or may represent a washout of early effects over time. However, neurodevelopment is not the only outcome of relevance to these compounds. Lapillonne et al. report that low levels of DHA and AA are associated with retinopathy of prematurity (ROP), chronic lung disease, late-onset sepsis, and potentially necrotizing enterocolitis in preterm neonates (40).

Carnitine is another compound involved in fat metabolism in the neonate, playing a major role in the oxidation of long chain fatty acids. Although carnitine deficiency is rare in the enterally fed infant because of high levels in human milk and supplementation of formulas, it remains a concern in infants receiving long-term exclusive parenteral nutrition in which carnitine has not been supplemented. Carnitine supplements can be added to total parenteral nutrition (TPN) and are recommended in infants who receive TPN for greater than 3 weeks. However, routine carnitine supplementation of preterm infants from birth has no positive effect on growth, apnea, or length of hospital stay and thus is not indicated (41).

Protein Requirements

Protein requirements in humans are determined by a number of factors including protein quality and quantity, the amount of energy delivered, and the protein nutritional status of the subject. The latter is influenced by the degree of previous malnutrition, by the rate of catch-up growth, and potentially by inflammatory processes. The sick newborn infant is exposed to many of these influences. Additionally, they have a high basal requirement for protein accretion based on *in utero* nitrogen accretion rates (7). Adequate energy intake is important to promote optimal protein utilization, with a nonprotein calorie-to-gram nitrogen ratio of 200:1 considered ideal. Protein intake in the neonate has previously been limited to about 4 g/kg/d because of concerns regarding the inability of the immature kidney to excrete titratable acid, blood urea nitrogen (BUN), and ammonium ion. However, more recent data have confirmed that levels of 4.5 to 5 g/kg/d are tolerated without increased BUN levels or metabolic acidosis (42).

Protein requirements, in general, and branched-chain amino acid needs, in particular, are increased in adults with physiologic instability as a result of septic or surgical illness. The possibility that similar changes might occur in sick neonates has been investigated (11,22). Neither acute respiratory disease nor sepsis nor surgical ligation of the patent ductus arteriosus (PDA) results in increased protein requirements (11,22). At this time, increasing protein delivery routinely on the basis of illness or physiologic instability is not recommended. Conversely, practitioners frequently limit nutrient delivery during illness out of concern that high loads may be metabolically taxing. Up to 3 g of protein per kg body weight can safely be administered daily to sick preterm infants beginning in the first 24 hours after birth (43), and currently, recommendations are to advance to at least 3.5 g/kg daily as tolerated.

Term Infants

The full-term breastfed infant grows adequately and maintains normal serum and somatic (i.e., muscle) protein status on as little as 1.5 g/kg/d of protein. Although the protein content is low (1.1%), the quality of human milk protein is excellent because the spectrum of amino acids provides a unique "match" for the amino acid needs of the newborn. The protein content is predominantly lactalbumin, as opposed to casein, which makes for smaller curds and easier digestibility. Additionally, human milk is replete with nondietary nitrogen sources including nucleotides, which may enhance the immune system; immunoglobulins and other antimicrobial factors, which help protect the gut epithelium; growth factors, which stimulate intestinal growth; and enzymes (e.g., lipases), which aid digestion (44).

The term infant fed a cow's milk or soy-based infant formula may require a greater protein delivery rate in order to compensate for the less-than-ideal protein quality. Thus, the infant on cow's milk formula was thought to require closer to 2 g/kg/d and the infant on soy formula up to 2.7 g/kg/d of protein (45). Cow's milk protein is predominantly casein, although a number of cow's milk–based formulas are modified to be whey predominant. The soy formulas also promote adequate growth of lean body mass. However, these formulas contain a smaller percentage of available nitrogen as essential or semi-essential amino acids (18).

Recently, the need for and potential risk of increased protein in term formula has been investigated. A large trial in Europe randomized over 1,600 infants to conventional or low-protein term formula. These infants were followed out through childhood, and they found that BMI, body fatness, and obesity risk were decreased dramatically in the low-protein group, and in fact, each of these values were similar to the control group of breastfed infants (45).

Protein can also be delivered to the term infant by way of protein hydrolysate or individual amino acid formulas. These formulas are specifically designed to decrease the exposure of the infant to potentially antigenic cow's or soy milk proteins. Hydrolysis of cow's milk–based protein such that greater than 90% of the proteins have a molecular weight of 1,250 Da or less allows the formula to be used for treatment of cow's milk allergy. These formulas provide approximately 2.8 g/kg/d of protein at an energy delivery of 100 kcal/kg/d.

Preterm Infants

Recommendations for protein intake in preterm infants follow many of the same parameters as in term infants. However, the needs of the preterm infant appear to be greater than the term infant. Preterm infants require protein initiation immediately after delivery to prevent loss of endogenous stores (45). In addition, preterm infants build up early deficits in protein due to illness, or transition to enteral feeds, and therefore likely require higher amounts later to correct for early losses (45). Studies of the protein requirements and distribution (synthesis vs. breakdown) in extremely low-birth-weight (ELBW) infants demonstrate that an average of 3.2 g/kg of protein is necessary to counter the negative nitrogen balance of neonatal illness and to match the expected *in utero* protein accretion rate (45). Growth and developmental outcomes are improved when protein intakes closer to 4 g/kg/d are established early and maintained throughout hospitalization. Olsen et al. (42) have shown that infants fed 4.6 to 5.5 g/kg/d enterally have less decline in length z-scores.

Besides total protein delivery, studies have considered which amino acids may limit protein accretion in the preterm infant. The terms "essential" and "nonessential" amino acids have been replaced in the neonatal lexicon by "indispensable" or "limiting" and "dispensable" because they are more descriptive of the effects of amino acids on protein metabolism. Threonine and lysine are clearly indispensable because they cannot be synthesized *de novo* from products of carbon intermediary metabolism (46).

Finally, illnesses or medications that increase protein turnover or muscle breakdown will have an influence on protein delivery. Steroids used for the treatment of BPD cause negative nitrogen balance by increasing the rate of protein breakdown but have little effect on protein synthesis. Long-term effects of steroids on growth have been demonstrated (47). The influence of illness and inflammation on linear growth and FFM gains (markers of protein accretion) has also been recognized and documented (48,49). Increased markers of inflammation and illness continue to negatively influence linear growth out to 24 months corrected age for prematurity (48).

Many preterm infants receive protein initially as part of a regimen of parenteral nutrition. Intravenous amino acid solutions have advanced to the point of being specifically formulated for preterm infants. These amino acid solutions are designed to normalize the plasma amino acid profile of the healthy infant, promoting levels similar to those of a 1-month-old breastfed infant. Infants receiving early amino acid solutions have improved and positive nitrogen balance and better developmental scores at 18 months (43). For these reasons, current recommendations for amino acid delivery are to begin at 3 g/kg/d immediately after birth and increase by 0.5 to 1 g/kg/d to approximately 4 g/kg/d (43).

Preterm infants who begin enteral feeds in the first days after birth will be relatively protein restricted because they are typically given human milk or low amounts of preterm infant formula.

Although human milk from mothers delivering preterm is initially higher in protein compared to term human milk (50), the content is still relatively low and rapidly decreases postnatally to term levels. In addition, the infant initially will receive low volumes while slowly advancing enteral feeds. Fortification with a human milk fortifier assists with this low-protein issue, however, still may not be enough. More recently, individualized fortification with fortifiers and additional protein supplementation has been recommended (51). Infants receiving this individualized fortification have been shown to have improved weight and head circumference gains (51).

Mineral and Trace Element Requirements

Mineral and trace element requirements in newborns are influenced by the immature status of the kidney, the gestational age, and medications that affect mineral metabolism (52–54). In general, preterm infants require higher amounts of minerals than term infants. The daily needs of some minerals (e.g., sodium, potassium chloride) are determined by measuring serum levels, while others (e.g., calcium, phosphorus) are estimated from *in utero* accretion rates (7).

Calcium and Phosphorus

The majority of calcium and phosphorus in the newborn is found in bone, yet the roles of these two minerals in biochemical reactions are essential to life. Ionic calcium mediates activation of neural impulses in the central and peripheral nervous systems and muscle contractions in skeletal and cardiac muscle. Phosphorus is at the core of cellular energy metabolic function through its role in adenosine triphosphate (ATP). Hypocalcemia or hypophosphatemia can lead to significant impairment of organ performance and ultimately death. Thus, the regulatory mechanisms for both are set up to ensure a constant source of adequate serum concentrations and tissue delivery. Catabolism of bone reserves of the two minerals provides a ready source to maintain this delivery.

Term Infants

Eighty percent of calcium and phosphorus in the term infant was accreted in the last trimester of gestation. Human milk has relatively low amounts of calcium and phosphorus (Table 20.1), which is nevertheless adequate to meet the skeletal growth requirements of the fully mineralized term infant. Subsequent loss of bone mineralization in the term-born infant is termed rickets and is usually due to dysregulation of vitamin D metabolism or inadequate intake

TABLE 20.1

Average Concentration of Major Nutrients per 100 mL in Term, Preterm, and Fortified Preterm Human Milk (52–54)

Nutrients[a]	Term Milk[b]	Preterm Milk[c]	Fortified Human Milk[d]
Energy (kcal)	67	67	80
Protein (g)	1.1	1.6	2.7
Calcium (mg)	25	25	113
Phosphorus (mg)	14	15	63
Sodium (mg)	28	28	48
Potassium (mg)	47	50	88
Iron (mg)	0.08	0.09	1.0
Zinc (mg)	0.36	0.37	1.0
Copper (µg)	37	38	130

[a]Human milk varies considerably in nutrient concentrations as a function of maternal age, infant age, time of collection, and maternal nutritional status in the case of certain, but not all nutrients. Generally recognized averages are presented.

[b]Term milk values are at 1 month of infant age.

[c]Preterm milk values are at 3 weeks of infant age.

[d]Multiple fortifiers are available. Data are averaged across four products added to preterm milk with the goal of fortifying to 80 kcal/100 mL.

or synthesis of vitamin D. It is rarely due to inadequate calcium or phosphorus intake.

Preterm Infants

In contrast to term infants, preterm infants are at high risk of bone demineralization, a condition termed osteopenia of prematurity, because of failure to accrete the minerals *in utero* (53). Calcium and phosphorus are the most difficult minerals to maintain in positive balance in the preterm infant because of the large deficit from lack of intrauterine loading, the high requirements for adequate mineralization due to rapid growth, excessive losses as a result of calciuric diuretics and steroids, the limited solubility of these nutrients in TPN, and their low concentrations in unfortified human milk. A calcium-to-phosphorus (mg/mg) ratio between 1.6 and 2.0 appears to be optimal for mineralization, depending on the source of the minerals (52,53). In contrast to rickets in term infants, osteopenia of prematurity is predominantly due to lack of adequate dietary calcium and phosphorus and not as much due to vitamin D deficiency, since preterm infants are capable of synthesizing 1,25 di-hydroxy vitamin D. However, preterm infants born to mothers with very low vitamin D status can have vitamin D deficiency, which will contribute to their bone demineralization. Maternal risk factors for low vitamin D status in her infant include low vitamin D intake and limited sun exposure due to latitude of residence or clothing practices. The preterm infant requires between 120 and 200 mg of calcium/kg body weight, 60 to 140 mg of phosphorus/kg, and at least 400 to 1,000 IU of vitamin D daily (53).

Iron

The majority of total body iron found in the term infant is accreted during the third trimester. The fetus maintains a constant total body iron content of 75 mg/kg during the last trimester, increasing from a total body iron of 35 to 40 mg at 24 weeks' gestation to 225 mg at term. Preterm delivery results in disruption of this process, and premature infants, including the late preterm, are therefore born with lower iron stores than term infants (55,56). Small-for-dates infants are frequently born with low iron stores for their gestational age, presumably because of decreased placental iron transport (56). Infants of diabetic mothers are born with low stores because much of the fetal iron has been sequestered in the expanded red cell mass (56). These infants also appear to be low in total body iron, most likely as a result of reduced transport of iron by the diabetic placenta, such that the increased iron need of the infants of diabetic mothers exceeds the placental transport capacity (56). Table 20.2 outlines the iron requirements for newborns of various birth weight and gestational age categories (57).

Term Infants

The breastfed appropriate-for-dates newborn infant who benefitted from delayed cord clamping and grows at a rate prescribed by the WHO standard curve has sufficient total body iron to remain nonanemic for up to 6 months (59). The small-for-dates term infant has closer to a 2-month reserve and is at high risk for postnatal iron deficiency if not adequately supplemented with dietary iron (60). The estimated daily iron requirement for the formula-fed appropriate for gestational-age (AGA) term infant is 1 mg/kg/d (33), although this may be an overestimate (59) (Table 20.2).

The major *dietary* source of iron for the healthy, term infant is human milk or infant formula fortified with iron. Additional iron is supplied by the relatively large iron stores with which the term infant is born with a resultant steady decline in those stores over the first 6 months of life (61). Thus, although human milk has a low iron content (0.3 mg/L) compared to either iron-fortified infant formula (10 to 12 mg/L) or "low-iron" formula (4.5 mg/L), the iron may be more bioavailable (33) and the fully fetally endowed infant has enough iron for the first 4 postnatal months (59). Infants fed formulas containing either 4 or 7 mg/L remain iron sufficient (62).

Preterm Infants

The preterm infant that is not growth restricted as a fetus begins extrauterine life with the same iron stores per kilogram body weight as the term infant (approximately 12 mg/kg). Serum ferritin concentrations, which reflect iron stores, are slightly lower in preterm infants (55,56). However, the preterm infant is exposed to several stressors that perturb iron balance; with the result that by the time of hospital discharge, the infant may be iron deficient or iron overloaded. The range of iron status of the preterm infant at 40 weeks post-conception appears to be far wider than the term infant, although systematic studies are lacking.

The preterm infant frequently goes into negative iron balance because of blood lost during phlebotomy coupled with a rapid growth rate (and expansion of the red cell mass) during the convalescent period (see also Chapter 42). The daily enteral iron requirement for the preterm infant who does not receive recombinant erythropoietin is 2 to 4 mg/kg/d, with the greater requirement for the more preterm infant (57,63). Infants who receive recombinant erythropoietin require at least 6 mg/kg/d of iron (Table 20.1) (63). It is important to monitor iron status markers such as serum ferritin, hemoglobin, and reticulocyte count to modulate iron delivery (57).

The issue of when to begin iron supplementation in the preterm infant is controversial. Iron is necessary for normal growth and development of all tissues, including the brain. A rich literature supports the hypothesis that early iron deficiency results in neurodevelopmental sequelae at the time of the deficiency and persists well after iron has been repleted (64). Iron deficiency in preterm infants slows nerve conduction (65). Nevertheless, iron is also a potent oxidant stressor since it catalyzes the Fenton reaction to produce reactive oxygen species. Since preterm infants have immature antioxidant systems, there is concern that free iron (i.e., in excess of the total iron-binding capacity) can exacerbate diseases that may be related etiologically to oxidative stress, including BPD, NEC, neuronal injury, and ROP (66). Infants who receive parenteral iron are at risk for having free circulating iron and increased markers of oxidative stress (67). Because of these concerns, parenteral iron should be used very sparingly. Conversely, enteral iron doses of up to 18 mg/kg daily have been given without generation of measureable reactive oxygen species or other sequelae (66). Since infants are born with adequate iron stores, there is no need to begin iron supplementation in a sick, nongrowing preterm infant. Therefore, enteral iron supplementation should not be started before 2 weeks postnatal age (57). Conversely, delaying iron supplementation until after 2 months confers a high risk of iron deficiency in the postdischarge period (58).

Human milk should be used whenever possible in preterm infants. However, because of the low iron content of human

TABLE 20.2

Iron Dosing for Neonates Based on Gestational, Size for Dates, and Diet (57,58)

Gestational Age	Size for Dates	Diet	Daily Iron Dose (mg/kg of Body Weight)
Term	AGA	Breastfed	0
Term	AGA	Formula	1
Term	SGA	Breastfed	1–2
Preterm >30 wk	AGA	Mixed	2
Preterm <30 wk	AGA	Mixed	3–4
Preterm; treated with rhEpo	AGA	Mixed	6

Data from Domellöf M. Meeting the iron needs of low and very low birth weight infants. *Ann Nutr Metab* 2017;71(Suppl 3):16; and Domellof M, Georgieff MK. Postdischarge iron requirements of the preterm infant. *J Pediatr* 2015;167:S31; PMC4571199.

milk and the rapid growth rate of these infants, additional iron supplementation is required. Additionally, those who receive recombinant human erythropoietin should be supplemented earlier with iron sulfate to have an adequate erythropoietic response. Preterm infant formulas are iron fortified and should provide adequate amounts to the larger preterm infant. However, preterm infants less than 30 weeks' gestation may well need enteral iron supplementation in addition to their preterm formula or fortified human milk to bring their total dose closer to 4 mg/kg/d. Those with serum ferritin concentrations below 76 μg/L may require additional iron, as that level in newborns has been associated with neurologic sequelae (65).

Zinc

Zinc is nutritionally essential for term and preterm infants (54,68). It plays a major role in gene regulation, tissue growth and differentiation, neural function, and immune competency. Zinc deficiency causes a classic dermatitis, increases the risk of infection, and reduces neural functioning. If prolonged, zinc deficiency affects long-term neurodevelopment.

Like iron, zinc is accumulated by the fetus largely in the third trimester, and the term newborn relies on stored zinc as well as zinc in maternal milk to meet postnatal requirements. This combination of sources is adequate for up to 4 to 6 months of age after which another source is required.

The preterm infant is at higher risk for zinc deficiency because of lower fetal loading, although the requirement is typically easily addressed with enteral and parenteral solutions (54,68). The preterm infant requires 1.4 to 2.5 mg of enteral zinc per kilogram body weight daily or 400 μg/kg parenterally. Zinc deficiency is relatively rare in the preterm infant with an uncomplicated hospital course. Nevertheless, assessment of zinc status in a preterm infant with otherwise unexplained growth failure can reveal that the etiology is zinc deficiency. In contrast to the healthy preterm infant, infants with short bowel syndrome or with significant fluid losses from the gastrointestinal track, for example, from an ileostomy or colostomy following bowel resection, are at higher risk for zinc deficiency (54).

Other Trace Elements

Six additional trace elements are considered nutritionally essential for the human infants: copper, selenium, chromium, manganese, molybdenum, and iodine (54). Excellent reviews of trace element requirements in newborns exist in the literature (52,54). Table 20.3 summarizes the daily requirements, biologic utility, and effects of deficiency of these elements in newborn infants (54,68,69). Most trace elements are accreted during the last trimester. Thus, the AGA term infant is fully replete and needs modest dietary intake of these elements. Both human milk and infant formula ensure adequate intakes. The preterm infant or the term infant on prolonged TPN would rapidly go into negative balance of any of these elements if not provided with an exogenous source (54). Infants should receive neonatal trace elements while on TPN. Preterm infant formulas and preterm human milk appear to supply adequate amounts of trace elements to the enterally fed premature infant (54).

Vitamins

Vitamin requirements in newborn infants are most easily conceptualized by considering water- and fat-soluble vitamins separately. An extensive review of all of the vitamins and their deficiencies is beyond the scope of this chapter, and the reader is referred to sources dedicated to this subject (33). This section will deal primarily with vitamins that are of particular relevance to neonates and to those with a specific risk for deficiency.

Water-Soluble Vitamins

Term newborns are rarely deficient of water-soluble vitamins in the B group (33). As with all humans, neonates need a daily source of vitamin C and folate. These are provided in adequate concentrations in human milk, infant formulas, and multivitamin preparations added to parenteral nutrition. The AAP has stated that term breastfed infants do not need supplemental water-soluble vitamins during the first 6 months unless there are extenuating circumstances (44). Preterm infants also do not appear to need supplemental water-soluble vitamins once they are taking an adequate amount of formula or fortified human milk. The minimum amount of enteral feeds needed to maintain vitamin sufficiency varies among the formulas and the human milk fortifiers available.

TABLE 20.3

Daily Enteral (E) and Parenteral (P) Requirements per kilogram Body Weight, Function and Clinical Effects of Deficiency of Selected Trace Elements (54,68,69)

Element	Daily Requirement	Biologic Function	Major Effects of Deficiency
Copper	E: 100–230 μg/kg P: 40 μg/kg	Electron transport Iron transport Brain development Antioxidant	Anemia (pancytopenia) Osteopenia Oxidant stress
Chromium	E: 0.03–1.25 μg/kg P: 0.05–0.3 μg/kg	Glucose regulation Insulin sensitivity	None reported in newborns
Iodine	E: 10–55 μg/kg P: 10 μg/kg[a]	Thyroid hormone Brain development	Hypothyroidism Growth failure Poor neurodevelopment
Manganese	E: 1.0–15 μg/kg P: 1.0–2.0 μg/kg	Antioxidant Neurotransmission Bone formation	Oxidant diseases Poor neurodevelopment Osteopenia
Molybdenum	E: 0.3–3 μg/kg P: 0.25 μg/kg	RedOx enzymes	None reported in newborns
Selenium	E: 5–10 μg/kg P: 2–10 μg/kg	Thyroid synthesis Antioxidant	Hypothyroidism Oxidant stress diseases Myopathy

[a]Reduce to 1 μg/kg if disinfectants with iodine are routinely used.

Fat-Soluble Vitamins

Fat-soluble vitamin deficiencies are also rarely a problem for term, healthy newborns fed human milk or infant formula. Nevertheless, certain groups of term and preterm infants are at risk for vitamin D deficiency (33,70). These include breastfed infants whose mothers are vitamin D deficient as a result of their diet (vegan) or whose mothers completely protect their own skin from sunlight. Their infants must also be exposed to less than 30 minutes of sunlight per day to be at greatest risk. The AAP recommends that all infants receive 400 IU of vitamin D daily (33,71).

Virtually all infants receive vitamin K in the delivery room to prevent hemorrhagic disease of the newborn. The prevalence of this condition is very low, but the neurologic consequences are so disastrous and preventable that the current recommendation is to continue to give vitamin K at birth. Once gut flora are established in the first 2 postnatal days, vitamin K deficiency is exceedingly rare (33).

Whereas infants are not wholly dependent on dietary sources for vitamin D (it can be synthesized *de novo* from sterol precursors by 1 week of age) and vitamin K (supplied by gut bacteria), vitamins E and A must be provided in the diet. The term infant who consumes human milk or infant formula receives an adequate amount of each, assuming that there are no impediments to fat absorption, such as cystic fibrosis or short bowel syndrome. In infants with those conditions, a water-soluble A and E preparation should be utilized and serum levels monitored.

There are significant issues with fat-soluble vitamins, particularly vitamins A and E, in preterm infants less than 34 weeks' gestation because of their relatively poor absorption of fats. As with term infants, vitamin K and, most likely, vitamin D are not major problems, although preterm infant formulas are supplemented with more vitamin D than are term formulas. Even the most premature infants are capable of synthesizing the active vitamin D metabolite by 1 week of age (72). Nevertheless, because of their increased risk for osteopenia of prematurity, premature infants may benefit from additional vitamin D if they show biochemical signs of vitamin D deficiency (53).

Vitamin A deficiency in growing mammals results in significant tissue fibrosis, particularly of the lung and liver. Preterm infants have low vitamin A levels and hepatic stores (73). Moreover, preterm infants with respiratory distress syndrome who have low cord blood vitamin A concentrations are more likely to develop BPD (73). A Cochrane review affirms that routine vitamin A supplementation of preterm infants reduces the risk for chronic lung disease (74). The risks are relatively small, but include intramuscular injections three times a week for 4 weeks in infants with little muscle mass, and the relatively remote possibility of vitamin A toxicity. Enteral vitamin A is poorly absorbed prior to 34 weeks post-conceptional age and thus is less reliable than parenteral strategies to improve vitamin A levels in extremely preterm infants (73).

Ever since it was noted that vitamin E deficiency causes hemolytic anemia, subsequent studies have assessed vitamin E's relationship to diseases that may involve oxidative stress in preterm infants such as BPD and ROP (75). Phospholipid membranes are at high risk for oxidative stress. If not adequately protected by circulating antioxidants such as vitamin E, selenium, and superoxide dismutase, membranes will be damaged, with subsequent cell death. Thus, it was hoped that vitamin E supplementation of the preterm infant who has an immature antioxidant system might prevent or ameliorate established BPD or ROP. Studies along those lines have been disappointing. A systematic review of trials of vitamin E supplementation to prevent the occurrence or progression of ROP has not shown a significant effect (75). Moreover, high vitamin E levels following supplementation appear to increase the risk of sepsis (75). Nevertheless, it is important to consider vitamin E deficiency in the diagnosis of hemolytic anemia in the preterm infant.

Preterm infant formulas are supplemented with vitamins E and A. For most infants fed the preterm infant formula with higher vitamin E and A concentrations, serum levels remain in the normal range. However, routine assessment of these levels in the high-risk infant less than 1,500 g may be prudent, since it is likely that the deficiency state is not advantageous to the growing infant.

NUTRIENT DELIVERY

Almost all term infants and some preterm infants more than 33 weeks' gestation will feed orally on demand immediately after birth. However, ill term infants and preterm infants who are not physiologically mature or who are unstable, and a significant number of late preterm infants will require alternate forms of nutrient delivery. The first decision revolves around whether the infant can be fed enterally or if supplemental parenteral nutrition is indicated. If long-term parenteral nutrition is anticipated, decisions will need to be made whether a central catheter should be placed or whether the nutrients should be given through a peripheral vein. If the infant is to be enterally gavage-fed, the practitioner has multiple options with respect to tube placement, rate of feeding advancement, and drip versus bolus approaches. Most of these approaches in preterm infants have been evaluated with respect to efficacy and safety through systematic reviews.

Parenteral Nutrition
Indications

The enteral route remains the preferred way to nourish babies. Parenteral nutrition is indicated in all infants in whom enteral nutrition is contraindicated or delivers less than 75% of total protein and energy requirements. Current recommendations are that trophic feeds, preferably of the infant's own mother's milk, are started on day 1 regardless of the degree of illness, in conjunction with prompt delivery of a parenteral solution that includes protein. Initiation of parenteral nutrition within 24 hours of birth is one factor associated with higher weight, length, and occipitofrontal circumference percentiles at discharge and reduced long-term morbidity (76). Furthermore, early enteral feedings in preterm infants promote ongoing maturity of the intestinal tract, reduces villous atrophy as a result of disuse, and kindles gut hormone activity (77). Thus, infants who still require moderate respiratory support still should receive low volume, often called "trophic" feeds supplemented with full parenteral nutrition. A recent Cochrane review of early trophic feedings versus enteral fasting for very preterm infants failed to show any risk (or benefit) to the practice. In particular, there was no effect of trophic feeding on the incidence of NEC, feeding intolerance, or growth rates (77).

Routes of Delivery

The decision whether to supply parenteral nutrition centrally or peripherally requires weighing the benefits versus the risks. Parenteral nutrition administered through a central line allows for greater energy delivery because solutions with dextrose concentrations more than 12.5% or osmolarity more than 1,000 mOsm/L can be administered. Dextrose concentrations of that magnitude and calcium infusions are poorly tolerated by peripheral veins and cause a high rate of venous sclerosis. Skin sloughs are likely to occur if the solution extravasates from the vein. For the same reasons, many intensive care nurseries will not allow or will limit the amount of calcium to be run through a peripheral venous line. This practice is sound but effectively limits the amount of calcium and phosphorus that can be delivered to a preterm infant already at great risk for osteopenia of prematurity.

The risks of central TPN relate primarily to the risk of central venous line placement and maintenance, with risks of venous thrombosis and catheter-related blood stream infections.

One risk of peripheral TPN is undernutrition. The infant receiving maximal concentrations of dextrose (D12.5%), amino acids (3.0 g/kg/d), and intravenous fat (3.5 g/kg/d) at an average fluid rate of 150 mL/kg/d will receive approximately 95 nonprotein kcal/kg/d. Although this amount of intake meets the daily resting energy expenditure of the premature infant (65 kcal/kg/d), there are insufficient "extra" calories to sustain weight gain at an intrauterine velocity. Thus, long-term peripheral TPN will result in preterm infants slowly falling away from the growth curve. Calcium delivery will also be constrained, either because of an absolute contraindication (in some nurseries) or because of osmolarity issues. Each day on peripheral TPN results in a larger deficit calcium balance and a higher risk of osteopenia of prematurity. Iron balance can become negative since intravenous iron is rarely utilized in neonates. Docosahexaenoic acid (DHA) balance is at risk because the preterm infant cannot synthesize it prior to 33 weeks' gestation.

Infants who are not expected to tolerate oral feedings within a week of starting parenteral nutrition should have a central line placed and be maintained on central parenteral nutrition. Central venous catheters may be umbilical venous catheters placed soon after birth, peripherally inserted central catheters and rarely in NICUS, surgically placed tunneled catheters (e.g., Broviac).

Nutritional Management

If parenteral nutrition is indicated, it should be started immediately after delivery and stabilization, since dextrose solutions alone cannot meet the resting energy requirements or the protein requirements of the neonate. Dextrose delivery should typically begin between 4 and 6 mg/kg/min and can be advanced as tolerated by following serum glucose concentrations. Glucose infusion rates of more than 12.5 mg/kg/min have been discouraged because of the significant negative effect on the respiratory quotient and concerns about increasing adiposity. However, in the few small studies that exist, increased caloric intake is associated with increased fat-free mass gains (28,31), and some of the long-term negative effects of hyperglycemia may be related to caloric restriction used as a therapy for the hyperglycemia (78). Insulin is useful in treating the hyperglycemia seen in ELBW infants in the first week of life, in whom glucose intolerance may necessitate decreasing dextrose delivery to unacceptably low rates that do not meet resting energy expenditure (<7 mg/kg/min). While it must be utilized carefully due to the risk of hypoglycemia, a recent study showed decreased mortality in those preterm infants with hyperglycemia that were treated with insulin (79).

Protein in the form of amino acid solutions designed for newborns should be administered within the first several hours after birth. There are few contraindications to early protein delivery, and there is evidence that amino acid solutions improve nitrogen balance (43). At energy intakes above resting energy expenditure (65 kcal/kg/d), the main determinant of positive nitrogen balance is the nitrogen intake. The goal is to achieve *in utero* nitrogen accretion rates while compensating for nitrogen losses as a result of illness. This appears to be possible with amino acid delivery rates of 4.0 g/kg/d (43). Although protein requirements may be higher as a result of prior malnutrition, diseases that increase nitrogen turnover, or catch-up growth, it is rarely practical to give more than 4.0 g/kg/d of parenteral amino acids. Studies demonstrate that administration of amino acids is safe for all infants on day 1 to 2. Most infants can be safely started on 3 g/kg/d and advanced by 1 g/kg/d to a maximum of 4.0 g/kg/d, thus ensuring that they will be on full protein delivery within 24 to 48 hours. Very unstable preterm infants and those with renal insufficiency as a result of

indomethacin administration, surgery, a PDA, or shock may need to be advanced more slowly.

Intravenous fats provide a low-volume source of calories and shift cellular metabolism toward less carbon dioxide production, perhaps improving the respiratory load of the infant. They can be utilized starting immediately after birth and are important in preventing essential fatty acid deficiency (80). Serum triglyceride levels are often monitored during intravenous fat therapy. Intravenous fat solutions can be started at a delivery rate of 1 to 2 g/kg/d and advanced to a maximum of 3.5 g/kg/d. Total intravenous fat calories should be less than 60% of the diet and typically are in the 30% to 40% range. Since fat incorporation into cells is dependent on insulin, fat intolerance in VLBW infants is more likely to be manifested by hypertriglyceridemia or, interestingly, hyperglycemia, requiring a slower rate of advancement (0.5 g/kg/d) or interruption of fat delivery. Fat emulsions are predominantly 20% solutions and are generally infused over no fewer than 16 hours to allow for clearance from the serum. It is important to run them separately from other solutions, so as not to disturb the stability of the emulsion. The solutions can be joined with the amino acid–containing solution with a Y-connector near the infusion point on the infant. Most commercially available intravenous fat solutions are soybean oil based. Concerns have been raised with the abnormal lipid profile that these induce and that cholestasis is a consequence of prolonged administration. Newer intravenous lipid emulsions that do not have soybean oil as their sole source of fatty acids have been utilized predominantly in Europe and recently become available in the United States. These products utilize various combinations of soybean oil, olive oil, MCT, and fish oil (SMOF). In early studies, they show promise in normalizing the fatty acid profile and reducing or treating severe TPN cholestasis. Double-blind RCTs assessing these preparations in preterm infants suggest that they are safe and well tolerated while promoting a more beneficial fatty acid profile and lower rates of cholestasis and/or sepsis (80). A systematic review recommended larger-scale trials to determine long-term outcome effects (80). While the SMOF trials have been prospective, beginning at the initiation of TPN, another lipid emulsion that is exclusively fish oil based has been used (in combination with other lipid emulsions) to treat infants with existing severe TPN cholestasis usually in the setting of short bowel syndrome (81). The results have been encouraging in reversal of cholestatic liver failure in neonates who had initially received exclusive soybean oil lipid emulsions (81). Both of these lipid strategies, along with variations of their respective themes, are becoming more common as the products become increasingly available in the United States (82).

Since infants initially undergo a free water diuresis before a salt diuresis, sodium needs remain low until after day 3 of life. Thereafter, sodium and potassium requirements increase rapidly, and serum concentrations should be monitored at least daily while infants are on intravenous solutions. Requirements may approach 10 mEq/kg/d for each if there are excessive urinary losses. Chloride is the usual anion for both sodium and potassium; however, these cations also can be given as acetates, allowing for fine tuning of acid–base balance. Amino acid solutions have an inherent chloride and acetate load.

Calcium and phosphorus balance are difficult to maintain in TPN nourished preterm infants. Because of solubility issues, calcium concentrations more than 16.6 mEq/L with a concomitant phosphorus concentration of 8.3 mM are rarely obtained. In an infant receiving 150 mL/kg/d, these values are equivalent to a calcium delivery of 50 mg/kg/d and a phosphorus delivery of 25 mg/kg/d—far less than the *in utero* accretion rate. Strategies to increase calcium retention and bone mineralization have been largely unsuccessful but have included infusing calcium in one line and phosphorus in another and alternate infusions of higher doses

TABLE 20.4

Nutritional Monitoring of Neonates during Transition: Special Phases

Nutrient	Circumstance	Assessment Tool	Frequency	Action Value(s)
Carnitine	Prolonged TPN	Serum [Free Carnitine]	Weekly after 2–4 wk of TPN	<20 µM/L
Copper	Overload with prolonged TPN + cholestasis	Serum [Copper]	Weekly after 2 wk of TPN	<20; >70 µg/L
Zinc	Overload with prolonged TPN or renal failure; deficiency post–GI surgery	Serum [Zinc]	Weekly after 2 wk of TPN post–GI surgery	<70; >130 µg/L
Manganese	Overload with prolonged TPN + cholestasis	Serum [Manganese]	Weekly after 2 wk of TPN or direct bilirubin > 2.0	>2.0 µg/L

of the two minerals. Monitoring of serum phosphorus and calcium levels while on TPN is important. Infants are prone to hypocalcemia in the first 72 hours as a result of transient hypoparathyroidism and hypophosphatemia. Both calcium and phosphorus should be added early during TPN therapy. Calcium delivery without phosphorus delivery should be avoided because of the likelihood of severe hypophosphatemia. This complication tends to occur in the first 72 to 96 hours because of the focus on the diagnosis and treatment of neonatal hypocalcemia. More acidic TPN solutions appear less likely to cause calcium–phosphorous precipitation.

Infants on TPN receive 0.2 mL/kg body weight of a neonatal trace element solution that supplies 0.02 mg/kg of copper, 0.3 mg/kg of zinc, 5 µg/kg of manganese, and 0.17 µg/kg of chromium. This supplement should be added with initiation of TPN and given daily. Selenium at 2 µg/kg should be added after 2 weeks of TPN (54,69,83). Although zinc, copper, chromium, manganese, or selenium levels in infants on TPN are not routinely monitored, the practitioner should be aware that preterm infants in particular have low stores of these trace elements and that deficiencies have been described (83,84). Certain medical conditions such as short bowel syndrome or enterostomies characterized by high fluid loss can increase zinc loss from the gastrointestinal tract, resulting in low plasma zinc concentrations and growth failure. Routine monitoring of zinc status is indicated in those conditions. While not ideal, measurement of plasma zinc concentrations is the most readily available test. Plasma levels less than 70 µg/dL should be addressed by increasing the amount of zinc in the TPN. In contrast, certain medical conditions (e.g., cholestasis or renal disease) can alter zinc (and copper) metabolism and result in overload (Table 20.4). These elements should be removed during overload conditions. Plasma levels can be monitored weekly or bi-weekly and the elements reinstituted in the TPN after levels return to normal. Water- and fat-soluble vitamins are added as a pediatric multivitamin solution to match the recommended parenteral dosing guidelines (83). This supplement should be added at initiation of TPN and given daily.

Complications of TPN

Administration of parenteral nutrition remains an inexact science. Because it is not the normal mode of nutritional delivery, it is not surprising that complications occur. For the most part, complications can be divided into those associated with catheters and those related to the nutrients themselves.

Intravenous lipids have been previously associated with hypoxia, pulmonary hypertension, hyperbilirubinemia, cholestasis, and infection (85). Infants with respiratory disease have minimally lower PaO_2 values when given intravenous lipids, most likely because lipids can uncouple hypoxic vasoconstriction. Normally, to optimize ventilation/perfusion matching, the pulmonary vasculature supplying a poorly oxygenated alveolar area will constrict. This effect is reduced by the infusion of lipids, most likely mediated by serotonin. Trials that have assessed whether early administration of intravenous lipids causes or protects preterm infants from chronic lung disease have had mixed results. Overall, given the prevalence of early and profound growth failure in infants with severe lung disease, it seems prudent to start lipids early in life.

Free fatty acids can displace bilirubin from albumin-binding sites, prompting some practitioners to limit the dose of lipids to very small preterm infants; however, clinical studies have demonstrated adequate albumin binding of bilirubin and no effect on serum bilirubin levels (85). There are no reports of fat emulsions increasing the incidence of kernicterus. Theoretically, chylomicrons can be taken up by the reticuloendothelial system and interfere with fighting infection. Fat emulsions are also good media for fungi, including *Candida albicans* and *Malassezia furfur*. Whether these risks clinically outweigh the benefits of higher energy intake for small preterm infants has not been studied. At this time, it is likely that intravenous lipids improve the survival of infants through better growth.

As noted above, neonates who receive TPN for more than 3 weeks are at greatest risk for cholestasis, particularly those with short bowel syndrome, NEC, and sepsis. Remaining NPO appears to increase the risk greatly, thus prompting various investigations into the role of small enteral feedings to protect and stimulate the gut. Small amounts of trophic feeds may reduce the prevalence of cholestasis by stimulating bile flow via cholecystokinin. Reduced bile flow from prolonged TPN is also associated with gallstones. In rare cases, prolonged TPN with no enteral intake will lead to cirrhosis. While the exact cause of cholestasis is unknown, current research has focused less on the role of amino acids and more on the role of abnormal fatty acid profiles induced by intravenous soybean emulsions. Thus, a large amount of research effort is being exerted to devise more optimal intralipid solutions (80,81).

Parenteral amino acids also are associated with toxicity. Excessive amino acid delivery will lead to increased serum BUN and ammonia levels as a result of the newborn infant's relatively immature renal and hepatic status. Previous concerns about parenteral amino acids being the cause of cholestasis appear to have been unfounded, and recent research shows they are typically tolerated as discussed above.

Aluminum toxicity is worth considering in infants who have been on TPN for more than 3 weeks. The largest contamination comes from the calcium and phosphorus salts that are added (86). The risk to the neonate is twofold. Aluminum accumulates in the bones of infants on TPN in which it is avidly taken up because of underlying osteopenia of prematurity (86). Of greater concern is the possibility that aluminum will cross the blood–brain barrier and induce an acute or chronic encephalopathy, as has been described in adult patients (86). Reduced renal capacity for excreting aluminum appears to be a necessary setting for this to occur, but it is not unusual for preterm infants to have a significant measure of renal insufficiency after treatment with indomethacin. Some have proposed that aluminum toxicity may be a factor in the poorer neurodevelopment of preterm infants (86). Since the body has no need for aluminum, manufacturers are being pressured to reduce the aluminum content of their solutions (86).

Monitoring TPN Efficacy and Toxicity

Careful monitoring of growth is indicated for any infant on TPN or partial parenteral nutrition. Weight should be measured daily and length and head circumference weekly. Protein status can be assessed in two ways: somatic protein deposition (arm muscle area, FFM, linear growth) and serum protein status (serum albumin, prealbumin, and BUN). The former provides a longitudinal view of protein accretion, although the latter reflects a more rapidly turned-over pool of protein. Prealbumin, also known as transthyretin, has a half-life of 1.9 days and can be measured if there is uncertainty regarding the need for higher protein intake. Like most rapidly turned-over proteins, prealbumin acts as an acute-phase reactant and will rise rapidly with stress, infection, and glucocorticosteroid administration, rendering it useless as a nutritional marker. Serum BUN can be used in a similar way to crudely judge nitrogen balance as long as there is no renal insufficiency. Serum BUN concentrations less than 4 mg/dL indicate inadequate protein intake. Serum albumin, which has a half-life of 21 days, could be monitored every 2 to 4 weeks. However, with more aggressive nutritional strategies utilizing early amino acid introduction and fortification, following these values has become less common.

It is important to monitor infants on parenteral nutrition because of the toxicities associated with its administration (Tables 20.4 to 20.6). At the least, infants on TPN should have a set of electrolytes and a serum glucose checked daily until stable and then a few times per week. Glucocorticosteroids increase the likelihood of both glucose and fat intolerance in preterm infants. ELBW infants and infants with sepsis are prone to hypertriglyceridemia, even if they have tolerated intravenous fat previously. Periodic monitoring of triglyceride levels may be indicated in high-risk groups. An elevated triglyceride level may be a sign of intolerance, and the lipid dose should not be advanced or potentially should be decreased or held for a brief interval.

Calcium status must be monitored carefully in the first days of postnatal life because hypocalcemia is commonly seen in ill newborns. Preterm infants, growth-restricted infants, and infants of diabetic mothers appear particularly prone to hypocalcemia. Infants receiving large amounts of citrated blood products, such as those who are postoperative, who are on ECMO, or who have disseminated intravascular coagulopathy, will require large amounts of calcium. Similarly, maintenance of normophosphatemia is important for normal metabolism. Therefore, serum calcium, phosphorus, and magnesium should be monitored daily in the first week of life, or until stable, and then weekly thereafter (Tables 20.5 and 20.6).

Bone mineralization is problematic for the preterm infant on long-term parenteral nutrition; therefore, close monitoring is indicated. Unfortunately, this can be quite difficult. Although osteopenia of prematurity is predominantly as a result of deficient

intakes of calcium and phosphorus, the serum levels of these minerals will be maintained at the expense of the bones. Thus, serial measurements of calcium are not useful in monitoring this complication. Serum alkaline phosphatase is an indirect measure of osteopenia because its level will increase with the bone remodeling that takes place to supply the serum calcium pool. The level should be monitored weekly to biweekly, particularly in preterm and growth-restricted infants. The level may be difficult to interpret, since the alkaline phosphatase will rise with cholestatic liver disease (a complication of parenteral nutrition itself) and

TABLE 20.5

Nutritional Monitoring of Neonates during Initial Illness

Nutrient	Assessment Tool	Frequency	Action Value(s)
Protein	BUN[a]	Daily–qod	<5 mg/dL
	Prealbumin[b]	Twice weekly	<5 mg/dL or reduction by 10% from previous
	Length	Weekly	<1 cm/wk
Energy	Serum [Glucose]	Daily	<70; >150 mg/dL
	Serum [Triglycerides]	Biweekly if on TPN	>200 mg/dL
	Weight	Daily	<15–18 g/kg
Calcium	Serum [Ca]	Daily × 3 d	<6.5; >10.0 mg/dL
	Serum ionized [Ca]	Daily × 3 d	<4.0; >6.0 mg/dL
Phosphorus	Serum [Phosphorus]	Daily × 3 d	<3.5; >8.5
Magnesium	Serum [Mg]	Daily × 3 d[c]	<1.3; >3.0 mEq/L
Iron	[Hemoglobin]	At birth; prn phlebotomy	Variable based on FiO$_2$ need
	Serum [Ferritin]	At birth	<40 µg/L
Vitamin A	Serum [Retinol]	At birth[d]	<20 µg/L
Vitamin E	Serum [Tocopherol]	At birth[e]	<6; >14 mg/L

[a]Assumes adequate renal function.
[b]Assumes no glucocorticosteroid therapy in prior 2 weeks.
[c]Longer if impaired renal function.
[d]If at risk for chronic lung disease.
[e]If actively dosing with vitamin E.

TABLE 20.6

Nutritional Monitoring of Neonates during Stable Growth in Hospital

Nutrient	Assessment Tool	Frequency	Action Value(s)
Protein	Length	Weekly	<1 cm/wk
Energy	Weight	Daily	<15–8 g/kg/d
	Length	Weekly	<1 cm/wk
	Head Circumference[c]	Weekly	<1 cm/wk
Bone mineralization	Alkaline Phosphatase	Weekly, biweekly	>450 IU/L
	Serum [Phosphorus]	Weekly, biweekly	<4.5 mg/dL
	X-ray	Only if fracture is suspected	Demineralization on x-ray indicates >33% bone loss
Iron	[Hemoglobin]	Weekly	Variable based on FiO$_2$ need
	% Reticulocytes	Weekly[d]	<3% if anemic
	Serum [Ferritin]	Weekly[e]	<100 µg/L
Vitamin A	Serum [Retinol]	Weekly until 34 wk postconception	<20 µg/dL
Vitamin E	Serum [Tocopherol]	Weekly until 34 wk postconception[e]	<6; >14 mg/L

[a]Assumes adequate renal function.
[b]Assumes no glucocorticosteroid therapy in prior 2 weeks.
[c]Only sensitive to severe malnutrition.
[d]If anemic.
[e]If actively dosing with vitamin E.

with intestinal injury (such as NEC). Fractionating the alkaline phosphatase level into its bone and nonbone components can be done but may take weeks depending on whether the laboratory has the capability to perform the fractionation. As with monitoring of most other biomarkers, the most important aspect of the alkaline phosphatase to follow is the trend. Rising alkaline phosphatase levels generally mean aggressive bone remodeling and an increased risk of osteopenia. Strategies to increase calcium and phosphorus delivery should be considered.

The incidence and severity of hepatic toxicity from parenteral nutrition have been on the decline but still complicate the courses of infants who are strictly NPO and on TPN. The toxicity is typically cholestatic in nature, with an initial rise in serum bile acids followed by an increase in the direct bilirubin, alkaline phosphatase, and gamma glutamyl transferase. Transaminase elevations are seen only in very severe cases. Total and direct bilirubin concentrations will typically be monitored in all newborns in the first week of life. Infants on prolonged TPN should have direct bilirubin measured weekly. If it is elevated, the remaining liver function tests should be assayed and followed weekly as well.

Trace minerals are rarely deficient in infants on TPN because of supplementation. Nevertheless, the importance of maintaining normal zinc status for growth and protein utilization (54,68) makes it wise to consider checking the serum zinc concentration if the infant is not growing adequately or has physical signs of zinc deficiency. Trace metals can also accumulate with cholestasis. Levels should be monitored and supplements adjusted.

With the exception of vitamins E and A, vitamin status generally need not be checked in infants on TPN. Most vitamin assays are cumbersome and are a poor reflection of total body load. Serum vitamin E and A levels also do not necessarily reflect total body stores. Nevertheless, the association of low serum retinol (circulating vitamin A) levels with an increased risk for BPD in the VLBW infant suggests that monitoring may be appropriate (73). An initial measurement in all infants less than 1,500 g with respiratory disease should indicate the degree of risk. Infants with levels less than 20 µg/dL should be supplemented and their levels followed weekly. The methodologies for assaying vitamin A (high-performance liquid chromatography or fluorometry) are the same as for vitamin E, and the values for both can be obtained simultaneously. As with vitamin A, it is important to keep vitamin E concentrations in the normal range, as an insufficient concentration has been associated with anemia, although toxic levels increase the risk of sepsis (75).

Enteral Nutrition

Oral Feeding

The goal for infants prior to discharge from the hospital is full oral feedings, preferably by breast (see also Chapter 18). Oral feedings come naturally to infants born at term but can be more problematic for the healthy premature infant. These infants rarely show any interest in oral feeding until approximately 32 weeks' gestation and rarely have a mature, safe feeding pattern until 34 weeks' gestation (87). Prior to that age, coordination of sucking, swallowing, and breathing is difficult; the issue is predominantly one of inappropriate swallow–respiration interfaces rather than suck–swallow interactions (87). Breastfed premature infants have longer periods of sucking with fewer obstructive apnea and desaturation spells than comparably sized bottle-fed infants (44). This may relate to the more metered rate of milk flow. It is important to note that preterm infants are frequently exposed to pacifiers to stimulate nonnutritive sucking, which improves gastric motility and likely increases the flow of important gastrointestinal hormones (88). It is unclear whether this nonnutritive sucking at an earlier postconceptional age affects the success of breastfeeding at 34 weeks' gestation, but a Cochrane review of the subject found a significant decrease in length of hospital stay and an earlier transition from tube feedings to bottle feedings in preterm infants (89).

A strong case can be made for feeding human milk to the preterm infant, either by gavage tube or by breastfeeding, because of its superior performance with respect to immune status, protection from NEC, establishing a normal microbiome and neurodevelopment, among other advantages (90,91). In order to successfully breastfeed the premature infant, the mother needs to be available to begin the process as the infant nears 33 weeks' gestation. Before that point, it is important that she maintains her milk supply. The intensive care nursery can help by providing a place to nurse, electric breast pumps, storage containers, and a freezer for storing the milk. An organized program with an informed leader is quite useful in timing the introduction of actual breastfeeding and in overseeing the progress made by the individual infant. With such a program, the majority of preterm infants whose mothers desire to nurse can successfully breastfeed at the time of discharge.

Preterm infants who are bottle fed also require close observation as they transition from gavage to nipple feeds. There is an energy cost to bottle feeding. Gavage feedings require less energy to process, and excessive oral feedings may tire an infant and reduce weight gain velocity. Typically, once-per-day attempts at bottle feeding can begin around 33 weeks' gestation. If the infant shows no interest or has significant obstructive apnea, it may be prudent to wait several days before attempting again. The frequency of feedings can be increased as the infant shows more aptitude. Once the infant has advanced to full oral feedings, it is important to see whether weight gain can be maintained on an ad libitum on-demand schedule prior to discharge. Consistency in feeding personnel can improve the infant's performance, and having the mother give most of the feedings is ideal. Adopting a cue-based feeding program, in which personnel pay attention to the feeding cues exhibited by the infant, may reduce the number of episodes in which the infant refuses to feed because of fatigue and aversion.

Oral aversion is a significant problem in infants who have been NPO or require mechanical ventilation for long periods of time. Symptoms include behaviors such as tongue-thrusting, head-turning, pooling of milk in the mouth, and occasionally breath-holding apneic spells. A barium swallowing study with fluoroscopy can help identify whether the problem is anatomical or is a result of discoordination, immaturity, or neurologic pathology. For infants with severe cases, the worst course is to force oral feedings. The involvement of an occupational or speech therapist can be invaluable in desensitizing the oral area and promoting safe feeding habits (92). Occasionally, preterm infants may not feed effectively until 48 weeks' postconceptional age (93).

Gavage Feeding

Gavage feedings are indicated for infants who can be fed enterally but not orally. For the most part, this approach is used in premature infants who are neurologically immature with the full expectation that they will feed orally. Infants who will not be candidates for oral feeds because of either anatomical or neurologic conditions can have gastrostomy tubes placed. Gavage feedings are most frequently accomplished by placing a naso- or orogastric tube and bolusing feedings intermittently; continuous transpyloric tube feeds are utilized occasionally to ensure nutrient delivery. Infants can receive feeds by continuous drip or by bolus; a Cochrane review affirms that there is no evidence that one is advantageous over the other (94).

Oro- or nasogastric tube feedings can be initiated using a soft silastic 5- or 8-Fr catheter. The tube is most commonly placed into the stomach prior to a feeding and usually kept in place for up to 7 days before replacement. The contents of the stomach are aspirated to ensure that the tip of the tube is still in the stomach before each feed. There is no evidence that routinely checking for residuals from the previous feeding prevents any complication. The feeding is allowed to run in by gravity or pushed in via a syringe. Feedings in infants with very slow gastric emptying times can have a 3-hour volume titrated in over 1 hour or more.

Bolus gastric gavage feedings can be given on a schedule between every 1 and 4 hours. Smaller infants may not tolerate excessive stomach distention with large-volume feedings and may exhibit respiratory compromise. They may need to be fed small amounts on a more frequent schedule. Infants less than 1,000 g can be fed on a bolus schedule of every 1 to 2 hours or with continuous drip feedings. Infants may be fed on this schedule until they weigh 1,250 to 1,500 g, after which every 3-hour feeds are more appropriate. Nevertheless, larger infants who are not tolerating bolus feedings, remain on ventilators, or have severe apnea and bradycardia may tolerate drip feedings. Term infants who require gavage feedings may do best on an every 3- to 4-hour schedule.

Tube placement and maintenance may cause significant problems in the infant. Tubes can be malpositioned in the airway instead of in the stomach. Placement of the tube can cause significant vagal stimulation that results in apnea or bradycardia. The presence of an indwelling tube can cause apnea and bradycardia either by excessive vagal stimulation or, more commonly, by upper airway obstruction. Although nasogastric tubes are more stable, they appear to cause more problems with airway obstruction. Gastric and esophageal perforations are rare but must be considered if there is a significant change in the infant's behavior or physical examination.

Gavage feedings can also be given through a transpyloric tube. The advantages of this type of feeding include ensured nutrient delivery and a smaller chance of gastroesophageal reflux (GER) and aspiration pneumonia. There are significant mechanical and nutritional disadvantages to this approach. The mechanical problems include the difficulty of placing the tube, although this becomes easier with practice. Although rare, the most devastating complication of transpyloric feedings is intestinal perforation and peritonitis.

Transpyloric feedings also pose significant nutritional risks (95). Bypassing the stomach decreases fat digestion and absorption, since up to 50% of fat processing takes place in the stomach by the lingual and gastric lipase enzymes. Additionally, secretion of gut hormones such as cholecystokinin and gastrin are dependent in part on stomach distention by a meal. Potassium accretion may be impaired. Bacterial colonization of the normally sterile intestine may be a significant risk since the normal mechanism by which the stomach acid kills bacteria has been bypassed. A Cochrane review confirmed a higher rate of gastrointestinal disturbance and mortality with transpyloric feedings (95).

Initiation of gavage feedings through any of the tubes mentioned above requires a careful assessment of the infant. The stable infant more than 1,500 g birth weight can typically be fed within hours of birth, although if the infant is less than 35 weeks' gestation, it is prudent to gradually advance the strength and volume of feedings. Advancement at a rate of 20 mL/kg body weight per day appears to be safe as long as the infant shows no signs of feeding intolerance. A Cochrane review of rapid (30 to 35 mL/kg daily) versus slow (15 to 20 mL/kg daily) rates of advancement revealed that more rapid rates were associated with a shorter time to regain birth weight and to achieve full enteral feedings without an increase in any morbidity including NEC (96). Infants with birth weights more than 1,500 g can be started on every 3-hour feedings; infants between 1,000 and 1,500 g on every 2-hour feedings; and infants less than 1,000 g on every 1-hour, 2-hour, or continuous-drip feedings. Although low-volume feedings are better tolerated from a respiratory standpoint, the gastric emptying time of the preterm infant is often between 60 and 90 minutes. Therefore, it is likely that gastric preaspirates will be present in an infant fed every hour or by continuous drip. The availability and ease of administration of parenteral nutrition make a strong argument for being conservative with feeding advancement in preterm infants.

Low Volume (Trophic) Feeds
Early initiation and slow advancement of feedings may benefit an infant who has been ill and likely had an ileus. There is no evidence that delaying the introduction of enteral feedings beyond 4 days or using dilute formulations after birth reduces the risk of NEC (97,98). The trend in the last 20 years has been to start with trophic feeds of less than 24 mL/d in preterm infants. A Cochrane review of 9 trials (754 subjects) concluded that there was no evidence that early trophic feedings affect feeding tolerance or growth rates (77). It should be noted, however, that the trials included in the review were mainly infants with birth weights greater than 1,000 g and of greater than 28 weeks' gestation (77). Trophic feedings can be considered more as "oral medication" than as true feedings because little is gained nutritionally from them.

WHAT TO FEED NEWBORN INFANTS

What one decides to feed infants is dependent on understanding the developmental physiology of the newborn gastrointestinal tract, the requirements of the infant for normal growth and body composition, and the available mechanisms of nutrient delivery. It is not surprising that term infants will thrive on different amounts and types of foods than will preterm infants and that allowances in both groups must be made for the effect of illness on nutrient requirements.

Term Infants
Human Milk
Human milk is species-specific food for human beings (Table 20.1) (44). As such, it represents the best choice of food for the newborn infant. Substitute feedings, usually made from an animal milk base, have been available for hundreds of years and have been highly refined in the past century. Nevertheless, no manufactured food can match the content of human milk for several reasons. Human milk is delivered fresh and has no "shelf life." This simple property allows live cells, growth factors, enzymes, and immune factors to remain intact and active. Formulas, which are designed to have a shelf life of 1 to 2 years (depending on the type of formulation), do not incorporate many of these factors because they would be unstable and would degrade over time.

There are few absolute contraindications to breastfeeding. Infants with galactosemia should not be breastfed nor should infants whose mothers are using illegal drugs. The exception is opioid using mothers who are encouraged to breast feed their infants, in order to decrease the severity of neonatal abstinence syndrome. Mothers with active tuberculosis and mothers in high-income countries who have human immunodeficiency virus (HIV) should also not breastfeed. In resource poor countries, exclusive breast feeding up to 6 months of age is recommended for infants born to HIV positive mothers, when no alternatives are available. Mothers who are taking certain medications (e.g., amethopterin, bromocriptine, cimetidine, clemastine, cyclophosphamide, ergotamine, gold salts, methimazole, phenindione, thiouracil) should not breastfeed. Complete lists of maternal medications that contraindicate breastfeeding are available. LactMed, a free database by the U.S. National Library of Medicine provides information on medicines used during lactation, potential effects on breast fed infants and possible alternatives to these drugs. Temporary disorders, such as maternal mastitis or engorgement, are not contraindications to breastfeeding.

Infant Formula
Many women choose formula feeding instead of breastfeeding for their infants. Infant formulas promote growth and development when used as an alternative to breastfeeding, but their performance remains short of human milk. They should be given for the first year (33). Formula manufacturers continuously attempt to improve their products, with the goal of matching human milk composition or performance. These are likely to remain unfulfilled quests. Most infant formulas are cow's milk based and are formulated at 20 cal/oz. Alternatives include soy-based formula and elemental formulas.

Carbohydrates provide approximately 40% to 45% of the calories in formula. The most commonly used cow's milk–based formulas contain lactose as the primary carbohydrate, whereas the soy formulas contain either sucrose or glucose polymers.

The protein in formula provides approximately 10% of the total calories. Cow's milk protein is casein predominant, which has a higher curd tension than whey. Formula manufacturers have increasingly processed the cow's milk protein to make the formulas whey predominant. The ratio in human milk is 70:30 (91). Soy formulas contain soy proteins, which also support normal linear growth and muscle accretion. The protein content of soy formulas is higher than that of cow's milk formula. Soy formulas contain phytic acid, which may bind divalent cations (Ca, Mg) in the formula. For this reason, the calcium content of soy formulas is greater than that of cow's milk formulas. Both bone mineralization and linear bone growth in term infants fed soy formulas appear to be adequate. Soy formulas are not suitable for preterm infants (see section on preterm infants below).

Fat constitutes 40% to 55% of calories in infant formula and is usually a blend of vegetable oils, such as corn, coconut, soy, or palmolein. Vegetable oils are added to cow's milk–based formulas because babies do not tolerate butterfat well. Formula manufacturers have added DHA and AA to their infant formulas.

Substantial alterations need to be made to whole cow milk to create a formula that a newborn infant will tolerate and thrive on. Whole cow milk is highly osmolar, low in calcium, high in phosphorus, low in vitamins A and D, and very low in bioavailable iron. Significant adjusting of all of these nutrients, in addition to the protein and fat manipulations, is necessary before an infant formula is safe for newborns.

Soy formulas are indicated for infants with galactosemia or lactase deficiency and infants whose mothers choose a vegetarian diet for their family (99). On the other hand, there is no evidence that soy formula prevents atopic disease. Soy formulas do not relieve colic and are not indicated for premature infants (see "Preterm Infants" section) (99).

Elemental and casein hydrolysate formulas continue to make up a larger part of the infant formula market despite their high cost. Their main use has been in the treatment and prevention of allergy because 90% of the protein fragments are less than 1,250 Da molecular weight. These low molecular weight fragments are less antigenic than cow's milk protein. In spite of this, anaphylaxis to these formulas can occur. Additionally, the rate of true cow's milk protein allergy in newborns is less than 3%. All hydrolysate formulas promote adequate growth and nitrogen retention. Hydrolysates are not indicated for refeeding infants after gastroenteritis or for treating colic. They are more osmolar than standard cow's milk or soy formulas and thus possess a potential risk to the intestinal epithelium, particularly in the preterm infant.

Preterm Infants

Human Milk

Mothers who deliver preterm initially produce milk that has a higher protein content, higher caloric density, higher calcium content, and higher sodium content than milk from mothers who deliver at term (50). To a certain extent, these higher concentrations match the increased needs for these nutrients in preterm infants. The composition of preterm human milk changes during the first few weeks postnatally and becomes more like term human milk thereafter.

Human milk provides multiple nutritional advantages for the low-birth-weight (LBW) infant (50,91). In spite of these advantages, feeding unsupplemented human milk to preterm infants poses several nutritional problems, particularly for the infant less than 1,500 g (91). Preterm infants fed unsupplemented human milk have slow growth rates and higher rates of hyponatremia and osteopenia (91). These findings suggest that despite the altered content of preterm human milk, there is still not enough energy, protein, calcium, phosphorus, and sodium to sustain adequate growth and bone mineralization. Thus, human milk delivered to all infants less than 1,500 g should be fortified with products that increase the caloric, protein, sodium, and calcium density of the milk (91). These products induce better growth and bone mineralization than unsupplemented preterm human milk when fortified to an assumed caloric density of 24 kcal/oz.

There is great variability in the milk expressed by mothers delivering preterm. Therefore, monitoring of nutritional status and customizing the supplementation are critically important in preterm infants fed fortified human milk. In particular, growth rates, serum sodium concentrations, and bone mineralization status (serum alkaline phosphatase concentration) should be assessed with regularity in these infants. Inadequate weight gain (<20 g/kg/d consistently over 1 week) can be treated by giving the infant more hind milk in the diet or with increased fortification. Poor linear growth can be partially addressed by adding calories and/or protein to the milk. Persistent increases in serum alkaline phosphatase concentrations despite fortification may necessitate adding some feedings of preterm infant formula.

Care must be taken in handling human milk to protect its important nutritional and immunologic advantages. Fresh human milk is best but is often impractical, particularly if the mother is not regularly available. Fresh milk can be kept refrigerated up to 24 hours but must then be frozen. Although live cells are destroyed by deep freezing, proteins, including the all-important lipase enzyme that improves fat absorption from 50% to greater than 90%, remain largely intact. Suboptimal freezing results in fat breakdown. Rewarming frozen human milk can be dangerous as microwaving heats milk unevenly and can cause esophageal or gastric burns. It is more prudent to thaw an aliquot of milk for the entire shift or day and dispense it once it has been warmed in a water bath.

With the acceptance of own mother's milk as the gold standard basis for feeding preterm infants, inevitably the question of the role of donor milk in preterm nutrition has arisen (89). In theory, donor milk that has been screened and pasteurized could retain many of the nutritional compositional advantages of own mother's milk, including proteins and fats that are species specific. The former would reduce the preterm's exposure to cow milk protein, and the latter would include some amount of LC-PUFAs. Nevertheless, other components such as live cells and lactase are lost in processing. The donor milk may be compositionally more like term milk and will not have the specific maternal antibodies that are generated through skin-to-skin care with her infant. Own mother's milk convincingly protects the preterm infant from NEC (91,100). This effect is also present with donor milk but is associated with slower growth, perhaps due to underestimation of the nutrient content and inadequate fortification (100). It is becoming increasingly common for NICUs to offer donor milk to preterm infants through the period of highest NEC risk, while others prescribe it for all infants. Additionally, there are now human milk–derived fortifier products available which allow for preterm infants to receive an exclusive human milk diet fortified to various caloric concentrations. These products may also reduce the risk of NEC when provided to high-risk infants, however remain expensive and therefore difficult to obtain for all infants. However, use is increasing across the United States, and increasing research is focused on the short- and long-term benefits of these products.

Human milk post-discharge can also form the basis for post-discharge nutrition. Many preterm infants will go home on a mixture of feedings; breastfeeding, bottle feeding of pumped human milk and intermittent feedings with preterm discharge formulas. The main concern is that infants with birth weights less than 1,500 g will have large accrued deficits at the time of discharge (10,48). Feedings with pumped human milk or preterm discharge formulas offer an opportunity for supplementation of the nutrients most likely to be in deficit: energy, protein, calcium, phosphorus, and iron. Fortification of bottled human milk can be accomplished through the addition of powdered formula (either a preterm discharge formula or a term formula) to own mother's milk. The number of fortified or supplemented bottle feedings per day should be titrated against the individual patient's nutrition monitoring panel, including standard anthropometrics and serum indices of bone mineralization and iron status.

Preterm Infant Formulas

Formulas specifically designed for the preterm infant represent an alternative to human milk in the nutrition of these infants. Preterm formula compared with fortified donor breast milk results in not only a higher rate of short-term growth but also a higher risk of developing necrotizing enterocolitis (101). Prior to the introduction of these formulas in the late 1970s through mid-1980s, preterm infants were fed various formulations intended for infants with very different intestinal maturity, nutrient assimilation capability, and nutritional requirements. The science that went into developing preterm infant formulas carefully measured the nutrient needs of the preterm infant based on the reference fetus (7) and the digestive and absorptive capabilities. When these two factors were considered together, a unique formulation for preterm infants evolved. For the most part, the preterm infant formulas are designed with the physiology of the less than 34-week gestational-age infant in mind. Infants more than or equal to 34 weeks whose mothers choose not to breastfeed are typically started on term infant formulas. If they show signs of intolerance (e.g., diarrhea, excessive gas, abdominal distention), relative lactase insufficiency as a result of immature intestinal development should be suspected, and a preterm formula can be used.

The carbohydrate source for preterm infant formulas is a combination of lactose and glucose polymers. The lactose content is reduced compared to term infant formulas because of the relatively lower lactase concentration found in the preterm intestine. Glucose polymers are easily digested and are low osmolar.

The protein source is cow milk that has been made whey predominant. The concentration of protein is quite high, delivering up to 4.5 g/kg/d when the formula is fed at a typical volume of 150 mL/kg/d. This high rate of delivery is designed to match the intrauterine accretion of nitrogen (46,102). Protein intakes at this rate maintain reasonable muscle mass accretion and support normal serum albumin and prealbumin concentrations.

As in term formulas, the fat blend is derived from vegetable oils. However, preterm infant formulas contain between 10% and 50% of the fat content as MCTs. The necessity of MCT remains controversial (27). Addition of MCT was stimulated by the finding that lingual and gastric lipases are particularly effective at hydrolyzing fatty acids of this length and because long-chain fatty acids require an adequate bile salt pool for absorption. As discussed previously, preterm infants have low bile salt pools, which contributes to their higher fat malabsorption rate. Excessive MCT are not indicated, as they are poorly utilized for fat storage. They are an excellent source of energy, with the excess being excreted in the form of dicarboxylic acids. As a result of the GRAS determination of LC-PUFAs in infant formula, preterm infant formulas contain DHA and ARA, an important addition given the rapid decline in LC-PUFA balance in preterm infants less than 33 weeks' gestation.

The sodium and potassium contents of preterm infant formulas are higher than term formulas to compensate for renal tubular immaturity. Levels of trace elements are likewise higher. The preterm infant formulas contain the most calcium and phosphorus of any formula available. The current formulations, when fed at a volume of 150 mL/kg/d, will provide approximately 225 mg/kg/d of calcium and 110 mg/kg/d of phosphorus. This is well in excess of intrauterine accretion rates, allowing these formulas to be utilized to provide catch-up bone mineralization for those infants who have been on prolonged parenteral nutrition or dilute formulas. In spite of this high content, many premature infants less than 1,500 g have evidence of osteopenia of prematurity at the time of discharge. Preterm infant formulas are supplemented with iron in recognition of the fact that preterm infants are born with low iron stores compared to term infants and that a rapid expansion of the red cell mass when catch-up growth ensues places a large stress on maintaining iron balance.

The preterm infant formulas are replete with water- and fat-soluble vitamins. Both formulations have higher vitamin D, E, and A concentrations compared to term formulas because of the poor fat absorption in preterm infants and the concern about the consequences of deficiency states in the infants. Vitamin A and E serum levels in preterm infants fed preterm infant formula with higher vitamin A and E concentrations demonstrate that additional supplementation with vitamins is not necessary once the infant is consuming at least 150 mL/kg body weight daily.

Techniques for the initiation, advancement, and maintenance of preterm infant formula feedings vary widely. Most infants will be on parenteral nutrition while their feedings are advanced. Although opinions vary greatly regarding whether formula volume or strength should be increased first, one should keep in mind that 1 mL of fully advanced peripheral parenteral nutrition (D12.5%, 3.0 to 4.0 g/kg/d of amino acids, 3.5 g/kg/d of lipids) is equivalent to approximately three-quarter strength formula. Thus, volume-for-volume substitution of TPN with dilute formula will reduce the caloric delivery to the infant, while substitution with full-strength formula, either 20 kcal/oz or 24 kcal/oz, will advance caloric intake. While most NICUs do not dilute breast milk and very few use diluted formula, a Cochrane review demonstrated that initiating feeds in LBW infants with dilute formula resulted in more rapid attainment of adequate energy intake (97). This occurred in spite of no differences in feeding tolerance.

Other Formulas

Although a large number of other formulas have been used for preterm infants, none are specifically designed to meet the nutritional needs of these infants. Any potential advantage of these formulas must be weighed against some fairly serious nutritional shortcomings or side effects. For example, soy formulas were used extensively in the late 1970s and early 1980s for preterm infants because they do not contain lactose and because of the concern that the preterm infant's intestine was particularly permeable to translocation of antigenic milk proteins. However, calcium absorption from soy formulas is poor because the phytates in soy bind divalent cations. The incidence of osteopenia and rickets in preterm infants who are fed soy formulas is too high to justify recommending these products for this population.

Similarly, the possibility of using elemental or casein hydrolysate formulas for preterm infants has been suggested. The attractiveness of these formulas stems from their more elemental nature, thus presenting less of a digestive challenge to the immature preterm intestine. Unfortunately, these formulas are a poor nutritional match for the preterm infant from a fat-soluble vitamin and mineral standpoint. The vitamin E and A contents of the hydrolysates are one-quarter to one-half that of premature infant formula. The significantly lower vitamin D levels, lower calcium levels, and poor calcium-to-phosphorus ratio (1.4:1) place the preterm infant at high risk for osteopenia of prematurity. Finally, the osmolarity of these formulas ranges from 290 to 330 mOsm/L at 20 kcal/oz, 25% higher than the preterm infant formulas, which have osmolarities of 210 to 220 mOsm/L at 20 kcal/oz and 250 to 270 mOsm/L at 24 kcal/oz. Hyperosmolarity is considered a risk factor for NEC in preterm infants. As currently formulated, elemental or casein hydrolysate formulas are not recommended for routine use in preterm infants.

Preterm Discharge Formulas

Fortified breast milk or follow-up formulas for preterm infants should be utilized to continue the process of catch-up growth in the postdischarge period. This process is incomplete at the time of discharge with significant energy, protein, and mineral deficits present (103). Growth restriction may continue for years afterward (48). Prior to their introduction, the formula-fed preterm infant was usually switched to a formula designed for term infants prior to discharge from the hospital. This made sense from a digestive standpoint because most intestinal capacities are similar to term by 34 weeks postconception, and preterm infants rarely leave the hospital prior to that age. Nevertheless, this practice neither did not take into account the large deficits in muscle stores, fat stores, and bone mineralization that occur in many of these infants (10,48,103) nor did they take into account the high rates of growth in preterm infants in the first year.

Follow-up formulas represent a hybrid between preterm and term infant formulas. The ones marketed in the United States are powders designed to be diluted to 22 cal/oz but can be prepared at various concentrations. At the 22 kcal/oz concentration, they have a 50% higher calcium and vitamin D content than cow's milk–based formula for term infants. The carbohydrate content is a blend of lactose and glucose polymers, and the fat blends contain MCT oil in a manner similar to preterm infant formulas. There is less vitamin A and less sodium than in preterm infant formulas, but more vitamin A and D than in term formulas. The recommendation has been to give these formulas for at least the first 6 months postdischarge, although the manufacturers state that the formulas are safe for the entire first postnatal year. In spite of promising preliminary studies, a recent Cochrane review failed to show that these formulas promote better growth rates and mineral status than does term formula in the preterm infant at follow-up (104). This is an important concept because of the large nutritional deficits that are accrued by the preterm infant in the NICU and the association between poor in-hospital growth and neurodevelopmental disability (16,48). The protein–energy deficit at hospital discharge is calculated at 25 g of protein and 1,000 kcal/kg of body weight (e.g., 50 g of protein and 2,000 kcal of energy for the average 2 kg premature infant at discharge) (101).

An alternative approach has been to continue to feed the discharged patient premature infant formula (104). Two problems arise with this solution: the formulas are not available commercially, and the improved fat digestive capacity of the infant after 34 weeks post-conception raises the possibility of excessive vitamin A absorption. Moreover, the preterm infant formulas were designed for the special physiology of the less than 1,500 g, less than 34-week postconceptional-age infant.

SPECIAL CONDITIONS THAT AFFECT NEONATAL NUTRITIONAL REQUIREMENTS

The Effect of Neonatal Illness on Nutritional Requirements

Most studies of neonatal nutritional requirements have dealt with defining the needs of the healthy growing term or preterm infant. Nevertheless, adults and older children who are ill undergo profound changes in metabolism, including the ability to absorb and utilize nutrients, based on the type and degree of illness. Cerra et al. (105) have investigated the independent effects of surgery, trauma, and sepsis on adult metabolism and have found consistent changes in protein–energy requirements. Each incident increases cellular oxygen consumption and promotes more negative nitrogen balance; sepsis has the most profound effects. Cytokines such as tumor necrosis factor (TNF-alpha), interleukin-6 (IL-6), and interleukin-1 (IL-1) appear to be important mediators of the response (105). These are elevated in preterm and term infants with sepsis (106). The adult studies suggest that energy and amino acid delivery must be significantly modified in sick patients. In particular, these patients appear to require higher energy delivery and more protein to remain in neutral or positive nitrogen balance. Fewer studies have assessed these issues in preterm and term newborns, but some of the metabolic effects of acute lung disease, chronic lung disease, CHF, and sepsis have been studied. Recent research has also shown associations with early illness and decreased long-term gains in FFM and length, which are both markers of protein accretion (48,49). These findings, specifically for length gains, persist until at least 24 months corrected age (48) and may suggest an association between inflammation and suppression of the growth hormone axis. In addition to the metabolic changes associated with illness, nutrition is often withheld during times of acute illness. This early accumulation of nutritional deficits is at least in part responsible for the long-term consequences poor growth and neurodevelopment (107). The conclusions of these studies support the concept that simply supplying the nutrients normally required by the healthy newborn will not be sufficient for infants with these illnesses.

Overall Approach Based on Stage of Illness in Preterm Infants

In 1995, the Canadian Pediatric Society proposed a novel approach to neonatal nutrition, primarily designed for premature infants but adaptable for term infants (108). This approach acknowledged that nutritional needs of premature infants change based on the metabolic demands of the phase of their illnesses. The initial "transition" phase is characterized as the time of neonatal illness and physiologic instability. Although defined as the first 10 postnatal days, the timing is flexible based on the duration of neonatal illness. The sick premature infant is likely to be relatively insulin resistant and to have increased circulating counterregulatory (gluconeogenic) hormones, including cortisol and glucagon. Vasopressor therapy with dopamine, dobutamine, or epinephrine may have effects similar to the endogenous hormones. These factors, combined with the release of cytokines during illness, place the infant in a catabolic rather than anabolic state. Under such circumstances, growth factors are down-regulated and growth is unlikely. Premature infants typically show weight loss, linear growth suppression, and lack of head growth during their period of illness (16,48). The nutritional strategy for this first phase is incompletely defined. Principles from the adult critical care would suggest that energy delivery should at least meet resting energy expenditure to prevent further glycogen, muscle, and fat breakdown for gluconeogenesis. Once resting energy expenditure has been met in the stable, growing infant (approximately 60 kcal/kg/d), additional calories are channeled for growth, with a cost of about 2.5 kcal/g of weight gain. However, in the insulin-resistant sick infant with down-regulated growth factors, it is uncertain if increased caloric provision will result in improved growth and there are very few randomized trials to answer this question. Moreover, carbohydrates, with their respiratory quotient of 1.0, generate more carbon dioxide than an equivalent caloric intake of fat. The major source of nutrition during illness is often parenteral with a minimal contribution from enteral feedings. Administration of protein from birth is beneficial during this period to reduce the degree of negative nitrogen balance. The safety and efficacy of 3 g of protein/kg body weight on day 1 of postnatal life have been established, and this has become the standard for neonatal nutritional therapy (43). The use of specialized protein blends to replace particular amino acids lost during illness has not yet been studied extensively.

After the initial illness has resolved, the infant enters the in-hospital growth period, which is characterized by physiologic stability and an anabolic state. The goal during this period is to match intrauterine growth rates and mineral accretion and to recover ground lost during the period of nutritional restriction and catabolism during the period of illness (16,48). For the preterm infants less than 34 weeks postconception, nutrient delivery should be adjusted to take into account digestive and absorptive immaturities. The preferred diet is fortified own mother's milk, but fortification of donor milk and premature infant formulas also address these issues.

Preterm infants in the postdischarge phase are also anabolic and growing. Compared to the in-hospital growth phase, their physiology is characterized by a mature absorptive and digestive system similar to that of the term infant. Unlike the term infant, however, these infants have accrued large energy, protein, and mineral deficits (16,48), and their growth indices are frequently below the tenth percentile for their age adjusted for prematurity. Premature infant discharge formula and fortification/supplementation of human milk after hospital discharge would appear to be indicated based on the projected nutrient deficits accrued during the hospitalization. The premature infant discharge formulas have increased energy, protein, calcium, phosphorus, iron, vitamin A, and vitamin D compared to term infant formulas.

In summary, a triphasic system seeks to customize nutritional delivery for the preterm infant based on physiology and nutrient needs. Better definition of specific nutrient needs (e.g., amino acids, growth factors) for each phase and the development of noninflammatory formulas to be delivered enterally during transition or periods of medical instability are indicated.

Specific Disease Effects on Nutrient Requirements

Whether acute lung disease, such as hyaline membrane disease, increases the oxygen consumption of the infant in direct proportion to the degree of respiratory illness remains debated (21). Unlike in adults, however, nitrogen balance in newborns appears to be unaffected by acute respiratory illness. The mean protein requirement to maintain neutral nitrogen balance during respiratory disease is 1.5 to 2.0 g/kg/d. Severe respiratory illness is associated with a higher incidence of hypocalcemia and hypoglycemia. There appears to be no indication to increase protein delivery beyond what would normally be given; for example, 4 g/kg daily.

In contrast to acute respiratory disease, significant chronic lung disease increases the resting energy expenditure by up to 30% (21), and infants with BPD will require greater energy intakes to grow adequately. Protein requirements have not been extensively studied in infants with BPD, but those who are treated with steroids have increased muscle breakdown, more negative nitrogen balance, and reduced linear growth velocity (47,48). Clearly, malnutrition plays an important role in the genesis of the disease and the rate of recovery (109).

CHF has a profound effect on resting energy expenditure. Infants with CHF as a result of structural heart disease may require up to 150 kcal/kg/d on the basis of both an increased metabolic rate and malabsorption as a result of intestinal edema. The protein requirement of infants with CHF has not been studied, although it is clear many fail to thrive and have reduced muscle mass. This may occur in part because of restricted protein intake (due to fluid restriction) and increased protein breakdown during a systemic inflammatory response induced by the surgery and its complications. It is prudent to increase the protein delivery commensurate with the increase in energy delivery, maintaining a 25 to 30 kcal:g protein ratio. Persistent cyanosis causes an additional nutritional stress by increasing the infant's need for iron. Since many of these infants have secondary polycythemia, there must be enough iron in the diet to support augmented erythropoiesis. Failure of a cyanotic infant to maintain an elevated hemoglobin may be as a result of iron deficiency, which can be screened for with a ferritin concentration and by assessing the red cell indices for microcytosis.

The effect of sepsis on neonatal nutritional status has not been thoroughly evaluated. Relatively small sample studies demonstrate that septic infants have increased TNF and IL-6 levels associated with negative nitrogen balance, but their levels are not nearly as high as seen in septic adults (11,22,106). Sepsis increases oxygen consumption (109)—although this may be a nonspecific response to illness, as it is seen in other nonseptic states. No studies have assessed whether nutritional interventions, for example, more protein or energy delivery, alter this physiologic condition. The roles of infection and inflammation on neonatal nutritional status and nutrient requirements clearly need greater study in light of the finding that the number of days on antibiotics is associated with poorer linear growth and neurodevelopmental outcome (48).

NUTRITIONAL MONITORING (TABLES 20.4 TO 20.7)

Any plan to nourish newborn infants should include plans for monitoring the nutritional status of the infant and the response to nutritional therapy. Assessment of nutritional status may include reviewing the dietary history, physical measurement, and interpretation of biomarkers obtained from the infant. A distinction should be made between biomarkers and bioindicators (110). A biomarker can give information about the status of the nutrient (e.g., serum ferritin concentration <40 µg/L indicates iron stores <5th percentile for age in a term infant (111), whereas a bioindicator can give information about the impact of a nutrient on a relevant health function (e.g., a serum ferritin concentration <76 µg/L

TABLE 20.7			
Nutritional Monitoring of Neonates after Discharge			
Nutrient	**Assessment Tool**	**Frequency**	**Action Value(s)**
Protein	Length	Monthly	Reduced velocity based on WHO standards
Energy	Weight	Variable	Reduced or increased velocity based on WHO standards
	Weight for length	Monthly	Asymmetric growth
	Head circumference[a]	Monthly	Reduced or increased velocity based on WHO standards
Bone mineralization	Alkaline phosphatase	At 4 wk postdischarge if indicated[b]	>450 IU/L
	Serum [Phosphorus]	At 4 wk postdischarge if indicated[b]	<4.5 mg/dL
	X-ray	Only if fracture is suspected	Demineralization on x-ray indicates >33% bone loss
Iron	[Hemoglobin]	At 4 wk postdischarge	Hemoglobin <105 g/L
		At 6 mo postterm[c]	
	Serum [Ferritin]	At 4 wk postdischarge	<30 µg/L at 4 wk; <12 µg/L at 6 mo
		At 6 mo postterm[c]	

[a]Only sensitive to severe malnutrition.

[b]Indications include active bone disease at discharge, severe osteopenia, on calciuric diuretics, on glucocorticosteroids as outpatient.

[c]Check iron status in premature infants and small-for-dates term infants earlier than in full-term AGA infant.

indicates a risk to brain function) (65). The distinction between biomarkers and bioindicators is important in deciding when to intervene nutritionally (110). Being two standard deviations from a population norm does not necessarily imply medical pathology. Conversely, as with the example of newborn ferritin concentration, medical pathology due to deficiency may exist at a level well above the lower cut off for population norms. Future research linking growth curves (see below) and other nutritional biomarkers to long-term relevant health outcomes is critical in order to determine whether interventions are effective (110).

Practically, for the healthy term infant, periodic plotting of the infant's weight, length, and head circumference on a standard growth curve is standard. The WHO curves now provide a standard, as opposed to reference growth curves for term infants around the world (12). The assessment of these parameters at birth provides a metric of the quality of fetal growth and also provides a starting point for postnatal monitoring. Small-weight-for-dates infants should be assessed for signs and symptoms of intrauterine growth restriction (e.g., hypoglycemia) that may compromise long-term outcomes. Signs of intrauterine wasting may also be present in some appropriate-weight-for-dates infants and will manifest as having an inappropriately low weight for their length. These infants are also at risk for neonatal symptomatology and long-term deficits (See Chapter 26).

Similarly, appropriate curves can be utilized to judge the relationship of growth and nutritional health of preterm infants (112). Before 40 weeks' gestation, there are two commonly used curves that have plotted cross-sectional data of infants born prematurely and more recently have been stratified by sex (15,17). These curves extend from 22 weeks' gestation to 42 weeks' gestation and are thought to resemble the growth of the fetus *in utero*. After this time, the WHO released standard curves developed from infants born at full term, breastfed, and growing "ideally" can be used (12). These curves were not generated from data of preterm infants; however, given the AAP goal of growing the preterm infant similarly to the *in utero* fetus and term infant, it may be the appropriate curve for the post-discharge preterm infant. When using this curve, preterm infants should be plotted at their age adjusted for prematurity. More outcome-based research is needed to clarify which pattern of growth will lead to the best metabolic, growth, and neurodevelopmental outcomes for these infants (5,111,112).

Recent efforts to come up with a working definition of malnutrition in preterm infants speak to this issue (111). Attempts to provide a better definition of malnutrition include monitoring z-score trajectory instead of percentiles with the goal of using a decline in z-score to project catch-up weight gain and establish a reasonable target of grams per day (113). Researchers are questioning whether assessing weight gain on a per kilogram body weight basis makes sense (114). Grams/day eliminates the problem that growth velocity varies with gender and age. Moreover, grams/kg varies with the number used in the denominator, that is, assumes that the weight reflects an appropriate, not water-weight-driven number (114). Ultimately, optimal growth patterns in preterm infants remain unknown. That ultimate pattern has to be informed by long-term health outcomes, that is, neurodevelopment and metabolic risk, and applies to optimal rates of catch-up growth as well (115).

The importance of monitoring protein–energy status in the hospitalized newborn cannot be overemphasized. It is state of the art for NICUs with substantial numbers of nutritionally at-risk infants to have Nutrition Support Services that review the infants' status daily and provide nutritional recommendations. Ideally, these nutrition support teams should include a registered dietician, a doctor of pharmacy, and a physician. All should have a background or additional training in neonatal nutritional principles. Such teams have a positive effect on the nutritional status of preterm infants at discharge (116).

Daily weights and weekly length and head circumference measurements should be routinely performed and charted. The effect of manipulating protein–energy delivery should be reflected in the rate of weight gain; however, interpretation of protein-energy status from weight measurements can be complicated by fluid retention or dehydration. Length measurements are the least reliable because of the difficulty in obtaining reproducible numbers but are important in terms of assessing protein accretion, which in turn is related to neurodevelopmental outcome (48). A more accurate method of length assessment is the routine use of an infant length board. Assessments of energy requirements can also be made by indirect calorimetry to estimate resting energy expenditure. These measurements require special equipment and provide only a brief (usually 20 minutes) glimpse into energy utilization. The daily energy expenditure is extrapolated from the short-term measurement with the potential errors introduced by the extrapolation. Stable isotope techniques such as double-labeled water are the province of research institutions and are not used for clinical monitoring. Similarly, dual-photon absorptiometry x-ray (DEXA) has been used in research studies to assess fat and lean body mass. More recently, air displacement plethysmography has become available as a method of body composition measurement in infants as small as 1 kg and has been validated for use in the preterm population (117). This method is quick (measurement takes 1 to 2 minutes) and noninvasive; however, it requires infants to be stable off of respiratory support and central lines. Given that this tool is most useful during periods of growth later in the hospitalization and postdischarge, most infants can tolerate the short measurement without support. Skinfold measurements and calculation of the arm fat area, as well as weight for length assessments, are additional inexpensive and noninvasive methods of assessing the infant's relative fat status.

Protein status can be assessed by measurements of somatic or serum proteins or the serum BUN and creatinine concentrations in the absence of renal disease. The BUN will reflect recent nitrogen intake, while the serum creatinine level indexes muscle mass. Low values are valid screening markers of poor somatic protein status. Somatic protein status is also reflected in the arm muscle area, which is calculated from the arm circumference and the skinfold thickness. The somatic muscle pool turns over relatively slowly, and serial measurements, like those of length, do not provide acute information with respect to recent nutritional manipulations. Serum proteins have various half-lives and thus give differential time information. Serum prealbumin (transthyretin) concentrations reflect recent protein intake and predict subsequent weight gain velocity. The half-life of the protein is 1.9 days; therefore, a weekly assessment of the serum prealbumin is useful. In contrast, serum albumin has a half-life of 10 to 21 days, can be used as a marker of chronic protein status, and can be assessed monthly if needed. It is not responsive to recent manipulations in protein delivery. Frequent routine assessment of fat free mass is another potential method of measurement of protein accretion and has become more plausible with the availability of infant air displacement plethysmography (117,118).

Rapidly changing glucose, mineral, and electrolyte status is best monitored with serum levels. Sodium and potassium levels should be followed in infants on who are on TPN or are receiving diuretics. Similarly, infants on TPN should have their serum glucose concentrations monitored. In the first days after birth, sick infants should have serum calcium, magnesium, and phosphorus levels assessed.

Chronic calcium and bone mineralization status should not be monitored solely with serum calcium and phosphorus levels because they will usually be in the normal to low-normal range. The serum alkaline phosphatase concentration is an indirect measurement of bone mineralization since it is closely tied to rapid bone turnover. An infant who is becoming osteopenic will have more rapid bone turnover and will have a higher serum alkaline phosphatase and lower phosphorus levels (119). A rapidly rising weekly alkaline phosphatase level is often indicative of active osteopenia. X-ray changes demonstrating demineralization are late findings and indicate that the bones are at least 33% demineralized. An elevated urinary excretion of phosphorus is also found during osteopenia of prematurity (119).

In general, it is unnecessary to routinely monitor trace element or vitamin status in the healthy, growing premature infant. However, higher-risk infants should be monitored periodically, depending on the micronutrient in question and the disease state of the infant. If one chooses to treat infants less than 1500g who are at high risk for BPD with Vitamin A (74), the infants most likely to benefit are those with low vitamin A status, as indexed by a serum retinol concentration of <20 microgram/dl. Concomitant vitamin E measurements can also be obtained. Weekly vitamin A and E levels should be followed in infants treated for deficiency.

The use of recombinant human erythropoietin has made monitoring of iron status an important consideration in the preterm infant. The iron status of the premature infant can fluctuate widely; infants who have received multiple transfusions have extremely high ferritin concentrations. Conversely, the meager iron stores of those who receive few or no transfusions will be rapidly consumed by erythropoiesis. Those treated with recombinant erythropoietin experience a decrease in their ferritin levels (63). They are likely to need iron supplementation earlier than premature infants who have been transfused. Reference values for ferritin have been published for neonates (55,56). Since iron has a narrow therapeutic-to-toxic ratio, better norms for assessing iron status in preterm infants are needed. Table 20.6 illustrates typical monitoring during the preemie growth phase of the hospital stay.

Nutritional monitoring does not end with hospital discharge since the preterm infant carries forward nutrient deficits accrued in the unit and remains on special formulations and supplements for variable time periods post-discharge. Nutrients at particular risk include energy, protein, calcium/phosphorus, and iron. While there are no official recommendations for post-discharge monitoring, Table 20.7 presents suggestions.

REFERENCES

1. Sammallahti S, Pyhala R, Lahti M, et al. Infant growth after preterm birth and neurocognitive abilities in young adulthood. *J Pediatr* 2014;165:1109.
2. Lewandowski AJ, Lamata P, Francis JM, et al. Breast milk consumption in preterm neonates and cardiac shape in adulthood. *Pediatrics* 2016;138(1):e20160050.
3. Balasuriya CND, Evensen KAI, Mosti MP, et al. Peak bone mass and bone microarchitecture in adults born with low birth weight preterm or at term: a cohort study. *J Clin Endocrinol Metab* 2017;102(7):2491.
4. Spector LG, Johnson KJ, Soler JT, et al. Perinatal risk factors for hepatoblastoma. *Br J Cancer* 2008;98(9):1570.
5. Raiten DJ, Steiber AL, Carlson SE, et al.; Pre-B Consultative Working Groups. Working group reports: evaluation on the evidence to support practice guidelines for nutritional care of preterm infants- the Pre-B Project. *Am J Clin Nutr* 2016;103:648S.
6. Raiten DJ, Raghavan R, Porter A, et al. Executive summary: evaluating the evidence base to support the inclusion of infants and children from birth to 24 mo of age in the Dietary Guidelines for Americans—"the B-24 Project". *Am J Clin Nutr* 2014;99(3):663S.
7. Ziegler EE, O'Donnell AM, Nelson SE, et al. Body composition of the reference fetus. *Growth* 1976;40:239.
8. Johnson MJ, Wootton SA, Leaf AA, et al. Preterm birth and body composition at term equivalent age: a systematic review and meta-analysis. *Pediatrics* 2012;130(3):E640. doi: 10.1542/peds.2011-3379.
9. Bell KA, Matthews LG, Cherkerzian S, et al. Associations of growth and body composition with brain size in preterm infants. *J Pediatr* 2019;214:20.
10. Ehrenkranz RA, Younes N, Lemons JA, et al. Longitudinal growth of hospitalized very low birth weight infants. *Pediatrics* 1999;104:280.
11. Ramel SE, Brown LD, Georgieff MK. The Impact of neonatal illness on nutritional requirements-one size does not fit all. *Curr Pediatr Rep* 2014;2(4):248.
12. WHO. Child growth standards based on length/height, weight and age. *Acta Paediatr Suppl* 2006;450:76.
13. Maguire JL, Salehi L, Birken CS, et al. Association between total duration of breastfeeding and Iron deficiency. *Pediatrics* 2013;131(5):e1530.
14. Papageorghiou AT, Ohuma EO, Altman DG, et al. International standards for fetal growth based on serial ultrasound measurements: the Fetal Growth Longitudinal Study of the INTERGROWTH-21st Project. *Lancet* 2014;384(9946):869.
15. Olsen IE, Groveman SA, Lawson ML, et al. New intrauterine growth curves based on United States data. *Pediatrics* 2010;125(2):e214.
16. Ehrenkranz RA, Dusick AM, Vohr BR, et al. Growth in the neonatal intensive care unit influences neurodevelopmental and growth outcomes of extremely low birth weight infants. *Pediatrics* 2006;117(4):1253.
17. Fenton TR, Chan HT, Madhu A, et al. Preterm infant growth velocity calculations: a systematic review. *Pediatrics* 2017;139(3):e20162045.
18. Ross Pediatrics. *Composition of feedings for infants and young children. Ross Ready Reference*. Columbus, OH: Ross Products Division, Abbott Laboratories, 1996.
19. Motil KJ. Meeting protein needs. In: Tsang RC, Zlotkin SH, Nichols B, et al., eds. *Nutrition during infancy*, 2nd ed. Cincinnati, OH: Digipub, 1997:83.
20. Stocker FP, Wilkoff W, Mietinen OS, et al. Oxygen consumption in infants with heart disease. *J Pediatr* 1972;80:43.
21. Dani C, Poggi C. Nutrition and bronchopulmonary dysplasia. *J Matern Fetal Neonatal Med* 2012;25(suppl 3):37.
22. Mrozek JD, Georgieff MK, Blazar BR, et al. Effect of sepsis syndrome on neonatal protein and energy metabolism. *J Perinatol* 2000;20:96.
23. Bauer J, Maier K, Linderkamp O, et al. Effect of caffeine on oxygen consumption and metabolic rate in very low birth weight infants with idiopathic apnea. *Pediatrics* 2001;107(4):660.
24. Heinig MJ, Nommsen LA, Peerson JM, et al. Energy and protein intakes of breast-fed and formula-fed infants during the first year of life and their association with growth velocity. The DARLING study. *Am J Clin Nutr* 1993;58:152.
25. Lindquist S, Hernell O. Lipid digestion and absorption in early life: an update. *Curr Opin Clin Nutr Metab Care* 2010;13(3):314.
26. Sauer PJJ, Dane HF, Visser HKA. Longitudinal studies on metabolic rate, heat loss, and energy cost of growth in low birth weight infants. *Pediatr Res* 1984;18:254.
27. Klein CJ. Nutrient requirements for preterm infant formulas. *J Nutr* 2002;132(6 suppl 1):1395S.
28. Costa-Orvay JA, Figueras-Aloy J, Romera G, et al. The effects of varying protein and energy intakes on the growth and body composition of very low birth weight infants. *Nutr J* 2011;10:140.
29. Hay WW Jr. Fetal and neonatal glucose homeostasis and their relation to small for gestation age infants. *Semin Perinatol* 1984;8:101.
30. Collins JW Jr, Hoppe M, Brow K, et al. A controlled trial of insulin infusion and parenteral nutrition in extremely low birth weight infants with glucose intolerance. *J Pediatr* 1991;118:921.
31. Ramel SE, Gray H, Christiansen E, et al. Greater early gains in fat-free mass, but not fat mass, are associated with improved neurodevelopment at 1 year corrected age for prematurity in very low birth weight preterm infants. *J Pediatr* 2016;173:108.
32. Ramel SE, Long JD, Gray H, et al. Neonatal hyperglycemia and diminished long-term growth in very low birth weight preterm infants. *J Perinatol* 2013;33(11):882.
33. American Academy of Pediatrics. In: Kleinman R, ed. *Pediatric nutrition handbook*, 7th ed. Elk Grove Village, IL: AAP, 2013.
34. Innis SM. Polyunsaturated fatty acid nutrition in infants born at term. In: Dobbing J, ed. *Developing brain and behaviour. chapter: The role of lipids in infant formula. the role of lipids in infant formula*. San Diego, CA: Academic Press, 1997:103.
35. Martin CR, Dasilva DA, Cluette-brown JE, et al. Decreased postnatal docosahexaenoic and arachidonic acid blood levels in premature infants are associated with neonatal morbidities. *J Pediatr* 2011;159(5):743.
36. Koletzko B, Baker S, Cleghorn G, et al. Global standard for the composition of infant formula: recommendations of an ESPGHAN coordinated international expert group. *J Pediatr Gastroenterol Nutr* 2005;41(5):584.
37. Jensen CL, Heird WC. Lipids with an emphasis on long-chain polyunsaturated fatty acids. *Clin Perinatol* 2002;29:261.
38. Jasani B, Simmer K, Patole SK, et al. Long-chain polyunsaturated fatty acid supplementation in infants born at term. *Cochrane Database Syst Rev* 2017;(3):CD000376.
39. Moon K, Rao SC, Schulzke SM, et al. Long-chain polyunsaturated fatty acid supplementation in preterm infants. *Cochrane Database Syst Rev* 2016;(12):CD000375.
40. Lapillonne A, Moltu SJ. Long-chain polyunsaturated fatty acids and clinical outcomes of preterm infants. *Ann Nutr Metab* 2016;69(suppl 1):35.
41. Kumar M, Kabra NS, Paes B. Carnitine supplementation for preterm infants with recurrent apnea. *Cochrane Database Syst Rev* 2004;(4):CD004497.
42. Olsen IE, Harris CL, Lawson L, et al. Higher protein intake improves length, not weight, z-scores in preterm infants. *J Pediatr Gastroenterol Nutr* 2014;58:409.

43. Embleton ND, van den Akker CHP. Protein intakes to optimize outcomes for preterm infants. *Semin Perinatol* 2019;43(7):151154.

44. Section on Breastfeeding. Breastfeeding and the use of human milk. *Pediatrics* 2012;129(3):e827.

45. Koletzko B, Demmelmair H, Grote V, et al. Optimized protein intakes in term infants support physiological growth and promote long-term health. *Semin Perinatol* 2019;43(7):151153.

46. Rigo J. Protein, amino acid and other nitrogen compounds. In: Tsang R, Uauy R, Koletzko B, et al., eds. *Nutritional requirements of the premature infant*. Cincinnati, OH: Digipub, 2005:45.

47. Tijsseling D, Ter Wolbeek M, Derks JB, et al. Neonatal corticosteroid therapy affects growth patterns in early infancy. *PLoS One* 2018;13(2):e0192162.

48. Ramel SE, Demerath EW, Gray HL, et al. The relationship of poor linear growth velocity with neonatal illness and two year neurodevelopment in preterm infants. *Neonatology* 2012;102:19.

49. Ramel SE, Gray H, Larson Ode K, et al. Body composition changes in preterm infants following hospital discharge: a comparison to term infants. *J Pediatr Gastroenterol Nutr* 2011;53(3):333.

50. Mimouni FB, Lubetzky R, Yochpaz S, et al. Preterm human milk macronutrient and energy composition: a systematic review and meta-analysis. *Clin Perinatol* 2017;44(1):165.

51. Radmacher PG, Adamkin DH. Fortification of human milk for preterm infants. *Semin Fetal Neonatal Med* 2017;22(1):30.

52. Koletzko B, Poindexter B, Uauy R. Recommended nutrient intake levels for stable, fully enterally fed very low birth weight infants. In: Koletzko B, Poindexter B, Uauy R, eds. *Nutritional care of preterm infants: scientific bases and practical guidelines*, vol 110. Basel, Switzerland: Karger, 2014:297.

53. Mimouni FB, Mandel D, Lubetsky R, et al. Calcium, phosphorus, magnesium and vitamin D requirements of the preterm infant. In: Koletzko B, Poindexter B, Uauy R, eds. *Nutritional care of preterm infants: scientific bases and practical guidelines*, vol 110. Basel, Switzerland: Karger, 2014:140.

54. Domellof M. Nutritional care of premature infants: microminerals. In: Koletzko B, Poindexter B, Uauy R, eds. *Nutritional care of preterm infants: scientific bases and practical guidelines*, vol 110. Basel, Switzerland: Karger, 2014:121.

55. Lorenz L, Peter A, Poets CF, Franz AR. A review of cord blood concentrations of iron status parameters to define reference ranges for preterm infants. *Neonatology* 2013;104(3):194.

56. Siddappa AJ, Rao R, Long JD, et al. The assessment of newborn iron stores at birth: a review of the literature and standards for ferritin concentrations. *Neonatology* 2007;92:73.

57. Domellöf M. Meeting the iron needs of low and very low birth weight infants. *Ann Nutr Metab* 2017;71(suppl 3):16.

58. Domellof M, Georgieff MK. Postdischarge iron requirements of the preterm infant. *J Pediatr* 2015;167:S31.

59. Georgieff MK, Krebs NF, Cusick SE. The benefits and risks of iron supplementation in pregnancy and childhood. *Annu Rev Nutr* 2019;39:121.

60. Berglund S, Westrup B, Domellof M. Iron supplements reduce the risk of iron deficiency anemia in marginally low birth weight infants. *Pediatrics* 2010;126(4):e874.

61. Ziegler EE, Nelson SE, Jeter JM. Iron stores of breastfed infants during the first year of life. *Nutrients* 2014;6(5):2023.

62. Lonnerdal B, Hernell O. Iron, zinc, copper and selenium status of breastfed infants and infants fed trace element fortified milk-based infant formula. *Acta Paediatr* 1994;83:367.

63. Carnielli VP, Da Riol R, Montini G. Iron supplementation enhances response to high doses of recombinant human erythropoietin in preterm infants. *Arch Dis Child Fetal Neonatal Ed* 1998;79(1):F44.

64. Georgieff MK. Iron assessment to protect the developing brain. *Am J Clin Nutr* 2017;106(S):1588S.

65. Amin SB, Orlando M, Eddins A, et al. In utero iron status and auditory neural maturation in premature infants as evaluated by auditory brainstem response. *J Pediatr* 2010;156(3):377.

66. Braekke K, Bechensteen AG, Halvorsen BL, et al. Oxidative stress markers and antioxidant status after oral iron supplementation to very low birth weight infants. *J Pediatr* 2007;151(1):23.

67. Pollak A, Hayde M, Hayn M, et al. Effect of intravenous iron supplementation on erythropoiesis in erythropoietin treated premature infants. *Pediatrics* 2001;107:78.

68. Terrin G, Berni Canani R, Di Chiara M, et al. Zinc in early life: a key element in the fetus and preterm neonate. *Nutrients* 2015;7:10427.

69. Darlow BA, Austin NC. Selenium supplementation to prevent short-term morbidity in preterm neonates. *Cochrane Database Syst Rev* 2003;(4):CD003312.

70. Taylor SN, Wagner CL, Fanning D, et al. Vitamin D status as related to race and feeding type in preterm infants. *Breastfeed Med* 2006;1(3):156.

71. Bouillon R. Comparative analysis of nutritional guidelines for vitamin D. *Nat Rev Endocrinol* 2017;13(8):466.

72. Hillman L, Hoff N, Salmons SJ, et al. Mineral homeostasis in very premature infants: serial evaluation of serum 25 hydroxy vitamin D, serum minerals and bone mineralization. *J Pediatr* 1985;106:970.

73. Schwartz E, Zelig R, Parker A, et al. Vitamin A supplementation for the prevention of bronchopulmonary dysplasia in preterm infants: an update. *Nutr Clin Pract* 2017;32(3):346.

74. Darlow BA, Graham PJ. Vitamin A supplementation to prevent mortality and short and long-term morbidity in very low birthweight infants. *Cochrane Database Syst Rev* 2007;(4):CD000501.

75. Brion LP, Bell EF, Raghuveer TS. Vitamin E supplementation for prevention of morbidity and mortality in preterm infants. *Cochrane Database Syst Rev* 2003;(4):CD003665.

76. Klevebro S, Westin V, Stoltz Sjöström E, et al. Early energy and protein intakes and associations with growth, BPD, and ROP in extremely preterm infants. *Clin Nutr* 2019;38(3):1289.

77. Morgan J, Bombell S, McGuire W. Early trophic feeding versus enteral fasting for very preterm or very low birth weight infants. *Cochrane Database Syst Rev* 2013;(3):CD000504.

78. Ramel SE, Rao R. Hyperglycemia in extremely preterm infants. *Neoreviews* 2020;21(2):e89.

79. Zamir I, Tornevi A, Abrahamsson T, et al. Hyperglycemia in extremely preterm infants—insulin treatment, mortality and nutrient intakes. *J Pediatr* 2018;200:104.

80. Vlaardingerbroek H, Veldhorst MA, Spronk S, et al. Parenteral lipid administration to very-low-birth-weight infants—early introduction of lipids and use of new lipid emulsions: a systematic review and meta-analysis. *Am J Clin Nutr* 2012;96(2):255.

81. Nandivada P, Fell GL, Gura KM, et al. Lipid emulsions in the treatment and prevention of parenteral nutrition-associated liver disease in infants and children. *Am J Clin Nutr* 2016;103(2):629S.

82. Kapoor V, Malviya MN, Soll R. Lipid emulsions for parenterally fed preterm infants. *Cochrane Database Syst Rev* 2019;(6):CD013163.

83. Greene H, Hambidge K, Schanler R, et al. Guidelines for the use of vitamins, trace elements, calcium, magnesium, and phosphorus in infants and children receiving total parenteral nutrition: report of the Subcommittee on Pediatric Parenteral Nutrient Requirements from the Committee on Clinical Practice Issues of the American Society for Clinical Nutrition. *Am J Clin Nutr* 1988;48:1324.

84. Zemrani B, McCallum Z, Bines JE. Trace element provision in parenteral nutrition in children: one size does not fit all. *Nutrients* 2018;10(11):1819.

85. Ghassan SA, Mahmmoud AF, Mai N, et al. Intravenous lipids for preterm infants: a review. *Clin Med Insights Pediatr* 2015;9:25.

86. Fortenberry M, Hernandez L, Morton J. Evaluating differences in aluminum exposure through parenteral nutrition in neonatal morbidities. *Nutrients* 2017;9(11):1249.

87. Commare CE, Tappenden KA. Development of the infant intestine: implications for nutrition support. *Nutr Clin Pract* 2007;22(2):159.

88. Berseth CL. Feeding methods for the preterm infant. *Semin Neonatol* 2001;6(5):417.

89. Foster JP, Psaila K, Patterson T. Non-nutritive sucking for increasing physiologic stability and nutrition in preterm infants. *Cochrane Database Syst Rev* 2016;(10):CD001071.

90. Brown JVE, Walsh V, McGuire W. Formula versus maternal breast milk for feeding preterm or low birth weight infants. *Cochrane Database Syst Rev* 2019;(8):CD002972.

91. Bhatia J. Human milk and the premature infant. *Ann Nutr Metab* 2013;62(suppl 3):8.

92. Prabhakar V, Hasenstab KA, Osborn E, et al. Pharyngeal contractile and regulatory characteristics are distinct during nutritive oral stimulus in preterm-born infants: implications for clinical and research applications. *Neurogastroenterol Motil* 2019;31(8):1.

93. Dalgleish SR, Kostecky LL, Blachly N. Eating in "SINC": safe individualized nipple-feeding competence, a quality improvement project to explore infant-driven oral feeding for very premature infants requiring noninvasive respiratory support. *Neonatal Netw* 2016;35(4):217.

94. Premji SS, Chessell L. Continuous nasogastric milk feeding versus intermittent bolus milk feeding for premature infants less than 1500 grams. *Cochrane Database Syst Rev* 2011;(11):CD001819.

95. Watson J, McGuire W. Transpyloric versus gastric tube feeding for preterm infants. *Cochrane Database Syst Rev* 2013;(2):CD003487.

96. Oddie SJ, Young L, McGuire W. Slow advancement of enteral feed volumes to prevent necrotising enterocolitis in very low birth weight infants. *Cochrane Database Syst Rev* 2017;(8):CD001241.

97. Basuki F, Hadiati DR, Turner T, et al. Dilute versus full-strength formula in exclusively formula-fed preterm or low birth weight infants. *Cochrane Database Syst Rev* 2019;(6):CD007263.

98. Alyahya W, Simpson J, Garcia AL, et al. Early versus delayed fortification of human milk in preterm infants: a systematic review. *Neonatology* 2020;117(1):24.

99. Bhatia J, Greer F. Use of soy protein-based formulas in infant feeding. *Pediatrics* 2008;121(5):1062.

100. Cacho NT, Parker LA, Neu J. Necrotizing enterocolitis and human milk feeding: a systematic review. *Clin Perinatol* 2017;44(1):49.

101. Quigley M, McGuire W. Formula versus donor breast milk for feeding preterm or low birth weight infants. *Cochrane Database Syst Rev* 2014;(4):CD002971.

102. van Goudoever JB, Vlaardigerbroek H, van den Akker CH, et al. Amino acids and proteins. In: Koletzko B, Poindexter B, Uauy R, eds. *Nutritional care of preterm infants: scientific bases and practical guidelines*, vol 110. Basel, Switzerland: Karger, 2014:49.

103. Cooke RJ, Griffin IJ, McCormick K, et al. Feeding preterm infants after hospital discharge: effect of dietary manipulation on nutrient intake and growth. *Pediatr Res* 1998;43:355.

104. Young L, Embleton ND, McGuire W. Nutrient-enriched formula versus standard formula for preterm infants following hospital discharge. *Cochrane Database Syst Rev* 2016;(12):CD004696.

105. Cerra FB, Siegel JH, Coleman B, et al. Septic autocannibalism: a failure of exogenous nutritional support. *Ann Surg* 1980;192:570.

106. Harris MC, D'Angio CT, Gallagher PR, et al. Cytokine elaboration in critically ill infants with bacterial sepsis, necrotizing enterocolitis, or sepsis syndrome: correlation with clinical parameters of inflammation and mortality. *J Pediatr* 2005;147(4):462.

107. Ehrenkranz RA, Das A, Wrage LA, et al. Early nutrition mediates the influence of severity of illness on extremely LBW infants. *Pediatr Res* 2011;69(6):522.

108. Canadian Paediatric Society and Nutrition Committee. Nutrient needs and feeding of premature infants. *CMAJ* 1995;152:1765.

109. Poindexter BB, Martin CR. Impact of nutrition on bronchopulmonary dysplasia. *Clin Perinatol* 2015;42(4):797.

110. Combs GF Jr, Trumbo PR, McKinley MC, et al. Biomarkers in nutrition: new frontiers in research and application. *Ann N Y Acad Sci* 2013;1278:1.

111. Goldberg DL, Becker PJ, Brigham K, et al. Identifying malnutrition in preterm and neonatal populations: recommended indicators. *J Acad Nutr Diet* 2018;118:1571.

112. Rabner M, Meurling J, Ahlberg C, et al. The impact of growth curve changes in assessing premature infant growth. *J Perinatol* 2014;34(1):49.

113. Rochow N, Raja P, Liu K, et al. Physiologic adjustment to postnatal growth trajectories in healthy preterm infants. *Pediatr Res* 2016;79:870.

114. Fenton TR, Senterre T, Griffin IJ. Time interval for preterm infant weight gain velocity calculation precision. *Arch Dis Child Fetal Neonatal Ed* 2019;104:F218.

115. Pfister K, Ramel SE. Linear growth and neurodevelopmental outcomes. *Clin Perinatol* 2014;41(2):309.

116. Loÿs CM, Maucort-boulch D, Guy B, et al. Extremely low birthweight infants: how neonatal intensive care unit teams can reduce postnatal malnutrition and prevent growth retardation. *Acta Paediatr* 2013;102(3):242.

117. Ramel SE, Gray HL, Davern BA, et al. Body composition at birth in preterm infants between 30 and 36 weeks gestation. *Pediatr Obes* 2015;10(1):45. doi: 11111/j.2047-6310.2013.00215.x.

118. Roggero P, Gianní ML, Amato O, et al. Evaluation of air-displacement plethysmography for body composition assessment in preterm infants. *Pediatr Res* 2012;72(3):316.

119. Koo WW. Laboratory assessment of nutritional bone disease in infants. *Clin Biochem* 1996;29:429.

21 Radiology

Jeremy B. Jones

MODALITIES USED IN NEONATAL IMAGING

The most frequently used imaging studies in neonatal units are chest and abdominal x-rays, cranial ultrasounds, and brain magnetic resonance imaging (MRI). These modalities will be explained before going on to consider some of the less frequently used neonatal imaging modalities.

X-Rays

X-rays are an excellent tool in the neonatal unit. They are used daily to check tube positions, assess lung parenchyma, assess causes of respiratory deterioration, and review bowel gas patterns. Some pedants may claim that the correct term for a chest x-ray is, in fact, a chest radiograph. The x-ray, they argue, should only be used to refer to the radiation that emanates from the x-ray machine and not to the image that we use to make clinical decisions. They forget that language is dynamic and that the vast majority of people use "x-ray" to refer to the radiation beam and the image. While some pedantry is appropriate, life is too short to worry about a narrow use of the word "x-ray."

In the neonatal population, several tests are performed portably in the neonatal unit:

- A chest x-ray may be performed for one of many indications including line and tube placement, difficulty breathing, suspected lung disease or infection, increasing oxygen requirement or follow-up of prenatal abnormalities (Fig. 21.1A).
- An abdominal x-ray may be performed in the preterm neonate where there is suspicion of necrotizing enterocolitis (NEC) (Fig. 21.1B) or in a neonate with abdominal distension, vomiting, altered bowel habit, or failure to pass meconium.
- X-ray for peripheral line placement should include the limb in which the line was inserted as well as the tip's expected location.
- Clavicle/arm x-ray may be performed after a challenging delivery where there is a concern for a fracture (Fig. 21.1C).

Safety

The image obtained during an x-ray examination is the result of firing a radiation beam through a patient so that some of the radiation hits a detector of some sort. The amount of radiation that makes it to the detector is dependent on what it passes through.

In most countries, there is strict legislation around the use of radiation in medical imaging. The referrer should only request appropriate examinations, and the radiology team must employ techniques to ensure that the dose to the patient is as low as reasonably achievable (known as the ALARA principle). Keeping the dose low is particularly important in the neonatal population, where the risk of radiation-induced neoplasms in later years is higher.

Depending on the hospital, radiographers, technologists, or radiologists may be involved in the process of justifying the types of studies that can be performed. There may be limitations on who is allowed to request particular investigations.

Request

Gestation, birth history, and clinical concern should be part of a minimum clinical dataset when making a request. Mention any lines and tubes as well as the clinical state of the patient and urgency of the request. A good request allows prompt justification and appropriate prioritization (recognizing that the radiographic staff are likely covering an entire hospital, not just the neonatal unit). It also provides the baseline clinical information used for the formal report.

Acquisition

In the past, the detector was a cassette filled with film. It required manual processing and resulted in an image on physical film. Things have changed over the last 20 years, and we have moved away from physical film to a digital environment. Those changes started with a hybrid technique termed computed radiography. After exposure, the detector was taken to a physical reader which created a digital image that was saved to PACS. The detector could only be used a second time once it had been read and reset. This type of system will still be present in some hospitals, but digital radiography has replaced it in many.

Digital radiography systems use a digital detector wirelessly linked to the x-ray machine. In many cases, this means that an image can be reviewed on the machine immediately. The radiographer or technologist will perform any relevant post-processing before sending a copy of the image to PACS.

It is best practice to remove as much monitoring as possible because it will interfere with interpretation. Most additional hardware can be removed to take an x-ray in most neonates. Where the neonate is preterm or sick, there is a balance between removing as much from the x-ray field as possible and the clinical safety of the patient.

Review

Once the image is on PACS, it is ready for review using a computer-based PACS client. It is worth remembering that reviewing the resultant picture in a bright environment with a standard relatively small monitor will not optimize the viewing experience.

You can optimize the assessment of an x-ray by reviewing it in a side office with the light off, and the door closed rather than on a computer-on-wheels, laptop, or tablet in the ward environment. Being comfortable using some of the standard tools available in the PACS client will also optimize your review experience, for example, the use of zoom, pan, and windowing.

Windowing describes the process of changing the brightness and contrast of the image. An x-ray image is made up of thousands of pixels each of which has a value. The value assigned to each pixel represents the amount of radiation that passed through the patient at that point. The numbers of different values are much higher than the number of grays that a computer monitor can display. Therefore, windowing of the image is used to change the values that can be seen, allowing improved visualization of a pneumothorax or to assess the lung parenchyma behind the heart, for example.

Report

In most neonatal units, all x-rays are reported by a radiologist. The radiologist will have the benefit of a large, dedicated, calibrated monitor and easy access to any previous studies on the system. However, they will have access to limited clinical information. Even where a neonatal electronic patient record is in use, it is unlikely that the radiologist will have access to it. The quality and relevance of any radiology report will be dependent on the clinical information provided. The clinical team may know that the patient

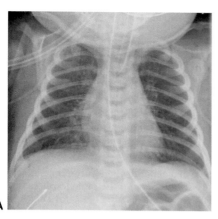 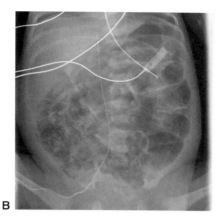 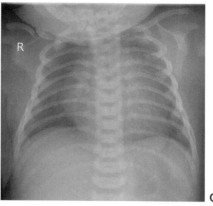

FIGURE 21.1 A selection of x-rays. A: Neonatal pneumonia with normally positioned ET and NG tubes. (Courtesy of Dr Jeremy Jones, Radiopaedia.org, rID: 23898.) **B:** Pneumoperitoneum secondary to NEC. (Courtesy of Dr Alice Spencer, Radiopaedia.org, rID: 67382.) **C:** Birth-related clavicular fracture in shoulder dystocia. (Courtesy of Dr Derrick Chansiongpen, Radiopaedia.org, rID: 40213.)

is a 32-week preterm neonate on CPAP with an acute deterioration in respiratory function. However, the report will be limited if the only clinical information available for the reporting radiologist is "acute deterioration."

Ultrasound

Ultrasound is an exceptional tool in the right hands. It is portable and works brilliantly in little people where the distance between the transducer and the anatomy or pathology is small. Moreover, it doesn't involve the use of radiation, which is useful in the neonatal population.

In the neonatal context, cranial ultrasound is the most frequently performed ultrasound examination. It is a great test to evaluate the neonatal brain at the cot-side. It is performed using the anterior fontanelle as a natural window through the otherwise impenetrable calvarium. The posterior and mastoid fontanelles allow additional views of the brain parenchyma and cerebrospinal fluid (CSF) spaces.

In the neonatal unit, the most commonly performed ultrasound is of the head. However, there are several reasons to perform an ultrasound:

- Cranial ultrasound in both the preterm and term population (Fig. 21.2A and B)
- Abdominal ultrasound for assessment of solid organs, abdominal distension, and in some cases, assessment of NEC (Fig. 21.2C)

- Soft tissue ultrasound for assessment of lumps, collections, or vascular malformations
- Echocardiography

Request

Depending on the neonatal unit, there may be clinical staff in the department who can perform a cranial ultrasound. In units where clinical staff perform the ultrasound, images are often only saved on the ultrasound machine and not sent to PACS. In this situation, there is not a requirement for a formal request. However, where images are saved to PACS, a radiology request is usually required to marry the patient demographics, clinical history, and pictures together.

If the ultrasound is to be performed by radiology staff, a radiology request should include gestation and birth history, current clinical state and in the context of cranial ultrasound, whether there is any history of focal neurology or seizures. Summarizing any previous imaging is helpful because the staff reviewing the radiology request may not have access to previous imaging, especially if the neonatal unit does not send all images to PACS.

Acquisition

Acquiring pictures using ultrasound takes skill and appropriate training and practice. It requires knowledge of anatomy and pathology in the scanned region and a proper understanding of how to optimize the scan using the probes and machine available.

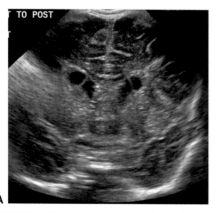 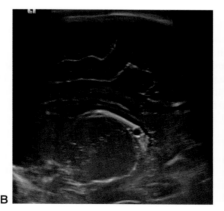 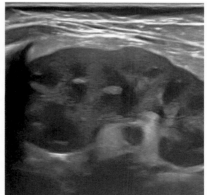

FIGURE 21.2 Ultrasound examples of some incidental findings. A: Connatal cysts. (Courtesy of Dr Tim Luijkx, Radiopaedia.org, rID: 56662.) **B:** A choroid plexus cyst. (Courtesy of Dr Jeremy Jones, Radiopaedia.org, rID: 27209.) **C:** Tamm-Horsfall protein causing increased echogenicity at the base of the renal pyramids. (Courtesy of Dr Tim Luijkx, Radiopaedia.org, rID: 62378.)

Probe Selection

Choosing the correct probe is the start of any procedure. Probes on an ultrasound machine come in a variety of shapes and sizes; although if the scanner is one dedicated for the neonatal environment, it may have a smaller selection than a portable machine from the radiology department. In general terms, there will be three types of probe:

- Linear probe
- Curvilinear probe
- Sector (phased array) probe

Linear probes have a rectangular surface. They tend to work at higher frequencies and create high-resolution pictures close to the surface of the body. The high-resolution makes them excellent for seeing structures near the probe in great detail, for example, vessels, subcutaneous lumps, or collections.

Curvy probes have a curved surface. They tend to work at slightly lower frequencies, which allow a picture that has a wider field of view and a greater depth of field. They are excellent for imaging a deeper cavity like the abdomen.

Sector (phased array) probes also have a rectangular surface but generally, a smaller footprint than the linear probes. They have a large depth of field and are useful for scanning areas with a small acoustic window, for example, the anterior fontanelle or between ribs.

Review

Ultrasound is a dynamic imaging modality, and the images saved to the system are only a representation of the images seen at the time of the study. As such, a standard set of images must be saved as well as additional images to represent any areas of abnormality.

Standard Image Set for Cranial Ultrasound

The image set for cranial ultrasound includes a set of coronal images through the frontal lobes, caudothalamic grooves, third ventricle, lateral ventricle atria, and finally, parieto-occipital region. The right side of the brain should always be on the left of the screen to correlate with any other radiologic imaging, for example, a coronal MRI sequence. Sagittal imaging should always have the front of the head on the left and the back on the right. This standard imaging plane correlates to a sagittal MRI sequence. The first sagittal image is a midline view followed by imaging of both sides of the brain. The first image is the caudothalamic groove, followed by lateral ventricle and parenchyma. Additional images of abnormalities can be included as well as additional views through the posterior or mastoid fontanelles.

Ultrasound is a dynamic process, but saving a standard collection of images allows others to review images and be confident that they represent a complete examination.

Report

All ultrasounds performed by a radiologist or sonographer will result in images saved to PACS and the generation of a report detailing findings. If the ultrasound is performed by staff from the neonatal unit, a report should be added to the patient's notes. It is worth remembering that it is unlikely that radiology will be able to review reports of examinations that are performed by neonatal staff with reports that are saved to the patient notes.

Magnetic Resonance Imaging

The frequency of MRI use in the neonatal population is dependent on several factors, including the location of the neonatal unit in relation to the scanning facilities and the ability for the MRI department to provide a timely and high-quality service.

MRI brain is the dominant MRI study performed in the neonatal population. In most centers, the protocol in the neonatal population will be different from standard brain imaging for older children. MRI studies performed in the neonatal period include the following:

- MRI brain for assessment of structure and pathology, predominantly in the term population but also in the preterm neonate or where there is a known antenatal abnormality
- MRI brain and spine for assessment of confirmed or suspected spinal dysraphism
- MRI neck for assessment of ligamentous structures and brachial plexus in children following a traumatic delivery

Safety

MRI makes use of a powerful magnet to align water molecules in the body. The MRI magnet is always on, and the radiographers or technologists who run the MRI have a responsibility for safety in the scanning environment. The scanning environment is a restricted environment that includes the scan room, and the places that lead into it. Anyone who enters the scan room must have completed a safety questionnaire and removed any metallic objects from the person or clothing.

Magnetic objects in the scan room may become projectile because they are forcefully attracted to the magnet. They can accelerate rapidly, resulting in severe harm and even death. The force on an object attracted to the magnet can be much higher than what is controllable by a person resulting in objects being pulled out of hands or pockets. Objects may also heat or explode in the MR environment.

Objects in the scanning environment are classified as MR Safe, MR Conditional or MR Unsafe:

- MR Safe items pose no safety hazard in the MR environment
- MR Conditional items may only enter the scanner room under particular conditions which will be determined by the manufacturer and enforced by the radiology staff
- MR Unsafe items should not enter the MRI scanner room

In addition to the static, always-on magnet, there are gradient coils which are used to alter the magnetic field around the patient slightly. It is the rapid switching of the gradient coils that results in the loud noise associated with MRI scanning. The sound in the scanner room can reach 100 decibels, so wearing hearing protection is mandatory for the patient and any clinical staff.

The aligned water molecules behave differently based on their environment. The MRI scanner can detect that behavior by applying a radiofrequency (RF) pulse to a body-part and reading the response. This emitted RF pulse is tiny, and the receiving coil must be as small as possible and as close to the patient as possible. Some vendors have specific neonatal coils, while others make use of more generic coils. Coil elements will need to surround the body part that is being examined (usually brain and spine).

Request

When requesting MRI, it is vital to provide as much clinical history as possible. The request must include gestation and birth history as well as clinical state at delivery and clinical course since birth. Additional information from blood tests, previous imaging, or other tests (cerebral function monitoring or electroencephalography) is also beneficial.

Remember that some imaging such as cranial ultrasound or echo performed on the unit may not be available to the radiology staff. The information included in a request allows the team to determine the urgency of the study and plan the sequences performed. Ultimately, it also affects report writing. Some digital request portals will include MRI Safety questions; they must all be answered. A separate form is required for any staff members entering the scanning room on the day.

Acquisition

During the scan, it is likely that the clinical team will want to monitor the neonate, and in some situations, the child will be intubated. It is vital that before the examination, it is clear that MR Safe equipment is available for monitoring or ventilation. Using standard equipment can be dangerous and result in significant harm, for example, using standard ECG monitoring equipment can result in severe burns at contact areas.

Scanning any patient requires that the scanned body part is placed within the center of the MRI scanner bore. Caring for a sick and potentially unstable patient in the middle of an MRI bore can be challenging. A member of the clinical team with experience looking after neonates in the MRI scanner should be present. Any team member who will potentially enter the scan room will have to complete an MRI safety questionnaire.

The RF signals used to create the pictures during an MRI deposit heat within the subject. However, in most cases, the scanner room will be cooled and the team must ensure that the room temperature is appropriate for scanning and the neonate is swaddled as required. Bubble wrap and heated gel bags can be helpful.

The MRI scan is composed of multiple sequences. The two primary sequences are as follows:

- T1: used to assess anatomy where fat is bright and fluid is dark
- T2: used to evaluate pathology where both fat and fluid are bright (Fig. 21.3A)

In addition to the T1 and T2 sequences, some sequences display different information:

- PD: a sequence with some T1 and T2 features often acquired alongside T2
- FLAIR: a T2-weighted sequence where fluid is dark and fat is bright
- STIR: a T2-weighted sequence where fat is dark and fluid is bright
- DWI (diffusion-weighted imaging): a sequence that highlights areas where water molecules cannot diffuse normally, especially useful in recent ischemia/infarction (Fig. 21.3B)
- SWI (susceptibility-weighted imaging): a sequence that highlights blood or calcification as areas of signal dropout (Fig. 21.3C)

Most sequences produce a set of slices through an image volume with a slice thickness of 3 to 5 mm. Some sequences will create a set of slices where the slice thickness and the in-plane resolution is the same. These volume sequences allow manipulation and reformatting into any plane after the scan is complete.

Short sequences such as a diffusion sequence may only take a minute. Volume sequences may take 5 minutes or longer. Most standard neonatal MRI protocols include axial and sagittal T1, axial T2, DWI, SWI, and a coronal sequence.

MR Spectroscopy (MRS) can be used to measure the relative concentration of metabolites in brain tissue. *N*-Acetylaspartate (NAA), choline, creatine, and lactate are the most useful metabolites to measure along with their relative ratios both in the thalamus and basal ganglia. There is growing evidence that MRS is more sensitive and specific for determining abnormal outcome than standard sequences (1).

A radiologist may review the images at the time of acquisition and consider addition sequences to answer specific questions.

Review

Unlike most other imaging modalities, MRI provides a multitude of different sequences in different planes. Looking at MRI takes practice because as well as recognizing what normal is, you need to understand what that normal looks like across multiple different sequences and at multiple gestations.

Report

The majority of neonatal MRI is of the brain. The guidelines produced by the British Association of Perinatal Medicine (BAPM) (2) suggest that neonatal brain imaging should be double read by two radiologists who have experience with neonatal head imaging. Double reading may be primary double-read before verification, a double-read at the center within 24 hours of the study, review at a clinicoradiologic meeting with an expert, or potentially a review by an external radiologist through the use of local imaging networks.

The BAPM have suggested that neonatal brain reports should always include comment on the following: cortical grey matter, white matter, deep grey matter, brainstem, and cerebellum. Any congenital abnormality will be contained in the report along with a description of any hemorrhage, including its location.

Remember that a 1-minute read on the workstation is a bit like giving a clinical opinion from the end of the bed. The 15-minute dedicated review in optimal reading conditions without disturbance will be more accurate and is more akin to a complete physical examination with chart review. Always wait for a formal verified report before making clinical decisions or having discussions with parents or other personnel.

Fluoroscopy

Fluoroscopy, like plain radiography, uses x-rays to create pictures. However, the radiation dose involved is generally much lower, and

THE NEWBORN INFANT

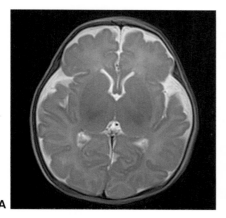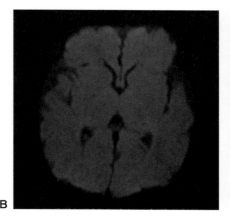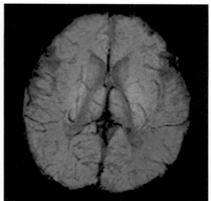

FIGURE 21.3 Examples of some different MRI sequences. All have been obtained in the axial plane in a newborn term neonate. **A:** T2 weighted imaging where CSF is bright. **B:** DWI (b 800) showing no diffusion restriction. **C:** SWI demonstrating that signal dropout occurs in normal vessels. There is no parenchymal or extra-axial hemorrhage in this case. (Courtesy of Dr Ian Bickle, Radiopaedia.org, rID: 52599.)

they are used continuously or in short pulses to assess the patient, usually after injection of a contrast agent.

Fluoroscopic examinations in the neonatal population are often used to assess the GI or GU tract:

- Upper GI contrast study to assess rotation in a neonate with a bilious vomit (Fig. 21.4A)
- Upper GI contrast study to assess esophageal continuity in a neonate with suspected tracheoesophageal fistula
- Lower GI contrast study to assess for causes of failure to pass meconium looking specifically for microcolon, filling defects, and altered caliber (Fig. 21.4B)
- Micturating cystourethrogram (MCUG) for the assessment of the posterior urethra (in boys) and assessment of presence and severity of vesicoureteric reflux (Fig. 21.4C)
- Cloacogram in a child with a cloacal abnormality to determine the connections and locations of the genitourinary sinus

Safety

Fluoroscopy examinations use x-rays and are therefore subject to the same considerations about the safe use of radiation. Fluoroscopic examinations are usually performed by a pediatric radiologist. The patient will need to be transported to the fluoroscopy room, which is usually in the radiology department. Transportation from the neonatal unit to the radiology department may only be a push down the corridor in an incubator. However, in some units, it will require transport to a locoregional center. Adequate contact details must be on the request.

Request

The requirements of the request for a fluoroscopic study are similar to that of an x-ray. You must provide an appropriate history to allow justification of the examination. You will also need to liaise with the radiology department and whoever transports the baby to determine when the test can be performed.

Acquisition

A radiologist will almost certainly perform the procedure. The neonate will need to be removed from the incubator and placed on the fluoroscopy bed. ECG tabs and leads may need to be moved or removed. Anyone staying with the child will need to wear a lead coat.

Contrast (usually an iodinated nonionic contrast media) is injected via an NG tube or catheter and is visible on a monitor using low-dose x-rays. The route and volume of contrast used will depend on the procedure.

Review

The radiologist will likely be able to give a verbal report at the time of the study. Fluoroscopy is a dynamic procedure, and a set of images will be saved to PACS that are representative of the imaging findings. Only a selection of images will be saved to PACS, not the complete procedure.

Report

The radiologist will review all the saved images after the examination is complete and will issue a report that takes into consideration the clinical context. A good quality request and thorough discussion of the case is vital in maximizing the usefulness of the report.

Computed Tomography

Computed tomography (CT) is the workhorse of imaging in the adult population. However, it is used sparingly in the pediatric population and used very infrequently in the assessment of neonates. Several features make CT less useful in neonatal imaging including its reliance on x-rays, its relatively high radiation dose, its reduced inherent contrast in neonates, and the fact that it is not portable.

CT is excellent for assessment of the heart and major vessels in children with congenital cardiac disease. It can also be helpful to gain additional information about the lungs, for example, a patient with progressive lobar overinflation requiring assessment for potential surgical intervention or in patients with congenital pulmonary abnormalities. It may be used if there is a need for emergent cross-sectional neuroimaging and an MRI cannot be arranged in a timely fashion, or where the neonate could potentially deteriorate during the time an MRI would take to perform. In the majority of other situations, alternative imaging modalities outshine CT in this population.

Nuclear Medicine

There are very few indications for nuclear medicine in the neonatal population. A radioactive material (usually technetium) is bound to a molecule that is absorbed or excreted by a body system. The bound radiotracer is injected into the patient (gut, urinary tract, or blood vessel) and is later detected where it is absorbed or excreted. For example, mebrofenin is taken up by the

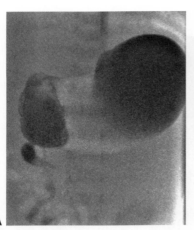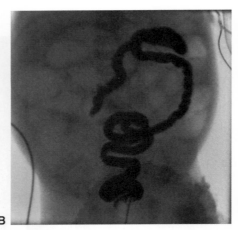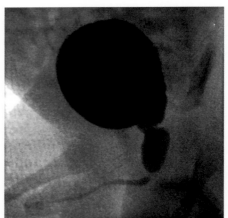

FIGURE 21.4 **A:** Single AP image of a stomach and duodenum. The duodenum is in an abnormal position and does not cross midline. This is malrotation with volvulus. (Courtesy of A. Prof Frank Gaillard, Radiopaedia.org, rID: 7909.) **B:** Single image from a lower GI contrast study with microcolon in a case of meconium ileus. (Courtesy of Dr Jeremy Jones, Radiopaedia.org, rID: 62785.) **C:** Single excretory image from an MCUG in a neonate with a dilated posterior urethra in posterior urethral valves. (Courtesy of A. Prof Frank Gaillard, Radiopaedia.org, rID: 5964.)

liver and excreted into the bile. Binding mebrofenin to technetium is helpful to determine biliary excretion in patients with suspected biliary atresia.

CATHETERS AND SUPPORT DEVICES

Assessment of the position of lines and tubes is one of the most frequent reasons to perform imaging in the neonatal period. These may relate to ventilation, feeding, or vascular access, or be larger bore tubes inserted into body cavities.

The Babygram

A combined chest and abdominal radiograph should only be performed for the assessment of line and tube positions. It is not optimized for chest or abdominal radiography, both of which require different parameters when taking an x-ray. Lung parenchyma will be difficult to assess, pneumothoraces will be more difficult to detect, and bowel assessment for mural gas or perforation will also be more difficult than a dedicated examination. If you want information about the chest, get a chest x-ray. If you want to assess the abdomen, get an abdominal x-ray.

Endotracheal Tube

Endotracheal (ET) tube placement is frequent among the patients on the neonatal unit, and assessment of tube position is vital for the safe care of patients. Ensuring that the tip ET tube is above the carina is vital with the ideal position being a tip 1 cm from the carina (**Fig. 21.5A**). Another useful guide is to position the tip of the tube between the top of the 1st thoracic vertebra and the bottom of the 2nd thoracic vertebra. In preterm babies, it may lie slightly closer to the carina. Tube tip position is dependent on the position of the head with lateral position and downward chin position resulting in a tube tip position higher than a neutral position.

Bronchial intubation most commonly occurs into the right main bronchus (**Fig. 21.5B**). The ET tube with deviate to the right at the level of the carina with the tip projected over the right main bronchus. The right lung may be hyperinflated, but the left will be underinflated or collapsed.

Remember that variant anatomy may result in a right upper lobe bronchus that arises from the distal trachea and that a low-lying tube may cause partial obstruction of the aberrant bronchus and upper lobe collapse.

It is worth recognizing that while very rarely missed clinically, esophageal intubation can be misinterpreted as tracheal unless image review is thorough and ET tube position is accurately assessed

(Fig. 21.5C). In esophageal intubation, the esophagus will be distended, and the ET tube will usually not be projected over the trachea.

Enteric Catheters

Enteric catheters include nasogastric, oral–gastric, and jejunal feeding tubes. In the majority of neonates, a NG tube insertion is straight forward and results in the tip below the diaphragm over the stomach. Resistance to advancement and catheter looping or retrograde coiling may occur at any level, even with a normal pharynx and upper GI tract. Radiographs for enteric catheters should cover the neonate's neck, chest, and upper abdomen.

It is vital to check the course of the tube, remembering that the tube should travel down the midline of the chest, over the vertebral bodies, and bisecting the diaphragm just to the left of the midline, and should continue distally across the expected location of the gastroesophageal junction with the tip lying over the stomach (which usually has a gas bubble).

A looped catheter in the esophagus would suggest esophageal atresia (**Fig. 21.6A**). A catheter that bisects the diaphragm in the midline but whose tip sits above the expected position of the hemidiaphragm would be suggestive of a congenital diaphragmatic hernia (CDH) (**Fig. 21.6B**), while a catheter coursing to the right in the upper abdomen would suggest situs inversus or heterotaxy (**Fig. 21.6C**). After traversing the stomach and entering the duodenum, a jejunal feeding tube that does not course back across the lumbar spine would suggest bowel malrotation.

Radiographic interpretation of enteric catheters must also exclude tracheal insertion and traumatic injury. Tracheal insertion is diagnosed radiographically when the catheter courses ipsilateral to the chin and within the intrathoracic trachea and right or left main bronchial silhouettes. Traumatic injury to the pharynx or esophagus during enteric catheter insertion may result in an atypical catheter location, pneumomediastinum, subcutaneous emphysema, pleural effusion, or a combination thereof.

Vascular Access

The lines and tubes used in neonates are tiny and the radiation doses used to image the neonate are also small. As such, it can be difficult to see the catheters and their tips at times. There are a couple of techniques that can be used to help accurately identify the tip of a catheter or line. The first and simplest option is to get the radiographer to save a second copy of the image to PACS with an edge-enhancement algorithm applied to the image. This makes it much easier to see the lines and tubes and determine the tip position. The edge enhancement produced by the x-ray

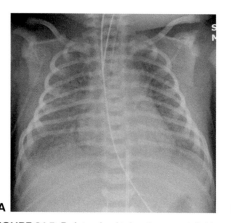
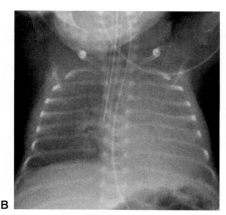
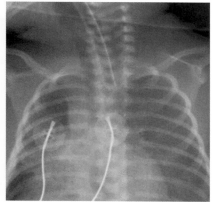

FIGURE 21.5 Endotracheal tube placement. A: Meconium aspiration with an ET tube slightly low, just above carina. (Courtesy of Dr Jeremy Jones, Radiopaedia.org, rID: 23901.) **B:** RDS with granular background appearance and an ET tube tip down the right main bronchus with secondary left lung collapse. (Courtesy of Dr Jeremy Jones, Radiopaedia.org, rID: 62755.) **C:** ET tube tip in the esophagus. The position of the head displaces the trachea to the right, confirming esophageal location. (Courtesy of Dr. Radswiki, Radiopaedia.org, rID: 11635.)

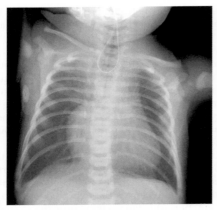
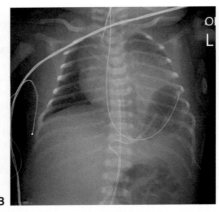
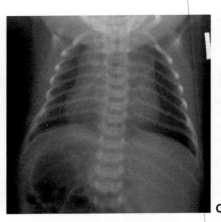

FIGURE 21.6 A: NG tube looped in a distended upper esophageal pouch in esophageal atresia. (Courtesy of A. Prof Frank Gaillard, Radiopaedia.org, rID: 7917.) **B:** NG tube tip projected in the lower left chest in a congenital diaphragmatic hernia. A malpositioned UVC in the left portal vein is also projected over the left hemithorax because the left lobe of the liver has also herniated through the defect. (Courtesy of Dr Jeremy Jones, Radiopaedia.org, rID: 23653.) **C:** The NG tube courses to the right after it bisects the diaphragm in a patient with heterotaxy. (Courtesy of Dr. Hani Salam, Radiopaedia.org, rID: 13992.)

machine may be better than the corresponding edge enhancement produced in PACS. It may be worth testing locally to determine which is the best option. In some departments, it might be worth considering the default position of always saving a standard and edge-enhanced picture to PACS.

The second option is to inject a small volume of iodinated contrast into the line, take the x-ray, and then flush the line afterward. The iodinated contrast agent will be determined by the local protocol as will the volume of contrast used.

Complications of correctly positioned catheters can include perforation, hemorrhage, in-situ thrombus, and thromboembolism. Complications of malposition may include cannulation of the incorrect vessel, incorrect final position (high, low, or within a branch vessel). The imaging appearances and risks associated with malposition depend on the type of vascular access.

Umbilical Artery Catheter

The umbilical arterial catheter (UAC) is easily recognizable on the abdominal radiograph because of the anatomy of the vessel that it occupies. Each umbilical artery is in continuity with the internal iliac arteries. As such, the umbilical artery catheter will enter at the umbilicus, descend caudally and laterally before turning cranially, and then tracking toward the midline (iliac artery) before ascending in the aorta (**Fig. 21.7A**). The tip should be in the supramesenteric thoracoabdominal aorta between T6 and T11 (**Fig. 21.7B**). Thoracic and lumbar spine

landmarks are used radiographically to confirm appropriate positioning. A tip too low may predispose to altered blood flow in the branch vessels and in-situ thrombus formation. UACs can potentially track into mesenteric and renal aortic branch arteries. They can track into the contralateral common iliac artery and lower extremity arterial tree although this is extremely rare (**Fig. 21.7C**).

Umbilical Vein Catheter

An umbilical vein catheter (UVC) inserted via the umbilical vein will be directed toward the right heart via the portal system. The umbilical vein will intersect the left portal vein and bridge between the portal and hepatic veins via the patent ductus venosus before ascending in the inferior vena cava toward the inferior cavoatrial junction (IVC-right atrial junction) at the level of the diaphragm. Several position failures can occur (**Fig. 21.8A and B**). A UVC tip is too low when the tip is projected over the liver. The line cannot be used to its full potential because some medications cannot be given through a line in a low position.

The tip is too high when it is either in or has passed through the right atrium (**Fig. 21.8C**). If the line has passed through the right atrium, it may be sitting in the superior vena cava, the left atrium (through a patent foramen ovale or atrial septal defect), right ventricle, or even a pulmonary vein. Leaving a line in this position risks cardiac arrhythmias and possibly thrombosis depending on the size terminal vessel.

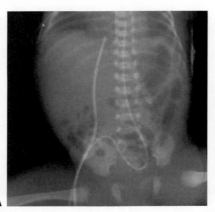
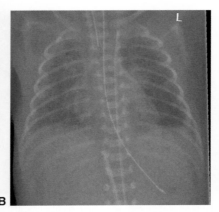
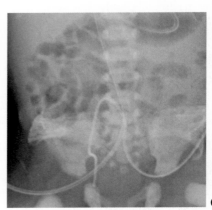

FIGURE 21.7 UAC positions. A: Appropriate positions of UVC and UACs. The patient is slightly rotated to the right. The descending loop to the internal iliac artery is clearly seen. (Courtesy of Dr. Radswiki, Radiopaedia.org, rID: 12048.) **B:** UAC position is too high. (Courtesy of Dr Jeremy Jones, Radiopaedia.org, rID: 56769.) **C:** The UAC tip has tracked into the internal iliac artery and descended into the femoral artery. (Courtesy of Dr Vinay V Belaval, Radiopaedia.org, rID: 66975.)

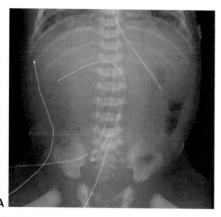
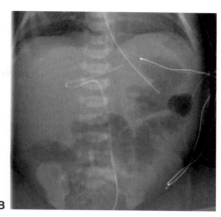
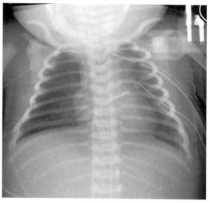

FIGURE 21.8 UVC positions. A: Malpositioned UVC with tip in the right portal vein. (Courtesy of Dr Jeremy Jones, Radiopaedia.org, rID: 27465.) **B:** UVC with tip in the left portal vein and a loop extending back toward the right portal vein. (Courtesy of Dr Jeremy Jones, Radiopaedia.org, rID: 24122.) **C:** UVC with tip extending across a patent foramen ovale into the left atrium. (Courtesy of Dr. Radswiki, Radiopaedia.org, rID: 12343.)

Occasionally, the line may get diverted into the portal system where the umbilical vein intersects the left portal vein. The line can end up in a branch of the left portal vein, the right portal vein, main portal vein, or even the superior mesenteric vein. These line positions risk thrombosis.

Peripheral Intravenous Central Catheter

Peripheral intravenous central catheter (PICC) insertion into upper or lower limbs is possible. PICCs are made out of silicone and polyurethane, the latter being a much stiffer product. Whichever type of catheter is used, the tip should always be positioned outside the cardiac silhouette. If the tip encroaches on the silhouette, it should be withdrawn appropriately (3).

An upper limb PICC is typically inserted in a peripheral upper limb vein such as the brachial or basilic vein. It should extend through the axillary vein and subclavian vein into the superior vena cava. Tip position will vary depending on arm abduction and adduction. An upper extremity PICC line could extend into an ipsilateral thoracodorsal vein, internal jugular vein, contralateral brachiocephalic vein, or the azygous vein.

Cephalic and lower limb PICC insertion is also possible but much less common. Cephalic PICC should have a similar final position as an upper limb PICC. A lower limb PICC is usually inserted via the common femoral vein. The expected path of the femoral and iliac vessels is toward the midline as the line extends cranially. Its course should be relatively straight until it reaches the iliac confluence at the IVC. A lower extremity PICC line could potentially extend into a lumbar or renal vein. When this happens, the tip of the line will usually be visible on the abdominal radiograph with angulation at (or near) the tip. A PICC should have a smooth course and should not deviate. Use of a line with its tip in a branch vessel such as the lumbar plexus can be catastrophic.

Other Vascular Catheters

Central access can also be achieved using jugular access. This can be as an external line or as a tunneled line. Tunneled lines are either Hickman lines or Broviac lines. ECMO catheters are also inserted via the neck vessels. These are larger bore lines, often with external metallic circumferential reinforcement. The ECMO catheter position will depend on the circuit being used, either venovenous (V-V) or venoarterial (V-A).

Intercostal Catheters

Intercostal thoracic catheters (chest tubes) are placed in the neonate for management of pleural effusions and pneumothoraces. Regardless of the source of pleural fluid, the thoracic catheter should be directed posteriorly for simple effusions since the neonate will be in a supine position and fluid will collect dependently.

A thoracic catheter should be directed anteriorly for management of pneumothorax. Ideally, it is directed toward the anteroinferior medial pleural space, where most air will collect in a supine neonate. Initial and serial radiographs are obtained, monitoring catheter positions and the amount of fluid or pleural air present. A persistent effusion or pneumothorax may suggest catheter malposition, catheter dysfunction, or loculation. Further assessment with ultrasound will help to confirm catheter location, exclude loculations and septations, as well as plan any additional imaging or intervention.

CHEST IMAGING

A chest x-ray is almost always the first investigation in a neonate with chest pathology. Ultrasound is an excellent problem-solving tool and allows assessment of an effusion, detection of a pneumothorax, or characterization in the rare case of a neonatal mediastinal mass. CT may be helpful in very specific situations where a lung parenchymal abnormality needs additional characterization following chest radiography.

There are many causes of respiratory compromise in the neonatal population, and it is helpful to consider the likely diagnoses based on clinical history and patterns of imaging findings. These groups are a somewhat artificial separation of pathology but are helpful to describe the commonest causes of neonatal respiratory compromise.

The Unwell Newborn Preterm Neonate

The preterm neonate is particularly at risk of respiratory distress syndrome because of lack of surfactant. This does not mean that respiratory distress syndrome cannot occur in the term neonate or that RDS is the only cause for an unwell newborn preterm neonate. However, it is the commonest cause for respiratory compromise in this group.

Respiratory Distress Syndrome

Respiratory distress syndrome is also known as hyaline membrane disease, neonatal respiratory distress syndrome, lung disease prematurity and surfactant-deficiency disorder.

Respiratory distress syndrome results from a lack of surfactant in the alveoli of the neonate and results in reduced lung compliance compared to the normal term neonate. The alveoli are in a permanent state of complete or partial collapse leading to reduced lung expansion and volume (**Fig. 21.9A**). The failure of alveolar expansion results in increased opacification of the lungs. This is usually evidenced by partial alveolar opacification seen as ground-glass change shadowing. In the absence of additional treatment, these ground-glass changes are usually bilateral and symmetric.

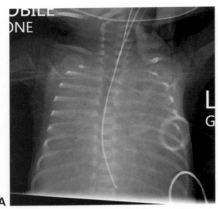
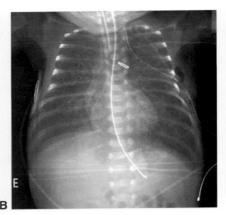
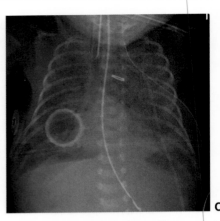

FIGURE 21.9 A 24-week neonate with RDS. A: Initial imaging with low-volume lungs. **B:** One day later following surfactant and PDA closure. Hyperexpanded lungs with virtually no airspace or interstitial opacities. **C:** Same day following a reduction in ventilator settings, lung volumes have reduced and patchy ground-glass change is more apparent. (Courtesy of Dr Jeremy Jones, Radiopaedia.org, rID: 23969.)

Treatment with exogenous surfactant instilled via an ET tube may complicate the picture. Where exogenous surfactant reaches collapsed alveoli, they will partially or completely inflate (**Fig. 21.9B**). Partial inflation may potentially result in a mixed picture with areas of normal expansion and persistent areas of ground-glass change.

In patients who have an ET tube placed, ventilator settings may result in a complete change of the radiographic picture. With a cuffed tube, titration of ventilator settings will result in a wide range of appearaces, from enlarged lucent lungs (**Fig. 21.9C**) to collapsed lungs that appear almost completely nonaerated.

A malpositioned tube may result in unilateral aeration and contralateral collapse. It is worth remembering that changes from a malpositioned tube may persist after it has been repositioned resulting in these changes in the context of a correctly positioned tube.

The Unwell Newborn Term Neonate

In our slightly stylized environment, respiratory distress in the newborn term neonate is the result of a heterogeneous group of disorders. The clinical history may help to stratify the likely diagnosis, for example, meconium aspiration syndrome in delivery complicated by thick meconium-stained liquor. While it is helpful to consider these classical associations, it is worth remembering that there are many more potential causes.

Transient Tachypnea of the Newborn

The dominant feature of transient tachypnea of the newborn (TTN) is fluid overload, which resolves over 24 to 72 hours. It is the analogue to heart failure in the adult population, and its features are similar. Fluid overload results in fluid in abnormal locations, for example, alveolar, interstitial, and pleural fluid. Alveolar fluid causes airspace opacification, which may be patchy at first and more confluent as alveolar filling increases. In most cases, this is perihilar, but it is not uncommon to see more generalized and even asymmetric opacities.

There may also be interstitial edema which is seen as smooth peribronchial thickening extending radially from the hila and interstitial lines peripherally. In some cases, there may also be pleural effusions with fissural fluid and cardiomegaly. Pleural fluid in the supine neonate may be difficult to appreciate and is seen as a peripheral opacity between the lung edge and the internal aspect of the ribs.

Meconium Aspiration

Meconium aspiration syndrome is the result of aspiration of meconium during birth that results in multifocal distal lung collapse and associated pneumonitis. The imaging findings reflect this background pathogenesis with multifocal atelectasis, streaky

(sometimes described as ropey) linear opacities radiating from the hila to the periphery, hyperinflation, air trapping, and potentially air leak. The findings are usually bilateral and symmetric. Pleural effusions are rare and likely point to an alternate diagnosis.

Neonatal Infection

Exposure to pathogens *in utero* (e.g., TORCH infections), at delivery (e.g., group B streptococcus), and postdelivery (e.g., rhinovirus, respiratory syncytial virus, influenza, enterovirus; *Staphylococcus*, *Escherichia coli*, *Enterococcus*; *Candida*) may result in neonatal infection.

Chest radiograph appearances are heterogeneous. There may be patchy or confluent air space opacification as well as granular, coarse, or fine interstitial patterns. On a chest x-ray, infection shares many imaging features with RDS, MAS, and TTN (**Fig. 21.10A and B**). However, there are some features that make an infection more likely than an alternate diagnosis (**Fig. 21.10C**). These include patchy distribution, persistent or progressive opacities, hyperinflation, and pleural effusions.

Recognizing normal mediastinal and lung contours is key to identifying small areas of abnormality. This is particularly true when an area of air space opacification abuts another structure resulting in a loss of the normal silhouette. A classic example of this is lower lobe collapse or consolidation resulting in loss of part of the normal diaphragmatic contour. Recognizing loss of a normal silhouette is key to correctly determining what part of the lung is abnormal.

Acute Lung Collapse

While meconium aspiration syndrome may cause subsegmental collapse, there are other causes of collapse, including aspiration of milk or mucus. These may cause obstruction of segmental or main bronchi leading to larger areas of collapse. If there is unilateral collapse or solitary complete/segmental collapse, think about a cause of lung collapse other than meconium aspiration.

Pleural Effusion

Fluid in the pleural space in a neonate may be congenital (e.g., hydrops, chylothorax) or acquired (e.g., iatrogenic injury, postoperative, infection, heart failure). In a supine neonate, it is unusual to see a blunted costophrenic angle. It is much more common to see generalized increased density of the hemithorax and thickening of the pleural space laterally at the lung–rib interface. Mediastinal shift will depend on the size of the effusion and underlying cardiopulmonary conditions. Ultrasound is useful to confirm an effusion and assess for septation and loculation. Effusions will also be visible on CT and MRI, although these are not usually used for primary assessment.

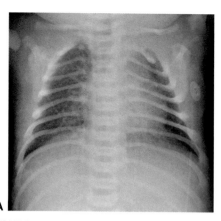 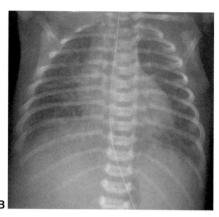 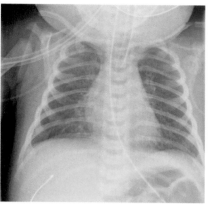

FIGURE 21.10 These three cases have similar, but distinct chest radiograph appearances in term neonates. The clinical history becomes very important in making the correct diagnosis. **A:** Transient tachypnea of the newborn with vascular prominence and a slightly enlarged heart. (Courtesy of Dr Jeremy Jones, Radiopaedia.org, rID: 23899.) **B:** Meconium aspiration syndrome with linear opacities that extend from the hila. (Courtesy of Dr Jeremy Jones, Radiopaedia.org, rID: 62746.) **C:** Neonatal pneumonia with interstitial and alveolar opacities. (Courtesy of Dr Jeremy Jones, Radiopaedia.org, rID: 23898.)

Acute Deterioration in the Ventilated Neonate

In a ventilated neonate, the cause of an acute change in respiratory effort or evidence of respiratory decompensation is wide. It may be the result of complications of mechanical ventilation, clinical deterioration related to the original reason for ventilation, or a second pathologic process. The commonest causes of complications secondary to mechanical ventilation are those related to tube position, pressure, or infection.

Tube-Related Complications

Tube-related complications are usually the result of a tube tip that is too close to the carina, or within the main bronchus. This commonly results in appropriate aeration of the intubated lobe or segment with the collapse of the lobes or segments that are not intubated. This is covered in more detail in the section that relates to the ET tube position.

Pressure-Related Complications

Pressure-related complications of mechanical ventilation are the result of gas moving from the tracheobronchial tree and alveoli into spaces where it should not be. Gas can escape into the mediastinum, pulmonary interstitium, or pleural space causing pneumomediastinum, pulmonary interstitial emphysema (PIE), and pneumothorax.

Pneumomediastinum

The dominant cause of pneumomediastinum in the neonate is as a complication of mechanical ventilation. On the x-ray (or potentially the CT), gas is seen as linear lucencies within mediastinal structures. On a chest x-ray, this is most frequently seen as a lucent line outlining the mediastinum, one or both sides, extending toward the neck. The challenge of diagnosis here is an artifact of imaging called the Mac effect. This is an observation artifact where the human eye fails to adequately assess the junction between the lung and mediastinum and instead adds a dark band which can be misinterpreted as gas.

In the context of mechanical ventilation, pneumomediastinum can be seen in concert with PIE and pneumothorax.

Pulmonary Interstitial Emphysema

PIE describes the situation where gas has escaped from the tracheobronchial tree into the pulmonary interstitium that surrounds the bronchovascular bundles that extend throughout the lung. It is seen as branching linear lucency that often starts in the hilar regions and branches peripherally. It is the result of a tear in the bronchus and secondary gas dissection of the bronchial interstitium. The gas that extends all the way to the mediastinum will result in pneumomediastinum. PIE may be seen in conjunction with pneumothorax also although there is no direct communication between the interstitial gas and the pleural space (Fig. 21.11A–C).

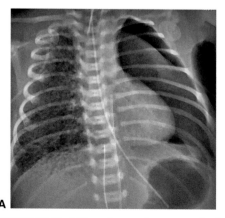 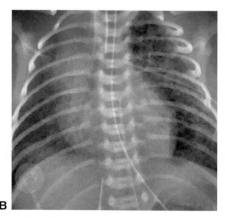 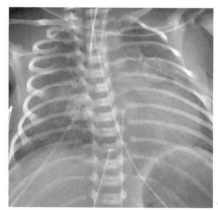

FIGURE 21.11 A 33-week-gestation neonate intubated and ventilated for treatment of RDS. Increased oxygen requirement with acute deterioration. **A:** Initial chest radiograph showing a large left-sided pneumothorax with multiple gas lucencies on the right consistent with PIE. **B:** Following chest tube placement and pneumothorax decompression, there is expansion of the left lung and left-sided PIE is also demonstrated. **C:** Less than 24 hours later following titration of ventilatory pressures, the previously demonstrated lucencies have resolved. (Courtesy of Dr Hisham Alwakkaa, Radiopaedia.org, rID: 58838.)

THE NEWBORN INFANT

Pneumothorax

Pneumothoraces may be a pressure-related complication in a mechanically ventilated neonate. These may occur in neonates ventilated via an ET tube but can also occur secondary to CPAP or other external modes of oxygen delivery that also involve the use of positive end-expiratory pressure. There is a correlation between the pressures achieved and the rate of pneumothorax, and also between earlier gestation neonates and pneumothorax, neither of which is surprising. It is worth noting that pneumothoraces are not only seen in mechanically ventilated neonates.

Neonates are supine when their x-ray is taken, and therefore, the gas collects dependently anteriorly in the chest. This means that small amounts of gas are difficult to appreciate on a neonatal chest radiograph, and we need to wait until a larger volume of gas has collected to see the deep sulcus sign. This describes the depression of the diaphragm laterally as gas collects in this region.

When pneumothoraces are large, it is possible to see a more classical lateral collection of gas within the pleural space. Whenever a large pneumothorax is visible, it is vital to assess the mediastinal position. Hyperexpansion of the hemithorax with mediastinal shift should trigger consideration of tension pneumothorax, even if a chest drain is in position.

Pulmonary Hemorrhage

Risk factors include respiratory stress and states of high pulmonary blood flow. Chest radiography will show progressive coalescent air–space opacification, potentially evolving to complete lung opacification, depending upon the severity of hemorrhage.

Respiratory Distress and a Big Heart

Determining the cause for a large heart on a chest x-ray usually involves additional examination with ultrasound in the form of an echocardiogram. CT with contrast is helpful in congenital heart disease to define the anatomy and aid surgical planning. Functional information with echocardiography and MRI may also be required.

There are a large number of potential causes of cardiomegaly. This includes congenital heart disease, cardiomyopathy, pericardial effusion, and aortic abnormalities.

Congenital Heart Disease

Broadly, this group of structural cardiac abnormalities can be split into four groups: right-sided obstruction, left-sided obstruction, left-to-right shunt, and admixture lesions. In all structural heart disease, cardiomegaly may be present. Echocardiography and CT are almost always required in the workup.

Right-Sided Intracardiac Obstructive Lesions

These lesions are distinguished radiographically by oligemia and variable degrees of cardiomegaly. This group includes Ebstein anomaly (Fig. 21.12A), tricuspid atresia, tetralogy of Fallot, and pulmonary atresia and stenosis (Fig. 21.12B). They are distinguished by a mechanical or functional obstruction involving the tricuspid valve, right ventricular outflow tract, pulmonary valve, or a combination thereof. The obstruction leads to diminished antegrade pulmonary blood flow, accentuated by an obligatory intracardiac right-to-left shunt.

Left-Sided Intracardiac Obstructive Lesions

These lesions will demonstrate variable pulmonary venous congestion. Heart size may range from normal to markedly enlarged. If an intracardiac shunt is present, there may be a component of increased pulmonary vascularity. This group includes cor triatriatum, congenital mitral stenosis and atresia, hypoplastic left heart syndrome, and congenital aortic stenosis. These lesions result in decreased systemic aortic perfusion. An intracardiac left-to-right shunt may be present to unload the left heart.

Morphologic Admixture Lesions

This group of CHD lesions are defined by structural abnormalities that lead to direct admixture of deoxygenated and oxygenated blood. Cyanosis is the hallmark as a result of the admixture. Lesions include double-inlet ventricle (single ventricle), transposition of the great arteries, double-outlet right ventricle, and truncus arteriosus. Associated septal, pulmonary, aortic, and coronary anomalies may be present, depending upon the lesion.

Left-to-Right Shunt Lesions

Excessive left-to-right shunting may occur in the setting of intracardiac or extracardiac shunts. Intracardiac shunts include atrial and ventricular septal defects (Fig. 21.12C) and a PDA. Intrathoracic, extracardiac shunts include pulmonary venous anomalies. Shunting leads to increased pulmonary blood flow, coinciding with the fall in pulmonary vascular resistance. The ensuing respiratory distress and tachypnea (without cyanosis) will lead to a chest radiograph, which is distinguished by variable cardiomegaly, central pulmonary artery enlargement, and pulmonary over circulation although this depends on the location and size of the shunt.

Cardiomyopathy

Cardiomyopathy will have variable appearances on a chest x-ray, which can include cardiomegaly with or without signs of heart failure, for example, pulmonary venous congestion, interstitial edema, or pleural and pericardial effusions.

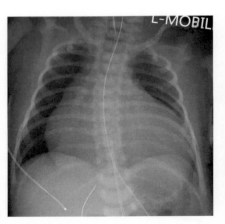 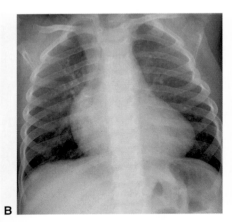 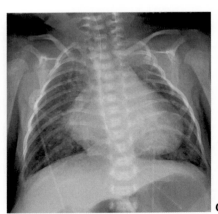

FIGURE 21.12 Three cases of cardiomegaly. Two demonstrate a right-sided obstructive pathology and the third highlights cardiomegaly secondary to admixture. **A:** Ebstein anomaly with massive cardiomegaly but very little in the way of pulmonary plethora. (Courtesy of Dr Jeremy Jones, Radiopaedia.org, rID: 24348.) **B:** Pulmonary stenosis with peripheral pruning. (Courtesy of Townsville radiology training, Radiopaedia.org, rID: 17885.) **C:** VSD in a patient with trisomy 18. (Courtesy of Dr Alexandra Stanislavsky, Radiopaedia.org, rID: 29396.)

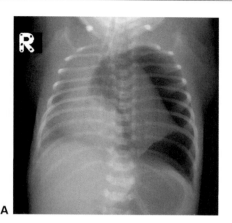 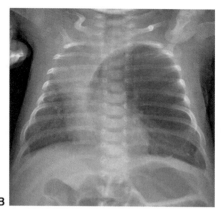 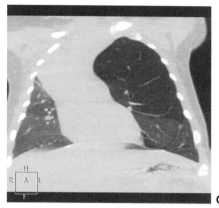

FIGURE 21.13 The importance of looking for a lung edge. A: Tension pneumothorax with hyperexpansion of the hemithorax and mediastinal shift. (Courtesy of Dr Pir Abdul Ahad Aziz, Radiopaedia.org, rID: 60602.) **B:** A very similar appearance but without a lung edge. This time, appearances are of congenital lobar overinflation. **C:** CT in the same case. (Courtesy of Dr Kewal Arunkumar Mistry, Radiopaedia.org, rID: 35577.)

Pericardial Effusion

Pericardial effusion results in the expansion of the pericardium with fluid. This is usually postoperative or potentially from cardiomyopathy or iatrogenic trauma following line insertion. It may be challenging to confidently diagnose a pericardial effusion on chest radiography alone. An echocardiogram will confirm fluid in the pericardial sac. Other pericardial diseases include pneumopericardium or congenital absence of the pericardium which can result in altered cardiac contour.

Vascular Abnormalities

Aortic abnormalities that cause cardiomegaly are the result of proximal intraluminal obstruction. These include aortic arch hypoplasia, interrupted aortic arch, or coarctation of the aorta, all of which result in chest radiograph appearances indistinguishable to left-sided obstructive heart disease. Other aortic and branch vessel abnormalities may result in an abnormal cardiomediastinal contour but will not usually cause cardiomegaly in isolation.

The Hyperexpanded Lucent Hemithorax

The hyperexpanded lucent hemithorax is an important differential to consider. Hyperexpansion may be seen as a definite difference in lung volumes, by the increased distance between ribs on the affected side and by mass effect, for example, mediastinal shift.

The most acute and life-threatening underlying abnormality is a tension pneumothorax (**Fig. 21.13A**). There will likely be a

concomitant clinical disturbance. A lung edge may or may not be seen. If it is, there will be no lung markings distally.

Focal hyperexpansion and lucency, often in the left upper zone, will make congenital lobar overinflation (CLO) more likely (**Fig. 21.13B and C**). This will likely develop over a series of films with increasing lucency and mass effect. CT will be helpful to confirm the diagnosis and define the overinflated segment if surgical intervention is considered.

The final main cause for hyperexpansion and lucency is congenital pulmonary airway malformation (CPAM) and is a heterogeneous group of conditions that have variable imaging findings from a microcystic mass to a complex mass containing large cysts. They only need cross-sectional imaging (with CT) if surgical management is being considered. In many cases, unless there is repeated superimposed infection, surgical management is not required.

Respiratory Distress with Abnormal Prenatal Imaging

Developmental anatomical abnormalities impacting neonatal pulmonary function include agenesis, hypoplasia, bronchopulmonary foregut malformations, and CDH.

CDH is the most commonly seen and represents a diaphragmatic developmental defect leading to herniation of abdominal viscera and mesentery into the thoracic cavity. Chest radiography may demonstrate ipsilateral chest opacification, contralateral cardiomediastinal shift, and decreased or absent intra-abdominal bowel gas (**Fig. 21.14A**). With a left CDH and gastric herniation, an enteric tube will overlie the left hemithorax (**Fig. 21.14B and C**).

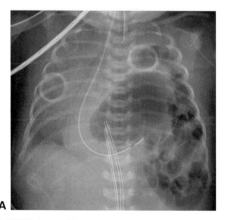 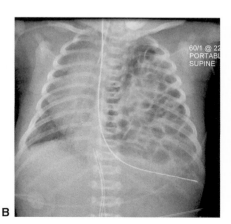 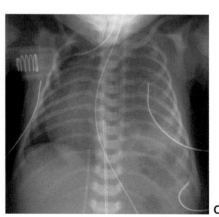

FIGURE 21.14 Three examples of left-sided diaphragmatic hernias. A: CDH containing stomach and small bowel. (Courtesy of Dr Jeremy Jones, Radiopaedia.org, rID: 27205.) **B:** Containing gas-filled small bowel only. (Courtesy of A. Prof Frank Gaillard, Radiopaedia.org, rID: 6351.) **C:** Loss of a normal left hemidiaphragm but without gas-filled loops of bowel in the defect. (Courtesy of Dr Jeremy Jones, Radiopaedia.org, rID: 62743.)

When air has reached bowel loops, herniation of bowel loops will readily be identified in the chest.

Unilateral pulmonary agenesis with bronchovascular atresia is a primary developmental abnormality, often associated with other congenital anomalies. Chest radiography will show complete hemithorax opacification with ipsilateral cardiomediastinal shift. Pulmonary hypoplasia has multiple possible extrinsic etiologies leading to abnormal pulmonary development, in addition to intrinsic developmental errors. These include *in utero* renal agenesis and oligohydramnios (e.g., Potter syndrome), neuromuscular disorders, skeletal dysplasias (leading to a small thorax), and CDH. A postnatal chest radiograph will demonstrate reduced unilateral or bilateral lung volumes associated with hemidiaphragm elevation and rib crowding. If unilateral, ipsilateral cardiomediastinal shift will also be present.

Bronchopulmonary foregut malformations are a spectrum of tracheobronchial tree developmental anomalies including bronchial atresia, bronchial cysts, and sequestration as well as CPAM (mentioned above).

Respiratory Distress in the Established Preterm Neonate

Mechanical ventilation pressure, high oxygen tension, and low surfactant in high-risk neonates with immature lungs can lead to inflammation with secondary irreversible bronchopulmonary damage, bronchial stenosis, and parenchymal cysts and fibrosis (bronchopulmonary dysplasia). PIE may be seen during mechanical ventilation, and its presence increases the likelihood of subsequent development of BPD. Clinically, the neonate will require supplemental oxygen for at least 28 days, to a corrected age of 36 weeks. Radiography can confirm the diagnosis: coarse reticular interstitial opacities, cystic lucencies, hyperinflation, and heterogeneous aeration with atelectasis. CT 3D airway reconstructions (e.g., virtual bronchoscopy) may define the extent of parenchymal disease and noninvasively define bronchial stenoses with potential tracheomegaly.

ABDOMINAL IMAGING

The breadth of pathology that can potentially occur within the abdominal cavity is huge and is split between gastrointestinal and genitourinary pathology.

An abdominal x-ray is a useful tool in the initial assessment of a neonate with vomiting, abdominal distension, or where there is suspicion of NEC in a preterm neonate. It will allow assessment of bowel gas pattern and determine whether gas has reached the large bowel and rectum. It will help to assess areas of bowel dilatation in cases of obstruction and may demonstrate bowel-gas displacement in the case of a mass. Remember that fluid-filled bowel

loops will not be visible on the x-ray. Anatomy textbooks suggest that small bowel tends to sit centrally and large bowel peripherally, in the neonate it can be difficult to distinguish small bowel from large bowel based on gas pattern.

The abdominal x-ray can also be helpful for assessing the bowel wall in NEC to look for mural gas and portal venous gas as well as perforation. Where additional information is required, ultrasound is invariably the next step. Ultrasound will visualize fluid-filled bowel, characterize a mass, and further assess the bowel wall.

Anatomic and functional evaluation is essential for investigating urogenital abnormalities. X-rays are not useful in this context and ultrasound is the most useful modality. A MCUG may be used to assess vesicoureteral reflux and exclude posterior urethral valves (PUVs). Renal scintigraphy is reserved for functional evaluation of the kidneys and rarely used in neonates.

The Vomiting Neonate

There is a broad range of potential causes for vomiting in a neonate. Assessment of the vomitus for bile is important because it is likely to alter the urgency of further investigation. Bile in the vomit suggests obstruction after the ampulla, and while there are a variety of causes, the most important diagnosis to exclude is malrotation and volvulus. An abdominal x-ray is often the first test and is helpful to exclude obstruction.

For assessment of malrotation and volvulus, an upper GI contrast study is performed and contrast is injected via an NG tube placed in the distal stomach. The radiologist will look for normal contrast passage in the duodenum and a normal duodenojejunal (DJ) flexure position.

Malrotation is defined by a low-lying DJ flexure. This predisposes to volvulus which is one of the causes of bilious vomiting. Volvulus may occasionally be seen as a corkscrew appearance on fluoroscopy. However, if there is complete obstruction, this will not be seen. Instead, ultrasound is helpful because it can visualize the volved segment (Fig. 21.15A–C). Other causes of proximal bowel obstruction include duodenal and jejunal atresia or external compression of the duodenum. Again, ultrasound is helpful either on the neonatal unit or as an adjunct to fluoroscopy.

Ultrasound can also be useful to assess the pylorus in the rare case of neonatal pyloric stenosis causing gastric outlet obstruction or in cases of a normal upper GI contrast study.

Failure to Pass Meconium

In neonates who fail to pass meconium and have an anus (Fig. 21.16A), bowel gas pattern on an abdominal x-ray will act as a starting point. The differential is between atresia, meconium ileus,

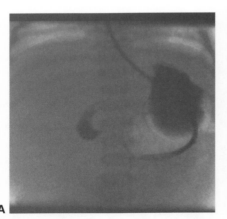
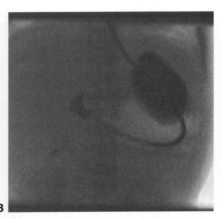
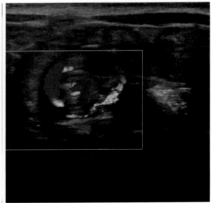

FIGURE 21.15 **An upper GI contrast study and ultrasound in a vomiting neonate. A:** The contrast study shows a tapered duodenum. **B:** A later image highlights a trace of contrast in the right lower quadrant, but no contrast between. **C:** An ultrasound performed on the table shows the swirl of the vascular pedicles of the volved bowel which is causing the obstruction and is not visible on the upper GI contrast study. (Courtesy of Dr Jeremy Jones, Radiopaedia.org, rID: 35352.)

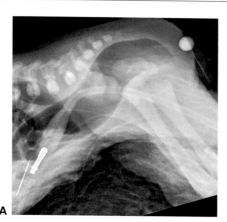
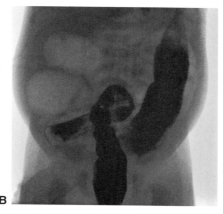
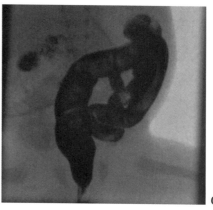

FIGURE 21.16 Several causes of failure to pass meconium. A: Anal atresia with a suspended lateral to visualize the distance between the rectal gas and the expected site of the anus to determine a high or low atresia. (Courtesy of Dr Jeremy Jones, Radiopaedia.org, rID: 30845.) **B:** Dilated descending colon in a patient with Hirschsprung disease. (Courtesy of Dr Jeremy Jones, Radiopaedia.org, rID: 62788.) **C:** Multiple filling defects on the lower GI contrast study with meconium plug syndrome. The contrast study was therapeutic relieving the obstruction. (Courtesy of Dr Jeremy Jones, Radiopaedia.org, rID: 62794.)

meconium plug, and Hirschsprung disease. Distended gas-filled bowel centrally, with an absence of peripheral gas, will confirm a likely underlying reason for failure to pass meconium. A lower GI contrast study is the next test to perform in conjunction with surgical discussion. Contrast instilled into the rectum will identify reversal of the normal colonic–rectal ratio in Hirschsprung disease (**Fig. 21.16B**). It will identify meconium plugs in the left colon in meconium plug disease (**Fig. 21.16C**). The contrast examination will help to wash out the meconium plugs and will act as treatment as well as a diagnostic test. In atresia and meconium ileus, the colon will not have been used normally and will, therefore, be small. The contrast study will identify a microcolon in these cases and will not be helpful therapeutically.

Perforation

Bowel perforation may occur *in utero* or postnatally. *In utero* perforation occurs most typically in the setting of bowel obstruction (e.g., meconium ileus, bowel atresia) and/or ischemia. The radiographic and sonographic hallmarks for *in utero* perforation are peritoneal calcifications, corresponding to intraperitoneal spillage of enteric meconium and secondary sterile peritonitis. Calcification may be present in the scrotum because of the patent processus vaginalis. Nonsealed *in-utero* perforations will lead to postnatal pneumoperitoneum.

Bowel perforations that occur exclusively in the postnatal period may occur in the setting of high-grade bowel obstruction and NEC. Perforations will result in pneumoperitoneum, peritonitis, and potentially intra-abdominal fluid and fluid collections. On AP radiographs, free air may be seen around bowel loops ("Rigler sign") and the falciform ligament ("football sign"), while on lateral decubitus, view gas is seen anterior to the liver edge. Sick preterm neonates may not tolerate being turned on their side for a decubitus film, and in such cases, a lateral shoot-through can be helpful to confirm pneumoperitoneum if there is doubt.

Necrotizing Enterocolitis

Necrotizing enterocolitis (NEC) occurs almost exclusively in the preterm neonate. Abdominal radiography may show dilated loops of small bowel and associated wall thickening. Serial radiographs will show a relatively static appearance of bowel gas. Pneumatosis intestinalis is seen as curvilinear lucency in the bowel wall (**Fig. 21.17A**) and portal venous gas as branching lucency over the liver. Both are helpful signs for confirming NEC. The treatment-altering imaging finding is pneumoperitoneum (**Fig. 21.17B and C**) confirming perforation, see above. Sonography may demonstrate bowel wall thickening, decreased or absent bowel perfusion, bowel wall echogenic foci (corresponding to pneumatosis), portal venous gas, and pneumoperitoneum. If there is mucosal sloughing, regions of wall thinning will be demonstrated.

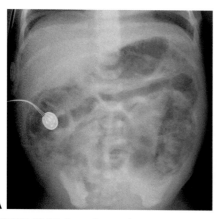
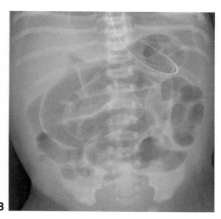
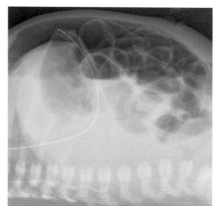

FIGURE 21.17 Several examples of NEC. Preterm neonate with bowel wall thickening and mural gas. A: NEC with perforation. (Courtesy of A. Prof Frank Gaillard, Radiopaedia.org, rID: 6355.) **B:** Rigler's sign on the frontal radiograph with gas seen on both sides of the bowel wall. **C:** Lateral shoot through confirms the free gas in the same case. (Courtesy of Dr Jeremy Jones, Radiopaedia.org, rID: 62793.)

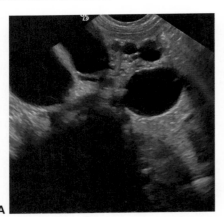
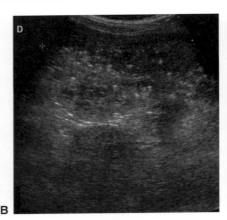
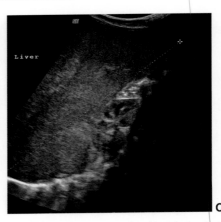

FIGURE 21.18 A selection of renal and pararenal masses. A: Multiple cysts of variable size and no normal renal parenchyma in a case of multicystic dysplastic kidney. (Courtesy of A. Prof Frank Gaillard, Radiopaedia.org, rID: 8528.) **B:** A classical microcystic appearance in ARPKD. (Courtesy of Dr Hani Salam, Radiopaedia. org, rID: 9487.) **C: C:** Grossly enlarged liver. The remainder of the ultrasound shows splenomegaly confirmed with CT. Neonatal neuroblastoma with hepatosplenomegaly. (Courtesy of Dr Hani Salam, Radiopaedia.org, rID: 9564.)

Abdominal Mass

Abdominal distension in the neonate may be the result of distended bowel loops with fluid or gas, or secondary to peritoneal fluid in ascites. However, when there is a palpable mass, the differential is smaller.

Cystic Kidney Disease

There are two main groups of neonatal renal cystic disease: cystic–dysplastic kidney disease (CDKD) (**Fig. 21.18A**) and polycystic kidney disease (PKD) (**Fig. 21.18B**). CDKD is a type of renal dysplasia in which there is variable connective tissue and cyst replacement of normal renal parenchyma. Cysts do not communicate with the collecting system. Ultrasound will show cysts along with echogenic parenchyma. The important step is to distinguish whether the CDKD is a mild form of the disease in which there is the preservation of some degree of identifiable renal parenchyma and function versus a severe form of the disease (e.g., multicystic dysplasia) in which there is complete replacement of renal parenchyma and absence of function. Renal scintigraphy at an appropriate age is useful to distinguish reduced versus absence of renal function.

PKD includes two entities: autosomal recessive polycystic kidney disease (ARPKD) and autosomal dominant polycystic kidney disease (ADPKD). Both may be diagnosed prenatally with fetal ultrasound. If undetected prior to birth, ARPKD will typically present during the neonatal period, while ADPKD will more commonly present later. Sonographic features for ARPKD include enlarged echogenic kidneys, dilated renal tubules, and "small cysts." Should ADPKD be detected during the neonatal period, renal sonography will typically show an enlarged echogenic kidney with micro- and macrocysts, associated with renal contour distortion (secondary to the cysts).

There may be additional findings in ARPKD. It is associated with periportal fibrosis and ectatic intrahepatic bile ducts. It also manifests with pancreatic cysts.

Solid Renal Masses

Neonatal renal masses are relatively rare. Diagnostic considerations would include mesoblastic nephroma, nephroblastomatosis, Wilms tumor, rhabdoid tumor, and clear cell sarcoma. Further radiologic imaging should proceed with MRI where available or with contrast-enhanced CT if MRI is not possible (**Fig. 21.18C**).

Hepatomegaly

Hepatomegaly may be secondary to hepatic congestion (e.g., right heart obstructive lesion) or obstructive jaundice. However, rarely, hepatomegaly may be the result of a hepatic mass (e.g., hepatic infantile hemangioma). Depending upon the sonographic features, CT or MRI with angiographic imaging is an appropriate next radiologic step for a hepatic mass (**Fig. 21.19A–C**).

Obstructive Jaundice

The workup of obstructive jaundice starts with an ultrasound. Using this approach, biliary atresia and choledochal cysts are both diagnosed with high accuracy, along with the exclusion of other

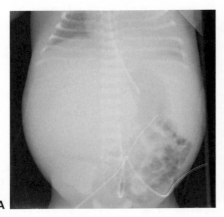
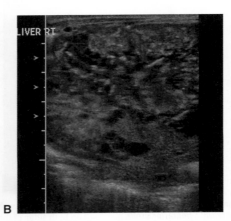
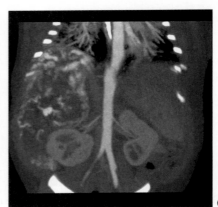

FIGURE 21.19 Multimodality imaging in a neonate with abdominal distension secondary to hepatomegaly and infantile hepatic hemangioma. A: Abdominal x-ray confirms liver enlargement and bowel displacement. **B:** Ultrasound shows an extremely disordered architecture. **C:** CT highlights very abnormal vascular supply and shunting. (Courtesy of A. Prof Frank Gaillard, Radiopaedia.org, rID: 8253.)

differential possibilities (e.g., bile plug). In the rare case where biliary atresia is suspected, further investigation with MRI and nuclear scintigraphy (the HIDA scan) can be helpful to confirm the diagnosis.

Obstructive Uropathy

Pelviureteric junction obstruction (PUJO) and PUVs are two anatomical obstructive uropathies in the neonate for which radiologic imaging is critical. PUJO occurs as stenosis at the transition between the renal pelvis and ureter and may be caused by intrinsic errors in ureteral development versus extrinsic compression (e.g., crossing vessels). PUVs are congenital obstructing urethral membranes (of connective tissue and muscle) located in the posterior urethra. Both PUJO and PUVs may be diagnosed pre- or postnatally. On neonatal ultrasound, PUJO manifests as hydronephrosis transitioning at the PUJ associated with diminished or absent ureteral jets. Renal function may be diminished; renal scintigraphy may show delayed washout of the radiotracer. PUVs are distinguished on ultrasound by a dilated "keyhole" posterior urethra associated with bladder wall thickening, likely ureteric dilatation and pelvicaliectasis, and potentially, renal dysplasia. An MCUG will show a dilated posterior urethra with abrupt caliber change between the posterior and anterior urethra, associated with bladder wall thickening, bladder neck hypertrophy, vesicoureteral reflux, and potentially a bladder diverticulum (Fig. 21.20A–C). Other rarer causes of bladder outflow obstruction include giant ureteroceles that obstruct the urethral orifice.

Renal Infection

Pyelonephritis (PN) may occur in the neonate and when it does, is often related to underlying urogenital structural or functional abnormalities (e.g., obstruction, reflux). Imaging is not necessary for the diagnosis but is useful to assess urogenital structure and function. Ultrasound findings in pyelonephritis are wide and include focal or multifocal echogenicities corresponding to regions of infection, associated with diminished or absent blood flow. Perinephric fluid or phlegmon may be present. MCUG can be used to determine whether there is obstruction or reflux, and a DMSA scan can be used to evaluate renal parenchymal scarring and determine split function.

Abnormal Renal Ultrasound

Some neonatal renal pathology may be asymptomatic and discovered while performing a renal ultrasound. The findings may be relevant in the context of other findings, for example, a duplex kidney in obstructive uropathy or nephrolithiasis in a metabolic abnormality, but sometimes, these findings are incidental and unrelated to a neonate's current clinical state.

Renal Developmental Abnormalities

Embryologic development of the kidney and upper and lower collecting system is a coordinated process in which a ureteral bud and mesodermal cells form a primitive metanephros in the pelvis with a ventral hilum. The developing kidney undergoes "relative ascent" to the expected retroperitoneal fossa with a 90-degree rotation. The bladder develops from ventral cloaca; during fetal development, the allantois (caudal end of the yolk sac) connects the bladder to the umbilicus. Abnormal progression of urogenital development can lead to a spectrum of anomalies including renal agenesis, hypoplasia, and dysplasia; ureteropelvic duplication; renal ectopia and fusion; urachal anomalies; and the bladder exstrophy–epispadias complex.

Nephrolithiasis

Secondary medullary nephrocalcinosis in the neonate may result from a variety of etiologies, including medications (e.g., furosemide), endocrine disorders, ARPKD, and renal tubular acidosis. It is depicted on ultrasound as renal pyramid coalescent hyperechogenicity. Large calcifications will typically demonstrate posterior shadowing. Tamm-Horsfall proteins are physiologically excreted in the neonatal period and may also cause focal echogenicity at the base of the renal pyramids. This may mimic nephrolithiasis but is a normal and transient finding.

NEUROIMAGING

Hypoxic-Ischemic Injury

HII of the brain is defined as irreversible cellular and parenchymal brain damage resulting from cerebral hypoperfusion and hypoxemia. The pattern of brain injury depicted by radiologic imaging will vary depending upon the degree of brain maturity (e.g., preterm vs. term infant), duration of hypoxia, and timing of imaging (4).

Ischemia will result in edema with associated mass effect. The amount of mass effect will depend on the volume of ischemic tissue and the tissue involved (subcortical white matter edema will cause more mass effect than basal ganglia edema). Ultrasound and MRI can both be used to detect changes in echogenicity (ultrasound) and signal (MRI) in the ischemic tissue, and also the secondary signs of mass effect with effacement of sulci and lateral ventricles. Patterns and extent of injury are useful for determining prognosis (5).

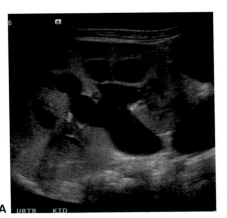
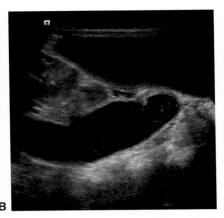
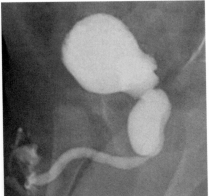

FIGURE 21.20 Multiple images from the same patient with posterior urethral values and bilateral hydroureteronephrosis. A: Hydronephrosis. **B:** Dilated tortuous ureters. **C:** MCUG with dilated bullet-shaped posterior urethra. (Courtesy of Dr Andrew Dixon, Radiopaedia.org, rID: 10432.)

THE NEWBORN INFANT

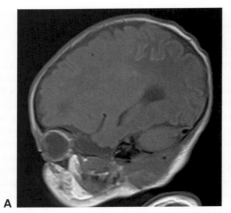
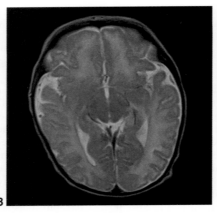
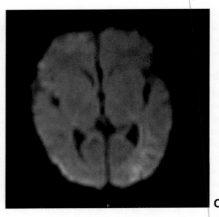

FIGURE 21.21 Watershed distribution HII. A: Sagittal T1 image with linear T1 hyperintensity of cortex highlighting laminar cortical necrosis. **B:** Abnormal T2 hyperintensity in the left posterior white matter. **C:** Diffusion restriction (b 800) confirming ischemic etiology. (Courtesy of Dr Jeremy Jones, Radiopaedia.org, rID 73219.)

Depending on the severity of ischemic and cell death, the amount of edema may be small and difficult to appreciate using ultrasound (6). With DWI, MRI will detect ischemic change almost immediately (7) with a corresponding decrease in ADC values. By day 6 to 7, DWI will have pseudonormalized meaning that the ADC values are normal despite an ischemic insult (this occurs later in cooled infants).

Term HII

In term babies, there are two main patterns of injury associated with hypoxic–ischemic injury (8). Where there is a mild-to-moderate insult (so called "chronic-partial"), the pattern seen is ischemia in the parasagittal watershed region and subcortical white matter (**Fig. 21.21A–C**). Metabolically less active areas are sacrificed as cerebral autoregulation seeks to preserve blood flow to the metabolically more active regions of the brain.

In neonates with severe global hypoperfusion and ischemia, regulatory measures cannot adequately compensate flow to the high metabolic regions. There is ischemic of the deep grey matter, cerebellum, and perirolandic cortex (**Fig. 21.22A–C**). In prolonged and profound hypoxia, global cortex and white matter involvement may be seen (See chapter 49).

Preterm HII

In a preterm infant, chronic HI can act alone or with inflammation to cause cellular damage to the poorly vascularized, watershed periventricular white matter, which results in periventricular leukomalacia (PVL) (**Fig. 21.23A and B**). Susceptible regions are white matter

dorsal and lateral to the lateral ventricles, centrum semiovale, optic radiations, and acoustic radiations. Inflammation and tissue necrosis can lead to cavitation, cyst formation, and parenchymal destruction. Cysts may coalescence to form larger cysts. Alternatively, cysts may dehisce into the adjacent ventricles forming porencephalic cysts. Progressive parenchymal destruction leads to loss of white matter, thinning of the corpus callosum, ex-vacuo ventriculomegaly, and irregular margins of the ventricles. These changes usually evolve over 4 to 10 weeks after extremely preterm birth (**Fig. 21.23C**).

With severe ischemia, in addition to features of PVL, there will likely be an HII pattern similar to term infants. In the preterm neonate, there will likely be less involvement of the basal ganglia and perirolandic cortex. A preterm infant with hypoxia of any degree may present with concomitant germinal matrix (GM) hemorrhage (See chapter 50).

Neonatal Arterial or Venous Stroke

Occasionally, imaging will demonstrate ischemia that does not correlate with HII as the result of generalized reduction in cerebral perfusion. Instead, the imaging highlights ischemia within an arterial territory, for example, a middle cerebral artery. Where territorial ischemia is identified, it is important to perform vascular imaging to identify a causative thrombus or dissection. Venous infarction secondary to venous thrombosis and altered venous draining pressures will present as focal areas of infarction outwith a defined arterial territory. MR venography is useful to identify venous sinus or cortical vein thrombosis.

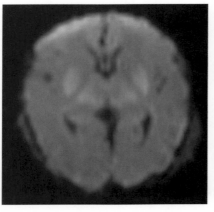
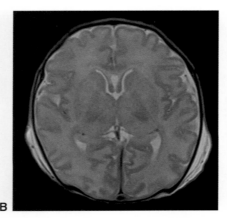
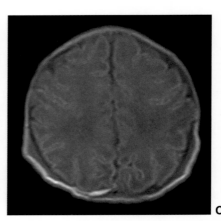

FIGURE 21.22 Profound hypoxic ischemic injury following cardiac arrest on day 1 of life. A: Diffusion abnormality centered on the basal ganglia. **B:** Grossly abnormal basal ganglia and white matter. **C:** Trace of right posterior subdural blood (T1 hyperintensity) not uncommon following delivery. (Courtesy of Dr Jeremy Jones, Radiopaedia.org, rID 73220.)

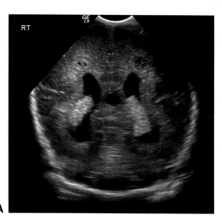
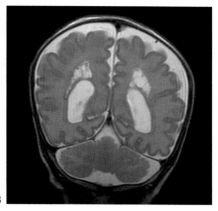
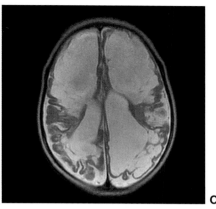

FIGURE 21.23 A: US with hyperechogenic periventricular white matter and cyst formation. **B:** MRI from the same patient confirming periventricular cysts. (Dr Hani Salam, Radiopaedia.org, rID: 14000.) **C:** Severe cystic encephalomalacia and porencephaly secondary to PVL. (Courtesy of Dr Gagandeep Choudhary, Radiopaedia.org, rID: 13145.)

Intracranial Hemorrhage

ICH in a neonate is an emergent condition for which imaging serves as a critical role in diagnosis and management. The cause of hemorrhage and clinical considerations differ between the preterm and term infant and imaging strategies and therefore different.

Preterm Hemorrhage

In a preterm infant (<34 weeks), the most common cause of intracranial hemorrhage is GM hemorrhage. The GM is a highly vascular subependymal region adjacent to the caudothalamic groove. It contains proliferating neuron and glial cell precursors, and its fragile capillaries are highly susceptible to physiologic stressors that impact cerebral blood flow autoregulation, for example, hypoxia, hypertension, hypotension, metabolic acidosis, and reperfusion. Depending on the maturity of the GM capillaries and the severity and duration of physiologic stress, the capillaries can rupture resulting in localized hemorrhage. Coagulopathy and fibrinolytic abnormalities are additional risk factors compounding a GM hemorrhage (9).

Localized hemorrhage at the caudothalamic groove is classed as grade I hemorrhage (Fig. 21.24A). Larger hemorrhages may extend into the lateral ventricles (grade II) (Fig. 21.24B) and potentially cause ventricular dilatation (grade III) (Fig. 21.24C). All grades of GM hemorrhage may be associated with periventricular venous infarction and secondary hemorrhage (ex-grade IV). Periventricular hemorrhagic infarction will often result in porencephaly.

Head ultrasound is performed in the preterm infant during the first week of life to screen for intracranial hemorrhage. Timing (e.g., day 1, 3, or 7) of the ultrasound will depend upon the clinical course and risk factors. Blood is depicted as coalescent echogenicity within the GM at the caudothalamic groove, ventricle, and parenchyma. Follow-up imaging proceeds with ultrasound and/or MRI as dictated by the initial imaging findings and clinical course. If no hemorrhage is detected during the initial screening period, additional surveillance imaging is typically performed with ultrasound.

Term Hemorrhage

In the term infant, intracranial hemorrhage may be the result of birth-related trauma. However, it is rare that it is large enough to cause symptoms and is usually low-volume, subdural, and posteriorly located.

Aside from birth-related hemorrhage, it is most commonly related to accidental or non-accidental trauma, the latter more correctly termed abusive head trauma (Fig. 21.25A–C). Other less common etiologies include the hemorrhagic transformation of cerebral infarction or rarely, hemorrhage into an aggressive, malignant congenital intracranial tumor (10). It is important to keep in mind that while these causes of ICH are infrequent in the preterm infant, they nonetheless may occur.

CT is the initial modality of choice to accurately and timely diagnose a traumatic ICH and associated potential fractures, mass effect, and midline shift. MRI can be used to assess associated parenchymal change after a decision about immediate management has been made.

Acute hemorrhage is hyperdense on CT, but a similar density to grey-matter by 14 days. On MRI, acute hemorrhage will be T1

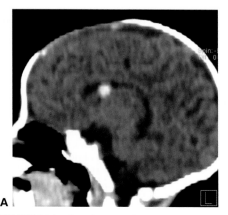
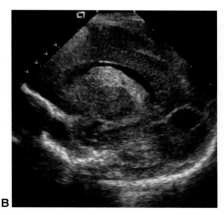
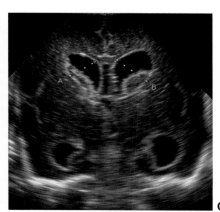

FIGURE 21.24 Germinal matrix hemorrhage. A: Grade I hemorrhage depicted on CT. (Courtesy of Dr Ahmed Abdrabou, Radiopaedia.org, rID: 24800.) **B:** Grade II on a sagittal US through the lateral ventricle. (Courtesy of Dr. Radswiki, Radiopaedia.org, rID: 11452.) **C:** Grade III coronal US. The temporal horns are dilated and a good sign to highlight ventricular dilatation. (Courtesy of A. Prof Frank Gaillard, Radiopaedia.org, rID: 8355.)

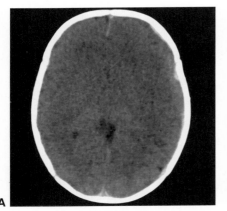 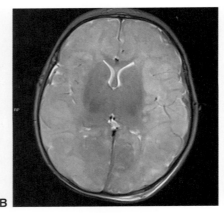 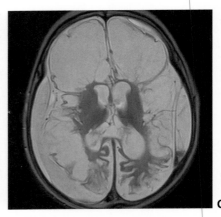

FIGURE 21.25 Hemorrhage and parenchymal injury in NAI. A: Small left-sided subdural hemorrhage with interhemispheric extension. Associated severe cerebral edema. **B:** MRI T2 sequence confirming the severe parenchymal edema and ventricular effacement. **C:** Imaging sequela with extensive cystic encephalomalacia (Courtesy of Dr Jeremy Jones, Radiopaedia.org, rID: 69537.)

hyperintense, T2 hypointense and will demonstrate signal dropout on SWI. CT is the only modality that can be used to determine the age of haemorrhage. Acute blood is hyperdense and will remain hyperdense for up to 7–10 days (11).

Correctly determining the location of hemorrhage is important. The most common location for extraaxial hemorrhage is subdural and may be convexity, interhemispheric, tentorial, or posterior fossa. Subdural hemorrhage that is not low volume and posteriorly located is concerning for inflicted injury, especially if there is interhemispheric extension. Subdural collections may also contain serum and CSF resulting in mixed density collections.

Subarachnoid hemorrhage is identified where blood extends into sulci or basal cisterns. It is far less common than subdural hemorrhage but may coexist where trauma is the cause. Extradural hemorrhage is very rare because the middle meningeal artery has not been incorporated into the calvarium in the neonatal period, and it is therefore mobile and not injured even if the skull is fractured. Intraventricular and intraparenchymal hemorrhage is also possible.

The mass effect caused by bleeding is the major immediate concern along with the parenchymal compression and herniation that occurs. If there is any concern for abusive head trauma, local child protection protocols must be instigated along with appropriate imaging which includes a skeletal survey and MRI brain and spine.

Neurocutaneous Syndromes

Among a large number of neurocutaneous disorders, tuberous sclerosis complex (TSC), Sturge-Weber syndrome, and PHACE syndrome commonly lead to radiologic imaging in a neonate (12).

Tuberous Sclerosis Complex

TSC is an autosomal dominant multisystem disorder, and it is the extracranial manifestations of the disease, that typically lead to a suspected diagnosis. These include cardiac rhabdomyomas, arterial aneurysms and stenotic–occlusive disease, renal cysts, and rarely retinal hamartomas and cutaneous lesions.

MRI is the investigation of choice for assessment of the brain in patients with suspected TSC. Intracranial manifestations in a neonate include cortical tubers, subependymal hamartomas, subependymal giant cell tumors, and white matter lesions. Early calcification may be present in the subependymal hamartomas and is demonstrated using SWI.

Sturge-Weber Syndrome

Sturge-Weber syndrome is defined by a cutaneous capillary malformation (in the trigeminal nerve distribution) and an intracranial leptomeningeal capillary–venous malformation, associated with enlargement of the ipsilateral choroid plexus and deep medullary veins. Involvement is typically unilateral. Additional features include gyriform cortical calcifications, brain hemiatrophy, and skull thickening. However, these are not typical in a neonate. MRI with arterial- and venous-phase MRA provides a comprehensive assessment of the intracranial vascular malformation.

PHACE Syndrome

PHACE syndrome is composed of posterior fossa malformations (e.g., Dandy-Walker malformation), hemangiomas, arterial anomalies (e.g., cervical and cerebral agenesis, hypoplasia, or dolichoectasia), cardiac anomalies and coarctation of the aorta, eye anomalies, and ventral, midline developmental defects. Head and neck infantile hemangiomas are commonly found; intracranial, thoracic, and extremity hemangiomas are also possible. Multisystem MRI with MRA is the modality of choice for complete cardiovascular and noncardiovascular evaluation.

Congenital Malformations

In many cases, neonates with congenital malformations will have had an antenatal diagnosis established by prenatal ultrasound and/or MRI. These include neural tube defects (open and closed), midline malformations, posterior fossa abnormalities, and neuronal migration abnormalities (**Fig. 21.26A–C**). In some cases, diagnosis is first suspected following birth, by a combination of the clinical presentation and an initial ultrasound examination. In both scenarios, postnatal MRI with multiplanar T1- and T2-weighted sequences in addition to DWI sequences provide the most comprehensive approach for evaluating and accurately characterizing these anomalies. CT may complement the workup, by providing a more detailed depiction of potential concomitant defects involving the calvarium and/or skull base (e.g., cephalocele).

Congenital Infection

Transplacental and transvaginal transmitted infections that can impact the CNS include Toxoplasmosis gondii, Rubella, Cytomegalovirus, and Herpesvirus (TORCH infections). The neurologic manifestation of disease may include intrauterine growth restriction, microcephaly, seizures, low muscle tone, and sensorineural hearing loss. Other systemic non-neurologic manifestations may also occur (e.g., bone, cardiac, and ophthalmic congenital abnormalities). MRI is the favored imaging modality to identify the associated brain abnormalities. These include calcification (areas of signal dropout on SWI), cortical malformations and white matter lesions, hydrocephalus, and volume loss with ex vacuo dilatation. The pattern and constellation of these findings along with cultures, titers, and other non-neurologic imaging findings will support the diagnosis (13).

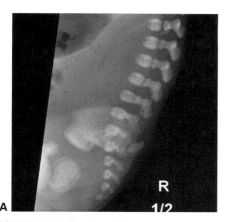
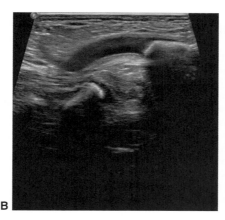
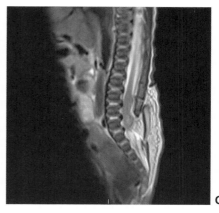

FIGURE 21.26 Newborn baby with hard lump in the midline at the lumbosacral junction. A: X-ray confirms an additional bony element superficial to the posterior elements. **B:** US demonstrates a neural tube defect with bone and cartilage. **C:** MRI confirms the defect and completes with assessment of the cord and neural placode. (Courtesy of Dr Jeremy Jones, Radiopaedia.org, rID: 73221.)

Congenital Masses

Benign and malignant congenital masses in the brain or spine are uncommon in the neonatal population. In some instances, prenatal ultrasound and MRI have detected a mass. Postnatal ultrasound of the brain and/or spine can be performed at the bedside to confirm the mass and evaluate for potential secondary complications (e.g., hydrocephalus). They can also be used to assess for associated anomalies (e.g., anorectal and genital malformations, spinal dysraphism). In other instances, non-specific symptoms may lead to the diagnostic evaluation. These include increased head circumference, vomiting, seizures, hypotonia, and constipation. If a mass is identified, further assessment with MRI is required.

Benign Intracranial Cysts

Common benign congenital cystic lesions in a neonate include arachnoid cyst, choroid plexus cyst (CPC), epidermoid, and dermoid. Arachnoid cysts (filled with clear CSF) will appear anechoic on ultrasound, of CSF density on CT, and T1 hypointense, T2 hyperintense on MRI. No enhancement will be present. When these extraaxial cysts are of sufficient size, they may cause local mass effect on the developing brain and may also result in scalloping of the inner table of the calvarium. A CPC is also sonolucent but may have an echogenic rim because of the surrounding choroid plexus. On CT, the CPC (with lipid-laden histiocytes) will appear iso- to hyperdense and on MRI, be T1 iso- to hyperintense and T2 hyperintense. Rim or nodular enhancement may be seen. Epidermoids (composed of cellular debris, keratin,

water, and cholesterol) are hypointense on CT and iso- to slightly hyperintense on T1- and T2-weighted MR imaging, reflecting the fluid and lipid contents. Calcification is not common. Although not common, rim enhancement may be seen on MRI. While an intracranial off-midline location is most prevalent (e.g., cerebellopontine angle, fourth ventricle, and sellar–parasellar locations), epidermoid may less commonly develop in the spine. An intracranial dermoid is almost exclusively midline (e.g., sellar, parasellar, frontonasal, midline posterior fossa). In distinction to the other intracranial cysts, it is composed primarily of fat (e.g., liquid cholesterol) and dermal appendages; its wall is thick and often calcified. The lesion will have fat attenuation on CT and have T1 hyperintense and heterogeneous T2 hypo- or hyperintense signal on MRI. The fatty elements will be hypointense on fat-suppression sequences. These lesions are typically uncomplicated in a neonate and, as such, show no enhancement. In both epidermoid and dermoid, a dermal sinus tract is possible and can be defined both on CT and MRI.

CNS Tumors

Neonatal brain tumors are rare, but when they occur tend to be supratentorial, in contradistinction to most pediatric brain tumors (14). They can be broadly grouped as germ cell tumors (with teratoma being the commonest neonatal tumor of the brain and spine) (Fig. 21.27A), choroid plexus tumors, embryonal tumors (embryonal tumors with multilayered rosettes, atypical teratoid/rhabdoid tumor AT-RT [Fig. 21.27B], and medulloblastoma), astrocytic

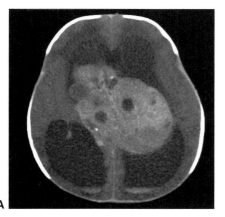
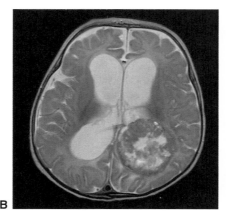
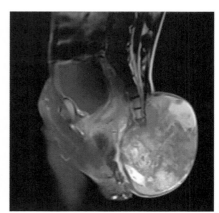

FIGURE 21.27 A: A 8-day old with a large head. The huge midline congenital mass with solid and cystic components causing hydrocephalus is an immature teratoma. (Courtesy of Dr Hani Salam, Radiopaedia.org, rID: 8336.) **B:** Large left-sided aggressive tumor with irregular margin and associated hydrocephalus. This was confirmed to be an AT-RT pathologically (Courtesy of Dr Fabien Ho, Radiopaedia.org, rID: 59091.) **C:** Sacrococcygeal teratoma on a sagittal T2 MRI with a large buttock mass. (Courtesy of Dr Ashutosh Gandhi, Radiopaedia.org, rID: 20644.)

tumors, and neuronal and mixed neuronal-glial tumors (15). Intraspinal (extradural) neuroblastoma may also be encountered in a neonate. Symptoms and secondary imaging findings (e.g., midline shift, hydrocephalus) will be reflective for the tumor size and degree of compression and displacement of these structures.

Teratomas most commonly are sacrococcygeal teratoma (SCT) but may also present as intraspinal, extradural masses in the lumbar and thoracic spine (**Fig. 21.27C**). Imaging of spinal tumors also aims to define secondary sequelae (e.g., localized mass effect and abdominopelvic extension in an SCT). Primary pre- and postcontrast radiologic characteristics of brain and spine congenital tumors depend upon the tumor histology. The majority of teratomas (with ectoderm, mesoderm, and endoderm germ layers) have benign, mature histology, presenting as a cystic lesion containing fat, fluid, soft tissue, and calcium—all readily distinguished on ultrasound, MRI, and CT. Less commonly, teratomas will have immature cellular neuroectodermal elements and present as a heterogeneous solid mass (e.g., intracranial teratoma). In a similar manner to these malignant teratomas, CT density, MRI signal, and enhancement pattern of the intracranial neuroepithelial tumors will vary based upon the degree of tumor cellularity and tissue necrosis. Tumor vascularity, arterial supply, and venous drainage can all readily be defined with MRI and CT to assist surgical planning.

REFERENCES

1. Thayyil S, Chandrasekaran M, Taylor A, et al. Cerebral magnetic resonance biomarkers in neonatal encephalopathy: a meta-analysis. *Pediatrics* 2010;125:e382. doi: 10.1542/peds.2009-1046
2. BAPM. Fetal and Neonatal Brain Magnetic Resonance Imaging: Clinical Indications, Acquisitions and Reporting. A Framework for Practice. Available from: https://www.bapm.org/resources/33-fetal-neonatal-brain-magnetic-resonance-imaging-clinical-indications-acquisitions-and-reporting
3. BAPM. Use of Central Venous Catheters in Neonates. A Framework for Practice. Available from: https://www.bapm.org/resources/10-use-of-central-venous-catheters-in-neonates-revised-2018
4. Cabaj A, Bekiesińska-Figatowska M, Mądzik J. MRI patterns of hypoxic-ischemic brain injury in preterm and full term infants—classical and less common MR findings. *Pol J Radiol* 2012;77:71.
5. Rutherford MA, et al. Assessment of brain tissue injury after moderate hypothermia in neonates with hypoxic-ischaemic encephalopathy: a nested substudy of a randomised controlled trial. *Lancet Neurol* 2010;9(1):39. doi: 10.1016/S1474-4422(09)70295-9
6. Salas J, Tekes A, Hwang M, et al. Head ultrasound in neonatal hypoxic-ischemic injury and its mimickers for clinicians: a review of the patterns of injury and the evolution of findings over time. *Neonatology* 2018;114:185. doi: 10.1159/000487913
7. Vermeulen RJ, Fetter WPF, Hendrikx L, et al. Diffusion-weighted MRI in severe neonatal hypoxic ischaemia: the white cerebrum. *Neuropediatrics* 2003;34:72. doi: 10.1055/s-2003-39599
8. Ghei SK, Zan E, Nathan JE, et al. MR imaging of hypoxic-ischemic injury in term neonates: pearls and pitfalls. *Radiographics* 2014;34:1047. doi: 10.1148/rg.344130080
9. Ballabh P. Intraventricular hemorrhage in premature infants: mechanism of disease. *Pediatr Res* 2010;67:1. doi: 10.1203/PDR.0b013e3181c1b176
10. Hong HS, Lee JY. Intracranial hemorrhage in term neonates. *Childs Nerv Syst* 2018;34:1135. doi: 10.1007/s00381-018-3788-8
11. Bradford R, Choudhary AK, Dias MS. Serial neuroimaging in infants with abusive head trauma: timing abusive injuries. *J Neurosurg Pediatr* 2013;12:110. doi: 10.3171/2013.4.PEDS12596
12. Vézina G. Neuroimaging of phakomatoses: overview and advances. *Pediatr Radiol* 2015;45(suppl 3):S433. doi: 10.1007/s00247-015-3282-3
13. Kwak M, Yum MS, Yeh HR, et al. Brain magnetic resonance imaging findings of congenital cytomegalovirus infection as a prognostic factor for neurological outcome. *Pediatr Neurol* 2018;83:14. doi: 10.1016/j.pediatr-neurol.2018.03.008
14. Bodeliwala S, Kumar V, Singh D. Neonatal brain tumors: a review. *J Neonatal Surg* 2017;6:30. doi: 10.21699/jns.v6i2.579
15. Shekdar KV, Schwartz ES. Brain tumors in the neonate. *Neuroimaging Clin N Am* 2017;27:69. doi: 10.1016/j.nic.2016.09.001

Health Care–Associated Infections

Joseph B. Cantey and Rebekah C. Gardea

INTRODUCTION

Infants cared for in the neonatal intensive care unit (NICU) are at high risk for health care–associated infections (HAIs), including infections caused by multidrug resistant organisms (MDROs). Preterm infants are at increased risk for infection for a variety of reasons including fragile mucocutaneous barriers, the need for indwelling support devices such as vascular catheters and endotracheal tubes, and prolonged hospital stays. In addition, the innate and adaptive immune system is immature in preterm infants relative to older children (see Chapter 48). As a result, infants in the NICU are not only at higher risk for acquiring HAIs, they are less equipped to deal with infections once they occur. Thus, the prevention of HAIs is of paramount importance for NICU personnel.

HAIs are defined by the National Healthcare Safety Network (NHSN) and the International Nosocomial Infection Control Consortium (INICC) as infections occurring more than 72 hours after admission (1,2). The NHSN/INICC definition of HAI therefore excludes early-onset sepsis, which occurs in the first 72 hours of life following perinatal exposure to organisms in the amniotic fluid or genital tract. In contrast to early-onset sepsis, late-onset infection is acquired from the NICU environment or the infant's own microbiome (3,4). Over the past quarter-century, the incidence of HAI in the NICU has steadily decreased across all gestational ages (Fig. 22.1) (5–11). However, HAIs remain a significant cause of morbidity and mortality among preterm infants. In the United States, the NHSN uses specific surveillance definitions to further divide HAIs into site-specific diseases, including primary bloodstream infection (BSI), urinary tract infection (UTI), ventilator-associated events (VAEs), and surgical site infections (SSIs). These HAI events are then stratified by five birth weight categories (≤750 g, 751 to 1,000 g, 1,001 to 1,500 g, 1,501 to 2,500 g, and ≥2,501 g). Gestational age and birth weight are closely correlated; NHSN uses birth weight classification rather than gestational age in their reporting. NHSN HAI definitions are complex and frequently updated, and coordination with infection control and prevention specialists is highly recommended for prospective surveillance within the NICU.

HEALTH CARE–ASSOCIATED INFECTIONS

Central Line–Associated Bloodstream Infections

Central line–associated bloodstream infections (CLABSIs) are the most common HAI in the NICU (12). Central venous catheters are used extensively for critically ill infants in order to administer fluids, nutrition, and medication. Central line use is measured by line-days, and CLABSIs are reported as events per 1,000 line-days (13). The longer a catheter remains in place, the higher the risk for CLABSI (14). Each manipulation of the central line (e.g., accessing and recapping the hub, infusing fluids or medications, changing tubing or dressings, and insertion and removal) also increases the risk of infection if proper technique is not strictly followed. The catheters of preterm infants are manipulated more than once an hour on average, and the number of line-days per patient is significantly longer for NICUs than other pediatric settings (15). Therefore, strategies to keep central line dwell time to a minimum are needed to reduce the rate of CLABSIs. In addition to dwell time, risk factors for CLABSIs in the NICU include low birth weight and degree of prematurity. The most preterm infants have the most impaired mucosal and innate immunity, and they also require the longest dwell times for their central lines.

Most organisms responsible for CLABSI are gram positive. Coagulase-negative staphylococci (CoNS) are the most common cause of late-onset sepsis overall in the NICU (50% to 70% of cases) and the most commonly implicated in CLABSI (3). The near-ubiquitous presence of CoNS on skin and oral mucosa, in conjunction with its ability to form biofilms on catheters, makes CoNS an effective colonizer of central lines. *Staphylococcus aureus* (methicillin susceptible and methicillin resistant) is the second most common cause of CLABSIs (10% to 15%), and that proportion may be increasing as effective central-line bundle techniques have decreased CoNS CLABSIs. Gram-negative pathogens and *Candida* species account for a minority of CLABSI, but the case-fatality rate for these pathogens greatly exceeds that of gram-positive organisms. Both gram-negative and *Candida* BSIs are more common in the setting of extreme prematurity or intra-abdominal pathology (16).

CLABSIs in the NICU are preventable, and NHSN data show that significant improvements have been made over the last decade. Effective strategies to prevent CLABSIs in the NICU mirror central line bundles in other care settings, with a few notable exceptions (Table 22.1). Providers should avoid placing unnecessary central venous catheters; only infants with an anticipated need for prolonged intravenous administration of fluids or medications should receive central lines (17). Using a small pool of providers with specific training on insertion techniques to obtain access has been associated with decreased risk for CLABSIs (18). Once catheters are *in situ*, every effort should be made to minimize dwell times. This means focusing on advancing feeding to the point where fluid and calorie requirements can be met enterally. However, depending on the rate of feeding advancement in a given NICU, this requires an average 7 to 10 days from birth to achieve. Central line bundles that focus on prompt removal of central lines when 120 mL/kg/d of enteral feeds has been achieved can effectively reduce CLABSIs (19).

The selection of catheter type can affect CLABSI risk. Umbilical venous catheters (UVCs), peripherally inserted central catheters (PICCs), or tunneled central catheters are all in common use in the NICU. UVCs are convenient and relatively simple to insert, but the CLABSI risk per line-day is higher with UVCs compared to other catheters, particularly beyond 4 to 7 days of dwell time. In contrast, PICC lines have a more constant CLABSI risk per line-day (20). Observational studies support exchanging UVCs for PICC lines if central access is needed beyond approximately age 7 days (range, 4 to 10 days), but the optimal timing of exchange has not been determined (21,22).

The best antiseptic for skin cleansing prior to insertion of central lines in neonates has not been determined; as a result, there is wide variability in the agents used for skin cleansing in NICUs. Chlorhexidine gluconate (CHG) is widely accepted as the most effective cleansing agent to be used prior to central line insertion. However, its use is not FDA approved in infants age less than 2 months due to the infant's increased body surface area and fragile skin, increasing the chance of systemic absorption of CHG (23,24). CHG has also been associated with dermatitis and burns in premature infants, with risk increasing in proportion to prematurity (25). Ten percent povidone–iodine (PI) has been used as a cleansing agent for hospitalized infants, but a recent study

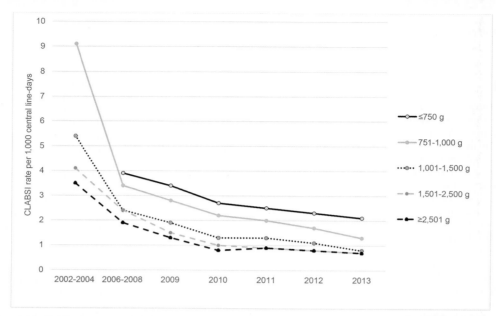

FIGURE 22.1 Decrease in central line–associated bloodstream infections (CLABSIs) reported to the National Healthcare Safety Network from 2002 to 2013, stratified by birth weight.

conducted by Kieran et al. (25) indicated that premature infants (mean gestational age, 27 weeks) receiving PI as a cleansing agent may experience thyroid dysfunction and dermatitis. Trials conducted comparing CHG to PI do not show a significant difference in catheter-tip colonization between the two products (24–27).

Ventilator-Associated Events

The term "ventilator-associated events" (VAEs) replaced "ventilator-associated pneumonia" (VAP) in NHSN surveillance in 2013 and was extended to the NICU setting in 2016 (28). VAEs are defined by a period of stability or improvement on mechanical

TABLE 22.1	
Evidence-Based Strategies to Prevent Central Line–Associated Bloodstream Infections in the Neonatal Intensive Care Unit	
	Recommendations
Insertion	• Hand hygiene before catheter insertion
	• Maximal sterile barrier precautions for catheter insertion
	• Skin preparation before insertion. Note: No specific recommendation for chlorhexidine given concern for systemic absorption or skin irritation in preterm infants. Many centers use chlorhexidine for older infants; povidone–iodine may be used for younger or more preterm infants.
	• No preferred site for insertion (in contrast to older children and adults, where femoral sites are avoided if possible)
Maintenance	• Disinfect catheter hubs and connectors before accessing catheter
	• Perform dressing changes *only* if loose or soiled (in contrast to older children or adults, where dressing changes are performed at least every 7 days)
	• Two-person sterile technique for dressing changes
Removal	• Daily "line-rounds" where need to continue central venous catheter is assessed
	• Remove catheter promptly once no longer required

ventilation for at least 2 calendar days, followed by clinical deterioration including need for increased oxygen ($\geq$25% from baseline) or mean airway pressure ($\geq$4 cm H_2O). In adults, VAP is now a subcategory of VAEs in which there is a positive respiratory diagnostic test for infection. A variety of acute illnesses among ventilated neonates can result in a VAE, and VAP is an important subset of those events. However, diagnosis of VAP in neonates is challenging since bacterial colonization of the upper airways is common and preterm infants can have changing radiographic findings due to bronchopulmonary dysplasia or atelectasis rather than infection. The NHSN discontinued reporting neonatal VAP in 2014, so VAP surveillance criteria do not currently exist for NICU infants. However, preliminary data suggest that extension of the adult VAE-subset VAP criteria to neonates may be feasible if nonspecific (29,30).

The greatest risk factor for VAP is the duration of endotracheal intubation. Endotracheal tubes allow bacteria to bypass most innate airway defenses and reach the distal airways and alveoli. Neonatal endotracheal tubes are usually uncuffed or microcuffed because the cricoid bone, the narrowest aspect of the upper airway, provides a natural cuff. In the absence of the seal provided by a cuff, however, gastric and oral secretions can reach the lower airway. Prematurity, as with CLABSIs, is another primary risk factor for neonatal VAEs due to the concomitant lung immaturity. Extremely low-birth-weight infants (ELBW, <1,000 g) are more likely to be intubated and require longer durations of mechanical ventilation than do more mature infants; as a result, ELBW infants have the highest incidence of VAEs per 1,000 ventilator days (5–11).

Other risk factors include the frequency of reintubation, either due to deterioration on noninvasive support or as a result of unplanned extubation, and pharmacologic acid suppression with proton pump inhibitors or H2 blockers (31). Notably, acid-blocking medication has also been associated with increased risk for other HAIs including CLABSI (32). The underlying medical condition leading to intubation does not seem to affect VAE rates; risks for VAE among infants with meconium aspiration, congenital anomalies, hypoxic–ischemic encephalopathy, and respiratory distress syndrome are similar (33).

The organisms associated with VAP in neonates are most commonly gram negative, although gram-positive organisms such as

TABLE 22.2

Evidence-Based Strategies to Prevent Ventilator-Associated Pneumonia in the Neonatal Intensive Care Unit

	Recommendations
Maintenance	• Head of bed elevation ($\geq$30 degrees) • Lateral positioning after feeding has been associated with decreased aspiration • Oral care. Chlorhexidine, sterile water, colostrum, expressed breast milk have been studied. (No formal preference for chlorhexidine in neonates due to safety concerns among more preterm infants, including skin irritation, systemic absorption.) • Change breathing circuit only when malfunctioning or visibly soiled
Removal	• Daily evaluation for readiness to extubate • Sedation should be kept to minimum amount necessary to prevent unplanned extubations

S. aureus and *Enterococcus* have been reported (34,35). Unfortunately, most epidemiologic studies are limited to upper respiratory cultures from sputum or tracheal aspirates, which makes distinguishing between pathogenic bacteria and colonizing flora a challenge. There is a paucity of studies utilizing bronchoscopy to obtain lower respiratory tract cultures. Both enteric (*Escherichia coli, Klebsiella, Enterobacter, Serratia*) and environmental (*Pseudomonas, Stenotrophomonas*) gram-negatives are common causes of neonatal VAP. CoNS or *Candida* recovered from cultures obtained from the upper airway are not usually pathogens and should not be routinely treated. However, endotracheal tube cultures may be used as evidence for *Candida* or MDRO colonization, which may affect future antibiotic selection, transmission-based precautions, or decolonization strategies.

Studies describing effective VAP prevention in neonates are limited, in part due to the difficulty with accurately assessing VAP in the NICU. Effective prevention bundles have largely used methods that have been successful in non-NICU settings (**Table 22.2**) (36). As with CLABSI prevention, the hallmarks of a successful VAP prevention bundle include minimizing duration and careful maintenance of indwelling hardware. Oral care is an important component of VAP prevention; preliminary data suggest that use of expressed colostrum or breast milk in neonatal oral care may be beneficial compared with sterile water (37). Sedation should be carefully addressed in order to minimize the risk of unplanned extubation while avoiding oversedation, which can result in prolonged mechanical ventilation (38). Finally, NICU providers should avoid obtaining routine cultures from the endotracheal tube. The upper airway is not sterile, and endotracheal tubes are rapidly colonized within hours of intubation. Therefore, culturing the endotracheal tube often forces providers to decide whether recovered organisms represent colonization or infection. Instead, endotracheal tube cultures should only be considered when pneumonia is suspected based on both clinical and radiographic findings and other sources of infection have already been considered (39).

Candidiasis

Candida infection is a major cause of morbidity and mortality in the NICU, especially among infants born $\leq$28 weeks of gestation. Rates of *Candida* colonization and invasive candidiasis vary greatly between NICUs due to differences in care practices. The incidence of candidiasis among ELBW infants ranged from 0% to 28% in one study of NICUs participating in the National Institute of Child Health and Human Development's Neonatal Research Network (40). *Candida* sp. colonizes the gastrointestinal tract and skin of infants after initial exposure. *Candida* may be transmitted horizontally following skin-to-skin contact or, less frequently, from

the maternal genital tract during labor and delivery (41). *Candida* colonization is a major risk factor for subsequent candidiasis, and infection is most often caused by the colonizing strain. Risk of infection is inversely proportionate to gestational age and birth weight. Other risk factors include prolonged central line requirements, intra-abdominal pathology, and acid-blocking medication. Finally, exposure to broad-spectrum antibiotic therapy, particularly third-generation cephalosporins or carbapenems, is a major risk factor for candidiasis. An NICU's rate of third-generation cephalosporin utilization is strongly correlated with the risk for invasive candidiasis within that NICU (42,43). This increased risk for candidiasis following cephalosporin exposure is seen among term infants as well; while the absolute risk is drastically lower, the odds ratio (approximately 1.5- to 2-fold increased risk) following cephalosporin exposure is the same as preterm infants (44).

In addition to the prevention techniques used to minimize CLABSI, candidiasis prevention should focus on minimizing exposure to broad spectrum antibiotics and acid-blocking medication. Prophylaxis with fluconazole given twice weekly either orally or intravenously reduces the risk for death or invasive candidiasis by approximately 50%. Fluconazole is usually well tolerated and has not been associated with subsequent increases in azole resistance with the NICU (45). Although fluconazole prophylaxis is not a substitute for standard precautions, CLABSI efforts, or effective antimicrobial stewardship, it can be used for NICUs who have ongoing candidiasis despite other efforts. Fluconazole prophylaxis is cost-effective if the incidence of candidiasis among at-risk infants exceeds 2.8% (46). Finally, there has been increased interest in probiotic therapy for a variety of indications, including prevention of candidiasis. Although low-quality evidence from prospective cohorts and clinical trials is promising, to date there has not been a large randomized controlled trial evaluating invasive candidiasis as a primary outcome (47).

MULTIDRUG-RESISTANT ORGANISMS

MDROs—pathogenic bacteria with intrinsic or acquired antibiotic-resistance genes—are increasingly common in the NICU setting (48). MDROs may be introduced horizontally by parents, visitors, or health care workers. They also may be generated *de novo* by antibiotic overuse within the NICU. Methicillin-resistant *S. aureus* (MRSA), vancomycin-resistant enterococci (VRE), and extended-spectrum β-lactamase-producing (ESBL) gram negative organisms are the most frequently reported causes of MDRO infections and outbreaks among NICUs. MRSA refers to *S. aureus* that carries the *mecA* gene, which confers resistance to beta-lactams including the semisynthetic penicillins such as oxacillin and nafcillin. MRSA accounts for approximately 25% to 30% of *S. aureus* infections in the NICU, but local epidemiology varies widely (49). MRSA and methicillin-susceptible *S. aureus* have comparable case fatality rates, but require drastically different therapies. MRSA is treated with vancomycin, while methicillin-susceptible *S. aureus* is best treated by oxacillin, nafcillin, or cefazolin; mortality actually increases when vancomycin is used (50). VRE is most frequently caused by *vanA* or *vanB* genes within *Enterococcus* species (most commonly *Enterococcus faecium*), which confer vancomycin resistance. VRE is generally treated with linezolid (51). ESBL-producing gram-negative organisms can carry a wide variety of resistance genes that can be encoded on plasmids or carried constitutively on the bacterial chromosome. ESBLs can range from those that hydrolyze cephalosporins or aminopenicillins all the way to carbapenemases, which can inactivate meropenem and other "last line of defense" antimicrobials (52). NICU outbreaks due to MDROs, and ESBL-producing gram-negative bacilli in particular, have increased steadily during the past 20 years (53). Infants with infections due to MDROs are at increased risk for morbidity and mortality, often because they are less likely to receive effective empiric antimicrobial therapy. Therefore, in order to optimally treat MDRO infection and prevent horizontal spread to other infants, active surveillance methods are critical.

Active surveillance involves prospectively obtaining samples from infants in the NICU to evaluate for colonization. The approach to screening is highly dependent on local epidemiology, which informs the cost–benefit of screening (52). Screening can be universal (e.g., all infants in the NICU) or targeted (e.g., screening for MRSA on admission from another NICU, or screening infants prior to cardiothoracic surgery). In addition, the number of MDROs screened for, number of sites sampled, and frequency of surveillance is dependent on local epidemiology (54). For example, an NICU with relatively a low rate of endemic MRSA and no VRE may screen monthly for MRSA and not at all for VRE. In contrast, an NICU experiencing a cluster of ESBL-producing *Klebsiella* infections may screen weekly for ESBL-producing gram negative colonization. In addition to epidemiologic information, screening identifies infants who should be placed in transmission-based precautions (see below), impacts future antimicrobial selection if a colonized infant were to develop signs of sepsis (e.g., vancomycin in lieu of oxacillin for an MRSA-colonized infant, or meropenem in lieu of gentamicin for an infant with ESBL-producing gram-negative colonization), and may allow targeted decolonization, as in the case of MRSA (54).

When an infant is identified as being colonized or infected with an MDRO, the infant should be placed in contact precautions and separated geographically from other infants. Infants infected or colonized with an MDRO should be cohorted, when possible, for staffing purposes. For example, if an NICU has three MRSA-colonized infants, then those infants should be placed in a 1:3 nursing assignment to minimize the risk of horizontal transfer to an MRSA-negative infant. For providers who must see both colonized and noncolonized infants (e.g., neonatologists), every effort should be made to examine the MDRO-colonized infants last.

Prevention of MDROs in the NICU relies on both infection prevention principles as well as antimicrobial stewardship. The most critical step in preventing MDRO transmission is hand hygiene. A randomized controlled trial of universal gown-and-glove usage demonstrated no additional benefit when hand hygiene compliance approached 100%, demonstrating the crucial importance of hand hygiene. In addition, adequate spacing of infants to prevent overcrowding is critical. The American Academy of Pediatrics' guidelines on perinatal care recommend 165 sq ft for single-infant rooms and at least 120 sq ft per infant in multipatient rooms (55). Understaffing—that is, elevated patient-to-nurse or patient-to-doctor ratios—has also been implicated in MDRO transmission (56,57). Increased provider workload combined with decreased work space is a dangerous combination that may reduce attention to hand hygiene and facilitate horizontal transfer of MDROs between infants. Understaffing and overcrowding conditions require support from NICU and hospital administration to alleviate, highlighting the importance of an ongoing dialogue between clinicians, hospital leadership, and infection preventionists (58).

VIRAL RESPIRATORY TRACT INFECTIONS

Another subset of common HAIs in NICUs is health care–associated viral respiratory tract infection, or HA-VRI. HA-VRI results from horizontal transmission between health care workers or family members and infants (59). Commonly implicated respiratory viruses include respiratory syncytial virus, influenza, parainfluenza, rhinovirus, and adenovirus (60). Some infants with HA-VRI may have overt respiratory symptoms such as rhinorrhea, cough, tachypnea, or hypoxia; others may present with nonspecific signs of late-onset sepsis, and a minority of infants with HA-VRI may have no symptoms at all (61). Studies that have systematically included respiratory viral testing in late-onset sepsis evaluations have found that 5% to 10% of sepsis is due to respiratory viruses (62–64).

Transmission risk for respiratory viruses within the NICU correlates closely with community transmission, and seasonal changes and community outbreaks can and should inform NICU policy regarding visitation (65). Family members and other visitors who have signs and symptoms of acute viral infection should be discouraged from visiting until their illness has resolved. Since asymptomatic viral shedding is relatively common, particularly during the winter, strict hand hygiene should be reinforced with all families (66). The majority of studies suggest that restricting younger children (age ≤ 12 years) from visiting during respiratory viral season—when respiratory syncytial virus and influenza viruses are circulating—can reduce the burden of HA-VRI (67,68).

ISOLATION PRECAUTIONS

Standard Precautions

Standard precautions are a set of practices that should be used with every patient contact, regardless of clinical setting or patient status (69). They include hand hygiene, personal protective equipment (PPE) for possible contact with blood or body fluids, along with respiratory hygiene, injection safety, safe medication storage and handling, environmental cleaning, and waste disposal. A full review of standard precautions can be found on the Centers for Disease Control and Prevention Web site (http://www.cdc.gov/infectioncontrol/) (69). However, hand hygiene is highlighted here as it is the single most critical step in the prevention of HAIs and MDRO colonization, and failure of hand hygiene is the most frequently implicated contributor to outbreaks (70). Hand hygiene refers to the use of either soap and water or an antiseptic waterless product (e.g., alcohol gel). In most cases, alcohol-based gels are more effective against pathogen transmission than soap and water when hands are not visibly soiled or greasy. CHG hand rubs may be effective against some organic soiling, and hand rub preparations that contain CHG or iodophors may provide residual antimicrobial activity (71). However, there are notable exceptions including contact with *Clostridioides difficile*, *Cryptosporidium*, and norovirus (72–74). Hand hygiene should be performed before and after patient contact, before and after performing procedures, and after removing gloves. Note that in the NICU setting, patient contact includes contact with the patient's immediate environment including the incubator or radiant warmer, monitor, lines, and other support devices in close proximity to the infant.

The most common cause of hand hygiene failure is noncompliance by health care staff, families, or visitors. However, there are other factors that have been associated with decreased effectiveness of hand hygiene. Complex or faceted rings, watches, bracelets, and even artificial nails can provide niches where pathogens can survive despite hand hygiene, and the use of these should be banned for caregivers in the NICU (75,76). Rings that are flat bands without grooves or facets are acceptable. Nail polish is acceptable if it is not chipped (77). Monitoring hand hygiene within the NICU is critical to maximize compliance and identify opportunities for education and feedback when compliance is suboptimal (78).

Transmission-Based Precautions

Transmission-based precautions include contact, droplet, and airborne precautions (Table 22.3). They are used in combination with standard precautions for patients with suspected or proven infection or colonization with certain pathogens (69). Contact precautions are indicated for conditions that can be spread through skin-to-skin contact, including MDRO colonization, and include PPE (gloves and gown, and a mask if splashes are anticipated) for all patient interactions. Droplet precautions are indicated for pathogens that can be transmitted by respiratory droplets (e.g., coughing or sneezing) and include the use of a face mask when entering patient space. Droplets have limited range and do not stay

TABLE 22.3
Standard and Transmission-Based Precautions and Common Indications in the NICU Setting

Type	Precautions	Sample Indications[a]
Standard	• Hand hygiene before and after patient contact, procedures, and after glove use • PPE for possible contact with blood or body fluid • Respiratory hygiene/cough etiquette • Safe injection practices • Safe medication practices • Cleaning and disinfection of the environment • Waste disposal	All patients
Contact	• Gown and gloves for all patient contact • Use disposable or dedicated patient-care equipment	MRSA VRE ESBL Most enteric pathogens HSV
Droplet	• Mask when entering patient spaces • Often combined with contact precautions	Respiratory viruses Pertussis
Airborne	• N95 or higher respirator with appropriate fit • Negative pressure room • Anteroom	*M. tuberculosis* Varicella Measles

[a]Full list of transmission-based precautions for clinical conditions and specific pathogens can be found at https://www.cdc.gov/infectioncontrol/pdf/guidelines/isolation-guidelines-H.pdf. (From Centers for Disease Control and Prevention. *Infection control*, 2019. https://www.cdc.gov/infectioncontrol/. Accessed September 27, 2019.)

HSV, herpes simplex virus.

airborne for long due to their weight; instead, they travel inches to feet and then land on environmental surfaces, where they can then be transmitted by contact. As a result, droplet precautions are usually combined with contact precautions. Finally, airborne precautions are used for pathogens that can be aerosolized and stay airborne for hours (e.g., measles, varicella, *Mycobacterium tuberculosis*.) Airborne precautions require the use of a respirator (N95 or higher) mask, an airborne isolation room with negative pressure air circulation, and an anteroom to prevent escape of airborne pathogens.

All patients on transmission-based precautions should be clearly identified as such, both in the electronic medical record as well as by use of signs/posters outside of patient spaces. In addition, NICU infants on transmission-based precautions should have their movement limited as much as possible. They should leave their spaces for medically necessary reasons only and should not be transferred from bed space to bed space (bays) or room-to-room (single-patient rooms). Finally, cleaning and disinfection of their areas, including frequently touched surfaces in the vicinity such as monitors, sinks, and computers, should be prioritized both during their NICU admission and promptly after discharge.

OUTBREAK MANAGEMENT

Outbreaks in the NICU setting require aggressive infection control processes above and beyond baseline infection prevention (52). Outbreak detection may be clinical, if a cluster of infants

experience a similar clinical illness (e.g., necrotizing enterocolitis, sepsis, or pneumonia) or are infected with a certain pathogen (e.g., ESBL-producing *Klebsiella pneumoniae* or VRE) (57). Outbreaks may also be detected through routine surveillance without overt clinical changes; for example, an NICU experiencing a sudden increase in the number of MRSA-colonized infants may be having an outbreak. Once an outbreak is recognized, several interventions should happen rapidly and concomitantly (58).

Hand hygiene should be immediately addressed, including reeducation of all staff and reinforcement of existing policy. Prospective audits should be performed to ensure compliance. All infants in the NICU should be clinically evaluated and screened to determine whether they are infected or colonized (cases) or unaffected (controls). Cases should then be promptly placed into the relevant transmission-based precautions and cohorted. The presence of understaffing or overcrowding should be investigated and immediately relieved if possible; this may require coordination with leadership to create additional space or bring in additional personnel as needed. Environmental cleaning processes should be audited, and reeducation of environmental services staff can be performed as needed. Finally, timely and transparent communication between neonatologists, nurses, hospital administration, infection control and preventionists, and patient families is critical.

APPROACH TO FAMILIES AND VISITORS

Family-centered care is a vital component of NICU care and has been associated with improved outcomes (79). However, the constant influx of families and visitors to the NICU can present opportunities for pathogen introduction. It is the responsibility of NICU personnel to find a balance between promoting family bonding while minimizing risk to the infant. Therefore, family and visitors with signs of respiratory or gastrointestinal illness should be discouraged from visiting the NICU until their illness has resolved (80). Hand hygiene should be taught and encouraged with each visit (81). Many NICUs will restrict visitation by younger children (e.g., age ≤12 years) during respiratory viral season, although studies evaluating the impact of such policies have shown mixed efficacy (68,82). Families of NICU infants should be encouraged to receive influenza and pertussis vaccines, and programs designed to facilitate vaccination have been successful (83,84).

There are limited data regarding the benefit of PPE use by families when their infant is placed in transmission-based precautions. If family members follow proper hand hygiene practices, transmission of MDROs from infants to family should not result in horizontal transmission to other infants in the NICU. In addition, there is increasing evidence that skin-to-skin contact (kangaroo care) promotes breast-feeding, attachment, and possibly long-term growth and development (85,86). Gowns limit skin-to-skin care and have been identified as a barrier to attachment and breast-feeding by surveyed families (87). Therefore, there is no recommendation at present for routine use of PPE by families (54). However, if family members and visitors have multiple infants being cared for in the NICU, it may be prudent for them to visit the infants on isolation precautions last. In addition, family members and visitors should also be reminded to avoid contact with other infants, including their surrounding bed space or medical equipment. This may be challenging in open bay units compared to NICUs with private rooms.

ANTIMICROBIAL STEWARDSHIP

Antimicrobial stewardship programs (ASPs) are closely intertwined with infection control and prevention efforts, particularly in the NICU setting. ASPs are critical for the prevention of MDRO emergence, and infection prevention reduces the use of antimicrobials and can inform selection of narrow-spectrum therapy (e.g., MRSA screening to drive vancomycin reduction) (88). In addition, there are mounting data supporting the adverse short- and long-term consequences of prolonged or unnecessary antimicrobial exposure during infancy, including increased risk for late-onset sepsis, necrotizing enterocolitis, atopic disease, obesity, and even death (89). Therefore, every NICU should have a multidisciplinary ASP that includes representatives from neonatology, infectious diseases, pharmacy, and nursing. Such ASPs in the NICU setting have been shown to be safe and effective (90). ASPs in the NICU setting are most successful when they include stakeholders or "champions" from neonatology to help direct meaningful interventions and metrics, facilitate the design and dissemination of interventions, and lead colleagues (91). The majority of providers strongly prefer recommendations that come from partners within their own specialty rather than from administration or outside specialists, so having a neonatologist as an ASP champion is vital (92).

Antimicrobial stewardship strategies include three main components. Prospective audit and feedback measures antimicrobial use and identifies common or high-use areas. Targeted interventions to safely reduce antimicrobial volume or spectrum are then designed and implemented, and additional data are collected to evaluate the safety and efficacy of those interventions. However, ASPs cannot be one size-fits-all, as there is significant variation in antibiotic prescribing between NICUs (93,94). Some of this variation is accounted for by case-mix index, inborn versus referral status, volume, and individual or NICU-level variations in practice management (95). A significant portion of antimicrobial use cannot be explained by objective measures, however (96). Therefore, ASPs must focus on local drivers of antimicrobial use that can be addressed with local stakeholders within a given NICU.

There are a variety of specific approaches that can be utilized within NICUs, depending on what prospective audit of antibiotic use reveals. Optimizing diagnostics can be critical. Appropriate cultures should be obtained prior to starting antibiotic therapy whenever possible. A minimum of 1 mL should be obtained for blood cultures, and samples of urine and cerebrospinal fluid should be obtained for culture when late-onset sepsis is considered (97,98). In contrast, samples of nonsterile sites such as skin, the upper respiratory tract, and mucosal surfaces should be obtained only when clinical suspicion for site-specific infection is high, and even then culture results should be interpreted cautiously.

When sepsis is considered, empiric therapy should be as narrow as possible while covering the likely pathogens. For late-onset sepsis (including suspected HAIs), oxacillin and gentamicin is usually sufficient if infants are known to be MRSA negative. Oxacillin is superior to vancomycin for the treatment of methicillin-susceptible *S. aureus*, and vancomycin-reduction programs that include MRSA screening have proven safe and effective (99). Although oxacillin does not generally provide adequate coverage for CoNS, infections with CoNS are not associated with mortality (100). Therefore, providers can confirm that CoNS infection is real (e.g., identified from ≥2 cultures) before changing from oxacillin to vancomycin. Gentamicin or an alternative aminoglycoside can be used for empiric treatment of BSI or UTI if meningitis is excluded, highlighting the importance of obtaining cerebrospinal fluid when late-onset sepsis is suspected. Finally, empiric antimicrobial therapy should be reevaluated as new information becomes available. Sterile cultures after 36 to 48 hours should prompt discontinuation of antimicrobials in the majority of cases. "Culture-negative" sepsis is not an appropriate indication for treatment if proper cultures have been collected before antibiotics were initiated (101); instead, alternative reasons for clinical illness, including viral infections or noninfectious conditions associated with prematurity, should be considered.

HUMAN MILK

Human milk is an important part of NICU care. Countless studies support the nutritional, immunologic, and developmental benefits of human milk for term and preterm infants, and NICUs increasingly are striving for exclusive human milk diets. This can be achieved with either mother's milk (expressed breast milk or direct breast-feeding) or with donor milk. There are several potential infectious complications with human milk use (Table 22.4). The only absolute infectious contraindications to breast milk in the United States are maternal human immunodeficiency virus or active brucellosis (102,103). In the United Kingdom, the British HIV association provides guidelines for safe breast feeding in women who are HIV positive, have undetectable viral loads and who wish to breast feed. Hepatitis C is also a consideration; although hepatitis C virus is not transmitted via breast milk, it can be transmitted by ingestion of maternal blood if mothers' nipples are cracked or bleeding (104). Several other conditions may preclude a direct latch on the breast due to breast infection; in these cases, expressed milk is still safe to use. Active (e.g., sputum-positive) maternal tuberculosis disease is a contraindication to close proximity to the infant and therefore to direct breast-feeding, but expressed breast milk is safe to use.

Notably, cytomegalovirus (CMV) can also be transmitted by human milk. In the era of CMV-safe blood transfusion methods (e.g., CMV seronegative donors; leukoreduction), breast milk is the predominant source of postnatally acquired CMV disease in the NICU setting (105). Freezing of breast milk reduces—but does not eliminate—CMV viral load; pasteurization inactivates CMV but also reduces the immunologic benefit of breast milk (106). However, in virtually all settings, the benefits of breast milk over infant formula outweigh the risks of postnatal CMV infection. A notable exception may be for the infant with newborn screening suggestive of severe combined immunodeficiency (SCID). CMV is capable both of causing severe disease among infants with SCID as well as decreasing the chance of successful engraftment of hematopoietic stem cell transplantation. Therefore, if suspicion for SCID is high, some experts recommend suspending breast-feeding until the diagnosis of SCID is definitively determined. However, preterm infants have relatively high rates of false-positive SCID screening (107), so NICU providers must weigh the risk of real T-cell dysfunction against the risk of withholding breast milk.

TABLE 22.4

Infectious Contraindications to Breast-Feeding or Human Milk Use

Breast milk contraindicated	Human immunodeficiency virus (HIV)[a]
	Hepatitis C IF cracked or bleeding nipples
	Active maternal brucellosis
Direct breast-feeding contraindicated but expressed breast milk safe	Breast infection:
	• Acute mastitis (bacterial or *Candida*)
	• Breast abscess
	• Herpetic outbreak
	Active maternal tuberculosis
Direct breast-feeding safe	All other common infectious diseases
	Maternal hepatitis B infection
	Maternal hepatitis C infection if no nipple bleeding

[a]Unless in a country where benefits of breast-feeding outweigh risk of HIV exposure.

REFERENCES

1. Centers for Disease Control and Prevention. National Healthcare Safety Network (NHSN), 2019. Available from: https://www.cdc.gov/nhsn/. Accessed September 29, 2019.
2. Rosenthal VD, Al-Abdely HM, El-Kholy AA, et al. International Nosocomial Infection Control Consortium report, data summary of 50 countries for 2010-2015: device-associated module. *Am J Infect Control* 2016;44(12):1495.
3. Stoll BJ, Hansen N, Fanaroff AA, et al. Late-onset sepsis in very low birth weight neonates: the experience of the NICHD Neonatal Research Network. *Pediatrics* 2002;110(2 Pt 1):285.
4. Stoll BJ, Hansen NI, Sanchez PJ, et al. Early onset neonatal sepsis: the burden of group B Streptococcal and *E. coli* disease continues. *Pediatrics* 2011;127(5):817.
5. National Nosocomial Infections Surveillance System. National Nosocomial Infections Surveillance (NNIS) System Report, data summary from January 1992 through June 2004, issued October 2004. *Am J Infect Control* 2004;32(8):470.
6. Edwards JR, Peterson KD, Mu Y, et al. National Healthcare Safety Network (NHSN) report: data summary for 2006 through 2008, issued December 2009. *Am J Infect Control* 2009;37(10):783.
7. Dudeck MA, Horan TC, Peterson KD, et al. National Healthcare Safety Network (NHSN) Report, data summary for 2010, device-associated module. *Am J Infect Control* 2011;39(10):798.
8. Dudeck MA, Horan TC, Peterson KD, et al. National Healthcare Safety Network (NHSN) report, data summary for 2009, device-associated module. *Am J Infect Control* 2011;39(5):349.
9. Dudeck MA, Horan TC, Peterson KD, et al. National Healthcare Safety Network report, data summary for 2011, device-associated module. *Am J Infect Control* 2013;41(4):286.
10. Dudeck MA, Weiner LM, Allen-Bridson K, et al. National Healthcare Safety Network (NHSN) report, data summary for 2012, device-associated module. *Am J Infect Control* 2013;41(12):1148.
11. Dudeck MA, Edwards JR, Allen-Bridson K, et al. National Healthcare Safety Network report, data summary for 2013, device-associated module. *Am J Infect Control* 2015;43(3):206.
12. Cantey JB. Healthcare-associated infections in the NICU: a brief review. In: McNeil JC, Campbell JR, Crews JD, eds. *Healthcare-associated infections in children*, 1st ed. Philadelphia, PA: Springer, 2018.
13. Mobley RE, Bizzarro MJ. Central line-associated bloodstream infections in the NICU: successes and controversies in the quest for zero. *Semin Perinatol* 2017;41(3):166.
14. Milstone AM, Reich NG, Advani S, et al. Catheter dwell time and CLABSIs in neonates with PICCs: a multicenter cohort study. *Pediatrics* 2013;132(6):e1609.
15. Mahieu LM, De Muynck AO, Ieven MM, et al. Risk factors for central vascular catheter-associated bloodstream infections among patients in a neonatal intensive care unit. *J Hosp Infect* 2001;48(2):108.
16. Greenberg RG, Kandefer S, Do BT, et al. Late-onset sepsis in extremely premature infants: 2000-2011. *Pediatr Infect Dis J* 2017;36(8):774.
17. Shahid S, Dutta S, Symington A, et al; McMaster University NICU. Standardizing umbilical catheter usage in preterm infants. *Pediatrics* 2014;133(6):e1742.
18. Sharpe E, Kuhn L, Ratz D, et al. Neonatal peripherally inserted central catheter practices and providers: results from the Neonatal PICC1 Survey. *Adv Neonatal Care* 2017;17(3):209.
19. Fisher D, Cochran KM, Provost LP, et al. Reducing central line-associated bloodstream infections in North Carolina NICUs. *Pediatrics* 2013;132(6):e1664.
20. Sanderson E, Yeo KT, Wang AY, et al. Dwell time and risk of central-line-associated bloodstream infection in neonates. *J Hosp Infect* 2017;97(3):267.
21. Butler-O'Hara M, D'Angio CT, Hoey H, et al. An evidence-based catheter bundle alters central venous catheter strategy in newborn infants. *J Pediatr* 2012;160(6):972.
22. Shalabi M, Adel M, Yoon E, et al. Risk of infection using peripherally inserted central and umbilical catheters in preterm neonates. *Pediatrics* 2015;136(6):1073.
23. Lee A, Harlan R, Breaud AR, et al. Blood concentrations of chlorhexidine in hospitalized children undergoing daily chlorhexidine bathing. *Infect Control Hosp Epidemiol* 2011;32(4):395.
24. Garland JS, Alex CP, Uhing MR, et al. Pilot trial to compare tolerance of chlorhexidine gluconate to povidone-iodine antisepsis for central venous catheter placement in neonates. *J Perinatol* 2009;29(12):808.
25. Kieran EA, O'Sullivan A, Miletin J, et al. 2% chlorhexidine-70% isopropyl alcohol versus 10% povidone-iodine for insertion site cleaning before central line insertion in preterm infants: a randomised trial. *Arch Dis Child Fetal Neonatal Ed* 2018;103(2):F101.
26. Garland JS, Alex CP, Mueller CD, et al. A randomized trial comparing povidone-iodine to a chlorhexidine gluconate-impregnated dressing for prevention of central venous catheter infections in neonates. *Pediatrics* 2001;107(6):1431.
27. Lai NM, Lai NA, O'Riordan E, et al. Skin antisepsis for reducing central venous catheter-related infections. *Cochrane Database Syst Rev* 2016;7:CD010140.
28. Network NHS. Pediatric Ventilator-Associated Event (PedVAE), 2019. Available from: https://www.cdc.gov/nhsn/pdfs/pscmanual/pedvae-current-508.pdf. Accessed September 26, 2019.
29. Cocoros NM, Priebe GP, Logan LK, et al. A pediatric approach to ventilator-associated events surveillance. *Infect Control Hosp Epidemiol* 2017;38(3):327.
30. Karandikar MV, Coffin SE, Priebe GP, et al. Variability in antimicrobial use in pediatric ventilator-associated events. *Infect Control Hosp Epidemiol* 2019;40(1):32.
31. Chung EY, Yardley J. Are there risks associated with empiric acid suppression treatment of infants and children suspected of having gastroesophageal reflux disease? *Hosp Pediatr* 2013;3(1):16.
32. Romaine A, Ye D, Ao Z, et al. Safety of histamine-2 receptor blockers in hospitalized VLBW infants. *Early Hum Dev* 2016;99:27.
33. Tan B, Zhang F, Zhang X, et al. Risk factors for ventilator-associated pneumonia in the neonatal intensive care unit: a meta-analysis of observational studies. *Eur J Pediatr* 2014;173(4):427.
34. Erfani Y, Rasti A, Janani L. Prevalence of Gram-negative bacteria in ventilator-associated pneumonia in neonatal intensive care units: a systematic review and meta-analysis protocol. *BMJ Open* 2016;6(10):e012298.
35. Apisarnthanarak A, Holzmann-Pazgal G, Hamvas A, et al. Ventilator-associated pneumonia in extremely preterm neonates in a neonatal intensive care unit: characteristics, risk factors, and outcomes. *Pediatrics* 2003;112(6 Pt 1):1283.
36. Azab SF, Sherbiny HS, Saleh SH, et al. Reducing ventilator-associated pneumonia in neonatal intensive care unit using "VAP prevention bundle": a cohort study. *BMC Infect Dis* 2015;15:314.
37. Zhang Y, Ji F, Hu X, et al. Oropharyngeal colostrum administration in very low birth weight infants: a randomized controlled trial. *Pediatr Crit Care Med* 2017;18(9):869.
38. Lucas da Silva PS, de Carvalho WB. Unplanned extubation in pediatric critically ill patients: a systematic review and best practice recommendations. *Pediatr Crit Care Med* 2010;11(2):287.
39. Cantey JB. Optimizing the use of antibacterial agents in the neonatal period. *Paediatr Drugs* 2016;18(2):109.
40. Benjamin DK Jr, Stoll BJ, Gantz MG, et al. Neonatal candidiasis: epidemiology, risk factors, and clinical judgment. *Pediatrics* 2010;126(4):e865.
41. Bliss JM, Basavegowda KP, Watson WJ, et al. Vertical and horizontal transmission of Candida albicans in very low birth weight infants using DNA fingerprinting techniques. *Pediatr Infect Dis J* 2008;27(3):231.
42. Cotten CM, McDonald S, Stoll B, et al. The association of third-generation cephalosporin use and invasive candidiasis in extremely low birth-weight infants. *Pediatrics* 2006;118(2):717.
43. Saiman L, Ludington E, Dawson JD, et al. Risk factors for Candida species colonization of neonatal intensive care unit patients. *Pediatr Infect Dis J* 2001;20(12):1119.
44. Lee JH, Hornik CP, Benjamin DK Jr, et al. Risk factors for invasive candidiasis in infants >1500 g birth weight. *Pediatr Infect Dis J* 2013;32(3):222.
45. Ericson JE, Kaufman DA, Kicklighter SD, et al. Fluconazole prophylaxis for the prevention of candidiasis in premature infants: a meta-analysis using patient-level data. *Clin Infect Dis* 2016;63(5):604.
46. Swanson JR, Vergales J, Kaufman DA, et al. Cost analysis of fluconazole prophylaxis for prevention of neonatal invasive candidiasis. *Pediatr Infect Dis J* 2016;35(5):519.
47. Hu HJ, Zhang GQ, Zhang Q, et al. Probiotics prevent Candida colonization and invasive fungal sepsis in preterm neonates: a systematic review and meta-analysis of randomized controlled trials. *Pediatr Neonatol* 2017;58(2):103.
48. Siegel JD, Rhinehart E, Jackson M, et al; Health Care Infection Control Practices Advisory Committee. 2007 guideline for isolation precautions: preventing transmission of infectious agents in health care settings. *Am J Infect Control* 2007;35(10 suppl 2):S65.
49. Shane AL, Hansen NI, Stoll BJ, et al. Methicillin-resistant and susceptible Staphylococcus aureus bacteremia and meningitis in preterm infants. *Pediatrics* 2012;129(4):e914.
50. Kim SH, Kim KH, Kim HB, et al. Outcome of vancomycin treatment in patients with methicillin-susceptible Staphylococcus aureus bacteremia. *Antimicrob Agents Chemother* 2008;52(1):192.
51. Andersson P, Beckingham W, Gorrie CL, et al. Vancomycin-resistant Enterococcus (VRE) outbreak in a neonatal intensive care unit and special care nursery at a tertiary-care hospital in Australia—a retrospective case-control study. *Infect Control Hosp Epidemiol* 2019;40(5):551.
52. Ramirez CB, Cantey JB. Antibiotic resistance in the neonatal intensive care unit. *Neoreviews* 2019;20(3):e135.
53. Cantey JB, Milstone AM. Bloodstream infections: epidemiology and resistance. *Clin Perinatol* 2015;42(1):1, vii.
54. Akinboyo IC, Zangwill KM, Berg WB, et al. SHEA neonatal intensive care unit (NICU) white paper series: practical approaches to Staphylococcus aureus disease prevention. *Infect Control Hosp Epidemiol* 2020; 41(11): 1251.

THE NEWBORN INFANT

55. Kilpatrick SJ, Papile L. *Guidelines for perinatal care*, 8th ed. Elk Grove, IL: American Academy of Pediatrics, 2017.

56. Stapleton PJ, Murphy M, McCallion N, et al. Outbreaks of extended spectrum beta-lactamase-producing Enterobacteriaceae in neonatal intensive care units: a systematic review. *Arch Dis Child Fetal Neonatal Ed* 2016;101(1):F72.

57. Cantey JB, Sreeramoju P, Jaleel M, et al. Prompt control of an outbreak caused by extended-spectrum beta-lactamase-producing *Klebsiella pneumoniae* in a neonatal intensive care unit. *J Pediatr* 2013;163(3):672, e671.

58. Johnson J, Quach C. Outbreaks in the neonatal ICU: a review of the literature. *Curr Opin Infect Dis* 2017;30(4):395.

59. Quach C, Shah R, Rubin LG. Burden of healthcare-associated viral respiratory infections in children's hospitals. *J Pediatr Infect Dis Soc* 2018;7(1):18.

60. Poole CL, Camins BC, Prichard MN, et al. Hospital-acquired viral respiratory infections in neonates hospitalized since birth in a tertiary neonatal intensive care unit. *J Perinatol* 2019;39(5):683.

61. Shui JE, Messina M, Hill-Ricciuti AC, et al. Impact of respiratory viruses in the neonatal intensive care unit. *J Perinatol* 2018;38(11):1556.

62. Ronchi A, Michelow IC, Chapin KC, et al. Viral respiratory tract infections in the neonatal intensive care unit: the VIRIoN-I study. *J Pediatr* 2014;165(4):690.

63. Cerone JB, Santos RP, Tristram D, et al. Incidence of respiratory viral infection in infants with respiratory symptoms evaluated for late-onset sepsis. *J Perinatol* 2017;37(8):922.

64. Gonzalez-Carrasco E, Calvo C, Garcia-Garcia ML, et al. Viral respiratory tract infections in the neonatal intensive care unit. *An Pediatr (Barc)* 2015;82(4):242.

65. Rose EB, Washington EJ, Wang L, et al. Multiple respiratory syncytial virus introductions into a neonatal intensive care unit. *J Pediatr Infect Dis Soc.* 2020.

66. Birger R, Morita H, Comito D, et al. Asymptomatic shedding of respiratory virus among an ambulatory population across seasons. *mSphere* 2018;3(4):e00249-18.

67. Forkpa H, Rupp AH, Shulman ST, et al. Association between children's hospital visitor restrictions and healthcare-associated viral respiratory infections: a quasi-experimental study. *J Pediatr Infect Dis Soc* 2020;9(2):240.

68. Horikoshi Y, Okazaki K, Miyokawa S, et al. Sibling visits and viral infection in the neonatal intensive care unit. *Pediatr Int* 2018;60(2):153.

69. Centers for Disease Control and Prevention. Infection control, 2019. Available from: https://www.cdc.gov/infectioncontrol/. Accessed September 27, 2019.

70. Won SP, Chou HC, Hsieh WS, et al. Handwashing program for the prevention of nosocomial infections in a neonatal intensive care unit. *Infect Control Hosp Epidemiol* 2004;25(9):742.

71. World Health Organization. *WHO guidelines on hand hygiene in health care*. Geneva, Switzerland: WHO Press, 2009.

72. Blaney DD, Daly ER, Kirkland KB, et al. Use of alcohol-based hand sanitizers as a risk factor for norovirus outbreaks in long-term care facilities in northern New England: December 2006 to March 2007. *Am J Infect Control* 2011;39(4):296.

73. Oughton MT, Loo VG, Dendukuri N, et al. Hand hygiene with soap and water is superior to alcohol rub and antiseptic wipes for removal of *Clostridium difficile*. *Infect Control Hosp Epidemiol* 2009;30(10):939.

74. Sandora TJ, Bryant KK, Cantey JB, et al. SHEA neonatal intensive care unit (NICU) white paper series: practical approaches to Clostridioides difficile prevention. *Infect Control Hosp Epidemiol* 2018;39(10):1149.

75. Trick WE, Vernon MO, Hayes RA, et al. Impact of ring wearing on hand contamination and comparison of hand hygiene agents in a hospital. *Clin Infect Dis* 2003;36(11):1383.

76. Loveday HP, Wilson JA, Pratt RJ, et al. Epic3: national evidence-based guidelines for preventing healthcare-associated infections in NHS hospitals in England. *J Hosp Infect* 2014;86(suppl 1):S1.

77. Fagernes M, Lingaas E. Factors interfering with the microflora on hands: a regression analysis of samples from 465 healthcare workers. *J Adv Nurs* 2011;67(2):297.

78. Boyce JM. Current issues in hand hygiene. *Am J Infect Control* 2019; 47S:A46.

79. Franck LS, O'Brien K. The evolution of family-centered care: from supporting parent-delivered interventions to a model of family integrated care. *Birth Defects Res* 2019;111(15):1044.

80. Gupta M, Pursley DM. A survey of infection control practices for influenza in mother and newborn units in US hospitals. *Am J Obstet Gynecol* 2011;204(6 suppl 1):S77.

81. Chandonnet CJ, Boutwell KM, Spigel N, et al. It's in your hands: an educational initiative to improve parent/family hand hygiene compliance. *Dimens Crit Care Nurs* 2017;36(6):327.

82. Peluso AM, Harnish BA, Miller NS, et al. Effect of young sibling visitation on respiratory syncytial virus activity in a NICU. *J Perinatol* 2015;35(8):627.

83. Shah SI, Caprio M, Hendricks-Munoz K. Administration of inactivated trivalent influenza vaccine to parents of high-risk infants in the neonatal intensive care unit. *Pediatrics* 2007;120(3):e617.

84. Dylag AM, Shah SI. Administration of tetanus, diphtheria, and acellular pertussis vaccine to parents of high-risk infants in the neonatal intensive care unit. *Pediatrics* 2008;122(3):e550.

85. El-Farrash RA, Shinkar DM, Ragab DA, et al. Longer duration of kangaroo care improves neurobehavioral performance and feeding in preterm infants: a randomized controlled trial. *Pediatr Res* 2020;87(4):683.

86. Ghavane S, Murki S, Subramanian S, et al. Kangaroo Mother Care in Kangaroo ward for improving the growth and breastfeeding outcomes when reaching term gestational age in very low birth weight infants. *Acta Paediatr* 2012;101(12):e545.

87. Seidman G, Unnikrishnan S, Kenny E, et al. Barriers and enablers of kangaroo mother care practice: a systematic review. *PLoS One* 2015;10(5):e0125643.

88. Cantey JB, Patel SJ. Antimicrobial stewardship in the NICU. *Infect Dis Clin North Am* 2014;28(2):247.

89. Cantey JB, Pyle AK, Wozniak PS, et al. Early antibiotic exposure and adverse outcomes in preterm, very low birth weight infants. *J Pediatr* 2018; 203:62.

90. Cantey JB, Wozniak PS, Pruszynski JE, et al. Reducing unnecessary antibiotic use in the neonatal intensive care unit (SCOUT): a prospective interrupted time-series study. *Lancet Infect Dis* 2016;16(10):1178.

91. Cantey JB, Vora N, Sunkara M. Prevalence, characteristics, and perception of Nursery Antibiotic Stewardship Coverage in the United States. *J Pediatr Infect Dis Soc* 2017;6(3):e30.

92. Patel SJ, Saiman L, Duchon JM, et al. Development of an antimicrobial stewardship intervention using a model of actionable feedback. *Interdiscip Perspect Infect Dis* 2012;2012:150367.

93. Cantey JB, Wozniak PS, Sanchez PJ. Prospective surveillance of antibiotic use in the neonatal intensive care unit: results from the SCOUT study. *Pediatr Infect Dis J* 2015;34(3):267.

94. Shipp KD, Chiang T, Karasick S, et al. Antibiotic Stewardship Challenges in a referral neonatal intensive care unit. *Am J Perinatol* 2016; 33(5):518.

95. Mukhopadhyay S, Taylor JA, Von Kohorn I, et al. Variation in sepsis evaluation across a national network of nurseries. *Pediatrics* 2017;139(3).

96. Schulman J, Benitz WE, Profit J, et al. Newborn antibiotic exposures and association with proven bloodstream infection. *Pediatrics* 2019;144(5).

97. Puopolo KM, Benitz WE, Zaoutis TE; Committee on Fetus and Newborn; Committee on Infectious Diseases. Management of neonates born at ≥35 0/7 weeks' gestation with suspected or proven early-onset bacterial sepsis. *Pediatrics* 2018;142(6).

98. Puopolo KM, Benitz WE, Zaoutis TE; Committee on Fetus and Newborn; Committee on Infectious Diseases. Management of neonates born at ≤34 6/7 weeks' gestation with suspected or proven early-onset bacterial sepsis. *Pediatrics* 2018;142(6).

99. Chiu CH, Michelow IC, Cronin J, et al. Effectiveness of a guideline to reduce vancomycin use in the neonatal intensive care unit. *Pediatr Infect Dis J* 2011;30(4):273.

100. Cantey JB, Anderson KR, Kalagiri RR, et al. Morbidity and mortality of coagulase-negative staphylococcal sepsis in very-low-birth-weight infants. *World J Pediatr* 2018;14(3):269.

101. Cantey JB, Baird SD. Ending the culture of culture-negative sepsis in the neonatal ICU. *Pediatrics* 2017;140(4):e20170044.

102. Ceylan A, Kostu M, Tuncer O, et al. Neonatal brucellosis and breast milk. *Indian J Pediatr* 2012;79(3):389.

103. Saloojee H, Cooper PA. Feeding of infants of HIV-positive mothers. *Curr Opin Clin Nutr Metab Care* 2010;13(3):336.

104. Mast EE. Mother-to-infant hepatitis C virus transmission and breastfeeding. *Adv Exp Med Biol* 2004;554:211.

105. Josephson CD, Caliendo AM, Easley KA, et al. Blood transfusion and breast milk transmission of cytomegalovirus in very low-birth-weight infants: a prospective cohort study. *JAMA Pediatr* 2014;168(11):1054.

106. Bapistella S, Hamprecht K, Thomas W, et al. Short-term pasteurization of breast milk to prevent postnatal cytomegalovirus transmission in very preterm infants. *Clin Infect Dis* 2018;69(3):438.

107. Ward CE, Baptist AP. Challenges of newborn severe combined immunodeficiency screening among premature infants. *Pediatrics* 2013;131(4):e1298.

23 Pharmacology

Mark A. Turner

INTRODUCTION

This chapter describes the principles that support careful use of drugs in neonates by neonatal prescribers working in a Level 1, 2, or 3 neonatal unit. This chapter includes only one graph, but no complex equations, and focuses on drugs that have effects related to their concentrations in the circulation.

This chapter will allow the reader to understand the principles of pharmacology sufficiently to use drugs carefully and contribute to a formulary chapter about a drug; to understand the principles used to adapt dosing information to individual babies; and to recognize the nature and value of research about drugs.

This chapter is not a training in clinical pharmacology (1–3), does not provide dosage regimens (4–6), is not a tutorial in research (1,7,8), and does not cover vaccines or pre- or postoperative cardiac surgery. The chapter will signpost readers toward relevant resources and how to use them. One key text is Barker et al. (9)

KEY CONCEPTS IN PHARMACOLOGY

Drugs have specific effects resulting from interactions with specific receptors. The effect of a drug depends on the concentration available to the receptor. There are many determinant of a drug's circulating concentration. It is important to understand what happens to the drug between its administration and effect.

PHARMACOKINETICS

The pharmacokinetics (PK) of a drug is studied by assessing drug disposition, summarized as ADME: absorption, distribution, metabolism, and elimination. The following paragraphs are not referenced but key reviews are (10,11). ADME can vary between age groups, between individuals, and within individuals. These variations can make it difficult to predict the concentration and effects of a given dose of a drug in any one individual.

Absorption

Drugs can enter the circulation through a number of routes in addition to intravenous and intramuscular routes: buccal, for example, midazolam and sucrose; nasal, also useful for rapidly absorbed drugs such as midazolam; and gastric, rectal, and cutaneous. Specific factors may alter absorption by each route in the newborn period.

Gastric

Gastric pH is relatively high shortly after birth leading to higher bioavailability of oral penicillin in newborns. However, gastric pH reduces within days of birth. Delayed gastric emptying can lead to lower and slower peak concentrations of some drugs, for example, paracetamol.

Rectal

Rectal absorption can be unpredictable due to inconsistent placement of suppositories with respect to the skin/mucosal junction.

Cutaneous

The newborn skin is more absorptive than other age groups leading to increased uptake of iodine from skin preparation.

Pancreatic and Biliary Function

Altered function may lead to reduced uptake of lipophilic drugs and fat-soluble vitamins compared to older age groups.

Ocular

The systemic absorption of bevacizumab may cause unwanted effects.

The extent of absorption is described by the bioavailability, which is the fraction of unchanged drug that reaches the systemic circulation. Drugs that are absorbed from the intestines can be metabolized in the intestine or the liver. This "first-pass metabolism" reduces bioavailability.

Distribution

Following absorption, or administration, to the bloodstream, drugs move into different parts of the body called compartments. Physical compartments include not only the circulation and extravascular space but also bone, peritoneum, brain, and subarachnoid space. Physical or physiologic barriers can prevent drugs from reaching some compartments. For example, treatment of an infection within a compartment needs useful concentrations of antibiotics within that compartment. That is why we select specific antimicrobials with good penetration for meningitis or bone infection.

Water versus Fat Solubility

Some drugs are water soluble and will distribute to water in the body. Some drugs are fat soluble and so will distribute to fat in the body. The amount and distribution of fat and water in the body change with age and illness. Neonates, particularly preterm neonates, have much more water (and less fat) than people in other age groups. Distribution means that a proportion of a dose will be in the circulation and a proportion of the dose will be somewhere else. Compared to older populations given a similar dose, neonates will "lose" more water-soluble drug from the circulation. Neonates have lower circulating concentrations of water-soluble drugs than do older populations and may need higher doses corrected for size than older populations (e.g., gentamicin).

Apparent Volume of Distribution

The proportion of a dose of a drug that is in the circulation is described by the "apparent volume of distribution," V_d. The V_d is the volume of plasma that would be needed to hold all the drug in the body and still have the same concentration that is found in the plasma. If a drug is distributed to fat, then the body can contain much more drug than is found in the plasma. Clearly, V_d is a theoretical construct rather than a practical measurement. However, it is a useful construct when deciding which dose to give (see below).

Compartments

PK modeling also involves compartments. These "modeling" compartments are one way to describe the relationship between time and concentration. In a single compartment model, the decline in the concentration of the drug can be explained by a single variable. If the data cannot be explained by a single compartment, then the decline will be described by a combination of variables. Modeling compartments are not the same as physical compartments because it may not be possible to resolve all the influences of physical compartments from blood tests taken in a single compartment.

Protein Binding

Protein binding is an important influence on distribution. Free drug is in the circulation and can be active or move into other compartments. Bound drug cannot be active. The extent of protein binding depends on the concentration of protein (mainly albumin) and competition (mainly with bilirubin among neonates). Protein binding is clinically relevant for drugs that display high protein binding, rapid elimination, and no visible effects (i.e., drugs that are not titrated to effect). Examples include teicoplanin and vancomycin. Small changes in protein binding can have large effects on the circulating concentrations of these drugs. Ceftriaxone can displace bilirubin from albumin: this has been reported to cause kernicterus and is one of the reasons why ceftriaxone is contraindicated in neonates.

Metabolism

Liver

The liver transforms endogenous and exogenous chemicals in two phases. Phase 1 prepares the chemical through oxidation, reduction, or hydrolysis. Phase 2 involves conjugation with chemical moieties that promote water solubility and elimination of the conjugated chemical. The fetus and the neonate are not exposed to the same chemicals. Following birth, the capabilities of the liver change in line with what the body expects to metabolize. (See Table 23.1 for neonatal examples.)

Phase 1 reactions include oxidation by cytochrome P450 enzymes. This superfamily of enzymes is abbreviated as CYP and has many families and subfamilies. For example, CYP3A7 and CYP2C19 are prominent during fetal life, but their activities decrease rapidly after birth. CYP3A4 and CYP2C9 show increased activity in the months after birth.

Phase 2 reactions include glucuronidation and sulfation. Glucuronidation gradually increase after birth with increased expression of UGT1A and UGT2B. The association between chloramphenicol and "gray baby" syndrome results from the low expression of UGT2B at birth. "Gray baby syndrome" could have been prevented with a full understanding of how ontogeny affects drug metabolism. The current understanding of ontogeny informs the development of new drugs for neonates. SULT1A1 and SULT1A3 enzymes are essential for metabolism of catecholamines and iodothyronines, so are well expressed during fetal life.

Intestinal

Intestinal CYPs are active and can contribute to first-pass metabolism or affect the absorption of medicines. Intestinal metabolism

---

TABLE 23.1

Selected Considerations for Some Medicines Commonly Used on Neonatal Units

Drug	Aspects of ADME of Neonatal Relevance	Comments
Acetaminophen	Metabolized by UGT1A6 (shows gradual increase after birth) and sulfation (active before birth)	Toxicity is unlikely in the neonatal period
Caffeine	Metabolized by CYP1A2 (shows gradual increase after birth)	Half-life 72–96 h compared to 5 h in older children
Catecholamines	Rapidly metabolized	Titrate to effect
Codeine	CYP2D6, rapid metabolism to morphine in some babies/mothers	Unpredictable effects. Avoided in maternity services because of risks arising from rapid metabolism (not all of which is predicted by genotype)
Thiazides	Eliminated unchanged by kidneys	Reduced clearance because of low GFR
Furosemide	Eliminated by kidneys (unchanged) and following glucuronidation	Reduced clearance because of low GFR and low glucuronidation. Half-life may be as long as 24 h in premature neonates increasing the risk of effects on hearing with repeated doses
Fentanyl	CYP3A4 (gradual increase after birth). Relatively high V_d in neonates. Elimination is reduced by laparotomy	Accumulation and slow terminal elimination may increase adverse events and tolerance in chronic use
Fluconazole	Eliminated unchanged by kidneys	Reduced clearance because of low GFR
Gentamicin and other aminoglycosides	Eliminated unchanged by kidneys	Rapid increase in elimination in days after birth as GFR increases; steady increase after that with postmenstrual age
Ibuprofen	CYP2C9 and CYP2C8 (increase after birth)	Half-life shortens after birth. Genetic variation in the expression of each enzyme contributes to interindividual variation
Levetiracetam	Eliminated unchanged by kidneys, low protein binding, linear PK, limited adverse event profile (so far)	Ideal PK profile for neonates (if it works)
Midazolam	CYP3A4, limited production of 1-OH-midazolam for at least 3 mo after birth	Longer half-life than in older infants
Morphine	UGT2B7, which is not active soon after birth and gradually increases. Limited formation of the active metabolite morphine-6-glucuronide	Accumulation is likely and may increase risk of adverse events
Omeprazole	CYP2C19 limited metabolism for months after birth	Genetic variation associated with rate of metabolism
Phenobarbital	CYP2C9	
Phenytoin	CYP2C9 or CYP2C19, limited metabolism for months after birth	Dose increases from 5 mg/kg/d at birth to 8–10 mg/kg/d at 6 mo
Teicoplanin	Eliminated unchanged; high protein binding	
Vancomycin	Eliminated unchanged	
Warfarin	Need higher doses on a mg/kg basis than adults	Apparent differences in clearance between children and adults can be accounted for by using liver weight to standardize dosage rather than body weight. Pharmacogenomics can support dosing in adults but understanding is limited in neonates

Selection based on Hsieh EM, Hornik CP, Clark RH, et al. Medication use in the neonatal intensive care unit. *Am J Perinatol* 2014;31:811; Mesek I, Nellis G, Lass J, et al. Medicines prescription patterns in European neonatal units. *Int J Clin Pharm* 2019;41:1578; Flint RB, van Beek F, Andriessen P, et al. Large differences in neonatal drug use between NICUs are common practice: time for consensus? *Br J Clin Pharmacol* 2018;84:1313.

by cytochrome P450 is lower than other age groups. Less first-pass metabolism of orally administered morphine or propranolol in neonates may lead to higher than expected effects for a specific dose.

Endogenous

Atracurium spontaneously degrades in the circulation (Hofmann degradation) and is metabolized by esterases. Hepatic or other types of metabolism or elimination are not involved. This means that the concentration of atracurium is consistent during renal or liver failure.

Other

Nitric oxide is oxidized to nitrate by binding to oxyhemoglobin within erythrocytes to form methemoglobin. The activity of methemoglobin reductase (cytochrome b5 reductase) prevents the buildup of methemoglobin. Relatively low levels of methemoglobin reductase in neonates lead to the relatively high risk of methemoglobinemia during therapeutic use of inhaled nitric oxide.

Elimination

Elimination is the removal of chemicals from the body. In neonatal practice, most drugs are eliminated by the kidneys.

Renal elimination: Filtration depends on glomerular blood flow, as well as the characteristics of the drug, and is measured as glomerular filtration rate (GFR). Glomerular blood flow increases in the days after birth as part of adaptation to extrauterine life (see Chapter 38). This means that filtration increases during the first week after birth and the elimination of renally filtered drugs increases. This means that circulating concentrations will be less for the same dose so that we need to alter the dose of drugs after the first week.

Tubular absorption and reabsorption are also important. For example, creatinine is an imperfect marker of renal filtration in preterm neonates because tubular reabsorption in the first couple of weeks after birth leads to higher plasma concentrations than would be expected. It is important to note that trimethoprim can inhibit secretion of creatinine, so could be associated with higher than expected creatinine concentrations. Some labs use the Jaffe reaction to measure creatinine: some cephalosporins and high doses of furosemide interfere with this reaction so that these drugs could be associated with higher than expected creatinine concentrations. Some labs measure creatinine using enzymatic assays that are affected by flucytosine. Comparisons between labs need to account for the assay method.

In the renal tubules, organic anion transporters (OAT) and organic cation transporters (OCT) actively secrete many drugs including acids such as penicillins, cephalosporins, thiazides, furosemide, glucuronide, and sulfate conjugates of metabolized drugs and bases such as morphine, aminoglycosides, and catecholamines. However, passive reabsorption can also occur. The activity of OAT and OCT appears to develop more slowly than GFR so

that filtration appears to be more important for the elimination of these drugs in neonates than in older age groups. Since reductions in renal blood flow are relatively common in sick preterm neonates, the concentrations of drugs secreted by renal tubules may be higher than expected in oliguric babies.

The liver is also important for elimination. Following glucuronidation or sulfation, drugs pass into the bile and then to the intestine. In the intestine, bacteria can reverse Phase 2 reactions and the drugs can be reabsorbed (enterohepatic circulation). In neonates, the bile may not enter the intestines as readily (e.g., during conjugated hyperbilirubinemia with prolonged parenteral nutrition), and this could affect elimination and enterohepatic circulation of morphine and warfarin. This may lead to unexpected variation in the effects of these drugs.

Clearance and Volume of Distribution

The combination of metabolism and elimination reduces the concentration of drug in the circulation. The standard way to quantify this is called "clearance." Systemic clearance is the volume of plasma in the vascular compartment that is cleared of drug during a specific time period. The half-life is the time taken for a drug to reach half its initial concentration in the plasma. A rule of thumb is that a drug is completely eliminated five half-lives after the last dose. To be precise, this is the elimination half-life and is relevant when absorption and distribution have stopped being relevant after a dose. We occasionally see mention of the terminal half-life, which is the time taken for a drug to reach half its concentration after the initial halving. The terminal half-life is important when elimination is not the main determinant of the circulating concentration. For example, fentanyl (which is extensively lipid soluble so that the main determinant of circulating concentrations is release from fat rather than metabolism or elimination) or azithromycin (which is concentrated in macrophages and released to the circulation more slowly than it is eliminated).

Clearance and elimination half-life are related to the volume of distribution. A prolonged elimination half-life can result from lower clearance or higher volume of distribution.

Reliable drug therapy assumes ADME processes are consistent so that ADME can be brought into a steady state. In that steady state, the relationship between time after dose and the circulating concentration is consistent. This consistency allows stable predictions about the benefits and harms of drug therapy. As a rule-of-thumb, it takes three elimination half-lives for most drugs to come to steady state in a physiologically stable person. In a stable neonate, dosages adjustments should be done at steady state, that is, at least three elimination half-lives after the last dosage adjustment. **Figure 23.1** illustrates time–concentration curves for three hypothetical drugs given at the same dosage interval of 8 hours. The drug in black (elimination half-life 4 hours) attains steady state after the second dose because most of it is cleared

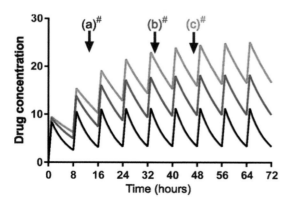

— (a) half-life 4 h
— (b) half-life 12 h
— (c) half-life 24 h

FIGURE 23.1 Time to steady state for three hypothetical drugs with different half-lives.

during the dosage interval. There is no accumulation between doses, so steady state can be reached quickly. The drug in blue attains steady state after the fifth dose because there is a significant amount of the drug in the circulation when the next dose is given. There is accumulation between doses, so steady state only happens when a balance between the dose and elimination occurs. This is even more marked for the drug in red. The practical importance of this is the need for loading doses when there is a long elimination or terminal half-life.

We have seen that gentamicin can have lower concentrations in neonates than expected in other age groups because of a greater volume of distribution. Gentamicin can also have higher concentrations than expected because of lower GFR. The actual concentration will reflect the net effect of these influences. It is not possible to estimate whether the V_d influences gentamicin concentrations more, less, or the same as GFR. The only way to make reliable predictions about the concentrations of gentamicin is to measure the circulating concentrations in neonates.

PHARMACODYNAMICS

Pharmacodynamics is the study of a drug's impact on the body. Rational pharmacotherapy involves knowing which receptors a drug acts on (intended and unintended targets) and how much of the drug is needed to have the desired effect. Receptors are identified and localized using in vitro methods based on healthy tissue or in vivo methods such as positron emission tomography (PET). Unfortunately, healthy tissue is almost impossible to obtain in preterm neonates, and PET methods have not been widely deployed to answer basic science questions in neonates. Therefore, assessments of pharmacodynamics in the newborn are based on incomplete data and rely heavily on extrapolation from older subjects, which are often flawed (e.g., see Chapter 31 for a discussion of adrenergic receptor distribution in preterm infants).

In the absence of robust data on receptor activity, pharmacodynamics must be based on endpoints that are clinically relevant and reliable. Convenient clinical endpoints are not necessarily clinically relevant (such as blood pressure measured through umbilical artery catheter (UAC) or peripheral arterial line, which is not closely correlated with brain function or injury) or reliable markers of drug effects (such as pain scores).

In practice, we assume that effects seen in older age groups are relevant to neonates. However, these assumptions may not hold because of age-specific differences in drug receptors. These difficulties mean that a lot of neonatal pharmacology is not well targeted or precise. Constant surveillance by the neonatal team is required. In parallel, we can support research that addresses that lack of knowledge about neonatal PD.

Ontogeny

Development is a central part of neonatology, with particular relevance to pharmacology. Illustrative examples of the effects of ontogeny have been given above and in Table 23.1. Development is most conveniently followed by measuring the gene expression of proteins that are relevant to PK or PD. However, many relevant proteins are not expressed in tissues that can be sampled easily. Changes in anatomy and physiology also affect PK. The traditional approach of using mg/kg to specify dosage regimens in pediatrics is a useful simplification based on an approximation to liver size. More accurate estimates of PK for many drugs can be obtained by using weight expressed by a power of ¾. Contemporary computerized approaches will make this approach easier to implement if more complex approaches can be shown to improve outcomes.

Targets of drugs can change with postmenstrual age, in nature, and in number. This is the main reason why it is essential to develop a specific understanding of the effects of drugs in neonates (12). For example, in adults, gamma-Aminobutyric acid (GABA)

inhibits neurones so that it is rational to use drugs that stimulate GABA receptors such as phenobarbital to treat seizures. In neonates, GABA can excite neurones rather than inhibit them so that it is rational to seek alternatives to phenobarbital (13).

Pharmacometrics: Describing PK and PD with Fancy Math

Time is a key variable in pharmacology: ADME means that drugs do not have constant concentrations. Most ADME processes transport or metabolize drugs and metabolites with "linear" kinetics. In this context, linear means that the rate of the process is proportional to the concentration of the drug (or metabolite). This situation is also described as first-order kinetics.

A few drugs saturate a key ADME process. This means that the rate of the process is limited by the maximum rate of the process, not the concentration of the drug. This situation is described as zero-order kinetics. Phenytoin saturates its metabolism by CYP2C9 and CYP2C19. This means that the proportion of phenytoin removed from the circulation per hour is lower at high concentrations and the circulating concentrations are not easy to predict. The complexities of using phenytoin in neonates are compounded by the switch between CYP2C9 and CYP2C19 after birth and because these enzymes are induced by phenytoin. The PK of phenytoin can be summarized as higher plasma concentrations reduce clearance and increase the elimination half-life.

Phenytoin illustrates a central principle of pharmacology: things change, so follow the rates of change, not just the concentrations of drugs. The need to pay attention to rates leads to mathematical models based on differential equations. These mathematical models are complex but powerful and are one of many justifications to include pharmacists and/or clinical pharmacologists in neonatal teams.

Noncompartmental descriptions record the concentrations (e.g., in blood) with time. This allows the computation of key parameters such as the time at which the maximum concentration appears and the maximum concentration itself (T_{max} and C_{max}); the time for half the drug to leave the circulation (half-life); and the area under the concentration curve (AUC), which can indicate the total amount of exposure to the drug. As noted above, most ADME processes are related to the concentration of the drug (or metabolite). Noncompartmental descriptions are quick and simple to build but are difficult to use in neonates because of the need to account for age (postnatal and postmenstrual). Noncompartmental descriptions do not account for compartments and need "rich" sampling—each study participant needs to contribute several data points. Accordingly, neonatal PK models take account of age and compartments, and can use "sparse" samples, that is, only two or three samples from each participant. These models can also account for renal impairment and other variables.

Neonatal PK models generally use "population PK" approaches. In PopPK approaches, the concentration of the drug is a variable that depends on a number of other variables. The math also accounts for the correlation between repeated concentrations taken from a single participant. PopPK models of drug concentration can be combined with models of physiology. This so-called physiologically based PK (PBPK) methodology can be used to assess the effects of different scenarios such as changes in renal blood flow or cardiac output.

The second key relationship is between the concentration of the drug and its effect. This allows identification of the optimal concentration through PK PD analysis. This depends on a clear understanding of the effect of a drug and a clear readout of the effect. In neonatology, we have a working understanding of the effects of antibiotics but we lack useful markers of the effects of most other drugs.

In combination, these mathematical approaches provide powerful ways to summarize and integrate understanding of the effects of drugs, known as modeling and simulation (14). This means that neonatal pharmacology is supported by a large amount of prior knowledge. Individual research projects or clinical applications do not need to start from the beginning. This is in contrast to traditional pharmacology that is based on building an independent set of information for each drug by rich sampling. Neonatal pharmacology can be based on finding what is needed to use existing knowledge. Research projects or clinical applications can be designed to target specific information rather than to build a comprehensive model.

SAFETY

All drugs have unintended effects. The whole neonatal team needs to be aware of what to look for in order to minimize avoidable harm. Drugs can cause harm due to an expected effect from a high dose (such as tachycardia with dopamine reducing ventricular filling time), an expected physiologic effect from prolonged exposure (such as hyperglycemia from a short course of corticosteroids or adrenal suppression with courses of corticosteroids that last several weeks), or from effects that are not expected from physiology (such as immune-mediated reactions to antibiotics or Steven-Johnson syndrome). Immune-mediated reactions are very rare in neonates but may become more prominent if biologics and stem cell therapies are introduced to neonatal practice.

Historically, disasters in neonatal drug safety have driven regulation of drugs (15). Examples include the use of diethylene glycol to solubilize sulfanilamide in the 1930s and gray baby syndrome and chloramphenicol in the 1960s. More recent examples include ceftriaxone (precipitation with calcium), kaletra (toxicity of the excipient propylene glycol), and codeine (genetic variation in CYP2D6 associated with toxic concentrations in some neonates). These problems were identified from reports made by professionals about unexpected events.

Adverse events that could be related to an administered drug need to be assessed to capture the event; the effects of the event on the baby (severity); the likelihood that the drug caused the event (causality); the effects of the event on the care given to the baby (seriousness). This assessment is then used to analyze the event to decide whether a change in management is needed: either to treat the effects or change drug therapy. This assessment and analysis are done implicitly on every neonatal unit every day. A formal process can clarify the situation and promote multidisciplinary collaboration. An unusual event should be reported to national pharmacovigilance reporting systems.

Long-term safety of drugs given in neonatal units is important but understudied. It is essential to develop a working understanding of the balance between benefits and risks of drugs given to neonates. This understanding depends on systematic evaluation of long-term effects of drugs (16).

FORMULARY SECTION

A formulary section provides the information needed by prescribers and other staff to use drugs safely in a specific facility. Each drug has a separate section in the facility's formulary. Pharmacists or clinical pharmacologists may write formularies in some health care facilities. However, these professionals are not available universally; so, this section aims to provide essential background for medical professionals who are involved in drafting, or reviewing neonatal formularies.

Standard reference books about dosing (4–6) are useful for prescribers but do not replace a local formulary that provides prescribers and staff who administer drugs with information that is tailored to local circumstances. Companies and regulators work hard to include reliable develop information about each drug in a license or marketing authorization. Labels, or product information leaflets, can be very useful when drafting formularies but are often underutilized by prescribers on neonatal units. A formulary

implies some background information about pharmacology that is not repeated in every formulary chapter. This background information is provided in the previous section of this chapter.

Consistency in use and dosage of drugs is important to build safety (e.g., antimicrobial stewardship), to contain costs, and to build confidence among the team. A formulary is an essential tool to promote rational pharmacotherapy. Drugs go to the heart of medical and nursing practice. Formulary development requires many skills including teamwork and management of human factors, change, and risk.

Contents of a Formulary Section
Indications

Given the risks and uncertainties involved in administering drugs to sick and premature neonates, it is essential to have clearly defined indications. Indications should be based on a thorough understanding of the condition and the effects of the drug on the condition. If we do not know what we are expecting to treat, and the expected effects, it is difficult to know when to start or stop a drug. Ideally, indications are supported by an evidence-based balance between benefit and risks that takes account of appropriate formulations and dosing. However, in neonates, we are left with a lack of information about benefits, dosing and formulation, and a range of unquantifiable risks.

Potential approaches to a drug with incomplete information include the following:

- Do not give the drug (according to the precautionary principle, do not expose people to risks that you do not understand).
- Give the drug without any controls (or at the sole discretion of individual clinicians).
- Give the drug in a controlled way:
  - As part of a safety study
  - As part of an RCT
  - With extra monitoring
- Give the drug according to some sort of protocol that ensures there is a need that is proportionate to the risks arising from the drug and the uncertainties. An example for paracetamol could be to specify the indication: not for procedural pain; when there is persistent pain and a defined cause for pain; and when there is a need to spare morphine. These conditions could be operationalized as scenarios when paracetamol is indicated, for example, within 7 days of a laparotomy, give paracetamol before increasing morphine above 10 µg/kg/h, if the pain score is high, etc.

The decision about each indication will be modulated by the team's views on the following:

- The risks of not treating the condition in question balanced against other risks
- The risks of the drug for example, fairly benign long term, balanced against other risks
- The importance of burden and welfare as a component of comparisons between options
- The utility of endpoint assessments (will we know whether the drug works or does harm)

Defining an indication can take a lot of work by the team that needs sensitive management. The team needs to acknowledge how its inherent biases will inform the discussion and may color individual comments (e.g., clinicians vary in how they approach the ethical requirement to do no harm vs. treat the person/family in front of you). We also need a view on what to say to families when evidence is uncertain. In some cases, such as postnatal corticosteroids, some units explain the risks and benefits. Each unit will need to find its own approach to telling families about uncertainty. It is important for all team members to accept the team decision, following a rational discussion based on principles and explicit reasoning and some attempt to recognize and manage risks.

THE NEWBORN INFANT

Contraindications

These can be absolute or relative.

Dosage Regimen

In principle, we decide dosage regimens by identifying: (a) the target; (b) the concentration needed to have the desired effect on the target while minimizing unwanted effects; and (c) the dose needed to get to the concentration that is needed to have the effect. These principles can be applied readily to neonatal antibiotic therapy (17). However, for most drugs, this approach is difficult in neonates because of problems with identifying the target and the PKPD relationship. In practice, neonatal dose identification is often based on assuming that a concentration that is useful in adults will be useful in neonates. Then, we can work out how to get to that concentration.

The formulation (dosage form) is important because its properties define the physical availability of the drug (18). Bioavailability depends on absorption, which can be affected by age, development, and illness. Dosing handbooks provide state-of-the-art information about distribution, metabolism, and elimination in neonates. These can be synthesized into a dosing regimen by considering the following:

- Loading dose—a loading dose is needed if there is a long elimination half-life (leading to delayed steady state) or a large volume of distribution (the medicine disappears from the circulation so the whole body needs to be filled up with the drug before it can work).
- Dose amount—this needs to have the desired effect in most babies at steady state and can be influenced by absorption, distribution, and clearance.
- Timing—this is directly influenced by clearance but absorption and distribution will affect the attainment of steady state. Continuous infusion may be useful if the effects are dependent on the duration of exposure to a specific concentrations or clearance is rapid.

Compatibility

Incompatibilities arise from the expected and unexpected physicochemical effects of mixing drugs, including nutrition (19). These can be assessed *in vitro*. Standard dosing books (4–6) contain this information for many drug combinations, but local practice will need to inform each unit's formulary. Consistent attention is required to prevent avoidable incompatible infusions (20).

Drug–drug Interactions

These are the pharmacologic effects (on receptors or ADME) of using more than one drug at a time. Neonatal examples include the effects of fluconazole on omeprazole and warfarin (inhibition of CYP2C9). In general, clinically significant drug–drug interactions are rare in neonates, so should be reported to pharmacovigilance authorities when they occur.

Method of Administration

Staff who administer drugs need a standardized process that is based on unit policies and equipment. These instructions need to take account of human factors, reconstitution (including the displacement volume that arises during reconstitution of some drugs and can make a significant difference to concentrations of drugs within vials, with implications for how much fluid is removed from the vial), consequences of dilution, and stability.

Availability

Ensuring that a drug is available on a neonatal unit is a complex task that is almost universally underappreciated by physicians. Neonatal pharmacists are modest people who do not draw attention to the vast amount of work they do to ensure drugs are available. The process that leads to a drug of suitable quality being available is long and susceptible to disruption. Pinch points include sourcing raw materials, manufacturing, transport, procurement, purchasing, and storage (21). Each of these steps can be disrupted by environmental, policy, and random factors (including human error) that are independent of the needs of neonates. The potential for disruption is addressed by stringent quality standards.

Selection of Drugs used in a Unit

It is essential to minimize the number of drugs used in a unit (e.g., antibiotics). Costs need to be considered: no health care system has limitless resources. Many drugs have marginal increases in benefits, or marginal reductions in harms, compared to other drugs. The selection of drugs should be addressed in a systematic way, similar to defining indications as described above.

SPECIAL POPULATIONS

Renal Failure

Identify renal failure in a timely way, bearing in mind the inadequacy of creatinine as a marker of acute kidney injury in neonates. Avoid nephrotoxic drugs (e.g., gentamicin and vancomycin). Make dosage adjustments for relevant drugs (as per standard dosing guides that should be based on data or PBPK studies)

Hepatic Failure

Identify hepatic failure in a timely way, bearing in mind the nonspecific and insensitive signals from "liver function tests." Avoid hepatotoxic drugs (e.g., acetaminophen). Make dosage adjustments for relevant drugs (e.g., morphine).

Hypothermia

Hypothermia decreases clearance and can increase or decrease V_d. Underlying illness will also affect these parameters, for example, reduced renal clearance due to poor perfusion and acute tubular necrosis (22). Hypothermia can also affect PD. The affinity of m-opioid receptors for morphine appears to be reduced during hypothermia so that higher doses may be needed initially.

Sepsis

Distribution and elimination can vary during phases of sepsis (23). These changes are rapid and can be difficult to match during neonatal therapeutics.

ECMO

The ECMO circuit increases V_d, particularly if drugs bind to the plastic (e.g., fentanyl and midazolam). Clearance can also be affected, in relation to the underlying disease (24).

PRESCRIBING

Good prescribing involves attention to the indication; the patient—their needs and comorbidities; the drug—knowledge about its benefits and risks; clear prescriptions; monitoring the patient; and clear communication with professionals and the family. Background knowledge ideally comes from a formulary shared by a unit but can come from the label/SmPC, dosing handbooks, and academic literature. Background information can be used to build a model of what is likely to be effective and safe, and which adverse effects can be used to monitor doses.

Adapting to the Baby in Front of You

Applying information about one or more drugs to the needs of a baby with complex medical issues requires making judgments on the basis of a thorough understanding of information relating to more standard situations (25). The available background information limits the judgments to the specificities of the case in hand rather than to broader issues. In difficult cases, clinical judgment should be explicit with clearly defined goals that are used to specify and monitor treatment. As far as possible, dosage adjustments should be anticipated. The alternative of implicit judgments may work some of the time. However, implicit judgments hinder consistent care and will not be capable of handling all the components of the most complex decisions.

Individualizing Care

Approaches to individualizing care include the following:

- Titrate to effect—this can be used when there is a clear and reliable, clinically relevant endpoint. Examples include treatment of hypotension (guided by target blood pressure) and treatment of hypothyroidism (guided by TSH concentrations)
- Therapeutic drug monitoring (TDM)—this can be used when there is a convenient and reliable drug assay and a clear relationship between drug concentrations and effects. It is particularly useful if there is a narrow therapeutic index (the concentrations that cause harm are similar to the concentrations that cause benefit) or if there is wide variation in clearance between individuals (so that it is difficult to predict whether an effective dose has been administered) or if adverse effects are not apparent to clinicians. Examples include aminoglycosides, glycopeptides, and phenobarbital. TDM can be done after a single dose, or as a "spot" sample, to check for toxicity. TDM can also be done to inform dosage at steady state, in which case the samples should be taken at steady state. Application of pharmacometric techniques can provide dosing information before steady state if estimates of key parameters such as clearance are available. TDM can also be done if the clinical condition changes.
- Work with clinical pharmacists/clinical pharmacologists—these professionals are skilled in reconciling patient needs and multiple drugs and can bring valuable expertise to complex situations (and simple situations).

The future of individualized care, or personalized medicine, has many opportunities. Application of pharmacometrics could provide drug regimens that are tailored to each baby's genome and clinical needs (26). Personalized medicine depends on a rich understanding of the biology of disease, precise disease endpoints, and good understanding of the effects of drugs. Currently, neonatal medicine lacks these characteristics so that impactful neonatal personalized medicine is likely to be deferred.

PREGNANCY

Medication is an essential element of contemporary maternity care, and standard texts are available to support health care professionals (27). Medicines are often used in normal pregnancy: analgesia, hypnotics, laxatives, and antireflux. Infection is common during pregnancy: UTI; PPROM; GBS; and sepsis. Chorioamnionitis is a special case. Maternal immunization has important public health benefits. Some treatments target fetal complications such as arrhythmias. Other treatments address maternal illness: intercurrent (transplant, mental health, essential hypertension, HIV/AIDS, endocrine) and conditions arising during pregnancy, most notably preeclampsia. In all these cases, neonatologists need to be aware of the potential impact of medicines on the fetus and newborn. Close teamwork with perinatal colleagues is essential. This includes the obstetricians involved as well as specialists in maternal health. Similar to the situation on the neonatal unit, consistent use of a limited formulary by the multidisciplinary team is central to safe, effective, and efficient care.

The principles of drug use in pregnancy include the approach to good describing noted above. In addition, the specific features of drug disposition during pregnancy should be accounted for (28,29). Benefit–risk assessment during pregnancy needs to account for the fetus and potential long-term effects on the child (30). The need for complex judgments is recognized in FDA guidance for

the content of drug labels (31). Since 2015, the FDA has required drug labels to include summaries of the evidence that contributes to assessment of risk. This was a move away from a categorical approach, for example, "Category A, adequate and well-controlled studies have failed to demonstrate a risk to the fetus in the first trimester of pregnancy (and there is no evidence of risk in later trimesters)."

Teratogenesis is assessed during drug development of licensed products using proxy models, but this does not usually relate to effects of medicines in the second half of pregnancy. When mother or fetus suffers from a significant illness, the harms arising from the condition being treated should drive the benefit–risk assessment. From the neonatal perspective, it is important to monitor postnatally for neonatal complications. All neonates requiring treatment need a thorough history about mother's intake of drugs (both prescribed and recreational) and other substances that may have pharmacologic effects (including herbs and products used in all health care traditions).

LACTATION

A few drugs are clearly contraindicated in lactating mothers. In most cases, careful assessment of the drug and the family allow a balance between benefits and risks. A lack of information in the label does not mean that the situation is dangerous. In the US, drug labels now provide risk summaries relating to lactation, rather than categories, as for pregnancy (31). There are a number of sources for information about specific drugs. (27)

SYSTEMS NEEDED TO SUPPORT GOOD PRESCRIBING AND ADMINISTRATION

A systematic review found that among neonatal intensive care units, medication error rates ranged from 5.5 to 77.9 per 100 medication orders. Prescribing and medication administration errors were the most common medication errors. Anti-infective agents were most commonly involved with medication errors (32). Medication errors can be reduced by prescribing and administering medicines appropriately. Good administration involves ensuring that the right patient receives the right drug by the right route at the right dose and frequency, with comprehensive documentation. While individuals have responsibility for their actions, organizations are responsible for the systems and conditions that individuals work in. Organizations need to provide safe working environments (avoiding disturbances during prescribing and administration); a neonatal clinical pharmacy service; regular training; appropriate technology such as pumps that can only be operated according to preprogrammed instructions; a comprehensive system for managing medication errors (reporting, evaluating, feedback, practice change) that does not demotivate staff; an environment that promotes safe checking and questioning (a horizontal hierarchy); and up-to-date information that is available at the point of care (e.g., a unit formulary as described above).

These approaches have been evaluated in neonatal care in a systematic review (33). The median rate of error reduction was 73% overall, 85% for interventions relating to prescribing and 52% for interventions relating to administration. The most important theme was the need for education and support for staff before and during any change in practice.

RESEARCH ABOUT DRUGS IN NEONATES

Why Study Drugs in Neonates?

There is marked variation in the use of medicines (34,35) and their dosages (36). This suggests that some of the drugs are not needed and some are given at doses that are too high or too low. If we want all babies to do well, we should know which medicines are useful and the dosages with the best balance between benefit and risk. Half of babies on NICU are exposed to at least one off-label medicine (37). This means that there is a lack of high-quality data that has been scrutinized by regulators who are independent of the pharmaceutical companies and health care professionals. In addition, the development of a dosage form that is suitable for neonates is complex and needs expert input (18).

How Can We Study Drugs in Neonates?

There are two broad approaches. One approach is driven by curiosity in specific contexts. This leads to studies that meet specific needs and can include single-centre studies using samples of convenience and large, multicentre studies that compare interventions designed according to the available evidence. This approach has led to many advances and underpins much "evidence-based medicine." The curiosity-driven approach has not provided the information we need for rational drug therapy in neonates. An alternative approach is to take a programmatic approach. This approach starts by defining the natural history of the targeted condition, develops appropriate definitions and endpoints for clinical trials, investigates PK and PD before defining a dose, and learns about the effects of the optimal dose before designing large trials to define the benefit risk profile of the drug in a specific indication. Regulators require pharmaceutical companies to complete a program of research before a drug can be marketed. These requirements stem from the history of therapeutic catastrophes before drug development was regulated. The public sector (academics and other clinicians) can also follow a programmatic approach (38). Key growth points in the design and conduct of clinical trials have been summarized (26). Many therapeutic uncertainties in neonates could be addressed by a partial programmatic approach that fills specific gaps.

It is important to remember that neonates can participate in more than one study, under some circumstances (39).

There is an urgent need for research about drugs used during pregnancy: neonatal health care professionals should advocate for, and contribute to, these studies (40).

How Can Individuals and Units Contribute to Research about Drugs?

The most important contribution is to support studies by recruiting participants and ensuring that high-quality data are collected. It is essential that the whole neonatal team is involved in research projects. Nurses and parents are essential collaborators at every step of designing and conducting studies, including the setup of a study in a unit (8). Studies can be observational, such as disease registries, or interventional when a new or existing drug is evaluated. It is important to report unusual adverse drug reactions to regional or national surveillance systems in order to detect unanticipated side effects.

The context for research is also important. All members of the neonatal team can identify gaps in knowledge about research and build demand for appropriate studies. Education about drug development and the need for research is important for all professional groups. Units can contribute to effective networks. This can mean joining master protocols (7) and surrendering some clinical autonomy as part of the research effort (e.g., agreeing to similar approaches to standard care). Studies should be designed to contribute directly to drug development. For example, in addition to studies that explore associations between disease and biomarker, we need to validate biomarkers (i.e., demonstrate precision, repeatability, links to clinically important outcomes, responsiveness to drugs etc.) (41,42).

Other key issues in research include how to assure access to drugs once they are on the market (21), particularly formulations that are appropriate to neonates (18); global needs for appropriate drugs; health technology assessments to ensure value for money;

and comparative effectiveness studies to ensure the most appropriate management strategies are followed.

■ SUMMARY

Drugs help but can also harm. The effects of drugs differ with the gestational and postmenstrual age of each neonate. The effects of the body on each drug also vary with time and between individuals. There are many uncertainties in neonatal pharmacotherapy and the underpinning science. We need to choose and use drugs wisely, in a considered, team-based way. Most neonatal drug use is an informal experiment. Whenever possible, we should join well-designed research studies and report unusual adverse events.

REFERENCES

1. Mulberg A, Murphy M, Dunne J, et al. *Pediatric drug development*, 2nd ed. Hoboken, NJ: Wiley-Blackwell, 2013.
2. Derendorf H, Schmidt S. *Rowland and Tozer's clinical pharmacokinetics and pharmacodynamics: concepts and applications*. Philadelphia, PA: Lippincott Williams and Wilkins, 2019.
3. Yaffe S, Aranda J. *Neonatal and pediatric pharmacology: therapeutic principles in practice*, 4th ed. Philadelphia, PA: Lippincott Williams and Wilkins, 2010.
4. Takemoto C. *Pediatric & neonatal dosage handbook*. Hudson, OH: Lexi-Comp, 2018.
5. Nederlands Kenniscentrum Farmacotherapie bij Kinderen. Kinderformularium. Available from: https://www.kinderformularium.nl. Last accessed December 18, 2020.
6. Ainsworth S. *Neonatal formulary: drug use in pregnancy and the first year of life*, 8th ed. Oxford, UK: Oxford University Press, 2020.
7. England A, Wade K, Smith PB, et al. Optimizing operational efficiencies in early phase trials: The Pediatric Trials Network experience. *Contemp Clin Trials* 2016;47:376.
8. Turner MA. Clinical trials of medicines in neonates: the influence of ethical and practical issues on design and conduct. *Br J Clin Pharmacol* 2015;79:370.
9. Barker C, Turner M, Sharland M. *Prescribing medicines for children*. London, United Kingdom: Pharmaceutical Press, 2019.
10. van den Anker J, Reed MD, Allegaert K, et al. Developmental changes in pharmacokinetics and pharmacodynamics. *J Clin Pharmacol* 2018;58(suppl 10):S10.
11. Ward RM, Benjamin D, Barrett JS, et al. Safety, dosing, and pharmaceutical quality for studies that evaluate medicinal products (including biological products) in neonates. *Pediatr Res* 2017;81:692.
12. Wang J, Avant D, Green D, et al. A survey of neonatal pharmacokinetic and pharmacodynamic studies in pediatric drug development. *Clin Pharmacol Ther* 2015;98:328.
13. Pressler RM, Mangum B. Newly emerging therapies for neonatal seizures. *Semin Fetal Neonatal Med* 2013;18:216.
14. Neely M, Bayard D, Desai A, et al. Pharmacometric modeling and simulation is essential to pediatric clinical pharmacology. *J Clin Pharmacol* 2018;58(suppl 10):S73.
15. Hawcutt DB, O'Connor O, Turner MA. Adverse drug reactions in neonates: could we be documenting more? *Expert Rev Clin Pharmacol* 2014;7:807.
16. Marlow N, Doyle LW, Anderson P, et al. Assessment of long-term neurodevelopmental outcome following trials of medicinal products in newborn infants. *Pediatr Res* 2019;86:567.
17. Le J, Bradley JS. Optimizing antibiotic drug therapy in pediatrics: current state and future needs. *J Clin Pharmacol* 2018;58(suppl 10):S108.
18. O'Brien F, Clapham D, Krysiak K, et al. Making medicines baby size: the challenges in bridging the formulation gap in neonatal medicine. *Int J Mol Sci* 2019;20:2688.
19. Kalikstad B, Skjerdal A, Hansen TW. Compatibility of drug infusions in the NICU. *Arch Dis Child* 2010;95:745.
20. Hani C, Vonbach P, Fonzo-Christe C, et al. Evaluation of incompatible coadministration of continuous intravenous infusions in a pediatric/neonatal intensive care unit. *J Pediatr Pharmacol Ther* 2019;24:479.
21. Iyengar S, Hedman L, Forte G, et al. Medicine shortages: a commentary on causes and mitigation strategies. *BMC Med* 2016;14:124.
22. Pokorna P, Wildschut ED, Vobruba V, et al. The impact of hypothermia on the pharmacokinetics of drugs used in neonates and young infants. *Curr Pharm Des* 2015;21:5705.
23. Roberts JA, Lipman J. Antibacterial dosing in intensive care: pharmacokinetics, degree of disease and pharmacodynamics of sepsis. *Clin Pharmacokinet* 2006;45:755.
24. Raffaeli G, Pokorna P, Allegaert K, et al. Drug disposition and pharmacotherapy in neonatal ECMO: from fragmented data to integrated knowledge. *Front Pediatr* 2019;7:360.

25. WHO. *Guide to good prescribing—a practical manual*. Geneva, Switzerland: World Health Organization, 1994.

26. Balevic SJ, Cohen-Wolkowiez M. Innovative study designs optimizing clinical pharmacology research in infants and children. *J Clin Pharmacol.* 2018;58(suppl 10):S58.

27. Briggs G, Freeman R, Towers C, et al. *Drugs in pregnancy and lactation*, 12th ed. Philadelphia, PA: Lippincott Williams and Wilkins, 2021.

28. Pariente G, Leibson T, Carls A, et al. Pregnancy-associated changes in pharmacokinetics: a systematic review. *PLoS Med* 2016;13:e1002160.

29. Kazma JM, van den Anker J, Allegaert K, et al. Anatomical and physiological alterations of pregnancy. *J Pharmacokinet Pharmacodyn* 2020;47(4):271.

30. Rasmussen-Torvik LJ, Zumpf KB, Betcher HK, et al. Interpreting the pharmacoepidemiology literature in obstetrical studies: a guide for clinicians. *Semin Perinatol* 2020;44:151225.

31. FDA. *Pregnancy, lactation, and reproductive potential: labeling for human prescription drug and biological products—content and format guidance for industry.* 2014.

32. Alghamdi AA, Keers RN, Sutherland A, et al. Prevalence and nature of medication errors and preventable adverse drug events in paediatric and neonatal intensive care settings: a systematic review. *Drug Saf* 2019;42:1423.

33. Nguyen MR, Mosel C, Grzeskowiak LE. Interventions to reduce medication errors in neonatal care: a systematic review. *Ther Adv Drug Saf* 2018;9:123.

34. Hsieh EM, Hornik CP, Clark RH, et al. Medication use in the neonatal intensive care unit. *Am J Perinatol* 2014;31:811.

35. Mesek I, Nellis G, Lass J, et al. Medicines prescription patterns in European neonatal units. *Int J Clin Pharm* 2019;41:1578.

36. Metsvaht T, Nellis G, Varendi H, et al. High variability in the dosing of commonly used antibiotics revealed by a Europe-wide point prevalence study: implications for research and dissemination. *BMC Pediatr* 2015;15:41.

37. Flint RB, van Beek F, Andriessen P, et al. Large differences in neonatal drug use between NICUs are common practice: time for consensus? *Br J Clin Pharmacol* 2018;84:1313.

38. Turner MA, Portman RJ, Davis JM. Regulatory science in neonates: a framework that supports evidence-based drug therapy. *JAMA Pediatr* 2017;171:721.

39. Davis JM, Baer GR, Portman R, et al. Enrollment of neonates in more than one clinical trial. *Clin Ther* 2017;39:1959.

40. Turner MA, Kenny L, Alfirevic Z. Challenges in designing clinical trials to test new drugs in the pregnant woman and fetus. *Clin Perinatol* 2019;46:399.

41. Ewen JB, Sweeney JA, Potter WZ. Conceptual, regulatory and strategic imperatives in the early days of EEG-based biomarker validation for neurodevelopmental disabilities. *Front Integr Neurosci* 2019;13:45.

42. Shores DR, Everett AD. Children as biomarker orphans: progress in the field of pediatric biomarkers. *J Pediatr* 2018;193:14.

THE NEWBORN INFANT

24 Anesthesia and Analgesia

Sally H. Vitali

INTRODUCTION

Pain perception and physiologic responses to pain and stress occur in neonates of all gestational ages. In addition to their vital role in reducing suffering, anesthesia and analgesia have important short- and long-term clinical, physiologic, psychological, and neurodevelopmental consequences for the neonate. In the short term, anesthesia and analgesia control the stress response in the perioperative period and improve the outcome of infants after surgery (1–3). Appropriate analgesia and sedation are proven means of reducing catabolism associated with surgery and recovery from surgery, illness, and injury. Human and animal studies have found compelling evidence that early pain and stress affect nociception and behavioral responses to pain later in life (4). Given that critically ill preterm neonates have been reported to experience an average of 11.4 painful procedures per day during their stay in neonatal intensive care units (NICUs), pain and its management may have profound implications for the short- and long-term health and development of these babies (5).

As neonatal pain management has become more of a defined objective in the NICU, more than 40 scoring systems have been validated to quantify the magnitude of responses to pain and drive the use of pharmacologic and nonpharmacologic pain control methods (6). One strategy that has had the most direct and quantifiable success in reducing the amount of pain in neonates is the reduction in the number of painful procedures performed (5). When painful procedures are unavoidable, the use of pharmacologic and nonpharmacologic therapies for pain has increased but evidence of significant variability in practice still exists (7). More recently, the choice of anesthetics and analgesics in neonates has been complicated by a growing body of animal data revealing the potential neurotoxicity of nearly all of the medications used for these purposes. Interpretation of these data and its translatability to the human is difficult, and effective nonneurotoxic alternatives for pain control and sedation are lacking.

In this chapter, the field of neonatal anesthesia and analgesia is reviewed, the relevant pharmacokinetic and pharmacodynamic data are summarized, and practical considerations for the most commonly used agents are highlighted.

PAIN PERCEPTION

At the foundation of our understanding of the neonatal pain experience and efforts to control pain is evidence that nociceptive pathways are present and functional even in preterm newborns.

Nociceptive pathways develop structure and function during gestation; their activity and function mature after birth as their organization and transcriptional program continue to develop. The density of nociceptive nerve endings in newborn skin, labeling of specific proteins (e.g., GAP43) produced by axonal growth cones, reflex activity and receptive fields of primary afferent neurons, and development of synapses between primary afferents and interneurons in the dorsal horn of the spinal cord indicate the anatomic and functional maturity of the peripheral pain system during fetal life (8,9). Cellular and subcellular organization in the dorsal horn, with maturation of primary afferent terminations, occurs later in gestation and postnatally (10,11). In the dorsal horn, various neurotransmitter and neuromodulatory substances associated with pain (e.g., substance P, somatostatin, calcitonin gene–related peptide, vasoactive intestinal peptide, met-enkephalin, glutamate) appear during early gestation (12).

Myelination of the nociceptive nerve tracts in the spinal cord and central nervous system is completed during the second and third trimesters of gestation. Development of the fetal neocortex begins at 8 weeks of gestation, and the full complement of neurons is present by 20 weeks. Dendritic processes in the cortical neurons arborize and then synapse with incoming thalamocortical fibers by 24 to 26 weeks of gestation (13). Functional maturity of the cerebral cortex is suggested by fetal and neonatal electroencephalographic patterns, cortical somatosensory-evoked potentials, studies of regional cerebral metabolism, early behavioral development, and the specific behavioral responses of neonates to painful stimuli (14). Studies using functional magnetic resonance imaging (fMRI) show that term neonates and adults have similar patterns of increased brain activity after a noxious stimulus to the foot, further demonstrating early maturity of nociceptive pathways (15).

Endorphinergic cells in the anterior pituitary are responsive to corticotrophin-releasing factor stimulation *in vitro* and show increased β-endorphin production during fetal and neonatal life. Endogenous opioids and other hormones (e.g., catecholamines, steroid hormones, glucagon, growth hormone) are secreted by the human fetus in response to stress, leading to catabolism and other complications (6,16). Significant changes in cardiovascular parameters, transcutaneous partial pressure of oxygen, and palmar sweating have been observed in neonates undergoing painful clinical procedures. These physiologic changes are closely associated with behavioral responses of newborns to pain. Neonatal behavioral responses are characterized by simple motor responses, precise changes in facial expression associated with pain, highly specific patterns of crying activity, and a variety of complex behavioral changes. These patterns form the basis for the pain scoring systems that have been developed, validated, and employed in the care of the term and preterm newborn.

Long-Term Effects of Neonatal Pain and Its Treatment

The developing nervous system of the neonate is vulnerable to insults that modulate neurodevelopment. These insults include not only the repeated stressors and pain necessitated by resuscitation and life support in the NICU but the medications used to prevent and treat pain. Many studies in preterm infants and animal models have provided evidence that repeated painful interventions in the neonatal period contribute to hyperalgesia that is more profound and long-lasting than seen in nonneonates (17). Poorer developmental outcomes have been associated with increased exposure to procedural pain in both human preterm infants and animal models (18).

At least 50 studies in a number of different immature animal models have documented the neurotoxic effect of most anesthetic and analgesic agents used in neonates (19). Many outcome studies of preterm and term infants who have undergone major surgery (and therefore major anesthesia) in the neonatal period provide some evidence that neurodevelopmental outcomes are adversely impacted by early anesthesia, but these data are confounded by many other complicating factors in these infants including the surgery itself and the multiple painful stressors in the NICU (20).

Recently, a large international multicenter trial (General Anesthesia compared to Spinal anesthesia, GAS) followed neurodevelopmental outcomes after inguinal herniorrhaphy during infancy using either awake regional anesthesia or general anesthesia with sevoflurane. There were no differences in 5-year neurodevelopmental outcome between the two groups (21). While this study

venipuncture, and subcutaneous injection in term and preterm infants (75,76). The analgesic effects of sucrose appear to be opioid receptor mediated because its antinociceptive properties in rats can be reversed with naltrexone (77). Infant formula and its components (protein, fat, sucrose, but not lactose) also have shown antinociceptive properties. In a randomized controlled trial, breast-feeding has been shown to reduce pain associated with newborn heel stick as much as sucking glucose on a pacifier (78).

Facilitated tucking, by holding the neonate's extremities flexed and close to the trunk, swaddling, and rocking have been shown to improve heart rate and pain scores after heel lance or injection (79). Skin-to-skin contact provides analgesia during single heel lance or injection (80). Nonnutritive sucking, enhanced by the use of a pacifier, reduces the physiologic response to pain and is synergistic with the effects of intraoral glucose or sucrose (79). These nonpharmacologic techniques to reduce pain should be sought whenever possible because of their effectiveness coupled with a rarity of both short-term side effects and long-term potential toxicity. Importantly, most of these studies have evaluated pain responses to a single painful episode. More study is required for all of these techniques to determine their short- and long-term effects when used repeatedly in infants during a longer stay in the NICU.

SEDATION

The goals of sedation in the intensive care unit include analgesia for painful conditions and procedures and compliance with controlled mechanical ventilation via endotracheal tube and routine care. The ideal agent would not have hemodynamic or pulmonary side effects and would not be associated with the production or accumulation of toxic metabolites. It would have a short duration of action, would have a high therapeutic index, would not lead to tolerance and dependence, and would not cause any long-term effects on pain response or neurodevelopment. Unfortunately, no agent meets this ideal standard. Opioids have become exceedingly popular due to their relatively high toxic-to-therapeutic ratio, reported lack of side effects, and potent analgesic properties. Although opioids (reviewed above) are considered the mainstay of sedation in the intensive care setting, tolerance to their sedating effects may occur rapidly, and adequate sedation for prolonged periods can be ensured only by administration of adjuvant sedative agents.

Benzodiazepines

The benzodiazepines have a variety of desirable clinical effects that include hypnosis, anxiolysis, anticonvulsant activity, anterograde amnesia, and muscle relaxation. Benzodiazepines have no analgesic effects and in the presence of a painful stimulus may produce hyperalgesia and agitation. These problems usually do not occur if benzodiazepines are combined with opioids. Benzodiazepines act through GABA receptors to inhibit neuronal activity. Benzodiazepines have cardiovascular and respiratory depressant effects that are more profound in term and preterm infants when compared with older children. The respiratory depression and hypotension caused by benzodiazepines are synergistic with the similar effects of potent opioids. This combination should be used with extreme caution in neonates and only with close monitoring in an intensive care unit.

Commonly used benzodiazepines are lorazepam and diazepam, which may be given enterally or parenterally and dosed intermittently, and midazolam, which has a much shorter half-life, is given parenterally, and may be given intermittently or as a continuous infusion.

Midazolam may be used as premedication for specific invasive procedures in doses of 0.05 to 0.2 mg/kg, for short-term sedation by continuous infusion (<12 hours) at rates of 0.025 to 0.05 mg/kg/h, or for longer-term sedation of the intubated patient at rates

starting at 0.05 mg/kg/h. After 12 hours, metabolites that have longer half-lives begin to accumulate, and midazolam's duration of action is prolonged. The pharmacokinetics of midazolam in neonates are characterized by rapid redistribution and elimination half-life of 6.5 hours, which is significantly longer than the elimination half-life reported for older infants and children. Lorazepam and diazepam also have longer half-lives in infants than in older children and adults and should only be used in settings where infants can be monitored closely for their respiratory depressant effects that may persist for many hours.

A clinical trial of midazolam for long-term sedation of neonates demonstrated worsened neurologic outcomes (death, IVH, or periventricular leukomalacia) when compared to a group sedated with morphine infusion (81). Midazolam boluses are known to cause hypotension in preterm infants, and this hypotension is likely the cause of the increased brain injury (82). A meta-analysis of three randomized controlled trials of midazolam infusion for sedation of term and preterm infants found a significantly longer NICU stay in the midazolam group (83). Because of the tendency for desaturations, hypotension, and decreased cerebral blood flow velocity in preterm infants, the AAP recommended that midazolam should not be used for intubation premedication in preterm infants (84). In addition to hypotension and respiratory depression, reported side effects include myoclonic jerks (particularly in preterm infants) and nausea and vomiting.

As with opiates, chronic benzodiazepine use leads to tolerance and dependence. In patients of all ages, benzodiazepine withdrawal is characterized by many of the same features as opiate withdrawal such as retching and vomiting, sweating, agitation, increased startle, yawning, and sneezing, but also manifests with an increased risk of seizures. After prolonged intravenous therapy with midazolam, another unique withdrawal syndrome has been described in infants and characterized by agitation; poor visual tracking; constant choreoathetoid and dyskinetic movements of the face, tongue, and limbs; and depression of consciousness (85,86). When it is used for chronic sedation as an infusion for longer than 3 to 5 days, midazolam must be weaned while monitoring withdrawal scores. Once midazolam dosing is low enough to be converted safely to lorazepam or diazepam, these intermittent medications may be used for the weaning process. Recently, midazolam infusions have been associated with the development of ICU delirium in adults and children, but only small case series have reported this phenomenon in the NICU (87).

Like other GABA agonists, benzodiazepines have been associated with neuronal apoptosis in fetal and neonatal animal models, mediated predominately via the GABA receptor (88,89). The applicability of these data to humans is not clear, but further tempers enthusiasm for its use in preterm infants, particularly in high doses or during prolonged administration.

Barbiturates

Phenobarbital has long been used as an anticonvulsant in newborns and children, although its routine use for sedation has been discouraged because of several drawbacks. Phenobarbital has hyperalgesic effects and may increase the requirement for analgesia, and rapid tolerance to its sedative action invariably occurs. It has a prolonged elimination half-life in neonates (5 to 6 days), and it may increase the risk of IVH in premature neonates (90). Phenobarbital has no specific antagonist, and prolonged use is associated with microsomal induction of hepatic enzymes and with a withdrawal syndrome. Its advantages in neonates include increased bilirubin metabolism, relatively mild cardiovascular and respiratory depression, and familiarity with its usage in preterm and term neonates. In ventilated preterm neonates, the changes in mean arterial pressure and intracranial pressure associated with endotracheal suctioning were blunted with phenobarbital therapy (91).

A neonatal dose–response study found increasing degrees of sedation and feeding difficulties with increasing serum phenobarbital concentrations. These responses were greater in preterm neonates than in term neonates (92).

Pentobarbital is a shorter-acting barbiturate than phenobarbital, with a half-life of 19 to 34 hours in adults. It may be useful as an adjunct for sedation to safely maintain the airway of the intubated infant and child for whom tolerance has led to rapid escalations of narcotic and benzodiazepine infusions and boluses of these medications are no longer having a sedative effect. Pentobarbital is associated with both tolerance and withdrawal. Pentobarbital causes more hypotension than do most other sedatives used in the infant and child; slower bolus infusions over 15 to 30 minutes reduce this side effect. Pentobarbital is mixed in propylene glycol, and continuous infusions may precipitate metabolic acidosis and nephrotoxic effects, particularly in patients susceptible to renal injury.

Chloral Hydrate

Chloral hydrate is used frequently as a sedative for short procedures in neonates and infants. Although not practical for use in premature or sick newborns because of the lack of intravenous formulation, chloral hydrate has been used for many decades in term infants because of its lack of cardiovascular and respiratory side effects when used at usual therapeutic doses. Higher doses may be required after repeated use in neonates because of the slow development of tolerance, and repeated doses can be irritating to the enteral mucosa. Former preterm infants had significantly more bradycardia when sedated with chloral hydrate at term postconceptual age. The preterm infants also had a prolonged duration of sedation compared with term infants (93). Oxyhemoglobin desaturation after chloral hydrate for MRI was correlated with age in term infants and postconceptual age in former preterm infants (94). An infant who received several doses of chloral hydrate (165 mg/kg of chloral hydrate over 16 hours) developed the toxic reactions of respiratory depression and lethargy, suggesting a need for moderation in dosing (95).

The sedative action of chloral hydrate may be mediated by generalized neuronal depression, similar to other halogenated hydrocarbons. A precise mechanism of action is unknown, and there is no specific antagonist. The pharmacokinetics of chloral hydrate are not clearly defined in neonates. Onset of clinical effects after oral dosage occurs at 30 minutes, and its duration of action is usually 2 to 4 hours, depending on the exact doses used.

Ketamine

Ketamine is a dissociative anesthetic that has been used as an induction agent for anesthesia, analgesic for conscious sedation, premedication before induction of anesthesia, and sedative for critically ill patients. There is a broad range of experience with this agent in older patients but limited experience in infants and newborns. Ketamine has been used to provide anesthesia in the spontaneously breathing, nonintubated newborn and causes less neonatal neurobehavioral depression than does thiopental after maternal administration for vaginal delivery (96). Ketamine produces reliable serum levels within 1 minute when administered intravenously or within 5 minutes when administered intramuscularly, and it is rapidly redistributed, with awakening occurring in 10 to 15 minutes. In neonates, the elimination half-life is significantly longer than 130 minutes, which has been reported in older children and adults (97).

Ketamine is a potent stimulator of the cardiovascular system, presumably by means of central sympathetic effects and inhibition of catecholamine reuptake (98). Compared with isoflurane, halothane, and fentanyl, ketamine had the least effects on mean arterial pressure in ill preterm neonates undergoing surgery (99).

Pulmonary vascular resistance does not appear to be altered in infants with or without preexisting pulmonary hypertension (100). For critically ill patients with moderate hypovolemia, low doses of ketamine (i.e., 0.5 to 1 mg/kg) are safer than barbiturates as rapid induction agents before tracheal intubation.

Ketamine's mechanism of action is NMDA receptor blockade. During brain development in animal models, blockade of NMDA receptors can trigger apoptosis. Ketamine has been shown to cause neuronal apoptosis in a large number of newborn rodent and nonhuman primate animal studies, and this apoptosis is dose and duration dependent (101). Intranasal ketamine has been studied to facilitate delivery room intubation of preterm neonates, and neurodevelopmental outcomes at 2 years were not different for those receiving ketamine compared to control preterm infants who did not receive ketamine (102). Extrapolating from the animal data, however, use of ketamine in high doses or for prolonged periods in term and preterm neonates should be avoided.

Clonidine

Clonidine is an α2-adrenoreceptor agonist and, via activation of receptors in the locus coeruleus of the brain, leads to decreased sympathetic outflow and a resulting antihypertensive effect. In addition to antihypertensive actions, clonidine has both sedative and antinociceptive effects. The mechanisms for these effects are less well understood, but both appear to be mediated through α2-receptor action because they are blocked by α2-antagonist drugs (103). Animal data have shown that the same potassium channels activated by µ opioid receptor agonists are also activated by α agonists, and these effects seem to be mediated via different G proteins (104).

Clonidine has been used as a component of epidural anesthesia because of its synergistic effects with local anesthetics. In addition, oral or transdermal administration at initial doses of 5 µg/kg/d is useful as an adjunct for sedation of the critically ill infant and child. Transdermal delivery is limited in the neonate because the smallest patch (TTS-1 providing 100 µg/d) can be halved for the 10-kg child but cannot easily be quartered. An oral suspension of clonidine is not commercially available but can be prepared by guidelines in the literature; dosing of 5 µg/kg/d divided into two or three times per day is effective. Doses that provide sedative and analgesic effects without accompanying hypotension are easily achievable. The mild antihypertensive effect contributes to the usefulness of clonidine in combating narcotic, benzodiazepine, and barbiturate withdrawal syndromes.

Several groups have reported using clonidine in the management of neonatal abstinence. Small randomized controlled trials have shown that clonidine added to oral tincture of opium therapy or as a single agent compared with opiate treatment alone significantly shortened the length of therapy for NAS (105,106). Abrupt discontinuation of clonidine after long-term use may be associated with tachycardia, hypertension, irritability, tremor, and decreased sleep, and weaning is therefore recommended.

Dexmedetomidine

Like clonidine, dexmedetomidine is an α2-adrenoreceptor agonist that induces sedation via reduction of sympathetic outflow from the locus coeruleus. Dexmedetomidine also has analgesic effects that are mediated by increased release of substance P from the spinal cord. Unlike clonidine, dexmedetomidine is delivered as a continuous intravenous infusion. Like clonidine, dexmedetomidine has also been used as an adjunct for epidural and caudal anesthesia. Dexmedetomidine lacks the respiratory depressant effects of most sedatives and can be used in both intubated and extubated patients. Side effects of dexmedetomidine are predominantly hemodynamic and related to its adrenoreceptor actions (hypotension and bradycardia related to sympatholysis and hypertension related to vasoconstriction), are attenuated by avoiding bolus dosing of the drug, and resolve with reducing the infusion rate or discontinuance.

Continuous infusion of dexmedetomidine for sedation during mechanical ventilation in term and preterm infants has been studied by two groups and found to be safe and effective (107,108). The plasma clearance for dexmedetomidine is slower and the half-life longer in preterm infants compared with term infants and children (108). The addition of dexmedetomidine to low-dose fentanyl infusion improved the hormonal stress response to cardiac surgery in infants (3). Recently, the use of dexmedetomidine infusions for sedation during mechanical ventilation in the PICU and NICU has increased as intensivists attempt to avoid deliriogenic agents such as midazolam. Like clonidine, abrupt discontinuation of dexmedetomidine infusions for prolonged intubation has been reported to lead to withdrawal symptoms (tachycardia, hypertension, irritability, tremor, or decreased sleep) in the pediatric population, and therefore weaning or transition to clonidine for weaning is recommended (109).

Dexmedetomidine has been found to be neuroprotective in animal models of hypoxic–ischemic injury (110,111) and perinatal excitotoxic brain injury (112,113). Animal studies have also shown that dexmedetomidine may protect the infant brain from other neurotoxic anesthetic medications (114). The long-term effects of chronic α2-adrenoreceptor stimulation in term and preterm infants have not been evaluated.

SUMMARY

The proper approach to sedation and analgesia includes an individualized regimen, which ensures efficacy with careful consideration of the important pharmacokinetic and pharmacodynamic differences in the neonatal population. Analgesia and sedation are needed for neonates undergoing the painful and/or stressful procedures required for therapy in the operating room or NICU, and effective sedative and analgesic techniques are available that can be used in a variety of clinical circumstances. Given the burgeoning animal data regarding the potential neurotoxicity of almost all of the anesthetics, reliable pain scoring must be performed regularly to ensure that infants' pain and stress are adequately controlled but that doses and duration of sedatives and analgesics are not higher than needed. The number of painful procedures that infants are exposed to must also be controlled to the minimum required for safe and effective treatment, and nonpharmacologic therapies to control pain employed whenever possible. Finally, future studies of the safety and efficacy of analgesic and sedative medications in preterm and term infants should follow long-term neurodevelopmental outcomes in order to better inform our use of these medications.

REFERENCES

1. Anand KJ, Hansen DD, Hickey PR. Hormonal-metabolic stress responses in neonates undergoing cardiac surgery. *Anesthesiology* 1990;73:661.
2. Anand KJS, Hickey PR. Halothane-morphine compared with high-dose sufentanil for anesthesia and postoperative analgesia in neonatal cardiac surgery. *N Engl J Med* 1992;326:1.
3. Naguib AN, Tobias JD, Hall MW, et al. The role of different anesthetic techniques in altering the stress response during cardiac surgery in children: a prospective, double-blinded, and randomized study. *Pediatr Crit Care Med* 2013;14:481.
4. Taddio A, Katz J. The effects of early pain experience in neonates on pain responses in infancy and childhood. *Paediatr Drugs* 2005;7:245.
5. Roofthooft DW, Simons SH, Anand KJ, et al. Eight years later, are we still hurting newborn infants? *Neonatology* 2014;105:218.
6. Cong X, McGrath JM, Cusson RM, et al. Pain assessment and measurement in neonates: an updated review. *Adv Neonatal Care* 2013;13:379.
7. Carbajal R, Rousset A, Danan C, et al. Epidemiology and treatment of painful procedures in neonates in intensive care units. *JAMA* 2008;300:60.

8. Reynolds ML, Fitzgerald M, Benowitz LI. GAP-43 expression in developing cutaneous and muscle nerves in the rat hindlimb. *Neuroscience* 1991;41:201.
9. Fitzgerald M. A physiological study of the prenatal development of cutaneous sensory inputs to dorsal horn cells in the rat. *J Physiol* 1991;432:473.
10. Rizvi TA, Wadhwa S, Mehra RD, et al. Ultrastructure of marginal zone during prenatal development of human spinal cord. *Exp Brain Res* 1986;64:483.
11. Pignatelli D, Ribeiro-da Silva A, Coimbra A. Postnatal maturation of primary afferent terminations in the substantia gelatinosa of the rat spinal cord. An electron microscopic study. *Brain Res* 1989;491:33.
12. Anand KJ, Carr DB. The neuroanatomy, neurophysiology, and neurochemistry of pain, stress, and analgesia in newborns and children. *Pediatr Clin North Am* 1989;36:795.
13. Anand KJ, Hickey PR. Pain and its effects in the human neonate and fetus. *N Engl J Med* 1987;317:1321.
14. Klimach VJ, Cooke RW. Maturation of the neonatal somatosensory evoked response in preterm infants. *Dev Med Child Neurol* 1988;30:208.
15. Goksan S, Hartley C, Emery F, et al. fMRI reveals neural activity overlap between adult and infant pain. *Elife* 2015;4:e06356.
16. Anand KJ. Hormonal and metabolic functions of neonates and infants undergoing surgery. *Curr Opin Cardiol* 1986;1:681.
17. Walker SM. Biological and neurodevelopmental implications of neonatal pain. *Clin Perinatol* 2013;40:471.
18. Vinall J, Grunau RE. Impact of repeated procedural pain-related stress in infants born very preterm. *Pediatr Res* 2014;75:584.
19. Kuratani N. The cutting edge of neonatal anesthesia: the tide of history is changing. *J Anesth* 2015;29:1.
20. Morriss FH Jr, Saha S, Bell EF, et al. Surgery and neurodevelopmental outcome of very low-birth-weight infants. *JAMA Pediatr* 2014;168:746.
21. McCann ME, deGraaf JC, Dorris L, et al. Neurodevelopmental outcome at 5 years of age after general anaesthesia or awake-regional anaesthesia in infancy (GAS): an international, multicenter, randomized, controlled equivalence trial. *Lancet* 2019;393:664.
22. http://www.fda.gov/Drugs/DrugSafety/ucm532356.htm
23. Anand KJ, Sippell WG, Schofield NM, et al. Does halothane anaesthesia decrease the metabolic and endocrine stress responses of newborn infants undergoing operation? *Br Med J (Clin Res Ed)* 1988;296:668.
24. Anand KJ, Sippell WG, Aynsley Green A. Randomised trial of fentanyl anaesthesia in preterm babies undergoing surgery: effects on the stress response. *Lancet* 1987;1:62.
25. Gruber EM, Laussen PC, Casta A, et al. Stress response in infants undergoing cardiac surgery: a randomized study of fentanyl bolus, fentanyl infusion, and fentanyl-midazolam infusion. *Anesth Analg* 2001;92:882.
26. Friesen RH, Lichtor JL. Cardiovascular effects of inhalation induction with isoflurane in infants. *Anesth Analg* 1983;62:411.
27. Gregory GA. The baroresponses of preterm infants during halothane anaesthesia. *Can Anaesth Soc J* 1982;29:105.
28. Lunn JK, Stanley TH, Eisele J, et al. High dose fentanyl anesthesia for coronary artery surgery: plasma fentanyl concentrations and influence of nitrous oxide on cardiovascular responses. *Anesth Analg* 1979;58:390.
29. Young CJ, Apfelbaum JL. Inhalational anesthetics: desflurane and sevoflurane. *J Clin Anesth* 1995;7:564.
30. Loeckinger A, Kleinsasser A, Maier S, et al. Sustained prolongation of the QTc interval after anesthesia with sevoflurane in infants during the first 6 months of life. *Anesthesiology* 2003;98:639.
31. Hickey PR, Hansen DD, Wessel DL, et al. Pulmonary and systemic hemodynamic responses to fentanyl in infants. *Anesth Analg* 1985;64:483.
32. Hickey PR, Hansen DD, Wessel DL, et al. Blunting of stress responses in the pulmonary circulation of infants by fentanyl. *Anesth Analg* 1985;64:1137.
33. Ross AK, Davis PJ, Dear GD, et al. Pharmacokinetics of remifentanil in anesthetized pediatric patients undergoing elective surgery or diagnostic procedures. *Anesth Analg* 2001;93:1393.
34. Scott CS, Riggs KW, Ling K, et al. Morphine pharmacokinetics and pain assessment in premature newborns. *J Pediatr* 1999;135:423.
35. Bellu R, de Waal K, Zanini R. Opioids for neonates receiving mechanical ventilation: a systematic review and meta-analysis. *Arch Dis Child Fetal Neonatal Ed* 2010;95:F241.
36. Willschke H, Bosenberg A, Marhofer P, et al. Epidural catheter placement in neonates: sonoanatomy and feasibility of ultrasonographic guidance in term and preterm neonates. *Reg Anesth Pain Med* 2007;32:34.
37. Dohms K, Hein M, Rossaint R, et al. Inguinal hernia repair in preterm neonates: is there evidence that spinal or general anesthesia is the better option regarding intraoperative and postoperative complications? A systematic review and meta-analysis. *BMJ Open* 2019;9:e028728.
38. McCann ME, Withington DE, Arnup SJ, et al. Differences in blood pressure in infants after general anesthesia compared to awake regional anesthesia (GAS Study-A prospective randomized trial). *Anesth Analg* 2017;125(3):837.
39. Somri M, Matter I, Parisinos C, et al. The effect of combined spinal-epidural anesthesia versus general anesthesia on the recovery time of intestinal

function in young infants undergoing intestinal surgery: a randomized, prospective, controlled trial. *J Clin Anesth* 2012;24:439.

40. Shenkman Z, Hoppenstein D, Litmanowitz I, et al. Spinal anesthesia in 62 premature, former-premature or young infants—technical aspects and pitfalls. *Can J Anaesth* 2002;49:262.

41. Mahe V, Ecoffey C. Spinal anesthesia with isobaric bupivacaine in infants. *Anesthesiology* 1988;68:601.

42. Goeller JK, Bhalla T, Tobias JD. Combined use of neuraxial and general anesthesia during major abdominal procedures in neonates and infants. *Paediatr Anaesth* 2014;24:553.

43. Di Pede A, Morini F, Lombardi MH, et al. Comparison of regional vs. systemic analgesia for post-thoracotomy care in infants. *Paediatr Anaesth* 2014;24:569.

44. Cook B, Doyle E. The use of additives to local anesthetic solutions for caudal epidural blockade. *Paediatr Anaesth* 1996;6:353.

45. Fellmann C, Gerber AC, Weiss M. Apnoea in a former preterm infant after caudal bupivacaine with clonidine for inguinal herniorrhaphy. *Paediatr Anaesth* 2002;12:637.

46. Bouchut JC, Dubois R, Godard J. Clonidine in preterm-infant caudal anesthesia may be responsible for postoperative apnea. *Reg Anesth Pain Med* 2001;26:83.

47. Lonnqvist PA. Regional anaesthesia and analgesia in the neonate. *Best Pract Res Clin Anaesthesiol* 2010;24:309.

48. Butler-O'Hara M, LeMoine C, Guillet R. Analgesia for neonatal circumcision: a randomized, controlled trial of EMLA cream versus dorsal penile nerve block. *Pediatrics* 1998;101:E5.

49. Howard CR, Howard FM, Fortune K, et al. A randomized, controlled trial of a eutectic mixture of local anesthetic cream (lidocaine and prilocaine) versus penile nerve block for pain relief during circumcision. *Am J Obstet Gynecol* 1999;181:1506.

50. McIntosh N, van Veen L, Bramayer H. Alleviation of the pain of heelstick in preterm infants. *Arch Dis Child* 1994;70:F177.

51. Abad F, Diaz-Gomez NM, Domenech E, et al. Oral sucrose compares favourably with lidocaine-prilocaine cream for pain relief during venepuncture in infants. *Acta Paediatr* 2001;90:160.

52. Gradin M, Eriksson M, Holmqvist G, et al. Pain reduction at venipuncture in newborns: oral glucose compared with local anesthetic cream. *Pediatrics* 2002;110:1053.

53. Biran V, Gourrier E, Cimerman P, et al. Analgesic effects of EMLA cream and oral sucrose during venipuncture in preterm infants. *Pediatrics* 2011;128:e63.

54. Allegaert K, de Hoon J, Verbesselt R, et al. Maturational pharmacokinetics of single intravenous bolus of propofol. *Paediatr Anaesth* 2007;17:1028.

55. Rigby-Jones AE, Nolan JA, Priston MJ, et al. Pharmacokinetics of propofol infusions in critically ill neonates, infants, and children in an intensive care unit. *Anesthesiology* 2002;97:1393.

56. Welzing L, Kribs A, Eifinger F, et al. Propofol as an induction agent for endotracheal intubation can cause significant arterial hypotension in preterm neonates. *Paediatr Anaesth* 2010;20:605.

57. Parke TJ, Stevens JE, Rice AS, et al. Metabolic acidosis and fatal myocardial failure after propofol infusion in children: five case reports. *BMJ* 1992;305:613.

58. Committee on Safety of Medicines/Medicines Control Agency. Propofol (Diprivan) infusion: sedation in children aged 16 years or younger contraindicated. *Curr Probl Pharmacovigilance* 2001;27:10.

59. Anand KJ, Willson DF, Berger J, et al. Tolerance and withdrawal from prolonged opioid use in critically ill children. *Pediatrics* 2010;125:e1208.

60. Arnold JH, Truog RD, Scavone JM, et al. Changes in the pharmacodynamic response to fentanyl in neonates during continuous infusion. *J Pediatr* 1991;119:639.

61. Arnold JH, Truog RD, Orav EJ, et al. Tolerance and dependence in neonates sedated with fentanyl during extracorporeal membrane oxygenation. *Anesthesiology* 1990;73:1136.

62. Dewhirst E, Naguib A, Tobias J. Chest wall rigidity in two infants after low-dose fentanyl administration. *Pediatr Emerg Care* 2012;28:465.

63. Walker SM. Neonatal pain. *Paediatr Anaesth* 2014;24:39.

64. Grunau RE, Whitfield MF, Petrie-Thomas J, et al. Neonatal pain, parenting stress and interaction, in relation to cognitive and motor development at 8 and 18 months in preterm infants. *Pain* 2009;143:138.

65. Anand KJ, Hall RW, Desai N, et al. Effects of morphine analgesia in ventilated preterm neonates: primary outcomes from the NEOPAIN randomised trial. *Lancet* 2004;363:1673.

66. Collins E. Maternal and fetal effects of acetaminophen and salicylates in pregnancy. *Obstet Gynecol* 1981;58(suppl):57S.

67. Howard CR, Howard FM, Weitzman ML. Acetaminophen analgesia in neonatal circumcision: the effect on pain. *Pediatrics* 1994;93:641.

68. Shah V, Taddio A, Ohlsson A. Randomised controlled trial of paracetamol for heel prick pain in neonates. *Arch Dis Child Fetal Neonatal Ed* 1998;79:F209.

69. Wong I, St John-Green C, Walker SM. Opioid-sparing effects of perioperative paracetamol and nonsteroidal anti-inflammatory drugs (NSAIDs) in children. *Paediatr Anaesth* 2013;23:475.

70. Allegaert K, Naulaers G, Vanhaesebrouck S, et al. The paracetamol concentration-effect relation in neonates. *Paediatr Anaesth* 2013;23:45.

71. Ceelie I, de Wildt SN, van Dijk M, et al. Effect of intravenous paracetamol on postoperative morphine requirements in neonates and infants undergoing major noncardiac surgery: a randomized controlled trial. *JAMA* 2013;309:149.

72. Moffett BS, Wann TI, Carberry KE, et al. Safety of ketorolac in neonates and infants after cardiac surgery. *Paediatr Anaesth* 2006;16:424.

73. Dawkins TN, Barclay CA, Gardiner RL, et al. Safety of intravenous use of ketorolac in infants following cardiothoracic surgery. *Cardiol Young* 2009;19:105.

74. Aldrink JH, Ma M, Wang W, et al. Safety of ketorolac in surgical neonates and infants 0 to 3 months old. *J Pediatr Surg* 2011;46:1081.

75. Harrison D, Bueno M, Yamada J, et al. Analgesic effects of sweet-tasting solutions for infants: current state of equipoise. *Pediatrics* 2010;126:894.

76. Stevens B, Yamada J, Ohlsson A. Sucrose for analgesia in newborn infants undergoing painful procedures. *Cochrane Database Syst Rev* 2016;7:CD001069.

77. de Freitas RL, Kubler JM, Elias-Filho DH, et al. Antinociception induced by acute oral administration of sweet substance in young and adult rodents: the role of endogenous opioid peptides chemical mediators and mu(1)-opioid receptors. *Pharmacol Biochem Behav* 2012;101:265.

78. Carbajal R, Veerapen S, Couderc S, et al. Analgesic effect of breast feeding in term neonates: randomised controlled trial. *BMJ* 2003;326:13.

79. Pillai Riddell RR, Racine NM, Gennis HG, et al. Non-pharmacological management of infant and young child procedural pain. *Cochrane Database Syst Rev* 2015;12:CD006275.

80. Johnston C, Campbell-Yeo M, Disher T, et al. Skin-to-skin care for the procedural pain in neonates. *Cochrane Database Syst Rev* 2017;2:CD008435.

81. Anand KJ, Barton BA, McIntosh N, et al. Analgesia and sedation in preterm neonates who require ventilatory support: results from the NOPAIN trial. Neonatal outcome and prolonged analgesia in neonates. *Arch Pediatr Adolesc Med* 1999;153:331.

82. McPherson C, Grunau RE. Neonatal pain control and neurologic effects of anesthetics and sedatives in preterm infants. *Clin Perinatol* 2014;41:209.

83. Ng E, Taddio A, Ohlsson A. Intravenous midazolam infusion for sedation of infants in the neonatal intensive care unit. *Cochrane Database Syst Rev* 2017;(1):CD002052.

84. Kumar P, Denson SE, Mancuso TJ. Premedication for nonemergency endotracheal intubation in the neonate. *Pediatrics* 2010;125:608.

85. McLellan I, Douglas E. Midazolam withdrawal syndrome. *Anaesthesia* 1991;46:420.

86. Bergman I, Steeves M, Burckart G, et al. Reversible neurologic abnormalities associated with prolonged intravenous midazolam and fentanyl administration. *J Pediatr* 1991;119:644.

87. Groves A, Traube C, Silver G. Detection and management of delirium in the neonatal unit: a case series. *Pediatrics* 2016;137:e20153369.

88. Jevtovic-Todorovic V, Hartman RE, Izumi Y, et al. Early exposure to common anesthetic agents causes widespread neurodegeneration in the developing rat brain and persistent learning deficits. *J Neurosci* 2003;23:876.

89. Young C, Jevtovic-Todorovic V, Qin YQ, et al. Potential of ketamine and midazolam, individually or in combination, to induce apoptotic neurodegeneration in the infant mouse brain. *Br J Pharmacol* 2005;146:189.

90. Kuban KCK, Leviton A, Krishnamoorthy KS. Neonatal intracranial hemorrhage and phenobarbital. *Pediatrics* 1986;77:443.

91. Ninan A, O'Donnell M, Hamilton K, et al. Physiologic changes induced by endotracheal instillation and suctioning in critically ill preterm infants with and without sedation. *Am J Perinatol* 1986;3:94.

92. Gilman JT, Gal P, Duchowny MS, et al. Rapid sequential phenobarbital treatment of neonatal seizures. *Pediatrics* 1989;83:674.

93. Allegaert K, Daniels H, Naulaers G, et al. Pharmacodynamics of chloral hydrate in former preterm infants. *Eur J Pediatr* 2005;164:403.

94. Litman RS, Soin K, Salam A. Chloral hydrate sedation in term and preterm infants: an analysis of efficacy and complications. *Anesth Analg* 2010;110(3):739.

95. Laptook AR, Rosenfeld CR. Chloral hydrate toxicity in a preterm infant. *Pediatr Pharmacol (New York)* 1984;4:161.

96. Hodgkinson R, Marx GF, Kim SS, et al. Neonatal neurobehavioral tests following vaginal delivery under ketamine, thiopental, and extradural anesthesia. *Anesth Analg* 1977;56:548A.

97. Cook DR. Newborn anaesthesia: pharmacological considerations. *Can Anaesth Soc J* 1986;33:S38.

98. Lundy PM, Lockwood PA, Thompson G, et al. Differential effects of ketamine isomers on neuronal and extraneuronal catecholamine uptake mechanisms. *Anesthesiology* 1986;64:359.

99. Friesen RH, Henry DB. Cardiovascular changes in preterm neonates receiving isoflurane, halothane, fentanyl, and ketamine. *Anesthesiology* 1986;64:238.

100. Hickey PR, Hansen DD, Cramolini GM, et al. Pulmonary and systemic hemodynamic responses to ketamine in infants with normal and elevated pulmonary vascular resistance. *Anesthesiology* 1985;62:287.

101. Dong C, Anand KJ. Developmental neurotoxicity of ketamine in pediatric clinical use. *Toxicol Lett* 2013;220:53.

102. Elaouf C, Le Moing AG, Fontaine C, et al. Prospective follow-up of a cohort of preterm infants <33 WG receiving ketamine for tracheal intubation in the delivery room: neurological outcome at 1 and 2 years. *Arch Pediatr* 2018;25(4):295.

103. Drew GM, Gower AJ, Marriott AS. Alpha 2-adrenoceptors mediate clonidine-induced sedation in the rat. *Br J Pharmacol* 1979;67:133.

104. Suresh S, Anand KJS. Opioid tolerance in neonates: a state-of-the-art review. *Paediatr Anaesth* 2001;11:511.

105. Agthe AG, Kim GR, Mathias KB, et al. Clonidine as an adjunct therapy to opioids for neonatal abstinence syndrome: a randomized, controlled trial. *Pediatrics* 2009;123:e849.

106. Bada HS, Sithisarn T, Gibson J, et al. Morphine versus clonidine for neonatal abstinence syndrome. *Pediatrics* 2015;135(2):e383.

107. O'Mara K, Gal P, Wimmer J, et al. Dexmedetomidine versus standard therapy with fentanyl for sedation in mechanically ventilated premature neonates. *J Pediatr Pharmacol Ther* 2012;17:252.

108. Chrysostomou C, Schulman SR, Herrera Castellanos M, et al. A phase II/III, multicenter, safety, efficacy, and pharmacokinetic study of dexmedetomidine in preterm and term neonates. *J Pediatr* 2014;164:276.e1.

109. Shutes BL, Gee SW, Sargel CL, et al. Dexmedetomidine as single continuous sedative during noninvasive ventilation: typical usage, hemodynamic effects, and withdrawal. *Pediatr Crit Care Med* 2018;19:287.

110. Ma D, Hossain M, Rajakumaraswamy N, et al. Dexmedetomidine produces its neuroprotective effect via the alpha 2A-adrenoceptor subtype. *Eur J Pharmacol* 2004;502:87.

111. Zhu YM, Wang CC, Chen L, et al. Both PI3K/Akt and ERK1/2 pathways participate in the protection by dexmedetomidine against transient focal cerebral ischemia/reperfusion injury in rats. *Brain Res* 2013;1494:1.

112. Paris A, Mantz J, Tonner PH, et al. The effects of dexmedetomidine on perinatal excitotoxic brain injury are mediated by the alpha2A-adrenoceptor subtype. *Anesth Analg* 2006;102:456.

113. Degos V, Charpentier TL, Chhor V, et al. Neuroprotective effects of dexmedetomidine against glutamate agonist-induced neuronal cell death are related to increased astrocyte brain-derived neurotrophic factor expression. *Anesthesiology* 2013;118:1123.

114. Andropoulos D. Effect of anesthesia on the developing brain: infant and fetus. *Fetal Diagn Ther* 2018;43:1.

THE NEWBORN INFANT

25 The Preterm Infant

Jayashree Ramasethu

INTRODUCTION

A preterm birth is defined as one occurring before 37 completed weeks of gestation or fewer than 259 days from the first date of a woman's last menstrual period (LMP) (1).

Preterm births have been known since antiquity. Dionysus, the Greek god of fertility and wine, was thought to be preterm and require special care in a warm, humid cave (2). Hippocrates (c.460 to c.370 BCE) described causes of preterm birth as premature rupture of membranes, placental insufficiency, maternal diseases during pregnancy, young or advanced maternal or paternal age, multiple pregnancy, and maternal psychological problems. Hippocrates set the duration of normal pregnancy at 280 days or 9 months and the lower limit for survival at 182 days or 26 weeks, with the intensity of crying at birth predicting survival (2). Over the millennia, humans have tried to save preterm infants, using commonsense approaches like warmth and feeding by any means possible. Stories abound of babies surviving after being wrapped in cotton wool and fed with droppers and spoons. Although Stephane Tarnier is credited with inventing the first incubator for premature infants, based on a chicken incubator, modern perinatal care was born only when Pierre Budin, a Parisian obstetrician, focused on more comprehensive care of preterm infants. Professor Budin wrote *Le Nourrison*, a series of 10 lectures for medical students published in 1901, which was translated into "The Nursling: The Feeding and Hygiene of Premature and Full-Term Infants" in English in 1907. Budin's observations were perceptive and his recommendations on providing warmth, incubator care, use of maternal breast milk, managing cyanotic spells, and involving the mother in the baby's care remain relevant today (3).

Since the time of Budin in the late 1800s, progress in modern medicine has enhanced the survival of all neonates, including preterm infants substantially in high-income countries. However, globally, an estimated 2.5 million newborns die in the first 28 days of postnatal life. The vast majority of deaths occur in low- and middle-income countries (LMIC). Eighty percent of deaths occur in low birth weight infants, and two-thirds in preterms (4). In the United States, disorders related to prematurity and low birth weight account for 17% of infant deaths and are among the five leading causes of infant deaths (5). Disparities in survival of preterm infants occur not only between high- and low-income countries, but within high-income countries due to racial and socioeconomic inequalities. In the United States in 2018, infants born to non-Hispanic black women had the highest mortality related to short gestation and low birth weight (247.5 per 100,000 live births), compared to rates of 62.1 for babies born to white women and 80.6 for babies born to Hispanic women (5).

PREVALENCE

Accurate global estimates of preterm birth are prevented by inadequate national civil registration of live births and vital statistics, particularly in LMIC, as well as by misclassification of preterm births. Previous global estimates indicated that 1 in 10 live births worldwide was born preterm, and this figure is still fairly accurate although there are significant variations between countries. A more recent systematic review and modeling analysis estimated 10.6% (uncertainty interval 9.0 to 12.0) of live births worldwide were preterm in 2014, equating to 14.84 (12.65 to 16.73 million) live preterm births (6). Twelve million (81%) of these preterm infants were born in south Asia and sub-Saharan Africa (Table 25.1). Five countries, India, China, Nigeria, Bangladesh, and Indonesia, accounted for 6.6 million (55%) of preterm births. In Europe, preterm birth rates were estimated to be 8.7% (uncertainty interval 6.3 to 13.3). In the United States, the preterm birth rate was 10.02% in 2018, with significant racial and ethnic differences; the rate of preterm births among African American women was 14%, 50% higher than the rate of 9.09% among White women. The preterm birth rate was lowest among non-Hispanic Asian mothers (8.57%) (7).

Preterm delivery is a frequent complication of multiple gestation. In the United States, the 2018 twin birth rate was 32.6 per 1,000 births. Sixty percent of twins are born preterm, with almost 20% being born at less than 34 weeks of completed gestation. Among triplets and higher order multiples, rates of preterm birth approach 97% to 100% (7,8). Many of these multiple gestations are conceived through assisted reproductive technology (ART) (8), but even singleton pregnancies conceived through *in vitro* fertilization +/− intracytoplasmic sperm injection are at increased risk of preterm birth (9).

CLASSIFICATION

Preterm infants are classified by the WHO as extremely preterm (< 28 weeks of gestational age [GA]), very preterm (29 to 32 weeks of GA), and moderate to late preterm (32 to 37 weeks of GA) (10) (see Chapter 1). This last group is frequently divided into moderately preterm infants (32 to 33 weeks of GA) and late preterm infants (LPI) (34 weeks and 0 days to 36 weeks and 6 days of GA) (Table 25.2). In addition, infants are often classified by birth weight. Low birth weight infants (birth weight <2,500 g) may be term or preterm. Very low birth weight (VLBW, birth weight ≤1,500 g) and extremely low birth weight (ELBW, birth weight ≤1,000 g) infants are usually preterm, except for rare VLBW term infants with extreme intrauterine growth restriction. Table 25.3 shows the distribution of preterm births in the different categories in the United States.

Globally, it is estimated that 4.1% of preterm infants are born at <28 weeks of GA, 11.3% at 28 to 32 weeks, and 84.7% are born at 32 to <37 weeks of GA (6). International comparisons in rates of preterm birth in different categories are difficult to make because of differences in registration practices across countries. Differences in country- and institution-specific policies on viability, particularly at lower GA can influence whether an extremely preterm birth is recorded as a stillbirth or as a live birth. In a large population-based study involving more than 9 million births in 27 European countries, the United States, Canada, and Japan, very preterm birth (<32 weeks) rates ranged from 4.0 to 11.9 per 1,000 live births, with some, but not all, of the variability being accounted for by differences in registering babies born at 22 to 23 weeks of GA (11). These differences are likely to be more severe in LMIC, where thresholds of viability may be set at 28 weeks or more (8,12).

ASSESSMENT OF GESTATIONAL AGE

Traditionally, the first day of the LMP has been used to determine the estimated due date or the expected date of delivery (EDD) with

THE NEWBORN INFANT

TABLE 25.1

Estimated Preterm Birth Rates and Number of Preterm Births in 2014

	Estimated Preterm Birth Rate[a] (%)	Estimated Number of Preterm Births	Proportion of Global Preterm Births (%)
Asia	10.4	7,847,643	52.9
Sub-Saharan Africa	12.0	4,182,440	28.2
Latin America and the Caribbean	9.8	1,062,800	7.2
North Africa	13.4	773,687	5.2
Europe	8.7	690,931	4.7
North America	11.2	491,297	3.3
Oceania	10.0	64,227	0.4
Global	10.6	14,835,606	100

[a]Preterm births per 100 live births.

Reprinted from Chawanpaiboon S, Vogel JP, Moller A-B, et al. Global, regional, and national estimates of levels of preterm birth in 2014: a systematic review and modelling analysis. *Lancet Glob Health* 2019;7(1):e37. Copyright © 2019 Elsevier, with permission.

TABLE 25.3

Preterm Births in the United States in 2018 by race and Hispanic origin of mother

Gestational Age in Weeks	All Races	White	Black	Hispanic
<28	0.66	0.44	1.51	0.62
28–31	0.91	0.76	1.60	0.84
32–33	1.18	1.07	1.79	1.09
34–36	7.28	6.83	9.23	7.17
Total <37	10.02	9.09	14.13	9.73

Data expressed as percentage of total births.

Data from Centers for Disease Control. Final data for 2019 *National Vital Statistics Reports* 2019;68(13).

the EDD being 280 days after the first day of the LMP, assuming that ovulation occurred 14 days after the LMP. However, this does not account for inaccurate recall of the LMP, irregularities in cycle length, or variability in the timing of ovulation. If pregnancy resulted from ART, the ART-derived GA is used to assign the EDD. For instance, the EDD for a pregnancy that resulted from *in vitro* fertilization is assigned using the age of the embryo and the date of transfer.

In the absence of ART, ultrasound measurement of the embryo or fetus in the first trimester (up to and including 13 weeks and 6 days of gestation) with measurement of the crown–rump length is the most accurate method to establish or confirm GA with an accuracy around ±5 to 7 days (13). GA assessment by ultrasonography in the first part of the second trimester (between 14 weeks 0 days and 21 weeks 6 days of gestation) is based on a composite of fetal biometric measurements and has an accuracy of ±7 to 10 days. GA assessment by ultrasonography in the third trimester (28 weeks and 0 days of gestation and beyond) is the least reliable method, with an accuracy of ±21 to 30 days. The Best Obstetric Estimate—a combination of dating by the LMP and early ultrasound, rather than dating by LMP alone—is recommended for clinical care, research, and surveillance purposes (13). Other techniques of GA assessment during pregnancy such as measurement of fundal height, date of quickening, or recording of fetal heart tones have not been found to be reliable.

After birth, assessment of GA is performed by clinical examination of the infant (Chapter 17). Compared to term infants, preterm infants have heads that appear disproportionately larger than their bodies, thinner skin, softer cartilage in the pinnae, and fewer creases in the soles of their feet. Several scoring systems have been devised for more precise estimation of GA at birth, considering external

physical characteristics and neurologic signs of maturation (14). The Dubowitz score, based on a combination of 11 physical criteria and 10 neurologic signs, identified GA to within 5 days of LMP in the original study (15), but a recent review of several studies noted that when compared to ultrasound dating, the Dubowitz score dated 95% of pregnancies within ±2.6 weeks (14). The commonly used New Ballard score includes six neuromuscular and six physical criteria and includes evaluation of extremely preterm infants (16) (Fig. 17.3). Compared with ultrasound, the Ballard score overestimated GA (0.4 weeks) and dated pregnancies within ±3.8 weeks (14).

While these scoring systems offer the best accuracy, they take 15 to 20 minutes to perform and considerable skill and may not be realistic in low-resource areas where only 1 to 2 staff are caring for multiple infants or centers in LMIC, where assessment of GA may be performed by traditional birth attendants or community-based health workers. Among several anthropometric measures, a simple screening test such as measuring the length of the foot using a plastic ruler has been advocated to be used as a screening test to differentiate preterm from term infants in these situations but does not necessarily differentiate the preterm infant from the term small for GA newborn (17).

PROBLEMS OF PREMATURITY AND MANAGEMENT

Immaturity of structure and function makes the preterm infant susceptible to a multitude of problems that involve every organ system in the body and could fill more than one textbook. Table 25.4 lists the common problems in preterm infants and the chapters in this book that provide a detailed description of the pathophysiology and management of these conditions. The rest of this chapter will present an overview of these issues.

Before Delivery
Antenatal Corticosteroids

Administering corticosteroids to the mother before anticipated preterm birth is one of the most important measures to improve neonatal outcomes. Antenatal corticosteroids enhance fetal lung maturity and reduce the risk and severity of respiratory distress syndrome (RDS) by about 60%. They also produce reductions in need for mechanical ventilation, risk of intraventricular hemorrhage (IVH), necrotizing enterocolitis (NEC), and neonatal death (18). Antenatal corticosteroid therapy is recommended for all women between 24 and 34 weeks of gestation (and should be considered in women between 23 weeks 0 days and 23 weeks 6 days of gestation) who are at risk of preterm birth within 7 days and are most effective when administered at least 24 hours prior to delivery (19). Common regimens are two doses of betamethasone 12 mg given by intramuscular injection 24 hours apart or four doses of dexamethasone 6 mg given by intramuscular injection 12 hours apart. In retrospective analyses, compared to dexamethasone, antenatal betamethasone has been associated with reduced risk

TABLE 25.2

Classification of Preterm Infants

Nomenclature	Gestational Age in Completed Weeks
Extremely preterm	<28 wk and 6 d
Very preterm	29 wk and 0 d to 31 wk and 6 d
Moderately preterm	32 wk and 0 d to 33 wk and 6 d
Late preterm	34 wk and 0 d to 36 wk and 6 d
Low birth weight	≤2,500 g
Very low birthweight	≤1,500 g
Extremely low birth weight	≤1,000 g

wk, weeks; d, days.

TABLE 25.4				
Problems of Preterm Infants				
	Early Problems	**Chapter Number**	**Late Complications**	**Chapter Number**
At birth	Delayed transition	15		
	Perinatal depression	16		
General	Thermoregulation	25		
Respiratory system	Respiratory distress syndrome	28	Bronchopulmonary dysplasia	29
	Pulmonary hemorrhage	28	Sudden infant death syndrome	27
	Apnea of prematurity	27		
Cardiovascular system	Hypotension	31		
	Patent ductus arteriosus	31		
Gastrointestinal system	Feeding problems and nutritional support	19	Metabolic bone disease	20
	Gastroesophageal reflux	20	TPN cholestasis	37
	Necrotizing enterocolitis	36	Short gut syndrome	36
Renal	Fluid and electrolyte imbalance	19		
	Acute kidney injury	38		
Hematologic	Anemia of prematurity	42		
	Neutropenia	43		
	Thrombocytopenia	44		
	Hyperbilirubinemia	45		
Infectious disease	Early-onset sepsis	47		
	Hospital-acquired infection	22		
Central nervous system	Intraventricular hemorrhage	50	Neurodevelopmental delay	9
	Cerebellar hemorrhage			
	Periventricular leukomalacia			
	White matter injury			
	Retinopathy of prematurity	58		

for neonatal death with trends of decreased risk for IVH and severe retinopathy of prematurity (ROP), but either steroid is preferable to none at all. Repeated regular courses of antenatal steroids are not recommended as they are associated with growth impairment and developmental delay. However, in specific circumstances, clinicians may opt to give a course of "rescue steroids" if preterm birth remains likely and a prior course of steroids was some weeks ago (e.g., a likely preterm delivery at 27 weeks where steroids were last given at 23 to 24 weeks). The administration of antenatal steroids has been associated with significantly higher survival rates and survival without major morbidities even in periviable infants 22 to 25 weeks of GA, although survival without major morbidities remains low at 22 and 23 weeks (20).

Antenatal steroids have also been recommended for women at risk of late preterm singleton births (at a gestation between 34 weeks 0 days and 36 weeks 6 days) within the next 7 days (but before 37 weeks of gestation), with definite evidence of preterm labor or definitive plan for preterm delivery (21). The antenatal late preterm steroids trial found that treatment with two doses of antenatal betamethasone was associated with significant decrease in need for respiratory support within the first 72 hours (11.6% in the betamethasone group vs. 14.4% in the placebo group) and significant decreases in the rates of severe respiratory morbidity but was associated with increased rates of hypoglycemia in the newborn (24% in the betamethasone group vs. 14.9% in the placebo group) (22).

Antenatal steroids have been included in the United Nations list of lifesaving commodities for women and children and have been recommended by the WHO for women at risk for preterm birth. However, the Antenatal Corticosteroids Trial (ACT), a cluster randomized trial in rural and semiurban areas that included almost 100,000 women in six LMIC (Argentina, Guatemala, India, Pakistan, Kenya, and Zambia), did not show the expected reduction in neonatal mortality; there was an excess of 3.5 neonatal deaths per 1,000 women exposed to steroids and an increase in the risk of maternal infection (23). Therefore, the role of antenatal steroids in LMIC remains uncertain, particularly where assessment of GA and care for preterm infants and their mothers may be suboptimal. Further efficacy trials are required in low-resource settings to inform practice.

Magnesium Sulfate

Observations of lower rates of cerebral palsy in preterm infants born to mothers who had received magnesium sulfate for tocolysis or prevention of seizures in preeclampsia led to numerous trials of magnesium for neuroprotection of the fetus. Meta-analysis of the trials showed significant decreases in rates of cerebral palsy in preterm infants born to mothers who received magnesium sulfate prior to delivery. It is now recommended by the WHO and several professional societies for women in preterm labor for fetal neuroprotection (24). The GA cutoff for administration of magnesium sulfate for women in preterm labor is variable; it is <30 weeks in Australia, New Zealand, and the United Kingdom and <32 weeks in Canada; no GA is specified in the United States. The WHO recommends magnesium sulfate in all women in preterm labor up to 33 weeks and 6 days. Magnesium sulfate is postulated to prevent injury to progenitor oligodendrocytes by acting as an N-methyl-D-aspartic acid (NMDA) receptor antagonist, reducing calcium influx into cells, decreasing free radical activity, and attenuating cytokine or excitatory amino acid–induced cell damage (24).

Other measures that may have an impact on the survival and outcomes of preterm infants are the use of tocolysis for the short-term prolongation of pregnancy to allow for the administration of antenatal steroids and the appropriate use of selected antibiotics to prevent infection in preterm premature rupture of membranes (25).

Place of Delivery

For over 40 years, delivery of VLBW or very preterm infants has been recommended to be at level 3 perinatal units, which have the staffing levels and equipment to manage these fragile and complex newborns in the most appropriate manner. Birth outside a level 3 hospital has been associated with increased likelihood of neonatal or predischarge death (26,27). In a study of 72,431 VLBW infants, birth at a hospital with 10 or fewer deliveries of VLBW infants per year was associated with the highest risk-adjusted probability of death (15.3% [95% CI, 14.4% to 16.3%]), death or severe IVH (17.5% [95% CI, 16.5% to 18.6%]), and death or NEC (19.3% [95% CI, 18.1% to 20.4%]) (28). An observational cohort study in England showed that in extremely preterm infants <28 weeks GA, birth in a nontertiary hospital followed by a transfer to a higher level of care within 48 hours was associated with decreases in mortality but significantly higher odds of severe brain injury (2.32, 1.78 to 3.06; number needed to treat [NNT] 8) and significantly lower odds of survival without severe brain injury (0.60, 0.47 to 0.76; NNT 9) (29). When high-risk preterm deliveries occur outside a tertiary center, the presence of a skilled dedicated retrieval team improves the quality of neonatal resuscitation by increasing intubation success, achieving earlier vascular access and decreasing rates of hypothermia (30).

Mode of Delivery

The optimal method of delivery for preterm infants is undecided. Although spontaneous vaginal births do occur, preterm birth may be indicated in conditions like preeclampsia, fetal growth restriction, premature rupture of membranes, chorioamnionitis, etc. In these situations, cesarean deliveries may be performed because of fear of prolonged induction or concern for fetal intolerance of labor. The overall rate of preterm cesarean deliveries is increasing and now approaches 50%, particularly for very preterm infants. Some guidelines recommend cesarean delivery for fetal indications like persistently abnormal fetal heart tracing or biophysical profile or fetal malpresentation for preterm infants beyond 25 weeks of GA, and to consider C-section at GA 23 weeks and 0 days to 24 weeks and 6 days, but not before 23 weeks (31). It is unclear if delivery by C-section improves neonatal outcomes in preterm infants in cephalic presentation (32), whereas significant decreases in neonatal mortality and severe IVH have been noted in extremely preterm singletons in breech position delivered by C-section (33). There are increased maternal risks with C-section at these early gestations including the need for a classical C-section, with potential increased risk of uterine rupture in subsequent pregnancies, so decisions have to be individualized.

At Delivery

Delayed Cord Clamping and Cord Milking

At birth, approximately a third of the baby's blood is in the placenta. Delaying cord clamping (DCC) by 30 to 180 seconds to allow transfusion of placental blood into the newborn has been shown to be beneficial for the preterm newborn. When compared to immediate cord clamping, DCC has been associated with improved blood pressure, decreased use of blood transfusions, decreased rates of NEC and IVH, and decreased mortality in preterm infants (34). Although DCC has been associated with reduction in IVH, it does not appear to impact severe grades of IVH. One recent large controlled trial of delayed versus immediate cord clamping in preterm infants <30 weeks GA showed that the mortality in the DCC group was 6.4% versus 9% in the immediate clamping group (p = 0.03 in unadjusted analysis), but after post hoc adjustments for multiple secondary outcomes, the differences were not significant (35). Concerns about potential delays in resuscitation led to trials of umbilical cord milking, where the cord is milked three times from

the placenta toward the baby prior to clamping. Meta-analysis of five small trials found umbilical cord milking to be beneficial (36), but a recent randomized controlled trial showed increased rates of severe IVH in very preterm infants 23 to 27 weeks of GA who had received cord milking in interim analysis, and the trial was halted early (37). DCC until the onset of ventilation has been shown to improve cardiovascular function in preterm lambs (38). Assisting ventilation in preterm infants prior to clamping the umbilical cord appears to be physiologically sound but is fraught with challenges, and there is little evidence at present about whether providing respiratory support to preterm infants before cord clamping improves outcomes (39). At the time of writing, supporting preterm infants to transition while attached to placental circulation for 1 to 3 minutes during delayed cord clamping is recommended (unless the infant is asphyxiated) but milking the cord is not. A number of resuscitation platforms have been introduced, which support initial care of the newborn with thermoregulation and respiratory support without the need for immediate cutting of the cord.

The "Golden Hour"

Problems and interventions in the first hour of life, now frequently called the golden hour (40,41), have immediate and perhaps long-term consequences, particularly for the very preterm newborn. Resuscitation and stabilization in the first minutes after birth in a preterm infant, particularly in an extremely preterm infant, should be a carefully coordinated and choreographed event, using all available evidence and expertise to make the transition as smooth as possible. The presence of infection due to chorioamnionitis or chronic fetal hypoxemia due to placental insufficiency may predispose the preterm newborn infant to delayed transition at birth. In addition to possible surfactant deficiency, the extremely preterm infant has weak chest muscles that limit ventilation, and a poor respiratory drive. Very preterm infants often require assisted ventilation and oxygen to establish lung aeration and a functional residual capacity. Immature thin skin with minimal subcutaneous fat, and evaporation of amniotic fluid from the surface may cause hypothermia within minutes. Table 25.5 delineates the elements of the golden hour, and Figure 6.6 provides a flowchart of management of infants' ≤32 weeks of gestation in the first hour of life. Although many interventions in the golden hour pertain to the very preterm infant, the principles of rapid stabilization of respiratory status, prevention of hypoglycemia, and temperature control are applicable to larger preterm infants as well. Preparations should be made prior to the delivery to have the necessary equipment and a team of members experienced in neonatal resuscitation who can work together in a coordinated manner to stabilize the infant efficiently and effectively. Although several actions need to be performed simultaneously or in quick succession, the need to be gentle and supportive to the fragile infant cannot be

TABLE 25.5

Components of the Golden Hour

1	Delayed cord clamping	Infection prevention
2	Respiratory support	
3	Prevention of hypothermia/thermal support	
4	Cardiovascular support	
5	Nutritional support and prevention of hypoglycemia	
6	Laboratory and radiologic investigations	
7	Treatment of suspected infection	
8	Communication with the family	
9	Documentation	

Note: Antenatal counseling and team/equipment preparation occur prior to the golden hour.

overemphasized. Implementation of golden hour protocols have been shown to decrease rates of hypothermia, hypoglycemia, and time to completion of stabilization and decrease rates of bronchopulmonary dysplasia (BPD) and late-onset sepsis (42,43).

Temperature Control

The newborn infant does not shiver and relies on nonshivering thermogenesis to regulate body temperature in the normal range. Brown adipose tissue (BAT) is a uniquely mammalian tissue that plays a key role in thermogenesis in the human newborn (44). BAT accumulates in fetal life, with volumes peaking at the time of term birth. Deposits of this capillary and mitochondrial rich tissue envelop the kidneys and adrenal glands and are present in the interscapular region and the mediastinum. It was previously thought that BAT involutes during neonatal life and disappears after infancy, until studies using positron emission tomography showed it was still present in adults, sparking considerable research on its role in lipid metabolism and prevention of obesity. In the newborn, cutting the umbilical cord at birth and exposure to the colder extrauterine environment stimulates the release of catecholamines, specifically norepinephrine, which, via β-adrenergic receptors in BAT causes fatty acid oxidation and thermogenesis. Mitochondria in BAT express a unique protein, UCP 1, uncoupling protein, or thermogenin that promotes free flow of protons across the inner mitochondrial membrane, thereby uncoupling oxidation from adenosine diphosphate phosphorylation, producing heat from metabolic fuels like glucose and free fatty acids. The optimal response of BAT to norepinephrine is dependent on thyroid hormone. BAT contains a 5'-monoiodothyronine deiodinase that deiodinates T4-T3 locally.

The preterm infant is poorly equipped to maintain temperature after birth. Heat loss from the body occurs through evaporation of amniotic fluid that covers the surface of the infant at birth, through conduction on contact with cold surfaces, via convection currents around the body and through radiation to the surrounding surfaces (Fig. 16.2). The preterm infant has a large surface area in relation to body weight, little insulating fat, decreased deposits of brown fat, thin immature skin that leads to increased evaporative losses, lower glycogen stores, and often delays in establishing enteral or parenteral nutrition. The necessity for close observation of respiratory status by the neonatal team, application of monitoring devices and therapeutic procedures may inadvertently worsen heat loss.

The WHO classifies hypothermia as mild for a core body temperature for newborns between 36°C and 36.4°C, moderate as 32°C to 35.9°C, and <32°C as severe (45). Hypothermia on admission to the NICU is a common problem both in high income and in LMIC, particularly in the smallest and most immature infants. Despite decreases, nearly 4 in 10 VLBW infants were cold on admission to one of the 1,112 NICUs in the Vermont Oxford Network between 2009 and 2016 (46). Hypothermia on admission to the NICU has been related to increased mortality with a 28% increase in mortality with each 1°C decrease in temperature, and increased risks of RDS, IVH, and late-onset sepsis (47,48). Routine precautions to prevent hypothermia in delivery rooms include increasing the ambient temperature, drying the infant thoroughly after birth, removing wet linens, and wrapping the infant (including the head) in dry prewarmed blankets, prewarming surfaces, and preventing draughts. In VLBW infants, the use of plastic wraps or bags to quickly cover the baby to reduce evaporative heat loss (without drying the baby) has been shown to decrease the risk of hypothermia when compared to conventional methods (49). Exothermic chemical mattresses containing sodium acetate gel that can be activated to produce heat have been used to prevent hypothermia but can cause hyperthermia in preterm newborns (50).

Following transfer to the NICU or special care nursery, the very preterm infant is usually nursed in an incubator or a radiant warmer. Over 60 years ago, Silverman showed the improved survival of preterm infants in incubators when normothermia was maintained (51). Incubators have become increasingly sophisticated, providing automated servocontrolled temperature settings, humidity controls, weighing scales, and phototherapy options, and their costs have also escalated to that of mid-size cars. Infants are nursed in a neutral thermal environment, the range of ambient temperature required for an infant to maintain a normal body temperature with minimal metabolic stress. The neutral thermal environment is dependent on age and weight with smaller and younger infants requiring a higher ambient temperature to maintain core temperature between 36.5°C and 37.5°C with the mean core and skin temperature fluctuating less than 0.2°C and 0.3°C, respectively (52). Incubators provide the benefit of a closed environment with regulated humidity, important for the extremely preterm infant who has significant insensible water loss through the thin, nonkeratinized, gelatinous skin in the first weeks of life (53). However, they do have a low-grade hum, with sound levels inside the closed incubator ranging from 53 dB to 68 dBA, which exceed the current recommended maximum sound level of 45 dBA for noise levels in the NICU (54). Open warmers provide easy access to the infant for care and procedures but are associated with increased insensible water loss and a need for increased fluid intake (55).

In resource-limited environments, few facilities have access to incubators. Even in regional referral hospitals, open warmers are preferred to incubators for reasons of cost and ease of maintenance, particularly for disinfection between patients (56). One small trial of cot nursing using heated water–filled mattresses showed increased rates of hyperthermia in infants weighing 1,300 to 1,500 g, when compared to incubator care (57). There have been several attempts to produce low-cost/low-tech incubators for LMIC. The NeoNurture, a low-cost incubator built of used car parts, made it to the 50 Best Inventions of 2010 in Time magazine, but did not find acceptance in the community (www.designthatmatters.org). Low-cost warmers using phase change materials can keep infants warm for short periods of time and may be used as an addition to skin to skin care, for transporting infants or help correct hypothermia (58).

Early bathing soon after delivery is common practice in many communities but should be avoided in preterm infants in whom it can result in significant heat loss. The WHO recommends a "warm chain" a series of 10 interlinked steps to prevent hypothermia in the newborn. This includes warming the delivery room, immediate drying, skin to skin care, early and exclusive breast-feeding, postponing bathing, appropriate clothing and bedding, placing mother and baby together and in institutions, warm resuscitation, warm transportation, and training and raising awareness.

Kangaroo mother care (KMC) was introduced in Bogota, Colombia in 1978 as an alternative to incubators for low birth weight infants. KMC has four components—early, continuous, and prolonged skin to skin contact (SSC) between the newborn and the mother, exclusive breast-feeding, early discharge from the health facility, and close follow-up at home. Meta-analysis of numerous trials performed since its inception has shown that KMC is effective in decreasing the incidence of hypothermia in LBW infants and is associated with lower mortality (59).

Respiratory Problems

Lung development starts in the human fetus at about 4 to 6 weeks of gestation as a ventral outpouching of the primitive foregut into the surrounding ventral mesenchyme. Further branching of the airway forms the bronchial tree with the first 16 airway generations being completed by 16 weeks in humans, and further branching occurring by 16 to 24 weeks. Histologically, lung development and maturation has been divided into four stages. The pseudoglandular stage (5 to 17 weeks in human fetus) is too immature to support gas exchange. The canalicular stage (between 16 and 25 weeks) is characterized by rapid expansion of the respiratory tree with development of terminal bronchioles, respiratory bronchioles, and alveolar ducts, accompanied by vascularization and angiogenesis along the airway. During the terminal saccular stage (24 weeks to late fetal period), there is thinning of the interstitium, increasing formation of a capillary and lymphatic network, and differentiation of alveolar epithelial cells into mature squamous Type 1 pneumocytes and secretory rounded Type II pneumocytes that synthesize and secrete surfactant, a complex substance that lowers surface tension and prevents atelectasis. Surfactant is a complex of dipalmitoylphosphatidylcholine, phosphatidylglycerol, and surfactant proteins A, B, C, and D. The alveolar stage is the last step of lung development and forms the bulk of the gas exchange surface. Alveolarization begins at about 20 weeks and is well established by 40 weeks (term gestation) but continues until 7 to 8 years of age in humans. Maturation of the surfactant system increases between 30 weeks and term in humans. See also Chapter 28.

Respiratory distress syndrome due to the deficiency of surfactant is the leading cause of respiratory insufficiency in preterm infants. RDS is characterized by labored breathing, grunting, retractions, and cyanosis with radiologic features of a diffuse ground glass opacification with an air bronchogram. In the presurfactant era, the respiratory distress typically worsened during the first few days after birth secondary to progressive atelectasis, and then, in surviving infants, improved gradually as the lungs started to produce surfactant. The incidence of RDS increases with decreasing GA, occurring in 80% of infants born at 28 weeks of GA and in 90% of infants born at 24 weeks of GA. The treatment of RDS comprises oxygen therapy, administration of exogenous surfactant, and assisted ventilation, in the form of either noninvasive ventilation using nasal continuous positive airway pressure (CPAP) or nasal intermittent positive pressure ventilation (NIPPV) or intubation and conventional or high-frequency ventilation.

Surfactant

The treatment of RDS has been revolutionized in recent decades by exogenous surfactant therapy, which, along with antenatal steroids to stimulate surfactant production may be credited with much of the increase in survival of extremely preterm infants. Animal-derived natural surfactants have been shown to be superior to synthetic surfactants, with faster weaning of respiratory support and shorter duration of ventilation, although newer synthetic surfactants are beginning to show promise (60). The administration of surfactant currently requires tracheal intubation, an invasive procedure with a risk of hypoxemia and bradycardia in vulnerable infants, and continued ventilation though an endotracheal tube may inflict barotrauma and volutrauma to the developing immature lungs.

A drive to avoid the potential risks of intubation for surfactant delivery led to several randomized multicenter trials examining the use of early CPAP with surfactant administration only in the presence of treatment failure in extremely preterm infants. This approach results in lower rates of BPD/death when compared to prophylactic or early surfactant therapy, and this is the current recommendation in the United States and Europe (61,62). Nevertheless, CPAP failure occurs in 45% to 50% of high-risk infants in the first week of life, with failure rates approaching 60% at 25 to 26 weeks of GA (63). If it is likely that respiratory support will be needed, early administration of surfactant followed by rapid extubation appears preferable to prolonged ventilation (Intubation–Surfactant–Extubation or INSURE).

Less invasive surfactant administration techniques in which spontaneously breathing preterm infants continue to receive CPAP without intubation and surfactant is administered by small diameter feeding tubes or vascular catheters placed directly into the trachea with visualization using a laryngoscope has been shown to result in less need for mechanical ventilation in infants with RDS, and a decrease in the composite outcome of death or BPD

at 36 weeks, lower incidence of BPD among the survivors, and a decreased incidence of IVH (64). While nebulized surfactants are tantalizing options, they have not reached mainstream use at the time of writing. A simpler approach, of dosing surfactant into the oropharynx on the basis that it will distribute over all air–surface interfaces (including the lungs) is another interesting, but as yet unproven approach.

Oxygen

Oxygen is lifesaving in infants with respiratory distress but may also be toxic, with risks of ROP and other oxidant injury. Five international randomized controlled trials to determine appropriate oxygen saturation targeting in extremely preterm infants demonstrated increased risks of death or major disability in infants in the 85% to 89% oxygen saturation target group versus 91% to 95% oxygen saturation group. The American Academy of Pediatrics now recommends a target oxygen saturation of 90% to 95% in ELBW infants (65), and the European consensus guidelines recommend 90% to 94% oxygen saturation targets, with alarm limits being set to 89% and 95% in preterm infants receiving oxygen (62).

Apnea of Prematurity

Immaturity of the respiratory control system results in respiratory pauses of variable duration in preterm infants. The decreased respiratory drive results in hypoventilation or cessation of respiration or apnea. Definitions of what is considered significant apnea vary. Generally, an apneic spell is defined as cessation of breathing for 20 seconds or longer, or a shorter pause of 10 to 15 seconds accompanied by bradycardia (<100 beats per minutes) or desaturation. Apnea may be classified as central (cessation of inspiratory effort), obstructive (upper airway obstruction in the pharynx or larynx with chest wall motion but without airflow), or mixed. The majority of events in preterm infants are mixed. Apnea of prematurity (AOP) is due to altered ventilatory responses to hypercapnia, hypoxia, and laryngeal afferents (66). Almost all preterm infants born at <28 weeks of GA exhibit AOP. The incidence of AOP decreases to 20% of those born at 34 weeks of GA, with few infants born at 35 to 36 weeks of GA being affected. The frequency of events decreases postnatally with maturation, with resolution of apnea at 40 weeks in 98% of preterm infants. However, AOP may not resolve until 43 weeks postmenstrual age in infants born at 24 to 26 weeks and those with BPD (67). AOP and its relation to sudden infant death syndrome are discussed in Chapter 27.

Continuous cardiorespiratory monitoring is standard in NICUs for infants born at less than 35 weeks of GA, with monitor alarms generally set at 20 seconds for apnea and 100 bpm for bradycardia. The duration of pulse oximetry is variable in NICUs, with some continuing to monitor infants until discharge and others discontinuing pulse oximetry after the infant has demonstrated stability in room air for variable periods of time. Xanthines and CPAP are used to treat AOP. Xanthines act through blockade of adenosine A_1 receptors and A_{2A} receptors with excitation of respiratory neural output, with resultant increased minute ventilation, decreased periodic breathing, and decreased hypoxic depression of breathing (68). Nasal CPAP splints open the upper airway and reduce the frequency and severity of apnea in preterm infants. Of the xanthines, caffeine is preferred to theophylline because of its longer half-life and higher therapeutic index. Drug levels do not need to be routinely monitored. Initiation of therapy before 3 days of age may be beneficial (68). Results of the Caffeine for AOP trial showed that caffeine treated infants had a shorter duration of mechanical ventilation; lower incidence of BPD, PDA, and severe ROP; and decreased neurodevelopmental disability at 18 months (69). However, follow-up of the VLBW patients in the study at 11 years of age showed that there was no difference in the combined rate of academic, motor, and behavioral impairments, but surprisingly, caffeine therapy was associated with a reduced risk of motor impairment (70). There are no definitive recommendations on when to discontinue xanthine treatment in preterm infants. Approaches include discontinuing caffeine after the infant has been event free for 5 to 7 days or when the infant is at 34 weeks postmenstrual age, with continued monitoring for events for 5 to 7 days after discontinuation.

Bronchopulmonary Dysplasia

In preterm infants born prior to 28 weeks of gestation, in addition to the deficiency of surfactant, there is insufficiency of the gas exchange surface, with only alveolar ducts and alveolar buds with which to breathe. In addition, the vascular and lymphatic components of the lung are poorly developed. Premature delivery and exposure to oxygen, positive pressure ventilation, sepsis, and inflammation all result in disruption of the normal development of the lung, resulting in chronic lung disease or BPD (71). Clinical criteria for BPD include an assessment of oxygen requirement at ≥28 days and at 36 weeks of postmenstrual age (PMA). Mild BPD is defined as the need for supplemental oxygen at ≥28 days but not at 36 weeks PMA, moderate BPD as the need for supplemental oxygen at 28 days and at 36 weeks PMA with the fraction of inspired oxygen being ≤0.30 at 36 weeks, and severe BPD as the need for supplemental oxygen at 28 days and at 36 weeks with the fractional inspired oxygen ≥0.3 or with mechanical ventilation (72). BPD affects a quarter of VLBW infants. Improvements in management of VLBW infants have resulted in stable rates of BPD, although increases in survival of the most immature infants have prevented the rates from declining substantially. The highest rates of BPD are in the smallest, most immature infants; 57% incidence in infants weighing 501 to 750 g, 32% at 751 to 1,000 g, 14% at 1,001 to 1,250 g, and 6% at 1,251 to 1,500 g being reported in the United States National Institute of Child Health (NICHD) Neonatal Network sites during the period 1997 to 2002, with significant intercenter variability in BPD rates, reflecting practice variations (73). Among the measures that decrease the incidence of BPD are noninvasive respiratory support, caffeine, and intramuscular Vitamin A. Noninvasive ventilation including nasal CPAP, nasal intermittent mandatory ventilation, and less invasive surfactant administration has been associated with reductions in the incidence of BPD in extremely preterm infants. Caffeine has a role in prevention of BPD, probably by reducing the requirement for mechanical ventilation and improving extubation success, in addition to a diuretic effect and potentially by direct anti-inflammatory activity. The role of Vitamin A in preventing BPD remains controversial. Vitamin A is essential for normal respiratory epithelial development and repair. Some studies have shown a reduction in BPD in preterm infants who received intramuscular Vitamin A, but the effect was modest. Due to the need for frequent IM injections, few units use Vitamin A. Trials of oral Vitamin A are under way. Treatment of BPD is primarily supportive with fluid management, nutritional support, judicious use of diuretics, and occasionally, postnatal steroids. (See Chapter 29 Bronchopulmonary dysplasia.) Infants with BPD are at increased risk for postneonatal mortality, higher rates of rehospitalization, asthma, pulmonary hypertension, growth failure, and neurodevelopmental delays (73).

Cardiovascular System

Major physiologic changes occur in the circulatory system during the transition from fetal to neonatal life. Clamping of the umbilical cord and loss of the low-resistance placental circulation result in increased systemic vascular resistance and an increase in left ventricular afterload. Aeration of the lungs leads to pulmonary arterial vasodilation and a decrease in pulmonary vascular resistance. The increase in systemic vascular resistance and decrease in pulmonary vascular resistance redirect right ventricular output into the pulmonary vascular bed, thus ensuring that left ventricular preload is maintained by adequate pulmonary vascular venous return. The right ventricular preload is dependent on systemic vascular return and the right ventricular afterload is low because of decreasing pulmonary vascular resistance. Flow across the ductus arteriosus becomes left to right within the first 24 hours of life. In term infants, flow through the ductus ceases within 48 hours because of ductal constriction secondary to increase in arterial oxygen tension and decrease in prostaglandin levels postnatally.

The extremely preterm infant has significant challenges in making these transitions after birth, with risk of hemodynamic instability (74). Systolic performance is impaired by inefficient contractility, diastolic performance is limited by poorly contractile collagen in the myocardium, and left ventricular filling is shortened by relative tachycardia. The thin walled and less muscular ductus arteriosus in preterm infants fails to constrict and remains patent longer. Left-to-right shunting across the ductus arteriosus and a patent foramen ovale causes pulmonary overcirculation and compromises systemic blood flow. Increased pulmonary venous return to the left atrium may result in increased left atrial pressure, pulmonary venous congestion, and pulmonary hemorrhage in some infants. Low systemic blood flow on the first day of life is common in infants <30 weeks of gestation, particularly if they are on mechanical ventilation with high mean airway pressures (75).

The major cardiovascular problems in preterm infants are hypotension and patent ductus arteriosus, but like term infants, they may also have congenital cardiac malformations and cardiac arrhythmias.

Hypotension and Circulatory Failure

Early hypotension, often occurring on the day of birth has been reported in 15% to 50% of extremely preterm infants. Antenatal steroids, delayed cord clamping, and noninvasive ventilation are all associated with higher blood pressures and lower incidence of hypotension. The definition of hypotension in a preterm newborn is controversial as is the management of low blood pressure (74,76). The "normal" mean blood pressure in the first few days of life is approximately equivalent to the GA (e.g., 25 mm Hg at 25 weeks GA, 27 mm Hg at 27 weeks GA, etc.) and rises subsequently. This has often been used as the threshold for intervention, although there is little evidence to support this. First, the accurate measurement of blood pressure should be emphasized. Compared with intra-arterial methods, measurement of systolic, diastolic, and mean arterial pressure by oscillometric methods are less accurate, particularly in neonates with mean arterial pressure <30 mm Hg (77). Hypotension after the first week of life in preterm infants is usually in association with sepsis or other severe illness.

Reliance on blood pressure alone to assess cardiovascular and circulatory stability in preterm infants is simplistic, since it does not take systemic vascular resistance and systemic blood flow into account, and these determine organ perfusion. Bedside measures used like prolonged capillary fill times, increasing acidosis or signs of reduced organ perfusion such as oliguria are helpful but may be late indicators. There is increasing expertise and use of bedside echocardiography to determine cardiac output and superior vena caval flow and near-infrared spectroscopy to measure cerebral blood flow. See Chapter 31.

If hypotension is felt to be associated with circulatory compromise, the most common intervention used in preterm neonates is volume expansion using 10 mL/kg of normal saline infused over 30 to 60 minutes. However, this provides only a transient rise in mean arterial pressure. The next intervention is the addition of inotropic support, usually with dopamine or dobutamine. Other medications like epinephrine, milrinone, vasopression, or hydrocortisone may be used, and each has its own efficacy and safety profile.

Patent Ductus Arteriosus

Spontaneous closure of the ductus arteriosus is delayed in preterm infants. A PDA is clinically diagnosed in 1/3 of infants less than 30 weeks of GA and in 60% of infants <28 weeks of GA. The median time to closure ranges from 71 days for infants born at <26 weeks of GA to 6 days for infants born at >30 weeks of GA (78). Left-to-right shunting across the PDA with resultant pulmonary congestion and systemic "steal" during this period may have a contributory role in the pathogenesis of IVH, BPD, NEC, and mortality, although cause–effect relationships are not established. Most preterm infants with PDAs have no early clinical signs. A long systolic murmur may be evident with a hyperdynamic precordium and bounding pulses, but these signs are not always present. Increased pulmonary blood flow is associated with increasing respiratory distress and increasing ventilator support or oxygen requirements. Echocardiography is the preferred tool for diagnosis and assessing the hemodynamic significance of the ductus arteriosus (79). See Chapter 31.

Treatment strategies for hemodynamically significant PDAs are variable and range from conservative management to pharmacologic prophylaxis/treatment and/or surgical ligation. Pharmacologic treatment is with indomethacin, ibuprofen, or paracetamol. Meta-analyses of PDA treatment have not shown consistent improvement in outcomes, but the trials have been weakened by open-label rescue treatment and by variation in timing and modalities of treatment (80). In a retrospective study of 39,096 VLBW infants born at 24 to 28 weeks of GA in 2007 to 2015 in 139 NICUS in 6 countries, treatment for PDA ranged from 13% to 77% with overall treatment rate of 45%. The relationship between the ratio of observed and expected PDA treatment and the primary outcome of death or severe neurologic injury was U shaped, showing that both high- and low-PDA treatment rates were associated with death or severe neurologic injury, whereas a moderate approach was associated with optimal outcomes (81). Targeted echocardiography may help identify and monitor hemodynamically significant PDAs, allowing definitive treatment in selected patients at highest risk (80), although whether this would translate to improved outcome is uncertain.

Fluids/Electrolytes/Nutrition

Clamping the umbilical cord abruptly discontinues the steady supply of glucose, protein, and other nutrients essential for growth and development the fetus was receiving constantly from the mother through the placenta. Unlike the term infant, the preterm infant has decreased glycogen stores, gluconeogenesis, and glycogenolysis, making the infant susceptible to hypoglycemia. Metabolic demands for maintaining temperature and for growth are increased. The incidence of hypoglycemia in preterm infants is reported to be 30% to 60%, particularly affecting those who are small for GA or have intrauterine growth restriction (82). In very preterm infants, increased insensible water loss through the immature thin skin (Fig. 19.4) can rapidly cause dehydration and hypernatremia. Immature renal function compounds these problems, with altered nephrogenesis, low glomerular filtration rates in the early days of life, and immature tubular function impacting fluid and electrolyte balances (83).

The mode of provision of nutrition for the preterm infant after birth is determined by GA and clinical illness. The very preterm infant or one who is critically ill often does not tolerate enteral nutrition and invariably requires parenteral alimentation, while more mature or stable infants may be managed with enteral nutrition. Immaturity of coordination of suck, swallow, and breathing patterns compromise breast- or bottle-feeding (84). Although much of the anatomical development of the gastrointestinal tract is complete by 20 weeks, increases in the absorptive area, functional and biochemical maturation impacting intestinal motility and digestion occur primarily in the third trimester, making the preterm infant susceptible to feeding intolerance (85). Increased gastric residuals, gastrointestinal dysmotility, and gastroesophageal reflux are common in preterm infants.

Optimal early nutrition, starting in the first few days of life, is essential for normal brain development and has the potential to improve neurodevelopmental outcomes in preterm infants (86). Early continuous glucose infusions provide a constant source of energy to the brain and vital organs and prevent hypoglycemia. The addition of amino acids from the day of birth prevents a catabolic state and is positively correlated with neurodevelopmental outcomes. Intravenous lipid emulsions provide a major energy source and essential fatty acids.

Early introduction of enteral feeding enhances intestinal motility, integrity, and growth. Very preterm infants are fed using nasogastric or orogastric tubes, with small aliquots of milk administered every 2 to 3 hours as bolus feeds or as a continuous feed. Volumes are increased gradually until full feeds are attained at a volume of 150 to 160 mL/kg/d; and volumes up to 180 to 200 mL/kg/d are usually well tolerated for infants receiving breast milk. Oral feeding, usually bottle feeding with occasional breast-feeding attempts, is generally initiated at 32 to 34 weeks of corrected gestation and advanced as tolerated. Early initiation of oral feeding has been associated with earlier discharges from the NICU.

In LMIC, the use of cup feeding is encouraged in preterm infants unable to breast-feed. The traditional "paladai," a metal cup with a spout, has been used in Southern India to cup feed infants for centuries. The modern NIFTY cup, made by a collaboration between PATH and Laerdal Global health has a similar design principle, is constructed of soft silicone, and is being widely used in parts of Africa to help preterm babies feed (https://www.path.org/articles/a-lifesaving-investment).

Maternal breast milk is the optimal food for feeding preterm infants because of its easy digestibility, excellent tolerance, and added immunologic and neurodevelopmental benefits (87). Banked pasteurized donor milk is increasingly used in NICUs when mother's milk is not available. However, human milk, and particularly donor milk, has inadequate levels of protein and minerals to meet the requirements of growing preterm infants and is often fortified with cow's milk or human milk–based fortifiers for appropriate growth in infants who weigh less than 1,800 g at birth (88). Very preterm infants require fortification of feeds postdischarge from the NICU for several months to maintain adequate growth. In LMIC, where milk fortifiers may be unavailable or too expensive to use, the volume of milk given may be increased to 200 to 300 mL/kg/d and many preterm infants are able to tolerate this and grow. Chapter 20 addresses both enteral and parenteral nutrition in the preterm infant.

Necrotizing Enterocolitis

NEC, a devastating inflammation of the intestine, leading to necrosis of the small intestine and colon occurs in 5% to 9% of extremely preterm infants. It presents with feeding intolerance, vomiting, lethargy, abdominal distension and tenderness, and occasionally, bloody stools. The classical radiologic features are pneumatosis intestinalis or portal venous gas. The disease may progress rapidly leading to intestinal perforation and/or gangrene, peritonitis, and death. Mortality is more than 50% in patients who require surgery, and short gut is not an uncommon outcome in survivors. Although the cause of NEC is not known, associations have been noted with prolonged antibiotic therapy suggesting that perturbations of the intestinal microbiome, or dysbiosis in preterm infants is the underlying cause (89). Associations have also been noted with red blood cell (RBC) transfusions, although it is unclear if the underlying severe anemia or the transfusion is the problem (90). The risk of NEC is lower in preterm infants fed maternal breast milk, and the use of probiotics to counteract intestinal dysbiosis is advocated in some countries (91).

Spontaneous Intestinal Perforation

Spontaneous intestinal perforation (SIP) is a serious complication that occurs in the first week of life in infants weighing <1,000 g and <28 weeks of gestation (92). Patients with SIP present with bluish discoloration of the abdomen and radiographs show pneumoperitoneum. While it may not be an entirely distinct process from that seen in NEC, SIP is an isolated perforation, usually in the antimesenteric border of the terminal ileum, a watershed area that is prone to local ischemia. A deficiency of the muscularis propria has been noted in a quarter of the cases. Risk factors associated with increased incidence of SIP in preterm infants include maternal preeclampsia, chorioamnionitis, *in utero* growth restriction, and postnatally, the use of indomethacin and steroids in the first week of life. Early enteral feeding may have a protective role in preventing SIP (92).

See Chapter 36 for further discussion of NEC and similar diagnoses.

Iron Deficiency

Preterm infants have low iron stores at birth, due to truncation of transplacental iron transport that occurs in the last trimester of pregnancy. Maternal iron deficiency in pregnancy, intrauterine growth restriction, maternal smoking, diabetes mellitus, and preeclampsia are additional causes of low fetal iron stores, which manifests as low ferritin levels in cord blood, while hemoglobin levels remain within the normal range (93). Without iron supplementation, iron stores in nontransfused preterm infant will sustain erythropoiesis only until about 2 months of age and stores may be depleted even earlier in ELBW infants. Iron deficiency during the perinatal period has an impact not only on hemoglobin levels but also on the developing brain, with immediate and long-term effects on neurodevelopment, some of which may not be reversed with repletion of iron stores. Prevention of iron deficiency is vital. Preterm infants should receive 2 to 4 mg of enteral iron per day, starting 2 to 4 weeks after birth. Infants receiving recombinant erythropoietin (EPO) therapy should receive at least 6 mg/kg/d. Intravenous iron is generally not recommended because of the risks of oxidative stress.

Hematologic Problems
Anemia of Prematurity

The hemoglobin level of preterm infants at birth increases with GA, rising from 14.5 g/dL at 24 weeks to 18 g/dL by 36 weeks (Table 42.3). After birth, hemoglobin levels decline in term and in preterm infants due to decreased endogenous EPO production in the first few weeks of life, reduced RBC life span, and increased plasma volume associated with growth. The decline leads to physiologic anemia in term infants by 3 months of age. In preterm infants, the decline results in a condition called anemia of prematurity, which is usually more severe, and is exacerbated by phlebotomy losses for laboratory investigations, particularly in very preterm infants or by oxidative hemolysis secondary to nosocomial infections. The nadir of hemoglobin levels may be as early as 6 weeks of age in a relatively well moderate or LPI. Anemia of prematurity is characterized by normochromic, normocytic anemia with low hemoglobin levels and disproportionately low reticulocyte counts. Recovery is signaled by increasing reticulocyte counts, followed by rising hemoglobin levels. The management of anemia of prematurity is primarily supportive, providing adequate nutrition and minimizing blood draws for laboratory investigations. Although the bone marrow is responsive to exogenous EPO, and treatment with EPO reduces the use of RBC transfusions, it has not been shown to eliminate the need for transfusions in critically ill preterm infants (94). Packed RBC transfusions are provided in critically ill preterm infants, but thresholds for transfusions remain controversial. Delayed cord clamping has been shown to increase hemoglobin levels in preterm infants and decrease the need for transfusions.

Thrombocytopenia

Platelet counts less than 150,000/μL occurs in 18% to 35% of all infants admitted to the NICU. Preterm infants are at increased risk of thrombocytopenia with rates approaching 70% to 80% in the most immature infants (95). Early-onset thrombocytopenia, occurring within 3 days of birth, is associated with maternal preeclampsia, intrauterine growth restriction, perinatal asphyxia, early-onset sepsis, or congenital infections such as cytomegalovirus. Thrombocytopenia occurring after the 3rd day (late onset) is usually secondary to late-onset bacterial sepsis, particularly Gram-negative or fungal sepsis, NEC, or central line–related vascular thrombosis. The evaluation and treatment of thrombocytopenia is discussed in detail in Chapter 44.

Neutropenia

Neutropenia is defined as an absolute neutrophil count less than 1,000/μL and severe neutropenia as less than 500/μL. Neutropenia is a frequent problem in VLBW infants in the NICU, affecting up to 50% of infants (96). In premature infants, early-onset neutropenia, noted at birth, is often secondary to pregnancy induced hypertension or placental insufficiency due to any cause and is particularly notable in preterm infants who are small for GA. This form of neutropenia recovers spontaneously within 3 to 4 days, and usually within a week. Late-onset neutropenia occurs in preterm infants with anemia, who have significant reticulocytosis at about 4 to 8 weeks of age and is probably secondary to the shift to erythropoiesis in the bone marrow. In this situation, neutropenia is not usually severe, there is no left shift and it resolves spontaneously. Both early- and late-onset sepsis, particularly with Gram-negative organisms and NEC, can be associated with severe neutropenia, which improves as the condition resolves.

Hyperbilirubinemia

Unconjugated hyperbilirubinemia is common in preterm infants, due to an increased bilirubin load, secondary to breakdown of senescent red cells that have a shorter life span in preterm infants, decreased hepatic uptake of bilirubin from plasma, and delayed bilirubin conjugation. High total bilirubin levels can result in increased mortality and bilirubin-induced neurologic dysfunction (BIND), a form of neurodevelopmental impairment associated with auditory neuropathic and visuomotor processing disorders (97). The preterm brain appears to be more susceptible to BIND due to additional risk factors such as hypoalbuminemia, infection, inflammation, or other central nervous system insults. Some preterm infants with modest total bilirubin levels can sustain long-term neurodevelopmental disability, termed low bilirubin kernicterus, making close monitoring and treatment of hyperbilirubinemia in preterm infants essential. Symptoms of bilirubin encephalopathy in preterm infants are subtle and may manifest simply as recurrent apnea or may be hard to distinguish from other symptoms in critically ill infants (98). Visual evaluation of jaundice is inaccurate, particularly in small preterm infants. Monitoring by blood testing is required, although increasingly transcutaneous bilirubin testing devices are being used to reduce blood sampling (99). Guidelines for phototherapy and exchange transfusion to decrease bilirubin levels and prevent BIND in preterm infants based on gestational and postnatal age have been developed by consensus in several countries (100,101). Table 45.7 is an example but practitioners are advised to adhere to intervention thresholds that apply in the country in which they are practising. In ELBW infants, aggressive early phototherapy reduces peak bilirubin levels and rates of neurodisability but has been associated with increased mortality (102), so phototherapy must be used judiciously in these infants.

Infectious Disease

Immunologic immaturity, including quantitative and qualitative deficiency of immunoglobulins, decreased cell-mediated immunity

TABLE 25.6

Incidence of Early-Onset Sepsis and Mortality in Preterm Infants in Comparison to Term Infants in the United States

Gestational Age in Weeks	Incidence of Early-Onset Sepsis per 1,000 Live Births	Mortality
≥37	0.5	1.6%
34–36	1.0	Data not reported
<34	6.0	Data not reported
<29	20	30%
22–24	32	50%

Data from Stoll, *Pediatrics* 2011; Stoll *JAMA* 2015; and Schrag, *Pediatrics* 2016.

and decreased complement levels together with immature mucosal barriers make the preterm infant particularly susceptible to bacterial sepsis, viral, and fungal infections (103). The incidence of early-onset sepsis defined as a positive blood or cerebrospinal fluid culture obtained within 72 hours of birth is much higher in preterm infants and is associated with a higher mortality than in term infants, with the most immature infants being extremely vulnerable (Table 25.6). In a study of 109 cases of EOS occurring among 5,313 VLBW infants over a 25 year period, 97% of the cases occurred in infants born to mothers with premature rupture of membranes or preterm labor or concern for intra-amniotic infection, with two cases of infection with listeriosis occurring in the context of unexplained fetal distress (104).

The clinical signs of EOS are nonspecific, with respiratory distress, hypothermia, tachycardia, and hypotension being the most common signs and often difficult to differentiate from the common noninfectious problems of prematurity (105). Apnea, lethargy, or irritability have also been noted. When risk factors for sepsis or clinical signs are present, drawing of blood for cultures, either from the umbilical cord at the time of delivery or from the infant after birth is essential for making an accurate diagnosis and for appropriate therapy. White blood cell counts and C reactive protein levels have inadequate sensitivity and specificity to rule in or rule out EOS. *Escherichia coli* are the most common bacteria isolated in preterm infants with EOS in the United States followed by Group B streptococcus (105). Ampicillin and gentamicin are the most commonly used empiric antibiotics while blood culture results are awaited, with changes in the antibiotic regimen being based on culture and sensitivity results (105,106). Recent data from a prospective surveillance study of EOS from 2015 to 2017 showed that only 22.2% of *E. coli* isolates were sensitive to ampicillin and 7.8% were resistant to both ampicillin and gentamicin (105). Guidelines have been recommended to reduce inappropriate and prolonged use of antibiotics in preterm infants (107). The risk of infection is significantly lower in preterm infants who are born by cesarean section with membrane rupture at delivery and without clinical chorioamnionitis, so empiric antibiotics could be avoided in these infants. The evaluation and management of infants with early-onset sepsis is discussed in detail in Chapter 47.

Late-onset sepsis or sepsis diagnosed after 72 hours of age is usually hospital-acquired infection, and the preterm infant is again vulnerable because of poor skin and mucosal integrity and the invasive procedures like endotracheal intubation and central line placements. The rate of infections is inversely proportional to GA, with LOS rates close to 40% in infants born at 24 weeks of GA and 8% in infants born at 28 weeks of GA (108). In LPIs, the incidence of LOS is reported to be 6.3 episodes per 1,000 NICU admissions (109). The most common infections are central line–associated bloodstream infections, ventilator-associated infections, skin and soft tissue infections, and urinary tract infections. Coagulase-neg-

ative staphylococci are the most common cause of catheter-associated bloodstream infections, while Gram-negative infections are seen with ventilator-associated pneumonia and urinary tract infections. In addition, outbreaks of disease with multidrug-resistant organisms are not uncommon in NICUs and disproportionately affect preterm neonates.

In LMIC, Gram-negative infections with *Klebsiella* and *Acinetobacter* predominate, with a high incidence of multidrug-resistant organisms even in infants with EOS (110,111). A study of EOS in 25 tertiary care NICUS in China showed that Gram-negative infections were responsible for 61.7% of EOS, with *E. coli* as the leading pathogen. Group B streptococcal infections accounted for only 2.5% of infections in China (112), but some centers in India have shown an increasing incidence of Group B streptococcal infection (113).

In addition to bacterial infections, the possibility of viral or protozoal infection should be considered in preterm infants. Congenital infections due to HIV, cytomegalovirus, rubella, herpes, syphilis, toxoplasma, malaria, and Chagas disease are covered in Chapter 46. Respiratory syncytial virus (RSV), influenza and parainfluenza viruses, and rhinovirus can result in escalation of respiratory support and prolong duration of stay in hospitalized infants or result in hospitalization of preterm infants who are at home (114,115). Rotavirus, adenovirus, and norovirus have been responsible for outbreaks of gastrointestinal illness in NICU patients and have been implicated in clusters of cases of NEC (116). Human parechovirus infections can present with sepsis-like syndromes, indistinguishable from bacterial infection, and with symptoms of meningoencephalitis (117).

Preterm infants born at less than 35 weeks GA are at increased risk of hospitalization, requiring ICU care or mechanical ventilation secondary to RSV infection (118). RSV immunoprophylaxis with palivizumab is recommended for preterm infants born at less than 29 weeks of GA who are less than 12 months old at the start of the season; for older preterm infants, RSV immunoprophylaxis is currently recommended in preterm infants of >29 weeks of GA only if they have evidence of chronic lung disease or congenital heart disease (119). Immunoprophylaxis reduces hospitalization rates and severity of illness.

Central Nervous System

There is a fourfold increase in the size of the brain in the third trimester of gestation with formation of sulci, gyri, development of neural circuitry, and myelination. Preterm infants are at increased risk of sustaining brain injury or dysmaturation and having altered neurodevelopment (see Chapters 9 and 50). The most important acquired brain lesions in preterm infants are germinal matrix/intraventricular hemorrhage (GM/IVH), cerebellar hemorrhage, and both cystic and diffuse white matter injury (WMI).

Germinal Matrix Hemorrhage/Intraventricular Hemorrhage

The germinal matrix is a richly vascularized collection of neuronal glial precursors, located over the head of the caudate nucleus and under the ventricular ependyma (120). It reaches its maximum volume around 25 weeks of gestation and then involutes gradually, disappearing by about 34 to 36 weeks of GA. The vasculature is composed of a network of thin walled capillaries that are prone to rupture and is connected to the deep Galenic venous system. Bleeding into the germinal matrix may break through the ependyma into the ventricles. Germinal matrix/intraventricular hemorrhage (IVH) occurs in 20% to 25% of VLBW infants, with the highest incidence and greatest severity in extremely preterm infants. IVH is rarely noted beyond 32 weeks of gestation. In addition to prematurity, hemodynamic instability, severe respiratory disease, pneumothorax, and chorioamnionitis are other risk factors.

IVH usually occurs in the first week of life, with 50% being noted on day 1 and 90% of lesions being identified by 72 hours of life. Progression of bleeding may occur within 1 to 3 days. IVH is usually asymptomatic or associated with subtle signs but major grades of IVH may have a catastrophic presentation with decerebrate posturing, apnea, bradycardia, and stupor accompanied by rapidly falling hematocrit and acidosis. Ultrasound scans are used for detection and classification of IVH, and current protocols recommend frequent scans on day 1, day 3, day 7, day 14, day 21, etc. for early detection of IVH and following progression (121). A detailed description of the classification of GM/IVH is given in Chapter 50 (121). Posthemorrhagic ventricular dilation (PHVD) may occur due to obstruction and hypersecretion of cerebrospinal fluid. This complication of IVH is more common with the severe grades of IVH and is associated with increased mortality and severe neurodevelopmental disability (122). Early intervention with serial lumbar punctures is recommended to reduce the need for ventriculoperitoneal shunts and to improve outcomes (123). Posthemorrhagic ventricular infarction is also associated with increased mortality and risk of neurodevelopmental disability (124). Treatment options for PHVD are discussed in Chapter 53.

The most important measure for prevention of IVH in the very preterm infant is administration of antenatal corticosteroids (18). Delayed cord clamping has been shown to reduce IVH but not severe IVH (34). In addition, a nursing intervention bundle consisting of maintaining the head in the midline, tilting the head of the incubator to 30 degrees, avoidance of flushing/rapid withdrawal of blood and avoiding sudden elevation of the legs was associated with reduced risk of developing new or progressive GM/IVH, cystic periventricular leucomalacia, and/or mortality when applied to very preterm infants during the first 72 hours of postnatal life (125).

Cerebellar Hemorrhage

The cerebellum increases in volume fivefold, and its surface area increases 30-fold between 24 and 40 weeks of gestation. Cerebellar hemorrhages are being increasingly recognized in extremely preterm infants when using the mastoid window to perform cranial ultrasound scans. The incidence of cerebellar hemorrhage in very preterm infants ranges from 2% to 9%; more hemorrhages are detected by brain MRI scans. The hemorrhages may be single, or several punctate lesions may be present in both cerebellar hemispheres or a large lesion in one hemisphere. Cerebellar hemorrhages are associated with motor problems as expected, but also with cognitive and behavioral deficits, and impaired language skills (126).

White Matter Injury

While parents and practitioners focus on IVH in the first 3 days of life in the preterm infant and heave a sigh of relief if there is none, there is a more insidious form of brain injury called WMI in preterm infants that is harder to detect and results in significant neurodevelopmental problems even in infants without IVH. Better neuroimaging techniques and advances in neuropathology have led to an understanding of WMI in the preterm brain. WMI is initiated by a combination of ischemia and inflammation, often due to maternal intrauterine infection or postnatal sepsis, leading to primary destructive disease and secondary maturational disturbances in the rapidly developing brain (127). WMI takes several forms. Cystic periventricular leukomalacia (PVL) consist of focal necrosis with significant destruction of axons and glia deep in the periventricular white matter and is associated with secondary loss of neurons and developing gray matter. These cysts evolve over days or weeks and may be visualized by cranial ultrasound scans. This type of injury has declined in the last decade and is seen in less than 5% of VLBW infants currently. Focal necrosis may also be microscopic (<1 mm in size) and evolve into glial scars, but these

are not detected by ultrasound scans. The most common form is diffuse WMI, which is characterized by chronic diffuse gliosis composed of activated astrocytes and microglia. Diffuse WMI targets the oligodendrocyte lineage with selective degeneration of preoligodendrocytes with impaired myelination as the end result. Since these dysmaturational events take place over a long period of time, there may a window of opportunity to intervene and provide "neurorestoration" by appropriate nutrition, minimizing pain and stress, and pharmacologic measures (127). Diffuse WMI is detected by MRI scans performed at term equivalent age, but subtle changes are recognized only by special techniques.

Vision and Retinopathy of Prematurity

Normal retinal vascular development in the fetus occurs mainly in the second and third trimesters *in utero*, reaching maturity by 36 to 40 weeks of GA. Oxygen tension is low in the fetus *in utero* and retinal angiogenesis proceeds at an orderly pace, stimulated by vasoactive factors, primarily vascular endothelial growth factor (VEGF), produced locally and insulin-like growth factor-1 (IGF-1), supplied by the mother through the placenta. The immature retinal vasculature is extremely sensitive to hyperoxia and other insults. After preterm delivery, when oxygen saturations rise to 80% to 100%, even in room air, compared to the 50% to 70% saturation *in utero*, retinal vascularization is inhibited by down-regulation of VEGF production, leading to vasoconstriction and a vaso-obliterative phase, which begins at birth and continues until around 32 weeks PMA. As the retina continues to grow and have an increased metabolic demand, the avascular area of the retina experiences relative hypoxia, which stimulates increased activity of VEGF, which with rising IGF-1 levels, results in excessive aberrant blood vessel growth at the interphase between the vascular and avascular retina, the vasoproliferative phase, which starts at about 30 to 32 weeks and peaks at 36 to 38 weeks. The neovascularization extends into the vitreous and results in hemorrhage, fibrous bands, macular dragging (see Fig. 58.18), and in severe cases, retinal detachment (128). The clinical spectrum of ROP ranges from spontaneous regression in milder stages to progression to bilateral retinal detachment and blindness. Prematurity and hyperoxia due to supplemental oxygen are major risk factors for ROP, but sepsis, blood transfusions, low postnatal weight gain, and lack of breast milk also play a role. ROP can be detected only by retinal examinations, which are performed at regular intervals to diagnose the condition and determine the severity of disease progression. Recommendations for screening vary in different countries. Table 52.2 shows American Academy of Pediatrics recommendations for age of first ROP screening, and Table 58.3 shows the stages of ROP. Figure 58.17 shows a schematic representation of the zones of the retina. Treatment of ROP is by laser photocoagulation or by injection of VEGF inhibitors like bevacizumab. Vitrectomy or scleral buckling may be performed for advanced ROP to salvage some vision (see Chapter 58).

In 2010, the annual incidence of blindness and visual impairment from ROP was estimated to be 32,200 cases worldwide, with the greatest burden in the middle-income countries, where the "third epidemic" of ROP is currently raging. In many LMIC, more mature and larger infants develop severe ROP, probably secondary to unregulated oxygen use. The National Neonatology Forum in India recommends screening infants born at <34 weeks of GA and or weighing <1,750 g, and also screening more mature (34 to 36 weeks of GA) and larger (1,750 to 2,000 g) infants if they have risk factors. Tele-ROP screening services are being developed to deal with the shortages in ophthalmologists trained in evaluating ROP, but equally important is the prevention of ROP by titrating oxygen use, prevention of infection, and optimizing care of preterm infants (129).

In addition to ROP, preterm infants are at risk for myopia and amblyopia and require close follow-up until school age.

Hearing

In large studies of children born extremely preterm, rates of severe or profound hearing loss are about 2.5%, which is almost 10 times higher than rates of hearing loss in term infants (130). Population studies show the rate of hearing loss is inversely proportional to GA, with an incidence of 2.46% in very preterm infants <32 weeks GA, 0.85% in moderately preterm infants, and 0.56% in LPIs, all significantly higher than 0.35% in term infants (131). Intracranial hemorrhage, seizures, and administration of ototoxic medications have been noted to be risk factors associated with hearing loss. Testing by automated auditory brain stem response (AABR) rather than by otoacoustic emissions (OAE) is recommended for screening newborn infants who are in the NICU for more than 5 days, and this will include many preterm infants. This population is at high risk for having auditory neuropathy spectrum disorder, with normal or near normal cochlear function, but absent or abnormal auditory nerve function, which is detected by AABR but not by OAE (132).

LATE PRETERM INFANTS

Although much attention has been paid to the survival and morbidity in extremely preterm infants, late preterm infants (LPI, 34 weeks and 0 days to 36 weeks and 6 days GA) constitute more than 70% of all preterm infants. There is increasing recognition that these infants are at increased neonatal mortality and morbidity and long-term sequelae compared to term infants. A review of 22 studies comparing 2,368,471 LPI to 27,007,204 term infants found that although the absolute incidence of neonatal morbidity and mortality was low in LPI, compared to term infants, LPI were more likely to have RDS (relative risk [RR] 17.3), IVH (RR 4.9), and death before 28 days of age (RR 5.9). They were also more likely to die in the first year of life (RR 3.7) and to suffer from cerebral palsy (RR 3.1) (133). Data from 12 institutions across the United States on 233,844 deliveries between 2002 and 2008 showed that 36.5% of 19,334 LPI were admitted to NICUS (134). RDS occurred in 10.5% of LPI compared to only 0.3% of infants born at 38 weeks. The odds of RDS decreased with each advancing week of gestation until 38 weeks. Transient tachypnea of the newborn due to delayed intrapulmonary fluid absorption due to developmentally regulated epithelial sodium channel expression occurred in 6.4% of LPI versus 0.4% at 38 weeks. Rates of persistent pulmonary hypertension (0.38% vs. 0.08% at 38 weeks) and pneumonia (1.5% vs. 0.1%) were also significantly greater in LPI. The need for respiratory support decreases with advancing GA.

Risks of early hypoglycemia in LPI range from 3 to 77 times that of term infants (133,134,135) and can occur in 16% of LPI, so routine screening for hypoglycemia is recommended. In addition, LPI have feeding difficulties, with suck swallow incoordination and often require tube feeding in the first few days of life or intravenous fluids or parenteral nutrition (133). Hyperbilirubinemia is more common in LPI with an increased need for phototherapy (OR 5.9; 95% CI 1.7 to 14.6) compared with term infants, and increased risk of severe jaundice and kernicterus (133,136).

In many institutions, LPI are managed like term infants and left in postnatal wards with their mothers without the close supervision and care they need. On the other hand, compared to extremely preterm infants, most LPI can survive with special care and have good outcomes, without needing expensive intensive care. LPIs are at increased risk for neurologic impairments, developmental difficulties, school failure, and behavioral and psychiatric problems, so long-term follow-up is essential (137).

SURVIVAL AND LONG-TERM OUTCOMES

The survival and outcomes of preterm infants are determined largely by where they are born and what resources are available or utilized to ensure their disability-free survival.

Advances in antenatal and neonatal care over the past few decades have enhanced the survival of preterm infants substantially. The GA at which infants are considered previable has decreased steadily over the years from 28 weeks to 25 weeks to 22 weeks in some countries. Before the 1960s and 70s, intensive care for VLBW infants was frequently considered experimental, with concerns about increasing salvage of children with significant handicaps. Stewart et al, in a review of outcomes for VLBW infants from developed countries showed that the mortality for VLBW infants decreased from 60% in 1946 to 1950 to about 35% by 1976 to 1977, with the proportion of healthy survivors trebling after 1960 while the proportion of handicapped children remained low at about 6% to 8% (138). The same study also showed that mortality rates for infants weighing ≤1,000 g (ELBW) ranged from 50% to 85% between 1966 and 1977. In a comparison of two cohorts of very preterm infants (GA <32 weeks) born in 1983 to those in 1996 to 1997 in the Netherlands, in hospital mortality decreased from 30% in the 1980s to 11% in the 1990s (139). Mortality in extremely preterm infants <27 weeks decreased from 76% to 33%. In the 1983 cohort, mortality was 100% for infants born at 24 and 25 weeks of GA and 60% for infants born at 26 weeks. Although the incidence of RDS was approximately 60% in both time periods, mortality from RDS decreased from 29% to 8%, but the incidence of BPD increased from 6% to 19%. Seventy-three percent of the very preterm infants in the 96 to 97 cohort were treated antenatally with glucocorticoids compared with 6% of the infants in 1983, and 42% of the 1996 to 1997 cohort received surfactant. In 1999, Hack and Fanaroff reviewed outcomes of ELBW infants born in the United Kingdom, Australia, United States, Canada, and Japan in the 1990s (140). At 23 weeks of GA, survival ranged from 2% to 35%, at 24 weeks 17% to 58%, and at 25 weeks 35% to 85% in different centers. Thirty percent of the few survivors born at 23 weeks were severely disabled. Their conclusion was that with the methods of care available at the time, the limits of viability had been reached at 23 to 24 weeks.

GA thresholds for intervention are now approaching 22 weeks. A review of 20-year trends from 1993 to 2012 in 34,636 extremely preterm infants, 22 to 28 weeks gestation, born at Neonatal Research Network centers in the United States, showed that survival of infants born at 23 weeks of GA increased to 33% and at 24 weeks of GA to 65% and 77% for infants born at 25 weeks of GA (108). These centers had achieved survival rates over 80% for infants born at 26 and 27 weeks and over 90% for infants born at 28 weeks by 1993. Survival for infants born at 22 weeks was only 7%. There was, encouragingly, a significant increase in survival without major morbidity, defined as one or more of NEC, infections, BPD, severe IVH, PVL, or ROP stage ≥ stage 3 in infants who survived to discharge, ranging from 20% in infants born at 26 weeks to 61% in infants born at 28 weeks of GA. For survivors born at 22 to 24 weeks, few escaped without major morbidity (0% to 8%).

It is interesting to note that even among high-income countries, survival of very preterm infants born between 24 and 29 weeks is variable, ranging from 78% to 93% among national and regional networks, with the greatest variance being noted at 24 weeks of GA (35% to 84% survival) and the lowest at 29 weeks of GA (92% to 98%) (141). Although this could be attributed to different philosophies of care or levels of intervention in the most immature infants (see Fig. 7.2 Gestational age thresholds for initiating care in three Northern European Countries), relative differences in survival followed a similar pattern at all GA.

Similar data about survival of preterm infants of different GA in LMIC is unavailable, with many papers reporting only on a sample of preterm births at the time of admission or birth, with little detail about the level of care offered to these infants, making assessments and comparisons impossible (142). It is estimated that 90% of infants born at < 28 weeks in resource-challenged countries die, compared to less than 10% mortality in these infants in high-income settings (12).

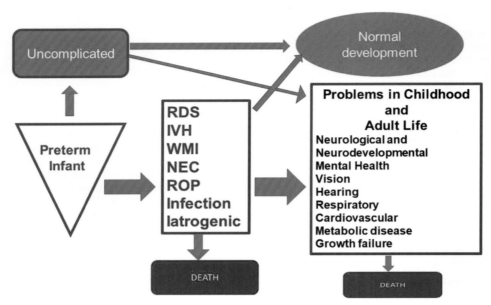

FIGURE 25.1 Sequelae of preterm birth. RDS, respiratory distress syndrome; IVH, intraventricular hemorrhage; WMI, white matter injury; NEC, necrotizing enterocolitis; ROP, retinopathy of prematurity. (Adapted by permission from Nature: Blencowe H, Lee ACC, Cousens S, et al. Preterm birth-associated neurodevelopmental impairment estimates at regional and global levels for 2010. *Pediatr Res* 2013;74(suppl 1):17. Copyright © 2013 Springer Nature.)

The increasing survival of preterm infants, sometimes at the limits of viability, always brings up the concern about long-term outcomes. Preterm birth has been associated with increased rates of cerebral palsy, cognitive, sensory and language impairments, seizure disorders, and growth abnormalities (143). Recent studies suggest that improvements in neonatal intensive care have resulted in decreases in rates of severe cerebral palsy from 16% to 12% and an increase in rates of mild cerebral palsy by 13%, together with increasing recognition of developmental coordination disorders, often not recognized until school age. The importance of parental education and socioeconomic status in long-term developmental outcomes remains paramount. Increased neurodevelopmental disability due to inadequate application of knowledge, insufficient resources, and iatrogenic disease is a major concern in middle-income countries with burgeoning neonatal intensive care units. This is exemplified by the increase in severe ROP, which is now a significant cause of blindness in these countries (129). In addition to neurodevelopmental sequelae, additional cardiovascular and respiratory consequences to preterm birth are being increasingly recognized in adulthood. **Figure 25.1** summarizes the sequelae of preterm birth.

ANTENATAL COUNSELING

The prospect of delivering a preterm infant fills parents with dismay and frequently, despair, particularly if the infant is extremely premature and periviable. Antenatal counseling prior to a preterm delivery is beneficial at all gestational ages to help parents to understand potential problems, the plan of care, and prognosis. In the case of an anticipated birth of an extremely preterm infant, shared decision making is appropriate after parents have been provided the most accurate information possible on the basis of all factors known to affect the outcome of the particular infant. National organizations provide guidelines on resuscitation of periviable infants (144,145), but thresholds for intervention vary, particularly in LMIC with limited resources. Each institution should have policies and procedures for antenatal counseling. Obstetric and neonatal providers may have different perspectives; it is important for a discussion to occur between them so that consistent information is provided to the parents. The primary goal of

antenatal counseling in these situations is to allow parents to make an informed decision regarding intervention and available options for care including comfort care. Counseling may be aided by the use of visual materials, which should take the family's intellectual and cultural attributes into consideration. GA alone is not an adequate predictor of outcomes. In the United States, the Eunice Kennedy Shriver NICHD Neonatal Research Network Extremely Preterm Birth Outcome model (also known as the NICHD calculator) provides estimates of survival and long-term outcomes based on GA, use of antenatal steroids, gender, and whether a singleton or part of a multiple gestation (146). A recent update of this model using data from babies born between 2006 and 2012 performed moderately well when applied to large U.S. cohorts and also demonstrated that hospital of birth contributed substantially to prediction outcome (147). The Canadian Neonatal Network provides up to date data on its website (www.canadianneonatalnetwork. org). While these tools provide estimates of outcomes, it should be emphasized that counseling should be individualized. Rational decision making is difficult in the midst of labor, medical interventions in the labor and delivery room and emotional turmoil, and parents may not be able to assimilate a lot of overwhelming statistics. Janvier et al state "We argue against trying to tell parents every fact we think might be relevant to their decision." Instead, they recommend that doctors should try to discern on a case-by-case basis, what particular parents want and need (148).

We should be humbled by the fact that over the millennia, some preterm babies have survived against all odds without the interventions of modern medicine, and more than a few have made tremendous contributions to the world (149). Isaac Newton, English mathematician, physicist, and astronomer acknowledged to be one of the greatest creative geniuses, was born 3 months premature in 1642. His mother remarked he was so small he could fit into a quart pot (150). Other preterm infants who became famous are Sir Winston Churchill, Prime Minister of the United Kingdom during the Second World War; Mark Twain, American novelist; the German astronomer and mathematician Johannes Kepler; Charles Darwin, English naturalist known for his contributions to the science of evolution; the French Emperor Napoleon Bonaparte; Anna Pavlova, world famous ballerina; Stevie Wonder, American singer and songwriter (who became blind because of ROP); and Wayde van Niekerk, born at 29 weeks and winner of the 2016 Olympic Gold Medal in the 400 m event. Even if not famous, the preterm infant has the potential to contribute much to society and to humanity.

REFERENCES

1. WHO: recommended definitions, terminology and format for statistical tables related to the perinatal period and use of a new certificate for cause of perinatal deaths. Modifications recommended by FIGO as amended. *Acta Obstet Gynecol Scand* 1977;56(3):247.
2. Malamitsi-Puchner A. Preterm birth in ancient Greece: a synopsis. *J Matern Fetal Neonatal Med* 2017;30(2):141.
3. Dunn PM. Professor Pierre Budin (1846-1907) of Paris, and modern perinatal care. *Arch Dis Child Fetal Neonatal Ed* 1995;73(3):F193.
4. UNICEF, WHO, World Bank Group. UN interagency group for child mortality estimation. In: *Levels and Trends in Child Mortality Report*, 2020. https://www.unicef.org/reports/levels-and-trends-child-mortality-report-2020
5. Ely DM, Driscoll AK. Infant mortality in the United States 2018: data from the period linked birth/infant death file. *Natl Vital Stat Rep* 2020;69:7:1.
6. Chawanpaiboon S, Vogel JP, Moller AB, et al. Global, regional, and national estimates of levels of preterm birth in 2014: a systematic review and modelling analysis. *Lancet Glob Health* 2019;7(1):e37.
7. Martin JA, Hamilton BE, Osterman MJK, et al. Births: final data for 2018. *Natl Vital Stat Rep* 2019;68:13:1.
8. Sunderam S, Kissin DM, Zhang Y, et al. Assisted reproductive technology surveillance—United States, 2016. *MMWR Surveill Summ* 2019;68(4):1.
9. McDonald SD, Han Z, Mulla S, et al. Preterm birth and low birth weight among in vitro fertilization singletons: a systematic review and meta-analyses. *Eur J Obstet Gynecol Reprod Biol* 2009;146(2):138.
10. WHO Preterm Birth. Available from: www.who.int
11. Delnord M, Hindori-Mohangoo AD, Smith LK, et al.; Euro-Peristat Scientific Committee. Variations in very preterm birth rates in 30 high-income countries: are valid international comparisons possible using routine data? *BJOG* 2017;124(5):785.
12. Blencowe H, Cousens S, Chou D, et al.; Born Too Soon Preterm Birth Action Group. Born too soon: the global epidemiology of 15 million preterm births. *Reprod Health* 2013;10(suppl 1):S2.
13. Committee on Obstetric Practice, the American Institute of Ultrasound in Medicine, and the Society for Maternal-Fetal Medicine. Committee opinion No 700: methods for estimating the due date. *Obstet Gynecol* 2017;129(5):e150.
14. Lee AC, Panchal P, Folger L, et al. Diagnostic accuracy of neonatal assessment for gestational age determination: a systematic review. *Pediatrics* 2017;140(6):e20171423.
15. Dubowitz LM, Dubowitz V, Goldberg C. Clinical assessment of gestational age in the newborn infant. *J Pediatr* 1970;77(1):1.
16. Ballard JL, Khoury JC, Wedig K, et al. New Ballard Score, expanded to include extremely premature infants. *J Pediatr* 1991;119(3):417.
17. Dagnew N, Tazebew A, Ayinalem A, et al. Measuring newborn foot length to estimate gestational age in a high risk Northwest Ethiopian population. *PLoS One* 2020;15(8):e0238169.
18. Roberts D, Brown J, Medley N, et al. Antenatal corticosteroids for accelerating fetal lung maturation for women at risk of preterm birth. *Cochrane Database Syst Rev* 2017;3:CD004454.
19. Committee on Obstetric Practice. Committee opinion No. 713: antenatal corticosteroid therapy for fetal maturation. *Obstet Gynecol* 2017;130(2):e102.
20. Ehret DEY, Edwards EM, Greenberg LT, et al. Association of antenatal steroid exposure with survival among infants receiving postnatal life support at 22 to 25 weeks' gestation. *JAMA Netw Open* 2018;1(6):e183235.
21. Society for Maternal-Fetal Medicine (SMFM) Publications Committee. Implementation of the use of antenatal corticosteroids in the late preterm birth period in women at risk for preterm delivery. *Am J Obstet Gynecol* 2016;215(2):B13. Erratum in: *Am J Obstet Gynecol.* 2017;216(2):180.
22. Gyamfi-Bannerman C, Thom EA, Blackwell SC, et al.; NICHD Maternal–Fetal Medicine Units Network. Antenatal Betamethasone for women at risk for late preterm delivery. *N Engl J Med* 2016;374(14):1311.
23. Althabe F, Belizán JM, McClure EM, et al. A population-based, multifaceted strategy to implement antenatal corticosteroid treatment versus standard care for the reduction of neonatal mortality due to preterm birth in low-income and middle-income countries: the ACT cluster-randomised trial. *Lancet* 2015;385(9968):629.
24. Chang E. Preterm birth and the role of neuroprotection. *BMJ* 2015;350: g6661.
25. Medley N, Poljak B, Mammarella S, et al. Clinical guidelines for prevention and management of preterm birth: a systematic review. *BJOG* 2018;125(11):1361.
26. Lasswell SM, Barfield WD, Rochat RW, et al. Perinatal regionalization for very low-birth-weight and very preterm infants: a meta-analysis. *JAMA* 2010;304(9):992.
27. Binder S, Hill K, Meinzen-Derr J, et al. Increasing VLBW deliveries at subspecialty perinatal centers via perinatal outreach. *Pediatrics* 2011;127(3):487.
28. Jensen EA, Lorch SA. Effects of a Birth Hospital's neonatal intensive care unit level and annual volume of very low-birth-weight infant deliveries on morbidity and mortality. *JAMA Pediatr* 2015;169(8):e151906.
29. Helenius K, Longford N, Lehtonen L, et al.; Neonatal Data Analysis Unit and the United Kingdom Neonatal Collaborative. Association of early postnatal transfer and birth outside a tertiary hospital with mortality and severe brain injury in extremely preterm infants: observational cohort study with propensity score matching. *BMJ* 2019;367:l5678.
30. McNamara PJ, Mak W, Whyte HE. Dedicated neonatal retrieval teams improve delivery room resuscitation of outborn premature infants. *J Perinatol* 2005;25(5):309.
31. American College of Obstetricians and Gynecologists; Society for Maternal-Fetal Medicine. Obstetric care consensus No. 6: periviable birth. *Obstet Gynecol* 2017;130(4):e187.
32. Kuper SG, Sievert RA, Steele R, et al. Maternal and neonatal outcomes in indicated preterm births based on the intended mode of delivery. *Obstet Gynecol* 2017;130(5):1143.
33. Grabovac M, Karim JN, Isayama T, et al. What is the safest mode of birth for extremely preterm breech singleton infants who are actively resuscitated? A systematic review and meta-analyses. *BJOG* 2018;125(6):652.
34. Rabe H, Gyte GM, Díaz-Rossello JL, et al. Effect of timing of umbilical cord clamping and other strategies to influence placental transfusion at preterm birth on maternal and infant outcomes. *Cochrane Database Syst Rev* 2019;9:CD003248.
35. Tarnow-Mordi W, Morris J, Kirby A, et al. Delayed versus immediate cord clamping in preterm infants. *N Engl J Med* 2017;377(25):2445.
36. Al-Wassia H, Shah PS. Efficacy and safety of umbilical cord milking at birth: a systematic review and meta-analysis. *JAMA Pediatr* 2015;169(1):18.
37. Katheria A, Reister F, Essers J, et al. Association of umbilical cord milking vs delayed umbilical cord clamping with death or severe intraventricular hemorrhage among preterm infants. *JAMA* 2019;322(19):1877.
38. Bhatt S, Alison BJ, Wallace EM, et al. Delaying cord clamping until ventilation onset improves cardiovascular function at birth in preterm lambs. *J Physiol* 2013;591(8):2113.
39. Meyer MP, Nevill E, Wong MM. Provision of respiratory support compared to no respiratory support before cord clamping for preterm infants. *Cochrane Database Syst Rev* 2018;3:CD012491.
40. Sharma D. Golden 60 minutes of newborn's life: Part 1: preterm neonate. *J Matern Fetal Neonatal Med* 2017;30(22):2716.
41. Shah V, Hodgson K, Seshia M, et al. Golden hour management practices for infants <32 weeks gestation age in Canada. *J Paediatr Child Health* 2018;23(4):e70.
42. Croop SEW, Thoyre SM, Aliaga S, et al. The Golden Hour: a quality improvement initiative for extremely premature infants in the neonatal intensive care unit. *J Perinatol* 2020;40(3):530.
43. Peleg B, Globus O, Granot M, et al. "Golden Hour" quality improvement intervention and short-term outcome among preterm infants. *J Perinatol* 2019;39(3):387.
44. Cannon B, Nedergaard J. Brown adipose tissue: function and physiological significance. *Physiol Rev* 2004;84(1):277.
45. WHO/RHT/MSM/97.2. *Thermal protection of the newborn: a practical guide.*
46. NICU by the numbers. Temperature at NICU Admission by year. public. vtoxford.org. Downloaded October 1, 2020.
47. Laptook AR, Salhab W, Bhaskar B; Neonatal Research Network. Admission temperature of low birth weight infants: predictors and associated morbidities. *Pediatrics* 2007;119(3):e643.
48. Wilson E, Maier RF, Norman M, et al. Effective Perinatal Intensive Care in Europe (EPICE) Research Group. Admission hypothermia in very preterm infants and neonatal mortality and morbidity. *J Pediatr* 2016;175:61.
49. McCall EM, Alderdice F, Halliday HL, et al. Interventions to prevent hypothermia at birth in preterm and/or low birth weight infants. *Cochrane Database Syst Rev* 2018;2:CD004210.
50. McCarthy LK, Molloy EJ, Twomey AR, et al. A randomized trial of exothermic mattresses for preterm newborns in polyethylene bags. *Pediatrics* 2013;132(1):e135.
51. Silverman WA, Fertig JW, Berger AP. The influence of the thermal environment upon the survival of newly born premature infants. *Pediatrics* 1958;22(5):876.
52. Sauer PJ, Dane HJ, Visser HK. New standards for neutral thermal environment of healthy very low birthweight infants in week one of life. *Arch Dis Child* 1984;59(1):18.
53. Kjartansson S, Arsan S, Hammarlund K, et al. Water loss from the skin of term and preterm infants nursed under a radiant heater. *Pediatr Res* 1995;37(2):233.
54. Marik PE, Fuller C, Levitov A, et al. Neonatal incubators: a toxic sound environment for the preterm infant? *Pediatr Crit Care Med* 2012;13(6):685.

THE NEWBORN INFANT

55. Baumgart S. Radiant energy and insensible water loss in the premature newborn infant nursed under a radiant warmer. *Clin Perinatol* 1982;9(3):483.

56. Narayanan I, Nsungwa-Sabiti J, Lusyati S, et al. Facility readiness in low and middle-income countries to address care of high risk/small and sick newborns. *Matern Health Neonatol Perinatol* 2019;5:10. doi: 10.1186/s40748-019-0105-9

57. Gray PH, Paterson S, Finch G, et al. Cot-nursing using a heated, water-filled mattress and incubator care: a randomized clinical trial. *Acta Paediatr* 2004;93(3):350.

58. May L, Nshimyiryo A, Kubwimana M, et al. Performance of a nonelectric infant Warmer in Rwandan health centers. *Glob Pediatr Health* 2019;6:2333794X19884820. doi: 10.1177/2333794X19884820

59. Boundy EO, Dastjerdi R, Spiegelman D, et al. Kangaroo mother care and neonatal outcomes: a meta-analysis. *Pediatrics* 2016;137(1):e20152238. doi: 10.1542/peds.2015-2238

60. Sardesai S, Biniwale M, Wertheimer F, et al. Evolution of surfactant therapy for respiratory distress syndrome: past, present, and future. *Pediatr Res* 2017;81(1-2):240.

61. Committee on Fetus and Newborn; American Academy of Pediatrics. Respiratory support in preterm infants at birth. *Pediatrics* 2014;133(1):171.

62. Sweet DG, Carnielli V, Greisen G, et al. European consensus guidelines on the management of respiratory distress syndrome—2019 update. *Neonatology* 2019;115(4):432.

63. Wright CJ, Sherlock LG, Sahni R, et al. Preventing continuous positive airway pressure failure: evidence-based and physiologically sound practices from delivery room to the neonatal intensive care unit. *Clin Perinatol* 2018;45(2):257.

64. Herting E, Härtel C, Göpel W. Less invasive surfactant administration (LISA): chances and limitations. *Arch Dis Child Fetal Neonatal Ed* 2019;104(6):F655.

65. Cummings JJ, Polin RA; Committee on Fetus and Newborn. Oxygen targeting in extremely low birth weight infants. *Pediatrics* 2016;138(2):e20161576.

66. Mathew OP. Apnea of prematurity: pathogenesis and management strategies. *J Perinatol* 2011;31(5):302.

67. Eichenwald EC; Committee on Fetus and Newborn, American Academy of Pediatrics. Apnea of prematurity. *Pediatrics* 2016;137(1). doi: 10.1542/peds.2015-3757

68. Dobson NR, Hunt CE. Caffeine: an evidence-based success story in VLBW pharmacotherapy. *Pediatr Res* 2018;84(3):333.

69. Schmidt B, Roberts RS, Davis P, et al.; Caffeine for Apnea of Prematurity Trial Group. Caffeine therapy for apnea of prematurity. *N Engl J Med* 2006;354(20):2112.

70. Schmidt B, Roberts RS, Anderson PJ, et al.; Caffeine for Apnea of Prematurity (CAP) Trial Group. Academic performance, motor function, and behavior 11 years after neonatal caffeine citrate therapy for apnea of prematurity: an 11-year follow-up of the CAP randomized clinical trial. *JAMA Pediatr* 2017;171(6):564.

71. Jobe AH. Mechanisms of lung injury and bronchopulmonary dysplasia. *Am J Perinatol* 2016;33(11):1076.

72. Jobe AH, Bancalari E. Bronchopulmonary dysplasia. *Am J Respir Crit Care Med* 2001;163(7):1723.

73. Van Marter LJ. Epidemiology of bronchopulmonary dysplasia. *Semin Fetal Neonatal Med* 2009;14(6):358.

74. El-Khuffash A, McNamara PJ. Hemodynamic assessment and monitoring of premature infants. *Clin Perinatol* 2017;44(2):377.

75. Osborn DA. Diagnosis and treatment of preterm transitional circulatory compromise. *Early Hum Dev* 2005;81(5):413.

76. Dempsey EM. What should we do about low blood pressure in preterm infants. *Neonatology* 2017;111(4):402.

77. Dionne JM, Bremner SA, Baygani SK, et al.; International Neonatal Consortium. Method of blood pressure measurement in neonates and infants: a systematic review and analysis. *J Pediatr* 2020;221:23.

78. Semberova J, Sirc J, Miletin J, et al. Spontaneous closure of patent ductus arteriosus in infants ≤1500 g. *Pediatrics* 2017;140(2):e20164258.

79. van Laere D, van Overmeire B, Gupta S, et al.; European Special Interest Group 'Neonatologist Performed Echocardiography' (NPE). Application of NPE in the assessment of a patent ductus arteriosus. *Pediatr Res* 2018;84(suppl 1):46.

80. El-Khuffash A, Weisz DE, McNamara PJ. Reflections of the changes in patent ductus arteriosus management during the last 10 years. *Arch Dis Child Fetal Neonatal Ed* 2016;101(5):F474.

81. Isayama T, Kusuda S, Reichman B, et al.; International Network for Evaluating Outcomes of Neonates (iNeo) Investigators. Neonatal intensive care unit-level patent ductus arteriosus treatment rates and outcomes in infants born extremely preterm. *J Pediatr* 2020;220:34.

82. Sharma A, Davis A, Shekhawat PS. Hypoglycemia in the preterm neonate: etiopathogenesis, diagnosis, management and long-term outcomes. *Transl Pediatr* 2017;6(4):335.

83. Filler G, Bhayana V, Schott C, et al. How should we assess renal function in neonates and infants? *Acta Paediatr* 2021;110(3):773. [Epub ahead of print].

84. Lau C. Development of infant oral feeding skills: what do we know? *Am J Clin Nutr* 2016;103(2): 616S.

85. Fanaro S. Feeding intolerance in the preterm infant. *Early Hum Dev* 2013;89(suppl 2):S13.

86. Cormack BE, Harding JE, Miller SP, et al. The influence of early nutrition on brain growth and neurodevelopment in extremely preterm babies: a narrative review. *Nutrients* 2019;11(9):E2029.

87. Bhatia J. Human milk and the premature infant. *Ann Nutr Metab* 2013;62(suppl 3):8.

88. Radmacher PG, Adamkin DH. Fortification of human milk for preterm infants. *Semin Fetal Neonatal Med* 2017;22(1):30.

89. Neu J. Necrotizing enterocolitis. *Semin Fetal Neonatal Med* 2018;23(6): 369.

90. Saroha V, Josephson CD, Patel RM. Epidemiology of necrotizing enterocolitis: new considerations regarding the influence of red blood cell transfusions and anemia. *Clin Perinatol* 2019;46(1):101.

91. Underwood MA. Impact of probiotics on necrotizing enterocolitis. *Semin Perinatol* 2017;41(1):41.

92. Olaloye O, Swatski M, Konnikova L. Role of nutrition in prevention of neonatal spontaneous intestinal perforation and its complications: a systematic review. *Nutrients* 2020;12(5):E1347.

93. Rao R, Georgieff MK. Iron in fetal and neonatal nutrition. *Semin Fetal Neonatal Med* 2007;12(1):54.

94. Ohlsson A, Aher SM. Early erythropoiesis-stimulating agents in preterm or low birth weight infants. *Cochrane Database Syst Rev* 2020;2:CD004863.

95. Christensen RD, Henry E, Wiedmeier SE, et al. Thrombocytopenia among extremely low birth weight neonates: data from a multihospital healthcare system. *J Perinatol* 2006;26(6):348.

96. Maheshwari A. Neutropenia in the newborn. *Curr Opin Hematol* 2014;21(1):43.

97. Bhutani VK, Wong RJ, Stevenson DK. Hyperbilirubinemia in preterm neonates. *Clin Perinatol* 2016;43(2):215.

98. Watchko JF. Bilirubin-induced neurotoxicity in the preterm neonate. *Clin Perinatol* 2016;43(2):297.

99. Nagar G, Vandermeer B, Campbell S, et al. Reliability of transcutaneous bilirubin devices in preterm infants: a systematic review. *Pediatrics* 2013;132(5):871.

100. Maisels MJ, Watchko JF, Bhutani VK, et al. An approach to the management of hyperbilirubinemia in the preterm infant less than 35 weeks of gestation. *J Perinatol* 2012;32(9):660.

101. Morioka I. Hyperbilirubinemia in preterm infants in Japan: new treatment criteria. *Pediatr Int* 2018;60(8):684.

102. Arnold C, Pedroza C, Tyson JE. Phototherapy in ELBW newborns: does it work? Is it safe? The evidence from randomized clinical trials. *Semin Perinatol* 2014;38(7):452.

103. Collins A, Weitkamp JH, Wynn JL. Why are preterm newborns at increased risk of infection? *Arch Dis Child Fetal Neonatal Ed* 2018;103(4):F391.

104. Mukhopadhyay S, Puopolo KM. Clinical and microbiologic characteristics of early-onset sepsis among very low birth weight infants: opportunities for antibiotic stewardship. *Pediatr Infect Dis J* 2017;36(5):477.

105. Stoll BJ, Puopolo KM, Hansen NI, et al. Early-onset neonatal sepsis 2015 to 2017, the rise of *Escherichia coli*, and the need for novel prevention strategies. *JAMA Pediatr* 2020;174(7):e200593.

106. Carr JP, Burgner DP, Hardikar RS, et al. Empiric antibiotic regimens for neonatal sepsis in Australian and New Zealand neonatal intensive care units. *J Paediatr Child Health* 2017;53(7):680.

107. Puopolo KM, Benitz WE, Zaoutis TE; Committee on Fetus and Newborn; Committee on Infectious Diseases. Management of neonates born at ≤34 6/7 weeks' gestation with suspected or proven early-onset bacterial sepsis. *Pediatrics* 2018;142(6):e20182896.

108. Stoll BJ, Hansen NI, Bell EF, et al. Trends in care practices, morbidity, and mortality of extremely preterm neonates, 1993-2012. *JAMA* 2015;314(10):1039.

109. Cohen-Wolkowiez M, Moran C, Benjamin DK. Early and late onset sepsis in late preterm infants. *Pediatr Infect Dis J* 2009;28:1052.

110. Investigators of the Delhi Neonatal Infection Study (DeNIS) Collaboration. Characterization and antimicrobial resistance of sepsis pathogens in neonates born in tertiary care centres in Delhi, India: a cohort study. *Lancet Glob Health* 2016;4(10):e752.

111. Johnson J, Robinson ML, Rajput UC, et al. High burden of bloodstream infections associated with antimicrobial resistance and mortality in the neonatal intensive care unit in Pune, India. *Clin Infect Dis* 2020:ciaa554. doi: 10.1093/cid/ciaa554. [Epub ahead of print].

112. Jiang S, Hong L, Gai J, et al.; REIN-EPIQ Study Group. Early-onset Sepsis among preterm neonates in China, 2015 to 2018. *Pediatr Infect Dis J* 2019;38(12):1236.

113. Sridhar S, Grace R, Nithya PJ, et al. Group B streptococcal infection in a tertiary hospital in India—1998-2010. *Pediatr Infect Dis J* 2014;33(10):1091.
114. Zinna S, Lakshmanan A, Tan S, et al. Outcomes of nosocomial viral respiratory infections in high-risk neonates. *Pediatrics* 2016;138(5):e20161675.
115. Goldstein M, Krilov LR, Fergie J, et al. Respiratory syncytial virus hospitalizations among U.S. preterm infants compared with term infants before and after the 2014 American Academy of Pediatrics Guidance on Immunoprophylaxis: 2012-2016. *Am J Perinatol* 2018;35(14):1433.
116. Civardi E, Tzialla C, Baldanti F, et al. Viral outbreaks in neonatal intensive care units: what we do not know. *Am J Infect Control* 2013;41(10):854.
117. Davis J, Fairley D, Christie S, et al. Human parechovirus infection in neonatal intensive care. *Pediatr Infect Dis J* 2015;34(2):121.
118. Anderson EJ, DeVincenzo JP, Simões EAF, et al. SENTINEL1: two-season study of respiratory syncytial virus hospitalizations among U.S. infants born at 29 to 35 weeks' gestational age not receiving immunoprophylaxis. *Am J Perinatol* 2020;37(4):421.
119. American Academy of Pediatrics Committee on Infectious Diseases; American Academy of Pediatrics Bronchiolitis Guidelines Committee. Updated guidance for palivizumab prophylaxis among infants and young children at increased risk of hospitalization for respiratory syncytial virus infection. *Pediatrics* 2014;134(2):415. Erratum in: *Pediatrics* 2014;134(6):1221.
120. Ballabh P. Intraventricular hemorrhage in premature infants: mechanism of disease. *Pediatr Res* 2010;67(1):1.
121. Parodi A, Govaert P, Horsch S, et al.; eurUS.brain group. Cranial ultrasound findings in preterm germinal matrix haemorrhage, sequelae and outcome. *Pediatr Res* 2020;87(suppl 1):13.
122. Shankaran S, Bajaj M, Natarajan G, et al.; Eunice Kennedy Shriver National Institute of Child Health and Human Development Neonatal Research Network. Outcomes following post-hemorrhagic ventricular dilatation among infants of extremely low gestational age. *J Pediatr* 2020. pii:S0022-3476(20)30979-3. doi: 10.1016/j.jpeds.2020.07.080. [Epub ahead of print].
123. El-Dib M, Limbrick DD Jr, Inder T, et al. Management of post-hemorrhagic ventricular dilatation in the infant born preterm. *J Pediatr* 2020. pii: S0022-3476(20)30978-1. doi: 10.1016/j.jpeds.2020.07.079. [Epub ahead of print].
124. Cizmeci MN, de Vries LS, Ly LG, et al. Periventricular hemorrhagic infarction in very preterm infants: characteristic sonographic findings and association with neurodevelopmental outcome at age 2 years. *J Pediatr* 2020;217:79.
125. de Bijl-Marcus K, Brouwer AJ, De Vries LS, et al. Neonatal care bundles are associated with a reduction in the incidence of intraventricular haemorrhage in preterm infants: a multicentre cohort study. *Arch Dis Child Fetal Neonatal Ed* 2020;105(4):419.
126. de Vries LS, Benders MJ, Groenendaal F. Progress in neonatal neurology with a focus on neuroimaging in the preterm infant. *Neuropediatrics* 2015;46(4):234.
127. Volpe JJ. Confusions in nomenclature: "Periventricular Leukomalacia" and "White Matter Injury"-identical, distinct, or overlapping? *Pediatr Neurol* 2017;73:3.
128. Hartnett ME. Advances in understanding and management of retinopathy of prematurity. *Surv Ophthalmol* 2017;62(3):257.
129. Vinekar A, Dogra M, Azad RV, et al. The changing scenario of retinopathy of prematurity in middle and low income countries: unique solutions for unique problems. *Indian J Ophthalmol* 2019;67(6):717.
130. Duncan AF, Matthews MA. Neurodevelopmental outcomes in early childhood. *Clin Perinatol* 2018;45(3):377.
131. Hirvonen M, Ojala R, Korhonen P, et al. Visual and hearing impairments after preterm birth. *Pediatrics* 2018;142(2):e20173888. doi: 10.1542/peds.2017-3888
132. Demirel CE. Neonatal hearing screening. In: Ramasethu J, Seo S, eds. *McDonald's atlas of procedures in neonatology*, 6th ed. Philadelphia, PA: Wolters Kluwer, 2020:482.
133. Teune MJ, Bakhuizen S, Gyamfi Bannerman C, et al. A systematic review of severe morbidity in infants born late preterm. *Am J Obstet Gynecol* 2011;205(4):374.e1-9.
134. Consortium on Safe Labor. Respiratory morbidity in late preterm births. *JAMA* 2010;304(4):419.
135. Committee on Fetus and Newborn; Adamkin DH. Postnatal glucose homeostasis in late-preterm and term infants. *Pediatrics* 2011;127(3):575.
136. Bhutani VK, Johnson L. Kernicterus in late preterm infants cared for as term healthy infants. *Semin Perinatol* 2006;30(2):89.
137. Woythaler M. Neurodevelopmental outcomes of the late preterm infant. *Semin Fetal Neonatal Med* 2019;24(1):54.
138. Stewart AL, Reynolds EO, Lipscomb AP. Outcome for infants of very low birthweight: survey of world literature. *Lancet* 1981;1(8228):1038.
139. Stoelhorst GM, Rijken M, Martens SE, et al. Leiden follow-up project on prematurity. Changes in neonatology: comparison of two cohorts of very preterm infants (gestational age <32 weeks): the project on preterm and small for gestational age infants 1983 and the Leiden follow-up project on prematurity 1996-1997. *Pediatrics* 2005;115(2):396.
140. Hack M, Fanaroff AA. Outcomes of children of extremely low birthweight and gestational age in the 1990's. *Early Hum Dev* 1999;53(3):193.
141. Helenius K, Sjörs G, Shah PS, et al. International Network for Evaluating Outcomes (iNeo) of Neonates. Survival in very preterm infants: an international comparison of 10 national neonatal networks. *Pediatrics* 2017;140(6):e20171264. doi: 10.1542/peds.2017-1264
142. Gladstone M, Oliver C, Van den Broek N. Survival, morbidity, growth and developmental delay for babies born preterm in low and middle income countries—a systematic review of outcomes measured. *PLoS One* 2015;10(3):e0120566.
143. McGowan EC, Vohr BR. Neurodevelopmental follow-up of preterm infants: what is new? *Pediatr Clin North Am* 2019;66(2):509.
144. Cummings J; Committee on Fetus and Newborn. Antenatal counseling regarding resuscitation and intensive care before 25 weeks of gestation. *Pediatrics* 2015;136(3):588.
145. Lemyre B, Moore G. Counselling and management for anticipated extremely preterm birth. *Paediatr Child Health* 2017;22(6):334.
146. Tyson JE, Parikh NA, Langer J, et al.; National Institute of Child Health and Human Development Neonatal Research Network. Intensive care for extreme prematurity—moving beyond gestational age. *N Engl J Med* 2008;358(16):1672.
147. Rysavy MA, Li L, Bell EF, et al. Eunice Kennedy Shriver National Institute of Child Health and Human Development Neonatal Research Network. Between-hospital variation in treatment and outcomes in extremely preterm infants. *N Engl J Med* 2015;372(19):1801.
148. Janvier A, Lorenz JM, Lantos JD. Antenatal counselling for parents facing an extremely preterm birth: limitations of the medical evidence. *Acta Paediatr* 2012;101(8):800.
149. Obladen M. Historical notes on immaturity. Part 2: surviving against the odds. *J Perinat Med* 2011;39(5):571.
150. Storr A. Isaac Newton. *Br Med J (Clin Res Ed)* 1985;291(6511):1779.

THE NEWBORN INFANT

26 The Small-for-Gestational Age Infant and IUGR

Bianca Carducci, Susan C. Campisi, Samia Aleem, and Zulfiqar A. Bhutta

INTRODUCTION

Perinatal and neonatal mortality and morbidity continue to be major global health challenges (1). Optimal growth during the first 1,000 days of life is paramount to not only survival but also thriving in childhood.

The prevalence of small-for-gestational age (SGA) births in developing countries was previously estimated at 32.4 million, or 27% of all births (2). More recently, a proxy indicator, low birth weight (LBW) estimated 20.5 million live births in 2015 were LBW (appropriate-for-gestational age [AGA] preterm neonates, term, and preterm SGA neonates), with the burden of such conditions greater in low- and middle-income countries (LMIC) (3,4). Though the definition of SGA varies, it is commonly defined as gender-specific birth weight below the 10th percentile for gestational age. Broader definitions include more than two standard deviations below the mean for weight and/or length (5). Often used synonymously, intrauterine growth restriction (IUGR) is identified perinatally, whereby estimated fetal weight (EFW) is below the recommended gender-specific weight for gestational age. Such condition is typically diagnosed through reduced fetal growth velocity measurements and or by the presence of compromised placental blood flow. This predisposition *in utero* can manifest into SGA at birth, with clinical and physiologic presentations of hypothermia, hypoglycemia, and asphyxia. However, it is important to note that not all growth-restricted fetuses will be SGA. Research into understanding the etiology of the SGA population has proved challenging. Risk factors are often classified as fetal, maternal, placental, and/or demographic in nature. As such, SGA infants are a heterogeneous population with specific postnatal management and care needs.

Although diagnosis perinatally and the prognosis of SGA infants have improved over the past decades, there are undoubtedly short- and long-term effects of SGA infants. Specifically, fetal growth restriction has been linked to childhood stunting and poorer intellectual performance, while long-term consequences include sequelae such as obesity, diabetes, and cardiovascular disease in adulthood.

DEFINITIONS OF IUGR AND SGA

Defining and differentiating IUGR and SGA has been an enduring challenge in clinical research and practice. Expert consensus has defined fetal growth restriction as abnormalities in biometric measures of fetal size, at a threshold of EFW less than 10th centile (6). In addition, IUGR is often diagnosed as early fetal growth restriction (<32 weeks) or late fetal growth restriction (≥32 weeks). At birth, as seen in **Figures 26.1 and 26.2**, SGA neonates can concomitantly be classified as preterm or term, as well as LBW or very LBW. Importantly, this chapter will focus on both preterm and term SGA neonates.

DIAGNOSIS

Multidisciplinary consensus on parameters for diagnosing IUGR is necessary for improved perinatal and neonatal outcomes for both IUGR/SGA neonates. The International Society of Ultrasound in Obstetrics and Gynecology Clinical Standards Committee recently agreed on best practice guidelines in fetal growth assessment, through biochemical, histologic, and clinical features. Estimation of fetal age and weight are prerequisites in determining appropriate gestational age and if warranted, further investigation. Fetal age is often assessed through last menstrual period and crown–rump length (before 14 weeks), while fetal weight can be estimated through ultrasonographic biometric parameters such as biparietal diameter (BPD), head circumference (HC), abdominal circumference (AC), and femur diaphysis length (FL). Given large intra- and interobserver variability, estimation of fetal weight should occur every 3 weeks and clinically interpreted using appropriate fetal growth and size reference standards.

The best reference standard to use to assess fetal growth remains controversial; it is unclear if a single growth reference is appropriate for use regardless of ethnic or country origin. Several longitudinal cohort studies have developed intrauterine fetal growth charts assuming optimal fetal growth in low-risk women (7,8). INTERGROWTH-21st was an international, multicentre, multiethnic, population-based project aiming to study growth, health, nutrition, and neurodevelopment from less than 14 weeks to 2 years of age (8). INTERGROWTH-21st was founded on scientifically robust methodology, whereby fetal growth in eight urban geographically defined sites (Brazil, China, India, Italy, Kenya, Oman, the United Kingdom, and the United States) was prospectively measured and allowed for the development of prescriptive standardized reference charts for fetal growth and fetal size (8). The WHO Multicenter Growth Reference Study included data from 10 countries (Argentina, Brazil, Democratic Republic of Congo, Denmark, Egypt, France, Germany, India, Norway, and Thailand). Although one growth chart was generated, there was significant variation between countries, based on ethnic distribution. Finally, the NICHD Fetal Growth Study included 12 sites in the United States; significant differences were noted in fetal growth by race and ethnicity leading to racial/ethnic-specific derived curves (7).

If IUGR is suspected, preliminary screening of maternal and familial history, maternal anthropometry (prepregnant and pregnant), and maternal nutritional status is key. Additionally, the Royal College of Obstetricians and Gynaecologists recommend the use of various Doppler velocities (uterine artery, umbilical artery, middle cerebral artery, cerebroplacental ratio, ductus venosus, and aortic isthmus), and cardiotocography for diagnosis (9). Intrauterine growth–restricted fetuses can be classified as early onset (before 32 weeks), later onset (after 32 weeks), or alternatively as asymmetrical (type I), symmetrical (type II), or mixed. The majority of IUGR cases (5% to 10%) are asymmetrical (late-onset) growth restriction, which occurs in the third trimester and is characterized by "head sparing." Ultrasound measures indicate that while AC decreases, normal BPD, HC, and femur length are observed. By contrast, insults that occur earlier during the cellular hyperplasia stage of fetal growth result in symmetrical IUGR (early-onset). Often due to genetic abnormalities or infections, symmetrical IUGR is less prevalent (0.5% to 1%) but has poorer prognosis. It is characterized by equally distributed decreases in BPD, HC, AC, and femoral length (10).

At birth, neonates can be further clinically examined using the Ponderal Index (PI) and Cephalization Index (CI). The PI is defined as an anthropometric measure (weight–length ratio) to diagnose impaired fetal growth using the formula (fetal weight in grams $\times$ 100/(length in centimeters)^3), whereby PI less than the

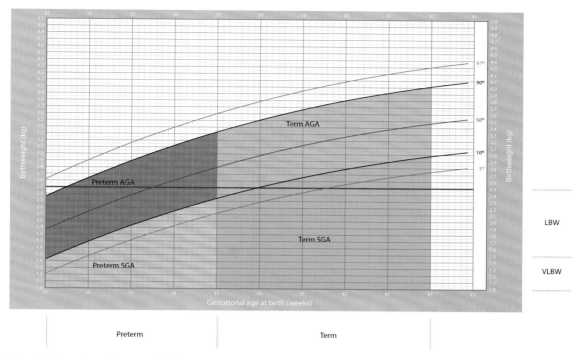

FIGURE 26.1 Classification of small-for-gestational age neonatal females. Adapted from Villar J, Cheikh Ismail L, Victora CG, et al. International standards for newborn weight, length, and head circumference by gestational age and sex: the Newborn Cross-Sectional Study of the INTERGROWTH-21st Project. *Lancet* 2014;384(9946):857.

10th percentile reflects poor fetal growth. The CI is defined as the ratio of HC to body weight, where a high CI indicates greater brain vulnerability (11). Newborns may be additionally classified as preterm, LBW, and/ or SGA, where the latter is often associated with early-onset IUGR. INTERGROWTH-21st also developed international newborn and postnatal prescriptive standards. These are complementary to World Health Organization (WHO) Child Growth Standards, which provide recommendations for growth and size and are particularly important when diagnosing growth-restricted infants (including preterm) postnatally (12,13).

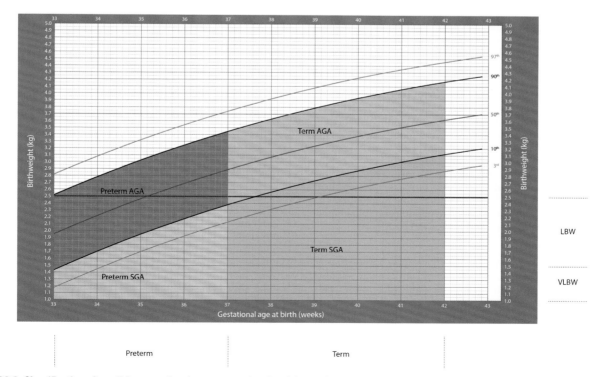

FIGURE 26.2 Classification of small-for-gestational age neonatal males. Adapted from Villar J, Cheikh Ismail L, Victora CG, et al. International standards for newborn weight, length, and head circumference by gestational age and sex: the Newborn Cross-Sectional Study of the INTERGROWTH-21st Project. *Lancet* 2014;384(9946):857.

THE NEWBORN INFANT

ETIOLOGY

First recognized in the late 1980s, the deceleration of fetal growth is a result of a complex interplay between maternal, placental, and fetal factors, both nutritional and nonnutritional (genetic, clinical diseases, social and environmental) in nature (14). In addition to these causes, a fetus may be exposed to other unfavorable conditions that can induce preterm birth. There is strong evidence to suggest that risk factors such as intrauterine infections (i.e., chorioamnionitis and bacterial vaginosis), systemic maternal infections (i.e., pneumonia and pyelonephritis), previous and current medical and obstetric history (i.e., past preterm birth, multiple pregnancy, uterus anomaly), premature prelabor rupture of membranes, hypertension in pregnancy, antenatal hemorrhage, and other miscellaneous causes (uterine malformation and cervical incompetence) are associated with preterm deliveries (15).

Maternal

Nutritional

Prepregnancy malnutrition and poor maternal weight gain during pregnancy has undoubtedly substantial implications for prematurity and SGA. According to the Institute of Medicine, maternal undernutrition is defined as a prepregnancy body mass index (BMI) of 18.5 kg/m², and it is recommended that a total of 12 to 18 kg (28 to 40 lbs) is gained during pregnancy for optimal outcomes (16). Available evidence on undernutrition and inadequate weight gain during gestation suggests that reduced intake of nutrients, including protein and micronutrients during the peri-implantation and placental development periods, results in poor nutrient availability for the fetus and growth restriction (17). Restriction of key micronutrients such as iron, folate, zinc, magnesium, calcium, vitamin A, vitamin D, and vitamin B$_{12}$ have been implicated in poor development of organs, alterations in hormonal regulation, body composition, and epigenetic gene function (18). In a LMIC context, this is more pronounced, whereby shorter interpregnancy intervals and adolescent pregnancies deplete maternal nutrient stores quicker and consequently nutrient competition with the fetus occurs (17). Moreover, numerous epidemiologic and experimental studies have suggested that preexistent or gestational diabetes is related to an increased risk of adverse fetal health outcomes including hypoglycemia, hyperbilirubinemia, polycythemia, and neonatal death (19).

Further, there is significant evidence to suggest that short maternal stature (<155 cm) is associated with reduced fetal growth, as well as an increased risk for preterm and LBW babies. A meta-analysis in LMIC by Kozuki et al. found maternal short stature was statistically significantly associated with term SGA, preterm SGA, and preterm AGA, where women under 145 cm in height had the highest adjusted risk term SGA—(risk ratio [RR] 2.03, 95% CI 1.76, 2.35; preterm AGA—RR 1.45, 95% CI 1.26, 1.66; preterm SGA—RR 2.13, 95% CI 1.42, 3.21) (20). Plausible mechanisms of action for this include reduced uterus size and lowered blood flow, which impedes physical growth of the fetus (21).

Environmental and Social

Various maternal environmental factors have been implicated in IUGR and SGA including maternal age, geography (i.e., developing country, and altitude), pollution, ethnicity and race, and socioeconomic status. Women of reproductive age under 16 years, or >35 years, have an increased risk of SGA babies. In addition, there is strong evidence to support the detrimental effects of maternal smoking and substance abuse on fetal growth and preterm birth (22). Some medications such as steroids, warfarin, anticonvulsants, antineoplastic agents, antimetabolite, and folic acid antagonists can result in IUGR.

Furthermore, a wide body of scientific evidence suggests that exposure to environmental pollutants during critical and time-sensitive periods of human development can impact growth. A meta-analysis on the maternal exposure of perfluorooctanoic acid (PFOA) on fetal growth indicated an inverse relationship, whereby a 1 ng/mL increase in serum or plasma PFOA was associated with a −18.9 g (95% CI −29.8, −7.9) difference in birth weight (23). Given this, The International Federation of Gynecology and Obstetrics, American College of Obstetricians and Gynecologists, the Royal College of Obstetricians and Gynecologists, the Endocrine Society, and the Society of Obstetricians and Gynecologists of Canada advise that all reproductive health professionals should advocate for the integration of environmental health within health care practice and educate patients on toxic environmental exposures (24).

Clinical Disorders

Several maternal conditions that diminish perfusion and/or damage the endothelial lining of the vascular system are associated with growth restriction of the fetus. This includes pregestational diabetes, hypertension, preeclampsia, chronic renal insufficiency (nephrotic syndrome, chronic renal failure, renal transplant, hemodialysis), autoimmune diseases (systemic lupus erythematosus and acquired thrombophilia), pulmonary disease (asthma, chronic obstructive pulmonary disease, cystic fibrosis), cardiac disease (cyanotic congenital heart disease, heart failure), and hematologic disorders (severe anemia, sickle cell anemia, b-thalassemia, hemoglobin H disease) (11).

Placental

Placental insufficiency due to reduced placental size and impedance in umbilical artery flow are important causes of growth restriction in fetuses. To cope with an abnormal blood flow pattern, and consequently compromised fetal oxygenation and nutrient delivery, fetal mechanisms redirect blood to the brain, as known as "brain sparing" (22). Redistribution of blood flow to vital organs and selective reductions in blood flow and oxygen supply to the peripheral musculature contributes to a 25% to 40% reduction in muscle mass observed in IUGR fetuses and neonates (25).

Other uteroplacental factors that can result in growth restriction and SGA include placenta previa and abruptio placentae (3). A recent systematic review and meta-analysis on singleton pregnancies with placenta previa observed a mild increased risk in the odds of IUGR/SGA neonates (OR 1.19, 95% CI 1.10 to 1.27) (26).

Fetal

There is a strong association between genetic and epigenetic factors modulating fetal growth malformations including chromosomal abnormalities (autosomal deletions, trisomy 13, 18, and 21), genetic syndromes due to disrupted imprinting (such as Bloom syndrome, Russell-Silver syndrome, Cornelia de Lange syndrome, Brachmann de Lange syndrome, mulibrey nanism syndrome, Rubinstein-Taybi syndrome, Dubowitz syndrome, Seckel syndrome, Johanson-Blizzard syndrome, Fanconi syndrome, Roberts syndrome, and De Sanctis-Cacchione syndrome), and polymorphisms in hormones that control endocrine homeostasis (insulin-like growth factor-1) (11). Furthermore, congenital anomalies (tracheoesophageal fistula, congenital heart disease, congenital diaphragmatic hernia, abdominal wall and neural tube defects) have been associated with IUGR (10).

Additionally, viral infections (rubella, cytomegalovirus, HIV, and herpes) and parasitic infections (toxoplasmosis, malaria, and syphilis), which increase cell death, have been associated with IUGR. Finally, metabolic and gene expression disturbances in key fetal hormones also have been implicated in IUGR, including insulin, insulin-like growth factor I and II, growth hormone, thyroid hormone, and glucocorticoids (27).

PATHOPHYSIOLOGY

Characteristically, there are unequivocal pathophysiologic differences and fetal adaptations in IUGR and SGA neonates. Anthropometrically, the body composition of IUGR fetuses and SGA newborns have been shown to be significantly different from AGA counterparts, in terms of lean body mass and adiposity. IUGR fetuses have a disproportionately low fat mass compared to lean mass, as well as impaired skeletal muscle development (28). This is attributed to various adaptations including structural changes in organ development, cardiovascular function, hormone regulation, and nutrient metabolism and utilization.

Poor lung development and redistribution of blood and oxygen away from peripheral tissues toward vital organs, have been recognized in IUGR/SGA neonates. In fact, recent studies have suggested that fetal oxygen deprivation impairs normal lung development, and consequently, makes the lungs more vulnerable to short- and long-term conditions such as neonatal respiratory distress, bronchopulmonary dysplasia (BPD), asthma and bronchiolitis. Additionally, key anabolic hormones (placental, pancreatic, thyroid, adrenal and pituitary) such as insulin-like growth factors I and II have been observed to be reduced in cord blood of IUGR infants. Reduced placental transport and fetal uptake of amino acids and glucose often occurs in IUGR fetuses. Deprivation of amino acids has been shown to limit cell division and protein accretion, ultimately down-regulating fetal growth of skeletal muscle mass. Given muscle fiber number is fixed at birth, compensation of muscle growth postnatally can only occur through muscle fiber size (25,29). Simultaneously, deficits in glucose transport due to reduced placental size and fewer glucose transporters, has been shown to result in fetal plasma hypoglycemia (29). Collectively, these adaptations allow fetal organs and tissues to maintain their energy-dependent function at the expense of body growth, which persists into childhood (25).

Epigenetic regulation of gene expression plays an important role in the risk and developmental origins of age-associated disorders. Disturbances in epigenetic pathways have been shown to contribute to the development of age-related diseases. The "Barker hypothesis" contends that malnourishment within the intrauterine environment programs the fetus toward a "thrifty phenotype." This hypothesis argues that inadequate nutrition *in utero* "programs" a number of fetal organ structures and associated fetal function, which lead to future disease. This programming includes alterations in homeostatic regulatory mechanisms that control appetite and energy output, resulting in increased food intake, increased fat deposition and ultimately, noncommunicable diseases such as cardiovascular, metabolic, and endocrine disease in adulthood (30).

Recent studies in humans and animals have shown that metabolic pathways involved in regulation of growth, body weight gain, and sexual maturation can influence epigenetic programming (31) with current and future generational impacts. In particular, phases of high developmental plasticity are susceptible to factors that affect metabolic programming, which can affect metabolic function throughout life. Significant DNA hypomethylation has been observed in the cord blood of infants with IUGR compared to AGA neonates, although there was no difference in telomere length (31,32).

COMMON COMPLICATIONS AMONG SGA NEWBORNS

Various complications have been observed in SGA neonates. However, it is important to recognize that the severity and temporality of each complication varies and is dependent on fetal and neonatal classification (SGA, LBW, prematurity, or any combination thereof).

Mortality

The relative risk (RR) of mortality during the neonatal period is significantly higher in premature SGA neonates (RR 15.42, 95% CI 9.11 to 26.12), as compared to SGA (RR 1.83, 95% CI 1.34 to 2.50) or prematurity (RR 6.82, 95% CI 3.56 to 13.07) alone (33).

Neonatal Brain Abnormalities (NBA)

Fetal growth restriction, and consequently brain sparing, has been considered a risk factor for various brain abnormalities such as periventricular leukomalacia (PVL), intraventricular hemorrhage (IVH), basal ganglia lesions (BGLs), and transient periventricular echodensities (TPE). Although several studies have indicated lower rates of IVH in SGA preterm infants compared to AGA preterm infants, higher rates of IVH have been noted in late preterm infants with IUGR compared to appropriately grown infants and in infants with history of placental insufficiency and abnormal umbilical artery Doppler flow patterns (34).

Some evidence suggests that growth-restricted infants born preterm have significantly more brain abnormalities as compared to matched AGA preterm infants (35,36). Growth-restricted infants appear to have deficits in morphologic neurostructure and function. Fetal studies (GA of 28 weeks and onward) using fetal magnetoencephalography to measure auditory and visual brain activity have demonstrated that IUGR fetuses have significantly slower visual evoked brain responses as compared to matched controls (37). Clinical studies have shown that being born SGA may result in a reduction of cortical and total brain volume, in both white and gray matter, decreased number of brain cells, delayed or decreased brain cell myelination, and compromised brain connectivity and integrity (34). Jiang et al. (38) revealed delayed brainstem maturation in preterm infants born SGA. Likewise, using MRI, Bruno et al. (39) found the thalamus and basal ganglion volumes to be reduced in growth-restricted preterm infants (34). Thus, there is mounting evidence that fetal growth restriction and being born SGA alters neurologic architecture.

Asphyxia

SGA infants are more likely to face complications related to birth asphyxia in the transition from *in utero* to *ex utero* life. In a large secondary analysis of an observational cohort of 115,502 women and their term neonates, SGA infants had higher rates of hypoxic neonatal morbidities, including the need for cardiopulmonary resuscitation within the first 24 hours of life, and hypoxic ischemic encephalopathy, as compared to AGA infants (40). A prospective study of greater than 91,000 women from nine maternal–fetal medicine units, found that a 5-minute Apgar score of less than 4 was significantly more common in term SGA infants, after adjustment for confounders (41). These findings were replicated in a retrospective study of 95,900 infants, which found that the odds of severe acidosis at birth, and a 5-minute Apgar score of less than 3 were significantly higher in SGA infants with birth weights less than 10th percentile (42). Term SGA infants are also more likely to be delivered via emergency cesarean section for nonreassuring fetal heart status and be admitted to the NICU, after controlling for confounders (41,42).

Hypoglycemia

SGA babies are highly prone to hypoglycemia in the first 24 hours of life; thus, careful blood glucose level monitoring is important for SGA infants (43). Preterm SGA and intrauterine growth-restricted neonates are especially vulnerable due to their lack of metabolic reserves of glycogen and associated comorbidities. Nearly 30% to 60% of these high-risk infants become hypoglycemic and require immediate intervention (44). Even late preterm SGA infants are at increased risk of hypoglycemia compared to late preterm AGA infants (45,46). See Chapter 41.

Hypothermia

Hypothermia has been well recognized as a grave risk to newborns, especially those born SGA. SGA infants have a greater body surface area relative to weight. This along with lower fat reserves, immature skin, and less subcutaneous fat puts them at higher risk of hypothermia and impaired thermoregulation (47). Hypothermia leads to increased oxygen consumption, metabolic acidosis, hypoglycemia, and increased peripheral vascular resistance (48). In infants with LBW, cold stress contributes to increased morbidity and mortality (49). Neonatal hypothermia has been associated with an increased risk of infection, respiratory distress syndrome (RDS), brain hemorrhage, and coagulation defects (49–51).

Respiratory
Respiratory Distress Syndrome and Bronchopulmonary Dysplasia

In numerous studies, there is evidence to support a reduced risk of RDS with being born SGA as compared to AGA counterparts, while the prevalence of BPD appears to be contingent on prematurity of the SGA newborn. Turitz et al. (52) determined that SGA is not associated with RDS or other adverse respiratory and neonatal composites. Similarly, other studies have also found a lower risk of RDS in SGA babies compared to AGA babies (46). Tannirwar et al. (53) found similar mortality rates in SGA and AGA infants, but respiratory morbidities such as RDS and BPD were more prevalent in AGA neonates (53). Conversely, some have determined that IUGR is a strong determinant of respiratory prognosis in preterm infants (54), whereby in preterm SGA infants, SGA was significantly associated with BPD, but not with an increased risk of mortality or RDS (55).

Cardiovascular

SGA infants have been found to exhibit higher rates of abnormalities in cardiac size and structural differences in terms of heart chambers and ventricles, accompanied by cardiac dysfunction (56–58). Aldana et al. determined that SGA infants possess abnormal cardiovascular structure and function, which increased with IUGR severity (59). As a result, these infants may have an increased risk of complications in the perinatal period and childhood and possibly an increased risk of adult cardiovascular disease (60).

Patent Ductus Arteriosus

Evidence on the association between SGA and or IUGR and patent ductus arteriosus (PDA) remains inconclusive due to the lack of consensus on definitions, including the uncertainty around "significant PDA." In a 2019 systematic review and meta-analysis, a significantly reduced rate of PDA was observed in the SGA/IUGR group when 47 studies were pooled (OR 0.82, 95% CI 0.70 to 0.96). However, upon subgroup and sensitivity analyses (based on refinement of definitions, i.e., hemodynamically significant PDA or PDA requiring treatment), this association was weakened and no longer significant (61). Regardless of whether or not being born SGA increases the risk of PDA, PDA may have a significant negative effect on cerebral oxygenation in preterm SGA neonates (62). In addition, it may be useful to note that PDA management did not differ between SGA and AGA infants. However, SGA infants had an increased risk of death or BPD regardless of their PDA status (63).

Gastrointestinal
Necrotizing Enterocolitis

The devastating disease of necrotizing enterocolitis (NEC) is associated significantly with prematurity, as well as SGA (64). A national population cohort study of 16,669 premature infants showed an increased risk of NEC in SGA infants (birth weight less than 10th percentile for the given gestational age) (OR 1.35, 95% CI 1.08 to 1.69) (65).

Renal

Premature infants, when born SGA, often have an increased risk of renal insufficiency. In a retrospective case–control study, preterm infants who were SGA were found to be compromised in terms of glomerular functions, though tubular functions were comparable to matched AGA counterparts (66).

Hematologic

SGA infants, both preterm and full term, are at a higher risk for improper excretion of bilirubin, leading to elevated total serum/plasma bilirubin (hyperbilirubinemia) and often present with jaundice 2 to 4 days after birth. If untreated, severe hyperbilirubinemia can potentially progress to sequelae such as bilirubin neurotoxicity. SGA infants (both preterm and term) should be monitored closely, especially within the first 24 to 48 hours after birth, as they are more likely to suffer from jaundice requiring phototherapy (67). In a 2017 study of 5,382 infants admitted into a neonatal intensive care unit in Norway, the use and duration of phototherapy was inversely associated with birth weight and gestational age, whereby there was a statistically significant difference in SGA neonates requiring phototherapy as compared to AGA neonates (68).

Decreased ferritin levels in the SGA neonate may result from impaired iron transport across the placenta or increased iron utilization during chronic hypoxia (due to placental insufficiency, which is a cause of IUGR) resulting in enhanced erythropoiesis in fetal life (69). SGA newborns have an increased risk of polycythemia at birth. Additionally, neutropenia is common in the first days of life and can be accompanied by thrombocytopenia (70,71).

Immune
Serious Infections, Sepsis, and Pneumonia

The altered immune system of term SGA infants including significantly higher umbilical cord plasmacytoid dendritic cell and natural killer cell count, as well as high IgM levels have been previously reported as compared to cord blood from term AGA infants (72). By contrast, very preterm SGA infants (≤32 weeks gestation) have been found to possess lower white blood cell and neutrophil counts than very preterm AGA infants at birth and 3 days postnatal (73). In addition, though late-onset sepsis is common in premature and SGA neonates, there are inconsistent findings in linking early sepsis with being born SGA (46).

The degree that SGA infants have been considered at risk for pneumonia is directly related to meconium aspiration and subsequent meconium aspiration syndrome (MAS) (74).

Retinopathy of Prematurity

Approximately 14% of preterm SGA infants develop complications associated with retinopathy of prematurity (ROP) (75). A recent systematic review and meta-analysis determined that, in preterm neonates, SGA was associated with increased odds of any stage of ROP, severe ROP and treated ROP (76). This finding may be due to the hypothesis that IUGR and low gestational age are both risk factors for retinopathy of prematurity. In a study modeling prethreshold ROP risk of preterm newborns with IUGR, low gestational age (23 to 24 weeks, OR 11.6, 95% CI 2.9, 47; 25 to 26 weeks, OR 8.1, 95% CI 2.1, 32) and severe growth restriction (birth weight Z-score < −2, OR 9.1, 95% CI 1.1, 76) were associated with an increased risk of prethreshold ROP (77).

POSTNATAL MANAGEMENT

Thermoregulation

The risk of cold stress is highest during the transition to *ex utero* life. Without appropriate precautions, a newborn's body temperature can rapidly drop by 2°C to 3°C within a few minutes (78). The WHO recommends setting the delivery room temperature to 25°C to prevent hypothermia (79). Heat loss by evaporation is greatest during the first few minutes of age and is inversely proportional to gestational age; this can be avoided by routine resuscitation methods, including wrapping in warm blankets, covering the infant's head and use of a radiant warmer (80,81). If the infant is otherwise clinically stable, performing these steps on the mother's chest allows preservation of the infant's temperature by skin-to-skin contact (48). In preterm infants, the additional use of polyethylene occlusive skin wrapping, warming mattresses, and incubators are recommended (48). The Heat Loss Prevention trial demonstrated that the use of an occlusive plastic skin wrap, placed around an undried newborn soon after birth, significantly reduced the incidence of hypothermia and led to higher temperatures on admission to the neonatal intensive care unit (82). Use of an exothermic chemical mattress allows prevention of heat loss via conduction by ensuring a warm surface for the infant (83). However, the combined use of the plastic wrap and chemical mattress leads to admission temperatures in the hyperthermic range, which could be detrimental (83). At this time, the Neonatal Resuscitation Program guidelines recommend the use of plastic wrap only in infants weighing <1,500 g. Careful monitoring during use of warming mattresses and occlusive wraps is required to prevent hyperthermia.

Heat loss continues to remain an important issue even after admission to the neonatal intensive care unit. The primary means of thermal control in the NICU is through radiant warmers and incubators. In double-walled incubators, the temperature of the inner wall remains stable despite environmental temperature fluctuations. Temperature should be servocontrolled to maintain an abdominal skin temperature of 36.5°C (84). Maintenance of a neutral thermal environment is improved when adequate humidity is present in the environment, which allows improved maintenance of body temperature and reduces transepidermal loss of fluid (85,86). In LMIC, emollient therapy (aquaphor or vegetable oils) is a common practice to prevent infections and heat loss in high-risk infants. However, a Cochrane meta-analysis examining the use of emollients in 3,089 preterm infants suggested no significant improvement in the prevention of infection or mortality (87).

Kangaroo Mother Care

Kangaroo mother care (KMC) was initially developed in the 1970s as an alternative technique to maintain infants' body temperature in low-resource areas (88). The major component of KMC is skin-to-skin contact between the mother and the infant, in which the infant is placed directly on the mother's chest. This role can be shared with other providers, especially the infant's father. There have been several randomized controlled trials (RCT) supporting the use of KMC. In a recent RCT analyzing neonatal outcomes of KMC, fewer infants died between enrollment and 28 days within the intervention group, as compared to the control group (hazard ratio: 0.70, 95% CI 0.51 to 0.96; p = 0.027) (89). There is compelling evidence to suggest that KMC is associated with a reduction in mortality, as well as a reduced incidence of infection, hypothermia, and shorter hospital length of stay. KMC also promotes breastfeeding, an increase in weight gain, and mother–infant attachment (88).

Nutrition

The specific nutritional management of growth-restricted newborns is described in Chapter 20. High-quality evidence suggests that breast milk should be recommended for both term and preterm infants, including those that are SGA and LBW. However, it is important to emphasize that growth-restricted infants are at high risk of hypoglycemia, and prolonged hypoglycemia has long-term effects on neurodevelopmental outcomes. These infants are at risk for hypoglycemia due to inadequate substrate supply available for glycogen synthesis; asymmetric growth restriction, with head preservation because of placental insufficiency further exacerbates this because of increased brain-to-bodyweight ratio. Additionally, these infants are unable to oxidize triglycerides and free fatty acids effectively (90). Infants are at highest risk for developing hypoglycemia during the first few days of age during the adaptation period to extrauterine life (91). In asymptomatic term infants, initial management with enteral feeds and close, frequent glucose monitoring is the current standard of treatment (92). This allows mothers and infants to remain together. In symptomatic term infants with whole blood glucose less than 40 mg/dL, immediate intravenous glucose treatment is recommended (92). See Chapter 41.

Summary of Postnatal Management Recommendations

- Prevention of hypothermia in the immediate postnatal period includes maintenance of the delivery room temperature at 25°C, covering the infant's head, and use of a radiant warmer.
- For premature infants, additional use of occlusive skin wrapping and warming mattresses are recommended.
- KMC involves skin-to-skin contact with a caregiver and has been shown to reduce mortality, infection, and promotes breastfeeding.
- Growth-restricted infants are at high risk of hypoglycemia that, if left uncorrected, may lead to neurodevelopmental impairments.
- Timely recognition and intervention with intravenous dextrose in cases of symptomatic or persistent hypoglycemia is of the essence.

DISCHARGE CRITERIA AND FOLLOW-UP CARE

Growth-restricted infants are considered high risk given their physiologic immaturity. Their discharge is dependent on meeting criterion as established by the American Academy of Pediatrics and other professional organizations (93). These include demonstration of physiologic stability, parental and home readiness, follow-up care with a trained health professional, and surveillance of growth and development. Infants should be able to maintain normal body temperature, without requiring extra layers, have sufficient oral intake to support weight gain of 30 g/day, and have mature respiratory control (93). Routine discharge care as recommended for healthy term infants is appropriate for growth-restricted infants as well. They should have routine immunizations administered, hearing and metabolic screens performed, and fundoscopic examination completed as indicated. For breastfeeding mothers, information on lactation should be provided. Depending on the infant's complexity and family status, some caregivers may benefit from home nursing visits (45). Those born prematurely, or with extremely LBW, will require closer follow-up and neurodevelopmental evaluations and would benefit from individualized discharge plans (45).

In order to ensure the safety of the SGA infant during vehicle transportation, the appropriate selection and use of car seats are necessary. Rear-facing car seats provide the best protection in a frontal crash and also support the infant's head (94). Infants should be placed in a car seat that is appropriate for their weight and should be used according to manufacturer recommendations. See Chapter 18 for car seat tests.

EARLY CHILDHOOD DEVELOPMENT ASSOCIATED WITH SGA

Catch-Up Growth

Catch-up growth (CUG) is commonly defined as accelerated growth during a defined period of time following a period of growth inhibition. CUG may occur at any stage of growth but has been most studied during the first 1 to 2 years of life, after intrauterine growth restriction. A recent systematic review found that a significant proportion of full-term SGA children achieved CUG, but CUG did not occur at a specific age (95). This review also identified challenges associated with comparing outcomes where there is both a lack of consensus on definitions used for SGA and CUG as well as multiple growth reference standards.

CUG has important advantages such as improved neurodevelopment, enhanced immune function, and final adult height (96). However, there are also certain disadvantages for those who experience CUG such as metabolic syndrome, type 2 diabetes mellitus/insulin resistance, hypertension, cardiovascular disease, and obesity, which are discussed below.

Cognition

There is a substantial body of literature regarding cognitive impairments observed in childhood as a result of being born SGA including IQ, memory, school performance, fluid intelligence, autism, and neurodevelopmental disorders (34); however, being born SGA has not been confirmed to be an independent risk factor for these cognitive deficits. Due to the heterogeneity of SGA pathologies, gestational age of participants in follow-up studies, and variation in neurocognitive outcomes and tools, mechanisms by which SGA pathologies impact cognitive function remain difficult to determine.

Recent neuroimaging techniques like whole-brain connectome multilevel analyses have allowed for a comprehensive neural map of connectivity to be generated and correlated to cognitive skills in children born with and without growth restriction (34). Findings suggest that children born IUGR (97) or preterm IUGR had poorer scores on neurodevelopmental and neuropsychologic assessments at 1, 6, and 10 years of age (Bayley Scale for Infant and Toddler Development, Behavior Rating Inventory of Executive Function, and Strength and Difficulties Questionnaire), and the scores were correlated to reduced network metrics, as compared to preterm controls (98,99). In addition, studies of brain metabolites in young children born SGA indicated that their brain chemistry was altered in comparison to children born AGA (100). Conversely, others have found no association of SGA with lower cognitive scores nor neurodevelopmental impairment but did see behavioral differences (101). It is also important to note that earlier CUG was determined to result in slightly higher IQ scores at age 4 (102).

Behavioral

There is conflicting evidence on low attention control in children born SGA compared to children born AGA. In a population-based prospective cohort study, hyperactivity, but not cognition or neurodevelopment deficits was significantly associated with being born premature SGA, in children at 5 years of age (101). Further, a longitudinal birth cohort study indicated that those born SGA, relative to those born AGA, were 3.6 times more likely to have Attention deficit and hyperactivity disorder (ADHD) symptoms, independent of gestational age (103). There is a stronger association between neonates born LBW or premature and disorders such as ADHD (104).

Motor

Again, there is a paucity of research regarding the risk associated with motor delay due to being born SGA. While some evidence indicates that children born SGA had similar motor skills to children born AGA despite cognitive and attention differences (105), other evidence indicates that males born SGA are at greater risk of fine motor delay (106).

Cerebral Palsy

IUGR has been thought to increase the risk of cerebral palsy (CP) due to the restriction of brain development (107), especially involving gray matter. In a recent systematic review, various CP registry cohorts in Europe, Canada, and Australia found SGA-term infants had an increased risk for developing CP, as compared to AGA counterparts. However, SGA infants frequently had other risk factors such as intrauterine infections, placental abnormalities, perinatal asphyxia, maternal gestational hypertension, birth defects, and delivery by emergency cesarean section (108,109). In fact, among term and late preterm neonates, marked fetal growth restriction was found to be associated with a four-fold increase in the risk of developing CP, though most were from normotensive pregnancies and diagnosis of birth asphyxia was not higher in growth-restricted neonates versus AGA neonates (34,110). Thus, the mechanism underlying the relationship between CP and SGA remains elusive.

LONG-TERM EFFECTS

Puberty

The hypothalamic–gonadal axis appears to be affected in children with early growth impairment, which has been attributed to fetal programming. In fact, rapid weight gain due to CUG in children born SGA predisposes this group to earlier puberty due to their tendency for increased central adiposity, and the mechanism is similar to precociousness resulting from obesity (111–113). SGA children who remain short begin puberty within a normal age range and follow a slightly faster puberty progression, often leading to earlier menarche in girls. This results in an inability to overcome their height difference during the pubertal growth spurt (114). CUG should be carefully monitored during infancy and childhood to prevent excessive rates of weight gain, which is presumably the cause of the issues later in life.

Metabolic and Cardiovascular Disease

Following the Barker hypothesis, several longitudinal cohort studies have suggested that children born SGA, who often exhibit CUG during school-age and adolescence, are predisposed to metabolic disease (defined as visceral obesity, dyslipidemia, impaired glucose tolerance or overt type 2 diabetes mellitus, and hypertension as a cluster) and other comorbidities (111). Early metabolic markers such as insulin resistance or reduced insulin sensitivity have been elucidated in the development of later life metabolic disease, though mechanisms have not been well delineated (115). In a study of 2,510 school-aged children from Colombia (aged 9 to 17.9 years), children born preterm SGA had a statistically significant higher odds of increased fasting glucose (OR 1.84, 95% CI 1.05 to 3.23) and metabolic disease (OR 1.52, 95% CI 1.04 to 2.41) as compared to term SGA or preterm AGA born children (116). However, a recent systematic review and meta-analysis of four studies of 3,655 children (including (116)) concluded that SGA status in preterm infants had no significant effect on childhood obesity after adjustment (OR 0.80, 95% CI 0.55 to 1.15, p-value: 0.226) (117).

The relationship between IUGR or SGA and cardiovascular morphology, function, and disease has been well studied (115). In a case–control study, SGA infants at 24 months of age showed a significantly impaired lower stroke volume, lower left ventricle volume and dimensions, aortic dimensions as well as vascular dysfunction. In fact, a marker for atherosclerosis, namely, artery intima–media thickness (cIMT), was also significantly greater in SGA infants as compared to AGA counterparts (118). Importantly, a nationwide longitudinal study (>2.6 million live births between

1987 and 2012) in Sweden has provided new evidence that infants born very SGA (>2 SD below the mean) as compared to AGA have a 2.69-fold increased risk for heart failure (95% CI 1.94 to 3.73), after adjustment for confounding variables (119). Thus, research over the last four decades has demonstrated that growth restriction in early life is a strong predictor of cardiovascular health.

REFERENCES

1. Lee AC, Kozuki N, Cousens S, et al. Estimates of burden and consequences of infants born small for gestational age in low and middle income countries with INTERGROWTH-21(st) standard: analysis of CHERG datasets. *BMJ* 2017;358:j3677.
2. Black RE. Global prevalence of small for gestational age births. *Nestle Nutr Inst Workshop Ser* 2015;81:1.
3. Carducci B, Bhutta ZA. Care of the growth-restricted newborn. *Best Pract Res Clin Obstet Gynaecol* 2018;49:103.
4. Blencowe H, Krasevec J, de Onis M, et al. National, regional, and worldwide estimates of low birthweight in 2015, with trends from 2000: a systematic analysis. *Lancet Glob Health* 2019;7:e849.
5. Rogol AD, Hayden GF. Etiologies and early diagnosis of short stature and growth failure in children and adolescents. *J Pediatr* 2014;164(5 suppl):S1.
6. Gordijn SJ, Beune IM, Thilaganathan B, et al. Consensus definition of fetal growth restriction: a Delphi procedure. *Ultrasound Obstet Gynecol* 2016;48(3):333.
7. Grantz KL, Hediger ML, Liu D, et al. Fetal growth standards: the NICHD fetal growth study approach in context with INTERGROWTH-21st and the World Health Organization Multicentre Growth Reference Study. *Am J Obstet Gynecol* 2018;218(2S):S641.
8. Papageorghiou AT, Ohuma EO, Altman DG, et al. International standards for fetal growth based on serial ultrasound measurements: the Fetal Growth Longitudinal Study of the INTERGROWTH-21st Project. *Lancet* 2014;384(9946):869.
9. Salomon LJ, Alfirevic Z, Da Silva Costa F, et al. ISUOG practice guidelines: ultrasound assessment of fetal biometry and growth. *Ultrasound Obstet Gynecol* 2019;53(6):715.
10. Figueras F, Caradeux J, Crispi F, et al. Diagnosis and surveillance of late-onset fetal growth restriction. *Am J Obstet Gynecol* 2018;218(2S):S790.
11. Sharma D, Shastri S, Sharma P. Intrauterine growth restriction: antenatal and postnatal aspects. *Clin Med Insights Pediatr* 2016;10:67.
12. Villar J, Ismail LC, Victora CG, et al. International standards for newborn weight, length, and head circumference by gestational age and sex: the Newborn Cross-Sectional Study of the INTERGROWTH-21st Project. *Lancet* 2014;384(9946):857.
13. Villar J, Giuliani F, Bhutta ZA, et al. Postnatal growth standards for preterm infants: the Preterm Postnatal Follow-up Study of the INTERGROWTH-21(st) Project. *Lancet Glob Health* 2015;3(11):e681.
14. Kramer MS. Determinants of low birth weight: methodological assessment and meta-analysis. *Bull World Health Organ* 1987;65(5):663.
15. Koullali B, Oudijk MA, Nijman TAJ, et al. Risk assessment and management to prevent preterm birth. *Semin Fetal Neonatal Med* 2016;21(2):80.
16. American College of Obstetricians and Gynecologists. ACOG Committee opinion no. 548: weight gain during pregnancy. *Obstet Gynecol* 2013;121:210.
17. Wu G, Bazer FW, Cudd TA, et al. Maternal nutrition and fetal development. *J Nutr* 2004;134:2169.
18. Christian P, Stewart CP. Maternal micronutrient deficiency, fetal development, and the risk of chronic disease. *J Nutr* 2010;140(3):437.
19. Barquiel B, Herranz L, Martinez-Sanchez N, et al. Increased risk of neonatal complications or death among neonates born small for gestational age to mothers with gestational diabetes. *Diabetes Res Clin Pract* 2020;159:107971.
20. Kozuki N, Katz J, Christian P, et al. Comparison of US birth weight references and the International fetal and newborn growth consortium for the 21st century standard. *JAMA Pediatr* 2015;169(7):e151438.
21. Rahman MM, Abe SK, Kanda M, et al. Maternal body mass index and risk of birth and maternal health outcomes in low- and middle-income countries: a systematic review and meta-analysis. *Obes Rev* 2015;16(9):758.
22. Ylijoki MK, Ekholm E, Ekblad M, et al. Prenatal risk factors for adverse developmental outcome in preterm infants-systematic review. *Front Psychol* 2019;10:595.
23. Johnson PI, Sutton P, Atchley DS, et al. The Navigation Guide—evidence-based medicine meets environmental health: systematic review of human evidence for PFOA effects on fetal growth. *Environ Health Perspect* 2014;122(10):1028.
24. Di Renzo GC, Conry JA, Blake J, et al. International Federation of Gynecology and Obstetrics opinion on reproductive health impacts of exposure to toxic environmental chemicals. *Int J Gynaecol Obstet* 2015;131(3):219.
25. Brown LD, Hay WW Jr. Impact of placental insufficiency on fetal skeletal muscle growth. *Mol Cell Endocrinol* 2016;435:69.
26. Balayla J, Desilets J, Shrem G. Placenta previa and the risk of intrauterine growth restriction (IUGR): a systematic review and meta-analysis. *J Perinat Med* 2019;47(6):577.
27. Finken MJJ, van der Steen M, Smeets CCJ, et al. Children born small for gestational age: differential diagnosis, molecular genetic evaluation, and implications. *Endocr Rev* 2018;39(6):851.
28. Priante E, Verlato G, Giordano G, et al. Intrauterine growth restriction: new insight from the metabolomic approach. *Metabolites* 2019;9(11):267.
29. Thorn SR, Rozance PJ, Brown LD, et al. The intrauterine growth restriction phenotype: fetal adaptations and potential implications for later life insulin resistance and diabetes. *Semin Reprod Med* 2011;29(3):225.
30. Ross MG, Beall MH. Adult sequelae of intrauterine growth restriction. *Semin Perinatol* 2008;32(3):213.
31. Roth CL, Sathyanarayana S. Mechanisms affecting neuroendocrine and epigenetic regulation of body weight and onset of puberty: potential implications in the child born small for gestational age (SGA). *Rev Endocr Metab Disord* 2012;13(2):129.
32. Gurugubelli Krishna R, Bhat BV, Bobby Z, et al. Are Global DNA methylation and telomere length useful biomarkers for identifying intrauterine growth restricted neonates? *J Matern Fetal Neonatal Med* 2019;1.
33. Katz J, Lee ACC, Kozuki N, et al. Mortality risk in preterm and small-for-gestational-age infants in low-income and middle-income countries: a pooled country analysis. *Lancet* 2013;382(9890):417.
34. Miller SL, Huppi PS, Mallard C. The consequences of fetal growth restriction on brain structure and neurodevelopmental outcome. *J Physiol* 2016;594(4):807.
35. Khazardoost S, Ghotbizadeh F, Sahebdel B, et al. Predictors of cranial ultrasound abnormalities in intrauterine growth-restricted fetuses born between 28 and 34 weeks of gestation: a prospective cohort study. *Fetal Diagn Ther* 2019;45(4):238.
36. Padilla-Gomes NF, Enriquez G, Acosta-Rojas R, et al. Prevalence of neonatal ultrasound brain lesions in premature infants with and without intrauterine growth restriction. *Acta Paediatr* 2007;96(11):1582.
37. Morin EC, Schleger F, Preissl H, et al. Functional brain development in growth-restricted and constitutionally small fetuses: a fetal magnetoencephalography case–control study. *BJOG* 2015;122(9):1184.
38. Jiang ZD, Li ZH. Mild maturational delay of the brainstem at term in late preterm small-for-gestation age babies. *Early Hum Dev* 2015;91(4):265.
39. Bruno CJ, Bengani S, Gomes WA, et al. MRI differences associated with intrauterine growth restriction in preterm infants. *Neonatology* 2017;111(4):317.
40. Chauhan SP, Rice MM, Grobman WA, et al. Neonatal morbidity of small- and large-for-gestational-age neonates born at term in uncomplicated pregnancies. *Obstet Gynecol* 2017;130(3):511.
41. Mendez-Figueroa H, Truong VT, Pedroza C, et al. Small-for-gestational-age infants among uncomplicated pregnancies at term: a secondary analysis of 9 Maternal-Fetal Medicine Units Network studies. *Am J Obstet Gynecol* 2016;215(5):628.e1.
42. Madden JV, Flatley CJ, Kumar S. Term small-for-gestational-age infants from low-risk women are at significantly greater risk of adverse neonatal outcomes. *Am J Obstet Gynecol* 2018;218(5):525.e1.
43. Bhat MA, Kumar P, Bhansali A, et al. Hypoglycemia in small for gestational age babies. *Indian J Pediatr* 2000;67(6):423.
44. Sharma A, Davis A, Shekhawat PS. Hypoglycemia in the preterm neonate: etiopathogenesis, diagnosis, management and long-term outcomes. *Transl Pediatr* 2017;6(4):335.
45. Mallick AK, Venkatnarayan K, Thapar RK, et al. Morbidity patterns of late preterm babies born small for gestation. *Indian J Pediatr* 2019;86(7):578.
46. Stewart B, Karahalios A, Pszczola R, et al. Moderate to late preterm intrauterine growth restriction: a retrospective, observational study of the indications for delivery and outcomes in an Australian perinatal centre. *Aust N Z J Obstet Gynaecol* 2018;58(3):306.
47. Doctor BA, O'Riordan MA, Kirchner HL, et al. Perinatal correlates and neonatal outcomes of small for gestational age infants born at term gestation. *Am J Obstet Gynecol* 2001;185(3):652.
48. Soll RF. Heat loss prevention in neonates. *J Perinatol* 2008;28(suppl 1):S57.
49. Day RL, Caliguiri L, Kamenski C, et al. Body temperature and survival of premature infants. *Pediatrics* 1964;34:171.
50. Silverman WA, Fertig JW, Berger AP. The influence of the thermal environment upon the survival of newly born premature infants. *Pediatrics* 1958;22(5):876.
51. Hill JR, Rahimtulla KA. Heat balance and the metabolic rate of new-born babies in relation to environmental temperature; and the effect of age and of weight on basal metabolic rate. *J Physiol* 1965;180(2):239.
52. Turitz AL, Gyamfi-Bannerman C. Is there a relationship between preterm small-for-gestational age and respiratory distress syndrome? *Am J Obstet Gynecol* 2016;214(1):S216.

THE NEWBORN INFANT

53. Tannirwar S, Kadam S, Pandit A, et al. Comparisons of mortality and pre-discharge respiratory morbidities in small for gestational age and appropri-ate-for gestational age premature infants-An Indian Experience. *Iranian J Neonatol* 2016;7(4):1.
54. Sasi A, Abraham V, Davies-Tuck M, et al. Impact of intrauterine growth restriction on preterm lung disease. *Acta Paediatr* 2015;104(12):e552.
55. Bianco-Miotto T, Craig JM, Gasser YP, et al. Epigenetics and DOHaD: from basics to birth and beyond. *J Dev Orig Health Dis* 2017;8(5):513.
56. Sehgal A, Doctor T, Menahem S. Cardiac function and arterial biophysical properties in small for gestational age infants: postnatal manifestations of fetal programming. *J Pediatr* 2013;163(5):1296.
57. Crispi F, Figueras F, Cruz-Lemini M, et al. Cardiovascular programming in children born small for gestational age and relationship with prenatal signs of severity. *Am J Obstet Gynecol* 2012;207(2):121.e1.
58. Altin H, Karaarslan S, Karatas Z, et al. Evaluation of cardiac functions in term small for gestational age newborns with mild growth retardation: a serial conventional and tissue Doppler imaging echocardiographic study. *Early Hum Dev* 2012;88(9):757.
59. Akazawa Y, Hachiya A, Yamazaki S, et al. Cardiovascular remodeling and dysfunction across a range of growth restriction severity in small for gestational age infants–implications for fetal programming. *Circ J.* 2016;80(10):2212.
60. Hobbins JC, Gumina DL, Zaretsky M, et al. Size and shape of the four-chamber view of the fetal heart in fetuses with an estimated fetal weight less than the tenth centile. *Am J Obstet Gynecol* 2019;221:495.e1.
61. Villamor-Martinez E, Kilani MA, Degraeuwe PL, et al. Intrauterine growth restriction and patent ductus arteriosus in very and extremely pre-term infants: a systematic review and meta-analysis. *Front Endocrinol* 2019;10:58.
62. Cohen E, Dix L, Baerts W, et al. Reduction in cerebral oxygenation due to patent ductus arteriosus is pronounced in small-for-gestational-age neo-nates. *Neonatology* 2017;111(2):126.
63. Aldana-Aguirre JC, Toye J, Shah PS, et al.; Canadian Neonatal Network Investigators. Patent ductus arteriosus and small for gestational age infants: treatment approaches and outcomes. *Early Hum Dev* 2019;131:10.
64. Juhl SM, Gregersen R, Lange T, et al. Incidence and risk of necrotizing entero-colitis in Denmark from 1994–2014. *PLoS One* 2019;14(7):e0219268.
65. Yee WH, Soraisham AS, Shah VS, et al. Incidence and timing of pre-sentation of necrotizing enterocolitis in preterm infants. *Pediatrics* 2012;129(2):e298.
66. Aly H, Ez El Din Z, Soliman RM, et al. Renal function in small for gesta-tional age preterm infants. *J Perinatol* 2019;39(9):1263.
67. Olusanya BO, Ogunlesi TA, Kumar P, et al. Management of late-preterm and term infants with hyperbilirubinaemia in resource-constrained set-tings. *BMC Pediatr* 2015;15:39.
68. Mreihil K, Benth JS, Stensvold HJ, et al. Phototherapy is commonly used for neonatal jaundice but greater control is needed to avoid toxicity in the most vulnerable infants. *Acta Paediatr* 2018;107(4):611.
69. Karaduman D, Ergin H, Kilic I. Serum ferritin, iron levels and iron bind-ing capacity in asymmetric SGA babies. *Turk J Pediatr* 2001;43(2):121.
70. Christensen RD, Yoder BA, Baer VL, et al. Early-onset neutropenia in small-for-gestational-age infants. *Pediatrics* 2015;136(5):e1259.
71. Christensen RD, Baer VL, Henry E, et al. Thrombocytopenia in small-for-gestational-age infants. *Pediatrics* 2015;136(2):e361.
72. Rathore DK, Nair D, Raza S, et al. Underweight full-term Indian neonates show differences in umbilical cord blood leukocyte phenotype: a cross-sectional study. *PLoS One* 2015;10(4):e0123589.
73. Troger B, Muller T, Faust K, et al. Intrauterine growth restriction and the innate immune system in preterm infants of </=32 weeks gestation. *Neonatology* 2013;103(3):199.
74. Joseph K, UdayKiran G, Reddy DR, et al. Incidence of meconium aspira-tion syndrome and associated risk factors in babies born to mothers with meconium stained amniotic fluid. *Int J Contemp Med Res* 2017;4(7):1457.
75. Narchi H, Skinner A, Williams B. Small for gestational age neonates—are we missing some by only using standard population growth standards and does it matter? *J Matern Fetal Neonatal Med* 2010;23(1):48.
76. Razak A, Faden M. Association of small for gestational age with retinopa-thy of prematurity: a systematic review and meta-analysis. *Arch Dis Child Fetal Neonatal Ed* 2020;105:270.
77. Lee JW, VanderVeen D, Allred EN, et al. Prethreshold retinopathy in premature infants with intrauterine growth restriction. *Acta Paediatr* 2015;104(1):27.
78. Baumgart S. Iatrogenic hyperthermia and hypothermia in the neonate. *Clin Perinatol* 2008;35(1):183.
79. World Health Organization. *Thermal protection of the newborn: a practi-cal guide.* Geneva, Switzerland: World Health Organization, 1997.
80. Hammarlund K, Sedin G. Transepidermal water loss in newborn infants. III. Relation to gestational age. *Acta Paediatr Scand* 1979;68(6):795.
81. Hammarlund K, Nilsson GE, Oberg PA, et al. Transepidermal water loss in newborn infants. V. Evaporation from the skin and heat exchange during the first hours of life. *Acta Paediatr Scand* 1980;69(3):385.
82. Vohra S, Roberts RS, Zhang B, et al. Heat Loss Prevention (HeLP) in the delivery room: a randomized controlled trial of polyethylene occlusive skin wrapping in very preterm infants. *J Pediatr* 2004;145(6):750.
83. Singh A, Duckett J, Newton T, et al. Improving neonatal unit admission temperatures in preterm babies: exothermic mattresses, polythene bags or a traditional approach? *J Perinatol* 2010;30(1):45.
84. Ringer SA. Core concepts: thermoregulation in the newborn, part II: pre-vention of aberrant body temperature. *NeoReviews* 2013;14(5):e221.
85. Harpin VA, Rutter N. Humidification of incubators. *Arch Dis Child* 1985;60(3):219.
86. Sedin G, Hammarlund K, Stromberg B. Transepidermal water loss in full-term and pre-term infants. *Acta Paediatr Scand Suppl* 1983;305:27.
87. Cleminson J, McGuire W. Topical emollient for preventing infection in preterm infants. *Cochrane Database Syst Rev* 2016;(1):CD001150.
88. Conde-Agudelo A, Belizan JM, Diaz-Rossello J. Kangaroo mother care to reduce morbidity and mortality in low birthweight infants. *Cochrane Database Syst Rev* 2011;(3):CD002771.
89. Mazumder S, Taneja S, Dube B, et al. Effect of community-initiated kan-garoo mother care on survival of infants with low birthweight: a ran-domised controlled trial. *Lancet* 2019;394(10210):1724.
90. Sabel KG, Olegard R, Mellander M, et al. Interrelation between fatty acid oxidation and control of gluconeogenic substrates in small-for-ges-tational-age (SGA) infants with hypoglycemia and with normoglycemia. *Acta Paediatr Scand* 1982;71(1):53.
91. Rosenberg A. The IUGR newborn. *Semin Perinatol* 2008;32(3):219.
92. Committee on Fetus and Newborn; Adamkin DH. Postnatal glucose homeo-stasis in late-preterm and term infants. *Pediatrics* 2011;127(3):575.
93. American Academy of Pediatrics Committee on Fetus and Newborn. Hos-pital discharge of the high-risk neonate. *Pediatrics* 2008;122(5):1119.
94. Bull MJ, Engle WA; Committee on Injury, Violence, and Poison Preven-tion and Committee on Fetus and Newborn, et al. Safe transportation of preterm and low birth weight infants at hospital discharge. *Pediatrics* 2009;123(5):1424.
95. Campisi SC, Carbone SE, Zlotkin S. Catch-up growth in full-term small for gestational age infants: a systematic review. *Adv Nutr* 2019;10(1):104.
96. Lundgren EM, Tuvemo T. Effects of being born small for gestational age on long-term intellectual performance. *Best Pract Res Clin Endocrinol Metab* 2008;22(3):477.
97. Al-Qashar F, Sobaih B, Shajira E, et al. Impact of intrauterine growth restriction and birth weight on infant's early childhood neurodevelop-ment outcome. *J Clin Neonatol* 2018;7(1):1.
98. Fischi-Gomez E, Munoz-Moreno E, Vasung L, et al. Brain network char-acterization of high-risk preterm-born school-age children. *Neuroimage Clin* 2016;11:195.
99. Munoz-Moreno E, Fischi-Gomez E, Batalle D, et al. Structural brain net-work reorganization and social cognition related to adverse perinatal con-dition from infancy to early adolescence. *Front Neurosci* 2016;10:560.
100. Simões RV, Cruz-Lemini M, Bargalló N, et al. Brain metabolite differences in one-year-old infants born at term and association with neurode-velopmental outcome. *Am J Obstet Gynecol* 2015;213(2):210.e1.
101. Graz MB, Tolsa J-F, Fumeaux CJF. Being small for gestational age: does it matter for the neurodevelopment of premature infants? A cohort study. *PLoS One* 2015;10(5):e0125769.
102. Varella MH, Moss WJ. Early growth patterns are associated with intelli-gence quotient scores in children born small-for-gestational age. *Early Hum Dev* 2015;91(8):491.
103. Heinonen K, Raikkonen K, Pesonen AK, et al. Behavioural symptoms of attention deficit/hyperactivity disorder in preterm and term children born small and appropriate for gestational age: a longitudinal study. *BMC Pediatr* 2010;10:91.
104. Serati M, Barkin JL, Orsenigo G, et al. Research review: the role of obstetric and neonatal complications in childhood attention deficit and hyperactivity disorder—a systematic review. *J Child Psychol Psychiatry* 2017;58(12):1290.
105. Tanis JC, Van Braeckel KN, Kerstjens JM, et al. Functional outcomes at age 7 years of moderate preterm and full term children born small for ges-tational age. *J Pediatr* 2015;166(3):552.
106. Jensen L, Piek J, Kane R, et al. Male infants and infants born small for gestational age are at risk of fine motor delay in infancy. *Physiotherapy* 2015;101:e678.
107. Michael-Asalu A, Taylor G, Campbell H, et al. Cerebral palsy: diagnosis, epidemiology, genetics, and clinical update. *Adv Pediatr* 2019;66:189.
108. Zhao M, Dai H, Deng Y, et al. SGA as a risk factor for cerebral palsy in moderate to late preterm infants: a system review and meta-analysis. *Sci Rep* 2016;6:38853.
109. Vollmer B, Edmonds CJ. School age neurological and cognitive outcomes of fetal growth retardation or small for gestational age birth weight. *Front Endocrinol (Lausanne)* 2019;10:186.
110. Blair EM, Nelson KB. Fetal growth restriction and risk of cerebral palsy in singletons born after at least 35 weeks' gestation. *Am J Obstet Gynecol* 2015;212(4):520.e1.

111. Mericq V, Martinez-Aguayo A, Uauy R, et al. Long-term metabolic risk among children born premature or small for gestational age. *Nat Rev Endocrinol* 2017;13(1):50.
112. Ong KK. Catch-up growth in small for gestational age babies: good or bad? *Curr Opin Endocrinol Diabetes Obes* 2007;14(1):30.
113. Ong KK, Ahmed ML, Emmett PM, et al. Association between postnatal catch-up growth and obesity in childhood: prospective cohort study. *BMJ* 2000;320(7240):967.
114. Hernandez MI, Mericq V. Impact of being born small for gestational age on onset and progression of puberty. *Best Pract Res Clin Endocrinol Metab* 2008;22(3):463.
115. Hong YH, Chung S. Small for gestational age and obesity related comorbidities. *Ann Pediatr Endocrinol Metab* 2018;23(1):4.
116. Ramirez-Velez R, Correa-Bautista JE, Villa-Gonzalez E, et al. Effects of preterm birth and fetal growth retardation on life-course cardiovascular risk factors among schoolchildren from Colombia: the FUPRECOL study. *Early Hum Dev* 2017;106–107:53.
117. Ou-Yang MC, Sun Y, Liebowitz M, et al. Accelerated weight gain, prematurity, and the risk of childhood obesity: a meta-analysis and systematic review. *PLoS One* 2020;15(5):e0232238.
118. Castagno M, Menegon V, Monzani A, et al. Small-for-gestational-age birth is linked to cardiovascular dysfunction in early childhood. *Am Heart J* 2019;217:84.
119. Carr H, Cnattingius S, Granath F, et al. Preterm birth and risk of heart failure up to early adulthood. *J Am Coll Cardiol* 2017;69(21):2634.

THE NEWBORN INFANT

Control of Breathing: Maturation and Associated Clinical Disorders

Nicole R. Dobson, Mark W. Thompson, and Carl E. Hunt

INTRODUCTION

The fetus makes breathing movements *in utero* that change in character and frequency throughout gestation. In addition to being important for lung development, the maturation of breathing control is essential for ensuring a successful transition from episodic fetal breathing to continuous postnatal breathing. Control of breathing is immature in infants born preterm and is progressively more immature the younger the gestational age at birth. As a consequence of this immaturity, clinical symptoms related to apnea, bradycardia, and intermittent hypoxia are common problems in the early weeks of life and may continue beyond term-equivalent age, especially in infants born extremely preterm. In this chapter, fetal breathing, initiation of breathing at birth, and immaturity of control of breathing in infants born preterm are first reviewed. We then describe the clinical manifestations of immature breathing, including respiratory pauses and periodic breathing, apnea, and apnea of prematurity (AOP) and potential adverse clinical consequences. Finally, we also review clinical disorders for which preterm infants are at increased risk after neonatal intensive care unit (NICU) discharge: sudden infant death syndrome (SIDS), brief resolved unexplained events (BRUEs) formerly identified as apparent life-threatening events (ALTEs), and sleep-disordered breathing (SDB) (obstructive sleep apnea).

MATURATION OF AUTONOMIC CONTROL OF BREATHING

Fetal Breathing

Studies in animal models and human fetuses have demonstrated a maturational progression in fetal breathing movements during gestation that can be altered by a variety of pharmacologic and physiologic inputs. In humans, fetal breathing movements have been characterized in response to maternal condition and as a potential indicator of overall fetal condition. Regardless of gestational age, fetal breathing is not a continuous process; significant periods of apnea lasting as long as 2 hours occur even in near-term fetuses and are generally more frequent and of longer duration at younger gestational ages (1). During periods of frequent respiratory motion, patterns of both regular and irregular breathing are documented by chest/abdominal wall movements and by Doppler sonography assessing tracheal fluid flow (2). Fetal breathing movements exhibit a circadian rhythmicity, with well-documented increases during certain periods of the day. Maternal condition, particularly maternal glucose status, can have significant effects on fetal breathing frequency, with well-documented increases in fetal breathing frequency after maternal glucose loading. This response to maternal glucose loading is most pronounced when the mother has been fasting (3).

Fetal breathing has some clinical utility when assessing fetal well-being. Several studies have documented diminished fetal breathing activity in association with poor fetal health, and this decreased activity, along with other measures of fetal well-being, can be helpful in guiding obstetric management (4). The fetal breathing pattern responds to a variety of pharmacologic and physiologic manipulations. Fetal breathing increases if the mother inhales CO_2 (5). Maternal hyperoxia does not alter fetal breathing movements or pattern in near-term normally grown fetuses, but growth-restricted fetuses exhibit an increase in respiratory rate with maternal hyperoxia (6). Tocolytics, indomethacin, and terbutaline increase fetal breathing movements when administered during preterm labor (7).

Animal studies augment the human ultrasound data and provide a clearer picture of the maturational development of breathing control. Fetal breathing activity in sheep starts early in gestation, arises from centrally mediated stimuli, and occurs primarily during periods of low-voltage electrocortical activity (REM sleep) (8). REM sleep constitutes about 40% of fetal life during the last trimester in sheep. Breathing also occurs during periods of high-voltage electrocortical activity (quiet sleep), but it is only episodic and generally associated with muscular discharges (9). Animal data have also confirmed that the fetal breathing pattern changes in response to physiologic derangements (i.e., hypercarbia, hypoxia, hyperoxia) (10,11). In response to hypercapnia, the fetus increases respiratory rate and tidal volume, suggesting intact central chemoreception. The fetal response to hypoxia appears to be centrally mediated and results in diminished neuronal activity and diminished or absent fetal breathing movements, but the peripheral chemoreceptors may also contribute to absence of the "adult" response to hypoxia of an increase in respiratory rate and tidal volume.

Initiation of Breathing at Birth

Despite the enhanced understanding of fetal maturation of breathing control, our understanding remains incomplete regarding factors responsible for initiating and maintaining a regular pattern at birth (12). Development and maintenance of respiration in the newborn are likely due to a complex interaction of sensory stimuli and both central and peripheral chemoreceptor inputs (Fig. 27.1). The basal level of fetal chemoreceptor discharge adapts to the fetal PaO_2, and the severalfold increase in PaO_2 at birth silences the chemoreceptors (13). During the fetal-to-neonatal transition, however, peripheral chemoreceptors may not be completely silenced, as evidenced by the fact that supplemental O_2 compared to room air at birth may delay onset of the first cry and of sustained ventilation thereafter. The degree of maturation in the central respiratory centers also appears to be important since the responses to respiratory stimuli in the term infant are more developed than are those in the preterm infant.

Neonatal Breathing

Studies in human and animal neonates have provided important insights into the understanding of respiratory rhythm generation (14). The control and maintenance of normal breathing largely reside within the respiratory control centers of the bulbopontine region of the brainstem. Neurons within this area respond to multiple afferent inputs to modulate their own inherent rhythmicity and provide efferent output to the respiratory control muscles. Multiple afferent inputs induce modulation of the central respiratory center efferent outputs to the lungs and respiratory and airway muscles. These afferent inputs are "categorized" by the respiratory control center; some inputs cause an instantaneous response in the control center output, while others only act to "shape" the respiratory response, resulting in small changes in muscular output, tidal volume, and airway tone (15). Among these inputs are signals from central and peripheral chemoreceptors, pulmonary stretch receptors, and cortical and reticuloactivating system neurons. These afferent inputs and resultant efferent outputs of the central respiratory center are summarized in Figure 27.1. Sleep state can also have a profound effect on respiratory pattern, although sleep state is often difficult to classify in preterm infants.

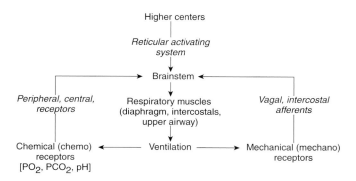

Higher centers

Reticular activating system

Brainstem

Peripheral, central, receptors

Respiratory muscles (diaphragm, intercostals, upper airway)

Vagal, intercostal afferents

Chemical (chemo) receptors [PO_2, PCO_2, pH]

Ventilation

Mechanical (mechano) receptors

FIGURE 27.1 Major factors influencing respiratory control. PCO_2, carbon dioxide partial pressure; PO_2, oxygen pressure. (Reprinted from Martin RJ, Miller MJ, Carlo WA. Pathogenesis of apnea in preterm infants. *J Pediatr* 1986;109:733. Copyright © 1986 Elsevier, with permission.)

In the adult, these multiple afferent inputs act upon neurons within the respiratory control center and provide a well-integrated response to perturbations in the system and characteristic respiratory patterns. For example, increased respiratory rate and depth will characteristically result from activation of central chemoreceptors in response to hypercarbia. In the newborn infant and especially in the preterm infant, however, these responses are less well organized and of lesser magnitude, and apnea with associated desaturation and/or bradycardia is a common result of this disorganized or immature response to multiple afferent inputs.

The central chemosensitivity to hypercarbia is diminished in infants born preterm and is unrelated to any mechanical limitations of ventilation (16). The slope of the CO_2 response curve increases significantly between 29 to 32 and 33 to 36 weeks of gestation, especially in infants without clinically evident apnea. The cause of this decreased sensitivity of central respiratory centers to CO_2 in preterm infants is related to central nervous system immaturity as indicated by decreased synaptic connections and incomplete dendritic arborization.

Preterm infants and full-term infants up to approximately 3 weeks' postnatal age have a characteristic biphasic response to hypoxia that is quite different than in older infants. In contrast to the sustained hyperventilation in older infants, preterm infants have only a transient hyperventilation lasting 30 seconds to a minute, followed by progressive ventilatory depression despite continued low inspired oxygen concentrations. The initial hyperventilatory response may be completely blunted in extremely premature infants. This initial transient hyperventilation is likely in response to peripheral chemoreceptor input, and the subsequent hypoxic depression appears to be at least primarily due to centrally mediated decreased peripheral chemoreceptor activity secondary to descending inhibition from the upper brainstem, midbrain, or higher structures (16).

In addition to maturation of central chemoreception, peripheral chemoreceptors progressively mature over the first weeks of life in both full-term and preterm infants, as manifested by the decrease in ventilation with hyperoxia and the hypoxic ventilatory response (13). The magnitude of the ventilatory depression occurring with acute hyperoxia is relatively blunted in infants born preterm, and the magnitude of the hypoxic ventilatory depression is greater in preterm infants with symptomatic AOP. However, it is still unclear to what extent, if any, immature or mature peripheral chemoreception is associated with apnea symptoms. Peripheral chemoreceptor activation plays a role in apnea termination, but excessive peripheral chemoreceptor activation may destabilize the respiratory pattern in AOP and exacerbate the extent of apnea and associated bradycardia and intermittent hypoxia. Carotid chemoreceptors may thus be important not only in stimulating arousal

from apnea-associated desaturation, and hence apnea termination, but also potentiating the risk of occurrence. The extent of apnea does seem to correlate with maturation of the ventilatory response to acute hypoxia, with less apnea and intermittent hypoxia present in the early weeks of life and increased apnea-related symptoms and intermittent hypoxia in the later weeks in association with maturation of carotid chemoreceptivity and greater sensitivity to acute hypoxia (13).

Both central and peripheral inputs are thus likely important in the onset and termination of apnea (16). The coordination of phasic and tonic inputs to determine breathing rhythms is not yet fully understood, but stable autonomic control of breathing appears to involve multiple phasic, random, and descending inputs. Upper airway reflexes also may play a role in inhibiting respiration, particularly in preterm infants. Multiple sensory afferent fibers exist within the upper airways, and stimulation of these fibers by various mechanisms can result in abnormal respiratory responses. Responses to upper airway afferent fiber stimulation can change markedly with maturation. Negative pressure in the upper airways in human infants results in depressed ventilation. This inhibition may contribute to the central apnea that often follows obstructed breaths (Fig. 27.2). As upper airway obstruction occurs, the infant makes respiratory efforts against this obstruction, and the resulting increased negative pressure in the upper airway may result in reflex inhibition of diaphragmatic contraction. Due to a blunted response to hypercarbia and hypoxic ventilatory depression, less mature preterm infants with apnea may be unable to recover spontaneously and hence be more likely to require active intervention.

Activation of laryngeal mucosal receptors can elicit strong airway protective reflexes in both full-term and preterm infants. This laryngeal chemoreflex can result in autonomic responses including apnea, bradycardia, hypotension, upper airway closure, and swallowing (16). Although this chemoreflex is an important contributor to aspiration-related apnea and bradycardia, there is no clear relationship to AOP.

Genetics of Control of Breathing

Recent genetic studies related to brainstem autonomic regulation have enhanced our understanding of normal development of respiratory regulation (17). Targeted gene inactivation studies in animals have identified multiple genes involved with prenatal brainstem development of respiratory control including arousal responsiveness. During embryogenesis, the survival of specific cellular populations constituting the respiratory neuronal network is regulated by neurotrophins, a multigene family of growth factors and receptors. Brain-derived neurotrophic factor (BDNF) is required for development of normal breathing behavior in mice, and newborn mice lacking functional BDNF exhibit ventilatory depression associated with apparent loss of peripheral chemoafferent input. Ventilation is depressed, and hypoxic ventilatory drive is deficient or absent.

Krox-20, a homeobox gene, appears to be required for normal development of the respiratory central pattern generator (18). *Krox-20* null mutants exhibit an abnormally slow respiratory rhythm and increased incidence of respiratory pauses, and this respiratory depression can be further modulated by endogenous enkephalins. Absence of *Krox-20* may result in the absence of a rhythm-promoting reticular neuron group localized in the caudal pons and could thus be a cause of life-threatening apnea.

Brainstem muscarinic cholinergic pathways are important in ventilatory responsiveness to carbon dioxide (CO_2). The muscarinic system develops from the neural crest, and the *ret* protooncogene is important for this development (17). *Ret* knockout mice have a depressed ventilatory response to hypercarbia, implicating absence of the *ret* gene as a cause of impaired hypercarbic responsiveness. Diminished ventilatory responsiveness to hypercarbia

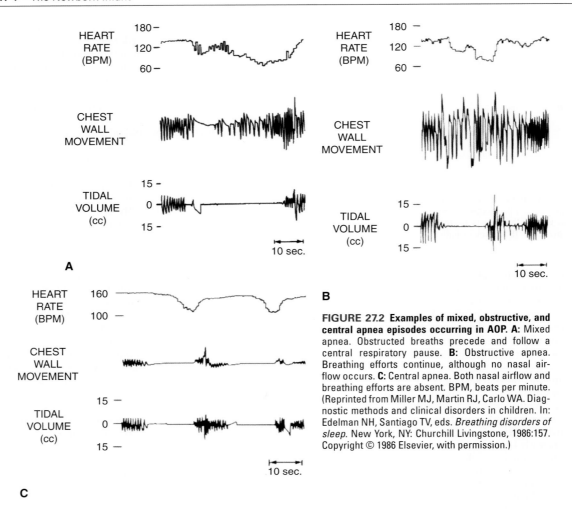

FIGURE 27.2 Examples of mixed, obstructive, and central apnea episodes occurring in AOP. A: Mixed apnea. Obstructed breaths precede and follow a central respiratory pause. **B:** Obstructive apnea. Breathing efforts continue, although no nasal airflow occurs. **C:** Central apnea. Both nasal airflow and breathing efforts are absent. BPM, beats per minute. (Reprinted from Miller MJ, Martin RJ, Carlo WA. Diagnostic methods and clinical disorders in children. In: Edelman NH, Santiago TV, eds. *Breathing disorders of sleep.* New York, NY: Churchill Livingstone, 1986:157. Copyright © 1986 Elsevier, with permission.)

has also been demonstrated in male newborn mice heterozygous for *Mash-1*. There is a molecular link between *ret* and *Mash-1*, and the latter is expressed in embryonic neurons in vagal neural crest derivatives and in brainstem locus coeruleus neurons, an area involved with arousal responsiveness.

Serotonin (5-HT) is a widespread neurotransmitter that affects cardiovascular control and modulates activity of the circadian clock. Serotonergic receptors in the brainstem are critical components of respiratory drive. Multiple genes are involved in the control of serotonin synthesis, storage, membrane uptake, and metabolism (17). Polymorphisms have been identified in the promoter region of the 5-HT transporter protein gene located on chromosome 17, and variations in the promoter region of the gene appear to have a role in serotonin membrane uptake and regulation. Several transporter polymorphisms have been described that may occur in greater frequency in SIDS than in control infants, but no data are available related to maturation of breathing control in preterm infants in general or to AOP in particular. Thus, there are no data on the potential role of serotonin-related polymorphisms in determining the extent of clinical manifestations of AOP. However, the greater concordance for AOP among monozygotic twins than same-sex dizygotic twins suggests a genetic contribution (19).

These studies illustrate potentially important genetic foundations of neonatal control of breathing. Further work is needed, however, to better understand the developmental regulation of these targeted genes and their influence on maturation of the fetal/neonatal respiratory centers and peripheral chemoreceptors.

CLINICAL MANIFESTATIONS OF IMMATURE BREATHING

Respiratory Pauses and Periodic Breathing

The clinical manifestations of immature autonomic regulation of respiration include brief respiratory pauses, apnea, bradycardia, and desaturation. Respiratory pauses occur commonly in both preterm and full-term infants and are typically manifested as periodic breathing. Periodic breathing is a pattern of regular breathing alternating with respiratory pauses persisting through at least three cycles of breathing. The pauses are at least 3 seconds in duration and may last for 5 to 10 seconds or more (20). The prevalence of periodic breathing has been reported to be as high as 80% in term infants and may approach 100% in extremely low-birth-weight preterm infants (21,22). The prevalence diminishes with increasing postnatal and postmenstrual age (PMA) and appears to reach a nadir by about 44 weeks of PMA (23). A recent study in 1,211 infants born less than 35 weeks' gestation using a novel computer algorithm to detect periodic breathing from bedside monitor chest impedance data revealed that preterm infants with higher gestational age spend more time in periodic breathing (24). Interestingly, the highest amount of periodic breathing occurred in infants 30 to 33 weeks of gestational age at around 2 weeks of chronologic age (**Fig. 27.3**) (24). Periodic breathing results primarily from immature central chemoreception, but the peripheral chemoreceptor response to intermittent hypoxia may also contribute to periodic breathing (16).

Periodic breathing is common, especially in preterm infants, but this respiratory pattern is likely not benign when associated with longer respiratory pauses or apnea, intermittent hypoxia, and/or bradycardia. Particularly in more immature preterm infants, minute ventilation can diminish significantly during episodes of periodic breathing, and oxygen saturation can decrease to hypoxemic levels in association with longer respiratory pauses and increased time spent in periodic breathing. The rate of decrease in oxygen saturation associated with respiratory pauses may also be related to baseline oxygenation, which in preterm infants may be adversely affected not only by reduced lung volumes but also by the extent of pulmonary disease. The intermittent respiratory pauses of periodic breathing are typically associated with intermittent hypoxia and heart rate decelerations or even bradycardia, and mounting evidence suggests that intermittent hypoxia may be associated with longer-term adverse consequences (discussed more in detail in later section) (25,26). The intermittent hypoxia and intermittent bradycardia associated with periodic breathing are typically not evident clinically and are documented only by review of continuous pulse oximeter recordings (27).

Periodic breathing appears to occur predominantly during REM sleep, but it also occurs during quiet sleep (20). During quiet sleep, periodic breathing is "regular" with consistent durations of the apneic and breathing periods, while during REM sleep, periodic breathing tends to be irregular with inconsistent cycle durations. Since more immature infants generally spend more time in sleep and more of this sleep time is characterized by periodic breathing, these infants may be experiencing significant amounts of intermittent hypoxia.

Apnea

In contrast to the shorter respiratory pauses observed with periodic breathing, cessations in ventilation lasting longer than 15 to 20 seconds are generally labeled as apnea, especially if associated with bradycardia and/or desaturation. The mechanism for bradycardia associated with apnea in preterm infants has not been fully elucidated (16). Some evidence suggests that this bradycardia is a consequence of apnea-related hypoxic stimulation of carotid chemoreceptors, but in some instances, the bradycardia occurs coincident with the apnea, suggesting a brainstem mechanism (**Fig. 27.4**). Bradycardia occurs more frequently with longer durations of apnea and usually follows the oxygen desaturation (28). Occasionally, bradycardia may follow apnea without desaturation. These events may be mediated by vagal nerve stimulation.

Apneic episodes are classified as central, obstructive, or mixed (29). Figure 27.2 demonstrates the respiratory patterns during these events. Central apneas result from lack of respiratory effort. Obstructive apneas (obstructed breaths) are also central in origin but are related to absence of neuromuscular control of upper airway patency rather than absence of inspiratory diaphragmatic stimulation. Obstructive apneas are characterized by cessation of inspiratory air flow into the lungs despite persisting respiratory effort. Mixed apneas represent a combination of absent respiratory effort (central apnea) and obstructed breaths.

There are multiple possible etiologic factors leading to symptomatic apnea in the preterm and full-term infant (**Tables 27.1 and 27.2**). Clinical and laboratory assessments are needed to rule out conditions for which specific treatment is indicated. There are no systematic prevalence data for symptomatic apnea in full-term infants, but most occurrences will have an identifiable medical cause (Table 27.2). In preterm infants less than 1,500 g at birth, approximately 70% will have at least one clinically observed episode of symptomatic apnea while in the NICU, and about 20% of these infants will have a specific medical cause (Table 27.1). The other 80% of preterm infants with symptomatic apnea do not have a specific pathologic cause other than immaturity of control of breathing, and by exclusion are then considered to have AOP, the most important and prevalent manifestation of respiratory control immaturity in preterm infants.

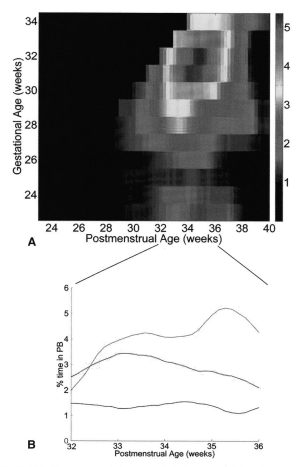

FIGURE 27.3 Percentage of time spent in PB per day of data, based on gestational and postmenstrual age. PB was analyzed during all times that chest impedance data were available and infants were not on mechanical ventilation for all infants <35 wk' GA (n = 1,211). (**A**) Heat map showing mean daily % time in PB, based on GA and PMA. The color scale goes from blue (mean 0% PB per day) to red (mean 5% PB per day). (**B**) Percent PB from 32 to 36 wk PMA in three GA groups, <27 wk (blue), 27–30 wk (green), and 31–34 wk (red).

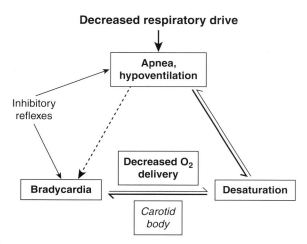

FIGURE 27.4 Proposed physiologic mechanisms by which apnea results in reflex bradycardia. This can occur secondary to hypoxemia or by stimulation of upper airway afferents. (From Martin RJ, Wilson CG. Apnea of prematurity. *Compr Physiol* 2012;2:2923. Copyright © 2012 American Physiological Society. Reprinted by permission of John Wiley & Sons, Inc.)

TABLE 27.1
Etiology of Apnea in Preterm Infants

Cause	Comment
Idiopathic	AOP, with immaturity of control of breathing; modified by sleep state
Central nervous system	Intracranial hemorrhage, seizures, depressant drugs, hypoxemia, hypothermia, hyperthermia
Respiratory	Pneumonia, obstructive airway lesions, respiratory distress syndrome, laryngeal reflex, phrenic or vocal cord paralysis, pneumothorax, hypoxemia, hypercarbia, nasal occlusion caused by phototherapy eye patches, tracheal occlusion caused by neck flexion
Cardiovascular	Heart failure, hypotension, hypertension, hypovolemia, increased vagal tone
Gastrointestinal	Abdominal distension, peritonitis. Apnea may increase the likelihood of GER following an apneic event. There is no evidence to support GER as the cause of apnea.
Infection	Pneumonia, sepsis, meningitis
Metabolic	Acidosis, hypoglycemia, hypocalcemia, hyponatremia, hypernatremia
Hematologic	Anemia

Adapted from Hunt CE. Apnea and sudden infant death syndrome in strategies. In: Kliegman RM, ed. *Pediatric diagnosis and therapy.* Philadelphia, PA: W.B. Saunders Co., 1996. Copyright © 1996 Elsevier, with permission.

Apnea of Prematurity
Pathophysiology

The maturation of cardiorespiratory control and the clinical course of premature infants with AOP parallel each other. AOP is a direct consequence of immaturity of brainstem respiratory control centers, but numerous factors contribute to the development of apnea, including altered ventilatory responses to hypercapnia and hypoxia (see "Neonatal Breathing" section, above). In addition, diaphragmatic fatigue may contribute to the development of AOP (28). It is not possible as part of routine clinical care to quan-

TABLE 27.2
Etiology of Apnea in Full-Term Infants

Cause	Comment
Intrapartum asphyxia	Hypoxemia, acidosis, brainstem depression
Placental transfer of central nervous system depressant	Narcotics, magnesium sulfate, general anesthetics
Airway obstruction	Choanal atresia, macroglossia–mandibular hypoplasia (Pierre Robin sequence), tracheal web or stenosis, airway mass lesions
Neuromuscular disorders	Absent or uncoordinated sucking/swallowing, uncoordinated sucking and breathing, congenital myopathies or neuropathies
Trauma	Intracranial hemorrhage, spinal cord transection, phrenic nerve palsy
Infection	Pneumonia, sepsis, meningitis
Central nervous system	Seizures, congenital central hypoventilation syndrome, Arnold-Chiari malformation, Dandy-Walker malformation

Adapted from Hunt CE. Apnea and sudden infant death syndrome in strategies. In: Kliegman RM, ed. *Pediatric diagnosis and therapy.* Philadelphia, PA: W.B. Saunders Co., 1996. Copyright © 1996 Elsevier, with permission.

tify the degree of immaturity of brainstem autonomic cardiorespiratory control systems. However, brainstem auditory maturation can be quantified by serial measurements of brainstem conduction time from the auditory-evoked response (wave VI interval) (30). The brainstem auditory nuclei are located in close proximity to the cardiorespiratory centers, and shortening of brainstem auditory conduction times occurs with advancing gestational age due to improved synaptic efficiency and myelination. Long brainstem conduction times for the auditory-evoked responses are strongly associated with clinical episodes of AOP. Since not all very-low-birth-weight (VLBW) preterm infants develop AOP and the severity varies among affected infants of the same gestational age, other genetic and/or environmental factors are also important. Twin modeling has been used to estimate the relative contributions of genetic and environmental influences in AOP (19). In this study, there was greater concordance for AOP among monozygotic twins than among same-sex dizygotic twins, suggesting a genetic contribution. Advanced model-fitting analysis revealed a strong genetic influence for AOP, and overall heritability was 87%. Genetic factors significantly contributed to susceptibility to AOP in males, but there was a combination of genetic and environmental factors in female infants. The importance of specific genetic risk factors and gene–environment interactions remains to be clarified.

Incidence and Diagnosis

Threshold criteria for diagnosis have not been objectively defined, and no established diagnostic test exists for AOP. Reported incidence data are therefore not based on standardized criteria for diagnosis and range from a low of less than 10% in preterm infants born at 34 weeks of gestation or more to approximately 60% at birth weights less than 1,500 g and to a high of greater than 85% among infants born at less than 28 weeks of gestation (31,32). A recent study analyzing bedside monitor chest impedance, electrocardiographic waveforms, and oxygen saturation data on 1,211 infants born less than 35 weeks' gestation showed that the number and duration of apnea events decreased with increasing gestational age and PMA (33). Clinical symptoms may manifest within the first day of life in spontaneously breathing infants, but the frequency of occurrence progressively increases after that. The peak incidence occurs 4 to 6 weeks after birth, a time course corresponding to increasing peripheral chemosensitivity and hence greater respiratory instability (see "Neonatal Breathing" section) (13,16,26).

Of the three types of apneic episodes (central, obstructive, or mixed), mixed apneas constitute the majority of AOP episodes (Fig. 27.2). Mixed episodes begin either with obstructed breaths or with central apnea, and multiple alternations between obstructed breaths and central apnea may occur within a single episode. The identification of individual episodes of AOP is typically based on bedside observations of prolonged apnea and clinically observed cyanosis or by detection of central apnea lasting at least 20 seconds using standard impedance-based cardiorespiratory monitoring, especially if there is accompanying bradycardia and/or oxygen desaturation sufficient to trigger a monitor alarm. To validate the clinical significance of monitor alarms, apparent episodes initially detected by alarm require visual confirmation. Visually confirmed episodes of apnea with associated heart rate decelerations and desaturation are classified as symptomatic episodes. No consensus-based threshold number of clinical episodes exists for a "diagnosis" of AOP, but most clinicians require at least one visually confirmed symptomatic episode unrelated to another medical cause (Table 27.1). The severity of AOP in individual patients and the threshold for initiating treatment are determined by the frequency and severity of subsequent clinically observed episodes, but clinical practice is quite variable. Since impedance-based cardiorespiratory monitors cannot directly detect obstructive apneas, episodes of AOP will not be detected by bedside monitoring until central apnea has persisted long enough to trigger a monitor alarm,

TABLE 27.5

Odds Ratio for SIDS in Infants Born Preterm Compared to Full Term

Gestational Age at Birth	Adjusted Odds Ratio (95% Confidence Intervals)	Postmenstrual Age at Death (Weeks; Mean ± SD)	Postnatal Age at Death (Weeks; Mean ± SD)
24–28	2.57 (2.08–3.17)	47.14 ± 8.8[a]	21.1 ± 9.1[a]
29–32	2.72 (2.38–3.10)	48.2 ± 8.7[a]	17.5 ± 8.6[a]
33–36	1.85 (1.72–1.99)	49.9 ± 8.7[a]	14.9 ± 8.6[a]
37–42	1.0	53.5 ± 8/7	14.6 ± 8.6

SIDS in preterm infants occurs at younger PMAs but older postnatal ages.

[a]$p < 0.05$ compared to 37 to 42 weeks of gestational age at birth.

SIDS, sudden infant death syndrome.

Adapted by permission from Nature: Malloy MH. Prematurity and sudden infant death syndrome: United States, 2005–2007. *J Perinatol* 2013;33:470. Copyright © 2013 Springer Nature.

BRIEF RESOLVED UNEXPLAINED EVENTS

A BRUE is diagnosed in an infant less than 1 year of age when the observer reports a sudden, brief, and now resolved episode characterized by at least one of the following: cyanosis or pallor; absent, decreased, or irregular breathing; marked change in tone (hyper- or hypotonia); or altered level of responsiveness (89). BRUEs were previously called ALTEs. Incidence rates for an ALTE varied from 0.5 to 10.0 per 1,000 live births. This 20-fold difference is likely related to different case definitions and methods of ascertainment. Infants born preterm are at increased risk for an ALTE (17). The incidence in preterm infants has been estimated to be in the range of 8% to 10%, with some studies reporting that up to 30% of infants experiencing an ALTE were less than 38 weeks' gestation at birth (23). Preterm infants thus are at increased risk for an ALTE, but it is unknown to what extent this might be related to persisting immature respiratory control and intermittent hypoxia, or to other mechanisms.

There are some important differences in the definition of a BRUE compared to an ALTE (89). Most important, a BRUE is only diagnosed when there is no explanation for the event. Second, BRUEs are divided into a low risk subgroup, for whom evaluation and management guidelines are included, and a high-risk subgroup for whom no guidelines are provided. To be low risk, there should be no history of prior episodes or clusters of episodes, the duration should be less than 1 minute and not requiring any resuscitation, and there should be no concerning historical features or physical exam findings. Of particular note, all preterm infants born less than 32 weeks of gestation and PMA less than 45 weeks are by definition classified as high risk. In a recent retrospective analysis of infants diagnosed with an ALTE, about 40% of infants previously diagnosed with an ALTE met the criteria for a BRUE, and about 20% of these were classified as low-risk BRUE (90). Adverse outcomes occurred in 9.2% of ALTE patients not meeting BRUE criteria, 2.9% in low-risk BRUE, and 9% in high-risk BRUE. In an administrative multicenter database, BRUE admissions declined after implementation of the BRUE clinical practice guideline, without an increase in recurrence or adverse outcomes (90). Prospective prevalence data for BRUE are not presently available.

SLEEP-DISORDERED BREATHING

Although estimates vary, as many as 4% or more of children have SDB, and infants born preterm are at increased risk for SDB (16). In a secondary study of 2,867 children, the odds ratio for SDB in children born preterm or low birth weight compared to term-born children was 1.74, 95% CI 1.30 to 2.32 ($p < 0.001$) (91). Other studies have reported as much as a 3 to 6 times greater frequency of SDB in children born preterm in population-based cohort studies (92). In a study of preterm infants born at 500 to 1,250 g and evaluated at school age, 9.6% had SDB, compared to 1% to 2% in a general population of same-age term-born children. In this report, SDB following preterm birth was associated with a history of chorioamnionitis and multiple gestations (93).

The mechanisms responsible for increased frequency of SDB with preterm birth are unclear. In a report of SDB and craniofacial development in preterm infants born at a mean gestational age of 31.5 ± 3.2 weeks, two-thirds had a narrow hard palate at 6 and 24 months of age, and 79% met the threshold polysomnographic definition for SDB (mean apnea–hypopnea index = 3.0) (94). By contrast, in a term-born control group, only 10% had a narrow hard palate and the mean apnea–hypopnea index was normal (0.5). Those children born preterm and with a narrow hard palate at 2 years of age had more sleep problems and a higher rate of developmental delay compared to children born preterm and without a narrow hard palate. These findings support the hypothesis that a narrow hard palate in preterm infants is associated with SDB-related sleep problems and neurodevelopmental delays (94). The persistence of a narrow hard palate after birth is thought to be an indicator of abnormal orofacial growth, but it is unclear to what extent the mechanism may be intrinsic versus related to postnatal severity of illness factors including intubation, or other acquired complications of preterm birth. Indeed, in a study of preterm infants at 8 to 11 years of age, cardiopulmonary resuscitation or intubation in the early neonatal period was associated with a two-fold to fourfold increased odds of SDB (95). In another recent retrospective report, SDB children born preterm and matched for age and severity of SDB with term-born children had increased parasympathetic tone during quiet sleep. This was suggested to be due to a more powerful parasympathetic response to changes in blood pressure related to increased work of breathing compared to full term–born children with similar SDB severity. Future studies need to determine whether known long-term morbidities affecting heart rate and cardiovascular control in children born preterm adversely affect risk for SDB. Follow-up studies are also needed to assess the longer-term effects of increased parasympathetic activity on cardiovascular outcomes (92). Finally, infants born preterm are also at increased risk for later obesity, but it is unknown to what extent obesity may also be a contributing factor to their increased risk of SDB (96). There is also a need in children born preterm to better understand the relationship between risk for SDB and neonatal intermittent hypoxia, neural plasticity, and both central and peripheral chemoreception.

DISCLAIMER

The views expressed in this chapter are those of the authors and do not necessarily reflect the official policy or position of the Department of the Army, Department of Defense, or the U.S. Government. Some authors are a military service member or a U.S. Government employee. This work was prepared as part of their official duties. Title 17 U.S.C. 105 provides that "Copyright protection under this title is not available for any work of the U.S. Government." Title 17 U.S.C. 101 defines a U.S. Government work as a work prepared by a military service member or employee of the U.S. Government as part of that person's official duties.

REFERENCES

1. Natale R, Nasello-Paterson C, Connors G. Patterns of fetal breathing activity in the human fetus at 24 to 28 weeks of gestation. *Am J Obstet Gynecol* 1988;158(2):317.
2. Kalache KD, Chaoui R, Marcks B, et al. Differentiation between human fetal breathing patterns by investigation of breathing-related tracheal fluid flow velocity using Doppler sonography. *Prenat Diagn* 2000;20(1):45.

3. Goodman JD. The effect of intravenous glucose on human fetal breathing measured by Doppler ultrasound. *Br J Obstet Gynaecol* 1980;87(12):1080.
4. Manning FA, Platt LD. Fetal breathing movements: antepartum monitoring of fetal condition. *Clin Obstet Gynaecol* 1979;6(2):335.
5. Ritchie JW, Lakhani K. Fetal breathing movements in response to maternal inhalation of 5% carbon dioxide. *Am J Obstet Gynecol* 1980;136(3):386.
6. Bekedam DJ, Mulder EJ, Snijders RJ, et al. The effects of maternal hyperoxia on fetal breathing movements, body movements and heart rate variation in growth retarded fetuses. *Early Hum Dev* 1991;27(3):223.
7. Hallak M, Moise K Jr, Lira N, et al. The effect of tocolytic agents (indomethacin and terbutaline) on fetal breathing and body movements: a prospective, randomized, double-blind, placebo-controlled clinical trial. *Am J Obstet Gynecol* 1992;167(4 Pt 1):1059.
8. Dawes GS. Breathing before birth in animals and man. An essay in developmental medicine. *N Engl J Med* 1974;290(10):557.
9. Rigatto H, Moore M, Cates D. Fetal breathing and behavior measured through a double-wall Plexiglas window in sheep. *J Appl Physiol (1985)* 1986;61(1):160.
10. Clewlow F, Dawes GS, Johnston BM, et al. Changes in breathing, electrocortical and muscle activity in unanaesthetized fetal lambs with age. *J Physiol* 1983;341:463.
11. Dawes GS, Gardner WN, Johnston BM, et al. Effects of hypercapnia on tracheal pressure, diaphragm and intercostal electromyograms in unanaesthetized fetal lambs. *J Physiol* 1982;326:461.
12. van Vonderen JJ, Roest AA, Siew ML, et al. Measuring physiological changes during the transition to life after birth. *Neonatology* 2014;105(3):230.
13. MacFarlane PM, Ribeiro AP, Martin RJ. Carotid chemoreceptor development and neonatal apnea. *Respir Physiol Neurobiol* 2013;185(1):170.
14. Bianchi AL, Gestreau C. The brainstem respiratory network: an overview of a half century of research. *Respir Physiol Neurobiol* 2009;168(1-2):4.
15. Haddad G. Respiratory control in the newborn: comparative physiology and clinical disorders. In: Mathew OP, ed. *Respiratory control and disorders in the newborn.* New York: Marcel Dekker, 2003:1.
16. Martin RJ, Wilson CG. Apnea of prematurity. *Compr Physiol* 2012;2(4):2923.
17. Hunt CE, Hauck FR. Gene and gene-environment risk factors in sudden unexpected death in infants. *Curr Pediatr Rev* 2010;6:56.
18. Fortin G, del Toro ED, Abadie V, et al. Genetic and developmental models for the neural control of breathing in vertebrates. *Respir Physiol* 2000;122(2-3):247.
19. Bloch-Salisbury E, Hall MH, Sharma P, et al. Heritability of apnea of prematurity: a retrospective twin study. *Pediatrics* 2010;126(4):e779.
20. Rigatto H. Breathing and sleep in preterm infants. In: Loughlin GM, Carroll JL, Marcus CL, eds. *Sleep and breathing in children, a developmental approach.* New York: Marcel Dekker, 2000:495.
21. Glotzbach SF, Baldwin RB, Lederer NE, et al. Periodic breathing in preterm infants: incidence and characteristics. *Pediatrics* 1989;84(5):785.
22. Ramanathan R, Corwin MJ, Hunt CE, et al. Cardiorespiratory events recorded on home monitors: comparison of healthy infants with those at increased risk for SIDS. *JAMA* 2001;285(17):2199.
23. Hunt CE, Corwin MJ, Weese-Mayer DE, et al. Longitudinal assessment of hemoglobin oxygen saturation in preterm and term infants in the first six months of life. *J Pediatr* 2011;159(3):377, e371.
24. Patel M, Mohr M, Lake D, et al. Clinical associations with immature breathing in preterm infants: part 2-periodic breathing. *Pediatr Res* 2016;80(1):28.
25. Hunt CE, Corwin MJ, Baird T, et al. Cardiorespiratory events detected by home memory monitoring and one-year neurodevelopmental outcome. *J Pediatr* 2004;145(4):465.
26. Di Fiore JM, MacFarlane PM, Martin RJ. Intermittent hypoxemia in preterm infants. *Clin Perinatol* 2019;46(3):553.
27. Rhein LM, Dobson NR, Darnall RA, et al. Effects of caffeine on intermittent hypoxia in infants born prematurely: a randomized clinical trial. *JAMA Pediatr* 2014;168(3):250.
28. Poets CF. Apnea of prematurity: what can observational studies tell us about pathophysiology? *Sleep Med* 2010;11(7):701.
29. Mathew OP. Apnea of prematurity: pathogenesis and management strategies. *J Perinatol* 2011;31(5):302.
30. Henderson-Smart DJ, Pettigrew AG, Campbell DJ. Clinical apnea and brainstem neural function in preterm infants. *N Engl J Med* 1983;308(7):353.
31. Barrington K, Finer N. The natural history of the appearance of apnea of prematurity. *Pediatr Res* 1991;29(4 Pt 1):372.
32. Hunt CE. Apnea and sudden infant death syndrome. In: Kliegman RM, Nieder ML, Super DM, eds. *Practical strategies in pediatric diagnosis and therapy.* Philadelphia, PA: WB Saunders, 1996:135.
33. Fairchild K, Mohr M, Paget-Brown A, et al. Clinical associations of immature breathing in preterm infants: part 1-central apnea. *Pediatr Res* 2016;80(1):21.
34. Bell EF, Strauss RG, Widness JA, et al. Randomized trial of liberal versus restrictive guidelines for red blood cell transfusion in preterm infants. *Pediatrics* 2005;115(6):1685.
35. Eichenwald EC; Committee on Fetus and Newborn, American Academy of Pediatrics. Apnea of prematurity. *Pediatrics* 2016;137(1).
36. Zagol K, Lake DE, Vergales B, et al. Anemia, apnea of prematurity, and blood transfusions. *J Pediatr* 2012;161(3):417, e411.
37. Lawson EE. Nonpharmacological management of idiopathic apnea of the premature infant. In: Mathew OP, ed. *Respiratory control and disorders in the newborn.* New York: Marcel Dekker, 2003:335.
38. Dobson NR, Hunt CE. Caffeine use in neonates: indications, pharmacokinetics, clinical effects, outcomes. *NeoReviews* 2013;14(11):e540.
39. Dobson NR, Hunt CE. Caffeine: an evidence-based success story in VLBW pharmacotherapy. *Pediatr Res* 2018;84(3):333.
40. Henderson-Smart DJ, De Paoli AG. Methylxanthine treatment for apnoea in preterm infants. *Cochrane Database Syst Rev* 2010(12):CD000140.
41. Henderson-Smart DJ, Steer PA. Caffeine versus theophylline for apnea in preterm infants. *Cochrane Database Syst Rev* 2010(1):CD000273.
42. Henderson-Smart DJ, Davis PG. Prophylactic methylxanthines for endotracheal extubation in preterm infants. *Cochrane Database Syst Rev* 2010(12):CD000139.
43. Schmidt B, Anderson PJ, Doyle LW, et al. Survival without disability to age 5 years after neonatal caffeine therapy for apnea of prematurity. *JAMA* 2012;307(3):275.
44. Schmidt B, Roberts RS, Davis P, et al. Long-term effects of caffeine therapy for apnea of prematurity. *N Engl J Med* 2007;357(19):1893.
45. Dobson NR, Patel RM, Smith PB, et al. Trends in caffeine use and association between clinical outcomes and timing of therapy in very low birth weight infants. *J Pediatr* 2014;164(5):992, e993.
46. Sreenan C, Lemke RP, Hudson-Mason A, et al. High-flow nasal cannulae in the management of apnea of prematurity: a comparison with conventional nasal continuous positive airway pressure. *Pediatrics* 2001;107(5):1081.
47. Dani C, Pratesi S, Migliori C, et al. High flow nasal cannula therapy as respiratory support in the preterm infant. *Pediatr Pulmonol* 2009;44(7):629.
48. Manley BJ, Dold SK, Davis PG, et al. High-flow nasal cannulae for respiratory support of preterm infants: a review of the evidence. *Neonatology* 2012;102(4):300.
49. Lemyre B, Davis PG, de Paoli AG. Nasal intermittent positive pressure ventilation (NIPPV) versus nasal continuous positive airway pressure (NCPAP) for apnea of prematurity. *Cochrane Database Syst Rev* 2002(1):CD002272.
50. Gerull R, Manser H, Kuster H, et al. Increase of caffeine and decrease of corticosteroids for extremely low-birthweight infants with respiratory failure from 1997 to 2011. *Acta Paediatr* 2013;102(12):1154.
51. Prins SA, Pans SJ, van Weissenbruch MM, et al. Doxapram use for apnoea of prematurity in neonatal intensive care. *Int J Pediatr* 2013;2013:251047.
52. Vliegenthart RJ, Ten Hove CH, Onland W, et al. Doxapram treatment for apnea of prematurity: a systematic review. *Neonatology* 2017;111(2):162.
53. Di Fiore JM, Poets CF, Gauda E, et al. Cardiorespiratory events in preterm infants: interventions and consequences. *J Perinatol* 2016;36(4):251.
54. Zhao J, Gonzalez F, Mu D. Apnea of prematurity: from cause to treatment. *Eur J Pediatr* 2011;170(9):1097.
55. Alvaro RE, Khalil M, Qurashi M, et al. CO(2) inhalation as a treatment for apnea of prematurity: a randomized double-blind controlled trial. *J Pediatr* 2012;160(2):252, e251.
56. Abu Jawdeh EG, Martin RJ. Neonatal apnea and gastroesophageal reflux (GER): is there a problem? *Early Hum Dev* 2013;89(suppl 1):S14.
57. Di Fiore J, Arko M, Herynk B, et al. Characterization of cardiorespiratory events following gastroesophageal reflux in preterm infants. *J Perinatol* 2010;30(10):683.
58. Poets CF. Gastroesophageal reflux and apnea of prematurity—coincidence, not causation. Commentary on L. Corvaglia et al.: A thickened formula does not reduce apneas related to gastroesophageal reflux in preterm infants (*Neonatology* 2013;103:98-102). *Neonatology* 2013;103(2):103.
59. Omari TI. Apnea-associated reduction in lower esophageal sphincter tone in premature infants. *J Pediatr* 2009;154(3):374.
60. Kimball AL, Carlton DP. Gastroesophageal reflux medications in the treatment of apnea in premature infants. *J Pediatr* 2001;138(3):355.
61. Terrin G, Passariello A, De Curtis M, et al. Ranitidine is associated with infections, necrotizing enterocolitis, and fatal outcome in newborns. *Pediatrics* 2012;129(1):e40.
62. Wheatley E, Kennedy KA. Cross-over trial of treatment for bradycardia attributed to gastroesophageal reflux in preterm infants. *J Pediatr* 2009;155(4):516.
63. Eichenwald EC, Aina A, Stark AR. Apnea frequently persists beyond term gestation in infants delivered at 24 to 28 weeks. *Pediatrics* 1997;100(3 Pt 1):354.
64. Dobson NR, Rhein LM, Darnall RA, et al. Caffeine decreases intermittent hypoxia in preterm infants nearing term-equivalent age. *J Perinatol* 2017;37(10):1135.
65. Lorch SA, Srinivasan L, Escobar GJ. Epidemiology of apnea and bradycardia resolution in premature infants. *Pediatrics* 2011;128(2):e366.

66. Hofstetter AO, Legnevall L, Herlenius E, et al. Cardiorespiratory development in extremely preterm infants: vulnerability to infection and persistence of events beyond term-equivalent age. *Acta Paediatr* 2008;97(3):285.

67. Hunt CE, Corwin MJ, Lister G, et al. Longitudinal assessment of hemoglobin oxygen saturation in healthy infants during the first 6 months of age. Collaborative Home Infant Monitoring Evaluation (CHIME) Study Group. *J Pediatr* 1999;135(5):580.

68. Ralston S, Hill V. Incidence of apnea in infants hospitalized with respiratory syncytial virus bronchiolitis: a systematic review. *J Pediatr* 2009;155(5):728.

69. Murphy JJ, Swanson T, Ansermino M, et al. The frequency of apneas in premature infants after inguinal hernia repair: do they need overnight monitoring in the intensive care unit? *J Pediatr Surg* 2008;43(5):865.

70. Sale SM. Neonatal apnoea. *Best Pract Res Clin Anaesthesiol* 2010;24(3):323.

71. Cote CJ, Zaslavsky A, Downes JJ, et al. Postoperative apnea in former preterm infants after inguinal herniorrhaphy. A combined analysis. *Anesthesiology* 1995;82(4):809.

72. Welborn LG, Hannallah RS, Luban NL, et al. Anemia and postoperative apnea in former preterm infants. *Anesthesiology* 1991;74(6):1003.

73. Cheung PY, Barrington KJ, Finer NN, et al. Early childhood neurodevelopment in very low birth weight infants with predischarge apnea. *Pediatr Pulmonol* 1999;27(1):14.

74. Sreenan C, Etches PC, Demianczuk N, et al. Isolated mental developmental delay in very low birth weight infants: association with prolonged doxapram therapy for apnea. *J Pediatr* 2001;139(6):832.

75. Janvier A, Khairy M, Kokkotis A, et al. Apnea is associated with neurodevelopmental impairment in very low birth weight infants. *J Perinatol* 2004;24(12):763.

76. Greene MM, Patra K, Khan S, et al. Cardiorespiratory events in extremely low birth weight infants: neurodevelopmental outcome at 1 and 2 years. *J Perinatol* 2014;34(7):562.

77. Pillekamp F, Hermann C, Keller T, et al. Factors influencing apnea and bradycardia of prematurity—implications for neurodevelopment. *Neonatology* 2007;91(3):155.

78. Poets CF, Roberts RS, Schmidt B, et al. Association between intermittent hypoxemia or bradycardia and late death or disability in extremely preterm infants. *JAMA* 2015;314(6):595.

79. Gozal D. Sleep-disordered breathing and school performance in children. *Pediatrics* 1998;102(3 Pt 1):616.

80. Hunt CE. Neurocognitive outcomes in sleep-disordered breathing. *J Pediatr* 2004;145(4):430.

81. Macey PM, Henderson LA, Macey KE, et al. Brain morphology associated with obstructive sleep apnea. *Am J Respir Crit Care Med* 2002;166(10):1382.

82. Hauck FR, Carlin RF, Moon RY, et al. Sudden infant death syndrome. In: Kliegman RM, Behrman RE, Jenson HB, et al., eds. *Nelson textbook of pediatrics*, 21st ed. Philadelphia, PA: Elsevier, 2019.

83. Task Force on Sudden Infant Death Syndrome; Moon RY. SIDS and other sleep-related infant deaths: updated 2016 recommendations for a safe infant sleeping environment. *Pediatrics* 2016;138(5).

84. Hunt CE, Darnall RA, McEntire BL, et al. Assigning cause for sudden unexpected infant death. *Forensic Sci Med Pathol* 2015;11(2):283.

85. United States Department of Health and Human Services (US DHHS), Centers of Disease Control and Prevention (CDC), National Center for Health Statistics (NCHS), Division of Vital Statistics (DVS). Linked Birth/Infant Death Records 1999-2002, 2003-2006, and 2007-2017, on CDC WONDER On-line Database. Available from: http://wonder.cdc.gov

86. Kinney HC, Haynes RL. The serotonin brainstem hypothesis for the sudden infant death syndrome. *J Neuropathol Exp Neurol* 2019;78(9):765.

87. Horne RSC. Cardiovascular autonomic dysfunction in sudden infant death syndrome. *Clin Auton Res* 2018;28(6):535.

88. Malloy MH. Prematurity and sudden infant death syndrome: United States 2005-2007. *J Perinatol* 2013;33(6):470.

89. Tieder JS, Bonkowsky JL, Etzel RA, et al. Brief resolved unexplained events (formerly apparent life-threatening events) and evaluation of lower-risk infants: executive summary. *Pediatrics* 2016;137(5).

90. Ramgopal S, Noorbakhsh KA, Callaway CW, et al. Changes in the management of children with brief resolved unexplained events (BRUEs). *Pediatrics* 2019;144(4).

91. Chen T, Hughes ME, Wang H, et al. Prenatal, perinatal, and early childhood factors associated with childhood obstructive sleep apnea. *J Pediatr* 2019;212:20, e10.

92. Thomas B, Thillainathan K, Delahunty M, et al. Cardiovascular autonomic control is altered in children born preterm with sleep disordered breathing. *J Pediatr* 2019;206:83.

93. Tapia IE, Shults J, Doyle LW, et al. Perinatal risk factors associated with the obstructive sleep apnea syndrome in school-aged children born preterm. *Sleep* 2016;39(4):737.

94. Huang YS, Hsu JF, Paiva T, et al. Sleep-disordered breathing, craniofacial development, and neurodevelopment in premature infants: a 2-year follow-up study. *Sleep Med* 2019;60:20.

95. Hibbs AM, Johnson NL, Rosen CL, et al. Prenatal and neonatal risk factors for sleep disordered breathing in school-aged children born preterm. *J Pediatr* 2008;153(2):176.

96. Vereen RJ, Dobson NR, Olsen CH, et al. Longitudinal growth changes from birth to 8-9 years in preterm and full term births. *J Neonatal Perinatal Med* 2020;13(2):223.

THE NEWBORN INFANT

28 Acute Pulmonary Disorders

Jeffrey A. Whitsett, Amy T. Nathan, Shawn K. Ahlfeld, Gloria S. Pryhuber, and Paul S. Kingma

INTRODUCTION

Successful adaptation to air breathing at the time of birth is the culmination of an orderly process of pulmonary cell growth and differentiation, leading to alveolar and capillary surfaces capable of providing oxygen and eliminating carbon dioxide. Failure to achieve adequate gas exchange at birth represents a major cause of perinatal morbidity and mortality. This chapter reviews the common disorders of neonatal respiratory adaptation, including respiratory distress syndrome (RDS), pulmonary meconium aspiration syndrome (MAS), pulmonary hypertension, pneumonia, air leak, pulmonary hemorrhage, transient tachypnea of the newborn (TTN), and other causes of acute respiratory dysfunction in the perinatal period. The clinical manifestations and therapy of these disorders are discussed in the context of the morphologic, biochemical, and physiologic factors critical to normal pulmonary growth, maturation, and function in the newborn.

HUMAN LUNG DEVELOPMENT

Human lung morphogenesis is divided into five distinct stages of organogenesis, which describe the histologic changes that the lung undergoes during development (1,2). These five stages are the embryonic, pseudoglandular, canalicular, saccular, and alveolar stages. Human lung development is initiated during the early embryonic period of gestation (3 to 7 weeks postconception, 5 to 9 weeks postmenstrual age) as a small saccular outgrowth of the ventral foregut called the respiratory diverticulum. During the subsequent pseudoglandular stage of lung development (5 to 17 weeks postconception), formation of the conducting airways (the tracheobronchial tree) occurs by elongation and repetitive branching of the primitive bronchial tubules. Vascularization of the surrounding mesenchyme with formation of the air–blood barrier (the alveolar–capillary membrane) occurs during the canalicular stage of lung development (16 to 26 weeks postconception). Cytodifferentiation of bronchiolar and alveolar epithelial cells is also initiated during this stage. Enlargement and expansion of the peripheral air spaces occur during the saccular stage of lung development (24 to 38 weeks postconception), resulting in the formation of primitive saccules. Formation of thin secondary alveolar septa and remodeling of the capillary bed occur during the alveolar stage of lung development (36 weeks postconception to 8 years of age), giving rise to the mature alveolar organization of the adult lung (Fig. 28.1).

The human lung is a derivative of the primitive foregut endoderm and the surrounding splanchnic mesoderm. The primitive respiratory diverticulum appears at 3 weeks of gestation as an enlargement of the caudal end of the laryngotracheal sulcus located in the median pharyngeal groove, which is an outgrowth of the ventral wall of the primitive esophagus. During the 4th week of gestation, the respiratory diverticulum enlarges and subdivides into the left and right primary bronchi (see Fig. 28.1A and B). The primitive lung grows caudally, expanding into the mesenchyme surrounding the primitive foregut, while the trachea becomes separated from the esophagus by a transient epithelial septum that is remodeled and replaced by a band of mesenchymal tissue called the tracheoesophageal septum. Between 4 and 5 weeks of gestation, the left and right primary bronchi subdivide to produce secondary, or lobar, bronchi (see Fig. 28.1C and D). Further subdivision of lobar bronchi into tertiary or segmental bronchi occurs during the 6th week of gestation, with the lung taking on a lobulated appearance as the segmental buds are formed (see Fig. 28.1E and F). The developing respiratory tract is lined by endodermally derived epithelium that forms the conducting airways and alveoli. The surrounding mesoderm is composed of mesenchymal cells that will differentiate into connective tissue components, including blood and lymphatic vessels, fibroblasts, smooth muscle cells, and cartilage.

Preacinar blood vessels first appear at the end of week 4. Pulmonary arteries arise from the sixth pair of aortic arches and grow into the mesenchyme, where they accompany the developing airways, segmenting with each bronchial subdivision (3,4). Pulmonary veins develop as outgrowths of the left atrium of the heart and subdivide several times before connecting to the pulmonary vascular bed. Intra-acinar vessels develop later, in parallel with alveolar formation.

The pseudoglandular stage of fetal lung development extends from about 5 to 17 weeks of gestation and is marked by the formation of the bronchial portion of the lung. This occurs through a process known as branching morphogenesis (5), during which the segmental tubules of the developing lung undergo repetitive lateral and terminal dichotomous branching to form the primitive bronchial tree (see Fig. 28.1G and H). By week 17 of gestation, the segmental bronchi have subdivided to produce approximately 23 generations of bronchial tubules ending in the terminal bronchioles. These bronchial tubules are lined initially by a pseudostratified columnar epithelium. A prominent basement membrane underlies the epithelium, and mesenchymal cells adjacent to these tubules differentiate into fibroblasts, which become organized in a circumferential orientation, perpendicular to the long axis of the tubules. As branching progresses, pseudostratified columnar epithelium is reduced to a tall columnar epithelium, especially in distal regions of the bronchial tree. During this period, cytodifferentiation of the airway epithelium occurs in a centrifugal direction with ciliated, nonciliated secretory, goblet, neuroendocrine, and basal cells appearing first in the more proximal airways. Cartilage, smooth muscle cells, nerves, and mucous glands are also found in the trachea during the pseudoglandular stage of development and extend as far as the segmental bronchi.

The canalicular stage of fetal lung development extends from week 16 to 24 of gestation. By the end of week 16, the terminal bronchioles have divided into two or more respiratory bronchioles that have subdivided into small clusters of short acinar tubules and buds lined by cuboidal epithelium. These structures undergo further differentiation and maturation to become the adult respiratory unit, or pulmonary acinus, consisting of the alveolated respiratory bronchiole, alveolar ducts, and alveoli. Clusters of acinar tubules and buds continue to grow by lengthening, subdividing, and widening at the expense of the surrounding mesenchyme (Fig. 28.2A). This peripheral growth is accompanied by the formation of intra-acinar capillaries, which align themselves around the air spaces, establishing contact with the overlying cuboidal epithelium. During this stage of lung development, type II epithelial cell differentiation occurs in acinar tubules with formation of intracellular multivesicular bodies and multilamellar bodies, the storage form of pulmonary surfactant phospholipids (6). Type I epithelial cell differentiation occurs in conjunction with development of the air–blood barrier, where endothelial cells of the developing capillary system come into close contact with the overlying epithelial cells.

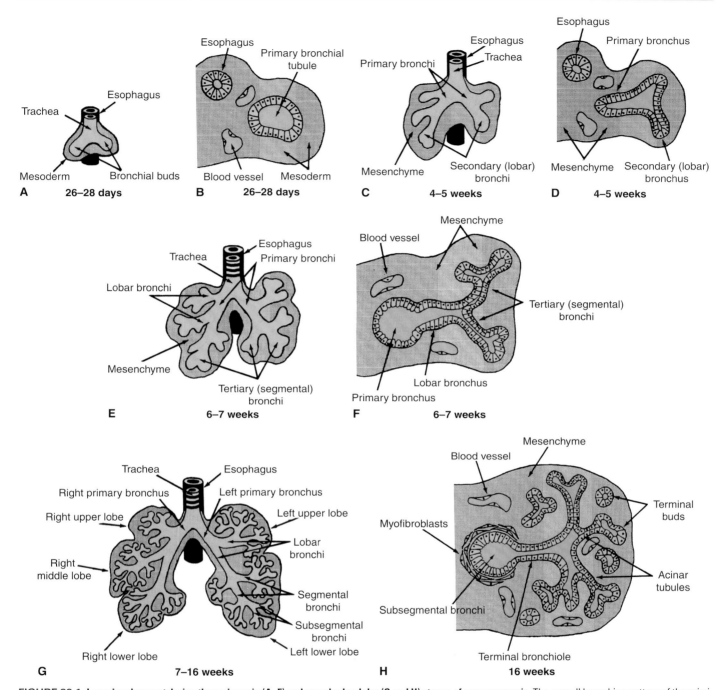

FIGURE 28.1 Lung development during the embryonic (A–F) and pseudoglandular (G and H) stages of organogenesis. The overall branching pattern of the primitive lung (*left panels*) results in the development of the bronchial tree. The histologic organization of the fetal lung becomes more complex as branching morphogenesis progresses through these stages (*right panels*).

During the saccular stage of fetal lung development, which extends from week 24 to 36 of gestation, the terminal clusters of acinar tubules and buds begin to dilate and expand into thin, smooth-walled, transitory ducts and saccules that later become the true alveolar ducts and alveoli of the adult (**Fig. 28.2B**). During this stage, there is a marked reduction in the amount of interstitial tissue. Intersaccular and interductal septa develop, which contain a delicate network of collagen fibers and the intra-acinar capillary bed. Near the end of this stage, elastin is deposited in regions in which future interalveolar septa will form. Increasing amounts of tubular myelin, the secretory form of pulmonary surfactant, are seen in the air spaces (6).

The alveolar stage, which extends from 36 weeks of gestation to between 2 and 8 years of age, is the last stage of lung development and is marked by the formation of secondary alveolar septa, which partition the transitional ducts and saccules into true alveolar ducts and alveoli (**Fig. 28.2C and D**). This process of alveolarization greatly increases the surface area of the lung available for gas exchange. At the beginning of this period, the secondary interalveolar septa consist of short buds or projections of connective tissue that contain a double capillary network and interstitial cells that are actively synthesizing collagen and elastic fibers. By 5 months of age, these secondary interalveolar septa have lengthened and thinned and now contain only a single capillary network.

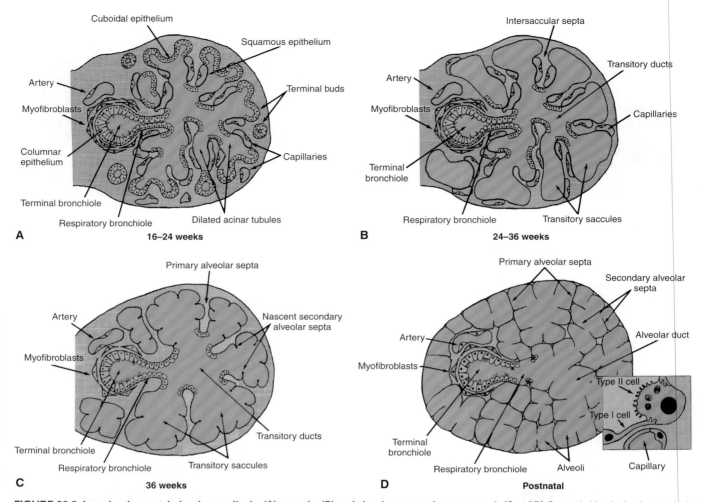

FIGURE 28.2 Lung development during the canalicular (A), saccular (B), and alveolar stages of organogenesis (C and D). Dramatic histologic changes in tissue organization occur during these periods. The adult alveolar epithelium is composed of squamous type I cells and cuboidal type II cells (inset).

Although definitive alveoli can be found in the human lung by 36 weeks of gestation, 85% to 90% of all alveoli are formed within the first 6 months of life (7). Overall the number of alveoli increases by about sixfold between birth and adulthood, that is, from an average of 50 million alveoli in the term lung to 480 million (range: 274 to 790 million) in the adult human lung (8). After the first 6 months of life, alveolar formation occurs at a slower pace until about 2 to 8 years of age, when further growth of the lung becomes proportional to growth of the body. The surface area available for gas exchange, and its diffusion capacity, increases linearly with body weight up to about 18 years of age (9). The conducting airways also increase in length and diameter, while airspace and capillary volumes increase coordinately at the expense of interstitial volume.

DEVELOPMENTAL ANOMALIES

Each of these stages of lung development includes distinct changes in tissue organization and cellular differentiation that are important for subsequent growth and maturation of the lung. Lung morphogenesis is determined by complex interactions among cells in the splanchnic mesenchyme and foregut endoderm that are regulated by multiple signaling pathways and transcriptional mechanisms (10). Structural and functional defects in lung development at birth can often be traced to arrested or aberrant development during one of these periods of organogenesis, often as a result of mutations in genes critical for patterning and growth of the lung such as the *GLI3* gene (Pallister Hall syndrome) (11);

a component of the Sonic Hedgehog signaling pathway, which in turn regulates *FOXF1* (mutations in which cause alveolar capillary dysplasia [ACD]), *TBX-4* (a transcription factor required for normal branching morphogenesis), and the fibroblast growth factor receptor, *FGFR2*, gene (Pfeiffer, Apert, and Crouzon syndromes) (12,13) that is required for FGF signaling. Mutations in NKX2.1, a transcription factor critical for growth and differentiation of the respiratory epithelium, cause pulmonary, central nervous system (CNS), and thyroid disorders.

Developmental anomalies of the lung occur through defective division and differentiation of the lung bud, of the left or right bronchial bud or of the trachea and esophagus. Pulmonary agenesis, tracheal and bronchial malformations, tracheoesophageal fistulas, ectopic lobes, bronchogenic cysts, and congenital pulmonary airway malformation (previously known as cystic pulmonary adenomatoid malformations [CPAM]) arise during the embryonic and pseudoglandular stages of lung development (14). Defects in lung growth and morphogenesis underlie common clinical disorders associated with pulmonary hypoplasia, such as congenital diaphragmatic hernia (CDH), and disorders associated with dysplasia, such as alveolar capillary dysplasia with misalignment of pulmonary veins (ACD/MPV) (14). Pulmonary hypoplasia can be caused by genes regulating growth, for example, *TBX-4*, *NKX2-1*, *FGFR-2*, and *FOXF1* (15–18). Reduction of space within the pleural cavity, usually as a consequence with another primary developmental defect such as CDH, and reduction in the amount of amniotic fluid (following prolonged premature rupture of membranes or fetal renal dysgenesis–agenesis) are secondary causes of lung growth abnormalities (14). RDS and bronchopulmonary dysplasia (BPD) are associated with premature birth at a time when biochemical functions (e.g., surfactant production) and the structure of the lung are still underdeveloped.

Hereditary–Genetic Causes of Acute Respiratory Failure in the Newborn

Mutations in the surfactant protein B (*SFTPB*), C (*SFTPC*), *ABCA3*, thyroid transcription factor-1 (*TTF-1*), and genes *NKX2-1*, *FOXF1*, and *TBX-4* are rare causes of acute respiratory failure in neonates (15–20). Hereditary SP-B and ABCA3 deficiency cause respiratory distress, generally in full-term infants, usually presenting within the first day of life. Respiratory failure progresses despite ventilatory support, surfactant replacement, or extracorporeal membrane oxygenation (ECMO), generally causing death from respiratory failure in the first months of life (20). Mutations in both *ABCA3* and *SFTPB* genes are inherited as autosomal recessive traits, resulting in the lack of surfactant in the airways, causing atelectasis and respiratory failure. While homozygous mutations in *ABCA3* are generally lethal in the neonatal period, several less severe mutations are associated with chronic lung disease in infancy and childhood and some have been treated by lung transplantation. Mutations in the *SFTPC* gene are generally inherited as autosomal dominant and cause both acute and chronic interstitial lung disease in newborns, infants, and adults. *SFTPC*-related lung disease is associated with the lack of SP-C protein in alveolar lavage and with folding mutations in the proSP-C protein that accumulates in alveolar type II cells causing cell injury. Hemizygous mutations or deletions in *NKX2-1*, the gene encoding the transcription factor TTF-1, cause variably penetrant lung disease, hypothyroidism, and CNS abnormalities (brain–lung–thyroid) syndrome, causing acute respiratory disease at birth or chronic respiratory disease in infancy (15). Recent genetic studies of newborn infants with acute respiratory failure caused by ACD/MPV identified mutations in the transcription factor, *FOXF1* (Forkhead orthologue F1) (18). Acinar–alveolar hypoplasia has been associated with mutations in *TBX-4* (19). At present, definitive diagnosis of these genetic disorders causing respiratory failure in newborn infants is best made by identification of the gene mutations by DNA sequencing.

THE SURFACTANT SYSTEM

The unique physical–chemical boundary between the alveolar gases and the highly solvated molecules at the apical surface of the respiratory epithelium generates a region of high surface tension produced by the unequal distribution of molecular forces among water molecules at an air–liquid interface. Surface-active material at this interface in the alveoli provides surface tension–lowering activity that contributes to the remarkable pressure–volume relationship that is characteristic of the lung. This surface-active material, called surfactant, has been subject to intense study in recent decades (6,21).

Deficiency or dysfunction of pulmonary surfactant plays a critical role in the pathogenesis of respiratory diseases in the newborn period. Pulmonary surfactant exists in a variety of physical forms when isolated from the alveolar wash of the lung. These physical forms include lamellated and vesicular forms and highly organized tubular myelin. Tubular myelin is highly surface active and, although it is composed predominately of phospholipids, its unique structure depends on Ca^{2+} and lung surfactant proteins A (SP-A), B (SP-B), and D (SP-D). Tubular myelin represents the major extracellular pool of surfactant from which a lipid monolayered/multilayered film is generated to produce an interface between the hydrated cellular surfaces and alveolar gas (**Fig. 28.3**). Lamellated and vesicular forms of surfactant represent nascent or catabolic

forms of surfactant material, respectively; the latter is taken up by type II epithelial cells and recycled. Surfactant proteins A, B, C, and D play important roles in the organization and function of the surfactant complex regulating surfactant homeostasis, and all have roles in innate immunity. Alveolar surfactant concentrations are tightly controlled by a variety of mechanisms that modulate lipid and protein synthesis, storage, secretion, and recycling (22).

Composition of Surfactant

Pulmonary surfactant is composed primarily of the phospholipids, phosphatidylcholine (PC), and phosphatidylglycerol (PG) (23). These lipid molecules are enriched in dipalmitoyl acyl groups attached to a glycerol backbone that pack tightly and generate low surface pressures. Rapid spreading and stability of pulmonary surfactant are achieved by the interactions of surfactant proteins and phospholipids. Surfactant is synthesized and secreted by type II epithelial cells in the alveolus. Synthesis of PC, surfactant proteins, and lamellar bodies, an intracellular storage form of pulmonary surfactant, increases with advancing gestation. Lamellar bodies are secreted into the lung liquid that contributes to the amniotic fluid. The measurement of amniotic fluid PC, dipalmitoylphosphatidylcholine (DPPC), PG, or the surfactant proteins has provided useful biochemical markers that predict lung maturation and the adequacy of lung function at birth (e.g., lecithin–sphingomyelin [L-S] ratio, lamellar body counts, and PG values). Surfactant function can be assessed by a variety of physical and physiologic tests that measure its ability to reduce surface tension at an air–liquid interface and to spread rapidly during dynamic compression and expansion. The Wilhelmy balance, Langmuir trough, pulsating bubble surfactometer, and a variety of animal models have been used to assess the efficacy of surfactant and surfactant replacements.

Control of Surfactant Synthesis and Secretion

The synthesis and secretion of pulmonary surfactant is a complex sequence that is closely linked to the morphologic and biochemical differentiation of alveolar type II cells in the peripheral respiratory epithelium. A basal rate of surfactant secretion occurs continuously, but surfactant secretion can be stimulated by β-agonists and purines or by mechanical distention of the lung or hyperventilation. Interactions between mesenchymal and epithelial cells, mediated by direct cell–cell contact or by paracrine factors, contribute to the differentiation process. Endocrine factors also modulate the differentiation of type II epithelial cells and the synthesis of surfactant components. *In vivo, in vitro,* and clinical data support the utility of antenatal glucocorticoids in prevention of respiratory distress morbidity and mortality in preterm infants (24).

Phospholipid Synthesis

PC is produced by type II epithelial cells using extracellular substrate, and the glycogen stores that accumulate in the pretype II cells of the fetal lung. Metabolic pathways producing PC depend on the production of phosphatidic acid and a glycerophosphate backbone; the latter is produced as an intermediate of the glycolytic pathway. The synthesis of PC involves the deacylation of phosphatidic acid and its reaction with cytidine diphosphocholine (CDP-choline) (22,23).

Disaturated forms of PC may be formed *de novo*, using disaturated acyl precursors or by remodeling of phospholipids by deacylation and reacylation reactions. Production of CDP-choline is critical to PC synthesis and is achieved by phosphorylation of choline and transfer to cytidine triphosphate in a reaction dependent on choline kinase and choline phosphate cytidylyltransferase. Acyl-transferases, for example, lysophosphatidylcholine acyltransferases (LPCATs), regulate the abundance and specificity of the acyl chain in PC. The activities of many of the enzymes in the

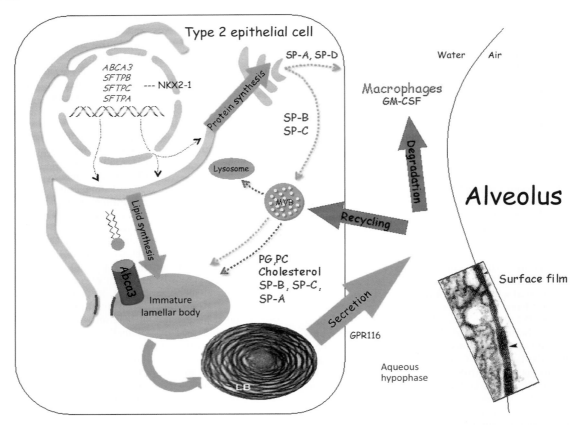

FIGURE 28.3 Surfactant synthesis and metabolism by type II alveolar epithelial cells. The hydrophobic surfactant proteins, SP-B and SP-C, and the phospholipid transporter, ABCA3, are synthesized in the endoplasmic reticulum (ER) and extensively modified during transit through the ER, the Golgi apparatus, and the multivesicular body (MVB) (*green dashed arrows*). The MVB then fuses with the lamellar body (LB), where final packaging of the surfactant proteins and phospholipids occurs before secretion into the alveolus (*green dashed arrows*). PC and PG are the most abundant surfactant lipids and are transported into the LB by ABCA3, located in the outer membrane of the LB. The hydrophilic surfactant proteins, SP-A and SP-D, are also synthesized in the ER, glycosylated in the Golgi apparatus, and then secreted into the alveolus (*solid green wide arrows*). After secretion, surfactant phospholipids and proteins are reorganized into a multilayered, bioactive, surface film at the air–fluid interface, which reduces surface tension in the alveolus. Secreted surfactant phospholipids and proteins are taken up by type II cells and are either catabolized within lysosomes or transported to the LB for recycling (*red arrows*). A fraction of the secreted surfactant proteins and phospholipids are also taken up and degraded by alveolar macrophages in a process requiring GM-CSF. (Diagram courtesy of Timothy Weaver, Cincinnati Children's Hospital Medical Center, Cincinnati, OH.)

synthetic pathway for PC increase with advancing gestation in the lung, generally increasing in the last third of gestation.

Glucocorticoid Enhancement of Pulmonary Maturation

A variety of hormonal factors influence the rate of production of the enzymes controlling PC synthesis in the developing lung (23). Glucocorticoids are the most clinically relevant and useful of these agents. Studies in fetal lambs and humans demonstrated that administration of glucocorticoid to the dam or mother resulted in precocious respiratory function in prematurely born offspring. The initial clinical studies of Liggins and Howie demonstrated that maternal administration of glucocorticoid decreased the incidence of respiratory distress in premature infants (25). Although the precise mechanisms by which glucocorticoids induce pulmonary maturation and lung function in premature infants have not been precisely identified, increased PC synthesis and morphologic remodeling of the alveolar architecture, including the thinning of interstitial components of the fetal lung, are observed after glucocorticoid treatment. Glucocorticoids regulate many genes that are associated with the differentiation of the fetal lung, functioning primarily by regulation of genes regulating pulmonary mesenchymal differentiation. The effects of glucocorticoids on cell differentiation are mediated primarily by activation of glucocorticoid receptor in lung mesenchyme to regulate gene transcription and mRNA stability, altering the abundance of the proteins synthesized by

pulmonary cells. Antenatal glucocorticoid therapy is standard care for prevention of RDS in preterm infants (24).

Other Hormonal Influences

Thyroid hormones that is, T_3, T_4, thyrotropin-releasing hormone (TRH), estrogens, prolactin, epidermal growth factor, β-adrenergic agents, and other agents that enhance cellular cyclic adenosine monophosphate (cAMP) levels influence pulmonary maturation or biochemical indices of pulmonary maturation (26). Both T_3 and T_4 increase the synthesis of phospholipids in mammalian lung but do not readily cross the placenta. None of the agents are currently used clinically to prevent RDS.

Surfactant Secretion

Surfactant is stored within type II cells in large lipid-rich organelles called lamellar bodies. Secretion of lamellar bodies occurs by a process of exocytosis that is regulated by a number of physical and hormonal factors. Stretch, the mode of ventilation, and the labor process enhance surfactant secretion and extracellular surfactant pool sizes at birth. Catecholamines and purinoceptor agonists (e.g., adenosine triphosphate) that activate protein kinases enhance phospholipid secretion by type II cells *in vitro*. Recent studies identified the role of a G protein–coupled receptor, GPR116, present on alveolar epithelial cells, that regulates surfactant lipid pool sizes by inhibiting surfactant secretion (27).

Hyperglycemia and hyperinsulinemia inhibit surfactant phospholipid secretion (28). Newly secreted surfactant enters the extracellular space and undergoes dramatic structural reorganization to form tubular myelin, a process dependent on SP-A, Ca^{2+}, phospholipids, and SP-B (6). Phospholipids must move from secreted lamellar bodies and tubular myelin to form monolayers and multilayers at the air–liquid interface, which reduce collapsing forces in the alveoli.

Surfactant Recycling and Catabolism

The process of inflation and deflation produces spent forms of surfactant phospholipids that are taken up by type II cells and reused or catabolized (6,29). Surfactant proteins B, C, and D enhance the reuptake of phospholipids in vitro. In the adult rabbit lung, the half-life of surfactant phospholipids is approximately 6 to 8 hours, and in newborn animals, the half-life is 3.5 days (29). The intracellular and extracellular pools of surfactant are generally larger in the newborn animal than in adults. SP-D regulates alveolar lipid structures and enhances reuptake by type II cells. SP-D regulates alveolar lipid structures and enhances reuptake by type II cells and is required for establishing the lower surfactant lipid pools characteristic of the more mature lung (30). A relatively small fraction of the alveolar surfactant pool is cleared by catabolism and alveolar macrophages, with most of the surfactant phospholipid recycled or catabolized by type II epithelial cells. Granulocyte–macrophage colony–stimulating factor (GM-CSF) and receptors play a critical role in the regulation of surfactant lipid and protein clearance, acting on the alveolar macrophage. Defects in GM-CSF signaling, caused by autoantibodies to GM-CSF or mutations in its receptors, inhibit alveolar macrophage–mediated degradation of surfactant lipids and proteins, leading to their accumulation in the postnatal lung, in turn, causing the syndrome of pulmonary alveolar proteinosis (PAP) (30). Exogenously administered surfactant phospholipid is reused efficiently by adult and newborn lungs (29). The effects of surfactant replacement therapy are therefore related both to the direct surface tension–lowering properties of surfactant introduced into the airway and to the recycling of the exogenously delivered phospholipids by type II cells.

The Role of Surfactant in Lung Disease

Quantitative and qualitative abnormalities of pulmonary surfactant contribute to the pathogenesis of lung disease in the newborn infant. Surfactant synthesis begins with the maturation of alveolar type II cells between 24 and 34 weeks of gestation in humans. Infants produce 4 mg/kg/d of surfactant PC, and this surfactant lipid remains in the lung with a half-life of approximately 110 hours (31). In preterm infants with RDS, alveolar surfactant pool sizes are 1 to 16 mg/kg. Term infant surfactant levels increase three- to fivefold above those values through an increase in synthesis and mobilization of surfactant lipids from type II cell intracellular pools (32). Surfactant pool sizes decrease to human adult levels of about 4 mg/kg by 1 week of age (33).

In premature infants, deficiencies in surfactant production and secretion decrease intracellular and extracellular pools of surfactant, leading to alveolar surfactant insufficiency, impaired pulmonary compliance, and atelectasis. Qualitative abnormalities of surfactant are also associated with many types of lung injury in infants and adults, where alveolar–capillary leak, hemorrhage, pulmonary edema, and alveolar cell injury fill the alveolus with proteinaceous material that inactivates surfactant. Serum and nonserum proteins, including albumin, fibrinogen, hemoglobin, and meconium, are potent inactivators of pulmonary surfactant in vivo and in vitro. In contrast, SP-A, SP-B, and SP-C act synergistically to stabilize the surface properties of phospholipids in the presence of these inactivating proteins.

Surfactant Replacement

The first successful surfactant replacement therapy in humans was reported by Fujiwara et al. in 1980 (34). Exogenous surfactants are routinely administered into the lungs of premature infants for treatment of RDS and meconium aspiration and are being tested for therapy of other lung diseases. Surfactant replacement is commonly used for prevention and treatment of RDS in preterm infants. Animal surfactant preparations containing phospholipids, SP-B, and SP-C (e.g., Survanta, Curosurf, Infasurf, BLES) and synthetic preparations composed primarily of phospholipids mixed with synthetic surfactant protein-like peptides are in widespread clinical use or are being studied, respectively (35,36). The surfactant preparations containing surfactant proteins provide highly surface active material to the alveolus. Surfactant replacement also contributes to the pool size of surfactant phospholipids, providing substrate for surfactant synthesis by means of the recycling pathways.

RESPIRATORY DISTRESS SYNDROME

Respiratory distress is a common cause of morbidity and mortality associated with premature birth. Recent data from the Vermont Oxford database reported an incidence of respiratory distress of approximately 86% in infants born between 22 and 33 weeks of gestation (37) although a definitive diagnosis of RDS is not readily identified in extremely preterm infants with respiratory insufficiency. The widespread use of antenatal glucocorticosteroids, early use of CPAP, and surfactant replacement in preterm infants makes definitive diagnosis of RDS related to surfactant deficiency challenging at present. The incidence and severity of RDS increase with decreasing gestational age. RDS is rare after 37 weeks of gestation but may occur in older infants with risk factors, including infants born by C-section, infants born to diabetic mothers with poor metabolic control, and infants born after fetal asphyxia, maternofetal hemorrhage, or pregnancies complicated by multiple births. The definitive diagnosis of RDS related to surfactant deficiency as a primary cause of lung dysfunction is virtually impossible at present.

Clinical Presentation

Infants with RDS typically present at birth with clinical signs of progressive respiratory distress that include tachypnea, grunting, retractions, poor aeration, diffuse crackles—rales, and cyanosis accompanied by increasing oxygen requirements. Physical findings are the result of diffuse atelectasis, an inability to maintain functional residual capacity and ventilation–perfusion (V/Q) imbalance. Chest radiographs are variable and may not reflect the degree of respiratory compromise but are typically characterized by diffuse atelectasis (as evidenced by homogeneous reticular–granular "ground glass" infiltrates or "white-out"), air bronchograms, and low lung volumes (Fig. 28.4).

The severity of RDS, the size and maturity of the infant at birth, and the type of therapeutic interventions determine the clinical course. The typical course of RDS is one of gradual decompensation and worsening respiratory failure followed by slow resolution. Initially, the infant presents with short, rapid respiration and expiratory grunting (exhalation against a partially closed glottis during exhalation to increase end expiratory pressure) in an attempt to maintain alveolar volume and functional residual capacity. The need for oxygen and ventilatory support often increases in the first 24 hours of age, peaks at approximately 2 to 3 days of age, and over several days gradually resolves. In uncomplicated RDS, typically seen in more mature infants, recovery occurs over several days, and generally after the first week of age infants no longer require oxygen or ventilatory support. The most premature infants are at greatest risk for severe RDS and frequently develop complications,

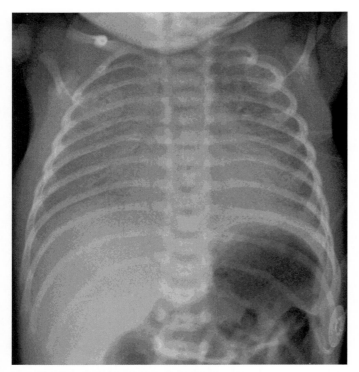

FIGURE 28.4 This premature infant presented with grunting, retractions, and cyanosis after delivery. The diffuse reticular–granular opacification, air bronchograms, and decreased lung volumes in the chest radiograph film indicate RDS.

including CNS hemorrhage, patent ductus arteriosus (PDA), air leak, infection, chronic lung disease, and BPD, which contribute to prolonged requirements for oxygen and ventilatory support.

Pathology

Pathologic findings early in the course of RDS include atelectasis, pulmonary edema, pulmonary vascular congestion, pulmonary hemorrhage, and evidence of direct injury to the respiratory epithelium (**Fig. 28.5**). Epithelial cell injury is especially evident in the bronchiolar region of the lung. Histologic findings include the

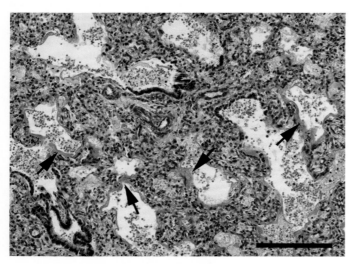

FIGURE 28.5 Dilated air spaces, hyaline membranes (*arrows*), and extensive atelectasis are seen throughout the lung of a premature infant born with severe RDS; scale bar = 200 μm. (Courtesy of Dr. Susan Wert, Cincinnati Children's Hospital, Cincinnati, OH.)

presence of hyaline membranes, the characteristic eosinophilic material derived primarily from bronchial and bronchiolar epithelial cell injury. Alveolar spaces are generally not inflated, and at autopsy the lungs of infants with RDS are often airless on passive deflation. Leukocytic infiltration is not observed early in the course of RDS unless there is concomitant infection. Inflammation, pulmonary edema, and hemorrhage are common pathologic features in RDS, especially if the clinical course is further complicated by PDA and congestive heart failure.

Pathophysiology

Avery and Mead first demonstrated the paucity of alveolar surfactant in the lungs of infants dying of RDS (38). In premature infants with RDS, quantitative and qualitative abnormalities of the pulmonary surfactant system are critical to the pathogenesis. Lack of pulmonary surfactant leads to progressive atelectasis, loss of functional residual capacity, alterations in ventilation–perfusion ratio, and uneven distribution of ventilation. RDS is complicated further by the relatively weak respiratory muscles and compliant chest wall of the premature infant, which impairs maintenance of functional residual capacity and alveolar ventilation. Diminished oxygenation, cyanosis, and respiratory and metabolic acidosis contribute to increased pulmonary vascular resistance (PVR). Right-to-left shunting through the ductus arteriosus, foramen ovale, and intrapulmonary ventilation–perfusion mismatch further exacerbate hypoxemia.

Prevention

Although the incidence of premature birth in the United States (approximately 10%) has not changed significantly in recent decades, due to advances in maternal and neonatal care the incidence of severe RDS has significantly decreased. Careful fetal monitoring, treatment of underlying maternal disorders, and avoidance of elective preterm delivery prior to 39 weeks' gestation have contributed to a decreased burden of RDS. However, the most notable intervention responsible for the significant reduction in both the incidence and severity of RDS has been the widespread use of antenatal steroids. Administration of glucocorticoids (dexamethasone or betamethasone) has decreased the incidence of RDS, as well as substantially improved the rates of severe intraventricular hemorrhage (IVH), necrotizing enterocolitis, neurodevelopmental impairment, and mortality. Although classically administered prior to 34 weeks of gestation, the American Congress of Obstetricians and Gynecologists (as well as other international advisory groups) presently recommends that for pregnancies prior to 37 weeks of gestation that are likely to deliver in the next 7 days, a course of maternal antenatal steroids be given to reduce the need for NICU admission and shorten the duration of respiratory support (39). Serial courses of steroids adversely impact growth and head circumference and are, therefore, discouraged. However, because the optimal window of neonatal benefit occurs between 48 hours and 7 days following the first dose, for women at less than 34 weeks' gestation who are threatening to deliver within 7 days and are at least 14 days beyond the initial course, a second "rescue" course of antenatal steroids can be considered (39). While antenatal glucocorticoids prevented RDS in preterm infants greater than 37 weeks' gestation, it is presently unclear whether this intervention is associated with long-term risk to the infants (40).

Treatment

Postnatal therapy of RDS begins immediately upon delivery with careful assessment and resuscitation. Before the infant is transferred from the delivery room to the appropriate site of care, adequate ventilation, oxygenation, circulation, and temperature must be assured. Although once considered standard of care, with widespread use of antenatal steroids and adoption of early noninvasive respiratory support, the benefits of prophylactic surfactant replacement have diminished. Early establishment and maintenance of functional residual capacity with nasal CPAP, early rescue surfactant replacement therapy, and avoidance of prolonged mechanical ventilation form the basis of contemporary care (41–43).

Assessment of Ventilation and Oxygenation

Adequacy of ventilation and oxygenation must be established as soon as possible to avoid pulmonary vasoconstriction, worsening ventilation–perfusion abnormalities, and atelectasis. Pulse oximetry provides a safe noninvasive assessment of tissue oxygenation that is now ubiquitous in neonatal care. Measurement depends on differential absorption of different wavelengths of light (red light at 660 nm and infrared light at 940 nm) by oxygenated and deoxygenated hemoglobin. The pulsatile nature of flow allows the instrument to differentiate absorption during systole from baseline absorption by tissue and nonpulsatile venous flow during diastole to estimate arterial oxygen saturation. Technologic enhancements have improved the accuracy of monitoring during motion and in low-flow states; however, oxygen saturation is still only accurate to approximately ±3%. An arterial saturation of 91% to 95% generally reflects an arterial PO_2 of around 50 to 80 mm Hg, but saturation levels are significantly impacted by proportion of fetal and adult hemoglobin, PCO_2, pH, and temperature.

Prior controversy regarding optimal oxygen saturation levels in extremely preterm infants has been mostly addressed by the Neonatal Oxygenation Prospective Meta-analysis (NeOProM) Collaboration, a prospectively designed meta-analysis of individual participant data from 4,965 infants in five randomized clinical trials. To balance the risk of mortality with risk of retinopathy of prematurity, supplemental oxygen should be titrated to maintain oxygen saturations 91% to 95%.

Adequate oxygen delivery obviously also depends on oxygen carrying capacity of the blood (primarily hemoglobin level) and hemodynamic status (see Chapter 31).

Optimal CO_2 range has not been fully defined, but it is accepted that avoidance of hypocarbia is important to prevent the development of cystic periventricular leukomalacia secondary to cerebral vasoconstriction at low CO_2 tensions. Higher CO_2 levels (50 to 60 mm Hg) are frequently tolerated in the extremely preterm infant if lowering the CO_2 level would require use of invasive ventilation or higher peak pressures, both of which are related to development of chronic lung disease.

Transcutaneous PO_2 monitoring can be used selectively in conjunction with pulse oximetry. Most devices contain oxygen (O_2) and CO_2 electrodes. Noninvasive PO_2 measurements continue to be helpful in certain situations, particularly if transcutaneous PCO_2 also is obtained. Calibration before use and correlation with an arterial sample are necessary, but the need for subsequent blood samples should be reduced.

Technical challenges mean that neither near-infrared spectroscopy nor end tidal CO_2 monitoring have yet been accepted as standard of care in preterm infants, but both are active areas of research.

Positive-pressure ventilation (via invasive mechanical ventilation or noninvasive support) and oxygen therapy may be required at any time and must be readily available. Close monitoring of pH, partial pressure of carbon dioxide (PCO_2), and oxygen saturation is critical in guiding ventilatory and supplemental oxygen requirements. Regardless of gestational age, infants with significant respiratory distress requiring substantial supplemental oxygen (>40%) to maintain oxygen saturation at 91% to 95% often benefit from nasal CPAP (5 to 10 cmH_2O).

The role of CPAP

Because invasive mechanical ventilation is associated with lung injury and development of chronic lung disease, avoidance of

endotracheal intubation and reliance on noninvasive ventilatory support has been widely adopted (41). Nasal CPAP stabilizes surfactant-deficient alveoli and improves both functional residual capacity and ventilation–perfusion matching. For infants with adequate respiratory effort, implementation of nasal CPAP in the delivery room reduces the need for mechanical ventilation. Over the past decade, several large multicentered randomized controlled trials comparing prophylactic surfactant and mechanical ventilation with nasal CPAP demonstrated that extremely preterm infants with RDS can be supported with nasal CPAP safely and effectively (43,44). Additionally, avoidance of mechanical ventilation is associated with a small but statistically significant reduction in death and chronic lung disease. Unfortunately, during these trials it was demonstrated that the majority of infants (30% to 50% within the first week of age) ultimately required mechanical ventilation. An approach that combines the judicious use of nasal CPAP with the known benefits of early rescue surfactant replacement is currently recommended. While no consensus has been reached, when the fraction of inspired oxygen exceeds 40% to 60% to maintain oxygen saturations at 91% to 95%, many advocate for surfactant treatment. Compared to bovine-derived products, the use of porcine-derived surfactant with a phospholipid dose of 200 mg/kg can be given less frequently and has been associated with slightly improved survival (45). Techniques to provide exogenous surfactant replacement therapy while avoiding mechanical ventilation are being increasingly adopted. Commonly referred to as INtubate SURfactant and Extubate (INSURE), one technique is to intubate for early rescue surfactant replacement therapy followed by extubation to CPAP once the infant is stable (usually within minutes to <1 hour). Avoidance of endotracheal intubation altogether can be achieved with a variation of the INSURE method, known as MIST (minimally invasive surfactant therapy) or LISA (less invasive surfactant administration), in which a small feeding tube is used to deliver intratracheal surfactant as the infant breathes spontaneously. Delivery of early rescue surfactant via the INSURE, MIST, or LISA method combined with nasal CPAP has been associated with reduced need for mechanical ventilation and may further reduce the risk of chronic lung disease (44).

Safe and effective care of infants with RDS requiring either invasive mechanical ventilation or noninvasive respiratory support requires careful attention. Nasal CPAP is most effectively delivered via nasal cannula or mask seeking to maintain distending pressure while avoiding soft tissue injury. Although there are many effective systems for CPAP, for its ease of use, widespread availability of materials, and oscillatory fluctuations in pressure, many have proposed use of bubble CPAP. Despite their ease of application and maintenance, especially in extremely preterm infants, the use of heated humidified high flow (HHHF) and RAM nasal cannula cannot reliably deliver constant distending pressure and should not be used as primary support (46). The optimal duration of nasal CPAP support is presently unknown. While data in infants are currently lacking, some propose maintaining preterm infants on nasal CPAP until a corrected gestational age of 32 to 24 weeks, when oxygen requirements and respiratory distress have resolved and normal work of breathing and growth are established (47).

Requirement for Intubation and Ventilation

In cases of ineffective respiratory effort, recurrent apnea, or severe respiratory failure, mechanical ventilation via an endotracheal tube is required. Intubation is a practical skill that cannot be taught by a textbook. Both oral and nasal intubation routes are widely used, with nasal intubation decreasing the risk of unplanned extubation but oral intubation being somewhat simpler and quicker. The endotracheal tube should allow a small leak between the tube and the glottis as too tight a tube may cause pressure necrosis. Optimal positioning for the tip of an endotracheal tube is in the middle of the trachea where it is least likely to dislodge upward out into the pharynx or downward into a bronchus. Immediately after intubation, the position of the tube should be confirmed by misting of the tube, auscultation of bilateral air entry, and CO_2 detection by colorimetry or direct measurement. Two common errors of tube placement (intubation of the esophagus and intubation of the right mainstem bronchus) cannot reliably be excluded by auscultation in extremely preterm infants, so a chest x-ray should be obtained to confirm optimal tube placement.

Pressure-limited ventilation has been the mainstay of neonatal care, but volume-targeted ventilation is increasingly used. Volume-targeted ventilation may be particularly helpful where significant changes in lung compliance are expected, such as following surfactant therapy. In such cases, pressure-controlled ventilation can rapidly cause inappropriately high tidal volumes and volutrauma.

Both pressure-limited and volume-limited approaches now generally include patient-triggered ventilation, where a rapidly responding sensor detects the onset of spontaneous respiratory effort and triggers the mechanical breath during early inspiration. Triggered modes are thought to increase infant comfort and decrease the need for sedation.

Regardless of the strategy, timely surfactant replacement can attenuate ventilator-induced lung injury of the surfactant-deficient lung. Avoidance of volutrauma with appropriate tidal volumes (usually 4 to 6 mL/kg) and prevention of atelectotrauma with appropriate positive end-expiratory pressure (usually 4 to 6 cmH$_2$O) is critical to reduce lung injury. Rapid changes in lung compliance following surfactant replacement must also be anticipated. As in all respiratory therapy, critical attention to adequacy of ventilation, as assessed by PCO$_2$, pH, and oxygen saturation, is required to adjust to the rapid changes in respiratory status occurring in these critically ill infants. Hyperventilation should be avoided, and the duration of mechanical ventilation should be minimized.

Other forms of ventilation such as high-frequency oscillatory or jet ventilators are often used in combination with exogenous surfactant for the treatment of RDS. High-frequency jet ventilation (HFJV) delivers high-flow, short-duration pulses of gas at rates of 150 to 600 breaths per minute. Exhalation is passive. HFJV can also be combined with conventional pressure-controlled ventilation as a hybrid mode. High-frequency oscillatory ventilation (HFOV) delivers smaller tidal volumes at high rates, with an active expiratory phase.

These therapies are often considered for treatment of severely affected infants whose ventilation has not been adequately supported by conventional ventilation and surfactant therapy. Randomized controlled trials examining the prophylactic use of high-frequency ventilation to reduce the risk of chronic lung disease in preterm infants have been inconsistent and do not appear to reduce chronic lung disease (48). Nitric oxide (NO) has also been used in the treatment of respiratory failure in term infants, but randomized trials of routine use in preterm infants have failed to show benefit (48,49).

Complications

Apnea, inadequacy of ventilation, atelectasis, mucous plugging, hyperaeration, or air leak may complicate the care of infants with RDS. CNS hemorrhage (most commonly IVH) and PDA represent significant clinical problems. PDA and subsequent congestive heart failure and pulmonary edema further compromise respiratory function, decreasing pulmonary compliance and perhaps inactivating pulmonary surfactant. Although the management of PDA remains highly controversial, hemodynamically significant PDA associated with RDS should be diagnosed and addressed promptly (see Chapter 31). Acute CNS hemorrhage is often associated with shock, pulmonary compromise, and pulmonary hemorrhage. Fluctuations in respiratory status may contribute to IVH and can be minimized by careful attention to respiratory care. Judicious use of intravenous fluid/nutrition during both the acute

and convalescent care of infants with RDS is critical to avoid fluid overload. Impaired pulmonary function and an increased risk of PDA are associated with excessive fluid administration.

Management of chronic lung disease, a frequent sequela of acute respiratory distress syndrome, is discussed in Chapter 29.

MECONIUM ASPIRATION SYNDROME

Meconium-stained amniotic fluid (MSAF) occurs in approximately 8% of deliveries at ≤37 weeks' gestation and 25% of live births at 41 weeks or greater (50,51). Of those with MSAF, 2% to 10% develop MAS defined as otherwise unexplained respiratory distress in newborns born through MASF (50,52). Changes in clinical practice to avoid gestation beyond 41 weeks have dramatically reduced the incidence of MAS. The cause, pathophysiology, and treatment of MSAF and MAS have been reviewed (50,52,53).

Meconium first appears in the fetal ileum between 10 and 16 weeks of gestation as a viscous green liquid composed of gastrointestinal secretions, cellular debris, bile and pancreatic juice, mucus, blood, lanugo, vernix, and approximately 72% to 80% water. Meconium passage between 20 and 34 weeks is infrequent, and MSAF rarely occurs before 38 weeks of gestation. The increased incidence of MSAF with advancing gestational age probably reflects the maturation of peristalsis in the fetal intestine. Intestinal parasympathetic innervation and myelination increase throughout gestation and may play a role in the increased incidence of passage of meconium in late gestation.

In utero passage of meconium is associated with fetal asphyxia and decreased umbilical venous blood PO$_2$. Experimentally, intestinal ischemia produces a transient period of hyperperistalsis and relaxation of anal sphincter tone, leading to the passage of meconium. The fetal diving reflex, which shunts blood preferentially to the brain and heart and away from the visceral organs during hypoxia, may enhance intestinal ischemia. The gasping respiratory efforts that accompany fetal asphyxia contribute to the entry of meconium into the respiratory tract.

Since passage of meconium can be induced by fetal hypoxia, meconium in amniotic fluid is a hallmark of fetal compromise and demands critical evaluation of fetal well-being. Abnormal fetal heart rate patterns predict infants at greatest risk of significant MAS and poor outcome. Perinatal morbidity is increased in newborns with MSAF associated with abnormal fetal heart rates, and these infants are at greatest risk for the MAS. Overall, neonatal outcomes of deliveries complicated by MSAF associated with fetal tachycardia or decreased fetal heart rate variability are similar to those of non–meconium-stained infants with similar abnormalities of fetal heart rate. In infants with normal fetal heart rate patterns, MSAF generally carries a low risk of perinatal morbidity that is comparable to deliveries with clear amniotic fluid.

Clinical Presentation

MAS describes a wide spectrum of respiratory disease, ranging from mild respiratory distress to severe disease and death despite mechanical ventilation. Severe disease increases with advancing gestational age with the incidence ranging from 0.1% at 37 to 38 weeks of gestation to 0.5% at 42 weeks (50). Severe MAS typically presents as respiratory distress, tachypnea, prolonged expiratory phase, and hypoxemia soon after birth in an infant heavily stained on the nails, hair, and umbilical cord with meconium or born through thick meconium. Major risk factors for MAS include fetal distress, nonreassuring fetal heart tracing, intrauterine growth restriction, cesarean section, and postmaturity. Infants with severe MAS often have an increased anteroposterior dimension of the thorax, a "barrel" chest, secondary to air trapping from obstructed airways. Persistent pulmonary hypertension of the newborn (PPHN) is more frequently observed in infants with severe MAS (see also Chapter 31). Less severe meconium aspiration may present with

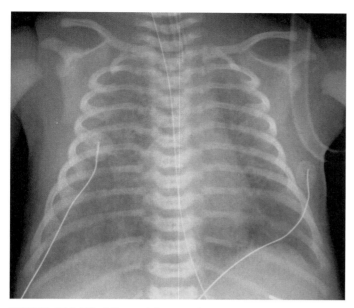

FIGURE 28.6 This full-term infant was born with fetal bradycardia and thick meconium in the amniotic fluid. Cyanosis and respiratory distress were evident within minutes of delivery. The chest radiograph film demonstrates coarse, irregular infiltrates; hyperinflation (left and right diaphragms at ribs 10 to 11); and right pleural effusion indicative of MAS. Endotracheal and nasogastric tubes are in position.

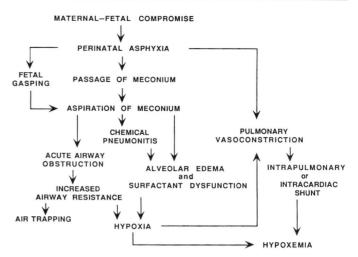

FIGURE 28.7 Pathogenesis of meconium aspiration syndrome.

pneumonitis of gradual onset with increased work of breathing and tachypnea that generally resolves over the first week of life.

The chest radiographs of infants with MAS vary but typically demonstrate coarse patchy infiltrates, with mixed areas of hyperaeration and consolidation (Fig. 28.6). Pleural effusions are detected in approximately 30% of infants with MAS. There is an increased risk of pneumothorax or pneumomediastinum, which occurs in approximately 25% of severely affected infants. Chest radiographs are abnormal in more than one-half of infants with meconium detected below the vocal cords, although fewer than 50% of the infants with abnormal radiographs have significant respiratory distress. Radiographic resolution of MAS occurs slowly, usually over 7 to 10 days. The severity of chest radiographic abnormalities may not correlate with the severity of clinical disease.

Pathology

Postmortem examination of lungs from infants with severe MAS reveals meconium, vernix, squamous cells, and cellular debris in the air spaces. An inflammatory response with polymorphonuclear leukocytes, macrophages, and alveolar edema may be present. Hyaline membrane formation, pulmonary hemorrhage, and necrosis of pulmonary microvasculature and parenchyma can occur. Platelet-rich microthrombi in small arterioles and increased muscularization of distal arterioles have been described in some infants dying of MAS.

Pathophysiology

Meconium in the amniotic fluid presents both a marker of fetal hypoxia with potential vascular effects in the lung and a chemical and mechanical cause of lung injury. The pulmonary abnormalities in meconium aspiration are related primarily to acute airway obstruction, decreased lung tissue compliance, and parenchymal lung damage (see **Fig. 28.7**). Instillation of meconium into adult rabbit and newborn dog tracheas causes acute mechanical obstruction of proximal and distal airways (54). A ball-valve mechanism produces partial airway obstruction causing air trapping, which results in increased anteroposterior chest diameter,

increased expiratory resistance, and increased functional residual capacity. Complete obstruction of small airways may result in regional atelectasis and ventilation–perfusion inequalities. Disruption of surfactant function by serum and nonserum proteins and fatty acids contributes to atelectasis, decreased compliance, and resulting hypoxia. Meconium is also toxic to pulmonary epithelial cells and may itself contain, and stimulate, the production of proinflammatory mediators including phospholipase A_2, IL-8, platelet-activating factor, and TNF-α.

In infants with severe MAS, pulmonary hypertension with right-to-left shunting contributes to the characteristically severe and sometimes refractory hypoxemia. Such clinical pulmonary hypertension correlates with increased muscularization of distal pulmonary vessels likely mediated by chronic intrauterine hypoxia. Perinatal asphyxia is a critical underlying factor in the pathogenesis of MAS, increasing the risks for pulmonary hypertension and meconium aspiration.

Prevention

The incidence of MAS has declined to about 0.1% to 1.8% of live births in developed countries, which has been attributed to reducing deliveries at ≥41 weeks and improved intervention for fetal distress. Antenatal diagnosis and treatment of fetal asphyxia is a focus for prevention of MAS. Clinical studies have not, however, supported the use of intrapartum prophylactic amnioinfusion in MSAF, although therapeutic amnioinfusion in cases of fetal heart tracing deceleration may improve outcome (55). Maternal risk factors for MAS include age ≥30 years, nulliparity, pregnancy-induced hypertension, and diabetes mellitus.

American Academy of Pediatrics and American Heart Association guidelines for delivery room management of infants born through MSAF have been revised multiple times since 2004 based on studies of interventions and outcomes including a randomized controlled study of over 2,500 babies showing no difference in MSAF-related morbidity with postdelivery nasopharyngeal or tracheal suctioning. As of 2015, intrapartum oro- and nasopharyngeal suctioning followed by routine intubation with suctioning of airway secretions immediately after delivery through MSAF is no longer recommended. The infant who is vigorous with good respiratory effort may stay with the mother for the initial steps of newborn care. Current US guidelines recommend that the nonvigorous infant with poor tone or inadequate respiratory effort should be resuscitated using the same approach used for infants without MSAF. Presence of meconium in the third trimester of pregnancy is strongly associated with fetal hypoxia and perinatal depression such that a team capable of neonatal resuscitation should be available for births of newborns with MSAF (56). Subsequent studies of outcome following adoption of the 2015 Neonatal Resuscitation Program (NRP) limiting airway suctioning of MSAF thus far have demonstrated fewer infants intubated at birth and no increase in severe MAS, but suggest a potential increase in needs for oxygen therapy, mechanical ventilation, and NICU care. Further evaluation of the change in management is needed. Studies do suggest that the risk and severity of MAS is greater when the consistency of meconium is thick versus thin in MSAF.

Treatment

Postnatal therapy for MAS begins with continuous observation and monitoring of infants at risk. Vigorous treatment of nonrespiratory sequelae of fetal stress and perinatal asphyxia, including temperature instability, hypoglycemia, hypocalcemia, hypotension, and decreased cardiac function are critical to promoting the fetal-to-newborn physiologic transition. Attention also needs to be given to the potential effects of multiorgan hypoxemia and ischemia, including reduced renal function, reduced production of clotting factors, hypoalbuminemia, cerebral edema, and seizures. From a respiratory standpoint, correction of hypoxemia and acidosis is indicated to prevent the pulmonary vasoconstriction and poor transition from fetal to neonatal circulation that is associated with MAS. Hyperventilation, hyperoxia, and infusion of bicarbonate to treat metabolic acidosis are no longer recommended in treatment of MAS. Chest physiotherapy and suctioning of particulate meconium may be useful if there is airway obstruction, and the infant maintains adequate oxygenation during such therapy. Continuous monitoring of oxygenation by transcutaneous oxygen monitoring or pulse oximetry and assessment of PaO_2, $PaCO_2$, and pH should be used to guide the application of oxygen therapy and mechanical ventilation.

The presence and severity of systemic hypotension should be noted and treated with volume resuscitation and vasopressors, while pulmonary hypertension should be evaluated by echocardiography in the hypoxemic infant with MAS. Labile and differential upper extremity as compared to lower extremity oxygen saturation measurements are common in severe MAS, especially with agitation, suggesting pulmonary hypertension and ductal shunting. Treatment of PPHN is covered separately in this chapter. Broad-spectrum antibiotics are routinely used in the therapy of MAS in infants with abnormal radiographic findings and respiratory distress: their efficacy in MAS, however, remains unlikely, and they may not be indicated once infection as cause of fetal stress has been ruled out (57). Treatment of acute MAS with glucocorticoids has not been shown to be beneficial. Mechanical complications, such as pneumothorax, should be anticipated, promptly recognized, and treated appropriately.

Surfactant treatment, inhaled nitric oxide (INO), additional pulmonary vasodilators, and high-frequency oscillatory or jet ventilation (HFOV/HFJV) (58) are frequently utilized to support some infants with MAS and may be used in combination. Meconium instilled into canine or piglet lungs or mixed with surfactant *in vitro* inactivates surfactant function, decreasing lung compliance and lung volumes and causing atelectasis and potential ventilation/perfusion (V/Q) mismatch. Meta-analyses of available studies support the use of surfactant therapy for MAS (59). More recent use of diluted surfactant in lung lavage in small studies of infants with MAS did not show any advantage of surfactant lavage as compared to bolus treatment. A study of surfactant function during and following whole body cooling, a therapy used in hypoxic–ischemic encephalopathy that often accompanies MAS, suggested improved surfactant function with hypothermic treatment (60,61). Current preclinical studies are testing intratracheal application of various agents in models of MAS, including recombinant superoxide dismutase, N-acetylcysteine (Mucomyst), selective inhibitors of NFkB, anti-IL8 antibody, and budesonide with or after surfactant, with mixed results, encouraging further study.

Ventilatory Support

Mechanical ventilation is frequently required for treatment of infants with severe MAS and must be managed carefully. The use of conventional ventilation and CPAP in MAS was reviewed (62). Although improvement in oxygenation was observed in patients with MAS treated with PEEP, further study of safety and efficacy of PEEP in MAS are needed. CPAP or PEEP may aggravate hyperinflation associated with MAS and should be used with care. However there is evidence that use of bubble CPAP as compared to head hood oxygen delivery reduced need for subsequent mechanical ventilation and reduced duration of oxygen therapy and incidence of pulmonary hypertension in the first 7 days following MAS (63). Pneumothorax and pneumomediastinum occur frequently during the course of MAS because of the ball-valve effect of meconium and may occur before or after the application of positive-pressure ventilation. Lengthening the expiratory time of the ventilatory cycle may reduce hyperinflation. Sedation, and occasionally muscle relaxation, is frequently required for infants intubated for MAS though care should be taken as instability can be increased by intubation and removal of the infant's respiratory drive.

HFOV has been studied alone and in combination with INO as treatment for MAS. Kinsella et al. (64) found that the response rate of infants with MAS to HFOV plus INO was greater than the response rate to either HFOV or INO with conventional ventilation alone. ECMO has been used successfully in rescue treatment of severe MAS refractory to conventional ventilatory therapy. The survival rate for babies with MAS treated with ECMO is above 95% (65).

PERSISTENT PULMONARY HYPERTENSION OF THE NEWBORN (SEE ALSO CHAPTER 31)

Normal transition to extrauterine life requires a shift from a state of high PVR and little blood flow to the pulmonary circulation to one of low PVR and ample perfusion to the lung. Failure of this transition results in PPHN, causing hypoxemia associated with significant morbidity and mortality. The incidence of PPHN is reported to be approximately 2 per 1,000 live births in the United States, with a mortality of 4% to 10% (66–68). The clinical presentation, updated classification, diagnosis, and treatment of pulmonary hypertension generally and of PPHN specifically was recently reviewed (69–73).

Pathophysiology of Perinatal Pulmonary Vasculature Adaptation

Fetal circulation *in utero* is characterized by PVR that exceeds systemic vascular resistance, resulting in right atrial and ventricular pressures exceeding left atrial and ventricular pressures. As a result of this pressure differential, more than one-third of the oxygenated blood returning to the fetus from the placenta through the inferior vena cava streams across the patent foramen ovale (PFO), is ejected from the left ventricle, and perfuses the head, neck, and upper body. Venous blood returning through the superior vena cava preferentially flows into the right ventricle and main pulmonary artery. A small amount of this deoxygenated blood, constituting approximately 10% to 15% of the cardiac output (74), perfuses the lungs, but because of elevated PVR, most is shunted across the PDA to mix with the blood in the aorta distal to cervical and subclavian arteries. Thus, the lower body is perfused with relatively less well-oxygenated blood than the head and neck. Because of the large right-to-left shunt at the PFO and the PDA, most of the cardiac output bypasses the lungs *in utero*. Mechanisms that maintain the fetal state of high PVR include relative acidosis and hypoxia, mechanical factors such as fluid-filled lungs, and vaso-constrictive mediators such as endothelin-1, platelet-activating factor, and products of the prostaglandin pathway (i.e., leukotri-ene and thromboxane) (75).

The "immediate" phase of postnatal transition is accomplished in the first minutes after birth when the fluid-filled fetal lungs are distended with air. Clamping of the umbilical cord separates the infant from the low-resistance placenta and increases sys-temic vascular resistance. A rapid decrease in PVR occurs with the mechanical distention of the lungs, allowing more oxygenated blood to perfuse the pulmonary vascular bed. Shear stress and oxygenation induce endothelial cell nitric oxide synthase (eNOS) and initiate synthesis of NO, a potent vascular smooth muscle cell relaxant. The entry of air into the alveoli increases the oxygen-ation of the pulmonary vascular bed, decreasing PVR. As a result, a marked increase in pulmonary blood flow occurs, and the rise in left atrial pressure prevents further shunting of blood across the PFO. Pulmonary vasoconstriction caused by postnatal persistent hypoxia, systemic acidosis, and decreased NO production contrib-utes to the pathophysiology of PPHN.

The "fast phase" of the transitional pulmonary circulation occurs from 12 to 24 hours after birth and accounts for the great-est reduction in PVR. The dramatic drop in PVR is associated with the production of vasodilators, such as prostacyclin and NO. Pros-tacyclin is produced in the neonatal lung in response to rhythmic distension of the lungs. Production of prostacyclin is dependent on the activity of cyclooxygenase. PPHN has been observed in infants of mothers receiving aspirin or nonsteroidal anti-inflammatory agents during pregnancy that inhibit cyclooxygenase activity.

The pulmonary vasodilation and increase in pulmonary blood flow occurring in response to oxygenation is dependent on NO. NO activates guanylate cyclase in vascular smooth muscle cells in turn activating cGMP-dependent protein kinase decreasing intra-cellular calcium, causing smooth muscle cell relaxation. Vascular effects of NO are confined primarily to the pulmonary vasculature because of the affinity of NO for hemoglobin and short half-life in circulating blood. Thus, inhaled NO (iNO) mediates pulmonary vasodilation without systemic hypotension.

The "final phase" of the neonatal pulmonary vascular transi-tion involves remodeling of the pulmonary vascular muscula-ture (76). In the normal fetal and term lung, fully muscularized, thick-walled preacinar arteries extend to the level of the terminal bronchioles. Intra-acinar and alveolar wall arteries are not mus-cularized. Within days after delivery, medial wall thickness of pre-acinar vessels smaller than 250 nm in diameter decreases, and within months, medial wall thickness of larger vessels decreases. Hypoxia at birth prevents the remodeling and regression of the smooth muscle of the preacinar bronchiolar arteries. *In utero*, or after birth, chronic hypoxia stimulates smooth muscle prolif-eration and differentiation causing abnormally thick and reactive arteriolar musculature. Extension of smooth muscle into small pulmonary vessels, increased abundant adventitial fibroblasts, and abnormal deposition of extracellular matrix are found in lungs of infants dying of MAS and PPHN.

Etiology of PPHN

PPHN has been classified into four main categories based on the etiology and anatomic pathology: *maladaption* of otherwise nor-mal vasculature (as seen in MAS or pneumonia); *maldevelop-ment* of pulmonary vasculature with normal lung parenchyma (as seen in premature closure of the ductus arteriosus); *hypoplasia* of both pulmonary parenchyma and vasculature (as seen in CDH), or disruptions of pulmonary vasculogenesis as seen in ACD; and *functional or intrinsic obstruction* (as seen with hyperviscosity) (Table 28.1). Identification of the causes of PPHN is helpful in pre-dicting severity and reversibility of the disease. Assessment of the clinical severity of PPHN helps determine the need for referral to

nurseries with extracorporeal membrane oxygenation (ECMO) and iNO capability.

Clinical Presentation

Clinically, PPHN presents as labile hypoxemia that is often dis-proportionate to the extent of pulmonary parenchymal disease. Infants with PPHN are commonly appropriate for gestational age and near term or term. Perinatal history frequently includes factors associated with perinatal hypoxia–ischemia. Clinical symptoms include tachypnea, respiratory distress, and often rapidly progres-sive cyanosis, particularly in response to stimulation of the infant. The cardiovascular examination may be normal or may reveal a right ventricular heave, closely split or single loud S2, and low-pitched systolic murmur of tricuspid regurgitation suggesting that pulmonary arterial pressure is equal to or greater than systemic arterial pressure. An oxygen saturation gradient of 10% between preductal (right arm) and postductal (lower extremity) sites sug-gests right-to-left shunting at the ductus arteriosus and is consis-tent with, although not required for, the diagnosis of PPHN. PPHN may occur without differential oxygen saturations if the ductus arteriosus is closed and mixing of cyanotic and oxygenated blood is occurring within the lungs or at other intracardiac sites. Differ-ential diagnosis of PPHN includes severe pulmonary parenchymal disease, such as severe MAS, RDS, pneumonia, sepsis or pulmo-nary hemorrhage, and cyanotic congenital heart disease (CCHD), such as transposition of the great arteries. Critical pulmonic steno-sis, hypoplastic left ventricle, ACD, or coarctation should be con-sidered in the differential diagnosis. Methods used to differentiate PPHN from pulmonary parenchymal disease or cardiac disease (Table 28.2) include comparison of pre- and postductal oxygen saturations and hyperoxia test. With exposure to 100% FiO_2, an increase in PaO_2 to greater than 150 suggests paren-chymal lung disease, whereas PaO_2 less than 50 or an increase of less than 20 mm Hg suggests CCHD or severe PPHN. Echocardiography pro-vides a key step in diagnosing PPHN and excluding structural con-genital heart disease. Findings consistent with PPHN include right ventricular (RV) hypertrophy with deviation of the intraventricu-lar septum to the left, tricuspid regurgitation, and right-to-left or bidirectional shunting at the PDA and/or PFO (77).

The oxygenation of infants with severe pulmonary parenchy-mal disease without PPHN generally improves after treatment with oxygen or mechanical ventilation. Infants with PPHN may have little or no parenchymal lung disease and may be easily ven-tilated but remain hypoxic despite high fraction of inspiratory oxygen (FiO_2). Ventilation and/or correction of metabolic acido-sis in infants with PPHN often improves oxygenation. In contrast, CCHD is usually associated with fixed, structural mixing of venous and arterial blood. In infants with CCHD, hypoxemia is generally unresponsive to increased FiO_2 and mechanical ventilation. Fixed hypoxia, refractory to supportive treatment, may also occur in cases of PPHN with severe remodeling of intrapulmonary arteri-oles.

Therapy of PPHN

Supportive medical management includes correction of metabolic acidosis and hypotension and treatment of underlying conditions such as sepsis. Specific therapy for PPHN is aimed at increasing pulmonary blood flow, decreasing right-to-left shunting, and reduc-ing V/Q mismatch. Supplemental oxygen and mechanical venti-lation are the primary therapeutic interventions for treatment of PPHN. Closure of the PDA is not useful; in fact, cardiac failure may occur after PDA closure as the right ventricle fails in the face of high pulmonary resistance. Shunting between the pulmonary and systemic circulations, such as through the ductus arteriosus or PFO, depends on the relative pressures of each system. Therefore, optimal therapy decreases pulmonary artery pressure while sup-porting systemic arterial pressure and cardiac output.

TABLE 28.1

Classification System for PPHN of the Newborn

Pathology	Associated Diseases	Proposed Mechanism	Prognosis
Functional vasoconstriction; normal pulmonary vascular development	Acute perinatal hypoxia Acute meconium aspiration Sepsis or pneumonia (especially group B streptococcus) Respiratory distress syndrome Hypoventilation CNS depression Hypothermia Hypoglycemia	Response to acute hypoxia, particularly in the presence of acidemia	Good; reversible
Fixed decreased diameter; abnormal extension and hypertrophy of distal pulmonary vascular smooth muscle	Placental insufficiency Prolonged gestation *In utero* closure of ductus arteriosus Aspirin Nonsteroidal anti-inflammatory agents Single ventricle without pulmonic stenosis Chronic pulmonary venous hypertension TAPVR Obstructive left-sided heart lesions Idiopathic diseases	Response to chronic hypoxia Excessive pulmonary blood flow *in utero* Elevated pulmonary venous pressure	Poor; fixed structural lesion
Decreased cross-sectional area of the pulmonary vascular bed	Space-occupying lesions Diaphragmatic hernia Lung dysgenesis Pleural effusions Congenital lung hypoplasia Severe intrauterine growth restriction Severe prolonged rupture of membranes Potter syndrome Thoracic dystrophies	Hypoplasia of alveoli and associated vessels	Poor; fixed structural lesion
Functional obstruction to pulmonary blood flow	Polycythemia Hyperfibrinogenemia	Increased blood viscosity	Good, unless chronic

CNS, central nervous system; TAPVR, total anomalous pulmonary venous return.

TABLE 28.2

Diagnostic Evaluation of Severe Neonatal Hypoxemia

Test	Method	Result	Suggested Diagnosis
Hyperoxia	Expose to 100% FiO_2 for 5–10 min	PaO_2 increases to >100 mm Hg PaO_2 increases by <20 mm Hg	Pulmonary parenchymal disease PPHN or CCHD
Hyperventilation–hyperoxia	Mechanical ventilation with 100% FiO_2 and respiratory rate 100–150 breaths/min	PaO_2 increases to >100 mm Hg without hyperventilation PaO_2 increases at a critical PCO_2, often to <25 mm Hg No increase in PaO_2 despite hyperventilation	Pulmonary parenchymal disease PPHN Cyanotic congenital heart disease or severe, fixed pulmonary hypertension
Simultaneous–preductal–postductal PO_2	Compare PO_2 of right arm or shoulder to that of lower abdomen or extremities	Preductal $PO_2 \geq 15$ + postductal PO_2	PDA with right-to-left shunt
Echocardiography	M-mode	Increased RVPEP and RVET	Right ventricular systolic time interval ratio (RVSTI = RVPEP/RVET > 0.5) predicts PPHN
	Venous contrast injection	Simultaneously appears in PA and LA	Patent foramen ovale
	Two-dimensional echocardiography	Deviation of intraatrial septum to left; rule out congenital heart defect	Increased pulmonary arterial pressure
	Doppler	Failure of acceleration of systolic blood flow between large main pulmonary artery and small peripheral pulmonary artery	Suggests right-to-left PDA or intracardiac shunt

LA, left atrium; PA, pulmonary artery; PDA, patent ductus arteriosus; PPHN, persistent pulmonary hypertension of the newborn; RVET, right ventricular ejection time; RVPEP, right ventricular ejection period.

Infants with severe PPHN are often sensitive to agitation. Stimulation should be minimized during the care of these infants. Transcutaneous and intravascular monitoring equipment and temporal clustering of interventions reduce agitation. Muscle relaxants (e.g., vecuronium) should be avoided since paralysis may further compromise ventilation, cause fluid retention, and has been associated with increased mortality (67). Sedation is often beneficial, but pharmacologic agents should be chosen to minimize systemic hypotension. Hypoxic–ischemic injury or sepsis increase the risk for systemic hypotension and may contribute to PPHN. The hematocrit should be maintained at or above 45%, and cardiac output should be supported with volume or pressors. Elevated right heart pressure with increased PVR, poor venous return secondary to high intrathoracic pressures during mechanical ventilation, and hypoxic–ischemic damage may contribute to myocardial dysfunction that can be responsive to dobutamine. Adrenergic agents are commonly used for refractory hypotension but should be used with caution, as they may contribute to pulmonary vasoconstriction. There is anecdotal evidence supporting the use of hydrocortisone for the treatment of refractory hypotension in the newborn with PPHN.

Respiratory and Metabolic Alkalosis during Treatment of PPHN

The often dramatic response of infants with PPHN to respiratory or metabolic alkalosis has led to their use in the care of infants with severe PPHN; however, the sometimes transient benefit of alkalosis must be balanced against the risk of lung injury, neurologic compromise from hypocapnic alkalosis, and cellular effects of infusion of hypertonic solutions. The degree of pulmonary parenchymal disease and risk of barotrauma may affect the clinical choice of inducing respiratory or metabolic alkalosis. Although it may be necessary to transiently raise arterial pH by increasing ventilation and alkali (sodium bicarbonate or THAM) to reverse severe pulmonary vasoconstriction, because of pulmonary and neurologic concerns (including sensorineural hearing loss), sustained hypocapnia and metabolic alkalosis are not advocated (78,79). Excessive mechanical ventilation with overdistension of the lung may increase right-to-left shunting. Pulmonary barotrauma associated with aggressive ventilation should be avoided, instead aiming to normalize ventilation, oxygenation, and pH. Hypocarbic alkalosis shifts the hemoglobin–oxygen dissociation curve and may compromise the release of oxygen at the tissue level. Importantly, both hyperoxia and hypocarbia may adversely affect cerebral blood flow. Corrections of hypoxemia and reversal of pulmonary vasoconstriction are the mainstays of treatment of PPHN: maintaining blood oxygen concentrations above physiologic levels may be harmful (80). Hyperoxia ($PaO_2 > 100$ mm Hg) does not further promote pulmonary vasodilation yet does increase oxidative stress and oxygen free radical production that may enhance pulmonary vasoconstriction and is better avoided. Adequate oxygenation with some buffer against intermittent hypoxia but avoidance of persistent hyperoxia is advised. A risk–benefit ratio exists between potential injury caused in pursuit of optimal blood gas results.

Nitric Oxide and High-Frequency Oscillatory Ventilation

Pharmacotherapy of PPHN was recently reviewed (81) and is a rapidly evolving field. iNO is useful for treatment of PPHN and is approved by the U.S. Food and Drug Administration (FDA) for this purpose (49,82–85). At low pharmacologic doses, less than 40 parts per million (ppm), iNO selectively dilates the pulmonary vasculature. Typical doses used to treat PPHN are 5 to 20 ppm. Avid binding to hemoglobin and a short half-life in the bloodstream prevent iNO from dilating systemic blood vessels. Because iNO is delivered as a gas, it preferentially dilates vessels of alveoli that are ventilated, thus improving V/Q matching. iNO combined with conventional ventilation increases oxygenation and decreases the oxygenation index (OI) in approximately 30% of infants with

PPHN. The likelihood of response to iNO was inversely related to the severity of parenchymal disease. In patients with moderate PPHN (alveolar–arterial oxygenation gradient, A-aDO$_2$ = 500 to 599), 15% of those treated with iNO, versus 58% of controls, progressed to severe PPHN (85). Approximately 25% of PPHN infants who lacked response to iNO improved when iNO was combined with HFOV, suggesting improved response to iNO if ventilation is optimized. The combined use of exogenous surfactant, HFOV, and iNO to enhance alveolar recruitment and perfusion may be useful in treatment of RDS and meconium aspiration. A systematic review of 17 randomized controlled trials in term or near-full term infants with hypoxic respiratory failure concluded that iNO reduced the need for ECMO, iNO improving oxygenation in approximately 50% of the infants (49). Caution in weaning infants from iNO is warranted to avoid recurrent pulmonary hypertension associated with abrupt cessation (86).

Pharmacologic Vasodilators Used to Treat PPHN

Although iNO is first-line therapy for PPHN, there are situations in which other agents should be considered. The expense of iNO and requirement for specialized equipment may limit its availability in low-resource settings. Patients who remain hypoxic may benefit from other pulmonary vasodilators. Infants requiring long-term therapy are often transitioned to oral medications. Arachidonic acid is converted by the enzyme cyclooxygenase to a class of prostanoids, which includes prostacyclin. Analogous to NO, prostacyclin increases cAMP, reducing intracellular calcium to relax smooth muscle cells. Prostacyclin and stable prostacyclin analogues, delivered by aerosolization, are used for treatment of pediatric pulmonary hypertension in infants and children. Epoprostenol is a synthetic prostacyclin analogue used to treat pulmonary hypertension in adults. Its rapid clearance requires administration by continuous intravenous infusion or by continuous nebulization. Aerosolized prostacyclin (87), prostaglandin E$_1$ (88) and iloprost (89,90) improved oxygenation in PPHN in limited studies. A systematic review of prostacyclins for treatment of pulmonary hypertension in neonates is under way (91).

Phosphodiesterase and endothelin receptor inhibitors have been considered for the treatment of PPHN. Phosphodiesterase inhibitors, for example sildenafil, which inhibits phosphodiesterases that degrade cGMP (PDE5), and milrinone, which inhibits PDE3 that degrades cAMP, cause vascular smooth muscle relaxation. For infants who have not responded to iNO, and have evidence of ventricular dysfunction, milrinone has theoretical benefits for the treatment of PPHN (92–95), although systemic hypotension may occur. A systematic review of the use of sildenafil in low-resource settings (either as single or adjuvant therapy) found improved oxygenation and reduced mortality, without additional benefit when used in conjunction with iNO; however, large-scale trials are needed to assess its effectiveness and ensure long-term safety of this approach (96). Systemic delivery of pulmonary vasodilators, such as sildenafil, function irrespective of ventilation and so may worsen ventilation–perfusion mismatch in cases of heterogenous lung disease. The US FDA published a warning about the use of sildenafil for the treatment of pediatric pulmonary hypertension (in patients >1 year of age) after a dose-escalation study showed higher mortality in a high-dose group (97). A subsequent FDA release clarified recognition of cases where risk: benefit ratio may be acceptable for use of the drug in individual patients.

Endothelin-1 activates the endothelium receptor A (ERA) causing vasoconstriction and smooth muscle cell proliferation in the pulmonary vasculature in response to hypoxia. ERA antagonists, such as ambrisentan, are in use in adult pulmonary hypertension (98) and are under investigation for treatment of neonatal PPHN (81,99). A multicenter study failed to show any additive benefit of bosentan when patients were also treated with iNO while a second suggested significantly improved oxygen index following bosentan therapy with or without iNO (100,101). A recent Cochrane review of endothelin receptor antagonists concluded that evidence was lacking to recommend their routine use (102).

Extracorporeal Membrane Oxygenation

ECMO has been useful for the treatment of severe PPHN refractory to medical management (49,85,103). ECMO describes prolonged (days to weeks) extracorporeal (out of body) cardiopulmonary support in which a membrane oxygenator supplies oxygen and eliminates CO_2 from the blood. ECMO aims to supports the patient's heart and lung function, while minimizing ongoing hyperoxic damage and baro/volutrauma, allowing the underlying disorder to improve. Bypass can be either venoarterial ("VA"—blood is removed from the right atrium and returned to the aorta, hence supporting both lung function and heart function) or venovenous (VV—blood is removed from and then returned to the right atrium, hence supporting only lung function). Management of an infant on an ECMO circuit requires a highly specialized multidisciplinary team approach best delivered at expert centers. Further discussion of the components of ECMO care is covered in Chapters 32 and 33.

A retrospective analysis of cases reported to the Extracorporeal Life Support Organization Registry from 2009 to 2015 reported a 74% survival rate for high-risk infants with the primary diagnosis of PPHN (93% for MAS), who were treated with ECMO (104). Prematurity, acidosis (pH ≤ 7.2), and hypoxia (SaO_2 ≤ 65%) prior to ECMO and need for 7 or more days of ECMO support were associated with increased mortality. For infants with PPHN, generally accepted indications for ECMO include hemodynamic instability or severe, persistent hypoxia with OI greater than 40 as (mean airway pressure [MAP] in $cmH_2O \times FiO_2 \times 100 \div PaO_2$) despite optimized medical management with mechanical ventilation and iNO (105).

Long-Term Outcome of PPHN

Most infants treated for PPHN have relatively few residual respiratory symptoms or neurologic or developmental sequelae by 1 year of age (106). However, a population-based report by Steurer et al. found that infants with PPHN had an added risk ratio (aRR) of 3.5 (95% CI 3.3 to 3.7) for postdischarge mortality or rehospitalization within 1 year of life compared with infants without PPHN. Even infants with only mild PPHN had an aRR of 2.2 (95% CI 2.0 to 2.5). Of infants with more severe disease, qualifying for iNO or ECMO, approximately 25% have chronic lung disease or recurrent reactive airway disease at 1 and 2 years of age. Of children with moderately severe PPHN, with OI of 24 ± 9 at study entry and randomized to receive iNO or placebo, approximately 13% had major neurologic abnormalities, 30% had cognitive delays, and 19% had hearing loss (68). There was no difference between iNO-treated and control infants, indicating that the severity of the disease process itself impacts long-term outcomes more than the therapies utilized. Infants with severe MAS, CDH, and PPHN are at increased risk for chronic pulmonary sequelae (107). Hearing, vision, and neurologic development should be followed closely in infants treated for PPHN. The risk of neurologic, growth, and pulmonary sequelae is greatest in infants with PPHN secondary to CDH (107).

TRANSIENT TACHYPNEA OF THE NEWBORN

TTN is a clinical syndrome of self-limited tachypnea affecting late preterm and term infants and is the most common etiology of neonatal tachypnea. It is postulated that TTN results from delayed clearance of fetal lung fluid due to immaturity or inactivity of lung epithelial sodium transport (ENaC and Na+-K+-ATPase), resulting in decreased pulmonary compliance and impaired gas exchange. Although likely underreported due to its high frequency and relatively benign course, TTN is estimated to complicate 3 to 6 per 1,000 infant births. Risk factors for TTN including twin gestation,

maternal asthma, late gestation prematurity, precipitous delivery, gestational diabetes, and cesarean delivery without labor are commonly present.

Clinical Presentation

Infants can exhibit mild respiratory distress or severe respiratory failure, making the clinical presentation of TTN highly variable. Physical examination is characterized by the onset of tachypnea upon or shortly after birth accompanied by retractions, occasionally expiratory grunting, and cyanosis; chest auscultation is generally unremarkable. Chest radiography may demonstrate prominent perihilar pulmonary vascular markings, hyperexpansion, and rarely, small pleural effusions or total opacification. The appearance of fluid in the minor intralobar pulmonary fissure is less common but pathognomonic. Metabolic acidosis and respiratory acidosis are uncommon. The diagnosis of TTN remains exclusionary. In late preterm and early term infants, it may be difficult to distinguish TTN from surfactant deficiency, meconium aspiration, and pneumonia, but rapid clinical recovery (usually within 6 to 12 hours) and the absence of radiographic findings characteristics of other lung disorders supports the diagnosis.

Pathophysiology

Normally, clearance of fetal lung fluid is facilitated by expression of epithelial sodium channels (ENaC) and sodium–potassium adenosine triphosphatase (Na+-K+-ATPase) that drive active sodium reuptake and interstitial fluid reabsorption. Lung sodium channel expression increases during development and is induced by glucocorticoids. Fetal hyperinsulinemia and the absence or shortening of active labor prior to birth are associated with TTN.

Treatment

TTN is self-limited, and treatment is supportive. Cyanosis is typically relieved by minimal (<40%) oxygen supplementation. When respiratory failure is present (as evidenced by severe retractions and/or expiratory grunting), nasal CPAP can be beneficial, and uncomplicated TTN generally requires brief (6 to 12 hours) positive-pressure support. Mechanical ventilation is rarely required and should prompt consideration for other disease processes, as should the need for increasing or persistent supplemental oxygen. The use of oral furosemide or nebulized racemic epinephrine to shorten the course of TTN is not based on evidence. When given early in the course of TTN, inhaled β2-agonists (salbutamol), presumably by facilitating lung fluid clearance by increasing expression and activation of ENaC and Na+-K+-ATPase channels, may improve oxygenation, shorten the duration of supplemental oxygen therapy, and expedite recovery (108). Regardless, usually within 24 to 72 hours, tachypnea improves and oxygen requirements resolve. Recent studies demonstrated improvement in respiratory outcomes of infants born near term by cesarean section by antenatal treatment with glucocorticoids (109). Further studies are needed to test whether antenatal steroids are indicated in these infants.

NEONATAL PNEUMONIA

Neonatal pneumonia remains a significant cause of morbidity and mortality in term and preterm infants worldwide, resulting in 150 to 500,000 infant deaths annually (110). Unique environmental exposures and deficits in innate host defense predispose the neonate (particularly premature and growth-restricted infants) to early pulmonary infections. Small size of conducting airways and immature ciliary and innate immune functions may contribute to impaired clearance of pathogens. Reduced recruitment and impaired phagocytic activity of neutrophils, paucity of alveolar macrophages, and deficiency of innate defense proteins and immunoglobulins likely contribute to lowered host immunity. Colonization with invasive bacteria, endotracheal intubation, ventilation-associated injury, and hyperoxia that damage the respiratory tract are additional predisposing factors. Despite improvements in care, the burden of neonatal pneumonia continues to be felt by developing countries disproportionately (111).

Neonatal pneumonia can be grouped into three main subtypes: congenital pneumonia (acquired transplacentally), early-onset pneumonia (<7 days of age, resulting from intrauterine infection or exposures during the birthing process), and late-onset pneumonia (>7 days of age, resulting from environmental or nosocomial exposures). A wide variety of pathogens, including viruses, bacteria, and fungi, causes neonatal pneumonia.

Congenital Pneumonia

Congenital neonatal pneumonia is usually present at birth and is acquired hematogenously through the placenta. Rubella, varicella–zoster, cytomegalovirus (CMV), herpes simplex virus (HSV), human immunodeficiency virus (HIV), adenovirus, and enterovirus are common causes of congenital pneumonia. Congenital pneumonia is usually part of a systemic illness, and the severity and duration of respiratory symptoms are variable. CMV is the most common neonatal viral infection. Seronegative mothers whose first infection occurs during the first half of pregnancy are most at risk; nearly half experience transplacental transmission. Although nearly one-third of seropositive mothers experience reactivation during pregnancy, transplacental transmission of CMV is uncommon.

Less commonly, congenital pneumonia results from transplacental spread of bacteria. *Treponema pallidum*, *Listeria monocytogenes*, and *Mycobacterium tuberculosis* are the most common bacterial pathogens. Maternal listeriosis classically presents with a flulike syndrome, with fever and chills occurring up to 2 weeks before preterm labor and delivery. Early-onset neonatal listeriosis presents soon after birth with respiratory distress and pneumonia. Transplacental transfer of *T. pallidum* most often occurs after the 20th week of gestation during primary or secondary maternal infection.

Early-Onset Pneumonia Acquired in the Perinatal Period

Early-onset neonatal pneumonia occurs in the first 7 days of age and is most commonly acquired vertically during the process of labor and delivery. Significant risk factors include prematurity, meconium-stained fluid, and chorioamnionitis. Infection results from organisms ascending from the genital tract after rupture of fetal membranes or acquired during passage of the infant through the birth canal. Respiratory symptoms are often present at delivery or have their onset in the first few hours or days. Despite the abundance and heterogeneity of organisms in the genital tract, only a few organisms commonly cause pneumonia.

The bacteria causing early-onset pneumonia mirror those responsible for early-onset neonatal sepsis and include Group B streptococcus (GBS), *Escherichia coli* (E. coli), *L. monocytogenes*, nontypeable *Haemophilus influenzae*, and Gram-negative enteric bacilli other than *E. coli*. Even with the advent of intrapartum maternal prophylaxis, GBS is responsible for nearly 45% of cases in term infants and remains the most common etiology. Representing nearly 30% of cases, *E. coli* is the second most common etiology. Risk and morbidity related to early-onset infection increases with the degree of prematurity, and premature infants are more likely to be infected with Gram-negative organisms (112). Although less common, other Gram-negative organisms (*Klebsiella*, *Enterobacter*, *Pseudomonas*, *Bacteroides*, *Citrobacter*, *Acinetobacter*, *Proteus*, and *Serratia*), Gram-positive organisms (non–group B *Streptococcus* species, *Staphylococcus*, *Enterococcus*), and *Candida* spp. are causes of early-onset neonatal pneumonia.

Late-Onset Pneumonia Acquired in the Postnatal Period

Late-onset neonatal pneumonia can be the result of pathogens acquired from the vaginal canal during birth or from subsequent environmental exposures. Bacteria, including GBS, *E. coli*, *Staphylococcus species*, nontypeable *H. influenzae*, and *Streptococcus pneumoniae* and viruses, including HSV, CMV, influenza, respiratory syncytial virus, and enteroviruses are common etiologies. Health care– or hospital-acquired pneumonia occurs almost exclusively in preterm and very low birth weight infants requiring respiratory support and is a separate entity with distinct etiologies as discussed below.

Late-onset viral pneumonia caused by CMV, HSV, and adenovirus typically manifests as systemic illness and pneumonitis. Postnatally, CMV is acquired through maternal secretion into breast milk. While term infants rarely exhibit systemic symptoms, preterm infants can develop life-threatening, overwhelming systemic decompensation associated with interstitial pneumonia (113). Although freezing breast milk prior to administering to preterm infants can reduce viral load, it has not been effective preventing the incidence of overwhelming systemic disease. Pneumonia caused by neonatal HSV most often accompanies disseminated disease in the first 3 weeks of age and up to one-third of the time occurs in the absence of skin lesions. The exposure most frequently occurs via contact with active lesions in the genital tract during birth and less frequently via contact with orolabial, oropharyngeal, or breast lesions postnatally. Infants often present with fever, lethargy, apnea, coagulopathy, and hepatocyte injury in addition to respiratory distress, which can be diffuse and severe (114). In the majority of cases, there is no known maternal history of disease. For mothers with active lesions at the time of delivery, there is a roughly 50% risk of transmission to the infant if it is a primary outbreak, in contrast to a less than 2% risk with secondary outbreaks. Congenital adenoviral pneumonia results from exposure in the birth canal to infected secretions. Disseminated disease is associated with severe respiratory failure and high mortality.

Interstitial pneumonitis caused by perinatal exposure to *Chlamydia trachomatis* usually occurs later (2 to 8 weeks of age) with upper respiratory tract symptoms, a staccato cough, and apnea. Antecedent conjunctival infection is common but not always observed. *Ureaplasma urealyticum* is a common inhabitant of the lower genital tract of women and in preterm birth is frequently associated with histologic evidence of chorioamnionitis; it has been associated with chronic lung disease in premature infants.

Ventilator-associated pneumonia (VAP) is an important health care–associated infection affecting preterm and very low birth weight babies and results in significant mortality and morbidity. It is postulated that seeding of the respiratory tract either directly via aspiration of enteric secretions or indirectly via nosocomial contamination of respiratory support equipment is the mechanism by which pathogenic bacteria enter. However, data informing the etiology, associated risk factors, and appropriate therapeutic strategies for VAP remain scarce. Gestational age, birth weight, duration of mechanical ventilation, and regional resources are important risk factors for development of VAP. A contemporary review of the literature including more than 1,000 neonates, relying on a combination of clinical and microbiologic diagnostic criteria, identified rates of VAP as low as 1.4 per 1,000 ventilator days (in resource-rich countries) to as high as 89 per 1,000 ventilator days (in resource-limited countries) (111). The most common pathogens isolated were enteric bacilli including *Pseudomonas*, Enterobacteriaceae (*Klebsiella* and *E. coli*), and *Staphylococcus* although microbiologic diagnosis can be challenging due to oral flora that contaminate endotracheal sampling. Nevertheless, bacterial signatures recovered from tracheal aspirates were strikingly consistent (111). Due to increased morbidity and mortality, many institutions have developed standardized protocols capable of lowering the incidence of VAP (115). Avoidance and minimization of mechanical ventilation, as well as proper hand washing techniques, form the basis of preventative strategies.

Pathologic Findings

Three common histopathologic patterns have been associated with neonatal pneumonia: hyaline membrane formation, suppurative inflammation, and interstitial pneumonitis. Hyaline membrane formation is a nonspecific response seen in lung injury associated with surfactant deficiency, pneumonia, and oxygen therapy. Damage to the alveolar epithelium results in cell necrosis and leakage of cell and serum proteins into the alveolar space. Hyaline membranes in neonatal pneumonia are often observed after GBS infection, but they are also associated with fatal pneumonia caused by *H. influenzae*, Gram-negative enteric organisms, and viral agents. Bacteria are commonly seen within the hyaline membranes (**Fig. 28.8**). Disruption of alveolar capillary permeability and cell injury results in leakage of proteins into the alveolus that further inactivate pulmonary surfactant, leading to atelectasis. The decreased compliance, atelectasis, and hypoxemia seen in pneumonia are often indistinguishable from findings in noninfected surfactant-deficient lungs in premature infants. The chest radiographic findings in RDS and neonatal pneumonia may be identical, although bronchopneumonia and pleural effusions are more common in GBS and other bacterial causes of neonatal pneumonia than in RDS (**Fig. 28.4**). Suppurative inflammation is an intense inflammatory response with necrosis of lung parenchyma, microabscess formation, and pneumatoceles. Pneumonia may be focal or may consolidate to produce large confluent abscesses. Interstitial pneumonitis is typically caused by a virus and characterized by interstitial inflammation, edema, mononuclear infiltration, and septal hyperplasia. Alveolar spaces may remain uninvolved, but in severe cases, a serous exudate containing desquamated pneumocytes and macrophages may be associated with hyaline membrane formation. Septal wall necrosis may occur, adding a component of hemorrhage to the inflammatory exudate.

Diagnosis of Neonatal Pneumonia

Diagnosis of neonatal pneumonia is largely based on clinical symptoms and remains difficult. Many studies of neonatal pneumonia have adopted the National Nosocomial Infection Surveillance system of the Centers of Disease Control and Prevention standard diagnostic criteria, which include radiographic evidence (new and persistent pulmonary infiltrates or effusions), evidence of compromised respiratory function (worsening gas exchange), and associated systemic symptoms (temperature instability, leukopenia or leukocytosis, increased respiratory secretions, and symptoms of cardiorespiratory distress) (116). Identification of a responsible pathogen is difficult, as neither blood culture nor culture from airway secretions is sufficiently sensitive or specific. Endotracheal suction can result in isolation of multiple organisms or organisms of unclear pathologic significance. Nevertheless, identification of a predominate organism and leukocytosis on tracheal aspirate analysis are often used to guide empiric therapy.

Treatment

In addition to appropriate respiratory support, antibiotic therapy directed against the identified or probable causative organism remains the cornerstone of treatment. Postnatal age, clinical circumstances, and local drug resistance patterns guide antimicrobial selection. Neonates presenting with early-onset and community-acquired late-onset neonatal pneumonia and sepsis are usually started on ampicillin and an aminoglycoside to provide coverage against GBS and Gram-negative organisms (including *E. coli* and *H. influenzae*). Acyclovir is often added, especially in instances of severe respiratory decompensation and coagulopathy with or without skin lesions) until the potential for HSV can be eliminated. For preterm infants that experience acute, significant respiratory decompensation in the face of interstitial pneumonia, consideration should be given for pneumonitis due to acquired CMV and treated with ganciclovir. If blood cultures (or viral PCR) identify a pathogen and antibiotic sensitivities, treatment can be further refined.

Though unit-specific strategies should rely upon local microbial and antibiotic-resistance patterns, infants developing VAP generally should be started on antimicrobial therapy capable of covering Gram-negative enteric bacilli (including *Pseudomonas* spp.) and *Staphylococcal* spp. (including methicillin-resistant *Staphylococcus aureus*). Tracheal aspirate culture may help tailor therapy, but due to lack of specificity and sensitivity, treatment will often be empiric and based on clinical response. Extensive supportive care, including oxygen, mechanical ventilation, and cardiovascular support, may also be required in treating an overwhelming infection. While surfactant therapy has also been advocated for treatment of neonatal pneumonia and appears promising, evidence to identify the benefits and harms remains insufficient (117).

AIR LEAKS

Air leaks include pneumothorax, pneumomediastinum, pneumopericardium, and pulmonary interstitial emphysema (PIE). During the era of neonatal care preceding widespread antenatal corticosteroid use, prophylactic surfactant replacement therapy significantly reduced the incidence of pneumothorax. In the present era, prompt administration of surfactant and avoidance of excessive tidal volumes during mechanical ventilation, as well as early selective surfactant replacement for infants not initially intubated, can significantly reduce the risk of air leak.

Pathophysiology

PIE, pneumomediastinum, pneumopericardium, and pneumothorax are closely related clinical entities. Air leaks are thought to begin with PIE in which alveoli rupture into the perivascular and peribronchial spaces. Air may remain trapped in the interstitium of the lung and manifest radiologically, or it can continue to dissect into the mediastinal, pericardial, or pleural spaces. Blebs on the surface of the lung rupture to cause pneumothorax.

Risk Factors

Spontaneous air leaks, the majority of which are asymptomatic, are common and have been reported to occur in 1% to 2% of all routine term deliveries (118). Meconium-stained fluid, RDS, mechanical ventilation, CPAP, and the need for positive pressure

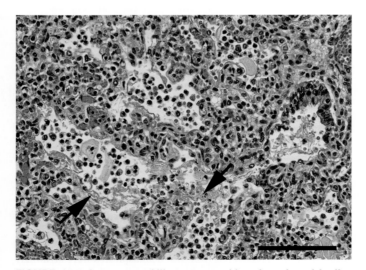

FIGURE 28.8 Acute neutrophilic response with atelectasis and hyaline membranes (*arrows*) are seen in lung tissue from a full-term infant who died of group B streptococcal pneumonia; scale bar = 100 μm. (Courtesy of Dr. Michael Baker, Cincinnati Children's Hospital, Cincinnati, OH.)

ventilation during resuscitation are important contributing risk factors (119). For very preterm infants suffering from RDS and managed primarily with nasal CPAP, roughly 5% to 7% will have a complicating air leak. In a large multicenter review of over 70,000 infants cared for in the Canadian Neonatal Network during the era of antenatal steroids, prophylactic CPAP, and early rescue surfactant replacement, the incidence of air leak followed a bimodal distribution: 4% of infants born at less than 32 weeks of GA, 2.6% of infants born at 32 to 36 weeks of GA, and 6.7% of infants born ≥37 weeks GA developed air leak (120). Risk factors for the entire cohort included worsening severity of respiratory distress, RDS, and surfactant replacement. Chorioamnionitis was significantly associated with air leak in early preterm infants (<32 weeks of GA). Male sex, MAS, and rupture of membranes greater than 24 hours were significantly associated with air leak in more mature infants (>32 weeks of GA). Infants that developed air leak suffered nearly twice the rates of death, BPD, and severe IVH and had longer lengths of hospital stay (120).

Radiographic Evaluation

Standard chest radiographic identification of radiolucent air in the pleural space, interstitium, or mediastinum remains diagnostic. While lung ultrasound is increasingly used, transillumination of the hemithorax remains a reliable, easily performed, and readily available method to emergently identify tension pneumothorax associated with critical clinical instability (121). Because neonatal chest radiographs are usually performed in the supine position, pleural air may accumulate in the anterior chest and may only be visible as a hyperlucent ipsilateral hemithorax. Cross-table lateral or decubitus radiography maybe needed for diagnosis. PIE is recognized by chest radiograph revealing radiolucent interstitial air juxtaposed to lung parenchyma in a "salt-and-pepper" pattern (**Fig. 28.9**). In a tension pneumothorax, the lung and mediastinal organs are displaced

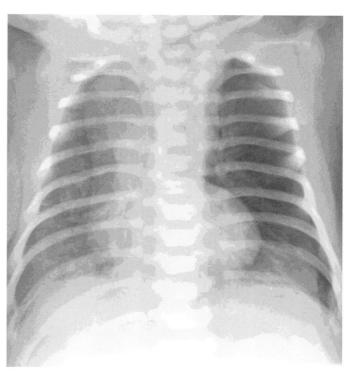

FIGURE 28.10 A full-term infant born by a difficult breech delivery presented shortly after birth with tachypnea, grunting, and retractions. An anteroposterior chest x-ray film demonstrates a tension pneumothorax on the left. The heart and mediastinum are compressed and shifted to the right. The left pleural air herniates across the midline. The left diaphragm is depressed and inverted.

away from the side of the pneumothorax (**Fig. 28.10**). The thymus may be outlined in pneumomediastinum, often referred to as a "sail sign" (**Fig. 28.11**). Pneumopericardium results in a characteristic outline of the heart by radiolucent air (**Fig. 28.12**).

Clinical Presentation

Infants with pneumothorax and pneumomediastinum often present with grunting, tachypnea, cyanosis, and retractions. Although some may have required positive pressure ventilation prior to symptom onset, many will have no preceding event. The clinical impact of the air leak correlates with its size and the extent of lung collapse or contralateral mediastinal shift. A shift of the trachea or point of maximal heart impulse and decreased breath sounds on the affected side may be found on clinical examination. Pneumothoraces fall into two major groups: spontaneous pneumothoraces and those associated with underlying pulmonary disease. Spontaneous pneumothoraces often occur within minutes of birth in otherwise healthy, full-term infants. Pneumothoraces associated with significant pulmonary disease frequently occur in the first several days after birth due to the need for respiratory support. Contrary to historical reports, compared to the general population, infants with spontaneous pneumothorax do not have a higher incidence of congenital urinary tract malformations (122). Routine renal ultrasonography is not warranted.

Treatment

Prompt recognition of air leak is essential for effective therapy. For infants requiring positive pressure ventilation, unexpected changes in clinical stability, including an abrupt increase in ventilatory and/or oxygen requirements as well as signs of cardiorespiratory instability (tachypnea, retractions, and oxygen desaturation) may indicate an air leak. Transillumination of the

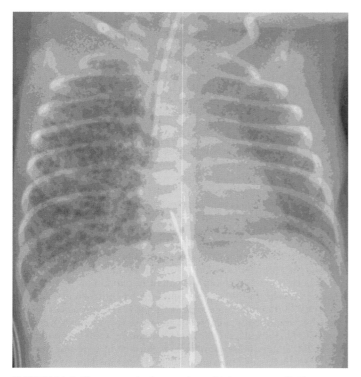

FIGURE 28.9 Chest x-ray of pulmonary interstitial emphysema (PIE). A premature infant with severe RDS requiring mechanical ventilation developed worsening respiratory acidosis and hypoxia refractory to increased ventilatory support. An anteroposterior chest x-ray film demonstrates a salt-and-pepper pattern resulting from radiolucent interstitial air surrounding compressed lung tissue.

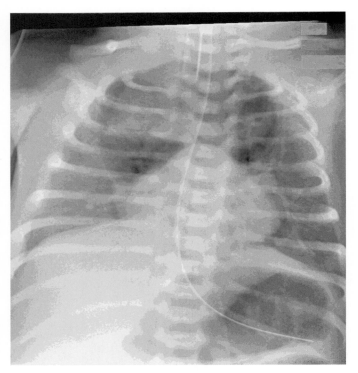

FIGURE 28.11 A term baby presented with tachypnea shortly after birth. An anteroposterior chest x-ray film demonstrates a pneumomediastinum with outline of the thymus.

thorax to identify an air leak can be useful for both the diagnosis and the response to therapy. Treatment of symptomatic tension pneumothorax requires immediate aspiration and frequently placement of a chest tube.

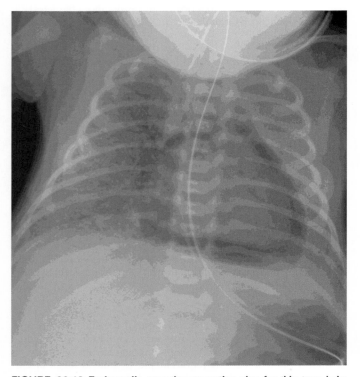

FIGURE 28.12 Tachycardia was the presenting sign for this term baby shortly after birth. An anteroposterior chest x-ray film demonstrates a pneumopericardium.

Treatment of a pneumothorax that is not under tension or causing cardiovascular compromise remains controversial. The majority of infants will remain clinically stable with mild respiratory compromise and frequently require only supplemental oxygen or observation alone. In infants not requiring drainage, the pneumothorax generally resolves within 1 to 3 days. For infants with associated respiratory failure and/or significant cardiorespiratory compromise requiring positive-pressure ventilation, the majority will need chest tube placement. In a single center, retrospective study of 136 infants that developed pneumothoraces while on the ventilator, only 14% of the babies had spontaneous resolution of their pneumothorax and did not require chest tube placement or needle thoracentesis (123). In term infants that do not require intubation, inhalation of 100% oxygen to displace nitrogen and facilitate resorption of the entrapped air ("nitrogen washout") has been suggested. Although animal data demonstrate accelerated resolution of pneumothoraces with a clear dose response with increasing concentrations of oxygen up to 50% (124), safety and efficacy in infants has never been studied in a controlled fashion. In two separate studies including 175 infants greater than 35 weeks of GA treated with the "nitrogen washout" compared to monitoring on room air, retrospective analysis failed to demonstrate a shortened time to resolution (125). Given the concerns associated with tissue injury caused by hyperoxia, use of the "nitrogen washout," particularly in premature infants at risk for retinopathy of prematurity, should be avoided.

Pneumomediastinum and pneumopericardium that do not cause cardiovascular compromise can be managed expectantly and resolve spontaneously. Tension pneumopericardium is a rare but life-threatening cause of cardiovascular compromise and must be drained surgically. PIE occurs most frequently in premature infants requiring mechanical ventilation for RDS (see **Fig. 28.9** for radiograph). Unilateral PIE can be managed by placing the infant with the affected side down for 24 to 48 hours. Selective bronchial intubation and/or high-frequency or jet ventilation have also been used to treat unilateral PIE. Careful attention to minimize lung injury by managing peak and mean inspiratory pressures may help prevent and treat PIE. In infants surviving PIE, BPD frequently develops.

PULMONARY HEMORRHAGE

Pulmonary hemorrhage typically affects extremely preterm infants and varies from a self-limited disorder to a massive, lethal hemorrhage. Studies examining surfactant replacement and respiratory support of ELBW infants in the modern era of neonatal care demonstrate that approximately 3% of preterm infants had pulmonary hemorrhage. A large database review of over 500,000 preterm infants noted an incidence of 86.9 per 1,000 extremely premature infants (126). Based on the observation that the hematocrit of lung effluent in pulmonary hemorrhage is lower than the hematocrit of blood, most affected infants likely suffer hemorrhagic pulmonary edema. Excessive pulmonary blood flow coupled with alveolar overdistension leading to rupture of pulmonary capillaries may underlie the pathogenesis. The role of surfactant replacement therapy in both the etiology and treatment of pulmonary hemorrhage remains unclear. In the original randomized controlled trials from the 1990s, surfactant replacement therapy was associated with a small but statistically significant increase in pulmonary hemorrhage (127). Recent clinical trials examining early support with nasal CPAP compared to prophylactic surfactant have not shown a significant increase in pulmonary hemorrhage associated with prophylactic surfactant replacement (128). In preterm infants of less than 34 weeks' GA, surfactant exposure, resuscitation requiring positive pressure ventilation, lack of antenatal steroids, and PDA are associated risk factors. For late preterm and term infants, risk factors include thrombocytopenia and/or coagulopathy, asphyxia, intrauterine growth restriction, infection, hypothermia, severe Rh hemolytic disease, and the need for respiratory support. The timing of presentation of pulmonary hemorrhage varies with gestational age. Hemorrhage occurred at a median age of 46 hours in infants less than 34 weeks of GA compared to 6 hours of age in infants greater than 34 weeks (129). Preterm infants suffered a higher mortality rate, nearly 50% compared to 25% mortality in late preterm/term infants (126,129). Extremely low birth weight infants that survive pulmonary hemorrhage are more likely to suffer neurodevelopmental impairment.

Clinical Findings

Massive pulmonary hemorrhage usually involves rapid deterioration of ventilatory function, progressive hypoxia, hypercarbia, and respiratory acidosis. The presence of bright red blood in the endotracheal tube is often noted. Chest radiographic findings depend on severity. Focal hemorrhage may be difficult to differentiate from atelectasis or pneumonia, while radiographs associated with significant pulmonary hemorrhage are often diffusely hazy or reveal patchy infiltrates. Because blood has tissue density, chest radiographs in large pulmonary hemorrhages may appear completely opacified.

Treatment

Early detection and aggressive supportive of massive pulmonary hemorrhage can improve outcomes. Positive-pressure ventilation and oxygen are critical components of therapy. The combination of increased MAP (often via high HFOV) and endotracheal administration of epinephrine (0.5 mL of 1:10,000 concentration, repeated after suctioning until hemorrhage resolves) have been proposed to facilitate tamponade. Anemia, thrombocytopenia, and coagulopathy should be aggressively corrected. Careful treatment of hypotension, hypoxemia, and acidosis is indicated. Based on the observation that pulmonary hemorrhage inactivates surfactant function, surfactant replacement therapy has been suggested as an important component of therapy. While no randomized controlled trials have assessed the benefits of surfactant replacement for the treatment of pulmonary hemorrhage, prospective open-label reports have shown promise. Several studies in VLBW infants suggest that prophylactic treatment with indomethacin, to facilitate closure of the ductus arteriosus, results in a 20% to 30% reduction in pulmonary hemorrhage (130,131).

REFERENCES

1. Whitsett JA, Kalin TV, Xu Y, et al. Building and regenerating the lung cell by cell. *Physiol Rev* 2019;99(1):513.
2. Swarr DT, Morrisey EE. Lung endoderm morphogenesis: gasping for form and function. *Annu Rev Cell Dev Biol* 2015;31:553.
3. Galambos C, deMello DE. Molecular mechanisms of pulmonary vascular development. *Pediatr Dev Pathol* 2007;10(1):1.
4. McCulley D, Wienhold M, Sun X. The pulmonary mesenchyme directs lung development. *Curr Opin Genet Dev* 2015;32:98.
5. Metzger RJ, Klein OD, Martin GR, et al. The branching programme of mouse lung development. *Nature* 2008;453(7196):745.
6. Whitsett JA, Wert SE, Weaver TE. Alveolar surfactant homeostasis and the pathogenesis of pulmonary disease. *Annu Rev Med* 2010;61:105.
7. Langston C, Kida K, Reed M, et al. Human lung growth in late gestation and in the neonate. *Am Rev Respir Dis* 1984;129(4):607.
8. Ochs M, Nyengaard JR, Jung A, et al. The number of alveoli in the human lung. *Am J Respir Crit Care Med* 2004;169(1):120.
9. Zeltner TB, Caduff JH, Gehr P, et al. The postnatal development and growth of the human lung. I. Morphometry. *Respir Physiol* 1987;67(3):247.
10. Morrisey EE, Hogan BL. Preparing for the first breath: genetic and cellular mechanisms in lung development. *Dev Cell* 2010;18(1):8.
11. Kang S, Graham JM Jr, Olney AH, et al. GLI3 frameshift mutations cause autosomal dominant Pallister-Hall syndrome. *Nat Genet* 1997;15(3):266.
12. Hajihosseini MK, Wilson S, De Moerlooze L, et al. A splicing switch and gain-of-function mutation in FgFR2-IIIc hemizygotes causes Apert/Pfeiffer-syndrome-like phenotypes. *Proc Natl Acad Sci U S A* 2001;98(7):3855.
13. Zackai EH, McDonald-McGinn DM, Stolle C, et al. Craniosynostosis with tracheal sleeve: a patient with Pfeiffer syndrome, tracheal sleeve and additional malformations in whom an FGFR2 mutation was found. *Clin Dysmorphol* 2003;12(3):209.
14. Gould S, Hasleton P. Congenital abnormalities. In: Hasleton P, ed. *Spencer's pathology of the lung*, 5th ed. New York, NY: McGraw-Hill, 1996:57.
15. Hamvas A, Deterding RR, Wert SE, et al. Heterogeneous pulmonary phenotypes associated with mutations in the thyroid transcription factor gene NKX2-1. *Chest* 2013;144(3):794.
16. Nogee LM. Genetic basis of children's interstitial lung disease. *Pediatr Allergy Immunol Pulmonol* 2010;23(1):15.
17. Wert SE, Whitsett JA, Nogee LM. Genetic disorders of surfactant dysfunction. *Pediatr Dev Pathol* 2009;12(4):253.
18. Sen P, Yang Y, Navarro C, et al. Novel FOXF1 mutations in sporadic and familial cases of alveolar capillary dysplasia with misaligned pulmonary veins imply a role for its DNA binding domain. *Hum Mutat* 2013;34(6):801.
19. Vincent M, Karolak JA, Deutsch G, et al. Clinical, histopathological, and molecular diagnostics in lethal lung developmental disorders. *Am J Respir Crit Care Med* 2019;200(9):1093.
20. Nogee LM. Genetic causes of surfactant protein abnormalities. *Curr Opin Pediatr* 2019;31(3):330.
21. Goss V, Hunt AN, Postle AD. Regulation of lung surfactant phospholipid synthesis and metabolism. *Biochim Biophys Acta* 2013;1831(2):448.
22. Perez-Gil J, Weaver TE. Pulmonary surfactant pathophysiology: current models and open questions. *Physiology (Bethesda)* 2010;25(3):132.
23. Batenburg JJ. Surfactant phospholipids: synthesis and storage. *Am J Physiol* 1992;262(4 Pt 1):L367.
24. Travers CP, Carlo WA, McDonald SA, et al. Mortality and pulmonary outcomes of extremely preterm infants exposed to antenatal corticosteroids. *Am J Obstet Gynecol* 2018;218(1):130.e1.
25. Liggins GC, Howie RN. A controlled trial of antepartum glucocorticoid treatment for prevention of the respiratory distress syndrome in premature infants. *Pediatrics* 1972;50(4):515.
26. Mendelson CR, Boggaram V. Hormonal control of the surfactant system in fetal lung. *Annu Rev Physiol* 1991;53:415.
27. Bridges JP, Ludwig MG, Mueller M, et al. Orphan G protein-coupled receptor GPR116 regulates pulmonary surfactant pool size. *Am J Respir Cell Mol Biol* 2013;49(3):348.
28. Nijjar MS, Khangura BS, Juravsky LI. The effect of maternal diabetes on the synthesis and secretion of phosphatidylcholine in fetal and maternal rat lungs in vitro. *Diabetologia* 1984;27(2):219.
29. Jobe A. Phospholipid metabolism and turnover. In: Pollin R, Fox W, Abman S, eds. *Fetal and neonatal physiology*. Philadelphia, PA: WB Saunders, 1992:986.
30. Trapnell BC, Nakata K, Bonella F, et al. Pulmonary alveolar proteinosis. *Nat Rev Dis Primers* 2019;5(1):16.
31. Bunt JE, Zimmermann LJ, Wattimena JL, et al. Endogenous surfactant turnover in preterm infants measured with stable isotopes. *Am J Respir Crit Care Med* 1998;157(3 Pt 1):810.
32. Cogo PE, Zimmermann LJ, Meneghini L, et al. Pulmonary surfactant disaturated-phosphatidylcholine (DSPC) turnover and pool size in newborn infants with congenital diaphragmatic hernia (CDH). *Pediatr Res* 2003;54(5):653.
33. Rebello CM, Jobe AH, Eisele JW, et al. Alveolar and tissue surfactant pool sizes in humans. *Am J Respir Crit Care Med* 1996;154(3 Pt 1):625.
34. Fujiwara T, Maeta H, Chida S, et al. Artificial surfactant therapy in hyaline-membrane disease. *Lancet* 1980;1(8159):55.
35. Owen LS, Manley BJ, Davis PG, et al. The evolution of modern respiratory care for preterm infants. *Lancet* 2017;389(10079):1649.
36. Johansson J, Curstedt T. Synthetic surfactants with SP-B and SP-C analogues to enable worldwide treatment of neonatal respiratory distress syndrome and other lung diseases. *J Intern Med* 2019;285(2):165.
37. Boghossian NS, Geraci M, Edwards EM, et al. Sex differences in mortality and morbidity of infants born at less than 30 weeks' gestation. *Pediatrics* 2018;142(6):e20182352.
38. Avery ME, Mead J. Surface properties in relation to atelectasis and hyaline membrane disease. *AMA J Dis Child* 1959;97(5, Part 1):517.
39. Committee opinion no. 677 summary: antenatal corticosteroid therapy for fetal maturation. *Obstet Gynecol* 2016;128(4):940.
40. Saccone G, Berghella V. Antenatal corticosteroids for maturity of term or near term fetuses: systematic review and meta-analysis of randomized controlled trials. *BMJ* 2016;355:i5044.
41. Committee on Fetus and Newborn; American Academy of Pediatrics. Respiratory support in preterm infants at birth. *Pediatrics* 2014;133(1):171.
42. Polin RA, Carlo WA; Committee on Fetus and Newborn; American Academy of Pediatrics. Surfactant replacement therapy for preterm and term neonates with respiratory distress. *Pediatrics* 2014;133(1):156.
43. Wright CJ, Sherlock LG, Sahni R, et al. Preventing continuous positive airway pressure failure: evidence-based and physiologically sound practices from delivery room to the neonatal intensive care unit. *Clin Perinatol* 2018;45(2):257.
44. Isayama T, Iwami H, McDonald S, et al. Association of noninvasive ventilation strategies with mortality and bronchopulmonary dysplasia among preterm infants: a systematic review and meta-analysis. *JAMA* 2016;316(6):611.

45. Singh N, Halliday HL, Stevens TP, et al. Comparison of animal-derived surfactants for the prevention and treatment of respiratory distress syndrome in preterm infants. *Cochrane Database Syst Rev* 2015;(12):CD010249.

46. Roberts CT, Owen LS, Manley BJ, et al. Nasal high-flow therapy for primary respiratory support in preterm infants. *N Engl J Med* 2016;375(12):1142.

47. Sahni R, Schiaratura M, Polin RA. Strategies for the prevention of continuous positive airway pressure failure. *Semin Fetal Neonatal Med* 2016;21(3):196.

48. Cools F, Offringa M, Askie LM. Elective high frequency oscillatory ventilation versus conventional ventilation for acute pulmonary dysfunction in preterm infants. *Cochrane Database Syst Rev* 2015;(3):CD000104.

49. Barrington KJ, Finer N, Pennaforte T. Inhaled nitric oxide for respiratory failure in preterm infants. *Cochrane Database Syst Rev* 2017;1:CD000509.

50. Fischer C, Rybakowski C, Ferdynus C, et al. A population-based study of meconium aspiration syndrome in neonates born between 37 and 43 weeks of gestation. *Int J Pediatr* 2012;2012:321545.

51. Rodriguez Fernandez V, Lopez Ramon YCCN, Marin Ortiz E, et al. Intrapartum and perinatal results associated with different degrees of staining of meconium stained amniotic fluid. *Eur J Obstet Gynecol Reprod Biol* 2018;228:65.

52. Balchin I, Whittaker JC, Lamont RF, et al. Maternal and fetal characteristics associated with meconium-stained amniotic fluid. *Obstet Gynecol* 2011;117(4):828.

53. Martin GI, Vidyasagar D. Introduction: proceedings of the first international conference for meconium aspiration syndrome and meconium-induced lung injury. *J Perinatol* 2008;28(suppl 3):S1.

54. Tran N, Lowe C, Sivieri EM, et al. Sequential effects of acute meconium obstruction on pulmonary function. *Pediatr Res* 1980;14(1):34.

55. Hofmeyr GJ, Xu H. Amnioinfusion for meconium-stained liquor in labour. *Cochrane Database Syst Rev* 2010;(1):CD000014.

56. Committee on Obstetric Practice. Committee opinion no 689: delivery of a newborn with meconium-stained amniotic fluid. *Obstet Gynecol* 2017;129(3):e33.

57. Kelly LE, Shivananda S, Murthy P, et al. Antibiotics for neonates born through meconium-stained amniotic fluid. *Cochrane Database Syst Rev* 2017;6:CD006183.

58. Hao LX, Wang F. Effectiveness of high-frequency oscillatory ventilation for the treatment of neonatal meconium aspiration syndrome. *Medicine (Baltimore)* 2019;98(43):e17622.

59. El Shahed AI, Dargaville P, Ohlsson A, et al. Surfactant for meconium aspiration syndrome in full term/near term infants. *Cochrane Database Syst Rev* 2007;(3):CD002054.

60. Autilio C, Echaide M, De Luca D, et al. Controlled hypothermia may improve surfactant function in asphyxiated neonates with or without meconium aspiration syndrome. *PLoS One* 2018;13(2):e0192295.

61. Giesinger RE, McNamara PJ. The impact of therapeutic hypothermia on pulmonary hemodynamics of meconium aspiration syndrome. *Am J Respir Crit Care Med* 2018;198(2):286.

62. Goldsmith JP. Continuous positive airway pressure and conventional mechanical ventilation in the treatment of meconium aspiration syndrome. *J Perinatol* 2008;28(suppl 3):S49.

63. Pandita A, Murki S, Oleti TP, et al. Effect of nasal continuous positive airway pressure on infants with meconium aspiration syndrome: a randomized clinical trial. *JAMA Pediatr* 2018;172(2):161.

64. Kinsella JP, Truog WE, Walsh WF, et al. Randomized, multicenter trial of inhaled nitric oxide and high-frequency oscillatory ventilation in severe, persistent pulmonary hypertension of the newborn. *J Pediatr* 1997;131(1 Pt 1):55.

65. Singh BS, Clark RH, Powers RJ, et al. Meconium aspiration syndrome remains a significant problem in the NICU: outcomes and treatment patterns in term neonates admitted for intensive care during a ten-year period. *J Perinatol* 2009;29(7):497.

66. Steurer MA, Jelliffe-Pawlowski LL, Baer RJ, et al. Persistent pulmonary hypertension of the newborn in late preterm and term infants in California. *Pediatrics*. 2017;139(1):e20161165.

67. Walsh-Sukys MC, Tyson JE, Wright LL, et al. Persistent pulmonary hypertension of the newborn in the era before nitric oxide: practice variation and outcomes. *Pediatrics* 2000;105(1 Pt 1):14.

68. Lipkin PH, Davidson D, Spivak L, et al. Neurodevelopmental and medical outcomes of persistent pulmonary hypertension in term newborns treated with nitric oxide. *J Pediatr* 2002;140(3):306.

69. Puthiyachirakkal M, Mhanna MJ. Pathophysiology, management, and outcome of persistent pulmonary hypertension of the newborn: a clinical review. *Front Pediatr* 2013;1:23.

70. Jain A, McNamara PJ. Persistent pulmonary hypertension of the newborn: Advances in diagnosis and treatment. *Semin Fetal Neonatal Med* 2015;20(4):262.

71. Simonneau G, Montani D, Celermajer DS, et al. Haemodynamic definitions and updated clinical classification of pulmonary hypertension. *Eur Respir J* 2019;53(1):1801913.

72. Rosenzweig EB, Abman SH, Adatia I, et al. Paediatric pulmonary arterial hypertension: updates on definition, classification, diagnostics and management. *Eur Respir J* 2019;53(1):1801916.

73. Abman SH, Hansmann G, Archer SL, et al. Pediatric pulmonary hypertension: guidelines from the American Heart Association and American Thoracic Society. *Circulation* 2015;132(21):2037.

74. Rasanen J, Wood DC, Weiner S, et al. Role of the pulmonary circulation in the distribution of human fetal cardiac output during the second half of pregnancy. *Circulation* 1996;94(5):1068.

75. Lakshminrusimha S, Steinhorn RH. Pulmonary vascular biology during neonatal transition. *Clin Perinatol* 1999;26(3):601.

76. Rabinovitch M. Structure and function of the pulmonary vascular bed: an update. *Cardiol Clin* 1989;7(4):895.

77. Mathew B, Lakshminrusimha S. Persistent pulmonary hypertension in the newborn. *Children (Basel)*. 2017;4(8):63.

78. Bifano EM, Pfannenstiel A. Duration of hyperventilation and outcome in infants with persistent pulmonary hypertension. *Pediatrics* 1988;81(5):657.

79. Hendricks-Munoz KD, Walton JP. Hearing loss in infants with persistent fetal circulation. *Pediatrics* 1988;81(5):650.

80. Farrow KN, Wedgwood S, Lee KJ, et al. Mitochondrial oxidant stress increases PDE5 activity in persistent pulmonary hypertension of the newborn. *Respir Physiol Neurobiol* 2010;174(3):272.

81. Steinhorn RH. Pharmacotherapy for pulmonary hypertension. *Pediatr Clin North Am* 2012;59(5):1129.

82. Roberts JD Jr, Fineman JR, Morin FC III, et al. Inhaled nitric oxide and persistent pulmonary hypertension of the newborn. The Inhaled Nitric Oxide Study Group. *N Engl J Med* 1997;336(9):605.

83. Davidson D, Barefield ES, Kattwinkel J, et al. Inhaled nitric oxide for the early treatment of persistent pulmonary hypertension of the term newborn: a randomized, double-masked, placebo-controlled, dose-response, multicenter study. The I-NO/PPHN Study Group. *Pediatrics* 1998;101(3 Pt 1):325.

84. Clark RH, Kueser TJ, Walker MW, et al. Low-dose nitric oxide therapy for persistent pulmonary hypertension of the newborn. Clinical Inhaled Nitric Oxide Research Group. *N Engl J Med* 2000;342(7):469.

85. Sadiq HF, Mantych G, Benawra RS, et al. Inhaled nitric oxide in the treatment of moderate persistent pulmonary hypertension of the newborn: a randomized controlled, multicenter trial. *J Perinatol* 2003;23(2):98.

86. Sokol GM, Fineberg NS, Wright LL, et al. Changes in arterial oxygen tension when weaning neonates from inhaled nitric oxide. *Pediatr Pulmonol* 2001;32(1):14.

87. Kelly LK, Porta NF, Goodman DM, et al. Inhaled prostacyclin for term infants with persistent pulmonary hypertension refractory to inhaled nitric oxide. *J Pediatr* 2002;141(6):830.

88. Sood BG, Keszler M, Garg M, et al. Inhaled PGE1 in neonates with hypoxemic respiratory failure: two pilot feasibility randomized clinical trials. *Trials* 2014;15:486.

89. Janjindamai W, Thatrimontrichai A, Maneenil G, et al. Effectiveness and safety of intravenous iloprost for severe persistent pulmonary hypertension of the newborn. *Indian Pediatr.* 2013;50(10):934.

90. Kahveci H, Yilmaz O, Avsar UZ, et al. Oral sildenafil and inhaled iloprost in the treatment of pulmonary hypertension of the newborn. *Pediatr Pulmonol* 2014;49(12):1205.

91. Shivanna B, Gowda S, Welty S, et al. Prostacyclins and analogues for the treatment of pulmonary hypertension in neonates. *Cochrane Database Syst Rev* 2018(2):CD012963.

92. Lakshminrusimha S, Porta NF, Farrow KN, et al. Milrinone enhances relaxation to prostacyclin and iloprost in pulmonary arteries isolated from lambs with persistent pulmonary hypertension of the newborn. *Pediatr Crit Care Med* 2009;10(1):106.

93. Kumar VH, Swartz DD, Rashid N, et al. Prostacyclin and milrinone by aerosolization improve pulmonary hemodynamics in newborn lambs with experimental pulmonary hypertension. *J Appl Physiol (1985)* 2010;109(3):677.

94. Lakshminrusimha S, Steinhorn RH. Inodilators in nitric oxide resistant persistent pulmonary hypertension of the newborn. *Pediatr Crit Care Med* 2013;14(1):107.

95. McNamara PJ, Shivananda SP, Sahni M, et al. Pharmacology of milrinone in neonates with persistent pulmonary hypertension of the newborn and suboptimal response to inhaled nitric oxide. *Pediatr Crit Care Med* 2013;14(1):74.

96. Kelly LE, Ohlsson A, Shah PS. Sildenafil for pulmonary hypertension in neonates. *Cochrane Database Syst Rev* 2017;8:CD005494.

97. Abman SH, Kinsella JP, Rosenzweig EB, et al. Implications of the U.S. Food and Drug Administration warning against the use of sildenafil for the treatment of pediatric pulmonary hypertension. *Am J Respir Crit Care Med* 2013;187(6):572.

98. Channick RN, Simonneau G, Sitbon O, et al. Effects of the dual endothelin-receptor antagonist bosentan in patients with pulmonary hypertension: a randomised placebo-controlled study. *Lancet* 2001;358(9288):1119.

99. Mohamed WA, Ismail M. A randomized, double-blind, placebo-controlled, prospective study of bosentan for the treatment of persistent pulmonary hypertension of the newborn. *J Perinatol* 2012;32(8):608.

100. Steinhorn RH, Fineman J, Kusic-Pajic A, et al. Bosentan as adjunctive therapy in persistent pulmonary hypertension of the newborn: results of the randomized multicenter placebo-controlled exploratory trial. *J Pediatr* 2016;177:90.

101. Maneenil G, Thatrimontrichai A, Janjindamai W, et al. Effect of bosentan therapy in persistent pulmonary hypertension of the newborn. *Pediatr Neonatol* 2018;59(1):58.

102. More K, Athalye-Jape GK, Rao SC, et al. Endothelin receptor antagonists for persistent pulmonary hypertension in term and late preterm infants. *Cochrane Database Syst Rev* 2016(8):CD010531.

103. Lazar DA, Cass DL, Olutoye OO, et al. The use of ECMO for persistent pulmonary hypertension of the newborn: a decade of experience. *J Surg Res* 2012;177(2):263.

104. Barbaro RP, Paden ML, Guner YS, et al. Pediatric extracorporeal life support organization registry international report 2016. *ASAIO J* 2017;63(4):456.

105. Lakshminrusimha S, Keszler M. Persistent pulmonary hypertension of the newborn. *Neoreviews* 2015;16(12):e680.

106. Ballard RA, Leonard CH. Developmental follow-up of infants with persistent pulmonary hypertension of the newborn. *Clin Perinatol* 1984;11(3):737.

107. Rosenberg AA, Kennaugh JM, Moreland SG, et al. Longitudinal follow-up of a cohort of newborn infants treated with inhaled nitric oxide for persistent pulmonary hypertension. *J Pediatr* 1997;131(1 Pt 1):70.

108. Moresco L, Bruschettini M, Cohen A, et al. Salbutamol for transient tachypnea of the newborn. *Cochrane Database Syst Rev* 2016(5):CD011878.

109. Sotiriadis A, Makrydimas G, Papatheodorou S, et al. Corticosteroids for preventing neonatal respiratory morbidity after elective caesarean section at term. *Cochrane Database Syst Rev* 2018;8:CD006614.

110. Hooven TA, Polin RA. Pneumonia. *Semin Fetal Neonatal Med* 2017;22(4):206.

111. Cernada M, Brugada M, Golombek S, et al. Ventilator-associated pneumonia in neonatal patients: an update. *Neonatology* 2014;105(2):98.

112. Shane AL, Sanchez PJ, Stoll BJ. Neonatal sepsis. *Lancet* 2017;390(10104):1770.

113. Lanzieri TM, Dollard SC, Josephson CD, et al. Breast milk-acquired cytomegalovirus infection and disease in VLBW and premature infants. *Pediatrics* 2013;131(6):e1937.

114. Kimberlin DW. Neonatal herpes simplex infection. *Clin Microbiol Rev* 2004;17(1):1.

115. Garland JS. Strategies to prevent ventilator-associated pneumonia in neonates. *Clin Perinatol* 2010;37(3):629.

116. Vergnano S, Buttery J, Cailes B, et al. Neonatal infections: case definition and guidelines for data collection, analysis, and presentation of immunisation safety data. *Vaccine* 2016;34(49):6038.

117. Deshpande S, Suryawanshi P, Ahya K, et al. Surfactant therapy for early onset pneumonia in late preterm and term neonates needing mechanical ventilation. *J Clin Diagn Res* 2017;11(8):SC09.

118. Steele RW, Metz JR, Bass JW, et al. Pneumothorax and pneumomediastinum in the newborn. *Radiology* 1971;98(3):629.

119. Smithhart W, Wyckoff MH, Kapadia V, et al. Delivery room continuous positive airway pressure and pneumothorax. *Pediatrics* 2019;144(3):e20190756.

120. Duong HH, Mirea L, Shah PS, et al. Pneumothorax in neonates: trends, predictors and outcomes. *J Neonatal Perinatal Med* 2014;7(1):29.

121. Cattarossi L, Copetti R, Brusa G, et al. Lung ultrasound diagnostic accuracy in neonatal pneumothorax. *Can Respir J* 2016;2016:6515069.

122. Al Tawil K, Abu-Ekteish FM, Tamimi O, et al. Symptomatic spontaneous pneumothorax in term newborn infants. *Pediatr Pulmonol* 2004;37(5):443.

123. Litmanovitz I, Carlo WA. Expectant management of pneumothorax in ventilated neonates. *Pediatrics* 2008;122(5):e975.

124. England GJ, Hill RC, Timberlake GA, et al. Resolution of experimental pneumothorax in rabbits by graded oxygen therapy. *J Trauma* 1998;45(2):333.

125. Clark SD, Saker F, Schneeberger MT, et al. Administration of 100% oxygen does not hasten resolution of symptomatic spontaneous pneumothorax in neonates. *J Perinatol* 2014;34(7):528.

126. Ahmad KA, Bennett MM, Ahmad SF, et al. Morbidity and mortality with early pulmonary haemorrhage in preterm neonates. *Arch Dis Child Fetal Neonatal Ed* 2019;104(1):F63.

127. Raju TN, Langenberg P. Pulmonary hemorrhage and exogenous surfactant therapy: a metaanalysis. *J Pediatr* 1993;123(4):603.

128. Wright CJ, Polin RA, Kirpalani H. Continuous positive airway pressure to prevent neonatal lung injury: how did we get here, and how do we improve? *J Pediatr* 2016;173:17.

129. Berger TM, Allred EN, Van Marter LJ. Antecedents of clinically significant pulmonary hemorrhage among newborn infants. *J Perinatol* 2000;20(5):295.

130. Alfaleh K, Smyth JA, Roberts RS, et al. Prevention and 18-month outcomes of serious pulmonary hemorrhage in extremely low birth weight infants: results from the trial of indomethacin prophylaxis in preterms. *Pediatrics* 2008;121(2):e233.

131. Kluckow M, Jeffery M, Gill A, et al. A randomised placebo-controlled trial of early treatment of the patent ductus arteriosus. *Arch Dis Child Fetal Neonatal Ed* 2014;99(2):F99.

THE NEWBORN INFANT

Bronchopulmonary Dysplasia

Robin H. Steinhorn and Jonathan M. Davis

INTRODUCTION

Bronchopulmonary dysplasia (BPD) has traditionally been defined as a form of chronic lung disease that develops in neonates treated with oxygen and positive-pressure mechanical ventilation for a primary lung disorder. Over the past 20 years, many new treatment modalities have been introduced, which has resulted in more neonates surviving and ultimately developing BPD. Despite a major shift toward the use of more noninvasive ventilation preterm neonates, approximately 15,000 new cases of BPD occur each year in the United States. BPD is associated with significant morbidity (both respiratory and neurodevelopmental) and mortality. The exact definition of BPD has been the subject of intense debate as investigators attempt to link the development of BPD with more meaningful short- and longer-term respiratory outcomes (e.g., asthma, respiratory infections). BPD remains an extremely important complication of neonatal intensive care and the most common form of chronic lung disease in neonates. In fact, BPD is the only major complication of prematurity that continues to increase in frequency (1).

The modern history of BPD began with Northway's observations in 1967 (2). This study documented the clinical course, radiographic findings, and histopathologic lung changes in a group of neonates who had received oxygen and ventilatory support for treatment of respiratory distress syndrome (RDS) and established the term BPD. Although Northway originally postulated that oxygen toxicity caused BPD, the exact mechanisms causing the lung injury appear to be multifactorial and continue to be the subject of significant investigation. Although treatment with positive-pressure ventilation appears to be important, factors such as oxygen toxicity, prematurity, genetic predisposition, infection, and inflammation also appear to play critical roles. The treatment of neonates with BPD is most often directed toward improving the pathophysiologic abnormalities after they occur. However, many different therapies are often used concurrently, even though adequate safety or efficacy data do not exist to justify their use.

This chapter reviews the definition and incidence of BPD, the pathogenesis, pathophysiologic changes, prevention and treatment strategies, and long-term outcome. This is particularly important since the optimal definitions, prevention, and treatment strategies have not been definitively established.

DEFINITION OF BPD

Following Northway's report (2), Shennan et al. proposed a BPD definition as oxygen requirement at 36 weeks of postmenstrual age (PMA), based on its ability to predict abnormal pulmonary outcomes at 2 years of corrected gestational age (CGA) (3). By 2000, survival was more common for neonates born at <1,000 g, and many of these neonates developed BPD even without significant initial lung disease. A workshop sponsored by the National Heart, Lung and Blood Institute (NHLBI) developed a more comprehensive definition for BPD, with a severity scale ranging from none to severe (4). A diagnosis of BPD was made after 28 cumulative days of supplemental oxygen and based on oxygen use at 36 weeks' PMA. A subsequent refinement in the definition included a "physiologic" test for oxygen requirement at 36 weeks' PMA; neonates were classified as having BPD if oxygen saturations were <90% within 60 minutes of a room air challenge test (5).

An NICHD workshop was held in 2016 and proposed a revised definition of BPD that removed the requirement for 28 days of supplemental oxygen, added a requirement for radiographic confirmation of parenchymal lung disease, and used a severity grading of I–III that incorporated newer modes of noninvasive ventilation (6) (Table 29.1). More than 30 years after the Shennan definition, there is still uncertainty on whether these definitions of BPD actually predict pulmonary outcomes later in infancy and childhood. These challenges are compounded by the dramatic evolution in populations at risk and newer respiratory treatment strategies. The number and survival of the smallest and most preterm neonates has increased, including those as young as 22 weeks' gestation (1). Respiratory care practices have also changed over the past two decades, as shown by the Prematurity and Respiratory Outcome Program (PROP) cohort of 765 surviving neonates born at <29 weeks' gestation (7). PROP investigators demonstrated that nearly half of their cohort was being treated with a nasal cannula at 36 weeks' PMA, including 12% receiving room air. This creates new problems for classifying BPD since it is not possible to differentiate if the flow was needed for treatment of apnea or lung injury. These classification challenges are compounded by difficulties in accurate data capture. A database maintained by National Perinatal Registry of the Netherlands found that only 67% of preterm neonates were correctly categorized according to the NHLBI Workshop definition (8). This was predominately due a 31% rate of false negative diagnoses, including 9% with severe BPD (sBPD). Newer proposed definitions have suggested quantifying oxygenation through assessment of oxygen dissociation curves or relying solely on the amount of positive pressure a neonate receives at 36 weeks' PMA (9,10).

The Severe BPD Collaborative group recently recommended that sBPD be further subclassified (11). Neonates only receiving nasal cannula oxygen at 36 weeks' PMA are classified as Type 1 and neonates still requiring mechanical ventilation as Type 2. The Canadian Neonatal Network provided further support for this concept by demonstrating that more sBPD (i.e., oxygen plus respiratory support at 36 weeks' PMA) better predicted serious respiratory morbidity at 18 to 22 months (12). However, because of the low incidence of type 2 sBPD at any single center, long-term outcomes remain poorly understood for this population. There is still a need for a clinical scale that captures the severity of BPD extending through the first year of life and beyond. Although one promising example is the chronic lung disease of infancy (CLDi) score, it is also based on clinical management such as supplemental oxygen, bronchodilators, and need for rehospitalization (13). More objective measures such as pulmonary function testing require sedation and are not yet practical outside of the research setting. A challenge for any classification system using longer term outcomes is to account for other environmental confounders such as smoking or viral infections.

Although early mortality prior to 36 weeks' PMA occurred in 3% of the PROP cohort (7), these highest-risk neonates have been inconsistently classified using existing definitions. The NICHD Workshop definition proposed a Grade IIIA BPD for neonates who died between 14 days of age and 36 weeks' PMA from respiratory failure not attributable to other neonatal morbidities (6). Further work is needed to better identify this population of neonates, so novel therapies can be used as soon as possible.

INCIDENCE/EPIDEMIOLOGY OF BPD

BPD is the most common complication of prematurity with the incidence increasing as gestational age decreases. Almost 50,000 extremely preterm neonates are born each year in the United States and approximately 35% develop BPD. The incidence of BPD

TABLE 29.1

NICHD Workshop Definition of Bronchopulmonary Dysplasia

	Invasive IPPV[a]	N-CPAP, NIPPV or NC ≥ 3 lpm	NC Flow 1–<3 lpm	Hood O₂	NC Flow <1 lpm
Grade I		21%	22%–29%	22%–29%	22%–70%
Grade II	21%	22%–29%	≥30%	≥30%	>70%
Grade III	>21%	≥30%			
Grade III(A)	Early death (between 14 d of postnatal age and 36 wk of PMA) due to persistent parenchymal lung disease and respiratory failure that cannot be attributable to other neonatal morbidities				

A diagnosis of BPD is assigned when a preterm neonate (<32 weeks' GA) has persistent parenchymal lung disease, radiographic confirmation of parenchymal lung disease, and at 36 weeks' PMA requires one of the above modalities for at least 3 consecutive days to maintain arterial oxygen saturation in the 90%–95% range.

[a]Excluding neonates ventilated for primary airway disease or central respiratory control conditions.

lpm, liters per minute.

Reprinted from Higgins RD, Jobe AH, Koso-Thomas M, et al. Bronchopulmonary dysplasia: executive summary of a workshop. *J Pediatr* 2018;197:300. Copyright © 2018 Elsevier, with permission.

varies widely between centers (approximately 20% to 75%) even after adjusting for potential risk factors (14). Similarly, data from global cohort studies demonstrate a wide prevalence rate of 11% to 50%, (15). For example, Japan had the lowest mortality but the highest rate of BPD and Spain had the highest mortality but a lower prevalence of BPD. These variations could be the result of population characteristics, perinatal health care delivery, case definitions, data quality and reliability, and/or care processes. This reinforces the urgent need for international multicenter clinical trials that are integrated with benchmarking and quality improvement activities.

PATHOGENESIS

The strongest risk factors for BPD are prematurity and low birth weight. While almost 80% of neonates born at 22 to 24 weeks of gestation develop BPD, it occurs in <20% of neonates born at 28 weeks of gestation (16). Other perinatal risk factors include intrauterine growth restriction, maternal hypertension, chorioamnionitis, male sex, race or ethnicity, intrauterine infection, and maternal smoking suggesting that lung development can be significantly impacted prior to birth (17). Maternal smoking during pregnancy may be the most important cause of abnormal *in utero* lung development and BPD (18). Genetic factors may also contribute to the development of BPD, particularly in more mature neonates with atypical disease. However, twin studies have not determined if a genetic component contributes to the development of BPD.

Postnatal risk factors are numerous and may depend on the nature of the injury, mechanisms of response, or the neonate's inability to respond appropriately to the injury process and "repair" the lung (**Fig. 29.1**). Although our understanding of the pathogenesis has improved, no treatment approach has unequivocally decreased the incidence of BPD. The NICHD Neonatal Research Network provides an online risk estimator (https://neonatal.rti.org/index.cfm) that uses antenatal and postnatal factors to estimate the risk for BPD according to postnatal day.

Barotrauma/Volutrauma

Although the initial phases of lung injury in BPD are the result of the primary disease process (e.g., RDS), superimposed mechanical ventilation appears to play an important role. Barotrauma describes the lung injury that occurs secondary to positive-pressure mechanical ventilation, although volutrauma from excessive tidal volume ventilation may be a more appropriate term. The role of volutrauma in BPD depends on several factors, including the structure of the tracheobronchial tree and the physiologic effects

PATHOGENESIS OF BPD

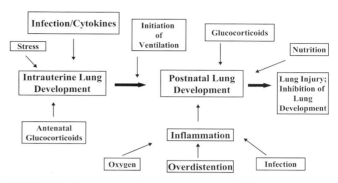

FIGURE 29.1 An overview of the pathogenesis of BPD showing prenatal and postnatal factors. (Reprinted from Jobe AH. Mechanisms of lung injury and bronchopulmonary dysplasia. *Am J Perinatol* 2016;33(11):1076. Copyright © 2016 Georg Thieme Verlag KG, with permission.)

of surfactant deficiency. When surfactant deficiency is coupled with an immature epithelium, surface tension forces are elevated, aeration is unequal, and most terminal alveoli are collapsed. The pressure needed to distend these poorly compliant saccules is high and is transmitted to the terminal bronchioles and alveolar ducts. In the preterm neonate, these airways are highly compliant and subject to rupture. Gas then dissects into the interstitium and pleural space, resulting in the development of pulmonary interstitial emphysema (PIE) and pneumothorax. These complications are strongly associated with the development of BPD, suggesting that ventilator-induced lung injury is important in the pathogenesis (19). Even with normal tidal volumes, ventilation of the immature or injured neonatal lung results in nonuniform inflation and relative overdistension of ventilated segments, especially in the presence of low functional residual capacity (FRC) due to surfactant deficiency. Excessive stretching of capillary endothelium and distal lung epithelium is associated with the release of reactive oxygen species (ROS), marked inflammatory changes in the lung, damage to cellular tight junctions, and increased permeability to serum proteins that may further inhibit surfactant function (20,21). This creates a vicious cycle that promotes cell damage and ultimately lung injury. This concept was reinforced by a recent Cochrane review, which indicated that volume-targeted ventilation was associated with reduced rates of death or development of BPD, pneumothoraces, hypocarbia, severe cranial ultrasound abnormalities, and duration of ventilation compared to pressure-limited ventilation (22).

While the widespread use of noninvasive ventilation, volume ventilation, and surfactant has reduced some complications of mechanical ventilation (reducing mean airway pressure and air leak while improving lung recruitment), BPD continues to increase, suggesting that barotrauma/volutrauma is only one of many factors involved in the pathogenesis of BPD.

Oxygen and Antioxidants

Under normal conditions, a delicate balance exists between the production of ROS and the antioxidant defenses that protect cells *in vivo*. ROS are molecules with extra electrons in their outer ring. They can act as important cell signaling molecules or can be toxic to living tissues (**Table 29.2**). Oxygen has a unique molecular structure and readily accepts free electrons generated by oxidative metabolism within the cell, producing ROS. Increased ROS production can occur under conditions of hyperoxia, reperfusion, or inflammation. Alternatively, ROS can increase because of an inability to quench production because of inadequate antioxidant defenses. Damage caused by ROS includes lipid peroxidation, mitochondrial injury, protein nitration, and unraveling of nucleic acids.

TABLE 29.2		
Free Radicals		
Radical	**Symbol**[a]	**Antioxidant**
Superoxide anion	O_2^-	Superoxide dismutase, uric acid, vitamin E
Singlet oxygen	$^1O_2$	β-Carotene, uric acid, vitamin E
Hydrogen peroxide	H_2O_2	Catalase, glutathione peroxidase, glutathione
Hydroxyl radical	OH·	Vitamins C and E
Peroxide radical	LOO·	Vitamins C and E
Hydroperoxyl radical	LOOH	Glutathione transferase, glutathione peroxidase

[a]L, lipid.

The preterm neonate may be more susceptible to ROS-induced injury because adequate concentrations of antioxidant enzymes (superoxide dismutase—SOD, catalase, and glutathione peroxidase—GPx) may be reduced at birth (Fig. 29.2) (23). These enzymes significantly increase later in gestation in a parallel maturation fashion to pulmonary surfactant. These developmental changes in the fetal lung allow proper ventilation by reducing surface tension and provide for the transition from the relative hypoxia of intrauterine development to the oxygen-rich extrauterine environment. Preterm birth can occur before the normal up-regulation of these antioxidant systems and placental transfer of other nonenzymatic antioxidants (e.g., vitamin E, ascorbic acid, glutathione, ceruloplasmin) and may result in an imbalance between oxidants and antioxidants and an increased risk of developing BPD (24). Clinical studies suggest that hyperoxia is involved in the pathogenesis of BPD. Askie and colleagues performed a meta-analysis examining outcome in preterm neonates randomized to receive lower (85% to 89%) compared to higher (91% to 95%) oxygen saturation targets (25). A total of 2,480 preterm neonates were randomized to the lower target range and 2,485 to the higher range and had a median gestational age of 26 weeks and a mean birth weight of 832 ±190 g. While the lower target range was associated with a higher risk of death and necrotizing enterocolitis, there was a significantly lower risk of retinopathy of prematurity

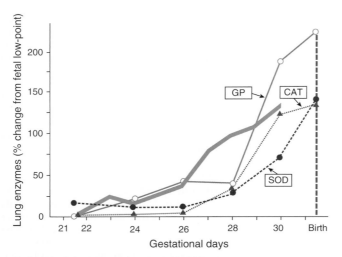

FIGURE 29.2 Developmental changes in antioxidant levels and activity during gestation. The increases in superoxide dismutase (*SOD*), catalase (*CAT*), and glutathione peroxidase (*GP*) late in gestation are similar to those seen for pulmonary surfactant (*dark, thick line*). (Reprinted by permission from Nature: Frank L, Groseclose EE. *Preparation for birth into an O₂-rich environment: the antioxidant enzymes in the developing rabbit lung. Pediatr Res* 1984;18:240. Copyright © 1984 Springer Nature.)

(needing treatment). While the lower target group had significantly lower use of oxygen at 36 weeks' PMA, there were no significant differences in the incidence of death or major disability between groups at 18 and 24 months' CGA, reinforcing the need to examine both short- and longer-term outcomes in preterm neonates. There had been concern that even brief periods of hyperoxia in the delivery room may be associated with an increased risk of significant lung injury. However, Oei and associates performed a meta-analysis of 504 preterm neonates <28 weeks of gestation who were resuscitated at the time of delivery with lower (≤0.30) or higher (≥0.60) inspired oxygen concentrations and could not find any differences in the overall risk of death or development of BPD (26).

Further evidence for the role of ROS in lung injury comes from animal studies demonstrating that exposure to chronic hyperoxia can induce oxidant injury, inflammation, and lung injury that has many features seen in preterm neonates developing BPD. Both epithelial and endothelial cells are extremely susceptible to oxidant injury, leading to increased permeability edema and cell dysfunction. Hyperoxia also impairs mucociliary function (increasing the susceptibility to infection), promotes inflammation, and inactivates antiproteases further complicating clinical outcome. The lungs of these animals also have evidence of differential gene expression as well as epigenetic changes suggesting that protein synthesis/function is significantly impacted in response to hyperoxia (27). These changes can be altered with supplementation with antioxidant enzymes, which have been shown to reduce cell damage, increase survival, and prevent lung injury from prolonged hyperoxia and mechanical ventilation (28,29). Although these studies all demonstrate that ROS are intimately involved in the development of acute and chronic lung injury in neonates, to date these results have not resulted in new medical therapies with antioxidant enzymes.

Inflammation

Marked inflammation in the lung appears to play an important role in the pathogenesis of BPD and allows many risk factors to be unified into a single common pathway. The initial stimuli activating the inflammatory process in the lung may be ROS, excessive stretch, infectious agents, or other stimuli that result in the attraction and activation of leukocytes. Inflammatory mediators and cellular responses have been found to be prominent in animal models of lung injury and in neonates who develop BPD (30). The role of inflammation is further supported by the attenuation of lung injury from a variety of causes in both animal and human models when administering early surfactant along with corticosteroids (31).

A variety of biomarkers associated with the inflammatory process have been identified in tracheal aspirates, serum, and urine, which have been consistently linked to the development of BPD (30). Bose et al. (32) analyzed serum samples from 932 extremely preterm neonates enrolled in the extremely low gestation age newborn (ELGAN) study and found that day 1 elevations in several cytokines, adhesion molecules, and proteases were associated with an increased risk of developing BPD. Ambalavanan et al. (33) analyzed serum from 1,067 preterm neonates with approximately 60% developing BPD. An early (<3 days of life) increase in levels of serum cytokines (both pro-inflammatory and anti-inflammatory) correlated with the development of BPD. The early detection of pro-inflammatory mediators suggests that *in utero* processes (e.g., chorioamnionitis, infection) associated with preterm labor and delivery initiate a fetal inflammatory response within the lung that continues after birth. All of these bioactive agents recruit and activate leukocytes, which can generate excessive ROS and reactive nitrogen species (by up-regulating nitric oxide synthases) and cause significant pulmonary damage.

As the cycle of injury continues with further production and accumulation of inflammatory mediators and ROS, significant injury to the lung can occur during a particularly critical period of rapid growth (i.e., six divisions from 24 to 40 weeks of gestation). This amplification phenomenon can be further exacerbated when there are inadequate concentrations and activity of anti-inflammatory agents such as Vitamin D and IL-10 (34). All of these studies clearly support the notion that this abnormal inflammatory process is a major contributing factor to the development of acute and chronic changes in the lungs of neonates with BPD.

Infection

Subclinical intrauterine infection and the ensuing inflammatory response have been implicated in the etiology of preterm labor and premature rupture of membranes. Significant basic science and epidemiologic evidence indicates that prenatal infection and inflammation are risk factors for the subsequent development of BPD, although not all studies are in complete agreement (30). While several investigators have found a lower incidence of RDS in preterm neonates born to mothers with chorioamnionitis (possibly due to an adaptive response to *in utero* stress), they also observed a significantly higher rate of BPD (35,36). This suggests that although intrauterine infection may accelerate lung maturation, the ensuing inflammatory response may also "prime the lung," causing progressive inflammation, lung injury, and subsequent inhibition of lung growth. Animal models have reinforced this concept with postnatal exposure to hyperoxia and mechanical ventilation further amplifying this injury process (37). However, a large meta-analysis of 59 studies did not definitively associate chorioamnionitis with an increased risk of developing BPD (38).

Ureaplasma urealyticum (UU) colonization in pregnant women has been implicated in the pathogenesis of preterm labor, premature rupture of membranes, and preterm delivery (39). In addition, the organism has been detected (by culture and polymerase chain reaction) in tracheal aspirates from high-risk neonates developing BPD suggesting that UU is an important factor in the pathogenesis (40). Glaser and colleagues studied 103 preterm neonates and found that 39% were colonized with *Ureaplasma* at the time of birth (41). Although colonization was not directly associated with the development of BPD, exposure was associated with neonates being ventilated for longer periods of time, having imbalanced inflammatory cytokine responses, and longer hospital stays. Although treating pregnant women who are colonized with azithromicin before birth or preterm neonates shortly after birth attenuates colonization, the development of BPD does not appear to be significantly impacted (42,43).

A number of investigators have focused on the early airway microbial metagenomic and metabolomic signatures in the pathogenesis of BPD. Lal and colleagues examined tracheal aspirates from neonates and identified specific pathways that were less abundant in the functional metagenome of the microbiota of neonates at high risk of developing BPD compared with lower risk neonates (44). This suggests that in extremely preterm neonates, the early airway microbiome may alter the metabolome and modify the risk of developing BPD. Pammi et al. demonstrated that increased microbial community turnover and changes in the relative abundance of different bacterial species in the airway microbiome were associated with increased severity of BPD, suggesting that microbial dysbiosis was involved in injury process (45). This could further contribute to our understanding of pathogenesis of wheezing and airway obstruction in preterm neonates with BPD.

Normal defense mechanisms against infection can be compromised in the preterm lung, especially when neonates are intubated and exposed to multiple courses of broad spectrum antibiotics. This makes them more susceptible to colonization and subsequent infection with a variety of infectious agents (e.g., virus, bacteria, fungi) that may increase the incidence and severity of BPD (30). Several large clinical studies have found a strong correlation between late-onset sepsis and the development of BPD, usually with organisms such as staphylococcus epidermidis (46,47).

These infections are associated with increased morbidity, mortality, and length of hospital stay and appear to contribute to the incidence and severity of BPD.

Nutrition

The nutritional status of the critically ill preterm neonate may also be important in the development of BPD. Adequate calories and essential nutrients for growth may be lacking during a period of significant stress. In addition, vital components for immunologic development and antioxidant defenses may be inadequate. Preterm neonates have increased nutritional requirements because of increased metabolic needs and rapid growth requirements. If these increased energy and protein needs are not met, the neonate will develop a catabolic state (e.g., negative nitrogen balance), which likely contributes to the pathogenesis of BPD. Inadequate nutrition interferes with normal growth and maturation of the lung and may potentiate the deleterious effects of oxygen, mechanical ventilation, infection, etc. This may explain why neonates who are small for gestational age and those with postnatal growth failure are more likely to develop BPD.

Human milk is well recognized to be highly beneficial for preterm neonates. Several studies (including a systematic review) have suggested that feeding human milk is associated with a lower risk of BPD in preterm neonates (48,49). Although the quality of evidence is low and it is unclear if the addition of human milk fortifiers alters the risk profile, the potential reduction in BPD is another reason why mother's own milk should be highly recommended for use in preterm neonates. Antioxidant enzymes may play a vital role in the protection of the lung and the prevention of BPD. Many of these enzymes have trace elements (e.g., copper, zinc, selenium) that are an integral part of their structure. Deficiencies in these elements may compromise lung defenses and predispose the lung to further injury. The repair of elastin and collagen is limited in animals that are undernourished and copper, zinc, and other elements may be necessary for this repair (50). Vitamin deficiency has also been postulated to be important in the development of BPD. While current feeding and hyperalimentation regimens appear to provide adequate amounts of vitamin E for preterm neonates, a relative decrease in the concentrations of other vitamins may be important in the pathogenesis of BPD (34). For example, concentrations of vitamin A (i.e., retinol) may be deficient in very preterm neonates (51,52). This vitamin is important in maintaining cell integrity and in tissue repair with deficiency associated with changes in the ciliated epithelium of the tracheobronchial tree (53). Systemic reviews of vitamin A supplementation suggest that the risk for developing BPD (oxygen requirement at 36 weeks' PMA) is attenuated in preterm neonates following intramuscular administration of vitamin A (54). However, it is unclear if this treatment approach significantly improves clinical pulmonary status later in infancy and childhood (55). Widespread shortages of the medication and significant increases in pricing have markedly reduced the use of vitamin A supplementation in preterm neonates without apparent increases in rates of BPD (56).

Large volumes of intravenous fluids are often administered to preterm neonates to provide adequate hydration and sufficient nutrition. Excessive fluid administration can be associated with the development of a patent ductus arteriosus (PDA) and pulmonary edema, which can lead to an increase in oxygen and ventilator requirements and the subsequent risk of BPD (57). Although early closure of the PDA using medical or surgical management has been associated with improvements in pulmonary function, these approaches have resulted in variable reductions in the development of BPD, leading many scientists and clinicians to question the validity of aggressive treatment of the PDA (58,59).

Genetics

A significant number of studies have been conducted in order to establish if genetic susceptibility is associated with an increased incidence and severity of BPD. Early studies observed that neonates were more likely to develop BPD if there was a strong family history of atopy and asthma. Nickerson and Taussig (60) found a positive family history of asthma in 77% of infants with RDS who subsequently developed BPD, compared with only 33% who did not. Lavoie et al. (61) studied 318 preterm twins of known zygosity who were ≤30 weeks of gestation and found that heritability factors contributed significantly to the development of BPD. By contrast, Parad et al. studied 250 sets of preterm twins (192 dichorionic, 58 monochorionic) born at <29 weeks' gestation (62). Their analysis failed to demonstrate that heritability was a major contributor to BPD risk in this population. Other investigators have conducted genome-wide association studies on independent groups of preterm neonates ≤28 weeks' gestation or analyzed single-nucleotide polymorphisms (SNPs) and have identified specific genes that appear to be associated with an increased risk for developing BPD (63,64). In the PROP cohort, 146 extremely preterm neonates with and without BPD underwent whole exome sequencing (65). The investigators tested for associations between BPD status and individual common variants, screened for rare variants exclusive to either affected or unaffected subjects, and tested the combined association of variants across gene loci. Marginal association with the development of BPD was observed for numerous common and rare variants. Pathway analysis implicated protein kinase A, MAPK, and neuregulin/epidermal growth factor receptor signaling, genes that may be important in respiratory epithelial cell differentiation. As significant advances occur in analyzing large amounts of genetic information, further delineation of risk factors in larger populations will be needed to more definitively identify neonates at high risk of developing BPD.

PATHOPHYSIOLOGY

Clinical Signs

Due to the widespread use of antenatal steroids and postnatal surfactant, BPD may develop after mild RDS that required minimal respiratory support. Development of BPD is usually associated with subsequent deterioration in lung function with increased respiratory support and/or oxygen requirements. Neonates with BPD are tachypneic, hypoxic, hypercarbic, and may display intercostal and subcostal retractions and use of accessory muscles. These neonates may grow poorly despite adequate caloric intake.

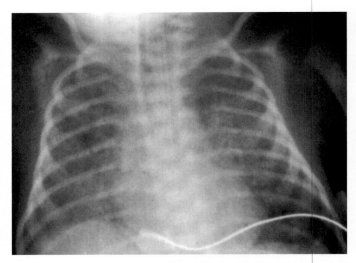

FIGURE 29.3 Typical chest radiograph of a neonate with early evidence of BPD. The bilateral hazy appearance represents inflammatory exudate, edema, and atelectasis.

Radiographic Changes

The first description of BPD in 1967 was based on characteristic radiographic abnormalities that described progression of lung injury toward an inhomogeneous appearance with marked hyperinflation, bleb formation, fibrosis, and cardiomegaly (2). Scoring systems have been difficult to validate for chest radiographs due to significant intra-observer variability and are seldom used in clinical practice. However, the 2018 NICHD Workshop definition of BPD did add a requirement for radiographic confirmation of parenchymal lung disease (Fig. 29.3) (6).

Computed tomography (CT) and magnetic resonance imaging (MRI) of the lung may provide more details of the structural lung disease in BPD and can reveal abnormalities that are not readily apparent on chest radiographs. CT scans are sometimes used in more severe cases to evaluate underlying parenchymal and airway pathology, although its use has been limited by concerns surrounding ionizing radiation exposure (Fig. 29.4). More recently, MRI imaging studies have revealed heterogeneous pulmonary pathology, including regions of decreased alveolarization,

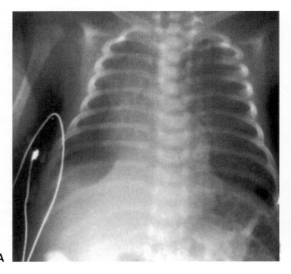
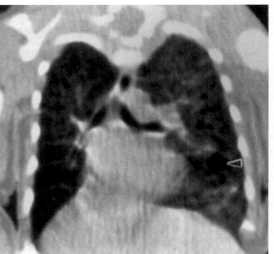

FIGURE 29.4 A: Chest radiograph of an older neonate with BPD, showing right-sided atelectasis and a shift of the mediastinum. The lung fields have a hazy appearance. **B:** Computed tomography scan on the same neonate. The major bronchi and areas of atelectasis are apparent. Fibrotic changes and a bleb are seen in the left lung (*arrow*).

cystic emphysema, fibrosis, and variable airway injury in neonates with BPD (66). MRI imaging may also be useful to further evaluate cardiac morphology in neonates with BPD-associated pulmonary hypertension (PH) (67). An increased pulmonary artery to aorta diameter ratio and left-ventricular eccentricity index were associated with BPD severity and clinical pulmonary outcomes during hospitalization and at discharge.

Changes in Pulmonary Mechanics

In the first few months of life, neonates with evolving BPD have reduced FRC primarily due to atelectasis. Neonates with more established BPD have decreased dynamic lung compliance due to lung fibrosis, lung interstitial fluid, and overdistension due to gas trapping. However, over the first 1 to 2 years of life, FRC values rise to above normal, most likely due to gas trapping and hyperinflation from small airway obstruction. BPD is consistently associated with increased airway resistance. Dynamic collapse of the small airways can occur, which leads to expiratory flow limitations including reduced forced expiratory flow (Fig. 29.5). The increased airway resistance in neonates with BPD may be partially reversible with bronchodilators, diuretic therapy, and inhaled or systemic corticosteroids.

As a result of the above changes, neonates with sBPD have hypoxemia and hypercapnia due to impaired ventilation-perfusion matching and alveolar hypoventilation. Recently, a bedside analysis of the "shift" of the oxyhemoglobin dissociation curve (accomplished through simultaneous measurement of inspired O_2 and peripheral saturation at a single point of time) was proposed as an objective test to quantify the degree of hypoxemia due to lack of alveolarization (9). The chronic hypercapnia and respiratory acidosis is often compensated by a rise in serum bicarbonate concentrations, which can be exacerbated by the administration of acetate in total parenteral nutrition as well as the use of diuretics.

Pulmonary Vascular Disease

Northway's original description of BPD highlighted that pulmonary vascular disease and right ventricular hypertrophy were associated with increased mortality (2). In contemporary studies of preterm neonates, PH is found in up to 40% of neonates with sBPD. Even neonates with mild or no BPD at 36 weeks' PMA are at risk for chronic PH (68). Clinical cohort studies have demonstrated a relationship between underperfusion of the placental villi and PH, suggesting that disruption of lung vascular growth likely begins antenatally (69). Recent prospective studies indicate that early echocardiogram evidence of pulmonary vascular disease and the need for mechanical ventilation at 7 days of life are each strongly associated with the development of BPD, PH, and late respiratory disease during childhood (70,71).

Echocardiography is the most common tool used to detect PH in preterm neonates. Screening is recommended at 36 weeks' PMA for neonates with moderate to sBPD or unexplained desaturation episodes (72). Echocardiography can provide qualitative assessment of elevated RV afterload, estimation of pulmonary hemodynamics including RV systolic pressure, and qualitative appraisal of RV morphology and function (73). However, echocardiography cannot always accurately assess the severity of PH and may be insufficient to differentiate etiologies of PH in preterm neonates. Cardiac catheterization remains the gold standard for the definitive diagnosis and assessment of PH in preterm neonates.

PATHOLOGY

Detailed morphometric studies have extensively characterized the lung pathology of neonates dying with BPD (74–76). The pathology of BPD provides insights into the effects of lung injury and subsequent repair processes in the developing lung as well as the timing of the injury. The original pathology reports of BPD described a continuous process through distinct stages of the disease, originating with an acute exudative phase and progressing to a chronic proliferative phase. This is still pertinent for adults who were born preterm and developed this form of BPD. These reports described a gross cobblestone appearance of the lungs, representing alternating areas of atelectasis, marked scarring, and regional hyperinflation (74). Typical histologic features of this BPD included squamous metaplasia of large and small airways, increased peribronchial smooth muscle and fibrosis, chronic inflammation, airway edema, and hyperplasia of submucosal glands. Parenchymal disease was characterized by volume loss from atelectasis and alveolar septal fibrosis alternating with overdistension or emphysematous regions (Fig. 29.6). Mesenchymal thickening with increased cellularity and destruction of alveolar septa with alveolar hypoplasia was present, suggesting a marked reduction in surface area available for gas exchange. Growth of capillary beds was reduced and small pulmonary arteries had hypertensive structural remodeling, which included smooth muscle hyperplasia and distal extension of smooth muscle growth into vessels that are normally nonmuscular.

Upper airways (i.e., trachea and main bronchi) of neonates with BPD can reveal significant lesions, depending on the frequency and duration of endotracheal intubation. Grossly, mucosal edema or necrosis can be focal or diffuse. The earliest histologic changes include patchy loss of cilia from columnar epithelial cells, which can then become dysplastic or necrotic, resulting in breakdown of the epithelial lining and decreased pulmonary clearance of mucous and other material. Ulcerated areas may involve the mucosa or extend into the submucosa. Infiltration of inflammatory cells into these areas may be prominent. Goblet cells can appear hyperplastic, indicating increased mucous production that can mix with cellular debris. Granulation tissue from the endotracheal tube can develop in the subglottis or more distally throughout the airway due to repeated suctioning. Significant narrowing of the trachea and main bronchi secondary to injury can lead to subglottic stenosis, tracheal cysts, polyps, and related lesions (less common due to a focus on noninvasive ventilation). Tracheomalacia often complicates the course of sBPD and can appear as marked redundancy of the posterior wall of the trachea due to chronic ventilation of the compliant preterm airway. Although neonates dying with BPD in the postsurfactant era have been described as having less severe distal airway injury, evidence of smooth muscle hypertrophy and alterations in extracellular matrix can still be seen (77). This may explain the increased rates of coughing and wheezing seen later in childhood.

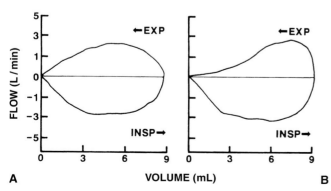

FIGURE 29.5 A: Normal flow–volume loop. **B:** Expiratory flow limitation as a result of dynamic collapse of small airways during expiration. INSP, inspiration; EXP, expiration.

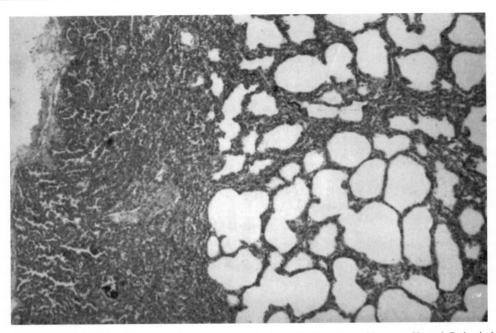

FIGURE 29.6 Light micrograph from a 1-year-old infant with BPD shows areas of atelectasis alternating with areas of hyperinflation (original magnification ×4).

Reductions in alveolar number were described in older neonates dying with BPD, but this pattern of "alveolar simplification" has become the most striking pathologic feature of current forms of BPD (**Fig. 29.7**) (78). The decreased alveolarization appears to be caused by impaired septation that can be directly influenced by growth factors, inflammation, vasculature growth, and the extracellular matrix. Neonates dying with BPD also have abnormal alveolar vasculature with disordered expression of growth factors (e.g., VEGF), and their receptors may contribute to these abnormalities. This impaired alveolar and vascular growth results in significant decreases in surface area for gas exchange and blood flow, which has important functional implications regarding late

cardiopulmonary sequelae (ventilation perfusion mismatching and PH). While much of our knowledge of lung growth and development in BPD has come from extensive study in animal models, examination of postmortem lung specimens has also contributed significantly to our understanding of the pathologic changes.

PREVENTION STRATEGIES

Avoidance of Mechanical Ventilation

Interest in minimizing lung injury in extremely preterm neonates has prompted recommendations to use noninvasive respiratory

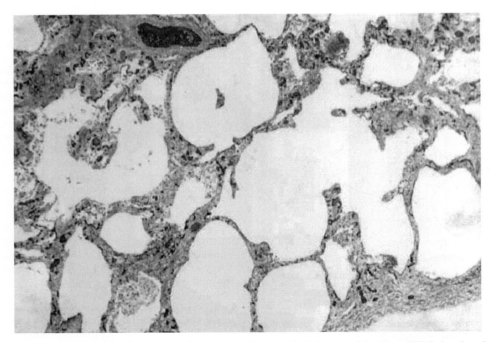

FIGURE 29.7 Lung histology from an infant dying in the postsurfactant era with the typical changes of the "New BPD," showing alveolar simplification and reduced septation (original magnification ×4; Courtesy of Dr. Steven Abman).

support if possible (79). Although nasal continuous positive airway pressure (NCPAP) remains the gold standard, nasal intermittent positive pressure ventilation (NIPPV) and high flow nasal cannula are being used more often, with modest evidence for their efficacy. Although instillation of exogenous surfactant has been shown to reduce mortality and air leak, it has not reduced the rates of BPD. To avoid the need for intubation, new techniques to deliver surfactant noninvasively have been developed including LISA (less invasive surfactant administration) and MIST (minimally invasive surfactant therapy) (80,81). A meta-analysis of six randomized trials involving 895 neonates showed that surfactant delivered using a thin catheter reduced the composite outcome of death or BPD compared with conventional surfactant delivery (82). Alternative administration routes have been proposed, such as nebulized surfactant or administration via a laryngeal mask airway. Administration of surfactant in the 2nd week of life has also been proposed as a strategy to overcome persistent surfactant dysfunction in high-risk neonates. One large trial demonstrated an approximately 20% reduction in the number of neonates requiring respiratory support at 40 weeks' PMA as well as a substantial decrease in the number of neonates who required home respiratory support during the first year of life in neonates receiving later doses of surfactant (83,84).

Oxygen

Balancing the risks and benefits of oxygen therapy is an important goal of neonatal intensive care. Administration of oxygen to preterm neonates is titrated to achieve target oxygen saturation ranges that are determined locally by each NICU. As discussed previously, an individual patient meta-analysis of five high-quality randomized controlled trials comparing high (91% to 95%) versus low (85% to 89%) oxygen saturation ranges found no difference in the primary composite outcome of death or major disability at 18 to 24 months CGA (25). In balance, the meta-analysis data favor the higher target ranges but will require clinicians to find other strategies to prevent and treat retinopathy of prematurity and BPD.

Vitamin A

With large randomized studies demonstrating that intramuscular vitamin A produced a small, but significant reduction of BPD in extremely preterm neonates, many NICUs adopted this approach (52). However, neurodevelopmental assessment of surviving neonates in the largest trial showed no difference between the groups at 18 to 22 months of age with long-term pulmonary outcomes not assessed. The use of vitamin A has been adopted into fewer than half of the neonatal units in the United States given the lack of availability, expense, and need for frequent intramuscular injections. Post hoc analysis of one of the multicenter randomized trials of inhaled NO suggested that neonates who received vitamin A in combination with iNO had better respiratory outcomes than preterm neonates who received either vitamin A or iNO alone (85).

Caffeine

Caffeine is perhaps the best-evaluated, most effective, and safest treatment for reducing the risk of BPD. The Caffeine for Apnea of Prematurity (CAP) trial demonstrated that caffeine administration reduced the risk of BPD and shortened the duration of mechanical ventilation and exposure to supplemental oxygen (86). A more recent systematic review found that earlier use of caffeine was more effective in reducing BPD than later use (87). Investigators from the Canadian Neonatal Network also demonstrated that the early use of caffeine was associated with improved neurodevelopmental outcomes compared with late caffeine in preterm neonates born at <29 weeks' gestation (88). Important questions about caffeine remain including (a) when should caffeine be started, (b) what is the optimal dose, (c) how long should treatment be continued, and (d) will early benefits correlate with improvements in long-term pulmonary outcomes.

Corticosteroids

Although administration of antenatal corticosteroids to women at risk for imminent preterm birth reduces mortality, RDS, intraventricular hemorrhage, and necrotizing enterocolitis, they have not been shown to reduce the rates of BPD (89). After birth, cortisol synthesis is decreased in preterm neonates, which may increase the risk of developing BPD. Corticosteroids are known to promote the synthesis of pulmonary surfactant and the expression of lung antioxidant enzymes, reduce pulmonary edema and inflammation, inhibit inflammatory cell infiltration and fibroblast proliferation, and reduce the risk for BPD (90). However, concerns about potential adverse effects of steroids (e.g., dexamethasone) on neurodevelopmental impairment led to a significant reduction in their use. However, a more recent systemic review by Doyle et al. suggested that initiating therapy after 7 days of age may facilitate extubation and reduce neonatal mortality without significantly increasing the risk of adverse long-term neurodevelopmental outcomes (91). However, there were concerns about the methodological quality of some of the studies and the potential for adverse effects from any exposure. The most prudent recommendations to be taken from this study include limiting the use of systemic corticosteroids to the highest risk neonates who cannot be weaned from mechanical ventilation, minimizing the dose, and limiting the treatment interval to as short a duration as possible.

Other attempts to prevent BPD have evaluated potentially less harmful corticosteroids and alternative routes of administration. In the large multicenter PREMILOC study, low-dose hydrocortisone prophylaxis was administered within 24 hours of birth for a total of 3 days. Although the trial stopped at 66% of planned recruitment, survival without BPD was better in the hydrocortisone compared to the placebo group (60% vs. 51%, $p = 0.04$) and neurodevelopmental outcomes were comparable at 2 years of age (92), (93). Although the most recent individual patient meta-analysis of four randomized trials (n = 982) reported that early low-dose hydrocortisone treatment significantly increased survival without BPD (OR 1.45, 95% CI 1.11 to 1.90, $p = 0.007$), there was an increased risk of intestinal perforation (when given with indomethacin) and late-onset sepsis (94). Other approaches to early steroid use have focused on inhaled delivery. Bassler et al. randomized extremely preterm neonates to receive inhaled budesonide versus placebo within the first 24 hours after birth until they no longer needed supplemental oxygen or other respiratory support (95). The risk of BPD, rates of reintubation, and the need for surgical closure of PDA was lower in the budesonide group. However, the mortality rate was higher in the budesonide group and follow-up at 2 years of age failed to demonstrate any significant benefits compared with placebo (96). Another trial randomized 265 very preterm neonates to early surfactant or a combination treatment with budesonide and surfactant (up to six doses) (97). Although the rates of death or BPD were reduced from 66% to 42% with the combination therapy, follow-up at age 2 to 3 years of age revealed no differences in neurodevelopmental impairment and little information about pulmonary outcomes.

Inhaled Nitric Oxide

Alterations in nitric oxide (NO) signaling have been observed in lung and vascular injury models of BPD (98). In addition, inhaled NO (iNO) has been shown to promote lung angiogenesis while reducing inflammation, oxidative stress, and apoptosis (99). However, based on large clinical studies, early prophylactic or rescue iNO in preterm neonates with respiratory failure did not reduce rates of BPD (100). However, it is possible that specific subgroups of neonates may benefit from iNO. Askie et al. conducted an individual patient meta-analysis in African American neonates and found a significant benefit from iNO treatment (relative risk for death or BPD of 0.77, 95% CI 0.65 to 0.91) (101). Racial differences in NO bioavailability and response due to genetic variations

THE NEWBORN INFANT

have been described in key genes in the NO regulatory pathway, suggesting that more study is needed in future trials.

MANAGEMENT OF BPD

Ventilator Strategies

Ventilator strategies need to evolve as neonates develop BPD, particularly when the disease is severe. Some clinicians support established BPD by continuing CPAP or other noninvasive modalities such as NIPPV. However, inadequate support may result in poor somatic growth, impaired lung development, and persistent ventilation/perfusion mismatch contributing to additional lung injury and the development of PH. The goals of care should focus on optimal mechanical ventilation to support adequate gas exchange, reduce the work of breathing, and optimize growth and healing of injured lungs. The BPD Collaborative Group reported data from eight U.S. academic centers and showed that 28% of neonates with sBPD were on invasive MV at a mean of 47 weeks' PMA (range 36 to 86 weeks) (11).

Severe BPD results in nonuniform ventilation in the lung with varying time constants in different parts of the lung. The respiratory system mechanics in these patients are explained by a two-compartment (fast and slow) model, rather than a linear one-compartment model typically seen in RDS (11). In addition, current data suggest that neonates with established BPD mainly have obstructive rather than restrictive disease and small airways are the primary contributor to the obstruction. Thus, the main goals of mechanical ventilation for sBPD are to maintain recruitment of alveoli and minimize air trapping. Lung volume is optimized through use of adequate tidal volumes (8 to 12 mL/kg), PEEP (8 to 15 cm H_2O), and support of spontaneous breaths through pressure support. It is important to note that one breath cycle consists of the inspiratory time added to the expiratory time (which is five times the time constant). Because of the higher time constants associated with BPD, the use of longer inspiratory times (e.g., 0.5 to 0.8 seconds) and slower ventilator rates (10 to 20 breaths/minute) is needed to allow adequate expiration and prevent air trapping.

Setting optimum PEEP is also important when overexpansion of the lungs is observed. Tracheobronchomalacia is commonly seen in neonates with sBPD and results in dynamic airway collapse and gas trapping, causing generation of intrinsic (inadvertent) PEEP. If the ventilator PEEP is set at less than the intrinsic PEEP, the neonate cannot generate enough inspiratory flow against the collapsed airway to trigger a respiratory cycle and will appear distressed and out of synchrony with the ventilator. Although intrinsic PEEP can be measured on contemporary ventilators through a bedside expiratory pause maneuver, bronchoscopy or dynamic CT scans have also been proposed as modalities to determine optimum PEEP.

The decision to perform a tracheostomy in a neonate with sBPD requires long-term specialized support and collaboration between care providers and family members. The goal of chronic ventilation is to optimize long-term survival and developmental outcome. For those neonates that ultimately receive a tracheostomy, improved growth and reduced need for sedation have been reported. Benefits may be greater if the procedure is not delayed beyond the first 4 months of life (102).

Oxygen

Supplemental oxygen is necessary to prevent intermittent or sustained hypoxemia. Recommended oxygen saturation targets are between 91% and 95% for neonates with BPD, including those with PH (72). Higher saturation levels of >95% have not been shown to improve short- or long-term outcomes. Two studies found that maintaining saturation targets of >95% after 32 weeks' PMA were associated with worse pulmonary outcomes and longer duration of oxygen exposure at term equivalent (103,104). Home oxygen

is used in up to 25% of extremely preterm neonates, which may shorten the length of hospital stay, but its impact on long-term outcomes has not been well studied. A retrospective cohort study compared propensity-matched neonates discharged with and without supplemental oxygen. Neonates on home oxygen had marginally improved weight z scores at 2 years and similar rates of neurodevelopmental impairment but were more likely to be rehospitalized for respiratory illness and more likely to use respiratory medications (105).

Nutrition

Slower postnatal growth is commonly observed in neonates with BPD compared with preterm neonates without lung disease. Longitudinal studies suggest that these growth deficits persist through the first year of life. The reasons for poor growth include a higher metabolic rate, failure to meet nutrient requirements, and any therapeutic interventions (e.g., fluid restriction, diuretics, corticosteroids) (106). If diuretics are used, maintenance of normal sodium and bicarbonate levels are needed to permit growth. Optimizing protein delivery is essential for adequate use of total calories for energy, with fats a source of calories that have a lower respiratory quotient and less production of carbon dioxide.

Reflux and microaspiration likely contribute to the development and severity of BPD. A three-fold higher tracheal pepsin concentration was found in preterm neonates who died or developed BPD compared to those who did not develop BPD (107). Although transpyloric feedings have been recommended to minimize aspiration, there is little evidence to support the safety and efficacy of antireflux medications and Nissen fundoplication for sBPD (108).

Medications

Many therapies for BPD are often used concurrently with inadequate studies to define safety (potential for significant side effects, especially from drug–drug interactions) and efficacy. Most studies have not evaluated long-term use and few have examined pulmonary and neurodevelopmental outcomes later in childhood. These medications should be used cautiously with specific goals and outcomes established prior to use (Table 29.3) (109). Inhaled bronchodilators (e.g., albuterol, ipratropium) are used in about

TABLE 29.3

Commonly Used Medications for Bronchopulmonary Dysplasia

Medication	Dosage
Diuretics	
Furosemide	0.5–1.0 mg/kg/dose IV or 1–2 mg/kg/dose PO; given every other day, daily, or twice daily
Chlorothiazide	10–20 mg/kg/dose PO every 12 h
Hydrochlorothiazide	1–2 mg/kg/dose PO every 12 h
Inhaled agents	
Albuterol	2.5 mg nebulized or 2 puffs every 4–12 h by MDI and spacer
Ipratropium bromide	75–175 µg by nebulizer every 6–8 h; 2–4 puffs (17 µg/puff) every 6–8 h by MDI and spacer
Systemic agents	
Caffeine citrate	LD 20 mg/kg; MD 5–10 mg/kg/dose IV or PO every 24 h
Dexamethasone	7–10 d course of dexamethasone beginning at 0.15 mg/kg/d (divided every 12 h) for 2–3 d, followed by 0.10 mg/kg/d for 2–3 d, 0.05 mg/kg/d for 2 d, and 0.02 mg/kg/d for 2 d (total of ~0.89 mg/kg over 10 d)
Sildenafil[a]	0.5 mg/kg PO every 8 h

[a]Increased risk of mortality may be seen with higher doses.

LD, loading dose; MD, maintenance dose; IV, intravenous; PO, oral; h, hour.

a third of neonates with evolving BPD to treat small airway disease. However, substantial interhospital variation in their use suggests that there is little agreement on their efficacy (110). More than half of all extremely preterm neonates receive diuretics such as furosemide during their hospitalization, with daily or intermittent dosing resulting in short-term improvements in pulmonary mechanics and oxygenation (109). However, the long-term benefits are less clear and risks are substantial including hypochloremic alkalosis and diminished bone growth and mineralization. The benefits of thiazide diuretics (with or without spironolactone) are even less compelling. Pharmacotherapy for PH should only be considered after optimization of lung disease and access to serial echocardiography and cardiac catheterization to monitor the response to therapy (72).

Systemic or inhaled steroids are commonly used to treat neonates with BPD, sometimes on a daily or every other day dosing schedule. In one single-center cohort, survival improved for neonates with sBPD with a comprehensive approach that reduced use of inhaled steroids and increased use of systemic steroids to more >80% of patients (primarily prednisone, 0.5 mg/kg every 48 hours) (111).

OUTCOMES

In general, while the severity of BPD has diminished for each gestational age and birth weight category, neonates with more severe forms of BPD are still at greater risk of developing significant short- and long-term morbidity and mortality compared to those surviving without BPD. Long-term outcomes of these extremely preterm neonates continue to be problematic despite significant shifts in treatment approaches (e.g., more noninvasive ventilation), with limited prevention options available. As the survival of extremely preterm neonates slowly increases and more long-term follow-up data are available, interpretation of results can become even more difficult since former preterm neonates who are now young adults were treated very differently than neonates being cared for at the present time.

Pulmonary Outcomes

Many survivors with BPD can develop increased wheezing, infections (e.g., upper and lower respiratory tract), pulmonary dysfunction, and PH leading to increased medical visits, treatments, and hospitalizations for respiratory illnesses. These problems are most prevalent in the early years of life and often improve by late childhood and early adult years. The impact of environmental, infectious, and genetic influences in addition to the prematurity confounds many of these long-term studies. This helps explain why many studies have demonstrated that these same morbidities are also present in extremely preterm neonates who did not have a diagnosis of BPD and who may or may not have received mechanical ventilation (17). With minimal drug and device development for the prevention and treatment of BPD, it is essential that more definitive short- and long-term pulmonary outcome measures are developed, validated, and accepted by global regulatory agencies.

Islam and colleagues conducted a comprehensive evaluation of the literature in order to examine long-term respiratory outcomes in infants with BPD (112). There was significant variation in study design, measurements, and end points used to document pulmonary outcomes in children and young adults. The authors found that neonates with more severe forms of BPD did have significant airway dysfunction, despite the fact that the "new BPD" is primarily characterized by alveolar simplification and limited airway injury. In a review of 14 studies examining adult survivors who had BPD, Gough et al. (113) found conflicting results with regard to long-term respiratory symptoms, ranging from an increased incidence in survivors with BPD to no statistical difference between groups.

In a subsequent study, Gough et al. (114) reported that adults with a previous history of BPD had wheezing and used asthma medications more often than those without BPD and term controls. More recently, Jackson et al. performed a retrospective analysis on 882 children born at <28 weeks' gestation who were followed at 12 and 24 months CGA and 10 years of age (115). A diagnosis of BPD was associated with significant increases in bronchodilator use at 12 months and 24 months CGA, but not with a diagnosis of asthma at 10 years. Although these data suggest that BPD is associated with wheezing in the first few years of life, these authors found that growth velocity and socioeconomic status were more significant predictors of a diagnosis of asthma in older children. Up to 50% of former preterm neonates with BPD require rehospitalization within the first 2 years of life (116). In addition, children born preterm with and without BPD have poorer lung function during early childhood compared with children born at term and are at higher risk for wheezing, asthma-like symptoms, and exercise intolerance (117). At 10 years of age, children with a history of BPD continue to display ventilation/perfusion abnormalities with prominent perfusion defects, suggesting the presence of residual alveolar-capillary impairment (118).

Among the most significant consequences of BPD is the need for tracheostomy and home ventilation. In a 10-year review, Overman et al. (119) reported a tracheostomy rate of 1.8% in neonates with birth weights of <1,000 g with 95% of these infants having a diagnosis of BPD as the major contributing factor. Cristea et al. (120) reported outcomes of 102 ventilator-dependent neonates with BPD, with 81% of these children ultimately surviving. Although the exact cause of death could not always be determined, 50% of neonates died while requiring chronic mechanical ventilation and 26% when only receiving oxygen via a tracheostomy collar. By 5 years of age, 97% of survivors had been weaned from mechanical ventilation and 97% were decannulated by 6 years of age.

Pulmonary Function

Numerous reports in early childhood, late childhood, adolescence, and in adults show improvement but continued impairment in pulmonary function over time for former preterm neonates who had a diagnosis of BPD. Filburn et al. (121) tested neonates with BPD longitudinally for the first 3 years of life with children continuing to demonstrate impaired pulmonary function (airway obstruction and air trapping) as well as diminished lung growth. Although in general there was a lack of catch-up growth, infants with greater somatic growth showed the most improvement in lung function. Doyle et al. studied 297 extremely preterm neonates at 8 and 18 years of age and compared them to term controls (122). The preterm group had evidence of significant airway obstruction at both ages. However, airway obstruction actually increased over time in those who had a diagnosis of BPD as well as those who were smokers. Thunqvist et al. studied 350 premature infants and term controls at 6 to 7 years of age (123). In neonates born at 22 to 24 weeks of gestation, 24% had FVC and 44% had FEV_1 below the lower limit of normal with sBPD only marginally contributing to pulmonary outcomes. Asthma-like disease was reported in 40% of the preterm group and 15% of controls.

Finally, Simpson et al. studied 163 preterm children (99 with BPD) and 58 term controls at 9 to 11 years of age (124). Former preterm neonates had pulmonary obstruction and hyperinflation as well as abnormal peripheral lung mechanics compared with term controls, with improvements in FEV_1 associated with higher gestational age and birth weight. Structural lung changes were found in 92% of former preterm neonates by chest CT scan. In view of the airway obstruction found in older children, it is reasonable to postulate that very preterm neonates (especially those with more sBPD) may be at higher risk for chronic obstructive pulmonary disease in later life.

Pulmonary Hypertension

PH is a very serious complication of BPD. As mentioned previously, impaired development of the alveolar and vascular compartments results in decreased alveolar and pulmonary vascular surface area leading to increased PVR, tricuspid regurgitation, right ventricular hypertrophy, and cor pulmonale. In a retrospective cohort study of 1677 preterm neonates born at <32 weeks of gestation with sBPD, PH occurred in 22% of patients (125). PH was associated with increased mortality, duration of mechanical ventilation, use of supplemental oxygen, need for tracheostomy, and repeated hospital readmissions following discharge. In a prospective study of very preterm neonates screened for PH using a broad echocardiographic-based definition, Mourani et al. demonstrated that the overall incidence of PH was 42% at 7 days of age and 14% at 36 weeks' PMA (70). While most late PH occurred in neonates with sBPD, preterm neonates with none, mild, and moderate BPD (9% to 10% in each group) also had evidence of late PH. These neonates also required more prolonged mechanical ventilatory support and oxygen supplementation. What is most important is that early development of PH was associated with later evidence of asthma, reactive airways disease, BPD exacerbation, bronchiolitis, pneumonia, or a respiratory-related hospitalization during follow-up (71).

Vayalthrikkovil performed serial echocardiograms in 126 very preterm neonates at 32, 36, and 40 weeks' PMA (126). Overall, 38% of neonates developed PH during their initial hospitalization. At 36 weeks' PMA, none of the neonates with mild BPD had PH, whereas 20% of moderate and 32% of sBPD infants had PH. Severe BPD and ventilator-associated pneumonia were independent risk factors for the development of PH. The presence of PH is also associated with reduced survival, suboptimal growth, and poor neurodevelopmental outcome in preterm neonates with BPD at 18 to 24 months CGA (127). However, long-term outcomes and impact of chronic therapy for preterm neonates with pulmonary vascular disease remain poorly understood. Preterm neonates developing PH as a complication of BPD are at very high risk of significant morbidity and mortality despite current treatment approaches, not only during the initial hospitalization but also following discharge.

Mortality

Determining BPD-specific mortality is difficult due to the number of comorbidities occurring in affected neonates. While most mortality in preterm neonates occurs in the first month of life, BPD is an important cause of late mortality prior to discharge. Eventov-Friedman et al. (128) reported that 15% of all deaths that occurred in the NICU happened after 30 days of age. Although BPD was the primary cause of death in only 8% of all mortalities, it was a contributing factor in 57% of late mortalities. In neonates with BPD who were ventilator dependent at the time of discharge, Cristea et al. (120) reported a 19% mortality rate during longitudinal follow-up. Finally, Altit et al. conducted serial echocardiograms in 52 neonates with BPD and PH of which 16 (31%) died at follow-up (129). The median time from the diagnosis of PH and death was 117 days. The severity of PH and underlying RV dysfunction at the time of diagnosis were associated with mortality. Although determination of pulmonary pressures is not always possible with screening echocardiography, examination of RV function and indirect measures of PH may permit identification of the highest-risk neonates who may benefit most from entry into applicable clinical trials.

Infection

Neonates with BPD are more susceptible to infection during their initial hospital stay and following discharge, especially in the first few years of life. BPD is an independent variable for late-onset sepsis, including an increased risk for *Candida* infections (130,131). This enhanced susceptibility to infection is a primary reason why neonates with BPD have higher rates of morbidity and mortality. Increased susceptibility to viral and bacterial infection in the first year following discharge is well documented in neonates with BPD (132,133). The severity of infection and risk of mortality are also greater once these viral infections develop. In a meta-analysis of 34 studies examining RSV infections, Szabo et al. (134) reported mortality rates for preterm neonates with BPD at 4.1% compared to 1.2% for preterm neonates without BPD and <1% for neonates who had been born at term.

Since there is a higher risk of RSV infection in preterm neonates with BPD, prophylaxis using Palivizumab has been recommended (135). Palivizumab is effective in preventing RSV-related hospitalization and need for ventilatory support in neonates with BPD. Although there has been significant debate about the cost-effectiveness of the treatment, in the United States RSV prophylaxis is currently recommended to begin for all neonates with BPD born at <29 weeks' gestation who are younger than 12 months CGA at the start of RSV season in the first year of life. During the 2nd year of life, palivizumab prophylaxis is recommended only for neonates with BPD who continue to require support with corticosteroids, diuretics, or supplemental oxygen during the 6-month period before the start of the second RSV season (136).

Neurodevelopment

Although all extremely preterm neonates are at risk for neurodevelopment impairment (NDI), those with BPD have more adverse motor function, worse cognitive development, and poorer academic progress than those without BPD. Nakanishi et al. studied 62 preterm neonates <28 weeks' gestation without BPD, 60 with BPD without PH, and 20 with BPD with PH (127). Multivariate analysis demonstrated that BPD with PH was an independent risk factor for developmental quotient <70 at 3 years of age. Other investigators have also demonstrated that neonates with BPD had worse motor function, cognitive development, and poorer academic performance than those without BPD (137). The need for special education, occupational therapy, speech therapy as well as poorer performance on standardized tests of intelligence, language, and perceptual organization were all significantly higher in neonates with more sBPD at 8 years of age, most likely representing an overall increase in disease severity (138). These effects may be explained by Lee et al. who studied 33 preterm neonates with BPD and 23 without BPD without evidence of focal abnormalities on conventional MRI at term-equivalent age (139). Preterm neonates with BPD had smaller white matter volumes than those without BPD as well as marked reductions in fractional anisotropy in the corpus callosum, corticospinal tract, and superior cerebellar peduncle. These changes suggest that abnormalities in the lung can mirror those occurring in the brain of high-risk neonates.

Growth

Neonates with BPD often grow poorly and are discharged below standard growth curves. Although neonates can grow steadily in the first 2 years of life (if given adequate nutrition to support catch up growth), they still lag behind neonates without BPD with respect to weight, length, and head circumference especially in neonates with more severe forms of BPD (106). Nakanishi et al. also found that in addition to neurodevelopmental delays, somatic growth was reduced in neonates with BPD compared to those without BPD, with further reductions in the group having BPD with PH (127). In childhood and early adulthood, BPD survivors are shorter and lighter with these deficiencies related to the severity of initial illness (122).

REFERENCES

1. Stoll BJ, Hansen NI, Bell EF, et al. Trends in care practices, morbidity, and mortality of extremely preterm neonates, 1993-2012. *JAMA* 2015;314:1039.
2. Northway WH Jr, Rosan RC, Porter DY. Pulmonary disease following respiratory therapy of hyaline-membrane disease. Bronchopulmonary dysplasia. *N Engl J Med* 1967;276:357.
3. Shennan AT, Dunn MS, Ohlsson A, et al. Abnormal pulmonary outcomes in premature infants: prediction from oxygen requirement in the neonatal period. *Pediatrics* 1988;82(4):527.
4. Jobe AH, Bancalari E. Bronchopulmonary dysplasia. *Am J Respir Crit Care Med* 2001;163:1723.
5. Walsh MC, Yao Q, Gettner P, et al. Impact of a physiologic definition on bronchopulmonary dysplasia rates. *Pediatrics* 2004;114(5):1305.
6. Higgins RD, Jobe AH, Koso-Thomas M, et al. Bronchopulmonary dysplasia: executive summary of a workshop. *J Pediatr* 2018;197:300.
7. Poindexter BB, Feng R, Schmidt B, et al. Comparisons and limitations of current definitions of bronchopulmonary dysplasia for the Prematurity and Respiratory Outcomes Program. *Ann Am Thorac Soc* 2015;12(12):1822.
8. van Rossem MC, van de Loo M, Laan BJ, et al. Accuracy of the diagnosis of bronchopulmonary dysplasia in a referral-based health care system. *J Pediatr* 2015;167(3):540.e1.
9. Svedenkrans J, Stoecklin B, Jones JG, et al. Physiology and predictors of impaired gas exchange in infants with bronchopulmonary dysplasia. *Am J Respir Crit Care Med* 2019;200(4):471.
10. Jensen EA, Dysart K, Gantz MG, et al. The diagnosis of bronchopulmonary dysplasia in very preterm infants: an evidence-based approach. *Am J Respir Crit Care Med* 2019;200:751.
11. Abman SH, Collaco JM, Shepherd EG, et al. Interdisciplinary care of children with severe bronchopulmonary dysplasia. *J Pediatr* 2017;181:12.e1.
12. Isayama T, Lee SK, Yang J, et al. Revisiting the definition of bronchopulmonary dysplasia: effect of changing panoply of respiratory support for preterm neonates. *JAMA Pediatr* 2017;171:271.
13. Gage S, Kan P, Oehlert J, et al. Determinants of chronic lung disease severity in the first year of life; A population based study. *Pediatr Pulmonol* 2015;50(9):878.
14. Lapcharoensap W, Gage SC, Kan P, et al. Hospital variation and risk factors for bronchopulmonary dysplasia in a population-based cohort. *JAMA Pediatr* 2015;169(2):e143676.
15. Shah PS, Lui K, Sjors G, et al. Neonatal outcomes of very low birth weight and very preterm neonates: an international comparison. *J Pediatr* 2016;177:144.e6.
16. Younge N, Goldstein RF, Bann CM, et al. Survival and neurodevelopmental outcomes among periviable infants. *N Engl J Med* 2017;376(7):617.
17. Jobe A. Mechanisms of lung injury and bronchopulmonary dysplasia. *Am J Perinatol* 2016;33:1076.
18. McEvoy CT, Spindel ER. Pulmonary effects of maternal smoking on the fetus and child: effects on lung development, respiratory morbidities, and lifelong lung health. *Paediatr Respir Rev* 2017;21:27.
19. Bahadue FL, Soll R. Early versus delayed selective surfactant treatment for neonatal respiratory distress syndrome. *Cochrane Database Syst Rev* 2012;(11):CD001456.
20. Davidovich N, Dipaolo BC, Lawrence GG, et al. Cyclic stretch-induced oxidative stress increases pulmonary alveolar epithelial permeability. *Am J Respir Cell Mol Biol* 2013;49:156.
21. Wu S, Capasso L, Lessa A, et al. High tidal volume ventilation activates Smad2 and upregulates expression of connective tissue growth factor in newborn rat lung. *Pediatr Res* 2008;63:245.
22. Klingenberg C, Wheeler KI, McCallion N, et al. Volume-targeted versus pressure-limited ventilation in neonates. *Cochrane Database Syst Rev* 2017;10:CD003666.
23. Frank L, Groseclose EE. Preparation for birth into an O_2-rich environment: the antioxidant enzymes in the developing rabbit lung. *Pediatr Res* 1984;18:240.
24. Auten RL, Davis JM. Oxygen toxicity and reactive oxygen species: the devil is in the details. *Pediatr Res* 2009;66:121.
25. Askie LM, Darlow BA, Finer N, et al. Association between oxygen saturation targeting and death or disability in extremely preterm infants in the neonatal oxygenation prospective meta-analysis collaboration. *JAMA* 2018;319(21):2190.
26. Oei JL, Vento M, Rabi Y, et al. Higher or lower oxygen for delivery room resuscitation of preterm infants below 28 completed weeks gestation: a meta-analysis. *Arch Dis Child Fetal Neonatal Ed* 2017;102(1):F24.
27. Perez M, Robbins ME, Revhaug C, et al. Oxygen radical disease in the newborn, revisited: oxidative stress and disease in the newborn period. *Free Radic Biol Med* 2019;142:61.
28. Auten RL, O'Reilly MA, Oury TD, et al. Transgenic extracellular superoxide dismutase protects postnatal alveolar epithelial proliferation and development during hyperoxia. *Am J Physiol Lung Cell Mol Physiol* 2006;290:L32.
29. Davis JM, Rosenfeld WN, Sanders RJ, et al. Prophylactic effects of recombinant human superoxide dismutase in neonatal lung injury. *J Appl Physiol* 1993;74:2234.
30. Wright CJ, Kirpalani H. Targeting inflammation to prevent bronchopulmonary dysplasia: can new insights be translated into therapies. *Pediatrics* 2011;128:111.
31. Venkataraman R, Kamaluddeen M, Hasan SU, et al. Intratracheal administration of budesonide-surfactant in prevention of bronchopulmonary dysplasia in very low birth weight infants: a systematic review and meta-analysis. *Pediatr Pulmonol* 2017;52(7):968.
32. Bose C, Laughon M, Allred EN, et al. Blood protein concentrations in the first two postnatal weeks that predict bronchopulmonary dysplasia among infants born before the 28th week of gestation. *Pediatr Res* 2011;69:347.
33. Ambalavanan N, Carlo WA, D'Angio CT, et al. Cytokines associated with bronchopulmonary dysplasia or death in extremely low birth weight infants. *Pediatrics* 2009;123:1132.
34. Mao X, Qiu J, Zhao L, et al. Vitamin D and IL-10 deficiency in preterm neonates with bronchopulmonary dysplasia. *Front Pediatr* 2018;6:246.
35. Villamor-Martinez E, Álvarez-Fuente M, Ghazi AMT, et al. Association of chorioamnionitis with bronchopulmonary dysplasia among preterm infants: a systematic review, meta-analysis, and metaregression. *JAMA Netw Open* 2019;2(11):e1914611.
36. Kim CJ, Romero R, Chaemsaithong P, et al. Acute chorioamnionitis and funisitis: definition, pathologic features, and clinical significance. *Am J Obstet Gynecol* 2015;213(4 suppl):S29.
37. Choi CW, Kim B, Hong JS, et al. Bronchopulmonary dysplasia in a rat model induced by intra-amniotic inflammation and postnatal hyperoxia: morphometric aspects. *Pediatr Res* 2009;65:323.
38. Hartling L, Liang Y, Lacaze-Masmonteil T. Chorioamnionitis as a risk factor for bronchopulmonary dysplasia: a systematic review and meta-analysis. *Arch Dis Child Fetal Neonatal Ed* 2012;97(1):F8.
39. Silwedel C, Speer CP, Glaser K. Ureaplasma-associated prenatal, perinatal, and neonatal morbidities. *Expert Rev Clin Immunol* 2017;13(11):1073.
40. Viscardi RM, Kallapur SG. Role of ureaplasma respiratory tract colonization in bronchopulmonary dysplasia pathogenesis: current concepts and update. *Clin Perinatol* 2015;42(4):719.
41. Glaser K, Gradzka-Luczewska A, Szymankiewicz-Breborowicz M, Kaweczynska-Leda N, et al. Perinatal *Ureaplasma* exposure is associated with increased risk of late onset sepsis and imbalanced inflammation in preterm infants and may add to lung injury. *Front Cell Infect Microbiol* 2019;9:68.
42. Kim SH, Chun J, Ko KH, et al. Effect of antenatal azithromycin for Ureaplasma spp. on neonatal outcome at ≤30 weeks' gestational age. *Pediatr Int* 2019;61(1):58.
43. Merchan LM, Hassan HE, Terrin ML. Pharmacokinetics, microbial response, and pulmonary outcomes of multidose intravenous azithromycin in preterm infants at risk for Ureaplasma respiratory colonization. *Antimicrob Agents Chemother* 2015;59(1):570.
44. Lal CV, Kandasamy J, Dolma K, et al. Early airway microbial metagenomic and metabolomic signatures are associated with development of severe bronchopulmonary dysplasia. *Am J Physiol Lung Cell Mol Physiol* 2018;315(5):L810.
45. Pammi M, Lal CV, Wagner BD, et al. Airway microbiome and development of bronchopulmonary dysplasia in preterm infants: a systematic review. *J Pediatr* 2019;204:126.e2.
46. Jung E, Lee BS. Late-onset sepsis as a risk factor for bronchopulmonary dysplasia in extremely low birth weight infants: a nationwide cohort study. *Sci Rep* 2019;9(1):15448.
47. Stoll BJ, Fanaroff AA, Wright LL, et al. Late-onset sepsis in very low birth weight neonates: the experience of the NICHD network. *Pediatrics* 2002;110:285.
48. Huang J, Zhang L, Tang J, et al. Human milk as a protective factor for bronchopulmonary dysplasia: a systematic review and meta-analysis. *Arch Dis Child Fetal Neonatal Ed* 2019;104(2):F128.
49. Villamor-Martínez E, Pierro M, Cavallaro G, et al. Mother's own milk and bronchopulmonary dysplasia: a systematic review and meta-analysis. *Front Pediatr* 2019;7:224.
50. O'Dell BL, Kilburn KH, McKenzie WN, et al. The lung of the copper-deficient rat: a model for developmental pulmonary emphysema. *Am J Pathol* 1978;91:413.
51. Shenai JP, Rush MG, Stahlman MT, et al. Plasma retinol-binding protein response to vitamin A administration in infants susceptible to bronchopulmonary dysplasia. *J Pediatr* 1990;116:607.
52. Darlow BA, Graham PJ, Rojas-Reyes MX. Vitamin A supplementation for preventing morbidity and mortality in very low birth weight infants. *Cochrane Database Syst Rev* 2016;(8):CD000501.
53. Anzano MA, Olson JA, Lamb AJ. Morphologic alterations in the trachea and the salivary gland following the induction of rapid synchronous vitamin A deficiency in rats. *Am J Pathol* 1980;98:717.
54. Araki S, Kato S, Namba F, et al. Vitamin A to prevent bronchopulmonary dysplasia in extremely low birth weight infants: a systematic review and meta-analysis. *PLoS One* 2018;13(11):e0207730.

55. Ambalavanan N, Tyson JE, Kennedy KA, et al. Vitamin A supplementation for extremely low birth weight infants: outcome at 18 to 22 months. *Pediatrics* 2005;115:e249.

56. Gawronski CA, Gawronski CH. Vitamin A supplementation for prevention of bronchopulmonary dysplasia: cornerstone of care or futile therapy? *Ann Pharmacother* 2016;50(8):680.

57. Sellmer A, Bjerre JV, Schmidt MR, et al. Morbidity and mortality in preterm neonates with patent ductus arteriosus on day 3. *Arch Dis Child Fetal Neonatal Ed* 2013;98:F505.

58. Liebowitz M, Clyman RI. Prophylactic indomethacin compared with delayed conservative management of the patent ductus arteriosus in extremely preterm infants: effects on neonatal outcomes. *J Pediatr* 2017;187:119.e1.

59. Hundscheid T, Onland W, van Overmeire B, et al. Early treatment versus expectative management of patent ductus arteriosus in preterm infants: a multicentre, randomised, non-inferiority trial in Europe (BeNeDuctus trial). *BMC Pediatr* 2018;18(1):262.

60. Nickerson BG, Taussig LM. Family history of asthma in infants with bronchopulmonary dysplasia. *Pediatrics* 1980;65:1140.

61. Lavoie PM, Pham C, Jang KL. Heritability of bronchopulmonary dysplasia defined according to the consensus statement of the National Institutes of Health. *Pediatrics* 2008;122:479.

62. Parad RB, Winston AB, Kalish LA, et al. Role of genetic susceptibility in the development of bronchopulmonary dysplasia. *J Pediatr* 2018;203:234.e2.

63. Hadchousel A, Durrmeyer X, Bouzigon E, et al. Identification of SPOCK2 as a susceptibility gene for bronchopulmonary dysplasia. *Am J Respir Crit Care Med* 2011;184:1164.

64. Floros J, Londono D, Gordon D, et al. IL-18R1 and IL-18RAP SNPs may be associated with bronchopulmonary dysplasia in African-American infants. *Pediatr Res* 2012;71:107.

65. Hamvas A, Feng R, Bi Y, et al. Exome sequencing identifies gene variants and networks associated with extreme respiratory outcomes following preterm birth. *BMC Genet* 2018;19(1):94.

66. Higano NS, Spielberg DR, Fleck RJ, et al. Neonatal pulmonary magnetic resonance imaging of bronchopulmonary dysplasia predicts short-term clinical outcomes. *Am J Respir Crit Care Med* 2018;198(10):1302.

67. Critser PJ, Higano NS, Tkach JA, et al. Cardiac MRI evaluation of neonatal bronchopulmonary dysplasia associated pulmonary hypertension. *Am J Respir Crit Care Med* 2020;201(1):73. doi: 10.1164/rccm.201904-0826OC

68. Arjaans S, Zwart EAH, Ploegstra MJ, et al. Identification of gaps in the current knowledge on pulmonary hypertension in extremely preterm infants: a systematic review and meta-analysis. *Paediatr Perinat Epidemiol* 2018;32(3):258.

69. Mestan KK, Gotteiner N, Porta N, et al. Cord blood biomarkers of placental maternal vascular underperfusion predict bronchopulmonary dysplasia-associated pulmonary hypertension. *J Pediatr* 2017;185:33.

70. Mourani PM, Sontag MK, Younoszai A, et al. Early pulmonary vascular disease in preterm infants at risk for bronchopulmonary dysplasia. *Am J Respir Crit Care Med* 2015;191(1):87.

71. Mourani PM, Mandell EW, Meier M, et al. Early pulmonary vascular disease in preterm infants is associated with late respiratory outcomes in childhood. *Am J Respir Crit Care Med* 2019;199(8):1020.

72. Krishnan U, Feinstein JA, Adatia I, et al. Evaluation and management of pulmonary hypertension in children with bronchopulmonary dysplasia. *J Pediatr* 2017;188:24.e1.

73. Levy PT, Jain A, Nawaytou H, et al. Risk assessment and monitoring of chronic pulmonary hypertension in premature infants. *J Pediatr* 2020;217:199. doi: 10.1016/j.jpeds.2019.10.034

74. Cherukupalli K, Larson JE, Rotschild A, et al. Biochemical, clinical, and morphologic studies on lungs of infants with bronchopulmonary dysplasia. *Pediatr Pulmonol* 1996;22:215.

75. Surate Solaligue DE, Rodríguez-Castillo JA, Ahlbrecht K, et al. Recent advances in our understanding of the mechanisms of late lung development and bronchopulmonary dysplasia. *Am J Physiol Lung Cell Mol Physiol* 2017;313:L1101.

76. Silva DM, Nardiello C, Pozarska A, et al. Recent advances in the mechanisms of lung alveolarization and the pathogenesis of bronchopulmonary dysplasia. *Am J Physiol Lung Cell Mol Physiol* 2015;309:L1239.

77. Ganguly A, Martin RJ. Vulnerability of the developing airway. *Respir Physiol Neurobiol* 2019;270:103263. doi: 10.1016/j.resp.2019.103263

78. Lignelli E, Palumbo F, Myti D, et al. Recent advances in our understanding of the mechanisms of lung alveolarization and bronchopulmonary dysplasia. *Am J Physiol Lung Cell Mol Physiol* 2019;317(6):L832. doi: 10.1152/ajplung.00369.2019

79. Committee on Fetus and Newborn. Respiratory support in preterm infants at birth. *Pediatrics* 2014;133(1):171.

80. Kribs A, Roll C, Gopel W, et al. Nonintubated surfactant application vs conventional therapy in extremely preterm infants: a randomized clinical trial. *JAMA Pediatr* 2015;169(8):723.

81. Dargaville PA, Aiyappan A, De Paoli AG, et al. Minimally-invasive surfactant therapy in preterm infants on continuous positive airway pressure. *Arch Dis Child Fetal Neonatal Ed* 2013;98(2):F122.

82. Aldana-Aguirre JC, Pinto M, Featherstone RM, et al. Less invasive surfactant administration versus intubation for surfactant delivery in preterm infants with respiratory distress syndrome: a systematic review and meta-analysis. *Arch Dis Child Fetal Neonatal Ed* 2017;102(1):F17.

83. Ballard RA, Keller RL, Black DM, et al. Randomized trial of late surfactant treatment in ventilated preterm infants receiving inhaled nitric oxide. *J Pediatr* 2016;168:23.e4.

84. Keller RL, Eichenwald EC, Hibbs AM, et al. The randomized, controlled trial of late surfactant: effects on respiratory outcomes at 1-year corrected age. *J Pediatr* 2017;183:19.e2.

85. Gadhia MM, Cutter GR, Abman SH, et al. Effects of early inhaled nitric oxide therapy and vitamin A supplementation on the risk for bronchopulmonary dysplasia in premature newborns with respiratory failure. *J Pediatr* 2014;164(4):744.

86. Schmidt B, Roberts RS, Davis P, et al. Caffeine therapy for apnea of prematurity. *N Engl J Med* 2006;354(20):2112.

87. Kua KP, Lee SW. Systematic review and meta-analysis of clinical outcomes of early caffeine therapy in preterm neonates. *Br J Clin Pharmacol* 2017;83(1):180.

88. Lodha A, Entz R, Synnes A, et al. Early caffeine administration and neurodevelopmental outcomes in preterm infants. *Pediatrics* 2019;143(1). doi: 10.1542/peds.2018-1348

89. Roberts D, Brown J, Medley N, et al. Antenatal corticosteroids for accelerating fetal lung maturation for women at risk of preterm birth. *Cochrane Database Syst Rev* 2017;3:CD004454.

90. Halliday HL, Ehrenkranz RA, Doyle LW. Early (<8 days) postnatal corticosteroids for preventing chronic lung disease in preterm infants. *Cochrane Database Syst Rev* 2010(1):CD001146.

91. Doyle LW, Halliday HL, Ehrenkranz RA, et al. An update on the impact of postnatal systemic corticosteroids on mortality and cerebral palsy in preterm infants: effect modification by risk of bronchopulmonary dysplasia. *J Pediatr* 2014;165(6):1258.

92. Baud O, Maury L, Lebail F, et al. Effect of early low-dose hydrocortisone on survival without bronchopulmonary dysplasia in extremely preterm infants (PREMILOC): a double-blind, placebo-controlled, multicentre, randomised trial. *Lancet* 2016;387(10030):1827.

93. Baud O, Trousson C, Biran V, et al. Association between early low-dose hydrocortisone therapy in extremely preterm neonates and neurodevelopmental outcomes at 2 years of age. *JAMA* 2017;317(13):1329.

94. Shaffer ML, Baud O, Lacaze-Masmonteil T, et al. Effect of prophylaxis for early adrenal insufficiency using low-dose hydrocortisone in very preterm infants: an individual patient data meta-analysis. *J Pediatr* 2019;207:136.e5.

95. Bassler D, Plavka R, Shinwell ES, et al. Early inhaled budesonide for the prevention of bronchopulmonary dysplasia. *N Engl J Med* 2015;373(16):1497.

96. Bassler D, Shinwell ES, Hallman M, et al. Long-term effects of inhaled budesonide for bronchopulmonary dysplasia. *N Engl J Med* 2018; 378(2):148.

97. Yeh TF, Chen CM, Wu SY, et al. Intratracheal administration of budesonide/surfactant to prevent bronchopulmonary dysplasia. *Am J Respir Crit Care Med* 2016;193(1):86.

98. Fujinaga H, Baker CD, Ryan SL, et al. Hyperoxia disrupts vascular endothelial growth factor-nitric oxide signaling and decreases growth of endothelial colony-forming cells from preterm infants. *Am J Physiol Lung Cell Mol Physiol* 2009;297(6):L1160.

99. Mercier JC, Olivier P, Loron G, et al. Inhaled nitric oxide to prevent bronchopulmonary dysplasia in preterm neonates. *Semin Fetal Neonatal Med* 2009;14(1):28.

100. Cole FS, Alleyne C, Barks JD, et al. NIH Consensus development conference statement: inhaled nitric-oxide therapy for premature infants. *Pediatrics* 2011;127(2):363.

101. Askie LM, Davies LC, Schreiber MD, et al. Race effects of inhaled nitric oxide in preterm infants: an individual participant data meta-analysis. *J Pediatr* 2018;193:34.e2.

102. Luo J, Shepard S, Nilan K, et al. Improved growth and developmental activity post tracheostomy in preterm infants with severe BPD. *Pediatr Pulmonol* 2018;53(9):1237.

103. Supplemental therapeutic oxygen for prethreshold retinopathy of prematurity (STOP-ROP), a randomized, controlled trial. I: primary outcomes. *Pediatrics* 2000;105(2):295.

104. Askie LM, Henderson-Smart DJ, Irwig L, et al. Oxygen-saturation targets and outcomes in extremely preterm infants. *N Engl J Med* 2003;349(10):959.

105. DeMauro SB, Jensen EA, Bann CM, et al. Home oxygen and 2-year outcomes of preterm infants with bronchopulmonary dysplasia. *Pediatrics* 2019;143(5). doi: 10.1542/peds.2018-2956

106. Poindexter BB, Martin CR. Impact of nutrition on bronchopulmonary dysplasia. *Clin Perinatol* 2015;42(4):797.

107. Farhath S, He Z, Nakhla T, et al. Pepsin, a marker of gastric contents, is increased in tracheal aspirates from preterm infants who develop bronchopulmonary dysplasia. *Pediatrics* 2008;121(2):e253.

108. McGrath-Morrow SA, Hayashi M, Aherrera AD, et al. Respiratory outcomes of children with BPD and gastrostomy tubes during the first 2 years of life. *Pediatr Pulmonol* 2014;49(6):537.
109. Bamat NA, Kirpalani H, Feudtner C, et al. Medication use in infants with severe bronchopulmonary dysplasia admitted to United States children's hospitals. *J Perinatol* 2019;39(9):1291.
110. Slaughter JL, Stenger MR, Reagan PB, et al. Inhaled bronchodilator use for infants with bronchopulmonary dysplasia. *J Perinatol* 2015;35(1):61.
111. Gien J, Kinsella J, Thrasher J, et al. Retrospective analysis of an interdisciplinary ventilator care program intervention on survival of infants with ventilator-dependent bronchopulmonary dysplasia. *Am J Perinatol* 2017;34(2):155.
112. Islam JY, Keller RL, Aschner JL, et al. Understanding the short- and long-term respiratory outcomes of prematurity and bronchopulmonary dysplasia. *Am J Respir Crit Care Med* 2015;192(2):134.
113. Gough A, Spence D, Linden M, et al. General and respiratory health outcomes in adult survivors of bronchopulmonary dysplasia. *Chest* 2012;141:1554.
114. Gough A, Linden M, Spene D, et al. Impaired lung function and health status in adult survivors of bronchopulmonary dysplasia. *Eur Respir J* 2013;10:1183.
115. Jackson WM, O'Shea TM, Allred EN, et al. Risk factors for chronic lung disease and asthma differ among children born extremely preterm. *Pediatr Pulmonol* 2018;53(11):1533.
116. Lombardi E, Fainardi V, Calogero C, et al. Lung function in a cohort of 5-year-old children born very preterm. *Pediatr Pulmonol* 2018;53(12):1633.
117. Sanchez-Solis M, Perez-Fernandez V, Bosch-Gimenez V, et al. Lung function gain in preterm infants with and without bronchopulmonary dysplasia. *Pediatr Pulmonol* 2016;51(9):936.
118. Kjellberg M, Sanchez-Crespo A, Jonsson B. Ten-year-old children with a history of bronchopulmonary dysplasia have regional abnormalities in ventilation perfusion matching. *Pediatr Pulmonol* 2019;54(5):602.
119. Overman AE, Meixia L, Kurachek SC, et al. Tracheostomy for infants requiring prolonged mechanical ventilation: 10 years' experience. *Pediatrics* 2013;131:e1491.
120. Cristea AI, Carroll AE, Davis SD, et al. Outcomes of children with severe bronchopulmonary dysplasia who were ventilator dependent at home. *Pediatrics* 2013;132:e727.
121. Filburn AG, Popova AP, Linn MJ, et al. Longitudinal measures of lung function in infants with bronchopulmonary dysplasia. *Pediatr Pulmonol* 2011;46:369.
122. Doyle LW, Anderson PJ. Adult outcome of extremely preterm infants. *Pediatrics* 2010;126:342.
123. Thunqvist P, Tufvesson E, Bjermer L, et al. Lung function after extremely preterm birth-A population-based cohort study (EXPRESS). *Pediatr Pulmonol* 2018;53(1):64.
124. Simpson SJ, Turkovic L, Wilson AC, et al. Lung function trajectories throughout childhood in survivors of very preterm birth: a longitudinal cohort study. *Lancet Child Adolesc Health* 2018;2(5):350.
125. Lagatta JM, Hysinger EB, Zaniletti I, et al. The impact of pulmonary hypertension in preterm infants with severe bronchopulmonary dysplasia through 1 Year. *J Pediatr* 2018;203:218.e3.
126. Vayalthrikkovil S, Vorhies E, Stritzke A, et al. Prospective study of pulmonary hypertension in preterm infants with bronchopulmonary dysplasia. *Pediatr Pulmonol* 2019;54(2):171.
127. Nakanishi H, Uchiyama A, Kusuda S. Impact of pulmonary hypertension on neurodevelopmental outcome in preterm infants with bronchopulmonary dysplasia: a cohort study. *J Perinatol* 2016;36(10):890.
128. Eventov-Friedman S, Kanevsky H, Bar-Oz B. Neonatal end of life care: a single center NICU experience in Israel over a decade. *Pediatrics* 2013;131:e1889.
129. Altit G, Bhombal S, Feinstein J, et al. Diminished right ventricular function at diagnosis of pulmonary hypertension is associated with mortality in bronchopulmonary dysplasia. *Pulm Circ* 2019;9(3):2045894019878598.
130. Makhoul IR, Sujov P, Smolkin T, et al. Epidemiological, clinical, and microbiological characteristics of late-onset sepsis among very low birth weight infants in Israel: a national survey. *Pediatrics* 2002;109:34.
131. Makhoul IR, Bental Y, Weisbrod M, et al. Candidal versus bacterial late-onset sepsis in very low birthweight infants in Israel: a national survey. *J Hosp Infect* 2007;65:237.
132. Akangire G, Manimtim W, Nyp MF, et al. Clinical outcomes among diagnostic subgroups of infants with severe bronchopulmonary dysplasia through 2 years of age. *Am J Perinatol* 2018;35(14):1376.
133. Pryhuber GS. Postnatal infections and immunology affecting chronic lung disease of prematurity. *Clin Perinatol* 2015;42(4):697.
134. Szabo SM, Gooch KL, Bibby MM, et al. The risk of mortality among young children hospitalized for severe respiratory syncytial virus infection. *Paediatr Respir Rev* 2013;13:S1.
135. Winterstein AG, Choi Y, Meissner HC. Association of age with risk of hospitalization for respiratory syncytial virus in preterm infants with chronic lung disease. *JAMA Pediatr* 2018;172(2):154.
136. American Academy of Pediatrics Committee on Infectious Diseases. Updated guidance for palivizumab prophylaxis among infants and young children at increased risk of hospitalization for respiratory syncytial virus infection. *Pediatrics* 2014;134(2):e620.
137. Cheong JLY, Doyle LW. An update on pulmonary and neurodevelopmental outcomes of bronchopulmonary dysplasia. *Semin Perinatol* 2018;42(7):478.
138. Short EJ, Klein NK, Lewis BA, et al. Cognitive and academic consequences of bronchopulmonary dysplasia and very low birth weight: 8-year-old outcomes. *Pediatrics* 2003;112(5):e359.
139. Lee JM, Choi YH, Hong J, et al. Bronchopulmonary dysplasia is associated with altered brain volumes and white matter microstructure in preterm infants. *Neonatology* 2019;116(2):163.

30 Surgical Management of the Airway and Lungs

Alison Maresh, Annie Harrington, Peter S. Midulla, and Vikash K. Modi

WORKUP OF AIRWAY OBSTRUCTION

It is critical to promptly evaluate and manage airway lesions in neonates. Initial symptoms often include noisy breathing and possible signs of increased work of breathing or distress. Desaturations are often a late sign of airway obstruction.

Clinical Examination

In some patients the cause of airway obstruction may be immediately obvious such as in an infant with micrognathia or other facial dysmorphisms. However, often diagnosis will require further investigation. An experienced practitioner can often isolate the site of the lesion by the type of noisy breathing. Nasal obstruction creates a different type of noise than palate/base of tongue obstruction. Stridor can be classified as inspiratory, expiratory, or biphasic. Inspiratory stridor is often associated with supraglottic and glottic obstruction; biphasic stridor is often associated with glottic, subglottic, and tracheal obstruction, while expiratory stridor is usually seen with tracheal or lower airway pathology. It should be noted that with smaller infants and preterm infants, noisy breathing that suggests obstruction may not be easily audible, especially in a noisy hospital environment. Auscultation over the upper airways with a stethoscope can be useful in evaluation.

Fiberoptic Evaluation

Flexible fiberoptic evaluation can be performed to assess the full supraglottic airway and is usually performed by an otolaryngologist. The standard pediatric flexible rhinoscope measures 2.2 to 2.7 mm in diameter and should be able to be easily passed transnasally in all but the smallest preterm infants (for comparison, a standard size 2.5 endotracheal tube [ETT] has an external diameter of 3.5 mm). Full assessment should include passage through both nostrils to assess for nasal lesions and patency, and passage into the nasopharynx to view the full supraglottic airway including the base of tongue, vallecula, supraglottis, and vocal folds. The goal is to assess for structural anomalies, abnormal lesions, signs of inflammation, as well as functional anomalies. This is a stimulating procedure that usually causes babies to cry and therefore may miss dynamic obstruction that occurs only during relaxation or sleep.

Drug-Induced Sleep Endoscopy

There are several techniques that can be used to assess the infant airway in the operating room if bedside assessment is unable to identify the pathology. Drug-induced sleep endoscopy (DISE) (1) is a valuable technique to evaluate for dynamic airway obstruction during sleep. It requires collaboration with anesthesia to provide a state of sleep with spontaneous ventilation. It can show changes in the airway tone, sleep-dependent laryngomalacia, and base of tongue collapse that cannot be seen during an awake bedside scope.

Direct Laryngoscopy and Bronchoscopy

Direct laryngoscopy and bronchoscopy (DLB) is the classic technique for evaluating the subglottic and tracheal airway and can better define lesions such as laryngeal cleft or tracheoesophageal fistula. A rigid bronchoscope is passed during direct laryngoscopy visualization to assess the larynx, subglottis, trachea, and mainstem bronchi (Fig. 30.1). In addition to evaluating for obstructive lesions, anatomic anomalies, and dynamic airway changes, it is standard during an airway evaluation under anesthesia to measure the size of the airway by assessing for a leak around a cuffless ETT. The Myer-Cotton scale grades subglottic stenosis (SGS) on a severity of 1 to 4 based on the age-adjusted expected airway size and the size ETT that fits in the airway with an air leak at less than 30 cm water (2).

Airway evaluation under anesthesia is a diagnostic technique, but interventions may be performed at the same time as further described in the individual pathology sections.

Initial Stabilization of the Airway

For babies in distress, stabilization of the respiratory status may need to occur whether or not the cause of obstruction has been fully evaluated. For anticipated difficult airway management, a multidisciplinary team including pediatric anesthesia and otolaryngology should be involved if possible given time and availability. Nasal cannula oxygen can be applied assuming patency of the nares. Pressure support can be administered transnasally with or without additional oxygen via high-flow nasal cannula (HFNC) or continuous positive airway pressure (CPAP). Intubation can be performed with caution as various obstructive pathologies may preclude classic direct laryngoscopy techniques. A laryngeal mask airway (LMA) can be helpful as placement may be performed without the need for direct laryngoscopy, and some types of LMAs can be used to facilitate fiberoptic intubation as long as the distal opening is not obstructed. Fiberoptic intubation may be also performed for infants with craniofacial dysmorphisms, classically in infants with micrognathia, macroglossia, or cervical spine abnormalities where direct laryngoscopy techniques are not possible.

For any intubation care should be taken to use a correct size ETT; a tube that is too small will result in a large leak and ventilation will be difficult, while a tube that is too large will cause glottic and subglottic trauma, which may result in long-term complications such as stenosis. A full-term infant has a subglottic diameter of about 4.5 to 5.5 mm. The size of an ETT refers to the inner diameter. The outer diameter of a 3.0 ETT is 4.3 mm and the outer diameter of a 3.5 ETT is 4.9 mm; hence these are appropriate tube sizes to consider for full-term infants, while 2.0 and 2.5 ETTs should be available for premature infants.

Often, a congenital anomaly may be identified during prenatal ultrasound assessment that suggests that the airway will be compromised at birth. Such abnormal lesions may include micrognathia, macroglossia, oral lesions such as an epignathus, fetal neck masses, or congenital high airway obstruction syndrome (CHAOS). In these cases, a multidisciplinary team may be appropriate to plan a strategy for airway management at birth. One option is to have a care team present at birth, which may be timed with induction or C-section. This team may include neonatal intensivists, pediatric anesthesia, pediatric surgery, and pediatric otolaryngology. If securing a safe airway on delivery is deemed particularly challenging, an ex utero intrapartum treatment (EXIT) procedure may be warranted. This involves a partial Cesarean section delivery with maintenance of uteroplacental circulation, which allows extra time for management of the airway. Airway management options include intubation, tracheotomy, establishing extracorporeal membrane oxygenation, or resection of an obstructing mass (3). Additional possible indications for an EXIT procedure may include mediastinal masses, congenital diaphragmatic hernia (CDH), severe congenital heart defects, congenital pulmonary airway malformation (CPAM), and bronchopulmonary sequestrations.

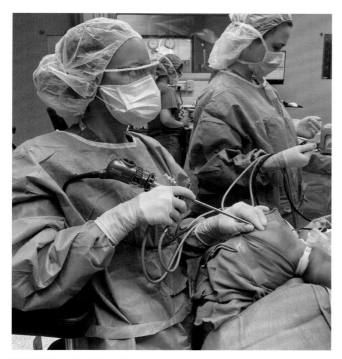

FIGURE 30.1 Technique for rigid direct laryngoscopy and bronchoscopy in an infant. (Image courtesy of Dr Alison Maresh.)

NASAL PATHOLOGY

Infants are obligate nasal breathers, and nasal obstruction warrants expeditious evaluation. The soft palate hangs below the posterior tongue and contacts the epiglottis; this facilitates a separation of the airway during feeding; however it makes breathing through the mouth difficult. The ability to breathe comfortably through the mouth develops with time, usually around 4 months of age. Complete nasal obstruction in a newborn will result in cyclical episodes of cyanosis and crying. The palate is elevated during crying, which allows for oral breathing; then, as the infant calms and stops crying, the palate relaxes and obstructs oral breathing causing recurrent obstruction, cyanosis, and crying. Partial obstruction of the nose causes nasal stertor, and depending on the severity of the obstruction, may result in signs of increased work of breathing. This is frequently particularly severe during feeding where there is both exertion and a complete reliance on nasal breathing.

Rhinitis

The most common reason for nasal obstruction is neonatal rhinitis. This can only be formally diagnosed after ruling out structural abnormalities by endoscopic evaluation. Findings include swollen mucosa with narrowed nasal cavities, sometimes with excess mucus. There are several potential causes including infection, reflux, trauma, and allergy; however, frequently it is idiopathic.

Infection is usually due to viral upper respiratory infections (URI) and is diagnosed based on associated viral symptoms and short temporal course with resolution of symptoms usually by 2 weeks. If symptoms seem to be from a URI but last longer with the presence of purulent secretions in the nose, it may have turned into a secondary bacterial rhinitis/adenoiditis and antibiotics may be warranted. Bacterial rhinitis may also be due to maternal transmission of chlamydia or syphilis during delivery, although this is rare.

Reflux rhinitis develops from inflammation of the delicate nasal mucosa from reflux material, which in infants frequently extends

into the nose. Traumatic rhinitis can develop from overaggressive suctioning or from nasal instrumentation with feeding tubes or cannulas for respiratory support. Allergic rhinitis may also be considered in infants. Environmental allergies are rare in younger infants as they develop from repeated exposure; however, food allergies can occur in young infants with first exposure and may manifest with nasal congestion and rhinorrhea. Cow's milk protein allergy is the most common food allergy. Allergy is frequently accompanied by additional symptoms of fussiness/crying, skin changes such as eczema, and stool changes such as excess mucus or blood.

Treatment for idiopathic rhinitis is largely observation. As long as the infant is breathing comfortably and able to feed well with good weight gain, it is not necessary to treat mild symptoms of nasal obstruction. For the more severely symptomatic infant, gentle saline drops, steam, saline nebulizers, and very limited judicious suctioning can help to manage the symptoms. Topical decongestion medications such as oxymetazoline and phenylephrine can be used carefully and only for short courses due to the risk of rebound congestion. Topical steroids can also be effective but again should be very limited in use due to high absorption and risk for iatrogenic adrenal insufficiency (4).

Nasolacrimal Duct Pathology

Obstruction of the nasolacrimal duct at the level of the nasal cavity can result in a nasolacrimal duct cyst (NLDC) and is another unusual cause for nasal obstruction. The duct opens anteriorly in the nose under the inferior turbinate. If the mucosal opening is not patent, a cystic mass will develop and can obstruct the nose (Fig. 30.2). These NLDCs can be unilateral or bilateral. The lacrimal sac will often cause another area of bluish swelling medial to the eye. Treatment involves unroofing the NLDC intranasally. Concurrent probing of the nasolacrimal system by ophthalmology can confirm full patency with visualization of the probe tip in the nose. Recurrence is rare.

Congenital Nasal Pyriform Aperture Stenosis

Congenital nasal pyriform aperture stenosis (CNPAS) causes bilateral nasal obstruction (but not total occlusion) anteriorly at the level of the nasal bony aperture with symptoms ranging from minimal intermittent noisy breathing to life-threatening obstruction. Inability to pass a small 5- or 6-Fr suction catheter or a pediatric-size

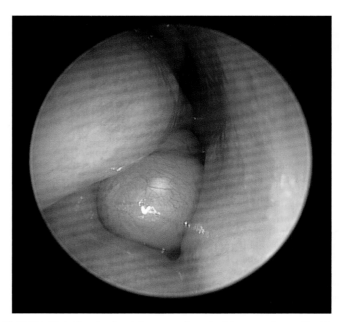

FIGURE 30.2 Nasolacrimal duct cyst viewed with a zero-degree Hopkins rod telescope. Note the cyst is inferior to the inferior turbinate and can result in near-total occlusion of the nasal cavity. (Image courtesy of Dr. Vikash Modi.)

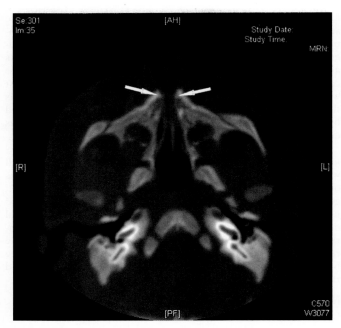

FIGURE 30.3 Axial CT scan without contrast demonstrating bilateral bony overgrowth of the nasal aperture (*arrows*) resulting in pyriform aperture stenosis. Note the posterior choanae are patent. (Image courtesy of Dr. Vikash Modi.)

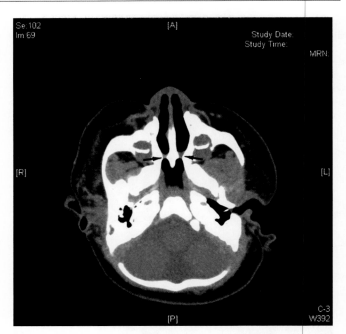

FIGURE 30.4 Axial CT scan without contrast demonstrating a mixed (bony and membranous) choanal atresia bilaterally (*arrows*). Note the anterior nasal pyriform is patent. (Image courtesy of Dr. Vikash Modi.)

flexible rhinoscope through the anterior aspect of the nares should causes suspicion for this pathology, which is confirmed by imaging (Fig. 30.3). There are no standard diagnostic criteria for the size of the pyriform aperture, although generally an opening less than 11 mm is consistent with CNPAS (5) while an opening less than about 6 mm is associated with need for surgical intervention (6). There is often an associated narrowing of the entire nasal cavity. If pyriform aperture stenosis is accompanied by a single central upper incisor, it may be part of solitary median maxillary central incisor (SMMCI) syndrome, which is associated with other midline defects including holoprosencephaly, endocrine abnormalities, congenital heart disease, and others warranting workup (7).

Treatment may include a trial of medication therapy with neosynephrine or oxymetazoline or with topical steroids; however due to concerns about rhinitis medicamentosa and adrenal suppression, long-term therapy should be used with extreme caution. If medical therapy is ineffective or infants are unable to be weaned off these medications, surgical intervention may be warranted. Surgery involves creating a sublabial incision to access the pyriform aperture and drilling the bony opening to widen it. The degree of opening is limited by the dental roots inferiorly and the nasolacrimal system posteriorly. As CNPAS is often accompanied by narrowing of the full nasal cavity, surgical opening of the pyriform aperture may also be accompanied by surgical reduction of the turbinates intranasally (8).

Choanal Atresia

Choanal atresia is the complete obstruction of the opening between the posterior nasal cavity and the nasopharynx. It can be unilateral or bilateral, and the nature of the barrier may be bony, membranous, or mixed (Fig. 30.4). In cases of bilateral choanal atresia there is complete nasal airway obstruction causing cyclic cyanosis in infants requiring intubation and urgent management. The incidence is between 1:5,000 and 1:7,000 births with female predominance (9). It may be an isolated anomaly or can be associated with a syndrome such as CHARGE syndrome. Given this possibility, genetic evaluation should take place, and preoperative cardiac assessment should be performed.

Treatment for the obstructed choana is surgical. Several approaches have been described without any identified benefit to any of the individual techniques (10). The most common technique is the endoscopic transnasal approach using various endoscopic instrumentation including drills and a microdebrider. Partial removal of the posterior septum decreases the incidence of restenosis. Postoperative stenting is controversial (11).

Nasal Septal Deviation

Due to intrauterine positioning the nose may appear asymmetric at birth. In the majority of cases this will straighten without intervention, although some do advocate for early taping to restore symmetry while the cartilage is still moldable. Management of traumatic dislocation of the septum is controversial, and intervention can be considered based on severity of symptoms.

Dermoids, Gliomas, and Encephaloceles

Nasal dermoids, gliomas, and encephaloceles are congenital lesions that may present with symptoms of obstruction and/or as a visible mass. Dermoids are congenital lesions that are lined with epithelium and contain dermal appendages. They may be a cyst, sinus, or fistula. They occur due to incomplete obliteration of neuroectoderm during development of the frontonasal process and can present as a mass anywhere from the glabella to the nasal tip, most commonly on the nasal dorsum (12). There may exist an intracranial extension, and MRI and CT imaging are recommended to better evaluate for this possibility (13).

An encephalocele is caused by the herniation of cranial contents through a defect in the skull base with communication of cerebrospinal fluid (CSF) within the mass. Encephaloceles tend to be bluish, compressible masses that transilluminate and can expand with crying, straining, or compressing the jugular vein. If the mass contains meninges, it is considered a meningocele; if it contains both brain and meninges, it is called a meningoencephalocele. Gliomas are masses of glial tissue that no longer communicate with the CSF; however, a small percentage will have a fibrous stalk that extends intracranially. They tend to be firm and do not change in size with straining or other maneuvers that elevate intracranial pressure. Imaging with MRI and CT again is critical both to define the external anatomy as well as to identify intracranial extension.

Surgical management of encephaloceles as well as gliomas and dermoids that have intracranial extension should be coordinated with neurosurgery and otolaryngology. Surgical management of lesions without internal connections may be deferred until the patient is older unless there is significant obstructive pathology. Delaying surgery until the child is bigger may provide more favorable cosmetic outcomes but must be balanced with the possibility of the lesion causing abnormal nasal development. Depending on the location and extent of the lesion the approach can be external, endoscopic, or via an open rhinoplasty approach (13). Recurrence is likely if the entire lesion and tract is not completely removed.

ORAL CAVITY/OROPHARYNX

Lesions of the Tongue

The tongue may be a source of airway obstruction in infants if it is too large, it is too posteriorly positioned as in infants with retro/micrognathia and glossoptosis, or there is an intralingual tumor, cyst, or other lesion. A large tongue is one of the hallmark features of Beckwith-Wiedemann syndrome (**Fig. 30.5**), which also includes findings of general overgrowth, abdominal wall defects, neonatal hypoglycemia, and predisposition to embryonal tumors (14). In addition to airway obstruction, macroglossia may cause feeding difficulty and eventual speech problems. If there are acute symptoms of airway obstruction a nasopharyngeal airway that bypasses the tongue base may be used temporarily. Tracheotomy may be necessary, and improvement can occur as patients get older. In some cases tongue reduction surgery can be considered (15). Trisomy 21 is associated with tongue protrusion; in most cases this is a relative enlargement due to a smaller oral cavity rather than true macroglossia. Progressive tongue enlargement can also occur in patients with mucopolysaccharidoses (16).

Focal lesions of the tongue are most commonly due to lymphatic malformations (LMs) or other vascular anomalies or congenital cysts. Foregut duplication cysts, epidermoid cysts, intralingual thyroglossal duct cysts (TGDCs), and vallecular cysts all can present in the tongue. Foregut duplication cysts are epithelial lined cysts that occur anywhere in the alimentary tract but may be present in the tongue. They appear in the anterior or ventral tongue and are more common in males (17). Epidermoid cysts, while common in the rest of the body, only rarely present in the oral cavity (18). Due to potential for growth and possible effects on breathing, feeding, and speech, surgical excision is recommended.

Posterior tongue cysts include intralingual TGDCs, which may rarely present in the base of tongue at the foramen cecum (**Fig. 30.6**), and vallecular cysts. TGDC are discussed in more detail in the "Neck" section below. Vallecular cysts are thought to be due to obstructed salivary glands and are mucus-filled cysts within the vallecula. Due to their posterior position, both of these types of lesions can only be seen with flexible laryngoscopy, thereby potentially delaying diagnosis, which often does not happen until after the development of symptomatic airway obstruction. Even smaller lesions should be managed aggressively to prevent obstruction due to potential for growth. Treatment is surgical marsupialization or excision via a suspension laryngoscopy approach; TDGCs may also be approached via a cervical transhyoid approach depending on the extent of the lesion (19).

Micrognathia

Micrognathia is the underdevelopment of the mandible and is often associated with Pierre Robin sequence (**Fig. 30.7A**). This is the association of micrognathia with glossoptosis, or inferior displacement of the tongue, and is also frequently associated with a cleft palate. It is thought to occur as cause and effect in which the underdeveloped mandible pushes the tongue backward and prevents the palatal shelves from fusing causing a cleft. It is associated with a genetic syndrome in 25% to 50% of cases, most frequently Stickler syndrome or 22q11 deletion syndrome; hence genetic evaluation is warranted (20,21).

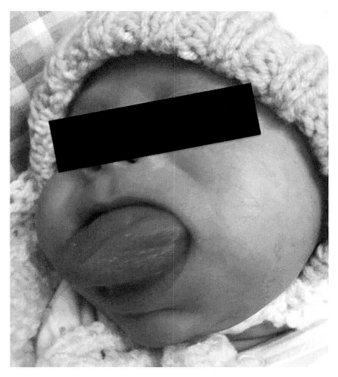

FIGURE 30.5 Macroglossia in an infant with Beckwith-Weidemann Syndrome. (Reprinted with permission from Johnson J. *Bailey's head and neck surgery*, 5th ed. Philadelphia, PA: Wolters Kluwer, 2013. Fig. 87.8.)

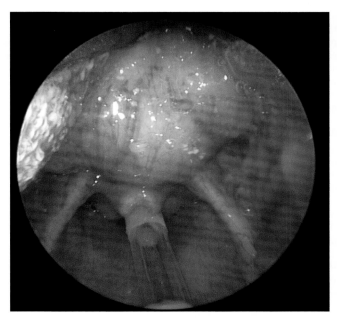

FIGURE 30.6 Endoscopic transoral view of a thyroglossal duct cyst located at the foramen cecum in the base of the tongue. Note there is displacement of the epiglottis posteriorly, which can lead to upper airway obstruction. (Image courtesy of Dr. Vikash Modi.)

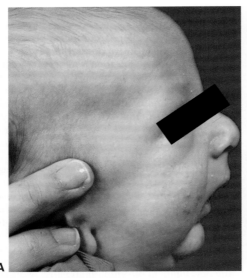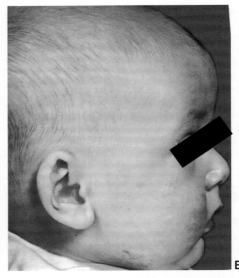

FIGURE 30.7 Pierre Robin sequence (isolated) in a 6-week-old boy. A: Preoperative image shows significant micrognathia (workup revealed upper airway obstruction). **B:** Postoperative image shows mandibular position improvement after bilateral mandibular distraction (and relief of airway obstruction). (Courtesy of J.P. Bradley. Reproduced from Chung KC. *Grabb and Smith's plastic surgery*. Philadelphia, PA: Wolters Kluwer, 2019.)

Feeding problems and airway obstruction are common. Obstructive symptoms may be temporized with prone positioning or a nasopharyngeal airway that bypasses the obstructing tongue base (22). As infants grow, due to craniofacial development, obstructive symptoms will often self-resolve, especially in nonsyndromic patients (23). Intervention for more symptomatic infants may involve tracheotomy; however, due to the morbidity of this intervention, alternative therapies have become more popular. Tongue lip adhesion, in which the anterior tongue is sutured to the lower lip for a period of several months, and mandibular distraction have both been shown to have successful outcomes. Mandibular distraction has the highest improvement in objective measures, such as severity of obstructive sleep apnea, and is appropriate for any level of severity of micrognathia (**Fig. 30.7B**) (24,25). Intubation is challenging in these patients as the tongue position precludes visualization of the glottis with direct laryngoscopy and glossoptosis worsens during sedation; therefore intubation is often carried out fiberoptically while the infant is awake. A stitch through the anterior tongue can assist with forward retraction and may be left in after surgery to help manage the airway during recovery.

Mucoceles

Mucoceles are pseudocysts originating from minor salivary glands and are usually located on the buccal surface of the lower lip. They are smooth round areas of swelling that can be sessile or pedunculated. They are unlikely to cause problems so observation is reasonable in younger infants, especially as some may spontaneously resolve. However, once infants grow teeth, they may traumatize the lesion, and eventual excision is often needed if there has been no resolution within a few months.

Dermoid Cysts, Ranulas, and Epulis

Within the floor of mouth the most common cystic masses include dermoid cysts and ranulas (**Fig. 30.8**). Dermoids are usually midline and will rarely recur if excised completely. Ranulas are pseudocysts that develop due to extravasation of saliva from salivary duct rupture and are usually located laterally in the floor of the mouth. It is possible for them to extend through the muscles of the floor of mouth into the neck in which case they

are known as plunging ranulas. Imaging with MRI or CT is recommended to examine the exact location and extent of the lesion, and classic findings will often confirm the diagnosis of ranula. Simple drainage or marsupialization of the cyst has a high rate of recurrence; however, these are safe options for an infant (26). Excision of the ranula along with the associated sublingual salivary gland is a more definitive surgery but is associated with higher risks of injury to the lingual nerve and submandibular duct (27,28).

Congenital epulis, also known as congenital granular cell tumor or gingival granular cell tumor of the newborn is a benign smooth fleshy mass that presents at birth along the alveolus. They are often pedunculated and are more common in females (29). They may be quite large causing feeding problems or, less commonly, airway obstruction. Surgical excision will confirm diagnosis, and recurrence is rare.

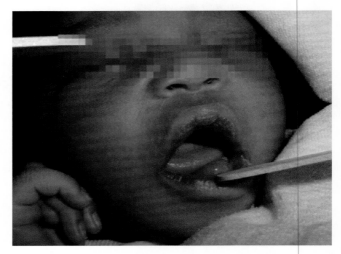

FIGURE 30.8 Newborn infant with ranula. (Courtesy of Dr. Shabnum Meer, with permission. From DeLong L, Burkhart NW. *General and oral pathology for the dental hygienist*, 3rd ed. Philadelphia, PA: Wolters Kluwer, 2018.)

LARYNX

Laryngomalacia

Laryngomalacia, in which supraglottic tissue prolapses during respiration causing airway obstruction, is the most common cause of stridor in an infant (**Fig. 30.9**). The stridor may present at birth but most commonly presents after a short period, usually around 2 weeks of age (30). Stridor is inspiratory and usually worse with feeding, agitation, and supine positioning. It is diagnosed with flexible laryngoscopy, in which prolapse of the supra-arytenoid tissues and/or epiglottis during respiration can be visualized. There are several potential causes including both anatomic anomalies with short aryepiglottic folds and excess supra-arytenoid tissue, as well as neurologic with hypotonia and decreased airway tone (31). There are frequently associated feeding issues including prolonged feeding times, frequent spitting up, coughing/gagging with feeds, and poor weight gain. Many patients can be observed and will outgrow their symptoms between 12 and 24 months of age. Reflux management can improve symptoms in some patients (32). In cases with severe respiratory or feeding symptoms surgery can be considered, both to rule out synchronous airway lesions that have a prevalence of 10% to 20% in patients with laryngomalacia (33) as well as to directly treat the laryngomalacia. Supraglottoplasty is an endoscopic procedure in which supraglottic tissues are altered, usually by cutting the aryepiglottic folds and trimming excess supra-arytenoid tissue. It has a high success rate and low complication rate; patients with comorbidities are more likely to require revision surgery or additional interventions such as tracheotomy (34).

Vocal Cord Pathologies

Vocal fold mobility disorders are the second most common cause of stridor in infants. Vocal fold mobility pathology may result from birth or other trauma, surgery that injures the vagus or recurrent laryngeal nerves (RLNs), intubation, or neurologic causes; if an underlying etiology cannot be identified it is considered idiopathic. The left RLN is particularly susceptible to injury due to its longer course under the aortic arch before coursing back up to the larynx through the tracheoesophageal groove, while the right RLN has a shorter course under the subclavian artery. Iatrogenic injury can occur during neck or thoracic/cardiac surgery. Intubation can cause vocal fold mobility pathology through several mechanisms including glottic injury causing cricoarytenoid joint fixation or posterior glottic stenosis or potentially via RLN injury by exerting pressure on the nerve as it travels in the tracheoesophageal groove. If there is no iatrogenic cause, then a neurologic evaluation should be performed including brain MRI to evaluate for such pathologies including Arnold-Chiari malformation, intraventricular hemorrhage, or hydrocephalus. Imaging should also include the neck and mediastinum to look for lesions that may be compressing the RLN. If no cause is identified, it is considered idiopathic.

Symptoms depend on wither the movement disorder is unilateral or bilateral and whether there is partial or complete paralysis (**Fig. 30.10**). Bilateral vocal fold paralysis usually causes stridor with significant airway compromise and may require urgent airway management. Unilateral vocal fold paralysis usually results in symptoms of dysphonia, aspiration/swallowing dysfunction, and inadequate cough. Spontaneous recovery is possible, and likelihood depends on the etiology. Following cardiac surgery recovery is about 35% likely with an average timeline to recovery of 6 months; however, recovery can occur years later (35). For patients with idiopathic paralysis, recovery is higher, around 50% to 70% (36).

Management of unilateral vocal fold paralysis depends on symptoms; many infants will be minimally symptomatic due to compensation from the normally functioning contralateral vocal fold. Aspiration and dysphonia are the most common symptoms that warrant consideration for intervention. For young infants, if there is a safe diet that can be tolerated, observation is preferred as recovery or compensation may occur with time. If there is no safe diet, then options include feeding tube placement or consideration for injection laryngoplasty in which an injectable material is used to medialize the affected vocal fold (37). This procedure is risky in small infants or infants with comorbidities as this does narrow the glottic inlet risking airway obstruction. There are additional surgical options for older pediatric patients including nerve reinnervation procedures (38).

Management of bilateral vocal fold paralysis also depends on symptoms; due to critical airway obstruction about 50% of patients will require tracheotomy (39). As recovery with time is possible, any surgical intervention that causes permanent destruction of the airway such as cordectomy or arytenoidectomy should be deferred. Other options for management in older children include cartilage grafting of the posterior cricoid to expand the airway or selective nerve reinnervation procedures (40,41).

Laryngeal Webs

Congenital laryngeal webs result from failure of the larynx to recanalize during embryogenesis and appear as tissue connection between the vocal folds anteriorly (42) (**Fig. 30.11**). It may be isolated or in association with a syndrome such as 22q11, so genetic evaluation is warranted (43). The Cohen grading system classifies laryngeal webs as type 1 if they obstruct less than 35% of the glottic opening, type 2 if they involve 35% to 50% of the glottic opening, type 3 for 50% to 75% obstruction, and type 4 involving up to 99% obstruction (44). Complete stenosis is also known as congenital high airway obstruction syndrome, or CHAOS, and is lethal without immediate tracheotomy. Respiratory symptoms include stridor or respiratory distress, and voice symptoms present as hoarseness or a high-pitched cry. If symptoms are mild, observation is reasonable. Surgical intervention with tracheotomy or endoscopic web division/excision may be warranted based on severity of respiratory symptoms or in older infants or children to improve voice. Endoscopic division of the web has high potential for restenosis especially with thicker webs, so stent placement may be needed (45).

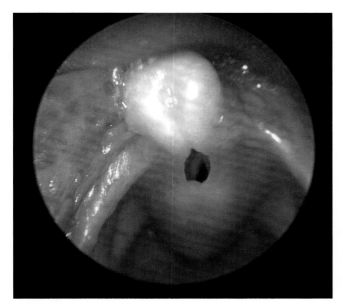

FIGURE 30.9 Endoscopic view of laryngomalacia in a newborn. Note the shortened aryepiglottic folds, which lead to a curled epiglottis. There is also anterior displacement of the arytenoids, which can lead to upper airway obstruction. The vocal folds can be barely visualized. (Image courtesy of Dr. Vikash Modi.)

Vocal cord paralyses

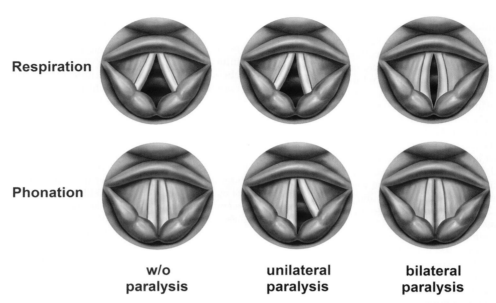

Respiration

Phonation

w/o paralysis   unilateral paralysis   bilateral paralysis

FIGURE 30.10 Unilateral and bilateral vocal cord paralysis. (Reproduced under a Creative Commons License from https://commons.wikimedia.org/w/index.php?curid=48281672)

Laryngeal Cleft

A laryngeal cleft occurs if there is a defect of the posterior larynx between the arytenoids into the pharynx. This defect may extend inferiorly through the cricoid cartilage into the trachea causing a connection into the esophagus. According to the Benjamin Inglis system, a type 1 cleft extends to the depth of the vocal folds, a type 2 cleft extends below the vocal folds into the cricoid cartilage, a type 3 cleft extends below the cricoid into the trachea, and a type 4 cleft extends into the thoracic trachea (**Fig. 30.12**) (46). Symptoms depend on the severity of the cleft, ranging from coughing with feeds to recurrent pneumonias to respiratory distress due to aspiration. Deeper clefts may also cause obstructive breathing symptoms such as stridor or apneas due to prolapse of the cleft edges into the airway. Type 3 and type 4 clefts can be lethal in infancy if not managed appropriately. There is associated tracheomalacia in the majority of cases, and about 20% of patients with a laryngeal cleft will have a tracheoesophageal fistula (47). There may be an associated syndrome such as Opitz-Frias syndrome, and genetic evaluation is warranted. A modified barium swallow study will show aspiration and suggest the possibility of a cleft; however, diagnosis can only be made with direct laryngoscopy under anesthesia. During this evaluation, probing of the interarytenoid area will confirm the presence of the defect and determine the extent of the lesion (**Fig. 30.12**). For more mild clefts thickening feeds may alleviate symptoms; however, if this doesn't work, then either feeding tube placement or cleft repair is necessary. Repair can be performed endoscopically with suture closure of the defect or via an open approach (48,49).

Laryngeal Stenosis

Laryngeal stenosis may be congenital or acquired and is most common in the subglottis. Congenital stenosis in the subglottis is usually due to abnormal recanalization of the cricoid cartilage, which is a complete cartilage ring just below the vocal cords. This may be seen as an elliptical cricoid in which the subglottis appears to have lateral shelves, or as a normally shaped cricoid ring that has a smaller lumen as is often seen in patients with trisomy 21. Acquired stenosis also usually occurs in the subglottis as this is

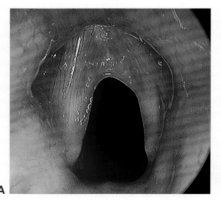
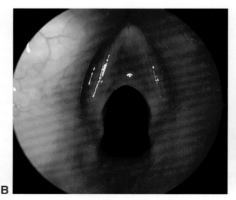
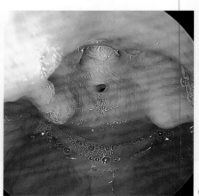

FIGURE 30.11 Endoscopic demonstration of the Cohen classification of laryngeal webs based on degree of laryngeal obstruction. A: Type 1, less than 35%. **B:** Type 2, 35% to 50%. **C:** Type 4, 75% to 100%. Type 3, not shown. (Images courtesy of Dr. Vikash Modi.)

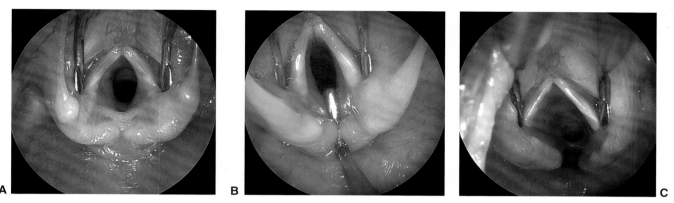

FIGURE 30.12 Endoscopic demonstration of the Benjamin-Inglis classification of laryngeal clefts. A: Type 1, extends to the level of the vocal folds. **B:** Type 2, extends below the level of the folds into the cricoid cartilage. **C:** Type 3, extends below the vocal folds, through the entire cricoid, and into the trachea. Type 4, not shown. (Images courtesy of Dr. Vikash Modi.)

the narrowest part of the infant airway and most vulnerable to injury from intubation (Fig. 30.13). The posterior glottis is also vulnerable to intubation injury from ulcerations from the posterior positioning of the ETT within the glottis. The frequency of SGS in neonates increased after the 1960s due to the introduction of prolonged intubation for respiratory support in neonates (50). The incidence of SGS is 0% to 2% of intubated neonates; factors associated with SGS include size of the ETT, duration of intubation, traumatic intubation, presence of infection while intubated, and gastroesophageal reflux (51,52).

Symptoms of SGS include biphasic stridor and recurrent croup. For premature infants that have been intubated since birth there may be failed trials of extubation or absence of an air leak around an appropriately sized ETT. Formal diagnosis is with direct visualization under anesthesia with laryngoscopy and bronchoscopy. It is standard to size the subglottic airway by identifying the largest size ETT that fits in the airway with a leak at less than 30 cm water. The Myer-Cotton staging system is the most common scale to assign severity of SGS by comparing the ETT size to expected airway size based on age. A grade 1 stenosis is lumen obstruction

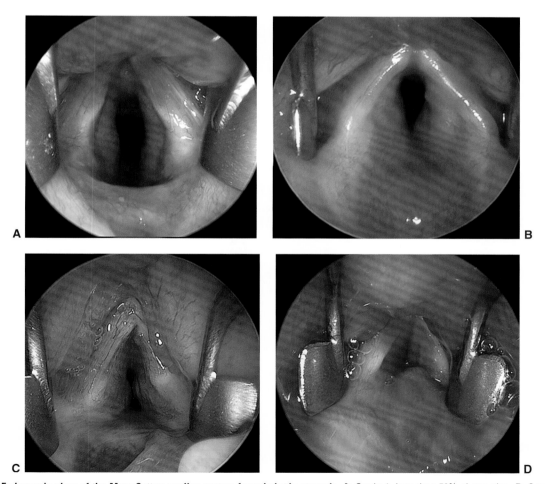

FIGURE 30.13 Endoscopic view of the Myer-Cotton grading system for subglottic stenosis. A: Grade 1, less than 50% obstruction. **B:** Grade 2, 51% to 70% obstruction. **C:** Grade 3, 71% to 99% obstruction. **D:** Grade 4, 100% obstruction. (Images courtesy of Dr. Vikash Modi.)

less than 50%, grade 2 is 51% to 70%, grade 3 is 71% to 99%, and grade 4 is complete stenosis (Fig. 30.13) (2).

Mild stenosis can often be observed, and mild symptoms often improve with growth. Intervention for more symptomatic patients may involve endoscopic or open surgical interventions. Endoscopic balloon dilation may be helpful for patients with more mild stenosis, especially if the stenosis scar is thinner or weblike (53). Open procedures are necessary for more severe stenosis, thicker/ dense scar, or in patients with multilevel disease (54). Open procedures include segmental resection of the stenosed airway or laryngotracheal reconstruction with airway framework expansion using rib cartilage grafts (55,56). Open procedures are rarely appropriate in smaller infants or patients with significant pulmonary or neurologic comorbidities, and therefore a tracheostomy is often needed until patients become open surgical candidates.

Subglottic cysts occur almost exclusively in premature infants with a history of intubation. They are the result of obstruction of native mucous glands due to subepithelial fibrosis after traumatic mucosal injury (57). Presenting symptoms include stridor, which is usually biphasic or recurrent croup. Diagnosis can only be made during DLB under anesthesia (Fig. 30.14). Treatment is endoscopic marsupialization with either cold knife technique or laser. There is a high recurrence rate after treatment, around 40% to 50%, and a planned second look to confirm resolution is recommended (58,59).

Airway Hemangioma

Infantile hemangiomas are the most common benign tumor of infancy and may present in the subglottis causing symptoms of airway obstruction including biphasic stridor and croup (**Fig. 30.15**). Airway hemangiomas (oral cavity, pharynx, larynx) are seen in about one-third of patients with facial segmental hemangiomas, so particular attention should be paid to the presence of airway symptoms in these patients (60). Subglottic hemangiomas follow typical growth patterns in which there is a proliferation phase for several months followed by involution. Diagnosis of subglottic hemangioma is made through direct visualization with laryngoscopy and bronchoscopy. MRI or CT imaging can fully evaluate the depth of the lesion. Hemangiomas in this area warrant treatment as the proliferation phase results in critical airway obstruction. Propranolol treatment is about 90% successful in treating

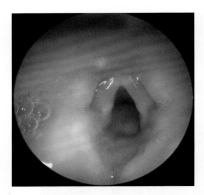

FIGURE 30.15 Endoscopic view of a subglottic hemangioma just deep to the vocal folds obstructing over 75% of the lumen. (Image courtesy of Dr. Vikash Modi.)

subglottic hemangiomas without need for surgical intervention (61). Endoscopic ablation and open surgical management are appropriate options for patients who fail propranolol therapy or if propranolol is otherwise contraindicated. Rarely, a tracheostomy will be needed.

▍TRACHEA

Tracheomalacia and Bronchomalacia

Intrinsic tracheomalacia (TM) refers to increased compliance of the trachea causing collapsibility, usually seen with dynamic changes with respiratory effort (**Fig. 30.16**). It may be associated with malacia of the distal bronchial airways as well, known as bronchomalacia. It may be an isolated finding, but it is commonly seen with other abnormalities such as esophageal atresia with or without tracheoesophageal fistula (EA/TEF) where tracheomalacia to some degree is considered a universal finding. Other associated pathologies include laryngeal cleft, cystic fibrosis, and trisomy 21 (62). Intrinsic tracheomalacia may be acquired in situations of prolonged intubation, with tracheostomy tubes with elevated cuff pressures, or in settings of chronic infection or inflammation. It

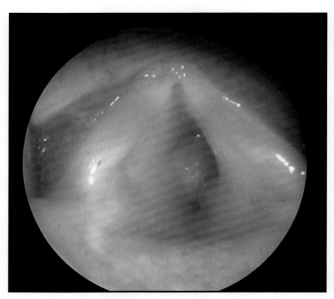

FIGURE 30.14 Endoscopic view of two subglottic cysts (larger on the left than right) just deep to the vocal folds obstructing the lumen. (Image courtesy of Dr. Vikash Modi.)

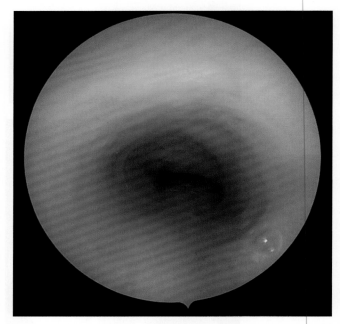

FIGURE 30.16 Endoscopic view of tracheomalacia in the distal 1/3 of the trachea. Note the flattened distal appearance of the trachea compared to the proximal more C-shape. (Image courtesy of Dr. Vikash Modi.)

is now appreciated as being common in prematurely born infants with severe bronchopulmonary dysplasia. In such infants, it often necessitates use of prolonged high PEEP to prevent airway collapse, especially during active expiration (See also Chapter 29).

Symptoms that should lead to suspicion for trachea–bronchomalacia (TBM) are variable including cough, which is often barking in nature, stridor, which is usually biphasic or expiratory, and recurrent pneumonias due to poor mucous clearance in the distal airways. Endoscopic evaluation under anesthesia should always be done with the infant spontaneously ventilating as the dynamic changes during the respiratory cycle will more clearly demonstrate the pathology.

Extrinsic causes of tracheomalacia are due to anomalies that compress on the airway deforming the cartilage such as a vascular ring or, less commonly, a mediastinal mass. Common vascular ring pathologies include aberrant right subclavian artery, double aortic arch, right aortic arch with persistent left ligament, Kommerell diverticulum, and pulmonary sling. Often the respiratory symptoms are the presenting findings leading to diagnosis (63). Some patients may also experience dysphagia. Any pulsatile compression of the airway identified during bronchoscopy should suggest a vascular ring pathology, which may be confirmed with CTA or MRA imaging.

Tracheomalacia may not require intervention and can be followed by observation only if the symptoms are mild; often patients will improve as they grow. Medical management involves optimizing clearance of secretions given the impaired cough clearance of patients with TM/TBM. Ipratropium bromide and saline nebulizers may be helpful to thin secretions, and chest physiotherapy can help with mucociliary clearance. For patients with more severe symptoms requiring continuous positive pressure ventilation, a tracheostomy is sometimes necessary for chronic ventilation until the patient outgrows the symptoms. Other surgical options for patients with severe, prolonged symptoms may be considered including external stent placement or tracheal resection if the area of malacia is segmental. The anterior airway can be fixed anteriorly via an aortopexy procedure, or the posterior aspect of the airway can be fixed posteriorly to the spine via a tracheopexy procedure to prevent collapse (64–66).

Tracheal Stenosis

Acquired tracheal stenosis usually occurs in the setting of intubation due to elevated pressures from a large ETT or inflated cuff. The trachea is a less common area of airway stenosis compared to the glottis and subglottis due to the relative larger diameter in infants and flexibility for some expansion due to the posterior membranous trachea. Acquired stenosis can also be due to iatrogenic framework disruption, most commonly with tracheotomy. Patients with mild pathology can be observed, and many will outgrow their symptoms. Patients with more severe symptoms warranting intervention may undergo endoscopic dilation or open repair either with resection of the stenosis or framework expansion with grafting.

Congenital tracheal stenosis usually presents in the form of complete tracheal rings in which there is an absence of the membranous trachea (**Fig. 30.17**). It is often described in 3 categories— complete, funnel shaped, or segmental (67). It usually presents with biphasic stridor and possible acute distress. Intubation may be difficult or impossible, and forced instrumentation of the airway may precipitate swelling and complete obstruction with the loss of ability to ventilate. Severe cases may necessitate extracorporeal membrane oxygenation (ECMO) until definitive surgical management. Surgical management is frequently warranted; often the severity of stenosis may worsen with time as the cartilage in the area of stenosis will not grow proportionally with the infant (68). If the length of the stenosis is less than 50% of the trachea, a primary resection may be performed. For longer segment stenosis, surgical intervention usually involves slide tracheoplasty (69) in which the trachea is overlapped to shorten the length but double the intraluminal volume. It is important to note that there is a high

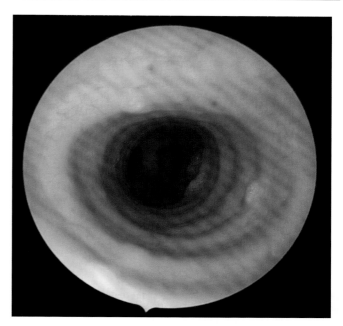

FIGURE 30.17 Endoscopic view of complete tracheal rings. Note the posterior trachealis is replaced with cartilaginous rings. (Image courtesy of Dr. Vikash Modi.)

association with vascular rings, especially pulmonary artery slings, and cardiac evaluation is warranted.

Tracheal Cartilaginous Sleeve

A tracheal cartilaginous sleeve involves the loss of segments between tracheal rings with a preserved posterior membranous wall (70). This results in abnormal tracheal growth, and many patients will require a tracheostomy. The majority of patients with a tracheal cartilaginous sleeve will have a craniosynostosis syndrome and should be evaluated by genetics. About 22% of patients with craniosynostosis syndromes will have a tracheal cartilaginous sleeve (71), and this airway pathology should be a consideration in all patients with this diagnosis.

■ NECK

Thyroglossal Duct Cysts

TGDCs are the most common midline congenital cyst in the neck, accounting for 75% of midline neck swellings. The thyroid gland begins its development during early gestation at the foramen cecum of the tongue and then descends along a ventral diverticulum, the thyroglossal duct, to its final position in the base of the neck. The tract usually disappears; however, sometimes there are persistent remnants from which a cyst may form. It usually appears as a painless round fluctuant midline swelling at or just below the hyoid, although it may be present anywhere from the foramen cecum within the tongue to the thyroid gland (**Fig. 30.18**). Presentation is usually during childhood but it may be visible at birth. Diagnosis is usually with ultrasound, which can assess the lesion directly, look for a tract, and confirm the presence of a normal thyroid gland, which is critical prior to surgical excision to rule out the lesion as ectopic thyroid. Any atypical appearance on exam or ultrasound may warrant additional imaging such as CT or MRI. While they are benign lesions, there is often a cosmetic deformity, there is a high risk of recurrent infections, and depending on location they may pose a risk to the airway with increasing size. Treatment is surgical excision. With simple cyst excision the risk of recurrence is 50%. The more appropriate surgery is called a Sistrunk procedure, in which the cyst is excised along with the tract, the central portion of the hyoid bone, and a

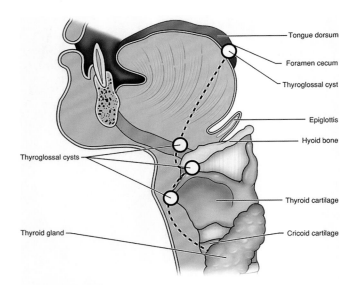

FIGURE 30.18 Tract of development of the thyroid tissue and various potential locations for both thyroglossal duct cysts and glandular ectopias. (Reprinted with permission from Sadler TW, ed. *Langman's medical embryology*, 11th ed. Philadelphia, PA: Lippincott Williams & Wilkins, 2006:279.)

portion of the intralingual tract toward the foramen cecum. This surgery has a recurrence rate of less than 15% (72–74).

Branchial Anomalies

Branchial anomalies are the most common congenital lesions of the lateral neck. Branchial clefts are ectodermal-lined recesses on the outside of the branchial arches. The first branchial cleft forms the external auditory canal; the second, third, and fourth clefts are obliterated during development. Abnormalities in the development/obliteration of these clefts leads to cysts (75%) or sinuses or fistulas (25%) in which there is an internal and/or external opening (75). These lesions are classically located anterior to the sternocleidomastoid muscle. First branchial clefts are rare (7%) and appear as lesions in or around the parotid or upper neck with the internal opening in the external ear canal or middle ear. Second branchial clefts are the most common (>90%) with an external opening in the mid neck region anterior to the sternocleidomastoid muscle and an internal opening in the tonsillar fossa. Third/fourth branchial cleft anomalies are rare (<5%) and located in the lower neck with an internal opening in the pyriform sinus next to the larynx, usually on the left side. Due to high risk of infection, especially in lesions with internal tracts, surgical excision is recommended. Failure to remove the entire tract results in recurrence (76). Third/fourth branchial cleft anomalies with an internal opening in the pyriform may be addressed by endoscopic obliteration of the pyriform sinus tract opening, which has been shown to prevent recurrence (77).

Vascular Anomalies of the Neck

Vascular anomalies refer to a number of benign lesions that can be either malformations or tumors. They are always present at birth but may not be immediately visible. They are frequently disfiguring and, depending on location and size in the head and neck region, may cause airway obstruction or feeding difficulties. Some types of high-flow lesions may cause cardiovascular compromise. Superficial lesions such as infantile hemangiomas (IH) may be diagnosed clinically by their appearance and growth patterns; however, while physical exam often give clues to the diagnosis, most lesions will require MRI imaging for confirmation. Many programs have a multidisciplinary team composed of specialists from radiology, interventional radiology, pediatric surgery,

otolaryngology, and dermatology to collaborate for diagnosis and treatment as multiple treatment options often exist for vascular anomalies and treatment may be multimodal.

Vascular anomalies are usually isolated lesions; however, in some cases they may be associated with a syndrome such as Sturge-Weber syndrome, Klippel-Trenaunay syndrome, and Rendu-Osler-Weber syndrome. PHACES syndrome (posterior fossa malformations, hemangiomas, arterial anomalies, coarctation of aorta and cardiac defects, eye abnormalities, and sternal defects) is a syndrome associated with infantile hemangioma and is important to recognize promptly due to the presence of cerebrovascular abnormalities with risk for ischemic stroke (78).

IHs are the most common vascular tumor, seen in about 4% to 10% of infants, and are more common in females and premature and low birth weight infants. They are not present at birth, appear in early infancy, grow and proliferate for several months, and then involute over a few years with replacement of the tumor endothelium with fibrofatty tissue (79). Complications related to head and neck IHs are based on size and location and may include ulceration/bleeding, abnormal vision development if around the eye, or airway compromise for those lesions found in the airway, particularly in the nose or subglottis. Airway hemangiomas (oral cavity, pharynx, larynx) are seen in about one-third of patients with facial segmental hemangiomas, so particular attention should be paid to the presence of airway symptoms in these patients (60). Propranolol has replaced surgery as the mainstay for treatment for IHs that are deforming or symptomatic (80).

Hemangiomas that are present at birth are called congenital hemangiomas and will either spontaneously involute shortly after birth (rapidly involuting congenital hemangioma, or RICH) or will not involute (noninvoluting congenital hemangiomas, or NICH).

Lymphatic malformations (LMs) are the most common vascular malformation, and are masses consisting of fluid-filled channels or spaces due to an abnormal development of the lymphatic system. Seventy-five percent occur in the head and neck (**Fig. 30.19**). They do not follow tissue planes and are known to envelop structures such as nerves and vessels, which adds complexity to management. They are categorized as macrocystic (cystic lesions are >2 cm), which are very soft and compressible, or microcystic (<2 cm), which can be quite firm. There are rare cases that spontaneously involute; however, most do not. Treatment options include surgical resection and/or sclerotherapy, and lesions that are more microcystic and invasive often require multiple treatments. LMs above the hyoid are more likely microcystic and infiltrative and subsequently difficult to treat while LMs below the hyoid tend to be more macrocystic and are more amenable to all treatment options (81–83).

Venous malformations are also frequently in the head and neck (40%) and often increase in size with the growth of the patient. They are composed of malformed venous channels and, similar to LM, they infiltrate surrounding structures. Stasis within venous channels may cause thrombi or phlebolith formation, which may cause pain. Small asymptomatic lesions can be observed; however, larger or symptomatic lesions require treatment. Sclerotherapy and surgery are options, and recurrence rates are often high. Surgery may be combined with preoperative glue embolization to improve structure identification for more complete surgery with lower risks of complications and recurrence (84,85).

Arteriovenous malformations (AVM) are high-flow vascular anomalies due to a localized shunt between the arterial and venous systems. They appear as a pulsatile lesion. They may be painful and are a risk for cardiac compromise. Treatment is usually embolization followed by surgical excision (86).

Cervical Dermoids

Cervical dermoids are the second most common midline congenital neck mass after TGDCs. They contain ectoderm and mesoderm.

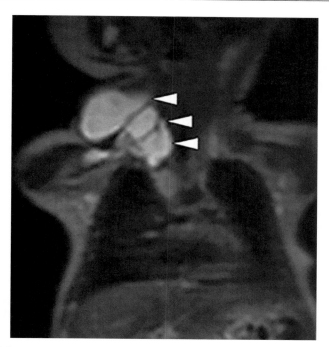

FIGURE 30.19 A right-sided neck lymphatic abnormality in a newborn. Coronal T2-weighted, fat-suppressed MRI demonstrates the multilocular fluid-filled mass (*arrowheads*) in the right neck and mediastinum. (Reprinted with permission from Lee EY. *Pediatric thoracic imaging*, 1st ed. Philadelphia, PA: Wolters Kluwer, 2018. Fig. 3.26B.)

While they are benign, there is a high risk for infection and growth. Surgical removal is standard, and recurrence is rare.

Fibromatosis Colli/Sternocleidomastoid Tumor

Fibromatosis colli, also known as sternocleidomastoid tumor of infancy, is a benign mass of the sternocleidomastoid muscle. It is actually a pseudotumor as it is a fibrotic swelling within the muscle. A physical exam shows a hard, fixed mass in the lateral neck, and frequently there is torticollis. It usually appears at weeks 2 to 4, is more common on the right side (75%), and is more common in males. There may be a history of traumatic delivery. It can be diagnosed with classic findings and an ultrasound. If there are any atypical features, additional imaging with possible biopsy is warranted. Treatment is conservative with physical therapy or passive stretching exercises if torticollis is present. Resolution usually occurs by 4 to 8 months of age (87,88).

Cervical Teratoma

Cervical teratomas are a rare cause of a fetal neck mass (**Fig. 30.20**). Most that present in infancy/childhood are benign. Small tumors may be asymptomatic; large tumors may cause significant deformity and potentially compress the airway. Large tumors are often diagnosed prenatally during fetal ultrasound, and given the potential for airway compromise, multidisciplinary planning for delivery is warranted with consideration for an EXIT procedure. Treatment is early surgical removal as they have aggressive local growth. Thyroid function should be tested pre- and postoperatively as the tumors often contain thyroid tissue. Serum alpha feta protein can be monitored as a marker for malignancy at follow-up.

CLEFT LIP AND PALATE

Cleft lip (CL) and cleft palate (CP) are the most common congenital craniofacial abnormalities (**Fig. 30.21**). Cleft lips develop due

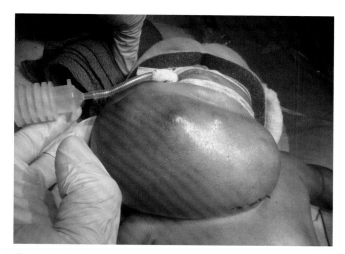

FIGURE 30.20 Cervical teratoma presenting as a neck mass in a newborn infant. (Image courtesy of Dr. Vikash Modi.)

to failure of the lateral and medial nasal prominences and the maxillary prominences to merge. There can be a unilateral or bilateral CL. CP is primary if it extends through the hard palate and alveolar ridge anterior to the incisive foramen, and is secondary if it starts posterior to the incisive foramen, which occurs when the palatine shelves fail to fuse. A submucous cleft palate is when there is intact mucosa in the midline, but the levator palatini muscles insert into the hard palate rather than interdigitating in the midline. This results in functional defects of the palate. CL/CP occurs in about 1 in 700 newborns, with the incidence varying according to geography and ethnicity with both genetic and environmental factors playing a role. There may be an associated syndrome in 30% of cases of CL/CP and 50% of cases of CP (89).

Diagnosis of CL/CP is possible prenatally by ultrasound. Airway symptoms are uncommon unless the cleft palate is part of Pierre Robin sequence, which also involves micrognathia and glossoptosis. There are significant effects on feeding and speech, and care usually involves a multidisciplinary team including otolaryngologists, plastic surgeons, maxillofacial surgeons, orthodontists, dentists, feeding specialists, speech therapists, and geneticists. Care by the cleft team continues throughout infancy and childhood due to continued issues related to feeding, speech, maxillofacial growth, and dentition.

Newborns with CP will often have feeding difficulties due to inability to generate the negative intraoral pressures that are necessary to suck. Feeding specialists should be involved early on, and this problem can be overcome using specialized equipment including a squeezable bottle and modified nipple along with parental education.

Cleft lip repair is usually undertaken around 3 months of age. There are several techniques with goals of creating muscular competence, symmetry, a straight lip margin, normal philtrum length, and normal Cupid's bow appearance. Secondary cleft rhinoplasty procedures may be needed in older patients to further correct the nasal deformities associated with CL.

Cleft palate causes significant speech problems due to air escape through an incompetent velopharynx. Feeding is also impaired with food and liquids often refluxing into the nose. Repair is usually performed around 9 to 12 months of age. Secondary soft palate cleft repair is successful at this age without future growth consequences; however, repair of hard palate clefts can potentially affect maxillofacial growth; despite this, due to the more concerning speech consequences of cleft palate, repair is still recommended at this age. There are multiple techniques that are used depending on the extent and width of the cleft with goals of creating separation from the nasal cavity and competence of the

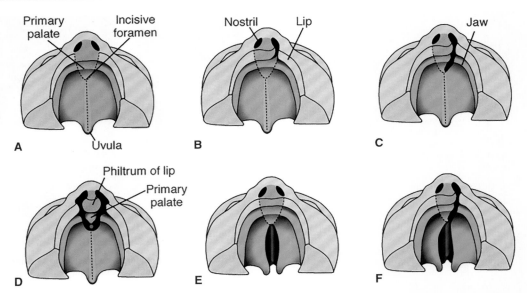

FIGURE 30.21 Classification of common types of cleft lip and palate. A: Normal. **B:** Unilateral cleft lip (type 1). **C:** Unilateral cleft lip and palate (type 2). **D:** Bilateral cleft lip and palate (type 3). **E:** Median cleft lip and palate (type 4). **F:** Not shown are slash-type defects (type 5). (Reprinted with permission from Sadler TW. *Langman's medical embryology,* 14th ed. Philadelphia, PA: Wolters Kluwer Health, 2018. Figure 17-28.)

velopharynx. Complications include fistula and persistent velopharyngeal dysfunction causing speech and communication difficulty. Additional interventions to improve velopharyngeal function are necessary in 15% to 45% of patients after cleft palate repair (90).

Ear and hearing problems in patients with cleft palate are essentially universal. Palatal musculature plays a role in eustachian tube function, and therefore patients with CP have eustachian tube dysfunction resulting in chronic effusions, recurrent ear infections, and hearing loss. These patients will need ear tube placement early on, usually concurrently with surgical repair of CL or CP, and audiologic monitoring is important throughout childhood.

▌ EAR

The external ear is developed from six auricular hillocks from branchial arches 1 and 2. Abnormalities in development can cause deformity in the size, shape, and position of the external ear. Microtia is graded based on the severity of the deformity. Grade 1 microtia involves a smaller than normal ear with present though possibly slightly altered cartilage structures. Grade 2 microtia involves significantly altered or absent cartilaginous landmarks of the ear, usually of the upper part of the ear. There is usually external auditory canal stenosis. Grade 3 microtia is when there is only a small peanut-shaped lobe, and the external ear canal is usually absent (**Fig. 30.22**). Grade 4 is rare, and involves complete absence of the external ear and ear canal, also known as anotia. Microtia has an incidence of 1 per 5,000 births although this varies by ethnicity. It is more common in males, and more common in the right ear (91).

Microtia may be isolated or may be associated with a syndrome such as Treacher Collins and the hemifacial microsomia syndromes. Genetic evaluation is always warranted. Acquired causes

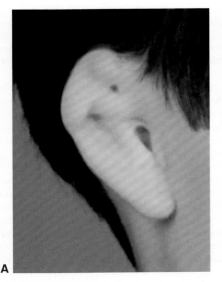
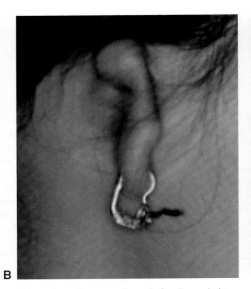
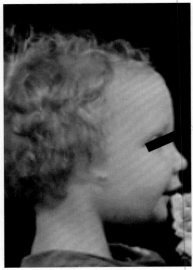

FIGURE 30.22 Microtia. The term microtia refers to a wide variety of presentations. **A:** Small conchal-type microtia. **B:** Lobular-type microtia. **C:** Almost complete anotia. (Adapted with permission from Chung KC, Gosain A. *Operative techniques in pediatric plastic and reconstructive surgery.* Philadelphia, PA: Wolters Kluwer, 2019.)

Developmentally, the immature myocardium has been shown to exhibit a higher basal contractile state and a greater sensitivity to changes in afterload (3). The intolerance of the immature myocardium to increased afterload may be attributable to differences in myofibrillar architecture, or immaturity of receptor development or regulation (22). Due to geometric, adaptive, and metabolic differences, the neonatal left and right ventricle also respond differently to afterload. When both ventricles are exposed to the same increase in afterload, the right ventricle experiences greater wall stress and therefore has a greater decrement in myocardial performance (23,24). The Frank-Starling law appears less applicable to the immature myocardium. The immediate postnatal period following the loss of the low-pressure system of the placenta and postoperative period following PDA ligation represent two clinical situations in which the neonatal myocardium is subjected to afterload stress. The net effect is impaired myocardial systolic performance and consequential poor systemic blood flow due to low cardiac output, oftentimes despite a normal systemic blood pressure. This problem is further compounded by any potential stressors such as hypoxia, anemia, and mechanical ventilation, which reduces venous return and causes pressure on the myocardium preventing effective contraction.

Control of Vascular Tone

After the transitional period, vascular tone is modulated by a balance between vasoconstrictors, for example, thromboxane, vasopressin, and vasodilators, for example, nitric oxide (NO) and prostaglandins. Immaturity of the central nervous system may also impact on transitional vascular changes.

Nitric Oxide

NO is produced by actions of nitric oxide synthase (NOS), present in abundance in smooth muscle tissue; it acts via cyclic guanosine monophosphate (cGMP) on calcium-sensitive potassium channels and myosin light-chain phosphatases to cause smooth muscle relaxation. Endotoxins and cytokines such as tumor necrosis factor alpha (TNF-α) and a variety of interleukins are potent stimulators of inducible NOS (iNOS) (25). Stimulation of iNOS in the setting of sepsis has been associated with high levels of circulating NO, which may contribute to profound dilatation and impaired delivery of blood to distal tissues due to low organ perfusion pressure in the presence of sepsis. In addition, excess NO leads to formation of free oxygen radicals leading to vascular wall damage.

Vasopressin

Vasopressin also plays an important role in regulating vascular tone postnatally; its vasoconstrictor effects are modulated through V1 receptors in many organs (excluding the lung, brain, and heart), which in turn increase calcium release from the sarcoplasmic reticulum, up-regulate adrenaline receptors on smooth muscle walls, and reduce NO synthesis. Its implication in shock has been studied in adults. Initially, vasopressin levels increase in response to shock to maintain vascular tone; however, as shock progresses, vasopressin stores are depleted and vascular tone is therefore compromised.

Prostaglandins

Prostaglandins are eicosanoids derived from cell membrane arachidonic acid by the actions of cyclooxygenase enzymes and play an important role of regulation of vascular tone. Prostaglandin E_2 (PGE_2), a vasodilator, and thromboxane A2, a vasoconstrictor are both implicated in the early regulation of vascular tone and may have a role in the pathogenesis of hypovolemia associated with shock.

ASSESSMENT OF THE CARDIOVASCULAR SYSTEM

Clinical Assessment of the Cardiovascular System

A healthy cardiovascular system is defined as one that ensures sufficient oxygen delivery to tissues to meet the metabolic needs of the cells. Assessment of the cardiovascular system begins with a comprehensive clinical history to identify relevant maternal, delivery-related, or postnatal factors that increase the risk of cardiovascular ill health. Continuous monitoring of heart rate and blood pressure, which are commonly used as surrogate markers of cardiac output, provides an objective and longitudinal assessment of cardiovascular well-being. Physical exam and investigations should be targeted toward assessing end-organ health and function as well as surrogate markers of the adequacy of oxygen delivery. For example, in the absence of primary central nervous system pathology, general observation of level of consciousness and tone can act as surrogate markers of cerebral perfusion. However, there is considerable variability in the normal range for many of the aforementioned hemodynamic measurements. In addition, many of the measurement tools are subject to operator-dependent variability and multiple confounding factors making single measurements unreliable (Table 31.1). The recommended approach is to perform a comprehensive appraisal of the cardiovascular system, which facilitates more holistic insights into illness severity and the pathophysiologic nature of disease, enabling a more targeted approach to therapeutic intervention.

Heart Rate

Tachycardia is often cited as a sensitive marker of low cardiac output based on the concept that stroke volume is relatively fixed due to limitations in the myocardial reserve. While there is some weak evidence of a direct correlation, many neonatal and animal studies have concluded that heart rate is not a major determinant of cardiac output in neonates. In a fetal ovine experimental paradigm,

TABLE 31.1

Clinical Indicators of Cardiovascular Health

Clinical Indicator	Pathophysiology	Confounding Factors
Tachycardia	Increasing HR may increase CO if stroke volume unchanged	Medications, pain, temperature, agitation
Systolic hypotension	Marker of decreased CO	Transitional circulation, left-to-right shunts
Diastolic hypotension	Marker of systemic vascular resistance and preload	Transitional circulation, left-to-right shunts
Increased capillary refill time	Vasoconstriction of skin	Wide range of normal
Pallor/acrocyanosis	Vasoconstriction of skin	Lighting, temperature, skin tone, anemia
Decreased level of consciousness	Decreased cerebral perfusion pressure	Sedative medications, meningitis, seizures
Decreased urinary output	Decreased renal perfusion pressure	Renal pathology, transitional changes
Elevated lactate	Anaerobic metabolism	Some IEM, hemolyzed samples, gluconeogenesis
Metabolic acidosis	Anaerobic metabolism	Bicarbonate loss
Low central venous saturation	Increased oxygen consumption	Catheter placement, peripheral shunts, necrotic tissue

HR, heart rate; CO, cardiac output; SV, stroke volume; IEM, inborn error of metabolism.

LVO remained stable despite wide variations in heart rate, suggesting that stroke volume may vary significantly to maintain an adequate cardiac output (26). In human preterm neonates, stroke volume also varies with changing heart rate. Echocardiography-based evaluations of cardiac output reaffirm this relationship; specifically, there is no difference in heart rate between patients with low systemic blood flow and those in whom the systemic blood flow is normal. Elevation in heart rate beyond 160 beats per minute, or a sustained elevation from baseline may indicate hypovolemia. However, many noncardiovascular factors can also influence heart rate. Elevated heart rate may be caused by pain, hyperthermia, and commonly used medications such as caffeine and atropine. Sinus bradycardia occurs commonly in sleep, and the neonate should respond with increased heart rate when awakened. Other factors that should be considered if the heart rate remains low include hypothermia, hypothyroidism, electrolyte imbalance, and some medications such as β antagonists (e.g., propranolol).

Blood Pressure

Blood pressure is used as a surrogate marker for blood flow because it is noninvasive and reproducible. In the absence of left-to-right shunt, outside of the transitional period low blood pressure represents either low cardiac output or low SVR. Both of these conditions can lead to inadequate organ perfusion. Typically, a cutoff of mean blood pressure (MBP) less than GA in completed weeks is used; however, most neonates after the first 72 hours of life will maintain their MBP greater than 30 mm Hg in the absence of a hemodynamically significant PDA.

In the transitional period, MBP and systemic blood flow are poorly correlated. Recent evidence suggests that SBP may correlate better with systemic blood flow (27). Currently, using an MBP less than gestational age in completed weeks has been shown to correctly capture only 71% of neonates with low systemic blood flow and falsely identify 12% of neonates as hypotensive (28) (see Hypotension section for more detail). Consideration of thresholds for SBP and diastolic blood pressure (DBP) may be more clinically useful as they drive a more pathophysiologic approach to diagnosis and treatment selection (Fig. 31.1).

Capillary Refill Time

Studies suggest that capillary refill time (CRT) in healthy neonates varies considerably. Central CRT of up to 4 seconds and peripheral CRT of up to 10 seconds have been documented in normal neonates. Comparative evaluations using Doppler echocardiography are inconsistent and have shown variable correlation between markers of systemic blood flow and central CRT (29).

The combination of central CRT of greater than 4 seconds and arterial lactate greater than 4, however, has been shown to correlate with low cardiac output.

Skin Color

The color of skin is modified by many factors including temperature, hemoglobin, skin translucency, oxygenation, jaundice, underlying pigmentation, and ambient factors such as environmental light. Interobserver variability of color assessment is high (30). When combined with other markers of low cardiac output, pallor and/or acrocyanosis may suggest peripheral vasoconstriction in skin vessels.

Urinary Output

In the absence of renal parenchymal disease and urinary retention, low urinary output can be a marker of cardiovascular compromise. Glomerular filtration is driven by the pressure gradient across the wall of the glomerular capillary. Renal perfusion pressure is generated by renal blood flow, which is dependent on cardiac output, systemic to pulmonary shunts and SVR. Like the adult kidney, the preterm kidney has the ability to autoregulate blood flow above an unknown threshold of renal perfusion pressure. Below that critical threshold, glomerular filtration (hence urinary output) decreases proportionally to prerenal blood pressure and hence renal blood flow.

In the preterm neonate, this relationship is obscured in the first week of life and caution must be used in relying on urinary output as a marker of renal perfusion. Urine output in preterm neonates follows a predictable pattern. There is minimal urine output in the prediuretic phase (birth to day 2) followed by an abrupt increase during the diuretic phase (days 1 to 5) and a gradual leveling out during the homeostatic phase. During this time, high urine output is not a reliable marker of adequate renal perfusion, though a significant decrease from baseline may be concerning (31).

Laboratory Markers

An increase in serum lactate may occur in clinical situations where anaerobic metabolism occurs when cellular oxygen delivery is compromised. This may occur due to inadequate oxygen content in the blood as occurs in significant anemia or hypoxemia, inadequate tissue blood flow, or a combination of the two. Hence, elevated arterial lactate may be a marker of low cardiac output particularly when used in combination with other clinical or echo markers of low systemic blood flow. Metabolic acidosis will also occur in conditions leading to tissue hypoxia and anaerobic metabolism; however, base excess is significantly

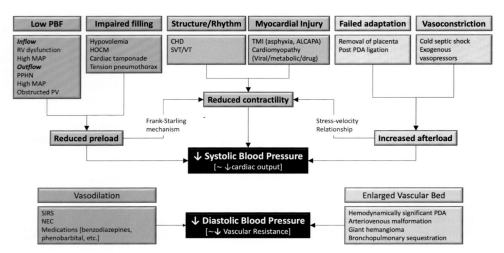

FIGURE 31.1 Physiologic approach to appraisal of low systolic and low diastolic blood pressure based on relevant disease states.

affected by bicarbonate loss and has been shown to correlate poorly with tissue perfusion.

In the absence of other clinical indices of cardiovascular health or cardiac output, elevated lactate has poor specificity (30). Lactate is produced as a result of increased gluconeogenesis, and in some inborn errors of metabolism. It is spuriously increased with sample hemolysis, and caution must be interpreted when catecholamines are being administered as sympathomimetic medications increase lactate via perfusion-independent mechanisms. Finally, lactate may be sequestered in damaged tissue and only when perfusion is improved will serum levels rise.

Mixed venous oxygen saturation (svO_2) is widely used in adult intensive care to measure tissue extraction of oxygen. Low svO_2 (<70%) is associated with negative outcomes in children, but neonatal studies are lacking (30). Poorly perfused organs in situations of low systemic blood flow extract as much oxygen as possible to optimize aerobic metabolism; hence, svO_2 will be low. Caution should be used interpreting svO_2 in disorders such as NEC as ischemic tissue does not extract oxygen, and therefore, high svO_2 may be misleading. In neonates, catheter positioning is difficult and acquiring a mixed svO_2, for which the optimal catheter position is the main pulmonary artery, is not typically possible. Central venous saturation, which is optimally acquired from the right atrium at the junction of the SVC or IVC, can be measured and changes in parallel with mixed svO_2. The absolute values of mixed and central svO_2 are not interchangeable, and central svO_2 is affected by catheter position. Due to differential blood flow to vital organs in conditions of shock, a catheter placed in the SVC will overestimate mixed svO_2, while one in the IVC will underestimate it. The presence of a high-volume peripheral shunt decreases systemic organ perfusion and increases PBF, hence leading to overestimation of svO_2. If catheter position is appropriate, changes in central svO_2 over time can be helpful in assessment of neonates with low cardiac output. If measurable, the difference between SVC and IVC PaO_2 may reflect ductal shunt volume. Elevated preductal LVO with high PaO_2 (due to pulmonary recirculation) may result in higher venous oxygen content in the SVC, while the postductal circulation has greater extraction due to lower overall blood flow.

The Importance of a Holistic Approach

In general, no individual marker of circulatory function should be used in isolation. Longitudinal monitoring of arterial pressure provides an objective and reliable surrogate of cardiovascular well-being; however, it should not be used as the sole basis to inform decision-making independent of other markers. The components of blood pressure, systolic and diastolic thresholds, may provide insights regarding the specific pathophysiologic process that may be useful in guiding treatment choices. Clinical and laboratory assessment should be combined with a compatible history before treatment decisions are made. Echocardiography or other measures of organ blood flow should be considered whenever possible.

Role of Targeted Neonatal Echocardiography

The approach to cardiovascular care in neonates was previously limited by the lack of reliable clinical tools to provide longitudinal information regarding cardiovascular well-being. The consequences include diagnostic assumptions, incorrect treatment choices, and limited ability for longitudinal evaluation. Targeted neonatal echocardiography (TNE) refers to the use of ultrasound by trained neonatologists to assess cardiovascular health, obtain physiologic information relevant to the clinical situation, formulate a diagnostic impression, make a therapeutic recommendation, and evaluate the response to treatment. It has now become the standard of care within many neonatal intensive care units (NICUs) throughout the world, and there is increasing evidence of its benefit to neonates. A variety of training and clinical models for

the application of cardiac ultrasound performed by neonatologists have evolved due to local needs, availability of cardiology consultation services, and clinical practice environment. In Australasia, where the discipline first evolved in the 1990s, most neonatal trainees learn cardiac imaging and are certified by the Australian Society of Ultrasound Medicine receiving the Certificate of Clinician Performed Ultrasound at the completion of training. This qualification includes dedicated basic and advanced training courses with a significant hands-on component, logging system, and mentoring by experienced neonatal echocardiographers (32). In North America, the Writing Group of the American Society of Echocardiography in collaboration with the European Association of Echocardiography and the Association for European Pediatric Cardiologists published TNE clinical practice guidelines and recommendations for training in 2011 (33). This consensus was followed by the recommendations for neonatologist-performed echocardiography (NoPE) in the United Kingdom subsequently endorsed by the European Society of Pediatric Research (34–36). Both guidelines were heavily influenced by pediatric cardiology and established basic and advanced training curriculums that involved a high level of expertise. The field of TNE has evolved in many centers to a program in which neonatologists with advanced training in both cardiac imaging and cardiovascular physiology provide diagnostic support and treatment advice to the primary neonatologist in a consultative capacity (37). The main limitation of this paradigm, however, is the extent of the training, which may delay a critical mass of trained clinicians acquiring core imaging skills essential to neonatal intensive care practice (38). For example, emergent assessment of patients with presumed pericardial effusions or catheter malposition may be lifesaving. Therefore, basic point-of-care cardiac ultrasound curriculums have been developed to enable training more providers in basic ultrasound applications.

It is essential that TNE evaluation of hemodynamics is comprehensive due to the complexity of neonatal cardiovascular physiology. Within the immediate postnatal period, it is difficult to determine whether hemodynamic instability is a result of intracardiac and extracardiac shunting, alterations in SVR and PVR, or a developmentally immature myocardium. The goals of TNE include longitudinal assessment myocardial function, systemic and pulmonary blood flow, shunts, organ blood flow, and tissue perfusion. TNE is usually performed by a neonatologist, is directed by a specific clinical question, and may provide hemodynamic information that either complements clinical findings or provides novel physiologic insights. The availability of real-time physiologic data is thought to help the attending physician provide more focused and targeted cardiovascular care. Combination of clinical examination and bedside echocardiography has been shown to improve clinical diagnosis and patient management in the adult population. There is some evidence that routine use of TNE in the neonatal unit may lead to identification of cardiovascular compromise, changes in management, and potentially improved short-term outcomes. TNE has enabled more targeted cardiovascular management, determining the type of inotropic agent most likely to be of benefit and monitoring treatment response. The provision of real-time information on cardiovascular performance and systemic hemodynamics, noninvasive nature of the technique, rapidity of data acquisition and report generation, and ability to perform longitudinal functional assessments have all contributed to in the increased utilization of functional echocardiography by neonatologists in the NICU. The use of this Hemodynamic Consultation model, in particular, enables individual TNE practitioners to acquire a high level of proficiency by repeated exposure to relatively uncommon problems, facilitates the introduction of "Precision Medicine" into neonatal cardiovascular care, and supports clinical operations. Many modern pediatric cardiology practices are not resourced to provide longitudinal assessment of cardiovascular physiology, and most North American NICUs are large, busy clinical practices. The complexity of cardiovascular physiology often requires a considerable time investment that may take away from the care of other patients. As the field of neonatology becomes increasingly advanced scientifically, to which TNE practitioners have and continue to contribute significantly, so too does the body of knowledge required to maintain competence in the field. Neonatology may benefit from gradual evolution in both hemodynamics and other areas (neonatal neurology, transport medicine, nutrition, etc.) just as other fields of medicine (e.g., internal medicine, pediatrics) have evolved to require both generalists and specialists.

There is growing evidence of the value of TNE in aiding diagnosis and guiding hemodynamic therapy in the NICU. Overall, the use of TnECHO has been associated with improved diagnostic clarity and a change in management in approximately 40% to 50% of cases (39–42). There are subpopulations of neonates in whom the diagnostic and therapeutic value of real-time physiologic assessment has direct clinical relevance. Infants with refractory hypoxemia or impaired tissue oxygen delivery may have complex, highly variable, and overlapping contributors to disease, each of which have different treatment approaches. In this patient population, TnECHO is associated with an 80% to 90% rate of change in management on the basis of refined physiologic precision (40). In the population of patients with a hemodynamically significant ductus arteriosus (HSDA) requiring surgical ligation, TnECHO-based clinical observations followed by natural history studies have led to an enhanced understanding of the role of afterload in postoperative cardiorespiratory instability. The subsequent identification of the importance of 1-hour postoperative LVO as a predictive marker of later decompensation has the capacity to identify at-risk neonates with high sensitivity and specificity (43,44) and a standardized TnECHO-based triaging model has been shown to reduce the frequency of surgical ligation without negative impact on outcomes (45). TnECHO-based research has, similarly, led to the development of a predictive score calculated on postnatal day 2 for later development of death or bronchopulmonary dysplasia (BPD) in infants with a conservatively managed ductus arteriosus (46) and identified a targeted approach to early ductal therapy which reduces the risk of pulmonary hemorrhage (47). Other important applications include identifying the mechanism of action of vasoactive medications (48), a refined understanding of the accuracy of clinical monitoring tools (49), and enhanced understanding of the hemodynamic antecedents of intraventricular hemorrhage (IVH) (49–51). Future research should continue to investigate "disease-specific" impact of TNE on relevant clinical outcomes.

Novel Methods for Assessment of the Cardiovascular System

There is increasing emphasis, in contemporary neonatal practice, on the importance and need to monitor minute by minute indices of physiologic stability to understand neonatal disease and enhance patient outcomes. Most of these newer devices are not used in routine clinical practice but they provide novel insights which will improve our understanding of neonatal hemodynamics, thus informing clinical practice.

Noninvasive Cardiac Output and Systemic Blood Flow Monitoring

Continuous cardiac output (CO) monitoring is a potentially valuable tool in the NICU in the management of a wide range of neonatal illnesses. In adults and older children, continuous CO measurement is frequently achieved by invasive methods, including thermodilution using a pulmonary artery catheter, an intraesophageal probe for continuous Doppler velocity flow assessment, or an arterial catheter for pulse contour analysis. Size constraints or suboptimal reliability preclude the use of these methods in preterm and term infants and in lieu, several noninvasive and semi-invasive modalities have been evaluated.

Detectable alterations in the electrical properties of the thorax have been used to estimate cardiac output. In children, bioimpedance estimates of cardiac output are unreliable when compared

with magnetic resonance imaging and direct Fick methods (52,53). Two newer electrical approaches, based on extensions of the theory of bioimpedance, are currently under evaluation. Electrical velocimetry is based on the principle that the conductivity of the blood in the aorta varies during the cardiac cycle. During systole, red blood cells align in the direction of flow, and the electrical current applied from external electrodes is easily conducted. In diastole, red blood cells assume a random orientation, which results in lower conductivity of the injected electrical current. Electrical velocimetry measures the peak rate of change in conductivity across the cardiac cycle and uses it to derive the mean aortic blood velocity index, from which left ventricular stroke volume is estimated using calculated aortic cross-sectional area and left ventricular ejection times (Fig. 31.2). Studies in small children have compared the cardiac output estimates of electrical velocimetry with transthoracic echocardiography (TTE). In a mixed population of children with repaired/unrepaired congenital heart disease, electrical velocimetry estimates of cardiac output had unacceptably high absolute and percentage bias compared with thermodilution and subxiphoid Doppler measurements (54,55). Noori et al. compared CO estimates of electrical velocimetry and TTE in healthy term neonates and found a mean difference of 4 mL/min (limits of agreement −234 to 242 mL/min) and an adjusted percentage bias of 31.6% (56). Grollmus et al. reported a similar 29% relative TTE–electrical velocimetry bias in a cohort of infants postoperatively from the arterial switch operation (57).

Transthoracic bioreactance is another newer method of noninvasive cardiac output monitoring (NICOM, Cheetah Medical, MA). In contrast to bioimpedance, which aims to detect changes in the amplitude of an applied electrical current, bioreactance estimates changes in the frequency of the current (the relative phase shift) between the input and output signals, which is induced by blood ejected into the aorta from the left ventricle. Stroke volume is estimated using the measured peak rate of change of the phase shift, ventricular ejection time, and a constant of proportionality that accounts for patient age, gender, and body size. Studies have reported variable reliability of NICOM-measured cardiac output. NICOM was compared with invasive measurements of CO using an aortic root catheter in anaesthetized beagles and demonstrated a bias of 63 ± 38 mL/min, a percent bias of 6.1%, and high responsiveness to pharmacologically induced changes in CO (58). By contrast, NICOM demonstrated poor reliability and responsiveness compared with pulmonary artery thermodilution measured CO in critically ill adults being treated with volume expansion (mean bias 0.9 L/min/m² and limits of agreement −2.2 to 4.1) (59). In a heterogeneous group of term and moderately preterm neonates, NICOM estimates of CO were strongly correlated with TTE (r = 0.95) but NICOM systematically underestimated CO by 31% ± 8% (60). In a cohort of extremely preterm infants undergoing patent ductus arteriosus (PDA) ligation, NICOM similarly underestimated CO relative to echocardiography (mean bias 39%, limits of agreement 8% to 69%), with increasing bias over time (61). Collectively, these studies suggest that NICOM is able to trend cardiac output over time, but it is not interchangeable with invasive or noninvasive measures. Use as a trending tool of CO in neonates likely requires initial and periodic calibration with echocardiography. Additional studies demonstrating adequate reliability are needed prior to independent use.

Noninvasive Cerebral Perfusion Imaging: Near Infrared Spectroscopy

Near infrared spectroscopy (NIRS) is a diffuse optical technique that measures variations of cerebral absorption and scattering within the spectral window of the near infrared range. It is sensitive to tissue chromophore (oxy and deoxyhemoglobin) concentrations and thus can be used to estimate regional cerebral oxygen saturation (rcSO₂), cerebral fractional tissue oxygen extraction (cFTOE), and cerebral blood volume. Neonates are ideal candidates for NIRS monitoring because the decreased thickness of the

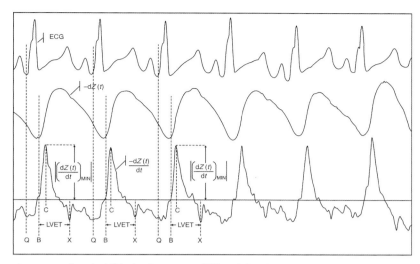

FIGURE 31.2 Surface ECG, impedance waveform [−dZ(t), also known as ΔZ(t)], and the electronically differentiated first time derivative of −dZ(t), −dZ(t)/dt, obtained from electrical velocimetry monitoring on a 25-day-old male (HR = 142 beats per minute, SV = 3.3 mL, CO = 0.47 L/min). The marker labeled "Q" on the ECG marks the beginning of ventricular depolarization and thus the onset of electromechanical systole. Shortly after aortic valve opening ("B"), the −dZ(t) waveform exhibits a significant upslope and, consequently, its time derivative, −dZ(t)/dt, exhibits a nadir ("C"). The amplitude at the point, which in the traditional presentation is depicted as a positive deflection, is the maximum slope or peak rate of change of the transthoracic electrical impedance during a particular cardiac cycle and measured beat to beat. The time to peak (rise time) of −dZ(t)/dt is concordant with the time to peak of −dv(t)/dt of the aortic blood velocity waveform. The magnitude at the peak of −dZ(t)/dt, that is $|$(dZ(t)/dt)$_{MIN}|$, is analogous to the magnitude $|$dv(t)/d$t|_{MIN}$ of this waveform. The first-time derivative of the impedance waveform, −dZ(t)/dt, exhibits a deflection at the time of aortic valve closure ("X"). The temporal interval between points B and X is defined as the left ventricular ejection time. (Reprinted from Norozi K, Beck C, Osthaus WA, et al. Electrical velocimetry for measuring cardiac output in children with congenital heart disease. *Br J Anaesth* 2008;100(1):88. Copyright © 2008 British Journal of Anaesthesia.)

neonatal skull permits deeper penetration of near infrared light. NIRS measurements are performed continuously and noninvasively at the bedside, without the need for general anesthesia.

The surveillance and prevention of early cerebral injury in neonates is one area where the clinical utility of NIRS in the NICU may be justified. Among very preterm neonates requiring respiratory support in the transitional period, cerebral hypoxia may occur in spite of an arterial oxygen saturation within the target range, as cerebral tissue oxygenation also depends on cerebral blood flow (influenced by open shunts during the transitional period), hemoglobin concentration, and cerebral oxygen consumption. Normative ranges of rcSO$_2$ and cFTOE during normal neonatal transition for term (62) and preterm (63) infants have been established. Lower rcSO$_2$ and higher cFTOE, both in the first minutes and days of life, herald the subsequent development of severe peri-IVH in very preterm infants (64,65), and accordingly potentially facilitates earlier identification of high-risk infants who may benefit from intervention to prevent cerebral injury. The recent SafeBoosc II trial reported that applying cerebral NIRS and implementing an algorithm to maintain rcSO$_2$ within a defined range (55% to 85%) resulted in a lower burden of cerebral hypoxia and hyperoxia (66). This intervention is currently being evaluated, in a follow-up trial, for its effect on improving survival without neurodevelopmental impairment among extremely preterm infants (67).

PATENT DUCTUS ARTERIOSUS

Pathophysiologic Continuum of the Ductal Shunt in Neonates

During normal transition at birth, clamping of the umbilical cord and the initiation of ventilation in air result in an increase in SVR and decrease in PVR. The ductal flow pattern, previously right to left *in utero*, becomes bidirectional and eventually left to right as PVR decreases below systemic arterial pressure. In unwell neonates, the ductal shunt is variable in direction, reflecting disordered pulmonary and/or systemic blood flow or perturbations in the programmed postnatal decrease in PVR. Consideration of the role of the ductus arteriosus should not be binary. The PDA may

play a supportive or neutral role in infants with persistent pulmonary hypertension of the newborn (PPHN), in whom there is a postnatal failure of vasorelaxation of the pulmonary arterioles (due to either abnormal fetal pulmonary development or maladaptive neonatal transition), resulting in persistently elevated PVR. In severe cases, PVR remains suprasystemic and the ductal shunt is from the pulmonary artery to the aorta, supporting the postductal systemic blood flow, albeit with deoxygenated blood that results in a difference in oxygen saturation between preductal and postductal circulations. Here, the PDA also results in reduced right ventricular (RV) afterload and may help preserve RV function. In mild cases of PPHN, the ductal shunt is bidirectional and may not contribute significantly to either pulmonary overcirculation or RV afterload reduction. Instead, the PDA may be an innocuous bystander, which provides a measure of the pressure gradient between the pulmonary and systemic circulations.

In preterm and a small minority of term infants whose PVR decreases at birth but in whom the ductus remains patent, a continuous left-to-right shunt develops. Shunt volume is determined by the pressure gradient between the pulmonary artery and aorta, and by the resistance to transductal flow, which is primarily influenced by ductal diameter and length. Determinants of PVR such as hypocapnemia, hyperoxia, or alkalosis may augment the shunt volume. A large shunt results in volume overload of the pulmonary artery, subsequent alveolar edema, reduced pulmonary compliance, and increased need for mechanical ventilation. Increased blood flow to the left heart results in increased end-diastolic volume of the left atrium and ventricle. Left ventricular dilatation occurs, and it compensates by increasing stroke volume. Impaired left ventricular diastolic compliance results in pressure loading of the left atrium and contributes to left atrial dilatation. Diastolic flow reversal from the descending aorta to the pulmonary artery via the PDA is common, as is absent or reverse end-diastolic flow in systemic arteries such as the celiac and superior mesenteric arteries. Diastolic "steal," combined with shorter diastolic times due to tachycardia and increased myocardial oxygen demand from left ventricular dilatation, may result in subendocardial ischemia.

THE NEWBORN INFANT

Clinical Importance of Patent Ductus Arteriosus in Preterm Infants: Severe Morbidities of Prematurity

One-third of very low birth weight (VLBW) infants and up to 65% of infants born at gestational age less than 28 weeks have PDA on the third day of life (68). Infants with persistent PDA have increased mortality, IVH, BPD, retinopathy of prematurity (ROP), and necrotizing enterocolitis (NEC) compared with infants without a PDA. Perinatal hemodynamic instability, cerebral ischemia, and subsequent reperfusion injury may contribute to the development of germinal matrix hemorrhage and subsequent extension into the cerebral ventricles (IVH) or periventricular hemorrhagic venous infarction. Most IVH occurs in the first week of life, coincident with the emergence of a left-to-right ductal shunt, which increases cerebral (preductal) blood flow and may contribute to reperfusion injury. Both the targeted and indiscriminate administration of prophylactic indomethacin reduce the incidence of all grades of IVH, possibly by mitigating the emergence of a significant ductal shunt (69).

PDA-induced pulmonary overcirculation and systemic hypoperfusion may contribute to increased BPD and NEC. Increased PBF results in pulmonary interstitial edema and greater need for invasive mechanical ventilation. Ventilator-induced lung injury promotes alveolar inflammation and ongoing need for respiratory support, a major risk factor for the development of BPD. Diastolic flow reversal in the abdominal aorta, celiac artery, and superior mesenteric artery (SMA) is common in infants with PDA, and this diastolic "steal" may contribute to intestinal hypoperfusion and an increased risk of NEC. While a causal relationship between PDA and IVH, BPD, NEC, and ROP has not been definitively established, a number of physiologic, observational, and randomized trials strongly support this association (68,70). The association of these morbidities with increased mortality and adverse neurodevelopmental outcome is the impetus behind the need to identify and potentially mitigate the multisystem effects of a pathologic ductal shunt.

Determining the Hemodynamic Significance of the Patent Ductus Arteriosus

For term neonates with PDA, treatment in infancy is considered if left heart volume loading and pulmonary overcirculation lead to feeding difficulty, inadequate weight gain, or pulmonary insufficiency. In the absence of these clinical findings, infants are permitted to grow to allow later catheter-device closure in lieu of an open surgical technique, and PDA closure is performed to prevent irreversible changes to the pulmonary arteriolar musculature and pulmonary hypertension (PH). The variability in timing of ductal closure in term infants highlights the pathophysiologic spectrum associated with PDA-related shunting.

By contrast, the clinical evaluation of the hemodynamic significance of PDA in preterm infants is more challenging due to the common coexistence of pulmonary disorders and immature oral feeding ability. Respiratory distress syndrome (RDS) and ventilator-induced lung injury result in pulmonary insufficiency that can be exacerbated by a significant ductal shunt. Myocardial diastolic dysfunction is also common in preterm infants (71) and reduces the infant's tolerance of left heart volume loading associated with a PDA. The clinical determination of the relative pathologic effect of the PDA and primary pulmonary disorders is also influenced by gestational age-based expectations and the evolution of an infant's respiratory and feeding physiology as he matures. The clinical hemodynamic significance of a PDA may therefore be considered to fall along a continuum between innocent bystander and prime pathologic contributor. Echocardiography is the primary method of PDA evaluation in preterm infants and requires assessments of the following: ductus arteriosus size and flow pattern, pulmonary overcirculation and left heart loading, and systemic arterial diastolic flow reversal ("systemic steal").

Assessment of the Ductus Arteriosus Size and Transductal Flow Pattern

Shunt volume is positively correlated with PDA radius; vessel size ≥ 1.5 mm on the first day of life predicts a subsequent symptomatic PDA (47) and correlates well with Doppler flow pattern in assessments of hemodynamic significance (72). For infants with birth weight near 0.5 kg, the 1.5-mm threshold may be insensitive and in lieu, PDA diameter may be indexed to weight (>1.5 mm/kg) or LPA diameter (PDA:LPA ratio >0.5), though unindexed ductal diameter is more strongly correlated with shunt volume (73).

The spectrum of PDA pulse-wave Doppler flow patterns reflects the varied and evolving status of a PDA as a barometer of pulmonary artery pressure versus primary pathologic contributor to left heart volume loading and pulmonary overcirculation. In severe neonatal PH, the ductal shunt is right to left when pulmonary artery pressure is suprasystemic and bidirectional (right to left in systole, left to right in diastole) when pulmonary artery pressure is approximately systemic. While a bidirectional ductal shunt is common in preterm infants on the first day of life, a persistent bidirectional ductal shunt has been associated with increased mortality, likely a surrogate marker of persistent PH due to severe pulmonary disease. The restricted or "closing" pattern of a PDA depicts a very high velocity ductal shunt (peak systolic velocity >2.0 m/s) and low peak systolic-to-minimum diastolic velocity ratio (<2.0) (**Fig. 31.3**). A hemodynamically significant PDA is characterized by an unrestrictive or "pulsatile" left-to-right flow pattern, with the highest peak velocity at the end of systole and very low diastolic velocity. While peak systolic velocity less than 1.5 m/s has been traditionally described as "unrestrictive," higher peak systolic velocities may be seen in infants with large unrestrictive ductal shunts, owing to very large shunt volumes or in the situation of a chronic funnel-shaped PDA, posttreatment, where there may be partial restriction at the pulmonary end.

Assessment of Pulmonary Overcirculation—Left Heart Loading

A large left-to-right ductal shunt is associated with increased pulmonary arterial blood flow, pulmonary venous return, left ventricular (LV) end-diastolic volume, and left-ventricular output. Pulmonary artery diastolic velocity, left atrial and LV chamber sizes, mitral valve Doppler velocities, and LV output provide surrogate estimates of pulmonary overcirculation and left heart volume and pressure loading, though they may be of reduced value in the presence of a large transatrial shunt. A large left-to-right ductal shunt delivers blood to the pulmonary artery throughout the cardiac cycle, resulting in more turbulent flow and increased antegrade diastolic flow in the main and branch pulmonary arteries. Left pulmonary artery diastolic velocity correlates with increased ductal shunting estimated by cardiac catheterization and a prolonged need for mechanical ventilation (74). Maximum left pulmonary artery diastolic velocity less than 0.2 m/s is suggestive of a small ductal shunt, while greater than 0.5 m/s is associated with a large shunt.

Infants with PDA have increased LV output and LV end-diastolic dimension (LVEDD), which are surrogates for increased LV end-diastolic volume. LVEDD can be compared to previously published normative values for LV chamber size for VLBW infants. LV output greater than 300 mL/kg/min is highly specific in predicting a symptomatic PDA (47). Left atrial dilatation occurs due to volume and pressure loading from increased pulmonary venous return and LV diastolic dysfunction. The relatively fixed transaortic diameter permits indexing of LA chamber size for comparison of the LA:Ao ratio between infants. LA:Ao greater than 1.4 has a high sensitivity for ductal significance (75); however, higher LA:Ao ratios (≥ 1.6) are more specific for a significant ductal shunt (76).

Mitral valve inflow Doppler indices and isovolumic relaxation time (IVRT) are affected by left atrium volume and pressure

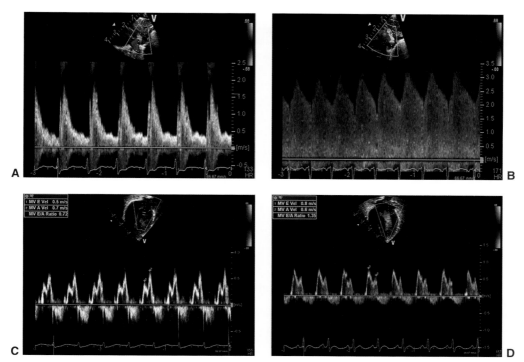

FIGURE 31.3 Pulse-wave Doppler interrogation of a PDA (A and B) and left ventricular inflow across the mitral valve (C and D). An unrestrictive left-to-right ductal shunt **(A)** has the Doppler profile of an arterial pulsation, with low diastolic velocity, while a restrictive shunt demonstrates high peak systolic and diastolic velocities and low systolic-to-diastolic peak velocity ratio. Left ventricular filling in diastole consists of early ("E") and late ("A," during atrial contraction) phases, with normal E:A ratio >1. Preterm infants with no PDA demonstrate normal inflow and an E:A ratio <1 due to prematurity-related decreased myocardial compliance and impaired early filling **(C)**. Large PDA is associated with left atrial pressure loading and increased early diastolic ventricular filling, resulting in a "pseudonormalized" E:A ratio >1.

loading associated with a large ductal shunt. In healthy term infants, the mitral valve E ("early") wave to A ("atrial") wave ratio (E:A) is greater than 1, signifying a predominance of early LV diastolic filling. The myocardium in preterm infants is less compliant resulting in impaired passive diastolic filling, reliance on atrial contraction for ventricular filling, and a resultant mitral valve E:A ratio less than 1. In the presence of a large ductal shunt, increased end-systolic left atrial pressure results in earlier mitral valve opening and a shortened IVRT (often <45 ms) (71) and increased early passive filling velocity and flow, with E:A greater than 1, termed "pseudonormalization" (Fig. 31.3).

Systemic Steal

Diastolic flow reversal in the abdominal aorta and splanchnic circulation due to a ductal shunt occurs when the aortopulmonary pressure gradient is greater than the diastolic pressure in the abdominal aorta or the specific end-organ arterial resistance. This diastolic "steal" in the abdominal aorta is one of the well-recognized and reliable indicators of a hemodynamically significant shunt in preterm infants, both clinically and on cardiac MRI (77). Celiac artery Doppler flow to LV output ratio (CAF:LVO) less than 0.1 is highly sensitive for the presence of a significant PDA (78). Infants with PDA may have reduced SMA blood flow, which may impair postprandial increases in intestinal perfusion. Although the middle cerebral artery (MCA) is supplied by preductal cardiac output, a large ductal shunt may result in reduced, absent, or reverse MCA diastolic flow, though the clinical sequelae of this are unknown. Reductions in diastolic flow associated with a PDA may be compensated for by increases in systolic blood flow. Echocardiography may assess arterial perfusion, but not vascular resistance. Reduced blood flow velocity and/or diastolic flow reversal in the splanchnic circulation improves immediately after PDA ligation.

Biomarkers

The potential role of biomarkers in the management of PDA may be to support the evaluation of PDA shunt volume and monitor the response to treatment. Given that echocardiography is the standard of care for PDA assessment to evaluate size and rule out ductal-dependent congenital lesions, biomarkers should not replace echocardiography as an initial step in PDA assessment.

In response to left heart pressure and volume loading, cardiac myocytes cleave pro-brain natriuretic peptide (BNP) into biologically active BNP and the inactive fragment amino-terminal pro BNP (NTpBNP). BNP inhibits the renin–angiotensin–aldosterone axis, vasodilates the pulmonary and systemic circulation, and promotes natriuresis and diuresis. While modalities to measure plasma BNP and NTpBNP concentrations are widely available, NTpBNP has the advantage of having a longer half-life (60 vs. 20 minutes).

Studies to date have predominantly investigated the ability of BNP and NTpBNP to discriminate among infants with versus without a hemodynamically significant PDA at various postnatal ages. Their broader clinical use in the NICU, however, has been hampered by the evaluation of many different testing kits (each with its own reference value range), significant uncertainty and heterogeneity in PDA management, and the absence of a gold-standard method of PDA severity staging, rendering the interpretation of results more challenging. These biomarkers have not been robustly investigated for their ability to predict neonatal outcomes and are therefore presently limited in clinical utility to being a method of screening for PDA to decrease the need for echocardiography.

The early identification of infants at high risk for developing a symptomatic PDA may be clinically useful in centers seeking to administer targeted treatment aimed at early ductal closure. In very preterm infants, elevations in plasma BNP and NTpBNP concentrations at birth and on the first day of life correlate with lower gestational and birth weight, but not the development of PDA.

TABLE 31.2

Relationship between Plasma BNP/NTpBNP Concentration in the First 3 Days of Life and a Diagnosis of hsPDA in Preterm Infants

Author (Year)	Bio-Marker	Mean or Median GA (wk)	No. Infants (No. with hsPDA)	Age (d) at Sample	Area under ROC (95% CI)	Threshold	Sensitivity (%)	Specificity (%)
Choi (2005)[a]	BNP	29	66 (23)	3	0.997 (0.99–1.00)	>1,100	100	95
Flynn (2005)[a]	BNP	28	20 (n/a)	3	N/A	>300	52	100
Czernik (2008)[b]	BNP	25	67 (24)	2	0.86 (0.75–0.96)	>550	83	86
El-Khuffash (2007)[c]	NTpBNP	27	48 (25)	3	0.87 (0.76–0.97)	>5,000	70	87
Farombi-Oghuvbu (2008)[c]	NTpBNP	30	49 (18)	3	0.98 (0.93–1.03)	>1,347	100	95
Nuntnarumit (2009)[c]	NTpBNP	29	35 (12)	3	0.96 (0.91–1.02)	>1,204	100	91
Ramakrishnan (2009)[c]	NTpBNP	28	56 (20)	3	0.90 (0.81–0.99)	>1,280	95	58
						>5,160	60	95
Martinovici (2011)[c]	NTpBNP	28	27 (12)	2	0.92 (0.67–0.99)	>1,182	89	100
				4	0.98 (0.84–1.00)	>591	91	100
Buddhe (2012)[d]	NTpBNP	27	69 (22)	3–5	0.98 (p < 0.001)	>697	96	90
Occhipinti (2014)[c]	NTpBNP	28	41 (32)	1	0.86 (0.74–0.98)	>1,165	71	100

BNP thresholds expressed in pg/mL; NTpBNP thresholds expressed in pmol/L. Studies reporting NTpBNP concentrations in pg/mL were converted to pmol/L (1 pmol/L = 8.457 pg/mL).

[a]Triage BNP test, Biosite Diagnostics.
[b]ADVIA Centaur analyzer, Siemens/Bayer.
[c]Elecsys proBNP, Roche Diagnostics.
[d]VITROS NTpBNP reagent pack, Ortho Clinical Diagnostics.

BNP, brain natriuretic peptide; GA, gestational age; hsPDA, hemodynamically significant patent ductus arteriosus; NTpBNP, amino-terminal pro brain natriuretic peptide; ROC, receiver operating curve.

After the second day of life, elevated concentrations predict hemodynamically significant PDA (Table 31.2), though the interpretation of widely varying cutoff values of BNP and NTpBNP is hampered by the use of different testing kits and diagnostic criteria for symptomatic PDA. Martinovici et al. found that plasma NTpBNP level less than 10,000 pg/mL measured on the second day of life had 89% sensitivity and 100% specificity for spontaneous ductal closure (79).

After the onset of clinical symptoms of suspected ductal shunting, plasma BNP/NTpBNP discriminate between infants with and without a hemodynamically significant PDA, as diagnosed by echocardiography. Chen et al. reported that a plasma BNP (Triage BNP assay, Biosite Diagnostics) cutoff value of 40 pg/mL had a 92% sensitivity, 46% specificity, 1.70 positive likelihood ratio (LR), and 0.17 negative LR for predicting a moderate-or-large PDA shunt as assessed by echocardiography (80). The low specificity and positive likelihood ratio reflect the large overlap in values among infants with and without a hemodynamically significant PDA. Higher cutoff values have lower sensitivity but higher specificity. A plasma BNP cutoff value of 200 pg/mL had a 59% sensitivity, 91% specificity, 6.91 positive LR, and 0.46 negative LR for predicting a moderate-or-large echocardiographic PDA shunt. These findings suggest that plasma BNP less than 40 pg/mL or greater than 200 pg/mL indicate a moderate likelihood of not having and having a hemodynamically significant PDA, respectively. In centers where access to echocardiography is limited, these cutoffs may be helpful for guiding administration of empiric pharmacologic therapy aimed at ductal closure. However, plasma BNP concentrations in the range of 40 to 200 pg/mL are poorly discriminatory and echocardiography is needed. A recent systematic review reported a summary sensitivity and specificity for the diagnosis of PDA of 0.88 (95% CI 0.76 to 0.95) and 0.92 (95% CI 0.81 to 0.97) for BNP (10 studies) and 0.90 (95% CI 0.79 to 0.96) and 0.84 (95% CI 0.77 to 0.90) for NTpBNP (11 studies) (81).

Management of PDA

Historical Perspectives and Current Trends

Despite over four decades and 60 randomized clinical trials of PDA treatment, neonatologists remain uncertain about "which PDA should be treated?" The broadly adopted approach to PDA management in the latter part of the 20th century was based on the then-accepted dogma that the ductal shunt was uniformly deleterious and exposure to PDA should be minimized (82). Early pharmacologic treatment and rescue surgical ligation were widely practiced with the singular focus of achieving PDA closure as quickly as possible. Trials of various approaches to PDA treatment have since demonstrated that pharmacotherapy facilitates earlier ductal closure but does not improve neonatal and neurodevelopmental outcomes, including early screening and treatment of asymptomatic PDA (1st or 2nd day after birth) (83–86) and treatment of symptomatic PDA (after the 3rd day of life) (87–91). Universal prophylaxis conclusively reduces all forms of IVH but without medium- or long-term benefit (92,93).

The lack of demonstrable improvement in neonatal outcomes in clinical trials has driven secular changes in management over the past decade, shifting the landscape of PDA treatment toward more selective treatment and even complete nonintervention (94,95). Among more mature preterm infants, decreased or more selective pharmacologic and surgical treatment has been associated with improved (or at least similar) neonatal outcomes (96,97). Periviable infants, however, have been reported to experience increased morbidity with decreased PDA treatment. Bixler et al. reported that PDA treatment declined, year-over-year, among all GA subgroups (p < 0.001) of a cohort of 61,520 preterm infants born at GA 23 to 30 weeks, but concomitant rates of BPD increased annually among infants born at GA 23 to 24 weeks (98). Furthermore, in a multicenter study of repeated measures, aggregated data from NICUs in the California Perinatal Quality Care Initiative, dose–response associations were identified between annual reductions in NICU-specific treatment and increased rates of all-cause mortality among the smallest ELGANs. While decreased PDA treatment was associated with decreased or unchanged mortality among infants born greater than 750 g, each percentage point decrease in pharmacologic treatment or surgical ligation was associated with a 0.21% (95% CI 0.06 to 0.35, p < 0.01) increase in mortality among infants with birth weight 400 to 749 g (99).

Redefining "Hemodynamically Significant" Using Major Clinical Outcomes

The lack of a standardized or validated definition of "hemodynamically significant PDA" among clinical trials has culminated in uncertainty regarding which infants with PDA should be considered for treatment. A systematic review of the definition of hemodynamically significant PDA used to establish inclusion criteria in clinical trials identified that studies used arbitrary cutoffs of select clinical and echocardiography parameters, unvalidated against important clinical outcomes (100). PDA diameter was used as the sole entry criterion in 15% of trials, a possible physiologic simplification based on a small cohort study that identified that a diameter of ≥1.5 mm on the first day of life predicted a later diagnosis of symptomatic PDA among moderately preterm infants (47). This "threshold" of ductal diameter has not been validated against neonatal outcomes and suffers from suboptimal imaging reliability (101–103), but it has nonetheless been used in most recent clinical trials as an inclusion criterion (86,89,91,104). The most commonly used echocardiography inclusion criteria were an increased left atrium to aortic root ratio (LA:Ao, a measure of left atrial dilatation, 60% of studies), the presence of diastolic flow reversal in the aorta (37% of trials), and more recently, combinations of indices, such as disturbed Doppler flow in the main pulmonary arteries (90) and Doppler evidence of systemic-to-pulmonary ductal shunting (105), though all of these parameters remain unvalidated and suffer from poor inter- and intraobserver reliability (73,101,102,106).

Studies to date have used simplified clinical and echocardiographic criteria to identify a hemodynamically significant PDA. Failure to define the spectrum of PDA-related hemodynamic disturbance may have resulted in diluted study populations underpowered for the target outcomes. The contemporary clinical decision to administer pharmacologic treatment should integrate a comprehensive echocardiography assessment of the hemodynamic significance of the PDA, rather than a simplified approach based on size. Therapy should target infants in whom the ductal shunt is estimated to be a primary pathologic contributor to current physiologic instability, compared with other concurrent pathologies (most commonly pulmonary immaturity and severe RDS related to prematurity). Ultimately, the valid definition of hemodynamic significance of the ductal shunt requires identifying an association with key clinical outcomes followed by demonstration that targeted treatment of such at-risk infants reduces the risk of morbidity.

A small number of studies have attempted to define hemodynamically significant PDA against clinical outcomes. Increasing PDA diameter and left ventricular dilatation have been associated with earlier time to successful extubation after surgical PDA ligation among ventilator-dependent ELGANs, suggesting that these echocardiography indices may accurately convey the severity of ductal shunting (and impact on pulmonary function) beyond the first 2 weeks of life (which is when ligation is most often performed) (107).

While individual echocardiography parameters are variably sensitive for PDA shunt volume (Table 31.3), their aggregation into a comprehensive PDA score permits the identification of clinically relevant echocardiography indices and avoids redundant measures. Several PDA scores have been reported and demonstrated strong predictive ability for neonatal and neurodevelopmental outcomes. Six echocardiography markers were combined in a PDA score that predicted severe neurologic disability or death in 2-day-old VLBW infants (108). El-Khuffash et al. enrolled 141 infants born at GA less than 29 weeks and prospectively derived a "PDA severity score," combining GA with four echocardiography characteristics estimated at 24 to 48 hours after birth to provide an accurate prediction of the composite outcome of death or BPD (AUC 0.92, 95% CI 0.86 to 0.97) (46). The score (Table 31.4)

TABLE 31.3

Echocardiography Parameters of Ductal Hemodynamic Significance

Parameter	Hemodynamic Significance		
	Mild	Moderate	Severe
Ductus arteriosus size and flow pattern			
PDA 2D diameter	<1.5 mm	1.5–2.5 mm	>2.5 mm
PDA Doppler			
Peak systolic velocity[a]	>2.5	1.5–2.5	<1.5
Peak systolic velocity: minimum diastolic velocity	<2	2–4	>4
Pulmonary overcirculation/left heart loading			
LV chamber size	No/mild dilatation	Moderate dilatation	Marked dilatation
Increased LA pressure			
LA:Ao	<1.5	1.5–2.0	>2.0
Mitral valve E:A ratio	<1	<1	>1
IVRT	>45 ms	30–45 ms	<30 ms
Systemic steal			
Abdominal aorta	No diastolic reversal	Diastolic reversal	Diastolic reversal
Celiac:aorta VTI ratio	—	—	<0.10

[a]Very large left-to-right ductal shunts may have higher peak systolic velocities (>1.5 m/s), indicating high shunt volume rather than flow restriction.

Ao, aorta; IVRT, isovolumic relaxation time; LA, left atrium; LPA, left pulmonary artery; LV, left ventricle; VTI, velocity–time integral.

had greater discriminatory ability than clinical indices alone and selected echocardiography indices for inclusion based on significant univariable association with the primary outcome.

A clinical trial is currently underway using the PDA severity score as entry criteria and evaluating whether early treatment of high-risk infants improves neonatal outcomes. In the absence of definitive data regarding the appropriate criteria for diagnosis or initiation of pharmacologic or surgical treatment for PDA, we present in the following section an overview of the therapeutic approaches used in contemporary practice.

Supportive Management—Strategies to Limit Shunt Volume

Conservative measures comprise treatment strategies aimed at reducing ductal shunt volume or improving an infant's physiologic tolerance of the ductal shunt without medical or surgical interventions to close it. Positive end-expiratory pressure (PEEP), target

TABLE 31.4

Clinical and Echocardiography PDA Score at 24–48 Hours of Life in Preterm Infants <28 Weeks Gestational Age and the Outcome of Death or Bronchopulmonary Dysplasia

Parameter	Standardized β Coefficient
Gestational age (completed weeks at birth)	−0.398
PDA diameter (2D) (mm)	0.079
Left ventricular output (mL/kg/min)	0.272
PDA peak velocity (m/s)	−0.163
Left ventricle a′ (cm/s)	−0.236

Area under the curve 0.92 (95% CI 0.86–0.97) for the outcome of death or bronchopulmonary dysplasia. A cutoff of 5 had a sensitivity of 92% and specificity of 87%.

Reprinted from El-Khuffash AF, James AT, Corcoran JD, et al. A patent ductus severity score predicts chronic lung disease or death before discharge. *J Pediatr* 2015;167(6):1354. Copyright © 2015 Elsevier. With permission.

oxygen saturations, diuretics, fluid restriction, and targeting high blood hematocrit are commonly used. Higher PEEP, administered via invasive or noninvasive mechanical ventilation, decreases systemic and pulmonary venous return, reducing pulmonary alveolar edema and left ventricular end-diastolic volume. An increase in PEEP from 5 to 8 cm H_2O has been demonstrated to significantly reduce echocardiographic indices of left-to-right ductal shunting (109). This may be due, in part, to mitigation of ductal shunting by mean airway pressure (MAP)-associated increases in PVR. Diuretics may be used to reduce pulmonary edema and work of breathing in infants with large left-to-right ductal shunts. Furosemide is the most commonly prescribed diuretic, and its use in preterm infants with PDA-associated volume overload has largely been extrapolated from older studies in infants with edema of varying etiologies, including congestive heart failure (CHF). However, furosemide increases renal prostaglandin production and may mitigate ductal constriction (110). The administration of furosemide to prevent fluid retention in preterm infants with PDA during treatment with indomethacin may result in excessive weight loss without a demonstrated benefit on PDA closure rates (111).

The rationale for the administration of other conservative treatments is based primarily on physiologic principles and is generally unsupported. Higher oxygen saturations may improve spontaneous ductal closure due to vasoconstrictive effects of higher arterial oxygen tension. However, recent large randomized trials comparing high versus low oxygen saturation targets in extremely preterm infants found no difference in the development of PDA (112). Similarly, while a higher hematocrit may increase PVR and mitigate left-to-right shunting across ventricular septal defects, randomized trials have found no difference in PDA development or management using strategies that increase hematocrit, such as liberal red cell transfusion practices or delayed cord clamping at birth (113). Fluid restriction has been reportedly used to reduce left heart volume loading in infants with PDA. While excessive fluid administration in the first days of life has been associated with higher rates of developing PDA, moderate fluid restriction does not improve pulmonary or systemic hemodynamics in infants with a PDA (114). Most importantly, to achieve a reduction in intravascular volume, daily fluid intake would have to be restricted beyond renal concentrating ability (typically <100 mL/kg/d), and this is not recommended due to reduced nutritional intake and somatic growth.

Ductal Closure Strategies

Pharmacotherapy—Prostaglandin Synthase Inhibitors

Ductal patency is promoted by the production of circulating prostaglandins catalyzed by the enzyme prostaglandin H_2 (PGH_2) synthase. PGH_2 synthase has both peroxidase (POX) and cyclooxygenase (COX) moieties that work in series to produce PGH_2, the precursor to PGE_2. Arachidonic acid is converted to PGH_2 by sequential reactions catalyzed by COX and POX. Inhibitors of COX, and more recently POX, which decrease circulating prostaglandins, constitute the dominant pharmacologic therapies targeting ductal closure.

Ibuprofen and indomethacin are the most commonly used COX inhibitors. Their efficacy in ductal closure wanes with decreasing gestational age, due to an immaturity-related absence of ductal intimal thickening, which is a necessary precursor for neointimal mound formation and subsequent anatomic closure after ductal vasoconstriction. The optimal timing of administration of COX inhibitor treatment for PDA remains uncertain. Prophylactic indomethacin reduces the risk of severe IVH, periventricular leukomalacia, pulmonary hemorrhage, symptomatic PDA, and PDA ligation in extremely low-birth weight infants, compared with later symptomatic treatment only (92). The use of prophylactic indomethacin declined after the publication of a large randomized trial that found no improvement in 18- to 24-month neurodevelopmental outcome (69). Nevertheless, improved neurodevelopmental

outcome has been demonstrated in later childhood, when psychological assessments are more reliable (115). The clear short-term benefits coupled with evidence of a lack of harm have led to its continued use in some centers. Ibuprofen prophylaxis, by contrast, facilitates early PDA closure but less reliably reduces IVH, rendering indomethacin the agent of choice for centers opting to administer universal prophylaxis (93). These data also suggest that indomethacin may have additional stabilizing effects on germinal matrix or modulates the risk of hemorrhage in alternative ways.

Targeted indomethacin prophylaxis, administered to infants with PDA greater than 1.5 mm in the first 6 hours of life, reduces symptomatic PDA and pulmonary hemorrhage and avoids the indiscriminate administration to infants who may have never developed PDA. Screening echocardiography also facilitates the identification of the small minority of infants with an entirely right-to-left shunt (indicating suprasystemic right ventricular pressures), in whom the PDA reduces right ventricular afterload and indomethacin prophylaxis is contraindicated (86).

For the treatment of symptomatic PDA, presurfactant era trials suggested that early treatment (in the first week of life) improved PDA closure rates and reduced pulmonary morbidity, such as the number of days of oxygen therapy and a more rapid wean of mechanical ventilation, but without demonstrating improvement in mortality, BPD, or other morbidities (87). Contemporary trials reported have no difference in mortality or severe neonatal morbidities among infants treated early for mildly symptomatic PDA compared with expectant management followed by late treatment (89,90). The recent exploratory PDA-TOLERATE study randomized extremely preterm infants with a moderate–large PDA during the second week of life to ibuprofen treatment or placebo and found no difference in the composite primary outcome of surgical ligation or open PDA at discharge (91). There were also no differences in secondary outcomes including mortality, NEC, or BPD, though among the subgroup ≥26 weeks GA at birth, infants in the intervention arm had increased late onset non–coagulase-negative Staphylococcus bacteremia and mortality (16% vs. 2%). In a secondary analysis, infants who were eligible but not enrolled in the study due to lack of physician equipoise (i.e., judged to be too ill to potentially receive placebo and/or wait until the second week of life for PDA treatment) had lower mortality and respiratory morbidity than enrolled infants, suggesting a potential benefit to earlier treatment among the highest risk infants (116).

COX inhibitor use in preterm infants is associated with reductions in cerebral and splanchnic blood flow. Adverse effects include oliguria, weight gain, gastrointestinal injury, transient dysfunction of platelet aggregation, and increased serum hyperbilirubinemia due to competitive binding of albumin. Their use is contraindicated in the setting of renal failure, NEC, intracranial (but not intraventricular) hemorrhage, and severe jaundice. Indomethacin should not be administered concurrently with systemic corticosteroids due to an increased risk of spontaneous intestinal perforation. Ibuprofen is as effective as indomethacin in achieving PDA closure, and ibuprofen-treated infants have lower risks of NEC and transient renal insufficiency (117). While early studies comparing ibuprofen and indomethacin identified an increased risk of BPD in ibuprofen-treated infants, a recent meta-analysis revealed no difference in BPD and earlier weaning from respiratory support with ibuprofen (117). Both oral and intravenous forms of ibuprofen are widely used, and intravenous formulations of indomethacin predominate. Indomethacin dosing of 0.2 mg/kg every 12 to 24 hours for three doses is a commonly used treatment regimen. Prolonged or higher total doses of indomethacin (more than 0.6 mg/kg) have been associated with increased risk of NEC without improvement in PDA closure rates (118). Oral and intravenous ibuprofen has similar rates of PDA closure and adverse effects and is typically administered in a 10-mg/kg initial dose, followed by two once-daily 5 mg/kg doses.

Acetaminophen is now an established pharmacologic therapy for PDA closure, with similar efficacy to ibuprofen and indomethacin, especially in more mature preterm infants (GA ≥ 27 weeks) (119). Its excellent safety profile, with a significantly lower incidence of gastrointestinal hemorrhage and renal insufficiency, makes it an attractive alternative to COX inhibitors as first-line therapy (119). One small clinical trial of universal prophylaxis in moderately preterm neonates demonstrated that intravenous acetaminophen resulted in earlier PDA closure (120). A common dosing regimen for treatment of symptomatic PDA or after echocardiography screening in the first week of life is 15 mg/kg/dose every 6 hours for 3 days. Among infants with moderate-or-large PDA after the first 2 weeks of life, treatment with oral acetaminophen (25 mg/kg load followed by 15 mg/kg/dose every 12 hours for preterm infants <32 weeks postmenstrual age) resulted in higher rate of ductal closure or constriction compared with placebo (63% vs. 25%, p = 0.0001) (121). Further trials in extremely preterm infants are needed to evaluate its use as potential synergistic treatment with COX inhibition, the optimal duration of therapy, and the comparative efficacy and adverse effects of oral versus intravenous preparations. In addition, as with pharmacotherapy with COX inhibitors, there is a paucity of evidence of improvement in neonatal outcomes with acetaminophen treatment.

Surgical PDA Ligation

Ligation is most commonly performed in an operating theatre or at the bedside in the NICU, via a left lateral thoracotomy, and with application of a clip or ligature to the PDA. Immediate surgical mortality is low. Surgical morbidity includes bleeding and vocal cord paresis, which occurs due to intraoperative injury to the left recurrent laryngeal nerve in 5% to 50% of infants. Other complications include bleeding, chylothorax, pneumothorax, and inadvertent occlusion of the left main bronchus, left pulmonary artery, or aorta. Inability to wean from mechanical ventilation is the most common indication for surgical ligation in infants with a persistent hemodynamically significant PDA, and ligation has been associated with earlier time to extubation. Severe refractory pulmonary hemorrhage, severe diastolic hypotension and end-organ hypoperfusion, and severe acute oxygenation failure are rare indications for urgent surgical ductal closure.

Surgical ligation has been associated with increased BPD, ROP and neurodevelopmental impairment in early childhood compared with infants treated medically, either with conservative management and/or pharmacotherapy (122). However, ligation may be a surrogate marker of illness severity (e.g., ventilator dependence) and was no longer associated with increased morbidity after controlling for confounding by indication (123). Nonetheless, these studies have been accompanied by a secular trend toward a permissive approach to the PDA. Treatment strategies that avoid or delay surgical ligation in infants who have failed pharmacologic treatment have reported improved neonatal and neurodevelopmental outcomes (96,97), or at least an absence of harm (124). Early routine ligation subjects many infants to the risk of surgery where the PDA may close spontaneously. A period of conservative management after failed pharmacologic closure may be considered to reduce the number of infants treated with surgery, though the optimal duration of "watchful waiting" is unknown. However, ligation has been associated with lower mortality compared with medical treatment alone (123,125). While the possibility of residual confounding necessitates caution in interpreting the finding of lower mortality, ligation may have an ongoing therapeutic role among high-risk infants with persistent large PDA.

Preoperative and Intraoperative Considerations: Adrenocortical insufficiency is common in preterm infants with PDA and adrenocorticotropin hormone (ACTH) stimulation testing may be performed preoperatively to inform steroid use in the case of postoperative instability. Infants with preoperative ACTH-stimulated serum cortisol responses less than 750 nmol/L are at increased postoperative risk of respiratory failure and hypotension. Intraoperatively, administering high-dose fentanyl (>10 μg/kg) during the induction phase of anesthesia reduces postoperative respiratory instability in preterm infants and results in lower biochemical stress responses in children undergoing cardiac surgery (126–128).

Postoperative Physiology and Management: PDA ligation results in an instantaneous increase in left ventricular (LV) afterload and decrease in LV preload, leading to a rapid decline in LV output. This manifests as an abrupt increase in diastolic and MBP. Over 40% of preterm infants experience a gradual postoperative decline in LV function and eventually display signs of a low cardiac output state, systolic hypotension, and secondary oxygenation and ventilation failure by 6 to 12 hours postoperatively. This clinical deterioration has been termed postligation cardiac syndrome (PLCS), is associated with increased respiratory morbidity (129), and appears to be primarily due to increased LV afterload, rather than reduced preload. Although reduced LV preload is detectable using echocardiography 1 hour postoperatively the patient is clinically asymptomatic; in addition, intraoperative volume expansion does not affect the need for postoperative inotropic agents, suggesting that LV preload is not a major determinant in the evolution of PLCS. By contrast, peak measures of LV afterload coincide with the clinical onset of PLCS. Milrinone prophylaxis, which causes significant afterload reduction along with mild lusitropy and inotropy, reduces the risk of PLCS in high-risk infants from 44% to 11%, corroborating the role of LV afterload as the major determinant of PLCS (43). Factors associated with an increased risk of PLCS include younger age (<28 days) and weight (<1,000 g) at the time of ligation. Postoperatively, preterm infants should remain invasively ventilated and adequate analgesia should be administered. Cessation of pulmonary overcirculation after interruption of the ductal shunt may result in a rapid improvement in pulmonary compliance. The potential need to reduce MAP and tidal volume should be anticipated and closely titrated to avoid pulmonary overdistention and associated impairment in systemic and pulmonary venous return.

The association of PLCS with adverse neonatal and neurodevelopmental outcomes highlights the potential importance of pathophysiology-driven preventative care in the postoperative period (129,130) (Fig. 31.4). At our center, we perform echocardiography at 1 hour postoperatively to estimate LVO. Infants with LVO less than 200 mL/kg/min receive an intravenous infusion of prophylactic milrinone at a starting dose of 0.33 μg/kg/min, administered with 10 mL/kg 0.9% sodium chloride to offset the reduction in SVR. In centers without access to echocardiography, the administration of prophylactic intravenous milrinone to infants based on perioperative risk factors may be considered. Care must be taken to ensure that milrinone is administered only to clinically stable infants demonstrating the expected postoperative immediate rise in DBP, normal or increased SBP, and stable oxygenation and ventilation status. Infants are typically hemodynamically stable in the immediate (<2 hours) postoperative period and demonstrate an abrupt increase in DBP, with normal SBP. The gradual development of isolated systolic hypotension, most commonly due to declining LV systolic function, may be managed with an intravenous infusion of dobutamine with isotonic volume expansion if preload compromised. Early hypotension (diastolic or combined) should prompt immediate evaluation of respiratory management, investigation for hemorrhage, obstruction to LVO (e.g., tension pneumothorax), pulmonary arterial hypertension, and etiologies of reduced SVR such as adrenal insufficiency or sepsis. Intravascular volume expansion and intravenous stress-dose hydrocortisone should be considered. Refractory diastolic hypotension may be treated with judicious use of an intravenous infusion of dopamine or epinephrine. Low postoperative cortisol concentrations have been associated with catecholamine-resistant hypotension and early glucocorticoid replacement should be administered to symptomatic infants.

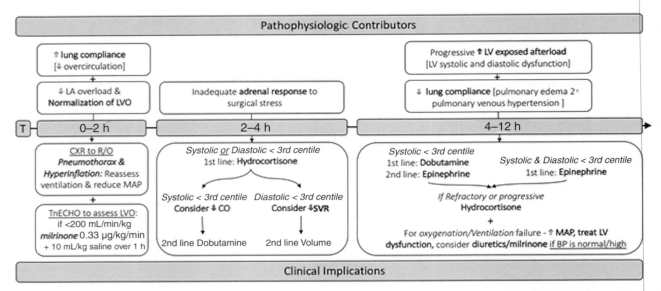

FIGURE 31.4 **Pathophysiologic contributors to cardiorespiratory instability following patent ductus arteriosus (PDA) ligation with associated clinical implications.** Early decompensation may be associated with impaired adrenal response. Supportive management may be required while awaiting the effect of hydrocortisone. Later decompensation is typically related to LV performance. T, time; CXR, chest x-ray; LA, left atrium; LV, left ventricle; LVO, left ventricular output; R/O, rule out; MAP, mean airway pressure; CO, cardiac output; SVR, systemic vascular resistance. (Reprinted from Weisz DE, Giesinger RE. Surgical management of a patent ductus arteriosus: is this still an option? *Semin Fetal Neonatal Med* 2018;23(4):255. Copyright © 2018 Elsevier. With permission.)

Catheter Device Closure—An Alternative to Surgical Ligation to Definitive PDA Closure

Catheter-based occlusion of a PDA is the procedure of choice among older infants and children owing to fewer complications, shorter recovery times, and lower costs compared with surgical ligation (131). Lack of availability of appropriately sized devices and delivery systems has historically limited the use of catheter-based occlusion among small preterm infants. In addition, the classic femoral arterial approach, requiring systemic heparinization, and the risk of arterial thrombosis were barriers to broad adoption.

Over the past decade, the availability of devices and delivery systems suited for very low weight infants, and new techniques for catheter guidance and device deployment have facilitated the use of catheter-based occlusion among VLWI at several pioneering sites around the world. Three devices are commonly used, all of which utilize a sheath size of as small as 4 Fr and have been evaluated in small–moderate sized case series. The Amplatzer Vascular Plug (AVP) II was approved by the US Food and Drug Administration (FDA) in 2007 and is limited by a minimum length of 6 mm, resulting in the potential for protrusion beyond the PDA causing occlusion of the left pulmonary artery or descending aorta. The Medtronic Micro Vascular Plug (MVP) received FDA approval in 2015 and lacks retention disks, making it suitable for the tubular PDAs of preterm infants. The Amplatzer Occluder II Additional Sizes (ADO II AS), also known as PICOLLO, is available in sizes ranging from 2 to 6 mm and was recently approved by the FDA after investigation in 192 infants, among whom 3 (1.5%) experienced serious adverse events (132).

Recently, a transvenous approach via the femoral vein, guided by intraprocedural TTE, has reported high procedural success (96% to 100%) and a relatively low risk of complications with minimal fluoroscopic exposure (133–135). Adverse event rates have been acceptable (<10%) and included device embolization (requiring retrieval) and partial left pulmonary artery obstruction (which may resolve with infant growth over time) (136). A limited number of retrospective studies have compared operative and neonatal outcomes among infants undergoing catheter-based occlusion versus surgical ligation, reporting earlier weaning from mechanical ventilation, reduced postoperative cardiorespiratory instability, and fewer procedural complications (137,138).

Although catheter-based occlusion appears promising as a method to achieve definitive PDA closure, there is a currently a paucity of evidence to support its use in lieu of ligation or any other approach to PDA management. Additional studies are necessary before clinicians trade the known risks of PDA ligation or conservative management with the lesser known risks of device closure.

PULMONARY HYPERTENSION

Introduction

PH is a serious cardiopulmonary disorder characterized by sustained elevation of pulmonary artery pressure, resulting in chronic exposure of the right ventricle to high afterload. It is defined as a mean pulmonary artery pressure (mPAP) greater than 25 mm Hg when measured by right heart catheterization or pulmonary artery peak systolic pressure greater than 35 mm Hg as measured by echocardiography. In physiologic terms, the relationship of mPAP with other pulmonary hemodynamic variables can be described by the equation, mPAP = (PBF × PVR) + PCWP, where PBF is pulmonary blood flow, PVR is pulmonary vascular resistance, and PCWP is pulmonary capillary wedge pressure, which is essentially the same as left atrial pressure. Hence, PH may result from an increase in PBF (e.g., ventricular and atrial septal defects, PDA), PVR (increased tone of resistance and precapillary arterioles), PCWP (left ventricular dysfunction), or a combination of these factors. In neonates, the most common reason for PHT is dysregulation of PVR, particularly in the immediate postnatal period.

PH is a common cause of admission to tertiary NICUs and is associated with significant patient mortality and morbidity. The etiology is diverse and may be broadly classified as acute or chronic (Fig. 31.5). While most research and clinical trials have focused on acute PH presenting in the immediate postnatal period, the burden of illness secondary to chronic PH in neonates is just beginning to be recognized. Although acute episodes of neonatal PH may occur late, most cases present as hypoxemia in the immediate postnatal period; this traditionally was referred to as PPHN or persistent fetal circulation (PFC). The former terminology is somewhat of a temporal misnomer as pulmonary arterial pressure only

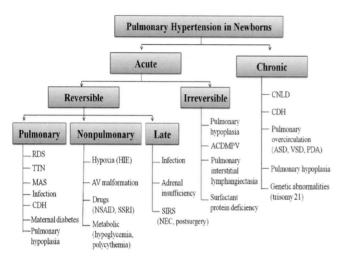

FIGURE 31.5 Pulmonary hypertension in neonates can be classified as acute or chronic and may arise from a variety of underlying disorders. RDS, respiratory distress syndrome; TTN, transient tachypnea of newborn; MAS, meconium aspiration syndrome; CDH, congenital diaphragmatic hernia; HIE, hypoxic–ischemic encephalopathy; AV, arteriovenous; NSAID, nonsteroidal anti-inflammatory drug; SSRI, selective serotonin reuptake inhibitors; SIRS, systemic inflammatory response syndrome; NEC, necrotizing enterocolitis; ACDMPV, alveolar capillary dysplasia with misalignment of pulmonary veins; CNLD, chronic neonatal lung disease; ASD, atrial septal defect; VSD, ventricular septal defect; PDA, patent ductus arteriosus.

normalizes by postnatal day 14; therefore, for the purpose of this chapter, we will refer to acute and chronic PH. Chronic neonatal lung disease (CNLD) is the most common acquired lung disease in neonates. It is a frequent complication of extreme premature birth and is the commonest cause of chronic PH in neonates. Even though both acute and chronic causes of PH are characterized by high PVR and mPAP, there are relevant distinctions in their pathophysiology, symptoms, and clinical course that require thoughtful consideration. For example, while acute PH is most commonly due to a disruption of the normal physiologic transition of the pulmonary circulation from fetal to postnatal life, chronic PH occurs much later and represents a secondary rise in PVR due to acquired or developmental lung disease. Given the relative high prevalence of these disorders in tertiary NICUs, it is imperative that clinicians caring for these babies familiarize themselves with the disease-specific physiology and associated hemodynamic alterations. Prompt recognition and early effective management are important for optimizing patient outcomes.

Acute Pulmonary Hypertension of the Newborn

Acute PH of the newborn (also described as PPHN) is a relatively common disorder of postnatal transition, accounting for up to 4% of all NICU admissions. Phenotypically, it is characterized by severe hypoxemic respiratory failure (HRF) presenting shortly after birth secondary to the failure of transition of the pulmonary circulation from a high resistance intrauterine to a low resistance extrauterine circuit. Although acute PH is often secondary to disorders of postnatal transition such as perinatal asphyxia, meconium aspiration syndrome (MAS), sepsis, or pulmonary hypoplasia (e.g., congenital diaphragmatic hernia), sometimes it represents a primary diagnosis when no other underlying pathology can be identified. The reported incidence of acute PH in high-income countries ranges from 1 to 2 per 1,000 live births with a mortality rate of approximately 10% (139). The incidence and burden of disease are likely to be much higher in low- and middle-income countries. Neonates who survive often require prolong cardiorespiratory support have a long hospital stay and are at a higher risk of long-term neurodisability (140,141).

Pathophysiology of Circulatory Derangements

Irrespective of the underlying etiology, the clinical phenotype in neonates with acute PH often remains the same and is primarily governed by the failure of normal postnatal decline in PVR. Persistence of high PVR is the hallmark pathophysiologic feature and the primary determinant of many of the secondary hemodynamic alterations, culminating in a vicious cycle of reduced PBF, hypoxemia, acidosis, ventilation–perfusion mismatch, and cardiac dysfunction. Although these hemodynamic disturbances are well appreciated, the physiologic cascade is poorly understood but is likely to vary between patients (**Fig. 31.6**) (142).

Significant or prolonged increase in right ventricular afterload may result in critically low PBF, which may be further aggravated by the presence of right ventricular dysfunction. Pulmonary hypoperfusion leads to ventilation–perfusion mismatch, worsening hypoxemia, and acidosis all of which induce vasoconstriction in the pulmonary vascular bed, further increase PVR, and may blunt the effect of pulmonary vasodilator therapies. The left ventricle is able to compensate for reduced preload by increasing its contractility and heart rate. The degree of compensation is variable but always occurs at an expense of increased myocardial oxygen consumption. Right ventricular dilatation, if present, causes the interventricular septum to deviate leftward, thereby further reducing the filling capacity and compliance of the left ventricle. In addition, contractile dysfunction of the right ventricle, by virtue of the shared myocardial fibers between the two ventricles, can also directly result in left ventricle systolic dysfunction. This phenomenon is termed as "ventricular-ventricular interaction" (143). Significant PH is also commonly associated with the presence of a PDA shunting blood from the pulmonary to systemic circulation (i.e., right-to-left shunt). While on one hand a right-to-left shunt across PDA can be beneficial in off-loading the pulmonary

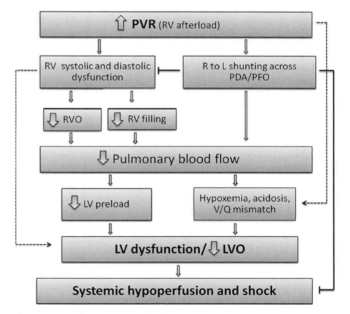

FIGURE 31.6 Circulatory pathophysiology in neonates with pulmonary hypertension. While in some neonates, high PVR may remain the only abnormality, others may suffer from associated alternations of varying severity resulting in a poorly understood vicious cycle of hypoxemia, V/Q mismatch, and cardiac dysfunction culminating in systemic hypoperfusion and shock. Although a right to-left shunt across PDA may off-load the pulmonary circulation and prevent RV failure and systemic hypoperfusion, it can also augment hypoxemia by its negative effect on reduced pulmonary blood flow. PVR, pulmonary vascular resistance; RV, right ventricular; R to L right to left; PDA, patent ductus arteriosus; PFO, patent foramen ovale; RVO, right ventricular output; LV, left ventricular; V/Q, ventilation/perfusion; LVO, left ventricular output.

circulation and thus protecting the neonatal right ventricle from failing as well as supporting the systemic perfusion, it may also potentiate the ongoing HRF through its contribution to reduced PBF. If uncorrected, the clinical picture may evolve into that of severe systemic hypoperfusion and shock.

Clinical Presentation

Central cyanosis and respiratory distress starting shortly after birth are the principal clinical features of acute PH in neonates. Cyanosis (hypoxemia) may remain partially or completely unresolved in spite of therapy with supplemental oxygen and artificial ventilation. A labile pulmonary vascular bed presenting clinically with worsening hypoxemia with handling is also a common finding. In the presence of a PDA shunting, deoxygenated blood from the main pulmonary artery to descending aorta (60% to 70% of cases), the oxygen saturation measured in the right arm (i.e., preductal) will be higher than those measured from lower limbs (i.e., postductal). The left arm should not be used for assessment of saturation gradient due to the known variability in the origin (preductal or postductal) of the left subclavian artery in the general population. A difference of at least 10% is considered as a sign of significant right-to-left ductal shunt, and may be diagnostic of PH, provided duct-dependent structural heart defects have been ruled out. While pre–post saturation gradient may be a specific sign of PH in neonates, it lacks sensitivity to rule out disease. The causes of absence of pre–post saturation difference despite significantly elevated pulmonary pressures include spontaneous ductus closure (approximately 20% to 30% cases of acute PH), net volume of right-to-left shunt across PDA being insufficient to cause significant postductal saturation gradient (e.g., bidirectional shunts, low circulatory volume, significant right ventricular systolic dysfunction with critically low right ventricular output), and severe anemia. Severe or prolonged PH is commonly accompanied by systemic hypotension. Infants initially demonstrate low SBPs (indicating low stroke volume), which may become more profound in later stages with clinical features of severe shock (pale skin color, prolong CRT, weak peripheral arterial pulsations, poor urine output). In severe disease, signs of circulatory failure may be present from the outset, especially in the presence of significant cardiac dysfunction.

Clinical Assessment and Investigations

A number of underlying etiologies can result in the clinical syndrome of acute PH. Birth asphyxia, MAS, and sepsis account for the majority of cases. A careful overview of the clinical scenario along with a focused history and clinical examination can often provide important clues to the underlying diagnosis. Clinical assessment will usually have to be quick and performed alongside early resuscitative measures to ensure timely stabilization. History of fetal distress, severe metabolic acidosis in cord gases, low Apgar score at 5 and 10 minutes after birth and clinical examination consistent with at least moderate encephalopathy are classical features suggesting a significant perinatal asphyxial event. Initial investigations will usually be targeted toward establishing adequacy of ventilation and evaluation for end-organ dysfunction as well as to assess severity of encephalopathy. Green colored amniotic fluid and/or green stained umbilical cord point toward MAS, which may be a primary diagnosis or may occur in the setting of significant perinatal asphyxia. Chest x-ray in MAS may demonstrate findings consistent with "air trapping" and chemical pneumonitis characterized by hyperexpansion and diffuse opacities scattered throughout the lung fields. The inflammation from aspirated meconium in MAS often worsens over the initial days before demonstrating signs of recovery. Other etiologies that may present with "green" colored amniotic fluid include *Listeria* sepsis and upper gastrointestinal obstructions, though the latter is not particularly associated with PH syndrome. Clinical features that may point toward an infective

cause include history of prolonged rupture of membranes, group B streptococcus (GBS) colonization, and signs suggestive of chorioamnionitis (including maternal tachycardia, maternal pyrexia, raised maternal white cell count, uterine tenderness, although in clinical practice often only one or two of these signs may be present). The clinical examination may reveal signs of septic shock (lethargy, poor perfusion, low blood pressure); chest x-ray may demonstrate bronchopneumonia and laboratory results show evidence of acute inflammatory response and/or consumptive coagulopathy (leukocytosis or leucopenia, thrombocytopenia, high C-reactive protein, abnormal coagulation profile). In cases of GBS pneumonia, the chest x-ray can be indistinguishable from RDS.

Other aspects of clinical history that may allude to relatively less common etiologies include maternal medical history (e.g., poorly controlled diabetes resulting in RDS); medication history (e.g., delayed transition from antenatal exposure to selective serotonin reuptake inhibitors; intrauterine closure of ductus arteriosus from maternal use of nonsteroidal anti-inflammatory drugs); antenatal serum screen (e.g., trisomy 21); antenatal ultrasounds revealing structural anomalies (e.g., congenital diaphragmatic hernia, arteriovenous malformations) and lack or excess of amniotic fluid (e.g., pulmonary hypoplasia resulting from severe long standing oligohydramnios; polyhydramnios in esophageal atresia). Clinical assessment of the infant may also provide important clues such as dysmorphisms (trisomy 21, 18, 13 or other genetic disorders); excessive oral secretions (tracheoesophageal fistula with esophageal atresia); scaphoid abdomen with heart sounds shifted to the right side of the chest (congenital diaphragmatic hernia); contractures with low muscle tone and decreased spontaneous movements (fetal akinesia syndrome); ruddy skin color (polycythemia); and detection of bruit on auscultation over scalp or liver (arteriovenous malformation).

Among the rarer genetic causes of severe PH, surfactant protein deficiency and alveolar capillary dysplasia with misalignment of pulmonary veins (ACDMPV) are seen most frequently. A family history positive for previous neonatal deaths from respiratory failure and/or consanguinity may point toward surfactant protein deficiency. Typically, chest x-ray demonstrates findings consistent with RDS. Infants with this condition often respond well to the first dose of intratracheal exogenous surfactant, and then again develop oxygenation failure and PH shortly thereafter. Subsequent doses of exogenous surfactant become progressively ineffective. In ACDMPV, infants often look well at birth with normal Apgar scores but minutes or hours later present with severe respiratory distress, hypoxemia, and acute PH which is unresponsive to medical management. ACDMPV is a rare genetic disorder characterized by maldevelopment of the capillary vascular bed around alveoli in the lungs. For both these disorders, definitive diagnosis can be made by lung biopsy or by genetic testing for known mutations—SFTPB, SFTPC, and ABCA3 gene mutation are the common mutations responsible for the former while the later disorder is often associated with mutations (FOX 1 gene) or deletion involving chromosome 16.

As noted above, a number of investigations may be required for neonates presenting with acute PH. While some investigations are standard for all cases, others will need to be individualized based on the index of suspicion. A list of investigations and their rationale is presented in Table 31.5.

Cyanotic Congenital Heart Defect versus Acute PH

Timely evaluation to rule out a critical cyanotic congenital heart defect (CHD) could be a decisive factor for infants suspected to have PH. Finding of severe cyanosis in the absence of respiratory distress in an otherwise comfortable appearing neonate is strongly suggestive of cyanotic CHD and should prompt clinical evaluation focused on the cardiovascular system as well as urgent consultation with a pediatric cardiologist. Particular clinical signs that

TABLE 31.5

Standard and Etiology-Specific Special Investigations for Neonates with PPHN

Investigations	Rationale	
Standard—should be considered in all cases of PPHN	• Blood culture, C-reactive protein	• Screen for sepsis
	• Complete blood count, blood group, blood glucose, serum electrolytes	• Evaluation for anemia, hypoglycemia, electrolyte disturbances
	• Serum lactate	• Assessment of systemic perfusion
	• ABG	• Screen for acidosis, hypercarbia
	• Chest x-ray (with nasal or oral gastric tube *in situ*)	• Confirm position of endotracheal tube
		• Rule out air leaks
		• Evaluation for parenchymal lung disease (e.g., RDS, MAS)
		• Rule out structural lung defects (e.g., CDH, esophageal atresia)
		• Abnormal heart shape (e.g., "snowman" shape in TAPVD; narrow mediastinum with egg shape heart in TGA; boot-shaped heart with apex "lifted" from the diaphragm in right ventricular hypertrophy)
	• Abdominal x-ray	• Confirm position of umbilical lines
	• Two-dimensional transthoracic echocardiogram	• Confirm diagnosis
		• Rule out CHD
Special cases—to be considered in specific circumstances	• ABG with hyperoxia test	• Screen for cyanotic heart defects
	• Liver, renal function tests, urinalysis, coagulation screen (INR, PT, APTT)	• Evaluate for end-organ dysfunction, coagulopathy (sepsis, birth asphyxia)
	• Electroencephalogram (12 lead or single channel amplitude integrated)	• Evaluation of background brain electric activity and screen for seizures (encephalopathy from birth asphyxia)
	• Serum ammonia, lactate, serum organic, and amino acids	• Metabolic screen
	• Genetic testing	• Presence of dysmorphic features
	• Karyotyping	• Suspicion of genetic causes of PPHN (surfactant protein deficiency, ACDMPV)
	• Screen for specific mutations	
	• Ultrasound, magnetic resonance imaging—brain	• Arteriovenous malformations (vein of Galen malformation)
		• Evidence of brain injury (birth asphyxia)
	• Chest CT scan	• Pulmonary lymphangiectasia
Pathology	• Lung biopsy	• ACDMPV; surfactant protein deficiency

ABG, arterial blood gas; INR, international normalized ratio; PT, prothrombin time; APTT, activated partial thromboplastin time; ACDMPV, alveolar capillary dysplasia with misalignment of pulmonary veins; RDS, respiratory distress syndrome; MAS, meconium aspiration syndrome; CHD, congenital diaphragmatic hernia; TAPVD, total anomalous pulmonary venous drainage; TGA, transposition of great arteries; CHD, congenital heart defect.

THE NEWBORN INFANT

should raise suspicion of a CHD include, but are not restricted to presence of a murmur, dampened lower limb pulsations, blood pressure in lower limbs (postductal) significantly lower than right arm (preductal), reverse differential cyanosis (i.e., preductal saturations lower than postductal by at least 10% indicating a "right-to-left" shunt of oxygenated blood across PDA; e.g., total anomalous pulmonary venous connections, transposition of great arteries), abnormal heart shape on chest x-ray, abnormal electrocardiogram, and "failed" hyperoxia test. Further, severe hypoxemia associated with cyanotic CHD is often associated with failure of response or worsening with pulmonary vasodilator therapy, relatively "fixed" oxygen saturations (i.e., absence of labile pulmonary vascular bed) and absence of systemic hypotension. Although a thorough clinical examination may provide important clues, given the low sensitivity and specificity of clinical signs, it can only be indicative at best. A hyperoxia test may also be equivocal in this setting. In addition, in certain congenital heart diseases, PH may coexist at presentation making clinical distinction even more challenging. A complete structural echocardiography assessment by an experienced pediatric cardiologist is the only definitive test. Ideally, all infants suspected to have acute PH should have an echocardiogram as soon as

possible to confirm the diagnosis and rule out CHD, but resources may not be available in many centers. Echocardiography assessment is mandatory in the setting of a presumptive diagnosis of PH when symptoms fail to resolve in spite of resuscitative measures and pulmonary vasodilator therapy or when treatment with extracorporeal membrane oxygenation (ECMO) is being considered. Failure of early recognition of cyanotic CHD and delay in appropriate treatment may worsen the prognosis (144). Further, therapeutic strategies used to reduce PVR may further compromise some patients with certain forms of heart defects, such as patients with cardiac lesions associated with excessive PBF (e.g., total anomalous pulmonary venous connection; double outlet right ventricle) and lesions with critical left sided outflow tract obstruction (e.g., hypoplastic left heart syndrome). It is our opinion that patients with a presumptive diagnosis of acute PH where the likelihood of cyanotic congenital heart disease may be high should be evaluated with a hyperoxia test, failing which an urgent evaluation by an experienced pediatric cardiologist must be organized. In such cases, it may be safer to maintain a PDA by intravenous infusion of prostaglandins until a duct-dependent CHD can be ruled out, especially if delays in cardiology consultation are anticipated.

Hyperoxia Test

Hyperoxia test is a clinical test designed to indicate the underlying pathology in neonates presenting with HRF, that is, parenchymal lung disease versus circulatory disorder. The rationale being that HRF when circulatory in origin (either due to severely low PBF or abnormal mixing of oxygenated and deoxygenated blood) will not improve in spite of treatment with 100% oxygen. On the other hand, in parenchymal lung disease, such treatment will result in appreciable improvement in oxygenation. To briefly review the basis for the hyperoxia test, at sea level barometric pressure is around 740 mm Hg. Subtracting around 40 mm Hg for water vapor means the pressure of inspired oxygen is roughly 7× the percentage of inspired oxygen (approximately 150 mm Hg in 21%, approximately 350 mm Hg in 50% oxygen). The normal alveolar–arterial oxygen gradient in the newborn is around 30 mm Hg when breathing 21% oxygen, and 300 mm Hg when breathing 100% oxygen. Therefore, a healthy term newborn will achieve a maximum arterial PO_2 of around 300 to 400 mm Hg if breathing 100% oxygen. The hyperoxia test is performed by first obtaining an arterial blood gas to measure preductal partial pressure of oxygen (PaO_2) at baseline with infant in room air or in lowest oxygen treatment tolerated. Then, 100% oxygen is provided continuously for at least 10 minutes and PaO_2 is remeasured. A posttreatment preductal PaO_2 of greater than 150 mm Hg indicates that HRF is unlikely to be circulatory in origin, while a PaO_2 of less than 50 mm Hg is highly suggestive of a critical cyanotic CHD, necessitating consideration to initiate prophylactic treatment with intravenous prostaglandin infusion to maintain ductal patency. PaO_2 between 50 and 150 mm Hg is considered equivocal. To minimize chances of erroneous result, it is important that care is taken to perform this test using optimal technique. The response to oxygen treatment must be established by measuring PaO_2 and not by using surrogate measures like pulse oximetry or transcutaneous oxygen measurements. Ideally, PaO_2 should be measured preductally as presence of "right-to-left" shunt across PDA can affect results. Finally, 100% oxygen must be provided with a face mask with good seal (or through endotracheal tube if infant receiving invasive ventilation) and not by nasal cannulae or "blow-by" as mixing with room air can reduce the actual oxygen content in inspired gas. Clinicians performing and interpreting this test should be aware that severe PH may be associated with profound reduction in PBF, which may result in a false-positive screen. Nevertheless, a positive hyperoxia test is considered a medical emergency and should prompt an immediate consultation with the regional pediatric cardiology service to rule out critical cyanotic CHD.

Approach to Management of Acute PH

Acute PH is one of the most challenging acute clinical scenarios managed in tertiary level NICUs. Early identification of at-risk neonates, prompt initiation and appropriate escalation of cardiorespiratory interventions, close clinical monitoring, judicious use of pulmonary vasodilators, and timely referral to suitable clinical care facility are key principles to ensure early stabilization and to optimize patient outcomes. Delays in recognizing the severity of disease and appropriate treatment may result in sudden catastrophic deterioration. The approach to intensive care for neonates with acute PH can be classified as: (a) general management, which includes resuscitation and postresuscitation care for "optimization" of patient's cardiorespiratory condition and (b) specific management including trial of pulmonary vasodilator therapies and assessment for eligibility for referral to regional ECMO centers.

General Management

For neonates presenting with HRF, timely stabilization and adjustment of intensive care support may result in resolution of HRF without the need for escalation to specific pulmonary vasodilator therapies. The resuscitation should be provided using the sequential A–B–C approach as recommended in standard neonatal resuscitation algorithms. This includes assessment and management of Airway—is the neonate apneic? Direct visualization of the oral cavity and perform suction if needed to clear potential sources of obstruction like excessive secretions, meconium, and blood; Breathing—are there signs of respiratory distress (mild, moderate, or severe)? Assessment of skin color (pink, cyanosis, pale)—is the neonate hypoxic (preductal oxygen saturation below 95%)?;—does oxygen saturation recover after administration of oxygen (establish amount of oxygen required to maintain normoxia) therapy?;—assess need and extent of positive pressure ventilatory support (apnea, significant respiratory distress, high oxygen requirement, and/or hypercapnia); Circulation—are there clinical signs of circulatory inefficiency (prolonged CRT, weak peripheral pulses, neonate appearing pale in color, tachycardia, and hypotension)? Obtain intravascular access and provide treatment with fluid boluses and/or inotropes as needed. By the end of initial resuscitation, the clinicians would have established the magnitude of clinical problem and the level of support required to correct each abnormality. It is important that throughout resuscitation and postresuscitation care quick regular reassessments of A–B–C are performed and treatments are titrated accordingly.

Postresuscitation, the clinical management should be broadened to identify clues for underlying etiology and establish adequacy of intensive care support being provided. This includes acquiring a detailed history, performing thorough clinical examination and organizing urgent investigations. The goal of ventilation strategy should be to establish adequate alveolar recruitment (qualitative assessment of chest x-ray) and carbon dioxide clearance (arterial blood gas), while avoiding lung hyperexpansion. Circulatory support should be titrated to maintain adequate systemic perfusion (indicated by the clinical signs highlighted above, metabolic acidosis on arterial blood gas and high arterial lactate). Other standard investigations as well as initiation of antibiotic treatment, if indicated, should be completed at the earliest. For neonates in whom HRF still persists, additional pulse oximetry should be applied to one of the lower limbs to assess pre- and postductal saturation difference. The possibility of cyanotic CHD and the need for hyperoxia test should be considered. The severity of HRF should be established by calculating the oxygenation index (OI) using the standard formula $OI = (FiO_2 \times MAP)/PaO_2$, where FiO_2 is the fraction of inspired oxygen, MAP is mean airway pressure, and PaO_2 is partial pressure of oxygen in arterial blood.

Specific Pulmonary Vasodilator Therapies

Specific pulmonary vasodilator therapies are usually indicated when likelihood of cyanotic CHD is considered low and HRF persists despite resuscitation with restoration of adequate ventilation and correction of circulatory derangements. Inhaled nitric oxide (iNO) is the only well tested and approved vasodilatory therapy for neonates with PH (145). A number of large scale randomized control trials and meta-analysis have shown that treatment with iNO reduces the need for ECMO in term and near-term neonates with HRF (146). It is recommended to initiate treatment at a dose of 20 parts per million (ppm) as it identifies the majority of "responsive" cases (147). Although some neonates may require 40 ppm, escalation of therapy beyond a dose of 40 ppm does not provide additional benefit and increases the risk of methemoglobinemia (148). iNO has been shown to improve clinical outcomes for neonates with HRF with an OI between 15 and 40. Although a trial of iNO may be appropriate for neonates in whom OI remains greater than 40 despite resuscitation and optimizing ventilatory management, it should not delay consultation with a regional ECMO center regarding suitability of transfer. An echocardiogram to confirm diagnosis and rule out cyanotic CHD is desirable in all infants with persistent HRF, but it is urgent for infants failing to respond to iNO or if ECMO is being considered.

Although widespread availability of iNO has significantly reduced the need for ECMO in patients with acute PH, both mortality and long-term morbidity rates have remained unchanged. Approximately 30% to 40% of infants with acute PH are either nonresponders or respond only transiently to treatment with iNO. The role of iNO use in premature infants has been controversial. Recent evidence suggests that the response rate in premature infants during the transitional period may be as high as 88% when PH is confirmed on echocardiography assessment (149). Of note, response is independent of gestational age. In addition, infants who positively responded to iNO were more likely to survive free of major morbidity (150). Additionally, the escalating cost and need for special delivery apparatus makes it a nonviable option in many centers in low- or middle-income countries world where both the incidence and mortality associated with PPHN are suspected to be higher. Several therapies are now available that can reduce PVR through alternate biologic pathways (151). The mechanism of action of some of these agents has been detailed elsewhere in this chapter. Although successful use of these agents has been reported in management of PPHN (152–154), their efficacy and safety has not been tested in large clinical trials (Fig. 31.7).

Role for Targeted Neonatal Echocardiography

Although acute PH is primarily a disorder of high PVR, it can be associated with a number of secondary hemodynamic alterations of varying severity. While in some patients high PVR may be the only abnormality, in others it may be complicated by reduced PBF, right and/or left ventricular dysfunction and low systemic blood flow. Further, HRF in neonates may result from exclusive

parenchymal lung disease, PH or a combination of both. In some patients, failure of improvement with vasodilator therapies may be because high PVR is truly unresponsive to treatment, while in others it may suggest lack of significant contribution of PH in ongoing symptoms. Further, therapies that do not lead to immediate clinical improvement in oxygenation are often deemed as a "failure." In our experience, TNE can facilitate identification of a subclinical response, where there are measurable improvements in cardiopulmonary indices even though clinical picture does not change immediately. In such situations prolonging treatment before deeming it ineffective or addition of synergetic therapy might be more beneficial than to discontinue the perceived "failed" treatment, although this requires further testing in systematic studies. Given the nonspecific nature of symptoms in neonates and low sensitivity and specificity of clinical signs, clinical integration of information obtained from a TNE can help establish diagnosis, define the true nature and severity of associated physiologic derangements and provide measures to monitor response to treatments, all of which may aid in enhanced clinical decision-making (Table 31.6).

Chronic Pulmonary Hypertension

Chronic neonatal PH is inextricably linked with developmental disorders of the lung, most commonly chronic lung disease (CLD), a frequent complication of infants born ≤1,000 g (extremely low birth weight, ELBW, infants) (see also Chapter 29). The pathophysiologic features of CLD that contribute to development of chronic PH include sustained pulmonary vasoconstriction and exaggerated vasoreactivity to hypoxemic episodes during early disease. After an ill-defined period of time this gets further complicated by

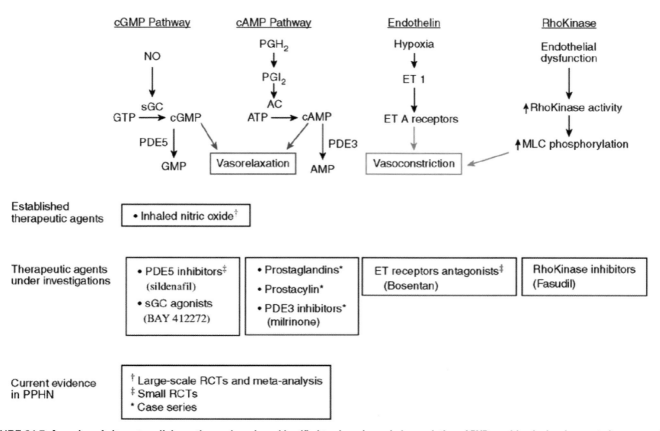

FIGURE 31.7 **A number of alternate cellular pathways have been identified to play a key role in regulation of PVR resulting in development of corresponding therapeutic agents.** iNO is the only established and approved therapy for neonates with PHT. While successful use with other agents has been reported, their efficacy and safety have not been tested in large randomized control trials. NO, nitric oxide; sGC, soluble guanylate cyclase; GTP, guanyl triphosphate; cGMP, cyclic guanyl monophosphate; PDE5, phosphodiesterase type 5; PGH2, prostaglandin; PGI2, prostacyclin; AC, adenyl cyclase; ATP, adenosine triphosphate; cAMP, cyclic adenosine monophosphate; PDE3, phosphodiesterase type 3; ET, endothelin; MLC, myosin light chain; RCT, randomized control trials.

THE NEWBORN INFANT

TABLE 31.6

Use of Targeted Neonatal Echocardiography in PPHN

Assessment of Pulmonary Artery Resistance and Pressure	Assessment of Impact on Left Heart Function and Systemic Circulation	Assessment of Right Heart Function and Pulmonary Blood Flow
Quantitative: calculation of right ventricular systolic pressure using modified Bernoulli equation from measurement of peak velocity of TR or Doppler of PDA flow	*LV preload*: subjective assessment of Doppler of pulmonary venous flow and Doppler of flow across mitral valve in diastole	*RV contractility*: quantitative evaluation using recently described indices—measurement of tricuspid annular plane systolic excursion, tissue Doppler-derived peak systolic myocardial velocity at the base of the right ventricle and fractional area change; qualitative assessment of right ventricular contractility and dilatation
Semiquantitative: monitor progress using serial measurements of Doppler-derived time intervals characteristics of systolic blood flow in main pulmonary artery—pulmonary artery acceleration time and its ratio with right ventricular ejection time	*LV contractility*: quantitative evaluation using well-established indices—fractional shortening, ejection fraction using Simpson biplane method, and mean velocity of circumferential fiber shortening corrected for heart rate; qualitative assessment of contractility	*Pulmonary blood flow*: quantitative measurement of right ventricular output and stroke distance in main pulmonary artery
Qualitative: estimation of right ventricular systolic pressure in comparison to systemic systolic pressure—interventricular septal positioning at end systole; pattern of blood flow across PDA and PFO	*Systemic blood flow*: quantitative measurement of left ventricular output and stroke distance in ascending aorta	

TR, tricuspid regurgitation; PDA, patent ductus arteriosus; PFO, patent foramen ovale; LV, left ventricle; RV, right ventricle.

characteristic developmental alterations in the pulmonary vascular bed—vascular hypoplasia and arterial wall remodeling exemplified by smooth muscle hyperplasia and distal extension into normally nonmuscular arteries, resulting in a "fixed" and often progressive elevation of PVR. The predisposing factors for early functional pulmonary vasoconstriction and progress to subsequent anatomic alternations as well as the severity of these changes and their relationship with postnatal age may be variable and remain poorly understood. Several recent studies have now reported a high prevalence (approximately 30% to 40%) of chronic PH in infants with established CLD, and the incidence of chronic PH is directly related to the severity of CLD, ranging from approximately 5% in those with mild CLD, 15% to 20% in moderate CLD and almost 60% in those with severe CLD. Although the majority of studies were based on retrospective review of clinical echocardiograms for signs of PH and had a variable postnatal age at assessment (mostly late), they suggest chronic PH to be a relatively common complication in CLD that may be independently associated with higher mortality, increased duration of need for respiratory support and longer hospitalization (155,156). Given the retrospective nature of the majority of published data, lack of long-term follow-up data, and the predominant reliance on late echocardiographic signs for diagnosis, the true incidence, severity, and prevalence of PH in formerly premature infants may be much higher.

Currently there is no approved therapy for chronic PH in neonates. In spite of minimal evidence, studies indicate that a wide variety of pulmonary vasodilator therapies are being used by clinicians to treat chronic PH, mostly late in the disease course (157). Therapeutic agents being used include oxygen, iNO, oral sildenafil (phosphodiesterase 5 inhibitor), bosentan (endothelin receptor antagonist), and prostacyclin. None of these can be recommended for use in neonates as their safety or efficacy in treating neonatal PH is not known, due to lack of therapeutic trials. It is our recommendation that preterm neonates with moderate or severe CNLD during their initial stay in NICU should be regularly *evaluated* using echocardiography for chronic PH. Neonates who demonstrate signs of PH should be followed up until discharge at regular intervals, and after, till disease resolves, to identify disease progression. Special attention should be given to identify, avoid and treat additional contributing factors such as ventilation with inadequate alveolar recruitment or hyperexpansion, hypercapnia, acidosis, chronic pulmonary overcirculation from significant left-to-right shunts, and periods of hypoxemia. Presence of progressive disease, especially in context of ongoing respiratory symptoms, may be considered as an indication for trial of specific

therapies, with close follow-up to establish efficacy and side effects in individual patients. Infants for whom chronic PH persists until discharge should be referred to a regional PH clinic for long-term follow-up, consideration for cardiac catheterization and/or cardiac MRI to confirm the diagnosis and eliminate CHD, and specific treatment.

HYPOTENSION

Definition

Blood pressure is used as a surrogate marker for blood flow because it is easily measurable through noninvasive and relatively reproducible techniques. Although it has been shown to correlate with blood flow in adults, the two are not equivalent and this relationship is poorly understood in neonates. Despite its limitations, blood pressure remains one of the few readily accessible measures of cardiovascular well-being. Attempts have been made to define limits of "normal" MBP in neonates, particularly at the time of transition when the neonatal brain is most commonly injured. It is known that infants at lower gestational agents are more likely to have lower blood pressure and values that gradually rise with advanced chronologic age (158). The most widely accepted definition of hypotension was generated by consensus opinion based on the observation that the majority of "healthy" preterm infants have a MBP greater or equal to their gestational age (GA) in weeks (159). This definition is problematic as it is based on limited normative data. It has been further refined by observational studies, although the sample size in each of these studies was low (Table 31.7). Some commentators suggest that hypotension be defined as MBP less than 30 regardless of gestanial or chronologic age based on observations of increased intracranial complications in some infants below this threshold (160). In addition, after the first 48 to 72 hours, most preterm neonates without a significant PDA will maintain their MBP greater than 30 mm Hg. In summary, the hierarchical importance of blood pressure as a symptom of cardiovascular well-being needs reconsideration within the context of enhanced methods to evaluate the adequacy of tissue oxygenation.

Blood Pressure and Cardiac Output

In the preterm neonate, particularly in the transitional period, there are multiple confounding physiologic differences that affect how blood pressure interacts with blood flow. Immediately after birth, there is a dramatic increase in left ventricular afterload

TABLE 31.7

Blood Pressure Thresholds at 3rd Percentile According to Postconceptual Age

Postconceptual Age (wk)	Systolic 3rd Centile	Mean 3rd Centile	Diastolic 3rd Centile
24	32	26	15
25	34	26	16
26	36	27	17
27	38	27	17
28	40	28	18
29	42	28	19
30	43	29	20
31	45	30	20
32	46	30	21
33	47	30	22
34	48	31	23
35	49	32	24
36	50	32	25

Adapted from Northern Neonatal Nursing Initiative. Systolic blood pressure in babies of less than 32 weeks gestation in the first year of life. *Arch Dis Child Fetal Neonatal Ed* 1999;80:38.

associated with the loss of the low resistance placental circulation. This is associated with a cascade of changes in both SVR and PVR to which the preterm myocardium must adapt. Blood pressure, which is the force exerted by arterial blood as it travels through the vessel in which it is measured, cannot reliably capture the complexity of these changes. Outside of the transitional period, the presence of left-to-right shunt continues to obfuscate the relationship between blood pressure and systemic blood flow.

It has been shown, using Doppler echocardiography of blood flow in the superior vena cava (SVC), that there is a weak relationship between blood pressure and blood flow in preterm neonates in the first 24 hours of life. In a group of 126 preterms at 5 hours of age, blood pressure and blood flow were oftentimes discordant; one of the two measures was low 42% of the time, but only 19% of babies had simultaneous low SVC flow and low blood pressure (50). Other studies in preterms less than 12 hours of age showed that the threshold of MBP less than GA correctly categorized only 71% of neonates with low SVC flow, while 12% of neonates with normal or high systemic blood flow were falsely identified as hypotensive. Using a MBP cutoff of 30 mm Hg in the first 12 hours of life translated into 64% of infants who were classified as hypotensive having either high or normal SVC flow (49). Low systemic blood flow is common in preterm infants. Evidence from prospective echocardiography evaluations identified low flow in 35% of infants born before 30 weeks and 61% of infants born before 27 weeks (161). The clinical relevance of low systemic blood flow is emphasized by its association with late-onset IVH. Hence, in practice, low systemic blood flow should be considered in all extremely preterm infants regardless of blood pressure; conversely, treating low blood pressure in the absence of other markers of end-organ underperfusion may lead to unnecessary intervention. Echocardiography is a useful tool to aid further characterization of these patients and determine patient populations at greatest risk of abnormal cardiovascular health and refined treatment choices based on actual physiology.

Impact on Neurodevelopmental Outcome

To be clinically relevant, the definition of an unacceptable blood pressure should consider its impact on outcomes. Though some studies have demonstrated an association between low blood pressure and intracranial hemorrhage, there has been no consistent link with impaired neurodevelopmental outcome (162). Some authors conclude that, based on current research, isolated hypotension does not warrant therapeutic intervention (163). An alternative interpretation of the current literature is that thresholds for intervention are overly simplistic and the approach to date, which is not physiology based, is imprecise and nonjudicious. Current research is flawed from several perspectives including heterogeneity in study methodology, lack of untreated controls, lack of standardization of the definition of hypotension, and failure to consider the heterogeneity of the underlying disease. Additionally, there is emerging evidence that cerebral blood flow in some preterm neonates may be governed by the same rules of autoregulation as in adults (164), adding another layer of complexity. Consideration of blood pressure alone with respect to short- and long-term brain-related outcomes, independent of cardiac output and cerebral perfusion, represents an oversimplification of the relationship. Though it is biologically plausible that dysregulation of cerebral blood flow, either by intrinsic or extrinsic factors such as vasoactive medications and rapid administration of fluid, may affect the risk of intracranial hemorrhage and white matter injury, this remains to be proven.

Etiology

Most clinicians predominantly use MBP to define hypotension. However, the individual components of SBP and DBP may provide additional information about the status of the cardiovascular system. By representing the force of blood exerted on the arterial wall in systole, SBP is reflective of the contractile force of the left ventricle propelling the blood forward. A low SBP is suggestive that stroke volume is diminished. DBP is the resting pressure of blood on the vessels and is reflective of both the SVR and volume status.

Systolic Hypotension

Stroke volume, the volume of blood ejected with each beat, is determined by three factors: ventricular preload, afterload, and contractility. The immaturity of the neonatal myocardium, particularly of the preterm infant, impairs its ability to adapt to dramatic changes in loading conditions. Additionally, the neonate is exposed to conditions, both pathologic and iatrogenic that can further impair systolic performance. Some common clinical examples of clinical situations in which a neonate may present with systolic hypotension can be found in **Table 31.8**. When a neonate with systolic hypotension has concomitant oxygenation failure, acute PH should be considered. The consequences of elevated PVR or impaired right ventricular performance include low effective PBF and therefore low left ventricular preload.

Cardiogenic shock may be caused by myocardial impairment. Arrhythmia is an important cause of cardiogenic shock, and it is important to rule out supraventricular tachycardia and ventricular arrhythmias when a neonate presents with unexplained cardiovascular dysfunction. Septic shock has a variable presentation in the neonate. "Cold" septic shock occurs when the compromised neonate attempts to compensate for insufficient cardiac output by increasing SVR; perfusion to the skin is sacrificed in an effort to maintain perfusion to vital organs. Among neonates with hypoxic–ischemic encephalopathy, right ventricular dysfunction, in particular, is a frequent contributor to low pulmonary and therefore systemic blood flow. This has been implicated as a contributor to deranged cerebral hemodynamics and abnormal brain outcome (6).

Diastolic Hypotension

The DBP primarily reflects vascular resistance. In the absence of extracardiac shunt, DBP reflects SVR, which is controlled by Poiseuille law in which the resistance of the circuit is inversely

TABLE 31.8

Common Factors Contributing to Systolic Hypotension

	Pathophysiology	Clinical Examples
Low preload	Decreased pulmonary blood flow	• Pulmonary hypertension • Mean airway pressure impairing pulmonary venous return • Obstructed pulmonary venous drainage
	Impaired diastolic filling causing obstructive shock	• Hypertrophic obstructive cardiomyopathy • Cardiac tamponade, tension pneumothorax
	Hypovolemia	• Acute hemorrhage • Transepidermal water loss (e.g., extreme preterms, skin abnormalities, gastroschisis)
High afterload	Failure of adaptation after change in loading conditions	• Loss of "low-resistance" placenta after birth • Ligation of a significant ductal shunt
	"Cold" septic shock Iatrogenic elevated systemic vascular resistance	• Vasoconstriction due to redistribution of blood to vital organs • Exogenous vasopressors • Hypothermia
Cardiogenic shock	Structural Ineffective cardiac rhythm	• Anatomic heart disease • Supraventricular tachycardia • Ventricular tachycardia (e.g., as with electrolyte imbalance)
	Impaired contractility due to myocardial injury	• Myocardial involvement after hypoxic ischemic injury • Viral or metabolic cardiomyopathy • Ischemic injury due to anomalous coronary arteries

proportional to radius to the 4th power. Hence, large vessel radius results in low SVR and low DBP and the converse. In the presence of an extracardiac shunt (e.g., ductus arteriosus, Vein of Galen malformation), both pulmonary and SVR may impact diastolic pressure, leading to the frequent finding of diastolic hypotension among preterm infants with a significant ductal shunt in the first postnatal week. Hypovolemia may also contribute to diastolic hypotension; however, compensatory vasoconstriction, in an effort to maintain organ perfusion pressure, typically occurs rapidly (Table 31.9). Sepsis presenting as diastolic hypotension is similar to the presentation of sepsis in adults. As part of the inflammatory response, there is a release of cytokines and alteration of endothelial function that are both associated with vasodilation and capillary leak. The consequences of these biologic effects include lower SVR and increased third space volume loss.

TABLE 31.9

Common Factors Contributing to Diastolic Hypotension

Pathophysiology	Clinical Examples
Enlarged vascular bed	• Patent ductus arteriosus • Bronchopulmonary sequestration, giant hemangioma, arteriovenous malformation
Vasodilation	• Systemic inflammatory response syndrome (necrotizing enterocolitis, septic shock) • Medication (phenobarbital, midazolam, morphine, etc.)
Hypovolemia[a]	• Capillary leak (necrotizing enterocolitis, septic shock) • Hemorrhage (intracranial, fetomaternal, etc.) • Transepidermal water loss • Excessive urine losses (physiologic diuresis, postobstructive diuresis, diabetes insipidus)

[a]Most neonates will adapt to hypovolemia by vasoconstricting to protect vital organs, resulting in systolic hypotension after adaptation.

Combined Systolic and Diastolic Hypotension

Both systolic and diastolic pressure becomes low as a common endpoint when the capacity of the circulatory system to compensate for ongoing hemodynamic stress is overwhelmed. The events leading up to severe hypotension may provide an indication of the underlying etiology (Fig. 31.8). When the underlying disease process is rapidly progressive, such as overwhelming septic shock, it may be difficult to determine the course of events. These neonates benefit from aggressive therapy and early echocardiography.

Clinical Presentations

Identifying the etiology of hypotension can be difficult as it is often multifactorial. In the setting of acute hemodynamic collapse, it is essential that duct-dependent systemic blood flow lesions be excluded. These include such disorders as coarctation of the aorta, hypoplastic left heart syndrome, and critical aortic stenosis and consultation with a pediatric cardiologist should be sought early. Prior to investigation of the cause and clinical relevance of systemic hypotension, it is important to ensure the accuracy of the test. Noninvasive blood pressure (NIBP) should be confirmed using the appropriate cuff size, and if an arterial line is present, waveform and correct zeroing should be verified. Oscillometric blood pressure readings can vary considerably based on a variety of factors, and it is prudent to consider the overall trend of blood pressure readings. This is particularly relevant because NIBP readings have been shown to differ systematically among preterm neonates over the first 4 weeks of postnatal life. Overestimation of systolic, and underestimation of diastolic pressure has been suggested in one study (165), but others have shown consistent overestimation by NIBP (166), no systematic difference (167), or an unpredictable difference (168), making the state of the literature difficult to interpret. The location of measurement may be important, particularly among babies with an open ductus. In the setting of a significant left-to-right ductal shunt, effective cardiac output to postductal sites (the typical location of an umbilical arterial line) may be diminished, and therefore, SBP may underestimate central nervous system (preductal) cardiac output. By contrast, significant

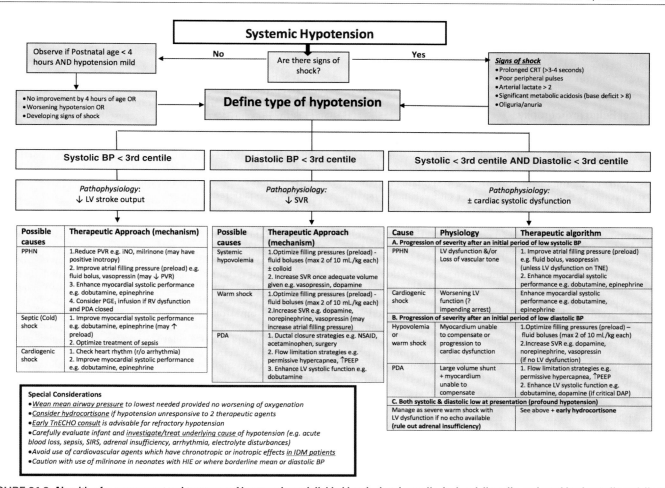

Systemic Hypotension

Are there signs of shock?

No → Observe if Postnatal age < 4 hours AND hypotension mild

Yes → **Signs of shock**
- Prolonged CRT (>3-4 seconds)
- Poor peripheral pulses
- Arterial lactate > 2
- Significant metabolic acidosis (base deficit > 8)
- Oliguria/anuria

- No improvement by 4 hours of age OR
- Worsening hypotension OR
- Developing signs of shock

→ **Define type of hypotension**

Systolic BP < 3rd centile

Pathophysiology: ↓ LV stroke output

Possible causes	Therapeutic Approach (mechanism)
PPHN	1. Reduce PVR e.g. iNO, milrinone (may have positive inotropy) 2. Improve atrial filling pressure (preload) e.g. fluid bolus, vasopressin (may ↓ PVR) 3. Enhance myocardial systolic performance e.g. dobutamine, epinephrine 4. Consider PGE₁ infusion if RV dysfunction and PDA closed
Septic (Cold) shock	1. Improve myocardial systolic performance e.g. dobutamine, epinephrine (may ↑ preload) 2. Optimize treatment of sepsis
Cardiogenic shock	1. Check heart rhythm (r/o arrhythmia) 2. Improve myocardial systolic performance e.g. dobutamine, epinephrine

Special Considerations
- *Wean mean airway pressure* to lowest needed provided no worsening of oxygenation
- *Consider hydrocortisone* if hypotension unresponsive to 2 therapeutic agents
- *Early TnECHO consult* is advisable for refractory hypotension
- *Carefully evaluate infant and investigate/treat underlying cause* of hypotension (e.g. acute blood loss, sepsis, SIRS, adrenal insufficiency, arrhythmia, electrolyte disturbances)
- *Avoid use of cardiovascular agents which have chronotropic or inotropic effects in IDM patients*
- *Caution with use of milrinone in neonates with HIE or where borderline mean or diastolic BP*

Diastolic BP < 3rd centile

Pathophysiology: ↓ SVR

Possible causes	Therapeutic Approach (mechanism)
Systemic hypovolemia	1. Optimize filling pressures (preload) - fluid boluses (max 2 of 10 mL/kg each) ± colloid 2. Increase SVR once adequate volume given e.g. vasopressin, dopamine
Warm shock	1. Optimize filling pressures (preload) - fluid boluses (max 2 of 10 mL/kg each) 2. Increase SVR e.g. dopamine, norepinephrine, vasopressin (may increase atrial filling pressure)
PDA	1. Ductal closure strategies e.g. NSAID, acetaminophen, surgery 2. Flow limitation strategies e.g. permissive hypercapnea, ↑PEEP 3. Enhance LV systolic function e.g. dobutamine

Systolic < 3rd centile AND Diastolic < 3rd centile

Pathophysiology: ± cardiac systolic dysfunction

Cause	Physiology	Therapeutic algorithm
A. Progression of severity after an initial period of low systolic BP		
PPHN	LV dysfunction &/or Loss of vascular tone	1. Improve atrial filling pressure (preload) e.g. fluid bolus, vasopressin (unless LV dysfunction on TNE) 2. Enhance myocardial systolic performance e.g. dobutamine, epinephrine
Cardiogenic shock	Worsening LV function (? impending arrest)	Enhance myocardial systolic performance e.g. dobutamine, epinephrine
B. Progression of severity after an initial period of low diastolic BP		
Hypovolemia or warm shock	Myocardium unable to compensate or progression to cardiac dysfunction	1. Optimize filling pressures (preload) – fluid boluses (max 2 of 10 mL/kg each) 2. Increase SVR e.g. dopamine, norepinephrine, vasopressin (if no LV dysfunction)
PDA	Large volume shunt + myocardium unable to compensate	1. Flow limitation strategies e.g. permissive hypercapnea, ↑PEEP 2. Enhance LV systolic function e.g. dobutamine, dopamine (if critical DAP)
C. Both systolic & diastolic low at presentation (profound hypotension)		
Manage as severe warm shock with LV dysfunction if no echo available (rule out adrenal insufficiency)		See above + early hydrocortisone

FIGURE 31.8 Algorithm for assessment and treatment of hypotension subdivided into isolated systolic, isolated diastolic, and combined systolic and diastolic categories.

right-to-left ductal shunt may augment UAC blood pressure and overestimate in a similar way (Fig. 31.9). Intermittent measurement of right arm pressure is recommended, particularly among acutely ill neonates. A clinical assessment of the neonate is then warranted to determine whether markers of low cardiac output are present.

The clinical history is often enlightening, as neonates may have previously identified risk factors for various causes of low cardiac output. In particular, history of dehydration or bleeding, risk factors for sepsis, and respiratory status including MAP and oxygenation are important. Neonates with a history of maternal diabetes represent a special group with significant risk of hypertrophic obstructive cardiomyopathy, and this should be considered highly in the differential diagnosis. Physical assessment should include heart rate, perfusion, pulses, color, and activity as well as urinary output. A cardiac exam to assess heart sounds and for murmur is important as are examinations of the abdomen and neurologic status to investigate for a source of hypotension. Laboratory markers of tissue perfusion such as metabolic acidosis, mixed venous saturation, and lactate may be helpful, as can chest radiography to assess for cardiomegaly, hyperinflation, and pneumothorax. If this assessment does not yield features concerning for either low cardiac output or a source of hypotension, consideration should be given to a period of close observation prior to initiating treatment for low blood pressure. If features consistent with low cardiac output are detected, the distinction between systolic and diastolic hypotension can allow for further clinical characterization of the

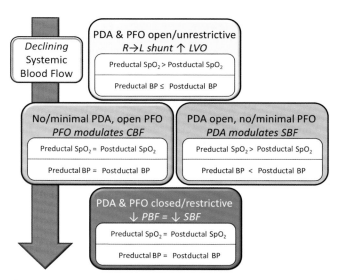

Declining Systemic Blood Flow

PDA & PFO open/unrestrictive
R→L shunt ↑ LVO
- Preductal SpO₂ > Postductal SpO₂
- Preductal BP ≤ Postductal BP

No/minimal PDA, open PFO
PFO modulates CBF
- Preductal SpO₂ = Postductal SpO₂
- Preductal BP = Postductal BP

PDA open, no/minimal PFO
PDA modulates SBF
- Preductal SpO₂ > Postductal SpO₂
- Preductal BP < Postductal BP

PDA & PFO closed/restrictive
↓ PBF = ↓ SBF
- Preductal SpO₂ = Postductal SpO₂
- Preductal BP = Postductal BP

FIGURE 31.9 Speculative relationship between oxygen saturation and blood pressure in pre- and postductal circulation among patients with acute pH. The relative magnitude of the shunt is the determinant of the relationship. Unrestrictive right-to-left shunt across the PFO augments preductal cardiac output; unrestrictive right-to-left shunt across the PDA augments postductal cardiac output. PBF, pulmonary blood flow; SBF, systemic blood flow; PDA, patent ductus arteriosus; PFO, patent foramen ovale; SpO₂, oxygen saturation; BP, blood pressure; LVO, left ventricular output.

underlying pathophysiology (Fig. 31.1). Among patients in whom myocardial dysfunction is identified, measurement of troponin is recommended. Both ischemic (e.g., related to asphyxia) and inflammatory (e.g., myocarditis) disease can be expected to result in elevated troponin while genetic/metabolic causes of cardiomyopathy are less likely to do so.

The Role of Echocardiography

In some neonates, there is a history and/or clinical symptoms consistent with a clear primary cause of hypotension. However, it must be recognized that all clinical measures of systemic blood flow are imperfect (see *Clinical Assessment of the Cardiovascular System*) including blood pressure (31). Neonates may have low systemic blood flow in the absence of clinical markers; the converse is also true. Direct assessment of cardiac output with echocardiography is often an invaluable addition to the process of diagnosis and treatment; it has been associated with management change in adult (169) and neonatal intensive care (40,42) and on neonatal transport (170).

In certain populations, such as the infant of a diabetic mother, twin-to-twin transfusion syndrome, and suspected pericardial effusion, echocardiography may demonstrate findings that may be uncovered only with a very high index of suspicion on clinical grounds. In other populations, such as a neonate with hypoxic–ischemic encephalopathy and concurrent acute PH, the physiology may be complex and direct visualization is the only way to appropriately target therapy. Echocardiography in neonates with diastolic hypotension can distinguish between hyperdynamic circulation, as with hypovolemia and warm septic shock, and a hemodynamically significant PDA. While SBP is a surrogate marker for decreased LV stroke volume, direct assessment of LVO, atrial filling or surrogate estimates of SVR may provide additional insights to the clinical assessment. Referral for TNE if available should be considered in the assessment of neonates with critically low or refractory low blood pressure at a minimum and may provide diagnostic clarity in many situations.

Management

The approach to treating a hypotensive neonate should be based on the presumptive etiology and may be aided by information obtained from TNE assessment. In general, as compared to a general pediatric or adult population, there is less emphasis on volume and more on appropriate selection of inotropic or vasopressor agents.

Volume

Treatment of hypotension usually begins with volume expansion, which is usually a crystalloid solution such as 0.9% saline. In clinical situations consistent with hypovolemia, irrespective of gestational age, volume expansion is the first line. Unless there is active hemorrhage or profound anemia, where packed red blood cells are indicated, clinical studies to date conclude that crystalloid and colloid have equivalent efficacy. Crystalloid is typically preferred as albumin may be associated with more fluid retention and an increased risk of impaired gas exchange (171).

For preterm infants with hypotension without antecedent hypovolemia, the role of volume is less certain. Rapid administration of crystalloid to hypotensive animals, without a history of hypovolemia, had no effect on cardiac output or arterial blood pressure (172). The neonatal literature is limited to small studies. Modest increases in both SVC flow and LVO have been documented in some infants with low systemic blood flow. These studies suggest that inadequate preload was a component of low cardiac output in these infants. However, many infants showed no benefit. Modest use of volume is likely to be advantageous in patients with impaired myocardial compliance such as septal or biventricular hypertrophy in the infant of a diabetic mother. Though it remains

biologically plausible that modest volume expansion has a positive effect on hemodynamics in some infants, caution must be exercised in nonhypovolemic preterm infants. Excess fluid intake is associated with increased morbidity and mortality (173). Additionally, volume expansion has no effect on cerebral oxygen delivery, unlike cardiotropic agents such as dopamine, which may provide a small increase in markers of cerebral oxygenation using NIRS (174). At present, 10 to 20 mL/kg of crystalloid remains an important part of the initial management of hypotension, if deemed clinically relevant, for the reasons outlined above. In addition, hypovolemia can be difficult to diagnose in practice, particularly in cases of concealed hemorrhage. If a trial of volume therapy is unsuccessful, early initiation of inotropic or vasopressor support should be considered.

Pharmacologic Interventions

There are fundamental differences in the development and activity of catecholamine receptors between preterm infants and adults. In animal studies, it has been shown that the myocardium of extremely low gestational age subjects has limited density of both α and β receptors which are maximally stimulated by small concentrations of catecholamines; however, these agents have a limited impact on stroke volume due to the preterm myocardium's limited ability to increase its contractile state. By contrast, the developing peripheral vasculature appears to have few $\beta 1$ receptors but many active $\alpha 1$ receptors (175). Thus, the balance of response to catecholamine stimulating agents is skewed toward peripheral vasoconstriction with a lesser increase or perhaps even a decrease in cardiac output. Additionally, cellular mechanisms by which calcium efflux is achieved differ between immature and adult patients. The sarcoplasmic reticulum in an adult makes up 1% to 5% of the cell volume and while coupling between the SR and sarcolemma are evident in the early myocyte, both the activity and ultrastructure of SR are developmentally regulated (176,177). The neonatal myocardium is relatively deficient in L-type calcium channels and fetal sheep demonstrate a decreased ability to store transported calcium due to an imbalance between calcium influx and efflux from the SR. Several studies suggest that this may be mediated by a greater density of calcium release channels in early development (176,178). This difference supports the hypothesis that the immature myocardium is more dependent on trans-sarcolemma calcium influx for contractility than the adult myocardium. Because calcium reuptake is important for muscle relaxation, immaturity of the SR may be a factor that contributes to the reduced ventricular compliance exhibited by preterm myocardium. The t-tubular system, which is important to rapid transit of calcium in the extracellular space, arises with increasing cell size and may also be immature at birth, particularly of preterm infants (177). As a result of these and other differences, caution must be exercised in extrapolating adult data to a preterm or term neonatal population; however, maintenance of serum calcium in the normal physiologic range is a reasonable precaution.

Dopamine is an adrenergic agent with variable and unpredictable effects in the developing human. Approximately 50% of dopamine's biologic activity is attributable to metabolism into downstream vasoactive catecholamines. Dopamine is converted to norepinephrine and then to epinephrine by the enzymes dopamine-beta-hydroxylase (DBH) and phenylethanolamine *N*-methyltransferase (PNMT) respectively. Among fetal sheep, activity of DBH, and therefore the metabolism of dopamine to norepinephrine, can be detected at a gestation equivalent to a 21-week human pregnancy (179). In several models, the development of DBH has been shown to precede PNMT, resulting in an earlier appearance of adrenal norepinephrine as compared to epinephrine and a potential skew toward a vasoconstricting rather than inotropic profile (180,181). Primate and human data also suggest that the maturation of this enzyme system may still be occurring for many neonates born at the earliest viable gestational ages (22 to 26 weeks) (181). While in animal models, dopamine improves renal and mesenteric blood flow at low doses, increases myocardial contractility via β adrenergic effects at moderate doses, and has predominantly vasoconstrictive α adrenergic effects at higher doses, among preterm neonates for whom there have been few studies on pharmacodynamics, this progression is less clear. There is variability between individual neonates in response to dopamine at similar doses. When exposed to dopamine at doses of 6 to 8 µg/kg/min, some neonates demonstrate an increase in LVO with a modest increase in MBP, whereas others demonstrated a reduction in LVO with a larger increase in MBP. This likely represents a difference in the balance of inotropic versus vasoconstrictive effect between individuals (182), which is independent of dose. The unpredictability of these effects is a concern. While dopamine has been consistently identified as superior to dobutamine at increasing blood pressure, echocardiography studies consistently suggest that the predominant mechanism is via peripheral vasoconstriction; more importantly, the increase in blood pressure is associated with little change in LVO (182) or superior vena cava flow. Caution should be used with dopamine in immature patients, particularly at higher doses. This is excepting specific disease states such as vasodilator septic shock when systemic vasoconstriction is the intended effect, and this may not be a relevant concern.

By contrast, *dobutamine*, a synthetic catecholamine with predominantly β-adrenergic activity (48,183), has been shown to increase cardiac output by augmenting stroke volume and may be more effective at improving systemic blood flow. It is a racemic mixture composed of two parts: the negative isomer is an α1-receptor agonist that increases myocardial contractility and SVR, while the positive isomer is a β1- and β2-receptor agonist that increases myocardial contractility and heart rate and decreases SVR. The net result is positive inotropy without major impact on peripheral circulation (184,185). In a blinded, randomized trial, SVC flow increased by 35% in infants receiving dobutamine as compared to a 1% decrease in infants receiving dopamine (48). PBF was also significantly higher in dobutamine-treated patients, suggesting it to be more advantageous as the primary agent in aPH (see PPHN subsection). The hemodynamic effects of dobutamine have been extensively studied. Animal models show a dose-dependent increase in heart rate and stroke volume, with increased cardiac output as a consequence (186–188). Studies in neonatal ovine and porcine models suggest that the vasodilating effects of dobutamine are more obvious in the systemic, rather than pulmonary circulation (188,189). In human neonates, the increase in cardiac output is determined mainly by increases in stroke volume (190), and the effects on arterial pressure are somewhat controversial (183,191–198). Importantly, dobutamine's effects on the peripheral circulation are neither potent nor reliable in situations that call for modification of vascular tone. Thus, among neonates with both impaired heart function and low systemic blood pressure (e.g., hypotension with asphyxia or myocarditis) that is either diastolic or combined, a more potent medication with both inotropic and vasoconstricting properties, such as epinephrine, may be a more appropriate first-line choice.

Epinephrine is an endogenous catecholamine produced by the adrenal gland in response to stressful stimuli. It is a potent stimulator of both α and β adrenoceptors with variable dose dependent effects. In animal models, epinephrine infusions have been shown to increase heart rate, stroke volume, and both SVR and PVR in a dose-dependent fashion (199). In human neonates, studies of the effects of epinephrine are limited; however, there is some evidence that while both epinephrine and dopamine increase blood pressure, epinephrine increases cardiac index and heart rate to a greater degree than dopamine (200). In addition to the aforementioned population who require an agent with combined vasopressor inotrope properties, epinephrine may play a role in

nonhypotensive patients. For patients with low cardiac output secondary to impaired LV systolic performance, but elevated blood pressure due to compensatory renovascular effects, low-dose epinephrine may have a positive inotropic effect which leads to improved systemic blood flow and a paradoxical normalization of blood pressure. Diseases in which epinephrine is commonly used include septic shock with cardiac dysfunction (e.g., cold shock), and diseases associated with severe cardiac dysfunction (e.g., myocarditis or ischemic cardiac injury in perinatal asphyxia). In patients with myocardial impairment secondary to acute PH, the combination of inotropy and vasoconstriction may improve right ventricular perfusion pressure and cardiac output (201). Caution is advised among patients with severe hypoxemia in the setting of aPH, however, because animal data suggest that epinephrine may also increase PVR and pulmonary artery pressure (202). Epinephrine also is associated with increase in serum lactate independent of tissue perfusion and, via stimulation of the gluconeogenesis pathway, an increase in serum glucose (203).

Norepinephrine may be a first-line therapy in vasodilatory shock in adult and pediatric patients; it is a precursor to epinephrine and is a potent alpha agonist. There are few published studies in neonates. Theoretically, norepinephrine may improve tissue perfusion pressure and cardiac function both directly by minor positive inotropy and, more importantly, indirectly via enhanced coronary flow in the presence of increased diastolic pressure. There is limited experience in term neonates suggesting that norepinephrine may be effective in some patients with shock refractory to dopamine and dobutamine (204), and small studies have suggested a greater increase in SVR as compared to PVR among patients with aPH (205). Caution, however, is recommended. The number of published patients is small, and there are animal data to suggest that norepinephrine may promote pulmonary vasoconstriction if administered with a high concentration of oxygen concurrently (206).

Vasopressin, increasingly used for specific indications, acts at V_1 receptors in the circulatory system to induce vasoconstriction of some vascular beds (e.g., splanchnic) but less so in others (e.g., renal, coronary, and cerebral). Variation in activity is primarily related to differences in endothelial V_1 receptor distribution (207). Stimulation of endothelial V_1 receptors triggers the release of NO and negates the vasoconstrictive effect of vasopressin (208). This is particularly relevant in the pulmonary vascular bed, in which a high density of endothelial V_1 receptor activity may counteract calcium-mediated signaling and results in net neutral vascular tone (207). In the kidney, it has osmotic effects by stimulation of the V_2 receptor and insertion of aquaporins in the collecting duct. In compensation, more proximal areas of the glomerulus modify sodium and chloride reabsorption in order to facilitate continued diuresis and considerable urinary sodium loss may occur. Although data are limited, there have been reports of successful vasopressin use in catecholamine-resistant shock (209–211). There is increasing interest in this agent as a treatment for aPH due to its selective vasoconstricting effects in the systemic vascular bed and concurrent vasodilating effects in the pulmonary vascular bed. Its use in this population to improve blood pressure and oxygenation has also been published (212–214).

Glucocorticoids have been shown in several studies to raise blood pressure within 2 to 6 hours in preterm neonates with refractory hypotension (215). The mechanism is thought to be multifactorial. Glucocorticoids induce the final enzyme involved in the transformation of norepinephrine to epinephrine and may therefore be involved in the up-regulation of epinephrine production. Additionally, in physiologic models, it has been shown that repetitive exposure uncouples catecholamine receptors from intracellular signaling mechanisms and thus down-regulates the response of catecholamine receptors to stimulus (216). This may be countered by corticosteroids, which increase adrenergic receptor expression (217).

Finally, preterm infants may be relatively unable to mount an adequate response in the face of stressful stimulus due to immaturity of enzyme systems in the extremely preterm adrenal gland. Hydrocortisone is the most well-studied glucocorticoid and is typically given in a dose of 2 to 4 mg/kg/d. A common regime is to give a loading dose of 2 mg/kg followed by 0.5 mg/kg every 6 hours. Although not specific to treatment of cardiovascular disease, early prophylactic hydrocortisone has been studied as an agent to prevent early mortality and/or reduce the risk of BPD with generally favorable outcomes (218–220). An individual patient meta-analysis demonstrated an increase in survival without BPD with an odds ratio of 1.45 (95% CI 1.11 to 1.9) for patients receiving 10 to 15 days of low dose hydrocortisone in the early postnatal period. Although neurodevelopment appears to be unaffected, based on 2-year outcome data available (221–223), longer-term data are sparse and both an increased risk of intestinal perforation when coadministered with indomethacin and an increased risk of late onset sepsis have been identified in hydrocortisone-treated patients (219).

Clinical Approach to Treatment

The approach to pharmacologic treatment should be individualized. Specifically, the choice of a specific agent should consider the presumed etiology, concurrent treatments, and the impact of other factors such as mechanical ventilation. It is prudent to first evaluate the clinical relevance of the hypotension, exclude measurement error, and ensure treatment is warranted (see above *Hypotension: Clinical Presentation*). Assessment of the SBP versus DBP may provide insights regarding the potential pathophysiologic nature of the hypotension (Fig. 31.8). The response to treatment should be thoroughly evaluated and agents that are associated with deterioration should be reconsidered. Progressive tachycardia may be related to disease progression; however, it is common for tachycardia to be a manifestation of excessive vasoconstriction, catecholamine toxicity (sinus tachycardia), or catecholamine-related arrhythmia (typically supraventricular tachycardia). New onset or worsening of elevated heart rate should prompt rethinking of drug choice.

Systolic Hypotension

Agents with positive inotropic properties should be used in neonates with low left ventricular stroke volume. Neonates with cardiogenic causes for hypotension, such as those with myocardial injury after hypoxic–ischemic encephalopathy, are best treated with inotropic agents such as dobutamine. Epinephrine is more potent and should be considered as second line in cases of severely depressed myocardial function. Long-term use may be associated with myocardial strain, and therefore, epinephrine should be weaned as soon as possible. It is uncommon for hypovolemia to be a significant contributor to cardiogenic shock and extra volume loading should be avoided unless there is a specific clinical indication. Arrhythmia should be ruled out and treated if present. Among neonates with central lines, pericardial effusion with tamponade should always be considered, particularly within the first 72 hours after line placement. Umbilical venous lines which are malpositioned, particularly crossing the patent foramen ovale into the left atrium, may be associated with significant left-to-right atrial shunt due to stenting, and this may contribute to low cardiac output. In both cases, moving the line is recommended and drainage of pericardial fluid may be required in some.

Septic shock presenting with evidence of poor perfusion or "cold shock" is treated similarly. Early antibiotics appropriate to the clinical situation should be a priority. The goal of therapy is to augment cardiac systolic function to overcome high SVR. This can be accomplished by using dobutamine and, if response is insufficient, epinephrine. Increasing preload with a 10- to 20-mL/kg of crystalloid may lead to improved cardiac output; however, further volume in the initial phase is not likely to be beneficial and may lead to delay in instituting inotropic support, which has

been demonstrated to be more effective. Neonates with sepsis are at risk of hematologic abnormalities such as thrombocytopenia and coagulopathy, and blood products may be needed to correct these. Oxygen carrying capacity should be maintained by optimizing hemoglobin.

In infants with profound hypoxemia, acute PH should be considered as low PBF causes insufficient venous return to the left ventricle and low stroke volume. This compromises preload, and therefore, cardiac output is impaired. The goal of therapy is to first improve atrial filling pressure. Treating the underlying disease process using interventions that will lower PVR (see section Acute PH) should be considered first line. After ensuring optimization of lung recruitments using targeted ventilation strategies and sedation, iNO should be considered. Milrinone is a useful adjunctive agent with pulmonary vasodilator and positive inotropic properties; however, caution is advised when administering milrinone to neonates with borderline mean or DBP as excessive systemic vasodilator may cause significant hypotension. Milrinone is not advisable in patients with hypoxic–ischemic encephalopathy, undergoing therapeutic hypothermia, as progressive hypotension is more likely due to impaired drug metabolism and clearance (224). Vasopressin is a plausible agent in neonates with acute PH and systemic hypotension as it increases SVR and may reduce PVR, modulating transductal resistance and reducing right–left flow across the ductus; the net consequence is increased left atrial preload, cardiac output, and SBP. Norepinephrine may be a logical alternative due to a greater increase in SVR than PVR; however, among patients with critical hypoxemia, even a small increase in PVR may not be tolerated and norepinephrine has been associated with paradoxically increased PVR in an animal model (225). There are no data to support the use of dopamine in patients with acute PH, and its greater increase in PVR as compared to SVR may lead to deterioration of oxygenation among patients with tenuous oxygenation. It is not advised in neonates with LV dysfunction where augmentation of LV afterload may further compromise myocardial performance.

Myocardial function should be assessed in infants with acute PH, particularly in refractory hypoxemia or hemodynamic instability. Agents that enhance systolic performance, such as dobutamine or epinephrine, are preferable in patients with RV dysfunction. Dobutamine has been shown to enhance RVO in preterms and may have some effect of dilating pulmonary vasculature. Epinephrine should be used more cautiously. Although epinephrine maintains the SVR:PVR ratio unchanged, its α-adrenergic effect may contribute to hypoxia. If right ventricular function is severely compromised leading to extremely low cardiac output and the PDA is closed, prostaglandin infusion should be considered both as an additional pulmonary vasodilator and to support the systemic circulation, but at the expense of lower postductal oxygen saturation and PaO_2. Caution must be used in infants with both acute PH and myocardial impairment as significant changes in loading conditions may not be tolerated.

Diastolic Hypotension

In clinical situations where the etiology is intravascular volume depletion (e.g., abdominal wall defects, acute blood loss), liberal use of volume is indicated. Acute hemorrhage requires replacement with packed red blood cells in volumes of 15 to 20 mL/kg; the rate of administration depends on the rate of blood loss and underlying disease process. If there is massive hemorrhage, consideration should be given to empiric use of platelets and/or clotting factors as well. Inotropic agents should be avoided, if possible, as hypovolemic neonates typically have hypercontractile left ventricles; increasing heart rate will decrease left ventricular filling time, further compromise coronary perfusion and worsen systemic blood flow. If pharmacologic support is required, agents with predominant vasopressor properties are recommended (**Fig. 31.10**).

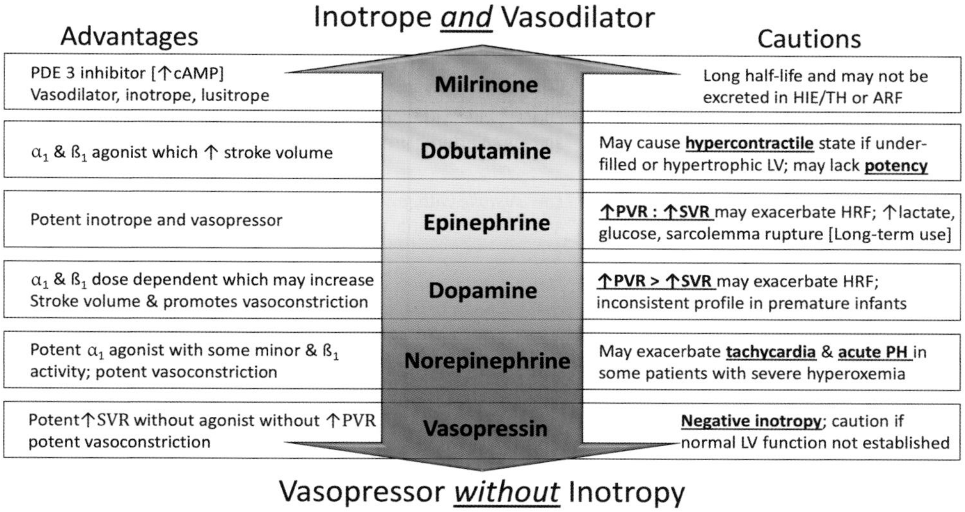

Inotrope _and_ Vasodilator

Advantages		Cautions
PDE 3 inhibitor [↑cAMP] Vasodilator, inotrope, lusitrope	**Milrinone**	Long half-life and may not be excreted in HIE/TH or ARF
α₁ & ß₁ agonist which ↑ stroke volume	**Dobutamine**	May cause **hypercontractile** state if under-filled or hypertrophic LV; may lack **potency**
Potent inotrope and vasopressor	**Epinephrine**	↑PVR : ↑SVR may exacerbate HRF; ↑lactate, glucose, sarcolemma rupture [Long-term use]
α₁ & ß₁ dose dependent which may increase Stroke volume & promotes vasoconstriction	**Dopamine**	↑PVR > ↑SVR may exacerbate HRF; inconsistent profile in premature infants
Potent α₁ agonist with some minor & ß₁ activity; potent vasoconstriction	**Norepinephrine**	May exacerbate **tachycardia** & **acute PH** in some patients with severe hyperoxemia
Potent↑SVR without agonist without ↑PVR potent vasoconstriction	**Vasopressin**	**Negative inotropy**; caution if normal LV function not established

Vasopressor _without_ Inotropy

FIGURE 31.10 Spectrum of drug activity from inotropes with vasodilator properties at one extreme to pure vasopressors at the other end. Selected advantages and cautions are described. PDE, phosphodiesterase; SVR, systemic vascular resistance; PVR, pulmonary vascular resistance; HIE, hypoxic–ischemic encephalopathy; TH, therapeutic hypothermia; ARF, acute renal failure; LV, left ventricle; HRF, hypoxic respiratory failure; PH, pulmonary hypertension.

If diastolic hypotension occurs in the setting of a hemodynamically significant PDA, specific treatment is required, which may be guided by TNE. These include both flow limitation strategies to minimize the impact of left-to-right shunt, and PDA closure using NSAIDs, acetaminophen, or surgical ligation (see section PDA) is indicated. In neonates with end-organ compromise due to low systemic blood flow, dobutamine may be considered to augment LV systolic function and improve organ perfusion. If flow modulation strategies are ineffective and organ perfusion pressure is compromised, judicious use of dopamine, which may improve diastolic pressure without driving left-to-right shunt, could be considered. This should be closely monitored due to an unpredictable dose–response relationship among preterm infants and a variable degree of end-organ vasoconstriction.

In infants with systemic inflammatory response syndrome, commonly due to sepsis or NEC, the etiology of hypotension is multifactorial and a combined approach is needed. Initial therapy is with crystalloid. As systemic vasodilation is a prominent component, early consideration of systemic vasoconstrictors such as dopamine is warranted. Many patients with warm shock have echocardiography evidence of a hypercontractile LV. One suggested approach is to give 10 to 20 mL/kg boluses of volume (to a maximum of 60 mL/kg) followed by initiation of dopamine. Critically ill neonates with sepsis and/or NEC may have significant 3rd space fluid losses of both fluid and salt making hemodynamic assessment intravascular volume status difficult; TNE may be beneficial in guiding cardiovascular decision-making in neonates who have failed to respond to aggressive volume replacement and/or a single inotrope. The use of more potent vasoconstrictors such as with epinephrine, norepinephrine, or vasopressin should be guided by TNE wherever possible. Intravenous hydrocortisone should be considered in refractory cases, but it must be recognized that it may take several hours to be effective. In some clinical situations, such as probable sepsis, NEC or SIRS early use of hydrocortisone may be warranted, although there are little data to support this approach.

Combined Systolic and Diastolic Hypotension

Combined hypotension occurs as the final common pathway, and there may be multiple contributors. Management should target the most likely underlying pathophysiology; echocardiography, which may be highly valuable in this population, is recommended whenever possible. The fundamental principles include establishing coronary perfusion pressure, supporting myocardial performance, and optimizing cardiac output. ***Distributive shock*** may occur among neonates with sepsis or perinatal asphyxia because severe endothelial dysfunction may lead to failure of normal compensatory vasoconstricting mechanisms for low cardiac output. Septic patients often have third-space losses which require ongoing fluid resuscitation, while patients with asphyxia commonly have renal failure and avoidance of excessive fluid is recommended. In both situations, vasopressor medications (e.g., norepinephrine, vasopressin) should be considered to correct coronary and organ hypoperfusion. ***Cardiogenic shock*** may result in profound hypotension due to failure of either the right or left ventricle or both for ischemic (e.g., asphyxia) and inflammatory (e.g., viral myocarditis) reasons. Epinephrine is the most appropriate first-line inotrope (Table 31.10). Prostaglandin to open the ductus arteriosus with alteration of the PVR:SVR ratio (e.g., manipulation of CO_2, target saturation thresholds) should be considered in situations where the function of one ventricle is substantially worse than the other. These infants can be treated like single ventricle physiology until function can be restored. ***Obstructive shock*** due to restricted PBF from acute PH typically requires pulmonary vasodilator therapy, avoidance of excess MAP, inotropic support for RV function (e.g., dobutamine or epinephrine), and a vasopressor to maintain coronary perfusion pressure (e.g., vasopressin) (Table 31.10). Milrinone should not be used when the patient is already hypotensive; however, it could be added at a later stage of the disease once systemic blood pressure has been restored to normal. Prostaglandin should be considered for patients with acute PH as a method to off-load the RV and provide perfusion to organs otherwise at risk of ischemia. ***Hypovolemic shock*** in the neonatal period is typically due to hemorrhage and should be treated with rapid emergency blood transfusion. Excess transepidermal water loss and post-ATN diuresis are uncommon causes of severe hypovolemia but should be considered in compatible situations and treated with crystalloid. If any vasoactive agent is to be used in hypovolemic shock, vasopressin is the typical first line due to its unique action in the kidney and, because it does not act via the β₁ receptor, it does not exacerbate tachycardia. Adrenal function should be evaluated and hydrocortisone considered early.

Role of TNE in Guiding Treatment

It is important in any neonate with a severe or refractory presentation to consider echocardiography as it is the only direct

THE NEWBORN INFANT

TABLE 31.10

Therapeutic Approach to Left and Right Ventricular Dysfunction According to Clinical Phenotype and Disease Severity

Echocardiography Findings	Management Principles	Clinical Phenotype	Suggested Management
LV systolic dysfunction	1. Support SBF 2. Positive inotropy 3. Maintain coronary perfusion	*Low systolic* with *normal diastolic* and mean arterial pressure	*Mild*: First-line **dobutamine** *Moderate/severe*: **milrinone** +/− low dose **epinephrine**
		Low systolic with *low diastolic* and/or mean arterial pressure	First-line **epinephrine** • Consider PGE (if restrictive DA) + maintenance of PVR > SVR
RV systolic dysfunction	1. Support PBF 2. Positive inotropy 3. Maintain coronary perfusion	*Normal oxygenation* with *low systolic* and *normal diastolic* and mean arterial pressure	*Mild*: First-line **dobutamine** *Moderate/severe*: **epinephrine** +/− **milrinone** • Consider PGE (if restrictive DA) • Hydrocortisone (if refractory)
		Normal oxygenation with *low systolic* and *low diastolic* and/or mean arterial pressure	*Mild*: First-line **dobutamine** *Moderate/severe*: **epinephrine** +/− **vasopressin** • Consider PGE (if restrictive DA); • **Vasopressin** or **norepinephrine** to augment diastolic and support coronary perfusion pressure • Hydrocortisone (if refractory)
		Hypoxic respiratory failure with *low systolic* and *normal diastolic* and mean arterial pressure	*Mild*: First-line **iNO** Second line: **dobutamine** or **milrinone** *Moderate/severe*: **iNO + milrinone**; Second line **epinephrine** (caution if critically hypoxemic) • Consider PGE (if restrictive DA) • Hydrocortisone (if refractory)
		Hypoxic respiratory failure with *low systolic* and *low diastolic* and/or mean arterial pressure	*Mild*: First-line **iNO** and **Vasopressin** Second line: **dobutamine** or **milrinone** (if BP normalized) *Moderate/severe*: **iNO + epinephrine** Second line **Vasopressin** or **norepinephrine** (VP preferred if tachycardia or critically hypoxemic) • Consider PGE (if restrictive DA) • Hydrocortisone (if refractory)

PGE, prostaglandin E; iNO, inhaled nitric oxide; LV, left ventricle; RV, right ventricle; PVR, pulmonary vascular resistance; SVR, systemic vascular resistance; SBF, systemic blood flow; PBF, pulmonary blood flow; DA, ductus arteriosus; VP, vasopressin.

measure of cardiac function that is available. It can be used to augment clinical suspicion by delineating the underlying physiology and identifying the relative contributions of preload, afterload, and contractility. Of particular importance is documenting the presence or absence of LV systolic impairment. Agents that increase afterload may cause further deterioration of LV function in neonates that have preexisting myocardial compromise. It is important to identify this physiology and adapt management to avoid doing harm. In addition, intravascular volume status may be difficult to determine in neonates with septic shock or acute hypovolemia and fluid overload has negative implications. Direct assessment of LV filling can guide fluid management. In neonates who present with profound hypotension, clinical clues to the underlying physiology may be impossible to determine. TNE is particularly useful in the setting of septic shock, as the determination of whether the patient is in a high versus low cardiac output state will enable a more physiologically appropriate treatment pathway. It is also important to recognize that the physiology is likely to change over time both as the disease state evolves and in response to treatment choices. TNE allows longitudinal monitoring, which will enable more focused reassessment and treatment decisions. For example when used in combination, dopamine and dobutamine produce supranormal cardiac output without changes in blood pressure (226). Careful titration of inotrope and vasopressor support should be guided by invasive arterial monitoring if possible, and frequent reassessments of biochemical markers of perfusion such as blood gas and lactate are appropriate.

SPECIAL CONSIDERATIONS

Mechanical Ventilation and Hemodynamics

The heart and lungs work closely together to ensure adequate tissue oxygen delivery. Interventions aimed at assisting one system may have beneficial or detrimental effects on the other. Mechanical ventilation induces changes in intrathoracic and intrapleural pressure and lung volumes, which may affect the major determinants of cardiovascular performance: atrial preload, ventricular afterload, heart rate, and myocardial contractility.

Impact on Atrial Preload

Systemic venous return depends on a driving pressure gradient between the extrathoracic great veins and the right atrium. In healthy spontaneously ventilated infants, the negative intrathoracic (and intrapleural) pressure generated by inspiration increases this gradient, enhancing systemic venous return. Diaphragmatic descent during inspiration simultaneously increases intra-abdominal pressure, augmenting the intra-abdominal great vein–to–right atrium gradient and promoting venous return from the lower extremities and abdomen (**Fig. 31.11**).

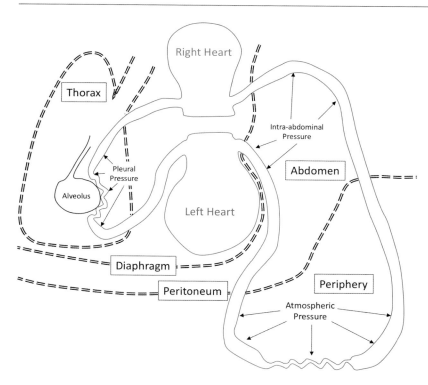

FIGURE 31.11 Model of the circulation, showing factors that influence systemic venous drainage. The right heart (RH) and intrathoracic great veins are subjected to pleural pressure (Ppl), which varies throughout the respiratory cycle. Intra-abdominal pressure increases with inspiratory diaphragmatic descent, and normalizes to atmospheric (Patmos) with expiration. Peripheral venous pressure is unaffected by respiration and so remains at atmospheric pressure throughout the respiratory cycle. Systemic venous drainage (*broken arrow*) depends on a driving pressure gradient between extrathoracic great veins (EGV) and the right atrium, and so during spontaneous respiration is maximized during inspiration as the pleural (and right atrial) pressure falls, and the intra-abdominal (and therefore EGV) pressure rises.

By contrast, invasive mechanical ventilation, which utilizes continuous positive airway pressure, may result in altered systemic venous return and cardiac output. Positive inspiratory intrapulmonary pressures are, depending on pulmonary compliance, transmitted to the pleural space and pericardium, resulting in a reduced pressure gradient between the extrathoracic great veins and right atrium. The subsequent reduced systemic venous return and right atrial preload results in reduced RV and left ventricular (LV) outputs. PEEP further prevents intrathoracic pressure from returning to atmospheric pressure during expiration and at high enough levels may impair cardiac output throughout the respiratory cycle. The reduction in cardiac output is partially offset by increased systemic arterial pressure in response to increased intrathoracic pressure. Intravascular volume expansion may augment cardiac output when high MAPs are needed (227).

In preterm infants with evolving CLD, the use of invasive mechanical ventilation necessitates careful titration of MAP. Heterogeneous areas of pulmonary atelectasis, hyperinflation, fibrosis, and disrupted alveolarization require sufficient airway pressure to maintain alveolar patency and ventilation along the compliant limb of the pressure–volume curve, without promoting overdistension that may impede systemic and pulmonary venous return. Segmental overdistention (e.g., secondary to asymmetric administration of surfactant) of the right middle lobe, which borders the right atrium, may impede systemic venous return in the absence of more diffuse hyperinflation.

The use of high-frequency modes of ventilation may have important effects on atrial preload compared with intermittent positive pressure ventilation (IPPV). Cardiac output is ultimately dependent on MAP, with similar outputs for both ventilation modes when the same MAP is used (228). However, in practice, high-frequency oscillatory or high-frequency jet ventilation are often initiated at higher MAP relative to IPPV, especially when used as a "rescue" mode of ventilation, and may be associated with reduced cardiac output (229). Additionally, it is biologically plausible that during the expiratory phase on conventional ventilation, there is an overall reduction in positive airway pressure enabling cardiac filling, whereas on high-frequency ventilation, the MAP is constant.

MAP should be titrated to the optimal balance of adequate oxygenation and cardiac output.

Initiation of Mechanical Ventilation, Premedication, and Intravascular Volume Status

The potential adverse effect of mechanical ventilation on atrial preload may be exacerbated at the time of endotracheal intubation. Premedication, often an opioid analgesic and neuromuscular blocker, is recommended to be used to optimize conditions associated with successful timely endotracheal tube placement. However, these medications may be associated with a decrease in systemic vascular tone and a subsequent reduction in systemic venous return. In infants with intravascular volume depletion (e.g., associated with severe hemorrhage, sepsis, or dehydration), the additive effects of increased intrathoracic pressure and premedication-induced peripheral blood pooling may precipitate an abrupt decrease in right atrial preload and acute circulatory collapse. Infants with pressure-passive PBF (e.g., cavopulmonary shunt), who are dependent on systemic venous return to maintain cardiac output, are at high risk of developing a low cardiac output state under these conditions.

Intrathoracic Pressure and Left Ventricular Function and Afterload

Blood is ejected into the aorta when left ventricular end-diastolic pressure, determined by the net interplay of pleural, pericardial, and left ventricular transmural pressures, exceed aortic pressure.

$$P_{\text{LV-End Diastole}} = P_{\text{LV-Transmural}} + P_{\text{Pericardial}} + P_{\text{Pleural}}$$

In spontaneously ventilating infants, the net pleural pressure is negative, and therefore, the left ventricular transmural pressure gradient is increased. However, in mechanically ventilated infants, the use of PEEP results in increased pleural pressure, with a resultant reduction in the left ventricular transmural pressure gradient (230,231). Mechanical ventilation with PEEP may be provided to infants with left ventricular dysfunction to reduce afterload, decrease volume loading via lower systemic and pulmonary venous return, and improve ventilation–perfusion mismatch caused by secondary pulmonary edema.

THE NEWBORN INFANT

Lung Volumes and Pulmonary Vascular Resistance

Lung volumes directly affect PVR, which is the main determinant of right ventricular afterload (232). PVR is minimized when lung volumes are at functional residual capacity (FRC), reflecting the optimal balance of the vascular resistances of intra- and extra-alveolar vessels (**Fig. 31.12**). In newborns with persistent PH, invasive mechanical ventilation may be used to target lung volumes at FRC, which facilitates ventilation (including the administration of iNO) and optimizes PVR.

Conversely, targeting changes in lung volume to modulate PVR may be a useful adjunct in the management of infants with congenital heart disease. Acyanotic shunts, such as PDA, may be modulated by modest increases in PEEP, with decreased ductal shunting when PEEP is increased from 5 to 8 cm H_2O (109), presumably due to a decrease in the ductal pressure gradient. In infants with univentricular physiology and excessive PBF (e.g., hypoplastic left heart syndrome), judicious use of PEEP to increase lung volumes and PVR may assist in improving conditions of low systemic blood flow.

Infant of Diabetic Mother

The risk of congenital anomalies and abnormal postnatal transition is increased in infants of a diabetic mother (IDM) and is estimated to be 2.5% to 12% (233). The incidence is thought to be greater for mothers on insulin at the time of conception or where there is poor glycemic control *in utero*. The phenotypic penetrance includes congenital heart disease, cardiac muscle hypertrophy disorders, and disturbances of cardiovascular adaptation

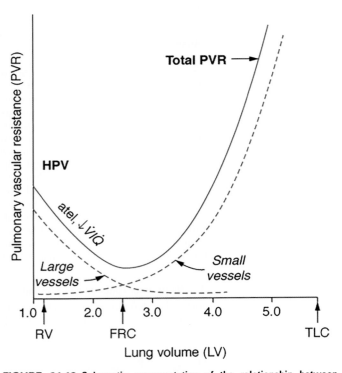

FIGURE 31.12 Schematic representation of the relationship between pulmonary vascular resistance (PVR) and lung volume. As lung volume increases from residual volume (RV) to total lung capacity (TLC), the alveolar vessels become increasingly compressed by the distending alveoli, resulting in increased resistance in the intra-alveolar vessels. The resistance of extra-alveolar vessels decreases with increasing lung volumes because they become less tortuous. The net effect of increasing lung volumes on the pulmonary vasculature produces the typical "U-shaped" curve, with its nadir (representing lowest PVR) at functional residual capacity (FRC). (Reprinted with permission from Flood P, Rathmell JP, Shafer S. *Stoelting's pharmacology & physiology in anesthetic practice*, 5th ed. Philadelphia, PA: Wolters Kluwer Health; 2014. Figure 24.29.)

after birth, which must all be considered in neonates presenting with oxygenation difficulty or hemodynamic instability after birth.

Structural Heart Disease

Congenital heart disease occurs in 5% of IDM mothers (234), with the highest risk occurring with the development of gestational diabetes and insulin resistance in the third trimester. The most common specific defects include ventricular septal defects, transposition of the great arteries, and aortic stenosis. The investigation and management of these defects should be conducted as for any neonate with suspected heart disease. Intravenous prostaglandin E1 is recommended for all patients with significant hypoxemia or cardiogenic shock, where there are ancillary clinical signs of structural heart disease.

Cardiovascular Adaptation after Birth

Closure of the ductus arteriosus and the postnatal decline in PVR are delayed in infants of diabetic mothers compared to healthy newborns, increasing their vulnerability to acute PH of the newborn (235). The pathologic nature of these changes is poorly understood. The management of acute PH or systemic hypotension in these patients should consider whether there is evidence of myocardial hypertrophy.

Hypertrophic Cardiomyopathy

An increase in cardiac muscle hypertrophy is an anabolic result of fetal hyperinsulinemia triggered by maternal hyperglycemia in the third trimester. Biventricular hypertrophic cardiomyopathy occurs in 12% of patients. Asymmetric septal hypertrophy, however, due to regional differences in insulin-like growth factor receptor density, occurs in 30% of IDM patients and is the most common form. Septal hypertrophy results in left ventricular outflow tract obstruction (LVOTO) in up to 5% of IDM neonates (236–238). In the absence of LVOTO, neonates are usually asymptomatic and identified on screening echocardiography (239). The dominant physiologic concern for neonates with hypertrophic cardiomyopathy is restrictive physiology with impaired left heart filling and consequently impaired cardiac output. Compensatory tachycardia reduces diastolic duration and therefore further compromises stroke volume. PH with limited left atrial preload, and high intrathoracic pressure from excessive ventilator settings, in this setting may be particularly problematic as high left atrial pressure is essential for forward flow into the poorly compliant hypertrophic ventricle; however, right-to-left ductal shunt may maintain systemic blood flow in situations were left ventricular outflow tract obstruction is severe. Low cardiac output in these patients is associated with lower cerebral resistance to compensate the low flow through carotid arteries (240,241). Myocardial hypertrophy should be considered in all IDM patients with clinical signs of low cardiac output. Liberal use of volume is recommended to improve atrial filling pressures and offset the negative impact of impaired myocardial compliance. Cardiovascular agents with chronotropic properties such as dopamine, dobutamine, or epinephrine are contraindicated as they will limit ventricular filling time leading to further compromise to cardiac filling. Augmenting afterload may improve LV end-systolic volume, which may be advantageous. Vasopressin is the ideal agent in this population. Increased SVR produces increased afterload and improves atrial filling pressures through systemic vasoconstriction. Negative inotropic properties for vasopressin have been postulated in adults but not yet demonstrated in the neonatal population. The antidiuretic properties of vasopressin may be advantageous; however, patients with normal renal function rapidly adapt and may develop significant natriuresis. Careful monitoring of serum and urine sodium concentrations may be helpful. In the acute period, many of these neonates have comorbid PH; although beta blockade is conceptually a good idea, there is a risk of exacerbating PH and precipitating a crisis of left heart filling and/or hypoxia. Once PH is controlled, a trial of esmolol, a rapid acting continuous infusion, could be considered if rate control is needed, particularly as an adjunct to wean off vasopressin and/or prostaglandin. Longer-acting beta blockers such as propranolol are used if symptoms persist, although the natural history for most patients is spontaneous resolution of symptoms and regression of the hypertrophy (242).

Hypoxic–Ischemic Encephalopathy

Neonates who have suffered hypoxic–ischemic injury often have multisystem end-organ injury. The cardiovascular consequences of this insult are less well delineated. Although therapeutic hypothermia (TH) improves long-term neurodevelopmental outcome in infants who have had moderate to severe hypoxic–ischemic brain injury, there is little evidence of how it modifies the cardiovascular course in either a beneficial or harmful way. It is important to consider, and wherever possible confirm, the physiologic contributors to cardiovascular instability enabling refinement of the medical decision-making process.

Etiology/Physiologic Considerations

In the setting of HIE, both the type and severity of the initial insult and TH impact on myocardial function, cardiac output, and cerebral blood flow (243) (**Fig. 31.13**). The scope and magnitude of the hemodynamic instability are influenced by multiple contributing factors including vasomotor tone (afterload), ischemia (myocardial function), and presence of PH (left heart preload). These symptoms may relate to primary myocardial injury, associated PH, adrenal injury, or a consequence of the induced hypothermia.

Primary Myocardial Injury
Evidence of cardiac ischemia on electrocardiogram assessment has been documented in 29% to 38% of neonates with perinatal

hypoxic injury (243). Mitral and tricuspid regurgitation are common and may be related to papillary muscle ischemic necrosis, and rarely, it may represent chordal rupture (244). Recent data suggest that the right ventricle is particularly vulnerable and may be an early indicator of abnormal brain magnetic resonance imaging (MRI), death, and abnormal neurologic outcome (6). The biologic rationale behind RV disease in this population is likely multifactorial. First, the dominant role of the RV during fetal life makes it the more metabolically active ventricle requiring of a higher blood supply during the transition (177). Among neonates with biventricular ischemia, there may be more detrimental effects on the RV. Its twofold higher ratio of circumferential radius to wall thickness results in a much greater wall stress for a similar increase in afterload as compared to the LV and the frequent coexistence of aPH places added afterload stress on the right side (23). Third, coronary perfusion to the RV versus the LV is more susceptible to derangement. The adult RV is perfused throughout the cardiac cycle due to low pulmonary to systemic arterial pressure during systole (245). In the neonatal period, high pulmonary artery pressure causes high central venous pressure and may compromise systolic flow. Diastolic flow becomes vulnerable when impaired PBF leads to low cardiac output and subsequently to low coronary root pressure. Because low aortic root pressure is typically associated with concurrent low LV end-diastolic pressure, a gradient is maintained and LV perfusion is relatively protected. Other factors, such as the impact of exposure to pathologically high SVR in the setting of an open ductus arteriosus, the influence of impaired RV preload in the setting of hemorrhage or hypovolemia, and the role of ventricular–ventricular interaction may also contribute.

Pulmonary Hypertension
A failure of the normal postnatal fall in PVR is commonly associated with hypoxic–ischemic injury and, like RV dysfunction, has

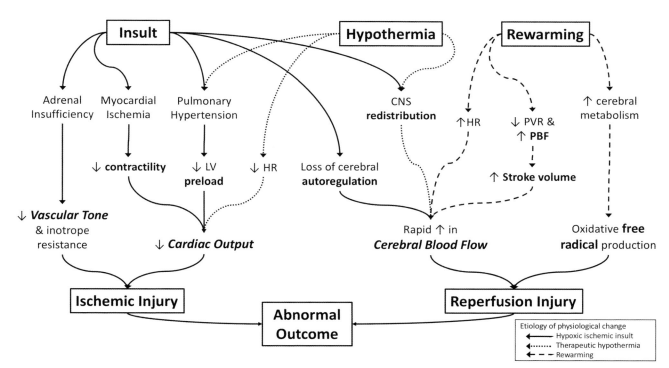

FIGURE 31.13 Interrelationship between contributors to ischemic injury resulting from initial insult, therapeutic hypothermia, and reperfusion injury on rewarming. The initial injury results in conditions that result in ischemia and systemic hemodynamic instability including adrenal insufficiency, transient myocardial ischemia, and pulmonary hypertension. Hypothermia modifies hemodynamic conditions and therapies for systemic underperfusion may transiently improve circulatory conditions. On rewarming, reversal of TH-induced bradycardia and pulmonary hypertension result in a rapid increase in cardiac output, hence cerebral blood flow. This may be especially detrimental due to the loss of cerebral autoregulation and CNS redistribution produced by the original injury. Resumption of cellular activity after transient suppression is a putative source of potentially damaging oxidative radicals. Both ischemia and reperfusion injury contribute to the degree of brain injury. PVR, pulmonary vascular resistance; PBF, pulmonary blood flow; LV, left ventricle; HR, heart rate.

been associated with abnormal brain MRI (246). Neonates with perinatal asphyxia have hypoxemia and acidosis, which promote elevated PVR. It is common for encephalopathic neonates to fail to establish respirations leading to delayed establishment of functional residual capacity and the consequent abnormally high PVR state (247). Associated conditions such as sepsis and MAS may also contribute (see section Acute PH). Induced hypothermia may lead to pulmonary vasoconstriction with consequential elevation of PVR and worsening of the efficacy of oxygenation. In an animal model, every 1 degree reduction in temperature is associated with a 1% to 2% increase in PVR (248). Appropriate medical control of oxygenation failure is recommended prior to initiating therapeutic hypothermia. Among patients with normal oxygenation but poor RV function, the increase in afterload may be poorly tolerated. Consideration of early echocardiography, particularly among hypotensive, severely asphyxiated or acidotic patients with quantitative assessment of RV disease is prudent. It is recommended to continue TH in the setting of acute PH, unless there is refractory hypoxemia despite pulmonary vasodilator treatments, for example, NO.

Adrenal Injury

In fetal sheep, it has been shown that, while blood flow to the gastrointestinal tract and kidneys is reduced during a period of asphyxia, blood flow to the heart and adrenal gland is increased. This compensation is maintained despite severe hypoxemia and acidosis (249) and is accompanied by a pronounced increase in ACTH and cortisol secretion (250). A stress-related cortisol surge is typical in asphyxiated neonates (251); however, lower concentrations of catecholamines have been found in term infants with moderate HIE as compared to mild HIE (252). This suggests that adrenal impairment may be associated with more severe injury. Imaging studies have shown that hypoxic–ischemic injury is associated with areas of hypo-echogenicity and diffuse enlargement (253) consistent with congestion and adrenal hemorrhage (254). Adrenal insufficiency has been reported in 30% of neonates with adrenal hemorrhage and may manifest as hypotension and/or hyponatremia (255).

Hemodynamic Effects of Therapeutic Hypothermia

Neonates undergoing TH demonstrate predictable changes in the cardiovascular system. The majority of neonates who have not sustained any cardiac injury have normal or mildly increased blood pressure. The latter is related to the increase in SVR associated with hypothermia-induced vasoconstriction. Hypothermia also causes a moderate reduction in heart rate due to prolongation of QT and RR intervals. These changes are generally well tolerated systemically, and clinically relevant tissue hypoperfusion rarely occurs. There is, however, a marked reduction in cardiac output to levels 60% to 70% of normal-term infants (256). This reduction is due to the decrease in heart rate, as LV systolic performance remains similar, both by conventional measures and on deformation by Tissue Doppler (257). The clinical relevance of this decrement in cardiac output is unknown. Deranged cerebral hemodynamics that reflect poor brain utilization of oxygen are seen among patients with impaired RV function (6) and may precede abnormal brain MRI (258,259). It remains to be seen, however, if therapeutic hypothermia modifies this relationship, and the optimal cerebral blood flow in this population is unknown.

It is important to weigh the adverse effects of TH against the overall neurologic benefits, particularly in borderline situations. The association of TH and increased PVR is an important consideration in neonates with acute PH. As TH improves neurodevelopmental outcome in neonates with moderate–severe HIE, an aggressive approach to the management of aPH is warranted. In medically refractory cases of acute PH, modification of target temperature by increments of 0.5°C to 1.0°C may improve the efficacy of oxygenation as vasoconstriction is less pronounced at temperatures closer to the normal range. In some rare situations, TH should be discontinued. In addition, avoidance of fever may have independent neuroprotective benefits.

Clinical Presentation

Symptoms vary between patients according to the underlying pathophysiology. These include systolic or combined systolic and diastolic hypotension, end-organ hypoperfusion, and/or apical systolic murmur. Hypotension following hypoxic–ischemic injury has been reported in 62% of neonates (243) and may be multifactorial. Neonates with low PBF may present with oxygenation failure; however, adequate oxygenation does not preclude severe disease. Perinatal asphyxia is relatively unique in that it is common for a neonate to have failed transition due to neurologic injury and absence of central drive in the presence of relatively little lung disease. As a result, the neonate may present with significantly elevated PVR in the absence of oxygenation failure due to intact ability to match ventilation to perfusion. The consequence may be underestimation or a complete failure to recognize RV disease unless the index of suspicion is high. Although less common, impaired LV function may present as left atrial hypertension and pulmonary edema. The elevation in SVR secondary to induced hypothermia may aggravate myocardial function in this situation.

In all neonates with hypoxic–ischemic injury, screening EKG is warranted to assess for transient myocardial ischemia. Echocardiography with quantification of RV performance should be considered for all HIE patients and is particularly important for neonates with hemodynamic instability and those with moderate to severe encephalopathy. Qualitative assessment of RV performance is poorly sensitive (260), and quantitative measures such as tricuspid annulus plane systolic excursion (TAPSE) and fractional area change (FAC) are associated with brain outcomes (6). The diagnosis of TMI is suspected on EKG and graded according to the appearance of T and Q waves and evidence of ST segment changes (Table 31.11). Serum biomarkers of myocardial ischemia are less specific in neonates than in adult populations but are associated with abnormal neurologic outcome. Troponin T, a cardiac specific marker of muscle injury, has been shown to be higher in neonates with severe HIE than controls. Troponin I is also elevated in neonates with asphyxia and may be a valuable marker of myocardial injury. CK-MB is significantly elevated in neonates with moderate to severe encephalopathy and begins to rise within 4 to 8 hours of injury (243).

Management

General Considerations

The approach to newborn care in the setting of hypoxia–ischemia where TH is initiated is complex with several modifying antecedent factors that affect the appropriate choice of therapy and the response of the neonate. Though limited evidence is available to

---

TABLE 31.11

EKG Grading of Transient Myocardial Ischemia

Grade	Severity	EKG Finding
I	Equivocal	Flat or inverted T wave in one lead only
II	Suggestive	Flat or inverted T wave in several leads + abnormal Q wave in any lead
III	Moderate	Flat or inverted T wave in several leads OR bundle branch block + abnormal Q + abnormal ST segments
IV	Severe	Classical segmental infarction pattern with abnormal Q waves + markedly elevated ST segments

Reprinted by permission from Springer: Barberi I, Calabro MP, Cordaro S, et al. Myocardial ischemia in neonates with perinatal asphyxia: electrocardiographic, echocardiographic and enzymatic correlations. *Eur J Pediatr* 1999;158:742. Copyright © 1999 Springer Nature.

TABLE 31.12

Effects of Therapeutic Hypothermia on Physiologic Determinants of Drug Pharmacokinetics (PK) and Pharmacodynamics (PD)

Physiologic Change	Pharmacologic Effect
Reduced activity of hepatic enzymes (e.g., CYP450)	Reduced clearance
Vascular redistribution toward essential organs (e.g., reduced blood flow to liver and kidneys)	Reduced clearance
Peripheral vasoconstriction	Smaller volume of distribution

Reprinted by permission from Nature: Zanelli S, Buck M, Fairchild K. Physiologic and pharmacologic considerations for hypothermia therapy in neonates. *J Perinatol* 2011;31:377. Copyright © 2011 Springer Nature.

guide dose adjustment, therapeutic hypothermia has physiologic effects that affect pharmacodynamics (PD) and pharmacokinetics (PK) of commonly used mediations that have effects on the cardiovascular system such as benzodiazepines, phenobarbital, and narcotics (251). These effects are listed in Table 31.12. Similarly, organ injury, particularly to the liver and kidney, due to hypoxia–ischemia may affect drug metabolism and excretion. For example, milrinone, which has renal clearance, may accumulate in neonates with acute kidney injury, exacerbating hypotension as a result of decreased SVR (224). Milrinone, therefore, is not recommended for babies undergoing TH for HIE and caution, in general, should be used when initiating and titrating medications. The pharmacodynamics and kinetics of cardiotropic medications in cooled and rewarming infants have not been delineated.

On rewarming, changes in vascular tone result in changes in blood pressure and volume of distribution and changes in organ perfusion affect metabolism and clearance. This may destabilize the cardiovascular system. Hypothermia-induced vasoconstriction is reversed, and there is a decrease in SVR; rewarming has been associated with a decrease in MBP of approximately 8 mm Hg (251). Drugs with a large volume of distribution will have an exaggerated effect on rewarming as drugs are mobilized from sequestered tissues. Metabolism and clearance will change as blood flow is redirected to renal and hepatic vascular beds and enzyme systems that are inhibited by cooling are up-regulated. These changes may require modification to cardiovascular support.

Management of Systemic Hypotension

Care of hypotensive neonates with cardiac dysfunction and HIE should be supportive as the majority of neonates improve over time. In light of dysregulated CBF and the association between high CBF and increased morbidity and mortality, volume should be avoided unless a clinical scenario compatible with hypovolemia, such as subgaleal hemorrhage, is present. Treatment should be targeted toward improving myocardial systolic performance without modulating SVR or PVR; early echocardiography, in particular for neonates with systolic or severe hypotension, is recommended. Positive inotropy, as with dobutamine, is the logical first-line approach for isolated systolic hypotension. If no improvement is seen with dobutamine of 5 to 10 μg/kg/min or diastolic hypotension is present, early transition to epinephrine is suggested. For severely affected neonates or those with refractory hypotension, adrenal injury should be considered and hydrocortisone, which has been associated with a lower requirement for catecholamine treatment in this population, may be indicated (261).

Infants with both HIE and acute PH may develop impairments in preload and myocardial performance that may both contribute to low systemic blood flow. Echocardiography is very valuable in these patients. iNO is the standard of care pulmonary vasodilator therapy, but it is essential to ensure adequate lung recruitment prior to intervention. Ventilation below functional residual capacity

is associated with areas of hypoxic vasoconstriction and tortuous capillaries, whereas over-distension results in compression of intra-alveolar capillaries. At both extremes of inflation pressure, PVR is exaggerated. Poor response may be seen in up to 40% of neonates (154). Dobutamine, or if very severe epinephrine, is a reasonable agent to support RV performance, and prostaglandin may be used in severe or refractory cases both to off-load the RV and facilitate post-ductal perfusion. Vasopressin is a biologic agent with dichotomous properties (see *Hypotension*) including systemic vasoconstriction without pulmonary vasoconstriction. There is evidence of benefit for neonates with acute PH (213), but it has not been formally studied in the specific population of neonates with HIE.

Role of Targeted Neonatal Echocardiography

The primary benefit of additional echocardiography information is to help refine the underlying physiology and differentiate the various causes of hemodynamic instability including LV or RV dysfunction and/or acute PH as outlined above. As previously described, quantitative RV assessment is important both because subjective assessment is unreliable and because abnormalities of measurements such as TAPSE and FAC at 24 hours of age have been associated with poor neurologic outcomes. It is typical for RV dysfunction to be dominant and to improve over time throughout the cooling period with most neonates normalizing by day 4 to 5 postnatal age (6). LV dysfunction is typically more subtle and most studies have showed conventional markers (e.g., fractional shortening, ejection fraction) within the normal range. Newer markers such as systolic strain and strain rate may identify deviations from normal; however, it remains unclear whether LV disease is primary or secondary to ventriculoventricular interaction with the RV (257,262). As previously described, biventricular outputs are lower for neonates undergoing TH; however, pathologically low output should be suspected if less than 90 mL/kg/min and clinical features of hypoperfusion are present.

Systemic Hypertension (See also Chapter 38)

Hypertension in neonates is uncommon with a reported incidence of 0.2% to 3%. The majority of neonates are asymptomatic. Measurement of blood pressure in neonates is subject to operator-dependent error; therefore, standardization of the methodology is imperative to improve diagnostic accuracy. Hypertensive emergency, considered in the setting of severely increased blood pressure and evidence of end-organ dysfunction, is rare in neonates. Specific signs of severe hypertension may include CHF, encephalopathy, seizures, and intracranial hemorrhaged or renal failure. Rarely, when afterload elevation is severe, left ventricular compensatory mechanisms fail and the neonate develops progressive pulmonary edema. These patients may also develop diastolic dysfunction, which may present with low systemic blood flow and pseudonormalization of blood pressure (263).

Etiology

There are two distinct populations of neonates who develop hypertension: (a) those with a single underlying etiology, typically born at term, and (b) those infants with hypertension associated with chronic disease that is likely multifactorial in the setting of extreme prematurity.

Vascular Disease

Vascular disease is a common reason for neonates to develop hypertension; this form may be severe. Included in this group are disorders of the renal vascular system such as renal vein thrombosis, renal artery fibromuscular dysplasia, and more proximal processes such as coarctation of the aorta. Renal parenchymal diseases and urologic conditions comprise a second large group of conditions affecting infants. The majority of these disorders are congenital such as polycystic or multicystic–dysplastic kidney disease or

TABLE 31.13

Categories of Disease Presenting as Hypertension in the Neonatal Period

Category	Select Examples
Vascular	Coarctation of aorta, renal vein thrombosis, renal artery stenosis, external compression of renal vessels
Renal Parenchymal	Polycystic or MCDK disease, UPJ obstruction, ATN, cortical necrosis, urinary obstruction (stones, tumors)
Endocrine	CAH, hyperaldosteronism, hyperthyroidism, neuroblastoma, pheochromocytoma
Neurologic	Pain, elevated intracranial pressure, seizures, subdural hematoma
Medications	Dexamethasone, methylxanthines, pancuronium, adrenergic agents
Multifactorial	Comorbid conditions of extreme prematurity: history of UAC, bronchopulmonary dysplasia, ductal shunt, nephrocalcinosis, medications

MCDK, multicystic-dysplastic kidney; UPJ, ureteropelvic junction; ATN, acute tubular necrosis; CAH, congenital adrenal hyperplasia; UAC, umbilical arterial catheter.

Adapted by permission from Springer: Dionne JM, Abitbol CL, Flynn JT. Hypertension in infancy: diagnosis, management and outcome. *Pediatr Nephrol* 2012;27:17. Copyright © 2012 Springer Nature.

TABLE 31.14

Standard Protocol for Optimizing Noninvasive Blood Pressure Measurement

Variable	Optimization Technique
Equipment	• Oscillometric device • Appropriately sized cuff (width to arm circumference ratio of 0.45–0.55)
Positioning	• Right upper arm cuff placement • Neonate in prone or supine position
Timing	• 1.5 h after an intervention or feed • Cuff placed and then left still for 15 min without handling • Asleep or quiet awake state • Three readings at 2-min intervals

Adapted from Nwankwo MU, Lorenz JM, Gardiner JC. A standard protocol for blood pressure measurement in the newborn. *Pediatrics* 1997;99:e10.

obstructive uropathy. Less commonly, infants with acquired renal injury such as acute tubular or cortical necrosis may develop hypertension (Table 31.13).

Hypertension in the Ex-Preterm Infant

Neonates born at extremely low gestational ages are at risk of hypertension both during their NICU stay and in the postdischarge period. These patients may be missed or diagnosis may be late as the onset is usually during the late rehabilitation phase of neonatal care. There are several risk factors. The most frequent is umbilical arterial catheterization (UAC) with increased risk proportional to duration of catheterization. This is thought to be due to thromboembolism; however, neonates remain at risk even in cases where a clot cannot be visualized on ultrasound. BPD is associated with a fivefold increase in hypertension when compared to controls. The precise mechanism is unknown; however, contributing factors may include PH, chronic hypoxemia and hypercapnia, steroid use, or changes in hormonal mediators such as angiotensin, antidiuretic hormone, and catecholamines. Recent evidence has highlighted an association between systemic hypertension and LV diastolic dysfunction (264,265). Some commentators have proposed a "postcapillary" PH phenotype that is clinically relevant from a treatment perspective as selective pulmonary vasodilators may have little benefit. There are little published mechanistic data in this patient population. Similarly, the presence of PDA has been associated with an increased risk (3.8-fold) (266). The mechanisms are not known. Commonly used medications, including dexamethasone and caffeine, also increase blood pressure.

Evaluation

In the acute phase of illness, blood pressure should be monitored every 4 hours at a minimum and adjusted to level of illness. The diagnosis is made when three separate systolic measurements done with appropriate equipment, positioning, and in a quiet neonate (Table 31.14) greater than the 95th percentile are documented. As the neonate reaches a stable convalescent phase, blood pressure should be monitored at a minimum every 12 hours and increased as needed. Investigation should be guided by a thorough history as many contributing factors can usually be readily identified. This should include a review of the pregnancy history to identify renal or another anomalies, history of UAC placement, comorbid

conditions, and medication exposure. Physical examination must include measurement of blood pressure in four limbs to rule out coarctation of the aorta and an abdominal exam for renal bruits and masses.

The investigative approach depends on the infant's clinical course; in most situations, thorough history and physical exam will provide direction. Renal function should be assessed with measurements of urea and creatinine along with electrolytes. Renal ultrasound with Doppler should be highly considered to assess for structural renal disease and renal vascular disease (Table 31.15).

TABLE 31.15

Initial Investigations for Hypertensive Neonates by Presenting Complaint: Investigations Useful in the Majority of Neonates

Diagnostic Test	Population	Assessing for
Urinalysis	All	Blood and protein for glomerular disease
CBC with platelet count	All	Evidence of thrombosis
Serum electrolytes, calcium urea, and creatinine	All	Renal failure (abnormal urea, creatinine): • Hyperkalemia • Hyponatremia (e.g., if volume overloaded)
Urinary protein:creatinine ratio	All	Evidence of renal parenchymal injury and as a baseline
Renal ultrasound with Doppler	All	Renal vein thrombosis, anatomic renal abnormalities, ± renal artery/aortic thrombus
Echocardiography	All	Aortic coarctation, myocardial function, valve regurgitation, pulmonary hypertension
Endocrine studies (thyroid, cortisol, urine VMA/HVA)	Select	If compatible symptoms of hyperthyroidism, CAH, neuroblastoma, etc.
Renin and aldosterone	Select	If hypokalemia or other electrolyte abnormality suggesting genetic disorder of tubules (RTA)

CAH, congenital adrenal hyperplasia; RTA, renal tubular acidosis; VMA, vanillylmandelic acid; HVA, homovanillic acid.

Adapted by permission from Springer: Dionne JM, Abitbol CL, Flynn JT. Hypertension in infancy: diagnosis, management and outcome. *Pediatr Nephrol* 2012;27:17. Copyright © 2012 Springer Nature.

Echocardiography should be performed to exclude primary cardiac conditions that are associated with systemic hypertension including coarctation of the aorta. In addition, echocardiography will provide insights into the impact of sustained hypertension on the heart. Specific findings suggestive of CHF include left ventricular systolic dysfunction without chamber dilation, concentric hypertrophy, dilated cardiomyopathy, left atrial dilation with ventricular diastolic dysfunction, and aortomegaly (267). Retinal complications of hypertension may be identified in childhood but are seldom present in the neonatal period.

Blood pressure assessment should be part of routine follow-up of all extremely preterm infants and those at risk due to renal or other systemic disease. Those infants with risk factors for development of hypertension including CLD, PDA, an history of systemic steroids, renal failure, and nephrocalcinosis or a disorder known to cause secondary hypertension should be followed closely over the first 6 months of life. Infants discharged home on antihypertensive medications should be considered for home blood pressure monitoring. There are no evidence-based recommendations for neonates. The majority of infants will not require escalation of treatment after 6 months of age unless there is a known cause of secondary hypertension. Preterm infants remain at increased risk of hypertension throughout their life and periodic monitoring, particularly in adolescence and adulthood is recommended.

Treatment

The approach to therapeutic intervention should be directed by the underlying cause. Modifiable factors contributing to hypertension including fluid overload and medications that induce hypertension should be addressed. Pharmacologic therapy in neonates is poorly studied, and management guidelines are typically based on previous experience or consensus opinion. Asymptomatic hypertension can be managed using oral or intermittent intravenous agents. In a retrospective cohort study, data were collected on the use of antihypertensive agents in neonates across 41 tertiary NICUs in United States (268). The most frequently used agents were vasodilators, most commonly hydralazine, followed by angiotensin inhibitors (captopril, enalapril) and calcium channel blockers (amlodipine). Beta-blockers such as propranolol were less frequently used. For long-term management, a calcium channel blocker is recommended. However, due to its long half-life, amlodipine takes 3 to 5 days to reach steady state and, therefore, is not ideal for rapid control of intermittent hypertension. For this purpose, hydralazine is a superior agent.

Management of hypertensive emergency should be by intravenous infusion. The choice of vasoactive agent should be guided by clinical experience, as there are limited pharmacologic data available in neonates. An intravenous infusion of a short-acting calcium channel blocker such as nicardipine may be particularly useful. Other drugs that have been used include sodium nitroprusside and short-acting beta-blockers such as esmolol; however, caution is advised with use of intravenous beta-blockers if there is concern for CHF due to its negative inotropic effects. Careful titration of blood pressure is needed to prevent an acute drop in organ perfusion pressure, which is most relevant for the brain. In pediatrics, the recommendation is to decrease blood pressure by no more than 25% to 30% over 6 to 8 hours (263); however, evidence-based recommendations for neonates have not yet been developed. Further studies are needed to investigate the impact of antihypertensive agents on developing organs. For example, animal data suggest that in the neonatal period, suppression of the renin–angiotensin system, as with angiotensin inhibitors, impairs renal development and leads to decreased nephron endowment (268). Some experts recommend avoidance of the use of ACE inhibitors until 44 weeks corrected GA to minimize the risk of this complication. The role of angiotensin receptor blockers is less clear.

Effusions

Acute pericardial effusions that develop in the postnatal period may have devastating consequences. Neonates with central venous catheter (CVC)-associated pericardial effusions have a mortality rate of 30% to 65% (269,270). Both peripherally inserted central catheters (PICCs) and umbilical venous catheters (UVCs) have been associated with moderate to large pericardial effusions. The precise incidence is difficult to estimate. One retrospective study estimated the incidence due to PICCs at 1.8/1,000 catheters with approximately 25% of cases first identified at autopsy (270). Other causes of acute effusions include bacterial or fungal infection and are extremely rare.

The mechanism by which CVCs lead to pericardial effusions is not well understood. When analyzed, the majority of effusions contain a similar composition as the infusate without significant contamination by blood. It is hypothesized that mechanical stress may contribute to myocardial necrosis followed by osmotic injury from hyperosmolar parenteral nutrition that then diffuses into the pericardial space (271). There may also be direct erosion of the catheter tip. The majority of effusions are associated with malpositioned catheters. The ideal position of a catheter tip is at the junction of the vena cava and the right atrium. This precise anatomic location on chest radiography varies between infants (272); in each infant, considerable movement of catheter tips occurs with arm movement (upper limb PICCs) and changes in girth or mummification of the cord (UVCs). Additionally, the pericardium extends over the proximal superior and inferior vena cava by approximately 1 cm in preterm and 2 cm in term infants and therefore infants with well-positioned CVCs remain at risk (269).

The presenting features of pericardial effusion include acute hemodynamic collapse in 61% of cases and unexplained hemodynamic instability in 36%. The majority of symptomatic effusions occurs early with a median time to presentation of 3 days but may occur at any time (271). Clinical signs are often nonspecific but may include cardiomegaly and distant heart sounds. The index of suspicion must remain high in all infants that acutely decompensate with CVCs in place. Emergency pericardial drainage is life-saving in this situation and should not be delayed in an arrest. Echocardiography is diagnostic and ultrasound-guided pericardiocentesis is indicated in symptomatic infants if available.

REFERENCES

1. Jain A, Mohamed A, El-Khuffash A, et al. A comprehensive echocardiographic protocol for assessing neonatal right ventricular dimensions and function in the transitional period: normative data and Z scores. *J Am Soc Echocardiogr* 2014;27(12):1293.
2. Evans N, Iyer P. Longitudinal changes in the diameter of the ductus arteriosus in ventilated preterm infants: correlation with respiratory outcomes. *Arch Dis Child Fetal Neonatal Ed* 1995;72:F156.
3. Rowland DG, Gutgesell HP. Noninvasive assessment of myocardial contractility, preload, and afterload in healthy newborn infants. *Am J Cardiol* 1995;75:818.
4. Schmidt MR, White PA, Khambadkone S, et al. The neonatal but not the mature heart adapts to acute tachycardia by beneficial modification of the force-frequency relationship. *Pediatr Cardiol* 2011;32:562.
5. Jain A, Mohamed A, Kavanagh B, et al. Cardiopulmonary adaptation during first day of life in human neonates. *J Pediatr* 2018;200:50.
6. Giesinger RE, El Shahed AI, Castaldo MP, et al. Impaired right ventricular performance is associated with adverse outcome following hypoxic ischemic encephalopathy. *Am J Respir Crit Care Med* 2019;200(10):1294.
7. Cheung YF, Wong KY, Lam BC, et al. Relation of arterial stiffness with gestational age and birth weight. *Arch Dis Child* 2004;89:217.
8. Reed KL, Sahn DJ, Seagnelli S, et al. Doppler echocardiographic studies of diastolic function in the human fetal heart: changes during gestation. *J Am Coll Cardiol* 1986;8:391.
9. Hooper SB, Polglase GR, te Pas AB. A physiological approach to the timing of umbilical cord clamping at birth. *Arch Dis Child Fetal Neonatal Ed* 2015;100:F355.
10. van Vonderen JJ, Roest AA, Siew ML, et al. Measuring physiological changes during the transition to life after birth. *Neonatology* 2014;105:230.

11. Yigit B, Tutsak E, Yıldırım C, et al. Transitional fetal hemodynamics and gas exchange in premature postpartum adaptation: immediate vs. delayed cord clamping. *Matern Health Neonatol Perinatol* 2019;5:5.

12. Smit M, Dawson JA, Ganzeboom A, et al. Pulse oximetry in newborns with delayed cord clamping and immediate skin-to-skin contact. *Arch Dis Child Fetal Neonatal Ed* 2014;99:F309.

13. Sommers R, Stonestreet BS, Oh W, et al. Hemodynamic effects of delayed cord clamping in premature infants. *Pediatrics* 2012;129:e667.

14. Usher R, Shephard M, Lind J. The blood volume of the newborn infant and placental transfusion. *Acta Paediatr* 1963;52:497.

15. Fogarty M, Osborn DA, Askie L, et al. Delayed vs early umbilical cord clamping for preterm infants: a systematic review and meta-analysis. *Am J Obstet Gynecol* 2018;218:1.

16. Noori S, Seri I. Pathophysiology of newborn hypotension outside the transitional period. *Early Hum Dev* 2005;81:399.

17. Mildenhall LF, Battin MR, Morton SM, et al. Exposure to repeat doses of antenatal glucocorticoids is associated with altered cardiovascular status after birth. *Arch Dis Child Fetal Neonatal Ed* 2006;91:F56.

18. de Vries WB, van der Leij FR, Bakker JM, et al. Alterations in adult rat heart after neonatal dexamethasone therapy. *Pediatr Res* 2002;52:900.

19. Lewandowski AJ, Lamata P, Francis JM, et al. Breast milk consumption in preterm neonates and cardiac shape in adulthood. *Pediatrics* 2016;138;e20160050.

20. Puglisi JL, Negroni JA, Chen-Izu Y, et al. The force-frequency relationship: insights from mathematical modeling. *Adv Physiol Educ* 2013;37:28.

21. Wiegerinck RF, Cojoc A, Zeidenweber CM, et al. Force frequency relationship of the human ventricle increases during early postnatal development. *Pediatr Res* 2009;65:414.

22. Anderson PA. The heart and development. *Semin Perinatol* 1996;20:482.

23. Reller MD, Morton MJ, Reid DL, et al. Fetal lamb ventricles respond differently to filling and arterial pressures and to in utero ventilation. *Pediatr Res* 1987;22:621.

24. Pinson CW, Morton MJ, Thornburg KL. An anatomic basis for fetal right ventricular dominance and arterial pressure sensitivity. *J Dev Physiol* 1987;9:253.

25. Titheradge MA. Nitric oxide in septic shock. *Biochim Biophys Acta* 1999;1411:437.

26. Kirkpatrick SE, Pitlick PT, Naliboff J, et al. Frank-Starling relationship as an important determinant of fetal cardiac output. *Am J Physiol* 1976;231:495.

27. Kharrat A, Rios DI, Weisz DE, et al. The relationship between blood pressure parameters and left ventricular output in neonates. *J Perinatol* 2019;39(5):619.

28. Kluckow M, Evans N. Relationship between blood pressure and cardiac output in preterm infants requiring mechanical ventilation. *J Pediatr* 1996;129:506.

29. Gale C. Question 2: is capillary refill time a useful marker of haemodynamic status in neonates? *Arch Dis Child* 2010;95:395.

30. de Boode WP. Clinical monitoring of systemic hemodynamics in critically ill newborns. *Early Hum Dev* 2010;86:137.

31. Miletin J, Pichova K, Dempsey EM. Bedside detection of low systemic flow in the very low birth weight infant on day 1 of life. *Eur J Pediatr* 2009;168:809.

32. Jacobs SE, Morley CJ, Inder TE, et al. Whole-body hypothermia for term and near-term newborns with hypoxic-ischemic encephalopathy: a randomized controlled trial. *Arch Pediatr Adolesc Med* 2011;165:692.

33. Mertens L, Seri I, Marek J, et al.; Writing Group of the American Society of Echocardiography, European Association of Echocardiography, Association for European Pediatric Cardiologists. Targeted neonatal echocardiography in the Neonatal Intensive Care Unit: practice guidelines and recommendations for training. Writing Group of the American Society of Echocardiography (ASE) in collaboration with the European Association of Echocardiography (EAE) and the Association for European Pediatric Cardiologists (AEPC). *J Am Soc Echocardiogr* 2011;24:1057.

34. Singh Y, Gupta S, Groves AM, et al. Expert consensus statement 'Neonatologist-performed Echocardiography (NoPE)'-training and accreditation in UK. *Eur J Pediatr* 2016;175:281.

35. de Boode WP, Singh Y, Gupta S, et al. Recommendations for neonatologist performed echocardiography in Europe: consensus statement endorsed by European Society for Paediatric Research (ESPR) and European Society for Neonatology (ESN). *Pediatr Res* 2016;80:465.

36. Singh Y, Roehr CC, Tissot C, et al.; European Special Interest Group "Neonatologist Performed Echocardiography". Education, training, and accreditation of neonatologist performed echocardiography in Europe-framework for practice. *Pediatr Res* 2018;84:13.

37. Hebert A, Lavoie PM, Giesinger RE, et al. Evolution of training guidelines for echocardiography performed by the neonatologist: toward hemodynamic consultation. *J Am Soc Echocardiogr* 2019;32:785.

38. Evans N, Kluckow M. Neonatology concerns about the TNE consensus statement. *J Am Soc Echocardiogr* 2012;25:242; author reply 242.

39. El-Khuffash A, Herbozo C, Jain A, et al. Targeted neonatal echocardiography (TnECHO) service in a Canadian neonatal intensive care unit: a 4-year experience. *J Perinatol* 2013;33:687.

40. Papadhima I, Louis D, Purna J, et al. Targeted neonatal echocardiography (TNE) consult service in a large tertiary perinatal center in Canada. *J Perinatol* 2018;38(8):1039.

41. Harabor A, Soraisham AS. Utility of targeted neonatal echocardiography in the management of neonatal illness. *J Ultrasound Med* 2015;34:1259.

42. Giesinger RE, Moore C, Louis D, et al. The impact of Targeted Neonatal Echocardiography on practice in the neonatal intensive care unit: a multicentre prospective observational study. *Annual Meeting of the Pediatric Academic Society*, 2016; Baltimore, USA.

43. Jain A, Sahni M, El-Khuffash A, et al. Use of targeted neonatal echocardiography to prevent postoperative cardiorespiratory instability after patent ductus arteriosus ligation. *J Pediatr* 2012;160:584.

44. Teixeira LS, McNamara PJ. Enhanced intensive care for the neonatal ductus arteriosus. *Acta Paediatr* 2006;95:394.

45. Resende MH, More K, Nicholls D, et al. The impact of a dedicated patent ductus arteriosus ligation team on neonatal health-care outcomes. *J Perinatol* 2016;36:463.

46. El-Khuffash AF, James AT, Corcoran JD, et al. A patent ductus severity score predicts chronic lung disease or death before discharge. *J Pediatr* 2015;167(6):1354.

47. Kluckow M, Evans N. Early echocardiographic prediction of symptomatic patent ductus arteriosus in preterm infants undergoing mechanical ventilation. *J Pediatr* 1995;127:774.

48. Osborn D, Evans N, Kluckow M. Randomized trial of dobutamine versus dopamine in preterm infants with low systemic blood flow. *J Pediatr* 2002;140:183.

49. Osborn DA, Evans N, Kluckow M. Clinical detection of low upper body blood flow in very premature infants using blood pressure, capillary refill time, and central-peripheral temperature difference. *Arch Dis Child Fetal Neonatal Ed* 2004;89:F168.

50. Kluckow M, Evans N. Low superior vena cava flow and intraventricular haemorrhage in preterm infants. *Arch Dis Child Fetal Neonatal Ed* 2000;82:F188.

51. Noori S, McCoy M, Anderson MP, et al. Changes in cardiac function and cerebral blood flow in relation to peri/intraventricular hemorrhage in extremely preterm infants. *J Pediatr* 2014;164:264.

52. Taylor K, La Rotta G, McCrindle BW, et al. A comparison of cardiac output by thoracic impedance and direct fick in children with congenital heart disease undergoing diagnostic cardiac catheterization. *J Cardiothorac Vasc Anesth* 2011;25:776.

53. Taylor K, Manlhiot C, McCrindle B, et al. Poor accuracy of noninvasive cardiac output monitoring using bioimpedance cardiography [PhysioFlow(R)] compared to magnetic resonance imaging in pediatric patients. *Anesth Analg* 2012;114:771.

54. Tomaske M, Knirsch W, Kretschmar O, et al.; Working Group on Non-invasive Haemodynamic Monitoring in Paediatrics. Cardiac output measurement in children: comparison of Aesculon cardiac output monitor and thermodilution. *Br J Anaesth* 2008;100:517.

55. Tomaske M, Knirsch W, Kretschmar O, et al.; Working Group on Noninvasive Haemodynamic Monitoring in Paediatrics. Evaluation of the Aesculon cardiac output monitor by subxiphoidal Doppler flow measurement in children with congenital heart defects. *Eur J Anaesthesiol* 2009;26:412.

56. Noori S, Drabu B, Soleymani S, et al. Continuous non-invasive cardiac output measurements in the neonate by electrical velocimetry: a comparison with echocardiography. *Arch Dis Child Fetal Neonatal Ed* 2012;97:F340.

57. Grollmuss O, Gonzalez P. Non-invasive cardiac output measurement in low and very low birth weight infants: a method comparison. *Front Pediatr* 2014;2:16.

58. Heerdt PM, Wagner CL, DeMais M, et al. Noninvasive cardiac output monitoring with bioreactance as an alternative to invasive instrumentation for preclinical drug evaluation in beagles. *J Pharmacol Toxicol Methods* 2011;64:111.

59. Kupersztych-Hagege E, Teboul JL, Artigas A, et al. Bioreactance is not reliable for estimating cardiac output and the effects of passive leg raising in critically ill patients. *Br J Anaesth* 2013;111:961.

60. Weisz DE, Jain A, McNamara PJ, et al. Non-invasive cardiac output monitoring in neonates using bioreactance: a comparison with echocardiography. *Neonatology* 2012;102:61.

61. Weisz DE, Jain A, Ting J, et al. Non-invasive cardiac output monitoring in preterm infants undergoing patent ductus arteriosus ligation: a comparison with echocardiography. *Neonatology* 2014;106:330.

62. Pichler G, Binder C, Avian A, et al. Reference ranges for regional cerebral tissue oxygen saturation and fractional oxygen extraction in neonates during immediate transition after birth. *J Pediatr* 2013;163:1558.

63. Binder C, Urlesberger B, Avian A, et al. Cerebral and peripheral regional oxygen saturation during postnatal transition in preterm neonates. *J Pediatr* 2013;163:394.

64. Alderliesten T, Lemmers PM, Smarius JJ, et al. Cerebral oxygenation, extraction, and autoregulation in very preterm infants who develop peri-intraventricular hemorrhage. *J Pediatr* 2013;162:698.
65. Baik N, Urlesberger B, Schwaberger B, et al. Cerebral haemorrhage in preterm neonates: does cerebral regional oxygen saturation during the immediate transition matter? *Arch Dis Child Fetal Neonatal Ed* 2015;100:F422.
66. Hyttel-Sorensen S, Pellicer A, Alderliesten T, et al. Cerebral near infrared spectroscopy oximetry in extremely preterm infants: phase II randomised clinical trial. *BMJ* 2015;350:g7635.
67. Hansen ML, Pellicer A, Gluud C, et al. Detailed statistical analysis plan for the SafeBoosC III trial: a multinational randomised clinical trial assessing treatment guided by cerebral oxygenation monitoring versus treatment as usual in extremely preterm infants. *Trials* 2019;20:746.
68. Sellmer A, Bjerre JV, Schmidt MR, et al. Morbidity and mortality in preterm neonates with patent ductus arteriosus on day 3. *Arch Dis Child Fetal Neonatal Ed* 2013;98:F505.
69. Schmidt B, Davis P, Moddemann D, et al. Long-term effects of indomethacin prophylaxis in extremely-low-birth-weight infants. *N Engl J Med* 2001;344:1966.
70. Chorne N, Leonard C, Piecuch R, et al. Patent ductus arteriosus and its treatment as risk factors for neonatal and neurodevelopmental morbidity. *Pediatrics* 2007;119:1165.
71. Schmitz L, Stiller B, Koch H, et al. Diastolic left ventricular function in preterm infants with a patent ductus arteriosus: a serial Doppler echocardiography study. *Early Hum Dev* 2004;76:91.
72. Condo M, Evans N, Bellu R, et al. Echocardiographic assessment of ductal significance: retrospective comparison of two methods. *Arch Dis Child Fetal Neonatal Ed* 2012;97:F35.
73. de Freitas Martins F, Ibarra Rios D, Resende MHF, et al. Relationship of patent ductus arteriosus size to echocardiographic markers of shunt volume. *J Pediatr* 2018;202:50.
74. Hiraishi S, Horiguchi Y, Misawa H, et al. Noninvasive Doppler echocardiographic evaluation of shunt flow dynamics of the ductus arteriosus. *Circulation* 1987;75:1146.
75. El Hajjar M, Vaksmann G, Rakza T, et al. Severity of the ductal shunt: a comparison of different markers. *Arch Dis Child Fetal Neonatal Ed* 2005;90:F419.
76. Iyer P, Evans N. Re-evaluation of the left atrial to aortic root ratio as a marker of patent ductus arteriosus. *Arch Dis Child Fetal Neonatal Ed* 1994;70:F112.
77. Broadhouse KM, Price AN, Durighel G, et al. Assessment of PDA shunt and systemic blood flow in newborns using cardiac MRI. *NMR Biomed* 2013;26:1135.
78. El-Khuffash A, Higgins M, Walsh K, et al. Quantitative assessment of the degree of ductal steal using celiac artery blood flow to left ventricular output ratio in preterm infants. *Neonatology* 2008;93:206.
79. Martinovici D, Vanden Eijnden S, Unger P, et al. Early NT-proBNP is able to predict spontaneous closure of patent ductus arteriosus in preterm neonates, but not the need of its treatment. *Pediatr Cardiol* 2011;32:953.
80. Chen S, Tacy T, Clyman R. How useful is B-type natriuretic peptide measurements for monitoring changes in patent ductus arteriosus shunt magnitude? *J Perinatol* 2010;30:780.
81. Kulkarni M, Gokulakrishnan G, Price J, et al. Diagnosing significant PDA using natriuretic peptides in preterm neonates: a systematic review. *Pediatrics* 2015;135:e510.
82. El-Khuffash A, Weisz DE, McNamara PJ. Reflections of the changes in patent ductus arteriosus management during the last 10 years. *Arch Dis Child Fetal Neonatal Ed* 2016;101:F474.
83. Hammerman C, Strates E, Valaitis S. The silent ductus: its precursors and its aftermath. *Pediatr Cardiol* 1986;7:121.
84. Kaapa P, Lanning P, Koivisto M. Early closure of patent ductus arteriosus with indomethacin in preterm infants with idiopathic respiratory distress syndrome. *Acta Paediatr Scand* 1983;72:179.
85. Weesner KM, Dillard RG, Boyle RJ, et al. Prophylactic treatment of asymptomatic patent ductus arteriosus in premature infants with respiratory distress syndrome. *South Med J* 1987;80:706.
86. Kluckow M, Jeffery M, Gill A, et al. A randomised placebo-controlled trial of early treatment of the patent ductus arteriosus. *Arch Dis Child Fetal Neonatal Ed* 2014;99:F99.
87. Gersony WM, Peckham GJ, Ellison RC, et al. Effects of indomethacin in premature infants with patent ductus arteriosus: results of a national collaborative study. *J Pediatr* 1983;102:895.
88. Merritt TA, Harris JP, Roghmann K, et al. Early closure of the patent ductus arteriosus in very low-birth-weight infants: a controlled trial. *J Pediatr* 1981;99:281.
89. Sosenko IR, Fajardo MF, Claure N, et al. Timing of patent ductus arteriosus treatment and respiratory outcome in premature infants: a double-blind randomized controlled trial. *J Pediatr* 2012;160:929.
90. Van Overmeire B, Van de Broek H, Van Laer P, et al. Early versus late indomethacin treatment for patent ductus arteriosus in premature infants with respiratory distress syndrome. *J Pediatr* 2001;138:205.
91. Clyman RI, Liebowitz M, Kaempf J, et al.; PDA-TOLERATE (PDA: TO LEave it alone or Respond And Treat Early) Trial Investigators. PDA-TOLERATE trial: an exploratory randomized controlled trial of treatment of moderate-to-large patent ductus arteriosus at 1 week of age. *J Pediatr* 2019;205:41.
92. Fowlie PW, Davis PG, McGuire W. Prophylactic intravenous indomethacin for preventing mortality and morbidity in preterm infants. *Cochrane Database Syst Rev* 2010;7:CD000174.
93. Ohlsson A, Shah SS. Ibuprofen for the prevention of patent ductus arteriosus in preterm and/or low birth weight infants. *Cochrane Database Syst Rev* 2019;6:CD004213.
94. Ngo S, Profit J, Gould JB, et al. Trends in patent ductus arteriosus diagnosis and management for very low birth weight infants. *Pediatrics* 2017;139:e20162390.
95. Lokku A, Mirea L, Lee SK, et al.; Canadian Neonatal Network. Trends and outcomes of patent ductus arteriosus treatment in very preterm infants in Canada. *Am J Perinatol* 2017;34:441.
96. Sung SI, Chang YS, Chun JY, et al. Mandatory closure versus nonintervention for patent ductus arteriosus in very preterm infants. *J Pediatr* 2016;177:66.
97. Wickremasinghe AC, Rogers EE, Piecuch RE, et al. Neurodevelopmental outcomes following two different treatment approaches (early ligation and selective ligation) for patent ductus arteriosus. *J Pediatr* 2012;161:1065.
98. Bixler GM, Powers GC, Clark RH, et al. Changes in the diagnosis and management of patent ductus arteriosus from 2006 to 2015 in United States Neonatal Intensive Care Units. *J Pediatr* 2017;189:105.
99. Hagadorn JI, Bennett MV, Brownell EA, et al. Covariation of neonatal intensive care unit-level patent ductus arteriosus management and in-neonatal intensive care unit outcomes following preterm birth. *J Pediatr* 2018;203:225.
100. Zonnenberg I, de Waal K. The definition of a haemodynamic significant duct in randomized controlled trials: a systematic literature review. *Acta Paediatr* 2012;101:247.
101. Hudson I, Houston A, Aitchison T, et al. Reproducibility of measurements of cardiac output in newborn infants by Doppler ultrasound. *Arch Dis Child* 1990;65:15.
102. Schwarz CE, Preusche A, Baden W, et al. Repeatability of echocardiographic parameters to evaluate the hemodynamic relevance of patent ductus arteriosus in preterm infants: a prospective observational study. *BMC Pediatr* 2016;16:18.
103. Skelton R, Evans N, Smythe J. A blinded comparison of clinical and echocardiographic evaluation of the preterm infant for patent ductus arteriosus. *J Paediatr Child Health* 1994;30:406.
104. Erdeve O, Yurttutan S, Altug N, et al. Oral versus intravenous ibuprofen for patent ductus arteriosus closure: a randomised controlled trial in extremely low birthweight infants. *Arch Dis Child Fetal Neonatal Ed* 2012;97:F279.
105. Aranda JV, Clyman R, Cox B, et al. A randomized, double-blind, placebo-controlled trial on intravenous ibuprofen L-lysine for the early closure of nonsymptomatic patent ductus arteriosus within 72 hours of birth in extremely-low-birth-weight infants. *Am J Perinatol* 2009;26:235.
106. Groves AM, Kuschel CA, Knight DB, et al. Echocardiographic assessment of blood flow volume in the superior vena cava and descending aorta in the newborn infant. *Arch Dis Child Fetal Neonatal Ed* 2008;93:F24.
107. Krishnappa S, Shah PS, Jain A, et al. Predictors of early extubation after patent ductus arteriosus ligation among infants born extremely preterm dependent on mechanical ventilation. *J Pediatr* 2019;214:222.
108. El-Khuffash AF, Slevin M, McNamara PJ, et al. Troponin T, N-terminal pro natriuretic peptide and a patent ductus arteriosus scoring system predict death before discharge or neurodevelopmental outcome at 2 years in preterm infants. *Arch Dis Child Fetal Neonatal Ed* 2011;96:F133.
109. Fajardo MF, Claure N, Swaminathan S, et al. Effect of positive end-expiratory pressure on ductal shunting and systemic blood flow in preterm infants with patent ductus arteriosus. *Neonatology* 2014;105:9.
110. Toyoshima K, Momma K, Nakanishi T. In vivo dilatation of the ductus arteriosus induced by furosemide in the rat. *Pediatr Res* 2010;67:173.
111. Lee BS, Byun SY, Chung ML, et al. Effect of furosemide on ductal closure and renal function in indomethacin-treated preterm infants during the early neonatal period. *Neonatology* 2010;98:191.
112. Saugstad OD, Aune D. Optimal oxygenation of extremely low birth weight infants: a meta-analysis and systematic review of the oxygen saturation target studies. *Neonatology* 2014;105:55.
113. Bell EF, Strauss RG, Widness JA, et al. Randomized trial of liberal versus restrictive guidelines for red blood cell transfusion in preterm infants. *Pediatrics* 2005;115:1685.
114. De Buyst J, Rakza T, Pennaforte T, et al. Hemodynamic effects of fluid restriction in preterm infants with significant patent ductus arteriosus. *J Pediatr* 2012;161:404.
115. Ment LR, Vohr BR, Makuch RW, et al. Prevention of intraventricular hemorrhage by indomethacin in male preterm infants. *J Pediatr* 2004;145:832.

116. Liebowitz M, Katheria A, Sauberan J, et al.; PDA-TOLERATE (PDA: TOLEave it alone or Respond And Treat Early) Trial Investigators. Lack of equipoise in the PDA-TOLERATE trial: a comparison of eligible infants enrolled in the trial and those treated outside the trial. *J Pediatr* 2019;213:222.

117. Ohlsson A, Walia R, Shah SS. Ibuprofen for the treatment of patent ductus arteriosus in preterm and/or low birth weight infants. *Cochrane Database Syst Rev* 2013;4:CD003481.

118. Herrera CM, Holberton JR, Davis PG. Prolonged versus short course of indomethacin for the treatment of patent ductus arteriosus in preterm infants. *Cochrane Database Syst Rev* 2007;2:CD003480.

119. Ohlsson A, Shah PS. Paracetamol (acetaminophen) for patent ductus arteriosus in preterm or low birth weight infants. *Cochrane Database Syst Rev* 2018;4:CD010061.

120. Harkin P, Harma A, Aikio O, et al. Paracetamol accelerates closure of the ductus arteriosus after premature birth: a randomized trial. *J Pediatr* 2016;177:72.

121. Kluckow M, Carlisle H, Broom M, et al. A pilot randomised blinded placebo-controlled trial of paracetamol for later treatment of a patent ductus arteriosus. *J Perinatol* 2019;39:102.

122. Madan JC, Kendrick D, Hagadorn JI, et al. Patent ductus arteriosus therapy: Impact on neonatal and 18-month outcome. *Pediatrics* 2009;123:674.

123. Weisz DE, Mirea L, Rosenberg E, et al. Association of patent ductus arteriosus ligation with death or neurodevelopmental impairment among extremely preterm infants. *JAMA Pediatr* 2017;171:443.

124. Chock VY, Goel VV, Palma JP, et al. Changing management of the patent ductus arteriosus: effect on neonatal outcomes and resource utilization. *Am J Perinatol* 2017;34:990.

125. Weisz DE, Mirea L, Resende MHF, et al. Outcomes of surgical ligation after unsuccessful pharmacotherapy for patent ductus arteriosus in neonates born extremely preterm. *J Pediatr* 2018;195:292.

126. Janvier A, Martinez JL, Barrington K, et al. Anesthetic technique and postoperative outcome in preterm infants undergoing PDA closure. *J Perinatol* 2010;30:677.

127. Anand KJ, Sippell WG, Aynsley-Green A. Randomised trial of fentanyl anaesthesia in preterm babies undergoing surgery: effects on the stress response. *Lancet* 1987;1:243.

128. Naguib AN, Tobias JD, Hall MW, et al. The role of different anesthetic techniques in altering the stress response during cardiac surgery in children: a prospective, double-blinded, and randomized study. *Pediatr Crit Care Med* 2013;14:481.

129. Ulrich TJB, Hansen TP, Reid KJ, et al. Post-ligation cardiac syndrome is associated with increased morbidity in preterm infants. *J Perinatol* 2018;38(5):537.

130. Bravo MC, Ybarra M, Madero R, et al. Childhood neurodevelopmental outcome in low birth weight infants with post-ligation cardiac syndrome after ductus arteriosus closure. *Front Physiol* 2019;10:718.

131. Lam JY, Lopushinsky SR, Ma IWY, et al. Treatment options for pediatric patent ductus arteriosus: systematic review and meta-analysis. *Chest* 2015;148:784.

132. Zanardo V, Vedovato S, Chiozza L, et al. Pharmacological closure of patent ductus arteriosus: effects on pulse pressure and on endothelin-1 and vasopressin excretion. *Am J Perinatol* 2008;25:353.

133. Zahn EM, Peck D, Phillips A, et al. Transcatheter closure of patent ductus arteriosus in extremely premature newborns: early results and midterm follow-up. *JACC Cardiovasc Interv* 2016;9:2429.

134. Morville P, Akhavi A. Transcatheter closure of hemodynamic significant patent ductus arteriosus in 32 premature infants by amplatzer ductal occluder additional size-ADOIIAS. *Catheter Cardiovasc Interv* 2017;90:612.

135. Sathanandam S, Justino H, Waller BR III, et al. Initial clinical experience with the Medtronic Micro Vascular Plug in transcatheter occlusion of PDAs in extremely premature infants. *Catheter Cardiovasc Interv* 2017;89:1051.

136. Nealon E, Rivera BK, Cua CL, et al. Follow-up after percutaneous patent ductus arteriosus occlusion in lower weight infants. *J Pediatr* 2019;212:144.

137. Rodríguez Ogando A, Planelles Asensio I, de la Blanca ARS, et al. Surgical ligation versus percutaneous closure of patent ductus arteriosus in very low-weight preterm infants: which are the real benefits of the percutaneous approach? *Pediatr Cardiol* 2018;39:398.

138. Sathanandam S, Balduf K, Chilakala S, et al. Role of transcatheter patent ductus arteriosus closure in extremely low birth weight infants. *Catheter Cardiovasc Interv* 2019;93:89.

139. Walsh-Sukys MC, Tyson JE, Wright LL, et al. Persistent pulmonary hypertension of the newborn in the era before nitric oxide: practice variation and outcomes. *Pediatrics* 2000;105:14.

140. Lipkin PH, Davidson D, Spivak L, et al. Neurodevelopmental and medical outcomes of persistent pulmonary hypertension in term newborns treated with nitric oxide. *J Pediatr* 2002;140:306.

141. Hosono S, Ohno T, Kimoto H, et al. Developmental outcomes in persistent pulmonary hypertension treated with nitric oxide therapy. *Pediatr Int* 2009;51:79.

142. Jain A, McNamara PJ. Persistent pulmonary hypertension of the newborn: physiology, hemodynamic assessment and novel therapies. *Curr Pediatr Rev* 2013;9:55.

143. Members ATF, Galiè N, Hoeper MM, Humbert M, et al. Guidelines for the diagnosis and treatment of pulmonary hypertension: the task force for the diagnosis and treatment of pulmonary hypertension of the European Society of Cardiology (ESC) and the European Respiratory Society (ERS), endorsed by the International Society of Heart and Lung Transplantation (ISHLT). *Eur Heart J* 2009;30:2493.

144. Brown KL, Miles F, Sullivan ID, et al. Outcome in neonates with congenital heart disease referred for respiratory extracorporeal membrane oxygenation. *Acta Paediatr* 2005;94:1280.

145. DiBlasi RM, Myers TR, Hess DR. Evidence-based clinical practice guideline: inhaled nitric oxide for neonates with acute hypoxic respiratory failure. *Respir Care* 2010;55:1717.

146. Finer NN, Barrington KJ. Nitric oxide for respiratory failure in infants born at or near term. *Cochrane Database Syst Rev* 2006;4:CD000399.

147. Tworetzky W, Bristow J, Moore P, et al. Inhaled nitric oxide in neonates with persistent pulmonary hypertension. *Lancet* 2001;357:118.

148. Salguero KL, Cummings JJ. Inhaled nitric oxide and methemoglobin in full-term infants with persistent pulmonary hypertension of the newborn. *Pulmon Pharmacol Ther* 2002;15:1.

149. Ahmed MS, Giesinger RE, Ibrahim M, et al. Clinical and echocardiography predictors of response to inhaled nitric oxide in hypoxic preterm neonates. *J Paediatr Child Health* 2019;55:753.

150. Baczynski M, Ginty S, Weisz D, et al. *Short and long term clinical outcomes of preterm neonates with refractory hypoxic respiratory failure following rescue treatment trial with inhaled nitric oxide.* Geneva, Switzerland: European Academy of Paediatric Societies, 2016:EAPS-1073.

151. Gao Y, Raj JU. Regulation of the pulmonary circulation in the fetus and newborn. *Physiol Rev* 2010;90:1291.

152. Steinhorn RH, Kinsella JP, Pierce C, et al. Intravenous sildenafil in the treatment of neonates with persistent pulmonary hypertension. *J Pediatr* 2009;155:841.

153. Mohamed WA, Ismail M. A randomized, double-blind, placebo-controlled, prospective study of bosentan for the treatment of persistent pulmonary hypertension of the newborn. *J Perinatol* 2012;32:608.

154. McNamara PJ, Shivananda SP, Sahni M, et al. Pharmacology of milrinone in neonates with persistent pulmonary hypertension of the newborn and suboptimal response to inhaled nitric oxide. *Pediatr Crit Care Med* 2013;14:74.

155. Slaughter JL, Pakrashi T, Jones DE, et al. Echocardiographic detection of pulmonary hypertension in extremely low birth weight infants with bronchopulmonary dysplasia requiring prolonged positive pressure ventilation. *J Perinatol* 2011;31:635.

156. del Cerro MJ, Sabate Rotes A, Carton A, et al. Pulmonary hypertension in bronchopulmonary dysplasia: clinical findings, cardiovascular anomalies and outcomes. *Pediatr Pulmonol* 2014;49:49.

157. Khemani E, McElhinney DB, Rhein L, et al. Pulmonary artery hypertension in formerly premature infants with bronchopulmonary dysplasia: clinical features and outcomes in the surfactant era. *Pediatrics* 2007;120:1260.

158. Northern Neonatal Nursing Initiative. Systolic blood pressure in babies of less than 32 weeks gestation in the first year of life. *Arch Dis Child Fetal Neonatal Ed* 1990;80:38.

159. British Association of Perinatal Medicine. Development of audit measures and guidelines for good practice in the management of neonatal respiratory distress syndrome. Report of a Joint Working Group of the British Association of Perinatal Medicine and the Research Unit of the Royal College of Physicians. *Arch Dis Child* 1992;67(10 Spec No):1221. PMID 1444567.

160. Miall-Allen VM, de Vries LS, Whitelaw GL. Mean arterial blood pressure and neonatal cerebral lesions. *Arch Dis Child* 1987;62:1068.

161. Paradisis M, Evans N, Kluckow M, et al. Pilot study of milrinone for low systemic blood flow in very preterm infants. *J Pediatr* 2006;148:306.

162. Dempsey EM, Barrington KJ. Treating hypotension in the preterm infant: when and with what: a critical and systematic review. *J Perinatol* 2007;27:469.

163. Dempsey EM, Al Hazzani F, Barrington KJ. Permissive hypotension in the extremely low birthweight infant with signs of good perfusion. *Arch Dis Child Fetal Neonatal Ed* 2009;94:F241.

164. Munro MJ, Walker AM, Barfield CP. Hypotensive extremely low birth weight infants have reduced cerebral blood flow. *Pediatrics* 2004;114:1591.

165. Werther T, Aichhorn L, Baumgartner S, et al. Discrepancy between invasive and non-invasive blood pressure readings in extremely preterm infants in the first four weeks of life. *PLoS One* 2018;13:e0209831.

166. Pichler G, Urlesberger B, Reiterer F, et al. Non-invasive oscillometric blood pressure measurement in very-low-birthweight infants: a comparison of two different monitor systems. *Acta Paediatr* 1999;88:1044.

167. Meyer S, Sander J, Gräber S, et al. Agreement of invasive versus non-invasive blood pressure in preterm neonates is not dependent on birth weight or gestational age. *J Paediatr Child Health* 2010;46:249.

168. König K, Casalaz DM, Burke EJ, et al. Accuracy of non-invasive blood pressure monitoring in very preterm infants. *Intensive Care Med* 2012;38:670.

169. Marcelino PA, Marum SM, Fernandes AP, et al. Routine transthoracic echocardiography in a general Intensive Care Unit: an 18 month survey in 704 patients. *Eur J Intern Med* 2009;20:e37.

170. Browning Carmo K, Lutz T, Berry A, et al. Feasibility and utility of portable ultrasound during retrieval of sick term and late preterm infants. *Acta Paediatr* 2016;105:e549.

171. So KW, Fok TF, Ng PC, et al. Randomised controlled trial of colloid or crystalloid in hypotensive preterm infants. *Arch Dis Child* 1997;76:F43.

172. Valverde A, Gianotti G, Rioja-Garcia E, et al. Effects of high-volume, rapid-fluid therapy on cardiovascular function and hematological values during isoflurane-induced hypotension in healthy dogs. *Can J Vet Res* 2012;76:99.

173. Bell EF, Acarregui MJ. Restricted versus liberal water intake for preventing morbidity and mortality in preterm infants. *Cochrane Database Syst Rev* 2001;3:CD000503.

174. Kooi EM, van der Laan ME, Verhagen EA, et al. Volume expansion does not alter cerebral tissue oxygen extraction in preterm infants with clinical signs of poor perfusion. *Neonatology* 2013;103:308.

175. Barrington KJ. Hypotension and shock in the preterm infant. *Semin Fetal Neonatal Med* 2008;13:16.

176. Mahony L. Maturation of calcium transport in cardiac sarcoplasmic reticulum. *Pediatr Res* 1988;24:639.

177. Smolich JJ. Ultrastructural and functional features of the developing mammalian heart: a brief overview. *Reprod Fertil Dev* 1995;7:451.

178. Mahony L, Jones LR. Developmental changes in cardiac sarcoplasmic reticulum in sheep. *J Biol Chem* 1986;261:15257.

179. McMillen IC, Mulvogue HM, Coulter CL, et al. Ontogeny of catecholamine-synthesizing enzymes and enkephalins in the sheep adrenal medulla: an immunocytochemical study. *J Endocrinol* 1988;118:221.

180. Verhofstad AA, Hokfelt T, Goldstein M, et al. Appearance of tyrosine hydroxylase, aromatic amino-acid decarboxylase, dopamine beta-hydroxylase and phenylethanolamine *N*-methyltransferase during the ontogenesis of the adrenal medulla: an immunohistochemical study in the rat. *Cell Tissue Res* 1979;200:1.

181. Wilburn LA, Goldsmith PC, Chang KJ, et al. Ontogeny of enkephalin and catecholamine-synthesizing enzymes in the primate fetal adrenal medulla. *J Clin Endocrinol Metab* 1986;63:974.

182. Zhang J, Penny DJ, Kim NS, et al. Mechanisms of blood pressure increase induced by dopamine in hypotensive preterm neonates. *Arch Dis Child Fetal Neonatal Ed* 1999;81:F99.

183. Subhedar NV, Shaw NJ. Dopamine versus dobutamine for hypotensive preterm infants. *Cochrane Database Syst Rev* 2003;3:CD001242.

184. Noori S, Seri I. Neonatal blood pressure support: the use of inotropes, lusitropes, and other vasopressor agents. *Clin Perinatol* 2012;39:221.

185. Seri I. Management of hypotension and low systemic blood flow in the very low birth weight neonate during the first postnatal week. *J Perinatol* 2006; 26(suppl 1):S8; discussion S22.

186. Al-Salam Z, Johnson S, Abozaid S, et al. The hemodynamic effects of dobutamine during reoxygenation after hypoxia: a dose-response study in newborn pigs. *Shock* 2007;28:317.

187. Hinds JE, Hawthorne EW. Comparative cardiac dynamic effects of dobutamine and isoproterenol in conscious instrumented dogs. *Am J Cardiol* 1975;36:894.

188. Cheung PY, Barrington KJ, Bigam D. The hemodynamic effects of dobutamine infusion in the chronically instrumented newborn piglet. *Crit Care Med* 1999;27:558.

189. Smolich JJ, Sano T, Penny DJ. Blunting of pulmonary but not systemic vasodilator responses to dobutamine in newborn lambs. *Pediatr Res* 2000;47:107.

190. Schranz D, Stopfkuchen H, Jungst BK, et al. Hemodynamic effects of dobutamine in children with cardiovascular failure. *Eur J Pediatr* 1982;139:4.

191. Martinez AM, Padbury JF, Thio S. Dobutamine pharmacokinetics and cardiovascular responses in critically ill neonates. *Pediatrics* 1992;89:47.

192. Robel-Tillig E, Knupfer M, Pulzer F, et al. Cardiovascular impact of dobutamine in neonates with myocardial dysfunction. *Early Hum Dev* 2007;83:307.

193. Stopfkuchen H, Queisser-Luft A, Vogel K. Cardiovascular responses to dobutamine determined by systolic time intervals in preterm infants. *Crit Care Med* 1990;18:722.

194. Stopfkuchen H, Schranz D, Huth R, et al. Effects of dobutamine on left ventricular performance in newborns as determined by systolic time intervals. *Eur J Pediatr* 1987;146:135.

195. Greenough A, Emery EF. Randomized trial comparing dopamine and dobutamine in preterm infants. *Eur J Pediatr* 1993;152:925.

196. Roze JC, Tohier C, Maingueneau C, et al. Response to dobutamine and dopamine in the hypotensive very preterm infant. *Arch Dis Child* 1993;69:59.

197. Klarr JM, Faix RG, Pryce CJ, et al. Randomized, blind trial of dopamine versus dobutamine for treatment of hypotension in preterm infants with respiratory distress syndrome. *J Pediatr* 1994;125:117.

198. Ruelas-Orozco G, Vargas-Origel A. Assessment of therapy for arterial hypotension in critically ill preterm infants. *Am J Perinatol* 2000;17:95.

199. Barrington K, Chan W. The circulatory effects of epinephrine infusion in the anesthetized piglet. *Pediatr Res* 1993;33:190.

200. Valverde E, Pellicer A, Madero R, et al. Dopamine versus epinephrine for cardiovascular support in low birth weight infants: analysis of systemic effects and neonatal clinical outcomes. *Pediatrics* 2006;117:e1213.

201. Jain A, McNamara PJ. Persistent pulmonary hypertension of the newborn: advances in diagnosis and treatment. *Semin Fetal Neonatal Med* 2015;20:262.

202. Cheung PY, Barrington KJ. The effects of dopamine and epinephrine on hemodynamics and oxygen metabolism in hypoxic anesthetized piglets. *Crit Care* 2001;5:158.

203. Pellicer A, Valverde E, Elorza MD, et al. Cardiovascular support for low birth weight infants and cerebral hemodynamics: a randomized, blinded, clinical trial. *Pediatrics* 2005;115:1501.

204. Tourneux P, Rakza T, Abazine A, et al. Noradrenaline for management of septic shock refractory to fluid loading and dopamine or dobutamine in full-term newborn infants. *Acta Paediatr* 2008;97:177.

205. Tourneux P, Rakza T, Bouissou A, et al. Pulmonary circulatory effects of norepinephrine in newborn infants with persistent pulmonary hypertension. *J Pediatr* 2008;153:345.

206. Lakshminrusimha S, Russell JA, Wedgwood S, et al. Superoxide dismutase improves oxygenation and reduces oxidation in neonatal pulmonary hypertension. *Am J Respir Crit Care Med* 2006;174:1370.

207. Garcia-Villalon AL, Garcia JL, Fernandez N, et al. Regional differences in the arterial response to vasopressin: role of endothelial nitric oxide. *Br J Pharmacol* 1996;118:1848.

208. Sai Y, Okamura T, Amakata Y, et al. Comparison of responses of canine pulmonary artery and vein to angiotensin II, bradykinin and vasopressin. *Eur J Pharmacol* 1995;282:235.

209. Meyer S, Gottschling S, Baghai A, et al. Arginine-vasopressin in catecholamine-refractory septic versus non-septic shock in extremely low birth weight infants with acute renal injury. *Crit Care* 2006;10:R71.

210. Meyer S, Loffler G, Polcher T, et al. Vasopressin in catecholamine-resistant septic and cardiogenic shock in very-low-birthweight infants. *Acta Paediatr* 2006;95:1309.

211. Bidegain M, Greenberg R, Simmons C, et al. Vasopressin for refractory hypotension in extremely low birth weight infants. *J Pediatr* 2010;157:502.

212. Mohamed A, Louis D, Surak A, et al. *Outcomes of preterm neonates treated with vasopressin for refractory pulmonary hypertension: case series.* Baltimore, MD: Pediatric Academic Society, 2016.

213. Mohamed A, Nasef N, Shah V, et al. Vasopressin as a rescue therapy for refractory pulmonary hypertension in neonates: case series. *Pediatr Crit Care Med* 2014;15:148.

214. Shivananda S, Ahliwahlia L, Kluckow M, et al. Variation in the management of persistent pulmonary hypertension of the newborn: a survey of physicians in Canada, Australia, and New Zealand. *Am J Perinatol* 2012;29:519.

215. Mizobuchi M, Yoshimoto S, Nakao H. Time-course effect of a single dose of hydrocortisone for refractory hypotension in preterm infants. *Pediatr Int* 2011;53:881.

216. Hausdorff WP, Caron MG, Lefkowitz RJ. Turning off the signal—desensitization of beta-adrenergic receptor function. *FASEB J* 1990;4:2881.

217. Higgins S, Friedlich P, Seri I. Hydrocortisone for hypotension and vasopressor dependence in preterm neonates: a meta-analysis. *J Perinatol* 2010;30:373.

218. Baud O, Maury L, Lebail F, et al. Effect of early low-dose hydrocortisone on survival without bronchopulmonary dysplasia in extremely preterm infants (PREMILOC): a double-blind, placebo-controlled, multicentre, randomised trial. *Lancet* 2016;387:1827.

219. Shaffer ML, Baud O, Lacaze-Masmonteil T, et al. Effect of prophylaxis for early adrenal insufficiency using low-dose hydrocortisone in very preterm infants: an individual patient data meta-analysis. *J Pediatr* 2019;207:136.

220. Watterberg K, Gerdes JS, Cole CH, et al. Prophylaxis of early adrenal insufficiency to prevent bronchopulmonary dysplasia. *Pediatrics* 2004;114:1649.

221. Baud O, Trousson C, Biran V, et al. Association between early low-dose hydrocortisone therapy in extremely preterm neonates and neurodevelopmental outcomes at 2 years of age. *JAMA* 2017;317:1329.

222. Ofman G, Perez M, Farrow KN. Early low-dose hydrocortisone: is the neurodevelopment affected? *J Perinatol* 2018;38:636.

THE NEWBORN INFANT

223. Renault A, Patkaï J, Dassieu G, et al. Hydrocortisone use in ventilated extremely preterm infants decreased bronchopulmonary dysplasia with no effects on neurodevelopment after two years. *Acta Paediatr* 2016;105:1047.

224. Bischoff AR, McNamara PJ, Giesinger RE. Milrinone use during therapeutic hypothermia is associated with adverse outcome among neonates with comorbid pulmonary hypertension and asphyxia. *Pediatric Academic Society Meeting*, 2018.

225. Lakshminrusimha S, Wiseman D, Black SM, et al. The role of nitric oxide synthase-derived reactive oxygen species in the altered relaxation of pulmonary arteries from lambs with increased pulmonary blood flow. *Am J Physiol Heart Circ Physiol* 2007;293:H1491.

226. Lopez SL, Leighton JO, Walther FJ. Supranormal cardiac output in the dopamine- and dobutamine-dependent preterm infant. *Pediatr Cardiol* 1997;18:292.

227. Dhainaut JF, Devaux JY, Monsallier JF, et al. Mechanisms of decreased left ventricular preload during continuous positive pressure ventilation in ARDS. *Chest* 1986;90:74.

228. Kinsella JP, Gerstmann DR, Clark RH, et al. High-frequency oscillatory ventilation versus intermittent mandatory ventilation: early hemodynamic effects in the premature baboon with hyaline membrane disease. *Pediatr Res* 1991;29:160.

229. Simma B, Fritz M, Fink C, et al. Conventional ventilation versus high-frequency oscillation: hemodynamic effects in newborn babies. *Crit Care Med* 2000;28:227.

230. Calvin JE, Driedger AA, Sibbald WJ. Positive end-expiratory pressure (PEEP) does not depress left ventricular function in patients with pulmonary edema. *Am Rev Respir Dis* 1981;124:121.

231. Peters J, Fraser C, Stuart RS, et al. Negative intrathoracic pressure decreases independently left ventricular filling and emptying. *Am J Physiol* 1989;257:H120.

232. Hakim TS, Michel RP, Chang HK. Effect of lung inflation on pulmonary vascular resistance by arterial and venous occlusion. *J Appl Physiol Respir Environ Exerc Physiol* 1982;53:1110.

233. Day RE, Insley J. Maternal diabetes mellitus and congenital malformation. Survey of 205 cases. *Arch Dis Child* 1976;51:935.

234. Narchi H, Kulaylat N. Heart disease in infants of diabetic mothers. *Images Paediatr Cardiol* 2000;2:17.

235. Seppanen MP, Ojanpera OS, Kaapa PO, et al. Delayed postnatal adaptation of pulmonary hemodynamics in infants of diabetic mothers. *J Pediatr* 1997;131:545.

236. Elmekkawi SF, Mansour GM, Elsafty MS, et al. Prediction of fetal hypertrophic cardiomyopathy in diabetic pregnancies compared with postnatal outcome. *Clin Med Insights Womens Health* 2015;8:39.

237. Maron BJ, Towbin JA, Thiene G, et al. Contemporary definitions and classification of the cardiomyopathies: an American Heart Association Scientific Statement from the Council on Clinical Cardiology, Heart Failure and Transplantation Committee; Quality of Care and Outcomes Research and Functional Genomics and Translational Biology Interdisciplinary Working Groups; and Council on Epidemiology and Prevention. *Circulation* 2006;113:1807.

238. Thorsson AV, Hintz RL. Insulin receptors in the newborn. Increase in receptor affinity and number. *N Engl J Med* 1977;297:908.

239. Reller MD, Kaplan S. Hypertrophic cardiomyopathy in infants of diabetic mothers: an update. *Am J Perinatol* 1988;5:353.

240. Kojo M, Ogawa T, Yamada K, et al. Multivariate autoregressive analysis of carotid artery blood flow waveform in an infant of a diabetic mother with cardiomyopathy. *Acta Paediatr Jpn* 1995;37:588.

241. Van Bel F, Van de Bor M, Walther FJ. Cerebral blood flow velocity and cardiac output in infants of insulin-dependent diabetic mothers. *Acta Paediatr Scand* 1991;80:905.

242. Way GL, Wolfe RR, Eshaghpour E, et al. The natural history of hypertrophic cardiomyopathy in infants of diabetic mothers. *J Pediatr* 1979;95:1020.

243. Armstrong K, Franklin O, Sweetman D, et al. Cardiovascular dysfunction in infants with neonatal encephalopathy. *Arch Dis Child* 2012;97:372.

244. Ranjit MS. Cardiac abnormalitites in birth asphyxia. *Indian J Pediatr* 2000;67:26.

245. Ryan JJ, Huston J, Kutty S, et al. Right ventricular adaptation and failure in pulmonary arterial hypertension. *Can J Cardiol* 2015;31:391.

246. More KS, Sakhuja P, Giesinger RE, et al. Cardiovascular associations with abnormal brain magnetic resonance imaging in neonates with hypoxic ischemic encephalopathy undergoing therapeutic hypothermia and rewarming. *Am J Perinatol* 2018;35(10):979.

247. Creamer KM, McCloud LL, Fisher LE, et al. Ventilation above closing volume reduces pulmonary vascular resistance hysteresis. *Am J Respir Crit Care Med* 1998;158:1114.

248. Rubini A. Effect of perfusate temperature on pulmonary vascular resistance and compliance by arterial and venous occlusion in the rat. *Eur J Appl Physiol* 2005;93:435.

249. Block BS, Schlafer DH, Wentworth RA, et al. Intrauterine asphyxia and the breakdown of physiologic circulatory compensation in fetal sheep. *Am J Obstet Gynecol* 1990;162:1325.

250. Davidson JO, Fraser M, Naylor AS, et al. Effect of cerebral hypothermia on cortisol and adrenocorticotropic hormone responses after umbilical cord occlusion in preterm fetal sheep. *Pediatr Res* 2008;63:51.

251. Zanelli S, Buck M, Fairchild K. Physiologic and pharmacologic considerations for hypothermia therapy in neonates. *J Perinatol* 2011;31:377.

252. Mialksoo M, Tal'vik TA, Paiu A, et al. [Function of the sympathetico-adrenal system and the acid-base equilibrium in newborn infants with a hypoxic lesion of the central nervous system]. *Zh Nevropatol Psikhiatr Im S S Korsakova* 1988;88:52.

253. Koplewitz BZ, Daneman A, Cutz E, et al. Neonatal adrenal congestion: a sonographic-pathologic correlation. *Pediatr Radiol* 1998;28:958.

254. Velaphi SC, Perlman JM. Neonatal adrenal hemorrhage: clinical and abdominal sonographic findings. *Clin Pediatr* 2001;40:545.

255. Mutlu M, Karaguzel G, Aslan Y, et al. Adrenal hemorrhage in newborns: a retrospective study. *World J Pediatr* 2011;7:355.

256. Hochwald O, Jabr M, Osiovich H, et al. Preferential cephalic redistribution of left ventricular cardiac output during therapeutic hypothermia for perinatal hypoxic-ischemic encephalopathy. *J Pediatr* 2014;164:999.

257. Nestaas E, Skranes JH, Stoylen A, et al. The myocardial function during and after whole-body therapeutic hypothermia for hypoxic-ischemic encephalopathy, a cohort study. *Early Hum Dev* 2014;90:247.

258. Wintermark P, Hansen A, Gregas MC, et al. Brain perfusion in asphyxiated newborns treated with therapeutic hypothermia. *AJNR Am J Neuroradiol* 2011;32:2023.

259. Wintermark P, Hansen A, Warfield SK, et al. Near-infrared spectroscopy versus magnetic resonance imaging to study brain perfusion in newborns with hypoxic-ischemic encephalopathy treated with hypothermia. *Neuroimage* 2014; 85(Pt 1):287.

260. Smith A, Purna JR, Castaldo MP, et al. Accuracy and reliability of qualitative echocardiography assessment of right ventricular size and function in neonates. *Echocardiography* 2019;36:1346.

261. Kovacs K, Szakmar E, Meder U, et al. A randomized controlled study of low-dose hydrocortisone versus placebo in dopamine-treated hypotensive neonates undergoing hypothermia treatment for hypoxic-ischemic encephalopathy. *J Pediatr* 2019;211:13.

262. Nestaas E, Stoylen A, Brunvand L, et al. Longitudinal strain and strain rate by tissue Doppler are more sensitive indices than fractional shortening for assessing the reduced myocardial function in asphyxiated neonates. *Cardiol Young* 2011;21:1.

263. Chandar J, Zilleruelo G. Hypertensive crisis in children. *Pediatr Nephrol* 2012;27:741.

264. Cao JY, Wales KM, Cordina R, et al. Pulmonary vasodilator therapies are of no benefit in pulmonary hypertension due to left heart disease: a meta-analysis. *Int J Cardiol* 2018;273:213.

265. Sehgal A, Alexander BT, Morrison JL, et al. Fetal growth restriction and hypertension in the offspring: mechanistic links and therapeutic directions. *J Pediatr* 2020;224:115.

266. Sahu R, Pannu H, Yu R, et al. Systemic hypertension requiring treatment in the neonatal intensive care unit. *J Pediatr* 2013;163:84.

267. Peterson AL, Frommelt PC, Mussatto K. Presentation and echocardiographic markers of neonatal hypertensive cardiomyopathy. *Pediatrics* 2006;118:e782.

268. Blowey DL, Duda PJ, Stokes P, et al. Incidence and treatment of hypertension in the neonatal intensive care unit. *J Am Soc Hypertens* 2011;5:478.

269. Sehgal A, Cook V, Dunn M. Pericardial effusion associated with an appropriately placed umbilical venous catheter. *J Perinatol* 2007;27:317.

270. Beardsall K, White DK, Pinto EM, et al. Pericardial effusion and cardiac tamponade as complications of neonatal long lines: are they really a problem? *Arch Dis Child Fetal Neonatal Ed* 2003;88:F292.

271. Nowlen TT, Rosenthal GL, Johnson DJ, et al. Pericardial effusion and tamponade in infants with central catheters. *Pediatrics* 2002;110:137.

272. Ades A, Sable C, Cummings S, et al. Echocardiographic evaluation of umbilical venous catheter placement. *J Perinatol* 2003;23:24.

32 Structural Cardiac Disease and Cardiomyopathies

David Blundell, Caroline Jones, and David S. Crossland

INTRODUCTION

Congenital heart disease is one of the most common group of structural abnormalities in newborn infants (1). In all populations and health care systems, it represents a significant cause of perinatal and infant mortality (2,3). It is testament to advances in antenatal and postnatal detection as well as the management of infants with congenital heart disease that survival is the expectation for many infants (3,4). In advanced health care systems, therefore, much of the focus has turned to reducing morbidity, improving long-term outcomes and the efficiency of the service. However, there remains a significant number of deaths associated with late diagnosis, complex variations of congenital heart disease, and congenital heart disease in association with other congenital abnormalities, prematurity, and low birth weight (5–8). These more complex infants represent a disproportionally high part of the work load and pose great challenges in terms of further improvements in survival within advanced health care systems. In less advanced health care systems or for those with limited access to health care, there remains considerable mortality associated with limited antenatal and postnatal diagnosis as well as poor access to neonatal cardiac surgery and intervention (9). The diagnosis and management of neonatal congenital heart disease and therefore outcomes are directly linked to the service that can be offered. Given the wide variety of potential treatment options and palliations in association with limited comparative trial data, management is not only specific to the health care system but also to unit practice within each health care system.

CLASSIFICATION OF CONGENITAL HEART DISEASE

Appropriate ways to classify congenital heart disease remain inconsistent and contentious. Clear classifications based on anatomical detail are well described, which outline the position of the heart within the chest, and sequential chamber analysis of the cardiac connections and cardiac abnormalities (10,11). Use of these anatomically descriptive systems is standard practice when making a final cardiac diagnosis. Although extremely useful for describing precise diagnosis and describing patient-specific anatomy, particularly due to the heterogeneous nature of congenital heart disease, these classifications are less useful when describing groups of patients or the clinical presentation of infants with Congenital heart disease (CHD). The subgroups mild (consisting of lesions that require observation only or a single curative procedure), moderate (lesions requiring repair and further observation throughout life with a likelihood of the need for further intervention), and severe (lesions that cannot be repaired and undergo palliative procedures, particularly single ventricle patients) are useful when describing the population of patients with congenital heart disease, and we will use those terms here in that setting. However, in terms of neonatal presentation, this classification is also limited as it does not take into account the severity of the neonatal presentation. For example, a patient with critical pulmonary stenosis (who following balloon pulmonary valvotomy would be considered mild CHD) presenting with severe cyanosis will be, at presentation, a much more significant clinical problem than patient with a single ventricle and balanced pulmonary blood flow (who has severe disease by this categorization). For this reason, when discussing the presentation of congenital heart disease and initial management, we will use terms that directly describe the clinical presentation

(such as cyanotic congenital heart disease, congenital heart disease presenting with/the potential to present with shock). It could be argued that describing presentation in this way is obsolete with expert fetal diagnosis and the availability of early diagnostic imaging. However, fetal diagnosis is by no means universal, and there are commonalities within each group not only with regard to presentation if the diagnosis is unknown but also the type and timing of different management strategies.

ETIOLOGY OF CARDIAC DISEASE

Embryology

Cardiogenesis is a complex process regulated by many genes and is also vulnerable to environmental and epigenetic factors. Multiple steps beginning in early gestation must occur in timely and sequential fashion to avoid development of a congenital heart lesion. The heart is the first human organ to function and begins to beat at day 21 and pump blood at day 24. One of the three primary germ layers, the mesoderm, begins to form the heart at day 18, and two strands (cardiogenic cords) form lumens, which become the endocardial tubes. Lateral folding causes their fusion creating the primitive heart tube where five distinct regions are formed, the truncus arteriosus, bulbus cordis, primitive ventricle, primitive atrium, and the sinus venosus. At this stage, venous blood from the sinus venosus and contractions pump the blood up toward the truncus arteriosus. This tube begins a craniocaudal folding process (morphogenesis) between days 23 and 28 creating an S shape with structures beginning to take their position. The truncus arteriosus twists and separates into the ascending aorta and main pulmonary artery. The bulbus cordis forms the right ventricle, and the primitive ventricle forms the left ventricle. The primitive atrium forms the atria and their appendages with the sinus venosus forming the posterior portion and coronary sinus (12). Alongside this process, the aortic arches develop in symmetrical pairs (six pharyngeal arches) connected to the cranial aspect of the primitive heart tube. Following this, the heart is partitioned initially by the interatrial and then the interventricular septum toward the end of the 5th week. The conotruncus (single outflow tract of the primitive heart tube) twists to create the aorta and pulmonary artery. The atrioventricular valves (mitral and tricuspid) are formed by cavitation of the atrioventricular cushion tissue and the semilunar valves (aortic and pulmonary) by cavitation of the truncoconal ridge (13). The mature heart is formed by day 50.

Cardiogenesis may be interrupted or modified at any stage in the pathway resulting in congenital heart disease. The following pathogenic mechanisms are known to cause patterns of congenital heart defects (14):

1. Defects in mesenchymal tissue migration—transposition of the great arteries (TGA), tetralogy of Fallot, truncus arteriosus, interrupted aortic arch, and doubly committed (subarterial) ventricular septal defect
2. Alteration of intracardiac blood flow—aortic or pulmonary valve stenosis, coarctation of the aorta, and pulmonary atresia with intact septum
3. Extracellular matrix defects (partial or complete atrioventricular septal defect)
4. Cell death abnormalities (muscular ventricular septal defect, Ebstein anomaly of the tricuspid valve)

TABLE 32.1

Recurrence Risk of Congenital Heart Disease in Selected Patient Groups

Defect	Recurrence Risk in Two Healthy Parents—One Child Affected	Recurrence Risk in Two Healthy Parents—Two Children Affected	Recurrence Risk if Mother Has CHD	Recurrence Risk if Father Has CHD
Overall	1–6	3–10	2–20	1–5
VSD	3	10	9–10	2–3
ASD	2–3	8	6	1–2
Coarctation of aorta	2	6	4	2–3
Aortic stenosis	2	6	15–20	5
Pulmonary stenosis	2	6	6–7	2
Tetralogy of Fallot	2–3	8	2–3	1–2
AVSD	3–4			
Ebstein	1	3		
HLHS	3	10		
Tricuspid atresia	1	3		
Pulmonary atresia	1	3		
TGA	1–2	5		
ccTGA	5–6			

ASD, atrial septal defect; AVSD, atrioventricular septal defect; ccTGA, congenitally corrected transposition of great arteries; HLHS, hypoplastic left heart syndrome; TGA, transposition of great arteries.

Adapted by permission from Nature: van der Bom T, Zomer AC, Zwinderman AH, et al. The changing epidemiology of congenital heart disease. *Nat Rev Cardiol* 2011;8:50. doi:10.1038/nrcardio.2010.166. Copyright © 2011 Springer Nature.

5. Abnormal targeted growth (partial or total anomalous pulmonary venous drainage [TAPVD], cor triatriatum)
6. Defective cardiac looping or laterality disturbance (left or right atrial isomerism [RAI])

Epidemiology

Congenital heart disease is the most common form of congenital abnormality accounting for a third of all abnormalities detected. The incidence of significant congenital heart disease has remained relatively consistent at around 9 cases per 1,000 live births and is present in 10% of stillborns. In preterm infants, the incidence is twice as high, with severe forms of congenital heart disease more prevalent. The combined impact equates to a higher mortality rate in those infants with congenital heart disease born prematurely. Globally, congenital heart diagnosis has increased by 10% every 5 years equating to 1.35 million new diagnoses worldwide each year (15). This is in part due to improved diagnostic capabilities in low- and middle-income countries and the increase in diagnosis of minor lesions (16). While the incidence of congenital heart disease is similar across all countries, this has a higher burden on those countries with young populations and a higher fertility rate (9). In a country with a fertility rate of about eight per woman, the population has to support four times as many children with congenital heart disease as in a country with a fertility rate of two. Countries with the highest fertility rates tend to have the lowest incomes per capita and more infants with congenital heart disease per wage earner, further accentuating the disparity. For many countries with high fertility rates, improving local health services and controlling infectious diseases (diarrheal illness, rheumatic fever, measles, rotaviral infection) are important but are mere "band-aids" compared to improving education, empowering women, and reducing birth rates (see Chapter 1).

Patterns in congenital heart disease globally continue to change due to an interplay between factors that are increasing incidence and those that are reducing it (4,17).

Screening programs and improved prenatal diagnosis have led to an increase in termination of pregnancy, particularly for those with complex and single ventricle lesions, thereby reducing their birth incidence (4). However, there is huge variability globally due to differing prenatal diagnosis rates and the heavy influence of individual, societal, cultural, and religious beliefs regarding the acceptability of termination of pregnancy. Despite this, as survival for congenital heart disease continues to improve this will impact on parental decision-making as to whether to proceed with a pregnancy, and with improved survival, even if the incidence at live birth is reduced the prevalence of each lesion within the population may increase. As more women with congenital heart disease survive to adulthood, they may choose to have their own children with an associated increased risk of giving birth to a baby with congenital heart disease (Table 32.1).

Frequently pinpointing why congenital heart disease has occurred in a particular pregnancy is challenging due to a complex interplay of genetic and environmental influences on cardiac development in early gestation. Around 30% of congenital heart disease arises in association with a chromosomal abnormality or single gene disorders (Table 32.2). For the other 70%, many are likely to have a genetic component to their disease that has not yet been identified on widely available genetic testing. In cases of nonsyndromic disease, less than 5% have a relevant family history. Certain forms of congenital heart disease such as hypoplastic left heart syndrome (HLHS) have a higher chance of recurrence (8% for HLHS and 22% for all other forms of congenital heart disease), suggesting a strong genetic component (21). Parental consanguinity (between first cousins) is associated with a two- to threefold increase in the chance of developing congenital heart disease in their offspring. Congenital heart disease in the most part occurs in "low-risk" pregnancies without an identifiable risk factor of family history. Environmental factors are known to play a role in congenital heart disease development with teratogens, alcohol, autoimmune disease, congenital infections, and smoking increasing the risk. The variable phenotypes and incomplete penetrance characteristic of CHD suggest that the interplay with environmental factors and epigenetic imprinting warrants further investigation (22).

Genetic Testing for Patients with CHD

Planning genetic investigation will depend on the clinical findings, type of CHD, and known associations. Some syndromic phenotypes are clearly recognizable at birth, whereas others may only become evident as a child develops when growth delay or learning difficulties are noted. Often, local guidelines will advise testing for particular types of CHD, for example, neonates with certain conotruncal abnormalities (e.g., tetralogy of Fallot, common arterial trunk,

TABLE 32.2

Congenital Disorders Associated with Congenital Heart Disease

Selected Disorders	Identified Gene(s)	Chromosome Location	% Heart Disease	Cardiovascular Anomalies
Autosomal dominant				
Alagille arteriohepatic dysplasia	Jagged 1, Notch 2	20p12, 1p11-12	100	Multiple PA stenosis and hypoplasia, PDA, ASD, VSD, renal artery stenosis, carotid aneurysm
Apert acrocephalosyndactyly	FGFR-2	10q26		VSD, hypoplastic PA
Beckwith-Wiedemann syndrome	H19, KCNQ10T1, CDK1C	11p15.5, 5q35.2-3	15 ?	HCM, ASD, VSD, TF, PDA
Cardiofacial cutaneous syndrome	KRAS, BRAF, MAP2K1, MAP2K1	12p12.1, 7q34 15q22.31 19p13.3		ASD, PS, HCM
CHARGE syndrome	CHD7, SEM3AE	8q12.1, 7q21.11	44	TF, ASD, VSD, DORV, PDA, PS
Costello syndrome	HRAS	11p15.5	44	HCM, PS, MVP, ASD, VSD, arrhythmia
de Lange syndrome CLLS1	NIPBL, SMC1A, HDAC8, RAD21, and SMC3	5p13.2, Xp11.22, Xq13.1, 10q25.2, 8q24.11	30	VSD, ASD, PDA, AS, EFE
DiGeorge/velocardiofacial syndromes	Multiple in DGCR including TBX1	22q11 DGCR	>50	TF, interrupted Ao arch, truncus arteriosus, right Ao arch
Goldenhar hemifacial microsomia/OAVS	Multiple	Multiple	4–33	TF, VSD, PDA, COARC
Hereditary hemorrhagic telangiectasia Osler-Weber-Rendu	ACVRL1, ENG, and SMAD4	12q13.3, 9q34.1, 18q21.2	100	Pulmonary and systemic AVM, arterial aneurysm telangiectasia
Holt-Oram heart–hand syndrome	TBX5	12q24.1	75	ASD-2, VSD or PDA in 2/3, HLHS, conduc. block, HLHS, TAPVC, truncus art
Juvenile polyposis hereditary telangiectasia JPHT	SMAD4 BMPR1A	18q21.2 10q23.2	15	Ao aneurysm, MVP, MR, AVM
Leopard syndrome	PTPN1, RAF1, BRAF, MAP2K1	12q24.13, 3p25.2, 7q34, 15q22.31	85	HCM, PS
Loeys-Dietz syndrome 1–4	TGFBR1, TGFBR2, SMAD3, TGF	Multiple	100	Ao aneurysm/dissection, cerebral and arterial aneurysm and tortuosity, MVP, MR, BAV, PS
Marfan syndrome	Fibrillin-1	15q21.1	Up to 100%	Ao aneurysm; AR, MR, TR, and prolapse
Myhre syndrome	SMAD4	18q21.2	63	ASD, VSD, PDA, AS, COARC, pericardial fibrosis
Neurofibromatosis type 1	NFI	17q11.2	Rare	PS, COARC, renal artery stenosis
Noonan syndrome types 1, 4, 8, NF type	PTPN11 (50%), SOS1 (28%), KRAS, NRAS, BRAS, RAF1, RITI, NF1, SOS2, LZTR1	12q24.13 (PTPN11)	50%–80%	PS/dysplasia, PDA, HCM, COARC
Rubinstein-Taybi type 1	CREBBP	16p13.3	35	VSD, PDA, ASD, COARC, PS, hemangioma, BAV
Saethre-Chotzen syndrome	TWIST, FGFR-3 and 22	7p21, 10q26	?	Various, subvalvar AS
Shprintzen-Goldberg craniosynostosis syndrome	SKI	1p36.33		Ao aneurysm, carotid and vertebral arterial tortuosity, MVP
Treacher-Collins syndrome	TCOF1, POLR1C, POLR1D	5q32-q33.1, 6p21.1, 13q12.2	11	ASD, VSD, PDA, Ao aneurysm
Tuberous sclerosis 1, 2	TSC1 (hemartin), TSC2 (tuberin)	9q34.13, 16p13.3	47%–67%	Rhabdomyomas, WPW, rarely Ao aneurysm
Williams-Beuren syndrome	ELN	7q11.23	75	Supravalvar AS, small aorta, BAV, AS, PS, stenoses of LCA, multiple PAs, cerebral and renal arteries, MVP, MR, ASD, VSD
Autosomal recessive				
Carpenter acrocephalopolysyndactyly 1,2	Type 1MEGF8 Type 2 RAB23	19q13.2 6p11.2	29	ASD, VSD, PDA, PS, VSD, TF, TGA, dextrocardia
Coffin-Siris fifth digit syndrome	ARID1A, ARID1B, SMARCA4, SMARCB1, or SMARCE1 gene	1p36.11, 6q25.3, 19p13.2, 22q11.23, 17q21.2	33	PDA, ASD, VSD, TF
Ellis-van Creveld syndrome	EVC, EVC2	4p16.2	80–99	ASD
Klippel-Feil syndrome	MEOX1, GDF6, GDF 3	17q21.31, 8q22.1,12p13.31	5–29	VSD, dextrocardia

THE NEWBORN INFANT

(Continued)

TABLE 32.2

Congenital Disorders Associated with Congenital Heart Disease (*Continued*)

Selected Disorders	Identified Gene(s)	Chromosome Location	% Heart Disease	Cardiovascular Anomalies
Mucopolysaccharidosis type 1	EVC	4p16.2	50–60	Single atrium, primum ASD, COARC, HLHS
Type 2	Iduronidase	4p16.3	>50	All types have valvular disease
Type 3D	Iduronate 2-sulfatase	Xq28		Coronary disease (type 2)
Smith-Lemli-Opitz syndrome 1 and 2	DHCR7	11q13.4	50	TF, COARC, pulmonary hypertension
Thrombocytopenia absent radius	RBM8A	1q21.1	15-22	VSD, PDA, ASD, TF, AV canal, COARC
Zellweger cerebrohepatorenal syndrome	Multiple PEX genes	Multiple peroxin-5,2, 6,12	?	VSD, ASD, PDA
Selected chromosomal disorders				
Trisomy 13—Patau syndrome		13	80	PDA, VSD, ASD, COARC, AS, PS
Trisomy 18—Edwards syndrome		18	90–100	VSD, polyvalvular, ASD, PDA
Trisomy 21—Down syndrome		21	40–50	AV canal, VSD, ASD1 and 2, PDA, TF
+8 Mosaicism		8	25	VSD, PDA, CoAo, PS
+9 Mosaicism		9	70	VSD, PDA, LSVC
XO Turners syndrome		X	>50	Bicusp AV, COARC, Ao aneurysm, AS, VSD
4p- Wolf syndrome		4p	33	VSD, ASD, COARC
5p- Cri-du-Chat syndrome		5p	20	VSD, PDA, ASD, PS
7q-		7q	20	
13q-		13q-	Common	
18q-		18q	25	VSD, ASD, PDA, PS
Ring 18		18	20	COARC, PA hypoplasia, HLHS, LSVC
10p trisomy		10p	30	AV canal, VSD, ToF
10q24 trisomy		10q24	50	
22+ Cat eye syndrome		22	40	TAPVC, TF
Fragile X		x	50	
Syndromes with unknown etiology			65–75	TF, DORV, ASD, VSD, PDA, COARC, AV canal
Asymmetric crying facies				
VACTERL association			10	VSD, ASD, TF
Nonrandom associations				
Cleft lip and palate			25	VSD, PDA, TGA, TF, SV
Diaphragmatic hernia			25	TF
Lung agenesis			20	PDA, VSD, TF, TAPVC
Omphalocele			20	TF, ASD
Intestinal atresia			10	VSD
Renal agenesis unilateral/bilateral			17/75	VSD

Ao, aortic; AR, aortic regurgitation; AS, aortic stenosis; ASD, atrial septal defect; ASD-1, primum atrial septal defect; ASD-2, secundum atrial septal defect; AV, aortic valve; AV canal, atrioventricular canal defect; AVM, arteriovenous malformation; BAV, bicuspid aortic valve; COARC, coarctation of the aorta; DORV, double-outlet right ventricle; EFE, endocardial fibroelastosis; HLHS, hypoplastic left heart syndrome; LCA, left coronary artery; LSVC, left superior vena cava; MR, mitral regurgitation; MVP, mitral valve prolapse; PAs, pulmonary arteries; PDA, patent ductus arteriosus; PS, pulmonary valve stenosis; TAPVC, totally anomalous pulmonary venous connection; TF, tetralogy of Fallot; TGA, transposition of great arteries; TR, tricuspid regurgitation; truncus art, truncus arteriosus; VSD, ventricular septal defect.

From Adam MP, Ardinger HH, Pagon R. *GeneReviews*. Available from: https://www.ncbi.nlm.nih.gov/books/NBK1116/. Accessed July 22, 2019; Muntean I, Togănel R, Benedek T. Genetics of congenital heart disease: past and present. *Biochem Genet* 2017;55(2):105. doi: 10.1007/s10528-016-9780-7; Lin AE, Alexander ME, Colan SD, et al. Clinical, pathological, and molecular analyses of cardiovascular abnormalities in Costello syndrome: a Ras/MAPK pathway syndrome. *Am J Med Genet A* 2011;155(3):486. doi: 10.1002/ajmg.a.33857. Ref. (18–20).

interrupted arch) should all be tested for 22q11.2 deletion (DiGeorge syndrome), or that where supravalvular aortic stenosis is identified, Williams syndrome should be excluded.

Karyotyping is typically the primary test to look for associated chromosomal rearrangements in association with CHD (aneuploidy or triploidy such as trisomy 21 [Down syndrome] or trisomy 18 [Edwards syndrome]). Increasingly array comparative genomic hybridization (array CGH or comparative microarray) is utilized, and this has higher resolution with the ability to diagnose microduplications and deletions (see also Chapters 10 and 56). For CHD, this will detect important copy number variants (CNVs) such as 22q11.2 deletion (DiGeorge syndrome). However, the clinician may need to be cautious in interpreting results (depending on laboratory reporting) and determine the relevance of the reported abnormalities to the noted phenotype as very small CNVs may be nonpathogenic. Where there are uncertain findings unaffected, parental samples may be required to establish whether this is inheritance of a benign CNV. Fluorescence *in situ* hybridization (FISH) is a method utilized to detect specific regions of DNA that may be deleted or duplicated, and is often used to detect DiGeorge, Williams, or Alagille syndrome. Single-gene disorders (such as Noonan or Alagille syndrome) require testing targeted at the specific gene such as Sanger or next-generation sequencing methods.

Laterality Disturbance (Heterotaxy Syndrome)

Laterality disturbance encompasses a spectrum of cardiac and extracardiac abnormalities that result from an abnormal arrangement of the thoracoabdominal organs across the left–right axis of

TABLE 32.3

TABLE 32.3

Common Abnormalities in Association with Laterality Disturbance

Left Atrial Isomerism	Right Atrial Isomerism
Cardiac abnormalities	
Atrioventricular or another septal defect	Atrioventricular septal defect
Partial or hemianomalous pulmonary venous drainage	Total anomalous pulmonary venous drainage
Abnormal p-wave axis (coronary sinus rhythm) or complete heart block	Transposition of the great arteries (TGA)
Ventricular noncompaction	Double outlet right ventricle (DORV)
Left heart obstruction—for example, aortic stenosis or coarctation of the aorta	Right heart obstruction—for example, pulmonary stenosis or pulmonary atresia
Bilateral superior vena cava	Bilateral superior vena cava
Interrupted IVC with azygos or hemiazygos continuation	
Extracardiac abnormalities	
Polysplenia (may still be nonfunctional)	Asplenia
Malrotation	Malrotation
Biliary atresia	

the body. Isomerism of the atrial appendages refers to the morphology of the atrial appendage, which is defined by their pattern of pectinate muscles (23). Using echocardiography both prenatally and postnatally, the position of the inferior vena cava and aorta are used to infer "normal atrial arrangement." Visualization of the appendage morphology may be possible in the neonate with good echocardiographic windows.

Three percent of congenital heart disease is associated with laterality disturbance, and anomalies are likely to be caused by complex multiple gene problems. Isomerism can be right (bilateral atrial appendages of right morphology) or left type (bilateral left atrial appendages). Though no cardiac or extracardiac anomaly is exclusive to one type, they do follow certain patterns (Table 32.3). Left atrial isomerism (LAI) may occur with normal intracardiac anatomy, and a significant proportion will have CHD amenable to surgery resulting in a biventricular circulation. This is in contrast to RAI that is almost universally associated with complex CHD meaning that frequently only univentricular palliation is possible. Sequential segmental echocardiographic evaluation is vital to fully describe the cardiac morphology in this group.

In addition, detailed pre- and postnatal assessment is required to look for the common associated extracardiac features (24) that may require treatment, such as penicillin prophylaxis for asplenia or consideration of a prophylactic Ladd procedure for malrotation.

SYMPTOMS, PHYSICAL EXAMINATION, AND INVESTIGATIONS

The symptoms and signs of individual lesions are outlined in Table 32.4, and their relevance to the presentation and management of CHD are discussed in the presentation section below.

Respiratory Symptoms of Cardiac Origin

Decreased lung compliance associated with increased pulmonary blood flow and pulmonary edema result in increased respiratory effort and rate. This can be due to either excessive pulmonary blood flow seen in patients with left-to-right shunts or due to pulmonary venous hypertension leading to pulmonary edema (irrespective of pulmonary blood flow). Pulmonary venous hypertension

can occur with pulmonary venous obstruction, obstruction to left atrial egress, or high left ventricular end-diastolic pressure due to impaired left ventricular function or left heart outflow obstructive lesions. These findings can be difficult to differentiate from a primary respiratory cause and warrant further assessment. Tachypnea in isolation can be seen in patients with cyanosis who have normal or reduced pulmonary blood flow.

Feeding Difficulties and Failure to Thrive

Failure to thrive and malnutrition are common systemic consequences and presenting signs of CHD, particularly in cyanotic infants or those with complex single ventricle lesions. Often, this has a multifactorial nature with high metabolic rate, inadequate calorie intake, swallowing difficulties, gastroesophageal reflux, and genetic factors impacting on feeding capabilities. Neonates with increased respiratory effort and rate invariably will struggle with the coordination of breathing and swallowing required to achieve effective feeding. This is compounded by the combined impact of the cardiac physiology, hypermetabolic state, and respiratory effort often necessitating the need for increased calorie intake for the infant to sustain growth. Additionally, for some infants, their cardiac physiology will impact on gastrointestinal functions causing malabsorption and/or gastroesophageal reflux or in severe cases severe hypoxemia and poor circulation resulting in necrotizing enterocolitis. Neonates with additional comorbidities, prematurity, or a syndromic diagnosis may have limitations in oromotor feeding skills and often will present with more marked feeding difficulty and failure to thrive. It is recognized that impaired nutritional status and growth negatively impacts on surgical recovery, neurodevelopment, and short- and long-term outcomes for the infant with CHD.

Desaturation and Cyanosis

Normal saturations in term infants are expected to be greater than 94% at 24 hours. Altitude can affect saturations, although even at 1,800 m a normal-term infant should expect saturations greater than 89% (26). Cyanosis is the clinical manifestation of reduced arterial oxygen saturations and is caused by an abundance of deoxyhemoglobin, typically over 5 g/dL. In a neonate with adequate hemoglobin levels, cyanosis becomes clinically apparent when the degree of oxygenation falls below 85%. However, in anemia, the deoxyhemoglobin levels may not be high enough for cyanosis to become clinically apparent. The appearance of cyanosis is of a blue or dusky tinge to the babies' skin color, often evident in the lips or tongue. As a clinical sign, cyanosis can be unreliable, with normal babies often having perioral or nail bed discoloration and cold infants can also appear blue or dusky. The widespread availability of pulse oximetry allows rapid identification of normal variants in color from true cyanosis. In some circumstances, formal assessment of the arterial blood gas may be required. Proven desaturation (whether or not this is diagnosed initially clinically or on pulse oximetry) requires immediate further assessment to ascertain the diagnosis and treatment plan to prevent the potential for further deterioration. The use of saturation monitoring as a screening tool and the investigation and management of patients presenting with desaturation are discussed below. The three physiologic causes of cyanosis should all be considered when approaching any baby with desaturation, namely:

1. Right-to-left shunting. Passage of deoxygenated blood from the systemic venous return to the systemic circulation can occur at the level of the systemic venous return, atrial septum, ventricular septum, or patent ductus arteriosus. This can occur due to abnormal cardiac connections or due to obstruction to flow at atrioventricular valves or pulmonary outflow leading to shunting at atrial and ventricular levels, respectively. This obstruction may be physical due to stenosis, atresia, or hypoplasia of a cardiac chamber or valve, poor compliance of that chamber

TABLE 32.4

Common Congenital Cardiac Lesions Are Arranged by How They Commonly Present in the Neonatal Period. Key Features of Anatomy Are Described As Well As Physical Examination, ECG, Radiographic, and Relevant ECHO Findings

Diagnosis	Anatomy	Physical Signs	CXR Findings	ECG	Neonatal Echo Assessment
Conditions causing early shock					
Hypoplastic left heart syndrome	Atresia/critical stenosis of aortic and mitral valves with resulting hypoplasia of the left ventricle and aortic arch	Single S_2, ↑respiratory work, tachycardia, ↓↓ perfusion, +/− SRM	↑Pulmonary arterial markings, cardiomegaly	↓LV force usually, develops RAE, RAD, RVH	Assessment of PDA and atrial communication vital to maintaining circulation
Coarctation of the aorta	Narrowing of the aorta. Commonly is distal to the left subclavian artery at the aortic isthmus. May be associated with hypoplastic aortic arch, left SVC, and/or BAV	Absent or ↓femoral pulses and leg BP SEM in back, +/− click, S_3, +/− Differential cyanosis (when PDA open)	↑Heart size, +/− pulmonary edema	+/− RVH, develops LVH, BVH	Posterior shelf noted, color Doppler flow turbulence Continuous wave Doppler demonstrates diastolic tail LV function assessment
Interrupted aortic arch	Arch is interrupted between ascending + descending thoracic aorta	Absent or ↓femoral pulses and leg BP +/− SEM, +/− PSM LSB Differential cyanosis (when PDA open)	↑Heart size, +/− pulmonary edema	+/− RVH, develops LVH, BVH	Site of arch interruption PDA size Anatomic type and size of VSD
Critical aortic stenosis	Primitive myxomatous valve often functionally bicuspid or unicuspid	↓Pulses and perfusion, SEM, click, S_3, single S_2	↑Heart size, pulmonary edema	LVH, T-wave abnormalities	Assessment of PDA Valve anatomy and degree of stenosis/regurgitation LV function assessment
Conditions causing early cyanosis					
Pulmonary atresia with VSD	Atretic pulmonary valve Ventricular septal defect with overriding aorta May be associated with major aortopulmonary collateral arteries (MAPCAs)	Single S_2 continuous murmur, LSB back, axillae	↓Pulmonary vascular markings Boot-shaped heart MAPCAs +/− ↑pulmonary vascular markings +/− Right arch	RAD and RVH	Assessment of PDA and MAPCAs supply to lungs Anatomic type and size of VSD
Pulmonary atresia with intact ventricular septum	Atretic pulmonary valve Frequently associated with hypoplastic right heart structures	Single S_2, soft SRM	↓Pulmonary vascular markings	LVH, ↓RV forces, +/− develops Q waves	Right-to-left interatrial shunt Assessment of PDA Hypertrophied RV Associated with coronary artery abnormalities.
Tetralogy of Fallot	Ventricular septal defect, overriding of the aorta, right ventricular outflow obstruction, right ventricular hypertrophy	Single S_2, SEM	↓Pulmonary vascular markings Boot-shaped heart +/− Right arch	Develops RAE, RAD, RVH	Assessment of right ventricular outflow tract and pulmonary anatomy Assessment of PDA flow Anatomic type and size of VSD
Double outlet right ventricle	The aorta and pulmonary artery arise from the RV with VSD May be Fallot type with PS, transposed great arteries, or both arteries unobstructed	↑S_2 loudness, ↑respiratory work	↑Heart size, ↑pulmonary vascular markings	LAD, develops RVH, BVH	Relationship of great arteries Assess pulmonary valve for stenosis
Pulmonary valve stenosis	Thickened dysplastic doming valve with fusion of leaflets, maybe bicuspid	SEM radiating to the back	Prominent MPA Normal/decreased pulmonary vascular marking	RAD, RVH	Assess degree of pulmonary valve stenosis May have right-to-left interatrial shunt Assessment of PDA
Conditions causing mixing with variable presentation					
Transposition of great arteries	Aorta arises from right ventricle, pulmonary artery arises from the left ventricle May be associated with VSD +/− hypoplastic aortic arch	Split S_2, +/− murmur, +/− ↑respiratory work	↑Pulmonary vascular markings, +/− Cardiomegaly with narrow mediastinum (i.e., "egg on a string")	Develops RAE, RAD, RVH	Assessment of site for mixing— ASD, VSD, PDA Great arteries are seen in parallel (rather than crossing) in parasternal long-axis view

TABLE 32.4

Common Congenital Cardiac Lesions Are Arranged by How They Commonly Present in the Neonatal Period. Key Features of Anatomy Are Described As Well As Physical Examination, ECG, Radiographic, and Relevant ECHO Findings (*Continued*)

Diagnosis	Anatomy	Physical Signs	CXR Findings	ECG	Neonatal Echo Assessment
Total anomalous pulmonary venous drainage	Pulmonary veins fail to drain to left atrium. Drain into venous system and right heart via ascending vein (supracardiac), descending vein (infracardiac), or via coronary sinus (cardiac)	Narrow S$_2$ split, +/− SEM, ↑respiratory work	↑Pulmonary venous markings, ↑diffuse interstitial markings "Snowman" sign	Develops RAE, RAD, RVH	Right-to-left interatrial shunt with volume loaded right heart. Confirm drainage ascending or descending vein to venous system. Dilated coronary sinus noted is cardiac drainage
Ebstein anomaly of the tricuspid valve	Spectrum condition, TV is displaced and rotated into RV, reducing the functional cavity. Variable amount of TV regurgitation	SRM, split S$_2$, hepatomegaly ↑respiratory work	Severe cases— ↑heart size ↓pulmonary arterial markings Normal in milder cases	RBBB, RAE	Right-to-left interatrial shunt. TV displacement and regurgitation. Pulmonary valve and arteries, may be "functional" or anatomical pulmonary atresia
Tricuspid atresia	Absent tricuspid valve with hypoplastic right ventricle. Ventricular septal defect. Arteries may be transposed or normally related	• Obstructed pulmonary flow Single S$_2$, SEM, ↑respiratory work • Unobstructed pulmonary flow Split S$_2$, heave, SRM, ↑respiratory work	↓Pulmonary arterial markings, +/− cardiomegaly ↑Pulmonary arterial markings, cardiomegaly	LAD	Right-to-left interatrial shunt. Assessment of VSD and PDA. Relationship of great arteries. Degree of pulmonary stenosis
Conditions causing left-to-right shunt					
Truncus arteriosus	Single arterial trunk leaves the heart overriding a large VSD. Truncal valve often dysplastic may be stenotic or regurgitant. Associated with right or interrupted aortic arch	Split S$_2$, multiple clicks, soft to loud SEM, +/− DRM, ↑respiratory work	↑Pulmonary arterial markings, cardiomegaly	Develops RAE, RAD, BVH	Anatomic type and size of VSD. Morphology and function of the truncal valve. Origin of the pulmonary arteries. Arch assessment
Complete atrioventricular septal defect	Ostium primum ASD, inlet VSD and common atrioventricular valve. Common valve is often regurgitant	Heave, harsh SRM, +/− S$_3$, +/− diastolic rumble, normal pulses ↑Respiratory work	↑Heart size (RV, LV, LA),↑pulmonary arterial markings	LAD, RBBB develops RAE, RVH, LVH, BVH	Assessment in 4CH of RV/LV size, valvular regurgitation. Arch assessment
Ventricular septal defect	Defects can be perimembranous, doubly committed subarterial or muscular	Heave, harsh SRM, +/− S$_3$, +/− diastolic rumble, normal pulses ↑Respiratory work	↑Heart size (RV, LV, LA),↑pulmonary arterial markings	Develops RAE, RVH, LVH, BVH	Identify number, size, and location of defects. Assessment of shunt velocity to estimate RV pressure
Patent ductus arteriosus	Persistence of the ductus arteriosus between the pulmonary artery and the aorta	Heave, ↑pulses, ↑pulse pressure, continuous or SRM ↑Respiratory work	↑Heart size (LV, LA),↑pulmonary arterial markings	Develops RVH, LVH, BVH	PDA size and shunt velocity to estimate PA pressure. Dimensions of LA and LV can give indication of shunt volume
Atrial septal defect	Defect can be primum defect, secundum defect, or sinus venosus defect	Hyperdynamic precordium, soft SEM, fixed split S$_2$, +/− diastolic rumble	↑Heart size (RV, normal LA, and LV), ↑pulmonary arterial markings	Develops RAD, RVH	Identify size, location of defect, and flow pattern. Confirm pulmonary venous anatomy

Non–duct-dependent lesions

Lesions with the potential to be duct dependent

Duct-dependent lesions

+/−, may or may not be present; ↓, decreased; ↑, increased; BAV, bicuspid aortic valve; BVH, biventricular hypertrophy; DRM, diastolic regurgitant murmur; LA, left atrium; LAD, left axis deviation; LSB, left sternal border; LV, left ventricle; LVH, left ventricular hypertrophy; PA, pulmonary atresia; PS, pulmonary stenosis; PSM, pansystolic murmur; RA, right atrium; RAD, right axis deviation; RAE, right atrial enlargement; RBBB, right bundle branch block; RV, right ventricle; RVH, right ventricular hypertrophy; S$_2$, second heart sound; S$_3$, third heart sound; SEM, systolic ejection murmur; SRM, systolic regurgitant murmur; TV, tricuspid valve; VSD, ventricular septal defect.

Data from *Paediatric Cardiology/Editors, Robert H. Anderson ... [et al.]; Illustrator, Gemma Price*, 3rd ed. Philadelphia, PA: Churchill Livingstone, 2010; Park MK, Myung K. *Park's pediatric cardiology for practitioners*, 6th ed. Philadelphia, PA: Elsevier Saunders, 2014. Ref. (25).

(due to impaired function or obstruction of the outflow), or to elevated downstream resistance (high pulmonary vascular resistance). When the ductus arteriosus is patent and the pulmonary vascular resistance is higher than the systemic vascular resistance, there will be right-to-left flow across the patent ductus arteriosus. If there is sufficient pulmonary venous return and forward flow of oxygenating blood into the systemic circulation, there will be differential cyanosis (i.e., higher saturations in the right arm than in the legs). This differential cyanosis is also seen in patients with aortic arch abnormalities when the systemic circulation distal to the aortic obstruction is dependent upon right-to-left flow through the ductus.

THE NEWBORN INFANT

2. Transposition physiology. In isolated transposition of the great arteries (TGA), desaturated systemic venous blood is directed to the aorta, and pulmonary venous return directed back to the pulmonary arteries leading to profound cyanosis. Transposition physiology is not limited to patients with isolated TGA, those with TGA and a potential site for mixing (e.g., ventricular septal defect) and also those with more complex TGA will also be desaturated due to intracardiac streaming of the blood with preferential flow of the systemic venous return into the aorta and pulmonary venous return into the pulmonary artery.

3. Pulmonary vein desaturation. A ventilation–perfusion mismatch from all causes prevents adequate oxygenation of pulmonary blood flow leading to pulmonary vein desaturation and therefore systemic desaturation. Although usually attributed to respiratory disease, significant pulmonary edema will lead to ventilation–perfusion mismatch and hence pulmonary vein desaturation, which can complicate the clinical differentiation of respiratory from cardiac causes of cyanosis.

Hyperoxia Test

The hyperoxia test is the response of the arterial PO_2 to administration of 100% oxygen and is often cited as a way of differentiating cyanotic heart disease from lung disease (see also Chapter 31). The infant is placed in 100% oxygen and a response in the preductal arterial PO_2 assessed. A posttreatment preductal PaO_2 of greater than 150 mm Hg indicates that hypoxia is unlikely to be circulatory in origin, while a PaO_2 of less than 50 mm Hg is highly suggestive of a critical cyanotic CHD (or in some cases severe Persistent pulmonary hypertension of the newborn (PPHN)), necessitating consideration to initiate prophylactic treatment with intravenous prostaglandin infusion to maintain ductal patency. PaO_2 between 50 and 150 mm Hg is considered equivocal. The basis of this investigation is that the high PO_2 is sufficient to improve the V/Q mismatch of lung pathology to allow high concentrations of dissolved oxygen in the pulmonary venous return (i.e., treats pulmonary vein desaturation) and a baby with transposition physiology or right-to-left shunting will not be able to increase their PaO_2 to the same extent because the physiology persists whatever the dissolved oxygen content of the pulmonary vein. Unfortunately, the test has significant limitations both practically and diagnostically. For a perfect test to be carried out, invasive preductal blood gas analysis is required, and delivery of 100% oxygen is difficult to supply to a nonventilated infant. Where there is an inconclusive test, infants will still need managing as though they may have congenital heart disease, until proven otherwise. In addition, the administration of 100% oxygen to certain groups of babies with congenital heart disease, particularly those with HLHS (who may present with cyanosis) can be detrimental. Coexistent pathologies may also mean the investigation is of limited value. A simple test of observing the response of the saturations to supplemental oxygen may provide a more pragmatic approach in many units where formal hyperoxia testing has been superseded by early availability of expert echocardiography.

Perfusion, Pulses, and Blood Pressure

Signs of diminished systemic circulatory output are common to many presentations and are not specific to reduced perfusion related to CHD. Individual clinical signs lack sensitivity to either a specific disease or an impaired circulation. However, when taken as a whole, the clinical assessment of circulatory output is an important tool for recognizing and then monitoring treatment of the impaired circulation. Suspicion of circulatory impairment and impending shock requires urgent assessment and early workup and management of all possible causes, including CHD. Poor feeding, irritability, listlessness, and reduced urine output may all be seen with circulatory compromise. Signs of poor peripheral skin

perfusion include prolonged capillary return, cool skin, and mottled skin. Palpation of the femoral and brachial pulses to assess pulse volume and quality should be undertaken. Pulse volume can be reduced in all cause of circulatory compromise, particularly with the development of shock. Weak pulses are associated with impaired cardiac output related to poor cardiac function or aortic stenosis and differential pulses (weak or absent femoral pulses and satisfactory pulses in the upper limbs) are observed in coarctation of the aorta. In some cases, these provide valuable information when compared to the dynamic pulses that are palpated in early sepsis or associated with a patent ductus arteriosus.

A variety of devices are used to measure blood pressure including Doppler measurement of systolic blood pressure, oscillometric devices, and direct invasive monitoring via percutaneously placed arterial lines, each with distinct advantages and disadvantages. Low blood pressure is a relatively late sign of impaired circulation due to all causes including CHD. There is potential for differential blood pressure in patients with aortic arch obstruction depending on whether the arterial supply limb used to measure the blood pressure is proximal (higher blood pressure) or distal (lower blood pressure) to the site of arch narrowing. It is therefore mandatory that the site of blood pressure recording is included as part of the neonatal chart. A consistent difference of greater than 20 mm Hg in the systolic BP between the right arm and either leg may be apparent in patients with coarctation of the aorta. While this clinical sign should be looked for when arch obstruction is suspected, limitations of non-invasive blood pressure measurement techniques, impracticalities of sitting two invasive arterial lines, and the lack of the differential in coarctation patients with an open arterial duct significantly limits this as a diagnostic technique. Although much of the emphasis is on low blood pressure, hypertension is an equally important sign when a cardiac problem is being considered. Older infants with arch obstruction may present with upper limb hypertension, and those with noncardiac causes of hypertension can present with impaired ventricular function and symptoms or signs of heart failure.

Cardiac Auscultation

Auscultation of the heart sounds and for murmurs is a necessary and ubiquitous part of routine neonatal examination and the assessment of babies with a suspected cardiac diagnosis. The different heart sounds and murmurs associated with individual CHD are outlined in Table 32.4. Importantly, the absence of a murmur does not preclude serious heart disease. The first and second heart sounds are identifiable in most settled infants using an appropriate size stethoscope, simultaneously palpating a pulse if necessary in order to differentiate between systole and diastole. Once the heart sounds have been identified, the periods of time between the heart sounds are focused on to identify systolic and diastolic murmurs, as well as additional heart sounds. The second heart sound is normally split due to the difference in timing of closure of the aortic valve (closes first) and the pulmonary valve. Prolongation of the splitting, or fixed splitting the second heart sound, is observed in atrial shunts, and a loud second heart sound can be identified in infants with a high pulmonary artery pressure. A third heart sound or gallop rhythm can be heard in patients with ventricular failure or dynamic circulations. Systolic murmurs are categorized by their volume (1–6) as well as their character (ejection systolic, pansystolic). The volume of diastolic murmurs is categorized 1 to 4 and always indicates underlying pathology. A continuous murmur is characteristic of a shunt at arterial level, in particular a patent ductus arteriosus. The presence and volume of a murmur are dependent in part on the pressure gradient between the chambers/vessels over which the turbulence occurs and can therefore evolve with time. For example, the pansystolic murmur of a small ventricular septal defect may not be heard until the normal drop in pulmonary vascular resistance has occurred and right ventricular pressure has fallen sufficiently to allow the left-to-right flow across the defect causing the murmur. By the same rationale, the loudness of a murmur is often not proportional to the severity of the lesion. Impaired cardiac function and low cardiac output will affect the volume of the murmur in patients with severe aortic or pulmonary stenosis resulting in a quieter ejection murmur than heard in those with less severe stenosis and good ventricular function. Large ventricular septal defects or a patent ductus arteriosus lead to equal pressure between the ventricles and great arteries and therefore often do not have a murmur from that lesion. Innocent murmurs are soft, systolic, heard in one area of the chest, do not radiate, and vary in intensity. Although they do not represent pathology and perhaps do not require investigation, differentiation from more significant lesions can often be difficult. Neonatal high heart rates and respiratory rates, or ventilator noises, can limit characterization of murmurs and recognition of the subtleties of abnormal heart sounds. Although as described and outlined in Table 32.4, the characteristics of a murmur can provide useful information when CHD is suspected, much of the data on the use of murmurs in isolation to detect congenital heart disease is based on the presence or absence of a murmur and not on the characteristics of that murmur (see Presentation section).

Chest X-ray

A chest x-ray is commonly carried out in any newborn presenting with respiratory symptoms or cyanosis. Its utility in the assessment of respiratory disease is well established (see Chapter 28). Although rarely diagnostic of specific cardiac lesions in the newborn period, it provides useful, rapid information as part of the workup for suspected cardiac disease where there is immediate clinical concern (cyanosis, increased respiratory effort). It is less useful in well babies presenting with a murmur. The "classical" cardiac silhouettes associated with specific lesions are shown in Table 32.4. Cardiomegaly is suggested by a cardiothoracic ratio greater than 0.6 in an anterior–posterior projection, although the cardiac border can be difficult to distinguish from the thymus. Poor quality films and those not taken in full inspiration can reduce accuracy. Increased pulmonary arterial and venous markings suggest increased pulmonary blood flow or, in particular, if there are prominent pulmonary venous markings, obstruction to pulmonary venous return either due to primary pulmonary vein obstruction or a raised left atrial pressure from left heart obstructive lesions or raised left ventricular end-diastolic pressure in the context of impaired left ventricular function (Fig. 32.1). Pulmonary edema is a late sign in left-to-right shunts.

In those presenting with cyanosis, decreased pulmonary vascular markings suggest impaired pulmonary blood flow either due to congenital heart disease or increased pulmonary vascular resistance. Cyanosis in association with increased pulmonary markings

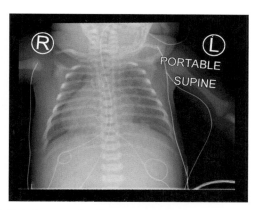

FIGURE 32.2 Dextrocardia. Chest x-ray demonstrating dextrocardia in a newborn with situs ambiguous, left atrial isomerism, unbalanced AVSD, and subaortic stenosis.

suggests common mixing with a net left-to-right shunt or transposition physiology with high pulmonary blood flow. The aortic arch position can be assessed as can the position of the heart within the chest (Fig. 32.2). Abnormalities in the bronchial branching pattern can be seen suggesting laterality disturbance. The chest x-ray may also reveal noncardiac lesions associated with congenital heart disease such as absence of the thymus or vertebral and rib abnormalities (Table 32.2).

Electrocardiography

A thorough examination of electrocardiography findings and arrhythmias is given in Chapter 34. The ECG, with care to ensure that the leads are placed in appropriate position, will also show the axis of the heart, the presence of ventricular hypertrophy and p wave axis, and conduction abnormalities associated with congenital heart disease (Table 32.4). Arrhythmias are discussed in Chapter 34.

Echocardiography

Two-dimensional Doppler and color Doppler echocardiography allows detailed, real-time, and immediate analysis of the cardiac and great vessel anatomy in small infants. The diagnosis of nearly all congenital heart disease is essentially now reliant upon this imaging modality. Neonates can be particularly good candidates for echocardiographic imaging with many having excellent imaging windows, and the safety of the technique is well established. Although fairly basic echocardiogram machines can provide the majority of the information, the use of small high-frequency probes and color analysis continues to improve the utility of this imaging modality. Doppler echocardiography demonstrates the direction and velocity of blood flow within the heart and vessels from which the pressure gradient can be derived. Color Doppler visualizes the anatomical point at which flow velocity changes in the setting of obstructive lesions as well as the flow across intracardiac shunts and the flow of valvar regurgitation (Fig. 32.3A). In addition to structural information, echocardiography allows immediate assessment of ventricular size, function, and myocardial thickness. More advanced echocardiographic techniques can be used to evaluate myocardial performance and diastolic function and assess cardiac output. Echocardiographic image acquisition can be limited in some infants, particularly those ventilated with high mean airway pressures resulting in a significant negative impact on the suitable windows. Complex extracardiac abnormalities with variations in aortic arch, pulmonary vein, or branch pulmonary artery anatomy may require additional cross-sectional imaging or occasionally cardiac catheterization to confidently delineate the pathology and reach a conclusive diagnosis.

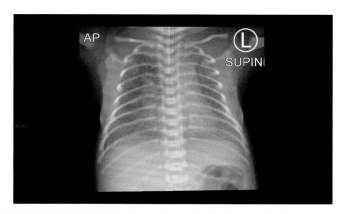

FIGURE 32.1 TAPVD. Chest x-ray demonstrating increased pulmonary vascular markings in a newborn with obstructed TAPVD with pulmonary veins draining into the SVC.

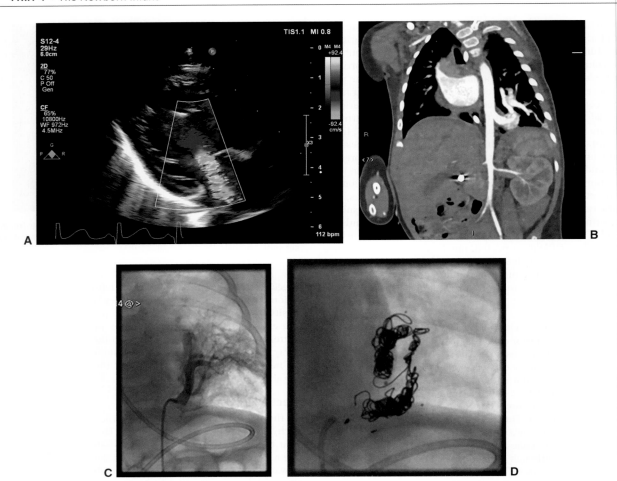

FIGURE 32.3 Unrecognized shunt. Images showing investigation hierarchy in congenital heart disease of a 4-week-old baby presenting with symptoms and signs of heart failure. **A:** Parasternal long-axis view showing a dilated left ventricle with annular stretch leading to mitral regurgitation. The suspected shunt could not be found on echocardiography, and therefore, a CT angiogram was carried out. **B:** CT angiogram which shows a large aortopulmonary collateral from the descending aorta to the left lung. **C:** Angiography with contrast injection directly into the large collateral vessel. **D:** This was embolized through the catheter with a series of coils and occlusion devices.

Delivering Structural Echocardiography

A prerequisite at all points in the care pathway for patients with known or suspected congenital heart disease (assessment following prenatal diagnosis, review of patients at risk of having CHD, as part of a pulse oximetry screening (POS) program, assessment of a murmur, assessment on the neonatal unit) is the availability and delivery of timely echocardiographic assessment. The majority of neonatal units now have ultrasound machines used to image a variety of organ systems. Many of these have the required probes for cardiac scanning, often as part of the increasing use of echocardiography by neonatologists to assess cardiac function, cardiac output, and the assessment of the arterial duct (Chapter 31). The widespread use of echocardiography for this functional assessment of babies with normal hearts has potential for inadvertent confusion and diagnostic delay in patients with suspected congenital heart disease. The causes of this are two-fold, the first is that the term echocardiogram is used for both a functional assessment and a full structural diagnostic study, and therefore, when a baby has a "normal" report, the echocardiogram may have been carried out only to look at the cardiac function and the presence or absence of a patent ductus arteriosus as opposed to confidently exclude congenital heart disease. The

second is that there is natural enthusiasm for those regularly carrying out functional echocardiography to extend their practice to assess babies with suspected congenital heart disease. However, the training, ongoing experience, and continuing professional development required to deliver accurate diagnostic structural echocardiography to a group of often unwell neonates who have the most to gain from early diagnoses and much to lose from delayed or missed diagnoses is very different from the equivalent professional skills required for functional assessment. Although gross abnormalities can be readily apparent (absence of the inlet valves, ventricular hypoplasia), other potentially lethal, yet entirely curable abnormalities, in particular abnormal pulmonary venous return and aortic arch obstruction, can be challenging to differentiate from structurally normal hearts with isolated pulmonary hypertension. Differentiation of the training requirements and roles when delivering echocardiography continues to be discussed with guidelines available for different health care systems (27). It should be noted that the majority of guidelines and training requirements refer to stable infants or those undergoing functional assessment. It remains vital that those carrying out structural echocardiography when CHD is suspected acutely are appropriately trained and are able to confidently exclude congenital heart disease. When providing or confirming a diagnosis, the clinician should also be clear in formulating an immediate management strategy and recognize when further advice or transfer to the cardiac center is required.

Cardiac Magnetic Resonance Imaging and Computerized Tomography

The excellent diagnostic quality of echocardiography in the infant allows the majority of cardiac problems to be diagnosed without additional cross-sectional imaging. However, where there is uncertainty after echo assessment, or complex abnormalities in extra-cardiac structures such the arch, pulmonary veins, or branch arteries are suspected, the anatomy can be clearly demonstrated using these modalities (Fig. 32.3B). Magnetic resonance imaging (MRI) and computerized tomography (CT) allow further appreciation of the anatomy and spatial relationships to other structures in the chest, facilitating more accurate interventional and surgical planning. CT angiography offers high-resolution imaging (down to 1 mm) of the cardiac chambers and vessels and is particularly useful for anatomical assessment of the pulmonary arteries to the peripheries, pulmonary veins, systemic-to-pulmonary collateral vessels, coronary arteries, and the aortic arch anatomy including assessment of laterality and vascular rings in infants. Modern CT scanners perform a detailed cardiac anatomical assessment in less than 1 second at radiation does approaching that of a chest x-ray. This often mitigates the need for ventilation in stable babies who can be scanned using a "feed and wrap" technique without sedation. MRI also provides anatomical detail but has the advantage of providing functional assessment, flow assessment, and tissue characterization of the ventricles and ventricular masses/cardiac tumors. MRI scan times are much longer (30 minutes to an hour for complete structural and functional assessment) and therefore often require general anesthetic, though some centers are increasingly advocating the use of feed and wrap techniques. However, further technologic developments to reduce scan times and post-processing techniques to decrease artifact from respiratory motion may remove the need for general anesthesia, increasing the scope of cardiac MRI in smaller patients.

Three-Dimensional (3D) Modeling and 3D Printing

The complete data set obtained from an MRI or CT scan can be used for 3D reconstruction of cardiac images allowing clear visualization of the cardiac anatomy and spatial relationships from all perspectives, potentially highlighting lesions that are less evident on conventional 2D imaging. This allows planning of interventional approaches and virtual dissection of the heart to plan intracardiac repair (Fig. 32.4). These data sets lend themselves ideally to 3D printing providing an anatomically accurate model of the heart allowing assessment of suitability for complex repair (e.g.,

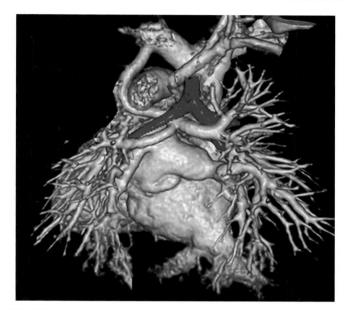

FIGURE 32.5 CT 3D reconstruction of neonate with hypoplastic left heart syndrome and anomalous pulmonary venous drainage. Spatial relationships of airway (colored *blue*) and position of ascending vein looping under the left main bronchus are clearly demonstrated.

the feasibility of tunneling ventricles to great arteries via the ventricular septal defect) simplifying and reducing surgical time, in some cases showing that the repair is possible and therefore avoiding single ventricle palliation (Figs. 32.5 and 32.6).

Diagnostic Cardiac Catheterization

Cardiac catheterization is carried out via sheaths placed in large vessels (usually femoral or jugular) and accurate pressure measurement and blood sampling carried out to calculate resistance and shunts with the catheters manipulated under fluoroscopy guidance. Contrast is injected to obtain angiographic images. MRI and CT imaging techniques have largely superseded both catheter-based hemodynamic assessment and catheter delivered angiography removing the morbidity from historically routine vascular puncture in neonates for cardiac assessment. In certain circumstances, the hemodynamic detail provided by invasive assessment is required, particularly where the relative implications of multiple potential causes for the infant's clinical state need to be differentiated (e.g., a patient with high pulmonary vascular resistance and an ongoing shunt or a postoperative cardiac patient with residual lesions). The main use of cardiac catheterization is now therapeutic rather than diagnostic (below) (Fig. 32.3C and D).

PRESENTATION, DIAGNOSIS, AND MANAGEMENT

Prenatal Diagnosis of Cardiac Disease

Fetal Echocardiography

The majority of congenital heart disease can be reliably diagnosed in the mid trimester and often earlier in specialist clinics within dedicated fetal echocardiographic programs. Initial detection rates are dependent on population access to the initial scan and the skills and ongoing training of sonographers who, following detection of abnormality, will refer on for detailed evaluation in the fetal cardiology clinic. Prenatal diagnosis is associated with improved preoperative condition that has translated into better postsurgical outcomes for certain lesions such as hypoplastic left syndrome (HLHS), coarctation of the aorta, and TGA (28,29). Following diagnosis and

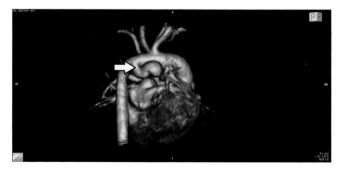

FIGURE 32.4 Reconstructed CT angiogram of the patient with a complex pulmonary atresia showing a highly tortuous duct (*arrow*) carried out as part of the assessment of pulmonary artery anatomy prior to consideration of ductal stenting.

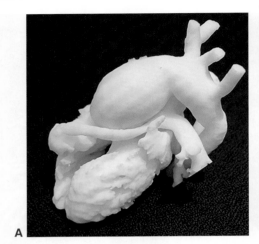
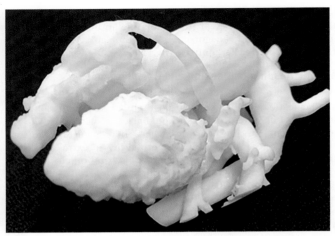

FIGURE 32.6 A and B: Printed model of a neonate with aortic atresia and VSD following palliation with the Norwood procedure. In figure B the model has been tilted and rotated to show the RV-PA shunt and descending aorta (**Fig. 32.5**).

counseling prenatal diagnosis provides the family with options on how to proceed with pregnancy; for complex lesions that cannot be repaired, this will include termination of pregnancy or choosing for compassionate care after birth. In those continuing with the pregnancy, this gives the family time to adjust and become informed about the CHD diagnosis and meet the team involved in postnatal care. Accurate diagnosis allows fetal cardiologists to formulate a perinatal management plan and, for some, delivery in a cardiac center where emergency treatment can be delivered promptly.

Population Prenatal Screening for Congenital Heart Disease

Most congenital heart disease will be diagnosed in "low-risk" pregnancies, and therefore, many countries worldwide have adopted anomaly screening programs. This scan is scheduled when echo windows are optimal at 18 to 24 weeks of gestation. Cardiac anatomy is assessed by visualizing the heart in cross-sectional views through the fetal thorax. Situs or laterality is assessed at the upper fetal abdomen, delineating the position of the descending aorta and inferior vena cava as well as the position of the fetal stomach, associated with usual atrial arrangement (situs solitus). The four-chamber cardiac view allows assessment of cardiac function, the atrioventricular valves and their offsetting (**Fig. 32.7**). The outflows and AV valves are identified as is the usual crossing arrangement of the great arteries (**Fig. 32.8**). The outflow valves in the fetus are very thin, mobile, and moving at high speed so can be difficult to see. Many screening programs will now include the "three-vessel view" or more importantly the "three-vessel and tracheal view" where the duct, superior vena cava, and transverse arch are identified in the upper mediastinum (30). When abnormalities in these views are identified, referral for detailed fetal echocardiography is made.

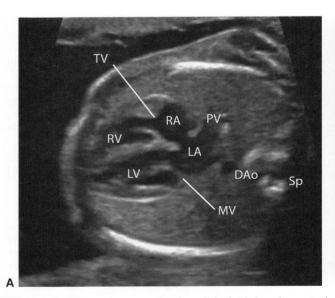
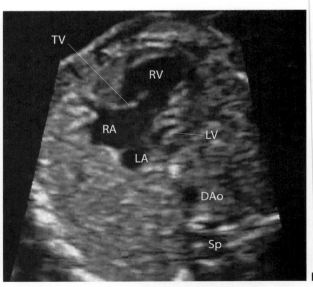

FIGURE 32.7 A: 4CH normal cross section through the fetal chest demonstrating a normal four-chamber view. The following structures are visualized: right and left atria (RA, LA); right and left ventricles (RV, LV); mitral (MV); and tricuspid valves (TV). Pulmonary veins (PV) can be seen entering the LA from the left and right sides. The descending aorta (DAo) lies in front of the fetal spine (Sp). **B:** 4CH HLHS four-chamber view in a fetus with hypoplastic left heart syndrome. There is small left atrium (LA) and rudimentary bright left ventricle (LV). The right atrium (RA) and right ventricle (RV) are the dominant structures separated by the tricuspid valve (TV).

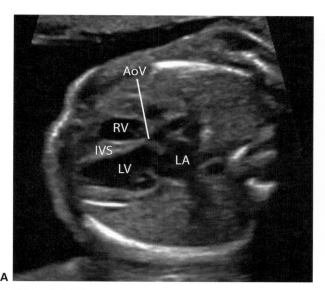 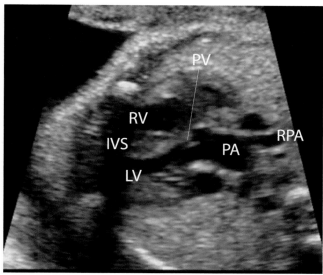

FIGURE 32.8 A: LVOT normal cross section through the fetal chest demonstrating a normal left ventricular outflow tract. The aorta valve (AoV) can be seen arising normally from the left ventricle (LV). The interventricular septum (IVS) is seen dividing the left and right ventricle (RV). Note the continuity between the septum and anterior wall of the aorta. The left atrium (LA) is connected to the LV by the mitral valve. **B:** Cross section through the chest of a fetus with transposition of the great arteries with intact ventricular septum. The vessel arising from the left ventricle (LV) is the main pulmonary artery (PA) that can be seen dividing; right pulmonary artery (RPA) is clearly visualized.

Prenatal Screening for Congenital Heart Disease in "High-Risk" Pregnancies

Introduction of early screening, particularly for nuchal translucency (NT) in the first trimester, will also identify fetuses at high risk for CHD (31). NT predicts CHD, and this risk increases with thickness measurement. Indication for fetal echocardiography varies by institution and resource, but this is usually greater than 99th centile for crown rump length (CRL) or an absolute value of greater than 3.5 mm. Transabdominal scanning in the fetal cardiology clinic can provide early diagnosis of severe forms of CHD at 13 to 14 weeks of gestation and transvaginal scanning at 10 to 12 may be offered weeks for high-risk groups.

Maternal, fetal, or familial factors that may increase the risk of the fetus being affected by CHD may be noted in early obstetric assessment and trigger referral for a specialist fetal echocardiogram in these pregnancies (Table 32.5). Many referrals will be for families affected by CHD in a previous pregnancy where thankfully often a detailed assessment reveals normal anatomy and provides welcome reassurance. Early assessments should be repeated at 18 to 24 weeks when windows are optimal to offer a further comprehensive assessment.

Fetal Cardiology Assessment

When abnormalities are suspected from the above detection programs, mothers are referred for detailed fetal cardiac assessment. This echocardiogram aims to detail the morphology and utilizes color-flow and pulsed- or continuous-wave Doppler to assess valve function and blood flow patterns in the great arteries and vessels. Cardiac function may be quantified using M Mode or other Doppler-derived indices (32,33) and fetal arrhythmia assessed using M mode. Documenting the movement at the atrial and ventricular walls allows assessment of AV conduction. It is recognized that even in specialist hands, some conditions remain challenging to reliably diagnose in the prenatal period such as coarctation of the aorta (34). Some specialist centers are beginning to use fetal MRI, particularly to look at extracardiac structures or delineate arch pattern or pulmonary venous anatomy (35). Following diagnosis at around 20 weeks, some forms of CHD evolve as gestation advances.

TABLE 32.5

Indications for Detailed Fetal Cardiac Assessment

Fetal	Maternal	Familial
Suspected abnormality at screening scan	CHD	Paternal CHD
Rhythm disturbance	Metabolic—pregestational diabetes, phenylketonuria	Previous fetus or sibling with CHD
Increased nuchal translucency		Inherited cardiac condition/cardiomyopathy (depending on type)
Extracardiac abnormality associated with CHD	Teratogens	
Chromosomal abnormality	Medications—for example, lithium, phenytoin, warfarin	Inherited genetic or chromosomal abnormality
Genetic syndrome		
Hydrops fetalis	Anti-Ro/SSA, anti-La/SSB often associated with maternal collagen vascular disease, for example, SLE, Sjögren's	
Pleural or pericardial effusion		
Monochorionic twins	Infections—for example, rubella, parvovirus	
Twin-to-twin transfusion syndrome	IVF	

When CHD is present, further identification of associated extracardiac abnormalities and ongoing assessment of fetal growth is undertaken. For many CHD lesions, fetal counseling encompasses the specific risk of underlying genetic or chromosomal abnormality. This is individualized by diagnosis. Options of invasive testing with chorionic villus sampling (>11 weeks) or amniocentesis (>15 weeks) are discussed (see Chapter 10). Details of potential surgical or interventional procedures and their immediate- and long-term outcomes are discussed as is any uncertainty in diagnosis or prognosis. Where severe disease is noted, particularly affecting the fetal right heart (systemic ventricle prenatally), for example, Ebstein anomaly of the tricuspid valve, there is a significant chance of intrauterine death. Where there are limited options or the family has chosen for compassionate care after birth, early involvement of the neonatal palliative care and parallel planning can provide time for the family to spend time with the baby either at home or in a specialist children's hospice environment.

Fetal Cardiac Intervention

Poor long-term outcomes of single ventricle CHD have encouraged clinicians to pursue fetal intervention, particularly where signs of evolving cardiac disease are noted early. Particular lesions whose progress may be delayed by fetal balloon dilation are outlet valve stenosis with the potential for reduced intrauterine growth of the subvalvar ventricle. Despite progress in technique, intrauterine fetal loss remains a significant risk (36).

Perinatal and Delivery Planning

Prenatal cardiac assessment allows perinatal planning to minimize risk to the baby, keep care close to home where possible, and optimize neonatal well-being, particularly where early intervention or surgery is necessary. For many biventricular conditions where there are well-developed and unobstructed outflow tracts (e.g., VSD, CAVSD), no changes are needed to routine obstetric and neonatal care. A period of observation to ensure normal saturations and establishment of feeding are needed postnatally, and arrangements should be made for early assessment in the cardiology clinic.

For infants with single ventricle CHD or duct-dependent physiology, delivery at or near a specialist cardiac center may be optimal. Early institution of a low-dose prostaglandin infusion can be safely administered in most neonatal units generally without the need for invasive ventilation. In contrast to those diagnosed postnatally, these neonates rarely need further Neonatal intensive care unit (NICU) support such as mechanical ventilation. Planning delivery at a specialist neonatal or cardiac center will often mean inducing labor near term (37). Normal vaginal delivery is possible for most CHD; only in a minority of cases will elective cesarean section be recommended for fetal cardiac reasons. Most commonly, this is where the fetal heart beat cannot be reliably monitored to assess fetal well-being, for example, in the fetus with complete heart block.

Very specific problems identified prenatally may require urgent or immediate intervention or surgery (see below).

Postnatal Detection of CHD

Screening and Opportunistic Checks

Particularly when antenatal detection is not available or limited, cardiology referral for postnatal screening should be considered for infants at higher risk of CHD, preferably by referral for echocardiography (Table 32.6).

Pulse Oximetry Screening for Critical Congenital Heart Disease

Despite advances in prenatal screening, a proportion of neonates will still go home with unrecognized critical congenital heart disease (CCHD). Routine newborn clinical examination will fail to

TABLE 32.6

Possible Teratogens for Congenital Heart Disease

Vitamin deficiency
Folate deficiency[a]
Environmental agents
High altitude,[a] organic solvents[a], dioxins[a], pesticides[a], irradiation
Drugs
Organic solvents
Ethanol,[a] folic acid antagonists ([a] trimethoprim,[a] sulfasalazine,[a] triamterene,[a] trimethadione,[a] phenytoin,[a] primidone,[a] phenobarbital,[a] carbamazepine,[a] methotrexate[a]), valproic acid,[a] lithium,[a] thalidomide,[a] retinoic acid,[a] antineoplastic agents (?), Coumadin,[a] amphetamine, cocaine
Metabolic factors
Maternal pregestational diabetes,[a] maternal phenylketonuria,[a] maternal obesity, homocysteine
Immune factors
Maternal autoimmune disease with anti-Ra anti-LA antibodies[b]
Infectious agents
Rubella,[a] influenza,[a] febrile illness,[a] mumps (?), cytomegalovirus (?)

[a]It is generally accepted that these prenatal factors increase the risk for congenital heart disease.

[b]Immune-mediated conduction block and myocarditis, no evidence to suggest increased incidence of structural abnormalities.

?, uncertain.

From Lage K, Greenway SC, Rosenfeld JA, et al. Genetic and environmental risk factors in congenital heart disease functionally converge in protein networks driving heart development. *Proc Natl Acad Sci U S A* 2012;109(35):14035. doi: 10.1073/pnas.1210730109; Feinstein JA, Benson DW, Dubin AM, et al. Hypoplastic left heart syndrome: current considerations and expectations. *J Am Coll Cardiol* 2012;59(1 suppl):S1. doi: 10.1016/j.jacc.2011.09.022; Jenkins KJ, Correa A, Feinstein JA, et al. Noninherited risk factors and congenital cardiovascular defects: current knowledge—a scientific statement from the American Heart Association Council on Cardiovascular Disease in the Young. *Circulation* 2007;115(23):2995. doi: 10.1161/CIRCULATIONAHA.106.183216; Jones KL. *Smith's recognizable patterns of human malformation/Kenneth Lyons Jones, Marilyn Crandall Jones, Miguel Del Campo*, 7th ed. Philadelphia, PA: Elsevier Saunders, 2013.Refs. (38–41).

identify 45% of cases of CCHD (42). Hospital stays following delivery have shortened in recent decades globally, and many neonates will be discharged home prior to complete transition to the postnatal circulation (with the ductus arteriosus remaining open). Those sent home with undiagnosed CCHD may then present in cardiovascular collapse following ductal closure and may die or suffer morbidity that may be lifelong. Efforts have been focused on identifying these infants who are often missed at prenatal anomaly screening and conventional newborn examination. Measuring oxygen saturations in the foot is an accurate, noninvasive, and reproducible test that will identify a newborn with CCHD that remains asymptomatic. In a meta-analysis including 437,000 newborns, the test had a sensitivity of 76.3% and specificity of 99.9% for detecting CCHD (43). After pulse oximetry screening (POS) was universally adopted in the United States, a review of 26 million newborns demonstrated mortality from CCHD fell by 33% (44). The decision not to provide POS in other countries such as the United Kingdom has been controversial in light of the evidence of improved survival. The national screening committee raised concern that false-positive tests could lead to over investigation of some healthy neonates, increased demand for echocardiography assessment and cause undue anxiety in some parents. Universal screening may have additional benefit as many newborns within the "false-positive group" were found to have other pathology such as sepsis or pneumonia following review on the neonatal unit (45). In targeted assessment of a newborn for suspected congenital heart disease, measurement of pre- and postductal saturations remains a useful tool with improved specificity in comparison with other noninvasive measurements such as four-limb blood pressure (46).

Postnatal Check, 6-Week Check, and Opportunistic Assessment

The schedule of postnatal review varies between health care systems. A standard postnatal check or predischarge check usually includes auscultation for cardiac murmurs and assessment of the femoral pulses. Heart murmurs are detected in between 1% and 2% of healthy term babies, though for many, this may reflect the transitional circulation or an innocent flow murmur. Neonatal echocardiography detects congenital heart disease in around 40% to 50% of these with a small but significant proportion requiring early surgery or intervention (47,48). The availability of neonatal echocardiography prior to discharge is limited in many units; therefore, further assessment is helpful to triage the urgency of referrals. Good practice should include evaluation of the murmurs character, intensity, location (where it is heard maximally), and any radiation (particularly to the back). Relevant clinical history should include any increased work of breathing, feeding difficulty, or failure to thrive. Where available, pre- and postductal saturations should be documented. Evidence of heart failure, respiratory distress, lower limb saturations of less than 95% (or >3% difference between pre- and postductal), or weak/absent femoral pulses should prompt urgent review. Four-limb blood pressure and chest x-ray are generally unhelpful in assessment of a neonate with a murmur (46). It would be advisable that neonates with a murmur remain in hospital for 24 hours to allow complete transition to the postnatal circulation. Some newborns without red flag symptoms or signs may be suitable for discharge and subsequent review in the cardiac clinic. Prior to discharge, parents should be aware of symptoms and signs to look out for that may prompt the need for more urgent review.

It is recognized that the newborn examination will continue to miss a significant proportion of neonates with CHD who are frequently initially asymptomatic and may not have a murmur (42). Neonatologists should be aware that advances in prenatal cardiac screening have changed the presentation of congenital heart disease in the postnatal period. Conditions that remain difficult to detect on prenatal examination such as coarctation, TAPVD, and valvular disease become a more probable "new" diagnosis for the infant presenting postnatally.

Clinical Presentation and Initial Management of CHD

Although we have chosen the headline groups of shock and cyanosis to describe presentation of critical congenital heart, there is considerable overlap in the way in which congenital heart disease presents and given the heterogeneous nature of each diagnosis, several different presentations within each headline diagnosis are possible. For example, critical left heart outflow obstruction with the potential to lead to shock may present with lower limb desaturation prior to the development of shock, particularly within a POS program. The initial management and approach to the infant, particularly where the diagnosis is not known antenatally is based on the clinical presentation as opposed to the final diagnosis. In addition to standard resuscitation and supportive care, early institution of prostaglandin to open or maintain patency of the arterial duct is required.

Prostaglandin

Prostaglandin E1 and E2 are produced by the placenta and act on the vascular smooth muscle in the prenatal duct maintaining its patency. Postnatal infusion of either prostaglandin E1 (alprostadil) or E2 (dinoprostone) will maintain patency of the duct and will also enlarge or reopen the constricting duct. Although there are some important adverse effects (below), prostaglandins are generally safe, particularly when compared with the potential life-threatening results of delayed treatment of critical CHD. The importance of early institution in newborns with suspected CHD cannot be overstated. Both medications are run as a continuous infusion due to their rapid metabolism and secure dedicated access should be

established. The initial dosing is dependent on the indication and clinical presentation. In cases with a prenatal diagnosis of CHD requiring postnatal patency of the arterial duct, otherwise well-cyanosed babies or an early postnatal diagnosis with a widely patent duct evident on echocardiogram a dose of 5 to 10 ng/kg/min is started. In less well neonates with suspected CHD, higher starting doses should be used (10 to 20 ng/kg/min). The dose should be titrated to clinical response or, if available, echocardiographic response. In unwell infants with clinical suspicion of CHD requiring ductal patency, the dose can be doubled every 20 minutes to a maximum of 100 ng/kg/min (49,50).

Apnea is a frequently observed side effect and is more common at higher doses, in unwell babies, and in premature infants. In stable babies, this can be managed by reducing the infusion to the lower end of the therapeutic range. Less well infants who have not shown a response will require ventilation. Pyrexia is often observed, and many babies without a definitive diagnosis will already be receiving treatment for possible infection. Tachycardia, vasodilation, and diarrhea may be seen though tend not to present a major clinical concern. Severe adverse effects such as disseminated intravascular coagulation are uncommon. Long-term intravenous prostaglandins can be used to allow time for growth of the infant before surgical intervention (see below). Cortical hyperostosis, gastric outlet obstruction syndrome, and vascular fragility are all reported following long-term use.

Oral dinoprostone is occasionally used when there is limited access to intravenous infusions or in some centers when there is a plan to maintain a patent duct for a longer period of time in lieu of intravenous prostaglandin. The initial oral dose is 20 to 40/kg initially given hourly, which can be gradually reduced to 4 hourly after a few days (50).

Oxygen Administration

An increase in the partial pressure of oxygen is one of the mechanisms by which the patent ductus arteriosus normally closes. In infants with congenital heart disease, there is therefore concern that giving oxygen will increase the speed of ductus arteriosus closure, which may be detrimental in duct-dependent lesions. However, the effect of oxygen is likely to be much less significant in terms of causing constriction of the patent ductus arteriosus in infants who are being started on prostaglandin, which should always be the case if significant congenital heart disease is suspected. However, oxygen causes significant reduction in pulmonary vascular resistance, and for patients with duct-dependent systemic circulations or obstruction to pulmonary venous return, the excess oxygen may have a deleterious effect by either reducing the systemic blood flow (by increasing the flow into the pulmonary arteries) or exacerbate pulmonary edema by decreasing the capillary pulmonary vascular resistance. Therefore, in babies presenting with suspected congenital heart disease, oxygen should be used with caution. This includes avoiding the hyperoxia test if there is rapid availability of echocardiography. Pragmatically administration of oxygen to a target saturation of 75% to 80% (consistent with the fetal ductal saturation) is a reasonable compromise until the diagnosis can be established.

Congenital Heart Disease Presenting Immediately after Birth

There are a number of congenital heart conditions that may present immediately after birth or in the first few hours of life that deserve special mention as prompt diagnosis and management is vital (Table 32.4). Although uncommon (as a group accounting for <1% of congenital heart disease), a degree of suspicion of these lesions needs to be maintained in babies presenting with suggestive signs immediately after birth who do not respond to conventional resuscitation. Those with complete or significant obstruction to pulmonary venous return (HLHS with intact or severely restrictive atrial septum or obstructed TAPVD) develop profound pulmonary edema, which may be hemorrhagic, associated with cyanosis, metabolic acidosis, and shock shortly after birth. The neonate with isolated TGA with restrictive atrial septum and arterial duct will be born with deep and persistent cyanosis leading to acidosis and circulatory compromise. Rapid diagnosis and intervention, particularly for those with TGA and intact atrial septum, result in immediate difference to the hemodynamic state. Further discussion with regard to the diagnosis and management of these patients is provided below.

Neonates with severe Ebstein anomaly of the tricuspid valve or tricuspid valve dysplasia require immediate NICU support and intensive medical management for the first few weeks of life. Mortality in this group remains high with a lack of good surgical options for the subset of patients presenting unwell immediately after delivery. Prenatal diagnosis is common in this group as chronic and severe tricuspid regurgitation *in utero* results in massive cardiomegaly and impaired forward flow through the right heart resulting in functional (pulmonary valve patent but not opening) or anatomical pulmonary atresia and underdeveloped lung arteries. In addition, persisting cardiomegaly from early gestation impacts on lung development, and right heart failure may result in fetal hydrops. Invariably those with severe disease require ventilation at birth. Prostaglandin is initiated in hypoxic newborns to provide ductal flow to the pulmonary arteries with deoxygenated blood bypassing the right side of the heart through the atrial sepal defect/patent foramen ovale. Early echocardiographic assessment is essential, and the decision as to whether there is anatomical or functional pulmonary atresia can be difficult. The usual high neonatal pulmonary artery resistance and the increased pulmonary artery pressure related to the open duct exacerbate the failing right sides ability to deliver forward flow through the pulmonary valve (functional atresia). Once the baby is stabilized, the prostaglandin may need to be stopped to reduce the pulmonary artery pressure related to ductal flow to assess whether there is forward flow through the pulmonary valve to differentiate functional from anatomical atresia. This is carried out in a setting where regular expert echocardiography can be undertaken and the prostaglandin restarted if required.

Rarely, CHD can have a significant impact on the airway presenting with respiratory distress immediately after birth. Absent pulmonary valve syndrome, with to and fro flow in the pulmonary artery, results in significant dilatation of the branch arteries *in utero*. Only postnatally does the significant bronchial compression become evident in some necessitating the need for positive pressure ventilation at birth.

Sustained fetal bradyarrhythmia due to complete heart block (with or without CHD) may result in the delivery of an unwell and hydropic neonate requiring maximal neonatal intensive care support. Chronotropic agents should be initiated, and early temporary pacing may be necessary (Chapter 34).

Presentation with Shock/Potential to Present with Shock in the First 2 Weeks

Neonates with critical left heart outflow obstruction either in isolation or in association with other cardiac lesions rely on right-to-left flow across the patient ductus arteriosus to provide the systemic circulation. As the ductus arteriosus begins to close in the first few hours to days of life, the systemic circulation becomes compromised, and the baby develops symptoms and signs of heart failure, which can progress rapidly to shock. Breathlessness develops due to pulmonary edema, and clinical signs of circulatory compromise including tachycardia and impaired perfusion. Those with critical aortic stenosis will have poor pulses and may have an ejection systolic murmur in the aortic area (**Fig. 32.9**). The murmur may be quieter or even absent when ventricular function is poor resulting in insufficient blood flow across the valve to produce the clinically

apparent murmur. Patients with aortic arch obstruction develop weak or absent femoral pulses, although pulses may be difficult to feel in all areas if the circulation is poor (**Fig. 32.10**).

Presentation of HLHS is variable. The neonate with a highly restrictive or intact atrial septum will present with deep cyanosis, pulmonary edema, and low cardiac output in the first few hours of life due to lack of egress of pulmonary venous return from the left atrium. More commonly, presentation is with signs of aortic arch obstruction. Irrespective of initial presentation, these patients can deteriorate rapidly; as the duct closes, there is excessive blood flow to the pulmonary circulation and limited retrograde flow to the coronary arteries leading to impairment of function of the systemic right ventricle. The vicious circle that this creates can be difficult to retrieve. The initial management of these babies is standard neonatal supportive care and to restore patency of the arterial duct with prostaglandin to allow provision of the systemic circulation from the right ventricle. Given the severe obstruction to cardiac outflow, these infants often have impaired cardiac function and commencement of intravenous inotrope should be considered. These infants are described in the section of infant presenting with heart failure, but there will also be cyanosis to various degrees due to the provision of systemic blood flow from the right ventricle through the ductus arteriosus in those with otherwise normally connected hearts or due to common mixing of systemic and pulmonary compulsory venous blood within the atrium or ventricles as part of the single ventricle circulation.

Other conditions presenting with heart failure or shock in the first few days of life include neonates with a primary myocardial problem with severely impaired ventricular function. This may be due to fetal and neonatal cardiomyopathy or neonatal myocardial infarction (see below). Sustained tachy- or bradyarrhythmia usually beginning in fetal life (see Chapter 34) has a variable impact on ventricular function depending on duration and ventricular rate. High output cardiac failure is noted in neonates with large systemic artery to systemic vein shunts such as vein of Galen malformations or hepatic shunting. Rarely, neonatal cardiac tamponade may occur in association with fetal hydrops.

Details of the findings of standard investigations are shown in Table 32.4; however, when critical left heart outflow obstruction is suspected, the most important investigation is early echocardiography.

Presentation with Cyanosis/Potential to Present with Cyanosis in the First 2 Weeks

The pathophysiology of cyanosis described previously provides the framework of the approach to any baby with desaturation. Specific diagnosis presenting with cyanosis and results of investigations are outlined in Table 32.4. Important information to differentiate a primary respiratory cause of cyanosis (pulmonary vein desaturation resulting from ventilation–perfusion mismatch), primary pulmonary vascular cause of cyanosis (right-to-left arterial and ductal shunting due to elevated pulmonary vascular resistance as seen in pulmonary hypertension of the newborn), and cardiac causes is obtained from the history, presentation, clinical assessment, investigations (including response to oxygen administration (hyperoxia test)), chest x-ray, and blood gases. Unfortunately, there is considerable limitation to these investigations in many infants leading to diagnostic uncertainty. Not least, this is due to the heterogeneous presentation of both respiratory and cardiac causes of cyanosis, overlap between diagnoses, and the potential for coexistence of diagnoses. For example, the oligemic chest x-ray seen in pulmonary hypertension of the newborn can be similar to a cardiac patient with obstruction to pulmonary blood flow and the pulmonary edema seen in patients with obstruction to pulmonary blood flow, in particular obstructed total anomalous pulmonary venous return, can be difficult to differentiate from the abnormalities seen

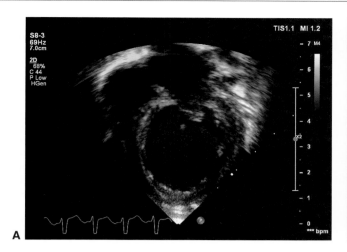

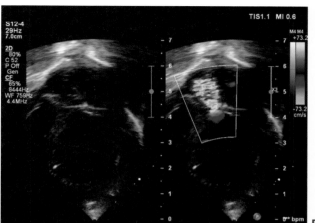

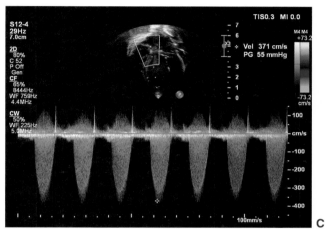

FIGURE 32.9 A: Apical four-chamber view shows a dilated ventricle with bright areas in the endocardium, which is endocardial fibroelastosis. **B:** Apical five-chamber view showing a small stenosed aortic valve with turbulence across it on color Doppler. **C:** Continuous wave Doppler across the aortic valve. The peak velocity is relatively low in keeping with the impaired ventricular function.

in respiratory disorders. Therefore, in any cases where there is doubt, early institution of prostaglandin to maintain patency of the arterial duct until a diagnosis confirmed is required. Patients with critical obstruction to or absence of pulmonary blood flow,

including Tetralogy of Fallot, pulmonary atresia with or without intact ventricular septum, and single ventricle patients with pulmonary outflow obstruction or pulmonary atresia, are dependent upon left-to-right flow across the patent ductus arteriosus

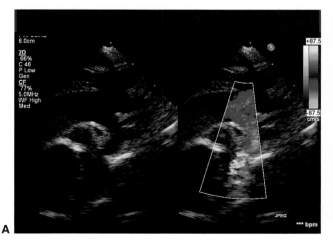

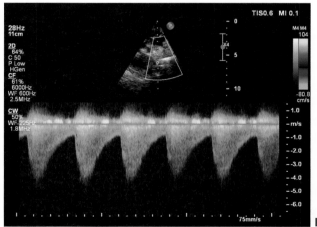

FIGURE 32.10 A: Suprasternal arch view showing juxtaductal coarctation with turbulent at the site of coarctation on color Doppler. **B:** Continuous wave Doppler in the suprasternal notch showing increased velocity through the site of coarctation and continued flow through the narrowing in diastole (sawtooth pattern).

THE NEWBORN INFANT

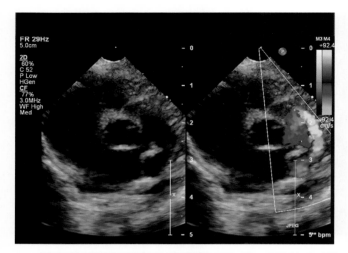

FIGURE 32.11 Parasternal short axis of a patient with pulmonary atresia, intact ventricular septum showing absent pulmonary valve, and blood supplied to the pulmonary arteries via the ductus arteriosus.

to supply pulmonary blood flow. As the ductus closes, therefore, these patients become increasingly cyanosed (**Fig. 32.11**).

Babies with TGA are dependent on mixing between the two parallel circulations. The most efficient position within the circulation this can occur is the atrial septum, and as described above,

although mixing can occur across a ventricular septal defect (if present) and the patent ductus arteriosus, both are limited as the pressure gradient between the systemic and pulmonary circulations tends to make this flow unidirectional rather than mixing.

The presentation of TAPVD is variable. The cyanosis in this setting is caused by right-to-left shunting at the atrial septum, and if there is high pulmonary blood flow and unrestricted flow (unobstructed TAPVD), this can be mild and not clinically apparent initially. Babies with obstruction to pulmonary venous return present with desaturation, pulmonary edema, and heart failure/shock (**Fig. 32.12**). This is particularly the case in infants with infradiaphragmatic TAPVD (obstructed at the liver) but also some patients with supracardiac TAPVD (obstructed due to compression of the ascending vein between the pulmonary artery and bronchus) and those with obstruction at the atrial septum. The pulmonary edema itself exacerbates the desaturation due to pulmonary vein desaturation in addition to right-to-left flow. Low cardiac output results from limitation of flow into the left ventricle. Signs of obstruction should prompt urgent assessment and transfer to a cardiac surgical center to facilitate early repair as medical management will rarely stabilize the circulation (see below).

The need to maintain patency of the arterial duct using prostaglandin is clear in critical obstruction to pulmonary blood flow to ensure left-to-right ductal flow into the pulmonary arteries. For neonates with TGA, maintenance of patency of the arterial duct allows a site for mixing, although perhaps more important is the left-to-right flow, which volume loads the left atrium potentially

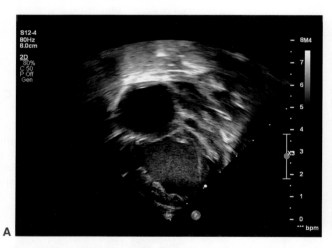

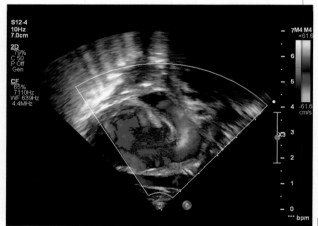

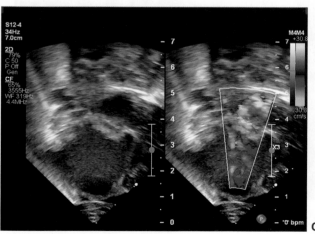

FIGURE 32.12 A: Apical four-chamber view of a 10-hour-old baby with severe cyanosis, acidosis, and pulmonary edema showing a hugely dilated right ventricle with a compressed slit-like left ventricle. **B:** Subcostal view. The pulmonary veins drain to the coronary sinus and into the right atrium. Usually, these patients do not present unwell; however, in this case, there was significant obstruction to right-to-left flow across the atrial septum **C.**

improving left-to-right flow at the atrial septum and improving effective systemic blood flow. Ductal patency is less important in patients with total anomalous pulmonary venous return and may exacerbate pulmonary edema in patients with obstructed pulmonary venous return. However, these patients will have significant pulmonary hypertension, and therefore, right-to-left flow at the duct will augment cardiac output. In neonates with severe pulmonary hypertension (Chapters 28 and 31), the same argument applies, preserving systemic flow by opening the duct albeit at the expense of desaturation in the lower limbs. There are known disadvantages of a widely patent ductus arteriosus in neonates with a primary respiratory problem due to unnecessary left-to-right flow at that level. However, in the first few hours and days of life, the high pulmonary vascular resistance in these babies will provide some protection from excessive pulmonary blood flow. Starting prostaglandin to maintain patency of the arterial duct is therefore potentially lifesaving with very little disadvantage in any baby in whom there is a suspicion of congenital heart disease while awaiting echocardiographic assessment and a definitive diagnosis.

Presentation with Heart Failure and/or Cyanosis beyond the First 2 Weeks of Life

The majority of critical left heart outflow obstruction and many cyanotic lesions described above will present in the first 2 weeks of life within the time scale of closure of the patent ductus arteriosus. Delayed closure of the ductus and therefore late presentation of these lesions must continue to be considered in infants developing breathlessness, signs of circulatory compromise, or cyanosis beyond the first 2 weeks. Prostaglandin infusion to open the arterial duct is less effective in older infants (usually requiring higher doses) and given the potential diagnoses in those presenting later is likely to be less useful. However, its use should still be considered in those with suggestive symptoms/signs up to about 4 weeks of age.

Less severe variations of the lesions described above including severe aortic stenosis, moderate coarctation of the aorta, tetralogy of Fallot (and variants), and unobstructed TAPVD can present at any time from birth with heart failure or desaturation. The timing is dependent on the degree of obstruction to pulmonary or systemic blood flow, whether the degree of desaturation is clinically apparent and the types of neonatal screening deployed prior to discharge.

When the pulmonary vascular resistance begins to fall (the timing of this may be variable), left-to-right shunting increases, and infants with these conditions begin to develop signs of heart failure associated with the increased pulmonary blood flow. Infants with left-to-right shunting at arterial level (truncus arteriosus, aortopulmonary window) tend to present earlier, sometimes within the first 2 weeks due to both systolic and diastolic flow into the pulmonary arteries (Fig. 32.3). Truncus arteriosus, in particular, can present with rapidly developing heart failure when there is associated regurgitation or stenosis of the truncal valve. Those with an isolated shunt at ventricular level (VSD, CAVSD, single ventricle without outflow obstruction) will present with these signs between 2 weeks and 2 months of age. However, some, particularly those with trisomy 21 and those with concomitant lung disease or airway problems, may not drop the pulmonary vascular resistance to the extent that the intracardiac shunt becomes apparent. A high index of suspicion therefore needs to be maintained to ensure that congenital heart disease is excluded in these cases. Other lesions presenting at this time with heart failure include congenital aortic and mitral regurgitation.

Presentation of Complex Congenital Heart Disease

Often, there is unnecessary anxiety about the presentation and initial management of complex congenital heart disease. Although the precise detail of the diagnosis and highly accurate anatomical information is vital for management at the cardiac center, the initial management is as described above. For example, although the final diagnosis maybe a complex single ventricle with coarctation of the aorta, the initial presentation and management will be as with isolated coarctation of the aorta (prostaglandin and referral for echocardiography).

Cardiology and Cardiac Surgical Diagnosis and Management

On arrival at the cardiac center, supportive measures and prostaglandin infusion continues until there is a definitive diagnosis. Echocardiography following a sequential segmental approach is often sufficient, but further cross-sectional imaging may be required to secure the final diagnosis and plan appropriate intervention or surgery.

Decision-Making at the Surgical Center

Perhaps, the antithesis of progress made in diagnostic imaging, cardiac intensive care, interventional cardiology, and cardiac surgery is the lack of a clear evidence base for many of the interventions available as well as their optimal timing. Unit preference and center volume play a part in the decision-making. For example, large surgical centers will be able to offer all three options described below for children with HLHS, whereas small units will tend to concentrate on a specific preferred palliation technique. In many units, treatment options will be discussed and final decisions made in multidisciplinary team meetings. Factors that impact on outcomes such as extracardiac comorbidities, prematurity, syndromic diagnoses, and birth weight/growth are integral to planning and deciding on future treatment. The team will need to take into account noncardiac interventions when looking at the care pathway of a complex neonate. Understanding the parent's wishes and concerns are a vital part of this team decision-making process. Available health care resources and the ability of the family to pay for care clearly dictate what treatment can be offered in some health care settings. This sadly means cardiac surgery or some treatment options will not be accessible. For infants, some decision-making relies on the role of visiting congenital heart teams offering the prospect of cardiac surgical repair. Where access to health care is limited, it is often unrealistic to offer treatment for infants with more complex and single ventricle lesions.

Exit Procedures

In antenatally recognized diagnoses, which are known to cause immediate cardiac, compromise following delivery requires careful planning of a procedure immediately after delivery can be considered. For those with TGA with intact atrial and ventricular septum, immediate septostomy can be carried out in the delivery room or on the neonatal unit using umbilical venous access and echocardiography to guide the procedure. More complex surgical procedures such as early relief of obstructed TAPVD and hybrid transatrial stenting in patients with HLHS intact atrial septum require the immediate availability of a cardiac surgical and interventional team. Practically cardiac surgical centers are often remote from delivery units. Success has been reported when arrangements are made for the infant to be delivered in the cardiac surgical center and moved immediately to the operating room for relief of critical intracardiac obstruction, which would otherwise cause demise soon after delivery (51).

Establishing Systemic Blood Flow
Aortic Stenosis

Patients with a diagnosis of severe or critical aortic stenosis require a detailed assessment of left ventricular size prior to planning intervention. In some cases, the left ventricle may be inadequate to support the systemic circulation, and a proportion of these patients will therefore need to be considered for single ventricle palliation. In the majority, where the left ventricular size is adequate, the initial management is focused on preserving the native aortic valve for as long as possible to delay (and in some cases avoid) aortic valve replacement. The options available are balloon aortic valvotomy carried out percutaneously or open surgical valvotomy. Although there is some controversy as to the preferred technique, and practices vary between the units, the most likely determinant of outcome from either procedure is the anatomy of the aortic valve, with small thickened unicuspid valves presenting much more of a challenge in terms of an optimal result than a well-developed fused trileaflet aortic valve. If the initial "valve sparing" procedure is unsuccessful or cannot be carried out, then consideration can be given to replacing the aortic valve. Small prosthetic valves and homografts can be used, although both have significant problems, particularly in terms of the longevity of the valve in a rapidly growing infant. The neonatal Ross procedure (replacing the native aortic valve with the patient's own pulmonary valve and positioning a right ventricle to pulmonary artery conduit to replace the autograft) can be used successfully, although requires long bypass time and surgical expertise and experience.

Coarctation of the Aorta
Surgery for neonatal coarctation of the aorta has evolved to be an almost "curative" procedure for the majority of infants with isolated coarctation. For discrete short segment coarctation, surgical removal of the area of coarctation with end-to-end anastomosis via lateral thoracotomy is the preferred technique and avoids the need for cardiopulmonary bypass (CPB). In neonates with a long segment coarctation or hypoplasia of the transverse arch, a subclavian flap can be deployed to augment the narrowed arch. The advantage of both techniques is native tissue will continue to grow with the baby. Postsurgical balloon dilation of the area of anastomosis is occasionally required. More complex coarctation with aortic arch hypoplasia or obstruction (often in association with other cardiac abnormalities) requires median sternotomy and CPB, while more extensive arch repair and reconstruction with homograft or pericardial patch is carried out.

Hypoplastic Systemic Outflow
In neonates with hypoplasia of the systemic outflow (in particular HLHS) or intracardiac obstruction of the systemic outflow (in particular single ventricle patients with subaortic obstruction), the native pulmonary valve and pulmonary artery are used to replace or augment the systemic flow and an alternative source for pulmonary blood flow deployed. The ascending aorta is connected directly to the pulmonary artery, which is disconnected from the branch pulmonary arteries (Damus-Kaye-Stansel procedure); this then allows ejection of blood from the ventricular mass through both outlet valves into the systemic circulation. For infants with aortic atresia, this allows vital retrograde flow into the small aortic root, perfusing the coronary arteries. An extension of this to include aortic arch reconstruction is known as the Norwood procedure. Prior to advent of this surgical technique, infants with HLHS did not survive. The three most commonly used surgical techniques are shown in **Figure 32.13**. The originally described Norwood procedure consisted of a Damus-Kaye-Stansel procedure, aortic arch reconstruction, and insertion of a systemic to pulmonary artery Gore-Tex shunt to provide pulmonary blood flow. Postoperative hemodynamic instability related to the systemic to pulmonary artery shunt has led to many units favoring placement of the shunt between the right ventricle and pulmonary artery (Sano modification) removing the diastolic connection between the systemic circulation and pulmonary artery. An alternative option is the hybrid Norwood procedure; here, the chest is opened, and Gore-Tex bands are placed on both branch pulmonary arteries to limit pulmonary flow. A stent is then placed in the arterial duct allowing maintenance of systemic circulation. While there are theoretical advantages to each of these procedures, there is no clear outcome difference between them (53,54).

Improving Intracardiac Mixing—Balloon Atrial Septostomy
Inability to deliver a robust way of mixing the systemic venous return and pulmonary venous return at atrial level to maintain satisfactory saturations in babies with TGA is historically one of the main causes of early mortality. Immediate improvement in survival of these infants was reported with the introduction of various techniques to establish this interatrial communication, which has now become standardized as balloon atrial septostomy (BAS). The procedure is particularly urgent in those with profound cyanosis with a small or absent atrial communication; however, the procedure is also considered to improve mixing in patients with transposition with ventricular septal defect or in patients with complex transposition to improve mixing and delay the need for surgery. BAS can be safely carried out under echo guidance on the neonatal unit shortly after delivery, and timely intervention is vital for the profoundly cyanosed neonate or those who are prenatally been identified to have an intact or highly restrictive atrial septum. The balloon catheter is passed into the right atrium via the umbilical or femoral vein and then into the left atrium. The balloon is inflated in the left atrium and pulled back sharply to tear open the foramen flap valve, creating an atrial septal defect and

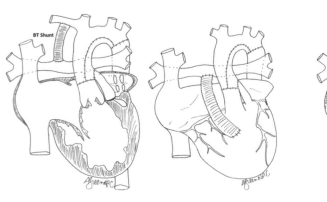
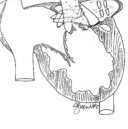

A Norwood Procedure with BT shunt   **B** Norwood Procedure with RV to PA shunt   **C** Hybrid Stage I Procedure

FIGURE 32.13 Diagram illustrating Norwood procedures and hybrid procedures. (Reproduced with permission from Nieves JA, Rudd NA, Dobrolet N. Home surveillance monitoring for high risk congenital heart newborns: improving outcomes after single ventricle palliation—why, how & results. *Prog Pediatr Cardiol* 2018;48:14. doi: 10.1016/j.ppedcard.2018.01. 004. Copyright © 2018 Elsevier. With permission. Ref. 52.)

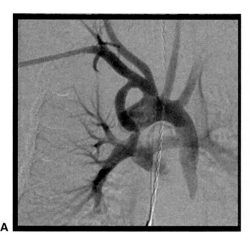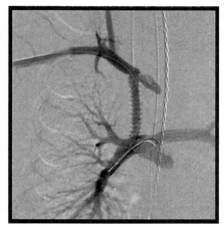

FIGURE 32.14 A: Digitally subtracted angiogram carried out through the right axillary artery puncture demonstrating a ductus arteriosus from the right subclavian artery in a patient with pulmonary atresia (the unusual origin of the duct had been predetermined by CT scanning). **B:** Angiogram showing a 3.5-mm stent within the ductus arteriosus inserted over the wire as the initial palliation to secure pulmonary blood flow.

often immediate improvement in oxygen saturation. Some centers prefer to avoid BAS in view of concerns about potential neurologic injury related to air or microclots as these will preferentially flow through the septostomy to the left-sided structures and aorta. However, the procedure remains potentially lifesaving in a subset of infants with profound cyanosis (55). Further indications for BAS include securing right-to-left flow in patients with tricuspid atresia or pulmonary atresia with intact ventricular septum and improving left-to-right flow in patients with obstructed pulmonary venous return from the left atrium egress obstruction.

Augmentation of Pulmonary Blood Flow

The use of a surgically placed anastomosis between the subclavian or other systemic artery and the pulmonary artery is a long established highly effective way of ensuring pulmonary blood flow in many types of congenital heart disease with no or limited flow to the pulmonary arteries. The initially described Blalock-Taussig Thomas shunt was used in older children with its use in newborn infants limited by the complexity of the anastomosis in small children and the excess pulmonary blood flow that resulted. The move to a Gore-Tex shunt provided more controlled pulmonary blood flow and has completely superseded the originally described shunt.

The shunt is used to augment or entirely provide pulmonary flow in neonates with pulmonary obstruction irrespective of the final destination (complete repair in patients with two good sized ventricles or as part of a staged single ventricle palliation strategy). Despite the immense success of the technique, significant concerns surround periprocedural instability due to the need for surgery itself (which may require CPB) and the diastolic flow through the shunt resulting in "steal" from the systemic circulation (56). These factors, and the desire to palliate increasingly high-risk neonates with complex cardiac anatomy and/or comorbidity, result in a significant early mortality after the procedure. An alternative increasingly utilized strategy to secure systemic to pulmonary artery flow is to stent the patent ductus arteriosus (**Fig. 32.14**) (57). Detailed analysis of the ductal morphology and pulmonary artery anatomy is undertaken prior to the ductal stent procedure to assess suitability as well as the intended approach (by the femoral, carotid, or axillary artery or transvenously through the heart into the aorta). Again, there have been no controlled trials comparing these two techniques. However, the results of ductal stenting as an alternative to systemic to pulmonary shunt are promising, and the increasing use of ductal stenting to augment point blood flow is apparent in many health care systems (**Fig. 32.15**).

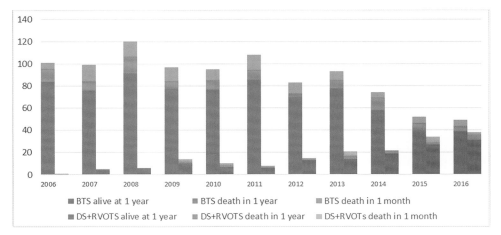

FIGURE 32.15 Data showing the frequency and the survival of patients undergoing BT shunt in the first month of life in the United Kingdom compared to the numbers undergoing ductal stenting or right ventricular outflow tract stenting. There has been a clear move away from BT shunts with compatible survival rates from the newer procedures. (Data from National Institute for Cardiovascular Outcomes Research (NICOR) [internet]. London, England: UCL, 2019. Available from: nicor4.nicor.org.uk/CHD/an_paeds.nsf/WBenchmarksYears?openview&RestrictToCategory=2015&start=1&count=500. Ref. 58.)

THE NEWBORN INFANT

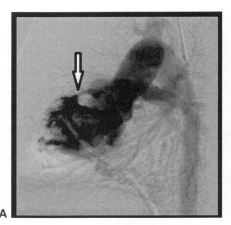
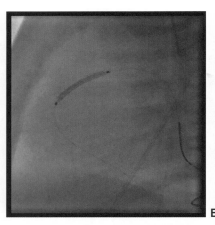
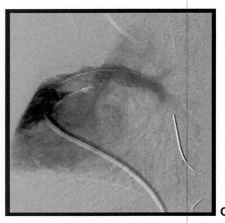

FIGURE 32.16 A: Lateral digitally subtracted angiogram in the right ventricle showing extremely tight infundibular narrowing (*arrow*) in a neonate with tetralogy of Fallot and severe cyanosis. The majority of contrast enters the aorta. **B:** A wire has been placed across the pulmonary outflow tract, and a stent passed over the wire into position across the muscular subpulmonary narrowing. **C:** The stent has been deployed with improved flow in the right ventricular outflow tract and into the pulmonary arteries.

For infants with significant desaturation or cyanotic spells as a result of subpulmonary and valvular obstruction (e.g., tetralogy of Fallot) who are considered too small for complete repair or in those with hypoplastic pulmonary arteries, stenting of the right ventricular outflow tract has become a valuable technique to improve pulmonary flow. The femoral vein or internal jugular vein is accessed percutaneously and the right ventricle outflow tract crossed with a wire over which the stent is passed and deployed across the outflow tract (**Fig. 32.16**). This improves forward flow, oxygen saturations and allows both growth of the pulmonary arteries and the infant, facilitating complete repair at a later stage (59,60).

Neonates with severe pulmonary stenosis presenting with cyanosis due to right-to-left flow across the atrial septum undergo balloon pulmonary valvotomy in the catheter laboratory usually with excellent results (**Fig. 32.17**). Echocardiography identifies patients with valvar pulmonary atresia that can be considered for radiofrequency perforation of the pulmonary valve followed by balloon pulmonary valvotomy. Prior to the procedure, careful assessment of the right ventricular size, function, and tricuspid valve are required to assess its potential ability to support the pulmonary

circulation. It is important to exclude coronary artery to right ventricular fistulae, which are common in this setting, as when the pulmonary valve obstruction is released and the right ventricle is decompressed, there can be immediate death due to loss of coronary perfusion pressure (**Fig. 32.18**).

Biventricular Repair
Timing of biventricular repair for many CHD lesions remains variable worldwide and depends on unit preference. In some conditions, there may be improved surgical results in more mature, heavier infants. However, for neonates with hypoxemia, delaying repair may have a deleterious effect on brain development with the potential to impact on neurodevelopment. For infants where definitive repair is deferred, this means a period of close observation, medical management, and regular visits to the cardiac clinic. Maintenance of good nutrition, supporting feeding, and promoting optimal growth are vital in this period. Many CHD infants have an imbalance in calorie intake and energy expenditure and will benefit from calorie-dense high-energy feeds. Oromotor skills may be limited, particularly in neonates with syndromic diagnoses or

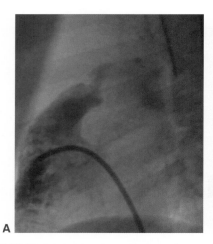
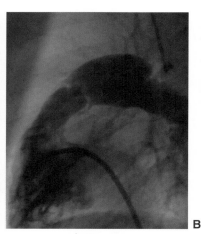
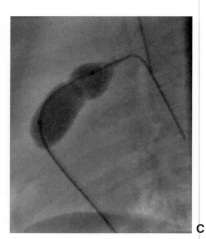

FIGURE 32.17 A: Lateral angiographic image from early in the contrast injection showing significant narrowing of flow through the pulmonary valve. **B:** Image from later in the injection cycle showing a thickened pulmonary valve. **C:** Balloon inflation across the pulmonary valve showing the waist on the balloon, which is abolished further balloon inflation pressure to relieve the stenosis.

and avoiding the need for any early intervention. Between 3 and 12 months of age, suitable single ventricle patients undergo a cavopulmonary anastomosis (connection of the superior vena cava to the pulmonary artery) removing pulsatile flow from the lungs. This is followed by total cavopulmonary (connection of the inferior vena cava to the pulmonary artery) anastomosis at between 2 and 5 years of age. Low pulmonary vascular resistance is vital for both these operations to work as pulmonary blood is provided by passive continuous flow from the systemic veins.

Cardiac Tumors

Cardiac tumors are rare at all ages. Rhabdomyomas are the commonest seen in neonates and constitute 45% to 80% of cardiac tumors noted in childhood. The majority are identified on prenatal scanning or sometimes as an incidental finding for echocardiography carried out for another reason. They are often multiple and are noted as well-circumscribed echo-bright, homogenous finely speckled lesions usually arising within the ventricles. Occasionally, large tumors can cause obstruction to the inflow valves, whereas even small lesions can obstruct outflow of cardiac chambers depending on position. Compression of the conduction system or the tumor providing an abnormal electrical connection between the atrium and ventricle can cause dysthymia. Rhabdomyomas regress over time, although neonatal surgery may occasionally be required to relieve obstruction (61). These tumors are frequently associated with the autosomal dominant condition tuberous sclerosis, with some studies suggesting that the condition was seen in 95% of fetuses or newborns with multiple rhabdomyomas (62).

OUTCOMES

Survival

In the majority of established congenital heart programs, the early survival for biventricular isolated congenital heart disease is approaching 100%. Although there is a mortality risk with any procedure or run of CPB, mortality in these conditions is often associated with noncardiac comorbidity as opposed to as a direct result of the intervention itself. Survival for infants with complex congenital heart disease, particularly single ventricle patients, continues to improve. For severe forms of congenital heart disease, in particular HLHS, the mortality is often dependent upon the case selection and underlying anatomy (63). For example, a well-grown baby with isolated HLHS with good ventricular function and no tricuspid regurgitation has a much better prognosis than an infant impaired ventricular function, significant tricuspid regurgitation, or a restrictive atrial septum. Comparison of unit outcomes based on survival alone may be misleading as case selection has a significant impact on reported survival.

Neurodevelopmental Outcomes

Even after excluding infants with chromosomal abnormalities and abnormality sequences associated with developmental delay, there is compelling evidence that many neonates with congenital heart disease have prenatally impaired brain development, with smaller brain volumes and reduced head circumference. These babies are at risk of developmental delay before presentation and subsequent intervention (64). There is a positive correlation between the severity of CHD and the degree of developmental delay noted in childhood. Preexisting problems with brain development partially explain this though there are considerable postnatal risks. Periods of severe hypoperfusion or cyanosis at presentation can cause neurologic injury as can low cardiac output states following surgical correction. Systemic emboli in patients with right-to-left shunting and TGA leading to stroke are well recognized. Considerable effort is made to maintain brain perfusion during CPB and to reduce cerebral metabolism with hypothermia. While short runs

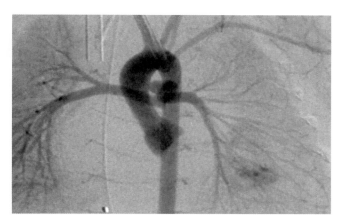

FIGURE 32.18 Digitally subtracted angiogram of a patient with pulmonary atresia intact ventricular septum who has deteriorated rapidly following presentation with cyanosis and was urgently cannulated on to VA ECMO. The angiogram was taken through the ECMO circuit. No coronary arteries can be seen arising from the aorta (coronary artery ostium atresia) with the only supply to the coronary arteries being from right ventricle to coronary artery fistulae. The patient was urgently listed for cardiac transplantation, which was successfully undertaken.

comorbidities where the insertion of a nasogastric or gastrostomy tube may be needed to feed or supplement oral intake. Regular input from dietetic services, cardiac specialist nurses, and speech and language therapists is invaluable in maintaining well-being and growth in this period prior to surgery. Infants with chronic left-to-right shunt may benefit from diuretic therapy to reduce pulmonary edema and breathlessness. There is little evidence to support the use of angiotensin-converting enzyme (ACE) inhibitors in this group.

Some units prefer to carry out an early biventricular repair in the neonatal period rather than palliate the infant with BT shunt or ductal stent. This minimizes the total number of procedures and avoids the risk of interstage mortality after the initial palliation. However, the surgery requires considerable expertise in small infants who may also be more vulnerable to CPB. Physiology necessitates early complete repair of other lesions such as obstructed TAPVD where the pulmonary venous confluence is anastomosed to the left atrium. The exacting timing of the arterial switch procedure for TGA remains controversial but should be performed in the first few weeks before the left ventricle becomes detrained in the subpulmonary position.

Surgical repair of systemic to pulmonary shunt lesions tend to be undertaken when infants begin to struggle with increasing breathlessness and difficulty feeding. For those with predominant shunting at ventricular level (VSD, CAVSD), this is usually carried out between 6 and 16 weeks of age depending on growth, other comorbidities, and clinical progress. Infants with significant comorbidities, small size, or prematurity may benefit from pulmonary artery banding (placed to limit pulmonary blood flow); this reduces breathlessness, facilitates growth, and delays the need for bypass surgery. Repair may be required within the first 2 weeks in neonates with truncus arteriosus and is particularly complicated for those with truncal valve stenosis or regurgitation.

Staged Single Ventricle Palliation
The initial management of single ventricle patients and surgical and interventional strategies for providing either systemic or pulmonary blood flow are described above. Patients with two unobstructed outflow tracts from the single ventricle will require pulmonary artery banding to limit pulmonary blood flow. A small subset develops the right amount of pulmonary obstruction from pulmonary valve or branch stenosis, creating a balanced circulation

of CPB with adequate brain protection seem to be safe in terms of gross neurologic and developmental outcome, more sensitive assessments that examine complex skills, such as attention, processing speed, and visual–spatial ability show impairments. Higher rates of attention deficit hyperactivity disorder have also been reported (65).

Long-Term Cardiac Outcomes

A proportion of infants will require further surgery and/or intervention following biventricular repair, with the staged palliation strategy for single ventricle patients described above. Patients with aortic valve abnormalities invariably require further repair or valve replacement following primary valvuloplasty or valvotomy. Any infants requiring placement of a right ventricle to pulmonary artery conduit (e.g., pulmonary atresia or truncus arteriosus) will need these replaced during childhood as they outgrow their conduit and/or conduit regurgitation develops. Following tetralogy of Fallot repair (particularly where a transannular patch has been used), regular monitoring is required to evaluate pulmonary regurgitation and right ventricular size and function with pulmonary valve replacement commonly needed in late teenage years or as young adults.

For neonates embarking on a single ventricle palliation strategy, long-term outcomes remain hugely variable depending on underlying anatomy, dominant ventricular morphology, and comorbidities. For patients with dominant RV morphology (HLHS) and particularly with high-risk findings or comorbidity, there is ongoing mortality risk throughout childhood. Published survival rates from fetal diagnosis (with intention to treat) to total cavopulmonary connection is around 70% in high volume, high performing centers (63,66). For patients (often with more favorable anatomy) reaching total cavopulmonary connection, reported long-term outcome is that 76% are alive 25 years from TCPC completion (67).

Although the age at death of the population of adults with congenital heart disease now approaches that of the normal population, these studies include all patients with congenital heart disease including minor congenital heart disease (68). For patients under ongoing follow-up, the median age of death is 48 years, and the development of heart failure in adults with congenital heart disease is a major concern (69). It is recognized that adults with congenital heart disease are likely to have additional problems with employment and life insurance and, in some studies, have lower health-related quality-of-life scores (70).

NEONATAL CARDIOMYOPATHY

Cardiomyopathies are primary disorders of the myocardium, which often result in impaired systolic and/or diastolic function and/or electrical disturbance. The disease can be isolated to the myocardium or occur as part of a systemic disease affecting other organ systems. There are many classification systems. A simplified clinically useful approach is based on clinical and echocardiographic findings broadly classifying neonatal cardiomyopathy into dilated cardiomyopathy (DCM) (including myocarditis), hypertrophic cardiomyopathy (HCM), and restrictive cardiomyopathy (RCM), although mixed pictures occur. Many other diagnoses including congenital heart disease, tachyarrhythmia, and metabolic derangement also have effects on cardiac function and the myocardium. These are better defined under their diagnosis with a description of the ventricular function as opposed to being given the diagnosis cardiomyopathy.

Epidemiology, Pathophysiology, and Etiology

Cardiomyopathy accounts for 1% of all cardiac disease and 10% of deaths in childhood from cardiac disease (71). It is important to exclude causes, which share phenotypical features of cardiomyopathy, particularly those that can be reversed following treatment

TABLE 32.7

Causes of Ventricular Failure to Be Excluded Before Diagnosis of Cardiomyopathy

Cardiac causes to be excluded
Anomalous origin of left coronary artery
Coarctation of the aorta
Critical aortic valve stenosis
Severe pulmonary hypertension
Tachycardia induced (incessant SVT or VT)
Work overload ("burnt out" shunts and valve regurgitation)

Potentially reversible causes to be excluded
Asphyxia
Bacterial sepsis (endotoxemia, exotoxemia)
Hormonal
Hyperthyroidism
Hypocalcemia
Hypoglycemia
Hypophosphatemia
Hypothermia
In utero sympathomimetic exposure
Maternal diabetes mellitus and other insulin excess
Myocardial ischemia
Pheochromocytoma
Polycythemia
Other electrolyte and metabolic disturbances
Viral (coxsackie, adenovirus, echo, CMV)
Hypertension

SVT, supraventricular tachycardia; VT, ventricular tachycardia.

of the underlying cause (Table 32.7). A higher proportion of cardiomyopathies presenting in the neonatal period and childhood have a genetic basis or underlying metabolic or neuromuscular disorder than adults, with 30% having an identifiable cause (Table 32.8) (72). Genetic testing can aid identification of the diagnosis and may guide prognosis. Once a genetic cause has been found, it is important that cascade genetic testing be performed on family members to identify other individuals who are at risk. This should ideally be done through a specific genetic or inherited cardiac conditions service (73).

DCM is characterized by a dilation of the left ventricular cavity and impaired systolic and diastolic function. The initial or ongoing myocyte damage can occur due to several factors including intrinsic disorders of the myocyte, which often have a genetic basis, inflammation and infection (myocarditis), toxin related, or energy deprivation from metabolic disorders or ischemia. This primary damage to the myocytes or myocyte function and resulting impaired ventricular function and reduced cardiac output lead to a neurohormonal response, which further exacerbates the myocardial changes that can continue even when the initial insult is transient (Fig. 32.19). Both the primary insult and resultant neurohormonal up-regulation drive a vicious circle of molecular and cellular changes with myocardial dysfunction, stunning, apoptosis, necrosis, and interstitial fibrosis exacerbating impaired systolic contractility and diastolic compliance.

HCM is characterized by primary ventricular hypertrophy, which is often asymmetrical, and although classically this asymmetry affects the mid and upper parts of the ventricular septum, any areas within either ventricle can be affected. Histologically, there may be hypertrophied but otherwise normal myocytes, although, in particular in those with genetic causes, there is usually myocardial disarray and fibrosis. The systolic function may be normal; however, there is often impaired diastolic function with

TABLE 32.8

Genetic Causes of Cardiomyopathy

Category	Cause	Gene Examples	Phenotype
Familial	Sarcomeric genes	*MYH7, MYBPC3, MYL2, MYL3, TNNT2, TNNI3, TNNC1, MYH6, TPM1, ACTC1,* etc.	HCM, DCM, RCM, LVNC
	Cytoskeletal genes	*TTN, CSRP3, TCAP, VCL, ACTN2, DES, LDB3, SGCD, MYPN, ANKRD1, BAG3, NEBL, NEXN,* etc.	HCM, DCM, RCM
	Desmosomal genes	*DSP, PKP2, DSG2, DSC2, JUP,* etc.	ARVC, DCM
	Nuclear envelope genes	*LMNA*	DCM
Metabolic	Fatty acid oxidation	*ACADVL, HADHA*	HCM
	Disorders (trifunctional protein, VLCAD, LCHAD)	*HADHB,* etc.	DCM, LVNC
	Carnitine abnormalities (carnitine acylcarnitine translocase deficiency, carnitine palmitoyltransferase deficiency) (CPTII)	*SLC25A20, CPT2*	DCM
	Mitochondrial disorders (including Kearns-Sayre syndrome, Barth syndrome, Friedreich ataxia)	Multiple genome mutations/deletion, *TAZ, FRDA, SCO2, SURF1, COX genes, ANT1,* etc.	HCM, DCM, LVNC
	Organic acidemias (propionic acidemia, etc.)	*PCCA, PCCB*	DCM
	Storage disorders (glycogen storage disorders, especially Pompe syndrome; mucopolysaccharidosis; Fabry disease, sphingolipidoses; hemochromatosis, Danon disease)	*PRKAG2, LAMP2, GLA, GAA, AGL,* etc.	HCM
Syndromic	RASopathies (Noonan, Costello, cardiofaciocutaneous, Noonan with multiple lentigines, etc.)	*PTPN11, RAF1, SOS1, KRAS, HRAS, BRAF, NRAS, MAP2K1, MAP2K2, CBL, SHOC2*	HCM
	Alström syndrome	*ALMS1*	DCM
Neuromuscular	Muscular dystrophies (Duchenne, Becker, limb girdle, Emery-Dreifuss, congenital muscular dystrophy, etc.), myotonic dystrophy, myofibrillar myopathy	*DMD, DMPK, EMD, LMNA, FHL1, FKRP, FLNC, LGMD2A, LGMD2B, LGMD2C, LGMD2D, LGMD2E,* etc.	DCM

ARVC, arrhythmogenic right ventricular cardiomyopathy; DCM, dilated cardiomyopathy; HCM, hypertrophic cardiomyopathy; LVNC, left ventricular noncompaction; RCM, restrictive cardiomyopathy.

Adapted from Ware SM. Evaluation of genetic causes of cardiomyopathy in childhood. *Cardiol Young* 2015;25(suppl 2):43. doi:10.1017/S1047951115000827. Copyright © 2015 Cambridge University Press.

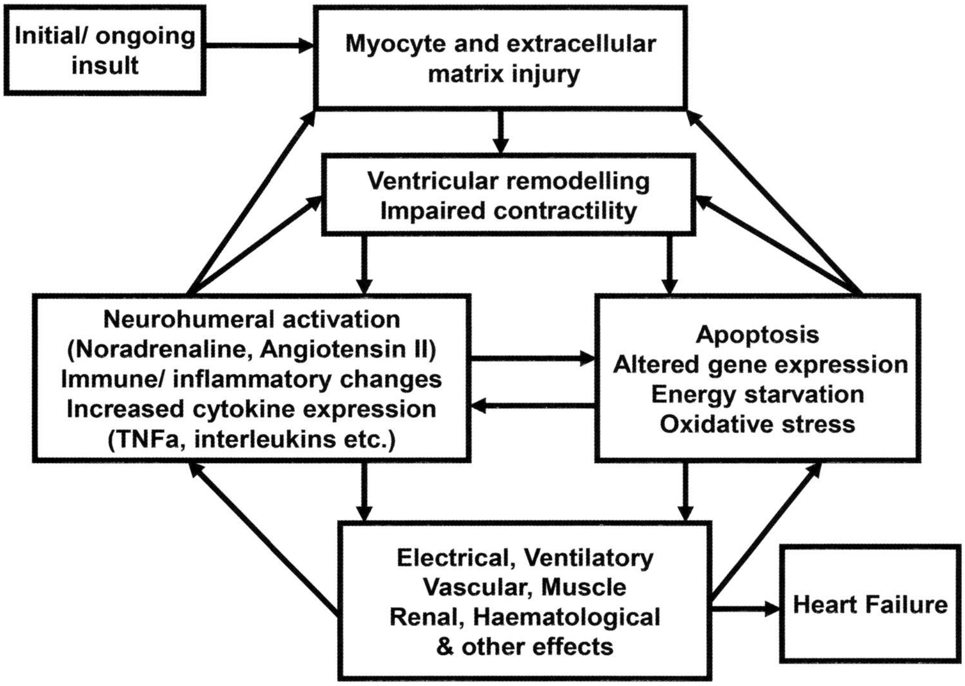

FIGURE 32.19 A schematic showing the vicious circle of ongoing myocardial damage associated with neurohormonal activation in patients with dilated cardiomyopathy.

THE NEWBORN INFANT

reduced ventricular filling and stroke volume, particularly when the severity of the hypertrophy is sufficient to lead to a reduction in cavity volume. Significant septal hypertrophy causes left ventricular outflow tract obstruction—hypertrophic obstructive cardiomyopathy (HOCM) and the turbulence through this can lead to systolic anterior motion of the mitral valve and mitral regurgitation. In addition to primary abnormalities of the myocytes, hypertrophy can be caused by deposition within the myocytes as observed in several metabolic diseases. External stimulus can lead to myocyte hypertrophy. This latter is observed in infants of diabetic mothers and other causes of hyperinsulinemia with high insulin levels leading to hypertrophy of the ventricular muscle. In this setting, the hypertrophy and therefore symptoms are dependent on the degree of insulin exposure and will regress following birth with restoration of normal glucose levels (74).

Noncompaction of the left ventricle is caused by intrauterine arrest of the normal compaction of the ventricular myocardium. This gives the ventricle the classical echo appearance of a spongy myocardium. Approximately 30% to 50% have a genetic basis (75). This can be classified as a separate entity with both DCM and HCM phenotypes observed.

RCM is characterized by impairment of diastolic function and therefore restriction of ventricular filling. In primary RCM, there is endocardial and epicardial fibroelastosis, although infiltrative causes are also described. Endocardial fibroelastosis may be apparent on echocardiography as a bright lining to the ventricle, although in neonates, this is more commonly associated with left heart outflow obstruction, in particular aortic stenosis, as opposed to an isolated disease (Fig. 32.20). In RCM, the atria become dilated, and the end diastolic pressure is elevated leading to pulmonary and systemic venous congestion. Often, right-sided heart failure is the predominant symptom. RCM is rare accounting for less than 10% of cardiomyopathies.

Clinical Approach to Neonatal Cardiomyopathy
Clinical Features and Investigations

Neonates present with signs of heart failure, which can vary from acute severe heart failure from birth to a more insidious onset. They may have difficulty in feeding, tachypnea, recession, a third heart sound (gallop rhythm), a systolic murmur from mitral regurgitation due to dilation of the mitral valve annulus, hepatomegaly, and signs of low cardiac output.

In HCM, there may be features secondary to the cause of the cardiomyopathy including macrosomia associated with high intrauterine insulin exposure or hypotonia and organomegaly due to underlying metabolic disease (Table 32.7).

Chest radiograph in DCM demonstrates cardiomegaly and pulmonary edema, although the heart may appear of normal size in HOCM and RCM.

The ECG is a particularly important investigation for cardiomyopathy. In DCM, there may be poor R-wave progression and signs of ventricular hypertrophy. In HCM, there will be prominent voltages in keeping with significant ventricular hypertrophy, and there may also be other ECG changes associated with specific diagnoses such as long-QT and short-QT syndrome, Brugada syndrome, and catecholaminergic polymorphic ventricular tachycardia (76). However, the most important aspects of the ECG are to look for potentially reversible causes, in particular ischemia due to coronary artery abnormalities and atrial and ventricular arrhythmia (below).

Echocardiography in DCM shows dilated ventricles, particularly affecting the left ventricle, and there may be associated mitral regurgitation. Myocardial trabeculation in the left ventricle should be sought suggesting noncompaction as a cause. In HCM, the ventricular wall appears thickened, which is often asymmetrical particularly affecting the septum. Left ventricular outflow tract

obstruction (HOCM) should be sought as should associated mitral regurgitation due to systolic anterior motion of the mitral valve. In RCM, the ventricular cavities appear small with biatrial dilatation. The most important part of the echocardiographic assessment is absolute exclusion of a structural or other reversible cause for the cardiomyopathy (Table 32.7).

Cardiac MRI can be used to help define the etiology, with differing causes displaying varying patterns of gadolinium distribution in the myocardium. The use of T1 and T2 mapping, along with gadolinium enhancement, can provide prognostic information and monitoring of treatment, indicating the degree of inflammation, fibrosis, and myocardial damage (77).

The troponin may be raised if there is acute myocyte damage in association with ischemia or inflammation. Biomarkers such as brain-type natriuretic peptide (BNP) and N-terminal brain-type natriuretic peptide (Nt-proBNP) are released in relation to the amount of stretch on a ventricle. These biomarkers are raised in heart failure and can be used as a guide to treatment.

Initial Management and Workup

Presentation and initial management of a baby with severe heart failure is as described in the above section on congenital heart disease. When the diagnosis is unknown prior to echocardiography, then these babies should all be started on prostaglandin, and usual supportive management until the diagnosis is confirmed. These will not be required for less severe presentations.

When faced with a baby with symptomatic heart failure and impaired ventricular function on echocardiogram, both structural and other reversible causes of that appearance must be excluded before a diagnosis of cardiomyopathy can be made. Particularly, important diagnoses and those that may be missed in this situation are summarized in Table 32.7 and include the following.

Anomalous Left Coronary Artery from the Pulmonary Artery

Anomalous left coronary artery from the pulmonary artery (ALCAPA) can present in neonates, although the timing of presentation is highly variable. Babies will present with varying degrees of heart failure depending upon the ventricular function and occasionally have symptoms of ischemia including becoming upset and seeming in pain with any activity including feeding, which is thought to represent angina. As part of the echocardiographic assessment of babies with poor cardiac function, particular attention should be given to the origins of both coronary arteries. As the pulmonary vascular resistance falls, there is diastolic flow from the anomalous left coronary artery into the pulmonary arteries causing ischemia. The area of impaired function is often well demarcated to the left ventricular free wall, and there may be bright ischemic papillary muscles of the mitral valve with significant mitral regurgitation. The left coronary artery may be seen entering the pulmonary artery with flow into (rather than away from) the pulmonary artery. If the coronary arteries cannot be clearly identified, CT scan is carried out to confirm or refute the diagnosis (Fig. 32.21). The ischemia will also be evident on the ECG and may progress to infarction. The anomalous left coronary artery is surgically relocated to the appropriate position, and if there has not been a complete infarct, the function often improves over time, although occasionally damage can be permanent.

Neonatal Myocardial Infarction

Although extremely uncommon, neonatal myocardial infarction presents immediately after birth often with signs of severe circulatory compromise. The postulated mechanism is coronary embolus (air, amniotic fluid, or thrombus), which may occur during separation from the placenta with right-to-left flow of the embolus across the patent foramen ovale. The ECG will

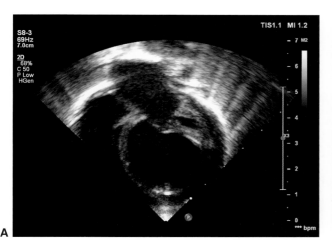
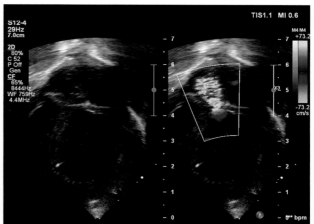
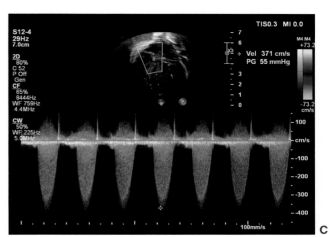

FIGURE 32.20 A: Apical four-chamber view shows a dilated ventricle with bright areas in the endocardium, which is endocardial fibroelastosis. **B:** Apical five-chamber view showing a small stenosed aortic valve with turbulence across it on color Doppler. **C:** Continuous wave Doppler across the aortic valve. The peak velocity is relatively low in keeping with the impaired ventricular function.

demonstrate ischemia with typical infarct patterns, and the echocardiogram shows extremely poor function of the areas of the myocardium supplied by the affected coronary artery. Although the coronary arteries are usually normal when the embolus has dissipated, cases are described of persistent coronary obstruction requiring thrombolysis.

Arrhythmia
Poor cardiac output secondary to very rapid atrial arrhythmia such as atrial flutter or reentry tachycardia are usually apparent from the absolute heart rate and the ECG. Incessant atrial tachycardia's can be more difficult to diagnose, and these should be actively sought as part of the workup for cardiomyopathy (see Chapter 34).

Myocarditis
Myocarditis can be difficult to differentiate from cardiomyopathy. Myocarditis is caused by inflammation of the myocardium secondary to a viral infection. Diagnosis by right ventricular percutaneous endomyocardial biopsy is performed by some centers in older children, although this is not performed in neonates due to the high procedural risk of cardiac perforation or tricuspid valve damage. However, opportunistic surgical biopsy may be carried out if the baby requires ECMO cannulation through an open chest or ventricular assist device insertion. Myocarditis may be categorized as fulminant and nonfulminant.

Fulminant viral myocarditis has a more severe presentation with high mortality rates early on in the disease. With improvements in intensive care and in particular the availability of ECMO, more patients are surviving this period, and if they can be supported through the acute period, complete recovery can be seen in 80% of those presenting in childhood. Nonfulminant myocarditis has an insidious progressive course and more often leads to the development of DCM with a higher risk of transplant or death (78). There is currently no evidence for any specific treatment options other than those already used for cardiomyopathy and heart failure, although some units continue to consider intravenous immunoglobulin and/or steroids for a presumed diagnosis of myocarditis (79).

Other Investigations
A thorough diagnostic workup of newly diagnosed cardiomyopathies should be undertaken to illicit any of the potential causes outlined in Table 32.7. A suggested workup is given in Table 32.9.

Management
In the acute setting, the aim of treatment should be to maximize cardiac output while reducing myocardial oxygen demands. The use of oxygen, ventilatory support, and sedation are important aspects of this management. The use of inotropes to support the cardiac output is often required and favored inotropes vary between units. As far as possible, inotrope selection should be

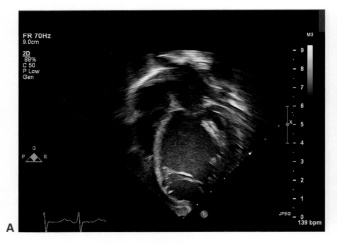

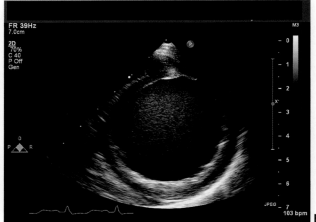

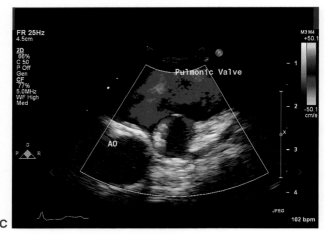

FIGURE 32.21 **A:** Apical four-chamber view shows a dilated left ventricle and echo bright mitral papillary muscles. **B:** Parasternal short axis with echo bright myocardium in the region of the left coronary artery supply. **C:** Parasternal short axis of the great arteries, the left coronary artery origins from the pulmonary artery. Note the retrograde flow through the coronary arteries into the pulmonary artery as opposed to forward flow into the coronary artery.

to encourage forward flow without excessive cardiac stimulation, and where possible, either inotropes which do not cause vasoconstriction or increase myocardial oxygen demands are preferred (in particular milrinone). There are some data from adult literature that prolonged use of alpha- and beta agonists in heart failure has detrimental effects and may reduce the chances of ventricular recovery and increase mortality. However, in unwell infants, it may not be possible to avoid these. Underlying metabolic abnormalities should be corrected where possible, and calcium infusion may be a valuable additional inotrope.

Fluid balance is important in acute decompensation. Cautious diuresis with loop or thiazide diuretics can reduce fluid overload, although excess volume depletion particularly in those acutely decompensated can lead to a reduction in cardiac output.

In cases with severe cardiopulmonary failure refractory to conventional therapy, venoarterial extracorporeal membrane oxygenation (ECMO) is deployed (see below).

In more stable infants, or once stability has been achieved in those presenting acutely, the mainstays of treatment are control of heart failure symptoms and management of any identified underlying cause. Diuretics improve symptoms related to pulmonary and systemic edema but have no effect on mortality or morbidity. There are excellent data from adults with cardiomyopathy that blocking the up-regulated neurohormonal pathway with ACE inhibitors, beta-blockers, and mineralocorticoid receptor agonists may lead to improvement in ventricular

function, improvement in symptoms, and improvement in survival. However, these data have not been replicated in children, and there is no clear evidence supporting their use in neonates. However, particularly given the quality of the data from the adult literature and the likely mechanism of up-regulation, the same pathways in continuing to exacerbate heart failure, these medicines are often also prescribed in children and neonates. Their use needs to be cautious and under expert guidance and not in babies who are decompensated. For occasional highly selected cases, placement of a pulmonary artery band in those with primary left ventricular dysfunction to increase right ventricular pressure and improve the component of left ventricular function contributed by the ventricular septum has been shown to lead to symptomatic improvement (80).

In those with HCM, in particular HOCM, beta-blockers are often used with extrapolated data from older children and adults, suggesting the potential for regression of the HCM, lower rates of potentially fatal arrhythmia, reduction in left ventricular outflow tract obstruction, and improved diastolic ventricular filling at lower heart rates. However, there are no clear data as to cardiac output improvement, survival advantage, or disease regression in neonates.

Outcomes

Cardiomyopathy presenting early has a more severe natural history than in the adult population, with the diagnosis having a

TABLE 32.9

Outline Investigation List for New Diagnoses of Ventricular Failure/Cardiomyopathy

Test

Influenza CFT (convalescent antibodies)
HIV
IgM parvovirus
IgM CMV
EBV VCA IgM
ASO
Based on symptoms and history—mycoplasma, HSV, HBV, HCV
PCR enterovirus and CMV
PCR enterovirus: stools
PCR in respiratory secretions
Throat swab C&S
Blood culture if pyrexial
Glucose
Lactate
TSH/FT4
Ca, PO_4
Vitamin D
Uric acid
CK
Total cholesterol
Triglyceride
Ferritin
Transferrin saturation
PTH
Ammonia
Transferrin isoforms
Acylcarnitines
Pompe screen
Cardiolipin (males)
Amino acids
Urine organic acids
Urine MPS screen
Muscle biopsy
Genetic testing—if dysmorphic, consanguinity, family history

large impact on survival rates. Five-year transplant free survival in childhood ranges is around 30% in RCM, 50% in DCM, and 90% in HCM. In a pediatric population, cardiac function can normalize in approximately 20% of patients with DCM, although biomarkers to reliably predict which infants with idiopathic cardiomyopathy will recover remain elusive (73).

MANAGEMENT OF SEVERE HEART FAILURE AND END-STAGE HEART FAILURE IN CHD AND CARDIOMYOPATHY

Despite optimum medical, interventional, and surgical management, some neonates are unable to maintain cardiac output either acutely for survival or sufficient for discharge home. A range of options is considered in these patients.

Extracorporeal Membrane Oxygenation

Venoarterial ECMO either via neck cannulation of the carotid artery and internal jugular vein or direct cannulation of the

systemic venous atrium and aorta has become an important part of the management of critically unwell neonates with heart failure from all causes. In some health care settings, the ability to provide ECMO has become a standard for neonatal cardiac surgical units (81). Venoarterial ECMO provides a complete bypass of both the heart and lungs providing cardiac output and oxygenation. ECMO can be used in a semielective manner in deteriorating cardiac patients or as part of an ECMO cardiopulmonary resuscitation (eCPR) service. Dedicated on-site trained teams are able to deliver ECMO extremely rapidly if sufficient cardiac output can be maintained during resuscitation while the baby is cannulated onto ECMO. ECMO is time limited with significant complications related to the ECMO circuit usually becoming apparent beyond 2 weeks. When a baby is established on ECMO, the immediate aim is to reverse the life-threatening condition. Once this has been achieved, cardiac ECMO essentially has three purposes:

1. **Bridge to decision**. Acute deterioration requiring ECMO may occur in the context of an undiagnosed or uncertain cause for that deterioration. ECMO allows time to investigate and manage causes of the deterioration (figure PA IVS no CA). For example, a patient deteriorates acutely before the cardiac diagnosis, and treatment options have been established, or a patient with shunt dependent pulmonary blood flow has an acute shunt occlusion. A decision can then be made as to the need for further cardiac intervention or cardiac surgery or whether other treatment options outlined below should be explored. In addition, further investigation of other organ systems can be undertaken and systemic abnormalities assessed so that an informed decision on the likely prognosis and appropriateness of continued active management can be decided.
2. **Bridge to recovery**. ECMO allows time to rest from the hemodynamic upset of CPB and the change in circulation that any cardiac intervention has caused. Patients presenting with cardiomyopathy due to presumed myocarditis may improve sufficiently with a period of ECMO to be weaned without the need for longer term mechanical support or cardiac transplantation.
3. **Bridge to transplant**. In some instances when there are no other mechanical support options for patients and they were unable to maintain sufficient cardiac output to wait for transplant, ECMO provides some time to wait for a suitable donor organ. Careful planning of the ECMO cannulation site and the way that the sites are looked after allows somewhat longer runs; however, the use of ECMO as a bridge to transplant is limited in view of the availability of donor organs.

Mechanical Support

The use of long-term ventricular assist devices has transformed the management of children and adults with heart failure from both congenital heart disease and, in particular, cardiomyopathy. The use of these devices has been extended to small children with a variety of cannula positioning techniques deployed, which essentially take blood from the pulmonary venous atrium or systemic ventricle and inject this into the aorta. Although the results of device use in infants less than 5 kg has a higher complication rate related to thrombus, complexities of anticoagulation in small infants and cannula size, these devices can provide an important way to maintain cardiac output in the medium term on the transplant waiting list.

Cardiac Transplant

Neonatal cardiac transplant for heart failure from end-stage congenital heart disease or cardiomyopathy can be carried out in designated centers with excellent results when compared to the very poor outcome for these patients otherwise (Fig. 32.22) (82). Careful consideration is given to the anatomical complexities, the

Pediatric Heart Transplants
Kaplan-Meier Survival by Diagnosis
Age: < 1 Year (Transplants: January 2005 – June 2017)

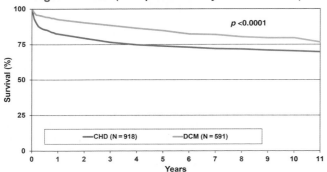

FIGURE 32.22 Kaplan-Meier curve showing the posttransplant survival of children undergoing heart transplant for congenital heart disease and cardiomyopathy under 1 year of age. (Rossano JW, Singh TP, Cherikh WS, et al. The International Thoracic Organ Transplant Registry of the International Society for Heart and Lung Transplantation: twenty-second pediatric heart transplantation report—2019; focus theme: donor and recipient size match. *J Heart Lung Transplant* 2019;38:1028.)

pulmonary vascular resistance (which needs to be sufficiently low to allow the donor right ventricle to function satisfactorily), the patient antibody status, and the family's wishes (in terms of the appropriateness of cardiac transplantation) and their ability to cope with the lifelong input that the child will require. Listing for cardiac transplant is not however synonymous with receiving a graft organ, and the wait for neonatal donor hearts can be significant. The availability of graft or organs is variable across different organ donation systems. In view of the lack of development of blood group antibodies in newborn infants, ABO incompatible transplant is often considered in these patients. Other methods used to increase the donor pool, depending upon each country's ethical approach and availability of the techniques, include donation after cardiac death and the use of donor organs from babies born with anencephaly.

Palliative Care and Comfort Care

In some cases, congenital heart disease can be such that no further palliation can be offered. These are often patients with extremely abnormal pulmonary arteries, patients with absent coronary arteries, or those who have significantly impaired ventricular function as part of a single ventricle diagnosis. There are also subgroups of patients with cardiomyopathy related to a systemic metabolic disease, which would continue after cardiac transplantation. In all of these patients, transplantation may be contraindicated/unrealistic in the timescale offered, not available in the health care system, or the parents may not wish to pursue this option. Depending upon the clinical state of the baby, a variety of options are explored with careful expert discussions with the family and appropriate support. Options include setting a ceiling of care and aiming for home if possible in relatively stable patients through to withdrawal of ventilatory support on the neonatal/cardiac unit (Chapter 8).

REFERENCES

1. Rankin J, Pattenden S, Abramsky L, et al. Prevalence of congenital anomalies in five British regions, 1991-99. *Arch Dis Child Fetal Neonatal Ed* 2005;90(5):374. doi: 10.1136/adc.2003.047902
2. Khoshnood B, Lelong N, Houyel L, et al. Prevalence, timing of diagnosis and mortality of newborns with congenital heart defects: a population-based study. *Heart* 2012;98(22):1667. doi: 10.1136/heartjnl-2012-302543
3. Oster ME, Lee KA, Honein MA, et al. Temporal trends in survival among infants with critical congenital heart defects. *Pediatrics* 2013;131(5):e1502. doi: 10.1542/peds.2012-3435
4. van der Bom T, Zomer AC, Zwinderman AH, et al. The changing epidemiology of congenital heart disease. *Nat Rev Cardiol* 2011;8(1):50. doi: 10.1038/nrcardio.2010.166
5. Alsoufi B, Manlhiot C, Mahle WT, et al. Low-weight infants are at increased mortality risk after palliative or corrective cardiac surgery. *J Thorac Cardiovasc Surg* 2014;148(6):2508. doi: 10.1016/j.jtcvs.2014.07.047
6. Curzon CL, Milford-Beland S, Li JS, et al. Cardiac surgery in infants with low birth weight is associated with increased mortality: analysis of the Society of Thoracic Surgeons Congenital Heart Database. *J Thorac Cardiovasc Surg* 2008;135(3):546. doi: 10.1016/j.jtcvs.2007.09.068
7. Massin MM, Astadicko I, Dessy H. Noncardiac comorbidities of congenital heart disease in children. *Acta Paediatr* 2007;96(5):753. doi: 10.1111/j.1651-2227.2007.00275.x
8. Patel A, Costello JM, Backer CL, et al. Prevalence of noncardiac and genetic abnormalities in neonates undergoing cardiac operations: analysis of The Society of Thoracic Surgeons Congenital Heart Surgery Database. *Ann Thorac Surg* 2016;102(5):1607. doi: 10.1016/j.athoracsur.2016.04.008
9. Hoffman JIE. The global burden of congenital heart disease. *Cardiovasc J Afr* 2013;24(4):141. doi: 10.5830/CVJA-2013-028
10. Paediatric Cardiology, Anderson RH, et al., eds., *Gemma Price*, 3rd ed. Philadelphia, PA: Churchill Livingstone, 2010.
11. Ezon DS. *Atlas of congenital heart disease nomenclature : an illustrated guide to the Van Praagh and Anderson approaches to describing congenital cardiac pathology.* Houston, TX: Ezon Educational Services, 2015.
12. Moorman A, Webb S, Brown NA, et al. Development of the heart: (1) Formation of the cardiac chambers and arterial trunks. *Heart* 2003;89(7):806. doi: 10.1136/heart.89.7.806
13. Anderson RH, Webb S, Brown NA, et al. Development of the heart: (2) Septation of the atriums and ventricles. *Heart* 2003;89(8):949. doi: 10.1136/heart.89.8.949
14. Clark EB. Pathogenetic mechanisms of congenital cardiovascular malformations revisited. *Semin Perinatol* 1996;20(6):465. doi: 10.1016/S0146-0005(96)80062-0
15. Van Der Linde D, Konings EEM, Slager MA, et al. Birth prevalence of congenital heart disease worldwide: a systematic review and meta-analysis. *J Am Coll Cardiol* 2011;58(21):2241. doi: 10.1016/j.jacc.2011.08.025
16. Liu Y, Chen S, Zühlke L, et al. Global birth prevalence of congenital heart defects 1970-2017: updated systematic review and meta-analysis of 260 studies. *Int J Epidemiol* 2019;48(2):455. doi: 10.1093/ije/dyz009
17. Bregman S, Frishman WH. Impact of improved survival in congenital heart disease on incidence of disease. *Cardiol Rev* 2018;26(2):82. doi: 10.1097/CRD.0000000000000178
18. Adam MP, Ardinger HH, Pagon R. *GeneReviews*. Available from: https://www.ncbi.nlm.nih.gov/books/NBK1116/. Accessed July 22, 2019.
19. Muntean I, Togănel R, Benedek T. Genetics of congenital heart disease: past and present. *Biochem Genet* 2017;55(2):105. doi: 10.1007/s10528-016-9780-7
20. Lin AE, Alexander ME, Colan SD, et al. Clinical, pathological, and molecular analyses of cardiovascular abnormalities in Costello syndrome: a Ras/MAPK pathway syndrome. *Am J Med Genet A* 2011;155(3):486. doi: 10.1002/ajmg.a.33857
21. Hinton RB, Martin LJ, Tabangin ME, et al. Hypoplastic left heart syndrome is heritable. *J Am Coll Cardiol* 2007;50(16):1590. doi: 10.1016/j.jacc.2007.07.021
22. Edwards JJ, Gelb BD. Genetics of congenital heart disease. *Curr Opin Cardiol* 2016;31(3):235. doi: 10.1097/HCO.0000000000000274
23. Uemura H, Ho SY, Devine WA, et al. Atrial appendages and venoatrial connections in hearts from patients with visceral heterotaxy. *Ann Thorac Surg* 1995;60(3):561. doi: 10.1016/0003-4975(95)00538-V
24. Ticho BS, Goldstein AM, Van Praagh R. Extracardiac anomalies in the heterotaxy syndromes with focus on anomalies of midline-associated structures. *Am J Cardiol* 2000;85(6):729. doi: 10.1016/S0002-9149(99)00849-8
25. Park MK, Myung K. *Park's pediatric cardiology for practitioners*, 6th ed. Philadelphia, PA: Elsevier Saunders, 2014.
26. Morgan MC, Maina B, Waiyego M, et al. Oxygen saturation ranges for healthy newborns within 24 hours at 1800 m. *Arch Dis Child Fetal Neonatal Ed* 2017;102(3):F266. doi: 10.1136/archdischild-2016-311813
27. Hébert A, Lavoie PM, Giesinger RE, et al. Evolution of training guidelines for echocardiography performed by the neonatologist: toward hemodynamic consultation. *J Am Soc Echocardiogr* 2019;32(6):785. doi: 10.1016/j.echo.2019.02.002
28. Franklin O, Burch M, Manning N, et al. Prenatal diagnosis of coarctation of the aorta improves survival and reduces morbidity. *Heart* 2002;87(1):67. doi: 10.1136/heart.87.1.67
29. Tworetzky W, McElhinney DB, Reddy VM, et al. Improved surgical outcome after fetal diagnosis of hypoplastic left heart syndrome. *Circulation* 2001;103(9):1269. doi: 10.1161/01.CIR.103.9.1269

30. Yagel S, Arbel R, Anteby EY, et al. The three vessels and trachea view (3VT) in fetal cardiac scanning. *Ultrasound Obstet Gynecol* 2002;20(4):340. doi: 10.1046/j.1469-0705.2002.00801.x

31. Hyett J, Perdu M, Sharland G, et al. Using fetal nuchal translucency to screen for major congenital cardiac defects at 10-14 weeks of gestation: population based cohort study. *Br Med J* 1999;318(7176):81. doi: 10.1136/bmj.318.7176.81

32. Rychik J, Ayres N, Cuneo B, et al. American society of echocardiography guidelines and standards for performance of the fetal echocardiogram. *J Am Soc Echocardiogr* 2004;17(7):803. doi: 10.1016/j.echo.2004.04.011

33. Lee W, Allan L, Carvalho JS, et al. ISUOG consensus statement: what constitutes a fetal echocardiogram? *Ultrasound Obstet Gynecol* 2008;32(2):239. doi: 10.1002/uog.6115

34. Familiari A, Morlando M, Khalil A, et al. Risk factors for coarctation of the aorta on prenatal ultrasound: a systematic review and meta-analysis. *Circulation* 2017;135(8):772. doi: 10.1161/CIRCULATIONAHA.116.024068

35. Lloyd DFA, Pushparajah K, Simpson JM, et al. Three-dimensional visualisation of the fetal heart using prenatal MRI with motion-corrected slice-volume registration: a prospective, single-centre cohort study. *Lancet* 2019;393(10181):1619. doi: 10.1016/S0140-6736(18)32490-5

36. Moon-Grady AJ, Morris SA, Belfort M, et al. International fetal cardiac intervention registry: a worldwide collaborative description and preliminary outcomes. *J Am Coll Cardiol* 2015;66(4):388. doi: 10.1016/j.jacc.2015.05.037

37. Peyvandi S, Nguyen TATT, Almeida-Jones M, et al. Timing and mode of delivery in prenatally diagnosed congenital heart disease—an analysis of practices within the University of California Fetal Consortium (UCfC). *Pediatr Cardiol* 2017;38(3):588. doi: 10.1007/s00246-016-1552-y

38. Lage K, Greenway SC, Rosenfeld JA, et al. Genetic and environmental risk factors in congenital heart disease functionally converge in protein networks driving heart development. *Proc Natl Acad Sci U S A* 2012;109(35):14035. doi: 10.1073/pnas.1210730109

39. Feinstein JA, Benson DW, Dubin AM, et al. Hypoplastic left heart syndrome: current considerations and expectations. *J Am Coll Cardiol* 2012;59(1 suppl):S1. doi: 10.1016/j.jacc.2011.09.022

40. Jenkins KJ, Correa A, Feinstein JA, et al. Noninherited risk factors and congenital cardiovascular defects: current knowledge—a scientific statement from the American Heart Association Council on Cardiovascular Disease in the Young. *Circulation* 2007;115(23):2995. doi: 10.1161/CIRCULATIONAHA.106.183216

41. Jones KL. *Smith's recognizable patterns of human malformation/Kenneth Lyons Jones, Marilyn Crandall Jones, Miguel Del Campo*, 7th ed. Philadelphia, PA: Elsevier Saunders, 2013.

42. Granelli ADW, Wennergren M, Sandberg K, et al. Impact of pulse oximetry screening on the detection of duct dependent congenital heart disease: a Swedish prospective screening study in 39,821 newborns. *BMJ* 2009;338:a3037. doi: 10.1136/bmj.a3037

43. Plana MN, Zamora J, Suresh G, et al. Pulse oximetry screening for critical congenital heart defects. *Cochrane Database Syst Rev* 2018;3(3):CD011912. doi: 10.1002/14651858.CD011912.pub2

44. Abouk R, Grosse SD, Ailes EC, et al. Association of US State implementation of newborn screening policies for critical congenital heart disease with early infant cardiac deaths. *JAMA* 2017;318(21):2111. doi: 10.1001/jama.2017.17627

45. Oddie S, Stenson B, Wyllie J, et al. UK consultation on pulse oximetry screening for critical congenital heart defects in newborns. *Lancet* 2019;394(10193):103. doi: 10.1016/S0140-6736(19)31515-6

46. Crossland DS, Furness JC, Abu-Karb M, et al. Variability of four limb blood pressure in normal neonates. *Arch Dis Child Fetal Neonatal Ed* 2004;89(4):F325. doi: 10.1136/adc.2003.034322

47. Ainsworth SB, Wyllie JP, Wren C. Prevalence and clinical significance of cardiac murmurs in neonates. *Arch Dis Child Fetal Neonatal Ed* 1999;80(1):F43. doi: 10.1136/fn.80.1.F43

48. Singh A, Desai T, Miller P, et al. Benefits of predischarge echocardiography service for postnatal heart murmurs. *Acta Paediatr* 2012;101(8):e333. doi: 10.1111/j.1651-2227.2012.02687.x

49. Akkinapally S, Hundalani SG, Kulkarni M, et al. Prostaglandin E1 for maintaining ductal patency in neonates with ductal-dependent cardiac lesions. *Cochrane Database Syst Rev* 2018;2(2):CD011417. doi: 10.1002/14651858.CD011417.pub2

50. Singh Y, Mikrou P. Use of prostaglandins in duct-dependent congenital heart conditions. *Arch Dis Child Educ Pract Ed* 2018;103(3):137. doi: 10.1136/archdischild-2017-313654

51. Hermuzi A, McBrien A, De Rita F, et al. Hybrid transatrial stent insertion for left atrial decompression in hypoplastic left heart syndrome with intact atrial septum. *Catheter Cardiovasc Interv* 2016;87(1):109. doi: 10.1002/ccd.26115

52. Nieves JA, Rudd NA, Dobrolet N. Home surveillance monitoring for high risk congenital heart newborns: improving outcomes after single ventricle

palliation—why, how & results. *Prog Pediatr Cardiol* 2018;48:14. doi: 10.1016/j.ppedcard.2018.01.004

53. Cao JY, Lee SY, Phan K, et al. Early outcomes of hypoplastic left heart syndrome infants: meta-analysis of studies comparing the hybrid and Norwood procedures. *World J Pediatr Congenit Heart Surg* 2018;9(2):224. doi: 10.1177/2150135117752896

54. Cao JY, Phan K, Ayer J, et al. Long term survival of hypoplastic left heart syndrome infants: meta-analysis comparing outcomes from the modified Blalock–Taussig shunt and the right ventricle to pulmonary artery shunt. *Int J Cardiol* 2018;254:107. doi: 10.1016/j.ijcard.2017.10.040

55. Doshia H, Venugopalb P, MacArthurc K. Does a balloon atrial septostomy performed before arterial switch surgery increase adverse neurological outcomes? *Interact Cardiovasc Thorac Surg* 2012;15(1):141. doi: 10.1093/icvts/ivr145

56. Dirks V, Prêtre R, Knirsch W, et al. Modified Blalock Taussig shunt: a not-so-simple palliative procedure. *Eur J Cardiothorac Surg* 2013;44(6):1096. doi: 10.1093/ejcts/ezt172

57. Bentham JR, Zava NK, Harrison WJ, et al. Duct stenting versus modified Blalock-Taussig shunt in neonates with duct-dependent pulmonary blood flow: associations with clinical outcomes in a Multicenter National Study. *Circulation* 2018;137(6):581. doi: 10.1161/CIRCULATIONAHA.117.028972

58. National Institute for Cardiovascular Outcomes Research (NICOR) [internet]. London, England: UCL, 2019. Available from: nicor4.nicor.org.uk/CHD/an_paeds.nsf/WBenchmarksYears?openview&RestrictToCategory=2015&start=1&count=500

59. Stumper O, Quandt D, Penford G. Stenting of the right ventricular outflow tract as initial palliation for Fallot-type lesions. In: *Atlas of Cardiac Catheterization for Congenital Heart Disease*. 2019;321. doi: 10.1007/978-3-319-72443-0_37

60. Quandt D, Ramchandani B, Stickley J, et al. Stenting of the right ventricular outflow tract promotes better pulmonary arterial growth compared with modified Blalock-Taussig shunt palliation in tetralogy of Fallot–type lesions. *JACC Cardiovasc Interv* 2017;10(17):1774. doi: 10.1016/j.jcin.2017.06.023

61. Padalino MA, Reffo E, Cerutti A, et al. Medical and surgical management of primary cardiac tumours in infants and children. *Cardiol Young* 2008;24(2):268. doi: 10.1017/S104795111300022X

62. Tworetzky W, McElhinney DB, Margossian R, et al. Association between cardiac tumors and tuberous sclerosis in the fetus and neonate. *Am J Cardiol* 2003;92(4):487. doi: 10.1016/S0002-9149(03)00677-5

63. Beroukhim RS, Gauvreau K, Benavidez OJ, et al. Perinatal outcome after prenatal diagnosis of single-ventricle cardiac defects. *Ultrasound Obstet Gynecol* 2015;45(6):657. doi: 10.1002/uog.14634

64. Mebius MJ, Kooi EMW, Bilardo CM, et al. Brain injury and neurodevelopmental outcome in congenital heart disease: a systematic review. *Pediatrics* 2017;140(1):e20164055. doi: 10.1542/peds.2016-4055

65. Marino BS, Lipkin PH, Newburger JW, et al. Neurodevelopmental outcomes in children with congenital heart disease: evaluation and management a scientific statement from the American Heart Association. *Circulation* 2012;126(9):1143. doi: 10.1161/CIR.0b013e318265ee8a

66. Liu MY, Zielonka B, Snarr BS, et al. Longitudinal assessment of outcome from prenatal diagnosis through Fontan operation for over 500 fetuses with single ventricle-type congenital heart disease: The Philadelphia Fetus-to-Fontan cohort study. *J Am Heart Assoc* 2018;7(19):e009145. doi: 10.1161/JAHA.118.009145

67. d'Udekem Y, Iyengar AJ, Galati JC, et al. Redefining expectations of long-term survival after the Fontan procedure: twenty-five years of follow-up from the entire population of Australia and New Zealand. *Circulation* 2014;130(11 suppl 1):S32. doi: 10.1161/CIRCULATIONAHA.113.007764

68. Khairy P, Ionescu-Ittu R, MacKie AS, et al. Changing mortality in congenital heart disease. *J Am Coll Cardiol* 2010;56(14):1149. doi: 10.1016/j.jacc.2010.03.085

69. Verheugt CL, Uiterwaal CSPM, van der Velde ET, et al. Mortality in adult congenital heart disease. *Eur Heart J* 2010;31(10):1220. doi: 10.1093/eurheartj/ehq032

70. Wotherspoon JM, Eagleson KJ, Gilmore L, et al. Neurodevelopmental and health-related quality-of-life outcomes in adolescence after surgery for congenital heart disease in infancy. *Dev Med Child Neurol* 2020;62(2):214. doi: 10.1111/dmcn.14251

71. Guimarães H, Costa S, Dória S, et al. Neonatal dilated cardiomyopathy. *Rev Port Cardiol* 2017;36(3):201. doi: 10.1016/j.repce.2016.10.017

72. Ware SM. Evaluation of genetic causes of cardiomyopathy in childhood. *Cardiol Young* 2015;25(suppl 2):43. doi: 10.1017/S1047951115000827

73. Lee TM, Hsu DT, Kantor P, et al. Pediatric cardiomyopathies. *Circ Res* 2017;121(7):855. doi: 10.1161/CIRCRESAHA.116.309386

74. Huang T, Kelly A, Becker SA, et al. Hypertrophic cardiomyopathy in neonates with congenital hyperinsulinism. *Arch Dis Child Fetal Neonatal Ed* 2013;98(4):F351. doi: 10.1136/archdischild-2012-302546

75. Towbin JA, Lorts A, Jefferies JL. Left ventricular non-compaction cardiomyopathy. *Lancet* 2015;386(9995):813. doi: 10.1016/S0140-6736(14)61282-4

76. McKenna WJ, Maron BJ, Thiene G. Classification, epidemiology, and global burden of cardiomyopathies. *Circ Res* 2017;121(7):722. doi: 10.1161/CIR-CRESAHA.117.309711

77. Patel AR, Kramer CM. Role of cardiac magnetic resonance in the diagnosis and prognosis of nonischemic cardiomyopathy. *JACC Cardiovasc Imaging* 2017;10(10 Pt A):1180. doi: 10.1016/j.jcmg.2017.08.005

78. Kuhl U, Schultheiss H-P. Myocarditis in children. *Heart Fail Clin* 2010;6(4):483, viii-ix. doi: 10.1016/j.hfc.2010.05.009

79. Dasgupta S, Iannucci G, Mao C, et al. Myocarditis in the pediatric population: a review. *Congenit Heart Dis* 2019;14(5):868. doi: 10.1111/chd.12835

80. Schranz D, Recla S, Malcic I, et al. Pulmonary artery banding in dilative cardiomyopathy of young children: review and protocol based on the current knowledge. *Transl Pediatr* 2019;8(2):151. doi: 10.21037/tp.2019.04.09

81. Congenital Heart Disease Standards and Specifications [internet]. London, England: NHS England, 2016. Available from: https://www.england.nhs.uk/commissioning/wp-content/uploads/sites/12/2016/03/chd-spec-standards-2016.pdf

82. International Society for Heart and Lung Transplantation (ISHLT). *J Heart Lung Transplant* 2019;38:1016.

33 Postoperative Management and Care of the Cardiac Surgical Patient

John M. Costello, Sinai C. Zyblewski, Jason R. Buckley, and Luke W. Schroeder

INTRODUCTION

Congenital heart disease (CHD) is the most common birth defect, occurring in approximately 8 per 1,000 live births. Approximately one-third of all patients with CHD undergo surgical or transcatheter intervention as neonates or in early infancy. This strategy limits the sequelae of prolonged cyanosis and heart failure. However, several factors complicate the perioperative care of neonates and young infants. Immaturity of many organ systems is associated with limited physiologic reserve. Neonates have limited myocardial contractile reserve, likely related to poorly organized contractile proteins and inefficient calcium delivery to myofilaments (1). Pulmonary functional residual capacity, fat and carbohydrate reserves, and ability to regulate temperature are all limited. Drug metabolism is altered by hepatic and renal immaturity, as well as total body water content.

This chapter provides an overview of the key issues, concepts, and strategies pertaining to the postoperative care of neonates and infants with CHD. A continuum of care is essential for achieving optimal outcomes for neonates with complex cardiac disease. The reader is referred to Chapter 32 for information regarding the presentation of critical CHD including prenatal diagnosis, preoperative evaluation and stabilization, and surgical strategy (e.g., palliation vs. primary complete repair). Cardiomyopathies and cardiac transplant are also discussed in Chapter 32. In this chapter, we provide an overview of cardiopulmonary bypass (CPB) and its sequelae. Common postoperative pathophysiologic states and early postoperative complications are reviewed. The general postoperative pathophysiology and management strategies described in this chapter are intended to provide a frame of reference for evaluation and management of this patient population. Subtle variations in cardiac anatomy and physiology exist following each major operative category, which must be fully appreciated when developing individualized management plans.

CARDIOPULMONARY BYPASS

An understanding of intraoperative events including the conduct of CPB is required to provide care for patients recovering from cardiac surgery. Most cardiac operations performed in neonates and infants require the use of CPB. The primary function of CPB is to temporarily replace the major functions of the heart and lungs while surgical interventions are performed on these organs. A typical CPB circuit used to perform these functions includes venous cannula(s) that drain systemic venous blood from the venae cavae or systemic venous atrium, a reservoir, a heat exchanger, a membrane oxygenator, a roller pump, a filter, and an arterial cannula to return blood to the aorta. Before initiation of CPB, the circuit is "primed" with standardized quantities of crystalloid solution, albumin, mannitol, sodium bicarbonate, heparin, calcium, and packed red blood cells. The patient is anticoagulated with heparin for the duration of CPB and cooled to a variable extent to minimize metabolic needs and oxygen consumption. Because hypothermia causes increased viscosity and red cell rigidity, hemodilution is used during hypothermic CPB.

To obtain a motionless heart for intracardiac repairs, the aorta is cross-clamped, and a potassium-rich cardioplegia solution is injected into the proximal ascending aorta. Asystole develops once the cardioplegia perfuses the coronary circulation. Myocardial protection is achieved through a combination of cardioplegia administration and hypothermia. Following placement of the aortic cross clamp, blood from aortopulmonary collateral vessels will continue to return to the left atrium. To eliminate the left atrial blood return and facilitate certain complex left heart operations, deep hypothermic circulatory arrest (DHCA) may be used. "Deep hypothermia" refers to cooling of the core temperature to 18°C to 20°C. During circulatory arrest, the CPB pump is shut off and the perfusion cannula may be removed from the surgical field, creating optimal conditions for an accurate repair. Circulatory arrest times longer than 45 to 50 minutes may be associated with increased postoperative neurologic complications (2). Regional perfusion techniques may be utilized to minimize or avoid the use of circulatory arrest, although evidence that such techniques improve neurodevelopmental outcomes is lacking (3). Following rewarming and weaning from CPB, the adequacy of the repair is assessed by some combination of vascular pressure measurements, cooximetry, and transesophageal echocardiogram. Once the surgeon is satisfied with the repair, protamine is administered to reverse the effect of heparin. Additional blood components and antifibrinolytic agents may be administered to control bleeding.

Exposure to CPB triggers a cascade of complex neurohumoral and inflammatory responses, which may impair myocardial, pulmonary, renal, and hematologic function. During CPB, formed elements of the blood are exposed to artificial surfaces and sheer stress. Ischemia reperfusion injury occurs, as does microembolization of gas bubbles and particulate matter. The release of endogenous catecholamines, vasopressin, and endothelin and activation of the renin–angiotensin–aldosterone axis occur, which contribute to elevation of systemic and pulmonary vascular resistances and fluid retention. A generalized inflammatory response develops, and the complement, coagulation, and fibrinolytic systems are activated. Capillary leak also occurs, related to fluid retention, the inflammatory response, and dilution of plasma proteins. White blood cells and platelets are also activated, leading to additional release of inflammatory mediators and proteolytic enzymes. Pulmonary leukosequestration occurs, as does oxygen free radical generation, and abnormal gas exchange and decreased pulmonary compliance may be evident. Platelet counts fall following CPB, and clotting factors are diluted, predisposing patients to bleeding. Myocardial dysfunction may occur, manifesting as a low cardiac output state.

Several pharmacologic agents and management strategies may be employed in the operating room to minimize these adverse effects of CPB. Mannitol is administered to the priming solution to induce osmotic diuresis and act as an antioxidant. Multiple small trials have shown that corticosteroid administration blunts the inflammatory response to CPB; however, data regarding impact on important clinical outcomes are conflicting (4–6). To aid in the removal of edema and to hemoconcentrate the infant's blood, ultrafiltration is typically used during rewarming on CPB. An additional technique known as modified ultrafiltration (MUF) may be used immediately following CPB. By removing fluid and inflammatory mediators, MUF may have favorable effects on hemodynamic indices, blood product requirements, and total body water balance.

POSTOPERATIVE CARE

Stabilization in the Intensive Care Unit Following Surgery

Following the operation, the intensive care unit (ICU) service should obtain a standardized handoff from the anesthesiologist and the surgeon. Included in this handoff are details about the anesthetic regimen, the operative findings, and surgical procedure performed, as well as duration of CPB, aortic cross-clamp, and circulatory arrest (if applicable). If performed, the results of the transesophageal echocardiogram and any pressure or cooximetry measurements should be communicated. Information regarding vascular access, pacing wires, chest drains, blood product utilization, and intraoperative arrhythmias or other complications should be discussed. Handoff should conclude with a summary statement that ensures a teamwide shared mental model of the patient's early postoperative management with attention to hemodynamic, ventilation, sedation, and analgesia goals.

Invasive hemodynamic monitoring is used in nearly all neonates and infants following cardiac surgery. One or more central venous lines are typically placed in the operating room. Sites for line placement are chosen depending upon the patient's anatomy, anticipated postoperative course, and clinician preference. Some clinicians prefer to avoid placement of central venous lines in the subclavian and jugular veins in patients with single ventricle physiology due to concerns for thrombosis of the systemic veins of the upper body. Intracardiac lines may be inserted by the surgeon prior to chest closure through the right atrial appendage to the right atrium ("RA line") or through the right upper pulmonary vein or left atrial appendage to the left atrium ("LA line").

A pulmonary artery catheter may be placed through an internal jugular or subclavian vein, the right atrium, or right ventricular outflow tract. These catheters are infrequently used in the current era but may be informative in selected patients at high risk for postoperative pulmonary hypertension, residual ventricular septal defects (VSDs), or residual right ventricular outflow tract obstruction.

Proper interpretation of intracardiac and vascular pressure measurements (markers of ventricular loading conditions) is beneficial for the detection of residual lesions, titration of volume administration, and the implementation of interventions that modify vascular tone. Interpretation of the atrial waveforms may provide insight into the presence of significant atrioventricular valve regurgitation or rhythm disturbances.

An arterial line facilitates continuous blood pressure monitoring and frequent arterial blood gas sampling. The waveform and pulse pressure may be informative as to the cardiac pathophysiology. For example, significant diastolic runoff may produce a wide pulse pressure in the presence of a systemic to pulmonary shunt, aortopulmonary collateral arteries, or severe aortic regurgitation. A narrow pulse pressure, along with tachycardia and hypotension, may signify cardiac tamponade. Patients who underwent repair of coarctation or aortic arch reconstruction should have four extremity blood pressure measurements taken to document any residual aortic arch gradient. Attention to coronary perfusion pressure can be particularly important in certain patient groups, such as those with Williams syndrome, pulmonary atresia with intact ventricular septum and right ventricular–dependent coronary circulation (RVDCC), residual aortic stenosis, and significant ventricular hypertrophy. Systemic blood pressures in general, and diastolic blood pressures in particular, that may be well tolerated in most other patients may be inadequate in patients noted above. Relative hypotension can lead to myocardial ischemia and subsequent cardiac arrest.

A variety of factors may contribute to erroneous data obtained from invasive monitoring, including inappropriate transducer height, and bubbles or clots in the catheters. Dampened arterial waveforms or pressures measured distal to stenotic arteries may give the false impression of hypotension. For example, arm blood pressure measurements in a patient who has, or had in the past, an ipsilateral Blalock-Taussig shunt may be diminished due to subclavian arterial stenosis or occlusion. Information obtained from invasive monitoring cannot be used in isolation, but when placed in the context of the overall clinical picture, can be very useful to guide management in the early postoperative period.

Complications associated with central lines are uncommon but include air embolus, thrombus, infection, bleeding, and arrhythmias (7). When using LA lines in patients with two-ventricular repairs, and with any central line in those with single ventricle physiology or intracardiac shunts, care must be taken not to inject air into the systemic circulation. Complications at the time of intracardiac catheter removal include retention and bleeding; the latter has been shown to occur more commonly with pulmonary artery catheters (8). When removing intracardiac lines, consideration should be given to coagulation status, surgical availability, having packed red blood cells at the bedside, and performing a limited echocardiogram to assess for an evolving hemopericardium.

Assessment of the heart rhythm is an important part of the initial evaluation following surgery. The heart rate and rhythm should be continuously monitored, and these data should be reviewable on a telemetry system. A 12-lead electrocardiogram is usually obtained in the immediate postoperative period to serve as a new baseline should the patient subsequently develop a tachyarrhythmia or myocardial ischemia. Atrioventricular synchrony is important for optimizing cardiac output. Temporary pacing wires may be placed before chest closure in the operating room. These pacing wires may be interrogated when attempting to clarify arrhythmia mechanism. They also may be used to pace-terminate certain tachyarrhythmias and are effective for pacing in the setting of junctional ectopic tachycardia (JET), heart block, or other bradyarrhythmias. Sensing and capture thresholds should be assessed regularly. These wires are quite safe and may be removed at the bedside when no longer clinically indicated.

Temperature should be monitored and regulated closely. High temperature increases metabolic demands and may adversely affect hemodynamics and neurodevelopmental outcomes, whereas hypothermia may increase systemic vascular resistance and cause bradycardia.

A directed physical examination should be performed to assess the cardiopulmonary status and adequacy of the surgical repair. Any murmurs or gallops should be noted, especially in the setting of surgical shunt placement, although dressings and chest tubes may limit the auscultatory findings. It is common to hear a friction rub in the first few days following cardiac surgery, usually due to accumulation of a small amount of fluid in the pericardial space. The liver span should be noted. Adequate chest rise and breath sounds should be noted bilaterally. The quality and symmetry of peripheral pulses and perfusion of the extremities are useful means of assessing the adequacy of the systemic circulation. Caution must be used when attempting to estimate the adequacy of cardiac output by assessing capillary refill or peripheral–core temperature gradients, as both have a poor correlation with cardiac index, systemic vascular resistance index, and lactate levels (9).

Chest tubes should be assessed for location and proper function. Attention should be given to the quality of chest tube drainage (i.e., sanguineous, serosanguineous, serous), which may evolve over time. In infants, the tubes may generally be removed when drainage falls to less than 20 to 30 mL/d and when there is no evidence for chylothorax or air leak (10). A CXR should be obtained upon admission to the ICU and daily for the first few days after surgery. Particular attention should be given to the location of all tubes and lines, as well as the heart size and lung fields.

The surgeon will occasionally leave the chest "open" after a Norwood procedure and other complex neonatal operations, with the skin closed using a Silastic patch, until hemodynamic stability can be achieved, bleeding controlled, and myocardial edema can decrease. The risk for mediastinitis may be increased when the chest is left open, and prophylactic antibiotics are typically continued during this time period (11). Delayed sternal closure may be performed in a few days in the operating room or in the ICU. Of note, much higher doses of narcotics are required during sternal closure when compared to many other ICU procedures. When the sternum is closed, respiratory compliance may decrease necessitating additional ventilatory support.

Cardiopulmonary interactions play an important role in the physiology of neonates and infants following cardiac surgery (12). Manipulations of $PaCO_2$, PaO_2, pH, and mean airway pressure may be used in the context of the patient's physiology to modulate hemodynamics. Mechanical ventilation and sedation are also useful to minimize oxygen consumption in patients with limited cardiopulmonary reserve. Respiratory acidosis may increase pulmonary vascular resistance, and efforts should be made in most cases to avoid it (13). Low functional residual capacity may predispose patients to atelectasis and increased pulmonary vascular resistance, whereas pulmonary overdistension may increase pulmonary vascular resistance and decrease cardiac output. More generous tidal volumes (e.g., 8 to 10 cc/kg) are often utilized after CPB when compared to those typically used in patients receiving mechanical ventilation for parenchymal lung disease.

Although early extubation policies have been reported for older infants and children, most neonates and young infants receive at least 12 to 24 hours of mechanical ventilation following congenital heart surgery. Criteria for extubation following cardiac surgery in neonates and infants include the presence of adequate cardiac output, appropriate neurologic status to maintain the airway, muscular strength to support respiratory pump function, acceptable gas exchange, and the absence of significant arrhythmias, bleeding, or fever.

Standard laboratory values need to be assessed in the early postoperative period. Electrolytes, including magnesium and ionized calcium levels, are monitored and corrected as needed. A complete blood count is initially obtained daily, and hemoglobin levels are monitored more frequently. In general, a hemoglobin level of 10 to 12 g/dL is appropriate for infants following a two-ventricular repair, and a hemoglobin level of 13 to 15 g/dL is reasonable for infants following a palliative operation with ongoing cyanosis. Relative anemia may place unnecessary workload on the myocardium, and transfusion of erythrocytes will improve oxygen delivery following pediatric cardiac surgery. An assessment of coagulation status (prothrombin and partial thromboplastin times (PTTs), and platelet count) is often obtained soon after CPB and repeated as clinically indicated.

In addition to the physical examination, several clinical parameters may be used to assess the adequacy of cardiac output and oxygen delivery in the immediate postoperative period. The presence of metabolic acidosis, as quantified by a base deficit or lactate level, suggests inadequate systemic cardiac output and requires investigation. Lactic acidosis develops when inadequate tissue oxygen delivery leads to anaerobic metabolism. Following congenital heart surgery, elevated lactate levels in infants and children upon admission to the ICU are associated with increased morbidity and mortality (14). Venous oxygen saturation may be measured to estimate cardiac output. Urine output and markers of renal function (blood urea nitrogen and creatinine) provide a good estimate of the systemic cardiac output. Oliguria may be seen for 12 to 24 hours after complex cases, but improvement should occur thereafter in most patients.

Near-infrared spectroscopy (NIRS) technology measures regional tissue oxygen saturation levels. Cerebral and renal NIRS are most commonly measured. Cerebral NIRS values tend to correlate with oxygen saturation measurements from the superior vena cava. The routine use of NIRS monitoring in the postoperative period is controversial, as no data exist to support any impact

on short- or long-term outcomes (15,16). NIRS data must be interpreted in the context of hemoglobin levels, patient state (e.g., sedated or agitated), and other factors that may influence systemic oxygen consumption (e.g., temperature).

Infants often receive inotropic support following CPB. Low-dose dopamine, epinephrine, or milrinone is the initial drug of choice at many centers. Inotropic support is discussed in more detail in the low cardiac output section below.

Infants may develop significant fluid retention following CPB, which may impair myocardial, respiratory, and gastrointestinal function. Strategies used to minimize this problem in the operating room, including the use of steroids and ultrafiltration, were discussed earlier. Despite the presence of total body fluid overload, intravascular volume depletion is common in the first few hours following surgery due in part to capillary leak, and one or more fluid boluses may be required. Diuretics are typically initiated 12 to 24 hours after surgery, as either bolus doses or continuous infusion. The correction of electrolyte disturbances, particularly hypokalemia, hyponatremia, and a hypochloremic metabolic alkalosis, is commonly necessary as diuresis occurs in the first few days following CPB.

Analgesia is provided for all patients following cardiac surgery. High-dose fentanyl is well tolerated and blunts the stress response in neonates following CPB (17). Morphine or other narcotics may also be used in the early postoperative period. Benzodiazepines or dexmedetomidine may be administered for amnesia and sedation. Continuous infusions of narcotics and sedative agents may be better tolerated when compared to intermittent boluses in hemodynamically labile infants. Neuromuscular blocking agents may be used in selected patients to eliminate ventilator dyssynchrony and minimize oxygen consumption in patients with labile hemodynamics.

Gastrointestinal tract motility is decreased following cardiac surgery. Contributory factors include the inflammatory effects of CPB, anesthesia, fluid retention, narcotics, and (in some cases) high central venous pressures or low cardiac output. If these considerations are anticipated to preclude the initiation of enteral nutrition for several days, then parenteral nutrition may be administered. Histamine-2 receptor antagonists may be administered to minimize the risk of upper gastrointestinal bleeding.

COMMON POSTOPERATIVE COMPLICATIONS

Low Cardiac Output

The product of heart rate and stroke volume determines cardiac output. Stroke volume is determined by preload, afterload, and contractility. Low cardiac output may thus be caused by abnormalities in one or more of these variables (Table 33.1). Transient low cardiac output, when defined as a cardiac index less than 2.0 L/min/m², occurs following approximately 25% of complex biventricular neonatal repairs (18). Signs of low cardiac output include tachycardia, hypotension, poor peripheral perfusion, poor urine output, and metabolic acidosis/elevated serum lactate levels. A detailed assessment must be undertaken to identify the cause in order to initiate proper and timely treatment.

A suboptimal surgical repair with significant residual intracardiac shunts, ventricular outflow or aortic obstruction, systemic or pulmonary venous stenosis, and/or valvular lesions may be the primary etiology for low cardiac output. Following neonatal cardiac surgery, the incidence of unplanned cardiac reinterventions during the same hospitalization as the initial operation is approximately 10% (19). Early identification of significant residual lesions requires an appreciation of the anticipated "normal" postoperative course, close attention to the physical examination and data obtained by various monitoring modalities, open communication with the cardiovascular surgeon, and a high index of suspicion. In

TABLE 33.1

Variables Impacting Cardiac Output

Variable	Abnormality	Common Etiologies
Heart rate	Tachycardia	Fever
		Pain
	Bradycardia	Hypothermia
		Sedation
	Arrhythmias	Heart block
		SVT (many types)
		Ventricular tachycardia/fibrillation
Preload	Decreased	Bleeding
		Excessive diuresis
		Capillary leak tamponade
	Increased	Fluid overload
Contractility	Decreased	Acidosis
		Electrolyte imbalance
		Hypothermia
		Myocardial injury (e.g., ventriculotomy, ischemia reperfusion injury, inflammation)
Afterload	↑ vascular resistance	Systemic hypertension
		Hypothermia
		Pain
		Pulmonary hypertension
	Ventricular outflow tract obstruction	Aortic arch obstruction
		Aortic stenosis
		Pulmonary stenosis
		Pulmonary artery stenosis

patients with a suspected residual lesion, cardiac imaging (usually starting with an echocardiogram) will be helpful to define the extent of the problem.

Treatment of low cardiac output in neonates differs in some respects from that in older children and adults due to differences in maturation-dependent cardiovascular physiology. Because neonates have a greater ratio of noncontractile to contractile myocardial mass, ventricular diastolic compliance is diminished. They also have a somewhat limited ability to increase stroke volume, which is relatively fixed at approximately 1.5 cc/kg. Thus, cardiac output is heart rate dependent in neonates. Heart rate may be optimized by pacing or by using intravenous infusions of chronotropic agents including dopamine or epinephrine. For patients with advanced second-degree or complete heart block, atrioventricular sequential pacing will increase cardiac output. Other postoperative arrhythmias are discussed in detail below.

Optimization of cardiac loading conditions is a key component to the management of low cardiac output. Attention to preload is paramount in this regard. As described by the Frank-Starling mechanism, augmentation of the end-diastolic volume increases the number of interactions between actin and myosin molecules, resulting in a larger stroke volume and thus higher cardiac output. Hypovolemia may result in decreased ventricular filling and lower cardiac output. Certain cardiac operations in neonates, such as repair of tetralogy of Fallot or truncus arteriosus, may result in impaired right ventricular compliance, and additional preload may be needed early after surgery to maintain cardiac output. Volume replacement should be guided by close attention to intracardiac filling pressures, arterial pressures, and physical examination findings including liver distention and peripheral pulses. The type and amount of fluid replacement is based upon the hematocrit, albumin level, and estimated percentage of volume loss. Boluses of fluid are typically given in aliquots of 5 to 10 mL/kg over several

minutes. A left atrial pressure above 14 to 16 mm Hg rarely produces an additional increase in cardiac output, and a left atrial pressure above 20 mm Hg may cause pulmonary edema. Of note, due to the large venous capacitance, right atrial pressures may not necessarily reflect the volume administered and should not be used in isolation to estimate preload.

Afterload, defined as the sum of forces that oppose systolic performance, is best quantified by systolic wall stress and vascular impedance, both of which are difficult to measure at the bedside. Elevated vascular resistance can significantly reduce stroke volume and the extent and velocity of wall shortening, resulting in decreased cardiac output and ventricular function. Increased vascular resistance is commonly seen following CPB in neonates (18). Physiologic factors such as hypoxia, acidosis, hypothermia, and pain may further increase systemic and pulmonary vascular resistance. Increased afterload may be due to residual right or left ventricular outflow tract obstruction. In the setting of decreased cardiac contractility, increased afterload may be a compensatory response necessary to maintain systemic blood pressure.

Vascular resistance, and thus afterload, can be pharmacologically decreased by vasodilatation of the systemic and pulmonary vascular beds. Systemic afterload reduction may be beneficial for patients with significant aortic or mitral valve regurgitation, left ventricular dysfunction, hypertension, or Norwood physiology. Afterload reduction in the pulmonary circulation may be beneficial for infants with tricuspid valve regurgitation, right ventricular dysfunction, and pulmonary hypertension. In addition to its inotropic properties, milrinone is a direct vasodilator of the systemic and pulmonary vascular beds. Milrinone has been shown to reduce the incidence of low cardiac output syndrome and infants and children undergoing complex two-ventricular repairs in a multicenter trial (20). Other vasodilators such as sodium nitroprusside, nitroglycerine, and nicardipine may be administered as infusions to reduce afterload. With the use of any vasodilators, volume augmentation may be necessary to fill the expanded vascular space and maintain adequate preload. Inhaled nitric oxide may be used as a selective vasodilator of the pulmonary vascular bed, thereby decreasing right ventricular afterload. Positive pressure ventilation may be used to reduce wall stress and left ventricular afterload (21).

Cardiac contractility is the load-independent ability of the myocardium to generate force. Contractility may be intrinsically impaired preoperatively. Intraoperatively, contractility may be depressed by medications, anesthesia, myocardial ischemia–reperfusion injury, an extensive ventriculotomy, or by myocardial resection. Postoperatively, hypoxia, acidosis, and certain pharmacologic agents may all compromise contractility. Myocardial contractility may be enhanced with pharmacologic agents. Several inotropic drugs are currently available, and each has its own characteristic effects that may be more suitable for use in various clinical situations.

Dopamine activates dopaminergic, alpha, and beta-receptors, depending on the dosage used. When prescribed at 1 to 5 µg/kg/min, dopamine preferentially dilates mesenteric and renal vessels, and increases renal blood flow. Dosing at 5 to 10 µg/kg/min tends to increase cardiac output with a mild increase in heart rate. Higher doses of dopamine (10 to 20 µg/kg/min) are usually avoided after cardiac surgery unless vasoconstriction is desired. Low-dose dopamine or epinephrine is the initial drug of choice to increase myocardial contractility at many centers.

Dobutamine, a synthetic catecholamine, acts primarily on myocardial beta-receptors. Contractility increases with infusion of dobutamine, but there may be less effect on heart rate or vascular tone than with dopamine.

Milrinone is a phosphodiesterase inhibitor that exerts a positive inotropic effect by increasing intracellular levels of cyclic AMP, leading to improving cardiac contractility. It also has lusitropic (enhancing myocardial relaxation) properties and acts as a direct vasodilator of the systemic and pulmonary vascular beds. Milrinone has been shown to improve hemodynamics in neonates with existing low cardiac output (22) and decrease the incidence of low cardiac output syndrome in patients less than 6 years of age undergoing a biventricular repair (20).

Epinephrine may also be used to augment myocardial contractility. When administered at 0.01 to 0.05 µg/kg/min, epinephrine primarily activates beta-1 cardiac receptors causing increased inotropy and beta-2 peripheral receptors causing reduced afterload. High-dose epinephrine (>0.1 µg/kg/min) is not frequently used because of marked alpha-adrenergic action and adverse effect on renal perfusion. Uncommonly, a neonate may have vasodilatory shock with inappropriately low systemic vascular resistance that is refractory to catecholamine infusions. In this setting, a vasopressin infusion may increase systemic vascular resistance, restore blood pressure and cardiac output, and reduce the requirement for inotropic agents (23).

Neonates with refractory low cardiac output, myocardial dysfunction, and impending cardiovascular collapse may benefit from reopening of the sternotomy incision in the ICU. The combination of edema of the myocardium and other mediastinal structures, and any fluid or blood collections around the heart, may contribute to poor ventricular filling and compliance. Reopening the chest will expand the mediastinal space until edema improves, and any fluid collections or blood clots can be easily removed.

In patients with excessive or prolonged inotropic or vasopressor needs following CPB, a state of relative adrenocortical insufficiency may exist (24). Myocardial beta-receptor down-regulation may occur in the perioperative period. Corticosteroids, probably acting by improving vascular tone and up-regulating adrenergic receptors, may facilitate weaning of high-dose catecholamine infusions (25).

Thyroid hormone plays an important role in the regulation of the cardiovascular system. Decreased levels of triiodothyronine (T_3) and thyroxine levels occur in some neonates following CPB (26). Clinical trials in such patients have found marginal benefits with thyroid hormone repletion following CPB (27,28).

Arrhythmias (See Also Chapter 34 for Overall Discussion of Arrhythmias)

Arrhythmias may compromise cardiac output following cardiac surgery. In addition to inappropriately fast or slow heart rates, arrhythmias often involve a loss of atrioventricular synchrony. When the atria contract against a closed atrioventricular valve during certain arrhythmias, cannon a-waves (i.e., an increase in amplitude of the atrial pressure waveform) are typically seen. Prolonged CPB and aortic cross clamp times and higher postoperative serum troponin levels are associated with the development of arrhythmias (29).

A specific arrhythmia diagnosis may often be obtained with a 12-lead electrocardiogram. If the mechanism remains unclear, an atrial electrogram may be obtained. To obtain an atrial electrogram, one technique is to connect the two-leg leads of the ECG to the temporary atrial pacing wires, and the two arm leads are placed on the patient's arms in the usual fashion. A rhythm strip of leads I, II, and III is then recorded. With this configuration, lead I will be a surface electrogram, and a sharp atrial electrogram (indicating atrial depolarization) is produced in leads II and III, which may be compared to the surface QRS complex in lead I to determine the relationship of P waves to the QRS complexes.

Nearly any type of arrhythmia may occur following infant CPB. Premature atrial complexes (PACs) are occasionally seen and may be related to central lines, electrolyte disturbances, or surgical incisions; they are usually benign. Reentrant forms of supraventricular tachycardia (SVT), such as atrial flutter and atrioventricular reentrant tachycardia, occasionally occur. Although rate-related aberrancy and antegrade conduction over accessory connections may occur, in most cases of SVT, the QRS complex in tachycardia is similar in morphology and axis to that seen on the baseline postoperative ECG. Note that the baseline QRS complex may be wide if a bundle branch block developed during surgery.

Atrial flutter is more likely to be seen following complex atrial baffling procedures. Atrial flutter is characterized by a rapid, regular atrial rate with variable atrioventricular conduction. Adenosine may be helpful diagnostically as the flutter waves will persist in the presence of atrioventricular block. Atrial flutter may be terminated using rapid atrial pacing or synchronized cardioversion.

Atrioventricular reentrant tachycardia may be seen in infants with accessory connections (i.e., Ebstein anomaly, L-looped ventricular inversion). Preexcitation (Wolff-Parkinson-White syndrome) may be present on the electrocardiogram in sinus rhythm. Atrioventricular reentrant tachycardia is characterized by retrograde P waves following the QRS complex in a one-to-one relationship and is terminated with adenosine, rapid atrial pacing, or synchronized cardioversion. Atrioventricular nodal reentrant tachycardia is uncommon in neonates. Retrograde P waves are typically hidden in the QRS complex. Termination may be achieved using adenosine, rapid atrial pacing, or synchronized cardioversion.

Ectopic atrial tachycardia is an uncommon form of SVT following congenital heart surgery. It is characterized by an automatic atrial rhythm with "warm up" and "cool down" behavior at its onset and termination. Treatment strategies include normalization of electrolytes and temperature, minimizing inotropic infusions, and administration of a variety of antiarrhythmic agents including beta-blockers and amiodarone.

Junctional ectopic tachycardia (JET) is a common type of SVT seen in the postoperative period in neonates and infants, particularly following repair of tetralogy of Fallot or VSDs (30). JET is an automatic rhythm originating from the bundle of His and, although thought to be caused by some form of trauma to the AV node during surgery, may occasionally be seen following cardiac surgical interventions distant from the AV node. Electrophysiologic characteristics of JET include a QRS morphology similar to that seen in sinus rhythm; atrioventricular dissociation with the ventricular rate faster than the atrial rate or 1:1 retrograde conduction; "warm up" behavior as seen with automatic arrhythmias; and failure to respond to adenosine, overdrive pacing, or cardioversion. Cannon a-waves will have variable amplitude in patients with JET if ventricular–atrial (V–A) dissociation is present, but a constant increased amplitude will be present if the junctional rhythm is conducted to the atria in a 1:1 retrograde pattern. A 12-lead ECG or interrogation of temporary atrial pacing wires will confirm the diagnosis. Although JET usually resolves spontaneously in the first few days following surgery, hemodynamic compromise may occur, particularly when the ventricular rate exceeds 170 to 180 beats per minute. Treatment is individualized based on the patient's heart rate and hemodynamic status. Strategies include fever control, provision of adequate analgesia to limit endogenous catecholamine release, minimizing the use of exogenous catecholamines, normalization of electrolytes and acid–base status, atrial pacing at a rate faster than the junctional rate, and mild hypothermia (31). If these measures are insufficient, medications to consider include amiodarone, esmolol, and procainamide. As these drugs have negative inotropic and chronotropic properties, close monitoring of hemodynamics and backup pacing capabilities are desirable.

Premature ventricular contractions (PVCs) may reflect myocardial irritability, electrolyte disturbances, or hypoxia. Lidocaine is often administered for frequent PVCs or nonsustained ventricular tachycardia (VT). VT is characterized by a fast, wide QRS complex that differs in morphology and axis compared to the postoperative baseline and has either 1:1 retrograde V–A conduction or V–A dissociation. The presence of complex ventricular ectopy or VT is suggestive of myocardial ischemia, and patients who had coronary manipulation as a component of their operation may warrant evaluation of myocardial function and coronary blood flow. Sustained VT with hemodynamic compromise may be terminated by synchronized cardioversion. Pharmacologic therapy, starting with either lidocaine or procainamide, may be considered for patients with hemodynamically stable VT. Ventricular fibrillation (VF) is characterized by a wide complex, irregular rhythm that requires immediate defibrillation, starting at 2 J/kg. Chest compressions should be performed during pulseless VT or VF until a perfusing rhythm is reestablished.

Surgical complete heart block is typically apparent when the patient is rewarmed following CPB but less commonly may develop in the first few days following surgery. Temporary atrioventricular sequential pacing is used for initial treatment. The capture threshold of the temporary ventricular pacing wire should be determined frequently in patients who have developed or are at high risk for complete heart block. If atrioventricular conduction does not return after a period of observation (typically at least 7 days), a permanent pacemaker is indicated to prevent low cardiac output and sudden death (32).

Pulmonary Hypertension

The contemporary practice of cardiac surgical intervention in early infancy has been associated with a decreased incidence of pulmonary hypertensive crises for patients with many complex congenital heart defects. However, this problem continues to complicate the postoperative course of selected patients in the current era. Pulmonary hypertension following CPB may be caused by a combination of preoperative, intraoperative, and postoperative factors (Table 33.2). Patients with obstructed pulmonary venous return, mitral stenosis, long-standing pulmonary hypertension, or left ventricular outflow obstruction (critical aortic valve stenosis or coarctation of the aorta) may have increased pulmonary vascular resistance. Down syndrome is also a risk factor for severe postoperative pulmonary hypertension (33). CPB is associated with increased pulmonary vascular resistance in infants and children (18,34,35). The conduct of CPB is associated with partial ischemia of the pulmonary vasculature, leading to endothelial cell dysfunction and decreased endogenous production of nitric oxide. CPB leads to increased plasma levels of catecholamines, endothelin-1, and other pulmonary vasoconstrictors. The presence of significant pulmonary hypertension soon after weaning from CPB is predictive of subsequent pulmonary hypertension in the ICU and the need for prolonged ventilatory support. Postoperatively, large residual left-to-right shunts, obstruction to pulmonary venous or distal pulmonary arterial blood flow, or left ventricular outflow tract obstruction may cause pulmonary hypertension. Noxious stimuli, particularly suctioning of the endotracheal tube, may trigger a pulmonary hypertensive crisis.

Pulmonary hypertension may manifest as low cardiac output following a biventricular repair, particularly when both septa are completely intact, or as excessive cyanosis in patients with palliated single ventricle physiology. The severity of pulmonary hypertension may be estimated noninvasively by Doppler interrogation of a tricuspid regurgitation jet using an echocardiogram. Pulmonary artery catheters, although not commonly used, provide direct and continuous measurement of pulmonary artery pressure following biventricular repairs.

A combination of relatively simple postoperative strategies should be sufficient to prevent the development of pulmonary hypertensive crises in many at-risk patients (Table 33.3) (36). Early definitive repair can reduce the incidence of postoperative pulmonary hypertension (37). Adequate oxygenation and ventilation are important in the early postoperative period to maintain low pulmonary vascular resistance, as is the maintenance of relatively normal lung volumes. Deep sedation and analgesia are also used to minimize the incidence of pulmonary hypertension crises. Fentanyl has also been shown to blunt the elevation in pulmonary artery pressure and pulmonary vascular resistance related to endotracheal suctioning (17).

All of the management strategies mentioned above regarding the prevention of pulmonary hypertension may be employed in the event of a pulmonary hypertensive crisis. Hyperventilation will typically reduce pulmonary artery pressure and pulmonary vascular resistance. The role of nonselective vasodilators used in the past to treat severe postoperative pulmonary hypertension has been replaced with inhaled nitric oxide. Nitric oxide diffuses to adjacent smooth muscle cells, where relaxation occurs by activation of guanylate cyclase, which increases intracellular guanosine 3′, 5′-monophosphate (cyclic GMP). Because inhaled nitric oxide is rapidly inactivated by hemoglobin, it acts as a selective pulmonary vasodilator. Multiple published studies report beneficial effects of inhaled nitric oxide in alleviating pulmonary hypertension following CPB in infants and children (38–40). Transient right ventricular dysfunction following repair of congenital heart defects may be exacerbated by pulmonary hypertension. Nitric oxide improves right ventricular ejection fraction and cardiac output while decreasing pulmonary artery pressure and vascular resistance in infants and young children following a biventricular repair (40). Side effects associated with nitric oxide include a rebound effect upon withdrawal of the drug, and

---

TABLE 33.2

Factors Contributing to Perioperative Pulmonary Hypertension in Infants with Complex Congenital Heart Disease

Preoperative
  Left-to-right shunts
  Obstructed pulmonary venous return
  Pulmonary hypoplasia (e.g., as seen in congenital diaphragmatic hernia, Ebstein anomaly, etc.)

Intraoperative
  Microemboli
  Pulmonary leukosequestration
  Excess thromboxane production
  Duration of CPB
  Endothelial injury

Postoperative
  Mechanical obstruction to pulmonary blood flow
  Residual left-to-right shunt
  Atelectasis
  Hypoxic pulmonary vasoconstriction
  Catecholamines (endogenous and exogenous)

TABLE 33.3

Critical Care Strategies for Treatment of Pulmonary Hypertension

Encourage	Avoid
1. Anatomic investigation	1. Residual anatomic disease
2. Right-to-left atrial pop off	2. Intact atrial septum
3. Sedation/analgesia	3. Agitation/pain
4. Moderate hyperventilation	4. Respiratory acidosis
5. Moderate alkalosis	5. Metabolic acidosis
6. Adequate inspired oxygen	6. Alveolar hypoxia
7. Normal lung volumes	7. Atelectasis or overdistension
8. Optimal hematocrit	8. Excessive hematocrit
9. Inotropic support	9. Low output and coronary perfusion
10. Pulmonary vasodilators	10. Pulmonary vasoconstrictors

TABLE 33.4

Etiologies of Cyanosis Following Palliative Cardiac Surgery

Category	Specific Etiologies
Inadequate pulmonary blood flow	• Stenosis or thrombosis in shunt or pulmonary arteries • Pulmonary hypertension • Pulmonary venous obstruction or left atrial outlet obstruction
Pulmonary venous desaturation	• Parenchymal lung disease • Pleural effusions • Systemic to pulmonary venous collateral vessels
Systemic venous desaturation	• Low cardiac output • Increased oxygen consumption • Anemia

methemoglobinemia. Sildenafil may be used to minimize rebound pulmonary hypertension and thus facilitate the weaning of inhaled nitric oxide (41,42).

Cyanosis

Excessive cyanosis following surgical repair or palliation may be caused by one or more anatomic or physiologic problems. In patients with palliated single ventricle physiology, excessive cyanosis may be attributable to *inadequate pulmonary blood flow*, *pulmonary venous desaturation*, and/or *systemic venous desaturation* (Table 33.4). Treatment of cyanosis is dictated by the underlying cause(s).

Bleeding

Excessive bleeding may occur from suture lines and/or abnormalities in the coagulation system following cardiac surgery. Excessive bleeding may be defined as greater than 5 mL/kg of blood from the chest tube in any given hour or greater than 3 mL/kg/h × 3 hours. Risk factors for postoperative bleeding include repeat sternotomy, cyanosis, and operations involving extensive suture lines in the aorta. Aminocaproic acid and tranexamic acid, both antifibrinolytic agents, may be administered intraoperatively to patients at risk for bleeding. The platelet count is usually maintained greater than 50,000 to 100,000/mL in the early postoperative period. Fresh frozen plasma may be administered for a prothrombin time (PT) of approximately 25 seconds or more, or for excessive bleeding. Hypertension might exacerbate bleeding and should be controlled. A prolonged PTT may be due to inadequate reversal of heparin, for which additional protamine administration may be considered. Bleeding may occur when intracardiac lines are removed as discussed earlier.

Cardiac tamponade may occur when significant bleeding is not evacuated by the chest tube(s). External compression of the heart by blood or blood clots leads to impaired ventricular filling, increased central venous pressure, tachycardia, a narrow pulse pressure, and eventually systemic hypotension. Tamponade is a clinical diagnosis, and although an echocardiogram may be helpful, surgical exploration should not be delayed while awaiting this test.

Cardiac Arrest

Cardiac arrest occurs in approximately 3% of all cardiac ICU admissions, and neonates and infants undergoing cardiac surgery are at greater risk (43). Algorithms exist for the management of cardiopulmonary arrest and will not be repeated here (44). A recent scientific statement from the American Heart Association summarizes the nuances of cardiopulmonary resuscitation in infants and children with cardiac disease (45). Patients having a cardiac arrest following congenital heart surgery have better survival rate when compared with other pediatric inpatients (46). The better survival rate may be attributed to a variety of factors unique to the cardiac

population, including the increased incidence of an acute ventricular arrhythmia, the absence of multiorgan system failure in the majority of cardiac patients, as well as the common presence of central venous access, arterial access, and epicardial pacing wires.

Need for Mechanical Cardiac Support

Mechanical circulatory support is used in approximately 2.4% of children undergoing cardiac surgery, and neonates and infants are at greater risk (47). ECMO is the most commonly used modality. Patients who cannot be weaned from CPB may be converted to an ECMO circuit before leaving the operating room. Once in the ICU, those neonates who develop refractory low cardiac output, severe cyanosis, arrhythmias, pulmonary hypertension despite maximal medical therapy, or have an unexpected cardiac arrest may be candidates for mechanical cardiopulmonary support. Mechanical support may be used as a bridge to myocardial recovery or cardiac transplantation. Venoarterial ECMO is used in nearly all neonates requiring mechanical support for primary cardiac failure, in contrast to neonates with primary respiratory failure who may be supported with venovenous ECMO. Relative contraindications to ECMO include multiorgan system failure, an irreversible or inoperable disease process, significant neurology impairment, uncontrolled bleeding, and extremes of size and weight (48). The decision to employ ECMO following cardiac surgery should ideally be made prior to the development of irreversible end-organ failure, as patients who have been placed on ECMO after extended efforts at medical management have been shown to do poorly (49).

A detailed overview of the intensive care management of patients on ECMO is beyond the scope of this chapter. However, several critical issues that are important for cardiac patients deserve comment. In those with biventricular physiology on ECMO, decompression of the left atrium and left ventricle are important to reduce myocardial wall stress and pulmonary edema. Left atrial hypertension may manifest as pulmonary edema on chest radiograph, and left ventricular distension may be evaluated by echocardiogram. Left heart decompression may be accomplished by increasing the ECMO flow rate, using low-dose inotropic agents and afterload reduction to improve myocardial ejection, and/or by decompressing the left atrium using surgical or transcatheter techniques (50).

The ventilator strategy used for cardiac ECMO patients is important to optimize the probability of myocardial recovery. In patients whose systemic ventricle is ejecting, even on full venoarterial ECMO flow, the coronary circulation is at least partially supplied by blood ejected from the heart. Thus, ventilator settings should be selected to maintain lung recruitment and minimize ventilation–perfusion mismatch, so that pulmonary venous blood, which eventually perfuses the myocardium, is adequately oxygenated. Cardiac ECMO runs are often short, and maintenance of open lungs is important to facilitate early weaning. This strategy contrasts with the typical initial ventilator management used in neonates and infants with primary respiratory failure on ECMO, which focuses on lung rest and avoidance of additional lung injury.

The use of ECMO in neonates with single ventricle physiology is challenging. As is the case prior to initiation of mechanical support, the physiology in these patients on ECMO is such that runoff of systemic arterial flow through a patent ductus arteriosus (PDA) or systemic to pulmonary shunt may lead to coronary ischemia, volume overload of the single ventricle, and systemic hypoperfusion. Thus, if a ductus arteriosus is present or the systemic to pulmonary shunt is present when ECMO is initiated, the flow on the ECMO circuit must be increased to compensate for systemic to pulmonary runoff. Complete occlusion of a systemic to pulmonary shunt at the time of ECMO cannulation will eliminate the runoff but may lead to pulmonary infarction and shunt thrombosis (51). Partial clipping of the shunt while on ECMO is a reasonable compromise, as the clips may be removed at the time of ECMO decannulation.

A high index of suspicion for residual lesions is necessary for any postoperative patient who is placed on ECMO. If transthoracic echocardiographic windows are poor, transesophageal echocardiography or CT angiography may be utilized in infants on ECMO to obtain diagnostic information. Cardiac catheterization may also be performed for patients on ECMO to evaluate for the presence of residual lesions that may be amenable to transcatheter or surgical intervention or to decompress the left heart via balloon septostomy (52).

Extracorporeal cardiopulmonary resuscitation (also known as "E-CPR" or "rapid-deployment ECMO") is useful to rescue patients who do not respond to conventional cardiopulmonary resuscitation. Current American Heart Association recommendations support the use of E-CPR for refractory cardiac arrest in children with underlying cardiac disease, provided that the cause of the arrest is potentially reversible and that the event occurs in an environment with established protocols, equipment, and expertise to implement ECMO rapidly (44,53).

Extracorporeal Life Support Organization registry data indicate that contemporary survival to hospital discharge following cardiac ECMO in neonates and infants is approximately 45% in neonates and 57% in children (54). When ECMO is utilized to facilitate cardiopulmonary resuscitation in neonates and children, survival to hospital discharge is 43% (54). In a recent multicenter analysis of patients receiving ECMO after a Norwood palliation, survival to hospital discharge was 43% (47). Inability to wean from ECMO within 3 to 5 days and the development of renal failure are ominous signs for pediatric cardiac patients. The intermediate-term survival is favorable for most neonates and infants who survive postpericardiotomy ECMO. Approximately one-third of such patients have neurodevelopmental issues, and significant deficits are present in approximately 10% (55). The etiology for these neurologic deficits is multifactorial. Quality of life for pediatric cardiac ECMO survivors is similar to that of other children with complex cardiac disorders (56).

Limited data are currently available regarding the use of ventricular assist devices in neonates and infants, and current outcomes are not encouraging. In one multicenter experience, 66% of patients weighing less than 5 kg died while being supported with a ventricular assist device (57). Young infants with CHD have particularly poor outcomes with ventricular assist device support (58). ECMO may be the preferred mode of ongoing mechanical circulatory support for these small patients, in contrast to older children who may benefit from transition to a ventricular assist device.

Pulmonary Complications

Pulmonary dysfunction occurs following CPB due to a variety of factors, including the diffuse inflammatory response, increased capillary permeability, fluid overload, and microemboli. In neonates and infants, decreased pulmonary compliance and increased alveolar–arterial oxygen gradient are commonly seen, and pulmonary vascular resistance may be elevated. A variety of strategies designed to counteract these adverse effects of CPB have been discussed earlier, including the use of MUF, corticosteroids, and methods to prevent and treat pulmonary hypertension.

Patients who cannot be weaned from mechanical ventilation or extubated in a timely fashion may have an underlying residual cardiac lesion and/or a noncardiac problem (19). Noncardiac reasons for difficult weaning are numerous and may include one or more of the following: abnormalities in respiratory drive (e.g., central nervous system injury, sedation), respiratory pump (e.g., critical illness polyneuropathy, phrenic nerve injury), gas exchange (e.g., parenchymal lung injury), or increased ventilatory load (e.g., overfeeding with increased carbohydrate load, increased dead space).

External compression of the central airways occasionally may complicate the perioperative course in neonates with CHD. For example, following aortic reconstruction (e.g., after the Norwood

operation or repair of interrupted aortic arch [IAA]), the aorta may cause extrinsic compression on the left mainstem bronchus. Some neonates with tetralogy of Fallot and absent pulmonary valve syndrome have significant pulmonary artery dilation that leads to tracheal and mainstem bronchial compression in the preoperative period, and tracheobronchial malacia may persist following surgery. Tracheal stenosis or tracheomalacia may develop postoperatively due to endotracheal tube-related mucosal injury. Stridor and other forms of upper airway obstruction will make intrathoracic pressure significantly more negative in the spontaneously breathing patient, and the resultant increased ventricular afterload may be poorly tolerated in the neonate with limited cardiac reserve.

The phrenic nerves are at risk for paresis or transection during cardiac surgery, and paralysis of a hemidiaphragm may make it difficult to wean neonates from mechanical ventilation. The diagnosis may be confirmed by ultrasound or fluoroscopy during spontaneous breathing. Diaphragmatic plication may be useful to facilitate weaning from the ventilator. The left recurrent laryngeal nerve, which arises from the left vagus nerve and loops underneath the aortic arch, may be injured during aortic arch surgery or PDA ligation, resulting in unilateral vocal cord paralysis. Postoperatively, such infants may have problems with maintenance of functional residual capacity and aspiration. Tracheobronchial ischemia, leading to obstruction of the lower airways, has been reported following unifocalization procedures in infants with pulmonary atresia, VSD, and MAPCAs. The tracheobronchial ischemia is probably related to interruption of peribronchial arterial blood supply during mobilization of MAPCAs (59).

The development of a postoperative chylothorax occurs in approximately 3.8% of cases following congenital heart surgery (60). A chylothorax may develop following thoracic duct injury, elevated systemic venous pressures, or thrombosis of the subclavian veins. The diagnosis is suspected when chest tube output becomes milky in appearance, significantly increases in volume, or is prolonged. Laboratory confirmation of chylothorax includes the presence of elevated pleural fluid triglyceride levels and lymphocyte counts. Treatment strategies initiate with chest tube drainage and dietary modification with defatted ("skimmed") breast milk and/or a medium chain triglyceride (MCT)–based formula. Prolonged drainage may lead to depletion of plasma proteins (albumin, coagulation factors, immunoglobulins) and lymphocytes, and consideration should be given to replacement with albumin, fresh frozen plasma, and/or intravenous immunoglobulins (IVIG). Additional treatment options are summarized in **Figure 33.1**. Embolization of abnormal lymphatic channels may be considered in selected patients with refractory chylothorax, but experience in neonates is limited (61).

Gastrointestinal Complications

Feeding problems, growth failure, and gastroesophageal reflux are all common in neonates and infants with complex CHD (62). Oropharyngeal dysphagia is particularly problematic in patients with certain genetic anomalies (e.g., DiGeorge syndrome), those who did not have the opportunity to acquire suck and swallow skills before surgery, and those experiencing prolonged oral-tracheal intubation. Postoperative nutrition algorithms have been published and may be utilized to decrease practice variation and optimize caloric intake (63). Nasogastric feedings may be initially utilized after surgery, and input from a speech therapist may be useful (63). In neonates for whom oropharyngeal dysphagia is anticipated to persist beyond hospital discharge, placement of a gastrostomy tube may be considered.

NEC may occur before or after congenital heart surgery, particularly in neonates with systemic to pulmonary runoff physiology (e.g., a single ventricle patient with a systemic to pulmonary artery shunt) (64). Because of bowel dysfunction related to anesthesia and narcotics, as well as the concern for NEC, total parenteral

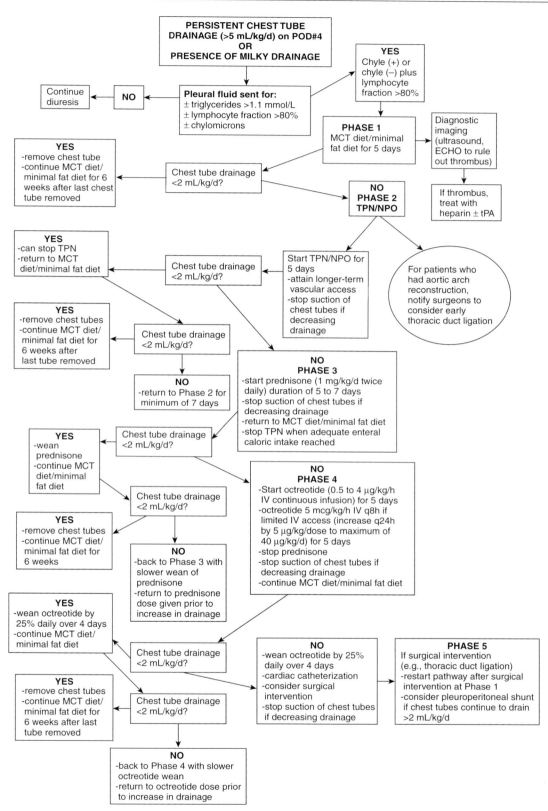

FIGURE 33.1 Care flow sheet for diagnosis and management of chylothorax. ECHO, echocardiogram; IV, intravenous; MCT, medium chain triglyceride formulae; NPO, nothing by mouth; POD, postoperative day; q8h, every 8 hours; q24h, daily; tPA, tissue plasminogen activator; TPN, total parental nutrition. (Reprinted from Chan EH, et al. Postoperative chylothorax after cardiothoracic surgery in children. *Ann Thorac Surg* 2005;80:1864, with permission.)

THE NEWBORN INFANT

nutrition may be administered for the first few days after cardiac surgery in neonates. In patients with heterotaxy syndrome, intestinal malrotation may exist and predispose afflicted patients to midgut volvulus. The elective performance of a Ladd procedure is such patients may be considered, but the risk–benefit ratio is uncertain (65,66).

Significant gastrointestinal bleeding due to peptic ulcers or gastritis is uncommon following cardiac surgery in neonates and infants. Histamine-2 antagonists are often administered until enteral feeding has been established.

Infectious Complications

A variety of factors predispose patients to infection following cardiac surgery. CPB generates a complex pro- and anti-inflammatory response; the latter contributes to a generalized state of immunosuppression (67). Neonates in particular may have prolonged perioperative ICU stays following cardiac surgery, during which they are exposed to a variety of indwelling catheters and tubes. Important risk factors for catheter-related bloodstream infection in children undergoing cardiac surgery include weight less than 5 kg, greater blood product exposure, and prolonged mechanical ventilation (68). Systematic interventions and guidelines exist for the prevention and management of catheter-related infections in infants and children (69,70).

Surgical site infections occur in approximately 2% of children recovering from cardiac surgery. Important risk factors include age less than 1 year, preoperative hospitalization, greater blood product exposure, prolonged CPB time, and delayed sternal closure (71). Comprehensive recommendations for surgical site infection monitoring and prevention have been published, although guidelines specific for infants and children are lacking (72,73). Prophylactic antibiotics that provide coverage for Gram-positive organisms (e.g., a first-generation cephalosporin) are administered in the early postoperative period, generally for the first 24 to 48 hours after surgery. Most surgical site infections may be treated with antibiotics; patients with mediastinitis typically also undergo surgical débridement.

Renal Insufficiency

Acute kidney injury is common after congenital heart surgery, and neonates and infants undergoing complex operations are at greater risk (74). Maintenance of adequate renal perfusion pressure is likely the most important preventative strategy. Renal perfusion pressure is calculated as mean arterial pressure minus central venous pressure. In general, a renal perfusion pressure of at least 40 mm Hg in neonates and 50 mm Hg in infants is desirable. Loop diuretics may be used to augment urine output in the early postoperative period. Spironolactone may be useful for its potassium sparing effect. Acute renal failure requiring dialysis occurs in 1% or less of children undergoing cardiac surgery, but affected patients have a mortality risk of at least 20% (75). Peritoneal dialysis or continuous venovenous ultrafiltration (CVVH) is typically used while awaiting recovery of renal function.

Neurologic Complications

A number of preoperative, intraoperative, and postoperative factors place neonates undergoing cardiac surgery at risk for suboptimal neurodevelopmental outcomes following cardiac surgery. Magnetic resonance imaging and proton magnetic resonance spectroscopy examinations obtained in fetuses with HLHS and d-TGA have demonstrated impaired metabolism and structural development of the brain (76). These findings may be related to abnormal in utero cerebral circulatory physiology. After birth, cyanosis, hemodynamic instability, and thromboembolism all may contribute to white matter injury and stroke in neonates with critical CHD (77). A longer duration of time between birth and surgery has been associated with decreased brain growth in neonates with

d-TGA (78). Exposure to CPB is associated with embolization of gas bubbles or thrombus. Longer periods of DHCA may be associated with an increased incidence of early postoperative seizures and new white matter injury (2,77). Longer circulatory arrest times and early postoperative seizures have been associated with neurologic deficits following the arterial switch and Norwood operations (79,80). In order to minimize the use of circulatory arrest, regional low-flow perfusion may be used for complex aortic arch reconstructions. However, a randomized clinical trial comparing regional perfusion low-flow and DHCA found no significant differences in neurodevelopmental outcomes (3). Other advances in the conduct of CPB, including a better understanding of the optimal hematocrit target on bypass, may lead to improved neurodevelopmental outcomes (81). For example, the incidence of early postoperative clinical seizures following DHCA was 8% in the Boston Circulatory Arrest Study (conducted between 1988 and 1992) but only 2% a decade later (2,82). Patients may be exposed to additional hypotensive or hypoxic episodes in the ICU following surgery, which may contribute to neurodevelopmental outcomes. Longer postoperative length of stay after neonatal cardiac surgery has also been associated with worse cognitive outcomes (83).

EARLY POSTOPERATIVE PHYSIOLOGY AND MANAGEMENT: SPECIFIC LESIONS

Palliation of the Neonate with a Functional Single Ventricle

Neonates who have cardiac anatomy unsuitable for a two-ventricular repair typically have atresia or significant hypoplasia of either of the atrioventricular valves, and/or significant hypoplasia of either ventricle. Most patients with single ventricle physiology undergo initial surgical palliation in the neonatal period. A superior cavopulmonary connection (i.e., bidirectional Glenn or hemi-Fontan operation) is then performed at 4 to 6 months of age, followed by a total cavopulmonary connection (i.e., Fontan operation) as toddlers. By rerouting superior and inferior vena cava blood flow directly to the pulmonary arteries, this surgical strategy volume unloads the single ventricle by separating the systemic and pulmonary circulations. Because Fontan physiology is characterized by passive pulmonary blood flow, this circulation is dependent on low pulmonary artery pressure, good ventricular function without hypertrophy, minimal atrioventricular valve regurgitation, and the absence of pulmonary artery distortion or pulmonary venous obstruction.

The aforementioned considerations dictate the surgical strategy in the newborn period. To limit ventricular hypertrophy and preserve myocardial performance, unobstructed systemic blood flow must exist, and if not present at birth, may be achieved using either a Norwood operation or Damus-Kaye-Stansel procedure. Pulmonary blood flow must be tightly regulated to prevent ventricular volume overload, atrioventricular valve regurgitation, and pulmonary artery hypertension. This usually requires the placement of a systemic to pulmonary artery shunt or a pulmonary artery band. Care must be taken with both procedures to minimize pulmonary artery distortion. Finally, pulmonary venous return must not be obstructed, as this may cause pulmonary artery hypertension. An atrial septectomys is required in some neonates, as is done during the Norwood operation.

Systemic to Pulmonary Artery Shunt

A systemic to pulmonary artery shunt may be used to provide a reliable and controlled source of pulmonary blood flow. A common type of systemic to pulmonary artery shunt is a modified Blalock-Taussig shunt, which entails surgical placement of a Gore-Tex tube graft between the subclavian or innominate artery and a pulmonary artery, typically without the use of CPB. This operation is widely used to palliate neonates with single ventricle physiology

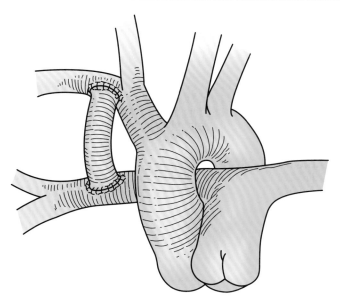

FIGURE 33.2 **The modified Blalock-Taussig shunt operation.** (Reprinted with permission from Wernovsky G, Bove EL. Single ventricle lesions. In: Chang A, Hanley FL, Wernovsky G, et al., eds. *Pediatric cardiac intensive care*. Baltimore, MD: Williams and Wilkins, 1998:271.)

and decreased pulmonary blood flow (**Fig. 33.2**), as well as selected neonates with two functional ventricles and obstructed pulmonary blood flow whose complete repair will be deferred. Another type of systemic to pulmonary artery shunt is a central shunt, which involves the placement of a Gore-Tex tube between the ascending aorta and pulmonary artery. Reasons for placing a central shunt include anatomical issues that preclude a modified Blalock-Taussig shunt or to promote growth of the central pulmonary arteries (84). A systemic to pulmonary artery shunt may be performed in isolation or as a part of a larger procedure, such as the Norwood operation for hypoplastic left heart syndrome (HLHS).

Several postoperative complications may occur following the placement of a systemic to pulmonary artery shunt. If the shunt is large relative to the size of the baby, pulmonary blood flow may be excessive, the systemic ventricle will be volume overloaded, and congestive heart failure may develop. By contrast, a relatively small shunt will result in excessive postoperative cyanosis. The average shunt diameter is 3.5 mm for a term neonate. Distortion or scarring of the pulmonary arteries may also develop at the shunt insertion site, which may manifest as cyanosis. Acute shunt thrombosis typically results in the rapid development of severe cyanosis. Thromboprophylaxis with aspirin early after placement of a modified Blalock-Taussig shunt has been associated with reduced mortality (85). Potential neurologic complications with this shunt include Horner syndrome, recurrent laryngeal nerve injury, and phrenic nerve injury. Hospital mortality following a modified Blalock-Taussig shunt is approximately 7%; patients at greater risk include those with pulmonary atresia with intact ventricular septum, functional single ventricles, a weight less than 3 kg, and those receiving preoperative mechanical ventilation (86).

PDA Stent

Stenting of the ductus arteriosus in the cardiac catheterization laboratory is an acceptable alternative approach to initial palliation for selected infants born with ductal-dependent blood flow. In infants with ductal-dependent systemic blood flow (i.e., HLHS), a PDA stent can be placed as part of the "hybrid procedure" (discussed further under the *Hypoplastic Left Heart Syndrome* section). A PDA stent can also be utilized for infants with ductal-dependent pulmonary blood flow with similar outcomes observed

when compared to a systemic to pulmonary artery shunt operation (87). The decision regarding whether to place a PDA stent or a systemic to pulmonary artery shunt is typically dependent on individual patient characteristics (i.e., patient weight, gestational age, comorbidities, PDA size/shape, pulmonary artery anatomy) and institutional preference.

Pulmonary Artery Band

In selected infants with functional single ventricles and unobstructed pulmonary and systemic blood flow, or occasionally in infants with two functional ventricles and pulmonary overcirculation, a restrictive band is placed on the main pulmonary artery, performed without CPB (**Fig. 33.3**). The purpose of this operation is to decrease the ratio of pulmonary to systemic blood flow (i.e., Qp/Qs) and thus limit symptoms of congestive heart failure, volume loading on the systemic ventricle, and the development of pulmonary vascular obstructive disease. Pulmonary flow (Qp) must be monitored following placement of the pulmonary artery band. A well-balanced circulation is associated with a systemic oxygen saturation of approximately 80% to 85%. However, as the pulmonary vascular resistance falls over time, pulmonary blood flow may increase, and signs of congestive heart failure will develop. If the pulmonary artery band migrates distally on the main pulmonary artery, distortion of the branch pulmonary arteries may develop. The band may be removed at the time of complete surgical repair or subsequent palliation.

Right Ventricular Outflow Tract Obstruction
Critical Pulmonary Valve Stenosis

In neonates with critical pulmonary valve stenosis, the pulmonary valve leaflets are thickened and fused to a variable extent, and their mobility is decreased. The pulmonary valve annulus may be

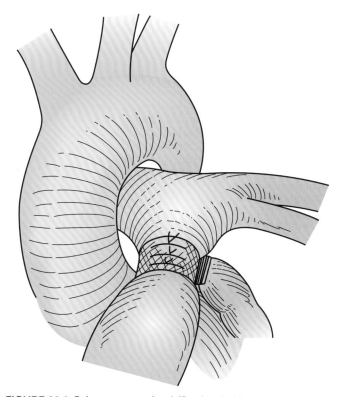

FIGURE 33.3 **Pulmonary artery band.** (Reprinted with permission from Wernovsky G, Bove EL. Single ventricle lesions. In: Chang A, Hanley FL, Wernovsky G, et al., eds. *Pediatric cardiac intensive care*. Baltimore, MD: Williams and Wilkins, 1998:271.)

hypoplastic, and the pulmonary arteries may be of normal size, stenotic, or dilated. The right ventricle is often hypertrophied and mildly hypoplastic. Significant tricuspid regurgitation and a right-to-left atrial shunt through the foramen ovale are often present after birth. Neonates with isolated critical pulmonary valve stenosis will develop significant cyanosis upon closure of the ductus arteriosus, and in such patients, a PGE$_1$ infusion should be administered to maintain ductal patency and adequate pulmonary blood flow. Most patients are candidates for a balloon valvuloplasty in the cardiac catheterization laboratory. Following this procedure, patients may have very poor right ventricular compliance, related to ventricular hypertrophy and (in some cases) myocardial ischemia and endocardial fibroelastosis. Significant cyanosis can result from right-to-left shunting through the foramen ovale. Such patients may require several additional days of a PGE$_1$ infusion to maintain ductal patency and provide adequate pulmonary blood flow while waiting improvement in ventricular compliance. Rarely, these patients may develop dynamic right ventricular outflow obstruction due to infundibular spasm ("suicide right ventricle") following balloon valvuloplasty, manifesting as cyanosis and low cardiac output. In this scenario, volume expansion and beta-blockers (relax contractility and promote ventricular filling by slowing the heart rate) are the initial treatments should infundibular spasm occur (88). Neonates who are unable to come off PGE$_1$ after several attempts may have a dysplastic valve, particularly poor right ventricular compliance, and/or inadequately sized right heart structures. In such patients, a surgical valvotomy and/or a systemic to pulmonary artery shunt may be considered. Placement of a stent in the ductus arteriosus during cardiac catheterization is an alternative strategy. Once the right ventricular compliance has improved, the systemic to pulmonary artery shunt (or the stented ductus arteriosus) may be surgically ligated or coil embolized.

Tetralogy of Fallot

Tetralogy of Fallot, the most common cyanotic congenital heart lesion, is comprised of an anterior malalignment VSD in a heart with two ventricles and aortic to mitral fibrous continuity. Anatomic details that need to be clarified at the time of diagnosis include the severity and location of right ventricular outflow tract obstruction, the pulmonary artery anatomy, the presence of additional VSDs, the sidedness of the aortic arch (rightward in 25%), and the coronary artery anatomy. The left coronary artery may arise from the right coronary artery and cross the right ventricular outflow tract in 5% of cases, and in such cases, the surgeon must be cognizant of it during right ventricular outflow tract reconstruction. DiGeorge syndrome is present in approximately 15% of patients with tetralogy of Fallot, and those with a right aortic arch are at higher risk. About 7% of patients with tetralogy of Fallot have trisomy 21.

In neonates with tetralogy of Fallot, a wide spectrum of presentation exists. Patients with a minimal degree of obstruction to pulmonary blood flow are usually asymptomatic and fairly well oxygenated (systemic saturations >85%) soon after birth. They are commonly observed in the hospital until the ductus arteriosus closes and then sent home to await elective surgical repair. These patients typically develop progressive right ventricular outflow tract obstruction and cyanosis. The timing of repair for these patients depends upon several variables including the development of increasing cyanosis, hypercyanotic spells ("TOF spells"), and institutional preference. Neonates with tetralogy of Fallot and severe right ventricular outflow tract obstruction or pulmonary atresia will develop excessive cyanosis (oxygen saturation <75% to 80%) upon closure of the ductus arteriosus. Such patients have ductal-dependent pulmonary blood flow and will require intervention during the initial hospitalization. Surgical options include a complete repair or a systemic to pulmonary shunt, depending

on the details of the anatomy and surgeon preference (89,90). In recent years, stenting of the ductus arteriosus or right ventricular outflow tract in the cardiac catheterization laboratory has become an acceptable palliative option, particularly for higher risk surgical candidates (91,92).

Neonates with tetralogy of Fallot and pulmonary stenosis who have a systemic to pulmonary artery shunt or ductal stent placed are at risk for developing pulmonary overcirculation. Total pulmonary blood flow from the shunt plus the native flow across the right ventricular outflow tract may be excessive. In this scenario, efforts to increase pulmonary vascular resistance may be useful. Supportive care is generally required for a few days until the circulatory system adapts to the new volume load. Acute shunt thrombosis and pulmonary artery distortion are also potential complications of this procedure.

Complete surgical repair of tetralogy of Fallot includes closure of the VSD and reconstruction of the right ventricular outflow tract and pulmonary arteries to reduce or eliminate obstruction to blood flow. The operation typically involves resection of muscle bundles in the right ventricular outflow tract, a pulmonary valvotomy or leaflet resection, and patch augmentation of the proximal pulmonary arteries. In patients with favorable anatomy, the operation may be accomplished using a transatrial–transpulmonary approach. However, right ventriculotomy with transannular patch is required in some cases to enlarge the right ventricular outflow tract. In neonates with tetralogy of Fallot and pulmonary atresia, a ventriculotomy is required if a complete repair is performed using a right ventricle to pulmonary artery conduit. Following complete repair of tetralogy of Fallot, residual lesions that may complicate the postoperative course include a VSD or significant right ventricular outflow tract obstruction.

One of the postoperative issues relatively unique to complex right heart reconstructions is the potential for the development of restrictive right ventricular physiology. In addition to tetralogy of Fallot, restrictive right ventricular physiology may also develop following surgical repair of pulmonary atresia or truncus arteriosus. Neonates are particularly at risk. Restrictive physiology has been defined as persistent antegrade flow from the right ventricle into the pulmonary artery during diastole as documented using pulsed Doppler echocardiography, suggesting that the right ventricle end-diastolic pressure is elevated (93). The primary underlying cause is impaired elastance of the right ventricle. A variety of factors are contributory as outlined in Table 33.5. Patients with

TABLE 33.5

Factors That May Contribute to Restrictive Right Ventricular Physiology Following Neonatal Right Ventricular Outflow Reconstruction

Risk Factor	Etiologies
Diastolic dysfunction	Poorly elastic, hypertrophied right ventricle; right ventriculotomy; right ventricular muscle bundle resection; myocardial ischemia–reperfusion injury; noncontractile VSD patch
Deceased right ventricular preload	Tricuspid stenosis
Myocardial ischemia	Injury to conal branch of coronary artery crossing RVOT

Inadequate coronary perfusion pressure |
| Volume load | Residual ventricular septal defect (VSD) or pulmonary regurgitation |
| Increased right ventricular afterload | Residual stenosis of the right ventricular infundibulum, pulmonary valve, or pulmonary arteries |

RVOT, right ventricular outflow tract; VSD, ventricular septal defect.

restrictive right ventricular physiology have increased right atrial filling pressure (e.g., 10 to 15 mm Hg) and systemic venous hypertension. Note that the right atrial pressures are not as elevated as one might expect due to high capacitance of the neonatal systemic venous circulation. Hepatic congestion, ascites, increased chest tube losses, and pleural effusions may develop. Because of the phenomenon of ventricular interdependence, changes in right ventricular diastolic function and septal position will in turn affect left ventricular compliance and function. Left ventricular preload and stroke volume are ultimately compromised. Restrictive right ventricular physiology may manifest with a low cardiac output state. Tachycardia, hypotension, poor perfusion, and a narrow pulse pressure may be present, along with oliguria and metabolic acidosis.

Anticipatory treatment for restrictive right ventricular physiology begins in the operating room (Table 33.6). Although any atrial septal defects (ASDs) are usually closed at the time of surgery in older patients, in neonates and young infants undergoing a two-ventricular repair involving right heart reconstruction, it is beneficial to leave a 3- to 4-mm atrial communication. In the face of diastolic dysfunction and increased right ventricular end-diastolic pressure, the resultant right-to-left atrial shunt will maintain preload to the left ventricle and therefore cardiac output. Patients may be mildly desaturated initially following surgery (SaO_2 85% to 95%), but as right ventricular elastance and function improves (usually within a few days), the amount of shunt decreases and both antegrade pulmonary blood flow and SaO_2 increase. If an atrial communication does not exist and significant and refractory restrictive right ventricular physiology develops in the early postoperative period, an atrial communication may be created in the cardiac catheterization laboratory.

Several other strategies must be used to manage restrictive right ventricular physiology, and each should be implemented with the overarching goal of maintaining adequate systemic oxygen delivery while minimizing myocardial oxygen consumption. As tachycardia and wall stress influence myocardial oxygen consumption, therapies that influence these variables need to be used

judiciously. Accordingly, avoiding fever with antipyretic therapy if the body temperature trends upward is advisable. Preload must be maintained despite elevation of the right-sided filling pressures. In selected cases, low-dose epinephrine (e.g., 0.02 to 0.05 µg/kg/min) may be beneficial provided that excessive tachycardia does not occur. Milrinone may be beneficial due to its inotropic, lusitropic, and vasodilatory properties; however, care must be taken to ensure that coronary perfusion pressure is adequate to avoid right ventricular subendocardial ischemia. Efforts are warranted to maintain low right ventricular afterload. Hypoxemia, hypothermia, and acidosis may contribute to elevated pulmonary vascular resistance and should be avoided (13). Hypo- or hyperinflation of the lung may also increase right ventricular afterload and impede pulmonary blood flow and promote pulmonary regurgitation. Higher airway pressures may also limit right ventricular preload. Thus, during mechanical ventilation, goals are to maintain functional residual capacity, limit mean airway pressure, and avoid hypoxia and respiratory acidosis. Using intermittent positive pressure ventilation, a short inspiratory time, a low positive end-expiratory pressure (PEEP) (e.g., 4 to 5 cm H_2O), and adequate tidal volume (e.g., 10 mL/kg) and FiO_2 are desirable for most patients. Any significant pleural effusions and other factors that may contribute to elevated pulmonary vascular resistance should be promptly addressed. Sedation and paralysis are often necessary for the first 24 to 48 hours to minimize the stress response and associated myocardial workload. Right ventricular compliance generally improves in a few days.

Loss of sinus rhythm may be poorly tolerated following tetralogy of Fallot repair. Loss of atrioventricular synchrony will increase right atrial pressure and compromise cardiac output and blood pressure. In the setting of restrictive right ventricular physiology, supraventricular arrhythmias may lead to the loss of the contribution of atrial systole to antegrade pulmonary blood flow. JET is the most common arrhythmia seen early following tetralogy of Fallot repair, whereas VT is (somewhat surprisingly) rarely seen in infants. Of note, a right bundle branch block pattern is common on the postoperative ECG but usually of little short-term significance.

Absent pulmonary valve syndrome, identified by the presence of rudimentary pulmonary valve leaflets and free pulmonary insufficiency, is a relatively rare lesion, present in approximately 3% of all patients with tetralogy of Fallot. This lesion is most notable for in utero development of aneurysmal dilation of the pulmonary arteries, which may occur due to the lack of a ductus arteriosus or due to the pulsatile blood flow pattern across the right ventricular outflow tract. When compared with infants with typical tetralogy of Fallot, there may be a higher incidence of DiGeorge syndrome in those with absent pulmonary valve. A nearly pathognomonic to-and-fro ("sawing wood") murmur is heard due to pulmonary annulus stenosis and free pulmonary insufficiency (Fig. 33.4). Such patients may have minimal if any respiratory symptoms and behave much like a "pink tet" or present with severe problems with oxygenation and ventilation soon after birth due to compression of the bronchi by the dilated pulmonary arteries. Intubation, mechanical ventilation (with judicious use of positive end-expiratory pressure), and deep sedation may be beneficial in neonates with symptomatic airway obstruction. Prone positioning may be advantageous as gravity will allow the pulmonary arteries to fall off the mainstem bronchi, thus permitting adequate gas exchange. Surgical repair is indicated in symptomatic neonates.

Surgical repair for tetralogy of Fallot with absent pulmonary valve syndrome includes a reduction pulmonary arterioplasty, VSD closure, and placement of a valved homograft in the right ventricular outflow tract (Fig. 33.5). Replacement of the dilated central pulmonary arteries with bifurcated valved pulmonary homograft is a surgical modification that has been associated with improved survival in symptomatic neonates. An alternative surgical approach includes translocation of the pulmonary artery anterior to the aorta (Lecompte maneuver) and away from the

TABLE 33.6	
Treatment Options for Restrictive Right Ventricular Physiology	
Physiologic Goals	**Specific Treatment Strategies**
Optimize ventricular preload	• Target right atrial pressure of 10–15 mm Hg • Drain ascites • Leave patent foramen ovale to preserve left ventricular preload • Maintain atrioventricular synchrony; treat arrhythmias
Inotropic support	• Judicious use of dopamine, milrinone and/or epinephrine
Lusitropy	• Milrinone
Optimize myocardial oxygen supply and demand	• Maintain coronary perfusion pressure • Heart rate control • Judicious use of inotropes
Maintain low right ventricular afterload	• Use lowest possible mean airway pressure to maintain FRC of lungs • Avoid acidosis • Drain pleural effusions, pneumothoraces, or hemothoraces
Minimize systemic oxygen consumption	• Maintain normothermia • Provide adequate sedation and analgesia • Consider muscle relaxant

FRC, functional residual capacity.

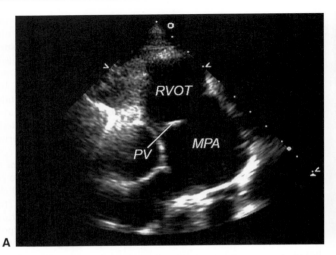

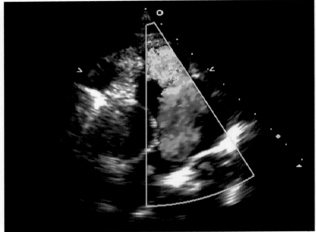

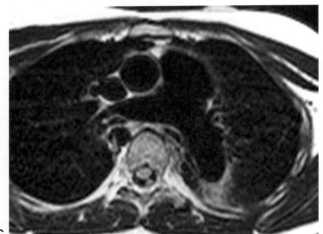

FIGURE 33.4 Tetralogy of Fallot with absent pulmonary valve. A: Two-dimensional echocardiogram from the parasternal long axis view demonstrating rudimentary pulmonary valve leaflets and aneurysmal dilation of the main pulmonary artery. **B:** Application of color Doppler during ventricular diastole revealing free regurgitation from the main pulmonary artery into the right ventricular outflow tract. **C:** Black blood axial magnetic resonance image in a patient with Tetralogy of Fallot with absent pulmonary valve syndrome. Note the dilated right and left pulmonary arteries with compression of the right and left mainstem bronchi (*arrows*). MPA, main pulmonary artery; PV, pulmonary valve; RVOT, right ventricular outflow tract. (Image courtesy of Dr. Cynthia Rigsby, MD, Department of Medical Imaging, Ann & Robert H. Lurie Children's Hospital of Chicago. Reprinted from Costello JM, Franklin WH. Preoperative and postoperative care of the infant with critical congenital heart disease. In: MacDonald MG, Seshai MMK, Mullett MD, eds. *Avery's neonatology pathophysiology & management of the newborn*, 6th ed., Philadelphia, PA: Lippincott Williams & Wilkins, 2005:710.)

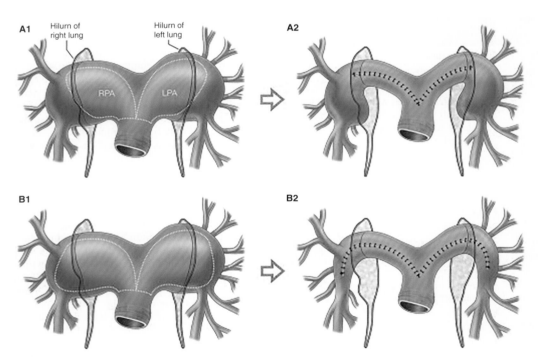

FIGURE 33.5 Pulmonary artery reduction surgery in absent pulmonary valve syndrome. Reduction of the proximally dilated pulmonary artery to the hilum only (A₁) with persisting posthilum dilation causing distal bronchial obstruction (A₂). Reduction of the pulmonary artery past the border of the hilum (B₁) relieves distal bronchial obstruction (B₂). (LPA, left pulmonary artery; RPA, right pulmonary artery.) (Reprinted from Yong MS, Yim D, Brizard CP, et al. Long-term outcomes of patients with absent pulmonary valve syndrome: 38 years of experience. *Ann Thorac Surg* 2014;97:1671. Copyright © 2014 The Society of Thoracic Surgeons. With permission.)

tracheobronchial tree. In addition to the aforementioned issues following tetralogy of Fallot repair, the postoperative course for infants with absent pulmonary valve syndrome may be significantly complicated by airway obstruction due to tracheobronchomalacia that persists even after plication and reduction of the aneurysmal pulmonary arteries. Some of these infants will require a tracheostomy and long-term positive-pressure ventilation until they "outgrow" the malacia.

Tetralogy of Fallot is associated with an atrioventricular canal defect in approximately 2% to 5% of cases. Evaluation and management strategies are similar to those used in simple tetralogy of Fallot with pulmonary stenosis. Given the aforementioned issues regarding right ventricular dysfunction following tetralogy of Fallot repair, the presence of residual tricuspid regurgitation following division of the common atrioventricular valve may be poorly tolerated.

Tetralogy of Fallot, Pulmonary Atresia, Major Aortopulmonary Collateral Arteries

In a subset of patients with tetralogy of Fallot with pulmonary atresia, the central pulmonary arteries may be diminutive and one or more major aortopulmonary collateral arteries (MAPCAs) are present. In approximately 15% to 25% of cases, there are no central pulmonary arteries. The MAPCAs are variable in number and usually arise from the descending aorta, although their origin may be from the ascending aorta, aortic arch, brachiocephalic vessels, or coronary arteries (Fig. 33.6). There may be multiple stenoses and diminished total cross-sectional area of the pulmonary vascular bed. In neonates with tetralogy of Fallot, pulmonary atresia, and MAPCAs, pulmonary blood flow may be quite variable depending upon the size and number of MAPCAs and the severity of stenoses within these vessels. True pulmonary arteries, MAPCAs, or both may supply blood to individual segments of the lungs. Generally, such patients are not dependent upon PGE_1 unless a major aortopulmonary collateral vessel arises from the ductus arteriosus. The physical examination may be notable for the presence of a widely radiating continuous murmur produced by the aortopulmonary collateral blood flow. Although cardiac CT or MRI provides

adequate visualization of central pulmonary arteries and the proximal course of important MAPCAs, cardiac catheterization is ultimately required to clarify distal pulmonary artery anatomy and identify all sources of pulmonary blood flow to each lung segment. As with other conotruncal defects, these infants should undergo genetic testing for DiGeorge syndrome.

Indications for initial surgical intervention in neonates with tetralogy of Fallot, pulmonary atresia, and MAPCAs include excessive cyanosis, refractory congestive heart failure, or diminutive central pulmonary arteries in need of a reliable source of blood flow to promote growth. In the absence of symptoms, elective surgical intervention may occur within the first few months of life to maximize the growth potential of the central pulmonary arteries. The ultimate goal of intervention is to optimize the effective cross-sectional area of the pulmonary arterial vascular bed, eliminate any MAPCAs that represent dual blood supply in order to minimize the risk of pulmonary vascular obstructive disease to lung segments, and thus limit right ventricular hypertension following eventual VSD closure. In situations where dual blood supply to a lung segment exists, the MAPCAs are coil occluded in the cardiac catheterization laboratory or ligated at the time of surgery to eliminate left-to-right shunting. Although primary complete repair in early infancy is possible in selected patients, in many cases, a staged series of surgical and transcatheter interventions are required, the timing and conduct of which must be individualized based on underlying anatomy and physiology at presentation. If the central pulmonary arteries are small but confluent, the initial operation must include the establishment of a reliable source of antegrade blood flow, which will promote growth of these vessels over time (Fig. 33.7). Options include placement of a systemic

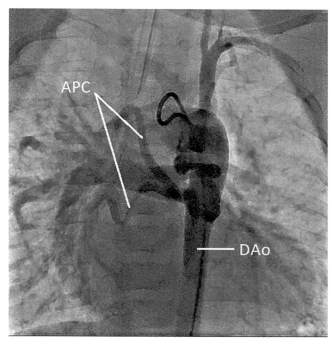

FIGURE 33.6 Angiogram in the descending aorta of tetralogy of Fallot with pulmonary atresia demonstrating major aortopulmonary collateral arteries. APC, aortopulmonary collateral arteries; DAo, descending aorta.

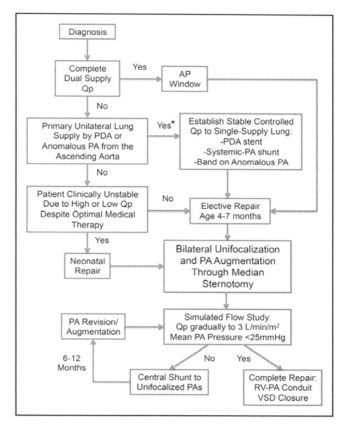

FIGURE 33.7 Treatment algorithm for the management of newborns with tetralogy of Fallot and major aortopulmonary collateral arteries. (Reprinted from Ma M, Mainwaring RD, Hanley FL, et al. Comprehensive management of major aortopulmonary collaterals in the repair of tetralogy of Fallot. *Semin Thorac Cardiovasc Surg Pediatr Card Surg Annu* 2018;21:75. Copyright © 2017 Elsevier. With permission.)

to pulmonary shunt, creation of an aortopulmonary window, or placement of a right ventricular to pulmonary artery (RV–PA) shunt (94). The latter approach may be advantageous in patients with abnormal aortic arch branching, which can complicate the proximal BT shunt anastomosis. Additionally, the RV–PA shunt decreases the risks associated with diastolic runoff (blood flow through the conduit occurs only during cardiac systole), and it provides easy antegrade transcatheter access to the distal pulmonary arteries for subsequent balloon angioplasty (94). If the central pulmonary arteries are absent, they can be constructed using pericardium or pulmonary allograft. Intervention for each MAPCA is customized depending upon its size, the presence or absence of proximal stenosis within the vessel, and a determination as to whether it represents redundant blood supply to individual lung segments. Redundant MAPCAs can be coil occluded in the cardiac catheterization laboratory or ligated at the time of surgery to eliminate left-to-right shunting and prevent the development of pulmonary vascular disease. If a MAPCA represents the sole source of pulmonary blood flow to a lung segment, the proximal end of the MAPCA is removed from its source and incorporated into the native or newly constructed central pulmonary arteries, such that blood flow to the lung is supplied from a single source (unifocalization procedure). Following unifocalization procedures, severe airflow limitation may occur secondary to tracheobronchial ischemia, which may originate from interruption of peribronchial arterial blood supply during mobilization of MAPCAs (59). Once the pulmonary vascular bed has been optimally recruited, intracardiac repair may be completed including VSD closure and (if not previously completed) right ventricular outflow tract reconstruction. The incidence of early postoperative right ventricular failure may be decreased by leaving the foramen ovale patent or placement of a fenestrated VSD patch in patients with an inadequate pulmonary vascular bed, both of which allow right-to-left shunting to preserve systemic cardiac output at the expense of mild postoperative cyanosis. An intraoperative flow study can help predict postoperative right ventricular pressure in order to determine suitability for intracardiac septation (95). The intermediate-term prognosis is guarded for this patient population secondary to pulmonary hypertension and right ventricular failure. Serial cardiac catheterizations with balloon angioplasty of the pulmonary arteries and reoperations (e.g., for conduit replacement) are often required.

Pulmonary Atresia with Intact Ventricular Septum

Pulmonary atresia with intact ventricular septum is an uncommon lesion characterized by a membranous or muscular obstruction of the pulmonary valve, associated with variable degrees of hypoplasia of the right ventricle and tricuspid valve. The left and right pulmonary arteries are usually of normal size. Right ventricle to coronary artery fistulae are present in nearly half of cases, particularly in those with more significant tricuspid valve and right ventricular hypoplasia (96). Coronary artery stenosis, interruptions, or ostial occlusions are present in one or more coronary vessels in 9% to 34% of patients. The myocardium supplied by these compromised coronary arteries is thus dependent on flow from the right ventricle through the coronary fistulae, a condition known as RVDCC (97).

By definition, neonates with pulmonary atresia and intact ventricular septum have ductal-dependent pulmonary blood flow. Complete intracardiac mixing occurs, as all systemic venous return to the right atrium flows through an obligatory atrial communication to the left atrium. The right ventricle is decompressed by tricuspid regurgitation or egress through the coronary fistulae to the aorta. If tricuspid regurgitation is limited, suprasystemic right ventricular pressure and marked right ventricular hypertrophy are usually present.

The initial echocardiogram should delineate the size and function of the tricuspid valve and right ventricle, and the anatomy of

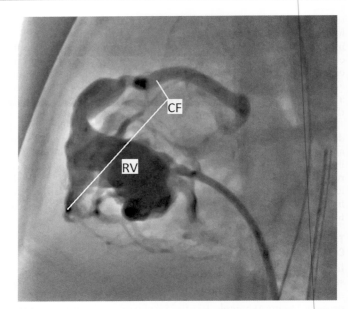

FIGURE 33.8 Angiographic injection in the right ventricle of a neonate with pulmonary atresia with intact ventricular septum demonstrating multiple fistulous connections to the coronary circulation. RV, right ventricle; CF, coronary fistula.

the right ventricular outflow tract. A judgment must be made as to whether the right heart structures are adequate (either presently or in the future) to support a two-ventricular circulation (98). Right ventricle to coronary artery fistulae may be identified by echocardiogram using color Doppler. Neonates with a tricuspid valve Z-score of ≤ −2.5 are very likely to have RVDCC (96). If coronary fistulae are seen by echocardiogram, the coronary anatomy should be precisely defined by cardiac catheterization (Fig. 33.8) (98). If stenoses, interruptions, or ostial occlusions exist such that a significant amount of myocardium is dependent upon flow from the right ventricle through the coronary fistulae, then surgical or transcatheter decompression of the right ventricle is contraindicated.

Provided that the tricuspid valve (Z-score > −2 to −3) and right ventricle are of reasonable size and there is no evidence for RVDCC, it is reasonable to pursue a two-ventricular repair (99). Right ventricular decompression may be accomplished by placement of a right ventricular outflow tract patch to encourage right ventricular growth and allow regression of right ventricular hypertrophy. The ASD is left open to allow for decompression of the right heart and maintenance of systemic cardiac output, and usually a systemic to pulmonary shunt is concurrently placed to ensure adequate pulmonary blood flow. Alternatively, in the subset of patients with membranous atresia, the right ventricle may be decompressed by transcatheter perforation of the pulmonary valve using a stiff wire or radiofrequency ablation catheter followed by balloon valvuloplasty (Fig. 33.9). At best, however, transcatheter intervention avoids the need for early surgical intervention in only approximately one-third of patients (100). If RVDCC exists, the initial operation is a systemic to pulmonary artery shunt as the first stage of single ventricle palliation (101). Placement of a PDA stent in the cardiac catheterization laboratory is an acceptable alternative initial palliation for selected patients with the caveat that this approach may increase the volume load on the left ventricle (102,103). Cardiac transplantation may be considered for the unusual patient with severe variants of RVDCC (e.g., those with coronary ostial atresia) and/or myocardial dysfunction that precludes single ventricle palliation (104). In this scenario, a systemic to pulmonary artery shunt, PDA stent, or prolonged PGE₁ infusion are all considerations as a bridge to transplantation.

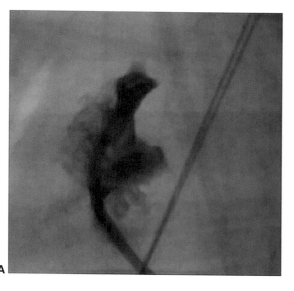

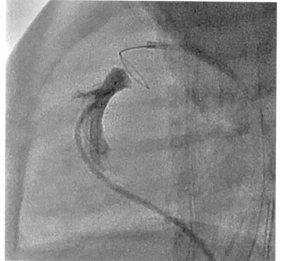

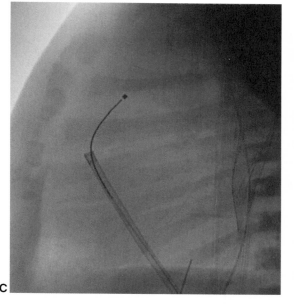

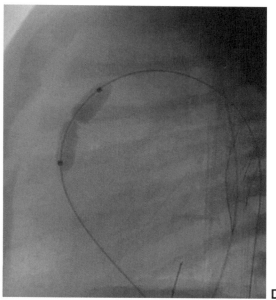

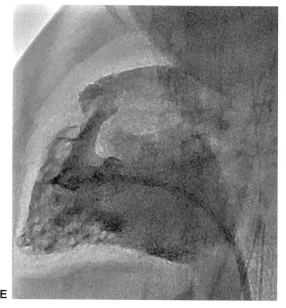

FIGURE 33.9 **Lateral projection angiograms obtained during therapeutic cardiac catheterization in a neonate with pulmonary atresia and intact ventricular septum. A:** Angiogram in the right ventricle demonstrating an adequate infundibulum and no antegrade flow across the pulmonary valve. **B:** Angiogram with the catheter tip in the right ventricular infundibulum. The snare wire in the main pulmonary artery was positioned retrograde through the descending aorta and ductus arteriosus and may be used as a target during subsequent perforation of the atretic pulmonary valve. **C:** A radiofrequency wire is used to perforate the atretic pulmonary valve. **D:** An angioplasty balloon is used to dilate the pulmonary valve. Note the waist in the balloon that defines the location of the pulmonary valve annulus. **E:** Right ventricular injection demonstrating antegrade flow through the pulmonary valve.

In patients palliated with a systemic to pulmonary shunt of ductal stent, there exists the potential for pulmonary overcirculation (high Qp/Qs), poor systemic perfusion, low diastolic blood pressure, and inadequate coronary perfusion. In this setting, maneuvers are indicated to increase pulmonary vascular resistance and thus "balance" the circulation, such as use of increased mean airway pressure and the avoidance of supplemental oxygen and respiratory alkalosis. Following placement of a right ventricular outflow patch in the neonatal period, supportive care as described above for patients with tetralogy of Fallot and restrictive right ventricular physiology may be necessary.

In shunted neonates with RVDCC, care should be taken to avoid excessive systemic vasodilation. Agents that increase systemic vascular tone such as norepinephrine or vasopressin may be utilized to maintain coronary perfusion pressure. Close ECG monitoring for ST segment changes is required, and if any signs of myocardial ischemia develop, prompt echocardiography should be obtained to evaluate for wall motion abnormalities. If RVDCC was unrecognized and a right ventricular outflow track was opened, myocardial ischemia, ventricular dysfunction, and arrhythmias are likely to develop immediately following the procedure (97). Recreation of pulmonary atresia by ligation of the main pulmonary artery may be performed in attempt to salvage such patients.

Following initial neonatal right ventricular decompression, palliated patients with pulmonary atresia and intact ventricular septum are evaluated for interval growth of right-sided heart structures and right ventricular compliance. During cardiac catheterization, test occlusions of the ASD and systemic to pulmonary shunt may be performed to determine whether cyanosis and systemic venous hypertension develop. If not, closure of the atrial communication and takedown or coil occlusion of the shunt are performed to separate the systemic and pulmonary circulations. One-and-one half ventricular repair (i.e., intracardiac repair in association with a superior cavopulmonary anastomosis) and Fontan palliation are options for older patients whose right heart has not developed adequately to support the entire circulation (105).

Mortality for patients with pulmonary atresia and intact ventricular septum in early infancy is approximately 10%, and patients with RVDCC or Ebstein anomaly are at greater risk (106). Using appropriate staged interventions in patients with pulmonary atresia and intact ventricular septum, 5-year survival rates greater than 80% may be achieved (105).

Ebstein Anomaly

Ebstein anomaly is a rare congenital heart lesion, representing less than 1% of all cases of CHD. The septal and posterior leaflets of the tricuspid valve are displaced into the anatomic right ventricle and variably adherent to the ventricular septum. The anterior leaflet may be fenestrated and redundant or "sail-like" and cause obstruction of the right ventricular outflow tract. The tricuspid valve chordae tendineae and papillary muscles may be abnormal, the true tricuspid valve annulus may be dilated, and tricuspid regurgitation may be severe (Fig. 33.10). The functional right atrium may be enlarged because of tricuspid regurgitation, and the fact that the inlet portion of the right ventricle is "atrialized" by the inferiorly displaced tricuspid valve leaflets. ASDs (commonly) and anatomic pulmonary valve stenosis or atresia (less common) are associated with Ebstein anomaly. Left-side heart abnormalities including ventricular noncompaction are occasionally present. One or more accessory conduction pathways may exist at the tricuspid valve annulus, creating the necessary substrate for atrioventricular reentrant tachycardia.

Many patients with Ebstein anomaly do not develop symptoms until adolescence or early adulthood, when a combination of right-sided congestive heart failure, cyanosis, arrhythmias, and sudden death may develop. However, newborns with severe Ebstein anomaly (i.e., severe tricuspid regurgitation, right ventricular hypoplasia, myocardial dysfunction, and severe cardiomegaly) may present with hydrops fetalis or severe cyanosis and heart failure soon after birth. Right-to-left shunting at the atrial level occurs and may be due to pulmonary hypertension, pulmonary valve stenosis or atresia, or right ventricular outflow tract obstruction by the sail-like anterior leaflet of the tricuspid valve. In some neonates, functional pulmonary atresia exists, which develops when the pulmonary artery pressure is greater than the pressure that the Ebsteinoid right ventricle can generate, and the pulmonary valve leaflets fail to open. Severe tricuspid regurgitation and extreme right atrial enlargement may result in pooling of venous return in the compliant right atrium with limited shunting across the ASD to the left atrium. The reduced preload to the left ventricle may contribute to underdevelopment of the left side of the heart and a low cardiac output state. Biventricular function may also be diminished by myocardial fibrosis. Neonates with Ebstein anomaly presenting with significant cyanosis (<75% to 80% systemic saturation) should initially receive PGE_1. The lungs may be compressed

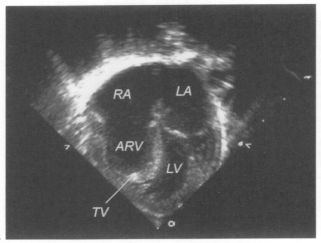
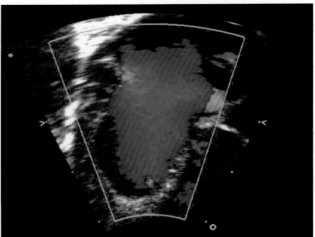

FIGURE 33.10 Ebstein anomaly of the tricuspid valve. A: Two-dimensional echocardiogram demonstrating severe Ebstein anomaly of the tricuspid valve in a neonate. Note the significant displacement of the tricuspid valve leaflets into the right ventricle. **B:** During ventricular systole, color Doppler demonstrating free retrograde flow (*blue color* Doppler) across the tricuspid valve annulus. ARV, atrialized right ventricle; LA, left atrium; LV, left ventricle; RA, right atrium; TV, tricuspid valve. (Reprinted with permission from Costello JM, Franklin WH. Preoperative and postoperative care of the infant with critical congenital heart disease. In: *Avery's neonatology pathophysiology & management of the newborn*, 6th ed., Philadelphia, PA: Lippincott Williams & Wilkins, 2005:710.)

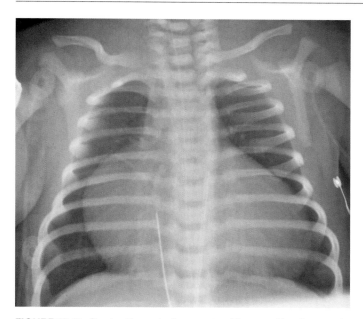

FIGURE 33.11 Chest radiograph of a neonate with severe Ebstein anomaly.

by severe cardiomegaly (Fig. 33.11), and thus, mechanical ventilation with judicious use of PEEP may be useful.

The size of the right atrium, anatomy, and function of the tricuspid valve and the right ventricular outflow tract are assessed by echocardiography (Fig. 33.10). Using echocardiographic measurements from the apical four-chamber view, the ratio of the right atrium and atrialized right ventricle to the area of the functional right ventricle, left atrium, and left ventricle (i.e., (RA + aRA)/(RV + LA + LV)) of greater than 1 is a strong independent predictor of mortality (107,108). Other predictors of mortality in the neonatal period include the presence of cyanosis, right ventricular outflow tract obstruction, and left ventricular systolic dysfunction (107–109).

Decision-making for symptomatic neonates with severe Ebstein anomaly is complex and requires a complete understanding of the evolving physiology. If pulmonary atresia is present, early consideration must be given to determining whether it is anatomic or functional. If functional atresia is suspected, discontinuation of PGE$_1$ may lead to ductal constriction. The resultant decreased pulmonary artery pressure may allow the pulmonary valve leaflets to open (110). Anatomic pulmonary atresia may warrant attempted balloon dilation or placement of a systemic to pulmonary shunt. In patients without pulmonary atresia, pulmonary vascular resistance may fall, and systemic to pulmonary runoff may occur through the ductus arteriosus leading to a low output state. Increased pulmonary venous return leads to elevated left atrial pressure, which may inhibit right-to-left atrial shunting and thus contribute to systemic venous hypertension. In this scenario, PGE$_1$ should be discontinued with the hope that ductal constriction will lead to decreased pulmonary artery pressure, thereby promoting increased antegrade flow across the right ventricular outflow tract and abating symptoms of heart failure. Persistent patency of a large ductus arteriosus may warrant surgical ligation, which may result in dramatic improvement. The judicious use of mechanical ventilation, supplemental oxygen, and inhaled nitric oxide may also facilitate a decline in pulmonary vascular resistance, thereby promoting antegrade flow across the right ventricular outflow tract (110,111). If cyanosis decreases, surgical intervention on the tricuspid valve can then be deferred.

For symptomatic neonates who fail medical management, there is no single reparative or palliative procedure that has been associated with widespread success. For neonates with both cyanosis and heart failure, one surgical option is to place a systemic to pulmonary artery shunt, over sew the tricuspid valve annulus, and perform an atrial septectomy as the first stage procedure toward Fontan palliation (112). Plication of the right atrium is usually necessary to reduce its size and volume and promote right-to-left shunting across the atrial septum. Alternatively, a two-ventricular repair may be attempted consisting of a reduction atrioplasty, fenestrated closure of the atrial septum, and complex tricuspid valvuloplasty (113). Heart transplantation may also be considered, but despite early listing, it may be difficult to medically manage these patients while waiting for a donor graft to become available. Despite aggressive care, a subset of neonates with severe Ebstein anomaly has persistent low cardiac output and profound cyanosis resulting in early mortality (111).

Neonates with Ebstein anomaly who require early surgical intervention are at significant risk for developing a low cardiac output state, and a number of factors may be contributory (111). In neonates with a ductus arteriosus or systemic to pulmonary shunt and tricuspid and pulmonary regurgitation, circular shunting may contribute to a low cardiac output state. A *circular shunt* implies ineffective circulation secondary to aortic blood flowing through the ductus arteriosus or aortopulmonary shunt, retrograde through the main pulmonary artery to the right ventricle and tricuspid valve, across the atrial communication and out the left ventricle and aorta, with resultant inadequate systemic blood flow (Fig. 33.12). Thus, blood may leave the aorta and return to

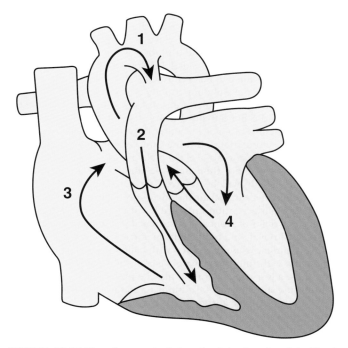

FIGURE 33.12 Line diagram depicting the "circular shunt" in Ebstein anomaly of the tricuspid valve with pulmonary insufficiency. There is ineffective blood flow from the aorta to the aorta (*1*), without traversing a capillary bed. This occurs through the PDA to the pulmonary artery (*2*) to the right ventricle through pulmonary insufficiency to the right atrium through the regurgitant tricuspid valve across the foramen ovale (*3*) to the left atrium and the left ventricle (*4*) and return to the aorta (*1*). (Reprinted from Wald RM, Adatia I, Van Arsdell GS, et al. Relation of limiting ductal patency to survival in neonatal Ebstein's anomaly. *Am J Cardiol* 2005;96:851. Copyright © 2005 Elsevier. With permission.)

THE NEWBORN INFANT

the aorta without crossing a capillary bed, creating a significant volume load and systemic steal (110). In this situation, an emergent reoperation may be required to ligate the ductus arteriosus, limit the shunt size, ligate the main pulmonary artery, or reduce tricuspid regurgitation with a valvuloplasty (110). Although the lungs may appear small on CXR, judicious airway pressures should be used and high mean airway pressures avoided, as overdistension of the lungs may increase pulmonary vascular resistance and limit left ventricular preload.

In general, good outcomes are achieved for neonates with Ebstein disease who do not require early intervention, intermediate outcomes for those in whom only a systemic to pulmonary shunt is performed, and suboptimal outcomes (mortality approaching 50%) for patients undergoing tricuspid valve repair or closure (right ventricular exclusion) (114,115). In one report, however, a conservative management strategy that recognized the potential pitfalls of prolonged ductal patency and the potential for circular shunting was associated with an overall neonatal mortality rate of 7% (110).

Left Ventricular Outflow Tract Obstruction
Critical Aortic Valve Stenosis

Aortic valve stenosis may present in a variety of ways, depending primarily upon the severity of stenosis. Neonates with a bicuspid aortic valve with no outflow tract obstruction and those with mild–moderate stenosis will be asymptomatic. At the other extreme, those with unrecognized critical aortic valve stenosis develop left atrial hypertension, pulmonary edema, and shock as the ductus arteriosus constricts. In patients with critical aortic valve stenosis, the systolic ejection murmur is typically softer than expected due to the low cardiac output state, and the gradient estimated by echocardiography may not correlate with the severity of the stenosis. In neonates with critical aortic valve stenosis, ductal-dependent systemic blood flow exists, and initiation of a PGE$_1$ infusion allows blood ejected from the right ventricle to provide systemic perfusion until an intervention can be performed.

Left ventricular systolic function is typically depressed in neonates with critical aortic valve stenosis. A careful assessment of the aortic valve and other left-sided heart structures is made by echocardiogram in order to judge whether they are adequate to support the systemic circulation following intervention and upon closure of the ductus arteriosus (116,117). Neonates with critical aortic valve stenosis who are thought to be suitable for a two-ventricle circulation usually will be referred for a balloon aortic valvuloplasty; although a surgical aortic valvotomy is an acceptable option (118,119). Reintervention rates are lower after surgical aortic valvotomy but relief of stenosis, postprocedural aortic insufficiency, long-term survival, and freedom from aortic valve replacement are relatively similar when compared with balloon valvuloplasty (120). In patients with important hypoplasia of multiple left-sided heart structures, a Norwood operation may be preferable.

Inotropic support may be administered for a few days following alleviation of critical aortic valve stenosis while awaiting recovery of left ventricular systolic function. The PGE$_1$ infusion may be discontinued immediately following the procedure or once left-to-right flow is seen at the ductal level by echocardiography. Note that the gradient across the aortic valve may be minimal immediately following intervention but will often increase as myocardial function and cardiac output improve. Approximately half of neonates with critical aortic valve stenosis who undergo balloon valvuloplasty require reintervention on the aortic valve during the first 5 years of life (120,121).

Critical Coarctation of the Aorta

A coarctation of the aorta is present when a significant narrowing exists in the thoracic aorta just distal to the left subclavian artery. A "posterior shelf" is present opposite the insertion site of the PDA. Coarctation of the aorta may exist in isolation or can be associated with aortic arch hypoplasia, a VSD, or other complex intracardiac lesions. A bicuspid aortic valve is present in at least 50% of cases. A coarctation of the aorta is deemed "critical" when ductal-dependent systemic blood flow exists, which represents only about 10% of cases.

Coarctation of the aorta may be suspected on physical examination by the detection of a brachial–femoral pulse discrepancy, which can be confirmed by measuring an arm–leg blood systolic pressure gradient. A systolic blood pressure gradient between the upper and lower extremities of greater than 10 mm Hg is clinically significant. In approximately 5% of infants with isolated coarctation of the aorta, the right subclavian artery will arise aberrantly from the descending thoracic aorta, distal to the coarctation, making the exam findings and blood pressure gradients described above unreliable.

In neonates with an unrecognized critical coarctation of the aorta, left atrial hypertension, and shock may develop upon constriction of the ductus arteriosus. In such patients, left ventricular systolic dysfunction develops due to the high afterload imposed on the left ventricle by the coarctation and resultant pulmonary hypertension. Occasionally, differential cyanosis will be present as the lower body is being perfused by deoxygenated blood from the ductus arteriosus. A PGE$_1$ infusion will reliably reopen the ductus arteriosus, allowing for improvement in myocardial and end-organ function prior to surgical repair.

In neonates and infants, coarctation may be adequately imaged in most cases by transthoracic echocardiogram. Occasionally, a cardiac MRI or CT scan may be useful to clarify details of the arch anatomy.

Several operative techniques are available for coarctation repair. These include resection with end-to-end anastomosis, patch aortoplasty, subclavian flap aortoplasty, and resection with *extended* end-to-end anastomosis. The later technique may be used to address aortic arch hypoplasia and appears to be associated with a low recoarctation rate (122). Due to a significant recoarctation rate and the potential for aneurysm formation, primary balloon angioplasty is generally not recommended in infancy.

Following repair of an isolated critical coarctation of the aorta, systemic hypertension may be seen. Four extremity blood pressure measurements should be obtained to evaluate for the presence of residual aortic arch obstruction. Neonates and infants are at lower risk for spinal cord ischemia or significant postoperative hypertension following coarctation repair when compared with older children and adults. As with any surgical intervention on the aortic arch, the phrenic and recurrent laryngeal nerves are at risk for injury. Diaphragmatic and vocal cord movement should be investigated if there is clinical suspicion for dysfunction. Mortality following repair of an isolated coarctation of the aorta is rare.

Hypoplastic Left Heart Syndrome

HLHS describes severe mitral and aortic valve stenosis or atresia, a diminutive left ventricle, ascending aorta, and aortic arch, and often a juxtaductal coarctation of the aorta. The left-sided heart structures are incapable of supporting the systemic circulation. An adequate ASD is also necessary to allow egress of the pulmonary venous blood flow from the left atrium to the right atrium.

At birth, most neonates with HLHS will have mild cyanosis and stable hemodynamics. A PDA is necessary to allow blood flow from the right ventricle to reach the systemic circulation, and shock will likely develop once the ductus arteriosus constricts. A PGE$_1$ infusion is thus indicated to maintain ductal patency. Echocardiography is used to clarify anatomic details. Genetic testing may identify Turner syndrome or other anomalies. Patients presenting with myocardial dysfunction may be treated with inotropic support to improve cardiac output and systemic oxygen delivery. However, care should be taken to avoid inotropic agents that increase systemic vascular resistance because this will favor pulmonary blood flow over systemic blood flow. Low-dose epinephrine, low-dose dopamine, or milrinone are reasonable inotropic agents for use in this setting.

Over the first few days of life, as pulmonary vascular resistance falls the ratio of pulmonary to systemic blood flow (Qp/Qs) will increase. This evolving physiology leads to right ventricular volume overload, as well as the potential for inadequate systemic perfusion and end-organ ischemia. The Qp/Qs may be calculated by the following equation, which is derived from the Fick principle: $Qp/Qs = (SaO_2-SvO_2)/(PvO_2-PaO_2)$, where SaO_2 = aortic saturation; SvO_2 = mixed venous saturation (estimated by the superior vena cava oxygen saturation); PvO_2 = pulmonary venous oxygen saturation (assumed to be >95% if not directly measured); and PaO_2 = pulmonary artery oxygen saturation (assumed equal to the aortic saturation). Most preoperative neonates will not have a central venous catheter positioned in the superior vena cava to measure SvO_2, and thus, the Qp/Qs cannot be precisely calculated. Determination of an absolute value for Qp/Qs is of less importance than having an appreciation for the physiologic disturbance that develops as these neonates become progressively overcirculated. Computer models of HLHS physiology demonstrate that that maximal oxygen delivery occurs at a Qp/Qs slightly less than 1.0 (**Figs. 33.13** and **33.14**) (123,124). These models also demonstrate that a SvO_2 < 40% or a SaO_2-SvO_2 difference of >40% is likely to be associated with a severe derangement in systemic oxygen delivery, related to either a high Qp/Qs or low cardiac output (124).

In the typical neonate with HLHS, interventions that lower the pulmonary vascular resistance, such as supplemental oxygen and hyperventilation, may increase Qp/Qs and should generally be avoided. Patients with pulmonary overcirculation (high Qp/Qs) and evidence of inadequate end-organ perfusion may be treated with hypoventilation or supplemental inspired carbon dioxide or nitrogen, with the intention of increasing pulmonary vascular resistance. These strategies require the concurrent use of a muscle relaxant or sedative to prevent compensatory hyperventilation.

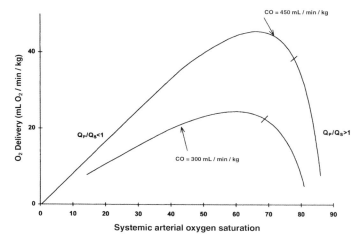

FIGURE 33.13 Systemic arterial oxygen saturation versus systemic oxygen (O₂) delivery in the theoretical newborn with hypoplastic left heart syndrome. A computer model was used to generate the curves by setting the cardiac output (CO) at 300 or 450 mL/kg/min and varying Qp/Qs from 0.2 to 10. The short line on each curve represents the point at which Qp/Qs = 1. As SaO₂ increases, oxygen delivery increases and reaches a peak, and then decreases rapidly. Peak oxygen delivery occurs at a Qp/Qs < 1. (Reprinted with permission from Barnea O, Santamore WP, Rossi A, et al. Estimation of oxygen delivery in newborns with a univentricular circulation. *Circulation* 1998;98:1407.)

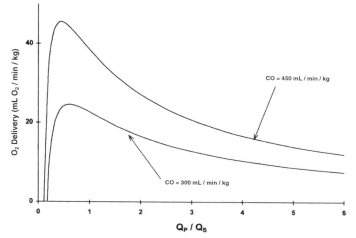

FIGURE 33.14 Systemic oxygen (O₂) delivery versus Qp/Qs in the theoretical newborn with hypoplastic left heart syndrome. A computer model was used to generate the curves by setting the cardiac output (CO) at 300 or 450 mL/kg/min. Note that increasing cardiac output can increase oxygen delivery, and that oxygen delivery decreases significantly once Qp/Qs exceeds 1. (Reprinted with permission from Barnea O, Santamore WP, Rossi A, et al. Estimation of oxygen delivery in newborns with a univentricular circulation. *Circulation* 1998;98:1407.)

Administration of subambient FiO_2 is an alternative strategy to increase PVR that has largely fallen out of favor given a neutral effect on systemic oxygen delivery (125).

A severely restrictive or intact atrial septum is present in 5% of neonates with HLHS, and these patients typically develop profound cyanosis, pulmonary edema, and shock almost immediately following delivery. Such patients develop pulmonary venous hypertension and lymphatic abnormalities in utero that persist following birth (126,127). The immediate management of these critically ill neonates involves emergent intervention to decompress the left atrium. A Brockenbrough atrial septoplasty (transcatheter, transseptal needle puncture followed by serial balloon dilation of the new ASD, and possibly stent placement) will serve to decompress the left atrium, increase pulmonary venous return and pulmonary blood flow, and alleviate cyanosis (128). Following atrial decompression, the patient may be medically managed for a few days with a PGE_1 infusion and diuretics to allow pulmonary vascular resistance to fall and pulmonary edema to improve prior to the Norwood operation. Survival rates between 53% and 80% following the Norwood operation have been reported with this strategy, which are better than results obtained with other management strategies for this lesion, but remain poor when compared with the outcomes of neonates without atrial obstruction who undergo the Norwood operation (129,130).

During the Norwood operation for HLHS, the distal pulmonary artery is over sewn, the proximal pulmonary artery and the aorta are anastomosed, and the aortic arch is reconstructed to allow for unobstructed systemic blood flow. An atrial septectomy is performed to allow pulmonary venous return to pass easily to the right atrium, and a systemic to pulmonary shunt is placed to provide pulmonary blood flow (**Fig. 33.15**). Following this operation, the single right ventricle pumps blood to the systemic circulation and coronary arteries via the reconstructed aorta (i.e., "neo-aorta") and to the pulmonary circulation via the shunt.

Historically, the modified Blalock-Taussig shunt was routinely used as the source of pulmonary blood flow during the Norwood operation. Given the concerns about diastolic runoff, volume loading, and coronary insufficiency associated with this shunt, in recent years, some surgeons place a right ventricular to pulmonary

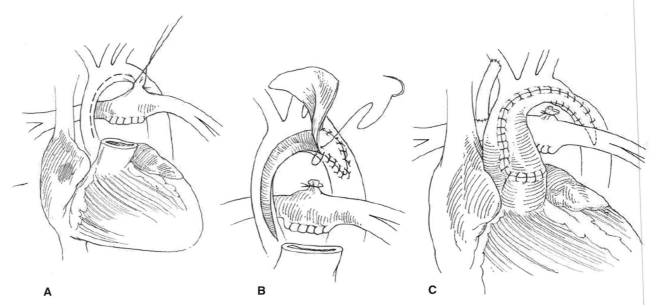

A   **B**   **C**

FIGURE 33.15 The stage I Norwood procedure. A: Initial steps include ligating and dividing the ductus arteriosus, detaching the distal portion of the main pulmonary artery, and incising the undersurface of the aortic arch. **B:** The hypoplastic aorta is augmented with a patch of homograft material. **C:** The augmented aorta is then connected (i.e., amalgamated) with the cardiac end of the main pulmonary artery stump. Pulmonary blood flow is supplied by a modified Blalock-Taussig shunt. Not shown is an atrial septectomy. (Reprinted with permission from Wernovsky G, Bove EL. Single ventricle lesions. In: Chang A, Hanley FL, Wernovsky G, et al., eds. *Pediatric cardiac intensive care.* Baltimore, MD: Williams and Wilkins, 1998:271.)

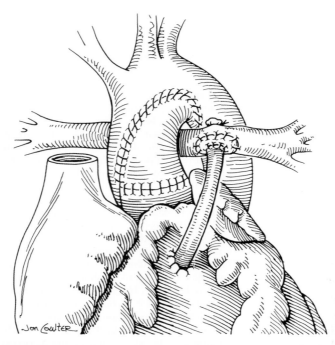

FIGURE 33.16 A completed Stage I Norwood procedure, in which pulmonary blood flow is supplied by a right ventricle–pulmonary artery conduit. (Reprinted with permission from Pizarro C, et al. Right ventricle to pulmonary artery conduit improves outcome after stage I Norwood for hypoplastic left heart syndrome. *Circulation* 2003;108 (suppl 1):II155.)

artery shunt to provide pulmonary blood flow. This modification was originally described by Dr. William Norwood but was applied successfully by Dr. Shunji Sano and colleagues and thus became known as the "Sano shunt" (**Fig. 33.16**) (131). The postoperative physiology following the Sano modification is somewhat different from the standard Norwood operation and deserves comment.

Patients with a Sano shunt tend to have higher diastolic blood pressure and improved coronary perfusion pressure (132). Due to the absence of diastolic runoff through a Blalock-Taussig shunt, infants with "Sano physiology" do not have pulmonary overcirculation (or a large Qp/Qs) and thus may benefit less from aggressive afterload reduction. In fact, excessive systemic vasodilation may lead to inadequate pulmonary blood flow and severe cyanosis (similar to the physiology of a patient with unrepaired tetralogy of Fallot). Risks related to this modification center upon the effects of performing a ventriculotomy in an infant with a single right ventricle and include myocardial dysfunction, arrhythmias, and false aneurysm formation. In a multicenter, randomized clinical trial, Norwood patients assigned to the right ventricular to pulmonary artery shunt group had higher 1-year transplant-free survival when compared to the modified Blalock-Taussig shunt group (133). However, subsequent follow-up of patients in this trial has revealed no significant differences in transplant-free survival.

Another alternative to the Norwood operation is a so-called "hybrid" procedure (134). This intervention entails transcatheter stenting of the ductus arteriosus, placement of bilateral pulmonary bands, and (typically) a balloon atrial septostomy during the neonatal period (Fig. 33.17). The aortic arch reconstruction is then performed concurrently with the bidirectional superior cavopulmonary connection at 4 to 6 months of age (i.e., a "comprehensive stage II palliation"). One advantage of the hybrid procedure is the avoidance of CPB in the neonatal period. Potential issues following this procedure include excessive or inadequate blood flow to the individual lungs depending on the relative tightness of each pulmonary artery band, the risk for the development of a "retrograde" coarctation in patients with a severely hypoplastic distal transverse aortic arch, and the potential that the ductal stent may incompletely cover the ductus arteriosus, which creates the substrate for right (systemic) ventricular outflow tract obstruction.

Ideally, the circulations will be balanced following the Norwood operation such that the Qp/Qs ratio will be approximately 1:1. Assuming an unrestrictive, surgically created ASD and unobstructed pulmonary venous blood flow, pulmonary blood flow

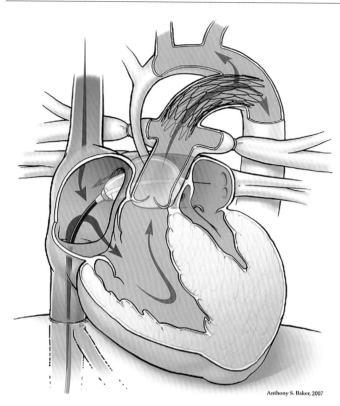

FIGURE 33.17 The hybrid stage 1 palliation. Branch pulmonary artery bands and a stent across the PDA are placed at one procedure, while the balloon atrial septostomy is performed as a separate procedure. (Reprinted from Galantowicz M, Cheatham JP, Phillips A, et al. Hybrid approach for hypoplastic left heart syndrome: intermediate results after the learning curve. *Ann Thorac Surg* 2008;85:2063. Copyright © 2008 The Society of Thoracic Surgeons. With permission; Courtesy of Dr. Mark Galantowicz.)

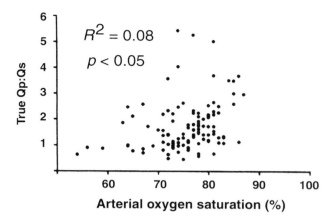

FIGURE 33.18 Regression analysis of SaO_2 against true Qp/Qs following the Norwood operation. SaO_2 is a poor predictor of Qp/Qs ($R^2 = 0.08$, $p < 0.05$). Variability in Qp/Qs is most pronounced at SaO_2 values in range of 65% to 85%, usual target range for patients after Norwood palliation. (Reprinted with permission from Taeed R, Schwartz SM, Pearl JM, et al. Unrecognized pulmonary venous desaturation early after Norwood palliation confounds Qp/Qs assessment and compromises oxygen delivery. *Circulation* 2001;103:2699.)

will be determined by the pulmonary vascular resistance and the resistance provided by the systemic to pulmonary artery shunt. Systemic blood flow will be determined by the systemic vascular resistance and, if present, any residual aortic arch obstruction. Excessive pulmonary blood flow with inadequate systemic perfusion, similar to that seen in a typical preoperative neonate with HLHS, was historically thought to be a major problem following the Norwood operation. Current understanding is that overcirculation is less of an issue, particularly if a Sano shunt or an appropriately sized Blalock-Taussig shunt has been placed. The ratio of systemic and pulmonary blood flow may be calculated by the modified Fick equation (discussed earlier). Note that calculating the Qp/Qs using only the arterial SaO_2 may be highly inaccurate without knowledge of SvO_2 and PvO_2 (**Fig. 33.18**). Pulmonary venous desaturation is common in the early postoperative period after the Norwood operation at some point, even in the absence of radiographic abnormalities on chest radiograph (135). In contrast to the preoperative period, after the Norwood operation, the provision of a judicious amount of supplemental oxygen may improve pulmonary venous oxygen saturation and ultimately systemic oxygen delivery.

Low cardiac output is a common problem following the Norwood operation. Contributory factors may include myocardial dysfunction, atrioventricular valve regurgitation, pulmonary overcirculation, coronary ischemia, residual aortic arch obstruction, or a combination of these factors. An anaerobic threshold is reached when the SvO_2 falls below 30% following the Norwood operation, and efforts to maintain SvO_2 above this value have been associated with very low early mortality (136). Inotropic support and afterload reduction may be beneficial for such patients.

Excessive cyanosis may occur following the Norwood operation. The differential diagnosis and management strategies are discussed previously in the postoperative cyanosis section.

Survival to hospital discharge rates of approximately 90% following initial surgical palliation for HLHS are currently achieved in high performing centers. Risk factors contributing to higher mortality following the Norwood operation include prematurity, genetic anomalies, significant atrioventricular valve regurgitation, the presence of multiple congenital anomalies, and a restrictive or intact atrial septum (137). Heart transplantation may also be considered as a primary management strategy for neonates with HLHS, although the limited donor pool results in a significant waitlist mortality, and complications inherent to heart transplant also need to be considered.

Interrupted Aortic Arch

IAA is classified by the location of the arch interruption in relation to the brachiocephalic vessels (**Fig. 33.19**) (138). IAA type B is the most common subtype (>50% of cases), and type C is rare. IAA is most commonly associated with a VSD but also is seen with a variety of other congenital cardiac malformations, including truncus arteriosus and d-TGA.

Neonates with an IAA will typically be stable at birth. Differential cyanosis will be present due to the fact that systemic blood flow to the lower part of the body is supplied by the ductus arteriosus. Those with an unrecognized IAA will present with shock, similar to a critical coarctation, upon constriction of the ductus arteriosus. Preoperative management strategies to balance the systemic and pulmonary circulations mimic those used in infants with HLHS. The cardiac anatomy can usually be clearly delineated by echocardiography. DiGeorge syndrome is present in approximately 60% of neonates with IAA type B (139).

Complete repair, including VSD closure and reconstruction of the aortic arch, is the preferred operation for newborns with IAA. If significant subaortic stenosis is present, a Norwood-type operation may be used to stage the patient for a future biventricular repair. Staged intervention may be considered as an alternative approach for high-risk neonatal patients. This pathway involves an initial "hybrid" operation, which includes stenting of the ductus arteriosus and pulmonary artery banding as a bridge to a complete repair later in infancy.

THE NEWBORN INFANT

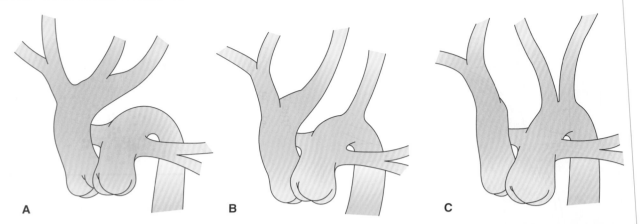

FIGURE 33.19 The three types of interrupted aortic arch. In type **A**, the interruption is at the aortic isthmus between the left subclavian artery and the ductus. In type **B**, the interruption is at the distal aortic arch between the left carotid and left subclavian arteries. In type **C**, the interruption is at the proximal aortic arch between the innominate and left carotid arteries. Type B is the most common form of this lesion. Type **C** is rare. (Reprinted with permission from Chang AC, Starnes VA. Interrupted aortic arch. In: Chang AC, Hanley FL, Wernovsky G, et al., eds. *Pediatric cardiac intensive care*. Baltimore, MD: Williams and Wilkins, 1998:243.)

Potential residual anatomic lesions following IAA repair include a VSD, subaortic obstruction, or aortic arch obstruction. Patients with respiratory compromise following surgery may have compression of the left mainstem bronchus by the reconstructed aortic arch.

Mixing Lesions
Transposition of the Great Arteries

In d-TGA, the aorta arises from the anatomic right ventricle and the pulmonary artery arises from the anatomic left ventricle. Approximately 40% of patients with d-TGA have an associated VSD, which occasionally is a malalignment-type defect. If anterior malalignment exists, there may be associated right ventricular outflow tract obstruction, aortic valvar stenosis, coarctation of the aorta or, rarely, an IAA. A posterior malalignment VSD is associated with left ventricular outflow tract obstruction, pulmonary stenosis, or atresia. Coronary artery branching abnormalities are present in approximately 30% of cases.

In this unique parallel circulation, deoxygenated systemic venous blood returns to the right heart and is pumped back to the systemic arterial circulation, and oxygenated pulmonary venous blood passes through the left heart and is pumped back to the lungs. Unless there is adequate mixing between these parallel circulations, severe cyanosis, metabolic acidosis, and death will occur. Such intercirculatory mixing represents *effective* pulmonary and systemic blood flows and may take place at the atrial, ventricular, or great artery level. Neonates with d-TGA and an intact ventricular septum are typically born with a patent foramen ovale (PFO) or ASD that allows some mixing at the atrial level. A PGE$_1$ infusion is routinely administered to open or maintain patency of the ductus arteriosus, which will increase effective pulmonary blood flow, provided that the pulmonary vascular resistance is lower than the systemic vascular resistance and that there is an adequate atrial communication.

If the PFO is restrictive, as assessed by echocardiography, and excessive cyanosis is present, an emergent balloon atrial septostomy should be performed to enlarge the atrial communication (Fig. 33.20). The balloon atrial septostomy may be performed at the bedside using echocardiographic guidance, or in the cardiac catheterization laboratory. In a minority of cases, excessive cyanosis may persist despite a technically successful balloon atrial septostomy. In this scenario, high pulmonary vascular resistance may limit effective pulmonary blood flow, and measures should

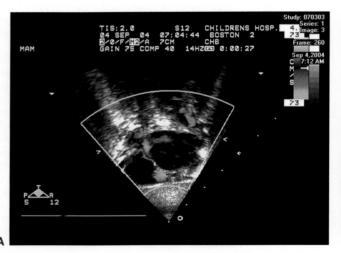
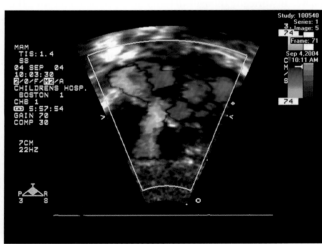

FIGURE 33.20 Restrictive atrial septum in a newborn with transposition of the great arteries. A: Two-dimensional echocardiogram with color Doppler from the subcostal window demonstrating a tiny patent foramen ovale with left-to-right flow across the atrial septum. **B:** Following successful balloon atrial septostomy, a wide communication now exists between the left and right atria. LA, left atrium; PFO, patent foramen ovale; RA, right atrium. (Reprinted with permission from Costello JM, Franklin WH. Preoperative and postoperative care of the infant with critical congenital heart disease. In: *Avery's neonatology pathophysiology & management of the newborn*, 6th ed., Philadelphia, PA: Lippincott Williams & Wilkins, 2005:710.)

be taken to lower pulmonary vascular resistance. Because the majority of systemic blood flow comes from the systemic venous circulation in d-TGA, neonates who remain excessively cyanotic following a balloon atrial septostomy may improve following interventions directed at increasing the mixed venous oxygen saturation. These include the use of sedatives and muscle relaxants to decrease oxygen consumption, and blood transfusion and use of inotropic agents to improve oxygen delivery.

Some clinicians recommend that a semielective balloon atrial septostomy be performed in patients with d-TGA and intact ventricular septum, even those without excessive cyanosis. Once the atrial septum is enlarged, PGE_1 can often be safely discontinued, thus avoiding complications related to that medication and the presence of a large ductus arteriosus (e.g., apnea, NEC). Furthermore, decompression of the left atrium and reduction in left-to-right ductal shunting may facilitate a decline in pulmonary vascular resistance prior to surgery. The major risks associated

with a balloon atrial septostomy include myocardial perforation or avulsion of the inferior vena cava from the right atrium during pullback of the balloon, both of which are rare.

Neonates with d-TGA, an intact ventricular septum, and no significant outflow tract obstruction typically are referred for an arterial switch operation. The arterial switch operation for such patients is ideally performed within the first few weeks of life before the left ventricle becomes deconditioned. The arterial switch operation involves transecting the aorta and pulmonary arteries above the semilunar valves, and anastomosing the aorta to the neoaortic root, such that the left ventricle ejects into the systemic circulation. The pulmonary artery is brought anterior to the aorta such that its branches drape over the aorta (Lecompte maneuver), and the pulmonary artery is anastomosed such that it receives blood from the right ventricular outflow tract. The coronary arteries are mobilized with a button of tissue around the ostia and reimplanted into the neo-aorta. The VSD (if present) is closed (Fig. 33.21).

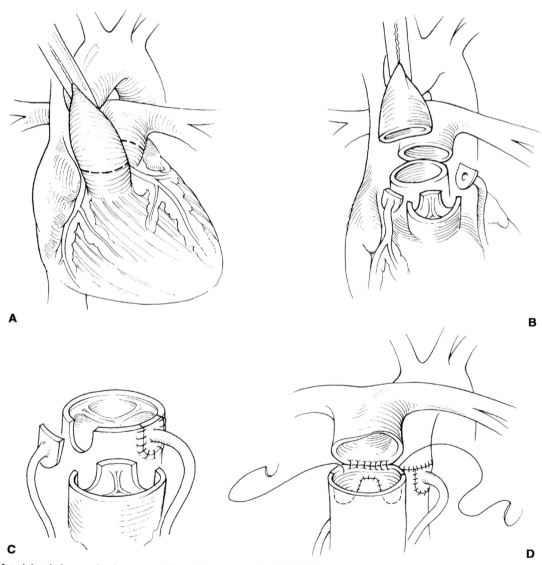

FIGURE 33.21 Arterial switch operation for transposition of the great arteries (TGA). A: The external anatomy is shown. The procedure is performed using cardiopulmonary bypass and either moderate or deep hypothermia with or without circulatory arrest. The *broken lines* show the sites of transection of the two great vessels. **B:** The aorta and main pulmonary arteries have been surgically transected, and the coronary ostia have been removed from the native aortic root. **C:** The coronary buttons are in the process of being transferred to the native aortic root. **D:** The coronary transfer has been completed, and the neoaortic root has been anastomosed to the ascending aorta. The coronary explantation sites on the neopulmonary root have been repaired with a patch and the neopulmonary artery is in the process of anastomosis to the distal pulmonary artery. Note, the distal pulmonary artery has been moved anterior to the ascending aorta as described by Lecompte. The procedure also involves closing the atrial septal defect and dividing the PDA. (Reprinted with permission from Wernovsky G, Jonas RA. Other conotruncal lesions. In: Chang A, Hanley FL, Wernovsky G, et al., eds. *Pediatric cardiac intensive care*. Baltimore, MD: Williams and Wilkins, 1998:289.)

Infants with d-TGA and intact ventricular septum who present for surgery after 1 to 2 months of age may undergo pulmonary artery band placement to "prepare" the left ventricle before the arterial switch operation (140). A systemic to pulmonary artery shunt is also placed at the time of the pulmonary artery band to ensure adequate pulmonary blood flow. These patients often develop transient biventricular failure (right ventricular failure due to the acute volume overload created by the shunt and left ventricular failure related to the acute increase in afterload from the pulmonary artery band) and low cardiac output following this operation (141). Inotropic support and measures to decrease pulmonary overcirculation are often required for several days until the hemodynamics stabilize. Once the left ventricle is prepared, the pulmonary artery shunt and pulmonary band are removed, and the arterial switch operation is performed.

Neonates with d-TGA, a moderate to large VSD, and no significant outflow tract obstruction generally are well oxygenated and thus do not require a PGE_1 infusion. Early congestive heart failure typically develops, and surgical repair is often performed within the first few weeks of life. Those who are referred for surgery *after* the first few months of life (typically from low- and middle-income countries) are at risk for having developed pulmonary vascular obstructive disease. Such patients may warrant a cardiac catheterization to assess pulmonary vascular resistance prior to surgery.

Neonates with d-TGA and a malalignment-type VSD may have significant left or right ventricular outflow tract obstruction. Those with right ventricular outflow tract obstruction (i.e., subaortic obstruction) may have an associated coarctation of the aorta or an IAA. Such patients may present with the very unique finding of reverse differential cyanosis, with low oxygen saturation in the right arm and high oxygen saturation in the leg. A PGE_1 infusion is indicated in such patients, followed by early surgical intervention. If the aortic valve is adequate for use as the neopulmonary valve, an arterial switch, and VSD repair is performed. If significant hypoplasia of the aortic valve precludes its use as the neopulmonary valve, a Damus-Kaye-Stansel procedure may be performed with placement of a systemic to pulmonary shunt or as a part of a complete repair including VSD closure and placement of a right ventricle to pulmonary artery conduit.

If significant left ventricular outflow tract obstruction exists, the classic surgical repair is the Rastelli procedure. This operation involves baffling the VSD to the aorta and placement of a right ventricle to pulmonary artery conduit (142). Another option is the Nikaidoh operation, which involves aortic root translocation into the surgically enlarged left ventricular outflow tract, VSD closure, and right ventricular outflow tract reconstruction (143).

The expected mortality for the arterial switch operation is very low, and many patients will have an unremarkable postoperative course. A period of early low cardiac output has been documented in approximately 25% of these patients (18). Coronary ischemia is very uncommon in the current era but may occur if there is kinking or stenosis of a coronary artery following reimplantation into the neo-aorta. Volume overload in the immediate postoperative period can cause cardiac distension that stretches the newly implanted coronary arteries, resulting in myocardial ischemia and/or infarction. Coronary insufficiency may manifest as low cardiac output with ischemic electrocardiographic changes or ventricular arrhythmias. Significant obstruction of the aortic or pulmonary anastomosis is unusual in the early postoperative period. Residual VSDs and ventricular outflow obstruction may be encountered in complex cases.

Tricuspid Atresia

Tricuspid atresia is present when there is agenesis of the tricuspid valve and an absent communication between the right atrium and right ventricle. The presentation is variable and depends primarily upon the presence and size of a VSD, whether the great arteries are normally related or transposed, and the degree of ventricular

TABLE 33.7

Classification System for Tricuspid Atresia

Type and Description	Frequency
Type I: Normally related great arteries	70%–80%
A. Intact ventricular septum with pulmonary atresia	
B. Small ventricular septal defect with pulmonary stenosis	
C. Large ventricular septal defect without pulmonary stenosis	
Type II: d-Transposition of the great arteries	12%–25%
A. Ventricular septal defect with pulmonary atresia	
B. Ventricular septal defect with pulmonary stenosis	
C. Ventricular septal defect without pulmonary stenosis	
Type III: l-Transposition of the great arteries	3%–6%

outflow tract obstruction (Table 33.7). These factors determine which neonates with tricuspid atresia will have ductal-dependent pulmonary blood flow, ductal-dependent systemic blood flow, or a "balanced" circulation in which ductal patency and neonatal surgery are not required. In tricuspid atresia, all of the systemic venous blood must pass through an obligate atrial communication to the left atrium, where it mixes with the pulmonary venous blood. In the presence of normally looped ventricles and normally related great arteries, the single left ventricle then ejects blood to the aorta, and through the VSD, if present, to the pulmonary artery. If the great arteries are transposed, the left ventricle pumps blood to the pulmonary artery (unless pulmonary atresia is present), and through the VSD to the aorta. Although essentially all patients with tricuspid atresia eventually undergo a Fontan operation, the type of initial palliation in the neonatal period depends upon the extent of cyanosis or systemic outflow obstruction. For example, neonates with tricuspid atresia, normally looped ventricles and normally related great vessels, a large VSD, and no or minimal right ventricular outflow tract obstruction (type I-C) will be well oxygenated and develop early heart failure. These patients are typically referred for pulmonary artery band placement. Those with a moderate size VSD and a moderate degree of right ventricular outflow tract obstruction (type I-B) may have a balanced circulation with an acceptable amount of cyanosis. Such patients may be discharged home with the expectation that a superior cavopulmonary connection will be performed within the first 6 months of life. Patients with tricuspid atresia and a small or absent VSD (type I-A or I-B) have ductal-dependent pulmonary blood flow. They require a PGE_1 infusion and typically undergo placement of a systemic to pulmonary artery shunt. Neonates with tricuspid atresia and transposed great arteries, a small or absent VSD (type II-A or II-B), and aortic arch obstruction have ductal-dependent systemic blood flow and may develop shock unless ductal patency is maintained. These patients initially undergo a modified Norwood operation.

The postoperative course following neonatal surgical palliation for tricuspid atresia depends upon the operation performed. Postoperative issues following a systemic to pulmonary artery shunt, a pulmonary artery band, and the Norwood operation are described in earlier sections of this chapter.

Total Anomalous Pulmonary Venous Return

In patients with total anomalous pulmonary venous return (TAPVR), all four pulmonary veins drain to a systemic vein or the right atrium. TAPVR results from a failure of the common pulmonary vein to fuse with the posterior surface of the left atrium early in fetal life. The pulmonary veins then decompress via the coronary sinus or primitive venous structures, which eventually lead to the right atrium, where mixing occurs with the systemic venous blood. TAPVR may be classified into supracardiac, cardiac, infracardiac, and mixed types, depending upon which primitive venous pathways are employed. Supracardiac TAPVR, the most common type, exists when all of the pulmonary veins come to a confluence behind the left atrium and drain via a vertical vein to the innominate vein or superior vena cava. Occasionally, the vertical vein is obstructed as it passes between the left mainstem bronchus and left pulmonary artery. Cardiac TAPVR exists when the pulmonary veins drain to the coronary sinus or right atrium. Obstruction is uncommon in cardiac TAPVR. In infracardiac TAPVR, the pulmonary venous confluence drains inferiorly through the diaphragm and into the portal or hepatic veins, where obstruction is common. Patients with mixed TAPVR have drainage to more than one site. An obligatory intracardiac (usually atrial) communication exists in neonates with TAPVR to allow some oxygenated blood to reach the left heart and systemic arterial circulation. TAPVR may be associated with significant intracardiac lesions, as is seen in patients with heterotaxy syndrome, or may exist as an isolated lesion.

The presentation of isolated TAPVR is primarily based upon the degree of obstruction (if any) between the pulmonary veins and the right heart. Most patients with infracardiac TAPVR and some with supracardiac TAPVR will have obstructed pulmonary venous pathways. In these patients, pulmonary edema, pulmonary hypertension, cyanosis, and significant respiratory distress are usually evident soon after birth. The clinical presentation and CXR may mimic those seen with neonatal pneumonia or respiratory distress syndrome, leading to delays in diagnosis. Stabilization for the neonate with obstructed TAPVR involves mechanical ventilation, sedation, and urgent surgical intervention. Hypoxemia may be abated somewhat by interventions that increase mixed venous oxygen saturation, including pharmacologic paralysis, correction of anemia, and inotropic support. Although neonates with obstructed TAPVR may be quite cyanotic, measures to lower pulmonary vascular resistance, including the use of hyperventilation and nitric oxide, are usually not beneficial. The use of PGE_1 infusion in such patients is generally not beneficial, as any left-to-right shunting at the ductus arteriosus may exacerbate pulmonary edema. Neonates with unobstructed isolated TAPVR and an adequate atrial communication will be mildly hypoxemic without overt clinical cyanosis at birth. CHF may develop in some of these patients within a few weeks to months. Surgical repair is usually electively performed within the first few days to weeks of life. In many patients with TAPVR, the cardiac anatomy can be clearly delineated by echocardiography. A subset of patients may benefit from a cardiac CT or MRI to clarify the pulmonary venous anatomy.

In infants with supracardiac and infracardiac TAPVR, the pulmonary venous confluence is anastomosed to the back of the left atrium using circulatory arrest, the primitive vertical vein is ligated, and the ASD is closed. If the pulmonary veins drain to the coronary sinus, surgical intervention involves unroofing of the coronary sinus, and closure of the ASD.

Postoperatively, pulmonary hypertensive crises may occur, in part related to abnormal muscularity of the pulmonary arteries and veins that develops in utero. Pulmonary edema and poor lung compliance may be evident. The left atrium may be small and poorly compliant, and rapid volume infusions may exacerbate pulmonary edema and pulmonary hypertension in this setting. Deep sedation and the judicious use of PEEP may be helpful in the early postoperative period to facilitate gas exchange. The pulmonary hypertension seen in some patients following repair of TAPVR is very responsive to inhaled nitric oxide (144). Approximately 10% of patients with TAPVR who undergo repair as neonates develop pulmonary venous stenosis later in infancy (145). This condition may be difficult to treat, particularly if bilateral pulmonary veins are involved.

Truncus Arteriosus

Truncus arteriosus is present when a single (common) arterial trunk gives rise to the aorta, at least one coronary artery and at least one pulmonary artery. A single semilunar ("truncal") valve

is always present, and an unrestrictive VSD is almost always present. About one-third of patients with truncus arteriosus have a 22q11.2 microdeletion (DiGeorge syndrome) (146). Several classification systems exist that may be used to describe the origins of the pulmonary arteries from the arterial trunk and the presence or absence of an IAA (147,148).

Newborns with truncus arteriosus will present with mild cyanosis due to obligatory complete intracardiac mixing. They do not require a PGE_1 infusion unless an IAA (about 10% of cases) or ductal origin of one of the pulmonary arteries is present. As pulmonary vascular resistance falls within a few weeks after birth, neonates with truncus arteriosus usually develop pulmonary overcirculation and congestive heart failure. These patients are also at risk for NEC. Supplemental oxygen should generally be avoided to minimize overcirculation. Congestive heart failure may be exacerbated in the presence of significant truncal valve insufficiency, which occurs in up to 50% of cases, or significant truncal valve stenosis (less common).

Surgical repair of truncus arteriosus is generally recommended in the newborn period. The operation involves VSD closure, removal of the pulmonary arteries from the arterial trunk, and placement of a conduit from the right ventricle to the pulmonary arteries. If present, surgical attention is also given to the IAA and/or truncal valve insufficiency. Care must be taken to identify the origin and course of the coronary arteries so that they are not injured during the operation.

Following repair of truncus arteriosus, infants are at risk for restrictive right ventricular physiology (see discussion about restrictive right ventricular physiology in earlier section on tetralogy of Fallot). Any residual branch pulmonary artery stenosis may exacerbate this physiology. To mitigate this issue, the surgeon may leave an atrial communication to decompress the right heart and maintain left ventricular preload and cardiac output, at the expense of mild postoperative cyanosis. The truncal valve functions as the aortic valve following surgical repair and may be stenotic or regurgitant. The severity of preoperative truncal valve stenosis usually is decreased in the postoperative period as the volume overload has been eliminated. Severe truncal valve insufficiency will be poorly tolerated in the postoperative period and may require a surgical valvuloplasty or replacement. Pulmonary hypertension may be problematic, particularly in patients referred for surgery beyond the neonatal period. The left ventricle is exposed to increased afterload following surgery due to the elimination of the low vascular resistance pulmonary circulation, and the effects of CPB, which may create temporary left ventricular failure. A residual VSD will add a volume load to the left ventricle and contribute to pulmonary hypertension. If an IAA was repaired, care must be taken to ensure that residual arch obstruction does not exist and exacerbate myocardial dysfunction and truncal valve insufficiency. A state of low cardiac output may exist related to one or more of the above problems. Operative mortality is less than 10% in the current era (149).

Left to Right Shunt Lesions
Atrial Septal Defect

ASDs may be present in isolation or with nearly any other type of congenital heart defect. ASDs are categorized by location and include secundum, ostium primum, and sinus venosus types. The most common type is the secundum ASD, which exists when there is a deficiency in the central portion of the atrial septum, in the region of the foramen ovale. Although secundum ASDs may become smaller and close spontaneously, particularly those that are less than 5 mm in diameter, the ostium primum and sinus venosus defects will always require surgical intervention. The ostium primum defects are located in the inferior region of the atrial septum and are almost always associated with an additional endocardial cushion abnormality. The sinus venosus defects are located at the junction between the superior (common) or inferior (rare) vena cava and the right atrium and are almost always associated with partial anomalous pulmonary venous return.

Isolated ASDs only rarely cause symptoms in infants, as significant left-to-right shunting does not occur until right ventricular compliance falls below left ventricular compliance, and this often takes years to occur. However, clinical judgment regarding the medical management and timing of surgical intervention is required in the infant with a large ASD and additional medical problems (e.g., chronic lung disease). The primary indication for surgery *in infancy* is the presence of symptoms secondary to left-to-right shunting.

Toddlers are typically referred for elective ASD closure if they have evidence of volume overload of the right ventricle. The rationale for elective intervention in early childhood is to prevent late complications including pulmonary vascular obstructive disease, thromboembolic events, arrhythmias, and right heart failure.

Secundum ASDs may be surgically closed primarily or with a pericardial or Gore Tex patch. A variety of devices may be used to close secundum ASDs in the catheterization laboratory. Primum ASDs typically require patch closure, and the commonly associated cleft in the mitral valve is usually sutured closed. Sinus venosus ASDs are typically associated with anomalous pulmonary venous drainage of the right pulmonary veins, which must be redirected to the left atrium.

Following ASD closure, most patients may be extubated in the operating room or catheterization laboratory. Atrial arrhythmias may occur following any ASD closure. There is an increased incidence of sinus node dysfunction following sinus venosus ASD repair that is usually transient. Postpericardiotomy syndrome may occur in the weeks following surgical ASD closure. Patients undergoing device closure are at risk for late device erosion into the aorta, which may manifest as pericardial tamponade.

Ventricular Septal Defect

VSDs may be found in a variety of complex congenital heart lesions or may exist in isolation. VSDs are categorized by location and size. VSDs may be located in the perimembranous, muscular, inlet, or conal (outlet, subarterial, supracristal) regions of the ventricular septum, and there may be more than one VSD present. Malalignment of the conal septum may exist, resulting in variable degrees of right or left ventricular outflow tract obstruction. Conal VSDs often develop involvement of the aortic valve over many years. The size of a VSD may be placed into clinical context by determining the diameter of the VSD in relation to the aortic annulus and by degree of restriction to blood flow as estimated by Doppler echocardiogram. Perimembranous and muscular VSDs may become smaller or close with time, particularly if the initial diameter of the VSD is less than 5 mm.

In patients with isolated moderate to large VSDs, congestive heart failure develops over time once an imbalance exists between systemic and pulmonary vascular resistance and a significant left-to-right shunt develops. Neonates with large VSDs will typically develop pulmonary overcirculation, left ventricular volume overload, and symptoms of congestive heart failure within the first several weeks to months of life as pulmonary vascular resistance falls. Any associated left ventricular outflow tract obstruction (e.g., coarctation of the aorta) will exacerbate this problem. Premature infants with left-to-right shunting at the ventricular or great artery level may develop congestive heart failure sooner due to decreased musculature in the pulmonary arterioles, which may allow for a precipitous drop in pulmonary vascular resistance.

A trial of medical management is reasonable in infants with moderate to large VSDs. Provision of adequate nutrition and administration of medications including loop diuretics and sometimes digoxin and/or angiotensin-converting enzyme inhibitors (ACE inhibitors) may allow surgery to be deferred for a few months in some patients. Supplemental oxygen and hyperventilation should generally be avoided, as they may cause pulmonary vascular resistance to fall and Qp/Qs to rise. Infants who continue to have failure to thrive or symptoms of CHF despite these measures are referred for surgical intervention.

The surgical approach to a VSD depends on its location. Perimembranous and inlet VSDs are approached through the right atrium, conal VSDs are approached through the pulmonary artery, and muscular VSDs may be approached through the atrium, although apical muscular defects often require a small ventriculotomy. Selected infants with large VSDs who are not thought to be candidates for primary repair because of patient size, the presence of multiple VSDs with anticipated difficult surgical exposure, or noncardiac comorbidities may be palliated with a pulmonary artery band.

The postoperative course following repair of large, isolated VSDs may be complicated by pulmonary hypertension, although this is quite uncommon in the current era of repair in early infancy. The incidence of a significant residual VSD, which also will cause pulmonary hypertension, is minimized with the routine use of transesophageal echocardiography. Data that would suggest a significant residual VSD include elevated left atrial and pulmonary artery pressures, a step-up of greater than 10% in oxygen saturation from the superior vena cava or right atrium to the pulmonary artery, the presence of low cardiac output syndrome, persistent cardiomegaly and increased pulmonary vascular markings on chest radiograph, and difficulty weaning from the ventilator. JET or surgical heart block may occur following repair of a VSD. Right bundle branch block occasionally occurs but does not appear to be of long-term significance.

Atrioventricular Septal Defect

The presence or absence of a common atrioventricular valve and the relative size of the inlet VSD characterizes the different types of atrioventricular septal defects, also known as endocardial cushion defects. In patients with an incomplete atrioventricular septal defect, an ostium primum ASD exists along with a cleft in the mitral valve. There is no VSD present. A transitional atrioventricular septal defect has an ostium primum ASD, dense attachments of the atrioventricular valve leaflets to the crest of the ventricular septum such that two functionally separate atrioventricular valves exist, and a small inlet VSD. A complete atrioventricular septal defect has a primum ASD, a common atrioventricular valve, and a large inlet VSD. Associated anomalies include a left superior vena cava to the coronary sinus, additional VSDs, and aortic arch obstruction. Uncommonly, right ventricular outflow tract obstruction is seen and such patients have features of tetralogy of Fallot and an atrioventricular canal. In most cases, the ventricles are balanced, such that both are of adequate size to support the full cardiac output following surgery. Occasionally, one of the ventricles is hypoplastic ("unbalanced"), precluding a two-ventricular repair. Such patients may be considered for a one and a half ventricular repair, the single ventricle pathway, or heart transplantation. There is an increased incidence of Down syndrome (trisomy 21) in patients with endocardial cushion defects, and such patients are predisposed to the early development of pulmonary vascular obstructive disease.

Patients with complete atrioventricular septal defects typically develop congestive heart failure within the first few weeks to months of life. The congestive heart failure will be exacerbated if significant atrioventricular valve regurgitation or aortic arch hypoplasia is present. A trial of medical management is indicated in symptomatic infants, as discussed above for patients with large VSDs. Surgical repair is generally indicated within the first 3 to

6 months of life to eliminate the symptoms of congestive heart failure, prevent the development of pulmonary vascular obstructive disease, and minimize the incidence of postoperative pulmonary hypertensive crises. Surgical repair is generally not performed in the newborn period, due in part to the difficulty with suturing the paper-thin atrioventricular valve leaflets. Infants with incomplete or transitional atrioventricular canal defects often follow the clinical course of patients with isolated ASDs, and these lesions are typically repaired sometime between 6 months and 4 years of age.

Complete atrioventricular septal defect repair may be accomplished using a one patch, two patch, or modified single-patch technique, dependent on patient anatomy and surgical preference (150). The common atrioventricular valve is divided to create separate right-sided and left-sided atrioventricular valves. Neonates with an atrioventricular septal defect and aortic arch obstruction represent a particularly challenging group of patients. A staged approach involving an initial repair of the aortic arch obstruction followed by delayed repair of the atrioventricular septal defect has been has been associated with more favorable outcomes when compared to a complete neonatal repair (151).

All of the postoperative concerns following VSD closure as discussed above also apply to the infant following atrioventricular canal repair. These include pulmonary hypertension, residual VSDs, and arrhythmias (specifically, JET and complete heart block). In addition, left-sided atrioventricular valve regurgitation may occur, causing ventricular volume overload, congestive heart failure, and pulmonary hypertension. Left-sided atrioventricular valve regurgitation may be suspected by auscultation and the identification of large ventricular waves on the left atrial line pressure tracing (if present) and further quantified by echocardiography. Inotropic support and afterload reduction may be beneficial in the early postoperative period when significant left-sided atrioventricular valve regurgitation is identified, and volume overload should be avoided. Mitral stenosis is less common but will cause elevated left atrial pressures and large atrial waves on the left atrial pressure tracing.

Incomplete and transitional atrioventricular canal defects typically are repaired with a patch closure of the ASD and, commonly, suture closure of the cleft in the mitral valve. The postoperative course is similar to that seen following ASD closure as described above.

Patent Ductus Arteriosus

The ductus arteriosus normally is functionally closed within the first hours to days of life. PDA may exist in isolation or with many other types of CHD. An isolated, large PDA will cause symptoms of congestive heart failure once the pulmonary vascular resistance falls, allowing a left-to-right shunt from the aorta to the pulmonary artery. Left atrial and left ventricular volume overload are present and pulmonary edema may develop. Diastolic runoff exists leading to a "steal" from systemic blood flow, which may contribute to mesenteric ischemia and thus predispose patients to NEC. PDAs are more common and cause more symptoms in premature infants. Small PDAs typically do not cause symptoms but are a long-term risk for bacterial endocarditis. Symptoms of congestive heart failure may be treated with diuretics, digoxin, and the provision of adequate nutrition. Approximately two-thirds of PDAs in premature infants will close following a course of indomethacin or ibuprofen (152). Surgical ligation may be considered for PDAs that do not respond to medical therapy in premature infants and symptomatic PDAs in any infant. Transcatheter closure of PDAs is now feasible in selected premature neonates (153). Older children with a continuous murmur but no symptoms may be referred for surgical or transcatheter PDA closure to minimize the risk of endocarditis. Most nonneonatal patients undergoing PDA closure may be extubated immediately after the procedure. Premature neonates

often develop a transient low cardiac output state following PDA ligation. Specific complications that are uncommonly encountered following surgical PDA closure are related to the injury of nearby structures, including the recurrent laryngeal and phrenic nerves. Following transcatheter closure, hemolysis or aortic or pulmonary artery obstruction may occur.

Aortopulmonary Window

An aortopulmonary window is an uncommon, typically large communication between the ascending aorta and pulmonary artery in the presence of two semilunar valves. This lesion usually exists in isolation, but may be associated with IAA, VSD, or other congenital heart defects.

Infants with large aortopulmonary windows will usually develop congestive heart failure at several weeks of life. Prompt surgical repair is indicated in most cases to eliminate the symptoms of congestive heart failure, prevent the development of pulmonary vascular obstructive disease, and minimize the incidence of postoperative pulmonary hypertension.

Although several surgical techniques may be used to repair an aortopulmonary window, currently the transaortic patch repair is favored by many surgeons (154). Any associated cardiac lesions are repaired during the same operation. Postoperative problems that may be encountered include pulmonary hypertension and residual left-to-right shunting. A related and somewhat rare lesion in which one pulmonary artery arises from the ascending aorta and the other from the right ventricle deserves special consideration. Preoperatively, the pulmonary artery that arises from the ascending aorta is exposed to systemic pressures, and the other pulmonary artery receives the entire cardiac output from the right ventricle. This unique combination of high pressure to one pulmonary vascular bed and high flow to the other predisposes these infants to having significant problems with pulmonary hypertension in the immediate postoperative period.

REFERENCES

1. Wiegerinck RF, Cojoc A, Zeidenweber CM, et al. Force frequency relationship of the human ventricle increases during early postnatal development. *Pediatr Res* 2009;65:414.
2. Newburger JW, Jonas RA, Wernovsky G, et al. A comparison of the perioperative neurologic effects of hypothermic circulatory arrest versus low-flow cardiopulmonary bypass in infant heart surgery. *N Engl J Med* 1993;329:1057.
3. Goldberg CS, Bove EL, Devaney EJ, et al. A randomized clinical trial of regional cerebral perfusion versus deep hypothermic circulatory arrest: outcomes for infants with functional single ventricle. *J Thorac Cardiovasc Surg* 2007;133:880.
4. Bronicki RA, Backer CL, Baden HP, et al. Dexamethasone reduces the inflammatory response to cardiopulmonary bypass in children. *Ann Thorac Surg* 2000;69:1490.
5. Pasquali SK, Li JS, He X, et al. Perioperative methylprednisolone and outcome in neonates undergoing heart surgery. *Pediatrics* 2012;129:e385.
6. Graham EM, Martin RH, Buckley JR, et al. Corticosteroid therapy in neonates undergoing cardiopulmonary bypass: randomized controlled trial. *J Am Coll Cardiol* 2019;74:659.
7. Costello JM, Clapper TC, Wypij D. Minimizing complications associated with percutaneous central venous catheter placement in children: recent advances. *Pediatr Crit Care Med* 2013;14:273.
8. Flori HR, Johnson LD, Hanley FL, et al. Transthoracic intracardiac catheters in pediatric patients recovering from congenital heart defect surgery: associated complications and outcomes. *Crit Care Med* 2000;28:2997.
9. Tibby SM, Hatherill M, Murdoch IA. Capillary refill and core-peripheral temperature gap as indicators of haemodynamic status in paediatric intensive care patients. *Arch Dis Child* 1999;80:163.
10. Bertrandt RA, Saudek DM, Scott JP, et al. Chest tube removal algorithm is associated with decreased chest tube duration in pediatric cardiac surgical patients. *J Thorac Cardiovasc Surg* 2019;158(4):1209.
11. Tabbutt S, Duncan BW, McLaughlin D, et al. Delayed sternal closure after cardiac operations in a pediatric population. *J Thorac Cardiovasc Surg* 1997;113:886.

12. Bronicki RA, Anas NG. Cardiopulmonary interaction. *Pediatr Crit Care Med* 2009;10:313.

13. Chang AC, Zucker HA, Hickey PR, et al. Pulmonary vascular resistance in infants after cardiac surgery: role of carbon dioxide and hydrogen ion. *Crit Care Med* 1995;23:568.

14. Charpie JR, Dekeon MK, Goldberg CS, et al. Serial blood lactate measurements predict early outcome after neonatal repair or palliation for complex congenital heart disease. *J Thorac Cardiovasc Surg* 2000;120:73.

15. Hirsch JC, Charpie JR, Ohye RG, et al. Near infrared spectroscopy (NIRS) should not be standard of care for postoperative management. *Semin Thorac Cardiovasc Surg Pediatr Card Surg Annu* 2010;13:51.

16. Tweddell JS, Ghanayem NS, Hoffman GM. Pro: NIRS is "standard of care" for postoperative management. *Semin Thorac Cardiovasc Surg Pediatr Card Surg Annu* 2010;13:44.

17. Hickey PR, Hansen DD, Wessel DL, et al. Blunting of stress responses in the pulmonary circulation of infants by fentanyl. *Anesth Analg* 1985;64:1137.

18. Wernovsky G, Wypij D, Jonas RA, et al. Postoperative course and hemodynamic profile after the arterial switch operation in neonates and infants. A comparison of low-flow cardiopulmonary bypass and circulatory arrest. *Circulation* 1995;92:2226.

19. Costello JM, Monge MC, Hill KD, et al. Associations between unplanned cardiac reinterventions and outcomes after pediatric cardiac operations. *Ann Thorac Surg* 2018;105:1255.

20. Hoffman TM, Wernovsky G, Atz AM, et al. Efficacy and safety of milrinone in preventing low cardiac output syndrome in infants and children after corrective surgery for congenital heart disease. *Circulation* 2003;107:996.

21. Pinsky MR, Summer WR, Wise RA, et al. Augmentation of cardiac function by elevation of intrathoracic pressure. *J Appl Physiol* 1983;54:950.

22. Chang AC, Atz AM, Wernovsky G, et al. Milrinone: systemic and pulmonary hemodynamic effects in neonates after cardiac surgery. *Crit Care Med* 1995;23:1907.

23. Rosenzweig EB, Starc TJ, Chen JM, et al. Intravenous arginine-vasopressin in children with vasodilatory shock after cardiac surgery. *Circulation* 1999;100:II182.

24. Wald EL, Backer CL, Dearani JA, et al. Total and free cortisol responses and their relation to outcomes after cardiopulmonary bypass in infants. *J Thorac Cardiovasc Surg* 2017;153:1155.

25. Shore S, Nelson DP, Pearl JM, et al. Usefulness of corticosteroid therapy in decreasing epinephrine requirements in critically ill infants with congenital heart disease. *Am J Cardiol* 2001;88:591.

26. Mainwaring RD, Healy RM, Meier FA, et al. Reduction in levels of triiodothyronine following the first stage of the Norwood reconstruction for hypoplastic left heart syndrome. *Cardiol Young* 2001;11:295.

27. Mackie AS, Booth KL, Newburger JW, et al. A randomized, double-blind, placebo-controlled pilot trial of triiodothyronine in neonatal heart surgery. *J Thorac Cardiovasc Surg* 2005;130:810.

28. Portman MA, Slee A, Olson AK, et al. Triiodothyronine supplementation in infants and children undergoing cardiopulmonary bypass (TRICC): a multicenter placebo-controlled randomized trial: age analysis. *Circulation* 2010;122:S224.

29. Pfammatter JP, Wagner B, Berdat P, et al. Procedural factors associated with early postoperative arrhythmias after repair of congenital heart defects. *J Thorac Cardiovasc Surg* 2002;123:258.

30. Hoffman TM, Bush DM, Wernovsky G, et al. Postoperative junctional ectopic tachycardia in children: incidence, risk factors, and treatment. *Ann Thorac Surg* 2002;74:1607.

31. Walsh EP, Saul JP, Sholler GF, et al. Evaluation of a staged treatment protocol for rapid automatic junctional tachycardia after operation for congenital heart disease. *J Am Coll Cardiol* 1997;29:1046.

32. Epstein AE, DiMarco JP, Ellenbogen KA, et al. ACC/AHA/HRS 2008 guidelines for device-based therapy of cardiac rhythm abnormalities: a report of the American College of Cardiology/American Heart Association Task Force on Practice Guidelines (Writing Committee to revise the ACC/AHA/NASPE 2002 guideline update for implantation of cardiac pacemakers and antiarrhythmia devices) developed in collaboration with the American Association for Thoracic Surgery and Society of Thoracic Surgeons. *J Am Coll Cardiol* 2008;51:e1.

33. Lindberg L, Olsson AK, Jogi P, et al. How common is severe pulmonary hypertension after pediatric cardiac surgery? *J Thorac Cardiovasc Surg* 2002;123:1155.

34. Wessel DL. Hemodynamic responses to perioperative pain and stress in infants. *Crit Care Med* 1993;21:S361.

35. Schulze-Neick I, Li J, Penny DJ, et al. Pulmonary vascular resistance after cardiopulmonary bypass in infants: effect on postoperative recovery. *J Thorac Cardiovasc Surg* 2001;121:1033.

36. Wessel DL. Managing low cardiac output syndrome after congenital heart surgery. *Crit Care Med* 2001;29:S220.

37. Bando K, Turrentine MW, Sharp TG, et al. Pulmonary hypertension after operations for congenital heart disease: analysis of risk factors and management. *J Thorac Cardiovasc Surg* 1996;112:1600.

38. Wessel DL, Adatia I, Giglia TM, et al. Use of inhaled nitric oxide and acetylcholine in the evaluation of pulmonary hypertension and endothelial function after cardiopulmonary bypass. *Circulation* 1993;88:2128.

39. Atz AM, Adatia I, Jonas RA, et al. Inhaled nitric oxide in children with pulmonary hypertension and congenital mitral stenosis. *Am J Cardiol* 1996;77:316.

40. Schulze-Neick I, Bultmann M, Werner H, et al. Right ventricular function in patients treated with inhaled nitric oxide after cardiac surgery for congenital heart disease in newborns and children. *Am J Cardiol* 1997;80:360.

41. Atz AM, Wessel DL. Sildenafil ameliorates effects of inhaled nitric oxide withdrawal. *Anesthesiology* 1999;91:307.

42. Namachivayam P, Theilen U, Butt WW, et al. Sildenafil prevents rebound pulmonary hypertension after withdrawal of nitric oxide in children. *Am J Respir Crit Care Med* 2006;174:1042.

43. Alten JA, Klugman D, Raymond TT, et al. Epidemiology and outcomes of cardiac arrest in pediatric cardiac ICUs. *Pediatr Crit Care Med* 2017;18:935.

44. de Caen AR, Maconochie IK, Aickin R, et al. Part 6: pediatric basic life support and pediatric advanced life support: 2015 international consensus on cardiopulmonary resuscitation and emergency cardiovascular care science with treatment recommendations. *Circulation* 2015;132:S177.

45. Marino BS, Tabbutt S, MacLaren G, et al. Cardiopulmonary resuscitation in infants and children with cardiac disease: a scientific statement from the American Heart Association. *Circulation* 2018;137:e691.

46. Jayaram N, Spertus JA, Nadkarni V, et al. Hospital variation in survival after pediatric in-hospital cardiac arrest. *Circ Cardiovasc Qual Outcomes* 2014;7:517.

47. Mascio CE, Austin EH III, Jacobs JP, et al. Perioperative mechanical circulatory support in children: an analysis of the Society of Thoracic Surgeons Congenital Heart Surgery Database. *J Thorac Cardiovasc Surg* 2014;147:658; discussion 664-5.

48. McMullan DM, Thiagarajan RR, Smith KM, et al. Extracorporeal cardiopulmonary resuscitation outcomes in term and premature neonates. *Pediatr Crit Care Med* 2014;15:e9.

49. Kulik TJ, Moler FW, Palmisano JM, et al. Outcome-associated factors in pediatric patients treated with extracorporeal membrane oxygenator after cardiac surgery. *Circulation* 1996;94:II63.

50. Eastaugh LJ, Thiagarajan RR, Darst JR, et al. Percutaneous left atrial decompression in patients supported with extracorporeal membrane oxygenation for cardiac disease. *Pediatr Crit Care Med* 2015;16:59.

51. Jaggers JJ, Forbess JM, Shah AS, et al. Extracorporeal membrane oxygenation for infant postcardiotomy support: significance of shunt management. *Ann Thorac Surg* 2000;69:1476.

52. Booth KL, Roth SJ, Perry SB, et al. Cardiac catheterization of patients supported by extracorporeal membrane oxygenation. *J Am Coll Cardiol* 2002;40:1681.

53. Kleinman ME, de Caen AR, Chameides L, et al. Part 10: pediatric basic and advanced life support: 2010 International Consensus on Cardiopulmonary Resuscitation and Emergency Cardiovascular Care Science With Treatment Recommendations. *Circulation* 2010;122:S466.

54. Barbaro RP, Paden ML, Guner YS, et al. Pediatric extracorporeal life support organization registry international report 2016. *ASAIO J* 2017;63:456.

55. Costello JM, Cooper DS, Jacobs JP, et al. Intermediate-term outcomes after paediatric cardiac extracorporeal membrane oxygenation—what is known (and unknown). *Cardiol Young* 2011;21(suppl 2):118.

56. Costello JM, O'Brien M, Wypij D, et al. Quality of life of pediatric cardiac patients who previously required extracorporeal membrane oxygenation. *Pediatr Crit Care Med* 2012;13:428.

57. Almond CS, Morales DL, Blackstone EH, et al. Berlin heart EXCOR pediatric ventricular assist device for bridge to heart transplantation in US children. *Circulation* 2013;127:1702.

58. Morales DLS, Zafar F, Almond CS, et al. Berlin heart EXCOR use in patients with congenital heart disease. *J Heart Lung Transplant* 2017;36:1209.

59. Schulze-Neick I, Ho SY, Bush A, et al. Severe airflow limitation after the unifocalization procedure: clinical and morphological correlates. *Circulation* 2000;102:III142.

60. Buckley JR, Graham EM, Gaies M, et al. Clinical epidemiology and centre variation in chylothorax rates after cardiac surgery in children: a report from the Pediatric Cardiac Critical Care Consortium. *Cardiol Young* 2017;27:1678.

61. Savla JJ, Itkin M, Rossano JW, et al. Post-operative chylothorax in patients with congenital heart disease. *J Am Coll Cardiol* 2017;69:2410.

62. Golbus JR, Wojcik BM, Charpie JR, et al. Feeding complications in hypoplastic left heart syndrome after the Norwood procedure: a systematic review of the literature. *Pediatr Cardiol* 2011;32:539.

63. Slicker J, Hehir DA, Horsley M, et al. Nutrition algorithms for infants with hypoplastic left heart syndrome; birth through the first interstage period. *Congenit Heart Dis* 2013;8:89.

64. McElhinney DB, Hedrick HL, Bush DM, et al. Necrotizing enterocolitis in neonates with congenital heart disease: risk factors and outcomes. *Pediatrics* 2000;106:1080.

65. Choi M, Borenstein SH, Hornberger L, et al. Heterotaxia syndrome: the role of screening for intestinal rotation abnormalities. *Arch Dis Child* 2005;90:813.

66. Yu DC, Thiagarajan RR, Laussen PC, et al. Outcomes after the Ladd procedure in patients with heterotaxy syndrome, congenital heart disease, and intestinal malrotation. *J Pediatr Surg* 2009;44:1089.

67. Allen ML, Peters MJ, Goldman A, et al. Early postoperative monocyte deactivation predicts systemic inflammation and prolonged stay in pediatric cardiac intensive care. *Crit Care Med* 2002;30:1140.

68. Costello JM, Graham DA, Morrow D, et al. Risk factors for central line-associated bloodstream infection in a pediatric cardiac intensive care unit. *Pediatr Crit Care Med* 2009;10:453.

69. Costello JM, Morrow DF, Graham DA, et al. Systematic intervention to reduce central line-associated bloodstream infection rates in a pediatric cardiac intensive care unit. *Pediatrics* 2008;121:915.

70. O'Grady NP, Alexander M, Burns LA, et al. Guidelines for the prevention of intravascular catheter-related infections. *Am J Infect Control* 2011;39:S1.

71. Costello JM, Graham DA, Morrow DF, et al. Risk factors for surgical site infection after cardiac surgery in children. *Ann Thorac Surg* 2010;89:1833.

72. Ban KA, Minei JP, Laronga C, et al. American College of Surgeons and Surgical Infection Society: surgical site infection guidelines, 2016 update. *J Am Coll Surg* 2017;224:59.

73. Araujo da Silva AR, Zingg W, Dramowski A, et al. Most international guidelines on prevention of healthcare-associated infection lack comprehensive recommendations for neonates and children. *J Hosp Infect* 2016;94:159.

74. Blinder JJ, Asaro LA, Wypij D, et al. Acute kidney injury after pediatric cardiac surgery: a secondary analysis of the Safe Pediatric Euglycemia After Cardiac Surgery Trial. *Pediatr Crit Care Med* 2017;18:638.

75. Madenci AL, Thiagarajan RR, Stoffan AP, et al. Characterizing peritoneal dialysis catheter use in pediatric patients after cardiac surgery. *J Thorac Cardiovasc Surg* 2013;146:334.

76. Limperopoulos C, Tworetzky W, McElhinney DB, et al. Brain volume and metabolism in fetuses with congenital heart disease: evaluation with quantitative magnetic resonance imaging and spectroscopy. *Circulation* 2010;121:26.

77. Beca J, Gunn JK, Coleman L, et al. New white matter brain injury after infant heart surgery is associated with diagnostic group and the use of circulatory arrest. *Circulation* 2013;127:971.

78. Lim JM, Porayette P, Marini D, et al. Associations between age at arterial switch operation, brain growth, and development in infants with transposition of the great arteries. *Circulation* 2019;139:2728.

79. Wypij D, Newburger JW, Rappaport LA, et al. The effect of duration of deep hypothermic circulatory arrest in infant heart surgery on late neurodevelopment: the Boston Circulatory Arrest Trial. *J Thorac Cardiovasc Surg* 2003;126:1397.

80. Bellinger DC, Wypij D, Rivkin MJ, et al. Adolescents with d-transposition of the great arteries corrected with the arterial switch procedure: neuropsychological assessment and structural brain imaging. *Circulation* 2011;124:1361.

81. Jonas RA, Wypij D, Roth SJ, et al. The influence of hemodilution on outcome after hypothermic cardiopulmonary bypass: results of a randomized trial in infants. *J Thorac Cardiovasc Surg* 2003;126:1765.

82. Menache CC, du Plessis AJ, Wessel DL, et al. Current incidence of acute neurologic complications after open-heart operations in children. *Ann Thorac Surg* 2002;73:1752.

83. Newburger JW, Wypij D, Bellinger DC, et al. Length of stay after infant heart surgery is related to cognitive outcome at age 8 years. *J Pediatr* 2003;143:67.

84. Barozzi L, Brizard CP, Galati JC, et al. Side-to-side aorto-GoreTex central shunt warrants central shunt patency and pulmonary arteries growth. *Ann Thorac Surg* 2011;92:1476.

85. Li JS, Yow E, Berezny KY, et al. Clinical outcomes of palliative surgery including a systemic-to-pulmonary artery shunt in infants with cyanotic congenital heart disease: does aspirin make a difference? *Circulation* 2007;116:293.

86. Petrucci O, O'Brien SM, Jacobs ML, et al. Risk factors for mortality and morbidity after the neonatal Blalock-Taussig shunt procedure. *Ann Thorac Surg* 2011;92:642.

87. Glatz AC, Petit CJ, Goldstein BH, et al. Comparison between patent ductus arteriosus stent and modified Blalock-Taussig shunt as palliation for infants with ductal-dependent pulmonary blood flow: insights from the Congenital Catheterization Research Collaborative. *Circulation* 2018;137:589.

88. Thapar MK, Rao PS. Significance of infundibular obstruction following balloon valvuloplasty for valvar pulmonic stenosis. *Am Heart J* 1989;118:99.

89. Al Habib HF, Jacobs JP, Mavroudis C, et al. Contemporary patterns of management of tetralogy of Fallot: data from the Society of Thoracic Surgeons Database. *Ann Thorac Surg* 2010;90:813.

90. Savla JJ, Faerber JA, Huang YV, et al. 2-year outcomes after complete or staged procedure for tetralogy of Fallot in neonates. *J Am Coll Cardiol* 2019;74:1570.

91. Sandoval JP, Chaturvedi RR, Benson L, et al. Right ventricular outflow tract stenting in tetralogy of Fallot infants with risk factors for early primary repair. *Circ Cardiovasc Interv* 2016;9:e003979.

92. Quandt D, Ramchandani B, Stickley J, et al. Stenting of the right ventricular outflow tract promotes better pulmonary arterial growth compared with modified Blalock-Taussig shunt palliation in tetralogy of Fallot-type lesions. *JACC Cardiovasc Interv* 2017;10:1774.

93. Cullen S, Shore D, Redington A. Characterization of right ventricular diastolic performance after complete repair of tetralogy of Fallot. Restrictive physiology predicts slow postoperative recovery. *Circulation* 1995;91:1782.

94. Bradley SM, Erdem CC, Hsia TY, et al. Right ventricle-to-pulmonary artery shunt: alternative palliation in infants with inadequate pulmonary blood flow prior to two-ventricle repair. *Ann Thorac Surg* 2008;86:183; discussion 188.

95. Ma M, Mainwaring RD, Hanley FL. Comprehensive management of major aortopulmonary collaterals in the repair of tetralogy of fallot. *Semin Thorac Cardiovasc Surg Pediatr Card Surg Annu* 2018;21:75.

96. Satou GM, Perry SB, Gauvreau K, et al. Echocardiographic predictors of coronary artery pathology in pulmonary atresia with intact ventricular septum. *Am J Cardiol* 2000;85:1319.

97. Giglia TM, Mandell VS, Connor AR, et al. Diagnosis and management of right ventricle-dependent coronary circulation in pulmonary atresia with intact ventricular septum. *Circulation* 1992;86:1516.

98. Giglia TM, Jenkins KJ, Matitiau A, et al. Influence of right heart size on outcome in pulmonary atresia with intact ventricular septum. *Circulation* 1993;88:2248.

99. Kwiatkowski DM, Hanley FL, Krawczeski CD. Right ventricular outflow tract obstruction: pulmonary atresia with intact ventricular septum, pulmonary stenosis, and Ebstein's malformation. *Pediatr Crit Care Med* 2016;17:S323.

100. Hasan BS, Bautista-Hernandez V, McElhinney DB, et al. Outcomes of transcatheter approach for initial treatment of pulmonary atresia with intact ventricular septum. *Catheter Cardiovasc Interv* 2013;81:111.

101. Powell AJ, Mayer JE, Lang P, et al. Outcome in infants with pulmonary atresia, intact ventricular septum, and right ventricle-dependent coronary circulation. *Am J Cardiol* 2000;86:1272.

102. McMullan DM, Permut LC, Jones TK, et al. Modified Blalock-Taussig shunt versus ductal stenting for palliation of cardiac lesions with inadequate pulmonary blood flow. *J Thorac Cardiovasc Surg* 2014;147:397.

103. Mallula K, Vaughn G, El-Said H, et al. Comparison of ductal stenting versus surgical shunts for palliation of patients with pulmonary atresia and intact ventricular septum. *Catheter Cardiovasc Interv* 2015;85:1196.

104. Rychik J, Levy H, Gaynor JW, et al. Outcome after operations for pulmonary atresia with intact ventricular septum. *J Thorac Cardiovasc Surg* 1998;116:924.

105. Jahangiri M, Zurakowski D, Bichell D, et al. Improved results with selective management in pulmonary atresia with intact ventricular septum. *J Thorac Cardiovasc Surg* 1999;118:1046.

106. Hirata Y, Chen JM, Quaegebeur JM, et al. Pulmonary atresia with intact ventricular septum: limitations of catheter-based intervention. *Ann Thorac Surg* 2007;84:574.

107. Celermajer DS, Bull C, Till JA, et al. Ebstein's anomaly: presentation and outcome from fetus to adult. *J Am Coll Cardiol* 1994;23:170.

108. McElhinney DB, Salvin JW, Colan SD, et al. Improving outcomes in fetuses and neonates with congenital displacement (Ebstein's malformation) or dysplasia of the tricuspid valve. *Am J Cardiol* 2005;96:582.

109. Yetman AT, Freedom RM, McCrindle BW. Outcome in cyanotic neonates with Ebstein's anomaly. *Am J Cardiol* 1998;81:749.

110. Wald RM, Adatia I, Van Arsdell GS, Hornberger LK. Relation of limiting ductal patency to survival in neonatal Ebstein's anomaly. *Am J Cardiol* 2005;96:851.

111. Atz AM, Munoz RA, Adatia I, et al. Diagnostic and therapeutic uses of inhaled nitric oxide in neonatal Ebstein's anomaly. *Am J Cardiol* 2003;91:906.

112. Starnes VA, Pitlick PT, Bernstein D, et al. Ebstein's anomaly appearing in the neonate. A new surgical approach. *J Thorac Cardiovasc Surg* 1991;101:1082.

113. Knott-Craig CJ, Overholt ED, Ward KE, et al. Repair of Ebstein's anomaly in the symptomatic neonate: an evolution of technique with 7-year follow-up. *Ann Thorac Surg* 2002;73:1786.

114. Shinkawa T, Polimenakos AC, Gomez-Fifer CA, et al. Management and long-term outcome of neonatal Ebstein anomaly. *J Thorac Cardiovasc Surg* 2010;139:354.

115. Luxford JC, Arora N, Ayer JG, et al. Neonatal Ebstein Anomaly: a 30-year institutional review. *Semin Thorac Cardiovasc Surg* 2017;29:206.

116. Rhodes LA, Colan SD, Perry SB, et al. Predictors of survival in neonates with critical aortic stenosis. *Circulation* 1991;84:2325.

117. Lofland GK, McCrindle BW, Williams WG, et al. Critical aortic stenosis in the neonate: a multi-institutional study of management, outcomes, and risk factors. Congenital Heart Surgeons Society. *J Thorac Cardiovasc Surg* 2001;121:10.

118. McCrindle BW, Blackstone EH, Williams WG, et al. Are outcomes of surgical versus transcatheter balloon valvotomy equivalent in neonatal critical aortic stenosis? *Circulation* 2001;104:I152.

119. Siddiqui J, Brizard CP, Galati JC, et al. Surgical valvotomy and repair for neonatal and infant congenital aortic stenosis achieves better results than interventional catheterization. *J Am Coll Cardiol* 2013;62:2134.

120. Hill GD, Ginde S, Rios R, et al. Surgical valvotomy versus balloon valvuloplasty for congenital aortic valve stenosis: a systematic review and meta-analysis. *J Am Heart Assoc* 2016;5(8):e003931.

121. McElhinney DB, Lock JE, Keane JF, et al. Left heart growth, function, and reintervention after balloon aortic valvuloplasty for neonatal aortic stenosis. *Circulation* 2005;111:451.

122. Kaushal S, Backer CL, Patel JN, et al. Coarctation of the aorta: midterm outcomes of resection with extended end-to-end anastomosis. *Ann Thorac Surg* 2009;88:1932.

123. Barnea O, Austin EH, Richman B, et al. Balancing the circulation: theoretic optimization of pulmonary/systemic flow ratio in hypoplastic left heart syndrome. *J Am Coll Cardiol* 1994;24:1376.

124. Barnea O, Santamore WP, Rossi A, et al. Estimation of oxygen delivery in newborns with a univentricular circulation. *Circulation* 1998;98:1407.

125. Tabbutt S, Ramamoorthy C, Montenegro LM, et al. Impact of inspired gas mixtures on preoperative infants with hypoplastic left heart syndrome during controlled ventilation. *Circulation* 2001;104:I159.

126. Rychik J, Rome JJ, Collins MH, et al. The hypoplastic left heart syndrome with intact atrial septum: atrial morphology, pulmonary vascular histopathology and outcome. *J Am Coll Cardiol* 1999;34:554.

127. Graziano JN, Heidelberger KP, Ensing GJ, et al. The influence of a restrictive atrial septal defect on pulmonary vascular morphology in patients with hypoplastic left heart syndrome. *Pediatr Cardiol* 2002;23:146.

128. Atz AM, Feinstein JA, Jonas RA, et al. Preoperative management of pulmonary venous hypertension in hypoplastic left heart syndrome with restrictive atrial septal defect. *Am J Cardiol* 1999;83:1224.

129. Vlahos AP, Lock JE, McElhinney DB, et al. Hypoplastic left heart syndrome with intact or highly restrictive atrial septum: outcome after neonatal transcatheter atrial septostomy. *Circulation* 2004;109:2326.

130. Hoque T, Richmond M, Vincent JA, et al. Current outcomes of hypoplastic left heart syndrome with restrictive atrial septum: a single-center experience. *Pediatr Cardiol* 2013;34:1181.

131. Sano S, Ishino K, Kawada M, et al. Right ventricle-pulmonary artery shunt in first-stage palliation of hypoplastic left heart syndrome. *J Thorac Cardiovasc Surg* 2003;126:504.

132. Maher K, Pizarro C, Gidding S, et al. Improved hemodynamic profile following the Norwood procedure with right ventricle to pulmonary artery conduit. *Circulation* 2002;106:II.

133. Ohye RG, Sleeper LA, Mahony L, et al. Comparison of shunt types in the Norwood procedure for single-ventricle lesions. *N Engl J Med* 2010;362:1980.

134. Galantowicz M, Cheatham JP, Phillips A, et al. Hybrid approach for hypoplastic left heart syndrome: intermediate results after the learning curve. *Ann Thorac Surg* 2008;85:2063; discussion 2070-1.

135. Taeed R, Schwartz SM, Pearl JM, et al. Unrecognized pulmonary venous desaturation early after Norwood palliation confounds Qp:Qs assessment and compromises oxygen delivery. *Circulation* 2001;103:2699.

136. Hoffman GM, Ghanayem NS, Kampine JM, et al. Venous saturation and the anaerobic threshold in neonates after the Norwood procedure for hypoplastic left heart syndrome. *Ann Thorac Surg* 2000;70:1515.

137. Tabbutt S, Ghanayem N, Ravishankar C, et al. Risk factors for hospital morbidity and mortality after the Norwood procedure: a report from the Pediatric Heart Network Single Ventricle Reconstruction trial. *J Thorac Cardiovasc Surg* 2012;144:882.

138. Backer CL, Mavroudis C. Congenital heart surgery nomenclature and database project: patent ductus arteriosus, coarctation of the aorta, interrupted aortic arch. *Ann Thorac Surg* 2000;69:S298.

139. Goldmuntz E, Clark BJ, Mitchell LE, et al. Frequency of 22q11 deletions in patients with conotruncal defects. *J Am Coll Cardiol* 1998;32:492.

140. Boutin C, Jonas RA, Sanders SP, et al. Rapid two-stage arterial switch operation. Acquisition of left ventricular mass after pulmonary artery banding in infants with transposition of the great arteries. *Circulation* 1994;90:1304.

141. Wernovsky G, Giglia TM, Jonas RA, et al. Course in the intensive care unit after 'preparatory' pulmonary artery banding and aortopulmonary shunt placement for transposition of the great arteries with low left ventricular pressure. *Circulation* 1992;86:II133.

142. Rastelli GC. A new approach to "anatomic" repair of transposition of the great arteries. *Mayo Clin Proc* 1969;44:1.

143. Nikaidoh H. Aortic translocation and biventricular outflow tract reconstruction. A new surgical repair for transposition of the great arteries associated with ventricular septal defect and pulmonary stenosis. *J Thorac Cardiovasc Surg* 1984;88:365.

144. Atz AM, Adatia I, Wessel DL. Rebound pulmonary hypertension after inhalation of nitric oxide. *Ann Thorac Surg* 1996;62:1759.

145. Yong MS, d'Udekem Y, Robertson T, et al. Outcomes of surgery for simple total anomalous pulmonary venous drainage in neonates. *Ann Thorac Surg* 2011;91:1921.

146. McElhinney DB, Driscoll DA, Emanuel BS, et al. Chromosome 22q11 deletion in patients with truncus arteriosus. *Pediatr Cardiol* 2003;24:569.

147. Jacobs ML. Congenital heart surgery nomenclature and database project: truncus arteriosus. *Ann Thorac Surg* 2000;69:S50.

148. Russell HM, Jacobs ML, Anderson RH, et al. A simplified categorization for common arterial trunk. *J Thorac Cardiovasc Surg* 2011;141:645.

149. Russell HM, Pasquali SK, Jacobs JP, et al. Outcomes of repair of common arterial trunk with truncal valve surgery: a review of the society of thoracic surgeons congenital heart surgery database. *Ann Thorac Surg* 2012;93:164.

150. Backer CL, Stewart RD, Bailliard F, et al. Complete atrioventricular canal: comparison of modified single-patch technique with two-patch technique. *Ann Thorac Surg* 2007;84:2038.

151. Shuhaiber J, Shin AY, Gossett JG, et al. Surgical management of neonatal atrioventricular septal defect with aortic arch obstruction. *Ann Thorac Surg* 2013;95:2071.

152. Van Overmeire B, Smets K, Lecoutere D, et al. A comparison of ibuprofen and indomethacin for closure of patent ductus arteriosus. *N Engl J Med* 2000;343:674.

153. Zahn EM, Peck D, Phillips A, et al. Transcatheter closure of patent ductus arteriosus in extremely premature newborns: early results and midterm follow-up. *JACC Cardiovasc Interv* 2016;9:2429.

154. Backer CL, Mavroudis C. Surgical management of aortopulmonary window: a 40-year experience. *Eur J Cardiothorac Surg* 2002;21:773.

Disorders of Heart Rhythm

Luciana Marcondes and Jonathan R. Skinner

Many cardiac arrhythmias can occur in neonates and infants, from benign to lethal. Management is guided by clinical status including comorbidities, cardiac function, and anatomy.

SINUS ARRHYTHMIA

In sinus arrhythmia, heart rate increases with inspiration and decreases with expiration. It is normal and relates to changes in vagal tone and cardiac filling pressures during respiration. It is more noticeable in children than in infants. The P wave morphology and axis do not change.

SINUS BRADYCARDIA

Sinus bradycardia is commonly associated with vagal stimulation (crying, straining or micturition, gastroesophageal reflux, or during endotracheal, nasogastric and orogastric intubation), but can be secondary to hypothyroidism, hypoxia, acidosis, hypoglycemia, raised intracranial pressure, and medications (e.g., beta-blockers). Intrinsic sinus node dysfunction is rare but may follow surgical repair of congenital heart disease (1).

SINUS TACHYCARDIA

The key features of sinus tachycardia are that the P wave morphology and axis are normal and do not change. Heart rate variability is usually more pronounced than in atrial tachycardias, so it is useful to assess telemetry recordings if the P waves are difficult to identify.

ATRIAL PREMATURE BEATS

Atrial premature beats (APBs, premature atrial complexes, or atrial ectopic beats) occur in up to 30% of newborns (2). The diagnosis is reliably assigned when there is an identifiable, early P wave with different morphology than the sinus P wave. It can be difficult to see the P wave if it is "buried" in the T wave, and a clue can be a T wave that looks different from that in sinus rhythm (Fig. 34.1A). If an APB arises very early, the AV node may be refractory and not conduct the beat (seen as a pause), or if one of the fascicles is refractory, it may be associated with a bundle branch block (Fig. 34.1B). When frequent, blocked APBs can result in bradycardia due to resetting of the sinus node with each premature atrial depolarization (Fig. 34.1C).

A central venous catheter tip can induce APBs by contacting an atrial wall; they will settle with catheter withdrawal. In infants, APBs might be secondary to electrolyte abnormalities, stimulant medications (e.g., dopamine, and caffeine), and after cardiac surgery. Very rarely APBs can be secondary to myocarditis or cardiac tumors.

In otherwise healthy infants, APBs generally do not warrant further evaluation, and spontaneous resolution occurs within weeks or months.

VENTRICULAR PREMATURE BEATS

Ventricular premature beats (VPBs, premature ventricular complexes, or ventricular ectopic beats) are seen on an ECG as early QRS complexes with a different morphology from the baseline sinus beats and without a preceding P wave (Fig. 34.2).

In neonates and infants, VPBs may not be much wider than normal QRS complexes. The morphology of the complexes can indicate the site of origin (e.g., right bundle branch morphology indicates origin in the left ventricle and vice versa).

VPBs are common in children and less common in infants (3). Isolated VPBs are usually benign but can be a worrying sign in an unwell infant, possibly indicating myocardial stress, hypoxia, or metabolic disturbance (4). Monomorphic beats are usually benign, but frequent polymorphic beats (with each having a different QRS morphology) may be a sign of incipient ventricular tachycardia (VT) or fibrillation. Stimulant medications such as adrenaline or caffeine can trigger VPBs, as can a central venous catheter inadvertently positioned in the ventricle.

Spontaneous resolution of benign monomorphic VPBs in neonates and infants is usually seen within a few months and treatment is rarely required. If they are very frequent, usually more than 10% beats over 24 hours, periodic echocardiographic monitoring is recommended to watch for ectopy-induced cardiomyopathy.

ACCELERATED IDIOVENTRICULAR RHYTHM

Accelerated idioventricular rhythm (AIVR) is not common, but might be underdiagnosed in neonates as it is usually asymptomatic. It is defined by a ventricular escape rhythm (wide QRS compared to baseline) at rates within 10% to 20% of the sinus rate (5). This likely represents enhanced automaticity, and there is some variation of the heart rate depending on autonomic tone. Ventriculo-atrial dissociation is usually seen (with the QRS complexes running faster than the P waves), but retrogradely conducted P waves are also a common finding (Fig. 34.3).

AIVR has a benign prognosis and will usually resolve spontaneously within weeks to months. Uncommonly, it can be associated with structural heart disease, electrolyte abnormalities, cardiac tumors, intracardiac catheters, maternal heroin and cocaine use, and respiratory distress (6).

TACHYARRHYTHMIAS

All neonates with tachyarrhythmias should have a 12-lead ECG (preferably during the tachycardia, and later in sinus rhythm), and echocardiography, to assess cardiac structure and function. Structural heart disease can be present in up to 25% of cases, most often Ebstein's anomaly of the tricuspid valve, corrected transposition of the great arteries (ccTGA or L-TGA), or hypertrophic cardiomyopathy (7). Cardiac tumors, myocarditis, and inherited channelopathies such as long QT syndrome (LQTS) rarely are predisposing causes for malignant ventricular arrhythmias.

SUPRAVENTRICULAR TACHYCARDIAS

Atrioventricular Reentrant Tachycardia

The most common type of fetal and neonatal supraventricular tachycardia (SVT) is atrioventricular reentrant (or reciprocating) tachycardia (AVRT). The tachycardia mechanism is a reentrant circuit via an accessory pathway that connects atrial and ventricular myocardium (8). The accessory pathway conducts only retrogradely (concealed accessory pathway), so the ECG in sinus rhythm is normal with no pre-excitation (no delta waves).

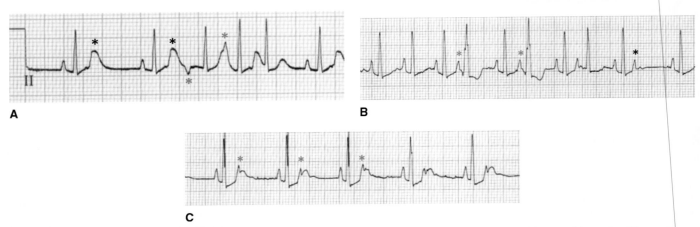

FIGURE 34.1 Atrial premature beats (APBs). A: The *green asterisk* indicates an APB, conducted with a longer PR interval (note the different P wave morphology). The *red asterisk* indicates an APB "buried" in the T wave. Note the different T wave morphology with the APB ("peaked") when compared to the usual, "rounded" T waves (*black asterisks*). **B:** APBs marked with *red asterisks* are followed by broader QRS complexes, indicating functional bundle branch block. The APB marked with a *black asterisk* does not conduct (blocked APB). Note the pause following a blocked APB due to resetting of the sinus node. **C:** Atrial bigeminy (every other beat is an APB; *red asterisks*). The APBs are not conducted, and with subsequent pause, there is resultant bradycardia.

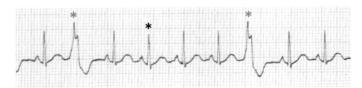

FIGURE 34.2 Ventricular premature beats (VPBs). *Red asterisks* indicate VPBs. Note the broad QRS complex with no preceding P waves, different than the baseline narrow QRS (*black asterisk*).

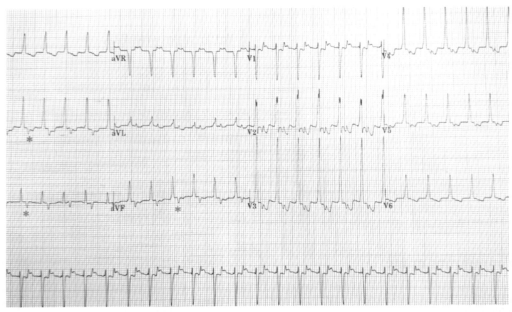

FIGURE 34.3 Accelerated idioventricular rhythm (AIVR) in a 3-week-old neonate. Note the "broad" QRS complexes. The heart rate is around 150 bpm, and P waves are marked with *red asterisks*. The P waves are negative in leads II, III, and AVF, indicating retrograde conduction from the ventricle to the atria (activation from low to high).

Orthodromic Atrioventricular Reentrant Tachycardia

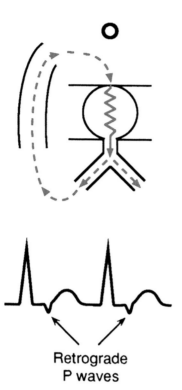

FIGURE 34.4 Schematic representation of the reentry circuit in atrioventricular reentrant tachycardia (AVRT). Antegrade conduction is over the AV node, and retrograde conduction is over the accessory pathway. (Modified from Lilly LS. *Pathophysiology of heart disease*, 6th ed. Philadelphia, PA: Wolters Kluwer, 2015.)

Antegrade conduction from the atria to the ventricles is over the AV node and His-Purkinje system, with retrograde conduction over the accessory pathway (Fig. 34.4). Since antegrade conduction is over the AV node and His-Purkinje system, there is usually a narrow QRS complex, except when there is rate-related functional bundle branch block (Fig. 34.5).

AVRT is characterized by abrupt onset and sudden termination, a relatively "fixed" heart rate, and retrograde P waves that are typically seen as a negative in leads II, III, and AVF. P waves are easier to identify if there is atrial dilatation (Fig. 34.6). In neonates and infants, heart rates are generally above 220 beats/min.

The clinical status of neonates and infants with AVRT depends on the ventricular rate, duration of tachycardia, underlying structural or functional heart disease, and additional comorbidities. In fortunate infants, the arrhythmia is noted incidentally during assessment for other reasons. Most common symptoms are irritability, poor feeding, restlessness, or respiratory difficulty. If the tachycardia is persistent, secondary dilated cardiomyopathy and heart failure may develop (tachycardia-induced cardiomyopathy). In fetal life, this can lead to hydrops and be life-threatening (9).

Wolff-Parkinson-White Syndrome

Some accessory pathways conduct impulses in both directions. During sinus rhythm, in addition to normal conduction over the AV node, there is antegrade conduction over the accessory pathway resulting in a short PR interval and wide QRS complex with characteristic delta wave, resulting from rapid depolarization of the ventricles via the accessory pathway (pre-excitation) (Fig. 34.7). The presence of pre-excitation and SVT defines Wolff-Parkinson-White (WPW) syndrome (10). Pre-excitation can be intermittent.

During SVT, antegrade conduction is typically over the AV node and His-Purkinje system (explaining the narrow complex in SVT), with retrograde conduction over the accessory pathway. This is known as orthodromic reentrant tachycardia. Rarely, antegrade conduction is over the accessory pathway and retrograde conduction is over the AV node, resulting in a wide QRS tachycardia (antidromic reentrant tachycardia), which may be difficult to distinguish from VT.

Some accessory pathways have the potential for very rapid antegrade conduction, and in the event of atrial fibrillation (AF), it can lead to ventricular fibrillation (11) (Fig. 34.8). Sudden death from pre-excited AF is a rare, but a well-recognized, event in WPW syndrome in children (12). It is extremely rare in neonates and infants.

WPW syndrome is usually sporadic but can be rarely inherited as an autosomal dominant trait associated with hypertrophic cardiomyopathy, sometimes with *PRKAG2* mutations (13).

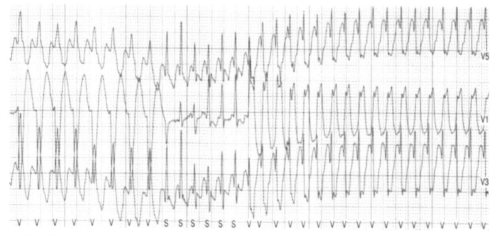

FIGURE 34.5 Holter recording showing AVRT with alternating left and right bundle branch blocks (there is left bundle branch block followed by narrow complex tachycardia and right bundle branch block). Note the heart rate in tachycardia during left bundle branch block is slower, indicating delayed retrograde conduction over a left-sided accessory pathway.

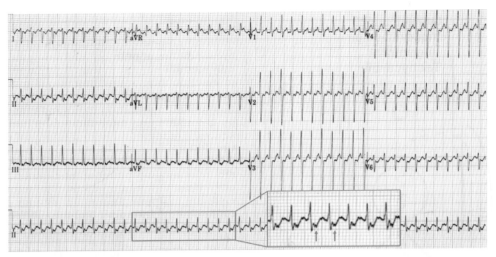

FIGURE 34.6 ECG from a 2-week-old neonate with a 1-week history of poor feeding and irritability. The ECG shows AVRT with narrow complex QRS and visible retrograde P waves (*red arrows*). Due to longstanding tachycardia, the atria were dilated, making visualization of the P waves easier.

Approximately 50% of infants with accessory pathway-mediated SVT, with or without WPW syndrome, appear to spontaneously lose accessory pathway conduction (and the potential for recurrent SVT) during the first year of life (14). Recurrence is possible in later childhood.

Permanent Junctional Reciprocating Tachycardia

This uncommon tachycardia tends to be slower than other SVT and be incessant, commonly resulting in tachycardia-induced cardiomyopathy.

The main ECG feature is a narrow complex tachycardia with deep, negative P waves in the inferior leads (II, III, and AVF), with a long RP interval (Fig. 34.9). The P wave axis reflects the retrograde activation pattern of the atria from low to high, through a slowly conducting accessory pathway typically in the right postero-septal area. Permanent junctional reciprocating tachycardia (PJRT) usually terminates transiently with vagal maneuvers, adenosine, atrial pacing, or electrical cardioversion, but commonly recurs.

Spontaneous resolution of PJRT is infrequent, and medical management aims for rate control if not complete rhythm control

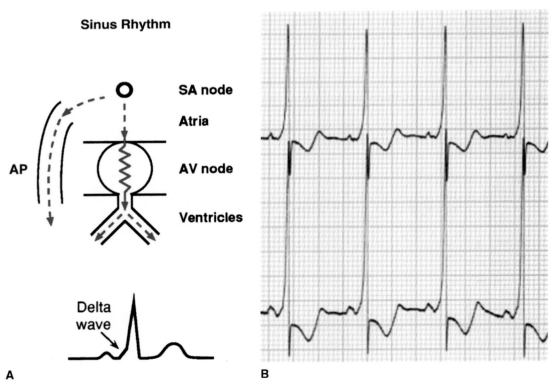

FIGURE 34.7 A: Schematic representation of pre-excitation (delta waves) due to concomitant antegrade conduction over the AV node and accessory pathway. **B:** ECG detail from infant with WPW syndrome. Note the short PR interval and initial "slurring" of the QRS complex, indicating slower myocardial activation over the accessory pathway (propagation of conduction over the accessory pathway to the ventricle is slower than via the specialized His-Purkinje conduction system). (**A:** Modified from Lilly LS. *Pathophysiology of heart disease*, 6th ed. Philadelphia, PA: Wolters Kluwer, 2015.)

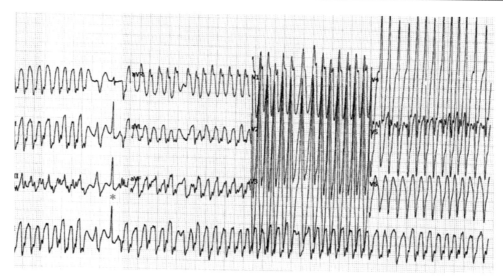

FIGURE 34.8 Pre-excited atrial fibrillation. Note the irregular broad complex tachycardia. There is some variation in the morphology of the QRS complexes, indicating different degrees of pre-excitation. A single narrow complex beat (*red asterisk*) represents one beat conducted over the AV node, called a capture beat.

of the tachycardia. Catheter ablation is the preferred treatment for older children but can be required in infancy (15).

Atrioventricular Nodal Reentrant Tachycardia

Atrioventricular nodal reentrant tachycardia (AVNRT) is the second most common SVT in children, however, it is uncommon in neonates and infants (8). The reentry circuit involves at least two "limbs" of the AV node, so-called fast and slow pathways. AVNRT is usually paroxysmal rather than incessant. Since the atrium and ventricle are depolarized at the same time from the AV node, P waves are not visible or are seen partly after the QRS (most noticeable in lead V1 as a "pseudo r wave") (16). It can be difficult to distinguish from AVRT, but management is similar.

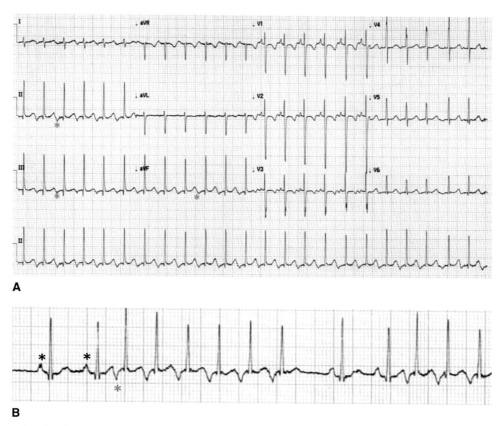

A

B

FIGURE 34.9 Permanent junctional reciprocating tachycardia (PJRT). A: the hallmark of PJRT is a narrow complex tachycardia with deep, negative P waves in leads II, III and AVF (*red asterisks*). Note the distance between the initial QRS to the following P wave is longer than the P wave to the subsequent QRS (long RP interval). **B:** Rhythm strip showing two sinus beats (*black asterisks*) followed by a "run" of PJRT with subsequent termination. Note the different morphologies of the retrograde P wave (*red asterisk*). Frequent recurrence or incessant tachycardia is characteristic of PJRT.

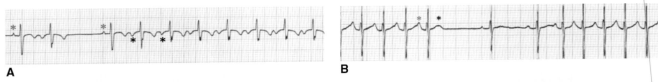

FIGURE 34.10 Ectopic atrial tachycardia (EAT). A: Run of EAT with sudden rather than gradual start. Note the clearly different P waves (*black asterisks*) compared to the baseline sinus P waves (*red asterisks*). **B:** EAT with P waves that are difficult to identify and are "buried" in the preceding T wave, distorting its shape ("peaked" P waves, *black asterisk*). Note the T wave morphology following tachycardia termination is "rounded" (*red asterisk*), with no P wave.

Ectopic Atrial Tachycardia

The most common mechanism of ectopic atrial tachycardia (EAT) is enhanced automaticity. Less common mechanisms include micro reentry or triggered activity (17). The tachycardia mechanism is independent of AV node conduction, therefore tachycardia can continue in the setting of AV block.

Since the atria are depolarized in an abnormal direction, the P-wave morphology is usually different from sinus rhythm, though distinct P waves can sometimes be difficult to identify. EAT can look like PJRT if the ectopic focus is from the right postero-septal area, and both EAT and PJRT can be incessant. Depending on the atrial rate and AV node conduction properties, there may be variable AV relationship (more atrial than ventricular complexes), which helps with the diagnosis. Heart rate is variable and there is usually gradual onset and termination ("warm up and cool down"); however, abrupt onset and termination can also be seen (Fig. 34.10). Transiently blocking AV conduction with vagal maneuvers does not terminate the tachycardia, but reveals rapid, nonconducted P waves. Adenosine is less predictable and may transiently terminate the tachycardia (18). EATs are generally not terminated by pacing or electrical cardioversion. It can be incessant and lead to tachycardia-induced cardiomyopathy (19). Spontaneous resolution is more likely in infants than older children (20).

Multifocal Atrial Tachycardia

Multifocal atrial tachycardia (MAT) or chaotic atrial tachycardia is uncommon in infants. It can occur in structurally normal hearts, as well as in association with pulmonary disease, structural heart disease (e.g., hypertrophic cardiomyopathy), RASopathies (Noonan and Costello syndromes), and catecholaminergic polymorphic tachycardia (CPVT) (21). It can be incessant and lead to ventricular dysfunction.

The ECG hallmark is the presence of an irregular tachycardia with at least three distinct P wave morphologies and variable PP, PR, and RR intervals (Fig. 34.11). Some QRS complexes might be broad due to functional bundle branch block. MAT cannot be terminated by pacing or electrical cardioversion.

Antiarrhythmic treatment might not be necessary if the infant is asymptomatic with normal ventricular function; and there is usually spontaneous resolution within a few months (22). If treatment is required, beta-blockers or amiodarone can be useful.

Junctional Ectopic Tachycardia

Junctional ectopic tachycardia (JET) is common after cardiac surgery but is otherwise a rare, often incessant, tachyarrhythmia due to abnormal enhanced automaticity around the AV node and His bundle. There is generally a narrow QRS morphology with variable ventricular rates. Typically, there is ventriculo-atrial dissociation with visible P waves slower and not "related" to each QRS (Fig. 34.12). Occasionally, there is retrograde atrial activation with 1:1 VA conduction.

Congenital JET is usually resistant to treatment, often requiring more than one antiarrhythmic medication, and due to tachycardia-induced cardiomyopathy, there is risk of significant morbidity and mortality (23). Recently, the addition of ivabradine as an adjunctive treatment has shown promising results (24).

Following cardiac surgery in infants, it can result in significant hemodynamic compromise. The presence of pacing wires can aid in the tachycardia diagnosis when P waves are not visible on the surface ECG (Fig. 34.12). Treatment strategies include reduction of exogenous catecholamines, fever control, hypothermia, synchronized pacing, and intravenous procainamide or amiodarone (25). This arrhythmia usually abates within a few days of surgery.

Atrial Flutter

Atrial flutter (AFL) is less common in neonates than AVRT but is also typically associated with a structurally normal heart. It can be incessant and lead to cardiomyopathy (26), and in the fetus, this may cause hydrops (27).

The arrhythmia substrate is macroreentry in the right atrium, typically involving the cavotricuspid isthmus (region between the inferior vena cava, tricuspid valve, and coronary sinus ostium) (Fig. 34.13). The atrial rate varies between 400 and 600 beats/min in neonates, and around 300 beats/min in older children. The AV node is not part of the tachycardia circuit, and there is often some degree of AV node block resulting in variable conduction, frequently with a 2:1 or 3:1 AV relationship (Fig. 34.14). The QRS complexes are usually narrow unless there is functional bundle branch block. The rare infant with 1:1 AV conduction will present with shock. With higher degrees of AV nodal block, a "saw tooth" pattern of continuous flutter waves is characteristically seen, often best in the inferior leads (II, III, and AVF). Esophageal recordings may demonstrate the atrial activity more clearly, or adenosine might be used to cause transient AV block and demonstrate the flutter waves (Fig. 34.14). Adenosine does not terminate the tachycardia.

Restoration of sinus rhythm can be attempted with esophageal overdrive pacing or synchronized electric cardioversion (0.5 to 1 J/kg initially). Recurrence is unusual. Antiarrhythmic medications may be required for refractory cases, and a second arrhythmia substrate is a more common finding in this situation (26).

Neonatal AFL has a good long-term prognosis once sinus rhythm is established, and chronic antiarrhythmic therapy is often not necessary (28).

Atrial Fibrillation

AF is recognized by an irregularly irregular ventricular rhythm. It is very rare in children and usually seen in patients with structural heart disease, cardiomyopathy, thyroid disease, and WPW syndrome. In neonates, there have been case reports of AF associated

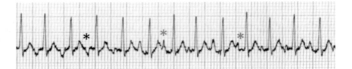

FIGURE 34.11 Rhythm strip from a 3-week-old neonate with multifocal atrial tachycardia in the context of significant respiratory distress. Note at least three different P wave morphologies (*black, red,* and *green asterisks*) and variable RR and PR intervals.

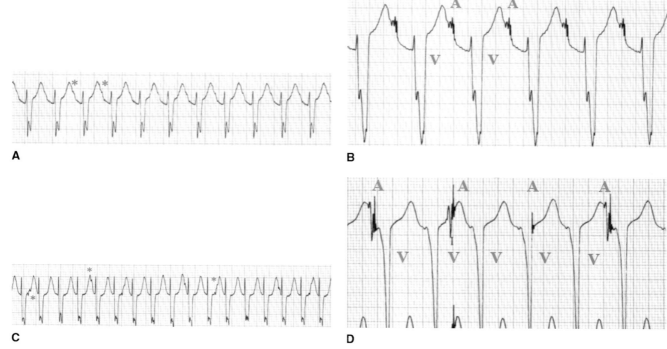

FIGURE 34.12 Surface rhythm strips and atrial rhythm strips depicting sinus tachycardia and junctional ectopic tachycardia (JET) following congenital heart surgery repair in a 3-month-old infant. The QRS complexes are broad, which is not uncommon following cardiac surgery. **A:** Rhythm strip depicting sinus tachycardia with P waves that are "buried" in the T waves (*red asterisks*). P waves can be difficult to identify during tachycardia. **B:** Atrial rhythm strip (speed increased to 50 mm/s). Atrial rhythm strips can be obtained by connecting the atrial temporary pacing wires to the ECG machine. This allows for recording of a direct intracardiac signal, which is easily identified as sharp deflections (*A*), compared to the QRS complexes (*V*). **C:** Rhythm strip depicting JET. Note the QRS complex is unchanged compared to the baseline in sinus tachycardia, and the P waves are not easily identified. Careful inspection reveals AV dissociation, with P waves that are not related to the QRS (*red asterisks*). **D:** Atrial rhythm strip can help with the diagnosis of JET by identifying the P waves (*A*) and demonstrating that the ventricular rate (*V*) is faster than the atrial rate and there is AV dissociation.

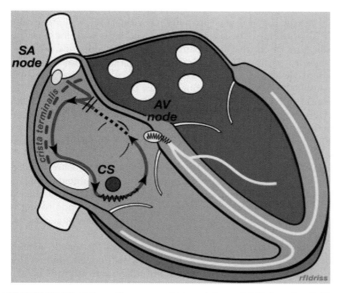

FIGURE 34.13 Schematic representation of the atrial flutter circuit. The circuit typically involves macroreentry in the right atrium, with the activation wave running through the cavotricuspid isthmus (are of slow electrical conduction between the inferior vena cava, the tricuspid valve, and the coronary sinus), up the interatrial septum and down the lateral wall (so-called typical counter clockwise flutter, the most common type). This propagation sequence gives the "saw tooth" appearance of the flutter waves on the ECG. (Reprinted from Mavroudis C, Deal BJ, Backer CL, et al. Arrhythmia surgery in patients with and without congenital heart disease. *Ann Thorac Surg* 2008;86:857.)

with other atrial arrhythmias and developing after treatment with digoxin (29). Synchronized electrical cardioversion (0.5 to 1 J/kg initially) is usually necessary to convert a sustained episode.

Treatments for Supraventricular Tachycardia

Acute Treatment

Treatment depends on the mechanism of tachycardia and hemodynamic status of the patient. If hemodynamically unstable, synchronized electrical cardioversion (0.5 to 1.0 J/kg initially) should be attempted without delay. It is usually very effective in terminating reentrant arrhythmias (e.g., AFL, AVRT) and less successful in automatic tachycardias (e.g., EAT).

In arrhythmias involving the AV node, such as AVRT, transiently slowing or blocking AV node conduction can terminate the tachycardia. Vagal maneuvers are often effective and in neonates and young infants can be achieved by the application of ice-cold damp cloth to the face, or facial immersion in iced water for 5 seconds (30). Ocular compression should never be used due to risk of eye damage.

Adenosine is the treatment of choice for most infants with SVT involving the AV node that is refractory to vagal maneuvers. Adenosine is an endogenous nucleoside that can transiently block AV node conduction, interrupting the SVT circuit. It also decreases sinus node automaticity, resulting in transient sinus bradycardia or sinus pause in addition to AV block. The effect of adenosine in EAT is less predictable; it can either have no effect or cause transient suppression (18). It is helpful to record an ECG during adenosine administration as it can provide useful information about the tachycardia mechanism even if the tachycardia does not terminate (e.g., unmask flutter waves or EAT).

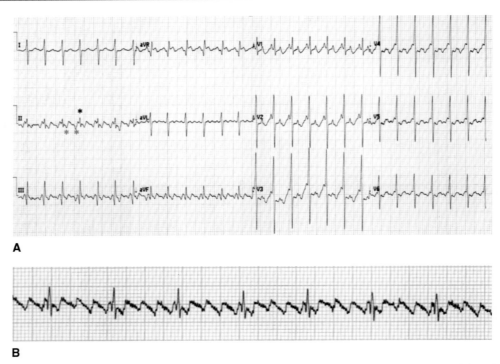

A

B

FIGURE 34.14 Atrial flutter in a 2-day-old neonate with structurally normal heart. A: Flutter waves are marked with *red asterisks* and are negative in leads II, III, and AVF. AV conduction is 2:1 (2 P waves for each QRS, marked with *black asterisk*). **B:** Administration of adenosine causes AV block, which does not terminate the tachycardia, but "unmask" the flutter waves, and the typical "saw tooth" appearance is easily recognized.

Adenosine is quickly metabolized by endothelial and red cells and has a very short half-life, so it must be given as a bolus followed by a rapid flush of normal saline or dextrose, preferably via a central venous line or large peripheral line. Since the usual recommended starting dose of 50 µg/kg is rarely effective, we recommend starting with at least 100 µg/kg, with doses at or above 150 µg/kg being required in most cases (31). If the initial dose fails, subsequent dose increments of 50 to 100 µg are recommended. Methylxanthines (e.g., theophylline and caffeine) are competitive antagonists to adenosine, and higher doses might be required.

Significant side effects are rare, but include AF, which can rarely lead to ventricular fibrillation in WPW syndrome. Adenosine can also paradoxically increase AV conduction in the setting of AFL due to a sympathetic response, so an external defibrillator should be readily available when administering adenosine.

Other antiarrhythmic agents can be used following transient termination of the arrhythmia, or for SVTs that do not involve the AV node (e.g., EAT). These might include beta-blockers (e.g., esmolol or propranolol), class I antiarrhythmics (e.g., procainamide or flecainide), digoxin, or class III antiarrhythmics (e.g., sotalol or amiodarone). For EAT, beta-blockers are often effective, and intravenous infusion of esmolol can be a good first-line therapy until the arrhythmia is controlled. However, class I or class III antiarrhythmic medications may be necessary to adequately suppress EAT, as well as refractory AVRT and AFL. Management of JET has been addressed in the previous section. With refractory SVT and poor ventricular function or hemodynamic compromise, management in an intensive care environment is essential. Extreme caution is needed with antiarrhythmics with negative inotropic effects, including amiodarone, sotalol, and beta-blockers. Except for adenosine, intravenous antiarrhythmic medications should be given as a slow infusion. Rapid bolus of intravenous verapamil has been associated with cardiovascular collapse and death in neonates and infants and should not be used to treat SVT in patients less than 1 year of age (32).

Chronic Treatment

Prophylactic antiarrhythmic therapy is prescribed for most infants with SVT, as there is approximately a 20% risk of recurrence. The risk diminishes after the first 6 to 12 months, and medications may be discontinued (33). The choice of antiarrhythmic medication is usually based on personal preference and institutional practice.

Digoxin may be used in patients with AVRT without evident WPW syndrome. The use of digoxin in patients with manifest preexcitation is controversial since digoxin can enhance antegrade accessory pathway conduction, allowing rapid conduction if the patient develops AF, potentially leading to a hemodynamically unstable VT or ventricular fibrillation. Digoxin has a narrow therapeutic index and serum level should be monitored. The risk of toxicity increases in the presence of electrolyte disturbances, particularly hypokalemia, hypoxemia, myocardial ischemia or inflammation, and concomitant use of drugs that decrease digoxin clearance such as amiodarone.

Beta-blockers are often used in AVRT and EAT. Care is necessary in using beta-blockers for children with significant lung disease due to the potential for bronchospasm. Hypoglycemia can occur in infants but is uncommon. Nevertheless, monitoring for side effects should take place when starting beta-blocker therapy in neonates and infants (34).

Other antiarrhythmic medications can be used, preferably under the direction of a pediatric cardiologist, due to their side effect profile. The most common antiarrhythmics used in the pediatric population include class IA agents (e.g., procainamide), IC (e.g., flecainide and propafenone), and class III (e.g., sotalol and amiodarone). Procainamide and flecainide have the potential advantage of measuring serum drug levels to help guide therapy. Amiodarone has an unusually long half-life and has many potential adverse effects; however, it is commonly used in infants with refractory SVT. Hypotension and bradycardia related to intravenous amiodarone are usually due to rapid infusion.

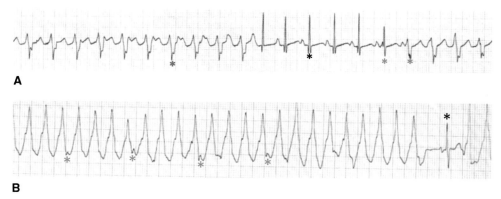

FIGURE 34.15 Rhythm strips of ventricular tachycardia. A: Initial part of the strip showing broad complex tachycardia, which terminates and subsequently restarts. The QRS complexes marked with *red asterisks* mark the onset of the tachycardia when the ventricular rhythm starts to "take over" the sinus rhythm. They have a morphology "in between" a broad complex (*green asterisk*) and a normal sinus QRS (*black asterisk*). They are called "fusion" beats and are only seen in ventricular tachycardia, because they represent combined activation from an ectopic beat coming from the ventricle and a sinus beat. **B:** Ventricular tachycardia with AV dissociation. P waves (marked with *red asterisks*) occur independent of the QRS. There is a normal sinus beat, marked with *black asterisk*, representing a capture beat.

Esophageal electrophysiology studies with programmed atrial stimuli can be used to determine probability of recurrence on medications or after medications have been discontinued. Rarely, radiofrequency or cryoablation is used in infants with SVT refractory to medications often with associated ventricular dysfunction (35).

Fetuses with SVT may be recognized *in utero*, and the tachycardia mechanism can usually be elucidated with fetal echocardiography. Incessant arrhythmia can lead to heart failure, hydrops, and fetal demise. Most common antiarrhythmic medications administered to the mother to treat sustained fetal SVT are digoxin, flecainide, and sotalol, alone or in combination (36).

VENTRICULAR TACHYCARDIAS

Wide-complex tachyarrhythmias may represent VT, antidromic reentrant tachycardia in WPW syndrome, or any SVT in the presence of rate-related or underlying bundle branch block (e.g., after cardiac surgery). In neonates and infants, the QRS complex in VT may be quite narrow, but it is always different than the baseline in sinus rhythm. While dissociation of the ventricles from the atria, with more ventricular complexes, is a hallmark of VT (V > A), there may be a 1:1 VA relationship if there is retrograde conduction. If identified, fusion beats, and capture beats can help with the diagnosis (Fig. 34.15). VT can be monomorphic (same QRS morphology in all beats) or polymorphic (variable QRS morphology). Polymorphic VT is very rare and sinister in neonates and should raise suspicion of cardiac ion channel or myocardial disease.

VT in neonates and infants can be associated with structural or functional heart disease, electrolyte abnormalities, intracardiac tumors (37), and inherited arrhythmia syndromes such as long QT syndrome (LQTS) and Catecholaminergic polymorphic ventricular tachycardia (CPVT). In the setting of a structurally normal heart, accelerated idioventricular rhythm (AIVR) is more common, with VT usually defined as heart rate above 20% of baseline sinus rhythm as previously discussed.

A rare type of monomorphic VT that can present in the neonatal period is fascicular tachycardia, or verapamil-sensitive tachycardia. The substrate involves reentry within the Purkinje system, most commonly at the left posterior fascicle (38). It can be incessant and lead to cardiomyopathy. Due to the close proximity of the tachycardia origin to the normal conduction network, the QRS complex is relatively narrow, and hence can be mistaken for SVT. The ECG hallmark is a regular tachycardia with right bundle branch block morphology and most commonly superior QRS axis (Fig. 34.16). The most successful treatment is with intravenous verapamil, as it is usually not responsive to other therapies. In infants, caution should be exercised when administering intravenous verapamil due to the risk of cardiovascular collapse, and infusion should be slow with close monitoring and resuscitation equipment readily available (39).

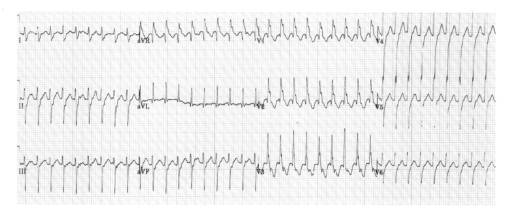

FIGURE 34.16 Fascicular VT in a 2-month-old infant. The typical appearance of the QRS complexes is right bundle branch block with superior axis (negative in leads II, III, and AVF). Note how narrow the QRS is in the inferior leads, which can look like SVT if only a single rhythm strip is recorded.

THE NEWBORN INFANT

Congenital LQTS is an inherited abnormality of ventricular repolarization that can cause polymorphic VT (torsades de pointes) and sudden death. At present, 17 LQTS-susceptibility genes have been identified. Most of these genes encode transmembrane ion channels or associated structural proteins, and around 75% of LQTS cases are due to pathogenic variants in the potassium channel encoding genes *KCNQ1* (LQTS type 1), *KCNH2* (LQTS type 2), and sodium channel encoding gene *SCN5A* (LQTS type 3) (40).

The diagnosis of LQTS is based on clinical and ECG criteria, and a scoring system has been developed (41) (Table 34.1). The QT interval should be corrected for heart rate, and this is usually done using the Bazzet formula (42), but many neonates have a QTc greater than 440 ms in the first week, so repeated ECGs are usually needed. Comprehensive family history should be obtained for possible events suggestive of an arrhythmia (e.g., sudden unexplained death, syncope with exercise or exertion, unexplained accidents, drowning, or seizures, particularly if nocturnal). Obtaining ECGs on parents and other family members of infants with a persistently prolonged QTc may help establish the diagnosis (43). Additionally, causes of acquired QT prolongation should be ruled out (see below).

A pathogenic variant in genetic diagnosis of LQTS can be obtained in about 80% of cases, the remainder 20% being classified as "genotype-negative" (40). Genetic testing through a cardiac genetic service is recommended in patients with a strong index of suspicion for LQTS, in the presence or absence of symptoms, and in family members of a genotype-positive proband (44).

Familial LQTS is most commonly recognized in the neonate (and fetus) due to relative sinus bradycardia, but a severe phenotype, including grossly prolonged QTc, torsades de pointes, 2:1 AV block, and bradycardia can occur due to a severe de novo mutation (Fig. 34.17). These neonates are at high risk of adverse cardiac events and mortality within the first year can exceed 60% (45).

Comprehensive management of patients with LQTS is beyond the scope of this publication but all patients must avoid QT prolonging medications/substances and manage times of risk of electrolyte disturbances. Other therapeutic interventions, such as beta-blockers, cervicothoracic sympathectomy, pacemakers, or implantable cardiac defibrillators are guided by individual risk assessment.

Acquired LQTS with risk of torsades de pointes can occur secondary to medications, electrolyte abnormalities (e.g., hypokalemia, hypocalcemia, or hypomagnesemia), endocrine abnormalities (e.g., hyperparathyroidism, hypothyroidism, or pheochromocytoma), or CNS disorders (e.g., encephalitis, head trauma, subarachnoid hemorrhage).

TABLE 34.1

Diagnostic Criteria for Long QT Syndrome

Electrocardiographic Findings[a]	Points
A. QTc[b]	
≥480 ms	3
460–479 ms	2
450–459 ms (in males)	1
B. QTc 4th minute of recovery from exercise stress test ≥480 ms	1
C. Torsade des pointes[c]	2
D. T wave alternans	1
E. Notched T waves in three leads	1
F. Low heart rate for age[d]	0.5
Clinical history	
A. Syncope[c]	
With stress	2
Without stress	1
B. Congenital deafness	0.5
Family history	
A. Family members with definite LTQS	1
B. Unexplained sudden cardiac death below age 30 among immediate family members[e]	0.5

[a]In the absence of medications or disorders known to affect these electrocardiographic features.
[b]QTc calculated by Bazett formula where $QTc = QT/\sqrt{RR}$.
[c]Mutually exclusive.
[d]Resting heart rate below the 2nd percentile for age.
[e]The same family member cannot be counted in A and B.
Score ≤1 point: low probability of long QT syndrome.
Score 1.5 to 3 points: intermediate probability of long QT syndrome.
Score ≥3.5 points: high probability of long QT syndrome.

Reprinted with permission from Schwartz PJ, Crotti L. QTc behavior during exercise and genetic testing for the long QT syndrome. *Circulation* 2011;124:2181.

Treatments for Ventricular Tachycardias
Acute Treatment

Because VT can be life threatening, it is safest to initially treat all wide complex tachycardias as VT. Treatment options depend on the hemodynamic status of the patient. If hemodynamically unstable, defibrillation (not synchronized cardioversion) should be promptly performed (1 to 2 J/kg initially).

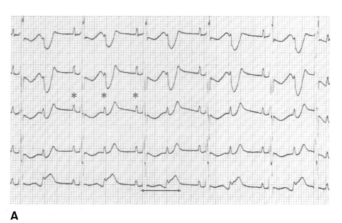

A

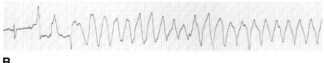

B

FIGURE 34.17 ECG and rhythm strip from a day 1 neonate with long QT syndrome type 2. A: Note the grossly prolonged QTc (over 600 ms, *red arrow*) with 2:1 AV block (P waves marked with *red asterisks*) due to the second P wave falling into the prolonged repolarization period. **B:** Typical polymorphic ventricular tachycardia in long QT syndrome known as "torsades de pointes," or twisting of the points, due to alternating QRS axis.

Hemodynamically stable monomorphic VT can be managed with antiarrhythmic medications such as beta-blockers, lidocaine, procainamide, or amiodarone. For torsades de pointes, treatment should include electrolyte optimization (particularly potassium and magnesium), magnesium sulfate, general anesthesia, and isoproterenol or cardiac pacing as the tachycardia is usually pause dependent.

Chronic Treatment

The type of VT, presence of underlying heart disease, and hemodynamic status should guide chronic antiarrhythmic therapy. Radiofrequency ablation can be performed in infants with refractory life-threatening VT (46). Internal cardiac defibrillators are reserved for infants at risk for recurrent life-threatening VT despite medication, such as severe forms of LQTS.

▌BRADYARRHYTHMIAS

Atrioventricular Block

First-Degree Atrioventricular Block

First-degree AV block is characterized by a PR interval above upper limits of normal for age and heart rate (47). Most commonly, this is due to enhanced vagal tone and seen during sleep. In neonates and infants, it can be secondary to antiarrhythmic medications (e.g., digoxin), hypothermia, hypothyroidism, or electrolyte disturbances. It can be associated with structural heart disease such as Ebstein's anomaly and atrioventricular septal defects, as well as mitochondrial disease (e.g., Kearns-Sayre syndrome), neonatal lupus, or familial progressive cardiac conduction disease.

In the absence of an underlying cause, first-degree AV block is generally well tolerated and requires no specific therapy.

Second-Degree Atrioventricular Block

Second-degree AV block is defined as intermittent failure of conduction of at least one nonpremature atrial depolarization to the ventricles. Second-degree AV block is classified into Mobitz type I (Wenckebach), Mobitz type II, 2:1 AV block, and high grade AV block (failure of conduction of at least two consecutive P waves).

The most common type is Mobitz type I (Wenckebach), in which there is progressive prolongation of the PR interval, before a single atrial beat fails to conduct (**Fig. 34.18**). The block is usually at the level of the AV node but can also be at or below the His bundle, usually associated with a wider QRS. It is generally due to enhanced vagal tone and is a common finding in children with structurally normal hearts, occurring at night, or during periods of increased vagal tone (e.g., bowel motion). It rarely progresses to more advanced conduction disease.

Mobitz Type II is recognized by intermittent failure of atrioventricular conduction, without an associated prolongation of the PR interval. It is usually pathologic and due to conduction block below the His bundle. It can occur following repair of congenital heart

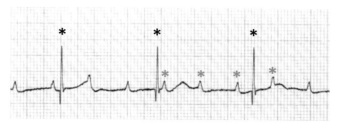

FIGURE 34.19 ECG detail from a neonate with complete heart block due to maternal auto-antibodies. The P waves (*red asterisks*) have no relationship with the QRS (*black asterisks*), and the atrial rate is faster than the ventricular rate. The QRS are narrow, suggesting a junctional escape rhythm.

disease. Pacemaker is generally indicated as there can be progression to higher grade AV block (48).

Second-degree 2:1 AV block is rare, and it can be seen either in the setting of increased vagal tone (as in Mobitz type I) or a manifestation of Mobitz type II; however, it is difficult to distinguish between the two in a single ECG as there is no opportunity to appreciate PR prolongation (Fig. 34.18). Longer rhythm strips or a Holter can be helpful. In neonates, 2:1 AV block can be associated with congenital heart disease such as ccTGA or maternal autoantibodies (see below). It can also be a feature of severe neonatal LQTS. Management depends on the underlying cause.

Third-Degree Atrioventricular Block

Third-degree or complete AV/heart block (CHB) is defined by the absence of conduction of all atrial impulses to the ventricles. The atrial rate is faster than the ventricular rate. The ventricular escape rhythm may arise from the AV node or His bundle (junctional escape rhythm), with a narrow QRS complex, or from the ventricle, resulting in a wide QRS complex. The ventricular rate is related to the origin of the escape rhythm, with junctional rhythms generally being faster than ventricular rhythms (**Fig. 34.19**).

CHB may be congenital or acquired. Acquired CHB in neonates and infants usually occur as a complication of cardiac surgery, particularly following repair of ccTGA, atrioventricular septal defects, tetralogy of Fallot, ventricular septal defects, or after cardiac catheterization. Rarely myocarditis has been implicated in young children (49).

Congenital CHB is frequently recognized *in utero*. It can be associated with cardiovascular malformations such as ccTGA, heterotaxy syndrome, and atrioventricular septal defects. Inherited progressive cardiac conduction disease has been linked to pathogenic variants in genes encoding cardiac connexins and ion channels, particularly *SCN5A*. Inheritance is generally autosomal dominant (50). Congenital myopathies can be associated with progressive conduction disease and CHB, but the onset is usually beyond infancy (51).

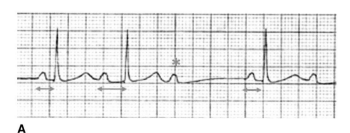

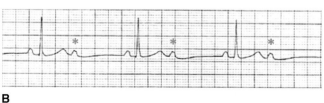

A

B

FIGURE 34.18 Second-degree AV block. A: Mobitz type I (Wenckebach). There is progressive PR prolongation (*arrows*) before a single P wave is blocked (*red asterisk*). The PR interval following the blocked beat is shorter than the interval preceding the blocked beat. **B:** 2:1 AV block with every other beat nonconducted (*red asterisks*). Both rhythm strips were obtained from the same patient at the same recording, so in this situation type I and 2:1 AV block share the same etiology (in this case increased vagal tone).

Isolated congenital CHB is estimated to occur in 1 of 20,000 live births (52). More than 90% are immune mediated and related to maternal autoantibodies (anti-Ro/SSA and/or anti-La/SSB) that cross the placenta and interact with the developing conduction system (53). These antibodies are associated with maternal connective tissue disease, particularly lupus and Sjögren syndrome, but many are asymptomatic and only have serologic evidence, so antibody testing is indicated in all mothers of neonates with isolated congenital CHB (54). Cardiomyopathy develops in about 10% of cases (48). Cardiac dilatation without ventricular dysfunction is a common finding and is likely related to longstanding compensatory increase in stroke volume.

Most infants tolerate the bradycardia well and do not require immediate intervention; pacing can usually be deferred for many years. Fetal diagnosis, fetal hydrops, ventricular fibroelastosis and delivery earlier than 32 weeks have been associated with increased mortality (52), as well as heart rates persistently below 55 bpm (55).

Medical therapy with isoproterenol or temporary cardiac pacing is helpful in the acute situation. Indications for permanent pacing include symptoms, ventricular rate less than 55 beats/min; or 70 beats/min in congenital heart disease, ventricular dysfunction, wide QRS escape rhythms; prolonged QTc intervals; complex ventricular ectopy or VT, and pauses longer than three times the basic cycle length (56).

Pacemaker implantation in infancy is usually done via an epicardial approach, due to the increased risk of venous occlusion. One center has reported favorable long-term outcomes with transvenous pacing in infants (57).

REFERENCES

1. Baruteau AE, Perry JC, Sanatani S, et al. Evaluation and management of bradycardia in neonates and children. *Eur J Pediatr* 2016;175:151.
2. Nagashima M, Matsushima M, Ogawa A, et al. Cardiac arrhythmias in healthy children revealed by 24-hour ambulatory ECG monitoring. *Pediatr Cardiol* 1987;8:103.
3. Southall DP, Richards J, Mitchell P, et al. Study of cardiac rhythm in healthy newborn infants. *Br Heart J* 1980;43:14.
4. Alexander ME, Berul CI. Ventricular arrhythmias: when to worry. *Pediatr Cardiol* 2000;21:532.
5. Levin MD, Stephens P, Tanel RE, et al. Ventricular tachycardia in infants with structurally normal heart: a benign disorder. *Cardiol Young* 2010;20:641.
6. Van Hare GF, Stranger P. Ventricular tachycardia and accelerated ventricular rhythm presenting in the first month of life. *Am J Cardiol* 1991;67:42.
7. Snyder CS, Fenrich AL, Friedman RA, et al. Usefulness of echocardiography in infants with supraventricular tachycardia. *Am J Cardiol* 2003;91:1277.
8. Ko JK, Deal BJ, Strasburger JF, et al. Supraventricular tachycardia mechanisms and their age distribution in pediatric patients. *Am J Cardiol* 1992;69:1028.
9. Jaeggi E, Ohman A. Fetal and neonatal arrhythmias. *Clin Perinatol* 2016;43:99.
10. Wolff L, Parkinson I, White P. Bundle branch block with short PR interval in healthy young people prone to paroxysmal tachycardia. *Am Heart J* 1930;5:685.
11. Bromberg BI, Lindsay BD, Cain ME, et al. Impact of clinical history and electrophysiologic characterization of accessory pathways on management strategies to reduce sudden death among children with Wolff-Parkinson-White syndrome. *J Am Coll Cardiol* 1996;27:690.
12. Etheridge SP, Escudero CA, Blaufox AD, et al. Life-threatening event risk in children with Wolff-Parkinson-White syndrome: a multicenter international study. *JACC Clin Electrophysiol* 2018;4:433.
13. Gollob MH, Green MS, Tang AS, et al. Identification of a gene responsible for familial Wolff-Parkinson-White syndrome. *N Engl J Med* 2001;344:1823.
14. Drago F, Silvetti MS, De Santis A, et al. Paroxysmal reciprocating supraventricular tachycardia in infants: electrophysiologically guided medical treatment and long-term evolution of the re-entry circuit. *Europace* 2008;10:629.
15. Kang KT, Potts JE, Radbill AE, et al. Permanent junctional reciprocating tachycardia in children: a multicentre experience. *Heart Rhythm* 2014;11:1426.
16. Jaeggi ET, Gilljam T, Bauersfeld U, et al. Electrocardiographic differentiation of typical atrioventricular node reentrant tachycardia from atrioventricular reciprocating tachycardia mediated by concealed accessory pathway in children. *Am J Cardiol* 2003;91:1084.
17. Seslar SP, Alexander ME, Berul CI, et al. Ablation of nonautomatic focal atrial tachycardia in children and adults with congenital heart disease. *J Cardiovasc Electrophysiol* 2006;17:359.
18. Engelstein ED, Lippman N, Stein KM, et al. Mechanism-specific effects of adenosine on atrial tachycardia. *Circulation* 1994;89:2645.
19. Bauersfeld U, Gow RM, Hamilton RM, et al. Treatment of atrial ectopic tachyeardia in infants < 6 months old. *Am Heart J* 1995;129:1145.
20. Salerno JC, Kertesz NJ, Friedman RA, et al. Clinical course of atrial ectopic tachycardia is age-dependent: results and treatment in children < 3 or > or =3 years of age. *J Am Coll Cardiol* 2004;43:438.
21. Baek SM, Chung H, Song MK, et al. The complexity of pediatric multifocal atrial tachycardia and its prognostic factors. *Korean Circ J* 2018;48(2):148.
22. Bradley DJ, Fischbach PS, Law IH, et al. The clinical course of multifocal atrial tachycardia in infants and children. *J Am Coll Cardiol* 2001;38(2):401.
23. Villain E, Vetter V, Garcia JM, et al. Evolving concepts in the management of congenital junctional ectopic tachycardia. *Circulation* 1990;81:1544.
24. Dieks JK, Klehs S, Muller MJ, et al. Adjunctive ivabradine in combination with amiodarone: a novel therapy for pediatric congenital junctional ectopic tachycardia. *Heart Rhythm* 2016;13:1297.
25. Walsh EP, Saul JP, Scholler GF, et al. Evaluation of a staged treatment protocol for rapid automatic junctional tachycardia after operation for congenital heart disease. *J Am Coll Cardiol* 1997;29:1046.
26. Texter KM, Kertesz NJ, Friedman RA, et al. Atrial flutter in infants. *J Am Coll Cardiol* 2006;48:1040.
27. Soyeur DJ. Atrial flutter in the human fetus: diagnosis, hemodynamic consequences, and therapy. *J Cardiovasc Electrophysiol* 1996;7:989.
28. Casey FA, McCrindle BW, Hamilton RM, et al. Neonatal atrial flutter: significant early morbidity and excellent long-term prognosis. *Am Heart J* 1997;133:302.
29. Radford DJ, Izukawa T. Atrial fibrillation in children. *Pediatrics* 1977;59:250.
30. Sreeram N, Wren C. Supraventricular tachycardia in infants: response to initial treatment. *Arch Dis Child* 1990;65(1):127.
31. Dixon J, Foster K, Wyllie J, et al. Guidelines and adenosine dosing for supraventricular tachycardia. *Arch Dis Child* 2005;90:1190.
32. Epstein ML, Kiel EA, Victorica BE. Cardiac decompensation following verapamil therapy in infants with supraventricular tachycardia. *Pediatrics* 1985;75:737.
33. Perry JC, Garson A Jr. Supraventricular tachycardia due to Wolff-Parkinson-White syndrome in children: early disappearance and late recurrence. *J Am Coll Cardiol* 1990;16:1215.
34. Léaute-Labrèze C, Boccara O, Degrugillier-Chopinet C, et al. Safety of oral propranolol for the treatment of infantile hemangioma: a systematic review. *Pediatrics* 2016;138(4):e20160353.
35. Saul JP, Kanter RJ, Abrams D, et al. PACES/HRS expert consensus statement on the use of catheter ablation in children and patients with congenital heart disease. *Heart Rhythm* 2016;13:251.
36. Donofrio MT, Moon-Grady AJ, Hornberger LK, et al. Diagnosis and treatment of fetal cardiac disease. A scientific statement from the American Heart Association. *Circulation* 2014;129(21):2183.
37. Perry JC. Ventricular tachycardia in neonates. *Pacing Clin Electrophysiol* 1997;20:2061.
38. Collins KK, Schaffer MS, Liberman L, et al. Fascicular and nonfascicular left ventricular tachycardias in the young: an international multicenter study. *J Cardiovasc Electrophysiol* 2013;24(6):640.
39. Kehr J, Binfield A, Maxwell F, et al. Fascicular tachycardia in infancy and the use of verapamil: a case series and literature review. *Arch Dis Child* 2019;104(8):789.
40. Giudicessi JR, Wilde AAM, Ackerman MJ. The genetic architecture of long QT syndrome: a critical reappraisal. *Trends Cardiovasc Med* 2018;28(7):453.
41. Schwartz PJ, Crotti L. QTc behavior during exercise and genetic testing for the long QT syndrome. *Circulation* 2011;124:2181.
42. Waddell-Smith K, Gow RM, Skinner JR. How to measure a QT interval. A standard approach in QT measurement improves communication between clinicians. *Med J Aust* 2017;207(3):107.
43. Priori SG, Wilde AA, Horie M, et al. HRS/EHRA/APHRS expert consensus statement on the diagnosis and management of patients with inherited primary arrhythmia syndromes. *Heart Rhythm* 2013;10(12):1932.
44. Ackerman MJ, Priori SG, Willems S, et al. HRS/EHRA expert consensus statement on the state of genetic testing for the channelopathies and cardiomyopathies. *Europace* 2011;13(8):1077.
45. Cuneo BF, Etheridge SP, Horigome H, et al. Arrhythmia phenotype during fetal life suggests long-QT syndrome genotype: risk stratification of perinatal long-QT syndrome. *Circ Arrhythm Electrophysiol* 2013;6(5):946.

46. Shebani SO, Ng GA, Stafford P, et al. Radiofrequency ablation on veno-arterial extracorporeal life support in treatment of very sick infants with incessant tachymyopathy. *Europace* 2015;17(4):622.

47. Davignon A, Rautaharju P, Boiselle E, et al. Normal ECG standards for infants and children. *Ped Cardiol* 1979–1980;1:123.

48. Baruteau AE, Pass RH, Thambo JB, et al. Congenital and childhood atrio-ventricular blocks: pathophysiology and contemporary management. *Eur J Pediatr* 2016;175(9):1235.

49. Batra AS, Epstein D, Silka MJ. The clinical course of acquired complete heart block in children with acute myocarditis. *Pediatr Cardiol* 2003;24(5):495.

50. Smits JP, Veldkamp MW, Wilde AA. Mechanisms of inherited cardiac conduction disease. *Europace* 2005;7(2):122.

51. Verhaert D, Richards K, Rafael-Fortney JA, et al. Cardiac involvement in patients with muscular dystrophies: magnetic resonance imaging phenotype and genotypic considerations. *Circ Cardiovasc Imaging* 2011;4(1):67.

52. Jaeggi ET, Hamilton RM, Silverman ED, et al. Outcome of children with fetal, neonatal or childhood diagnosis of isolated congenital atrioventricular block. A single institution's experience of 30 years. *J Am Coll Cardiol* 2002;39(1):130.

53. Buyon JP, Hiebert R, Copel J, et al. Autoimmune-associated congenital heart block: demographics, mortality, morbidity and recurrence rates obtained from a national neonatal lupus registry. *J Am Coll Cardiol* 1998;31:1658.

54. Waltuck J, Buyon J. Autoantibody-associated congenital heart block: outcome in mothers and children. *Ann Intern Med* 1994;120:544.

55. Schmidt KG, Ulmer HE, Silverman NH, et al. Perinatal outcome of fetal complete atrioventricular block: a multicenter experience. *J Am Coll Cardiol* 1991;17(6):1360.

56. Epstein AE, DiMarco JP, Ellenbogen, KA, et al. ACC/AHA/HRS 2008 Guidelines for device-based therapy of cardiac rhythm abnormalities. *Circulation* 2008;117:350.

57. Konta L, Chubb MH, Bostock J, et al. Twenty-seven years experience with transvenous pacemaker implantation in children weighing <10 kg. *Circ Arrhythm Electrophysiol* 2016;9(2):e003422.

THE NEWBORN INFANT

35 Development of Structure and Function of the Gastrointestinal Tract

Diomel M. de la Cruz and Josef Neu

The gastrointestinal (GI) tract is a combination of organs whose roles comprise not only digestion and absorption but also immune defense and neuroendocrine functions. In the human adult, the surface area of the intestine is similar to that of a tennis court, approximately 200 m², which is about 100 times that of the skin, which is approximately 2 m² (1). In addition to its massive absorptive surface area, the GI tract can also be considered the major immune organ of the body where a single layer of epithelial cells and gut-associated lymphoid tissue (GALT) interacts with a huge load of microbial and food antigens, seemingly knowing when to react against or tolerate antigens (1). The intestine contains neural tissue equivalent to that of the spinal cord and is also involved in exocrine and endocrine functions and communication with the central nervous system (CNS), the so-called gut–brain axis. Accordingly, the development of the GI tract during the fetal and neonatal period needs to be understood to optimize not only nutrition but also immunologic well-being and neurodevelopment during the early stages of life, which are considered to be one of the most critical windows for subsequent health.

ANATOMIC DEVELOPMENT AND ORGANOGENESIS

During the 2nd week of gestation, the primitive streak is formed and its subsequent migration forms the endoderm, mesoderm, and ectoderm (2–4). The alimentary canal is formed from the folding of the endoderm and splanchnic mesoderm by the 3rd to 4th week of gestation (5). The GI tract begins from three structures: the foregut, which is formed when the cranial portion of the yolk sac becomes enclosed within the embryo; the hindgut, which is the caudal part of the yolk sac enclosed in the embryo; and the midgut, which remains outside the embryo.

The boundaries of the foregut, midgut, and hindgut are consistent with the arterial supply of the alimentary canal. The foregut gives rise to the pharynx, oral cavity, esophagus, stomach, and upper duodenum. The midgut gives rise to the distal duodenum, jejunum, ileum, and proximal transverse colon. The hindgut develops into the distal transverse colon, descending colon, sigmoid colon, and rectum (4,6,7).

Esophagus

The esophagus averages 8 to 10 cm in length in the newborn. The esophagus is derived from the foregut during the 4th week of gestation. The respiratory system develops from a median diverticulum of the foregut, which elongates and becomes bifid, forming the lung buds. Elongation of the tracheal diverticulum creates separation of the trachea and the esophagus. The esophagus reaches its full length relative to the size of the fetus around the 7th week of gestation. Esophageal and tracheoesophageal abnormalities may develop during this phase. The tracheal diverticulum forms the primitive respiratory tract (8) (see Fig. 35.1).

By the 10th week of gestation, the esophagus has a single lumen. The epithelial lining is ciliated at this time but is then replaced by stratified, nonkeratinized squamous epithelium by the end of the first trimester.

Blood supply to the esophagus is subdivided. The cranial part of the esophagus is supplied by vessels originating from the inferior thyroid artery. The rest of the esophagus is supplied by bronchial vessels of the descending thoracic aorta. It may also receive blood supply from inferior phrenic and left gastric arteries (3).

Accordingly, nervous supply of the esophagus is subdivided into upper third and lower two-thirds. The upper third is innervated by the cervical sympathetic trunks, whereas the lower esophagus is innervated by the splanchnic nerves. Neurons begin to be identified in the esophagus around the 8th week of gestation.

Clinical Correlation

As mentioned, aberrations before the 7th week of gestation when the foregut is divided into respiratory primordium and esophagus result in esophageal malformations and tracheoesophageal fistulas. Esophageal atresia results from an interruption of recanalization of the primitive gut during the 8th week of gestation. Esophageal stenosis is a narrowing most commonly found in the lower thirds of the esophagus. Esophageal rings are another form of defect in the lower third characterized by concentric extension of esophageal tissue (9,10).

Failure to reestablish the esophageal lumen during embryonic development can also lead to abnormalities called esophageal duplication cysts (11). Gastrointestinal anomalies will be further discussed in Chapter 36.

Stomach

The stomach follows the esophagus caudally and is joined to the duodenum by the pylorus. On average, the newborn stomach has a capacity of 30 mL compared to 1 to 2 L in adults (2).

As with the esophagus, the stomach is derived from the primitive foregut and arises by the end of the 4th week of gestation. Prior to 6 weeks, the stomach is suspended to the dorsal body wall by the dorsal mesogastrium and to the ventral body wall by the ventral mesogastrium. At the beginning of the 6th week of gestation, the stomach undergoes two rotations (see Fig. 35.2): a first counterclockwise rotation that brings the dorsal stomach toward the left side of the fetus's abdomen and a second clockwise rotation that causes the former dorsal stomach to point caudally. At approximately 8 weeks, the formation of the stomach is complete. The final shape of the stomach can be divided into four regions: the cardia, the fundus, the body, and the antrum (5).

The epithelium of the stomach is initially a pseudostratified columnar epithelium. Later on, this is replaced by a cuboidal epithelium that contains gastric pits, which house effector cells of gastric secretion (5). Various cell types are found in the stomach. Parietal cells (involved in hydrochloric acid and intrinsic factor production) are mostly found in the fundus. Chief cells (pepsinogen secretion) are more commonly found in the fundus. G cells (gastrin secretion) and D cells (somatostatin and amylin secretion) are the most common neuroendocrine cells found in the stomach (1).

The blood supply to the stomach is largely from the celiac axis. The four major vessels are the right and left gastric and gastroepiploic arteries. Venous drainage is mostly via the portal system with the exception of esophageal veins, which drain the gastroesophageal junction.

Parasympathetic and enteric nervous systems provide neural innervation of the stomach. Sympathetic innervation, originating from the thoracic spinal cord, is mostly inhibitory in nature, while parasympathetic innervation derived mostly from brainstem and vagal nerves is stimulatory. Interestingly, the enteric nervous system is separate anatomically from the CNS.

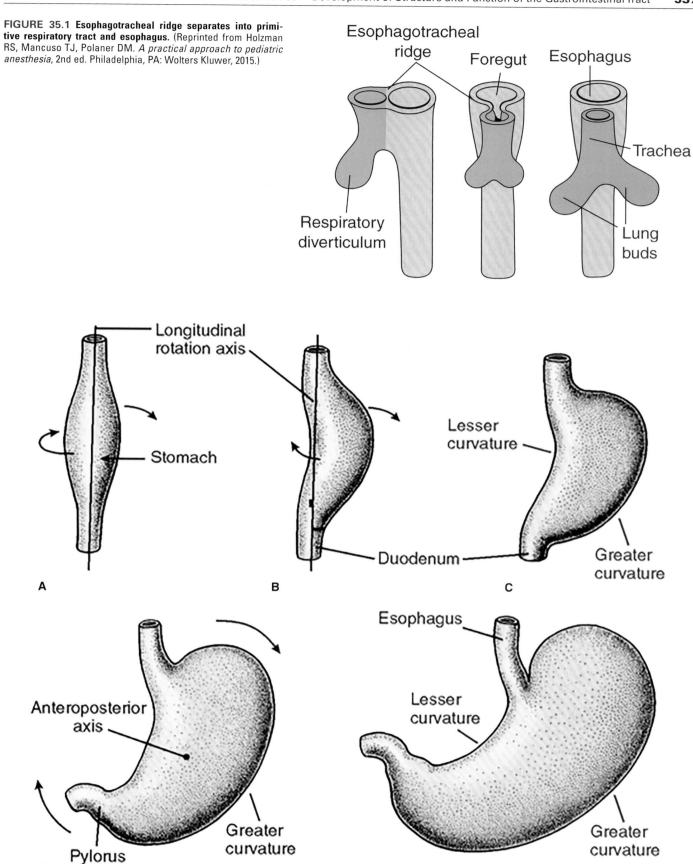

FIGURE 35.1 Esophagotracheal ridge separates into primitive respiratory tract and esophagus. (Reprinted from Holzman RS, Mancuso TJ, Polaner DM. *A practical approach to pediatric anesthesia*, 2nd ed. Philadelphia, PA: Wolters Kluwer, 2015.)

FIGURE 35.2 Depiction of the two rotations the stomach undergoes on the longitudinal and anteroposterior axis until its final position. (Reprinted from Sadler TW, Leland J, Sadler-Redmond SL. *Langman's medical embryology*, 10th ed. Philadelphia, PA: Wolters Kluwer, 2010.)

THE NEWBORN INFANT

Clinical Correlation

Failure of the mesentery to fixate the stomach can predispose to gastric volvulus. Gastric volvulus is a rare condition distinguished by a 180-degree rotation due to the laxity of the normal fixation of the stomach to the body (12–14). Abnormalities in the enteric nervous system are the primary hypotheses in the development of hypertrophic pyloric stenosis (15–17), which is further discussed in Chapter 36.

Intestine

During fetal life, the GI tract undertakes an immense expansion in length and size. From the 5th week to the 40th week of gestation, intestines elongate approximately 1,000-fold to a mean of 275 cm at birth (1). At the beginning of 6th week of gestation, the lengthening and maturation of the midgut contributes to the formation of the small and large intestines (see **Fig. 35.3**). The embryonic midgut gives rise to the distal duodenum, jejunum, ileum, and proximal colon. The gut herniates out of the abdomen from weeks 6 to 12 and reenters with a 270-degree rotation around the superior mesenteric artery. The shortening of the dorsal mesentery of duodenum fixes itself into a retroperitoneal position. This is complete by 20 weeks of gestation. The duodenal lumen obliterates during the 2nd month of gestation and recanalizes later on in development.

By the 16th week of gestation, fingerlike projections called villi are already formed in the small intestines. At this point, villi are also present in the large intestine but partially regress by the 29th week of gestation. Half of the growth in the length of the intestine occurs in the third trimester. Due to the microvilli covering the surface of the small intestinal epithelium, the intestinal surface affords the greatest interface between the outside environment and the internal milieu (3,5,18).

After mitotic cell division of intestinal epithelial cells in the crypts, migration to the villus occurs where they undergo differentiation. These actively absorbing cells are then sloughed from the villus tip to the intestinal lumen. Migration time is believed to be 2 days in an adult and around 4 days in an infant (1).

Numerous cell types are found in the small intestines including absorptive epithelium, goblet cells (involved in mucus secretion), Paneth cells (involved in secretion of defensins), and other cell types associated with the immune and neuroendocrine system. Enteroendocrine cells secrete hormones involved in satiety, motility, and secretion of digestive enzymes. In response to acid in the lumen, secretin is secreted by duodenal S cells, which then stimulates bicarbonate production from the liver, pancreas, and duodenal mucosal cells. Cholecystokinin is produced in response to fatty acids and amino acids, which stimulates contraction of the

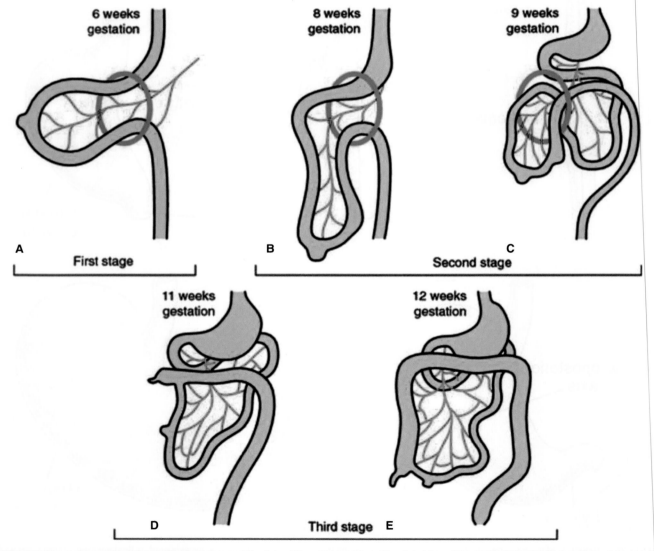

FIGURE 35.3 Three stages of small intestinal rotation and fixation of the mesogastrium. (Reprinted from Filston HC, Kirks DR. Malrotation—the ubiquitous anomaly. *J Pediatr Surg* 1981;16(4 suppl 1):614. Copyright © 1981 Elsevier. With permission.)

gallbladder and pancreatic exocrine function. Glucose-dependent insulinotropic peptide stimulates B cells in the pancreas to produce insulin in response to food intake.

The blood supply to the small intestine is chiefly from the superior mesenteric artery.

Neural innervation of the small intestines is principally from vagal neural crest cells that migrate craniocaudally from the 5th week to 12th week of gestation and form myenteric plexuses. Circular and longitudinal musculature of the small intestines appears at 6 and 8 weeks, respectively. Myenteric and submucosal innervations are noted by the 9th week of gestation. Although peristalsis can be noted early in gestation, myenteric muscle contractions are more coordinated by the 32nd week to 34th week of gestation. Maturity of myenteric muscle contractions appears only by 38 weeks of gestation.

Clinical Correlation

Fixation of the duodenum via the shortening of the dorsal mesentery is critical. Failure to achieve this process predisposes the infant to midgut volvulus and malrotation. Duodenal stenosis is due to the failure to recanalize the alimental canal during fetal life (12,13,19,20). Other abnormalities in the development of the midgut can include abdominal wall defects such as omphalocele and gastroschisis (21–23). More detail on these and other intestinal abnormalities will be discussed in Chapter 36.

Colon, Rectum, and Anus

The colon is composed of six different zones: the cecum, appendix, ascending colon, transverse colon, descending colon, and sigmoid colon. Two foremost functions of the colon are the absorption of water and electrolytes and elimination of feces.

The distal transverse colon, descending colon, sigmoid colon, and rectum all originate from the hindgut. During the 4th week of gestation, the cloaca is formed. The anorectal and urogenital canals arise during the 4th to 6th weeks of gestation from septation of the cloaca. By the 12th week of gestation, the anal canal, vaginal canal, and urethral canals are distinct (2,18,24).

Similar to the duodenum, the colon also undergoes a counterclockwise rotation during the 10th to 12th week. This 270-degree rotation determines the final position of the colon wherein the cecum is found in the right lower quadrant, transverse colon from hepatic to splenic flexure, and sigmoid colon connecting to descending colon at around the third sacral vertebra. The cecum is variably fixed and can be completely retroperitoneal or sometimes on a mesentery. The ascending and descending colons are retroperitoneal, but the transverse and sigmoid colons are on a mesentery (25,26).

The colon has unique muscular components when compared to the small intestine. One obvious difference is the presence of teniae coli. These teniae create haustrations that radiographically can identify large from small intestines. These may not be obvious in radiographs in infants. The mucosa of the colon also contains absorptive, goblet, endocrine cells within the crypts of Lieberkühn.

Vascular circulation of the colon is provided by the inferior and superior mesenteric arteries. The distribution of the two vessels has a watershed area around the midtransverse colon to the splenic flexure. The rectum is supplied by the iliac arteries in addition to the inferior mesenteric arteries.

Like the small intestine, the colon and rectum are innervated by the process of neural crest cell migration forming enteric ganglion cells. During the 4th week of gestation, spinal nerves from S2–S4 contribute to parasympathetic nervous supply, which influences motility and proprioception.

Clinical Correlation

Congenital intestinal aganglionosis (Hirschsprung disease) results from failed development and migration of the myenteric nervous

system. The sigmoid colon is the region most frequently affected, but the aganglionosis may be more extensive affecting more proximal regions of the colon (27). Other abnormalities in the development of the hindgut include imperforate anus, rectourethral or rectovaginal fistulas, and other anorectal malformations (25).

Pancreas

Within 30 days of gestation, the beginnings of the pancreatic bud and common bile ducts appear from the part of the gut that forms the second part of the duodenum. By 5 weeks of gestation, the main duct of the ventral pancreatic bud connects to the common bile duct at the ampulla of Vater. By the 6th week of gestation, the two pancreatic buds (dorsal and ventral) join and form the definitive pancreas. Failure of this process leads to an annular pancreas. The dorsal pancreatic bud gives rise to the head, body, and tail of the pancreas, whereas the uncinate process originates from the ventral bud (28,29).

The pancreas has crucial endocrine and exocrine functions. It is a central source for digestive enzymes such as chymotrypsin, trypsin, and peptidases. Pancreatic amylase and lipase are also important in carbohydrate and lipid digestion, respectively. The pancreas also plays a key role in glucose and metabolic homeostasis via the islets of Langerhans. Within the islets, alpha cells (involved in glucagon production), beta cells (insulin production), PP cells (for pancreatic polypeptides), and gamma cells (somatostatin production) are found. Somatostatin antagonizes the acid-stimulating effects of histamine and also prevents the release of other hormones including gastrin. This may slow down the process of digestion.

Liver and Biliary System

The liver, gallbladder, and bile ducts arise from the duodenal endoderm at the distal end of the foregut. The liver bud appears in the mid 3rd week of gestation on the ventral side of the duodenum. Within 30 days, the hepatic plate grows to give rise to the primitive liver. The gallbladder is formed from the hepatic diverticulum. Bile production begins by the 12th week of gestation. Because of the hematopoietic function of the liver in early gestation, the liver accounts for approximately 10% of total fetal body weight (28).

DIGESTION AND ABSORPTION

The GI tract's role in the absorption and digestion of nutrients is of paramount importance in the maintenance of a healthy neonate. The development of gastrointestinal digestion and absorption during the neonatal period should be understood in order to optimize nutrition delivery.

Carbohydrate Digestion

The digestion and absorption of complex carbohydrates and starches in human development is a well-defined sequence. First, they are hydrolyzed into oligosaccharides by processes in the mouth, stomach, and intestinal lumen (see Fig. 35.4). Hydrolysis is primarily achieved by the work of salivary and pancreatic amylases. At the brush border of the intestines, oligosaccharides are then further hydrolyzed into monosaccharides by the action of brush border hydrolases, namely, maltase, lactase, and sucrase (30). See **Figure 35.4**.

There is no great variation in amylase activity between term and preterm human milk. Comparatively, salivary amylase is lower in children than in adults. Salivary amylase activity increases shortly after term birth, while pancreatic amylase only begins to increase from 3 months until they reach adult levels by 2 years (31,32).

In the fetus, intestinal lactase levels are low between 2 and 3 weeks of gestation, and a relatively high concentration is achieved at around 37 weeks. Sucrase activity, while present in the fetal colon, disappears before birth. Postnatally, lactose absorption in premature infants at 30 weeks of gestation has been demonstrated. Colonic salvage of lactose is adequate by the second week

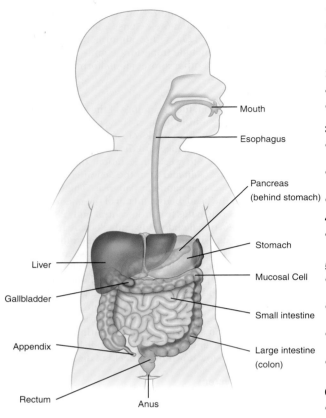

Mouth

Esophagus

Pancreas
(behind stomach)

Stomach

Mucosal Cell

Small intestine

Large intestine
(colon)

Liver

Gallbladder

Appendix

Rectum

Anus

1. Mouth
- Lingual lipase hydrolyzes triglycerides to diglycerides and free fatty acids.
- Salivary glands secrete salivary amylase, which breaks down alpha 1-4 bonds of complex sugars.

2. Stomach
- Lipid digestion occurs in the stomach through the action of gastric lipase.
- Protein digestion begins in the stomach via hydrochloric acid and pepsin.

3. Pancreas
- Pancreatic lipase is released into the intestine to break down triglycerides into monoglycerides, fatty acids, and glycerol.
- Pancreas secretes chymotrypsin, trypsin, and other enzymes for protein digestion.
- Pancreas secretes pancreatic amylase.

4. Liver
- Bile is produced in the liver, stored in the gallbladder, and released into the small intestine to aid in digestion of lipids.

5. Small Intestine
- In the small intestine, micelles are formed from fat digestion and diffuse into mucosal cells.
- Polypeptides are broken down into amino acids, dipeptides, and tripeptides by protein-digesting enzymes secreted by the pancreas.
- Pancreatic alpha amylase cleaves alpha 1-4 bonds of carbohydrates reducing them to simple sugars and oligosaccharides.
- Intestinal brush border disaccharidases and alpha-dextrinase convert disaccharides and oligosaccharides to monosaccharides.

6. Colon
- Small amounts of dietary protein are lost in fecal matter.
- Undigested carbohydrates are digested by colonic bacteria ("colonic salvage pathway").

7. Mucosal Cell
- Inside the mucosal cells, fatty acids are reassembled and incorporated into chylomicrons, which enter lymphatic vessels.
- Dipeptides and tripeptides enter the mucosal cell and are broken down into single amino acids.
- Glucose and galactose are actively transported into the cell by the sodium glucose transporter (SGLUT-1).

Blue—Lipid Digestion
Green—Protein Digestion
Red—Carbohydrate Digestion

FIGURE 35.4 Digestion of carbohydrates, proteins, and lipids.

after birth. In premature infants, lactose absorption compensated with colonic salvage to absorb short-chain fatty acids (SCFAs) has been demonstrated to be efficient (30).

Clinical Correlation
Many preterm formulas utilize partially hydrolyzed starches, such as corn syrup solids. One salient feature of premature infants' feeding is that their limitations of suck and swallow coordination necessitate tube feeding. These tubes bypass the oral cavity reducing the efficacy of any salivary amylase that may be secreted. Undigested starches would pass into the colon, where they would either leave the GI tract undigested or be subject to microbial digestion with production of hydrogen gas and SCFAs, which can be absorbed and used as a fat-based energy source. SCFAs, particularly butyrate, are involved in proliferation, differentiation, and turnover of colon epithelium and act as a fuel source to these cells, as well as affect immunity.

Lactose is the primary carbohydrate source in mammalian milk, and the activity of lactase is relatively low in the preterm infant's small intestine. Despite this relative lactase deficiency in preterm infants, symptoms of lactose intolerance do not seem to occur in this population (33). Many preterm infants have their feedings gradually advanced and thus do not receive large quantities of lactose abruptly. The amount of lactose intake is thus not likely to overwhelm the lactase-hydrolyzing capacity (30). Furthermore, the aforementioned microbial salvage pathways in the colon convert lactose into beneficial SCFAs. Studies wherein preterm infants received enteral feeds at 4 days of life had 100% and 60% more lactase activity at 10 and 28 days after birth compared to preterm infants who had their enteral feedings initiated at approximately 2 weeks after birth (34). For poorly understood reasons, lactase activity was higher in human milk–fed infants than those receiving formula at 10 days of life.

Protein Digestion
Protein digestion commences in the stomach and continues in the small intestines. Dietary proteins are broken down into amino acids and polypeptides. Two main sources of proteolytic enzymes that facilitate digestion are stomach and the pancreas. Pepsinogen from the stomach is activated into pepsin by acid. Fetuses can produce gastric acid and gastrin at the beginning of the second trimester or roughly around 4 months of gestation. Hydrochloric acid levels are found to be much lower in premature infants compared to those in term infants (35). Pancreatic proteases, like trypsin and chymotrypsin activated by enterokinase, hydrolyze dietary protein into small and medium peptides. These peptides are then absorbed by small intestinal enterocytes via cotransport with H+ ions. Once within the enterocyte, further hydrolysis of dipeptides and tripeptides into single amino acids occurs by way of cytoplasmic peptides, and are then exported into the bloodstream (36,37). See Figure 35.4.

Clinical Correlation

There are several developmental issues in the digestion and absorption of proteins in the preterm newborn including low gastric acid output and an inability to convert pancreatic proteases into an active form due to a lack of enterokinase. Gastric acid is necessary for intraluminal denaturation of proteins and to cleave pepsinogen into active pepsin. As preterm infants are known to have a reduced capability to produce gastric acid, they likely will be less able to initiate gastric protein digestion compared to term infants.

Cow's milk formula is often used in preterm infants if mother's milk is not available. Fortifiers derived from cow's milk are also commonly used to meet preterm infants' requirements. If preterm infants have decreased activity of enterokinase and other peptidases compared to term infants, should hydrolyzed formulas be used instead of formulas containing more native proteins? Mihatsch et al. compared hydrolyzed to standard preterm formula as to the time needed to reach full feeds in preterm infants (38). The group receiving the standard formula had a longer overall time to reach full feeds compared to those receiving the hydrolyzed formula. Although this result is of major interest, many hydrolyzed formulas may not be suitable for preterm infants because of their relatively low protein and mineral content.

Lipid Digestion

The largest component of dietary lipid is triglyceride, which requires two key processes for digestion, mediated by bile acids and lipases. First, triglycerides must undergo micellar emulsification, a process that involves the physical breakdown of molecules, followed by hydrolysis of triglycerides into monoglycerides and fatty acids for absorption.

Bile acids play an important role in the emulsification of lipids. They have hydrophilic and hydrophobic domains. Bile acids break down aggregates of triglycerides into smaller droplets to increase surface area to be acted upon by lipase. Pancreatic lipase hydrolyses triglycerides to free fatty acids and monoglyceride. Micelles are formed, which are even smaller aggregates of mixed lipids and bile acids. Micelles allow for a greater surface for interaction with small intestine brush border enterocytes for uptake. Free fatty acids and monoglycerides are taken up into the enterocytes by simple diffusion. See **Figure 35.4**.

In the very premature infant, lipid digestion and absorption are limited owing to lower bile acid concentration in the duodenum. Micellar solubilization is also less efficient leading to lower absorption of molecules. Digestion of long-chain triglycerides proceeds in the presence of bile salt–stimulated lipase, which is present in human milk.

Two types of pancreatic enzymes that are involved in lipid hydrolysis are found in adults: (a) pancreatic lipase and (b) pancreatic carboxylase esterase. Lipases show the lowest activity at birth and slowly increase to adult levels within the first 6 months. During the first week of life, lipase activity increases fourfold in a linear matter (39,40).

Clinical Correlation

As mentioned, term and preterm infants have a relative pancreatic insufficiency when compared to older children, with lower levels of pancreatic lipases noted at birth; these levels increase to near-adult levels by 6 months of life. Human milk exhibits esterolytic activity not shown in bovine milk (40). Bile salt–stimulated lipase present in human colostrum and term milk aids in the digestion of long-chain triglycerides (41,42). Bile acid levels measured in the duodenum, important for normal fat digestion and absorption, are also lower in preterm infants compared to those in term infants (39). This is due to decreased synthesis by the immature hepatocytes as well as lower ileal reabsorption.

Essential fatty acid deficiency occurs when there is inadequate intake of linoleic and linolenic acid. Under normal circumstances, these 18-carbon fatty acids are converted by desaturase and elongase enzymes into long-chain polyunsaturated fatty acids (LCPUFAs) with greater than 20 carbons. These LCPUFAs are required for formation of eicosanoids that in turn are critical in numerous metabolic processes as well as synthesis of CNS structures. Whether or not preterm human infants have the ability to complete this conversion of dietary essential fatty acids into LCPUFAs is a matter of debate. In the uterus, the fetus receives appreciable quantities of docosahexaenoic acid (DHA) via transfer from the mother. However, many of the currently used intravenous lipid solutions do not contain preformed DHA. Although preformed DHA as well as other LCPUFAs are present in human milk, and formulas are supplemented with DHA, many very preterm infants receive limited enteral nutrition for the first week or two after birth, hence do not receive the same quantities they would have received had they remained *in utero*, and develop a deficit.

New intravenous lipid preparations containing fish oil have become available. Studies show that lipid emulsions using formulations of soybean oil, olive oil, MCT, and fish oil are safe and well tolerated. There is also a growing body of data that indicates this decreases the degree of parenteral nutrition–associated liver disease (43). It is unclear if these contain the right balance of lipids for preterm infants.

Vitamins D, Calcium, Iron, and Phosphorus

Two-thirds of a fetus's accumulation of calcium occurs during the last trimester of pregnancy. Calcium accretion ranges from 90 mg/kg/d to a peak of 150 mg/kg/d by the 36th week of gestation (44). Intestinal absorption of calcium in the preterm infant increases with postnatal age. Infants absorb 50% to 80% of their dietary intake (45,46). Several calciotropic hormones—vitamin D, parathyroid hormone (PTH), parathyroid hormone–related peptide (PTHrP), growth hormone, calcitonin, insulin-like growth factors, and $1,25\text{-}(OH)_2$ cholecalciferol, all contribute to an elaborate mechanism in which calcium homeostasis is achieved.

Parathyroid hormone stimulates bone resorption of calcium and the conversion of 25-OH vitamin D to the more active $1,25(OH)_2$ vitamin D. Calcitonin lowers serum calcium by decreasing renal and bone calcium resorption. PTHrP stimulates placental calcium transfer in response to low PTH or hypocalcemia.

Vitamin D_3 is synthesized in the skin and can also be found in fish oils. Also known as cholecalciferol, it is converted to 24-OH vitamin D in the liver and subsequently converted to $1,25\,(OH)_2$ vitamin D.

Eighty percent of iron accretion in the term infant occurs between 24 and 40 weeks of gestation (47,48). Iron can be absorbed in the form of ferritin and hemoprotein, which is usually contained in the liver and muscles of red meat. This is not a typical source of iron in the neonate. Breast milk contains little heme iron (49). Neonates also obtain iron through the inorganic ferrous form. This can be delivered by dietary supplements or added into formula feeds (see Chapter 20). Iron absorption occurs in the enterocytes of the duodenum.

Clinical Correlation

Osteopenia of prematurity is a metabolic bone disease characterized by undermineralization of the skeleton of the premature infant. This is due to delayed or inadequate skeletal mineralization in the extrauterine environment. The etiology of this disorder is multifactorial, most likely a combination of decreased calcium and phosphorus delivery, vitamin D deficiency, bone toxicity, increased mineral needs, and increased calcium losses.

Iron deficiency anemia is a severe form of iron deficiency. Many studies have demonstrated early iron deficiency with cognitive deficits (50,51).

GASTROINTESTINAL MOTILITY

The maturation of the gastrointestinal motility hinges on a sophisticated coordination between the developing neuromuscular innervations and anatomic structures.

Gastrointestinal motility is influenced by several factors that include anatomic and physiologic changes, embryologic development, and maturation of the central and enteric nervous systems.

THE NEWBORN INFANT

Simply put, the neonatal gut facilitates the transit of food and luminal contents away from the airway and through the GI tract to enable the absorption of nutrients and the excretion of waste (52–54).

Peristalsis is first identified in the fetal period and continues to evolve and mature throughout the first postnatal year. Peristalsis is facilitated by gastric, duodenal, and midgut contractions. These contractions are modulated by the autonomic, central, and enteric nervous systems. The interstitial cells of Cajal, specialized muscle cells in the duodenum, play a role in triggering contraction. Motor function is also affected by endocrine and exocrine activity, which may result in excitatory or inhibitory modulation. These reflexes mature in frequency, sensitivity, and magnitude in accordance with postnatal age (55–57).

Sucking and Swallowing

The passage of a liquid bolus, sucking, is the adaptation of the neonatal oral cavity. The development of sucking, expression of milk from breast or bottle, begins *in utero* and continues after birth. As early as 15 weeks of gestation, oral and lingual movements are appreciated and continue to progress to coordinated sucks until 28 weeks. Preterm and term infants exhibit maturation of the sucking patterns postnatally. As the infant grows, the oral cavity may enlarge enough to be able to manage a food bolus, which usually commences around 3 to 4 months of age (58–60).

Swallowing, the propulsion of a liquid bolus through the pharynx to the esophagus, proceeds directly after sucking. Contraction of longitudinal and intrinsic lingual muscles, elevation of the tongue, and a peristaltic wave contribute to the propagation of the food bolus into the pharynx. This is followed by soft palate and laryngeal muscle elevation, closure of the nasopharynx and epiglottis. The swallowing center in the medulla is composed of two main regions that control the neural integration of this highly coordinated response—the nucleus tractus solitarius and the nucleus ambiguus (61–63).

Esophageal Peristalsis

In neonates, pharyngeal and esophageal sphincter functions have been characterized. On average, upper esophageal sphincter (UES) pressure increases over time from a newborn of an average of 17 mm Hg to approximately 53 mm Hg on adults. Correspondingly, the lower esophageal sphincter (LES) tone increases with maturation. Preterm infants may exhibit lower esophageal relaxation as early as 26 weeks of gestation (64,65).

Primary peristalsis is an integrated sequence that is dependent on swallowing. After swallowing, the UES relaxes and the esophageal body propagates the food contents until they reach the distal end where the LES relaxes to allow entry to the stomach. UES pressure is generated by contraction of the cricopharyngeal muscle. Reflexes mature as the infant ages along with coordination of the sequence of relaxation. During primary peristalsis, respiration is paused during swallowing to prevent the food bolus from entering the airway. This sequence can be initiated by swallowing, sucking, or local distention. Food is pushed into the stomach by the sequential contraction of circular muscle causing a peristaltic wave. This entire complex is an interface between afferent and efferent nerves, and effectors and receptors, which mature over the course of gestation. The LES pressure has two main components: the crural diaphragm and the smooth muscle sphincter. Both swallowing and peristaltic activity permit LES relaxation to allow passage of food into the stomach (66–68).

Gastric Motility

The stomach functions to temporarily store and mechanically break down food and facilitate passage into the duodenum. The stomach receives food boluses by relaxation mediated by the vagal nerve in the fundus. The antrum is responsible for the churning of food, along with initiating secretions to help with digestion, and emptying to the small intestines. Gastric emptying is known to be delayed during severe illness or stress. Gastric emptying is slow in the very preterm infant and matures over time. Several factors

such as medications, caloric density, and rate of tube feeding have been shown to affect gastric emptying (57,69,70).

Gastric emptying is also regulated by feedback from the duodenum. Once food reaches the duodenum, neural feedback promotes a decrease in fundal tone and suppressed antral contraction and stimulates pyloric contraction. Somatostatin, produced by delta cells found in the pyloric antrum, duodenum, and pancreatic islets, acts to decrease gastric acid production, inhibit pancreatic exocrine secretion, reduce splanchnic blood flow, and decrease gastrointestinal motility

Small Intestinal Motility

As early as 24 weeks of gestation, motor function of the small intestine has been identified. The small bowel has two principle responses—a fasting and a fed response. The fasting state is described as cyclical gut contractions in four phases. A state of quiescence is followed by contractions increasing in frequency and intensity, and then contractile waveforms migrating in sequence distally (migrating motor complex). The fourth phase is reappearance of quiescence. The migrating motor complex is triggered by the hormone motilin, whose effects are stunted in infants younger than 32 weeks of gestation. Initiation of small feeds accelerates maturation of the faster motor patterns. The second chief response is the fed response. During the fed response, muscle layers are disorganized, which results in churning and mixing of nutrients and secretions producing chime (71–73).

Colonic Motility

The colon serves as a temporary storage of fecal contents and as a conduit to move stool from small intestine to the rectum. Colonic responses usually manifest postprandial and with gastric distention.

The interstitial cells of Cajal mediate slow-amplitude activity that initiates colonic contractions that are very much distinct from the small intestine. The internal anal sphincter is maintained in tonic contraction to main continence. Reflex relaxation of the sphincter is typically triggered by feces distending the rectum. Colonic motility follows a circadian rhythm that usually begins upon waking and can occur cyclically throughout the day. (74) Information on colonic motility is limited in premature infants and needs to be further studied.

During defecation, rectal contraction positions fecal material into the anal canal, which then stimulates stretch receptors. Stretch receptors initiate a spinal reflex that leads to relaxation of the internal anal sphincter. By 26 weeks of gestation, the infant may present with normal anorectal pressure and inhibitory reflexes to defecation (75–77).

Clinical Correlation

Gastrointestinal motor function is complex and encompasses the ability to coordinate suck and swallow and still breathe, and move food down through the digestive absorptive pathways of the intestinal tract. Abnormal motility patterns may result in gastroesophageal reflux (GER) disease, feeding intolerance due to delayed gastric emptying, and poor passage of undigested–unabsorbed waste material from the intestinal tract.

Oral Feeding Skills

Under normal circumstances, aspiration of food does not occur because respiration is inhibited by the act of swallowing. Cardiorespiratory immaturity in preterm infants precludes this protective mechanism and necessitates feeding via enteral tubes inserted into the stomach via the nose or mouth. Usually, at a corrected gestational age of 33 to 34 weeks, most preterm infants begin to exhibit coordination comparable to full term infants.

Gastroesophageal Reflux

The movement of gastric contents into the esophagus can be a normal response in humans and may be quite frequent. This is termed

GER. On the other hand, GER disease (GERD) occurs when reflux causes distressing symptoms or complications such as aspiration pneumonia, esophagitis, or failure to thrive. Management of GERD is usually with feeding modification or antireflux medications.

GER is commonly blamed for apneas and bradycardia in preterm infants. Although apneic events are often associated with signs suggestive of reflux such as arching and coughing, studies have not been able to document a true causal relationship between GER and apnea (78). Infants with GERD have longer hospital stays than do infants without GERD.

Although GER symptoms are typically often treated with acid suppression medications such as H_2 antagonists (ranitidine, famotidine, nizatidine) and proton pump inhibitors (PPI; omeprazole, lansoprazole, esomeprazole), it is becoming clear that routine use of these medications may be associated with increased risk of necrotizing enterocolitis and late-onset sepsis thought to be at least partially due to a dysbiosis induced by alterations in the intestinal acid–base balance. This dysbiosis, in turn, is thought to contribute to increased inflammation in the intestine (79,80).

Abnormal Gastric and Intestinal Motility

Delays in gastric emptying are more common in preterm infants than term infants. The greater the caloric density of feeds, the lower is the speed of gastric emptying in infants born between 32 and 39 weeks of gestation. Of interest is the fact that during the last trimester *in utero*, the fetus swallows approximately 450 mL of amniotic fluid per day, which is low in caloric density. Since some preterm infants have difficulty tolerating high-caloric density feeds, one lowering fat or carbohydrate concentration may be a solution, but this may not meet the nutritional needs of these infants. Enteral feeding is a known stimulus that promotes intestinal motility. Enteral feeding of preterm neonates as early as 27 weeks of gestation can stimulate postprandial motor activity (81).

Promotility agents such as macrolides, erythromycin, and azithromycin, which are motilin agonists, are often used to promote gastric emptying. A meta-analysis on the use of erythromycin showed benefits with higher doses (82,83). However, they should be used very selectively and not routinely because of rare but associated complications related to arrhythmias and pyloric stenosis. Other drugs used in the management of hypomotility in the neonate include cholinergic agonists, prokinetic agents, opioid antagonists, cisapride (taken off the market in the United States and several other countries because of rare but serious tachyarrhythmias). It is important to remember that certain drugs such as opioids and magnesium sulfate as well as mydriatics used for ophthalmologic examinations can slow down intestinal motility.

INTESTINAL MUCOSAL BARRIER

The human intestine provides the largest interface of the body to the external environment and is a critical component of the innate immune system. Aside from its function in terms of absorption and digestion, the neonatal gut must adapt to a wide array of bacterial commensals and also microbial threats and pathogens. The neonatal gut transitions from being exposed to amniotic fluid flora to having a complex interaction with enteric microorganisms that include commensal and pathogenic microbes. Understanding the natural course of the developing gut is critical in comprehending the diseases in which the processes are disrupted (1,84). A breakdown in these barrier defenses leads to an imbalance between immune tolerance and exaggerated inflammatory response (85). It is apparent that certain microbial activity in the alimentary canal during development may influence an individual's propensity to acquire certain diseases such as sepsis, NEC, atopic disease, inflammatory bowel disease, and diabetes (86–88).

The intestinal barrier is composed of three primary layers of defense that include (a) cell–antigen interactions, (b) nonspecific mucosal defenses, and (c) specific cell–cell interactions.

Cell–Antigen Interactions

Antimicrobial peptides are proteins preserved by the innate immune system that contributes to antimicrobial defenses. They are usually produced by Paneth cells, although they can also be produced by epithelial cells in response to lipopolysaccharide stimulation. Antimicrobial peptides create pores in the bacteria's cell membrane eventually killing the organism (89,90).

Nonspecific Mucosal Defenses

The gut is protected from colonization by potentially pathogenic bacteria by a host of nonspecific barrier defenses, which includes digestive enzymes, peristalsis, immunoglobulins, and an intestinal mucosal layer. Digestive enzymes assist by eradicating pathogens. Peristalsis ameliorates bacterial stasis and antigen elimination. The intestinal mucosal layer functions as a barrier preventing microorganisms from attaching to epithelial lining, facilitating their removal. This protective layer is composed of water, immunoglobulins, albumin, mucins, and glycolipids. Mucins are produced in the goblet cells, which can up-regulate production when exposed to hormones, inflammatory mediators, lipopolysaccharide, flagellin A, and other microbial-derived factors (84,91,92).

Cell–Cell Interactions

Transcellular and paracellular pathways are crucial in the preservation of the intestinal barrier. These two main pathways regulate passage of substances through the epithelial membranes. The transcellular pathway achieves this goal via the endocytosis of molecules to enter the luminal border of the enterocyte. The paracellular pathway on the other hand uses sophisticated structures called tight junctions. Tight junctions have two mains functions (a) as a barrier and (b) maintenance of electrophysiologic polarity. As a barrier, the tight junctions selectively allow solutes to pass through intracellular space. Transmembrane proteins make up tight junctions, which impedes diffusion of lipids and proteins between the different basolateral and apical membranes (93–96).

Several neonatal exposures affect the intestinal barrier as shown in Table 35.1.

TABLE 35.1

Common Exposures and Effects on Intestinal Mucosal Barrier

Exposure	Effect
Delayed/poor enteral feeding	Villous atrophy
	↓ mucus production
	↓ digestive enzymes
	Poor peristalsis
	Delayed/abnormal bacterial colonization
	↑ intestinal permeability
Prematurity	↓ IgA
	↓ mucus production
	Abnormal inflammatory response
	Poor peristalsis
	↑ intestinal permeability to lactulose
Antibiotics	Abnormal bacterial colonization
H_2 blockers	↓ Gastric acidity
Sedatives, opiates, paralytics	Poor peristalsis
Indomethacin	↑ risk for perforations and enterocyte injury
Stress	↑ intestinal permeability
	Mucosal ischemia

REFERENCES

1. Neu J, Li N. The neonatal gastrointestinal tract: developmental anatomy, physiology, and clinical implications. *Neoreviews* 2003;4(1):7e.
2. Thomas D. Larsen's human embryology. *Osteopat Medizin* 2009.
3. O'Rahilly R, Müller F. Developmental stages in human embryos: revised and new measurements. *Cells Tissues Organs* 2010;192(2):73.
4. Zorn AM, Wells JM. Vertebrate endoderm development and organ formation. *Annu Rev Cell Dev Biol* 2009;25:221.
5. Moore KL, Mark G, et al. The developing human. *Clin Oriented Embryol* 2004.
6. Spence JR, Lauf R, Shroyer NF. Vertebrate intestinal endoderm development. *Dev Dyn* 2011;240(3):501.
7. San Roman AK, Shivdasani RA. Boundaries, junctions and transitions in the gastrointestinal tract. *Exp Cell Res* 2011;317(19):2711.
8. Khan S, Orenstein SR. Embryology, anatomy, and function of the esophagus. In: *Nelson textbook of pediatrics*. Philadelphia, PA: Elsevier, 2011.
9. Höllwarth ME. Esophageal atresia and tracheoesophageal fistula. In: *Pediatric surgery: diagnosis and management*. Berlin Heidelberg/New York: Springer, 2009.
10. Bruch SW, Coran AG, Kunisaki SM. Esophageal malformations. In: *Pediatric thoracic surgery*. Milan: Springer Verlag, 2013.
11. El-Gohary Y, Gittes GK, Tovar JA. Congenital anomalies of the esophagus. *Semin Pediatr Surg* 2010;19(3):186.
12. El-Gohary MA, Etiaby A. Gastric volvulus in infants and children. *Pediatr Surg Int* 1994;9:486.
13. Peitz HG. Volvulus in childhood. *Radiologe* 1997;37(6):439.
14. McIntyre RC Jr, Bensard DD, Karrer FM, et al. The pediatric diaphragm in acute gastric volvulus. *J Am Coll Surg* 1994;178(3):234.
15. Coppola CP. Pyloric stenosis. In: *Pediatric surgery: diagnosis and treatment*. New York: Springer International Publishing, 2014.
16. Mrad C, Chouikh T, Ghorbel S. Hypertrophic pyloric stenosis. In: *Pediatric surgery handbook for residents and medical students*. New York: Nova Biomedical, 2017.
17. Puri P, Kutasy B, Lakshmanadass G. Infantile hypertrophic pyloric stenosis. In: *Newborn surgery*, 4th ed. New York: CRC Press, 2017.
18. Polin RA. *Fetal and neonatal physiology*, Vol. 2. Philadelphia, PA: Elsevier Saunders, 2011.
19. Adams SD, Stanton MP. Malrotation and intestinal atresias. *Early Hum Dev* 2014;90(12):921.
20. Hong AR. Duodenal atresia. In: *Fundamentals of pediatric surgery*, 2nd ed. 2016.
21. Stoll C, Alembik Y, Dott B, et al. Omphalocele and gastroschisis and associated malformations. *Am J Med Genet A* 2008;146A:1280.
22. Christison-Lagay ER, Kelleher CM, Langer JC. Neonatal abdominal wall defects. *Semin Fetal Neonatal Med* 2011;16(3):164.
23. So S, Patterson C, Gold A, et al. Early neurodevelopmental outcomes of infants with intestinal failure. *Early Hum Dev* 2016;101:11.
24. Puri P, Höllwarth M. *Pediatric surgery: diagnosis and management*. Berlin Heidelberg/New York: Springer-Verlag, 2009.
25. Kluth D. Embryology of anorectal malformations. *Semin Pediatr Surg* 2010;19(3):201.
26. Holschneider AM, Fritsch H, Holschneider P. Anatomy and function of the normal rectum and anus. In: *Anorectal malformations in children: embryology, diagnosis, surgical treatment, follow-up*. Berlin Heidelberg/New York: Springer-Verlag, 2006.
27. Avansino JR, Levitt MA. Hirschsprung disease. In: *Fundamentals of pediatric surgery*, 2nd ed. Philadelphia, PA: Elsevier, 2016.
28. Ando H. Embryology of the biliary tract. *Dig Surg* 2010;27(2):87.
29. Mattei P. *Fundamentals of pediatric surgery*. New York: Springer International Publishing, 2011.
30. Kien CL. Digestion, absorption, and fermentation of carbohydrates in the newborn. *Clin Perinatol* 1996;23(2):211.
31. Hegardt P, Lindberg T, Börjesson J, et al. Amylase in human milk from mothers of preterm and term infants. *J Pediatr Gastroenterol Nutr* 1984;3(4):563.
32. Rossiter MA, Barrowman JA, Dand A, et al. Amylase content of mixed saliva in children. *Acta Paediatr Scand* 1974;63(3):389.
33. Antonowicz I, Lebenthal E. Developmental pattern of small intestinal enterokinase and disaccharidase activities in the human fetus. *Gastroenterology* 1977;72(6):1299.
34. Shulman RJ, Schanler RJ, Lau C, et al. Early feeding, feeding tolerance, and lactase activity in preterm infants. *J Pediatr* 1998;133(5):645.
35. DiPalma J, Kirk CL, Hamosh M, et al. Lipase and pepsin activity in the gastric mucosa of infants, children, and adults. *Gastroenterology* 1991;101(1):116.
36. Fairclough PD, Silk DB, Clark ML, et al. Proceedings: new evidence for intact di- and tripeptide absorption. *Gut* 1975;16(10):843.
37. Adibi SA, Morse EL, Masilamani SS, et al. Evidence for two different modes of tripeptide disappearance in human intestine. Uptake by peptide carrier systems and hydrolysis by peptide hydrolases. *J Clin Invest* 1975;56(6):1355.
38. Mihatsch WA, Franz AR, Högel J, et al. Hydrolyzed protein accelerates feeding advancement in very low birth weight infants. *Pediatrics* 2002;110(6):1199.
39. Boehm G, Braun W, Moro G. Bile acid concentrations in serum and duodenal aspirates of healthy preterm infants: effects of gestational and postnatal age. *Biol Neonate* 1997;71(4):207.
40. Tarassuk NP, Nickerson TA, Yaguchi M. Lipase action in human milk. *Nature* 1964;201:298.
41. Arora NK, Hall B, Maller DPR. Bile salt stimulated lipolytic activity of human milk. *Indian J Pediatr* 1982;49:575.
42. Freed LM, York CM, Hamosh P, et al. Bile salt-stimulated lipase of human milk: characteristics of the enzyme in the milk of mothers of premature and full-term infants. *J Pediatr Gastroenterol Nutr* 1987;6(4):598.
43. Kapoor V, Glover R, Malviya MN. Alternative lipid emulsions versus pure soy oil based lipid emulsions for parenterally fed preterm infants. *Cochrane Database Syst Rev* 2015;2015(12):CD009172.
44. Shaw JCL. Evidence for defective skeletal mineralization in low birthweight infants: the absorption of calcium and fat. *Pediatrics* 1976;57(1):16.
45. Hillman LS, Johnson LS, Lee DZ, et al. Measurement of true absorption, endogenous fecal excretion, urinary excretion, and retention of calcium in term infants by using a dual-tracer, stable-isotope method. *J Pediatr* 1993;123(3):444.
46. Schanler R, Atkinson S, Tsang R, et al. *Nutrition of the preterm infant—scientific basis and practical guidelines*. Cincinnati, OH: Digit Educ Publ Inc., 2005.
47. Singla PN, Gupta VK, Agarwal KN. Storage iron in human foetal organs. *Acta Paediatr Scand* 1985;74(5):701.
48. Widdowson EM, Spray CM. Chemical development in utero. *Arch Dis Child* 1951;26(127):205.
49. Collard KJ. Iron homeostasis in the neonate. *Pediatrics* 2009;123(4):1208.
50. Lozoff B, Jimenez E, Hagen J, et al. Poorer behavioral and developmental outcome more than 10 years after treatment for iron deficiency in infancy. *Pediatrics* 2000;105(4):E51.
51. Logan S, Martins S, Gilbert R. Iron therapy for improving psychomotor development and cognitive function in children under the age of three with iron deficiency anaemia. *Cochrane Database Syst Rev* 2001;(2):CD001444.
52. Mansfield LE. Embryonic origins of the relation of gastroesophageal reflux disease and airway disease. *Am J Med* 2001;111(suppl 8A):3S.
53. Sadler TW. *Langman's Essential Medical Embryology*. Philadelphia, PA: Wolters Kluwer Health/Lippincott Williams & Wilkins, 2012.
54. Miller JL, Sonies BC, Macedonia C. Emergence of oropharyngeal, laryngeal and swallowing activity in the developing fetal upper aerodigestive tract: an ultrasound evaluation. *Early Hum Dev* 2003;71(1):61.
55. Grundy D. The enteric nervous system. *Eur J Gastroenterol Hepatol* 2006;22(2):102.
56. Berseth CL. Gastrointestinal motility in the neonate. *Clin Perinatol* 1996;23(2):179.
57. Berseth CL. Motor function in the stomach and small intestine in the neonate. *NeoReviews* 2006;7(1):e28.
58. Bu'Lock F, Woolridge MW, Baum JD. Development of co-ordination of sucking, swallowing and breathing: ultrasound study of term and preterm infants. *Dev Med Child Neurol* 1990;32(8):669.
59. Rommel N, van Wijk M, Boets B, et al. Development of pharyngo-esophageal physiology during swallowing in the preterm infant. *Neurogastroenterol Motil* 2011;23(10):e401.
60. Mizuno K, Ueda A. The maturation and coordination of sucking, swallowing, and respiration in preterm infants. *J Pediatr* 2003;142(1):36.
61. Miller AJ. The neurobiology of swallowing and dysphagia. *Dev Disabil Res Rev* 2008;14(2):77.
62. Broussard DL, Altschuler SM. Central integration of swallow and airway-protective reflexes. *Am J Med* 2000;108(suppl 4a):62S.
63. Michou E, Hamdy S. Cortical input in control of swallowing. *Curr Opin Otolaryngol Head Neck Surg* 2009;17(3):166.
64. Staiano A, Boccia G, Salvia G, et al. Development of esophageal peristalsis in preterm and term neonates. *Gastroenterology* 2007;132(5):1718.
65. Omari TI, Miki K, Fraser R, et al. Esophageal body and lower esophageal sphincter function in healthy premature infants. *Gastroenterology* 1995;109(6):1757.
66. Singendonk MMJ, Rommel N, Omari TI, et al. Upper gastrointestinal motility: prenatal development and problems in infancy. *Nat Rev Gastroenterol Hepatol* 2014;11(9):545.
67. Sivarao DV, Goyal RK. Functional anatomy and physiology of the upper esophageal sphincter. *Am J Med* 2000;108(suppl 4a):27S.
68. Bowie JD, Clair MR. Fetal swallowing and regurgitation: observation of normal and abnormal activity. *Radiology* 1982;144(4):877.
69. Gariepy CE. Intestinal motility disorders and development of the enteric nervous system. *Pediatr Res* 2001;49:605.
70. Jadcherla SR, Klee G, Berseth CL. Regulation of migrating motor complexes by motilin and pancreatic polypeptide in human infants. *Pediatr Res* 1997;42(3):365.
71. Jones MP, Bratten JR. Small intestinal motility. *Curr Opin Gastroenterol* 2008;24(2):164.
72. Berseth CL. Gestational evolution of small intestine motility in preterm and term infants. *J Pediatr* 1989;115(4):646.

73. Al Tawil Y, Berseth CL. Gestational and postnatal maturation of duodenal motor responses to intragastric feeding. *J Pediatr* 1996;129(3):374.
74. Soffer EE, Scalabrini P, Wingate DL. Prolonged ambulant monitoring of human colonic motility. *Am J Physiol* 1989;257(4 Pt 1):G601.
75. Bharucha AE. Pelvic floor: anatomy and function. *Neurogastroenterol Motil* 2006;18(7):507.
76. Benninga MA, Omari TI, Haslam RR, et al. Characterization of anorectal pressure and the anorectal inhibitory reflex in healthy preterm and term infants. *J Pediatr* 2001;139(2):233.
77. Whitehead WE, Schuster MM. Anorectal physiology and pathophysiology. *Am J Gastroenterol* 1987;82(6):487.
78. Di Fiore JM, Poets CF, Gauda E, et al. Cardiorespiratory events in preterm infants: etiology and monitoring technologies. *J Perinatol* 2015;36(3):165.
79. Guillet R. Association of H2-blocker therapy and higher incidence of necrotizing enterocolitis in very low birth weight infants. *Pediatrics* 2006;117(2):e137.
80. Dalton J, Schumacher R. H2-blockers are associated with necrotizing enterocolitis in very low birthweight infants. *J Pediatr* 2012;161(1):168.
81. Jadcherla SR, Chan CY, Moore R, et al. Impact of feeding strategies on the frequency and clearance of acid and nonacid gastroesophageal reflux events in dysphagic neonates. *JPEN J Parenter Enteral Nutr* 2012;42(3):365.
82. Ng E, Shah VS. Erythromycin for the prevention and treatment of feeding intolerance in preterm infants. *Cochrane Database Syst Rev* 2008;(3):CD001815.
83. Ng PC, Lee CH, Wong SP, et al. High-dose oral erythromycin decreased the incidence of parenteral nutrition-associated cholestasis in preterm infants. *Gastroenterology* 2007;132(5):1726.
84. Neu J, Mackey AD. Neonatal gastrointestinal innate immunity. *NeoReviews* 2003;4(1):e14.
85. Fasano A, Shea-Donohue T. Mechanisms of disease: the role of intestinal barrier function in the pathogenesis of gastrointestinal autoimmune diseases. *Nat Clin Pract Gastroenterol Hepatol* 2005;2(9):416.
86. Tlaskalová-Hogenová H, Štěpánková R, Kozáková H, et al. The role of gut microbiota (commensal bacteria) and the mucosal barrier in the pathogenesis of inflammatory and autoimmune diseases and cancer: contribution of germ-free and gnotobiotic animal models of human diseases. *Cell Mol Immunol* 2011;8(2):110.
87. Abrahamsson TR, Jakobsson HE, Andersson AF, et al. Low diversity of the gut microbiota in infants with atopic eczema. *J Allergy Clin Immunol* 2012;129(2):434.
88. Johnson CL, Versalovic J. The human microbiome and its potential importance to pediatrics. *Pediatrics* 2012;129(5):950.
89. McElroy SJ, Weitkamp JH. Innate immunity in the small intestine of the preterm infant. *NeoReviews* 2011;12(9):e517.
90. Louis NA, Lin PW. The intestinal immune barrier. *NeoReviews* 2009;10(4):e180.
91. Martin CR, Caicedo RA, Walker WA. Development of the intestinal mucosal barrier. In: Walker WA, ed. *Gastroenterology and nutrition: neonatology questions and controversies*. Philadelphia, PA: Elsevier Saunders, 2012.
92. Dharmani P, Srivastava V, Kissoon-Singh V, et al. Role of intestinal mucins in innate host defense mechanisms against pathogens. *J Innate Immun* 2009;1(2):123.
93. Schneeberger EE, Lynch RD. The tight junction: a multifunctional complex. *Am J Physiol Cell Physiol* 2004;286(6):C1213.
94. Anderson JM, Van Itallie CM. Physiology and function of the tight junction. *Cold Spring Harb Perspect Biol* 2009;1(2):a002584.
95. González-Mariscal L, Betanzos A, Nava P, et al. Tight junction proteins. *Prog Biophys Mol Biol* 2003;81(1):1.
96. Groschwitz KR, Hogan SP. Intestinal barrier function: Molecular regulation and disease pathogenesis. *J Allergy Clin Immunol* 2009;124(1):3.

THE NEWBORN INFANT

36 Disorders of the Gastrointestinal Tract

Janice A. Taylor and Josef Neu

INTRODUCTION

In this chapter, the presentation, evaluation, assessment, and management of congenital structural anomalies of the gastrointestinal system, gastrointestinal dysfunction, and disorders that primarily occur in the premature population are discussed. There may be overlap of these diagnoses in patients encountered by the neonatologist, so these crossover situations will also be reviewed within the relevant context. It is important to note that even the most commonly encountered diagnoses, like reflux and necrotizing enterocolitis, do not always lend themselves to straightforward management solutions; these controversies will be addressed, knowing that the combination of bench-to-bedside research, expert opinion, and application of evidence-based medicine can be a fickle relationship. With advances in prenatal care, many congenital anomalies are diagnosed *in utero*, allowing for parents to have important conversations with health care providers and family members regarding expectations for the outcomes once the fetus is delivered, and what long-term prognoses to anticipate, including quality of life. The referral of these families to centers that provide complex fetal counseling is as appropriate as the timing of the referral, to accommodate for any multidisciplinary planning needs. While many disorders of the gastrointestinal system may lend themselves to surgical correction, it is not uncommon—and appropriate—that associated anomalies or concurrent comorbidities may result in a family's decision for palliative or comfort care for their newborn.

ANOMALIES OF THE ESOPHAGUS AND TRACHEA: ESOPHAGEAL ATRESIA/TRACHEOESOPHAGEAL FISTULA

During fetal life, the trachea and esophagus begin developing as one single lumen. This separates into two distinct lumens at approximately 4 to 8 weeks after conception. These are separated by a "wall." If this wall does not form properly, congenital anomalies of the esophagus and trachea may occur. Esophageal atresia (EA) pertains to an esophagus that ends in a blind pouch. Depending on the subtype of EA/TEF diagnosis, this atretic pouch can be proximal, distal, or both. Tracheoesophageal fistula (TEF) refers to the abnormal connection that develops between the trachea and esophagus. The separation of the trachea and esophagus is believed to be facilitated by signaling factors that include Noggin and sonic hedgehog (Shh), which are believed to be involved in the development of type C EA/TEF (1). The overall process of how EA/TEF develops is poorly understood, but it is generally agreed that it is multifactorial, the end result of the effects of genetic, embryologic, and environmental influences.

The worldwide prevalence of EA is 2.44 per 10,000 births, ranging between 1.77 and 3.68 per 10,000 births (2). Sixty percent of newborns with EA will have coexisting anomalies. These include vertebral anomalies (V), anal atresia (A), cardiac anomalies (C), tracheoesophageal fistula (T), renal anomalies (R), and limb anomalies (L), often referred to as the "VACTERL" association. The current definition of VACTERL is presence of at least three of the involved anomalies in the absence of a specific genetic diagnosis. Trisomy 21, trisomy 18, 22q11 deletion, and CHARGE (coloboma, heart defects, atresia choanae, growth retardation, genital abnormalities, and ear abnormalities) are the most common syndromic diagnoses, distinguishing the VACTERL

association from these clearer genetic syndromes. About 88.5% cases of EA and 77.8% cases of EA + TEF are likely not to meet the criteria for VACTERL (3). The types of EA/TEF anomalies are illustrated in Figure 36.1.

Diagnosis

Although the symptoms of EA/TEF may differ depending on the anomaly, some of the most common symptoms include frothy saliva from the mouth shortly after birth. This is often witnessed in the delivery room. Other symptoms include coughing or choking with feeding, vomiting, cyanosis, and respiratory distress.

Some cases can be diagnosed prenatally by ultrasound. Routine prenatal ultrasounds that are performed around 20 weeks' gestation ("anatomy scans") can detect these anomalies: polyhydramnios and a small or absent stomach bubble will arouse suspicion for EA/TEF. Magnetic resonance and amniotic fluid analyses may improve prenatal diagnostic accuracy over ultrasound (4). Such early diagnosis using these techniques can significantly improve postnatal outcomes by improving the clinical team's preparedness for the potential problems that might arise shortly after birth. For isolated EA/TEF, there is no current indication for prenatal intervention.

After birth, EA/TEF can be suspected on clinical evaluation. In addition to the symptoms mentioned previously, confirmation is accomplished by inserting a Salem sump or Replogle tube. If these tubes do not pass beyond approximately 10 cm and coil in the upper thoracic region, a diagnosis of EA with or without TEF should be considered. Radiographs as seen in Figure 36.2 can confirm the diagnosis. Absence of gas in the stomach suggests isolated EA, or EA/TEF without the distal TEF.

Management

Appropriate preoperative management of a neonate with EA/TEF is crucial. Once diagnosed, it is important for the infant to have nothing by mouth (NPO) and to start intravenous fluids. The infant's head should be positioned between approximately 30 and 40 degrees to prevent reflux of secretions into the esophagus and/or trachea. A Replogle tube should be used to prevent aspiration. It is important to also evaluate for concomitant anomalies in the VACTERL association such as congenital heart disease and anal, renal, and vertebral anomalies by thorough physical examination: echocardiogram, babygram, spinal ultrasound, and renal ultrasound. The echocardiogram is important not just to identify congenital cardiac defects but to confirm left-sided position of the descending aorta; this has significant implications for surgical repair.

Preoperative respiratory management must be carefully managed. When a TEF is present, it is preferable to have the baby breathing room air without the aid of noninvasive support or intubation. Positive pressure ventilation will preferentially pass into a distal TEF and into the stomach. Without a way to decompress the stomach with a proximal EA, there can be significant cardiorespiratory compromise and in extreme situations, gastric perforation. Additional attention to this must be paid if the baby also has imperforate anus or any evidence of proximal intestinal atresia. Thus, keeping the baby minimally agitated and on room air is of paramount importance. If the baby requires intubation or significant positive pressure, close attention must be paid to the abdomen for distention, and a histamine blocker or proton pump inhibitor should be started to help decrease the effects of gastroesophageal reflux (GER) from the TEF into the distal trachea. Intubation and

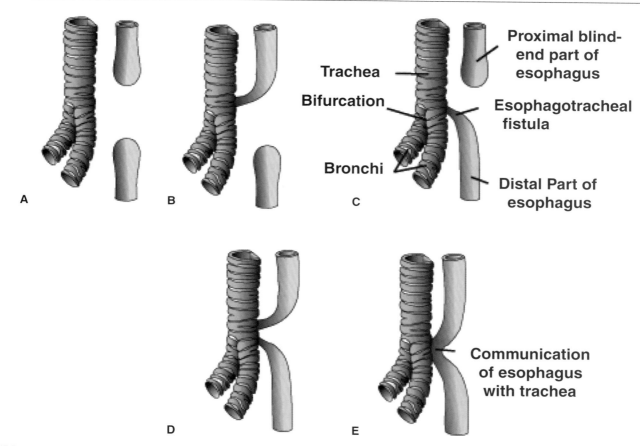

FIGURE 36.1 **Different types of esophageal atresia-tracheoesophageal anomalies. A:** Type A is pure esophageal atresia. **B:** Type B is a proximal tracheoesophageal fistula with distal esophageal atresia. **C:** Type C is a proximal esophageal atresia with distal tracheoesophageal fistula. **D:** Type D has proximal and distal tracheoesophageal fistulas. **E:** Type E is an isolated tracheoesophageal fistula. (Reprinted with permission from Sadler TW. *Langman's Medical Embryology.* 9th ed. Philadelphia, PA: Wolters Kluwer, 2003.)

THE NEWBORN INFANT

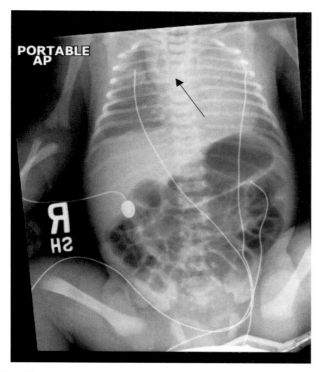

FIGURE 36.2 **Babygram in patient with newly diagnosed esophageal atresia with distal tracheoesophageal fistula.** Note Replogle coiled in proximal esophagus (*arrow*) and gas-filled stomach and bowel. (Photo courtesy of Janice Taylor, MD.)

need for significant positive pressure may be a driving force in the timing of operation.

Specific details of surgical repair of EA/TEF are beyond the scope of this chapter. Most of these repairs consist of fistula ligation and esophageal anastomosis through a right-sided thoracotomy. Thoracoscopic repair may be entertained based on the baby's comorbidities, size, and gestational age. The operation is often started with a bronchoscopy to evaluate for associated tracheomalacia, laryngeal cleft, proximal TEF, and position of distal TEF relative to the carina. This distal TEF takeoff is valuable information for the anesthesia and surgery teams when managing episodes of respiratory decompensation during surgery. The location of the distal TEF also helps to further plan intraoperatively for the gap length needed to traverse to create the esophageal anastomosis. There is usually a notion of this preoperatively, taking the number of vertebral bodies between the end of the proximal esophageal pouch and the carina as the anticipated greatest distance possible between the esophageal limbs.

In newborns with isolated EA, repair is still initiated with bronchoscopy to confirm the clinical and radiographic suspicions of lack of Replogle passage with a gasless abdomen. Gastrostomy tube placement is also performed so that the newborn may receive enteral feeds while awaiting esophageal reconstruction. The anastomosis of the proximal and distal ends of isolated EA is typically done in a delayed fashion to allow for growth of the patient, and for procedures to assess the gap length (the distance between the proximal and distal atretic ends of the esophagus) with patient growth, which are usually done with certain maneuvers to lengthen the esophagus. Thus, the patient may be approximately 2 to 3 months old before he or she is appropriate for esophageal reconstruction. Timing is critical, as the longer the gap, the higher likelihood of postoperative complications like anastomotic leak and stricture. The isolated EA is generally considered to be a long gap variant if the distance between the ends is at least three vertebral bodies long, or 3 cm; there is no standard method of measuring.

Operative and nonoperative options exist for esophageal lengthening, for which decisions are based on patient size, gap length, and the presence of comorbidities. Nonoperative methods to lengthen the esophagus and shorten the gap distance include, but are not limited to, spontaneous growth if the distance does not appear extensive on initial assessment but reconstruction is delayed due to patient factors, and interval bougienage. Access to the distal esophageal limb may be through the gastrostomy site. Operative methods to lengthen the esophagus include, but are not limited to, staged lengthening of the proximal and distal ends, placement of traction sutures, and use of stomach, small bowel, or colon.

Extubation of the patient after EA/TEF surgery should be done without haste. Reintubation should be performed by an experienced team member, to limit the risk of disrupting the fresh esophageal anastomosis if the esophagus is inadvertently intubated. Parenteral nutrition should be provided shortly after surgery. Enteral feeds may be initiated using a transanastomotic feeding tube, or by mouth, and is typically started after contrast study usually 1 week after surgery to confirm lack of anastomotic leak. The output of a chest tube placed during surgery will also help determine presence of a leak.

Postoperative Complications

Survival for EA/TEF is now approximately 90% in patients even with severe associated anomalies. The mortality of patients born with EA/TEF is more likely to be related to their cardiac, pulmonary, or renal anomalies, or prematurity related if the baby is not term. Regarding long-gap EA, this subset of patients is at increased risk of long-term morbidity due to the higher potential of anastomotic complications due to tension or need for replacement, patient size, or corrected gestational age, if they underwent delayed primary repair, or a combination of these factors.

Acute postrepair complications typically are related to the esophageal anastomosis. Anastomotic leak can be identified by the occurrence of frothy saliva or feeds in the chest tube. Postoperative esophagram to evaluate for this prior to initiating feeds is typically performed 1 week after surgery. The chest tube may be left in place for up to a day after initiating feeds, after negative esophagram.

Infants who develop anastomotic stricture may have dysphagia or respiratory distress with oral feeds. This may occur as early as 3 weeks after surgery. Esophagram will confirm suspicions. Strictures are typically treated with balloon dilation with use of fluoroscopy, and sometimes need to be addressed with serial dilations. Motility disorders are expected, with the distal esophageal limb having more abnormal motility than the proximal end. Swallowing function is normal in the oral phase. Dysmotility will manifest as reflux, dysphagia, foreign body impaction, and upper respiratory infections. There are no durable medical or surgical strategies for this, and often the child grows out of them after the first few years of life. Esophageal dilation may help if stricture appears to be a contributing factor, as well as finely chopped foods, teaching the child to chew well, acid suppression, and parental reassurance.

GASTROESOPHAGEAL REFLUX (GER) AND GASTROESOPHAGEAL REFLUX DISEASE (GERD)

GER and gastroesophageal reflux disease (GERD) refer to different entities and are often confused in neonatal intensive care. GER usually refers to a very common physiologic process involving retrograde passage of gastric contents into the esophagus. The physiology of GER/GERD is beyond the scope of this chapter, but we refer you to more detailed reviews that cover this topic in greater detail (5,6). In brief, GER occurs concomitant with transient lower esophageal sphincter relaxation, which involves a decrease in lower esophageal pressures than intragastric pressures. These are quite common in preterm infants (5,6).

When this process becomes associated with cardiorespiratory issues, aspiration pneumonia, injury to the esophagus, or other symptoms that cause concern, it is more commonly referred to as GERD (2). GERD is usually considered a clinically significant entity. Since the material that is refluxed into the esophagus is usually acid, this can be considered injurious to the esophagus if the acidity is high enough and if the quantity is large and rate of recurrence of reflux is often (7). Nevertheless, there remains considerable confusion as to the definition of GER/GERD as witnessed by large diagnostic and treatment variation across different NICUs (8). GERD is of concern because this diagnosis is associated with longer hospital stays and costs than those for infants without GERD (9). GER/GERD is a very common diagnosis in the NICU and is sometimes wrongfully based on soft clinical signs such as apnea, oxygen desaturation and bradycardia, feeding intolerance, poor growth, as well as nonspecific behavioral signs including arching, irritability, and apparent discomfort associated with feedings. The evidence that these signs are caused by GER is lacking (10–13). Its true incidence is unknown, as symptomatic versus benign GER/GERD is subjective despite standard definitions, and presentations can vary based on patient age and underlying conditions.

More definitive diagnostic techniques to evaluate GER in neonates include acid pH measurements and impedance measurements. The former is considered somewhat unreliable because preterm infants produce smaller amounts of acid during different stages of development, rendering this technique somewhat unreliable. Nevertheless, these techniques are not commonly used in the NICU setting (13–15). Use of esophagrams or swallow studies to diagnose pathologic reflux is less reliable, as these studies give a snapshot in time of the patient, whereas the pH probe with or without impedance is a 24-hour study.

In terms of certain putative conditions associated with GER and their treatment, there has been considerable controversy. Apnea and bradycardia have been very commonly treated with antireflux medications, agents that decrease stomach acid production, and even promotility agents. These have not been found to be beneficial and in fact can cause harm and are no longer recommended for this purpose (16–18). It has been hypothesized that GER may exacerbate chronic lung disease, but the evidence for this is weak at best (19,20). Feeding problems are commonly associated with GER. As mentioned previously, symptoms of discomfort with feedings are commonly associated with GER, but there is little evidence to support that these are causative. Nevertheless, there are studies that suggest that prolonged feedings by pump may be helpful for signs of feeding intolerance (21). Thickening of feedings is common but not supported by strong evidence (22). Positioning to left side down shortly after feeding showed less GER (23), but supine position remains the preferred position because of the concern for sudden infant death (24).

Once there is agreement that a patient has failed nonoperative management of GERD, the Nissen fundoplication is the most common intervention to address this. The Nissen fundoplication is the act of wrapping the fundus of the stomach in a 360-degree retrograde fashion around the distal esophagus, just above the gastroesophageal junction. It may be completed open or laparoscopically and is often done with gastrostomy tube placement to help the infant maintain enteral nutrition within the context of GER/GERD, recovery from surgery, and learning to take nutrition reliably by mouth. Particularly in infants who are neurologically intact and are expected to be able to feed by mouth, it is important to not make the fundoplication too tight, which would impair swallowing. Intraoperatively, size-appropriate bougies are inserted into the esophagus to assist in making the fundoplication an optimal wrap (25).

Large pediatric patient group studies have shown success rates of around 95% (26,27). Case-specific complications from fundoplication are gas bloat and retching, slipped wrap, leak, dysphagia, and persistence or recurrence of reflux. Gas bloat and retching can be addressed with changing rate or volume of feeds, or the type of feed. Slippage of the wrap can manifest as recurrence of reflux, and studying the wrap via contrast study can elucidate this further. Concern of leak or dysphagia may also be assessed with contrast study, to be able to visualize the operative area and extravasation of contrast in the case of a leak, or decreased flow through the region of the wrap in the case of dysphagia. Continued reflux can also be evaluated with a contrast study to determine tightness of the wrap. This can be managed with reinitiation of antireflux medications, revision surgery, postpyloric feeds, or manipulation of the feed type, rate, or volume. Revision fundoplication surgery should be not taken lightly, as subsequent interventions can lead to scarring, distortion of the anatomy, and devascularization, which can lead to continued problems with persistent reflux. In rare cases where pathologic reflux persists that results in aspiration pneumonia or respiratory distress, a gastroesophageal dissociation may be indicated. This would be an option in neurologically impaired patients who are not foreseen to take nutrition by mouth, as this surgical option permanently divides the stomach from the esophagus, with feeds being purely via a gastrostomy tube. The esophagus maintains continuity with the intestinal system via a limb of jejunum that is routed to the distal esophagus, but this is not a clinical scenario where normal oral feeding is tolerated.

Fundoplication to treat reflux is effective but arguably more intervention than is needed when one considers that the infant may be fed as effectively and with less intervention, if fed into the jejunum. Particularly with neurologically impaired infants, fundoplication carries a higher rate of complications. Nasojejunal or gastrojejunal feeds may be as durable an option without exposing the patient to the operative risks of fundoplication. Gastrojejunal feeding tubes may require future anesthetic needs to replace a dislodged tube, and they may pose an obstruction risk if the patient is too small. Single-center studies have evaluated outcomes of patients with fundoplication compared to gastrojejunal feeds and have found similar outcomes regarding reduction of aspiration (28,29). The choice of intervention must be based on not only physiologic factors of the infant but also access to care and social determinants of the family.

In summary, diagnosis and management of GER/GERD is a challenge. Many of the presentations that are considered diagnostic are not. It is to be remembered that many of the signs considered to be associated with GER/GERD are related to overall immaturity and will resolve in time. Pharmacologic therapies have been underwhelming in terms of benefit and may cause harm. Conservative management with optimal nutrition, feeding strategies along with reassurance, tends to be the safest approach in managing most of these infants. Surgery should be reserved for those who truly fail medical management, and enteral access options exist that may allow the infant to safely feed without needing maximum surgical intervention.

STOMACH AND UPPER INTESTINE

Hypertrophic Pyloric Stenosis

Pyloric stenosis is a form of gastric outlet obstruction caused by thickening and elongation of the pylorus. Prior to the description and development of the surgical procedure for pyloric stenosis by Conrad Ramstedt in 1912, most babies with this disorder died. Although hypertrophic pyloric stenosis was first described over a century ago, its cause remains enigmatic (30). Risk factors include

a high predominance in male sex (4:1 male: female), first-born child, prematurity between 28 and 36 weeks' gestational age, and postnatal erythromycin exposure (rate ratio of 29.8 in infants with exposure within the first 2 weeks of life, compared to infants with no exposure) (31). There is also a familial predisposition to occurrence of hypertrophic pyloric stenosis, although no specific genetic factor has been identified. It is more commonly seen in developed countries (30). Pyloric stenosis typically presents between 2 and 8 weeks after birth with nonbilious emesis. This is also true in preterm infants, where correcting for gestational age should not be considered. There is usually an associated history of changes in formula types or addition of acid suppression to help alleviate the emesis, without any effect. The infant typically still shows signs of hunger and interest in feeding after bouts of emesis.

Physical examination includes a palpable "olive" related to the elongated and thickened pylorus and possibly gastric peristalsis waves seen in the mid-upper abdomen, but these forms of diagnosis are becoming less common. The pylorus is often difficult to palpate in a crying infant who is also tightening his/her abdomen. Plain films do not aid in diagnosis of hypertrophic pyloric stenosis. The use of ultrasound is the standard to diagnose and is preferred to upper gastrointestinal imaging with contrast agents. The latter classically shows a "string sign," a narrow passage of contrast through the hypertrophied pylorus. Ultrasound has largely replaced upper GI contrast studies because of its high sensitivity and specificity and lack of exposure to radiation (**Fig. 36.3**). Muscle wall thickness greater than 3 mm and pyloric channel length longer than 14 mm confirm the diagnosis of hypertrophic pyloric stenosis. Passage of gastric fluid, or lack thereof, through the pyloric channel can also be observed on ultrasound.

Serum electrolytes should be checked to manage dehydration, and once the diagnosis is confirmed, to prepare the patient for surgery and anesthesia. Patients with hypertrophic pyloric stenosis will often present with a hypokalemic, hypochloremic metabolic alkalosis due to the long-term emesis. Urine examination may show evidence of paradoxical aciduria. The infant should be adequately resuscitated with isotonic fluids such that urine output and laboratory values normalize, particularly serum chloride

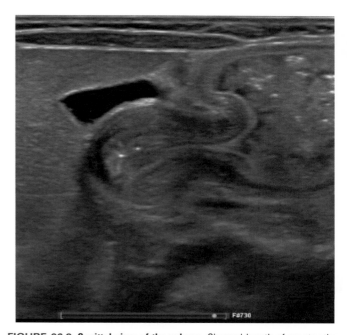

FIGURE 36.3 Sagittal view of the pylorus. Channel length of greater than 14 mm and wall thickness (not total pyloric diameter) of greater than 3 mm are minimal measurements to define hypertrophic pyloric stenosis. (Photo courtesy of Janice Taylor, MD.)

and bicarbonate. Surgery should be delayed until normalization of hydration and of serum electrolytes, as uncorrected hypovolemia may result in cardiovascular collapse on anesthetic induction and uncorrected serum bicarbonate may delay the ability to extubate the baby after surgery.

Surgical intervention is pyloromyotomy, which may be performed open or laparoscopically. The crux of the procedure is the creation of a longitudinal incision on the pyloric serosa, then spreading this incision open down through the muscle layers until the submucosal layer is visualized. The submucosa should have a bulging appearance. Both edges of the pyloromyotomy incision are grasped and moved independently, to confirm completeness of the pyloromyotomy. A leak check is then performed through an orogastric or nasogastric tube to confirm that the mucosa has not been violated. Feeding may be restarted soon after surgery, *ad libitum* or in a scheduled, graduated fashion (32). Repeat imaging studies are not necessary unless the patient has persistent emesis, to rule out incomplete myotomy. Of note, it is common for patients to still have some emesis after successful pyloromyotomy, particularly if the dimensions of the muscle are large.

DUODENAL OBSTRUCTION

Duodenal obstruction can present as the end result of a spectrum of anomalies of duodenal development: atresia, stenosis, and web. Workup and operative management have similarities among the presentations. The incidence of duodenal obstruction is 1 in 7,000 to 40,000 live births (33).

Duodenal atresia results from a lack of normal gut recanalization during fetal development, causing a complete obstruction. Although commonly seen with trisomy 21, and can be an isolated finding, duodenal atresia has been found to be associated with other congenital anomalies in over 50% of cases (34). It can be diagnosed prenatally; common findings on ultrasound include polyhydramnios in combination with a double bubble. The stomach is usually dilated. In the neonate, bilious or nonbilious emesis usually occurs shortly after feedings. Radiographically, the "double bubble" sign is diagnostic (**Fig. 36.4**).

The remainder of the abdomen is typically gasless. Management is surgical intervention to create a duodenoduodenostomy. Prior to surgery, echocardiogram should be performed to rule out associated cardiac anomalies; this is a particular concern with trisomy 21 patients. In the absence of other suspicious findings on plain films, no other imaging is typically needed preoperatively. After surgery, advancement of feeds may be slow as there is residual dysmotility of the proximal duodenum with stasis because of its dilated lumen. This resolves with time, and the infant may benefit from continuous feeds before transitioning to physiologic oral feeding.

When compared to duodenal atresia, duodenal stenosis and webs only partially obstruct flow of intestinal material. Notably, early imaging within the first 6 hours of life may yield results that suggest complete obstruction, as no distal intestinal air may be yet visualized. Duodenal stenosis is a narrowing typically of the second segment of the duodenum. The etiology is incomplete recanalization of the duodenum during embryonic/fetal life. This can be seen on upper GI radiography. A duodenal web is a thin membrane that also usually occurs in the second segment of the duodenum at the level of the ampulla of Vater. On upper GI radiography a duodenal web may be represented by a "wind sock" deformity, caused by distention of the dilated proximal duodenum that bulges into a nondilated distal segment (**Fig. 36.5**). Similar findings can be seen by sonography. It is important to note that duodenal stenosis and web are often associated with malrotation and annular pancreas. Malrotation can be identified on upper GI imaging. Definitive management for stenosis and webs is operative intervention, and the presence of annular pancreas does not necessarily affect the approach. If malrotation is confirmed, a Ladd procedure is performed at the time of correction of the duodenal obstruction. As with duodenal atresia, there may be some delay in ability to advance feeds due to dysmotility of the proximal dilated duodenum. This size decreases spontaneously with time.

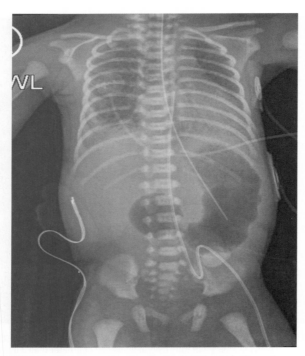

FIGURE 36.4 Babygram showing double bubble sign. There is no distal bowel gas pattern. (Photo courtesy of Janice Taylor, MD.)

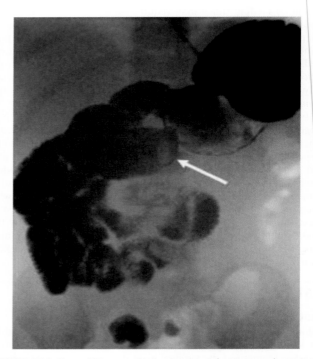

FIGURE 36.5 Upper GI image with duodenal web (*white arrow*) at point of proximal dilation. Bowel is decompressed distally. There is associated malrotation, as all of the small bowel remains to the right of midline. (Photo courtesy of Shawn D. Larson, MD, FACS.)

MALROTATION

Intestinal rotation anomalies are caused by absent or incomplete bowel rotation during embryologic life (see Chapter 35). These often lead to abnormal bowel fixation. Malrotation presents in around 1 in 2,500 live born infants (under 1 year of age); however, as an anatomic entity, it is much more common than this, occurring in 0.2% to 1% of the normal population (35). Several other anomalies such as diaphragmatic hernia, omphalocele, gastroschisis, and heterotaxy syndromes have a high association with malrotation; with the first three listed diagnoses, complete visceral rotation does not occur by definition.

Malrotation can be classified as true malrotation, atypical malrotation, and nonrotation. Regardless of the classification, the management is the same and is not affected by the esoteric nomenclature, as the problem is based on the narrow vascular pedicle supplying the small bowel; this was appreciated in one of the original papers discussing its embryology and anatomy (36). In classic malrotation, there is an abnormal position of the ligament of Treitz in the right upper quadrant or near-midline as seen by radiographic upper GI contrast study, with no identification of duodenal limb passing into the retroperitoneum on lateral views. The cecum may be found in an abnormal position in the mid or upper abdomen if contrast enema is obtained, but this finding is not pathognomonic for malrotation, as it can be associated with other anatomic variations.

Upper GI series is the standard imaging modality to diagnose malrotation with a sensitivity of 95% and specificity of 86% (37). False-negative rates are reported up to 15% for upper GI series (38). Abdominal ultrasound has been put forth as another method of diagnosing malrotation without radiation exposure. Findings on ultrasound consistent with malrotation are the abnormal relationship of the superior mesenteric vein (SMV) and superior mesenteric artery (SMA) (the vein is abnormally positioned to the left of the artery) and a swirl ("whirlpool") sign representing the twisting of these vessels in the setting of volvulus. Dilated and edematous bowel loops may also be seen. However, abnormal SMA/SMV position may be seen in normally rotated bowel, and malrotation exists with normal SMA/SMV relationships. Coupling this with a sensitivity of 86% and specificity of 75%, abdominal ultrasound is not yet viewed as a more ideal imaging choice to diagnose malrotation, over upper GI series (39).

The abnormal positioning of bowel results in a narrow mesenteric pedicle that can obstruct the SMA by twisting (volvulus), causing ischemia of the entire midgut. Commonly associated with this malrotation are aberrant adhesive peritoneal bands (Ladd bands) that can potentially overlay the duodenum and cause duodenal obstruction. One very clear classic diagnostic feature of malrotation with possible volvulus is bilious emesis. When an infant present with bilious emesis, this should be assumed to be malrotation with volvulus and thus a surgical emergency, until proven otherwise. Bilious emesis has been found to have a surgical etiology in almost 50% of cases (40). Obtaining a plain film study to evaluate the cause of the patient's emesis is nondiagnostic for malrotation: in infants, there is less ability to discern small bowel from large bowel based on the bowel gas pattern. Abdominal films exhibiting a gasless abdomen or dilated loops of bowel, while abnormal, do not specifically point to malrotation as the diagnosis. Free air seen on plain film studies could arise from a wide differential diagnosis, and should this be an initial finding, next steps should be discussed first with the surgical consultants. An upper GI contrast study should otherwise be done immediately. The potential devastating consequence of a delayed diagnosis of malrotation with volvulus is complete necrosis of the midgut, with high mortality rate if not intestinal failure. Findings diagnostic for malrotation on upper GI study include abnormal position of the ligament of Treitz to the right of the spine (Fig. 36.6) and proximal jejunal loops located in the right upper abdomen. With midgut volvulus, there is a cork-

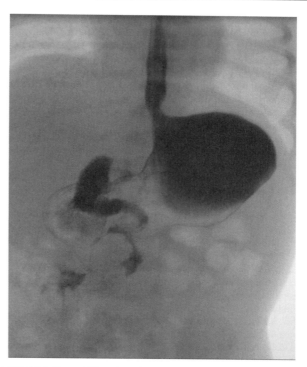

FIGURE 36.6 Upper GI imaging showing corkscrew formation of proximal small bowel on the right that does not cross midline in a 1-day-old with malrotation and volvulus. The baby had bilious emesis as the presenting finding. (Photo courtesy of Janice Taylor, MD.)

screw configuration of the duodenum with a tapered or beaked appearance (Fig. 36.6).

Operative intervention is the Ladd procedure, which involves detorsion of the bowel (typically 270 degrees in a counter-clockwise fashion), division of the Ladd bands, broadening of the small bowel mesentery to help prevent future volvulus, appendectomy, and the positioning of the small bowel on the right side of the abdominal cavity and colon on the left side. The incidental appendectomy is performed since its position would be on the left side of the body, possibly creating a situation of delayed diagnosis if the child developed appendicitis in the future. While feeds are often able to be initiated and advanced without delay after surgery, a prolonged ileus may also be experienced by the patient. Developing a postoperative ileus is not necessarily based on severity of malrotation or presence of volvulus, and resolution is eventually spontaneous.

LOWER GASTROINTESTINAL DISORDERS

Jejunoileal atresia, the commonest of the intestinal atresias, is thought to arise from necrosis and resorption of intestine during intrauterine life after a vascular insult. This can lead to segmental stenosis. Jejunoileal atresias have been reproduced by ligation of mesenteric vessels in utero in canine studies; analysis of the post-atretic intestinal content demonstrates bile salts, epithelial cells, and ingested lanugo hair in humans (35).

Frequency of jejunoileal atresia is estimated at 1 in every 5,000 to 10,000 live births (35). Over one-third of affected children are born prematurely; there is no sex predominance and usually there are no associated chromosomal abnormalities (<1%). When diagnosed prenatally, there is an often a suspicion for bowel obstruction, as polyhydramnios and dilated bowel loops are noted.

The neonate with jejunoileal atresia presents in the first days after birth with bilious emesis if the atresia is proximal. Nonbilious or bilious emesis and abdominal distention are typical

552 PART 4 • The Newborn Infant

findings with distal atresias. There is failure to pass meconium, and documentation by clinical staff must be specific about this, as recording mucus stools as true stools may be misleading and result in a delayed diagnosis of intestinal atresia. Atresias are classified as seen in **Figure 36.7**. Shortened bowel length is seen with types III and IV. There may be autosomal recessive associations with types IIIb and IV intestinal atresia, although a specific genetic code has not been identified to date. Surgery is required by all atresia types to restore bowel continuity.

More distal ileal atresias are characterized by numerous distended loops of bowel (**Fig. 36.8**). If *in utero* perforation has occurred, meconium may spill into the peritoneal cavity, become calcified, and be visualized with a typical distended abdomen with a speckled appearance. This is termed meconium peritonitis. Also, commonly seen on contrast enema is a microcolon, which results from a functionally unused or underutilized colon (**Fig. 36.9**).

Colonic atresias are seen in about 1 in 5,000 to 60,000 live births. The etiology colonic atresia is thought to be a vascular insult, similar to that of small bowel atresias. Hirschsprung disease can be associated with 2% of colonic atresia cases (41,42). Thus, on operative confirmation of colonic atresia, a suction rectal biopsy should be performed to diagnose a concurrent case of Hirschsprung disease.

The clinical suspicions of intestinal atresia are confirmed by contrast enema, possibly followed by upper GI study with small bowel follow-through. While abdominal x-rays alone may show multiple dilated loops of bowel that indicate the need for operative intervention, the contrast studies aid surgical planning. The infant

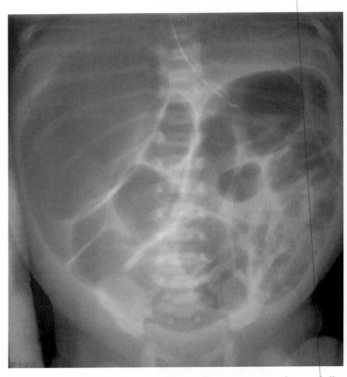

FIGURE 36.8 Abdominal x-ray with significant, numerous loops of distended bowel due to distal intestinal atresia. There is no rectal air. (Photo courtesy of Janice Taylor, MD.)

should be made NPO with gastric decompression if not already, once atresia is confirmed on imaging.

Surgery typically consists of primary anastomosis with possible tapering of the proximal dilated end to aid with motility and decreasing bowel caliber mismatch with the smaller, distal atretic limb. Patients with a type IIIb or IV jejunoileal atresia may also

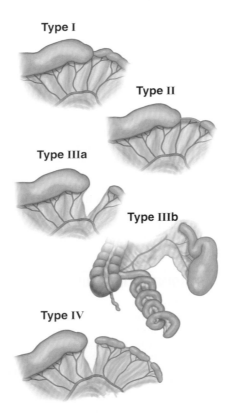

FIGURE 36.7 Classification of intestinal atresia types. Type I has a mucosal web but no lumenal or mesenteric defect. **Type II** has 2 blind bowel ends that are connected by a fibrous cord. **Type IIIa** has 2 blind ends with a mesenteric defect between the ends. **Type IIIb** is also called an "apple peel" or "Christmas tree" deformity; there is no superior mesenteric artery, thus no significant small bowel length. **Type IV** has multiple intestinal atresias present. (Reprinted from Frischer JS, Azizkhan RG. Jejunoileal atresia and stenosis. In: Coran AG, ed. *Pediatric surgery*, 7th ed. Philadelphia, PA: Saunders, 2012:1059. Copyright © 2012 Elsevier. With permission.)

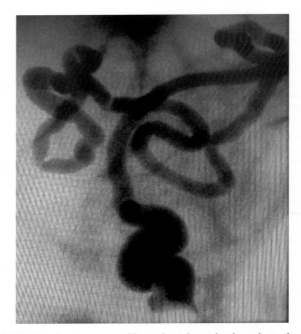

FIGURE 36.9 Contrast enema illustrating microcolon in patient who was diagnosed with a type IIIa ileal atresia. Note the normal caliber of the rectum, which can help rule out Hirschsprung disease if it were on the differential diagnosis. (Photo courtesy of Janice Taylor, MD.)

receive a gastrostomy tube at the first operation, as they are at high intrinsic risk of feed intolerance or short gut syndrome. For colonic atresias, it is generally recommended that the patient undergo colostomy with mucus fistula initially until rectal biopsy results return. Primary anastomosis in the setting of an undiagnosed distal process (i.e., Hirschsprung disease) has a high risk of complications like anastomotic leaks.

SHORT BOWEL SYNDROME

Short bowel syndrome (SBS), also referred to as short gut syndrome, is the clinical situation in which so much intestinal length has been removed that the patient requires parenteral nutrition. A patient may still be thought to have SBS if they require long-term parenteral nutrition (>3 months) for adequate nutrition regardless of intestinal length, as this would be a functional SBS scenario. SBS is the most common cause of intestinal failure in children, with an incidence of 1 to 30 per million (43). Typical causes of SBS in the neonatal population are necrotizing enterocolitis (35%), intestinal atresia (25%), gastroschisis (18%), and malrotation with volvulus (14%).

The ability to take all nutrition by mouth or enteral access, and not requiring any parenteral nutrition, is called enteral autonomy. The definition of acceptable bowel length to reach enteral autonomy is different in adults compared to pediatric patients, as the relative lengths of complete bowel length are so variable within pediatric age groups. There is no standard to date within the neonatal population for acceptable bowel length to be enterally autonomous, but minimum bowel lengths that are considered adequate for survival and weaning from parenteral nutrition are 10 to 15 cm small bowel length if the ileocecal valve is present, or 15 to 20 cm small bowel length if the ileocecal valve or colon are absent. A multicenter study showed that ≥41 cm of remaining small bowel was predictive of the ability to because enterally autonomous. For every 1-cm increase in residual small bowel, the odds of achieving enteral autonomy increased by 4% (44). Premature infants who have undergone massive small bowel resection for reasons like necrotizing enterocolitis are less likely to develop intestinal failure, as they are still in a developmental state; this is believed to be the background stimulus for the ability of their bowel to adapt.

Intestinal failure is the inability of the small bowel in SBS to absorb enough nutrients to allow patient growth, thus requiring parenteral nutrition. SBS is one cause of intestinal failure, as it is the state of having lost long lengths of bowel, either due to surgery or *in utero* accidents like intestinal atresia. Intestinal failure can also be the result of motility disorders or luminal pathology, exclusive of SBS. Intestinal adaptation describes the global process of the lengthening of intestinal villi, increased smooth muscle thickness and protein content, and deepening of crypts, allowing the goal of enteral autonomy to be attained (45). Adaptation can take up to 2 years. The prognosis of patients with intestinal failure is 50% will wean from parenteral nutrition, 25% will require small bowel transplant with or without liver transplant, and 25% will die from the underlying disease process or complications related to intestinal failure like liver disease, sepsis, and loss of venous access for parenteral nutrition (45).

Intestinal rehabilitation is the organized, long-term, surgical, and medical management of promoting intestinal adaptation in patients with SBS and intestinal failure. This can involve manipulating how nutrition is administered, surgical intervention to increase bowel length and therefore absorptive capabilities, and medications to affect secretions, motility, absorption, and bacterial load. Intestinal rehabilitation promotes optimization of enteral autonomy to avoid liver damage that results from parenteral nutrition, to avoid intestinal/liver transplant, and can also be taken from the perspective of improving growth as much as possible

so that a patient has greater bowel transplant potential. Even if a patient fails the intestinal rehabilitation process from the standpoint of avoiding transplant, there is often less liver damage and decreased transplant mortality in these patients because they have been otherwise optimized.

Surgical Management

Surgical management of SBS is headlined by two main operations: the Bianchi (or LILT, longitudinal intestinal lengthening and tapering) and the STEP (serial transverse enteroplasty) (46,47). Both are lengthening procedures, with the goal of increasing surface area and length of time that the lumen is exposed to nutrients. The patient's native bowel needs to be adequately vascularized, and the bowel needs to be at least 4 to 5 cm in diameter for the patient to be a candidate. Upper GI contrast study with small bowel follow-through is the study of choice to determine whether a patient's anatomy makes them a candidate for lengthening. If there is less than 100 cm of small bowel, and particularly if it is dilated, the patient is likely to benefit from a bowel lengthening surgery. Dysmotility may not be affected by lengthening operations. As the goal of the surgeries is lengthening to improve absorptive capacity, the small bowel is the focus, not the colon.

The Bianchi procedure consists of dividing the small bowel lumen in half longitudinally, then reanastomosing the ends together in an antegrade fashion. Care must be taken to keep the bowel vascular supply evenly distributed, as the bowel limb in question will be divided down the center of the mesentery (**Fig. 36.10**). There are multiple staple lines created; thus, anastomotic leak is a common

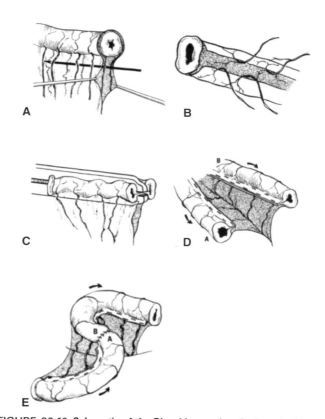

FIGURE 36.10 Schematic of the Bianchi procedure for intestinal lengthening. A: *Dividing the mesentery longitudinally, defined by the direction of the arrow.* **B:** *Mesentery after division, as seen from the mesenteric side of the bowel.* **C:** *Stapled division of the bowel limb into two limbs.* **D:** *The newly divided limbs,* arrows *defining antegrade direction.* **E:** *Bowel following end-to-end anastomosis of the newly divided limbs,* arrows *define antegrade direction.* (Reprinted from Coran AG, Caldamone A, Adzick NS, et al., eds. *Pediatric surgery*, 7th ed. Philadelphia, PA: Elsevier, 2012.)

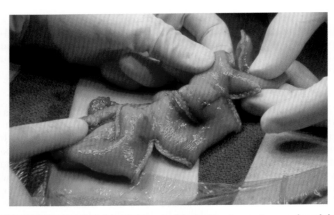

FIGURE 36.11 Dilated small bowel after stapling to create more length in the STEP (serial transverse enteroplasty) procedure. (Photo courtesy of Janice Taylor, MD.)

complication. Worsening dysmotility, bowel ischemia, and repeat dilation of the bowel are other postoperative complications.

The STEP procedure consists of serial stapling of the dilated length of small bowel in such a way to create a step-like, "zigzag" configuration of the bowel (**Fig. 36.11**). It is considered technically easier to perform compared to the Bianchi, with staple-line leaks being the main complication. While the bowel may dilate again after surgery with this technique as well, a repeat STEP may be performed, whereas a repeat Bianchi cannot be performed on bowel that has previously undergone a Bianchi. Motility after STEP may show some improvement compared to the Bianchi, and in some cases, the resulting bowel length may be doubled with the STEP.

Medical Management

Improvements in nonoperative management of pediatric SBS have decreased mortality from 50% to 10% over the past 40 years (48). Medical management may certainly be concurrent with surgical procedures, or be the sole method of management if the patient is not an operative candidate. Focusing on improving enteral feeds has been found to improve direct bilirubinemia, even normalize it (49). Medical management of SBS may be thought of as feeding methods, nutritional absorption, managing bacterial overgrowth, and growth factors.

Feeding access is often needed with SBS patients, as the rate of feeds needs to be controlled to prevent dumping. To help facilitate adaptation and tolerance, feeds are typically started at a slow rate and then increased every 2 to 3 days. Feed advancement is also dictated by the amount of stool output, as this can also be an indication of malabsorption. Evaluating stool for reducing substances and fecal fats can help alter feeding schedules when carbohydrate or fat malabsorption is found; abnormal stool studies can also be impetus for formula modification. There is no established method of feed advancement; rates of advancement vary among and within physician groups. Continuous or bolus feeding is another feeding method option that can affect nutrition malabsorption and intolerance. Continuous feeds provide a lower volume of feeds per hour compared to bolus feeds; bolus feeds are more physiologic. SBS babies who are continuously fed tend to have better fluid and nutrition absorption since the enterocytes are not as overwhelmed as with bolused large volumes. While a long-term goal should be transition to bolus feeds and/or oral feeding, the overriding motivation in advancing enteral feeds is for the patient to be free of parenteral nutrition. Finally, the type of feed given can have significant outcomes for the patient. Breast milk and elemental feeds are more easily absorbed in neonates, but more complex formulations may stimulate intestinal adaptation to a higher degree. A patient's

formula type may need to be intermittently evaluated if a potential change is indicated based on trends in growth and stool output.

While neonates may already be on parenteral nutrition prior to feed initiation due to other medical factors or recovery from surgery, it is important to note that parenteral nutrition may need to be continued or added back to their feed regimen if the patient is not tolerating or growing appropriately with enteral feeds. Lipid reduction should be attempted as a hepatoprotective maneuver (e.g., 1 g/kg/d for 2 to 3 d/wk), being mindful that aggressive lipid reduction can impact neurodevelopment. Standard lipid formulations are soybean oil-based, which are high in proinflammatory omega-6 fatty acids: greater than 1 g/kg/d is associated with intestinal failure-associated liver disease (IFALD). IFALD manifests as liver dysfunction that ranges from cholestasis and steatosis to fibrosis and end-stage liver failure (50). Alternatives to standard lipid formulas consist of different fatty acids or other fat sources that result in greater hepatoprotection. Formulations currently in use are Omegaven, which is high in omega-3 fatty acids, and SMOFlipid, which is made of soybean oil, medium-chain triglycerides, olive oil, and fish oil. Parenteral nutrition may be weaned or cycled as they are shown to have improved growth on gradually increasing volumes of enteral nutrition.

Nutritional absorption in SBS is measured in terms of weight, length, head circumference, vitamin deficiencies, and stool/urine output. For neonates, goal weight gain is 20 to 30 g/d. Total body sodium depletion can be seen even with appropriate caloric intake and results in poor growth and failure to thrive. Urine sodium less than 10 mEq/L is concerning for this and is best supplemented orally with sodium chloride or sodium bicarbonate replacements. Gastric hypersecretion can inhibit nutrient absorption, which can be seen in as many as 50% of SBS patients (51). It results in high output and low pH and tends to occur in the earlier postoperative period after extensive small bowel resection. Gastric hypersecretion can be treated with proton pump inhibitors or H2 antagonists, which helps to both decrease output and normalize pH.

Small intestine bacterial overgrowth can occur in up to 60% of SBS patients and is due to poor motility, which results in stasis and bowel dilation (52). Bacterial overgrowth can result in abdominal pain, worsening already poor motility, mucosal ulceration, mucosal bleeding, and sepsis. The treatment for suspected overgrowth is largely empiric, with oral antibiotics. Many regimens exist, and while there is no standard, the typical course is for 7 days monthly, alternating antibiotic choice to avoid resistance. Commonly chosen antibiotics are metronidazole, amoxicillin/clavulanic acid, neomycin sulfate, sulfamethoxazole/trimethoprim, and rifaximin (53,54). Probiotics and fecal transplant have been investigated to treat bacterial overgrowth of the intestine, but there are no proven therapies to date.

Administration of growth factors to promote intestinal adaptation in SBS is a focus of much bench-to-bedside research. Promising animal models incorporate the use of epidermal growth factor (EGF), heparin-binding EGF, growth hormone, and glutamine (55). Glucagon-like peptide 2 (GLP-2) is the most commonly researched factor for SBS, and as of this writing, has a commercial analog approved for treatment of SBS in adults and children over the age of 1 year: teduglutide. GLP-2 is released after meals by cells in the ileum and right colon. It promotes enzymatic activity, as well as absorption by slowing gastric transit times. Teduglutide has shown a significant reduction in parenteral nutrition needs of patients. While there is approval for use in children, concerns of increasing intestinal malignancy risk exist.

Outcomes of Intestinal Rehabilitation and Transplant

Sixty percent of pediatric patients listed for intestinal transplant have SBS. A 2008 study looking at the care needs of pediatric SBS found that the mean total cost of care per child over 5 years was $1,619,851 ± $1,028,985 (56). Almost half of this amount was from the first year of care due to inpatient admissions. Multidisciplinary intestinal rehabilitation programs bring specialists together to provide an organized approach to SBS patients and include gastroenterologists, surgeons, pharmacists, dieticians, nurses, social workers, and speech therapists. These programs have been shown to help streamline care for this population of complex patients and affect outcomes, specifically reducing morbidity and mortality.

Long-term survival rates of greater than 90% have been self-reported from intestinal rehabilitation groups, with likewise self-reported mortalities from 6.4% to 37.5% (57). Forty to eighty percent of SBS patients cared for by multidisciplinary groups will be transitioned to full enteral autonomy. While many intestinal rehabilitation programs will care for patients with multiple causes of their intestinal failure, the impact of improvement in care with reduction in line sepsis, weaning of parenteral nutrition, reversal of liver disease from parenteral nutrition, improved overall coordination of care, and more appropriate timing of referral for intestinal and multivisceral transplant has been reported (58–60). No standard exists to guide exact timing of referral for intestinal transplant, but pretransplant management by a multidisciplinary intestinal rehabilitation team has been shown to improve post-transplant survival.

Referral to an intestinal transplant center should be made when a patient is not able to wean off parenteral nutrition, developing IFALD, experiencing loss of vascular access sites for parenteral nutrition, and having repeated sepsis due to central line needed for parenteral nutrition (61). Patients with SBS who have not yet achieved these parameters but are at high risk based on their hospitalization trends or etiology of SBS may benefit from early referral so that a relationship and expectations may be established with the family and the transplant team. Evaluation of the Intestinal Transplant Registry revealed that the indications for intestinal transplant has not changed since data were first collected in the 1980s (62). Intestinal transplant has historically possessed a high associated mortality, but improvements in immunosuppression and critical care have resulted in 1-year survival of 80% and 5-year survival approaching 60% when including multivisceral transplants (62). Predictors for improved survival based on the registry were young age, admission for the transplant as an outpatient, and when liver was also transplanted. Cause of death after transplant has not changed over time: sepsis (50%), rejection (13%), and cardiac related (8%) (62). Intestinal transplant case volumes have decreased over time, a possible result of the positive impact that intestinal rehabilitation programs are making on SBS and other intestinal failure patients.

IMPERFORATE ANUS

Although imperforate anus is usually clinically evident at the time of birth, it can also be frequently diagnosed prenatally by ultrasound. Features on ultrasound include dilation of the proximal bowel, although it is sometimes possible to see actual anal atresia on the ultrasound. Its incidence is approximately 1 in 5,000 births, with a slight male predominance (63). Imperforate anus is sometimes associated with trisomies 18 and 21; imperforate anus without fistula is most seen with trisomy 21. Most cases of imperforate anus are sporadic. The anatomic details of imperforate anus patients can vary significantly and have major implications for their management and long-term outcomes. As with EA/TEF, VACTERL associations must be investigated.

Radiographic visualization can be very helpful but does not solely dictate operative management; the prime factors are physical exam and any other associated defects. Lateral prone x-ray ("invertogram") may be useful for neonatal operative planning and should be ordered in conjunction with the surgery team recommendations. Examination of the opening expressing meconium relative to where the anal musculature is positioned is critical

information for surgical planning. The presence of a skin bridge overlying the anal area ("bucket handle") suggests a distal fistula. Beads of meconium in the midline of the perineum leading to the scrotum can also be a clue to a lower defect. If the buttocks are flat or there are sacral abnormalities, a more complex imperforate anus variant may be present, and this may also be a harbinger of poor continence, as underdeveloped buttocks are associated with poor fecal continence and sensation.

Once any associated VACTERL anomalies have been addressed, preoperative care of these infants consists of NPO, gastric decompression, and intravenous fluids. Empiric antibiotics outside of perioperative administration are not typically needed.

Surgical management often first involves a colostomy and mucus fistula if primary creation of a neorectum and anus (posterior sagittal anorectoplasty, PSARP) is not indicated based on anatomy variant or patient comorbidities. If surgical intervention is staged, it is important to obtain fluoroscopy via the mucus fistula for presurgical planning to determine whether associated genitourinary anomalies such as fistulas exist (**Fig. 36.12**). If the infant is premature, a staged repair is typically performed even if the anatomy would otherwise be amenable to a primary PSARP, allowing the baby time to grow with a temporary colostomy, until a more optimal size is reached to complete the PSARP. Likewise, if the patient has physiologically significant cardiac defects discovered during the VACTERL workup, this may drive the decision for colostomy first instead of complicated primary PSARP.

Imperforate anus occurs on a spectrum that may affect the patient's fecal continence throughout life; this is due to the associated underdevelopment of the pelvic floor musculature and innervation. While the more common malformations for each gender (rectourethral fistula in males, rectovestibular fistula in females) have a high rate of overall success with continence and quality of life, these patients will still tend to be constipated. Lower malformations such as perineal fistulas, rectourethral bulbar fistulas, rectovestibular fistulas, short channel (<3 cm) cloacas, and rectal atresia can experience fecal continence rates of 35% to 80%, and 39% to 75% will experience constipation (64). Higher, more

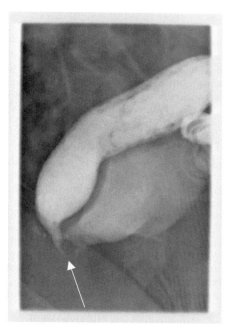

FIGURE 36.12 Distal colostogram done for the next stage of reconstruction for imperforate anus (posterior sagittal anorectoplasty, PSARP). In this image of a male infant, the fistula to the prostatic urethra is seen at the *arrow*. (Photo courtesy of Janice Taylor, MD.)

complex forms of imperforate anus (long-channel cloacas >3 cm, rectobladder neck fistulas, rectourethral prostatic fistulas) will see lower rates of fecal continence (4% to 25%) and thus constipation (18% to 43%), correlating with a more underdeveloped pelvic floor (64). It must also be kept in mind that patients born with lower malformations will have a higher likelihood of having voluntary bowel movements, even in the setting of fecal incontinence, compared to patients born with higher malformations. Constipation may present as the inability to pass stool, or as encopresis because of overflow fecal incontinence. Close follow-up by the pediatric surgery team is necessary to ensure that a reliable bowel regimen is maintained. These patients often need to be on a life-long bowel regimen, so being followed by a clinical team that understands the implications of noncompliance is important for success with fecal continence. Children born with imperforate anus tend to achieve toilet training for stool later than children with normal anorectal anatomy, so parental reassurance is part of the long-term management. Biofeedback and pelvic floor physical therapy are useful adjuncts for managing fecal incontinence starting with the older child.

FUNCTIONAL IMMATURITY OF THE COLON

There are several entities associated with dysfunction of the colon. Here, we will briefly summarize small left colon syndrome, meconium plug syndrome, and differentiate it from meconium ileus, and briefly mention the iatrogenic effect of antenatal magnesium administration.

Small Left Colon Syndrome

Small left colon syndrome is characterized by an abrupt intestinal caliber transition at or near the splenic flexure that causes typical signs of intestinal obstruction evidenced in the first couple of days after birth. It is most commonly seen in infants whose mothers have gestational diabetes, accounting for nearly half of the cases (65). Although the pathogenesis is not entirely clear, it is hypothesized that in the pregnant diabetic, there is hypoglycemia-induced release of glucagon in the infant, and this interferes with development of the intestinal muscularis (66).

Diagnosis is made using a contrast enema, which typically shows an abrupt transition at the splenic flexure with narrowing of the left colon. The radiographic appearances may have some similarities to Hirschsprung disease, but the latter usually has an absence of rectal gas. Furthermore, if there is a doubt, rectal biopsy showing ganglion cells will help rule out Hirschsprung. Management is usually conservative in that symptoms of small left colon syndrome usually resolve in the first 24 to 48 hours after birth, putatively due to normalization of these infants' endogenous insulin output and passage of meconium.

Meconium Plug versus Meconium Ileus

Meconium plug syndrome is different than meconium ileus in that the obstructive meconium in the latter is usually found in the ileum rather than in the colon. In meconium plug syndrome, contrast enema may demonstrate a small left colon. The rectum is usually normal in size whereas that in Hirschsprung disease is often narrowed. Contrast enemas may be both diagnostic and therapeutic because they can induce passage of the meconium plug.

Meconium ileus is usually of much greater consequence than meconium plug syndrome partially because of its high association with cystic fibrosis. Meconium ileus occurs when thick viscid meconium becomes congealed because of various chemical processes related to cystic fibrosis and obstructs the distal ileum. Approximately 20% of infants with cystic fibrosis present with meconium ileus at birth. The manifestations of meconium ileus can be severe when the meconium distended segments give rise to prenatal volvulus, ischemic necrosis, and perforation with extrusion of meconium into the peritoneum, causing meconium peritonitis.

Frequently, neonates whose mothers received magnesium sulfate for the treatment of preeclampsia or for neuroprotection may have slow intestinal transit times. Magnesium is known to produce intestinal atony and fecal impaction (67). This subsequent hypomotility may lead to increased water absorption and formation of fecal plugs. This neonatal iatrogenic hypermagnesemia may result in the formation of fecal plugs and difficulty passing stools. It has been implicated in the pathophysiology of spontaneous intestinal perforations (68).

HIRSCHSPRUNG DISEASE

Hirschsprung disease is a congenital disorder characterized by absence of ganglion cells of the myenteric and submucosal plexus of a segment of the rectum and the colon. It is the result of incomplete distal migration and maturation of ganglion cells in the intestinal system. In rare instances, the entire bowel length including the small intestine can be aganglionic. Complete aganglionosis results in a clinical picture of intestinal failure for which intestinal transplant may be the only option for long-term survival. Recently, it has been recognized that skip segments may occur in Hirschsprung disease, and that the transition zone appreciated on intraoperative examination and biopsies—the portion of bowel that exhibits the transition from ganglionated to aganglionated—may not always occur in singular fashion. While rare, it is necessary to consider skip segments of aganglionosis in a patient with Hirschsprung disease who continues to behave obstructed even after definitive surgical intervention (69,70).

The incidence of Hirschsprung disease is 1 in every 5,000 live births with approximately a 2.5 to 5.1 male predilection. Some of the cases appear to be familial, and multiple mutations have been identified. For example, families in which Hirschsprung disease runs may have a higher likelihood of having longer segment disease. Seven percent of Hirschsprung patients will have trisomy 21 (71). Patients with multiple endocrine neoplasia 2A (MEN 2A) may also have a higher risk of having Hirschsprung disease, related to RET proto-oncogene mutations.

The segment of intestine that is aganglionic lacks the signal to relax. Because of this, the neonates with this disease typically present with failure to pass meconium in the first days after birth and have abdominal distention. Rectal exam may result in an explosive, watery stool. These history and examination findings are particularly relevant to term infants who have not passed meconium. Premature infants may still have immature bowel function, and thus, delayed passage of meconium is not a symptom of Hirschsprung disease. When conventional radiographs are done during the early phases of workup, there is usually very significant gaseous distention of numerous loops of bowel, which cannot necessarily be distinguished from other forms of lower intestinal obstruction. If the baby's presentation is that of bilious emesis with or without abdominal distention, upper GI series should be performed first to rule out malrotation with volvulus before proceeding with enema studies, as the consequences of a delayed diagnosis of volvulus can be devastating. Neonates who present with Hirschsprung-associated enterocolitis may also have findings of diffuse bowel wall edema on plain films. This may also be accompanied by physical examination findings of abdominal distension with tenderness, and in some instances, erythema of the abdominal wall.

Fluoroscopic imaging may be helpful in the diagnosis of Hirschsprung disease but rectal biopsies are the gold standard and needed for definitive diagnosis (Fig. 36.13). Contrast enemas consistent with Hirschsprung disease will have a reversed rectal: sigmoid size ratio; normally, the rectum has more capacity than the sigmoid, so it will be of larger diameter compared to the sigmoid. In Hirschsprung patients, the sigmoid colon is more dilated than the rectum, and the area where the lumen narrows is where the transition from the ganglionated bowel to aganglionic bowel

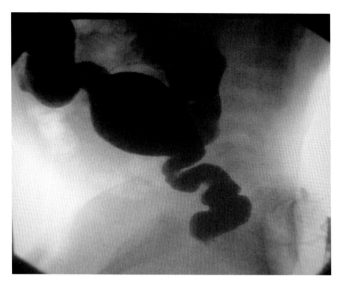

FIGURE 36.13 Contrast enema in a patient with Hirschsprung disease. Note that the caliber of the rectum is less than the distended proximal sigmoid. Diagnosis was confirmed with suction rectal biopsy. (Photo courtesy of Janice Taylor, MD.)

occurs. In these cases, it is important to remember that the dilated bowel is the histologically normal bowel, as the distal aganglionic segment will lack the ability to distend with contrast. If the aganglionic segment is long, the contrast enema results may be difficult to interpret. This reinforces the need for rectal biopsies being the diagnostic standard.

Bedside suction rectal biopsies may be reliably performed on the neonate without requiring anesthesia. The specimens are processed using permanent methods, not frozen sampling, to yield more definitive results. Features consistent with Hirschsprung disease are lack of ganglion cells and hypertrophic nerve fibers. Hypertrophic nerve fibers will stain positive for acetylcholinesterase. Calretinin immunostaining is also used and is negative in Hirschsprung patients. While these pathologic results will confirm the diagnosis of Hirschsprung disease, the length of affected bowel segment will be determined during operative intervention.

While awaiting surgery, the neonate may require rectal irrigations to help decrease abdominal distention and the risk of Hirschsprung-associated enterocolitis. Rectal irrigations are instillations of normal saline or water into the rectum and colon with a catheter; the fluid is then actively aspirated through the catheter. This is different from enemas, where the fluid instilled can dwell and will be expelled by the patient's ability to have a bowel movement; Hirschsprung patients lack this ability. Based on the patient's presentation, broad-spectrum antibiotics with anaerobic coverage may be indicated. Feeding the patient may still be appropriate based on their response to rectal irrigations. If the patient is not tolerating feeds, parenteral nutrition is indicated until after surgery.

Operative management of Hirschsprung disease in the newborn period may be a primary pull-through surgery. This is dependent on whether the patient presents with enterocolitis, or how dilated the bowel is. Temporary ostomy at the level of ganglionated bowel is an appropriate temporizing procedure. Diversion with an ostomy may also be an appropriate plan with the neonate who has other significant comorbidities. There are different ways in which the pull-through surgery may be performed, but the goals are similar: removal of aganglionic bowel with anastomosis that provides the patient with the least risk of complications related to continence and enterocolitis. During the operation, segments of bowel are sent to pathology for immediate processing to determine the

level at which ganglion cells exist. **Figure 36.14** shows a bowel specimen from a pull-through surgery. Bowel is sampled for pathology above the transition zone, to ensure that the proximal portion of colon that is anastomosed to the area of the anus above the dentate line has normal histology.

Following pull-through surgery or ostomy, feeds are typically reinitiated with return of bowel function. For primary pull-through patients, there should be no medications or instrumentation in the anus after surgery to prevent complications related to disruption of the new suture line. Once the neonate is discharged from the hospital, close follow-up with the pediatric surgery team is recommended, to ensure consistent stooling without concerns for Hirschsprung-associated enterocolitis. Enterocolitis is still possible after successful surgery because the most distal portion of bowel above the dentate line, to where the proximal bowel is sutured, will not have ganglion cells. As the infant gets older and the diet is advanced in an age-appropriate fashion, episodes of enterocolitis may still occur, requiring antibiotics, rectal irrigations, and/or hospital admission. Rectal dilations may also be needed for a period of time. These issues tend to improve and resolve as the patient ages beyond the toddler years. Should concerns of recurrent enterocolitis persist, or recurrent constipation, rebiopsy may need to be entertained to rule out need for revision surgery or the rare diagnosis of Hirschsprung disease with skip segments of aganglionosis. In older children, anorectal manometry, motility studies, and biofeedback can be useful diagnostic and treatment adjuncts in patients with history of Hirschsprung disease but who have persistent issues with constipation and bowel distention after corrective surgery.

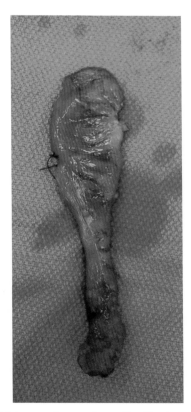

FIGURE 36.14 Intraoperative specimen after Hirschsprung's pull-through surgery. Note the relative larger caliber of bowel at the upper part of the specimen (proximal, ganglionated) compared to the lower part of the photo (distal, aganglionic). The area where the dilated bowel becomes more decompressed is the transition zone. (Photo courtesy of Janice Taylor, MD.)

ABDOMINAL WALL DEFECTS

Abdominal wall defects consist of gastroschisis and omphalocele, and their presentations are on a spectrum. While their defining physical features are of incomplete abdominal wall development, the defects can have a significant impact on gastrointestinal function. Prenatal diagnosis for both is typically made at the 20-week anatomy ultrasound; both conditions are also associated with elevated maternal alpha-fetoprotein levels. Both gastroschisis and omphalocele patients will have malrotation by default since the bowel does not complete the normal rotational patterns during early fetal life. Survival past the newborn period is dependent on associated systemic defects and access to care.

Gastroschisis

Gastroschisis occurs in approximately 4 in 10,000 live births (72). Its incidence is increasing worldwide without a defined cause, and young maternal age is a consistent factor (73,74). While gastroschisis is not commonly associated with multiple birth defects, it is often associated with jejunoileal atresias. The incidence of associated atresias has been reported to be between 10% and 20% (75). The umbilical defect is to the right of the umbilical cord, and there is no biologic covering on the exposed bowel. An inflammatory rind, or "peel," is often seen adhered to the serosa; this is believed to develop from exposure of the bowel to amniotic fluid, although bowel is commonly also observed to appear grossly normal without these inflammatory changes. Other than the bowel, stomach and bladder may also be herniated out the defect. Herniation of the liver is associated with a larger defect size and correlates with a poor prognosis.

Vaginal delivery is acceptable, and decision for cesarean section should be made based on maternal and fetal factors aside from the gastroschisis. Following delivery, the lower half of the baby should be placed in a sterile bag with warm saline-soaked gauze to cover the exposed bowel (**Fig. 36.15**). The baby's assessment in the NICU should be made in conjunction with a member of the pediatric surgery team. Appearance of the bowel and size of the abdominal wall defect will be the driving factors behind method of closure. Wound management in patients with large defects is often drawn from experience with omphalocele (76). Intravenous access is needed, and the baby should be kept adequately hydrated to counter fluid losses. Placement of the bowel in a silo, with sequential reduction of the bowel back into the abdomen, may be done at bedside. Findings concerning for perforation, ischemia, or small abdominal defect relative to exposed bowel may require operative management. Even if identified at birth, atresias associated with gastroschisis are not managed definitively until several weeks after abdominal closure, when the bowel has had time to become less edematous, and contrast studies are performed to rule out additional atresias. If the defect size is amenable and the bowel is of appropriate caliber that it may all be reduced primarily, sutureless closure may be considered (77).

Once the gastroschisis defect has been closed and bowel continuity confirmed, enteral feeds may be introduced. This may take upward of 3 weeks to initiate, so parenteral nutrition is required in the meantime. Whether or not bowel length is foreshortened, or if an associated bowel atresia exists, infants born with gastroschisis may have an element of dysmotility. The reasons for this are not clear but may be related to the inflammatory changes of the bowel as manifest by the overlying peel formation, and bowel of infants born with gastroschisis has been found to possess decreased concentrations of interstitial cells of Cajal (78). Gastroschisis-associated intestinal dysmotility is a described entity, and as such, advancement of feeds may be a slow process. Methods to promote successful feed advancement may be as banal as deliberate, gradual increases of enteral feed rate to allow for intestinal adaptation with feed exposure. Gabapentin has shown some success

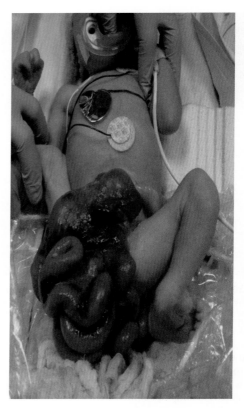

FIGURE 36.15 Newborn with gastroschisis. Note the edematous, matted appearance of the bowel. (Photo courtesy of Janice Taylor, MD.)

with improving feed intolerance in infants born with abdominal wall defects (79). If the infant with gastroschisis was born with an associated intestinal defect such as an atresia and has since been placed back into bowel continuity but persists with feed intolerance, evaluation may be needed to determine whether the patient needs additional intervention for anastomotic revision or tapering enterostomy. Intolerance of enteral feeds and documentation of poor motility in the absence of a surgical etiology may necessitate input from specialists in intestinal failure.

Omphalocele

Omphalocele is an abdominal wall defect that occurs in 1 to 4 cases per 10,000 live births worldwide (80). Ratio of occurrence based on gender is 2:1 male:female. The omphalocele layers are made up of amnion, Wharton jelly, and the peritoneum. Through the layers, the bowel and other abdominal organs may be observed (**Fig. 36.16**). Care is taken to not disrupt the omphalocele sac during delivery. Fetal diagnosis of omphalocele is not an absolute indication for cesarean section; vaginal delivery should be planned unless maternal or other fetal factors dictate otherwise. The defect typically has the umbilical cord protruding from it, compared to gastroschisis, which occurs to the right of the umbilical cord. While considered in the same general category of defects types as gastroschisis, the associated defects and implications of management are much different.

When associated with other defects, the affected systems are often cardiac (40% incidence), nervous (33%), musculoskeletal (25%), genitourinary (20%), and respiratory (4.5%) (74). Chromosomal anomalies associated with omphalocele are trisomy 13, 18, and 21; up to 90% of infants with trisomy 18 will have an omphalocele (81). Beckwith-Wiedemann syndrome also has a strong association with omphalocele. Omphalocele is also associated with the rare conditions of cloacal exstrophy and Pentalogy of Cantrell.

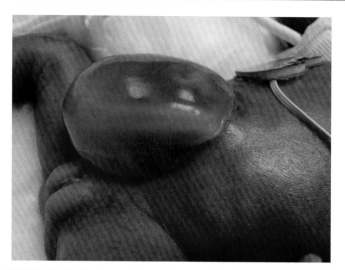

FIGURE 36.16 Newborn with omphalocele defect. (Photo courtesy of Moiz Mustafa, MD.)

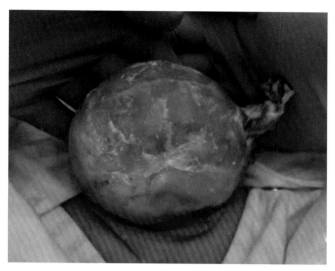

FIGURE 36.17 Appearance of omphalocele after over 1 week of topical sclerosis therapy ("paint and wait"). Silvadene was used in this case; some residual white substrate can be seen on its surface. (Photo courtesy of Moiz Mustafa, MD.)

Thus, the neonate with omphalocele should undergo chromosomal studies, abdominal ultrasound, echocardiogram, and possibly also spinal ultrasound following delivery. Additional workup based on routine postnatal laboratory values and physical exam findings should also be performed. The severity of these will often dictate the timing of surgical management of the omphalocele, as the omphalocele is often the less physiologically significant part of the neonate's presentation. Mortality of isolated omphalocele is approximately 5%; mortality can be as high as 50% if associated with cardiac defects (82).

As with gastroschisis, infants with omphalocele may be appropriately considered for vaginal delivery. There has not been proven benefit when delivered by cesarean section, but studies have not specifically addressed this as it applies to giant omphaloceles (80). Following delivery, the patient should be assessed by the pediatric surgery team to help determine any necessary resuscitation parameters and to begin a plan of care with the neonatology team. The size of the omphalocele and whether its covering is intact are the major factors that guide surgical management. If larger than 4 cm in diameter, it may be categorized as a "giant" omphalocele, although this label may also be reserved for those with liver in the sac. There is no standardized definition of giant omphaloceles (80). Likewise, ruptured omphalocele presentations must be managed with the newborn's specific clinical findings in mind.

The most common treatment of omphalocele is the "paint and wait" method of management (**Fig. 36.17**). This allows for scarring and/or epithelialization of the sac to occur while managing the comorbidities, attempting gradual reduction of the sac contents into the abdominal cavity for eventual closure, or as the main goal of initial treatment, with planned closure at a much later date. During the initial phases of eschar formation, the neonate may require parenteral nutrition, as bowel function may not be optimal. Advancing with enteral feeds should take into consideration the potential dysfunction of the bowel and any nonoperative reduction maneuvers that may produce feed intolerance. Delayed fascial closure may occur acceptably as far as 2 to 5 years' age, as waiting tends to decrease the likelihood of ventral hernias. Patients born with giant omphaloceles may require multiple-staged operations to close their fascia. Mesh or biologic materials may be necessary to achieve closure. Complex abdominal wall closure techniques like component separation have been found to be successful in these patients (83). Few infants are appropriate for primary closure based on omphalocele size or comorbidities.

"Paint and wait" management consists of coating the omphalocele with a substance that will promote eventual epithelialization. Historically, mercury was used but was associated with significant toxicity. Silver sulfadiazine is a commonly used topical treatment with minimal side effects, as is bacitracin or Betadine solution (84). If tolerated by the infant, as eschar forms on the omphalocele, and the infant is physiologically stable, gradual compression of the defect with gauze or elastic wraps (i.e., ACE) help achieve abdominal domain. Dressings should be done daily and provides an opportunity for involvement by the newborn's family unit. Epithelialization may take several weeks to achieve. If surgical closure is not planned during the neonatal admission, close outpatient follow-up with the pediatric surgery team is recommended to determine timing of surgery.

NECROTIZING ENTEROCOLITIS

Necrotizing enterocolitis (NEC) is an unfortunately common and destructive disease in neonates (85). Over the past 50 to 60 years until approximately the last decade, the incidence of NEC did not decrease, but recent evidence from one large data base suggests a small decrease, with an approximate 7.6% prevalence in very low birth weight infants, with slightly more than half with medical NEC and the rest with surgical NEC (86). The estimated rate of death associated with NEC ranges between 20% and 30%, with the highest rate among infants requiring surgery (87).

The term "necrotizing enterocolitis" is an umbrella term that describes several forms of intestinal injury. Unfortunately, this lack of a discrete definition can be very detrimental for our ability to understand pathophysiology and treatment. The categorization of NEC into three stages is becoming less helpful as we care for more immature babies who almost all exhibit some of the findings of what is been termed as Stage 1 disease (88). Here, instead of focusing on the umbrella term "NEC," some of the entities that have been categorized as such will be discussed separately in order emphasize the fact that a more refined definition of the entities we are currently calling "NEC" is necessary if we are to develop clearer targets for development of sensitive and specific biomarkers of disease and preventative and therapeutic strategies. We will start with for want of a better term, "classic NEC."

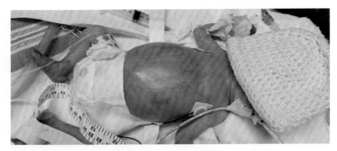

FIGURE 36.18 Premature infant with necrotizing enterocolitis. Note the distention of the abdomen, discoloration, dilated veins, and shiny skin tone. (Photo courtesy of Janice Taylor, MD.)

"Classic NEC"

For want of a better term, the majority of cases of what we term NEC present between corrected gestational ages of 28 to 32 weeks (85,89,90). Clinical signs include bloating and discoloration of the abdomen, feeding intolerance and emesis, bloody stools, and lethargy (Fig. 36.18).

A somewhat outdated system has been utilized for staging the severity of NEC that was first described by Bell in 1978 and subsequently refined (88,91). This system includes three stages. However, the three stages are highly unreliable and lead to considerable confusion. For example, Stage 1 is highly nonspecific wherein criteria include feeding intolerance, abdominal distension, and other nonspecific signs that are evidenced in many extremely- or very low birth weight preterm infants. Stage 2 criteria rely largely on radiographic findings such as pneumatosis intestinalis, which may also be difficult to detect and often bubbly lucencies caused by feces may mimic this finding. Occasionally fixed loops of bowel are seen, which if persistent over a period of 24 to 48 hours may indicate an area of necrotic intestine. Specific biomarkers for NEC are being evaluated, but currently, the ones commonly used are relatively nonspecific measures such as C-reactive protein, platelet count, white blood cell count, and shifting white cell differential counts toward more immature cells.

Criteria for stage 3 include signs of a perforated viscus, usually evidenced by a pneumoperitoneum on radiograph. Spontaneous intestinal perforations, which are a different disease entity than NEC, may prompt placement of a peritoneal drain rather than direct visualization of the bowel. Hence, whether intestinal necrosis is actually present may not be determined and the patient's diagnosis frequently is coded as NEC (92). Currently, as with several other diseases seen in neonatal intensive care such as bronchopulmonary dysplasia and sepsis, we are still struggling with defining this disease in a classic form.

Radiographic Features

Intraperitoneal gas, portal venous gas, and pneumatosis intestinalis are considered as important and diagnostic features of NEC. It must be remembered that intraperitoneal gas may represent spontaneous intestinal or gastric perforation as well and is not diagnostic. **Figure 36.19** shows a baby with portal venous gas and intestinal distension without clear pneumatosis intestinalis. Pneumatosis intestinalis consists of gas bubble collections in the bowel wall and is considered a diagnostic sign for NEC. Although not proven, it is thought that the gas is produced by bacteria in the bowel wall. **Figure 36.20** shows both portal venous gas and pneumatosis intestinalis on radiograph. Sonography is also being used to attempt to diagnose NEC, but its efficacy remains unproven.

Pathophysiology

An exhaustive discussion of the various theories pertaining to the pathophysiology of NEC is beyond the scope of this chapter. Here is included a summary of factors that are considered some of the most important antecedents in the pathophysiology of "classic" NEC.

The first of these factors is intestinal immaturity, that relates to barrier function, motility, immune defenses, and vascular

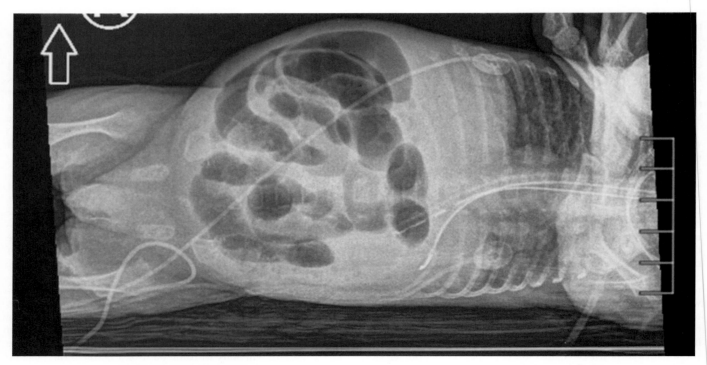

FIGURE 36.19 Left side down radiograph showing portal venous gas in a baby subsequently taken to surgery who had necrotizing enterocolitis. (Photo courtesy of Josef Neu, MD.)

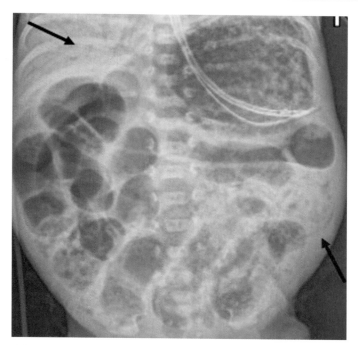

FIGURE 36.20 Radiograph showing portal venous air and diffuse and linear air in the bowel wall—pneumatosis intestinalis -*arrows*). (Photo courtesy of Josef Neu, MD.)

development, which all likely play a role. In conjunction with these immaturities, a combination of environmental factors that favor "dysbiosis" of the microbial ecosystem also likely contributes to a "perfect storm" scenario that culminates in uncontrolled intestinal and systemic inflammatory response—"NEC" (89,93–95).

Medical and Surgical Interventions

Medical intervention includes bowel rest, abdominal decompression, intravenous nutrition, and broad-spectrum intravenous antibiotics. Indications for surgery may include intestinal perforation, deteriorating clinical condition including shock, and/or deteriorating laboratory studies such as increasing inflammatory mediators, hyponatremia, and decreasing platelets. Exploratory laparotomy with resection of necrotic bowel is a broad goal, with the hope that NEC totalis (necrosis of most of the bowel) is not encountered, which is not a survivable finding. Operative intervention may require serial explorations if there are concerning segments of bowel that are not definitively necrotic on initial exploration. These serial explorations allow for the neonate to recover from the initial damage control operation with additional resuscitation. Should the patient survive, subsequent repeat laparotomies allow the surgery and neonatology teams to make decisions about excision of additional bowel, long-term management of anticipated short gut syndrome, or comfort care, depending on the patient's clinical course. Birth weight, gestational age, and surgical intervention contribute to patient mortality from NEC. Overall mortality from NEC is 25% to 30%. Death after nonoperative management of NEC around 20%, with lower mortality associated with heavier birth weight (96). If surgical intervention is needed, there is up to a 50% to 70% death rate, with many infants in this group having NEC totalis (97).

Complications and Morbidities Associated with NEC

Common complications of NEC include those that are short term, frequently seen while the babies are still in the NICU. These include failure to thrive, strictures, and adhesions causing obstructive symptoms, cholestasis, and SBS. Longer-term problems include

significant neurodevelopmental delays (98). The specific etiology for developmental delays remains unclear, and long-term studies evaluating this relationship are needed.

Prevention of NEC

With the advent of modern neonatology since the early 1960s, intestinal problems seen in preterm infants that have been termed NEC have been highly prevalent. One of the few modalities that appear to have a strong evidence base to prevent NEC is human milk feeds; however, this is not a singularly preventative measure against NEC. Clearly, to prevent this disease, we need to have a better definition with clearer clinical and laboratory-based delineation of the different diseases that are being termed NEC. This is a very fertile area for investigation.

The following are forms of intestinal injury commonly termed "NEC":

Cardiogenic Ischemic Intestinal Injury

Congenital heart disease is a risk factor for intestinal injury in term and preterm infants. Mesenteric ischemia is commonly associated with intestinal necrosis. Some examples of heart disease associated with intestinal ischemia are hypoplastic left heart syndrome, interrupted aortic arch, and truncus arteriosus. A better term for this type of intestinal injury than NEC would be "cardiogenic ischemic necrosis" of the intestine (99). Features that would distinguish NEC from cardiogenic ischemic injury would be the corrected gestational age and presence or absence of physiologically significant congenital heart disease. Meta-analyses have shown that the risk in babies with congenital heart disease of developing NEC as well as mortality is higher. The medical and surgical management of the intestinal ischemia in both patient populations regardless of etiology of intestinal ischemia is the same. However, the need for intestinal surgery is lower in babies with cardiogenic ischemic intestinal injury than in those with classical NEC (99).

Food Protein–Induced Enterocolitis Syndrome

The findings of abdominal distension, bloody stools, discoloration of the abdomen and pneumatosis intestinalis are very frequently coded as NEC. However, it is increasingly clear that some of these cases are related to protein in the feeds, and thus can be ameliorated when the inciting food protein eliminated (100,101). Although food protein–induced enterocolitis (FPIES) has been primarily described in infants outside of the neonatal age range, the similar presentation seen in neonates has raised suspicion that this is one of the several imposters for "NEC." FPIES appears to be a still poorly understood non–immunoglobulin E-mediated syndrome resulting in hypersensitivity to food antigens (100). FPIES has likely been called "NEC" in many infants but very likely represents a disease with a distinct pathogenesis. At this juncture, it appears that from a clinical perspective, these babies more often present with bloody stools and may have eosinophils in their differential white blood cell count, but a clear delineation from many of the cases termed NEC with use of sensitive and specific biomarkers is lacking.

FPIES may still occur in breast-fed infants. Since mothers' milk may not always be devoid of the sensitizing agent, it is possible to see this in exclusively breast-fed babies and at a minimum, temporary treatment with extensively hydrolyzed or amino acid formulas, and/or altering the mother's diet may be the best form of treatment and/or prevention in those infants who are disposed to this form of intestinal injury.

Spontaneous Intestinal Perforation

SIP is seen more commonly in extremely low birth weight infants (102). It is usually not accompanied by extensive intestinal inflammation or necrosis and most commonly presents as a distended abdomen that is caused by a discrete perforation, usually of the ileum, within the first week after birth. Radiographically, this often presents with free air in the peritoneal cavity—a "pneumoperitoneum."

Concomitant administration of postnatal steroids and prophylactic indomethacin has been shown to significantly increase the risk of development of SIP (103). The pathophysiology of SIP includes focal thinning or absence of intestinal muscularis propria (104). Many of these babies are unstable and extremely preterm and peritoneal drainage is often done without direct visualization of the intestine. Thus, it is likely that many cases of SIP have been misdiagnosed as NEC, creating considerable artifact in data sets where NEC is considered as a study variable.

Enterocolitis Associated with Other Intestinal Anomalies

Babies recovering from gastroschisis repair may develop an enterocolitis-like syndrome. The pathophysiology of this is poorly understood, but poor motility and microbial overgrowth are likely components.

Babies with Hirschsprung aganglionosis may develop an enterocolitis, which is the greatest cause of mortality in this disease. Presenting symptoms include abdominal distension, explosive diarrhea, vomiting, fever, and lethargy. The pathophysiology of this disease is also unclear, but as with gastroschisis, associated enterocolitis also may result from poor motility and microbial overgrowth.

REFERENCES

1. Billmyre KK, Hutson M, Klingensmith J. One shall become two: Separation of the esophagus and trachea from the common foregut tube. *Dev Dyn* 2015;244:277.
2. Nassar N, Leoncini E, Amar E, et al. Prevalence of esophageal atresia among 18 international birth defects surveillance programs. *Birth Defects Res Part A Clin Mol Teratol* 2012;94:893.
3. Guptha S, Shumate C, Scheuerle AE. Likelihood of meeting defined VATER/VACTERL phenotype in infants with esophageal atresia with or without tracheoesophageal fistula. *Am J Med Genet A* 2019;179:2202.
4. Spaggiari E, Faure G, Rousseau V, et al. Performance of prenatal diagnosis in esophageal atresia. *Prenat Diagn* 2015;35:888.
5. Omari TI, Barnett C, Snel A, et al. Mechanisms of gastroesophageal reflux in healthy premature infants. *J Pediatr* 1998;133:650.
6. Gulati IK, Jadcherla SR. Gastroesophageal reflux disease in the neonatal intensive care unit infant: who needs to be treated and what approach is beneficial? *Pediatr Clin North Am* 2019;66:461.
7. Poets CF, Brockmann PE. Myth: gastroesophageal reflux is a pathological entity in the preterm infant. *Semin Fetal Neonatal Med* 2011;16:259.
8. Jadcherla SR, Slaughter JL, Stenger MR, et al. Practice variance, prevalence, and economic burden of premature infants diagnosed with GERD. *Hosp Pediatr* 2013;3:335.
9. Khalaf MN, Porat R, Brodsky NL, et al. Clinical correlations in infants in the neonatal intensive care unit with varying severity of gastroesophageal reflux. *J Pediatr Gastroenterol Nutr* 2001;32:45.
10. Dhillon AS, Ewer AK. Diagnosis and management of gastro-oesophageal reflux in preterm infants in neonatal intensive care units. *Acta Paediatr* 2004;93:88.
11. Golski CA, Rome ES, Martin RJ, et al. Pediatric specialists' beliefs about gastroesophageal reflux disease in premature infants. *Pediatrics* 2010;125:96.
12. Snel A, Barnett CP, Cresp TL, et al. Behavior and gastroesophageal reflux in the premature neonate. *J Pediatr Gastroenterol Nutr* 2000;30:18.
13. Funderburk A, Nawab U, Abraham S, et al. Temporal association between reflux-like behaviors and gastroesophageal reflux in preterm and term infants. *J Pediatr Gastroenterol Nutr* 2016;62:556.
14. Vandenplas Y, Rudolph CD, Di Lorenzo C, et al. Pediatric gastroesophageal reflux clinical practice guidelines: joint recommendations of the North American Society for Pediatric Gastroenterology, Hepatology, and Nutrition (NASPGHAN) and the European Society for Pediatric Gastroenterology, Hepatology, and Nutrition (ESPGHAN). *J Pediatr Gastroenterol Nutr* 2009;49:498.
15. Mitchell DJ, McClure BG, Tubman TRJ. Simultaneous monitoring of gastric and oesophageal pH reveals limitations of conventional oesophageal pH monitoring in milk fed infants. *Arch Dis Child* 2001;84:273.
16. Wheatley E, Kennedy KA. Cross-over trial of treatment for bradycardia attributed to gastroesophageal reflux in preterm infants. *J Pediatr* 2009;155:516.
17. Kimball AL, Carlton DP. Gastroesophageal reflux medications in the treatment of apnea in premature infants. *J Pediatr* 2001;138:355.
18. Ho T, Dukhovny D, Zupancic JAF, et al. Choosing wisely in newborn medicine: five opportunities to increase value. *Pediatrics* 2015;136:e482.
19. Akinola E, Rosenkrantz TS, Pappagallo M, et al. Gastroesophageal reflux in infants < 32 weeks gestational age at birth: lack of relationship to chronic lung disease. *Am J Perinatol* 2004;21:57.
20. Nobile S, Noviello C, Cobellis G, et al. Are infants with bronchopulmonary dysplasia prone to gastroesophageal reflux? a prospective observational study with esophageal pH-Impedance monitoring. *J Pediatr* 2015;167:279.
21. Jadcherla SR, Chan CY, Moore R, et al. Impact of feeding strategies on the frequency and clearance of acid and nonacid gastroesophageal reflux events in dysphagic neonates. *J Parenter Enteral Nutr* 2012;36:449.
22. Corvaglia L, Aceti A, Mariani E, et al. The efficacy of sodium alginate (Gaviscon) for the treatment of gastro-oesophageal reflux in preterm infants. *Aliment Pharmacol Ther* 2011;33:466.
23. Loots C, Kritas S, van Wijk M, et al. Body positioning and medical therapy for infantile gastroesophageal reflux symptoms. *J Pediatr Gastroenterol Nutr* 2014;59:237.
24. American Academy of Pediatrics Committee on Fetus and Newborn. Hospital discharge of the high-risk neonate. *Pediatrics* 2008;122:1119.
25. Ostlie DJ, Miller KS, Holcomb GW III. Effective Nissen fundoplication length and bougie diameter size in young children undergoing laparoscopic Nissen fundoplication. *J Pediatr Surg* 2002;37:1664.
26. Fonkalsrud EW, Ashcraft KW, Coran AG, et al. Surgical treatment of gastroesophageal reflux in children: a combined hospital study of 467 patients. *Pediatrics* 1998;101:419.
27. Rothenberg SS. Two decades of experience with laparoscopic Nissen fundoplication in infants and children: a critical evaluation of indications, technique, and results. *J Laparoendosc Adv Surg Tech A* 2013;23:791.
28. Wales PW, Diamond IR, Dutta S, et al. Fundoplication and gastrostomy versus image-guided gastrojejunal tube for enteral feeding in neurologically impaired children with gastroesophageal reflux. *J Pediatr Surg* 2002;37:407.
29. Stone B, Hester G, Jackson D, et al. Effectiveness of fundoplication or gastrojejunal feeding in children with neurologic impairment. *Hosp Pediatr* 2017;7:140.
30. El-Gohary Y, Abdelhafeez A, Paton E, et al. Pyloric stenosis: an enigma more than a century after the first successful treatment. *Pediatr Surg Int* 2018;34:21.
31. Lund M, Pasternak B, Davidsen RB, et al. Use of macrolides in mother and child and risk of infantile hypertrophic pyloric stenosis: nationwide cohort study. *BMJ* 2014;348:g1908.
32. Adibe OO, Iqbal CW, Sharp SW, et al. Protocol versus ad libitum feeds after laparoscopic pyloromyotomy: a prospective randomized trial. *J Pediatr Surg* 2014;49:129.
33. Cragan JD, Martin ML, Moore CA, et al. Descriptive epidemiology of small intestinal atresia, Atlanta, Georgia. *Teratology* 1993;48(5):441.
34. Mustafawi AR, Hassan ME. Congenital duodenal obstruction in children: a decade's experience. *Eur J Pediatr Surg* 2008;18(2):93.
35. Adams SD, Stanton MP. Malrotation and intestinal atresias. *Early Hum Dev* 2014;90:921.
36. Dott NM. Anomalies of intestinal rotation: their embryology and surgical aspects: with report of five cases. *Br J Surg* 1923;11:251.
37. Torres AM, Ziegler MM. Malrotation of the intestine. *World J Surg* 1993;17:326.
38. Dilley AV, Pereira J, Shi ECP, et al. The radiologist says malrotation: does the surgeon operate? *Pediatr Surg Int* 2000;16:45.
39. Orzech N, Navarro OM, Langer JC. Is ultrasonography a good screening test for intestinal malrotation? *J Pediatr Surg* 2006;41:1005.
40. Mohinuddin S, Sakhuja P, Bermundo B, et al. Outcomes of full-term infants with bilious vomiting: observational study of a retrieved cohort. *Arch Dis Child* 2015;100:14.
41. Kim PC, Superina RA, Ein S. Colonic atresia combined with Hirschsprung's disease: a diagnostic and therapeutic challenge. *J Pediatr Surg* 1995;30:1216.
42. Arca MJ, Oldham KT. Atresia, stenosis, and other obstructions of the colon. In: Coran AG, Adzick NS, Krummel TM, et al., eds. *Pediatric surgery*, 7th ed. Philadelphia, PA: Elsevier, 2012.
43. DiBaise JK, Young RJ, Vanderhook JA. Intestinal rehabilitation and the short bowel syndrome: part 1. *Am J Gastroenterol* 2004;99:1386.
44. Khan FA, Squires RH, Litman HJ, et al. Predictors of enteral autonomy in children with intestinal failure: a multicenter cohort study. *J Pediatr* 2015;167:29.
45. Warner BW. Intestinal failure. Stay Current: Pediatric Surgery. GlobalCastMD 2017. Available from: https://www.globalcastmd.com/episodes/intestinal-failure
46. Bianchi A. Intestinal loop lengthening—a technique for increasing small intestinal length. *J Pediatr Surg* 1980;15:145.

47. Kim HB, Lee PW, Garza J, et al. Serial transverse enteroplasty for short bowel syndrome: a case report. *J Pediatr Surg* 2003;38:881.

48. Jaksic T, Gutierrez IM, Kang KH. Short bowel syndrome. In: Coran AG, Adzick NS, Krummel TM, et al., eds. *Pediatric surgery*, 7th ed. Philadelphia, PA: Elsevier, 2012.

49. Javid PJ, Collier S, Richardson D, et al. The role of enteral nutrition in the reversal of parenteral nutrition-associated liver dysfunction in infants. *J Pediatr Surg* 2005;40:1015.

50. Lilja HE, Finkel Y, Paulsson M, et al. Prevention and reversal of intestinal failure-associated liver disease in premature infants with short bowel syndrome using intravenous fish oil in combination with omega-6/9 lipid emulsions. *J Pediatr Surg* 2011;46:1361.

51. Hyman PE, Everett SL, Harada T. Gastric acid hypersecretion in short bowel syndrome in infants: association with extent of resection and enteral feeding. *J Pediatr Gastroenterol Nutr* 1986;5:191.

52. Kaufman SS, Loseke CA, Lupo JV, et al. Influence of bacterial overgrowth and intestinal inflammation on duration of parenteral nutrition in children with short bowel syndrome. *J Pediatr* 1997;131:356.

53. Quigley EM, Quera R. Small intestinal bacterial overgrowth: roles of antibiotics, prebiotics, and probiotics. *Gastroenterology* 2006;130:S78.

54. Oliveira SB, Cole CR. Insights into medical management of pediatric intestinal failure. *Semin Pediatr Surg* 2018;27:256.

55. McMellen ME, Wakeman D, Longshore SW, et al. Growth factors: possible roles for clinical management of the short bowel syndrome. *Semin Pediatr Surg* 2010;19:35.

56. Spencer AU, Kovacevich D, McKinney-Barnett M, et al. Pediatric short-bowel syndrome: the cost of comprehensive care. *Am J Clin Nutr* 2008;88:1552.

57. Fullerton BS, Hong CR, Jaksic T. Long-term outcomes of pediatric intestinal failure. *Semin Pediatr Surg* 2017;26:328.

58. Cowles RA, Ventura KA, Martinez M, et al. Reversal of intestinal failure-associated liver disease in infants and children on parenteral nutrition: experience with 93 patients at a referral center for intestinal rehabilitation. *J Pediatr Surg* 2010;45:84.

59. Stanger JD, Oliveira C, Blackmore C, et al. The impact of multi-disciplinary intestinal rehabilitation programs on the outcomes of pediatric patients with intestinal failure: a systematic review and meta-analysis. *J Pediatr Surg* 2013;48:983.

60. Javid PJ, Oron AP, Duggan CP, et al. The extent of intestinal failure-associated liver disease in patients referred for intestinal rehabilitation is associated with increased mortality: an analysis of the Pediatric Intestinal Failure Consortium database. *J Pediatr Surg* 2018;53:1399.

61. Ching YA, Gura K, Modi B, et al. Pediatric intestinal failure: nutrition, pharmacologic, and surgical approaches. *Nutr Clin Pract* 2007;22:653.

62. Grant D, Abu-Elmagd K, Mazariegos G, et al. Intestinal transplant registry report: global activity and trends. *Am J Transplant* 2015;15:210.

63. Levitt MA, Pena A. Anorectal malformations. *Orphanet J Rare Dis* 2007;26:33.

64. Levitt MA, Peña A. Imperforate anus and cloacal malformations. In: Holcomb GW, Murphy JP, eds. *Ashcraft's pediatric surgery*, 5th ed. Philadelphia, PA: Elsevier, 2010.

65. Davis WS, Campbell JB. Neonatal small left colon syndrome. Occurrence in asymptomatic infants of diabetic mothers. *Am J Dis Child* 1975;129:1024.

66. Stewart DR, Nixon GW, Johnson DG, et al. Neonatal small left colon syndrome. *Ann Surg* 1977;186:741.

67. Lu JF, Nightingale CH. Magnesium sulfate in eclampsia and pre-eclampsia: pharmacokinetic principles. *Clin Pharmacokinet* 2000;38:305.

68. Rattray BN, Kraus DM, Drinker LR, et al. Antenatal magnesium sulfate and spontaneous intestinal perforation in infants less than 25 weeks gestation. *J Perinatol* 2014;34:819.

69. Coe A, Avansino JR, Kapur RP. Distal rectal skip-segment Hirschsprung disease and the potential for false-negative diagnosis. *Pediatr Dev Pathol* 2016;19:123.

70. Shenoy A, De Los Santos Y, Johnson KN, et al. Distal rectal skip segment Hirschsprung disease: case report and review of literature. *Fetal Pediatr Pathol* 2019;38:437.

71. Friedmacher F, Puri P. Hirschsprung's disease associated with Down syndrome: a meta-analysis of incidence, functional outcomes and mortality. *Pediatr Surg Int* 2013;29:937.

72. Kilby MD. The incidence of gastroschisis. *BMJ* 2006;332:250.

73. Castilla EE, Mastroiacovo P, Orioli IM. Gastroschisis: international epidemiology and public health perspectives. *Am J Med Genet C Semin Med Genet* 2008;148c:162.

74. Frolov P, Alali J, Klein MD. Clinic risk factors for gastroschisis and omphalocele in humans: a review of the literature. *Pediatr Surg Int* 2010;26:1135.

75. Snyder CL, Miller KA, Sharp RJ, et al. Management of intestinal atresia in patients with gastroschisis. *J Pediatr Surg* 2001;36:1542.

76. McClellan EB, Shew SB, Lee SS, et al. Liver herniation in gastroschisis: incidence and prognosis. *J Pediatr Surg* 2011;46:2115.

77. Petrosyan M, Sandler AD. Closure methods in gastroschisis. *Semin Pediatr Surg* 2018;27:304.

78. Zani-Ruttenstock E, Zani A, Paul A, et al. Interstitial cells of Cajal are decreased in patients with gastroschisis associated intestinal dysmotility. *J Pediatr Surg* 2015;50:750.

79. O'Mara KL, Islam S, Taylor JA, et al. Gabapentin improves oral feeding in neurologically intact infants with abdominal disorders. *J Pediatr Pharmacol Ther* 2018;23:59.

80. Islam S. Advances in surgery for abdominal wall defects: gastroschisis and omphalocele. *Clin Perinatol* 2012;39:375.

81. Khan FA, Hashmi A, Islam S. Insights into embryology and development of omphalocele. *Semin Pediatr Surg* 2019;28:80.

82. Ayub SS, Taylor JA. Cardiac anomalies associated with omphalocele. *Semin Pediatr Surg* 2019;28:111.

83. Levy S, Tsao K, Cox CS Jr, et al. Component separation for complex congenital abdominal wall defects: not just for adults anymore. *J Pediatr Surg* 2013;48:2525.

84. van Eijck FC, Aronson DA, Hoogeveen YL, et al. Past and current surgical treatment of giant omphalocele: outcome of a questionnaire sent to authors. *J Pediatr Surg* 2011;46:482.

85. Neu J, Walker WA. Necrotizing enterocolitis. *N Engl J Med* 2011;364:255.

86. Han SM, Hong CR, Knell J, et al. Trends in incidence and outcomes of necrotizing enterocolitis over the last 12 years: a multicenter cohort analysis. *J Pediatr Surg* 2020;55:998.

87. Fitzgibbons SC, Ching Y, Yu D, et al. Mortality of necrotizing enterocolitis expressed by birth weight categories. *J Pediatr Surg* 2009;44:1072; discussion 5.

88. Bell MJ, Ternberg JL, Feigin RD, et al. Neonatal necrotizing enterocolitis: therapeutic decisions based upon clinical staging. *Ann Surg* 1978;187:1.

89. Pammi M, Cope J, Tarr PI, et al. Intestinal dysbiosis in preterm infants preceding necrotizing enterocolitis: a systematic review and meta-analysis. *Microbiome* 2017;5:31.

90. Gordon PV, Clark R, Swanson JR, et al. Can a national dataset generate a nomogram for necrotizing enterocolitis onset? *J Perinatol* 2014;34:732.

91. Walsh MC, Kliegman RM. Necrotizing enterocolitis: treatment based on staging criteria. *Pediatr Clin North Am* 1986;33:179.

92. Swanson JR, Attridge JT, Gordon PV. Potential confounder of NEC clinical trials. *J Perinatol* 2009;29:256; author reply 7–8.

93. Neu J. Necrotizing enterocolitis: the mystery goes on. *Neonatology* 2014;106:289.

94. Bazacliu C, Neu J. Pathophysiology of necrotizing enterocolitis: an update. *Curr Pediatr Rev* 2019;15:68.

95. Neu J, Pammi M. Necrotizing enterocolitis: the intestinal microbiome, metabolome and inflammatory mediators. *Semin Fetal Neonatal Med* 2018;23:400.

96. Hull MA, Fisher JG, Gutierrez IM, et al. Mortality and management of surgical necrotizing enterocolitis in very low birth weight neonates: a prospective cohort study. *J Am Coll Surg* 2014;218(6):1148.

97. Stanford A, Upperman JS, Boyle P, et al. Long-term follow-up of patients with necrotizing enterocolitis. *J Pediatr Surg* 2002;37(7):1048; discussion 1048.

98. Bazacliu C, Neu J. Necrotizing enterocolitis: long term complications. *Curr Pediatr Rev* 2019;15:115.

99. Siano E, Lauriti G, Ceccanti S, et al. Cardiogenic necrotizing enterocolitis: a clinically distinct entity from classical necrotizing enterocolitis. *Eur J Pediatr Surg* 2019;29:14.

100. Lenfestey MW, de la Cruz D, Neu J. Food protein-induced enterocolitis instead of necrotizing enterocolitis? a neonatal intensive care unit case series. *J Pediatr* 2018;200:270.

101. Caubet JC, Cianferoni A, Groetch M, et al. Food protein-induced enterocolitis syndrome. *Clin Exp Allergy* 2019;49:1178.

102. Donahue L. Spontaneous intestinal perforation. *Neonatal Netw* 2007;26:335.

103. Paquette L, Friedlich P, Ramanathan R, et al. Concurrent use of indomethacin and dexamethasone increases the risk of spontaneous intestinal perforation in very low birth weight neonates. *J Perinatol* 2006;26:486.

104. Gordon PV. Understanding intestinal vulnerability to perforation in the extremely low birth weight infant. *Pediatr Res* 2009;65:138.

THE NEWBORN INFANT

37 Hepatobiliary Disorders

Björn Fischler, Afrodite Psaros Einberg, and Maria Magnusson

INTRODUCTION

The liver of the newborn is presented with metabolic demands that are not fully matched by functional maturation. While the fetus can largely depend on glucose transfer from the mother over the placenta, the newborn must rapidly gain independent control over glucose hemostasis. When available glycogen stores are spent during the first 12 hours of life, glucogenesis is required.

Another important function of the liver is bile formation and secretion to the gut. Bile acids are the driving force of bile secretion. There are immaturities at all levels of this system, that is, bile acid synthesis, pool size, and intraluminal concentrations at birth with a gradual improvement during the first year of life.

The liver is involved in detoxification of both endogenous and exogenous substances; the latter are often referred to as xenobiotics. To transform these substances into water-soluble compounds, in order to have them excreted in urine, several sophisticated hepatic systems are used. Their capacity is age dependent; for example, the different enzymes in the cytochrome P450 system show a very complex ontogeny, with a gradual maturation not only during early life but actually throughout childhood and adolescence.

The liver of the newborn is vulnerable to age-specific diseases that may be of infectious, immunologic, metabolic, or genetic etiology. The main clinical types of liver and biliary diseases in this age group described in this chapter are neonatal liver failure, neonatal cholestasis, viral infections, and vascular diseases.

SIGNS OF LIVER DISEASE

Liver disease is often either asymptomatic or subclinical in its presentation. This is true both for neonates and older children and adults. In such cases, liver involvement may only be discovered by abnormalities in biochemistry or imaging procedures. The available biochemical tests used to detect liver disease in daily clinical practice include markers for hepatocyte turnover, cholestasis, hypersplenism (as an indirect sign of portal hypertension), synthetic function, and malignancy, as depicted in Table 37.1 (1).

Overt clinical signs suggesting liver disease in a neonate include jaundice, ascites, and hepatomegaly. Encephalopathy, which in toddlers and older children would suggest ongoing liver failure, is usually hard to define in neonates.

The most important and widely available imaging technique is ultrasonography. It can give clinically relevant information regarding gross anatomy, echogenicity of the liver, focal abnormalities, obvious bile duct problems, vascular abnormalities, and the existence of ascites. For further and more detailed studies, magnetic resonance imaging is preferred, in particular to visualize the bile tree in detail. Computerized tomography (CT) is mainly of specific use for detailed studies of vascular abnormalities.

Liver biopsy is sometimes needed for precise diagnosis, in particular in the workup of cholestatic neonates. The diagnostic yield is good, but great care should be taken to ensure the lowest possible risk of complications, in particular bleeding (2).

NEONATAL LIVER FAILURE

Neonatal liver failure is a rare but often dramatic disease state. The management of such patients demands thorough knowledge of differential diagnostics and possible therapies, as well as the existence of an infrastructure involving teams not only for pediatric hepatology but also for neonatal intensive care and liver transplantation. Although some improvements in the outcome have been reported the last decades, survival rates are still below those seen in acute liver failure of older children or adults (3,4).

Neonatal liver failure is defined as biochemical liver abnormality occurring within the first 28 days of life, with concomitant deficiency of hepatic synthetic function, measured as vitamin K–resistant INR at or above 2.0. In comparison to acute liver failure of older children, neonates are more often prone to hypoglycemia and coagulopathy. With regard to timing of onset, at least two distinct groups of neonatal liver failure can be defined, one with prenatal liver disease and one with peri- or postnatal disease. This distinction can be of help when deciding on diagnostic procedures. The prenatal causes include congenital infections, neonatal hemochromatosis (NH), which is currently believed to be caused by gestational alloimmune liver disease (GALD), and hemophagocytic lymphohistiocytosis (HLH). Peri- or postnatal diseases include metabolic liver disease of various types, certain infections, vascular abnormalities causing shunts, and liver failure secondary to asphyxia or endocrine deficiency such as hypocortisolism. Of 42 patients with neonatal liver failure in a review from King's College, London, UK, 17 were described as having NH, 10 had viral infections, 6 had hematologic conditions, 5 had metabolic disease, and the remaining had miscellaneous or undetermined etiologies (3).

Gestational Alloimmune Liver Disease

These patients present with apparent liver failure already at birth, and there are usually clear signs of an intrauterine onset. Thus, the liver will appear as cirrhotic on imaging studies, preferably ultrasonography; there are often ascites and hypoalbuminemia. Since these patients were previously described to have iron depositions in extrahepatic organs, such as pancreas, spleen, or heart and markedly elevated levels of ferritin in serum, the term NH was coined and treatment was directed toward reducing the iron storage. However, survival without liver transplantation was very poor. It was also noted that mothers giving birth to one such patient ran a risk of 95% to 100% of having equally sick offspring in consecutive pregnancies. Assuming that this might be primarily an alloimmune disease, Whitington et al subsequently showed that by treating the mother with intravenous immunoglobulins (IVIGs) during subsequent pregnancies, this seemingly very repetitive pattern could effectively be broken. Further studies strongly suggested that the fetal liver injury of this so-called GALD was mediated by formation of a complement C5b-9 complex. GALD is thereby thought to be the cause of NH. However, not all cases with GALD exhibit full NH features. Index patients with neonatal liver failure and signs of extrahepatic iron deposition could reasonably effectively be treated with exchange transfusion or plasmapheresis, in combination with IVIG (4–6). Early identification and treatment is necessary, while on the other hand, diagnostic procedures are either unspecific or complicated to achieve (7). Thus, an elevated serum level of ferritin is a common feature also in HLH and in certain mitochondrial depletion diseases. The identification of extrahepatic iron storage demands either a biopsy, for example, from the lip to demonstrate iron deposition in salivary glands, which may be problematic in a very sick neonate with coagulopathy. Alternatively, some authors suggest that iron deposition in the heart or pancreas could be visualized by MRI studies, but this demands specific programs and infrastructure to perform such investigation in this situation.

THE NEWBORN INFANT

TABLE 37.1

Biochemical Markers Used to Detect and Characterize Liver Disease in Clinical Practice

Type of Marker	Test
Hepatocyte turnover	AST, ALT
Cholestasis	Conjugated bilirubin, gamma-GT, ALP, total bile acid level
Synthetic function	Albumin, prothrombin time measured as INR, other coagulation factors
Hypersplenism	Platelets, leukocytes, hemoglobin
Malignancy	Alpha-fetoprotein, CA19-9

Viral Infections

The most common viral cause for neonatal liver failure is herpes simplex virus (HSV). Both type 1 and 2 infections have been described in these patients, and they can occur in association with either primary or secondary maternal infections. In fact, clinical signs in the mother are reported only in a minority of cases.

These patients often present with very severe liver involvement, which is unfortunately part of a multisystemic disease (3,4). Survival is therefore quite poor, despite the possibility to treat with the effective antiviral compound acyclovir. Since such treatment is relatively nontoxic and the chances of survival after a fulminant HSV infection is low, it is widely suggested that acyclovir treatment should be considered for all neonates with liver failure.

Other important viral infections causing neonatal liver failure include cytomegalovirus (CMV), parvovirus B19, and HSV type 6. To some extent, these may be treatable with antiviral medications.

The more traditional hepatitis viruses, such as hepatitis A, B, and C rarely cause neonatal liver failure. Thus, although vertical transmission from mother to infant of hepatitis B and C virus infection, respectively, may very well occur, it usually results in subclinical, but chronic, infections. By contrast, hepatitis E virus infection carries a high risk (20%) of resulting in acute liver failure in pregnant women, and if transmitted to the fetus results in a very high proportion of stillbirths or early deaths due to neonatal liver failure. This dramatic pattern has so far only been reported from endemic areas, for example, the Indian peninsula (8).

Mitochondrial Disorders

These patients usually present during the first weeks to months of life. Neonatal liver failure may be isolated or part of a broader multiorgan profile, including involvement of the central nervous system (CNS) and peripheral muscular dysfunction. The typical biochemical feature of mitochondrial disease, such as elevated lactate levels in serum is less obvious or absent in the isolated cases of liver disease. Specific metabolic disruptions in mitochondrial function, detected in muscle biopsies, are often also absent or unspecific in isolated liver disease. Currently, the clinically most important diagnostic tool is the detection of mutations in specific genes for mitochondrial diseases, in particular the so-called mitochondrial depletion syndromes. These tools, which are mostly based on high-throughput new-generation sequencing techniques, can be used to detect mutations in important genes such as POLG, DGUOK, MPV17, and TRMU (9). Rapid response to testing is of clinical importance, since liver transplantation may be contraindicated for patients with certain mutations, due to the very poor survival rates secondary to severe extrahepatic diseases, in particular from the CNS.

Other Metabolic Conditions Causing Neonatal Liver Failure

Galactosemia often results in severe liver disease, with the possibility of liver failure within the first week of life. Early initiation of galactose-free diet will resolve this, but the patients are also prone to potentially life-threatening episodes of *E. coli* sepsis that must be detected and treated promptly. Patients with galactosemia are to a very large extent identified within neonatal screening programs.

Tyrosinemia results in liver failure that classically presents during the first months of life and commonly includes extrahepatic features such as renal tubular acidosis and rickets. The combination of pharmacologic treatment with nitisinone and a diet low in tyrosine and phenylalanine is very effective. Currently, many countries have added neonatal screening for this disease in their regular programs, so that many patients will be discovered and started on treatment before the development of severe liver disease.

NEONATAL CHOLESTASIS

Bile acids constitute the main, but not exclusive driving force for the bile flow. Decreased or obstructed bile flow at any level from the hepatocyte to the junction of the extrahepatic biliary tree and the duodenum is referred to as cholestasis. There are two main pathophysiologic consequences of cholestasis. Firstly, the lack of bile acids in the gut causes fat malabsorption, which results in deficiency of fat-soluble vitamins and in malnutrition. Secondly, the retention of hepatotoxic bile acids in the liver causes progressive injury of the hepatocytes and if left untreated will result in the development of cirrhosis and subsequent risk for liver failure.

When described in general text books of medicine, jaundice and pale stools are regarded as the main clinical signs of cholestasis. However, neither of these is actually an obligate finding. Thus, there could be anicteric cholestasis, particularly in infants, and the stool color may be either normal or pale. Symptoms and signs such as pruritus, dark urine, unexplained bleeding, and steatorrhea can be cholestatic manifestations. The increased risk of bleeding is most often caused by vitamin K deficiency, secondary to the malabsorption. Biochemically, elevated serum levels of conjugated bilirubin, gamma-glutamyl transpeptidase (G-GT), alkaline phosphatase (ALP), and fasting bile acids indicate cholestasis (10,11).

In neonates, there is an immaturity in the enterohepatic circulation of bile acids, resulting in a state of so-called physiologic cholestasis (12). This may last for at least the first half year of life, and during this period, there is an increased vulnerability to develop cholestasis. The term neonatal cholestasis is often used to describe nonphysiologic cholestasis in infants from birth to the age of 6 months.

A large and continuously growing number of defined causes for neonatal cholestasis have been identified (Table 37.2). They were previously classified as either extrahepatic or intrahepatic in origin. In the first group, biliary atresia (BA) is by far the most common. The second group, which includes many different diseases, is referred to as intrahepatic neonatal cholestasis. The term neonatal hepatitis has often been used for the intrahepatic group in some literature. However, while this might be an adequate term considering the histologic picture, it is also confusing because it implies an infectious etiology, which is evident in only a minority of cases.

The most common causes of intrahepatic neonatal cholestasis include alpha-1-antitrypsin deficiency (AATD), different viral infections, and a group of genetic cholestatic disorders, including progressive familial intrahepatic cholestasis (PFIC) of different types and Alagille syndrome (10). Most other etiologies are rare, but some of them are important to detect because they indicate the need for specific treatments. This is true for some of the identified inborn errors of metabolism, as well as for cystic fibrosis (CF) and hormone deficiencies (10).

The incidence of neonatal cholestasis is difficult to establish, since mostly referred patients are reported and this would

TABLE 37.2

Most Common Causes for Cholestasis in Term Infants, with Estimated Proportions of the Total Number

Disease	Proportion of Total
Biliary atresia	30%
Infections	15%
α_1-Antitrypsin deficiency	10%
Alagille syndrome	5%
Progressive familial intrahepatic cholestasis (PFIC), different types	5%
Other rare inborn errors of metabolism	3%
Chromosomal aberrations	2%
Miscellaneous: endocrine deficiencies, cystic fibrosis, asphyxia, and common bile duct lithiasis	5%
Idiopathic	25%

underestimate the number of mild cases. However, the generally accepted figure in term infants is between 1 in 2,500 and 5,000 (11). For BA, which is easier to define more strictly, there are a number of population-based studies available, suggesting an incidence of 1 in 8,000 to 20,000 infants (13).

Biliary Atresia

BA is considered to be an inflammatory obliteration of the hepatic or common bile duct at any point from the porta hepatis to the duodenum. It is a heterogeneous disorder, with a subgroup of 10% to 20% presenting with associated anomalies of the heart, gastrointestinal (GI) tract, and/or genitourinary tract, while the rest have isolated BA (14).

The etiology and pathogenesis of BA is still unclear. Previous studies suggest either an alteration in the remodeling of the so-called ductal plate during the first trimester of fetal life, an association to different viral infections (Table 37.3), immunologic mechanisms, alterations in the vascular system, and toxic insults (14). Repeated cases in the same family are uncommon, and monozygotic twins are most often discordant for the disease. The data on ethnic differences in the incidence are contradictory, but higher incidences have indeed been reported from South East Asia (13).

Reovirus type 3 has been linked to BA in serologic studies (15). A condition resembling BA was described in weanling mice infected by reovirus 3. However, results of studies utilizing polymerase chain reaction (PCR) to detect reovirus RNA in the liver tissue of these patients are divergent (16). There is currently no obvious clinical relevance in humans of these findings.

Based on animal investigations on rotavirus A, studies in humans on the related rotavirus C have suggested an association to BA. Rotavirus C RNA was detected by PCR in liver tissue from such patients and in some cases also in stool samples (17). Several groups have subsequently described in detail the development of a BA-like disease in a murine model infected with rhesus type rotavirus, but these models did not replicate the particular finding of progressive fibrosis that is a hallmark in human BA. Very recently, a modified such model was shown to express features of fibrosis (18).

Such experimental models would be needed to possibly find therapeutic improvements for human BA. Meanwhile, it has been suggested from Taiwan that the introduction of universal vaccination against rotavirus infection might impact the incidence of BA, possibly by lowering the overall rate of this infection (19). However, later studies from United States and South Korea could not corroborate these findings (20).

CMV infection has been linked to BA in several case reports (21). We have described an association between ongoing CMV infections, defined by the detection of CMV-IgM in serum in 38% of BA patients at the time, which was significantly higher than the 6% found in age-matched controls without any liver disease (22). Other studies suggest the rate of BA patients with ongoing CMV infection to be anywhere between 10% and 74%. The group at Kings College, London, the United Kingdom, studied patients with "CMV-IgM-positive BA" more closely and found that they had distinctively different histopathologic features, including more pronounced inflammation and that their outcome with regard to survival with native liver was significantly worse than BA patients without ongoing CMV infection (23). In a descriptive follow-up, they reported that patients with CMV-IgM-positive BA who had received antiviral treatment against the infection had a better outcome than those who had not been treated. However, this was not a randomized controlled trial. (24).

Thus, several different viral infections have been associated with BA, but it is yet unclear whether, for example, CMV plays a role in the pathogenesis and/or natural history of BA or if it is just "an innocent bystander." It has been suggested that this or other viruses could nonspecifically trigger an abnormal series of events that eventually causes bile duct obliteration. The initial viral lesion might occur several months before the clinical picture is obvious, that is, in intrauterine life. This could explain the variable results in studies trying to detect the presence of virus or its nucleic acid in the liver at the time of clinical presentation.

Patients with BA most commonly present at the age of 2 to 6 weeks with jaundice and pale stools, although presentation at birth can indeed occur. Compared to infants with intrahepatic cholestasis, a normal birth weight, a firm and enlarged liver, and apart from the jaundice a rather healthy baby are more commonly found signs. However, none of these signs, nor any of the suggested biochemical markers, such as the serum G-GT, is 100% specific for BA (11,14).

To visualize the lack of biliary excretion to the gut in BA, hepatobiliary scintigraphy is often used (14). In patients with BA, there is a good hepatic uptake of the isotope without any sign of excretion to the gut within 24 hours. However, the specificity of this method is questioned, because patients with severe intrahepatic cholestasis will sometimes lack excretion (11).

A needle liver biopsy, on the other hand, as interpreted by an experienced pathologist, will show a histologic pattern specific for BA in 90% to 95% of the true cases (11).

In patients with a liver histology suggesting BA, a laparotomy with an intraoperative cholangiogram is considered to be the diagnostic gold standard (11).

The prognosis of BA if untreated is very poor, with 100% mortality before 2 years of age. However, the portoenterostomy procedure, as first described by Kasai, has improved the situation (14).

TABLE 37.3

Possible Viral Etiologies for Biliary Atresia

Virus	Animal Model	Serology Findings in Patients	Detection in Liver by PCR in Patients	Clinical Implication
Reovirus	+	+	Highly variable	None
Rotavirus	+++	−/+	Highly variable	Vaccination?
Cytomegalovirus	+	+++	Highly variable	Antiviral treatment?

If performed by experienced surgeons, it is successful also in the very long run in approximately one-third of the patients, while one-third will need a liver transplantation early, often during the second half of the first year of life, because of a rapid progression to liver cirrhosis and liver failure. In fact, BA is the most common indication for pediatric liver transplantation. The remaining one-third will in most cases need a liver transplantation, but later, during the first two decades of life. The long-term outcome depends on the age at portoenterostomy. Thus, the group of patients operated on before 2 months of age generally do better than those treated later (14). The other proven predictor of outcome is the level of centralization, that is, centers with a higher case load have higher rates of survival with native liver (14).

The nutritional treatment of BA includes supplementation with the fat-soluble vitamins A, D, E, and K. A high total energy intake, including high levels of medium chain triglycerides (MCT), and of branched chain amino acids is also recommended (10).

The risk of developing bacterial cholangitis is highest in the first year postoperatively. The question of prophylaxis against cholangitis is still unsolved. Trimethoprim–sulfamethoxazole is most widely used, but there may be a risk of selecting more virulent bacteria if continuous prophylaxis is used.

Pruritus is common in all children with chronic cholestasis, and it may severely disturb daily life. The exact mechanism for the pruritus is not known. There is no clear cut correlation between the serum bile acid levels, which are thought to reflect the degree of cholestasis, and the grade of pruritus. Pruritus treatment with ursodeoxycholic acid has been attempted with some success in cholestatic children. Other drugs such as rifampicin, cholestyramine, and phenobarbital have also been tried with varying success (10).

The use of corticosteroids after Kasai procedure for BA is heavily debated. The rationale would be that such treatment could weaken the inflammatory response that is suggested to be of pathogenetic importance and thereby improve the bile flow. Some earlier uncontrolled studies suggested this to be beneficial. Two independent randomized controlled studies have been reported, one from the United Kingdom and one from the United States (14). While the former concluded that some, although quite modest, positive effects of steroid treatment was seen, this was not the case in the latter. In fact, the study from the US suggested a negative outcome with regard to side effects, including growth retardation (25). The use of steroids thus remains controversial, but some centers tend to use it, one argument being that we so far have no other adjunctive treatment for this very problematic situation.

Alpha-1-antitrypsin Deficiency

AAT-deficient individuals are classified according to the protease inhibitor (Pi) type, which is determined by agarose electrophoresis (26). AATD was first correlated to early onset pulmonary emphysema but later also to neonatal cholestasis and juvenile liver cirrhosis. The most common deficiency type is designated PiZZ. In a Swedish population-based study of 200,000 newborns, Pi type ZZ was found in 1 in 1,600 babies of whom 10% had neonatal cholestasis (26).

The mechanism for the liver disease in AATD, and the reason why only a minority of deficient individuals will develop this is still unclear. The accumulation of abnormal AAT in the endoplasmic reticulum (ER) of the liver cells is of pathogenetic importance. Molecular mechanisms responsible for this accumulation include a folding defect (27), as well as a loop-sheet polymerization causing an altered tertiary structure. It has been postulated that the susceptibility to liver disease in AATD is associated to other, yet unknown factors of genetic or environmental origin (27).

Liver disease in AATD often starts with neonatal cholestasis (10). The clinical and histologic picture is often indistinguishable from other causes of neonatal cholestasis, including BA (10,11). While liver biopsy in patients with AATD will show the presence of diastase-resistant globules in the hepatocytes, this finding is not specific to AATD and can be found in the biopsies of patients with liver disease of other causes too.

At present, there is no specific pharmacologic treatment for the liver disease in AATD. Enzyme replacement therapy, which has been attempted in patients with pulmonary emphysema, would probably not help the situation. For patients with neonatal cholestasis caused by AATD, the treatment is supportive, including substitution with fat-soluble vitamins.

The outcome for these patients is very variable. In Sveger's group of 14 prospectively followed cholestatic infants with AATD, almost one-third eventually died, one-third had consistently elevated transaminases, and one-third normalized their transaminases (27). Similarly, severe outcome results were reported by other groups (28). A subgroup of the patients with poor prognosis will progress early and rapidly to liver failure, that is, within the first 1 to 2 years of life. Another subgroup will progress slower, that is, liver failure will appear around 10 to 15 years of age. The long-term outcome is hard to predict in the early course of the disease.

Liver transplantation is in the long run the only alternative for AATD patients with end-stage liver disease. Transplantation will not only replace the diseased liver but also ensure normal levels of properly functioning AAT. This is because the transplant recipient will express the normal Pi phenotype of the donor (28).

Alagille Syndrome (Syndromic Paucity of Intrahepatic/Interlobular Bile Ducts)

This syndrome was described by Alagille et al. in 1975 (29). The fully developed syndrome included the following five features: chronic cholestasis starting in infancy, characteristic box-shaped facies, vertebral arch defects, posterior embryotoxon, and cardiovascular abnormalities (30). However, all features are not expressed in all patients. This multisystemic disease was shown to be inherited in an autosomal dominant fashion, but with a variable expression. Later studies revealed that a majority of the defined patients have a mutation in the *JAG1* gene, whereas a smaller group has mutation in the *Notch 2* gene. The Notch signaling system is very central for embryonic differentiation, for example, in the heart and vasculature, as well as in bile duct development.

Patients with Alagille syndrome are often growth retarded. However, treatment with growth hormone (GH) seems nonbeneficial, suggesting GH insensitivity. A subgroup of the patients has been described as having mild mental retardation. However, in a standardized test for cognitive and academic achievements, the Alagille patients did not differ from children with other chronic liver diseases (31).

When presenting with neonatal cholestasis, the peculiar facies is not always evident. Furthermore, the initial liver histology does not always show the later typical pattern with a decreased ratio of interlobular bile ducts to number of portal areas (30), and the hepatobiliary scintigraphy, if performed, may often lack excretion to the gut (11). There is a risk that these patients are subjected to laparotomy because BA cannot be ruled out. Biochemically, apart from increased cholestatic markers, there are no specific diagnostic signs at early age, although the serum levels of cholesterol are generally very high (32).

The long-term prognosis is variable. In 80 patients studied by Alagille et al, the mortality was 26% (30). The cause of death was liver involvement in five of them, severe cardiovascular abnormalities in six and nonspecified infections in seven. In other descriptive studies, the risk of cerebrovascular incidents was pointed out (32). There are also case reports on the development of hepatic malignancies quite early in life.

Interestingly, despite the fact that a large proportion of these patients develop chronic cholestasis, which, for example, can lead to debilitating pruritus, growth failure, and severe metabolic bone disease, it seems evident that a certain proportion may in the long run improve with subsiding cholestasis. The reason for this is not entirely clear, but it seems that the paucity of intrahepatic bile ducts in early years may improve, that is, bile duct development matures with time.

Progressive Familial Intrahepatic Cholestasis

This disease was first described in an Amish family named Byler and was initially referred to as Byler disease (33). Stepwise developments in genetics have resulted in a long and still growing list of different types of PFIC. The following clinical and biochemical criteria for PFIC were suggested several decades ago and are still relevant:

1. Chronic unremitting cholestasis with onset in infancy
2. Exclusion of anatomic and metabolic etiologies, including inborn error of bile acid biosynthesis
3. Typical biochemical markers of cholestasis, including increased serum levels of bile acids and ALP, but low to normal levels of serum G-GT in most cases

The liver histology at onset is often nonspecific with giant cell hepatitis. Later on, a pattern of paucity of the intrahepatic bile ducts may develop.

The original patients with Byler disease were in the late 1990s shown to have mutations in the gene encoding for the FIC protein. This disease, which often is called PFIC type 1, has a multisystemic feature; for example, there is often involvement of the GI canal and pancreas. Furthermore, in the sickest patients, who are subjected to liver transplantation, some extrahepatic symptoms prevail, and there is unfortunately a high risk to develop liver disease posttransplantation. Two other types, that is, PFIC type 2 (mutation in the gene encoding for bile salt export pump [BSEP]) and PFIC type 3 (mutation in the gene encoding for multidrug-resistant protein [MDR]) were also genetically characterized some 20 years ago. The additionally defined types of PFIC have been genetically characterized quite recently, all with the use of new-generation sequencing techniques. Some important examples include PFIC phenotypes with mutation in the genes encoding for the tight junction protein 2 (TJP2), the nuclear bile acid receptor FXR, and the myosin 5b (Myo 5b) protein. Thus, at least six different diseases with PFIC phenotypes have to date been defined. Extrahepatic involvement seems evident for Myo 5b disease with microvillus disease of the small gut and to some extent also in TJP2 disease with lung involvement. For PFIC type 2/BSEP disease, an important aspect is the extremely increased risk for early onset hepatocellular carcinoma (HCC), which for patients with certain mutations can be as high as 15% (34).

Different variants of surgical procedures to block the enterohepatic circulation of bile acids have been tried in PFIC patients, in particular those with types 1 and 2. Such procedures seem successful in alleviating cholestasis and actually stopping progression to liver cirrhosis in a proportion of the patients, and it can considered as early as in infancy (34,35). However, in other patients, where progression to decompensated cirrhosis and/or HCC is evident, liver transplantation remains the only viable option.

Viral Infections

The most common viral cause of intrahepatic neonatal cholestasis is CMV infection. As such, it has mostly been described within the framework of multisystemic disease in newborns with congenital CMV infection. Since this is defined by the detection of ongoing CMV infection at the age of 2 weeks or younger, such patients are mostly prone to be discovered in the intensive care unit or at early postnatal follow-up. Apart from various forms of liver involvement,

that is, cholestasis and/or hepatosplenomegaly and/or elevated transaminases, patients with symptomatic congenital CMV often have involvement from the CNS, chorioretinitis, and can develop deafness or impaired hearing. (See Chapter) In addition, bone marrow depression can occur. The use of antiviral treatment is indicated for symptomatic congenital CMV infection. In patients with ongoing CMV infection and cholestasis presenting after 2 weeks of age, the distinction between pre- and perinatal infection cannot be made. However, if stored Guthrie cards, sampled at 3 days of age and used for metabolic screening, are available, they can be used to detect CMV DNA by PCR. A positive such analysis would suggest congenital/prenatal CMV infection (36).

Although two of the more classic viruses causing hepatitis, that is, hepatitis B and C viruses can be transmitted from mother to infant quiet efficiently, neither one seems to cause cholestasis in the neonate, but rather a chronic but subclinical infection.

Other Causes for Neonatal Cholestasis

Neonatal cholestasis may occur in conjunction with several systemic diseases. One example is the case of septicemia. In fact, bacterial endotoxins have been showed to induce cholestasis in several experimental systems (37). Other nonviral infectious causes for neonatal cholestasis include congenital syphilis and toxoplasmosis. The rapid detection and subsequent treatment of these underlying causes usually results in resolution of cholestasis.

Neonatal cholestasis may also be associated to perinatal asphyxia. However, the relative frequency of this, when compared to the number of asphyxiated newborns, seems quite low, and it seems much less common than the more widely recognized pattern with grossly elevated transaminases after severe asphyxia. The hepatologic outcome in asphyxiated newborns with cholestatic features is reported to be benign, possibly suggesting that major diagnostic procedures in these often critically ill newborns might be avoided (38).

A large number of different inherited metabolic diseases may manifest as neonatal cholestasis. For example, several inborn errors of bile acid synthesis have been described (39). In these disorders, an enzymatic block causes accumulation of potentially hepatotoxic compounds in the liver. Additionally, the decrease in bile acids excreted to the gut causes fat malabsorption. These diseases share some important features with, for example, PFIC 2, including the paradoxically low or normal gamma-GT level in serum despite ongoing cholestasis. Although very rare, these disorders should be screened for in patients with neonatal cholestasis, because they can be very effectively treated with oral bile acids (39).

Isolated or combined forms of hormonal deficiencies can present with neonatal cholestasis (10,40). Cortisol, thyroid hormone, and probably also GH seem to be of importance to uphold a normal bile flow. Consequently, deficiencies may result in retention of bile and its bile acids, causing cholestasis. Prompt diagnosis and initiation of substitution(s) will in almost all cases result in resolution of cholestasis, and the development of chronic liver disease in these cases is very uncommon. In one report, 7 of 20 (35%) patients with congenital hypopituitarism presented with cholestasis as the major clinical feature (40).

Certain chromosomal abnormalities, in particular trisomy 21 (Down syndrome), are associated to neonatal cholestasis. In a population-based study, 8 out of 206 (4%) newborns with trisomy 21 had cholestasis, that is, a 100-fold increase in incidence when comparing to term infants. Other organ involvement from the GI tract, heart, and bone marrow was associated with an increased risk for cholestasis. The prognosis of cholestatic patients was guarded, that is, two with concomitant bone marrow disease succumbed early, one developed chronic liver disease, whereas cholestasis resolved in the remaining five (41).

Studies on the embryology of the liver have revealed that the intrahepatic bile duct system is derived from hepatocyte precursor cells surrounding the portal vein branches like a sleeve (42). The concept of this sleeve is referred to as the ductal plate, and the remodeling of the ductal plate is thought to be essential for the normal development of the intrahepatic biliary tree. If the remodeling does not occur or is incomplete, this will result in diseases entitled ductal plate malformations. These disorders, for example, *congenital* hepatic fibrosis and Caroli disease and other forms of genetically defined ciliopathies, can occasionally present with neonatal cholestasis (43).

CF, which is a genetic multiorgan disease involving mainly lungs, pancreas, and the GI tract, may present with neonatal cholestasis (44). Interestingly, extrahepatic symptoms may not be present at this early stage. Although cholestasis usually resolves with time, these children are at risk for development of CF-associated chronic liver disease.

Cholestasis Related to Extreme Prematurity and Total Parenteral Nutrition

The incidence of cholestasis is much higher in extremely preterm than in term babies. For example, we identified an incidence of up to 14% in a population-based observational study of infants born before 30 weeks of gestational age, suggesting a 350-fold elevation in the rate of cholestasis compared to term infants (45). The underlying causes of cholestasis are often completely different from those seen in term infants. Thus, the main risk factors for development of cholestasis in this specific group are low gestational age, the use of total parenteral nutrition, lack of enteral feeding, surgical abruptions of the gut most often secondary to necrotizing enterocolitis, and septicemias. This cholestatic situation of these patients is sometimes referred to as TPN-associated cholestasis or intestinal failure–associated liver disease (IFALD). The outcome with regard to cholestatic liver disease is usually good if gut continuity and enteral feedings are ensured. However, in the subgroup where this is not possible, the risk of developing end-stage liver disease and subsequent multiorgan failure is evident.

TPN-associated cholestasis may also occur in term infants after surgery for severe malformations. If gut continuity and improved intestinal function cannot be obtained and the need for TPN becomes chronic, the risk of progressive IFALD is evident. This development can often be balanced, for example, by procedures increasing the functional capacity of the intestine and the use of alternative fat emulsions for TPN, such as those based on fish oil or olive oil instead of the traditional ones based on soy (45). However, if intestinal failure prevails and liver disease progresses, a proportion of these patients must be considered for combined intestine and liver transplantation, preferably before multiorgan failure has developed.

Diagnostic Considerations in Neonatal Cholestasis

The detection of conjugated hyperbilirubinemia is decisive to establish ongoing cholestasis. Serum levels of conjugated bilirubin above 20 μmol/L (1.2 mg/dL), with the ratio of conjugated to total bilirubin being above 20%, are strongly suggestive. In fact, all jaundiced infants aged 2 weeks or above should be subjected to blood sampling for total and conjugated bilirubin in serum. Once cholestasis is established, some stepwise diagnostic procedures are needed (10,11):

- Step 1
  - Identify treatable disorder or complication and define the severity of the liver involvement.
  - Check prothrombin time (measured as international normalized ratio [INR]), if clearly pathologic, give intravenous vitamin K to avoid life-threatening bleeding.
  - Consider bacterial cultures of blood, urine, and other fluids, especially if infant is clinically ill.

  - Check remaining liver function tests, hemoglobin, platelets, white blood cells, cortisol, TSH, T3, T4, and glucose to detect other treatable diseases.
  - Test for alpha-1-antitrypsin level, viral infections, in particular CMV and other herpes virus infections and toxoplasma.
  - Perform ultrasonography, in particular to detect choledocal cysts, multiple spleens, and situs inversus (which occurs in some 10% to 20% of BA cases).
- Step 2
  - In patients with acholic stools, a percutaneous liver biopsy is suggested to rule in or rule out the possibility of BA.
  - Consider investigations for Alagille syndrome, such as echocardiogram to detect malformations, ophthalmology consultation for posterior embryotoxon, and X-ray investigation for butterfly vertebrae.
  - In patients with normal colored stools but no improvement of cholestasis and negative outcome of investigations suggested above, the use of next-generation genetic sequencing tools is strongly suggested (9).

In individuals who belong to patient groups with a known increased risk for cholestasis, such as extremely preterm infants or patients with trisomy 21, step 2 could be modified or in many cases omitted.

Management of Cholestasis

Regardless of the nature of the underlying disease, all patients with cholestasis are at risk for malabsorption of fat-soluble vitamins (A, D, E, K), and these should all be substituted. Furthermore, to avoid poor weight gain and growth, an increased overall intake of calories and also of MCT fats are indicated (10). Additionally, the use of the choleretic bile acid compound ursodeoxycholic acid is also advocated, since it may often reduce the cholestasis.

VIRAL HEPATITIS AND VERTICAL TRANSMISSION

Hepatitis C Virus

Hepatitis C virus (HCV) infection is a blood-borne disease affecting the liver. Chronic HCV infection is an important global health issue, affecting an estimated 71 million people worldwide (46). Among them, around 6 million are children (47). The majority of HCV-infected individuals are unaware of their infection status (46,48). Chronic HCV infection is usually asymptomatic the first 20 years but might eventually progress into liver cirrhosis and HCC (48). The introduction of highly effective and safe direct acting antiviral (DAA) treatment has revolutionized the treatment outcome of HCV infection, which is now considered a relatively easy-to-treat disease.

Antenatal Screening

No country has yet implemented general antenatal HCV screening of pregnant women. Only pregnant women considered to be at risk (e.g., previous or present drug use, blood transfusion before 1992) are currently tested. The reason for not including HCV in antenatal screening programs is lack of interventions to prevent HCV vertical transmission (HCV-VT). Direct-acting antiviral treatment regimens are not currently approved for use in pregnancy. The only way to eliminate the risk of HCV-VT is to eradicate the infection in fertile women, which is possible with the new treatment options.

Vertical Transmission

HCV can be transmitted from a chronically infected mother to her child during pregnancy or delivery. HCV-VT is nowadays the most common route of HCV transmission in children. The risk of HCV-VT in children of HIV-negative mothers is estimated to be around 5% (range 1% to 10%) (49). HIV coinfection doubles the risk of HCV-VT.

THE NEWBORN INFANT

The exact time point of transmission is difficult to determine, but around one-third of all cases are thought to occur during pregnancy and the rest during delivery (50). Clinical factors associated with an increased risk of HCV-VT are coinfection with HIV, high maternal viral load, prolonged rupture of membranes, and fetal scalp monitoring during labor. Delivery mode or breast feeding have not been shown to influence the risk, and mothers with HCV infection are not discouraged from vaginal delivery or breastfeeding (49).

Despite viral exposure of the fetus during delivery, the rate of HCV-VT is low compared to the vertical transmission rate of other viral infections, such as HIV and hepatitis B virus (HBV). The reason for the comparatively low risk of HCV vertical transmission remains unclear, but various immunologic factors have been suggested to play a protective role. Previous in vitro studies have shown that vertical exposure to HCV induces virus-specific cell-mediated immune responses in uninfected children of mothers with HCV infection (51).

Management of Children Born of HCV-Infected Mothers

All children of HCV-infected mothers are recommended to be tested for anti-HCV at the age of 18 months, when passively transferred maternal antibodies have disappeared. The rate of spontaneous clearance after perinatal transmission is calculated to be around 20%, and the median time of clearance is 15 months after infection (52). In children, HCV infection is considered to be less progressive, maybe due to lack of certain adult risk factors such as alcohol consumption. Clinical symptoms are rare during childhood, even though moderately elevated liver transaminases are common. However, some children and adolescents do develop an advanced liver disease with progressive fibrosis and even cirrhosis (52,53).

Vaccination

There is no available prophylactic hepatitis C vaccine.

Treatment

DAA treatment is approved for children above the age of 12 years. The treatment is considered as safe in these children as in adults. Twelve weeks of oral treatment will eradicate the virus in almost 100% of cases (54).

Hepatitis B Virus

An estimated 257 million people are infected with chronic HBV globally, with the highest prevalence in Africa and Asia. Only 9% of the infected individuals are diagnosed, mainly due to the asymptomatic early course of infection and lack of access to affordable testing in rural areas (46). HBV is transmitted by blood and body fluids. The highest risk of developing chronicity is infection at birth (90%), and the risk declines with time to around 50% by the age of 5 years and 5% in adult age.

Antenatal Screening

Testing for HBV is included in antenatal screening programs of pregnant women in most Western countries; however, access to antenatal testing is very low in several low-income countries with high prevalence of HBV infection (46).

Vertical Transmission

The overall risk of vertical transmission of HBV from mother to child during delivery is around 90% without postpartum vaccination (55). Mothers who are HBeAg positive are at higher risk of transmitting the infection. All children born of HBV-infected mothers should receive postpartum vaccination prophylaxis.

In countries where antenatal HBV screening is not implemented, a birth dose of HBV vaccine is recommended for all babies, regardless of maternal viral status. The birth dose is considered the cornerstone of HBV prevention in children according to the WHO. However, globally, only 39% of babies were given the birth dose in 2015 (46).

Caesarean section has not been shown to reduce the risk of transmission. HBV-infected women can breastfeed their infants. Amniocentesis and other invasive procedures should be avoided in highly viremic women if possible (56).

Management of Children Born of HBV-Infected Mothers

Early vaccination of the baby within 24 hours after birth reduces the risk of infection to almost 0% in children born of HBeAg-negative mothers and to 20% in HBeAg-positive mothers. Immunoglobulin should be administered in addition to vaccine to children born of HBeAg-positive mothers, mothers coinfected with hepatitis D, or in case of premature delivery (before gestation week 34) or low birth weight (<2 kg). In many countries, immunoglobulin is given to all children born of HBV-infected mothers. Pregnant women with high viral titers (>200,000 IU/mL) are recommended antiviral treatment from the third trimester in order to reduce the risk of vertical transmission (57,58).

Children born of mothers with chronic HBV infection should receive the first vaccine dose within 24 hours, the next dose at 1 month of age, and thereafter 2 to 3 more doses depending on the nature of the local vaccination program. After completing vaccination series, these children should be tested for HBsAg, antiHBc, and antiHBs, to rule out chronic infection and ensure immunity, respectively.

Vaccination

Universal hepatitis B vaccination has been implemented in most pediatric vaccination programs. Between 1990 and 2015, the HBV vaccine coverage in infants increased from 1% to 84% (1). The vaccine is normally given in a three-dose regime with a 90% protective antibody response.

Treatment

Children with chronic HBV infection and elevated transaminases can be offered antiviral treatment that will lower the viral load but seldom eradicate the infection. Approved treatment options for children are either intramuscular pegylated interferon treatment for 1 year or oral nucleoside analogs (NUCs) with fewer side effects but longer treatment duration. The approved oral treatment options for children are either entecavir from 2 years of age or tenofovir from the age of 12 years (58).

CONGENITAL PORTOSYSTEMIC SHUNTS

Congenital portosystemic shunts (CPSS) are rare vascular malformations that cause shunting of splanchnic blood from the portal system into the systemic circulation and thereby bypass the liver (59). These vascular shunts are formed secondary to disturbed remodeling of embryologic vessels from the 4th to 6th week of gestation until the first days after birth when the ductal hepatic vein normally closes (60). The prevalence of CPSS is estimated 1/30,000 to 1/50,000, and the first case was described by Abernethy in 1793 (59,61,62). CPSS is associated with increased risk of severe complications from several organs.

Definitions

These shunts can be anatomically very different. Originally, CPSS was divided into intrahepatic and extrahepatic shunts. The intrahepatic shunts could be of various types. The extrahepatic shunts were classified as Abernathy type 1, where an end-to-side portal vein-inferior vena cava shunt causes a complete diversion of all portal blood to the systemic circulation ("complete absence of the portal vein") and Abernathy type 2, where a side-to-side shunt causes partial diversion of portal blood from some intrahepatic

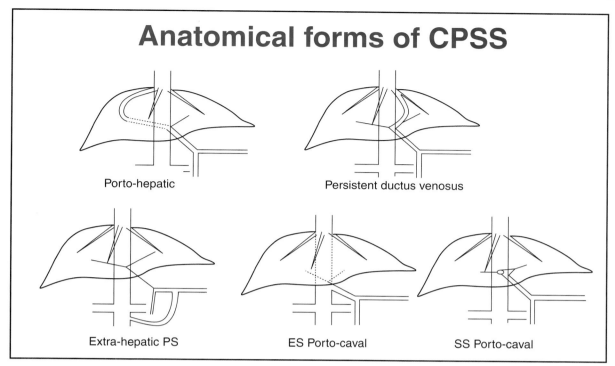

FIGURE 37.1 Anatomical forms of congenital portosystemic shunt (CPSS). The portohepatic shunt and patent ductus venosus are considered intrahepatic shunts. The bottom three diagrams are considered extrahepatic shunts. Note the minimal or absent portal venous flow owing to the large portosystemic communication. ES, end-to-side; PS, portosystemic; SS, side-to-side. (Reprinted with permission from McLin VA, Abella SF, Debray D, et al. Congenital portosystemic shunts: current diagnosis and management. *J Pediatr Gastroenterol Nutr* 2019;68:615.)

portal vein branches into the systemic circulation (63,64). With improved imaging techniques and treatment modalities, these classifications are not valid anymore, and several new classifications are suggested (59,65–67). A schematic overview of anatomical forms of CPSS is shown in **Figure 37.1** (68).

Clinical Presentation and Complications

CPSS may be diagnosed incidentally on antenatal ultrasound scans as part of standard monitoring of pregnancies, often around 25 weeks of gestation (69). Indirect signs of CPSS on conventional antenatal ultrasound are abnormal intrahepatic tubular structure, enlarged hepatic vein, and congestive heart failure (70). About 13% to 66% of the children with prenatally diagnosed CPSS have intra-uterine growth retardation (IUGR) (69,71,72). Other concomitant malformations include cardiac, intestinal, vascular, renal, and/or musculoskeletal malformations. CPSS has also been reported in the following syndromes: trisomy 21, Noonan, trisomy 18, Turner, Bannayan-Zonana, Leopard, Cornelia de Lange, Holt-Oram, Goldenhar, Costello, Adams-Oliver, and Wolf-Hirschhorn (69,73,74).

In the neonatal period, shunting can lead to galactosemia, hyperammonemia, and hyperinsulinemia (with prolonged hypoglycemia), increased bile acid levels, and unconjugated hyperbilirubinemia due to reduced hepatic degradation. Deficiency of nutrients, trophic factors, and oxygen secondary to the deprivation of blood flow into the liver are considered to be the underlying mechanism when development of liver atrophy, neonatal cholestasis, increased transaminases, and coagulopathy occurs. CPSS-associated cardiac malformations, pulmonary hypertension (PH), hypoxemia, cutaneous hemangiomas, and thrombocytopenia may also be presenting signs leading to diagnosis in the neonatal period (59,67,70,71,73,75–77). It should be noted that increased vascular resistance to blood flow through the liver due to neonatal cholestasis of other origin can cause secondary shunting through the

ductus venosus or other shunts, and this condition needs to be differentiated from CPSS (68).

On the other hand, CPSS can be asymptomatic and go unnoticed until later in life when found, unintentionally on ultrasound for some unrelated indication or due to the development of associated complications from different organ systems. The main complications are hepatic encephalopathy (HE), liver nodules, PH, and hepatopulmonary syndrome (20).

HE can occur in all age groups, and all types of shunts but may go undiagnosed due to vague symptoms; the latter is particularly true in neonates (59). HE is associated with hyperammonemia, but symptoms do not clearly correlate with the ammonia level (59,68,78,79).

Liver nodules have been described from 3 months of age but are more common later in childhood and adulthood. Liver nodules include focal nodular hyperplasia, regenerative hyperplasia, adenomas, hepatocellular cancer (HCC), hepatoblastoma, and sarcoma. The malignant tumors have only been reported in extrahepatic CPSS and not in intrahepatic CPSS. HCC is more common in males and adenoma in females (59,68).

PH may be the presenting sign of CPSS in all age groups and cause dyspnea, fainting, and progressive right heart failure, which may lead to sudden death, even in infancy (59,67,78). Shunting of vasoconstrictive substances, microthromboses, and high cardiac output are suggested to contribute to the condition (80). Hepatopulmonary syndrome cause chronic hypoxemia, may occur in combination with PH, and is overrepresented in patients with CPSS and polysplenia (59,67,78).

Evaluation

If antenatal screening ultrasound examination reveals suspicion of CPSS, color Doppler should be performed to characterize the shunt. Associated malformations ought to be evaluated. Fetal echocardiography is recommended in case of concomitant cardiac malformation, and signs of poor hemodynamic tolerance need to be assessed, including biventricular dilatation with cardiomegaly, pericardial effusion, and tricuspid insufficiency. Genetic analysis should be discussed in severe IUGR and/or congenital malformations. Fetal growth and cardiac tolerance need to be followed during the pregnancy (67,69).

All patients with incidental finding of CPSS, neonatal cholestasis, unexplained galactosemia, and/or hypoglycemia or any sign of other systemic complication of CPSS should be examined with blood tests and imaging studies (59,68). The extent of evaluation, however, needs to be personalized, especially in antenatally diagnosed intrahepatic CPSS which often close spontaneously.

Blood Tests

Full blood count, gamma-GT, bilirubin, transaminases, fasting serum total bile acids, blood glucose (especially in neonates), ammonium, blood manganese, coagulation factors (INR, fibrinogen, antithrombin and/or protein C), and α-fetoprotein should be analyszed (59,68,69,77).

Imaging Studies

Abdominal Doppler color ultrasonography is the first-line imaging technique in CPSS. Angio-computed tomography or MRI with contrast can further characterize the shunt and lesions and rule out liver hemangioma. Portovenography with balloon occlusion test is used to search for hypoplastic portal vessels, which may not be visualized with other techniques and to measure pressure in the portal venous system. This test is important to evaluate conditions for shunt closure. Liver biopsy can be performed during angiography if indicated (64,67,68).

Echocardiography is advised to identify cardiac malformations and cardiopulmonary complications of CPSS. Contrast-enhanced transthoracic cardiac echocardiography is used to diagnose hepatopulmonary syndrome. In PH, right heart catheterization is added to measure pulmonary pressures and vascular resistance (59,67,68,78).

Brain MRI is proposed in CPSS with neurologic symptoms to look for the hyperintense T1 signal of the globus pallidus which is associated with HE (59,68,78,79). Per-rectal scintigraphy may be used to quantify the degree of shunting, although the reliability has been questioned (59,67).

Additional Evaluation

Physical examination (including signs of clubbing, palmar erythema, telangiectasia, and hyperemic lips in cardiopulmonary involvement, signs of associated syndromes), percutaneous O_2 saturation, capillary blood gases, neurocognitive testing, proteinuria, liver histology, and liver tumor histology when indicated should be performed (59,68).

Treatment and Outcome

Most small intrahepatic CPSS diagnosed in the antenatal or neonatal period close spontaneously within the first 2 years of life, often within the first months (67,71). Neonatal cholestasis in intrahepatic CPSS has been shown to be a predictor of spontaneous shunt closure, but not for patent ductus venosus (77).

In most cases, a wait-and-see approach with regular follow-up can be undertaken the first 2 years of life in asymptomatic patients. However, it is recommended to close extrahepatic shunts upstream of the portal vein very early in life to prevent development of portal vascular hypoplasia and to close patent ductus venosus to restore intrahepatic portal vasculature. Early closure should always be performed if complications to CPSS occur, if technically possible and if procedure-related risks are tolerable for the patient (68).

After 2 years of age, it is recommended to close remaining CPSS to prevent complications, since spontaneous closure rarely occurs after this time (59,68,76).

Shunt closure is usually performed by placing an occlusive device or coil in the shunt via interventional radiology. If this is not possible, due to anatomical reasons, surgery is indicated. A two-step approach can be used when there is a high risk of severe portal hypertension after closure. With this technique, banding of the shunt is performed a few months before surgical closure to let the intrahepatic portal branches adjust to increasing blood flow (59). Liver transplantation is rarely required in CPSS but can be considered in patients with multiple shunts and severe complications of CPSS (59,68).

Complications of shunt closure include thrombotic complications, portal hypertension, and device migration. Anticoagulation may be used to prevent thrombosis. There are also risks related to anesthesia and interventions in patients with PH and cardiac disease that must be considered (59).

Shunt closure improves most complications of CPSS including bile acid and ammonia levels, HE, benign tumors, hepatopulmonary syndrome, and heart failure (59,67,68,78). PH may be stabilized but not cured after shunt closure (80).

LIVER TRANSPLANTATION

Liver transplantation was originally developed in young pediatric patients with end-stage liver disease more than 50 years ago. However, survival was quite poor until modern immunosuppression, in particular the calcineurin inhibitors, came into use in the 1980s. Further surgical innovations, for example, the use of partial or split liver grafts and also the developments to use not only deceased donors but also healthy, live adult donors, have improved the situation dramatically. For example, patients with BA, which is currently the main indication for pediatric liver transplantation, have a long-term survival of 80% to 90% after this procedure.

Neonatal liver transplantation is technically more demanding than the same treatment in, for example, a 1-year-old, and the outcome is still not as good. Still, in selected cases with neonatal liver failure, long-term survival of 50% to 70% has been reported (3). Regardless of age at liver transplantation, the current notion is that lifelong immunosuppression is needed to avoid graft failure.

REFERENCES

1. Arnell H, Fischler B. Laboratory evaluation of hepatobiliary disease. In: D'Antiga L, ed. *Pediatric hepatology and liver transplantation*, 1st ed. Switzerland, Springer Nature 2019:57.
2. Dezsőfi A, Baumann U, Dhawan A, et al. Liver biopsy in children: position paper of the ESPGHAN Hepatology Committee. *J Pediatr Gastroenterol Nutr* 2015;60:408.
3. Shanmugam NP, Bansal S, Greenough A, et al. Neonatal liver failure: aetiologies and management—state of the art. *Eur J Pediatr* 2011;170(5):573.
4. Taylor SA, Whitington PF. Neonatal acute liver failure. *Liver Transpl* 2016;22:677.
5. Whitington PF. Gestational alloimmune liver disease and neonatal hemochromatosis. *Semin Liver Dis* 2012;32(4):325.
6. Taylor SA, Kelly S, Alonso EM, et al. The effects of gestational alloimmune liver disease on fetal and infant morbidity and mortality. *J Pediatr* 2018;196:123.
7. Heissat S, Collardeau-Frachon S, Baruteau J. Neonatal hemochromatosis: diagnostic work-up based on a series of 56 cases of fetal death and neonatal liver failure. *J Pediatr* 2015;166:66.
8. Khuroo MS, Kamili S, Khuroo MS. Clinical course and duration of viremia in vertically transmitted hepatitis E virus (HEV) infection in babies born to HEV-infected mothers. *J Viral Hepat* 2009;16:519.
9. Nicastro E, D'Antiga L. Next generation sequencing in pediatric hepatology and liver transplantation. *Liver Transpl* 2018;24:282.
10. Fischler B, Lamireau T. Cholestasis in the newborn and infant. *Clin Res Hepatol Gastroenterol* 2014;38(3):263.
11. Fawaz R, Baumann U, Ekong U, et al. Guideline for the evaluation of cholestatic jaundice in infants: joint recommendations of the North American Society for Pediatric Gastroenterology, Hepatology, and Nutrition (NASPGHAN) and the European Society for Pediatric Gastroenterology, Hepatology, and Nutrition (ESPGHAN). *J Pediatr Gastroenterol Nutr* 2017;64:154.

12. Suchy FJ, Balistreri WF, Heubi JE, et al. Physiologic cholestasis: elevation of the primary serum bile acid concentrations in normal infants. *Gastroenterology* 1981;80:1037.

13. Jimenez-Rivera C, Jolin-Dahel KS, Fortinsky KJ. International incidence and outcomes of biliary atresia. *J Pediatr Gastroenterol Nutr* 2013;56:344.

14. Betalli P, Davenport M. Biliary atresia and other congenital disorders of the extrahepatic biliary tree. In: D'Antiga L, ed. *Pediatric hepatology and liver transplantation*, 1st ed. Springer Nature, 2019:129.

15. Morecki R, Glaser J, Cho S, et al. Biliary atresia and reovirus type 3 infection. *N Engl J Med* 1982;307:481.

16. Steele MI, Marshall CM, Lloyd RE. Reovirus 3 not detected by reverse transcriptase-mediated polymerase chain reaction analysis of preserved tissues from infants with cholestatic liver disease. *Hepatology* 1995;21:697.

17. Riepenhoff-Talty M, Gouvea V, Evans M, et al. Detection of group C rotavirus in infants with extrahepatic biliary atresia. *J Infect Dis* 1996;174:8.

18. Mohanty SK, Lobeck I, Donnelly B, et al. Rotavirus reassortant induced murine model of liver fibrosis parallels human biliary atresia. *Hepatology* 2020;71(4):1316.

19. Lin YC, Chang MH, Liao SF. Decreasing rate of biliary atresia in Taiwan: a survey, 2004-2009. *Pediatrics* 2011;128:e530.

20. Lee JH, Ahn HS, Han S, et al. Nationwide population-based study showed that the rotavirus vaccination had no impact on the incidence of biliary atresia in Korea. *Acta Paediatr* 2019 ;108:2278.

21. Hart MH, Kaufman SS, Vanderhoof JA, et al. Neonatal hepatitis and extrahepatic biliary atresia associated with cytomegalovirus infection in twins. *Am J Dis Child* 1991;145:302.

22. Fischler B, Ehrnst A, Forsgren M, et al. The viral association of neonatal cholestasis in Sweden, a possible link between cytomegalovirus infection and extrahepatic biliary atresia. *J Pediatr Gastroenterol Nutr* 1998;27:57.

23. Zani A, Quaglia A, Hadzić N, et al. Cytomegalovirus-associated biliary atresia: An aetiological and prognostic subgroup. *J Pediatr Surg* 2015;50:1739.

24. Parolini F, Hadzic N, Davenport M. Adjuvant therapy of cytomegalovirus IgM + ve associated biliary atresia: prima facie evidence of effect. *J Pediatr Surg* 2019;54:1941.

25. Alonso EM, Ye W, Hawthorne K, et al. Impact of steroid therapy on early growth in infants with biliary atresia: the multicenter steroids in biliary atresia randomized trial. *J Pediatr* 2018;202:179.

26. Sveger T. Liver disease in alpha-1-antitrypsin deficiency detected by screening of 200,000 infants. *N Engl J Med* 1976;294:1316.

27. Teckman JH, Perlmutter DH. Difference in ER degradation of alpha-1-ATZ protein in protected and susceptible hosts. *Gastroenterology* 1995;108:1263.

28. Ruiz M, Lacaille F, Berthiller J, et al. Liver disease related to alpha1-antitrypsin deficiency in French children: The DEFI-ALPHA cohort. *Liver Int* 2019;39:1136.

29. Alagille D, Odièvre M, Gauthier M, et al. Hepatic ductular hypoplasia associated with characteristic facies, vertebral malformations, retarded physical, mental, sexual development, and cardiac murmur. *J Pediatr* 1975;86:63.

30. Alagille D, Estrada A, Hadchouel M, et al. Syndromic paucity of interlobular bile ducts (Alagille syndrome or arteriohepatic dysplasia): review of 80 cases. *J Pediatr* 1987;110:195.

31. Helps S, Caulfield C, Chadwick O, et al. Cognitive and academic status of children with Alagille syndrome. *J Pediatr Gastroenterol Nutr* 1998;26:576.

32. Kamath BM, Baker A, Houwen R, et al. Systematic review: the epidemiology, natural history, and burden of Alagille syndrome. *J Pediatr Gastroenterol Nutr* 2018;67:148.

33. Whitington PF, Freese DK, Alonso EM, et al. Progressive familial intrahepatic cholestasis (Byler's disease). In: Lentze M, Reichen J, eds. *Pediatric cholestasis—novel approaches to treatment.* Dordrecht, The Netherlands: Kluwer, Academic press, 1992:165.

34. Bull LN, Thompson RJ. Progressive familial intrahepatic cholestasis. *Clin Liver Dis* 2018;22:657.

35. Arnell H, Papadogiannakis N, Zemack H, et al. Follow-up in children with progressive familial intrahepatic cholestasis after partial external biliary diversion. *J Pediatr Gastroenterol Nutr* 2010;51:494.

36. Fischler B, Rodensjö P, Nemeth A, et al. Cytomegalovirus DNA detection on Guthrie cards in patients neonatal cholestasis. *Arch Dis Child Fetal Neonatal Ed* 1999; 80:130.

37. Clements WD, Erwin P, McCaigue MD, et al. Conclusive evidence of endotoxaemia in biliary obstruction. *Gut* 1998;42:293.

38. Vajro P, Amelio A, Stagni A, et al. Cholestasis in newborn infants with perinatal asphyxia. *Acta Paediatr* 1997;86:895.

39. Jahnel J, Zöhrer E, Fischler B, et al. An attempt to determine the prevalence of two inborn errors of primary bile acid synthesis: results of a European survey. *J Pediatr Gastroenterol Nutr* 2017;64:864.

40. Leblanc A, Odièvre M, Hadchouel M, et al. Neonatal cholestasis and hypoglycemia: possible role of cortisol deficiency. *J Pediatr* 1981;99:577.

41. Arnell H, Fischler B. Population based study of incidence and clinical outcome of neonatal cholestasis in patients with Down syndrome. *J Pediatr* 2012;161:899.

42. Van Eyken P, Sciot R, Callea F, et al. The development of intrahepatic bile ducts in man. *Hepatology* 1990;8:1586.

43. Rock N, McLin V. Liver involvement in children with ciliopathies. *Clin Res Hepatol Gastroenterol* 2014;38:407.

44. Leeuwen L, Magoffin AK, Fitzgerald DA, et al. Cholestasis and meconium ileus in infants with cystic fibrosis and their clinical outcomes. *Arch Dis Child* 2014;99:443.

45. Teng J, Arnell H, Bohlin K, et al. Impact of parenteral fat composition on cholestasis in preterm infants: a population based study. *J Pediatr Gastroenterol Nutr* 2015;60:702.

46. WHO. Global hepatitis report, 2017. Available from: https://www.who.int/hepatitis/publications/global-hepatitis-report2017/en/

47. Gower E, Estes C, Blach S, et al. Global epidemiology and genotype distribution of the hepatitis C virus infection. *J Hepatol.* 2014;61(1 suppl):S45.

48. Thrift AP, El-Serag HB, Kanwal F. Global epidemiology and burden of HCV infection and HCV-related disease. *Nat Rev Gastroenterol Hepatol.* 2017;14(2):122.

49. Benova L, Mohamoud YA, Calvert C, et al. Vertical transmission of hepatitis C virus: systematic review and meta-analysis. *Clin Infect Dis* 2014;59(6):765.

50. Mok J, Pembrey L, Tovo PA, et al. When does mother to child transmission of hepatitis C virus occur? *Arch Dis Child Fetal Neonatal Ed* 2005;90(2):F156.

51. Psaros Einberg A, Brenndorfer ED, Frelin L, et al. Neonatal exposure to hepatitis C virus antigens in uninfected children born to infected mothers. *J Pediatr Gastroenterol Nutr* 2018;66(1):106.

52. European Paediatric Hepatitis C virus network. Three broad modalities in the natural history of vertically acquired hepatitis C virus infection. *Clin Infect Dis* 2005;41:45.

53. Bortolotti F, Verucchi G, Camma C, et al. Long-term course of chronic hepatitis C in children: from viral clearance to end-stage liver disease. *Gastroenterology* 2008;134:1900.

54. Balistreri WF, Murray KF, Rosenthal P, et al. The safety and effectiveness of ledipasvir-sofosbuvir in adolescents 12-17 years old with hepatitis C virus genotype 1 infection. *Hepatology* 2017;66:371.

55. Dunkelberg JC, Berkley EM, Thiel KW, et al. Hepatitis B and C in pregnancy: a review and recommendations for care. *J Perinatol* 2014;34:882.

56. Society for Maternal-Fetal Medicine, Dionne-Odom J, Tita AT, et al. Hepatitis B in pregnancy screening, treatment, and prevention of vertical transmission. *Am J Obstet Gynecol* 2016;214:6.

57. European Association for the Study of the Liver, Electronic address: easloffice@easloffice.eu, European Association for the Study of the Liver. EASL 2017 Clinical Practice Guidelines on the management of hepatitis B virus infection. *J Hepatol* 2017;67(2):370.

58. Terrault NA, Lok ASF, McMahon BJ, et al. Update on prevention, diagnosis and treatment of chronic hepatitis B: AASLD 2018 hepatitis B guidance. *Hepatology* 2018;67(4):1560.

59. Bernard O., et al. Congenital portosystemic shunts in children: recognition, evaluation, and management. *Semin Liver Dis* 2012;32:273.

60. Collardeau-Frachon S, Scoazec JY. Vascular development and differentiation during human liver organogenesis. *Anat Rec (Hoboken)* 2008;291:614.

61. Abernethy J. Account of two instances of uncommon formation in the viscera of the human body: from the Philosophical Transactions of the Royal Society of London. *Med Facts Obs* 1797;7:100–108.

62. Ono H., et al. Clinical features and outcome of eight infants with intrahepatic porto-venous shunts detected in neonatal screening for galactosaemia. *Acta Paediatr* 1998;87:631.

63. Morgan G, Superina R. Congenital absence of the portal vein: two cases and a proposed classification system for portasystemic vascular anomalies. *J Pediatr Surg* 1994;29:1239.

64. Ponziani FR, et al. Congenital extrahepatic portosystemic shunt: description of four cases and review of the literature. *J Ultrasound* 2019;223:349.

65. Blanc T, et al. Congenital portosystemic shunts in children: a new anatomical classification correlated with surgical strategy. *Ann Surg* 2014;260:188.

66. Kanazawa H, et al. The classification based on intrahepatic portal system for congenital portosystemic shunts. *J Pediatr Surg* 2015;50:688.

67. Franchi-Abella S, et al. Congenital portosystemic shunts: diagnosis and treatment. *Abdom Radiol (NY)* 2018;43(8):2023.

68. McLin VA, et al. Congenital portosystemic shunts: current diagnosis and management. *J Pediatr Gastroenterol Nutr* 2019;68:615.

69. Francois B, et al. Prenatally diagnosed congenital portosystemic shunts. *J Matern Fetal Neonatal Med* 2018;31:1364.

70. Han BH, et al. Congenital portosystemic shunts: prenatal manifestations with postnatal confirmation and follow-up. *J Ultrasound Med* 2013;32:45.

71. Francois B, et al. Outcome of intrahepatic portosystemic shunt diagnosed prenatally. *Eur J Pediatr* 2017;176:1613.

72. Gorincour G, Droulle P, Guibaud L. Prenatal diagnosis of umbilicoportosystemic shunts: report of 11 cases and review of the literature. *AJR Am J Roentgenol* 2005;184:163.

73. Sokollik C, et al. Congenital portosystemic shunt: characterization of a multisystem disease. *J Pediatr Gastroenterol Nutr* 2013;56:675.

74. Perez-Garcia C, et al. Adams-Oliver syndrome with unusual central nervous system findings and an extrahepatic portosystemic shunt. *Pediatr Rep* 2017;9:7211.

75. Weigert A, et al. Congenital intrahepatic portocaval shunts and hypoglycemia due to secondary hyperinsulinism: a case report and review of the literature. *J Med Case Rep* 2018;12:336.

76. Paganelli M, et al. Predisposing factors for spontaneous closure of congenital portosystemic shunts. *J Pediatr* 2015;167:931.

77. Beattie W, et al. Characterization of the coagulation profile in children with liver disease and extrahepatic portal vein obstruction or shunt. *Pediatr Hematol Oncol* 2017;34:107.

78. Baiges A, et al. Congenital extrahepatic portosystemic shunts (Abernethy malformation): an international observational study. *Hepatology* 2020;71(2):658.

79. Hanquinet S, et al. Globus pallidus MR signal abnormalities in children with chronic liver disease and/or porto-systemic shunting. *Eur Radiol* 2017;27:4064.

80. Uike K, et al. Effective shunt closure for pulmonary hypertension and liver dysfunction in congenital portosystemic venous shunt. *Pediatr Pulmonol* 2018;53:505.

38 Renal Disease

Suhas M. Nafday, Craig B. Woda, Jeffrey M. Saland, Joseph T. Flynn, David Askenazi, and Luc P. Brion

INTRODUCTION

Neonatal nephrology has changed due to the increasing survival of extremely low birth weight (ELBW, <1,000 g) infants. Widespread use of invasive procedures in these infants has created new challenges in fluid overload/hypovolemia, electrolyte anomalies, high/low blood pressure (BP), and acute kidney injury (AKI) management. Furthermore, an early diagnosis of congenital anomalies of the kidney and urinary tract (CAKUT) or AKI allows for rapid determination of the best medical and/or surgical treatment, preventing or at least delaying the evolution toward chronic kidney disease (CKD) and end-stage renal disease (ESRD).

DEVELOPMENTAL PHYSIOLOGY

Fetal urine is a key component of amniotic fluid production and helps drive appropriate lung development (1,2). Ultrasound (US) studies of bladder volumes demonstrate that the rate of urine production in a normal fetus is approximately 5 mL/h at 20 weeks of gestational age (GA) and gradually increases to about 40 to 50 mL/h by 40 weeks of GA (1,3).

Embryology

In humans, three pairs of kidneys arise from the intermediate mesoderm; the nonfunctional *pronephros* at 3 weeks of gestation, followed by the intermediate *mesonephros* at 4 weeks (which has little function and eventually becomes part of the male epididymis and urinary bladder), and finally the definitive mammalian kidney or *metanephros* at 5 to 6 weeks of gestation. Although the pronephros and mesonephros involute quickly, absence of these primitive structures leads to renal agenesis.

Within the metanephric kidney, the developmental process initially occurs as the ureteric bud (UB), an offshoot of the wolffian duct, which extends and invades into a mass of cells known as the metanephric mesenchyme (MM). Reciprocating inductive signaling between the UB tip and the mesenchymal cells leads to repetitive morphogenic branching of the UB and eventual formation of the ureter, renal pelvis, calyces, and collecting tubules (4). In contrast, the cells of the MM differentiate into renal epithelium, through *mesenchymal-to-epithelial transition*, to become the glomerulus, proximal tubule, loop of Henle, and distal convoluted tubule. Thus, nephronogenesis (the formation of new nephrons) and branching morphogenesis occur simultaneously and influence the development of each other.

Since the UB invades the central aspect of the MM, nephrons develop and mature in a centrifugal pattern (2,5,6). Thus, deep juxtamedullary nephrons develop and mature before the cortical nephrons. The full complement of approximately 1 million nephrons per kidney in the human is achieved by 35 to 36 weeks of GA, or at a body weight of about 2,300 g (2). When birth occurs before this age, nephronogenesis continues after birth but may not reach a full complement, especially in babies with intrauterine growth restriction (IUGR). Furthermore, evidence suggests that ELBW infants and small-for-GA (SGA) infants may have fewer nephrons (7) and consequently are at increased risk for CKD and hypertension (HTN) long term.

Blood vessels arise in a synchronous fashion alongside tubular development. Evidence suggests that blood vessels in the kidney may arise through a combination of metanephric mesenchymal progenitor cells differentiating into endothelial cells (vasculogenesis) or infiltration of the MM by preformed vessels (angiogenesis) (8). Vascular progenitor cells within the MM express vascular endothelial growth factor (VEGF) receptor 2 (VEGFR2, Flk-1), and VEGF helps direct the movement of these cells toward the developing nephron. This process occurs early in development since the first glomerulus is noted by approximately 9 weeks of embryonic life.

Molecular Biology of Renal Development

Close examination of the cells located at the UB tip demonstrates high expression of rearranged in transfection (RET) (9), a tyrosine kinase receptor. The cells of the MM secrete high amounts of glial cell–derived neurotrophic factor, which preferentially binds to RET leading to overall migration and invasion of the UB into the MM (9–11). Studies in humans (12) with absent or mutated RET result in renal agenesis, whereas overexpression of RET results in multicystic kidney disease (MCKD) (13). In addition to RET, the UB also expresses bone morphogenic protein (BMP) 4 and 7, members of the transforming growth factor family, with loss of BMP resulting in kidney agenesis (14). Whether BMP may become a viable factor capable of leading to nephron repair in patients with renal disease is still unclear and actively being explored.

Metanephric mesenchymal cells adjacent to the UB tip are referred to as the cap mesenchyme and include the self-renewing nephron progenitor cells, expressing key transcription regulators working in a coordinated and synergistic fashion, such as Lim1, Eya1, Pax2, Sall1, Meox, Cited1, WT1, and Six2 (14). Loss of function in one or more of these factors leads to either renal agenesis or renal hypoplasia. Several human syndromes with associated renal dysplasia such as Townes-Brocks, branchiootorenal, and renal coloboma are related to mutations in Sall1, Eya1, and Pax2, respectively. Furthermore, some transcription factors have different temporal effects with regard to overall kidney development such that expression of WT1 in later phases, for instance, promotes podocyte differentiation needed for appropriate glomerular function (15).

All the components of the renin–angiotensin–aldosterone system (RAAS) are present in the metanephros early in gestation. Angiotensin 2 receptors (AT2R) are detected in the UB tip cells and the adjacent mesenchymal cells with activation of AT2R by angiotensin II (AII) leading to UB branching and elongation of the collecting duct. At 20 weeks of gestation, AT2R begin to regress, whereas mRNA of AT1R increases and subsequently persists throughout the remainder of metanephric development. Disruption of the RAAS system using pharmacologic agents results in complications such as renal medullary hypoplasia, hydronephrosis, renal dysplasia, duplicated renal collecting system, and renal tubular dysgenesis (16). This helps explain fetal anuria and oligohydramnios, leading to pulmonary hypoplasia, in a mother taking an ACE inhibitor during pregnancy. Furthermore, ACE inhibition leads to urinary concentrating defects secondary to atrophy of the renal papilla as well as reduced medullary microvessels that prevent appropriate functioning of the countercurrent multiplier system (17).

PHYSIOLOGY

Renal Blood and Plasma Flow

Low rates of fetal and neonatal renal blood flow (RBF) exist, whether normalized to body weight, surface area, or kidney weight. RBF is mainly determined by a combination of cardiac output (CO) and the degree of renal vascular resistance (RVR). RBF in the human fetus, estimated by Doppler ultrasonography, increases in parallel with fetal weight from 20 mL/min at 25 weeks of GA to more than 60 mL/min by 40 weeks of GA; it reaches adult levels by 2 years of age (18–21). Developmental changes in both CO and RVR contribute to a postnatal increase in RBF from 2% to 5% of the CO in the fetus to 9% in the 1-week-old full-term infant, 12% at 45 days postnatal age, and 20% to 25% in the adult.

While the predominance of blood flow in early fetal life is distributed primarily to the medulla and inner cortex, renal maturation is accompanied by a redistribution of blood flow toward the outer cortex (21–24) (**Fig. 38.1**). The maturational increase in overall RBF results more from a decrease in RVR (25) than by the rise in CO (25–27). Thus, at maturity, about 93% of RBF goes to the cortex (which constitutes about 75% of the renal mass), whereas only 7% is distributed to the renal medulla and perirenal fat.

RVR, localized both at the afferent and efferent glomerular arterioles, is much higher in the newborn than in the adult (25). Interestingly, the postnatal fall in RVR occurs at a time when the systemic vascular resistance increases about sixfold (25). Increases in vasodilatory humoral factors, such as nitric oxide, in

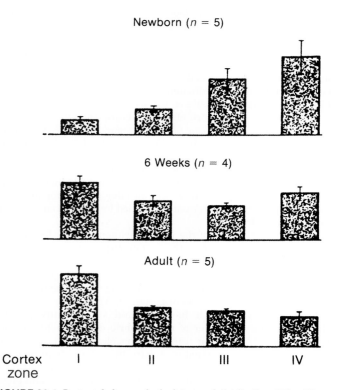

FIGURE 38.1 Postnatal changes in the intrarenal distribution of blood flow. Relative rates of blood flow per glomerulus in the four cortical zones of the canine kidney. Zone I represents the most superficial region, and zone IV represents the deepest. The total height of the bars in each age group is equal. At birth, the blood flow to the superficial cortex was lowest, with most blood flow perfusing the deep cortex. By 6 weeks of age, this pattern was reversed. Maturation is accompanied by an increase in blood flow to the outer cortex, due primarily to a decrease in renal vascular resistance. (From Aperia A, Broberger O, Herin P, et al. Renal hemodynamics in the perinatal period: a study in lambs. *Acta Physiol Scand* 1977;99:261. Copyright © 1977 Scandinavian Physiological Society. Reprinted by permission of John Wiley & Sons, Inc.)

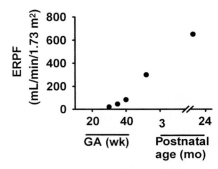

FIGURE 38.2 Developmental changes in effective renal plasma flow (ERPF), calculated from the renal clearance of para-aminohippurate (PAH) and corrected for the fraction of PAH extracted by the kidney. The ERPF, used to estimate RBF, increases rapidly between 30 and 40 weeks of GA, reaching adult values by 24 months of postnatal life. (Adapted with permission of American Society for Clinical Investigation, from Rubin MI, Bruck E, Rapoport MJ. Maturation of renal function in childhood: clearance studies. *J Clin Invest* 1949;28:1144; permission conveyed through Copyright Clearance Center, Inc.)

combination with a decrease of the vasoconstrictive RAAS mediate, at least in part, the developmental reduction in RVR. Ultimately, the balance of afferent and efferent arteriolar resistances determines not only the RVR and RBF but also the hydrostatic pressure within the glomerulus and level of glomerular filtration rate (GFR).

Effective renal plasma flow (RPF) has traditionally been calculated from the secretion of organic acid para-aminohippurate (PAH) within the S2 segment of the proximal convoluted tubule (PCT) and ultimate renal clearance of this molecule. RPF increases rapidly between 30 and 40 weeks of GA, reaching adult values by 1 to 2 years of life (19) (**Fig. 38.2**). The low calculated RPF in premature infants is likely related to immature PCT acid secretory pathways in combination with fewer nephrons having established vasa recta to allow for appropriate PAH delivery to the basolateral aspect of PCT cells.

Renin–Angiotensin–Aldosterone System

The RAAS, pivotally involved in BP regulation as well as in sodium and water homeostasis, is very active in the fetus and newborn (28–30) (**Fig. 38.3**). Plasma renin activity (PRA), the ability of a subject's plasma to generate angiotensin I from angiotensinogen, is elevated in fetal life (60 ng/mL/h at 30 weeks of GA) and decreases by term (to about 10 to 20 ng/mL/h) (31). Although there is a significant decrease in PRA with advanced gestation, PRA at term is 3 to 5× higher than adult levels (31–33). As expected, the high levels of renin in neonates are associated with elevated circulating levels of AII and aldosterone compared with those in adults (34–36). The effect of AII on glomerular hemodynamics depends on relative activation of AT1R and AT2R, which mediate, respectively, vasoconstriction and vasodilatation of the efferent arteriole.

Prostaglandins

Prostaglandin (PG) synthesis from arachidonic acid is mediated by the enzyme cyclooxygenase (COX), which is the inhibitory target of various nonsteroidal anti-inflammatory drugs (NSAIDs) (37). Two isoforms of COX exist; COX-1 has been proposed to participate in glomerulogenesis (38), whereas COX-2 regulates renal perfusion and glomerular hemodynamics (39). PGs, particularly PGE2 and PGI2 (prostacyclin), synthesized by the endothelial cells of both the afferent and efferent arterioles, help buffer against circulating vasoconstrictive agents and thus maintain effective RBF and GFR. Urinary excretion of PGE2 and PGI2 metabolites in the premature infant is five times that noted at term and 20 times that measured in older children (40), presumably reflecting a high rate of renal synthesis.

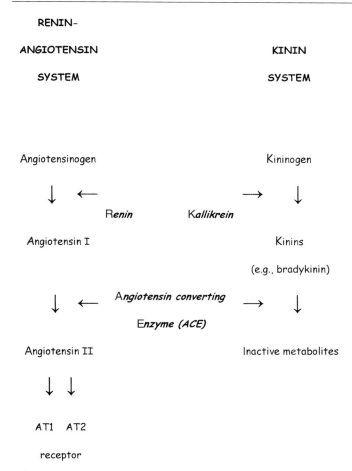

FIGURE 38.3 Relationship between the renin–angiotensin and kinin systems. See text for details.

Maternal administration of indomethacin, a nonselective COX inhibitor, increases fetal RVR and reduces fetal RBF, GFR, and urine output, ultimately leading to oligohydramnios (41–44). Postnatal administration of a PG synthase inhibitor to preterm infants (45), to close a patent ductus arteriosus (PDA), may also compromise renal function, leading to a reduction in RBF, GFR, and urine volume.

The Adrenergic System

Circulating catecholamine levels, particularly norepinephrine, are very high just before and immediately after birth (46) and fall to adult values within a few days of life. The high catecholamine levels act directly to increase afferent arteriolar tone and indirectly, via stimulation of renin and AII release, to increase efferent resistance, possibly contributing to the maintenance of the high RVR characteristic of the neonatal kidney (47). The fetal and neonatal kidneys also demonstrate enhanced sensitivity to catecholamines compared to those of adults, related in part to developmental differences in adrenergic receptor density (48).

Dopamine and Dopamine Receptors

Dopamine typically has a biphasic response in normal adults with low concentrations, through binding to dopaminergic receptors, producing marked vasodilation and increased RBF but high concentrations, via their effects on alpha-adrenergic receptors, resulting in vasoconstriction. Yet, fetal and neonatal kidneys have a blunted response to low-dose dopamine (49) through limited generation of the vasodilatory second messenger cyclic adenosine monophosphate (cAMP) (50) and a low density of renal dopamine-1–like receptors (51). In contrast, intrarenal dopamine

infusions in neonatal animals lead to marked vasoconstriction (52), given the abundance of α-adrenoceptors present (53).

Atrial Natriuretic Factor

Atrial natriuretic factor (ANF), released from atrial cardiocytes, has multiple functions within the mature kidney such as antagonizing renal vasoconstriction, increasing GFR, and inhibiting renin secretion, ultimately promoting tubular sodium excretion (54). However, the natriuretic and diuretic response to systemically infused ANF in the newborn is blunted compared to that in adults (55–57), likely a reflection of ineffective production of the second messenger cyclic GMP. Furthermore, while ANF receptors are present on near-term fetal glomerular membranes, ANF-binding capacity increases sevenfold between fetal and adult life (58).

Glomerular Filtration

The first glomerulus is detected as early as 9 weeks of gestation, and GFR in the human fetus begins immediately thereafter (59). GFR averages approximately 8 to 10 mL/min/1.73 m^2 at 28 weeks and increases to 25 mL/min/1.73 m^2 by 34 weeks of GA. After 34 weeks of GA, the GFR increases by three- to fourfold within 1 week (60), coinciding with completion of nephronogenesis (**Fig. 38.4**). Interestingly, an infant born prematurely at 28 weeks of GA shows little increase in GFR until the infant is about 6 weeks old, that is, until a postmenstrual age of 34 weeks is attained and nephronogenesis has been completed (61). Of note, GFR continues to increase rapidly during the first 4 months of life, followed by a slower rise to adult levels by 2 years of age (18,62,63).

At birth, the more mature glomeruli in the juxtamedullary cortex are nearly as large as glomeruli in the adult kidney and have a higher GFR than do the more recently formed superficial glomeruli. The rise in overall GFR is mainly due to an increase in single nephron GFR (SNGFR) of superficial nephrons through an increase in glomerular surface area and in glomerular hydrostatic pressure related to enhanced perfusion of the renal cortex (21,64) (**Fig. 38.1**).

Autoregulation of Renal Blood Flow and Glomerular Filtration Rate

Autoregulation is an important mechanism that allows for maintenance of constant RBF and GFR over a given range of mean arterial

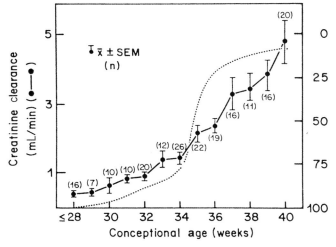

FIGURE 38.4 Changes in GFR (mL/min), estimated by creatinine clearance, and nephrogenic activity in the kidney cortex (%) are plotted as a function of postgestational age in the human infant. There is a temporal relationship between the accelerated rate of increase in GFR and completion of nephrogenesis after 34 weeks of gestation. (Reprinted with permission from Arant BS. Neonatal adjustments to extra uterine life. In: Edelman CM Jr, ed. *Pediatric kidney disease.* Boston, MA: Little, Brown and Company, 1992:1021.)

THE NEWBORN INFANT

pressures (MAP) accomplished primarily by changes in the RVR at the level of the afferent and efferent arterioles. Although MAP (i.e., 20 to 60 mm Hg) in the fetus and neonate is less than the lower limit of autoregulatory range defined for adults (i.e., 80 to 150 mm Hg), evidence suggests that the fetus and newborn are able to autoregulate RBF appropriately in the setting of their low arterial pressure (65–67) due to a combination of renal afferent arteriole dilation with subsequent constriction of the efferent arteriole. The latter effect is due, at least in part, to enhanced renal sympathetic tone, renin release, AII generation, activation of the AT1R, and activation of hormones such as AVP and endothelin (68,69).

Tubuloglomerular Feedback

Tubuloglomerular feedback (TGF) serves to maintain a constant rate of filtration so that appropriate water and salt are delivered to distal segments of the nephron. A stimulus (e.g., low tubular flow or low chloride delivery) at the macula densa is transmitted to the afferent arteriole of the nephron leading to changes in SNGFR. For example, low urinary flow in the thick ascending limb of Henle promotes decreased vascular resistance within the afferent arteriole, resulting in improved glomerular blood flow, higher glomerular capillary hydrostatic pressures, and ultimately an improvement in GFR. Although GFR is known to increase with maturation, the mechanisms underlying TGF are present early on and unaltered during growth (70,71). Intact RAAS appears to be critical for this signaling pathway, and NO may additionally play a modulatory role (72).

Tubular Handling of Electrolytes

The axial and polarized (apical vs. basolateral) distribution of transport proteins along sequential segments of the nephron allows the kidney to reabsorb the bulk of glomerular filtrate proximally and then, in more distal segments, adjust the solute and water content of the urine to maintain homeostasis. The kidney of the full-term, but not necessarily preterm, infant is uniquely suited to meet its developmental stage-specific metabolic demands.

Sodium (Na)

Full-term infants are in a state of positive sodium balance, a requisite for appropriate somatic growth, achieved predominately through enhanced tubular reabsorption of sodium. FENa, the fractional excretion of Na, in the full-term newborn generally averages about 0.2% (73). The tendency of the full-term neonatal kidney to retain significant amounts of filtered Na may become problematic, however, under conditions of salt loading leading to a rise in serum Na levels, abnormal increases in weight, and generalized edema (74).

In contrast to full-term infants, FENa may be as high as 20% in premature infants less than 30 weeks of GA with urinary Na losses exceeding dietary Na intake (75,76). Even with formula designed for preterm infants or use of fortified breast milk, premature infants are at risk for a negative Na balance (i.e., hyponatremia of prematurity) and loss of body weight. They may require up to 10 mEq/kg/d of supplemental Na following birth to maintain a normal serum sodium concentration and remain in positive balance.

Sodium is freely filtered at the glomerulus with the reabsorptive capacity of Na increasing in the proximal tubule following birth. Clearance studies in preterm infants (77–81) suggest that the percent of filtered sodium reabsorbed by the proximal tubule increases by about 5% between 28 and 34 weeks of GA. Unfortunately, premature infants represent a state of functional imbalance in glomerulotubular feedback whereby the reabsorptive Na capacity of the proximal tubule lags behind increases in GFR (79,82).

The fractional reabsorption of Na in the loop of Henle increases by about 20% during postnatal development (83), consistent with functional maturation of this nephron segment and increased abundance of the furosemide- and bumetanide-sensitive apical Na-K-2Cl tri-transporter and basolateral Na/K ATPase pump (84,85). Similarly, studies in premature infants demonstrate an increase

of more than 15% in distal Na uptake between 28 and 34 weeks of GA (78–81). This maturational increase in distal Na reabsorption in early life may help explain the sodium retention observed with sodium loading.

Distal sodium reabsorption occurs in the cortical collecting duct (CCD) by apical sodium entry into principal cells through the amiloride-sensitive epithelial sodium channel (ENaC) and its extrusion at the basolateral membrane by the Na-K-ATPase. In the fully differentiated nephron, the cellular effects of aldosterone induce increases in the density of apical ENaC channels and stimulation of Na-K-ATPase activity (86,87), which drives enhanced sodium absorption. Although high levels of aldosterone prevail through early postnatal life (36,88), clearance studies in premature infants (36,89) reveal a blunted responsiveness of the immature kidney to aldosterone. Given that the density of aldosterone binding sites and receptor affinity appear to be similar in immature and mature kidneys (90), the early hyposensitivity to aldosterone represents a postreceptor phenomenon. The resulting relative hypoaldosteronism in the premature infant results in an inability to conserve sodium, manifested clinically by weight loss and hyponatremia. In addition, the sodium wasting, characteristic of the preterm infant, may also be a result of a paucity of ENaC in the urinary membrane of the distal nephron. As a result, the premature infant is unable to conserve sodium, manifested clinically by weight loss and hyponatremia.

Urinary sodium excretion during maturation is regulated by the RAAS, renal sympathetic innervation, ANF, dopamine, and glucocorticoids. Direct stimulation of renal nerves in fetal and newborn sheep leads to Na retention (91), a response qualitatively similar to that observed in adult animals and attributed to norepinephrine acting on α-adrenergic receptors (92). In contrast, studies in newborns indicate a relatively poor natriuretic response to ANF (56,93) as well as dopamine (94–96) compared to their adult counterparts. Circulating levels of glucocorticoids, including cortisol and corticosterone, surge in many species during or just before the period of weaning (97,98). Both endogenous gluco- and mineralocorticoids bind to the mineralocorticoid receptor with equal affinity (99). Although blood glucocorticoid concentrations are approximately 100-fold higher than aldosterone concentrations, the metabolism of cortisol into inactive derivatives by 11β-hydroxysteroid dehydrogenase type 2 (11-β-HSD2) within the CCD protects the mineralocorticoid receptor from glucocorticoids. The presence of ENaC, mineralocorticoid receptor, and low levels of 11-β-HSD2 (in the CCD) suggests that glucocorticoids may act as sodium-retaining steroids during early postnatal life (100,101).

Potassium (K)

Potassium is transported actively across the placenta from mother to fetus (102), and thus, fetal K is maintained at levels more than 5 mEq/L even in the face of maternal K deficiency (102,103). Unlike adults, who are in net zero balance, growing infants maintain a state of positive potassium balance reflected by their higher plasma K values. These levels average 5.2 mEq/L from birth to age 4 months, ultimately decreasing to 4.2 mEq/L by 3 years of age (104). Under normal circumstances, K retention by the newborn kidney is appropriate and a requirement for growth.

Potassium is freely filtered at the glomerulus with approximately 50% of the filtered K reabsorbed along the proximal tubule in both newborns and adults (83). Up to 40% of the filtered load of K reaches the superficial distal tubule of the newborn, in contrast to about 10% in mature animals, providing evidence for functional immaturity of the loop of Henle (83,105). Urinary potassium excretion is derived almost entirely from secretion in distal segments of the nephron, including the CCD. In the adult nephron, K secretion occurs by the principal cells of the CCD in association with the electrochemical reabsorption of sodium ions through apical ENaC. The low rates of K excretion characteristic of the newborn kidney appear to be due to a paucity of small-conductance (SK) and calcium-activated maxi-K channels within the urinary membrane of the CCD in combination with reduced delivery of tubular sodium (in full-term infants) in the setting of low dietary Na intake. The developmental expression of immunodetectable renal outer medullary potassium (ROMK) channels, the molecular correlate of the SK channel (106–108), and, shortly thereafter, the maxi-K channel (109) immediately precedes the appearance of baseline and flow-stimulated potassium secretion, respectively, in the CCD.

Chloride (Cl)

Chloride is freely filtered into the glomerular ultrafiltrate and predominately reabsorbed in the proximal tubule through a paracellular pathway. Compared to adults, the neonate has a high transepithelial resistance that limits the overall paracellular reabsorption of Cl within the proximal tubule (110,111). This elevated tubular resistance is due to a combination of proteins known as occludins and claudins, which interact between the epithelial cells forming a tight barrier. Studies show that the neonatal proximal tubule contains not only the occludin and claudins (claudin 1, claudin 2, claudin 10, and claudin 12) found in adults but also claudins 6, 9, and 13, which likely represents the reason for the tighter membrane and decreased proximal Cl uptake (112).

Calcium (Ca)

A state of positive calcium balance, characteristic of full-term infants and growing individuals, is sustained by the coordinated interaction of bone, intestine, and kidney. Calcium balance is rarely positive in the first weeks of life in very preterm infants. Calcium represents the most abundant mineral in the body and plays a diverse role as a major constituent of bone and teeth, as well as in neuromuscular activity and intracellular signal transduction. Urinary excretion of Ca is inversely related to GA and varies directly with both urine flow and sodium excretion (113). High rates of Ca excretion may contribute, in part, to early neonatal hypocalcemia, which is commonly seen in the first 24 to 48 hours of life (114). The urinary calcium-to-creatinine ratio in full-term infants ranges up to 1.2 mg/mg during the first week of life but may exceed 2 mg/mg in premature neonates (113,115). In children more than 2 years of age, the ratio decreases to approximately 0.2 mg/mg, which persists through adult life (116).

Approximately 50% of filtered Ca is reabsorbed along the superficial proximal tubule, yet only 1% of filtered Ca is excreted in adults suggesting that, in the adult, a large portion of filtered calcium is reabsorbed at sites beyond the proximal tubule or in deep nephrons (83). The fractional reabsorption of Ca in the loop of Henle, like that for sodium, potassium, and chloride, is low in newborn rats, increasing significantly with advancing postnatal age (83,117). Furosemide, through its effect on inhibiting the apical thick ascending loop of Henle (TALH) tri-transporter leading to loss of the luminal positive charge, increases urinary Ca excretion resulting in an enhanced risk of promoting nephrocalcinosis (NC) and nephrolithiasis. Absorption in both the proximal tubule and TALH is predominantly coupled to Na absorption and is a passive process through paracellular means. Of interest, Ca absorption in the TALH occurs through tight junctions containing Paracellin-1, which when mutated leads to familial syndromes such as hypomagnesemic hypercalciuria and NC (118).

The principal hormones that regulate renal Ca excretion in the adult are parathyroid hormone (PTH), 1,25-dihydroxyvitamin D, and calcitonin. Under normal conditions, a reduction in serum Ca results in the release of PTH from the parathyroid glands. PTH enhances serum Ca by direct effects on the nephron and indirectly through the PTH-induced synthesis active 1,25-dihydroxyvitamin D stimulating intestinal Ca absorption. In mature animals, PTH decreases urinary Ca excretion by stimulating Ca reabsorption in the cortical TALH and distal convoluted tubule

(119–121). Although PTH-responsive adenylate cyclase has been found in preterm and full-term newborns (122,123), the administration of exogenous PTH has minimal effects on renal calcium or phosphorus handling (124). Thus, it has been suggested that neonatal hypocalcemia may be as a result of end-organ unresponsiveness to PTH. Of note, renal production of 1,25-dihydroxyvitamin D increases rapidly after birth, provided that the concentration of the substrate, 25-hydroxyvitamin D, is adequate (125).

Systemic calcium homeostasis is controlled, in large part, by the extracellular G protein–coupled calcium-sensing receptor (CaSR), located on parathyroid and kidney cells in which it senses the extracellular Ca concentration and in turn alters the rate of PTH secretion and renal Ca reabsorption in the TALH and early distal nephron (29,126). There is little expression of CaSR in the fetal kidney but steady-state abundance of CaSR mRNA and protein increase significantly during the first week of life (127).

Phosphate (Pi)

Inorganic phosphate (Pi) is critical for appropriate growth and development given that it is a major component of bone, muscle, and membrane phospholipids as well as critical for many cellular processes that involve ATP. The plasma Pi concentration in infants is 4.5 to 9.3 mg/dL and decreases to 3.0 to 4.5 mg/dL in adulthood (128), achieved mainly through enhanced Pi reabsorption by the kidneys early in life. The fractional reabsorption of Pi increases from 85% of the filtered load at 28 weeks of GA to almost 99% at term, decreasing thereafter to approximately 85% between 3 and 20 months of age (129). The high renal reabsorptive capacity for Pi early in life allows the full-term infant to sustain a state of net positive phosphate balance (129).

Ninety percent of plasma Pi is freely filtered at the glomeruli with ten percent being protein bound. Pi entry into the PCT cells is coupled to sodium and is dependent on the electrochemical gradient delivered by the basolateral Na/K ATPase pump. While three Na^+-P_i (NaPi) cotransporters have been described, the expression of the NaPi-2 transporter is highly influenced by dietary Pi intake and hormones such as PTH and growth hormone. NaPi-2 expression is also significantly greater in juvenile animals, under normal conditions, and decreases with advancing age (130). Furthermore, the phosphaturic effect of PTH is blunted early in life despite the normal circulating PTH levels in the immediate postnatal period, a response mediated, in large part, by the presence of growth hormone (131) preventing the PTH-induced internalization of apical Na^+-P_i cotransporters in the PCT. Whether neonates display a blunted response toward circulating FGF23, another phosphaturic hormone with comparable levels between adults and neonates, remains unknown at this time. Interestingly, a defect in NaPi-2c, the growth-related Pi transporter in humans, is linked to hereditary hypophosphatemic rickets with hypercalciuria (HHRH) (132), while a mutation in NaPi-2a has been observed in siblings with features of Fanconi syndrome and phosphaturia (133). Overall, the high intrinsic rate of Pi reabsorption measured in neonatal proximal tubules has been attributed to an abundance of a growth-related sodium–phosphate cotransporter in the luminal membrane (134), a high membrane fluidity of the immature nephron that increases the transport activity of the NaPi cotransporter (135), a low intracellular phosphate concentration (136), and the favorable hormonal milieu prevailing in the perinatal period (135,137). Nephron heterogeneity may also explain, in part, the limited urinary phosphate excretion observed in the rapidly growing animal. Because deep nephrons reabsorb more phosphate than do cortical nephrons (138,139), and nephronogenesis begins in the juxtamedullary region, the kidney of the immature animal may contain a relatively greater number of functioning nephrons with a high capacity for phosphate reabsorption.

The renal tubule of the preterm infant, however, has limited ability to reabsorb phosphate. The tubular reabsorption of Pi (at normal serum Pi levels) is 56% in preterm infants born at 23 to 25 weeks of GA and 3 to 5 weeks postnatal, increases to 85% at 26 to 31 weeks of GA at 3 to 5 weeks postnatal, and reaches almost 90% at 35 to 37 weeks of postmenstrual age (140). Thus, high phosphaturia in preterm infants may result in a net negative Pi balance and osteopenia of prematurity if sufficient Pi intake is not provided.

Magnesium (Mg)

Over 95% of filtered Mg is reabsorbed by the mature nephron, regulated by a number of hormones including PTH, calcitonin, glucagon, and AVP (see (141) for review). Micropuncture analysis shows that the proximal tubule of the adult reabsorbs only about 10% of the filtered Mg, whereas that of the developing animal reabsorbs about 60% of the filtered load (85). Overall, the avid retention of Mg within the PCT by the immature kidney likely contributes to the elevated plasma Mg levels noted during early postnatal life. From a clinical perspective, administration of the loop diuretic furosemide also inhibits Mg absorption, similar to that seen with Ca, and increases magnesium excretion as a result of the inhibition of the apical tri-transporter and modification of the transepithelial voltage within the TALH.

Glucose

The PCT is responsible for reclaiming all the glucose filtered at the glomeruli. Two Na-dependent glucose transporters (SGLT) exist on the apical surface of the PCT cells: a high-affinity but low-capacity SGLT1 localized in the S3 segment and a low-affinity but high-capacity SGLT2 found in the S1 and S2 segments. Since SGLT1 is also present within the intestine, a defect in SGLT1 produces prolific neonatal watery diarrhea (142). A mutation within SGLT2 leads to familial glucosuria (143). Premature infants of less than 34 weeks of GA have a higher urinary glucose concentration and lower maximal reabsorption of glucose than do full-term infants and older children (144). While the neonatal proximal tubule possesses both high- and low-affinity Na-coupled glucose transporters, the developmental rise in tubular glucose uptake is due to a maturational increase in the number of both SGLT1 and SGLT2 cotransporters (145). Studies also suggest a three- to fourfold developmental increase in the activity of the basolateral Na-K ATPase pump in the postnatal period that helps drive transcellular glucose reabsorption (146,147).

Organic Acids

Organic acids, including PAH (see discussion of RBF) and endogenously produced uric acid, are eliminated by filtration and proximal tubular secretion. Organic acids are transported from the peritubular circulation across the basolateral surface of the proximal tubule to the tubular fluid. The renal clearance of organic acids is low in the neonate, even when corrected for body size, and increases gradually with age (148,149). As discussed previously, the limitation in tubular excretion of weak acids may be due, in part, to the preponderance of blood flow to the juxtamedullary region, bypassing tubular secretory sites. Additional variables that may account for the limited clearance of organic acids include the low GFR, limited energy for transport, and restricted expression of organic anion transporter proteins (150).

Amino Acids

The renal reabsorption of many amino acids, including threonine, serine, proline, glycine, and alanine, is lower in newborns compared to that in adults, often resulting in aminoaciduria (151,152). This does not appear to be a generalized defect in amino acid reabsorption, because other filtered amino acids (e.g., methionine, isoleucine, leucine, and tyrosine) are reabsorbed more completely in the newborn. The transient limitation in net transtubular reabsorption of amino acids characteristic of the neonate most likely arises from intrinsic differences in activity and transport capacity of these discrete transport systems.

Acid–Base

The fetal kidney in the second half of pregnancy is able to acidify the urine (153), although the acid–base state of the full-term newborn is characterized by metabolic acidosis with respiratory compensation generally occurring within 24 hours following birth (154). The normal range for serum bicarbonate is lower for preterm infants (16 to 20 mmol/L) and full-term infants (19 to 21 mmol/L) than that for children and adults (22 to 28 mmol/L).

The concentration of bicarbonate in plasma is determined predominately by the renal bicarbonate threshold, which is lower in preterm and term infants than in adults (155,156). The low bicarbonate threshold characteristic of the newborn is considered to reflect nephron heterogeneity and/or a low fractional reabsorption of bicarbonate in the PCT of immature kidneys. In the adult nephron, proximal tubular bicarbonate reabsorption is mediated by the presence of an apical Na-H exchanger (NHE) and carbonic anhydrase (which facilitates the interconversion of carbonic acid to water and carbon dioxide). Evidence suggests that the low neonatal bicarbonate reabsorption is a product of reduced carbonic anhydrase activity as compared to mature kidneys (157,158) with improved proximal tubular bicarbonate reabsorption postnatally resulting from an increase in NHE activity as well as carbonic anhydrase abundance within this segment (157,159,160). Specifically, the amount of NHE3, the major isoform found within the adult proximal tubule apical membrane, is significantly reduced in neonates (161,162).

The renal response to acid loading increases with advancing gestational and postnatal ages. When compared to adult subjects given a comparable acid load, the infant exhibits a larger fall in blood pH and bicarbonate concentration, a smaller and slower fall in urine pH, and much smaller increase in urinary titratable acid and ammonium excretion (163,164). Premature infants born at 34 to 36 weeks of GA exhibit rates of net acid excretion and ammonium generation that are about 50% lower compared to those in term infants. Thus, net acid excretion increases to levels observed in term newborns only after 3 to 4 weeks of age (164). By the end of the second postnatal week, urinary pH values of 5 or lower are consistently observed in term infants (165). The rates of ammonia synthesis and excretion are low in the neonate and in response to acid loading do not increase to mature values until 2 months of age (165). Of note, phosphate loading, administration of cow's milk (which is rich in protein and phosphate) instead of breast milk, or high-protein feeding enhances the ability of the newborn to excrete titratable acids and ammonia (166).

The final site of urinary acidification is the renal collecting duct. Functional immaturity of this segment and particularly the acid–base transporting intercalated cells therein may further limit the ability of the neonate to effectively eliminate an acid load (167). Postnatal differentiation of intercalated cells has been shown to include changes in the morphology and function of these specialized cells with an increase in their density along the CCD.

Urinary Concentration and Dilution

The fetal metanephric kidney produces large amounts of hypotonic urine that contribute significantly to the volume and composition of amniotic fluid (168). While urine osmolality early in life is typically one-fifth that achieved by the adult (168), the fetal nephron is able to concentrate urine under conditions of stress, such as that induced by maternal water deprivation (169), hemorrhage (170), or infusion of vasopressin (AVP) (171). After fluid deprivation for 12 to 24 hours, the maximal urine osmolality achieved in premature and full-term newborns is 600 and 800 mOsm/kg, respectively (172). The kidney's maximal urinary concentrating ability (approximately 1,200 mOsm/kg) in both children and adults is generally not attained until at least 6 to 12 months of age (173).

Urinary concentration requires a corticomedullary osmotic gradient, the pituitary release of AVP, and the ability of the collecting duct principal cells to increase its water permeability in response to AVP. The limited urinary concentrating ability of the infant appears to be due primarily to an inability to generate a corticomedullary osmotic gradient in combination with a diminished responsiveness of the distal nephron to AVP (174).

The capacity to concentrate urine has been directly related to elongation of the loops of Henle and their penetration into the medulla (175). Unfortunately, the inner medulla and renal papillae are poorly developed in the immature kidney. In addition to anatomic maturation of the loops of Henle, urinary concentration requires the generation of a high interstitial solute concentration gradient in the medulla, which is underdeveloped early in life (176). Generation of the corticomedullary osmotic gradient necessitates the postnatal maturation of several processes involved in urinary concentration including sodium chloride reabsorption by the TALH as well as urea sequestration by the principal cells of the inner medullary collecting duct (in the presence of ADH). Furthermore, the functionally limited countercurrent multiplier system in the immature kidney prevents the appropriate buildup and maintenance of a medullary gradient needed for effective urinary concentration. Thus, preterm infants can dilute the urine to 70 mOsm/kg and full-term infants can dilute urine to 50 mOsm/kg as do adults. Nevertheless, the neonate has limited ability to excrete a water load due to low distal delivery of tubular fluid, presumably due to low GFR, which improves during the first month of life.

Antidiuretic Hormone (or Arginine Vasopressin)

Antidiuretic hormone (ADH), or AVP, was noted to have vasoconstrictive properties when first discovered. The limited ability of the immature kidney to concentrate urine is not a result of an inability to synthesize and secrete ADH. In fact, circulating levels of ADH are elevated in preterm and term infants and decrease rapidly in term infants within 24 hours of birth (177). Studies in human infants (178) indicate a qualitatively appropriate response to osmolar or volume stimuli known to affect ADH release. Furthermore, exogenous administration of ADH or 1-des-amino-8-d-AVP (DDAVP) to healthy 1- to 3-week-old newborns leads to a response, albeit of shorter duration and reduced magnitude than that observed at 4 to 6 weeks (179). Cumulative evidence suggests that the blunted sensitivity of the fetal and neonatal kidneys to AVP and limited concentrating ability of the neonatal animal is not a result of a paucity of V2 receptors (receptor to which ADH binds in the collecting duct) (180), or a lack of aquaporin channels involved in water transport across renal tubule epithelia (181), or efficiency of coupling to second messengers (adenylate cyclase and protein kinase A activity) (182) but is limited primarily by the poorly developed corticomedullary osmotic gradient.

CLINICAL EVALUATION OF RENAL DISEASES

Early diagnosis of a renal anomaly may help to prevent complications, including those related to the kidney itself (e.g., progressive loss of renal function as a result of systemic hypertension, obstructive or reflux uropathy, or infection) and those related to systemic disorders (shock, hypothermia, respiratory failure, hypoxemia, congenital metabolic disorders), therapy (nephrotoxic drugs), or other organs (e.g., cerebral hemorrhage, seizures or congestive heart failure [CHF] secondary to hypertension, ventricular arrhythmia secondary to hyperkalemia, urosepsis). In this section, clinical and laboratory features that should raise suspicion of a renal abnormality are reviewed and an approach to establish the correct diagnosis is presented.

Incidence of Renal and Urinary Tract Malformations

Use of prenatal US is a good screening tool in detecting congenital malformations of the urinary tract (approximately 80% detection rates). However, accuracy of ultrasonography is operator dependent, and kidney visualization may be limited by high maternal body mass index. The frequency of urinary tract malformations is 1% to 2% by prenatal US screening (183). Unfortunately, many abnormalities are missed even by expert sonographers. Prenatally detected renal malformations should result in a careful examination for further anomalies. In about one-third of the cases, renal malformations are within the category of associated malformations, which include multiple nonsyndromal malformations, chromosomal aberrations, and nonchromosomal syndromes (183).

Review of Prenatal/Family History

It is imperative to review details of the present pregnancy and pertinent family history along with details of prenatal US while evaluating an infant with renal abnormalities. The risk of renal or urinary tract malformation or renal failure is increased by maternal diabetes and by certain medications or drugs, including ACE inhibitors, angiotensin receptor blockers, nonselective NSAIDs, and selective COX-2 inhibitors. ACE inhibitor fetopathy is characterized by fetal hypotension, anuria–oligohydramnios, growth restriction, pulmonary hypoplasia, renal tubular dysplasia, and hypocalvaria (184). Maternal cocaine abuse and polydrug abuse are associated with higher incidence of genitourinary malformations with odds ratio varying from 5 to 6.1, respectively (185).

Maternal diabetes, especially in poorly controlled cases, is associated with a higher incidence of urogenital malformations and neonatal renal vein thrombosis (186). The risk for renal or urinary tract malformations is higher in an infant of a diabetic mother with a caudal regression syndrome or a femoral hypoplasia–unusual facies syndrome. Fetal alcohol syndrome is associated with unilateral renal agenesis, renal hypoplasia, ureteral duplication, and hydronephrosis (187). A high maternal serum or amniotic alpha-fetoprotein (AFP) concentration may be associated with mild fetopathy, oligohydramnios from fetal oligoanuria (188). Among many causes, polyhydramnios may be the first clue to the diagnosis of a nephrogenic defect of urinary concentration, whereas fetal hydrops may be the first sign of congenital nephrotic syndrome.

Positive family history should be sought for hereditary diseases, including renal cystic disease, tubular disorders, and nephrotic syndrome. There is a 9% frequency of asymptomatic renal malformations—most often unilateral renal agenesis—in the first-degree relatives of infants with agenesis or dysgenesis of both kidneys or agenesis of one kidney and dysgenesis of the other (189). The clinician should keep in mind that some autosomal dominant diseases have variable penetrance or time of presentation (e.g., adult-type polycystic kidney disease [PKD]) and that a new mutation may occur. Additionally, a history of prior fetal loss should be carefully reviewed, preferably with an autopsy review.

Prenatal Sonography

Prenatal sonography for diagnosis of CAKUT should include assessment of kidney size, echogenicity, structural malformations; ureters; bladder size, shape, and thickness; ascites; other organs; and amniotic fluid volume. Table 38.1 provides important prenatal findings with possible causes. Patients with CAKUT may get prenatal genetic screening, but in utero management options are limited, with little evidence of benefit from shunting of obstructed systems or installation of artificial amniotic fluid (190).

Physical Examination

Special attention should be paid to a detailed physical examination that includes focusing on the presence of dysmorphic features/anomalies, evaluating volume status in a newborn with suspected

TABLE 38.1

Elements of Prenatal Urologic Ultrasonographic Diagnosis

Parameter	Comment	Possible Causes
Hydronephrosis	Variable severity; may include pelviectasis and/or caliectasis	Obstruction, reflux
Caliectasis	Intrarenal dilation; more indicative of significant pathologic process	Obstruction, reflux
Pelvic anteroposterior diameter	Measured in the coronal plane, variable; in extremes may predict clinical outcome; caution should be exercised in overreliance on these measurements	Increased obstruction, reflux
Renal parenchyma	Echogenicity should be less than that of the liver or spleen; lucent medullary pyramids should be seen	Increased echogenicity in dysplasia, obstruction. ARPKD
Urothelial thickening	Increased thickness of pelvic lining	Variable dilation as with reflux or occasionally obstruction
Duplication	Separation of renal pelvic sinus echoes when no hydronephrosis seen	Possible associated reflux or obstruction; look for dilated ureter and ureterocele
Cystic structures, renal	Simple cysts rare	MCDK, ADPKD
Cystic structures, intravesical	May be very large and fill bladder, thin walled	Ureterocele
Urinoma	Fluid collection around kidney; perinephric or subcapsular	Obstruction
Bladder filling	Fill and void cycles may be demonstrated over time	Urine production
Bladder wall thickness	Must be interpreted in context of bladder filling	Obstruction, neurogenic dysfunction
"Keyhole sign"	Dilated posterior urethral; difficult to image	Posterior urethral valves
Oligohydramnios	Markedly reduced amniotic fluid; usually considered as no pocket of fluid <2 cm	Poor urine output due to obstruction and/or renal failure

ARPKD, autosomal recessive polycystic kidney disease; MCDK, multicystic dysplastic kidney.

Reprinted from Peters CA. Perinatal urology. In: Walsh PC, Retik AB, Vaughan ED, et al., eds. *Campbell's urology*, 8th ed. Philadelphia, PA: WB Saunders, 2002. Copyright © 2002 Elsevier. With permission.

renal disease, measuring BP accurately, and undertaking a careful abdominal/systemic examination.

Any dysmorphic feature should alert the provider to underlying renal abnormalities, especially the presence of vertebral, cardiac, limb, or anorectal anomalies suggesting a possible VACTERL syndrome, aniridia, hemihypertrophy, abnormalities of external genitalia, or limb deformities. The most typical sequence related to kidney disease is the oligohydramnios sequence, that is, Potter syndrome, which may result from prolonged leakage of amniotic fluid or from intrauterine oligoanuria. Fetal deformation caused by severe oligohydramnios includes Potter facies, which is characterized by a redundant, wrinkled skin, flat nose, low-set ears, bilateral skin folds arising at the inner canthi, receding chin, and malposition of the hands and feet. Lung hypoplasia results from fetal compression as a result of the oligohydramnios and, in some cases, massive abdominal distention. Readers are referred to Chapter 39 for more details. Upper urinary tract anomalies may be associated with several isolated anomalies (e.g., abnormal vertebrae—agenesis, ectopic, horseshoe kidney, duplication, and anorectal malformations—agenesis, duplication, VUR, hypospadias, ureteropelvic junction obstruction (UPJO), neurogenic bladder). In contrast, isolated single umbilical artery (191) or preauricular pits (sinuses) do not warrant renal ultrasonography. Several limb anomalies are part of syndromes or sequences associated with renal or urinary tract malformations, such as skeletal dysplasia, caudal regression syndrome, radial aplasia, femoral hypoplasia, rocker bottom feet, compression deformation, polydactyly, syndactyly, and hemihypertrophy.

Measurement of Blood Pressure

Neonatal BP measurement directly through an indwelling umbilical artery catheter (UA) provides the most accurate method of measuring BP, except for minor artifacts from air bubbles or blood clots in the tubing (192). The most commonly used indirect method of BP measurement is the oscillometric technique, which directly measures MAP based on the oscillations of the arterial wall; systolic and diastolic BP are then back-calculated from the MAP using manufacturer-specific algorithms. These devices are usually sufficiently accurate for routine clinical use.

Selection of a proper-sized cuff is crucial for correct indirect BP measurement. As discussed in the 2017 American Academy of Pediatrics Clinical Practice Guideline on Childhood Hypertension (AAP CPG), the length of the cuff bladder should be 80% to 100% of the arm circumference, and the width of the cuff should be one-third the length of the upper arm as measured between the olecranon and acromion (192). If BP is measured in the calf, it is important to use a wide enough cuff; cuffs designed for use in the upper arm may be too narrow, resulting in a falsely high BP reading. Calf BPs are generally the same as upper arm BPs in neonates, and this similarity may persist for as long as the first 6 months of life. Standardized protocol for measuring BP in neonates includes 3 successive BP readings at 2-minute interval with the infant lying supine or prone, measurement in right arm using appropriately sized cuff, the infant asleep or in a quiet-awake state, and preferably 1.5 hours after feeding or medical intervention.

Zubrow et al. (193) examined BPs obtained in over 600 infants of varying birth weights (BWs) and GAs admitted to 14 NICUs. They found that BP at birth is closely correlated with GA and BW (Figs. 38.5 and 38.6).

There is then a predictable increase in BP over the first 5 days of life that is independent of these factors. Thereafter, BP continues to rise gradually, with the most important determining factor in the Zubrow study being postmenstrual (postconceptual) age (Fig. 38.7). Dionne et al. (194) have summarized available BP data on preterm neonates and have published a table of BP values that has been recommended for use when categorizing an infant's BP as normal or elevated (Table 38.2). Satoh et al provide similar data for Japanese newborn infants (195).

Examination by Systems

Physical examination may show evidence of rash, respiratory failure, insufficient preload, shock, CHF, liver failure, bleeding diathesis, or encephalopathy. Signs of dehydration include weight loss, sunken fontanelle, and signs of hypovolemia. In newborn

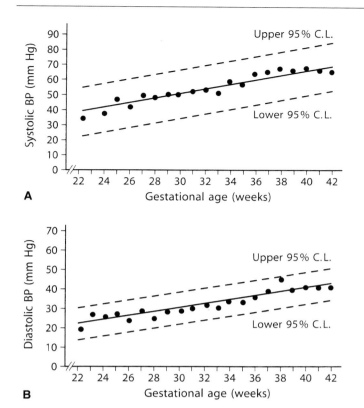

FIGURE 38.5 Blood pressure by gestational age. Linear regression between gestational age and mean systolic **(A)** and diastolic **(B)** BP, along with the upper and lower 95% confidence limits, which approximate mean ± 2 standard deviations. (Reprinted by permission from Nature: Zubrow AB, Hulman S, Kushner H, et al. Determinants of blood pressure in infants admitted to neonatal intensive care units: a prospective multicenter study. *J Perinatol* 1995;15:470. Copyright © 1995 Springer Nature.)

infants, generalized edema usually starts around the eyes, at the perineum, and on the lateral sides of the trunk. Edema may be a sign of fluid overload, AKI, or nephrotic syndrome, among other causes. Tachyarrhythmia, premature ventricular contractions, or abnormal QRS complexes on cardiac monitoring may be the first sign of hyperkalemia, which may be as a result of, or related to, renal immaturity or AKI. A small chest suggests hypoplastic lungs, which can be associated with renal and urinary tract malformations. Seizures or coma may be as a result of hypertension or complications of renal failure. Motor and sensory dysfunction of the lower limbs suggests an occult spinal dysraphism.

Abdominal examination may show distention, hepatosplenomegaly, peritonitis, pneumoperitoneum, or ascites. In a stable neonate, deep bimanual palpation should be done to assess the presence of a normal kidney in each flank. The examination is easiest soon after birth, before the bowel is filled with gas; later, it is facilitated by relaxation of the abdominal wall musculature obtained, for instance, by eliciting the sucking reflex. Several characteristics of the kidneys should be evaluated, including location (normally in the flank; an ectopic kidney may be located in the pelvis), size (the normal size for a 3.3 ± 0.5 [mean ± SD] kg infant is 4.2 to 4.3 ± 0.5 cm) (196), and long axis orientation (normally cephalocaudal). A horseshoe kidney may be suspected if the lower pole is closer to the midline than the upper pole. The consistency of a normal kidney is firm, in contrast to a cystic or a hydronephrotic kidney, which may be depressible. The surface normally is smooth, but large cysts can be palpated in multicystic or autosomal dominant polycystic kidneys.

Majority of abdominal masses are genitourinary in origin and may be as a result of a polycystic/multicystic kidney, renal vein

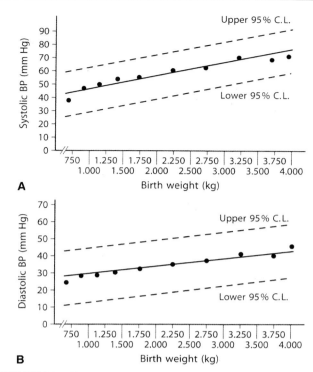

FIGURE 38.6 Blood pressure by birth weight. Linear regression between BW and mean systolic **(A)** and diastolic **(B)** BP, along with the upper and lower 95% confidence limits, which approximate mean ± 2 standard deviations. (Reprinted by permission from Nature: Zubrow AB, Hulman S, Kushner H, et al. Determinants of blood pressure in infants admitted to neonatal intensive care units: a prospective multicenter study. *J Perinatol* 1995;15:470. Copyright © 1995 Springer Nature.)

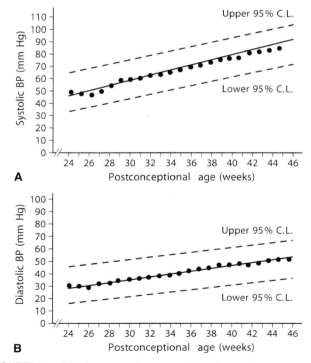

FIGURE 38.7 Blood pressure by postgestational age. Linear regression between postconceptual age and mean systolic **(A)** and diastolic **(B)** BP, along with the upper and lower 95% confidence limits, which approximate mean ± 2 standard deviations. (Reprinted by permission from Nature: Zubrow AB, Hulman S, Kushner H, et al. Determinants of blood pressure in infants admitted to neonatal intensive care units: a prospective multicenter study. *J Perinatol* 1995;15:470. Copyright © 1995 Springer Nature.)

THE NEWBORN INFANT

TABLE 38.2

Neonatal and Infant Blood Pressure Normative Data after 2 Weeks of Chronologic Age Based on Postmenstrual Age (Gestational Age + Chronologic Age)

Postmenstrual Age	50th Percentile	95th Percentile	99th Percentile
44 wk			
SBP	88	105	110
MAP	**63**	**80**	**85**
DBP	50	68	73
42 wk			
SBP	85	98	102
MAP	**62**	**76**	**81**
DBP	50	65	70
40 wk			
SBP	80	95	100
MAP	**60**	**75**	**80**
DBP	50	65	70
38 wk			
SBP	77	92	97
MAP	**59**	**74**	**79**
DBP	50	65	70
36 wk			
SBP	72	87	92
MAP	**57**	**72**	**77**
DBP	50	65	70
34 wk			
SBP	70	85	90
MAP	**50**	**65**	**70**
DBP	40	55	60
32 wk			
SBP	68	83	88
MAP	**49**	**64**	**69**
DBP	40	55	60
30 wk			
SBP	65	80	85
MAP	**48**	**63**	**68**
DBP	40	55	60
28 wk			
SBP	60	75	80
MAP	**45**	**58**	**63**
DBP	38	50	54
26 wk			
SBP	55	72	77
MAP	**38**	**57**	**63**
DBP	30	50	56

SBP, systolic blood pressure; MAP, mean arterial pressure; DBP, diastolic blood pressure.

Adapted by permission from Springer: Dionne JM, Abitbol CL, Flynn JT. Erratum to: Hypertension in infancy: diagnosis, management and outcome. *Pediatr Nephrol* 2012;27:159. Copyright © 2012 Springer Nature.

may be felt at another place in the abdomen), or renal hypoplasia or aplasia. Some abnormalities of the abdominal wall, such as bladder exstrophy, cloacal exstrophy, and prune belly syndrome, are associated with renal anomalies.

Anorectal anomalies or ambiguous genitalia, including severe hypospadias, should raise the suspicion of associated renal or urologic malformations. Percussion of the abdomen may disclose ascites or a large bladder. Neonatal ascites in the absence of hydrops fetalis may be as a result of the rupture of an obstructed urinary tract.

Urine Evaluation

With early feeding, most infants void within 24 hours after birth (including in the delivery room). Urine produced *in utero* normally is dilute, with an average osmolality less than 200 mOsm/kg. Higher osmolality *in utero* may result from obstructive urinary tract disease, poor tubular reabsorption of sodium, administration of oxytocin or indomethacin to the mother, or intrauterine asphyxia. Urine produced after birth usually is isotonic or hypertonic, probably as a result of increased release of oxytocin and ADH. In full-term infants, urine output after the first day of life increases progressively, in parallel with daily intake. In low BW (LBW, <2,500 g) and very LBW infants (VLBW, <1500 g), three phases occur in the early postnatal period: an oliguric phase, during which the urine output is always lower than the intake; a polyuric phase starting between 24 and 72 hours of age, during which the output exceeds the intake; and an adaptive phase, during which the kidney adjusts to the rate of fluid intake (197). A diuretic phase is observed in most infants, regardless of respiratory status or environment. The diuretic phase is associated with a high excretion of sodium and chloride, and, in much smaller amounts, potassium and bicarbonate (198). Urine output may be normal in patients with AKI, because some infants may present with nonoliguric renal failure. The neonate should be observed for dribbling or persistence of a large bladder after urination, suggesting either posterior urethral valves (PUV) or neurogenic bladder. Urination through an abnormal location suggests hypospadias, epispadias, ambiguous genitalia, or both. Additional discussion can be found in Chapter 39.

Urinalysis

The examination of a freshly voided urine specimen provides valuable information about the condition of the kidneys. Urine can be collected by attaching an adhesive plastic bag to the perineum, by expressing urine from cotton balls or gel-free diapers, or by bladder catheterization. Urine culture should be obtained by suprapubic bladder aspiration or by bladder catheterization. Urinalysis assesses the pH and the presence of protein, glucose, and blood and performs microscopic analysis for leukocyturia and hematuria, crystals, and casts and measurement of specific gravity and osmolality. Massive glycosuria may occur when glycemia is greater than 150 mg/dL (approximately 8.5 mmol/L), whereas mild glycosuria is common in VLBW infants even when glycemia is normal. A yellow-brown to green color may represent conjugated bilirubin. Presence of leukocyte esterase and nitrite may raise suspicion of urinary tract infection (UTI).

Assessment of Renal Function

Inulin clearance is the gold standard marker for assessing GFR in children and adults because it is freely filtered and not secreted or reabsorbed. Other markers include polyfructosan, radionuclides such as 99m technetium-diethylenetriaminepentaacetic acid (DTPA), and cystatin C (CysC) (199). GFR may be expressed in mL/min, mL/min/1.73 m^2 of BSA, mL/min/kg of body weight, or mL/min/kg of lean body mass. Which of these units is most appropriate for infants is controversial. Vieux et al. (199) have published reference values for GFR in very preterm infants (**Fig. 38.8**).

thrombosis, congenital or acquired hydronephrosis (e.g., as a result of a fungus ball or papillary necrosis), or a renal tumor. A suprapubic mass suggests bladder distention, which may result from lower urinary tract obstruction (suggested by dribbling), an occult spinal cord lesion (suggested by sphincter dysfunction), or deep sedation. In some patients, one or both kidneys cannot be palpated. This may be as a result of a less-than-optimal examination (e.g., absence of patient relaxation, bowel distention), unilateral renal agenesis, renal malposition (in which case the kidney

Parameter	3rd Percentile	10th Percentile	Median	90th Percentile	97th Percentile
27 wk GA					
Day 7	7.9	8.7	13.4	18.1	18.9
Day 14	10.7	11.5	16.2	20.9	21.7
Day 21	12.5	13.3	18.0	22.7	23.5
Day 28	15.5	16.3	21.0	25.7	26.5
28 wk GA					
Day 7	10.7	11.5	16.2	20.9	21.7
Day 14	13.5	14.4	19.1	23.8	24.6
Day 21	15.3	16.1	20.8	25.5	26.3
Day 28	18.3	18.7	23.9	28.1	29.4
29 wk GA					
Day 7	13.6	14.4	19.1	23.8	24.6
Day 14	16.4	17.2	21.9	26.6	27.4
Day 21	18.2	19.0	23.7	28.4	29.2
Day 28	21.2	21.6	26.7	30.9	32.2
30 wk GA					
Day 7	16.4	17.2	21.9	26.6	27.4
Day 14	19.3	21.1	24.8	29.4	30.3
Day 21	21.0	21.8	26.5	31.2	32.0
Day 28	24.0	24.4	29.6	33.8	35.0
31 wk GA					
Day 7	19.3	20.1	24.8	29.5	30.3
Day 14	22.1	22.9	27.6	32.3	33.1
Day 21	23.9	24.7	29.4	34.1	34.9
Day 28	26.9	27.3	32.4	36.6	37.9

FIGURE 38.8 **Reference values of GFR (mL/min/1.73 m²) in very premature infants during the first month of life.** (Reproduced with permission from Vieux R, Hascoet JM, Merdariu D, et al. Glomerular filtration rate reference values in very preterm infants. *Pediatrics* 2010;125:e1186. Copyright © 2010 by the American Academy of Pediatrics.)

In the clinical setting, GFR often is estimated by creatinine clearance or by using empirically derived formulae (200) using serum creatinine (SCr) concentration. Normal values for GA and postnatal age have been published (201) (**Figs. 38.9** and **38.10**). Initial values of SCr reflect a combination of maternal SCr and neonatal tubular reabsorption from leaky, immature tubules. In full-term infants, SCr decreases exponentially after birth (201), whereas in VLBW infants, it increases in the first 36 to 96 hours

of life and then gradually decreases. In the most immature infants, the increase in SCr is higher and the decrease is more gradual, probably as a result of a slower progression of glomerular function and a greater backflow across the immature tubular and vascular structures (201) (**Figs. 38.9** and **38.10**). Thus, the initial rise in SCr in these infants is not necessarily a sign of AKI. In case of CAKUT, the initial value of SCr may be normal and increase slowly, whereas CysC at birth reflects GFR. The value of SCr

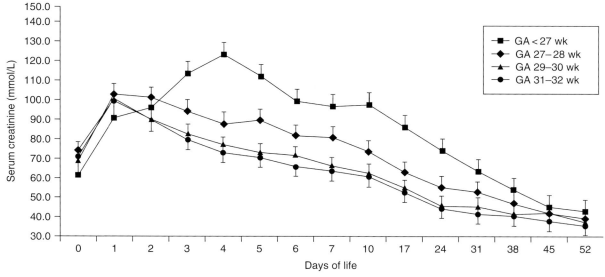

FIGURE 38.9 **Postnatal evolution of SCr (mmol/L) in preterm infants.** Values are given as mean and standard error. (Reprinted by permission from Springer: Gallini F, Maggio L, Romagnoli C, et al. Progression of renal function in preterm neonates with gestational age < or = 32 weeks. *Pediatr Nephrol* 2000;15:119. Copyright © 2000 Springer Nature.)

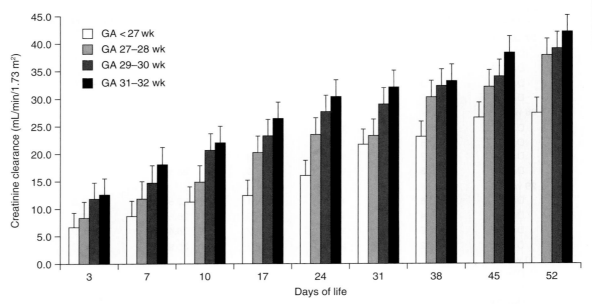

FIGURE 38.10 Postnatal evolution of creatinine clearance (mL/min/1.73 m²) in preterm infants. Values are given as mean and standard error. (Reprinted by permission from Springer: Gallini F, Maggio L, Romagnoli C, et al. Progression of renal function in preterm neonates with gestational age < or = 32 weeks. *Pediatr Nephrol* 2000;15:119. Copyright © 2000 Springer Nature.)

changes slowly when AKI develops or when it resolves. GFR may be adversely affected by nephrotoxic drugs (e.g., COX inhibitors), septicemia, and the use of diuretics (202).

A high value of blood urea nitrogen (BUN) can result from catabolism, dehydration, high protein load (e.g., oral, intravenous, gastrointestinal bleeding), or renal failure. A low value of BUN can result from extracellular fluid (ECF) expansion or decreased production of urea. The latter may be observed in association with anabolism, low protein intake, urea cycle disorder, liver failure, or liver immaturity.

Several serum and urinary biomarkers have been investigated for their role as noninvasive indicators of early AKI (203). They include urine biomarkers, for example, CysC, neutrophil gelatinase–associated lipocalin (NGAL), interleukin-18 (IL-18), and kidney injury molecule-1 (KIM-1). More data are needed before these biomarkers can be incorporated into clinical care. Importantly, premature infants have higher levels of urine biomarkers at baseline than do term infants; thus, evaluation of these novel biomarkers needs to be adjusted for GA.

The most common indication for the measurement of PRA is the evaluation of hypertension. See "Developmental Physiology" section and section on "Hypertension."

Immaturity of renal tubular acidification results in a significantly lower value of serum bicarbonate concentration in VLBW infants than that in full-term infants. In parallel, the serum base excess is often between −5 and −10 mEq/L in VLBW infants, compared with 0 to −5 mEq/L in full-term infants, and the anion gap is normally 15 to 22 mEq/L in premature infants, compared to 12 ± 2 mEq/L (<15 mEq/L) in full-term infants. In newborn infants, metabolic acidosis with high anion gap may result from lactic acidosis (asphyxia, hypoxia, shock, congenital heart disease, sepsis, or local tissue damage), an inborn error in metabolism (see Chapter 55), or renal failure. Metabolic acidosis with normal anion gap may result from renal tubular acidosis (RTA), gastrointestinal loss of bicarbonate, or cysteine chloride (in parenteral nutrition); a high urine pH may suggest distal renal tubular acidosis (see "Tubular Function").

The measurement of urinary and blood osmolality, urea, creatinine, and electrolytes is indicated for the differential diagnosis of polyuria and hyponatremia and for the early diagnosis of AKI.

Genetic, Biochemical, and Molecular Diagnostics

Readers are referred to Chapters 10 and 55, and reference (204).

Imaging of the Kidney and the Urinary Tract
Ultrasonography and Doppler Flow Analysis

US is performed to screen for CAKUT or as one of the first steps in the workup of AKI, hypertension, UTI, or hematuria. Indications for the performance of neonatal US are shown in Table 38.3.

US is a sensitive and reliable method for the detection of renal calcifications, including urolithiasis and nephrocalcinosis (NC). The bright foci are almost always located in the medulla, as white dots or white flecks, and diminish gradually over a period of months to years. NC rarely is seen in the pyelocalyceal system and does not influence kidney length in the first 2 years of life. Cortical NC is rare and develops within a few weeks of acute renal cortical necrosis and may be evident radiographically as a rim of cortical calcification (204,205). Diffuse cortical NC may be noted in primary hyperoxaluria (PH).

High-resolution images obtained with high-frequency linear array transducers allow excellent characterization of renal parenchymal architecture and pathologic conditions. In neonates, the US appearances are distinctive, because the renal cortex has echogenicity equal to or greater than that of the liver and spleen, whereas in older children, the cortex is hypoechoic relative to other organs. The differential diagnosis of US anomalies is presented in Table 38.4.

Blood flow through renal vessels can be assessed by Doppler US, which is indicated for the evaluation of hematuria, hypertension, and AKI, especially in a patient with a history of UA. Pulsed Doppler flow analysis, that is, duplex scanning, allows the measurement of blood flow velocity, which gives an assessment of RBF, and calculation of the ratio of end-diastolic minimum velocity to systolic peak velocity (i.e., diastolic-to-systolic ratio), thereby helping in the assessment of RVR.

Voiding Cystourethrogram

Vesicoureteric reflux (VUR) and bladder obstruction should be ruled out in patients with hydronephrosis, renal dysplasia, trabeculated bladder, bladder distention, or myelomeningocele. In a neonate with symptomatic UTI, US may be done initially to assess the presence of obstructive uropathy and signs of renal involvement;

TABLE 38.3

Indications for Ultrasonography to Rule Out Renal–Urinary Tract Malformations and/or Acquired Renal Disease in Newborn Infants

History
  Family history
    First-degree relative with Potter syndrome (bilateral renal agenesis/dysgenesis), autosomal dominant polycystic kidney disease
    Sibling with autosomal recessive polycystic kidney disease
  Abnormal prenatal ultrasonography (kidney, bladder, ascites)
  Oligohydramnios, unless normal postnatal renal function and oligohydramnios attributed to prolonged rupture of the membranes, postdate delivery, subacute fetal distress
Physical examination or evidence for other congenital anomaly
  Syndrome, sequence, or field defect
  Any part of a possible VATER syndrome (vertebral anomalies, anorectal anomalies, tracheoesophageal fistula)
  Preauricular pits, if family history
  Supernumerary nipples
  Congenital diaphragmatic hernia with additional anomalies
  Lung hypoplasia, symptomatic spontaneous pneumothorax
  Abnormal abdominal examination
    Abnormal kidney palpation
    Abdominal mass bruit
  Ascites
  Single umbilical artery
  Second- or third-degree hypospadias
  Ambiguous genitalia
Evidence for renal disease
  Renal failure, oligoanuria
  Systemic hypertension
  Urinary tract infection
  Hematuria
  Significant proteinuria
  Nephrotic syndrome
  Nephrocalcinosis and nephrolithiasis in preterm infants on prolonged diuretic therapy

TABLE 38.4

Renal Ultrasonographic Patterns in Newborn Infants

Normal appearance
  Prerenal failure
  Renal artery thrombosis
  Congenital renal disease, e.g., renal tubular acidosis
  Renal cystic disease (in which cysts develop late)
  Developing hydronephrosis or vesicoureteral reflux
Increased cortical echogenicity
  With increased corticomedullary differentiation in large kidneys
    Beckwith-Wiedemann syndrome
  With normal corticomedullary differentiation
    Prerenal failure
    Renal ischemia
    Mild renal dysplasia
    Congenital nephrotic syndrome, Finnish type
  With loss of corticomedullary differentiation in normal to small kidneys[a]
    Severe renal dysplasia
    Pyelonephritis, including renal candidiasis (often heterogeneous)
    Renal tubular dysgenesis/glomerular dysgenesis[b]
  With loss of corticomedullary differentiation in large kidneys[a]
    Renal vein thrombosis
      Edema results in decreased echoes
      Hemorrhage results in increased echoes
    Corticomedullary necrosis[c]
    Autosomal recessive polycystic kidney disease
    Renal glomerular dysgenesis/tubular dysgenesis
    Transient nephromegaly (benign)
    Contrast nephropathy
    Lymphangioma
    Mesoblastic nephroma[d]
Cysts(s)[e]
Increased medullary echogenicity
  Nephrocalcinosis
  Medullary cystic disease
  Tamm-Horsfall proteinuria, acute tubular necrosis
  Medullary sponge kidney
Intrapyelic echogenicity
  Renal candidiasis ("fungus ball")
  Lithiasis
Hydronephrosis

This list does not include findings shown by Doppler ultrasonography.

[a]Diffuse or heterogeneous hyperechogenicity of cortex or whole kidney.

[b]Renal size may be enlarged.

[c]Renal size may be normal or enlarged.

[d]Solid mass causing distortion of intrarenal collecting system, with occasional cystic areas corresponding to necrosis or hemorrhage.

[e]Absence of cysts visualized by ultrasonography does not rule out a renal cystic disease in a newborn infant. Some entities result in development of cysts later in life, whereas others (e.g., ARPKD) result in hyperechogenicity.

Modified from Slovis TL. Pediatric renal anomalies and infections. *Clin Diagn Ultrasound* 1989;24:157. Copyright © 1989 Elsevier. With permission.

US may be omitted if a third trimester prenatal US has excluded CAKUT (204,206). If no dilatation is seen and there is a good response to treatment, voiding cystourethrogram (VCUG) can be delayed. If US demonstrates an abnormal bladder, VCUG (using radio-opaque or US contrast) should be undertaken as soon as possible. The emergence of cassette-sized, high-frame rate (and high-detective quantum efficiency) digital radiography (DR) detectors may make it possible to get these studies using portable equipment soon.

Renal Radionuclide Scan

Mercaptoacetyltriglycine (MAG-3) scanning is frequently coupled with US providing a powerful combination for morphologic and functional renal assessment (207). It has a high protein binding and thus remains in the blood pool rather than being distributed in the extravascular space, as with 99mTc-DTPA. The renal extraction of MAG-3 is virtually double that of DTPA. In contrast, 99mTc-dimercaptosuccinic acid (DMSA) binds to the PCTs and is only minimally excreted into the urine; it is preferred for the analysis of renal morphology and differential function. Typical indications for radionuclide studies include renovascular hypertension, lack of visualization of a kidney by US, preoperative evaluation of the severity of urinary tract obstruction, and evaluation of differential renal function. However, due to immaturity of renal function in newborn

infants, many pediatric nephrologists and urologists will wait until the infant is at least 1-month post term corrected age before ordering such studies in order to obtain an interpretable result.

Magnetic Resonance Imaging

Magnetic resonance (MR) imaging, specifically functional MR urography, has been increasingly used because of its excellent delineation of anatomy with functional information and is achieved without ionizing radiation with additional advantage of nonnephrotoxic contrast medium, gadolinium chelate. This is especially helpful in the evaluation of renal tumors, renal abscess, ureteral ectopia, and genital anomalies. MRI T2-weighted images (which emphasize the difference in transverse relaxation times between different tissues) are independent of renal function and provide images in which water is bright, and with excellent contrast between normal and abnormal tissues (207). However, caution should be exercised in undertaking gadolinium-enhanced MRI in patients with AKI and in infants with CKD, since nephrogenic systemic fibrosis with gadolinium has been reported (208). Additionally, MRI appears to be more sensitive than US in detecting a tethered cord in a patient with bladder distention and lack of VUR or urethral stenosis on VCUG. Gadolinium-enhanced magnetic resonance (MR) angiography using a fast three-dimensional gradient echo sequence allows a good depiction of the major vessels.

Renal Pathology

Renal biopsy is indicated in nephrotic syndrome and may be indicated in PKD, hematuria, or persistent severe renal failure of unclear origin. Major contraindications to renal biopsy include bleeding diathesis, anticoagulant therapy, moderate or severe hypertension, solitary kidney, and intrarenal tumor (209). The technique involves visualization of the kidney using US, radioisotope, or radiopaque contrast. The most common complication is macroscopic hematuria, which occurs in 5% to 7% of biopsies.

ACUTE KIDNEY INJURY

The term AKI has replaced acute renal failure, primarily to highlight that this condition should be recognized early during the course of "injury" as opposed to waiting until the organ has failed. AKI occurs whenever there is a sudden deterioration in the ability of the kidneys to maintain proper homeostasis. This can be associated with an acute decrease in GFR (functional change) or anatomical change (i.e., acute tubular damage). AKI can be manifested as accumulation of uremic toxins, electrolyte abnormalities, or inability to maintain adequate fluid balance. Because the placenta fulfills the role of the kidney *in utero*, congenital malformations associated with limitation of renal function will not lead to renal dysfunction until delivery.

Pathophysiology and Differential Diagnosis of AKI in Neonates

With advancements in the field of critical care medicine and other fields of pediatrics, the etiology of AKI has changed in large tertiary centers, whereby less than 10% of those with AKI and those who receive continuous renal support have a primary renal diagnosis (210). Similarly, most neonates who develop AKI are born with normal kidney function, and the cause of AKI is inherent to the interventions, other organ failures, presence of sepsis/shock, or nephrotoxic medications. Primary renal diseases (such as congenital nephrotic syndrome or acute glomerulonephritis) are rare in newborn infants. However, many infants with renal failure in the neonatal ICU have congenital diagnosis (Table 38.5).

AKI is commonly multifactorial. Classically, the underlying cause of rising serum creatinine (SCr)/drop in urine output has been divided into prerenal azotemia, renal injury, and postrenal obstruction. As newer diagnostic techniques become available at the bedside, we will soon be able to also differentiate infants with AKI as having functional change (i.e., rise in SCr), structural (markers of tubular injury) damage, or both.

Prerenal Azotemia

Prerenal azotemia occurs in response to decreased RBF. Causes of prerenal azotemia are listed in **Table 38.6**. Renal hemodynamic

TABLE 38.5

Etiology of Congenital Acute Kidney Injury

Parenchymal malformation[a]
- Renal agenesis
- Renal hypoplasia
  - Simple hypoplasia
  - Oligonephronic hypoplasia
- Renal dysplasia
  - Multicystic
  - Hypoplastic
  - Aplastic
  - Associated with urinary tract obstruction or vesicoureteral reflux
- Nephron dysgenesis
  - Tubular dysgenesis: congenital hypernephronic nephromegaly with tubular dysgenesis = congenital tubular dysgenesis = isolated congenital renal tubular immaturity
  - Glomerular dysgenesis:
  - Secondary to maternal administration of indomethacin or angiotensin-converting enzyme inhibitors
- Polycystic kidney disease
  - Adult type (autosomal dominant)
  - Infant type (autosomal recessive)
  - Other

[a]May not cause acute renal failure until after the neonatal period.

changes associated with autoregulation of GFR decrease water and sodium losses, so as to maintain systemic volume expansion and BP.

In infants with prerenal azotemia and intact tubular function, tubular reabsorption of sodium and urea increases. This is reflected by low urine sodium concentrations (FENa < 1%), low urine urea concentration (FEUrea < 35%), and increased blood urea: creatinine ratio. These renal indices should be interpreted with caution when baseline tubular function is affected by prematurity, salt-losing state, or CKD. Utility of FEUrea to help differentiate prerenal insult from acute tubular necrosis is controversial. This period of renal hypoperfusion is critical to recognize and treat to prevent cellular damage. Correction of the underlying cause of hypoperfusion restores GFR unless renal hypoperfusion is severe enough to cause renal tubular and endothelial damage, that is, intrinsic AKI.

Intrinsic Acute Kidney Injury
Ischemic Acute Kidney Injury

Prerenal azotemia and ischemic AKI are a continuum of physiologic responses. Prolonged or severe hypoperfusion causes injury to renal parenchymal cells, particularly to tubular epithelium of the terminal medullary portion of the proximal tubule (S3 segment) and of the TALH. In contrast to prerenal azotemia, renal function abnormalities in intrinsic AKI are not immediately reversible. The severity of intrinsic AKI ranges from mild tubular dysfunction to acute tubular necrosis, renal infarction, and corticomedullary necrosis with irreversible renal damage. Prerenal azotemia and intrinsic acute tubular necrosis can be differentiated using several methods (Table 38.7).

The course of ischemic AKI may be subdivided into the early, initiation, extension, maintenance, and recovery phases (211) (Fig. 38.11). If restoration of RBF occurs during the prerenal azotemia stage, GFR can return promptly to normal. The initiation phase includes the original insult and the associated events resulting in a drop in GFR. The extension phase involves extensive inflammation, cellular apoptosis/necrosis, and the beginning of cellular repair. Tubular dysfunction with low GFR represents the maintenance phase. The duration of the maintenance phase depends on the severity and duration of the initial

TABLE 38.6

Differential Diagnosis of Acute Neonatal Kidney Injury

Asphyxia/hypoxia/ischemia (may lead to prerenal or intrinsic renal failure)

Systemic hypotension, shock, hypovolemia, severe dehydration

Renal artery vasoconstriction, e.g., nephrotoxins, endotoxin, endothelin

Reverse diastolic blood flow (preeclampsia, patent ductus arteriosus)

Prenatal/perinatal/postnatal asphyxia

Hypoxemia

Heart failure

Cardiopulmonary bypass surgery

Hyperviscosity, polycythemia

Severe anemia

Poor intravascular volume

Hypoalbuminemia

High abdominal pressure

Sepsis

Vascular

Arterial/arteriolar thrombosis/embolism/stenosis

Cortical/medullary necrosis, renal infarction

Venous thrombosis

Urinary tract obstruction

Urinary tract infection

Disseminated intravascular coagulation

Hemolytic–uremic syndrome

Preceded by bacterial infection (typically *E. coli*)

Atypical: may be familial

Genes encoding complement regulatory proteins

Cobalamin C disorder

Drugs

Antibiotics (aminoglycosides, amphotericin, acyclovir)

Nonsteroidal anti-inflammatory agents

Alpha-adrenergic agents

Angiotensin-converting enzyme inhibitors

Radiocontrast agents

Cyclosporine

Toxins

Hemoglobinuria

Myoglobinuria

Hyperoxaluria

Benzyl alcohol

Polysorbate

Ethylene glycol

Uric acid nephropathy

Glomerular disease

Membranous glomerulonephritis (IgG mediated)

Congenital syphilis

Diffuse mesangial sclerosis

insult. The recovery phase is characterized by the gradual restoration of GFR and tubular functions, which can take months to occur. Recognition of the different phases of intrinsic AKI is helpful in the diagnosis, clinical management, and prognostication of the disorder.

The pathophysiology of ischemic AKI includes damage of tubular epithelial cells, the innermost lining of the renal vascular system, and endothelial cells (212). Damaged endothelial and tubular cells also produce a systemic inflammatory response that leads to distant organ dysfunction in the brain, lung, heart, liver, bone marrow, and gastrointestinal tract (213) and may account for long-term fibrosis and ultimately CKD.

TABLE 38.7

Differential Diagnosis: Prerenal versus Intrinsic AKI^a

	Prerenal	Intrinsic
FENa (%)	≤1	>3
UNa (mmol/L)	≤20	>50
USG	>1,025	<1,014
U Osm (mOsm/kg)	≥500	≤300
U/P Osm^b	≥1.2	0.8–1.2
U/Pcr	High (>40)	Low (9.7 ± 3.6)
BUN/Pcr (mg/mg)	>30	<20
Renal failure index^c	Low (<1)	High (>4)
Ultrasonography^d	Normal	May be abnormal^d
Response to challenge^e	UO > 2 mL/kg/h	No↑UO

^{a}FENa is obtained by dividing sodium clearance by GFR and multiplying by 100. FENa and UNa are high (falsely suggesting an intrinsic renal failure) after diuretic administration, volume expansion, urinary excretion of nonabsorbable solutes (glycosuria, mannitol, glycerol, bicarbonate [in metabolic alkalosis]), adrenal insufficiency, or GA <28 wk. FENa increases transiently in normal full-term infants immediately after birth and in premature infants during the diuretic phase. FENa is also high in case of prolonged urinary tract obstruction and in chronic renal failure. Conversely, FENa and UNa are low (falsely suggesting prerenal failure) in acute renal failure due to severe vasoconstriction (e.g., indomethacin, radiocontrast nephropathy, sepsis, early phase of myoglobinuria), in acute urinary tract obstruction, and in some cases of nonoliguric ATN.

^{b}Although plasma osmolality can be estimated using the formula: Posm: $2 \times$ PNa (mEq/L) + gl (mg/dL)/18 + BUN (mg/dL)/2.8 where PNa is plasma sodium concentration, gl is glycemia, and BUN is blood urea nitrogen, the measured value of P osm is preferable, especially in critically ill patients, because of large differences in the case of sick cell syndrome (leaking cellular membranes), and in infants with a BW <1,000 g (Giacoia GP, Miranda R, West KI. Measured vs. calculated plasma osmolality in infants with very low birth weights. *Am J Dis Child* 1992;146(6):712.)

^{c}Renal failure index = UNa × Pcr/Ucr.

^{d}The ultrasonography in "intrinsic" renal failure may show increased echogenicity of the pyramids, which probably corresponds to precipitation of Tamm-Horsfall protein, signs of renal vein thrombosis, renal artery thrombosis, adrenal hemorrhage, hydronephrosis, cystic kidney disease, renal dysplasia, hypoplasia, or other pathology (see **Table 38.5**).

^{e}The challenge corresponds to the administration of 20 mL/kg of crystalloid (more should be given if there is evidence of hypovolemia) and/or 1 mg/kg of furosemide. Normalization of the urine output after such a challenge may correspond to a prerenal failure or to the polyuric phase following an oliguric renal failure. See text for additional comments.

FENa, fractional excretion of sodium; UNa, urinary sodium concentration; USG, urine specific gravity; U osm, urine osmolality; U/P osm, ratio of urine to plasma osmolality; U/Pcr, urine-to-plasma creatinine ratio; BUN/Pcr, ratio of blood urea nitrogen to plasma creatinine concentration; UO, urine output.

Nephrotoxic Acute Kidney Injury

Nephrotoxic AKI may result from pharmacologic agents, and less commonly from endogenous substances like hemoglobin, myoglobin, and uric acid. These toxins can cause AKI by decreasing renal perfusion (NSAIDs, diuretics, and ACE inhibitors), direct

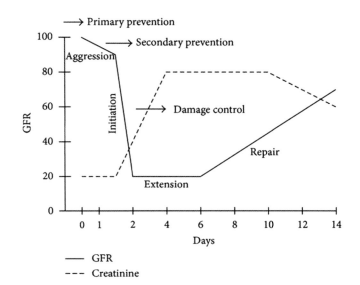

FIGURE 38.11 Stages of AKI.

tubular injury (aminoglycosides, cephalosporins, amphotericin B, rifampin, vancomycin, NSAIDs, contrast media, myoglobin/hemoglobin), interstitial nephritis, or tubular obstruction (acyclovir, uric acid). See **Table 38.8** for injury mechanisms and clinical picture (214).

Evaluation and Treatment of Nephrotoxicity

The ideal way to avoid nephrotoxicity is to seek avoidance of any nephrotoxic medication, and if it is absolutely necessary, then a multidisciplinary approach to seek dosage recommendations and monitoring of drug levels is helpful. Appropriate discussions should be undertaken among neonatology, pharmacy, and pediatric subspecialties such as nephrology and infectious diseases to discuss the necessity and alternative medications with lower renal injury profile that can be dispensed (214).

Obstructive Kidney Injury

The most common causes of obstructive induced kidney dysfunction in neonates are congenital malformations (PUV, urethral stricture, prune belly syndrome, cloacal anomalies, and imperforate prepuce). Acute obstruction may also result from neurogenic bladder, extrinsic compression, and intrinsic obstruction from renal calculi or fungal balls. Depending on the cause and associated damage to the kidneys, relief of the obstruction is imperative to restore renal function.

Evaluation of the Newborn with Abnormal Kidney Function

Infants who are at high risk to develop AKI, and those with signs or symptoms that suggest an impairment of one or more functions of the kidney should have the following reviewed:

- Evaluation of risk factors of AKI from the maternal or birth history.
- Evaluation of other factors that can predispose infants to AKI (i.e., cardiac disease, liver failure, nephrotoxic medications).
- Assessment for potential causes of AKI (decreased intake, increased losses, urinary tract symptoms, drug exposure, presence of sepsis, fever, rashes).

- Clinical exam findings: rash, fever, skin perfusion, heart rate, BP, audible renal bruits, abdominal mass and palpable bladder.
- Evaluation of fluid status (dehydration vs. fluid overload vs. euvolemia): vital signs, fontanelle, skin turgor, edema, mucous membranes, pulmonary crackles, cardiac murmurs/rubs, peripheral perfusion. Evaluation of fluid intake and output and daily weights.
- Estimation and tracking of cumulative fluid balance is essential.
- Laboratory/radiologic tests will depend on the history and physical exam. They include serum electrolytes, BUN, SCr, CysC, complete blood cell count, urinalysis, microbiology, urinary electrolytes, chest x-ray, electrocardiogram, serum albumin (to determine if appropriate oncotic pressure is present), and renal and bladder US and may include urine culture and full sepsis workup.
- Kidney biopsy is rarely necessary in neonates with AKI to make a diagnosis.

Diagnosis of AKI

Historically, neonatal AKI has been classically defined by oliguria/anuria and/or a persistent SCr elevation ≥ 1.5 mg/dL. Despite several concerns, SCr remains the most frequent measure of kidney function in neonates. At an NIH-sponsored workshop on Neonatal AKI in April 2013, one of the main focus questions was how to best define AKI. The neonatal AKI definition subgroup concluded the definition outlined in **Table 38.9** and is currently the best available definition. This neonatal AKI definition has been adapted for neonates from the 2012 KDIGO definition, with the following modifications included to account for the specific neonatal issues.

- Because SCr normally declines over the first week of life (201), each SCr is compared to lowest previous value.
- As SCr of 2.5 mg/dL represents GFR less than 10 mL/min/1.73 m² in neonates, this cutoff is used to define stage 3 AKI (as opposed to 4.0 mg/dL in adults).
- Many NICUs do not monitor strict urine output, and instead weigh diapers several times a day.

TABLE 38.8

Commonly Used Drugs Known to Cause Nephrotoxicity in Neonates and Summary of Injury Mechanisms and Clinical Picture	
Medication	**Proposed Mechanism of Injury and Salient Clinical Features**
Aminoglycosides	Mechanism: Primarily directly toxic to the proximal tubules (transport in the tubule, accumulate in lysosome, intracellular rise in reactive oxygen species and phospholipidosis, cell death); tubular obstruction from dead cells sloughing into the tubule; intrarenal vasoconstriction; and local glomerular/mesangial cell contraction.
	Clinical: Gradual serum creatinine (SCr) rise, urine concentration defects (nonoliguria or polyuria), urine sodium, potassium, calcium and magnesium loss with hypokalemia ± hypomagnesemia.
Vancomycin	Mechanism: Unclear, possibly including proximal tubular injury with generation of reactive oxygen species.
	Clinical: Unclear clinical nephrotoxicity profile because recent studies have not convincingly demonstrated nephrotoxicity due to vancomycin alone.
Amphotericin B	Mechanism: Renal vasoconstriction and decreased glomerular filtration rate (GFR); distal tubular toxicity.
	Clinical: Renal potassium, magnesium, and sodium wasting; impaired urinary concentration with polyuria; distal renal tubular acidosis.
Acyclovir	Mechanism: Urinary precipitation, especially with low flow and hypovolemia, with renal tubular obstruction and damage and decreased GFR. May cause direct tubular toxicity (metabolites).
	Clinical: Oliguria; serum urea, potassium, and creatinine rise.
Nonsteroidal anti-inflammatory drugs	Mechanism: Decreased vasodilatory prostaglandin production causing afferent arteriole vasoconstriction and reduced GFR.
	Clinical: SCr, potassium and urea rise, decreased urine output/weight gain. Enhanced toxicity in settings of renal ischemia, hypovolemia. Also known to less commonly cause acute interstitial nephritis.
ACE inhibitors	Mechanism: Decreased angiotensin II production leading to reduction in GFR via dilation of the efferent arteriole.
	Clinical: Increase in SCr and potassium, especially in the setting of volume depletion of reduce renal blood flow (e.g., renal artery stenosis).
Radiocontrast agents	Mechanism: Toxicity to renal tubules with increase in reactive oxygen species; also likely intrarenal vasoconstriction.
	Clinical: SCr rise with renal enzymuria (urine β-2 microglobulin, mild proteinuria), may be nonoliguric.

TABLE 38.9

Neonatal AKI Definition

Stage	Serum Creatinine Criteria	UOP Criteria
1	SCr rise by ≥0.3 mg/dL w/in 48 h or SCr rise by ≥1.5–1.9 × reference SCr within 7 d	UOP >0.5 mL/kg/h and ≤1 mL/kg/h
2	SCr rise ≥2–2.9 × reference SCr	UOP >0.1 mL/kg/h and ≤0.5 mL/kg/h
3	SCr rise ≥2–2.9 × reference SCr ≥2.5 mg/dL or Receipt of dialysis	UOP ≤0.1 mL/kg/h

Baseline SCr will be defined as the lowest previous SCr value.

Hopefully, newer definitions based on other serum and urine AKI biomarkers will be developed that will need to be tested against clinical outcomes (such as mortality or development of CKD).

Incidence and Outcomes of Neonates with AKI

Growing evidence based on large cohort studies in critically ill children suggests that AKI is associated with increased mortality even after controlling for medical comorbidities, severity of illness scores, and patient demographics.

In 2017, the Neonatal Kidney Collaborative conducted a 24-center retrospective study in critically ill neonates admitted to the NICU over a 3-month period called the Assessment of Worldwide Acute Kidney Epidemiology in Neonates (AWAKEN). Using the Neonatal KDIGO AKI definition, they found that approximately 30% of the cohort had at least one episode of AKI. The incidence differed across the gestational age in a "U" distribution, with the rate of AKI of 43% in those less than 29 weeks of GA, 18% in those between 29 and 36 weeks of GA, and 37% in the those greater than 36 weeks of GA. The mortality in infants with AKI was 9.7% compared to 1.4% in infants who did not have AKI (215).

AKI in VLBW Infants

Koralkar et al. (216) published a prospective study on 229 VLBW infants admitted to a single institution. Utilizing a modified AKIN definition (Table 38.9), 18% of the cohort developed AKI. Infants with AKI were more likely to have lower BW, GA, and Apgar scores, as well as higher rates of assisted ventilation and inotropic support. Those with AKI had higher mortality after adjusting for multiple confounders. In a retrospective study, Viswanathan et al. (217) reported an incidence of 12.5% among ELBW infants, using a cutoff of SCr ≥1.5 mg/dL to define AKI, with 70% mortality in neonates with AKI compared to 22% in ELBW without AKI.

AKI in Critically Ill Infants

In 2013, Askenazi et al. (218) reported an incidence of 16% AKI in neonates with BW greater than 2,000 g, and 5-minute Apgar scores ≤7 with 78% mortality among infants with AKI. In infants receiving therapeutic hypothermia, 38% incidence of AKI was reported using AKIN definition with 14% mortality in a retrospective study. Those infants with AKI had a longer NICU stay and longer duration on mechanical ventilation (219). In infants receiving ECMO, those with AKI had 3.2 higher odds of death than did those without AKI. AKI in infants undergoing cardiopulmonary bypass (CPB) have been reported to increase the odds of death.

Long-Term Kidney Function Following AKI in the Neonatal Period

Preterm infants are at high risk of AKI during their initial hospitalization, and there is growing evidence to suggest that preterm infants are at risk of CKD (220). A recent meta-analysis showed that preterm infants are more likely to have albuminuria, ESRD, and low estimated GFR (eGFR) compared to their term peers

(221). Among the 489 children in the NIH-sponsored CKD in Children (CKiD) study, there was a high rate of LBW (17%), prematurity (<13%), SGA (15%), and ICU admission (41%), and these factors were associated with lower stature (222). Thus, as more extremely preterm infants survive and live into adulthood, the impact of CKD on preterm infants poses a tremendous health and economic burden.

The reasons leading to a high risk for CKD among preterm infants are unclear. One explanation is that preterm infants are born with a paucity of nephrons (223). The extrauterine environment may not be amenable to neoglomerulogenesis and/or proper glomerular development (224). Another explanation is that preterm infants are at risk for acute hypoxic, hyperoxic, ischemic, septic, and nephrotoxic events between birth and termination of glomerulogenesis (225). Although the exact etiology of the pathogenesis from AKI to CKD continues to be explored, most experts believe that endothelial damage leads to nephron dropout and interstitial fibrosis and, ultimately, CKD (226).

Management of AKI in Critically Ill Patients

The aims of the interventions should be to (a) reverse the underlying process/limit further kidney damage, (b) administer specific therapies to improve kidney function/limit renal injury, and (c) manage the consequences of impaired homeostasis.

Reverse the Underlying Process and Limit Further Damage

The clinician needs to uncover and treat the primary cause of renal dysfunction. In patients with prerenal azotemia, specific maneuvers to address hypovolemia, hypotension, shock, poor cardiac output, hyperviscosity, increased abdominal pressure (abdominal compartment syndrome), or low oncotic pressure may restore kidney function and limit further damage. In patients with bladder obstruction, placement of a bladder catheter is critical to assure adequate drainage. In neonates with sepsis or UTI, systemic antibiotic therapy is indicated. In those with nephrotoxin-associated AKI, all medications suspected of causing harm should be removed, if possible. The benefits of prescribing nephrotoxic drugs should be carefully balanced with the risk of further damage. In oliguric/anuric patients who have an adequate intravascular volume, conservative fluid provision will prevent fluid overload, while in those who have fluid overload, invasive therapy will be required (see below).

Administer Specific Therapies to Improve Kidney Function

There is currently not enough evidence to conclusively recommend a specific therapy to prevent or halt the progression of AKI. A systematic review failed to provide enough evidence to recommend routine use of low-dose dopamine for improving renal function and urine volume in critically ill neonates (227). Data from the AWAKEN cohort showed that despite the fact that infants who received caffeine were sicker, those who received caffeine had a much lower adjusted odds of developing AKI than did those who were not exposed to caffeine (number needed to treat = 4.3) (228). Theophylline has been shown in randomized trials to reduce the risk of AKI in neonates with hypoxic-ischemic encephalopathy (229).

Manage the Consequences of Impaired Homeostasis

Supportive treatment of infants with AKI should be aimed at maintaining homeostasis of all vital systems. Some patients may need major respiratory and cardiovascular support, and all such patients require adequate fluid and electrolyte balance and adjustment of the dosage of medications that are eliminated by the kidney. Early diagnosis, appropriate provision of fluids/electrolytes to match output, and avoiding further insults may help prevent progression of the complications associated with AKI.

THE NEWBORN INFANT

Fluid and Electrolytes

Fluid and electrolyte hemostasis is one of the essential roles of the kidneys. Thus, infants with AKI are at risk for electrolyte disturbance. Dependent on the underlying physiology, the infant may have a net positive or net negative electrolyte balance when kidney damage is present. For example, an oliguric or anuric baby may have a progressive rise in serum phosphorous or potassium. Infants with nephrotoxic AKI can have damaged tubules, which excrete large quantities of water and potassium. Shift of electrolytes from the intracellular to extracellular compartment provides for additional homeostatic function, which can help balance electrolytes; alternatively, damage to cells (e.g., during tumor lysis syndrome) can overburden an impaired kidney's ability to provide sufficient clearance.

Hyperkalemia

Patients with AKI often develop hyperkalemia, that is, a potassium concentration greater than 6.5 mEq/L. Factitious hyperkalemia can result from hemolysis or clot formation during sampling, that is, release of potassium from erythrocytes or platelets. If hyperkalemia is associated with hyponatremia, hypoglycemia, and hypotension, a diagnosis of adrenal insufficiency should be considered (see Chapter 40). This most often results either from congenital adrenal hyperplasia or from bilateral adrenal hemorrhage; the latter may be suspected on the basis of anemia with thrombocytopenia, jaundice, and bilateral abdominal masses and confirmed by US.

The treatment of hyperkalemia includes discontinuing any potassium intake, discontinuing any medication that could cause hyperkalemia (e.g., indomethacin, ACE inhibitors, potassium-sparing diuretics), and correcting hypovolemia using isotonic saline to promote tubular secretion of potassium. Hyperkalemic infants requiring red blood cell transfusions should receive either fresh or washed packed cells. Consultation with a pediatric nephrologist prior to transfusing a hyperkalemic infant is advised.

Simultaneous administration of several forms of therapy (**Table 38.10**) often is required for treating life-threatening hyperkalemia (230). These can be divided into therapies that remove potassium (cation-exchange resins, dialysis, and diuretics), those that decrease myocardial excitability (calcium), and those that shift potassium from the extracellular to the intracellular compartment (sodium bicarbonate, insulin/glucose, or albuterol).

If electrocardiographic changes are associated with hyperkalemia, administration of calcium chloride or calcium gluconate is indicated; this will rapidly, but only transiently, decrease myocardial cell excitability (**Table 38.10**). The administration of calcium should be followed immediately by at least one method to decrease the potassium concentration.

Several methods (**Table 38.10**) have been proposed to induce cellular uptake of potassium, including the combination of glucose and insulin, albuterol, bicarbonate, and exchange transfusion with washed packed cells. Glucose–insulin infusion is more efficient in correcting hyperkalemia than are bicarbonate or cation exchange resins, and equally efficient as albuterol. If glucose and insulin are infused, the initial ratio of glucose to insulin for VLBW infants should be approximately 2.2 g/U of insulin; the ratio should be adjusted (range 1 to 3 g/U of insulin) according to the evolution of the glycemia.

Albuterol increases cellular uptake of potassium by inducing Na^+/K^+ ATPase activity through cAMP, independently of the action of insulin or aldosterone, and by inducing an increase in serum insulin level. A randomized trial in preterm neonates showed that nebulized albuterol (400 µg every 2 hours) decreases potassium level by 0.7 mEq/L within 4 hours and by 1.1 mEq/L within 8 hours versus no significant change in the saline group (231).

Although sodium bicarbonate (1 mEq/kg) has been recommended for treating hyperkalemia, its efficacy in patients with renal failure is controversial. Bicarbonate administration will improve pH and decrease hyperkalemia by H^+/K^+ exchange in metabolic acidosis. However, correction of acidosis will also drop serum ionized calcium concentration, and repeated doses of bicarbonate may result in hypernatremia. The use of bicarbonate in preterm infants should be weighed against the potential risk for intraventricular hemorrhage (IVH).

Although cation-exchange resins offer the potential advantage of removing potassium permanently from the body rather than

TABLE 38.10

Treatment of Hyperkalemia in Renal Failure

Medication	Dose (IV Unless Otherwise Specified)	Mechanism	Onset of Action	Duration
Calcium chloride	0.25–0.5 mEq/kg over 5–10 min	Modifies myocardial excitability	1–3 min	30–60 mm
Calcium gluconate	0.5–1 mEq/kg over 5–10 mm			
Sodium bicarbonate	1 mEq/kg over 10–30 mm	Intracellular uptake of K	5–10 min	2 h
Glucose	0.5 g/kg/h	Intracellular uptake of K	30 min	4–6 h
+Insulin	1 U/2.2 g glucose (1–3)[a]			
Albuterol	4–5 µg/kg over 15–20 min[b]	Intracellular uptake of K	30–40 mm	>120 min
Cation exchange resin (Na/Ca polystyrene sulfonate)	1 g/kg intrarectally q6h[c]	Exchange of K for Na or Ca	1–2 h	6 h
Exchange transfusion[d]	2/3 washed RBCs reconstituted with 5% albumin	Uptake of K by RBCs	Minutes[e]	>12 h
Peritoneal dialysis	Use a dialysate with low K concentration	Dialysis	Minutes[e]	No limit
Hemo(dia)filtration		Filtration (and dialysis)	Minutes[e]	Days

[a]The preparation of an insulin drip requires saturating the plastic tubing with the insulin solution before infusing to the patient. The average ratio of glucose to insulin associated with maintenance of normal glycemia in VLBW infants is 2.2 ± 0.6 g/U (mean ± SD) (Lui).

[b]Since administration of albuterol may cause a transient increase in serum potassium concentration, it should not be used as the first medication to treat hyperkalemia (see text for details). The IV preparation is not available in the United States. Albuterol is also efficient by aerosol.

[c]Oral administration of polystyrene resin should be avoided in VLBW infants and those with poor peristalsis (risk for concretions) (Ohlson). Substantial load of calcium or sodium may result from the respective resin. The effect on potassium concentration is slower than that on glucose–insulin combination.

[d]Many blood banks do not wash red blood cells anymore.

[e]These techniques are both rapid and extremely effective in correcting potassium levels. The time to set them up may be the limiting factor; other techniques may be used to stabilize the infant initially.

Modified from Smith JD, Bia MJ, DeFronzo RA. Clinical disorders of potassium metabolism. In: Arieff AI, DeFronzo RA, eds. *Fluid, electrolyte, and acid–base disorders, Vol. 1*. New York, NY: Churchill-Livingstone, 1985:413. Copyright © 1985 Elsevier. With permission.

increasing cellular uptake, their use in neonates is not recommended because of low efficacy and safety. Side effects of these resins include sodium overload (if using sodium polystyrene sulfonate but not if using a resin with calcium instead of sodium), bowel obstruction, perforation, and bleeding. Some clinicians have used decanting methods to reduce the amount of potassium given to the patients by adding this resin to the formula, mixing, allowing it to sit, and then providing only the supernatant (the resin falls and remains at the bottom of the container) (232). Novel K chelating agents, Patiromer or Zirconium, have been developed and are being used in adults and children. Studies evaluating their efficacy and safety in neonates have not been performed. When medical management is not sufficient to control hyperkalemia, dialysis (a.k.a. renal support therapy [RST]) is indicated.

Other Electrolyte Disturbances

Metabolic acidosis develops rapidly in most infants with severe AKI. Administration of sodium bicarbonate is controversial, which may aggravate fluid overload. Hypocalcemia develops rapidly in almost all patients with severe AKI. It may result from hyperphosphatemia and increased deposition of calcium in injured tissues, skeletal resistance to PTH, which results from decreased hydroxylation of vitamin D and, in aminoglycoside-induced AKI, parathyroid dysfunction secondary to hypomagnesemia, which results from increased tubular loss. Hyperphosphatemia is as a result of tissue damage (e.g., severe asphyxia, shock, and rhabdomyolysis) and decreased urine excretion. Additionally, AKI usually causes hypermagnesemia, which may result from decreased excretion and from shift from the intracellular space.

During the oliguric phase, no intake of supplemental magnesium or phosphate should be provided, to limit both hypermagnesemia and hyperphosphatemia. Intravenous calcium may be required to treat severe hypocalcemia (low ionized calcium with either symptoms or electrographic changes) or hyperkalemia with electrocardiographic changes; however, additional intravenous calcium should not be given routinely until the plasma phosphate level has been reduced to normal, to limit the risk of ectopic calcification. The hyperphosphatemia is managed by the addition of phosphate binders (e.g., calcium carbonate) to feeds. This binds phosphate, rendering it insoluble and thereby reducing its absorption. Aluminum hydroxide is not used anymore as a phosphate binder because of the risk of neurotoxicity.

Fluid

Appropriate fluid balance should take into account the expected weight loss over the first week of life. In preterm infants, fluid restriction during the first weeks of life reduces the risk for PDA and necrotizing enterocolitis, and trends have been shown for decreased IVH and BPD (233).

Managing fluids in critically ill neonates with AKI can be very difficult. Infants with AKI may require fluid to correct intravascular volume to maintain adequate nutrition and hematologic indices and to provide appropriate medications. Infants with obstructive uropathy require increased fluid intake during the postobstructive diuresis. In an oliguric/anuric child, fluid excess can cause CHF, chest wall edema, and pulmonary failure. Therefore, prevention of fluid overload (by limiting crystalloid infusions) and maximizing nutritional supplement concentration should be undertaken. Severe fluid restriction limiting intake to insensible and gastrointestinal and renal losses is sometimes required but limits nutrition.

As fluid overload develops, the clinician must maximize medical therapy to prevent or treat further fluid accumulation. Consultation with a pediatric nephrology team that can perform RST must be done early because severe fluid overload makes placement of a peritoneal or hemodialysis catheter more difficult, and as fluid overload worsens, cardiopulmonary dysfunction increases the complexity and limits success of therapy.

Studies in children show that prevention and treatment of fluid overload are two of the most common reasons for initiation of RST. Fluid overload can be calculated as follows: [(fluid input in liters) − (fluid output in liters)]/NICU admission weight in kg. On stratification of the prospective pediatric continuous renal replacement therapy (ppCRRT) database to children less than 10 kg (n = 84), Askenazi et al. showed that patients with fluid overload greater than 20% at the time of continuous renal replacement therapy (CRRT) initiation had a 4.9 times higher odds of death than did those with fluid overload less than 10%. Those who were able to return to dry weight during CRRT had improved outcomes.

Studies in neonates on the impact of fluid overload have begun to show what is seen in children and adults, namely, that fluid overload is independently associated with mortality. Determination strategies to prevent and treat fluid overload are needed to improve outcomes in neonates with AKI (234).

Nutrition

One of the biggest challenges facing a clinician caring for an infant with AKI or CKD is nutrition. Malnutrition should be avoided. Protein and calories should be provided as recommended for age and degree of illness of the child. If CRRT (either via blood or peritoneum) is required, an additional 1 to 1.5 g/kg/d of protein should be given to replace extra losses from these therapies. If appropriate, providing only the amount of phosphorous that the kidneys can excrete is prudent. Breast milk or special formula that limits the amount of phosphorus is preferred; the latter can be used to increase caloric content of breast milk. If the infant cannot be fed, TPN should be initiated. If an infant cannot receive an adequate amount of calories and protein necessary due to concern about fluid accumulation, RST should be considered.

Adjustment of Medication Dosage

The interval of administration of medications with renal elimination (e.g., antibiotics, paralyzing agents, theophylline, antiepileptic drugs, and digoxin) should be adjusted to drug levels or actual renal function (spontaneous or RST) to avoid toxic levels. The latter might, in turn, increase the severity of the renal failure. Although there are insufficient data to calculate adjustment of dosage in newborn infants, predictions can be made based on serial drug levels or based on the relationship between SCr and the half-life of serum concentration of a particular drug. When possible, medications with minimal or no renal toxicity should be chosen.

Renal Support Therapy for Neonates

The phrase "renal support" may be better than "renal replacement" as some have suggested that clinicians should not wait to support critical organ function when the organ has "failed"; instead, the endeavor should be to support organ function when organ begins to affect critical functions, especially if those processes are likely to continue to deteriorate. When caring for critically ill patients, clinicians must consider the potential risks and benefits of providing an intervention versus an alternative intervention versus providing conservative management. Outcomes in infants with AKI who do not receive RST are staggeringly poor. The decision to initiate RST is often very difficult in infants with renal dysfunction because of the need for chronic therapy including kidney transplant in those with severe congenital kidney anomalies when the child reaches around 10 kg and lack of strong evidence about outcomes in neonates with AKI who receive RST.

However, recent advancements in provision of RST in neonates have greatly improved in the last few years. The use of machines that have much smaller extracorporeal volume greatly reduces the risks associated with the therapies and allows for smaller vascular access. Initiation of RST with these machines is for the most part uneventful, even in very small and very critically ill infants. These machines include the "The Newcastle Infant Dialysis Ultrafiltration

System" (NIDUS) (235), the Cardiac and Renal Pediatric Dialysis Emergency Machine (CARPEDIEM) (236), and the Aquadex machine (237,238).

As these devices become mainstream, there will be lower risks associated with performing RST and the risk/benefit ratio will allow for more judicious use and earlier intervention and will have a profound improvement in the care of critically ill neonates.

A multidisciplinary team discussion early in the course of AKI is critical to provide the family and team with adequate information to make informed decisions. Under this premise, input from neonatology and nephrology teams will provide important information about potential benefits/risks for each of the therapies available and the risk of not performing RST and only providing conservative management. Each individual family/patient deserves individual evaluation. The options for RST include peritoneal dialysis (PD) and hemodialysis (HD). Both modalities can be performed intermittently (8 to 10 hours a day for PD; 3 to 4 hours a day for HD) or continuously. Continuous support provided via an extracorporeal circuit is referred to as CRRT. Continuous therapies provide the advantage to be able to accomplish the necessary goals of therapy over a 24-hour period with less potential for hemodynamic instability secondary to sudden fluid shifts.

THROMBOEMBOLIC EVENTS LEADING TO AKI

Thromboembolic complications in the neonatal period leading to AKI are being increasingly recognized due to the increased use of invasive vascular catheterizations and possibly due to the lower concentrations of antithrombin, heparin cofactor II, and protein C along with a reduced fibrinolytic capacity in neonates. Numerous factors such as perinatal asphyxia, neonatal infections, maternal diabetes, central lines, trauma or surgery, and dehydration may contribute to thrombotic complications. Various genetic prothrombotic defects, particularly those affecting the physiologic anticoagulant systems, that is, antithrombin III, protein C, and protein S deficiency; the mutation of coagulation factor V Leiden (G1691A); and the factor II variant (G20210A), have been well established as risk factors of thrombotic events (239).

Renal Artery Thrombosis

The clinical presentation of renal artery thrombosis is a variable combination of hyperreninemic systemic hypertension, hematuria, thrombocytopenia, severe oligoanuric AKI (if the lesion is bilateral), and loss of femoral pulses and of blood flow to the lower extremities. Renal artery thrombosis is often but not always associated with a history of UAC. Although mechanical injury and alteration of blood flow in the relatively small arteries of neonates is the major stimulus, other contributing factors may include an immature fibrinolytic system, partly as a result of physiologic deficiency in protein C, or plasminogen, hemodynamic factors, and hereditary antithrombin III deficiency. The incidence of thrombi in infants with a UAC in place ranges between 24% and 95% (240). These thrombi may become symptomatic when massive or when embolism occurs.

Real-time US may be normal or show increased cortical echogenicity or nephromegaly. The diagnosis of renal artery thrombosis is confirmed by MR angiography or color Doppler sonography. MR angiography is superior to color Doppler sonography in the evaluation of renal vasculature.

AKI associated with bilateral renal artery thrombosis may require prolonged RST (e.g., PD). The indications for surgical treatment are not clear. Systemic anticoagulation, thrombolysis, and, if it fails, thrombectomy should be considered for patients with refractory hypertension and those with massive aortic thrombus resulting in major complications (e.g., compromised limb perfusion, renovascular hypertension, or anuria). The other patients usually can be treated with antihypertensive agents and

symptomatic management of the complications of AKI; heparinization may help limit further extension of the thrombus. Although renal artery thrombosis often results in localized or diffuse renal hypotrophy, renal function often improves to a level that is close to normal, and hypertension resolves in most patients within a few months.

Renal Venous Thrombosis

Neonatal renal venous thrombosis is an uncommon condition, usually seen in term or near-term appropriate or large-for-GA infants. It may be associated with polycythemia; severe perinatal asphyxia; severe dehydration, sometimes with shock; maternal diabetes; angiography for congenital cyanotic heart disease; adrenal hemorrhage and umbilical venous catheterization; and prothrombotic abnormalities (241) (Chapter 44). Suboptimal fibrinolysis in stressed newborn infants may be an important factor. Renal venous thrombosis presents clinically as the association of a unilateral or bilateral palpable flank mass with hematuria, proteinuria, and, in some cases, oligoanuria.

Renal US shows a typical image, characterized by enlargement of the kidney, loss of definition of the corticomedullary junction, abnormal focal or generalized increase in echo amplitude of the renal parenchyma, and decrease in the size and echo amplitude of the central echo complex (241). The diagnosis of renal venous thrombosis is confirmed by MR angiography or color Doppler sonography. In cases in which patency of the inferior vena cava (IVC) is unclear on MR angiography, color Doppler sonography should also be performed (241). Ultrasonography and Doppler studies will show whether the thrombosis extends to the IVC.

The acute complications of renal venous thrombosis include AKI, systemic hypertension, and disseminated intravascular coagulation. The lesion ultimately may result in renal atrophy.

Affected infants have been treated with supportive care or heparin anticoagulation with a good survival rate, but they usually lose some renal mass, with cortical or segmental atrophy or hypertension. Infants who do not have risks for increased bleeding should be considered for combined therapy with thrombolysis and anticoagulation, which has shown more promising results (242,243). The therapeutic decision should take into account the risk of disseminated bleeding and IVH, especially in preterm infants. The indications for surgery are not clear.

CHRONIC KIDNEY DISEASE AND END-STAGE RENAL DISEASE

Introduction

CKD and congenital AKI are conceptually difficult to separate, frequently overlap, and are often indistinguishable in the perinatal period. While the National Kidney Foundation defines "chronic" to mean ≥3 months' duration, it is reasonable to apply this term to infants with congenital conditions that will clearly persist (e.g., renal dysplasia, autosomal recessive PKD [ARPKD]). In other cases, the label of CKD or ESRD following either congenital or noncongenital AKI is deferred until the depth and persistence of renal injury is known. The levels of severity of pediatric CKD are outlined in Table 38.11. Structural kidney damage may be established by renal imaging, renal pathology, or examination of the urine (244).

Causes of CKD and ESRD

CAKUT are the predominant causes of CKD and ESRD in infancy. In particular, PUV and bilateral hypo-/dysplasia are most likely to result in moderate-to-severe CKD, while other forms of CAKUT may not manifest severe complications until later childhood, adolescence, or adulthood. Immediate mortality of infants with CAKUT depends primarily on the severity of respiratory failure associated

TABLE 38.11

Levels of Severity of CKD

Description	GFR (mL/min/1.73 m^2)
Structural kidney damage with normal or ↑ GFR	≥90
Structural kidney damage with mild ↓ GFR	60–89
Moderate ↓ GFR	30–59
Severe ↓ GFR	16–29
Kidney failure	<15 or dialysis

GFR, glomerular filtration rate.

Adapted from Hogg RJ, Furth S, Lemley KV, et al. National Kidney Foundation's Kidney Disease Outcomes Quality Initiative clinical practice guidelines for chronic kidney disease in children and adolescents: evaluation, classification, and stratification. *Pediatrics* 2003;111(6 Pt 1):1416.

with lung hypoplasia and pulmonary hypertension (245). Infants with severe pulmonary hypoplasia, often associated with typical Potter syndrome, die within the first postnatal hours or days. The presence of bilateral renal parenchymal disease is the major factor predicting poor renal function in cases with CAKUT. If prenatal assessment demonstrates severe urinary tract obstruction with oligohydramnios in a fetus without a lethal disease and without evidence for bilateral renal dysplasia (246), intervention may be indicated to alleviate oligohydramnios and thus limit or prevent lung hypoplasia. Comprehensive multidisciplinary evaluation is needed to assess the prognosis, to counsel the family, and to establish a therapeutic plan during pregnancy and delivery and after birth. Depending on GA, one may consider either intrauterine decompression of the urinary tract or elective preterm delivery after steroid administration to the mother. Serial determinations of urinary indicators appear more reliable in predicting long-term renal function than do single measurements (247). The reader is referred to Chapter 39 for the description of specific malformations.

Another significant cause of infantile CKD and ESRD is made up of a broad swath of rare disorders, often autosomal recessive in nature, such as congenital nephrotic syndrome, ARPKD, and primary hyperoxaluria (PH). Perinatal ischemia/renal injury may also induce CKD and ESRD; for example, renal cortical necrosis may be precipitated by fetal hemorrhagic events such as placental abruption or fetomaternal hemorrhage. Tumors or vascular anomalies are among other conditions that may rarely result in CKD or ESRD in this group.

Epidemiology and Outcomes

Defining infants with CKD and ESRD as those who reach the 3-month milestone noted above excludes fetal losses, many neonates who do not survive, and many who have multiple morbidities who may not be referred for RST or specific renal management. As such, it is likely that databases tracking ESRD underestimate the incidence in the neonatal period, while still providing useful estimates of the cohort of perinatal survivors who proceed to further treatment.

The US renal data system (USRDS) reported just 320 children in the United States with incident ESRD between the ages of 0 and 4 years old (the youngest group routinely tracked) for a rate of 14.5 per million during the year 2011. Within that group, most reached ESRD before 1 year of age (median age 0.6 years). In terms of outcomes, 90-day, 1-year, and 5-year survival from the diagnosis of ESRD was 96.3%, 89.2%, and 76%, respectively. The mortality rate was approximately 10 times higher for infants and children who were never placed on the transplant waitlist as compared to those who were. Mortality rate for HD patients was about three times higher than for those receiving PD.

Rarer Disorders Causing Nephrolithiasis and Urolithiasis

A variety of rare stone diseases may cause severe disease in infants and young children.

Primary Hyperoxaluria

PH represents a small group of autosomal recessive diseases leading to intrinsic production of oxalate (248). Type I PH results from functional deficiency of the hepatic peroxisomal enzyme alanine: glyoxylate aminotransferase (AGT). The diagnosis is strongly suggested by a high oxalate-to-creatinine ratio in a "spot" urine specimen, which is further corroborated by 24-hour quantitative analysis, and definitively diagnosed by molecular (genetic) testing. Historically, liver biopsy for enzyme activity was required; it is still occasionally used if genetic testing is inconclusive. Some patients with type I PH benefit from vitamin B$_6$ supplementation, and there is some phenotype–genotype correlation. Type II PH is caused by deficient hepatic glyoxylate reductase/hydroxypyruvate reductase (GRHPR) enzyme activity. Type III PH results from deficiency of 4-hydroxy-2-oxoglutarate aldolase, encoded by *HOGA1* (249). Additional clinical diagnostic testing includes measurement of urine glycolate and L-glyceric acid, the latter being elevated in most cases of type II PH.

Type I hyperoxaluria is the most common (50% to 60%), followed by type III (20% to 30%), with type II and unclassified PH accounting for the remainder. In general, type III is the mildest and type I the most severe. Presentation in the neonatal period is rare, but infantile oxalosis does occur and can present with anorexia, failure to thrive, vomiting, dehydration, and fever; some have already experienced ESRD with "crystalline" kidneys easily visualized on plain x-ray. Renal damage includes NC, urolithiasis, repeated obstruction, and AKI; there is a very elevated lifetime risk of ESRD. Extreme hydration is the most important intervention (>3 L/m^2/d) and has been demonstrated to greatly mitigate stone formation and risk of CKD and ESRD. Pyridoxine (in a subset of type II) as well as inhibitors of Ca-oxalate precipitation (citrates, pyrophosphates) is the supportive treatment recommended. For type I or II PH (both hepatic enzyme deficits), liver or combined liver–kidney transplantation remains a potential treatment at least for those individuals with ESRD and the most extreme oxalate production, usually those who presented during early infancy.

Cystinuria

Cystine derives its name from its original identification from bladder stones formed by individuals with cystinuria. Cystinuria is an autosomal recessive disease caused by a defective tubular reabsorption of cysteine; the majority of cases are caused by mutations in either of two genes coding subunits of that "cysteine" transporter (250). Stones may be massive and can completely fill spaces within the renal pelvis, ureters, and bladder (251). The transport defect actually includes other branched chain amino acids (BCAAs) transport such that urinary ornithine, arginine, and lysine are also elevated though these are not associated with kidney stones. These urinary levels are fully diagnostic, and gene testing is generally not necessary. Neonatal urinary screening programs are also feasible and have shown an average prevalence of approximately 1 in 7,000, with a range of 1:2,000 in England to 1:15,000 in the United States. Where neonatal screening is not performed, testing family members is important. Obligate carriers have a slightly elevated risk of kidney stones, and affected carrier siblings can be identified by intermediate urinary amino acid levels.

Therapy for cystinuria includes very high fluid intake, alkalization (urine pH must be >7.5 to significantly help), decreased dietary sources of BCAA (in older children and adults), and thiol drugs. These agents prevent the formation of cystine from spontaneous combination of cysteine molecules via binding of their active sulfhydryl groups. Treated patients may continue to have a large stone burden, but individual stone sizes are reduced and are more likely to pass without the need for surgery. Tiopronin and penicillamine are the most commonly used in severe cases but have significant potential side effects (hematologic) and are generally avoided in infants and young children when possible. Captopril is often suggested as a potential therapeutic as it also has a sulfhydryl group; its efficacy is questionable due to limited urinary excretion. Monitoring disease activity requires expertise; for example, thiols interfere with quantification of urinary cystine and measures of supersaturation. Access to urologic care and attention to radiation burden from radiology studies is clinically important.

Disorders of Purine and Pyrimidine Metabolism Associated with Nephrolithiasis

Several metabolic disorders of purine and pyrimidine metabolism may lead to nephrolithiasis in infancy. These disorders are generally associated with elevated uric acid production and excretion, but the kidney stones generally also contain Ca (252).

Classic Xanthinuria

It consists of two autosomal recessive disorders with overlapping genotypes; stones are predominantly uric acid (radiolucent). Serum uric acid levels are low. Patients may have symptoms of myopathy due to uric acid deposition, and type II patients may have neuropathy.

Lesch-Nyhan Syndrome

It results from deficiency of hypoxanthine guanine phosphoribosyltransferase (HGPRT). It is an X-linked disease with neurologic symptoms that do not present at birth but often become profound. Serum uric acid levels are extremely elevated due to overproduction, and infants generally present with copious and persistent pink, orange, or red urate crystals in the diapers. Brisk hydration and allopurinol are mainstays of treatment to avoid repeated uric acid stones. However, allopurinol leads to production of xanthine stones. Xanthinuria can be followed to titrate the dose. Disease prognosis is poor, predominantly due to neurologic degeneration.

Adenine Phosphoribosyltransferase Deficiency

Adenine phosphoribosyltransferase deficiency (ARPT) is an autosomal recessive disorder. Round brown stones and crystals consist of 2,8-dihydroxyadenine, which can be distinguished from uric acid only by infrared spectrophotometry. While some patients may present as early as the neonatal period, others do not present until adulthood. In addition to fluids to induce high urine output, a diet low in purines and allopurinol is helpful. Alkali therapy is not helpful as solubility is not affected below a pH of 9. ESRD can occur, but renal outcomes are quite variable.

Phosphoribosyl Pyrophosphate Synthetase Superactivity

It is an X-linked disease sometimes associated with sensorineural deafness. Affected males suffer extreme elevation of serum uric acid leading to uric acid stones, gout, and neurodevelopmental disease. Females may also exhibit (less extreme) symptoms. High fluid intake, allopurinol, low-purine diet, and alkalinization are helpful. Like Lesch-Nyhan, in some cases, allopurinol can lead to xanthine stones.

Hereditary Renal Hypouricemia

In patients with hereditary renal hypouricemia (HRH), increased renal excretion of uric acid leads to hypouricemia and nephrolithiasis. Two discrete molecular causes are known. The first is a defect in URAT1, a renal uric acid transporter, and the second a defect in GLUT9 (named for its similarity to glucose transporters, despite later appreciation of its importance in uric acid transport) (253).

Uromodulin-Associated Kidney Diseases

Uromodulin, the protein also known as Tamm-Horsfall protein, appears to have many functions, contributing to water impermeability, antimicrobial defense, and inhibition of stone formation,

to name a few. The human diseases resulting from mutation of *UMOD*, the gene coding for uromodulin, are familial juvenile hyperuricemic nephropathy, medullary cystic kidney disease type 2, and glomerulocystic kidney disease (254). These autosomal dominant tubulointerstitial diseases have some common and differing manifestations, but the relation between genotype and phenotype is complex and has not yet been clarified. Progressive loss of renal function occurs, though ESRD generally does not occur until young adulthood. In familial juvenile hyperuricemic nephropathy, hyperuricemia and gout are common though the urinary concentrating defect is mild and cysts are generally only microscopic. In medullary cystic disease type 2, the hyperuricemia and gout are less pronounced, but urinary concentration defects and corticomedullary cysts visible on imaging are likely. Glomerulocystic kidney disease is not clinically well defined.

Further Causes of Fanconi Syndrome
Nephropathic Cystinosis

In general, the prevalence of cystinosis is between 1:200,000 and 1:100,000 individuals, though some communities have much higher rates due to founder genetic effects (255,256). Described by Guido Fanconi, it is an autosomal recessive lysosomal disease resulting from mutation of *CTNS*, the gene coding cystinosin, a transporter of cystine from the lysosomes to the cytosol (where it is normally reduced to cysteine). As a result, cystine accumulates within the lysosome and ultimately causes cellular toxicity. The infantile, which is, nephropathic type of cystinosis, is the most severe form and is characterized by Fanconi syndrome with onset of symptoms generally between 6 and 12 months of age. Retinopathy may be detected within the first weeks of life, and characteristic corneal opacities (visible by slit-lamp exam) usually occur by 16 months of age. In the absence of treatment, renal failure generally occurs by 10 years of age.

Based on clinical suspicion, laboratory diagnosis can be made by measuring the cystine content of white blood cells; affected patients generally have concentrations of 3.0 to 23.0 nmol half-cystine/mg cell protein, whereas normal is under 0.2.

The treatment of cystinosis must include (a) symptomatic treatment of Fanconi syndrome, (b) symptomatic care of CKD and established extrarenal disease, and (c) cysteamine therapy to reduce ongoing renal and extrarenal damage. The first aspect includes alkalinization and supplementation of water, potassium, phosphate, vitamin D, and sometimes carnitine. The general management of CKD, ESRD, and transplantation is discussed elsewhere, but the second aspect must address common extrarenal manifestations of cystinosis including hypothyroidism, diabetes, and other endocrinopathies. Multisystem involvement may also lead to musculoskeletal, neurologic, hepatic, gastrointestinal, and bone marrow/hematologic diseases that need specific management (Table 38.12).

Cysteamine (β-mercaptoethylamine hydrochloride) is an oral medication that enters the lysosome and reacts with cystine to form cysteine, which can then exit the lysosome. Topical cysteamine is used to prevent corneal disease. In many patients, oral immediate-release cysteamine is poorly tolerated due to frequency of administration (every 6 hours), strong odor, and often nausea. Recently, an extended-release/microbead formulation of cysteamine was created with twice-daily dosing and fewer side effects; with demonstrated noninferiority, it is now in active clinical use, despite some controversy about an initial cost more than 30 times higher than the immediate release form (257). Treatment with either agent improves all aspects of disease, especially when initiated early, but the threat of progression toward renal failure or extrarenal disease is not eliminated. Importantly, patients receiving a kidney transplant require ongoing treatment to prevent extrarenal disease.

TABLE 38.12

Conservative Management of Infants with CKD

Problem	Usual Therapy	Comment
Acidosis	Alkali (Na citrate, NaHCO$_3$)	Correction of acidosis necessary to maintain anabolism and promote normal growth.
Anemia	Recombinant erythropoiesis-stimulating agent	Iron supplementation always necessary during erythropoietin treatment.
Anorexia	Nasogastric or gastrostomy feeds	Nearly all infants with CKD require supplemental feedings.
Hyperphosphatemia	Low-phosphate formula; phosphate binders	CaCO$_3$ most commonly used phosphate binder in infancy; sevelamer in powdered form is also used; avoid aluminum-containing binders.
Secondary hyperparathyroidism	Vitamin D analogues (paracalcitol, calcitriol)	Maintain serum intact PTH in normal range in predialysis; CKD patients; avoid calcium*phosphorous product >70.
Uremia	Protein-adjusted diet	Do not restrict protein intake below RDA for age; infants with congenital nephritic syndrome require increased protein intake; inability to provide RDA for protein without uremia should prompt consideration of renal replacement therapy.
Growth failure	Supplemental feedings; rHGH	Correction of all above problems must be achieved prior to instituting rHGH treatment.
Neurodevelopmental delay	"Early intervention" services	Most infants require some combination of physical, occupational, and speech/feeding therapies.
Immune function	Ig lost in nephrosis and via peritoneal dialysis	IVIg may be advised. Accelerated vaccination schedule, especially live vaccines, prior to transplant immunosuppression.
Urinary tract	Attention to maintaining a low pressure system UTI prophylaxis	Close collaboration with pediatric urology. Attention to incomplete voiding, reflux, anterograde obstruction.

CKD, chronic kidney disease; Ig, immunoglobulin; PTH, parathyroid hormone; RDA, recommended dietary allowance; rHGH, recombinant human growth hormone; IVIg, intravenous immune globulin; UTI, urinary tract infection.

Tyrosinemia

Hereditary tyrosinemia type I, that is, hepatorenal tyrosinemia (see Chapter 55), is an autosomal recessive disorder as a result of a deficiency in fumarylacetoacetate hydrolase (FAH or fumarylacetoacetase) (258). The disorder is uncommon but has historically had an increased incidence in the Saguenay–Lac-St. Jean region of the province of Québec, in Norway, and in Finland; specific mutations may also be found in Southern Europe and in the Ashkenazi Jewish population. Renal tubular dysfunction results from the accumulation of cytotoxic intracellular metabolites including succinylacetoacetate and succinylacetone. Tyrosinemia usually presents severely in newborns and infants, often with fatal consequences. While Fanconi syndrome may be present, signs are often overshadowed by other manifestations including liver failure, bleeding, or neurologic crisis; hepatocellular carcinoma is a longer-term risk. Carrier screening, prenatal diagnosis, and newborn screening are all employed to reduce the transmission of tyrosinemia. Treatment includes use of nitisinone (NTBC) and avoidance of phenylalanine and tyrosine in the diet (259). Some infants may require liver transplantation.

Fanconi-Bickel Syndrome

Fanconi-Bickel syndrome (FBS) is generally considered a GSD. This syndrome is caused by homozygous or compound heterozygous mutations within GLUT2, the gene encoding the most important facilitative glucose transporter in hepatocytes, pancreatic β cells, enterocytes, and renal tubular cells. It is characterized by the association of hepatomegaly secondary to glycogen accumulation, glucose and galactose intolerance, fasting hypoglycemia, Fanconi syndrome, and severely stunted growth (260). These severe systemic symptoms begin during early infancy. This differs significantly from GSD type Ia (glucose-6-phosphatase deficiency), which is associated with late onset of proximal tubular dysfunction in approximately 15% of the cases (261).

Galactosemia (Galactose-1-Phosphate Uridyltransferase Deficiency)

Galactosemia is an autosomal recessive disorder that results in intracellular accumulation of galactose-1-phosphate in various tissues, including the kidney (262). Galactose phosphate uridyltransferase is included in neonatal screening programs. Symptoms of the severe form often develop in the neonatal period, soon after initiating lactose (mild) intake, and include hypoglycemia, anorexia, vomiting, diarrhea, hepatomegaly, jaundice, and hypoprothrombinemia. Lactose intake leads to galactosuria, which produces a positive test for reducing substances, but no glucosuria. Removal of lactose and galactose from the diet results in rapid resolution. Hepatic and hematologic manifestations and, in some, sepsis, predominate the clinical picture to the extent that renal disease is overlooked in some sources. Nonetheless, tubulopathy is present and characterized by low molecular weight proteinuria, generalized aminoaciduria, and a significant defect in transport of phosphate, bicarbonate, and glucose (263).

Specific Aminoacidurias
Lysinuric Protein Intolerance

This is an autosomal recessive disorder of reabsorption of dibasic amino acids (lysine, arginine, and ornithine) in the renal tubule, and the gastrointestinal tract resulting from mutations of SLC7A, which encodes the γ+L amino acid transporter-1 (γ+LAT-1) (264). The urinary loss of these amino acids is quantitatively more significant than that seen in cystinuria and may lead to secondary hyperammonemia (due to lack of substrate); in contrast, urinary cystine levels are much lower than those of cystinuria. This disorder is extremely rare, except in Finland, where the prevalence historically reached 1:60,000 (265). Most breast-fed infants are asymptomatic, although some may develop symptoms of hyperammonemia during the neonatal period. Typically, infants manifest symptoms within 1 week of weaning or increase in the protein intake; most infants affected with this disorder develop nausea, vomiting, and mild diarrhea. Later on, patients can manifest severe multisystem complications. Treatment consists of a low-protein diet and citrulline supplementation (as substrate for the urea cycle); severe episodes of hyperammonemia may also be treated with additional cycle substrates.

Hartnup Disorder

It results from defective renal transport of neutral amino acids. Under conditions of a protein-replete diet, this disorder is asymptomatic. Tryptophan, a neutral amino acid, is a precursor of niacin and serotonin; thus, under protein-deficient conditions or malnutrition, the disease can manifest with pellagra-like symptoms, cerebellar symptoms, and psychosis. Neonatal screening and clinical awareness is particularly important in areas where dietary resources are chronically scarce or become acutely limited, for example, after natural or social disasters. Treatment centers on providing sufficient protein and supplementing niacin.

Iminoglycinuria

It is defined by urinary wasting of glycine, proline, and hydroxyproline due to a defective renal tubular imino transporter. The disease is generally considered asymptomatic, although potential associations with several disorders have been described anecdotally (266).

Dicarboxylic Aminoaciduria

It results from mutation in SLC1A1, the gene coding a transporter for anionic amino acids; urinary levels of glutamate and aspartate are marked. Association with neurologic or psychiatric conditions is not clear; this condition may be asymptomatic (267).

Other Genetic Causes of Nephrotic Syndrome

Diffuse mesangial sclerosis is a clinicopathologic entity that was first described in 1985 and is another common cause of congenital nephrotic syndrome. It is seen exclusively in infancy and appears to be transmitted in some families as an autosomal recessive trait (268). The onset varies between the second trimester of gestation and 33 months of age. Unlike CNF, infants with DMS appear normal at birth, with a normal BW and without enlarged placenta. Patients with DMS present with proteinuria (with or without nephrotic syndrome), sometimes hematuria, often arterial hypertension, and progressive chronic renal failure (CRF) leading to ESRD within a few months to 2 years from the onset. Because CRF develops rapidly in these patients, it is the major cause of death in the absence of dialysis and renal transplantation. Renal venous thrombosis is a frequent complication. Histologic examination of the glomeruli shows mesangial cells embedded in a periodic acid-Schiff–positive and silver-positive fibrillar network occluding the capillaries. Tubular changes are similar to those seen in CNF, and interstitial fibrosis is more pronounced than in CNF.

Treatment is supportive and consists of maintenance of electrolyte and water balance and adequate nutrition, prevention and treatment of infectious complications, use of ACE inhibitor and indomethacin, and management of renal failure. Bilateral nephrectomy has been considered at the time of transplant because of the potential risk of developing a Wilms tumor. DMS is reportedly resistant to steroid and immunosuppressive therapy, although there are some reported cases of patients responding to steroid and calcineurin inhibitor drugs.

Three genes are implicated in DMS: WT1, LAMB2, and PLCE1. WT1 gene is located on chromosome 11p13 and encodes a zinc finger transcription factor involved in kidney and gonadal development. LAMB2 is located on chromosome 3p21 and encodes laminin beta 2, a component of laminin that is an essential component of the basement membrane where it plays a key role in anchoring and differentiation of podocyte foot processes. PLCE1 gene is located on chromosome 10q23 and encodes for a protein PLCε1 that is a member of phospholipase family of enzymes that generates second messengers, which regulate various processes affecting cell growth, differentiation, and gene expression.

DMS can be associated with one of many genotypic disorders including the WAGR syndrome, Denys-Drash syndrome, Pierson syndrome, and Galloway-Mowat syndrome. Children with WAGR syndrome present with Wilms tumor (W), aniridia (A), genitourinary anomalies (G), and mental retardation (R) (269). Cytogenetic analysis revealed large deletions of the WT1 gene on chromosome 11p13 in these patients. Mutations of PAX6 on band 13 of chromosome 11 results in aniridia.

Children with Denys-Drash syndrome present with early-onset nephrotic syndrome, DMS rapidly progressing to ESRD, 46, XY male gonadal pseudohermaphroditism, and Wilms tumor (270). Germ line WT1 missense mutations located in exons 8 or 9 coding for zinc fingers 2 or 3 have been detected in nearly all patients with Denys-Drash syndrome. These mutations alter the binding of the WT1 protein to DNA. Abnormal expression of WT1 is associated in some patients with increased PAX2 gene, which encodes a transcription factor normally expressed early during development. Increased expression of PAX2 is associated with podocyte hyperplasia and may be responsible for the glomerular lesion seen in Denys-Drash syndrome. Several patients have incomplete forms of Denys-Drash syndrome (i.e., only two of the three signs of the triad), while others present with antenatal ESRD and Potter phenotype.

Pierson syndrome is an autosomal recessive disorder and is another cause of primary congenital nephrotic syndrome not caused by mutations of either WT1 or genes encoding proteins in the slit diaphragm. It is caused by homozygous or compound heterozygous mutations in the gene encoding laminin beta 2 (LAMB2) on chromosome 3p21 (271). Laminin beta 2 is normally expressed in the glomerular basement membranes and structures of the anterior eye. Patients with Pierson syndrome present with congenital nephrotic syndrome with DMS, ocular abnormalities with microcoria (narrow nonreactive pupils), and enlarged corneas (271).

DMS is also common in Galloway-Mowat syndrome, an autosomal recessive disorder that includes microcephaly, abnormal gyral pattern, developmental delay, and nephrotic syndrome. Renal pathology in this syndrome may show DMS, focal segmental sclerosis, mesangial proliferation, or basement membrane and tubular anomalies. In a consanguineous family with previously affected siblings, prenatal diagnosis may be suggested by demonstration of enlarged hyperechogenic kidneys with amniotic fluid at the upper limit of normal and normal amniotic fluid concentration of AFP. The cause of Galloway-Mowat syndrome is unknown, and genes for a variety of renal proteins have been excluded, including laminin β2, synaptopodin, glomerular epithelial protein 1, and nephrin. Nevertheless, the presence of some of these or other proteins in the kidney and brain suggests that the pathogenesis is related to developmental dysregulation in the formation of both organs.

Isolated diffuse mesangial sclerosis (IDMS) or nonsyndromic DMS is an autosomal recessive disorder presenting with the onset of nephrotic syndrome from a few days of life to 4 years of age. Mutations in PLCE1 gene are the main cause of IDMS and have been detected in 28.6% of families with IDMS. WT1 mutations have been identified in 9% of families with IDMS.

HYPERTENSION

Definition

As discussed earlier, several changes in BP occur normally in the first few weeks of life, making it difficult to define hypertension in neonates. Dionne et al. (194) have compiled available data on neonatal BP, and their summary table of BP values (Table 38.2) includes values for the 95th and 99th percentiles for infants of up to 44 weeks of PMA. Normative BP values for infants between 1 and 12 months of age can be found in the curves published in the Second Task Force report (272) (Fig. 38.12).

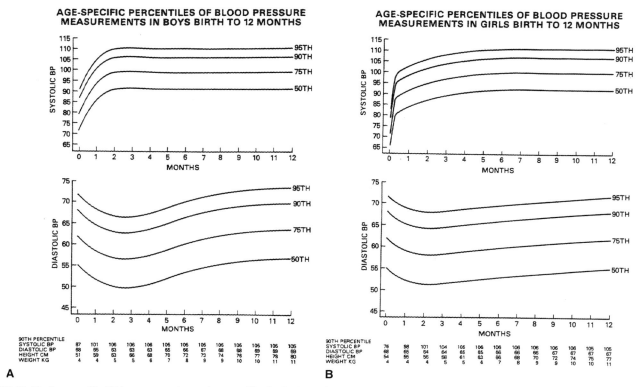

AGE-SPECIFIC PERCENTILES OF BLOOD PRESSURE MEASUREMENTS IN BOYS BIRTH TO 12 MONTHS

AGE-SPECIFIC PERCENTILES OF BLOOD PRESSURE MEASUREMENTS IN GIRLS BIRTH TO 12 MONTHS

FIGURE 38.12 Age-specific BP by sex up to 1 year. Age-specific distributions of systolic and diastolic BP for male **(A)** and female **(B)** infants between birth and 12 months of age. (Reprinted with permission from National Heart, Lung and Blood Institute. Task Force on Blood Pressure Control in Children. Report of the Second Task Force on blood pressure control in children—1987. *Pediatrics* 1987;79:1. Copyright © 1987 by the American Academy of Pediatrics.)

As with older children, the diagnosis of hypertension should not be made based on a single reading. If the infant is critically ill and continuous BP monitoring reveals sustained BP elevation over several hours, then hypertension should be diagnosed, and appropriate investigation and intervention should be initiated (273). For less critically ill infants still in the NICU, a pattern of elevated readings over 1 to 2 days should be sufficient to make the diagnosis of hypertension. For older infants who are being followed as outpatients, at least three elevated readings should be documented over 1 to 2 weeks before a diagnosis of hypertension is made (192).

Incidence

The incidence of diagnosed hypertension in neonates is very low, ranging from 0.2% in healthy newborns to between 0.7% and 2.5% in high-risk newborns (198). One representative study demonstrated a 1.3% prevalence of hypertension requiring treatment among infants admitted to a teaching hospital NICU. Similarly, the incidence of hypertension in the AWAKEN study was 1.8%—although another 3.7% were judged to have "undiagnosed" hypertension based upon post hoc review of BP data (274).

Certain categories of infants are at significantly higher risk, however. For example, hypertension is relatively common in patients with a history of UAC (3%) and those with BPD (as high as 43%) (275–279). Hypertension in neonates has also been associated with AKI, PDA, IVH, and SGA status. On the other hand, hypertension is so uncommon in otherwise healthy term infants that routine BP determination is not recommended (273).

Etiology and Pathophysiology

While numerous conditions may cause hypertension in the neonate or older infant (Table 38.13), the most important categories are renovascular hypertension, renal disease, and BPD.

Renovascular Hypertension

The most common cause of neonatal renovascular hypertension is aortic or renal thromboembolism related to UAC (275–277). Hypertension may develop either while the catheter is in place or long after its removal and may be associated with a history of AKI or hematuria. Hypertension associated with UAC is likely related to thrombus formation at the time of line placement, probably related to disruption of the vascular endothelium of the UA. Such thrombi may then embolize to the kidneys, causing areas of infarction and increased renin release (275–277). A systematic review analyzed 14 randomized clinical trials related to UAC and found high incidence of hypertension secondary to thrombi (276). One study using alternate assignments concluded that hypertension appeared with equal frequency among infants with high or low UAC placement (276). Congenital vascular anomalies responsible for neonatal renovascular hypertension include stenosis or hypoplasia of the renal artery and segmental intimal hyperplasia. All these conditions may involve the aorta and the renal arteries. Other causes of renovascular hypertension include neonatal renal arterial embolism in the absence of UAC, intramural hematoma of the renal artery, renal venous or arterial thrombosis, and external compression of the renal artery by a hydronephrotic kidney, adrenal hemorrhage, and urinoma.

Bronchopulmonary Dysplasia

Many infants with BPD develop hypertension. This phenomenon was first described in the mid-1980s by Abman et al. (278). Another retrospective study on long-term effects of BPD described a frequency of 28.6% of pulmonary hypertension (279). Over half of the infants with BPD who developed hypertension did not display it until after discharge from the NICU, highlighting the need for measurement of BP in NICU "graduates," whether or not they have lung disease. The more severe the BPD, the higher the

TABLE 38.13

Causes of Hypertension in Infancy

Renovascular	*Endocrine*
Thromboembolism	Congenital adrenal hyperplasia
Renal artery stenosis (FMD)	11β-hydroxylase deficiency
Mid-aortic coarctation	17α-hydroxylase deficiency
Renal venous thrombosis	11β-hydroxysteroid dehydrogenase deficiency
Compression of renal artery	Hyperaldosteronism
Abdominal aortic aneurysm	Hyperthyroidism
Idiopathic arterial calcification	*Medications/intoxications*
Congenital rubella syndrome	Infant
Renal parenchymal disease	Dexamethasone/corticosteroids
Congenital	Adrenergic agents
Autosomal dominant PKD	Vitamin D intoxication
Autosomal recessive PKD	Theophylline/aminophylline
Multicystic dysplastic kidney disease	Caffeine
Tuberous sclerosis	Pancuronium
Ureteropelvic junction obstruction	Phenylephrine eye drops
Unilateral renal hypoplasia	Maternal
Primary megaureter	Cocaine
Congenital nephrotic syndrome	Heroin
Acquired	*Neoplasia*
Acute tubular necrosis	Wilms tumor
Cortical necrosis	Mesoblastic nephroma
Interstitial nephritis	Neuroblastoma
Hemolytic–uremic syndrome	Pheochromocytoma
Obstruction (stones, tumors)	*Neurologic*
Pulmonary	Pain
Bronchopulmonary dysplasia	Intracranial hypertension
Pneumothorax	Seizures
Cardiac	Familial dysautonomia
Thoracic aortic coarctation	Subdural hematoma
Genetic	Opiate withdrawal
Single-gene disorders	*Miscellaneous*
Glucocorticoid-remediable aldosteronism	Fluid overload
Liddle syndrome	Total parenteral nutrition
Pseudohypoaldosteronism type II	Closure of abdominal wall defect
(Gordon syndrome)	Adrenal hemorrhage
Malformation syndromes	Hypercalcemia
Williams syndrome	Traction
Turner syndrome	ECMO
Neurofibromatosis	Birth asphyxia
Cockayne syndrome	

ECMO, extracorporeal membrane oxygenation; FMD, fibromuscular dysplasia; PKD, polycystic kidney disease.

likelihood of the development of increased BP. If severe hypertension develops, the risk of CHF and renal failure may outweigh the possible beneficial effects of steroids on the lung disease.

Renal Causes of Hypertension

Hypertension is a common complication of renal anomalies and diseases such as Ask-Upmark kidney (renal segmental hypoplasia), renal hypodysplasia, hydronephrosis, and AKI. It is well known that both autosomal dominant PKD (ADPKD) and ARPKD may present in the newborn period with severe nephromegaly and hypertension. The most severely affected infants with ARPKD are at risk for development of CHF as a result of severe, malignant hypertension. Bilateral nephrectomy may be lifesaving in such infants.

Although much less common than in PKD, hypertension has also been reported in infants with multicystic dysplastic kidneys (280). This is somewhat paradoxical, as such kidneys are usually thought to be nonfunctioning. Hypertension in such patients may be the result of another coexisting abnormality such as parenchymal scarring. Another possible explanation is increased renin production by macrophages within the dysplastic kidney.

Renal obstruction may be accompanied by hypertension, even when there is no compression of the renal artery. This has been seen for example in infants with congenital UPJO and sometimes may persist following surgical correction of the obstruction. Hypertension has also been described in infants with congenital primary megaureter. Ureteral obstruction by other intra-abdominal masses may also be accompanied by hypertension. The mechanism of hypertension in such instances is unclear, although the RAAS has been implicated. Finally, unilateral renal hypoplasia may also present with hypertension, although this is uncommon.

Hypertension from acquired renal parenchymal disease occurs less commonly in the NICU than does that as a result of congenital renal abnormalities. However, severe ATN, interstitial nephritis, or cortical necrosis may be accompanied by significant hypertension, usually because of fluid and sodium overload or hyperreninemia.

Genetic Causes of Hypertension

Genetic forms of hypertension that may present in the neonatal period fall into two broad categories, namely, hypertension resulting from a single-gene disorder and hypertension occurring as one feature of a malformation syndrome. Single-gene disorders affecting sodium transport and causing hypertension with reported cases in infancy include Liddle syndrome (mutation of the epithelial Na+ channel [ENaC]), glucocorticoid-remediable aldosteronism (GRA), and Gordon syndrome (pseudohypoaldosteronism [PHA] type II).

Malformation syndromes that may cause hypertension include Williams syndrome (renal artery stenosis), Turner syndrome (aortic coarctation), neurofibromatosis, and Cockayne syndrome. Usually, the hypertension in these syndromes presents beyond the neonatal period, but infantile presentations with hypertension have been described.

Other Causes of Hypertension

Coarctation of the thoracic aorta (see Chapter 32) has been reported in numerous case series of neonatal hypertension. Although usually easily detected in the newborn period based on decreased pulses and lower BPs in the lower extremities compared to the upper extremities, similarity of upper and lower extremity BP readings in early infancy means that echocardiography is needed for definitive diagnosis. Hypertension may persist or recur in these patients even after surgical repair of the coarctation. Repair early in infancy seems to lead to an improved long-term outcome compared to delayed repair.

Endocrine disorders, particularly congenital adrenal hyperplasia, hyperaldosteronism, and hyperthyroidism, constitute easily recognizable clinical entities that have been reported to cause hypertension in neonates. Several adrenal disturbances can induce hypertension directly; they should be differentiated from Liddle syndrome. A recent case series has implicated phthalate-induced activation of the mineralocorticoid receptor, mediated via inhibition of 11β-HSD2, as a possible explanation for unexplained cases of neonatal hypertension (281). In that study, many infants responded to spironolactone monotherapy, reinforcing the proposed mechanism of BP elevation. Hyperthyroidism is associated with systolic hypertension and sustained tachycardia and, sometimes, with episodes of supraventricular tachycardia.

Tumors, including neuroblastoma, Wilms tumor, and mesoblastic nephroma, may all present in the neonatal period and may produce hypertension, either because of compression of the renal vessels or ureters or because of production of vasoactive substances such as renin or catecholamines.

Neurologic causes of hypertension include intracranial hypertension, drug withdrawal, seizures, pain, and familial dysautonomia. Seizures are common complications of severe hypertension; in turn, BP may increase transiently during seizure episodes. Appropriate pain relief should be given before and after surgical procedures.

Iatrogenic causes of neonatal hypertension such as volume overload are usually obvious but important to consider and correct. If fluid restriction is not possible and severe hypertension with CHF is present, RST should be strongly considered.

If hypertension is induced by a medication, one may consider withholding it, decreasing the dose, or switching to an alternative medication. Dexamethasone may cause BP elevation relatively commonly; if this occurs, a decision must be made regarding the possible benefits of continued steroid treatment versus the risks of hypertension. Hypertension induced by pancuronium probably is mediated by release of catecholamines; BP may normalize after replacing pancuronium with vecuronium.

Hypertension develops in 11% to 92% of neonates receiving ECMO (282) and may result in serious complications, including intracranial hemorrhage and increased mortality. Despite extensive investigation, the exact pathogenesis of this form of hypertension remains poorly understood. Nicardipine infusions are commonly used to treat this form of hypertension.

Hypertension may develop after surgery, for example, after surgical repair of an abdominal wall defect. Hypertension is more frequent and more persistent in patients with omphalocele than in patients with gastroschisis (283). Hypertension appearing after primary closure for bladder exstrophy may be related to traction for skeletal immobilization.

Investigation

The first step in the evaluation is to determine whether the infant is indeed hypertensive or if the BP rises only during periods of agitation, pain, crying, feeding, or performance of procedures. As discussed earlier, only infants with persistent BP elevation should have the "diagnosis" of hypertension made and diagnostic workup initiated.

A relatively focused history should be obtained, paying attention to determining whether there were any pertinent prenatal exposures and to the particulars of the infant's nursery course and any concurrent conditions. The procedures that the infant has undergone (e.g., UAC) should be reviewed, and the medication list scrutinized. Easily identifiable causes of hypertension such as fluid overload or medication-induced hypertension should be identified and corrected.

The physical examination should similarly focus on identifying obvious problems that may be causing the BP elevation. The general appearance of the infant should be assessed, with particular attention paid to the presence of dysmorphic features. Careful cardiac and abdominal examinations should be performed. Table 38.14 lists physical exam findings associated with specific causes of hypertension.

Urinalysis and routine chemistries should be obtained (see Table 38.15). Hyponatremia may occur in renovascular hypertension due to unilateral disease because of increased natriuresis via the other kidney. If hypertension appears to be iatrogenic or secondary to drug withdrawal, specific therapy can be tried before additional investigations are performed. If no cause is evident, or if a renal or renovascular etiology is suspected, the workup usually will include US of the kidneys, adrenals, aorta, and bladder, with a flow study, that is, Doppler US, of the aorta and the renal arteries. An echocardiogram will be needed to confirm the diagnosis of aortic coarctation. Renal scans, angiography, MRI, or CT may be indicated in specific patients.

PRA should be obtained as part of the workup in most hypertensive infants. The PRA is most helpful if extremely low—in such cases, a single-gene disorder affecting renal sodium transport

TABLE 38.14

Physical Exam Findings in Hypertensive Infants

Finding	Probable Cause of Hypertension
Abdominal bruit	Renal artery stenosis
Ambiguous genitalia	Congenital adrenal hyperplasia
Bilateral flank masses	PKD; UPJ obstruction (bilateral); tumor
Bulging anterior fontanelle	Intracranial hemorrhage
Diminished LE pulses	Aortic coarctation
Edema	Fluid overload; congenital nephrotic syndrome
Elfin facies	Williams syndrome (renovascular)
Unilateral flank mass	UPJ obstruction; tumor
Widely spaced nipples; neck folds	Turner syndrome (coarctation)

LE, lower extremity; PKD, polycystic kidney disease; UPJ, ureteropelvic junction.

TABLE 38.15

Diagnostic Studies for Evaluation of Hypertensive Infants

Generally Useful	Useful in Selected Infants
BUN, creatinine	Abdominal/pelvic ultrasound
Calcium	Aldosterone
CBC and platelet count	Aortography
Chest x-ray	Cortisol (morning)
Electrolytes	Echocardiogram
Plasma renin	Nuclear scan (DTPA/MAG-3)
Renal ultrasound with Doppler	Renal angiography
Urinalysis (± culture)	Thyroid studies
	Urine VMA/HVA
	VCUG

BUN, blood urea nitrogen; CBC, complete blood count; DTPA, diethylenetriaminepentaacetic acid; HVA, homovanillic acid; MAG, mercaptoacetyltriglycine; VMA, vanillylmandelic acid; VCUG, voiding cystourethrogram.

should be suspected (see earlier). An elevated PRA is less helpful as it may be secondary to the administration of diuretics or adrenergic medications or to severe respiratory disease; mild elevations of PRA may be seen in normal infants.

Treatment

Treatment of neonatal hypertension should be tailored to the severity of the hypertension and the infant's overall clinical status. For example, critically ill infants with acute onset of severe hypertension should be treated with an intravenous agent administered by continuous infusion, as this will allow the greatest control over the magnitude and rapidity of the BP reduction. These infants should have their BP lowered by no more than 25% of the planned reduction over the first 8 hours to prevent cerebral ischemia (284). On the other hand, relatively well infants with mild hypertension may be treated with oral antihypertensive agents. Recommended doses for intravenous and oral antihypertensive drugs can be found in Tables 38.16 and 38.17.

Nicardipine has emerged as the most useful intravenous medication for management of severe neonatal hypertension. It can be precisely titrated to the desired antihypertensive effect and may be continued for prolonged periods of time without loss of antihypertensive efficacy. Alternative agents that may be given by continuous infusion include esmolol, hydralazine, labetalol, and sodium nitroprusside. Esmolol and labetalol may be contraindicated in infants with lung disease, and nitroprusside can only be used for limited time periods (usually <72 hours) because of the accumulation of thiocyanate (285). Intravenous agents that can be administered by intermittent bolus injection include hydralazine and labetalol. The intravenous ACE inhibitor enalaprilat has been reported to be effective in cases of severe neonatal hypertension; however, our anecdotal experience suggests that this agent may cause sudden, oliguric acute renal failure similar to that reported for oral enalapril, and given this, we do not recommend use of enalaprilat in neonates.

The choice of oral antihypertensive medications is more controversial. Whereas ACE inhibitors are considered the drugs of choice for adults and children with renal forms of hypertension and although there is a long history of their use in neonatal hypertension, many neonatologists and pediatric nephrologists have serious concerns about the potential major side effects such as excessive hypotension, AKI (286), and neurologic abnormalities.

Of the available vasodilators, the calcium channel blockers isradipine and amlodipine have found widespread use. Amlodipine is now commercially available as a suspension; isradipine may be compounded into a stable extemporaneous suspension. Older vasodilating agents such as hydralazine and minoxidil may also be useful in selected infants, or when the newer agents are not available.

Surgery is indicated for treatment of neonatal hypertension in a limited set of circumstances. In particular, hypertension caused by ureteral obstruction or aortic coarctation is best approached surgically. For infants with renal arterial stenosis, it may be necessary to manage the infant medically until it has grown sufficiently to undergo definitive repair of the vascular abnormalities. Infants with hypertension secondary to Wilms tumor or neuroblastoma will require surgical tumor removal, possibly following chemotherapy. Prophylactic removal of multicystic dysplastic kidneys because of the risk of development of hypertension is controversial.

TABLE 38.16

Intravenous Antihypertensive Agents

Drug	Class	Dose	Route	Comments
Diazoxide	Vasodilator (arteriolar)	2–5 mg/kg/dose	RAPID bolus injection	NOT RECOMMENDED
				Slow injection ineffective; duration unpredictable
Enalaprilat	ACE inhibitor	15 ± 5 µg/kg/dose Q8–24h	Bolus injection	NOT RECOMMENDED
				May cause prolonged hypotension and acute renal insufficiency
Esmolol	β-Blocker	Drip: 100–300 µg/kg/min	Continuous infusion	Very short acting; continuous infusion necessary
Hydralazine	Vasodilator (arteriolar)	Bolus: 0.15–0.6 mg/kg/dose Q4h	Bolus or continuous infusion	Tachycardia frequent side effect; must administer Q4h when given IV bolus
		Drip: 0.75–5.0 µg/kg/min		
Labetalol	α- and β-blocker	Bolus: 0.20–1.0 mg/kg/dose	Bolus or continuous infusion	Heart failure, lung disease relative contraindications
		Drip: 0.25–3.0 mg/kg/h		
Nicardipine	Ca²⁺ channel blocker	Drip: 0.5–4 µg/kg/min	Continuous infusion	May cause reflex tachycardia
Sodium nitroprusside	Vasodilator (arteriolar and venous)	Drip: 0.5–10 µg/kg/min	Continuous Infusion	Thiocyanate toxicity can occur with prolonged (>72 h) use or in renal failure

α, Alpha; ACE, angiotensin-converting enzyme; β, beta; Ca²⁺, calcium; IV, intravenous; kg, kilogram; µg, micrograms; mg, milligrams; Q, every.

TABLE 38.17

Oral Antihypertensive Agents

Drug	Class	Initial Dose	Interval	Maximum Dose	Comments
Amlodipine	Ca^{2+} channel blocker	0.06 mg/kg	QD–BID	0.6 mg/kg/d	May have slow/gradual onset of effect
Captopril	ACE inhibitor	0.01 mg/kg/dose	TID	2 mg/kg/d	1st dose may cause rapid drop in BP; monitor SCr and K$^+$
Chlorothiazide	Thiazide diuretic	5 mg/kg/dose	BID	30 mg/kg/d	Monitor electrolytes
Clonidine	Central α agonist	0.05–0.1 mg/kg/dose	BID–TID	Not established	May produce dry mouth and sedation; rebound HTN with abrupt discontinuation
Enalapril	ACE inhibitor	0.08 mg/kg/dose	QD–BID	0.58 mg/kg/d	Monitor SCr and K$^+$
Hydralazine	Vasodilator (arteriolar)	0.25–1.0 mg/kg/dose	TID–QID	7.5 mg/kg/d	Tachycardia and fluid retention common side effects
Hydrochlorothiazide	Thiazide diuretic	1 mg/kg/dose	QD	3 mg/kg/d	Monitor electrolytes
Isradipine	Ca^{2+} channel blocker	0.05 mg/kg/dose	TID-QID	0.8 mg/kg/d	Suspension may be compounded; useful for both acute and chronic HTN
Labetalol	α- and β-blocker	2 mg/kg/dose	BID	20 mg/kg/d	Monitor heart rate; avoid in infants with BPD
Minoxidil	Vasodilator (arteriolar)	0.1–0.2 mg/kg/dose	BID–TID	1 mg/kg/d	Most potent oral vasodilator; excellent for refractory HTN
Propranolol	β-Blocker	0.5–1.0 mg/kg/dose	TID	8–10 mg/kg/d	Monitor heart rate; avoid in infants with BPD
Spironolactone	Aldosterone antagonist	0.5 mg/kg/dose	BID	3.3 mg/kg/d	Potassium "sparing"; monitor electrolytes

α, alpha; ACE, angiotensin-converting enzyme; β, beta; BID, twice daily; BPD, bronchopulmonary dysplasia; Ca^{2+}, calcium; HTN, hypertension; K$^+$, potassium; kg, kilogram; mg, milligrams; QD, once daily; QID, 4 times daily; TID, 3 times daily.

Prognosis

The prognosis of neonatal hypertension depends on etiology, timing of the diagnosis, presence of complications, and response to therapy. Patients in whom hypertension is diagnosed on the basis of neurologic, cardiovascular, or renal decompensation have a high mortality rate. The mortality rate of patients with idiopathic calcification of the arteries or with massive aortic thrombosis remains high despite aggressive therapy. The long-term prognosis for newborn infants with thromboembolism of the renal artery or the aorta is good, often with progressive resolution of the hypertension within a year and only mild-to-moderate decrease in renal function. Hypertension in patients with BPD tends to resolve after 6 months of age. Hypertension in infants with underlying renal disease is likely to persist indefinitely. Infants who undergo repair of aortic coarctation are at risk for persistent or recurrent hypertension.

DIURETIC THERAPY IN NEONATES

The effects of diuretics on water and solute excretion are summarized in Table 38.18. Diuretics, especially furosemide, are commonly administered for CHF, fluid overload, or lung disease in VLBW infants. Small randomized trials have shown short-term benefit on preterm infants with or developing bronchopulmonary dysplasia (287,288).

TABLE 38.18

Effects of Various Types of Diuretics on Urine and Solute Excretion

Type of Diuretic	Site of Major Action	Elimination	FENa (%)	Volume	CH$_2$O	K$^+$	Ca^{2+}	Mg^{2+}	H$_2$PO$_4^-$	Cl	HCO$_3^-$
CA inhibitors	PCT	Secretion	3–6	+	+	+++	0,+	0,+	++	0	+++
Osmotic	Loop	Filtration	>10	+++	+	+	+	+	++	+	+
Loop	TAl > PCT^a	Secretion	15–30	+++	+, −^{b}	++	+++	++	++	+++	+,^{c}
Thiazides	DCT > PCT	Secretion	5–10	++	0	++	−,+^{d}	++	++	+++	+,−^{d}
Metolazone	DCT > PCT	Secretion	4–7	+++	0,−	0	−	+	+	+++	0
Spironolactone	CD	Metabolization	2–3	+	0	−	++	+	+	+	0
Other K-sparing	CD > DCT^e	Variable^f	2–3	+	0	−	−	−	+	+	+

Most of these studies were performed in adults.
^{a}Ethacrynic acid at usual doses does not have any significant effect on proximal tubule reabsorption. Note that ethacrynic acid is not recommended because of its ototoxicity.
^{b}Decreased CH$_2$O during water loading and increased CH$_2$O during dehydration.
^{c}Despite decreased reabsorption of bicarbonate related to the inhibition of carbonic anhydrase, the acute result is a "contraction" alkalosis. Chronic administration results in increased urine acidification in the distal part of the nephron (see text).
^{d}Thiazides may be associated with hypercalciuria after salt loading.
^{e}Amiloride causes mild metabolic acidosis by decreasing Na/H exchange, especially in the DCT.
^{f}Amiloride is not metabolized and acts on the luminal side. Triamterene is hydroxylated in the liver.
+, increase; 0, no change; −, decrease.
CA, carbonic anhydrase; CD, connecting tubule and collecting duct; CH$_2$O, free water clearance; DCT, distal convoluted tubule; FENa, fractional excretion of sodium; loop, thin Henle loop; PCT, proximal convoluted tubule; TAL, thick ascending loop of Henle.
Modified from Chemtob S, Kaplan BS, Sherbotie JR, et al. Pharmacology of diuretics in the newborn. *Pediatr Clin North Am* 1989;36:1231. Copyright © 1989 Elsevier. With permission.

THE NEWBORN INFANT

Loop diuretics are most commonly used because of their rapid and potent activity. Thiazides (or metolazone in case of renal failure) minimize bone calcium loss and may limit NC and nephrolithiasis in the absence of other diuretics or sodium load or replacement. During chronic therapy, the efficacy of a single diuretic decreases progressively, because of compensatory mechanisms that increase sodium reabsorption at other sites of the nephron. Thus, the combination of two diuretics with different sites of action has been suggested. Conflicting results have been reported in observational studies in the 21st century (288,289). Either randomized trials or observational studies with propensity score analysis are needed to assess short-term and long-term effects.

In many patients, fluid restriction should be initiated along with diuretic therapy. However, an effective circulatory volume and a normal BP should be established and maintained before considering diuretic administration. Hyponatremia is a common complication especially when thiazides are initiated without fluid restriction, because they do not impair urinary concentrating ability. Mild hyponatremia does not justify additional sodium intake; the latter may initiate the vicious cycle of diuretic–low serum sodium concentration–increased sodium intake–more hypertension or lung edema–more diuretic. However, potassium and chloride depletion should be prevented by KCl administration (except when using spironolactone). Both hypokalemia and hypochloremic metabolic alkalosis may occur during thiazide or loop diuretic administration, unless the patient has renal failure or appropriate preventive therapy is initiated. Acute thiazide or loop diuretic administration results in a "contraction" alkalosis because of a reduction of the ECF volume and a relatively low bicarbonate concentration in the urine. Metabolic alkalosis results from increased distal urine acidification (caused by hypokalemia, mineralocorticoid excess, and increased delivery of sodium to the distal convoluted tubule, in which protons are secreted in exchange for sodium). Severe metabolic alkalosis is associated with increased mortality. A short course of acetazolamide or arginine chloride (290–292) may be considered for severe metabolic alkalosis in patients with chronic respiratory failure; however, its efficacy remains to be determined.

One trial comparing thiazide with thiazide and spironolactone showed no difference in lung disease or electrolyte balance (293). Spironolactone may cause potassium retention and hyperkalemia and has antiandrogenic effect (294); long-term implication of the latter for neonates is not clear.

BACTERIURIA AND URINARY TRACT INFECTIONS

Bacteriuria in newborn infants can be either asymptomatic or associated with pyelonephritis or sepsis. Similarly, candiduria can be asymptomatic, cause hydronephrosis, or be part of a disseminated infection. Cystitis usually cannot be diagnosed on clinical grounds in newborn infants, except when associated with hematuria.

Frequency in Newborn Infants

The frequency of bacteriuria ranges between 0% and 2.0% in an unselected neonatal population and between 0.6% and 10% in a NICU population (295). UTI is an unusual occurrence during the first 3 days after birth; it typically presents in the 2nd week after birth in term infants and somewhat later in preterm infants. Risk factors for neonatal UTI include prematurity, male gender, and urinary tract anomalies. The higher incidence of neonatal males also appears to occur in preterm infants, although data are limited. Circumcision reduces the risk for UTI in infancy, especially in those with hydronephrosis (295–300). Breast-feeding is associated with a decreased risk for UTI (301).

Pathophysiology

UTIs in neonates usually represent upper tract infections (pyelonephritis) and are often associated with bacteremia. It is not clear whether neonatal UTIs are due to ascending infections with associated bacteremia because of high incidence of the associated urinary tract abnormalities or if they arise from hematogenous spread from a remote source. The same organism is found in urine and bloods in approximately one-third of neonates with UTI and bacteremia, and a substantial proportion also have meningitis (298). The risk of associated bacteremia is also common in preterm infants and decreases with increasing postnatal age.

The risk of UTI depends on bacteriologic factors (see Chapter 47) and host characteristics. The normal defense against UTI includes maintenance of an adequate flow of urine, complete emptying of the bladder, and presence of an anatomic barrier, that is, the bladder outlet. These defense mechanisms may be compromised by urinary tract obstruction, VUR (see Chapter 39), bladder dysfunction (e.g., neurogenic bladder), or manipulation (e.g., prolonged or repeated bladder catheterization). In the case of pyelonephritis, endocytosis of bacteria is performed by inflammatory cells and by proximal tubular cells.

Pathology

Acute pyelonephritis is characterized by the presence of polymorphonuclear leukocytes in the glomeruli, tubules, and interstitium. Some glomeruli are completely destroyed, whereas others are infiltrated with leukocytes and surrounded by fibrin. The tubules are necrotic and dilated, and their lumens are filled with leukocytes and bacteria. Suppuration may develop in the kidney, often with multiple abscesses, and in other parts of the genitourinary tract. Chronic or recurrent pyelonephritis is characterized by infiltration of inflammatory cells, loss or hyalinization of glomeruli, and atrophy of tubules, with obstruction of the lumen with colloid casts. The development of renal scars may not occur until after 1 year of life.

Clinical Presentation

The clinical presentation of UTI in newborn infants is nonspecific and may include one or more of the following signs:

- Growth failure and gastrointestinal symptoms. Failure to thrive, excessive weight loss, poor feeding, diarrhea, and vomiting are the most common clinical features of neonatal UTI.
- Jaundice. Hyperbilirubinemia is commonly the main clinical feature at presentation and may be the only sign of UTI. In neonates, UTI-associated hyperbilirubinemia is indirect and may be associated with hemolytic anemia, whereas in infants after 6 weeks of life, it is often conjugated hyperbilirubinemia and associated with anemia, elevated hepatic aminotransferases, and E. coli infection.
- Temperature instability or fever (temperature ≥38°C). UTI has been reported in 7.5% to 11% of febrile infants presenting to the emergency room during the first 8 to 12 weeks of life.
- Irritability, lethargy.
- Abnormal urination. This includes poor urinary stream, malodorous urine, and polyuria, which may lead to severe dehydration.
- Signs associated with bacteremia (e.g., respiratory distress) or with focal infection (e.g., mucocutaneous candidiasis, omphalitis).
- Hypertension. This may develop as a result of hydronephrosis associated with the UTI.

The clinical manifestations of UTI in preterm infants are similar to those of term infants, with the addition of apnea and hypoxia (301).

Laboratory Features
Urinalysis

Based on specimens obtained by bladder catheterization or suprapubic aspiration, only one-half of febrile outpatients with documented UTI during the first 3 months of life had an abnormal urinalysis. Invasive urine culture must always be performed in an infant in whom UTI is suspected. Microscopic demonstration of yeast cells in urine obtained by suprapubic aspiration or bladder catheterization is very suggestive of candiduria.

Urine Culture

Urine cultures in neonates should be obtained by suprapubic aspiration or by bladder catheterization (Table 38.19). There is no consensus about the magnitude of bacteria required to reach significance, though the commonly used adult threshold of 100,000 colony forming units/ml may be considered to be too high in the newborn. Agents most commonly responsible for neonatal UTI include E. coli and other Gram-negative rods such as Klebsiella, Enterobacter, Citrobacter, Proteus, Providencia, Morganella, Serratia, and Salmonella species. Common Gram-positive organisms causing UTI include Staphylococcus aureus and Enterococcus. The most common organism isolated in the newborn period is E. coli, accounting for up to 80% of infections in most large series. The incidence of early-onset group B Streptococcus infections has decreased as a result of the use of intrapartum antibiotic prophylaxis. Fungal infections, predominantly Candida species, occur more commonly in premature infants in the NICU (299).

Blood Culture

A blood culture should be obtained in all infants in whom a UTI is suspected since, as noted above, approximately one-third of newborns with UTI have an accompanying bacteremia. Approximately 1% of infants with UTI have meningitis; thus, clinicians should have a low threshold for a lumbar puncture, especially in ill-appearing infants or those with high fever (299).

Complications

Acute complications of UTI in newborn infants include bacteremia, abscess formation, VUR, urolithiasis, urinary tract obstruction, severe mineral imbalance, methemoglobinemia, and AKI, which may result from urinary tract obstruction or massive VUR. VUR usually decreases or disappears after treatment and may reappear at the time of recurrent infections. Intraparenchymal reflux is associated with a high risk of renal scarring (see Chapter 39). As many as one-third of infants with mycotic UTIs develop fungus balls, which may obstruct the renal pelvis or the bladder outlet (299). This obstruction may lead to the development of an abdominal mass, systemic hypertension, or anuria.

Pyelonephritis versus Bacteriuria

Pyelonephritis, which presents a high risk for renal scarring, should be differentiated from asymptomatic bacteriuria, which presents a low risk. Clinical and laboratory features suggesting the diagnosis of pyelonephritis include fever, an increase in blood leukocyte count with a left shift, an elevated sedimentation rate, an increase in the serum concentration of C-reactive protein, and renal tubular dysfunction. Unfortunately, none of these tests, alone or in combination, can reliably establish the diagnosis or predict the development of renal scars. Guidelines for the management of febrile UTI in children from the American Academy of Pediatrics (AAP) reaffirmed in 2014 advocate for a more selective and evidenced approach (300). AAP guidelines still recommend renal and bladder US, but in infants 2 to 24 months of age, VCUG should not be performed routinely after the first UTI. Rather, VCUG should be performed if US "reveals hydronephrosis, renal scarring, or other findings that would suggest either high-grade VUR or obstructive uropathy, as well as in other atypical or complex clinical circumstance." However, these guidelines are not applicable to neonates.

Given the high prevalence of associated urinary tract abnormalities, including obstructive anomalies such as UPJO or ureterovesical junction obstruction, and PUVs; malformations such as ectopic ureter; or renal conditions such as polycystic diseases and renal dysplasia, it is suggested to continue to obtain both renal US and VCUG in all neonates after an initial UTI (302). Infants with a BW less than 1,000 g may have a low incidence of underlying urinary tract abnormalities (303).

Imaging for UTI includes US, followed by VCUG or renal cortical scintigraphy (with 99mTc-DMSA), or both. Ultrasonography of the entire urinary tract may detect urinary tract malformations, hyperechogenic areas suggestive of pyelonephritis, and renal pyelectasis or ballooning during voiding, both suggestive of VUR. It has been suggested by some authors that radiographic imaging, particularly renal US, after a UTI in infants may not be useful if prenatal US has excluded the diagnosis of major structural anomalies. Alternatively, if the US is negative, the VCUG may be delayed for approximately 1 month, that is, after resolution of transient, low-grade, UTI-related VUR. Cortical defects observed on DMSA scans performed 1 month after a UTI are associated with pyelonephritis, VUR, and the development of renal scars. Because 99mTc-DMSA binds to the proximal tubules and is excreted only minimally into the urine, it yields excellent visualization of the parenchyma and detection of cortical defects. The presence of areas of decreased cortical uptake of DMSA is a reliable indicator of pathologic inflammatory changes of acute pyelonephritis.

Renal Function

Renal glomerular and tubular function should be assessed at the time of the diagnosis and during treatment and follow-up. Especially in patients with obstructive urinary tract disease, UTI can result in transient or permanent decrease in GFR or in tubular dysfunction, characterized by RTA, PHA, decreased urine concentrating ability, or increased N-acetyl-beta-D-glucosaminidase (NAG) enzymuria.

Treatment

Antibiotics are selected according to urine culture and to local epidemiology and antibiotic stewardship. The dose and interval of administration of the antibiotics may have to be adjusted according to drug levels and to GFR. A repeat urine culture should be obtained during treatment and after completion of the antibiotic therapy. In the case of failure to respond to treatment, US should be repeated, antibiotic therapy may have to be adjusted,

TABLE 38.19
Methods of Diagnosing Bacteriuria/UTI in Newborn Infants

Method	Bacteria/mL	Organism Species	Interpretation
Suprapubic aspiration	Any	One	Positive
Catheterization	1,000–10,000	One	Positive only if pt symptomatic or if dilute urine sample
	1,000–10,000	Two or more	Contaminated
	>10,000	One	Positive
Clean-catch	10,000–100,000	One	Positive only if pt symptomatic or if dilute urine sample
	10,000–100,000	Two or more	Contaminated
	>100,000	One	Positive

and a systemic infection or other foci should be ruled out. Low-dose antibiotic therapy may be indicated after the initial course until the VCUG or the DMSA scan is performed, at least in those patients with abnormal US.

Therapy for asymptomatic bacteriuria in the absence of bacteremia can be given orally after the first few days. It is possible that shorter courses for the treatment of asymptomatic bacteriuria may be adequate, but this has not been evaluated in newborn infants. Surgical intervention may be required for patients with severe VUR and those with urinary tract obstruction (see Chapter 39).

Long-Term Complications and Follow-Up

In patients with pyelonephritis or urinary tract anomalies, GFR, urinary concentrating ability, and tubular acidification should be assessed serially. Additionally, US may demonstrate the formation of urolithiasis. The development of renal failure, once a common complication of UTI in small children, is observed only rarely, except in patients with major urinary tract malformations and renal dysplasia. Infants at risk for chronic renal scarring need long-term follow-up by a nephrologist and a urologist, including repeat urine cultures and sequential isotopic scans, and they should be considered for prophylactic antibiotic therapy.

Prevention

Controversy over the medical benefits, harms, and ethical considerations for nonreligious male circumcision (NRC) is long-standing. Current practice in the United States is guided by the 2012 AAP evidence-based recommendations, which indicated that the health benefits of newborn male circumcision outweigh the risks and that the procedure's benefits justify access to this procedure for families who choose it. Specific benefits identified included prevention of UTIs, penile cancer, and transmission of some sexually transmitted infections, including HIV (296). In contrast in several European countries, NRC prior to the age of informed consent is considered either unethical or harmful.

Infants with neurogenic bladder associated with myelodysplasia often receive intermittent bladder catheterizations and anticholinergic medication. This may result in a lower frequency of long-term deterioration of the radiologic appearance of the kidney, despite a relatively high incidence of bacteriuria–UTI.

Among children 2 to 71 months of age with VUR after UTI, antimicrobial prophylaxis was associated with a substantially reduced risk of recurrence but not of renal scarring (304,305). A meta-analysis of subjects with VUR comparing trials with antibiotics alone or a combined approach with reimplantation surgery/chemoprophylaxis demonstrated a reduction of UTI in the combined approach only up to 2 years of age. Subsequently, the frequency of all forms of UTI was similar in these two groups (305). Prophylactic antibiotics include low-dose amoxicillin or cephalexin as a daily or twice-daily dose up to 6 weeks to 2 months of age and subsequently replaced by cotrimoxazole (1 to 2 mg/kg of trimethoprim component) or nitrofurantoin (1 to 2 mg/kg) given as a single evening dose. Neonatal VUR resolves or improves in a large majority of patients by 4 years without somatic growth restriction or hypertension (76% in low-grade and 59% in high-grade reflux) (306).

▌TUBULAR DYSFUNCTION

This section deals with some of the more common tubular and tubulointerstitial renal disorders that present in the neonatal period or in early childhood, with special emphasis on those disorders where early recognition allows prognostication or treatment that may modify or delay major complications. The reader is referred to other sources for discussion of a wide array of less common disorders that cannot be included here (307,308).

Hypercalciuria, Nephrocalcinosis, and Nephrolithiasis

Normal values of the urinary calcium-to-creatinine ratio in full-term infants are less than 0.86 mg/mg (2.42 mmol/mmol) between 5 days and 7 months (309). NC and nephrolithiasis may occur in infants with hypercalciuria, most often in preterm infants (see next section and Table 38.20). Prenatal development of nephrolithiasis should prompt evaluation of causes of maternal or inherited hypercalcemia. Hypercalciuria may result from hypercalcemia, increased calcium intake or ingestion, decreased tubular reabsorption (see sections on "Renal Tubular Acidosis" and "Salt Wasting Syndromes"), or increased bone calcium reabsorption or uptake. NC and nephrolithiasis also may result from the precipitation of

TABLE 38.20

Mechanisms of Nephrocalcinosis and Nephrolithiasis in Infancy

Hypercalciuria
  Increased calcium intake or absorption with/without hypercalcemia
    Excessive calcium intake (PO or IV)
    Rapid calcium infusion
    Hypervitaminosis D
    Fanconi syndrome if excessive vitamin D administration
    Phosphate depletion, low phosphate intake
    X-linked hypophosphatemia (during phosphate and vitamin D administration)
  Decreased renal tubular reabsorption
    Diuretics (loop diuretics, spironolactone, thiazides if sodium intake or extracellular volume is increased)
    Osmotic diuresis
    Distal renal tubular acidosis (RTA type I)
    Arthrogryposis multiplex congenita with renal and hepatic anomalies
    Bartter syndrome and related syndromes
    Autosomal dominant hypocalcemia
    Dent disease (hypercalciuric nephrolithiasis)[a]
  Increased bone reabsorption or decreased bone uptake
    Primary hyperparathyroidism (including neonatal familial hyperparathyroidism)
    Secondary hyperparathyroidism
    Acidosis
    Chronic corticosteroid therapy
    Hypophosphatasia
    Hyperthyroidism
  Idiopathic hypercalcemia
Other mechanisms
  Factors facilitating precipitation of calcium phosphate/oxalate
    Low urine output
    Alkaline urine
    Absence of inhibitors: citrate, inorganic phosphate, magnesium
    Oxaluria (primary or secondary)
  Other causes of nephrolithiasis
  Cystinosis
  Cystinuria
  Oxaluria (primary or secondary)
  Hyperuricemia
  Classical hereditary xanthinuria
  Adenine phosphoribosyltransferase deficiency (2,8-dihydroxyadenine lithiasis)
  Acyclovir
  Urinary tract infection
  Obstructive urinary tract malformations

[a]Youngest patient described is 1 year old.

calcium phosphate or oxalate in the absence of hypercalciuria (see "Primary Hyperoxaluria" [PH]).

Noncalcium substrate depositions can mimic the appearance of NC or result in nephrolithiasis. Such substrates include cystine, uric acid, xanthine, 2,8-dihydroxyadenine (see below), acyclovir, or melamine (310); an appearance of NC can also occur with UTI or may occur in association with UTI or with obstructive urinary tract malformations.

NC may be associated with or cause decreased renal tubular function, whereas nephrolithiasis may cause hematuria, colic, dysuria, UTI, obstruction, AKI, or CKD/ESRD.

Nephrocalcinosis in Preterm Infants

NC or nephrolithiasis, detected by US in up to 40% of preterm infants, occurs predominantly as a result of hypercalciuria, which itself is the aggregate result of a variety of intrinsic and external factors (310). Intrinsic risk factors for NC in preterm infants include lower BW and greater urinary Na losses, and possibly lower renal function as well (311). Clinical risk factors include the use of TPN, high Ca or low phosphorus intake, acidosis, and use of glucocorticoids and loop diuretics or spironolactone, as described below.

Hypercalciuria results from increased calcium intake or gastrointestinal absorption, decreased renal tubular calcium reabsorption, and abnormal regulation of bone mineral content (Table 38.20). Chronic use of intermittent calcium infusions is associated with recurrent periods of hypercalcemia and hypercalciuria, so continuous infusion is preferable. Intake of calcium and phosphorus should be individualized to serial serum levels and adjusted according to urine levels in patients with NC. High enteral calcium intake may be associated with hypercalciuria even in the absence of hypercalcemia. Insufficient phosphate intake may result in hypophosphatemia, hypercalcemia, hypercalciuria, and osteopenia of prematurity. Other risk factors for NC in preterm infants include furosemide, dexamethasone, methylxanthines, duration of mechanical ventilation, and acidemia. If diuretic therapy is required for extra renal disease (e.g., BPD), a thiazide or metolazone is preferable because it reduces calciuria (in the absence of other diuretics and of sodium supplementation). The effect of thiazides on established NC in preterm infants has not been assessed; however, in patients with X-linked hypophosphatemia (XLH), thiazide administration prevents its progression.

NC appears to resolve spontaneously in most cases, with a small percent of cases having persistent findings after 1 to 2 years of age; follow-up of renal function and growth is prudent (312). Long-term sequelae may be subtle and include RTA and a mild concentrating defect. Urolithiasis is quite uncommon.

Rarer disorders causing nephrolithiasis and urolithiasis, such as primary hyperoxaluria, cystinuria, xanthinuria, Lesch-Nyhan syndrome, adenine phosphoribosyltransferase deficiency, phosphoribosyl pyrophosphate synthetase superactivity, hereditary renal hypouricemia, and uromodulin-associated kidney diseases, are discussed in the online version of this book.

Fanconi Syndrome

Fanconi syndrome is defined by generalized dysfunction of the proximal tubule. The cardinal signs are glucosuria, hyperphosphaturia, and generalized (nonspecific) aminoaciduria. Other features, present inconsistently, include proximal RTA (pRTA); tubular proteinuria; increased urinary excretion of urate, sodium, potassium, and calcium; and decreased ability to concentrate the urine. The massive load of filtrate normally reabsorbed by the proximal tubule can lead to significant whole-body deficiencies when function is reduced even by fractions of a percent.

The clinical presentation of Fanconi syndrome includes normoglycemic glucosuria, polyuria, polydipsia, dehydration, and failure to thrive. Loss of phosphate may lead to rickets and other widespread bone disease. Loss of bicarbonate may lead to profound acidemia. Loss of potassium may be severe. Sodium, chloride, and bulk fluid losses may be profound and lead to chronic dehydration and failure to thrive. Serum amino acids and carnitine levels may be very low, and the sum effect of the loss of these micronutrients is often severe.

Prognosis depends on the underlying disorder. Treatment includes replacement, to the extent possible, of lost filtrate. Administration of sodium citrate or bicarbonate and, as required, water, potassium, phosphate, and carnitine may be required. Once rickets has developed, careful administration of vitamin D is required; excess vitamin D may result in hypercalciuria and NC. Indomethacin is used selectively in some patients.

Primary Fanconi Syndrome

It is extremely rare and usually sporadic, although autosomal recessive, autosomal dominant, and X-linked recessive transmission has been described. The genetic if not molecular origin of an autosomal dominant cause was elucidated in 2001 on chromosome 15q 15.3. The molecular basis of another form of inherited Fanconi syndrome has also been isolated. This defect disrupts mitochondrial metabolism in the proximal tubule and highlights the importance of energy metabolism to maintain tubular function; the specific dependence of proximal tubular cells on fatty acid metabolism and mitochondrial function is an important detail that informs the mechanism of many secondary causes (313,314).

Secondary Causes of Tubulointerstitial Disease and Fanconi Syndrome

Only some causes can be highlighted here (Table 38.21). Individually rare, but more common when considered as a group, is Fanconi syndrome secondary to metabolic defects that result directly or indirectly in impaired energy metabolism, such as mitochondrial cytopathies (see Chapter 55) (314–316). Another common mechanism of secondary Fanconi syndrome is damage to the proximal tubule due to storage diseases (cystinosis, glycogen storage diseases [GSD], Wilson disease). Other causes include tyrosinemia, multiple medications, heavy metal toxicity, or a variety of infections (317). Finally, a third type of mechanism involves diseases that cause cellular damage and dysfunction of renal tubules; examples include Lowe syndrome, Dent disease, various medications (e.g., platinum-containing chemotherapy, valproate, aminoglycosides, aspirin), heavy metal toxicity, or a variety of infections. Tubulointerstitial disease may manifest as the complete Fanconi syndrome or, more frequently, an incomplete set of dysfunctional tubular function. Approaches to treatment of these conditions are generally symptomatic, but in some cases, there may be specific metabolic interventions. For example, specific therapy for fructose intolerance, galactosemia, or tyrosinemia results in disappearance of the Fanconi syndrome. In many other diseases, treatment is much less effective.

Tubulointerstitial Disease and Fanconi Syndrome Related to Disorders of Energy Metabolism

The proximal tubule requires large energy consumption for normal function and is therefore sensitive to defects in energy metabolism. In addition to the renal manifestations, these disorders have a wide but often severe range of clinical presentation, including multiorgan dysfunction, lactic acidosis, hematologic disturbances such as pancytopenia, growth failure, liver failure, pancreatic insufficiency, myopathy, cardiomyopathy, and neurologic disturbances. A more detailed discussion of such disorders is found in Chapter 55. Often, the renal component may initially be relatively minor, even overlooked, only to be noticed as the renal phenotype worsens. Mitochondrial disease may be caused by defects in nuclear or mitochondrial genes, the latter of which is characterized by maternal inheritance (318). Secondary mitochondrial dysfunction may occur in diseases such as methylmalonic acidemia.

TABLE 38.21

Causes of Fanconi Syndrome in Infancy

Idiopathic	Secondary	
	Inherited disease of the metabolism (AR unless specified)	Acquired
Isolated	GRACILE syndrome	Renovascular accident in neonatal period
ARC syndrome (AR)	Cystinosis	Interstitial nephritis
	Fructose-1-phosphate aldolase deficiency	Medications: valproate, aminoglycosides, ifosfamide[a]
	Hepatorenal tyrosinemia type 1	
	Galactosemia	Renal transplantation
	Glycogenosis with Fanconi S (Fanconi-Bickel S)	Toluene, heavy metal poisoning
	Oculocerebrorenal (Lowe) syndrome (X-linked)	Vitamin D–deficiency rickets
	Vitamin D–dependent rickets	Dysproteinemia
	Disorders of the energy metabolism	Nephrotic syndrome
	Pearson syndrome (maternofetal transmission)	
	Cytochrome-c oxidase deficiency	
	Pyruvate carboxylase deficiency	
	Carnitine palmitoyltransferase I deficiency	

[a]Fanconi syndrome also has been reported after administration of other medications in older patients.
S, syndrome; AR, autosomal recessive; ARC, arthrogryposis, renal tubular dysfunction, and cholestasis.

Renal involvement most often consists of Fanconi syndrome, although some patients develop RTA, Bartter-like disease, chronic tubulointerstitial nephritis, nephrotic syndrome, or renal failure. Pathology may show cytoplasmic vacuolization of tubular cells and giant mitochondria.

Hereditary Fructose Intolerance

Hereditary fructose intolerance (HFI) is an autosomal recessive disorder resulting from deficiency in fructose-1-phosphate aldolase (aldolase B) (see Chapter 55) (319). Following ingestion of fructose, phosphate is "trapped" leading to ATP depletion. While this mechanism fits within the paradigm of impaired energy metabolism already described, this condition is singled out in this discussion as a one that is highly treatable (through fructose avoidance). While fructose is not part of a neonatal diet, sucrose is sometimes used for comfort during neonatal procedures. Typically, the diagnosis is strongly suggested by sudden onset of major systemic symptoms in an infant following first sucrose or fructose ingestion. Similarly, tubular dysfunction can be acute and short-lived, with hypoglycemia, hypophosphatemia, generalized hyperaminoaciduria, RTA, proteinuria, and phosphaturia, and transient fructosuria or glucosuria following an isolated ingestion of fructose (319). Removal of fructose and sucrose from the diet results in normalization of tubular function within 2 weeks.

Growth Restriction, Aminoaciduria, Cholestasis, Iron Overload, Lactic Acidosis, and Early Death Syndrome

Another example of a defect in energy metabolism leading to tubulopathy is the growth restriction, aminoaciduria, cholestasis, iron overload, lactic acidosis, and early death (GRACILE) syndrome, an autosomal recessive mutation in the *BCS1L* gene leading to reduced mitochondrial function (Complex III). Although somewhat heterogeneous, the disease is typically severe and characterized by fetal growth restriction, lactic acidosis, generalized aminoaciduria, cholestasis, and iron overload (320).

Storage Disorders Leading to Tubulointerstitial Kidney Disease

A large variety of rare disorders result in cellular or tissue deposition of abnormal metabolic products in the kidneys that can result in tubulointerstitial disease. A rare disease, cystinosis is considered the most common cause of Fanconi syndrome in children (320). Tyrosinemia, galactosemia, and other conditions are also well-known causes presenting in infants; Wilson disease presents

at an older age. A complete discussion is not possible, but clinicians should be alert to renal tubular dysfunction in the setting of many storage diseases.

Further causes of tubular damage such as nephropathic cystinosis, tyrosinemia, Fanconi-Bickel syndrome, and galactosemia are discussed in chapter 55.

Diseases Associated with Damage and Dysfunction of Tubular Cells

Lowe Syndrome

Oculocerebrorenal (OCRL) syndrome of Lowe is a rare X-linked disorder caused by mutations of the *OCRL1* gene (321). Deficiency in the *OCRL1* gene product, a phosphatidylinositol 4,5-bisphosphate (PIP2)-5-phosphatase, appears to affect membrane trafficking or function of the actin cytoskeleton. Of note, some subjects with a clinical diagnosis of Dent disease are also found to have mutation of *OCRL1*.

The phenotype includes major abnormalities in the eyes (including cataracts), nervous system (mental retardation), and kidneys (tubulopathy). Glomerular involvement develops progressively in childhood and eventually leads to renal failure in the second to fourth decade.

Although historically Lowe syndrome is held as an example of Fanconi syndrome, in fact the tubular dysfunction is selective, not generalized. There is universal elevation of low molecular weight protein in the urine, and most patients have generalized (modest) aminoaciduria. However, only half have RTA or NC, glucosuria is rare if seen at all, and urinary phosphate excretion is normal in most.

Treatment of the renal manifestations of Lowe syndrome address the individual's needs and may include alkali, carnitine supplementation, and, if needed, phosphate, potassium, or calcium. Some individuals require no specific treatment.

Autosomal Recessive Polycystic Kidney Disease and Nephronophthisis

ARPKD and juvenile nephronophthisis (NPH) present features of tubulointerstitial diseases that merit brief discussion here.

Histologically, the renal lesion of ARPKD involves fusiform dilatation of collecting tubules. While the more dramatic clinical manifestations may dominate the presentation, some patients present only with enlarged kidneys or hypertension and a quarter of patients demonstrate hyponatremia, presumably the result of tubular dysfunction. Particularly in infants and young children, polyuria and impaired urinary concentration are also often present, but other signs of tubular disease such as tubular proteinuria and aminoaciduria are typically absent (322).

NPH is a group of autosomal recessive disorders that manifest tubulointerstitial fibrosis and medullary cystic kidney disease and progress to ESRD (323). As other cystic kidney diseases, it is classified as a ciliopathy. Massive solute losses typical of Fanconi syndrome are largely absent, but patients manifest polyuria, polydipsia, and some degree of salt wasting and are at risk of dehydration. Often, children have significant CKD or ESRD when they are diagnosed. Low molecular weight proteinuria, aminoaciduria, and other markers of tubular disease are encountered out of proportion to the degree of reduced GFR (323,324). Associations with eye disorders (retinitis pigmentosa, congenital nystagmus, Leber amaurosis) as well as several syndromes (e.g., Meckel-Gruber) are well described.

Twelve neonates born to consanguineous parents from the Old Order Amish community with lethal nephronophthisis-3 have been described (325). Most patients presented with oligohydramnios, prematurity, cystic kidneys, low-set ears, small lungs with respiratory insufficiency, and cardiac anomalies. Occasional features included single lung, situs inversus, and absent bladder.

Arthrogryposis, Renal Tubular Dysfunction, and Cholestasis Syndrome

Autosomal recessive defects in *VPS33B* are the predominant cause of arthrogryposis, renal tubular dysfunction, and cholestasis (ARC) syndrome (326). VPS33B is involved in regulation of cell polarity, and its importance is corroborated by the fact that ARC also results from mutation in *VIPER* coding a product in the same regulatory pathway. Renal tubular dysfunction ranges from isolated RTA to complete Fanconi syndrome, and hepatic histology shows various combinations of cholestasis, intrahepatic biliary hypoplasia, giant cell hepatitis, lipofuscin deposition, and fibrosis. Platelet dysfunction carries a high risk of bleeding such that genetic diagnosis allows safer identification than does organ biopsy. Infants often suffer failure to thrive; a subset has dysgenesis of the corpus callosum or cardiac defects. Arthrogryposis results at least in part due to fetal position and oligohydramnios as well as neurogenic muscular atrophy.

DISEASES ASSOCIATED WITH SPECIFIC TUBULAR TRANSPORTERS AND CHANNELS

Nephrogenic Diabetes Insipidus

NDI is a rare inherited disease characterized by failure or incomplete renal response to AVP (327). The most common form of congenital NDI is an X-linked trait; is a result of mutations of *AVPR2*, which codes for the basolateral vasopressin V2R in the collecting duct; and accounts for approximately 90% of cases. Congenital NDI may also result from mutations in AQP2, coding for the apical aquaporin-2 water channels responsible for allowing ADH-dependent reabsorption of water in the CCD. Most cases with AQP2 mutation have autosomal recessive inheritance, though autosomal dominant inheritance is also documented.

Because infants do not have independent access to water despite polyuria, hypertonic dehydration results, with other symptoms frequently including unexplained fever, constipation, and failure to thrive. Pertinent laboratory findings include a persistently low urine osmolality, even during hypernatremic dehydration, without other tubular dysfunction. Severe episodes of dehydration with hypertonic encephalopathy can result in long-term neurologic problems and mental retardation. However, with preventative measures, most children with NDI are cognitively normal.

The differential diagnosis of NDI includes several entities causing polyuria (Table 38.22). In addition to molecular genetic analysis of *AVPR2* and *AQP2*, the diagnosis of NDI is confirmed by failure to concentrate the urine in response to administration of DDAVP, in contrast to patients with central diabetes insipidus, that is, ADH deficiency, who will respond. While primary extrarenal clinical manifestations are not known, V2R is distributed throughout the body, and differences, for example, in fibrinolytic responses can be demonstrated in male patients with AVPR2 versus AQP2 mutations or versus children without NDI at all (328). Female carriers of the X-linked NDI may have mild impairment of urine-concentrating ability with accompanying degrees of modest polyuria and polydipsia; however, these girls are quite unlikely to manifest clinical problems.

Therapy rests on three major strategies. These include increased water intake, decreased nonessential solute intake, and use of distal diuretics. The primary need is to provide sufficient water to support the profound defect in urinary concentrating ability. In many cases, the defect is so profound that overnight fluid therapy remains a requirement throughout early childhood to avoid significant dehydration. Older children and adults with congenital NDI often are found to have diminishing severity of the concentrating defect. However, during infancy and early childhood, the majority of children demonstrate failure to thrive and require feeding tubes to permit sufficient caloric and fluid intake to promote normal growth.

The effect of close attention to the renal solute load on polyuria must not be ignored. Even while increasing caloric intake, the multiplier effect of nonessential solutes on urinary volume must be considered. Renal solutes are derived principally from dietary NaCl and protein, while carbohydrates and fats have no renal residual (329). Excess solutes must be avoided because, for example, every

TABLE 38.22

Etiology of Nephrogenic Defect in Urinary Concentration

	Decreased Effect of Antidiuretic Hormone on Tubular Permeability to Water	Decreased Corticomedullary Concentration Gradient
Congenital	Nephrogenic diabetes insipidus	Medullary cystic disease, polycystic kidney disease
	Hypokalemia	Bilateral dysplastic kidneys
	Bartter syndrome and related syndromes	Urinary tract obstruction
	Pseudohypoaldosteronism	
	Proximal renal tubular acidosis	
	Duplication of the mitochondrial genome	
Acquired	Drug: PGE_2, PGE_1, amphotericin, lithium	Polyuria: water/osmotic diuresis
	Hypokalemia	Obstructive disease (before and after treatment)
	Hypercalcemia	Chronic/acute renal failure
		Pyelonephritis
		Nephrocalcinosis
		Medullary necrosis
		Malnutrition

PG, prostaglandin.

nonessential mOsm for an infant with a maximal urinary concentrating capacity of 80 mOsm/L will result in 5 to 10 times the obligatory urine output of an infant with normal concentrating capacity (approximately 500 mOsm/L in infants up to a few weeks old and 1,000 mOsm/L or more in infants older than 6 months). Thus, low-solute infant formulas suitable for CKD should be used, and reduction in sodium and protein intake in older children taking solids is required.

Finally, pharmaceutical treatment with thiazide diuretics, amiloride, and indomethacin is frequently required. Careful balance of kaliuresis and potassium retention is required; potassium supplements may be required. The mechanism of the distal diuretics is not entirely clear but likely involves secondary renal adaptation and altered expression of a variety of transporters throughout the nephron (330).

SALT WASTING SYNDROMES

Bartter Syndrome

Bartter syndrome results from one of several specific autosomal recessive defects in tubular transporters leading to polyuria and salt wasting. It results in hypokalemic metabolic alkalosis, hyperreninemic hyperaldosteronism with low normal BP, hyperplasia of the juxtaglomerular apparatus, and impaired urinary concentrating ability (331). Depending on the specific transporter defect and its role in normal renal function, patients may present prenatally (polyhydramnios), as neonates or during early infancy, later in childhood, and in rare circumstances, even later. An earlier name for this syndrome was "hyperprostaglandin E syndrome" due to the extreme, but secondary, PGE production.

Antenatal or neonatal Bartter syndrome is usually due to type I (SLC12A1, the Na-K-2Cl cotransport) or type II (KCNJ1 or ROMK channel) disease. Type III (CLCNKB, a basolateral chloride channel) and type IV (BSND, barttin, a requisite subunit of basolateral chloride channels) round out the disease types; the latter is associated with sensorineural hearing loss. A similar condition is due to a mutation in the *CaSR* causing autosomal dominant hypocalcemia with Bartter-like syndrome.

Antenatal manifestations lead to polyhydramnios and can precipitate preterm birth. Infantile Bartter syndrome can cause life-threatening volume depletion, hyponatremia, profound hypokalemic alkalosis, and renal failure. Infants often experience hypercalciuria/NC and may develop hypomagnesemia as well. A transient, unique, and counterintuitive feature of neonatal type II Bartter syndrome is hyperkalemia, which occurs in neonates up to 1 to 2 months of age because ROMK is the most important route of K secretion and due to immaturity; neonates have decreased flow-dependent K secretion to offset the loss of ROMK function (see "Developmental Physiology" section).

Treatment of Bartter syndrome is centered on replacement of Na, K, water, and, when necessary, magnesium. Many infants require feeding tubes to allow sufficient volume to be given. NSAID therapy, classically indomethacin but also with more specific inhibitors of COX-2, is effective in reducing urinary volume by counteracting secondary mechanisms resulting from the primary defect. A feared potential side effect of NSAIDs is gastrointestinal hemorrhage.

Renal Tubular Acidosis

The most general description of RTA is acidosis resulting from inadequate renal acidification or from renal bicarbonate wasting (332–337). RTA should be suspected based on a low anion gap metabolic acidosis with a low plasma bicarbonate (HCO_3^-) concentration for age, in the absence of diarrhea or cystine chloride supplementation in TPN. The differential diagnosis of decreased plasma bicarbonate includes respiratory alkalosis, with neonatal causes including CNS disease, hyperammonemia, and iatrogenic hyperventilation. Blood gas analysis is required to correctly classify acid–base disorders.

The diagnosis and classification of RTA have traditionally been made on the basis of functional studies. Four types of RTA have been described: classic distal, that is, type I; pRTA, that is, type II; hyperkalemic distal, that is, type IV, which is the most common type of RTA; and mixed proximal and distal, that is, type III (Table 38.23). Application of molecular biology techniques has opened a new perspective to understanding the pathophysiology of inherited cases of RTA. Clinical presentations of RTA may include failure to thrive, respiratory effort, vomiting, or serum biochemical disturbances. Correction of acidosis often results in catch-up growth and resolution of symptoms.

Diagnostic Evaluation

Diagnosis of RTA requires considering whether a patient is in a steady state or transient state—for example, during illness or in the midst of treatments that could alter the results of diagnostic testing. General considerations are uncovering competing causes of metabolic acidosis, measurement of BP, general renal function, and whether NC, UTI, or urinary tract malformations are present. Specific diagnosis of RTA centers on determining whether there is decreased ability to acidify the urine or whether a defect in bicarbonate reabsorption is present. Diagnostic tests and maneuvers include measurement of the urinary anion gap as a surrogate measure of renal ammonium excretion, urine–blood pCO_2 differential, tubular reabsorption of bicarbonate and phosphorus, urine citrate and calcium, or rarely, acid loading tests (337).

Proximal Renal Tubular Acidosis

pRTA or RTA type II is characterized by hyperchloremic metabolic acidosis as a result of impaired capacity of proximal tubule to reabsorb HCO_3 (332,334,336,337). While isolated pRTA is extremely rare, one inherited form results from loss of function of a Na^+/HCO_3^- cotransporter, reducing reabsorption. Most pRTA occurs as a manifestation of a generalized proximal tubular dysfunction (Fanconi syndrome), together with distal RTA (dRTA), that is, type III RTA.

Often described as threshold-dependent RTA, pRTA recapitulates the normal physiologic state, in which bicarbonate is not reabsorbed when its concentration exceeds the normal level. With pRTA, the threshold is lower than normal. Thus, just as in the normal state, urinary pH may vary depending on diet. The diagnosis of pRTA is suspected when the serum bicarbonate concentration is low for age and attributable to acidosis; the urinary pH may be "normal" but is inappropriately high (i.e., not low enough to demonstrate normal bicarbonate retention in the acidemic state). The diagnosis is confirmed either by the presence of a Fanconi syndrome or by measuring the urinary concentration of bicarbonate at various serum levels during a bicarbonate infusion. Alternatively, the serum bicarbonate can be raised to normal by administration of bicarbonate or citrate supplement, with subsequent observation of the serum bicarbonate level at which the urine becomes acid.

Treatment consists of the administration of sodium bicarbonate or citrate (typically 5 to 10 mEq/kg/d) and potassium citrate. In some patients, acidosis will persist despite administration of high doses of alkali; hydrochlorothiazide or occasionally an NSAID may be beneficial.

Distal Renal Tubular Acidosis

dRTA is defined by limited ability to acidify the urine due to defects in the distal nephron and is suspected when urinary pH fails to fall below 5.5 during metabolic acidosis (333,335). In contrast to pRTA, dRTA is almost always observed in children as a primary entity, which may be inherited as either a recessive or dominant form. Autosomal dominant dRTA has been associated with mutations in the *SLC4A1* gene encoding the Cl/HCO_3^- exchanger AEI. Most patients with autosomal recessive dRTA and nerve deafness have mutations in the *ATP6B1* gene encoding the B-1 subunit of H^+-ATPase. Autosomal recessive dRTA without deafness may result from mutations of the *ATP6VOA4* gene encoding the A-4 subunit of the H^+-ATPase (335).

Several diagnostic tests are of potential utility to diagnose dRTA. Normal distal acidification requires adequate ammonium (NH_4^+) excretion during acidosis. While ammonium can be measured, it is usually approximated by the urinary anion gap or urine net charge (urine Na+-K-Cl). If one's kidneys are responding appropriately to an acidosis, the excretion of cations, mainly in the form of (unmeasured) ammonium, in the urine is increased. This is accompanied by increased urinary excretion of chloride, leading to a negative urine anion gap unless RTA is present. However, neonates have large amounts of unmeasured urinary anions, so this method is unreliable in this age group (338). In an alkalinized state (i.e., following treatment for acidemia to a slightly elevated serum bicarbonate), the urine-minus-blood CO_2 partial pressures (U-B pCO_2) is a good indicator of distal tubular H+ secretion because secreted H+ combines with nonreabsorbed bicarbonate to produce CO_2. This can be measured by obtaining arterial blood and urine gases, which can be run in the same commercial machine.

In classic or type I RTA, there is no defect of potassium secretion, but NC and nephrolithiasis are common. The development of NC is attributed to the association of hypercalciuria, high urine pH, and hypocitraturia. The treatment includes the administration of sodium bicarbonate or citrate and potassium citrate. Administration of citrate is important for the prevention of nephrolithiasis. In general, the dose of alkali is lower than that required for pRTA, in the range of 2 to 4 mEq/kg/d.

Hyperkalemic Distal RTA

Hyperkalemic dRTA or type IV is the most common type of dRTA. It results from the association of defects in K+ and H+ secretion at the level of the collecting duct. Primary type IV RTA results from recessive mutation in the amiloride-sensitive ENaC found in principal cells of the distal nephron. Secondary cases of type IV RTA are more frequent and can be due to hypoaldosteronism or PHA (type I; or type II or Gordon syndrome, see below). Functionally, type IV RTA is also common in patients with obstructive uropathy as part of generalized distal tubular failure. Treatment of type IV RTA includes alkali therapy, limitation of potassium intake, and use of potassium-binding resins. Acquired causes of hyperkalemic RTA include ACE inhibitors and aldosterone receptor antagonists.

Mixed Renal Tubular Acidosis

In some disorders, both proximal and dRTA is present; this is known as mixed RTA or type III (see Table 38.23). VLBW infants during the first days or weeks of life have a mild degree of mixed tubular acidosis, with lower normal values of serum bicarbonate concentration and higher urine pH despite metabolic acidosis (see "Developmental Physiology"). Patients with carbonic anhydrase II deficiency exhibit autosomal recessive mixed RTA and develop osteopetrosis, growth restriction, mental retardation, and cerebral calcifications; such patients may require bone marrow transplantation in addition to alkali therapy.

TABLE 38.23

Etiology of Renal Tubular Acidosis in Infancy

Proximal RTA (Type 2)	Hyperkalemic RTA (Type 4)	Distal RTA (Type 1)	Mixed (Type 3)
Primary	Early childhood hyperkalemic RTA	With bicarbonate wasting in infancy and early childhood	Familial hyperparathyroidism with hypercalciuria and RTA (Nishiyama) VLBW infant
AR, AD sporadic transient		Sporadic	
		With cystic fibrosis	
Secondary			
Fanconi syndrome	1: Primary hypoaldosteronism, adrenal insufficiency	Hypergammaglobulinemia (i.e., maternal Sjögren syndrome)	Carbonic anhydrase II deficiency (with osteopetrosis) (AR)
Metachromatic leukodystrophy[a]			
Mitochondrial diseases	2–3: Hyporeninemic hypoaldosteronism[b] with chronic renal disease	Fetal alcohol syndrome	Hyperparathyroidism
		Toluene, amphotericin B, lithium	Nephrocalcinosis and Fanconi syndrome
Hereditary nephritis	4: Pseudohypoaldosteronism-1 with or without salt wasting	Hypercalcemic hyperthyroidism	Renal transplantation
Tetralogy of Fallot[a]	5: Partial unresponsiveness to aldosterone	Vitamin D intoxication	
Vitamin D deficiency	Tubulointerstitial disease	Nephrocalcinosis	
Vascular accident in	Urinary tract obstruction, UTI	Medullary sponge kidney	
NN period	Unilateral dysplastic kidney or RVT	Urinary tract obstruction	
Hereditary nephritis	Drugs (e.g., KCl, K-sparing diuretics, heparin, ACE inhibitors, PGSI, cyclosporine)	Carnitine palmitoyltransferase type I deficiency (1)	
Carbonic anhydrase inhibition	Toxins	Carbonic anhydrase II deficiency with osteopetrosis (AR)	
Carbonic anhydrase II deficiency with osteopetrosis (AR)		AR with sensorineural deafness: deficiency in B1 subunit of H+-ATPase	
Drugs and toxins: valproic acids, heavy metals		AR without sensorineural deafness: deficiency in A-4 subunit of H+-ATPase	
Deficiency in NBC-1 (pRTA with glaucoma)		AD: mutation of SLC4A1 gene: deficiency in Cl−/HCO$_3$− exchanger AE1	

Renal tubular acidification also may be deficient in the case of renal failure (i.e., normochloremic metabolic acidosis) or of acute diarrhea (hypochloremic metabolic acidosis) (see text).

[a]The only patients with this type of RTA were diagnosed after 12 months of age.

[b]Types 2 and 3, associated with hyporeninemic hypoaldosteronism, are seen mostly in adults.

ACE, angiotensin-converting enzyme; AD, autosomal dominant; AR, autosomal recessive; H+-ATPase, proton pump (ATPase); NBC-1, Na-HCO$_3$ cotransport NN, neonatal; PGSI, prostaglandin synthetase inhibitor; pRTA, proximal renal tubular acidosis; RTA, renal tabular acidosis; RVT, renal venous thrombosis; UTI, urinary tract infection; VLBW, very low birth weight.

Pseudohypoaldosteronism Type 1

PHA-1 consists of unresponsiveness of the collecting duct to mineralocorticoids (339). Autosomal dominant and recessive forms of PHA exist; both are characterized by severe neonatal salt wasting, hyperkalemia, and metabolic acidosis, manifesting as polyuria, dehydration, vomiting, and failure to thrive. More devastating presentations with hyperkalemic cardiac arrest or cardiovascular collapse may occur. Upon further investigation, patients may be found to have hypercalciuria and NC.

Types of PHA-1

Autosomal recessive PHA-1 results from a mutation of either one of the three subunits (α, β, γ) of ENaC. Because ENaC is present in many epithelia, this type of PHA-1 also causes respiratory symptoms (impaired mucociliary clearance), eczema or skin lesions (sweat glands), and possibly other subclinical alterations in secretory function. Autosomal dominant PHA-1, caused by loss-of-function mutations in the mineralocorticoid receptor gene (MLR), is milder than recessive PHA-1; its manifestations are limited to the kidney, and frequently, it clinically resolves over time. The core treatment of PHA-1 consists of administering large amounts of sodium chloride and limiting potassium intake. Potassium-binding resin is frequently utilized.

PHA-II or Gordon syndrome is an autosomal dominant cause of low-renin, low-aldosterone hypertension with hyperkalemia and mild metabolic acidosis. Clinical response to thiazide diuretics is usually good. Gordon syndrome results from mutations in WNK1 and WNK4, which are involved in tubular Na and K transport.

Tubular Defects Associated with Hypertension

These are discussed in the section on "Hypertension."

Familial Hypocalciuric Hypercalcemia

All three types of familial hypocalciuric hypercalcemia (FHH) (340,341) are autosomal dominant.

Genetic Disorders of Renal Phosphate Wasting (Table 38.24)

Hyperphosphaturia results from decreased proximal tubular reabsorption. Severe hyperphosphaturia may result from hyperparathyroidism or Fanconi syndrome, and mild hyperphosphaturia occurs after administration of diuretics (e.g., loop diuretics, carbonic anhydrase inhibitors, thiazides) or from drugs or toxins that are toxic to the proximal tubule. Other causes of hypophosphatemia (e.g., rickets and phosphate depletion) are discussed in Chapters 19 and 20.

X-Linked Hypophosphatemia

XLH (also called familial hypophosphatemic rickets or vitamin D–resistant rickets) is the most common disease associated with hyperphosphaturia in infancy and results from mutation of PHEX (342). This gene is most functionally expressed in the bone and leads to increased levels of FGF-23. While hypophosphatemia and decreased tubular reabsorption of phosphate can be noted in neonates, clinical signs, including bone deformations, usually appear after the first year of life. Treatment includes oral phosphate and 1,25-dihydroxyvitamin D (calcitriol). This therapy improves but does not cure the bone disease and induces iatrogenic NC, a potential risk for ESRD or hyperparathyroidism (342). Cinacalcet has been proposed as a potential treatment for secondary hyperparathyroidism. Burosumab, an anti-FGF-23 antibody therapy, was recently approved for specific treatment of XLH with marked benefit particularly in severely affected patients (343).

Three types of the much less common autosomal recessive hypophosphatemic rickets (AHRH) are described in Table 38.24.

Autosomal Dominant Hypophosphatemic Rickets

Autosomal dominant hypophosphatemic rickets (ADHR) is a rare autosomal dominant disease with variable penetrance. Patients generally have infantile onset of phosphate wasting, which can manifest low serum phosphorus concentration, rickets, osteomalacia, and lower extremity deformities. Additionally, patients demonstrate short stature, bone pain, and dental abscesses. ADHR results from mutations in a gene for the fibroblast growth factor (FGF) family, FGF23, rendering its protein product, now considered the prototypical phosphatonin, resistant to degradation. Treatment consists of administration of 1,25-dihydroxyvitamin D and phosphate supplementation.

Hypophosphatemic Rickets with Hypercalciuria

Hypophosphatemic rickets with hypercalciuria (HHRH) is an autosomal recessive disorder with rickets, bone pain, muscle weakness, failure to thrive, hypophosphatemia with hyperphosphaturia, normocalcemia with hypercalciuria, high plasma 1,25-dihydroxyvitamin D concentration, low PTH concentration, and elevated plasma alkaline phosphatase activity. The treatment consists of the administration of supplemental phosphate. HHRH results from mutation of SLC34A3, coding for a sodium-dependent phosphate transporter.

Vitamin D–Dependent Rickets

Vitamin D–dependent rickets type I (VDDR I) is an autosomal recessive disorder resulting from mutations in the 25-hydroxyvitamin D 1-alpha-hydroxylase gene (CYP27B1). In the untreated state, reduced 1,25-dihydroxyvitamin D results in hyperparathyroidism; this in turn results in phosphate wasting. Presentation is during infancy with typical signs of rickets, including hypotonia, tetany, irritability, motor retardation, deformations, and growth failure. Serum calcium and phosphate are low, PTH is elevated, and 1,25-dihydroxyvitamin D is very low or undetectable. This disorder should be differentiated from other causes for deficiency in 1-alpha-hydroxylase (e.g., Fanconi syndrome, RTA, or X-linked hypophosphatemia). Fortunately, 1,25-dihydroxyvitamin D (calcitriol) is available for oral dosing, and children with VDDR I respond very well to physiologic dosing.

Hereditary Vitamin D–Resistant Rickets

Hereditary vitamin D–resistant rickets (HVDRR) is also known as VDDR type II (VDDR II). Patients with this autosomal recessive disorder lack sensitivity of target organs to 1,25-dihydroxyvitamin D as a result of mutations of the vitamin D receptor (VDR) gene. Infantile presentation with rickets is usual; some will have alopecia. The pattern of alopecia may be very unusual with areas of total baldness, adjacent to normal hair, and regions of scant hair. Serum calcium and phosphate are low, but in contrast to VDDR-1, serum $1,25\text{-}(OH)_2$ vitamin D levels are very high, and treatment with high doses of oral calcium and supraphysiologic doses of calcitriol has only limited effect in most cases. However, in some patients, vitamin D analogs may partially or completely restore the responsiveness of the mutated VDR.

OTHER RENAL TUBULAR REABSORPTION DEFECTS

Glucosuria

The tubular handling of glucose in neonates is discussed above (see "Developmental Physiology" section). Glucose infusion in VLBW especially of early postnatal age is more likely to result in glucosuria due to lower glucose tolerance (hyperglycemia) and maturity-related differences in tubular reabsorption. In addition to glucosuria due to prematurity and that associated with Fanconi syndrome or broader dysfunction of the proximal tubule, glucosuria results from specific disorders of Na–glucose cotransporters (344). Congenital glucose–galactose malabsorption results from mutations in SGLT1, a renal/intestinal Na–glucose cotransporter; the predominant clinical finding in these neonates is severe, watery, acidic diarrhea, and dehydration with only mild glucosuria (SGLT1 mediates only a small proportion of renal glucose

TABLE 38.24

Genetic Disorders of Renal Phosphate Wasting

Diagnosis	Genetic Transmission	Gene	Protein	Pathophysiology	Treatment
Disorders with high fibroblast growth factor 23					
X-linked hypophosphatemic rickets (XLHR) = X-linked hypophosphatemia (XLH) = Familial hypophosphatemic rickets = Vitamin D–resistant rickets	X-linked dominant	PHEX	Fibroblast growth factor 23	Increased concentration of FGF23, hypophosphatemia, phosphaturia, bone deformations (>1 y of age), nephrocalcinosis, high PTH, ESRD	Oral phosphate; 1,25-dihydroxyvitamin D (calcitriol); cinacalcet for hyperparathyroidism; burosumab (anti-FGF23 antibody) (FDA approved for 6 mo and older)
Autosomal recessive hypophosphatemic rickets (AHRH 1)	Autosomal recessive	DMP1	Dentin matrix protein	Increase in FGF23	Phosphate; 1,25-dihydroxyvitamin D; consider burosumab
Autosomal recessive hypophosphatemic rickets (AHRH 2) overlaps with generalized arterial calcification of infancy = GAC1	Autosomal recessive	ENPP1	Ectonucleotide pyrophosphatase/ phosphodiesterase 1	Increase in FGF23, overlaps with GAC1: arterial, articular and organ calcifications beginning in infancy, pseudoxanthoma, myocardial ischemia, hearing loss, retinal angioid streaks, cardiovascular complications	Biphosphonates; cardiovascular treatment; phosphate; 1,25-dihydroxyvitamin D; consider burosumab
Autosomal recessive hypophosphatemic rickets (AHRH 3) = Raine syndrome	Autosomal recessive	FAM20C	Family with sequence familiarity 20C: GEF-CK	Phosphorylation defect presumably causing increase in FGF23; often lethal osteosclerotic bone dysplasia; nonlethal osteosclerosis with periosteal bone formation, ectopic calcifications, dental anomalies	Phosphate; 1,25-dihydroxyvitamin D; consider burosumab
Autosomal dominant hypophosphatemic rickets (ADHR)	Autosomal dominant	FGF23	Fibroblast growth factor 23	FGF23 resistance to proteolysis, phosphaturia in infancy, rickets, bone deformities	Phosphate; 1,25-dihydroxyvitamin D; consider burosumab
Other disorders					
Hypophosphatemic rickets with hypercalciuria (HHRH)	Autosomal recessive	SLC34A	Na-dependent phosphate cotransporter 2c (NaPi-2c)	Hyperphosphaturia, hypercalciuria, high 1,25 dihydroxy-vitamin D, low PTH, high alkaline phosphatase, bone pain, growth delay, nephrolithiasis	Oral phosphate; **should not be treated with calcitriol**
Vitamin D–dependent rickets type I (VDDR I)	Autosomal recessive	CYP27B1	25-hydroxy-vitamin D 1-alpha-hydroxylase	Very low to undetectable 1,25 dihydroxyvitamin D, high PTH, low Ca and P, hypotonia, tetany, irritability, motor retardation, deformations, and growth failure	1,25-dihydroxyvitamin D
Hereditary vitamin D–resistant rickets (HVDRR) = VDDR type II (VDDR II)	Autosomal recessive	VDR	Vitamin D receptor	Alopecia (variable), very high 1,25 dihydroxyvitamin D, rickets	Vitamin D analogs; calcium and calcitriol have limited effect

Also consider disorders with generalized proximal tubule dysfunction: Fanconi syndrome, Dent disease, Lowe syndrome, cystinosis.

FGF23, fibroblast growth factor 23; ESRD, end-stage renal disease; PTH, parathyroid hormone.

reabsorption). On the other hand, familial renal glucosuria results from mutation in *SGLT2*; while benign clinically, glucosuria is pronounced due to the fact that SGLT2 mediates 90% of glucose reuptake (up to 160 g/d) from the glomerular filtrate delivered to the proximal tubule. In a fascinating turn of events, an inhibitor of SGLT2 was developed and approved as an adjunctive treatment for patients with type 2 diabetes mellitus (345).

Specific Aminoacidurias

Details of specific aminoacidurias such as lysinuric protein intolerance, Hartnup disorder, iminoglycinuria, and dicarboxylic aminoaciduria are discussed in the online version of this book.

■ CONGENITAL NEPHROTIC SYNDROME

Nephrotic syndrome is defined by the association of marked proteinuria (more than 1 g/m²/d) with hypoalbuminemia (<2.5 g/dL), hyperlipidemia, and edema. A nephrotic syndrome is called congenital if it presents within the first 3 months of life and infantile when it presents between 3 months and 1 year of age. Two-thirds to as many as 85% of cases that occur in the first 3 months of age can be explained by mutations in the following four genes (346): NPHS1, which encodes nephrin and is responsible for CNF; NPHS2, which encodes podocin and is responsible for familial focal segmental glomerulosclerosis (FSGS); WT1, which encodes the transcription tumor suppressor and is responsible for the Denys-Drash syndrome; and LAMB2, which encodes laminin beta 2 and is responsible for the Pierson syndrome. In addition, mutations in the PCLE1 gene, which encodes phospholipase C epsilon, are responsible for the early-onset diffuse mesangial sclerosis (DMS). NPHS1 and NPHS2 mutations are the most common and account for 95% of cases.

Finnish Type (CNF or NPHS 1, OMIM 256300)

The incidence of CNF is estimated to be 1 per 8,200 births in Finland (347) but is considerably less frequent in other countries (e.g., 1:50,000 in North Americans). CNF should be suspected if there is a history of CNF in a sibling; hydrops fetalis or edema of the placenta, that is, placental weight greater than 25% of BW; or an elevated AFP or total protein concentration in the amniotic fluid. Because the disease begins *in utero* in all patients, an increased AFP (more than 10 SD above the mean amniotic fluid concentration during the second trimester) can be an early prenatal marker of the disease.

CNF is an autosomal recessive disorder in which both sexes are involved equally (347). It is caused mainly by mutations in the nephrin gene (NPHS1), mapped to chromosome 19q13.1, which encodes nephrin, a putative transmembrane protein belonging to the immunoglobulin superfamily of adhesion molecules and is phosphorylated by Src family kinases (347). Nephrin is specifically located at the slit diaphragm of the glomerular podocytes that forms the decisive size-selective filter of glomerular ultrafiltration barrier. In Finnish families, four main CNF haplotype categories have been observed. Analysis of non-Finnish families suggests that most patients with CNF share the same disease locus. More than 140 different NPHS1 mutations have been identified so far, caused by nonsense, missense, frameshift insertion/deletion, and splice-site mutations.

The natural history of the disease often includes prematurity (42%), small size for GA, and a large placenta. Signs of nephrotic syndrome (i.e., edema, proteinuria, hypoalbuminemia) are present in the first week of life in half of the cases but may not develop until the 3rd month of life. Complications include severe failure to thrive and ascites in all patients, severe bacterial infections (peritonitis, respiratory infections), hypothyroidism, pyloric stenosis, and thrombotic events. An increase in SCr or BUN may be observed, but none has frank uremia. Before availability of renal transplantation in young patients, the disease had a very high mortality with 50% of the patients dying by 6 months of life, and all of them by 4 years.

The proteinuria, initially very selective, that is, almost entirely albumin as a result of increased permeability of the glomerulus only for small proteins, increases progressively and becomes nonselective, corresponding to increased sieving coefficient and to tubular damage. Blood chemistry is significant for severe hypoalbuminemia and hypogammaglobulinemia, hypothyroxinemia (as a result of urine loss of thyroxine-binding globulin), a normal or mildly elevated SCr, and hyperlipidemia. Ultrasonography shows enlarged kidneys, increased echogenicity of the renal cortex, decreased differentiation between cortex and medulla, and poor visualization of the pyramids. Tubular dilations may be misinterpreted as other causes of cystic disease, including ARPKD. The diagnosis of CNF can be confirmed by linkage analysis or by renal biopsy. The latter shows irregularities of the glomerular basement membrane and thinning of the lamina densa, followed by fusion of the epithelial cell foot processes, all of which are similar to the findings in minimal-change, steroid-sensitive nephrotic syndrome.

Infants with CNF require intensive management, which includes repetitive administration of albumin and diuretics for ascites, thyroxin, anticoagulation, oral and parenteral hyperalimentation, and the treatment of multiple complications. Since the nephrotic syndrome is not an immunologic disease, it is always resistant to glucocorticoids and immunosuppressive drugs. These drugs can be harmful if given, as these infants are already highly susceptible to infections. Chronic renal insufficiency develops between 6 and 23 months of age. As a consequence, most patients eventually receive dialysis while waiting for transplantation. The aim of early management is to allow the infant to reach a sufficient size so that early transplantation can be performed. Because protein malnutrition, which leads to a negative nitrogen balance, is the prime factor affecting prognosis, a reduction of the urinary protein loss and subsequent protein catabolism is important. Aggressive therapy, including bilateral nephrectomy and peritoneal dialysis until transplantation when the infant reaches about 8 to 10 kg, allows normal growth and development, a patient survival rate of 97%, and a good graft survival rate. Recently, conservative management of CNF with captopril and indomethacin, and sometimes in combination with unilateral nephrectomy, has been described to significantly improve plasma albumin concentration, reduce the need for albumin infusion and duration of hospitalization, maintain normal growth, and allow delay of dialysis and transplantation for at least 3 years. It has also now become clear that not all NPHS1 mutations cause severe congenital nephrotic syndrome or a severe clinical course. Some are associated with ESRD occurring after the age of 20 years, others with partial or complete remission in childhood.

Increased amniotic fluid/maternal serum AFP concentration is helpful as a screening test in high-risk families; however, genetic linkage and haplotype analysis identify four haplotypes with up to 95% accuracy. Commercial tests are also available for NPHS1 mutations.

NPHS2 Mutation (OMIM 604766)

NPHS2 encodes an integral membrane protein, podocin, which is found exclusively in glomerular podocytes and is the causative gene for an autosomal recessive form of familial FSGS and a significant proportion of patients with childhood-onset steroid-resistant nephrotic syndrome. Although NPHS2 is responsible for most of the cases of nephrotic syndrome presenting between the ages of 4 and 12 months (29% to 35.2%), it has been found in infants presenting with congenital nephrotic syndrome (15% to 39%). However, disease severity is variable, and it may occur at birth, during childhood, or even later during adulthood.

Other Genetic Causes of Nephrotic Syndrome

Rarer genetic causes of nephrotic syndrome, including diffuse mesangial sclerosis (WAGR syndrome, Denys-Drash syndrome, Pierson syndrome, and Galloway-Mowat syndrome), are discussed in the online version of this book.

Congenital Nephrotic Syndrome and Congenital Infection

Nephrotic syndrome as a result of congenital infection is seen most commonly in congenital syphilis, in which case the lesion is characterized by epimembranous or proliferative glomerulopathy, with diffuse deposits of immunoglobulin and treponemal antigen along the glomerular capillaries and subepithelial electron-dense deposits. The condition responds very well to the administration of penicillin. The nephrotic syndrome associated with congenital toxoplasmosis is less common. Proteinuria may be present at birth or may develop during the first 3 months, in association with ocular and neurologic symptoms. The lesion is characterized by the deposition in the glomeruli of immunoglobulin, complement, and *Toxoplasma* antigen and antibody. It may respond to administration of pyrimethamine, sulfadiazine, and steroid. Congenital nephrotic or infantile nephrotic syndrome has also been reported in patients with congenital cytomegalovirus infection, rubeola virus, and human immunodeficiency virus.

128. Carpenter TO, Key LL. Metabolism of calcium, phosphorus, and other divalent ions. In: Ichikawa I, ed. *Pediatric textbook of fluids and electrolytes*. Baltimore, MD: Williams & Wilkins, 1990.

129. Hohenauer I, Rosenberg TF, Oh W. Calcium and phosphorus homeostasis on the first day of life. *Biol Neonate* 1970;15:49.

130. Woda C, Mulroney SE, Halaihel N, et al. Renal tubular sites of increased phosphate transport and NaPi-2 expression in the juvenile rat. *Am J Physiol* 2001;280(5):R1524.

131. Toverud SU, Boass A, Garner SC, et al. Circulating parathyroid hormone concentrations in normal and vitamin D-deprived rat pups determined with an N-terminal-specific radioimmunoassay. *Bone Miner* 1986;1:145.

132. Bergwitz C, Roslin NM, Tieder M, et al. SLC34A3 mutations in patients with hereditary hypophosphatemic rickets with hypercalciuria predict a key role for the sodium-phosphate cotransporter NaPi-IIc in maintaining phosphate homeostasis. *Am J Hum Genet* 2006;78(2):179.

133. Magen D, Berger L, et al. A loss-of-function mutation in NaPi-IIa and renal Fanconi's syndrome. *N Engl J Med* 2010;362(12):1102.

134. Neiberger RE, Barac-Nieto M, Spitzer A. Renal reabsorption of phosphate during development: transport kinetics in BBMV. *Am J Physiol* 1989;257:F268.

135. Segawa H, Kaneko I, Takahashi A, et al. Growth-related renal type II Na/Pi cotransporter. *J Biol Chem* 2002;277:19665.

136. Barac-Nieto M, Dowd TL, Gupta RK, et al. Changes in NMR-visible kidney cell phosphate with age and diet: relationship to phosphate transport. *Am J Physiol* 1991;261:F153.

137. Prabhu S, Levi M, Dwarakanath V, et al. Effect of glucocorticoids on neonatal rabbit renal cortical sodium-inorganic phosphate messenger RNA and protein abundance. *Pediatr Res* 1997;41:20.

138. Haramati A, Haas JA, Knox FG. Nephron heterogeneity of phosphate reabsorption: effect of parathyroid hormone. *Am J Physiol* 1984;246:F155.

139. Haas JA, Berndt T, Knox FG. Nephron heterogeneity of phosphate reabsorption. *Am J Physiol* 1978;234:F287.

140. Hellstrem G, Poschl J, Linderkamp O. Renal phosphate handling of premature infants 23–25 weeks gestational age. *Pediatr Nephrol* 2003;18:756.

141. Dai LJ, Ritchie G, Kerstan D, et al. Magnesium transport in the renal distal convoluted tubule. *Physiol Rev* 2001;81:51.

142. Wright EM, Turk E, Martin MG. Molecular basis for glucose-galactose malabsorption. *Cell Biochem Biophys* 2002;36:15.

143. Kanai Y, Lee WS, You G, et al. The human kidney low affinity Na+/glucose cotransporter SGLT2. Delineation of the major renal reabsorptive mechanism for D-glucose. *J Clin Invest* 1994;93:397.

144. Arant BS Jr. Developmental patterns of renal functional maturation compared in the human neonate. *J Pediatr* 1978;92:705.

145. You G, Lee WS, Barros EJ, et al. Molecular characteristics of Na(+)-coupled glucose transporters in adult and embryonic rat kidney. *J Biol Chem* 1995;270:29365.

146. Schwartz GH, Evan AP. Development of solute transport in rabbit proximal tubule. III. Na-K-ATPase activity. *Am J Physiol* 1984;246:F845.

147. Beck JC, Lipkowitz MS, Abramson RG. Characterization of the fetal glucose transporter in rabbit kidney: comparison with the adult brush border electrogenic Na-glucose symporter. *J Clin Invest* 1988;82:379.

148. Aperia A, Broberger O, Herin P, et al. Renal hemodynamics in the perinatal period: a study in lambs. *Acta Physiol Scand* 1977;99:261.

149. Horster M, Lewy JE. Filtration fraction and extraction of PAH during neonatal period in the rat. *Am J Physiol* 1970;219:1061.

150. Lopez-Nieto CE, You G, Bush KT, et al. Molecular cloning and characterization of NKT, a gene product related to the organic cation transporter family that is almost exclusively expressed in the kidney. *J Biol Chem* 1997;272:6471.

151. Brodehl J, Gellissen K. Endogenous renal transport of free amino acid in infancy and childhood. *Pediatrics* 1968;42:395.

152. Webber WA, Cairns JA. A comparison of the amino acid concentrating ability of the kidney cortex of newborn and mature rats. *Can J Physiol Pharmacol* 1968;46:165.

153. Vaughn D, Kirschbaum TH, Bersentes T, et al. Fetal and neonatal response to acid loading in the sheep. *J Appl Physiol* 1968;24:135.

154. Weisbrot IM, James LS, Prince CE, et al. Acid–base homeostasis of the new-born infant during the first 24 hrs of life. *J Pediatr* 1958;52:395.

155. Tuvdad F, McNamara H, Barnett HL. Renal response of premature infants to administration of bicarbonate and potassium. *Pediatrics* 1954;13:4.

156. Edelmann CM Jr, Rodriguez-Soriano J, Boichis H, et al. Renal bicarbonate reabsorption and hydrogen ion excretion in normal infants. *J Clin Invest* 1967;46:1309.

157. Brion LP, Zavilowitz BJ, Rosen O, et al. Changes in soluble carbonic anhydrase activity in response to maturation and NH4Cl loading in the rabbit. *Am J Physiol* 1991;261:R1204.

158. Fisher DA. Carbonic anhydrase activity in fetal and young rhesus monkeys. *Proc Soc Exp Biol Med* 1961;107:359.

159. Baum M, Quigley R. Maturation of proximal tubular acidification. *Pediatr Nephrol* 1993;7:785.

160. Schwartz GJ, Olson J, Kittelberger AM, et al. Postnatal development of carbonic anhydrase IV expression in rabbit kidney. *Am J Physiol* 1999;276:F510.

161. Twombley K, Gattineni J, et al. Effect of metabolic acidosis on neonatal proximal tubule acidification. *Am J Physiol Regul Integr Comp Physiol* 2010;299:R1360.

162. Baum M, Biemesderfer D, et al. Ontogeny of rabbit renal cortical NHE3 and NHE1: effect of glucocorticoids. *Am J Physiol* 1995;268:F815.

163. Hatemi N, McCance R. Renal aspects of acid–base control in the newly born. III. Response to acidifying drugs. *Acta Paediatr Scand* 1961;50:603.

164. Kerpel-Fronius E, Heim T, Sulyok E. The development of the renal acidifying processes and their relation to acidosis in low-birth-weight infants. *Biol Neonate* 1970;15:156.

165. Svenningsen NW, Lindquist B. Postnatal development of renal hydrogen ion excretion capacity in relation to age and protein intake. *Acta Paediatr Scand* 1974;63:721.

166. McCance RA, Widdowson EM. Renal aspects of acid–base control in the newly born. I. Natural development. *Acta Paediatr Scand* 1960;49:409.

167. Mehrgut FM, Satlin LM, Schwartz GJ. Maturation of HCO3 transport in rabbit collecting duct. *Am J Physiol* 1990;259:F801.

168. Robillard JE, Weitzman RE, Fisher DA, et al. The dynamics of vasopressin release: blood volume regulation during fetal hemorrhage in the lamb fetus. *Pediatr Res* 1979;13:606.

169. Ross MG, Sherman DJ, Ervin MG, et al. Maternal dehydration-rehydration: fetal plasma and urinary responses. *Am J Physiol* 1988;255:E674.

170. Gomez RA, Meernik JG, Kuehl WD, et al. Developmental aspects of the renal response to hemorrhage during fetal life. *Pediatr Res* 1984;18:40.

171. Woods LL, Cheung CY, Power GG, et al. Role of arginine vasopressin in fetal renal response to hypertonicity. *Am J Physiol* 1986;251:F156.

172. Polacek E, Vocel J, Neugebauerova L, et al. The osmotic concentrating ability in healthy infants and children. *Arch Dis Child* 1965;40:291.

173. Siga E, Horster MF. Regulation of osmotic water permeability during differentiation of inner medullary collecting duct. *Am J Physiol* 1991;260:F710.

174. Horster MF, Zink H. Functional differentiation of the medullary collecting tubule: influence of vasopressin. *Kidney Int* 1982;22:360.

175. Trimble ME. Renal response to solute loading in infant rats: relation to anatomical development. *Am J Physiol* 1970;219:1089.

176. Edelmann CM Jr, Barnett HL, Troupkou V. Renal concentrating mechanisms in newborn infants: effect of dietary protein, and water content, role of urea and responsiveness to antidiuretic hormone. *J Clin Invest* 1960;39:1062.

177. Hadeed AJ, Leake RD, Weitzman RE, et al. Possible mechanisms of high blood levels of vasopressin during the neonatal period. *J Pediatr* 1979;94:805.

178. Rees L, Forsling ML, Brook CGD. Vasopressin concentrations in the neonatal period. *Clin Endocrinol* 1980;12:357.

179. Svenningsen NW, Aronson AS. Postnatal development of renal concentration capacity as estimated by DDAVP-test in normal and asphyxiated neonates. *Biol Neonate* 1974;25:230.

180. Ostrowski NL, Young WS, Knepper MA, et al. Expression of vasopressin V1a and V2 receptor messenger ribonucleic acid in the liver and kidney of embryonic, developing, and adult rats. *Endocrinology* 1993;133:1849.

181. Bonilla-Felix M, Jiang W. Aquaporin-2 in the immature rat: expression, regulation, and trafficking. *J Am Soc Nephrol* 1997;8:1502.

182. Gengler WR, Forte LR. Neonatal development of rat kidney adenyl cyclase and phosphodiesterase. *Biochim Biophys Acta* 1972;279:367.

183. Wiesel A, Queisser-Luft A, Clementi M, et al.; EUROSCAN Study Group. Prenatal detection of congenital renal malformations by fetal ultrasonographic examination: an analysis of 709,030 births in 12 European countries. *Eur J Med Genet* 2005;48(2):131.

184. Cragan JD, Young BA, Correa A. Renin-angiotensin system blocker fetopathy. *J Pediatr* 2015;167(4):792.

185. Lutiger B, Graham K, Einarson TR, et al. Relationship between gestational cocaine use and pregnancy outcome: a meta-analysis. *Teratology* 1991;44:405.

186. Nasri HZ, Houde Ng K, Westgate MN, et al. Malformations among infants of mothers with insulin-dependent diabetes: is there a recognizable pattern of abnormalities? *Birth Defects Res* 2018;110(2):108.

187. Hofer R, Burd L. Review of published studies of kidney, liver, and gastrointestinal birth defects in fetal alcohol spectrum disorders. *Birth Defects Res A Clin Mol Teratol* 2009;85(3):179.

188. Petrikovsky BM, Nardi DA, Rodis JF, et al. Elevated maternal serum alpha-fetoprotein and mild fetal uropathy. *Obstet Gynecol* 1991;78:262.

189. Roodhooft AM, Birnholz JC, Holmes LB. Familial nature of congenital absence and severe dysgenesis of both kidneys. *N Engl J Med* 1984;310:1341.

190. Yulia A, Winyard P. Management of antenatally detected kidney malformations. *Early Hum Dev* 2018;126:38.

191. Deshpande SA, Jog S, Watson H, et al. Do babies with isolated single umbilical artery need routine postnatal renal ultrasonography? *Arch Dis Child Fetal Neonatal Ed* 2009;94(4):F265.

THE NEWBORN INFANT

192. Flynn JT, Kaelber DC, Baker-Smith CM, et al.; Subcommittee on Screening and Management of High Blood Pressure in Children. Clinical Practice Guideline for screening and management of high blood pressure in children and adolescents. *Pediatrics* 2017;140(3):e20171904. Erratum in: *Pediatrics* 2018;142(3).

193. Zubrow AB, Hulman S, Kushner H, et al. Determinants of blood pressure in infants admitted to neonatal intensive care units: a prospective multicenter study. *J Perinatol* 1995;15:470.

194. Dionne JM, Abitbol CL, Flynn JT. Hypertension in infancy: diagnosis, management and outcome. *Pediatr Nephrol* 2012;27:17. Erratum: *Pediatric Nephrol* 2012;27:159.

195. Satoh M, Inoue R, Tada H, et al. Reference values and associated factors for Japanese newborns' blood pressure and pulse rate: the babies' and their parents': longitudinal observation in Suzuki Memorial Hospital on intrauterine period (BOSHI) study. *J Hypertens* 2016;34(8):1578

196. Pinto E, Guignard JP. Renal masses in the neonate. *Biol Neonate* 1995;68(3):175.

197. Lorenz JM, Kleinman LI, Ahmed G, et al. Phases of fluid and electrolyte homeostasis in the extremely low birth weight infant. *Pediatrics* 1995;96:484.

198. Ramiro-Tolentino SB, Markarian K, Kleinman LI. Renal bicarbonate excretion in extremely low birth weight infants. *Pediatrics* 1996;98:256.

199. Vieux R, Hascoet JM, Merdariu D, et al. Glomerular filtration rate reference values in very preterm infants. *Pediatrics* 2010;125:e1186.

200. Schwartz GJ, Feld LG, Langford DJ. A simple estimate of glomerular filtration rate in full term infants during the first year of life. *J Pediatr* 1984;104:849.

201. Gallini F, Maggio L, Romagnoli C, et al. Progression of renal function in preterm neonates with gestational age < or = 32 weeks. *Pediatr Nephrol* 2000;15:119.

202. Su SW, Stonestreet BS. Core concepts: neonatal glomerular filtration rate. *NeoReviews* 2010;11:e714.

203. Kamianowska M, Szczepański M, Wasilewska A. Tubular and glomerular biomarkers of acute kidney injury in newborns. *Curr Drug Metab* 2019;20(5):332.

204. Song R, Yosypiv IV. Genetics of congenital anomalies of the kidney and urinary tract. *Pediatr Nephrol* 2011;26(3):353.

205. Karlowicz MG. Renal calcification in NICU patients. *NeoReviews* 2010;11:e696.

206. Preda I, Jodal U, Sixt R, et al. Value of ultrasound in evaluation of infants with first urinary tract infection. *J Urol* 2010;183:1984.

207. Epelman M, Daneman A, Donnelly LF, et al. Neonatal imaging evaluation of common prenatally diagnosed genitourinary abnormalities. *Semin Ultrasound CT MR* 2014;35(6):528.

208. Marckmann P, Skov L, Rossen K, et al. Clinical manifestation of gadodiamide-related nephrogenic systemic fibrosis. *Clin Nephrol* 2008;69(3):161.

209. Edelmann CM Jr, Churg J, Gerber MA, et al. Renal biopsy: indications, technique, and interpretation. In: Edelmann CM Jr, ed. *Pediatric kidney disease*, 2nd ed. Boston, MA: Little, Brown, 1992:499.

210. Hui-Stickle S, Brewer ED, Goldstein SL. Pediatric ARF epidemiology at a tertiary care center from 1999 to 2001. *Am J Kidney Dis* 2005;45:96.

211. Sutton TA, Fisher CJ, Molitoris BA. Microvascular endothelial injury and dysfunction during ischemic acute renal failure. *Kidney Int* 2002;62:1539.

212. Molitoris BA, Sutton TA. Endothelial injury and dysfunction: role in the extension phase of acute renal failure. *Kidney Int* 2004;66:496.

213. Awad AS, Okusa MD. Distant organ injury following acute kidney injury. *Am J Physiol Renal Physiol* 2007;293:F28.

214. Zappitelli M, Selewski DT, Askenazi DA. Nephrotoxic medication exposure and acute kidney injury in neonates. *NeoReviews* 2012;13:e420.

215. Jetton JG, Boohaker LJ, Sethi SK, et al. Incidence and outcomes of neonatal acute kidney injury (AWAKEN): a multicentre, multinational, observational cohort study. *Lancet Child Adolesc Health* 2017;1(3):184.

216. Koralkar R, Ambalavanan N, Levitan EB, et al. Acute kidney injury reduces survival in very low birth weight infant. *Pediatr Res* 2010;69:354.

217. Viswanathan S, Manyam B, Azhibekov T, et al. Risk factors associated with acute kidney injury in extremely low birth weight (ELBW) infants. *Pediatr Nephrol* 2012;27:303.

218. Askenazi DJ, Griffin R, McGwin G, et al. Acute kidney injury is independently associated with mortality in very low birth weight infants: a matched case–control analysis. *Pediatr Nephrol* 2009;24:991.

219. Selewski DT, Jordan BK, Askenazi DJ, et al. Acute kidney injury in asphyxiated newborns treated with therapeutic hypothermia. *J Pediatr* 2013;162(4):725.

220. Carmody JB, Charlton JR. Short-term gestation, long-term risk: prematurity and chronic kidney disease. *Pediatrics* 2013;131:1168.

221. Luyckx VA, Bertram JF, Brenner BM, et al. Effect of fetal and child health on kidney development and long-term risk of hypertension and kidney disease. *Lancet* 2013;382:273.

222. White SL, Perkovic V, Cass A, et al. Is low birth weight an antecedent of CKD in later life? A systematic review of observational studies. *Am J Kidney Dis* 2009;54:248.

223. Greenbaum LA, Munoz A, Schneider MF, et al. The association between abnormal birth history and growth in children with CKD. *Clin J Am Soc Nephrol* 2011;6:14.

224. Abrahamson DR. Glomerulogenesis in the developing kidney. *Semin Nephrol* 1991;11:375.

225. Rodriguez MM, Gomez AH, Abitbol CL, et al. Histomorphometric analysis of postnatal glomerulogenesis in extremely preterm infants. *Pediatr Dev Pathol* 2004;7:17.

226. Coca SG, Singanamala S, Parikh CR. Chronic kidney disease after acute kidney injury: a systematic review and meta-analysis. *Kidney Int* 2012;81:442.

227. Prins I, Plotz FB, Uiterwaal C, et al. Low dose dopamine in neonatal and pediatric intensive care: a systematic review. *Intensive Care Med* 2001;27:206.

228. Harer MW, Askenazi DJ, Boohaker LJ, et al. Association between early caffeine citrate administration and risk of acute kidney injury in preterm neonates: results from the AWAKEN study. *JAMA Pediatr* 2018;172(6):e180322.

229. Al-Wassia H, Alshaikh B, Sauve R. Prophylactic theophylline for the prevention of severe renal dysfunction in term and post-term neonates with perinatal asphyxia: a systematic review and meta-analysis of randomized controlled trials. *J Perinatol* 2013;33(4):271.

230. Kemper MJ, Harps E, Müller-Wiefel DE. Hyperkalemia: therapeutic options in acute and chronic renal failure. *Clin Nephrol* 1996;46:67.

231. Singh BS, Sadiq HF, Noguchi A, et al. Efficacy of albuterol inhalation in treatment of hyperkalemia in premature neonates. *J Pediatr* 2002;141:16.

232. Rivard AL, Raup SM, Beilman GJ. Sodium polystyrene sulfonate used to reduce the potassium content of a high-protein enteral formula: a quantitative analysis. *JPEN J Parenter Enteral Nutr* 2004;28:76.

233. Bell EF, Acarregui MJ. Restricted versus liberal water intake for preventing morbidity and mortality in preterm infants. *Cochrane Database Syst Rev* 2014;(12):CD000503.

234. Selewski DT, Gist KM, Nathan AT, et al. The impact of fluid balance on outcomes in premature neonates: a report from the AWAKEN study group. *Pediatr Res* 2019;85(1):79.

235. Coulthard MG, Crosier J, Griffiths C, et al. Haemodialysing babies weighing <8 kg with the Newcastle infant dialysis and ultrafiltration system (Nidus): comparison with peritoneal and conventional haemodialysis. *Pediatr Nephrol* 2014;29(10):1873.

236. Ronco C, Garzotto F, Brendolan A, et al. Continuous renal replacement therapy in neonates and small infants: development and first-in-human use of a miniaturised machine (CARPEDIEM). *Lancet* 2014;383(9931):1807.

237. Askenazi D, Ingram D, White S, et al. Smaller circuits for smaller patients: improving renal support therapy with Aquadex. *Pediatr Nephrol* 2016;31(5):853.

238. Menon S, Broderick J, Munshi R, et al. Kidney support in children using an ultrafiltration device: a multicenter, retrospective study. *Clin J Am Soc Nephrol* 2019;14(10):1432. doi: 10.2215/CJN.03240319.

239. Seligsohn U, Lubetsky A. Genetic susceptibility to venous thrombosis. *N Engl J Med* 2001;344:1222.

240. Brown EM, MacLeod RJ. Extracellular calcium sensing and extracellular calcium signaling. *Physiol Rev* 2001;81:239.

241. Seibert JJ, Northington FJ, Miers JF, et al. Aortic thrombosis after umbilical artery catheterization in neonates: prevalence of complications on long-term follow-up. *AJR Am J Roentgenol* 1991;156:567.

242. Manco-Johnson M, Nuss R. Neonatal thrombotic disorders. *NeoReviews* 2000;1:e201.

243. Weinschenk N, Pelidis M, Fiascone J. Combination thrombolytic and anticoagulant therapy for bilateral renal vein thrombosis in a premature infant. *Am J Perinatol* 2001;18:293.

244. Hogg RJ, Furth S, Lemley KV, et al. National Kidney Foundation's Kidney Disease Outcomes Quality Initiative clinical practice guidelines for chronic kidney disease in children and adolescents: evaluation, classification, and stratification. *Pediatrics* 2003;111(6 Pt 1):1416.

245. Glick PL, Harrison MR, Golbus MS, et al. Management of the fetus with congenital hydronephrosis. II. Prognostic criteria and selection for treatment. *J Pediatr Surg* 1985;20:376.

246. Hubert KC, Palmer JS. Current diagnosis and management of fetal genitourinary abnormalities. *Urol Clin N Am* 2007;34:89.

247. Elder JS, O'Grady JP, Ashmead G, et al. Evaluation of fetal renal function: unreliability of fetal urinary electrolytes. *J Urol* 1990;144:574.

248. Hoppe B, Beck BB, Milliner DS. The primary hyperoxalurias. *Kidney Int* 2009;75(12):1264.

249. Belostotsky R, Seboun E, Idelson GH, et al. Mutations in DHDPSL are responsible for primary hyperoxaluria type III. *Am J Hum Genet* 2010;87(3):392.

250. Mattoo A, Goldfarb DS. Cystinuria. *Semin Nephrol* 2008;28(2):181.

251. Kim SJ, Mock S, Stock JA. Cystine nephrolithiasis. *Urology* 2013;82(2):e7.

252. Cochat P, Pichault V, Bacchetta J, et al. Nephrolithiasis related to inborn metabolic diseases. *Pediatr Nephrol* 2010;25(3):415.

253. Dinour D, Gray NK, Campbell S, et al. Homozygous SLC2A9 mutations cause severe renal hypouricemia. *J Am Soc Nephrol* 2010;21(1):64.

254. Iorember FM, Vehaskari VM. Uromodulin: old friend with new roles in health and disease. *Pediatr Nephrol* 2014;29(7):1151.

255. Nesterova G, Gahl WA. Cystinosis: the evolution of a treatable disease. *Pediatr Nephrol* 2013;28(1):51.

256. Langman CB, Greenbaum LA, Sarwal M, et al. A randomized controlled crossover trial with delayed-release cysteamine bitartrate in nephropathic cystinosis: effectiveness on white blood cell cystine levels and comparison of safety. *Clin J Am Soc Nephrol* 2012;7(7):1112.

257. Morrow T. Do comparable efficacy & convenient dosing justify Procysbi's extremely high price? *Manag Care* 2013;22(7):71.

258. Scott CR. The genetic tyrosinemias. *Am J Med Genet C Semin Med Genet* 2006;142C(2):121.

259. de Laet C, Dionisi-Vici C, Leonard JV, et al. Recommendations for the management of tyrosinaemia type 1. *Orphanet J Rare Dis* 2013;8:8.

260. Santer R, Steinmann B, Schaub J. Fanconi-Bickel syndrome—a congenital defect of facilitative glucose transport. *Curr Mol Med* 2002;2(2):213.

261. Chou JY, Jun HS, Mansfield BC. Glycogen storage disease type I and G6Pase-beta deficiency: etiology and therapy. *Nat Rev Endocrinol* 2010;6(12):676.

262. Elsas LJ II, Lai K. The molecular biology of galactosemia. *Genet Med* 1998;1:40.

263. Bosch AM. Classical galactosaemia revisited. *J Inherit Metab Dis* 2006;29(4):516.

264. Camargo SM, Bockenhauer D, Kleta R. Aminoacidurias: clinical and molecular aspects. *Kidney Int* 2008;73(8):918.

265. Ogier deBaulny H, Schiff M, Dionisi-Vici C. Lysinuric protein intolerance (LPI): a multi organ disease by far more complex than a classic urea cycle disorder. *Mol Genet Metab* 2012;106(1):12.

266. Broer S, Bailey CG, Kowalczuk S, et al. Iminoglycinuria and hyperglycinuria are discrete human phenotypes resulting from complex mutations in proline and glycine transporters. *J Clin Invest* 2008;118(12):3881.

267. Bailey CG, Ryan RM, Thoeng AD, et al. Loss-of-function mutations in the glutamate transporter SLC1A1 cause human dicarboxylic aminoaciduria. *J Clin Invest* 2011;121(1):446.

268. Habib R, Gubler MC, Antignac C, et al. Diffuse mesangial sclerosis: a congenital glomerulopathy with nephrotic syndrome. *Adv Nephrol Necker Hosp* 1993;22:43.

269. Scott RH, Stiller CA, Walker L, et al. Syndromes and constitutional chromosomal abnormalities associated with Wilms tumour. *J Med Genet* 2006;43(9):705.

270. Mueller RF. The Denys-Drash syndrome. *J Med Genet* 1994;31:471.

271. VanDeVoorde R, Witte D, Kogan J, et al. Pierson syndrome: a novel cause of congenital nephrotic syndrome. *Pediatrics* 2006;118:e501.

272. Report of the Second Task Force on Blood Pressure Control in Children—1987. Task Force on Blood Pressure Control in Children. National Heart, Lung, and Blood Institute, Bethesda, Maryland. *Pediatrics* 1987;79:1.

273. U.S. Renal Data System NIoH, National Institute of Diabetes and Digestive and Kidney Diseases, Bethesda, MD. USRDS 2013 Annual Data Report: Atlas of Chronic Kidney Disease and End-Stage Renal Disease in the United States.

274. Kraut EJ, Boohaker LJ, Askenazi DJ, et al; Neonatal Kidney Collaborative (NKC). Incidence of neonatal hypertension from a large multicenter study [Assessment of Worldwide Acute Kidney Injury Epidemiology in Neonates-AWAKEN]. *Pediatr Res* 2018;84(2):279. Erratum in: *Pediatr Res* 2018;84(2):314.

275. Bauer SB, Feldman SM, Gellis SS, et al. Neonatal hypertension: a complication of umbilical-artery catheterization. *N Engl J Med* 1975;293:1032.

276. Rizzi M, Goldenberg N, Bonduel M, et al. Catheter-related arterial thrombosis in neonates and children: a systematic review. *Thromb Haemost* 2018;118(6):1058.

277. Durante D, Jones D, Spitzer R. Neonatal arterial embolism syndrome. *J Pediatr* 1976;89:978.

278. Abman SH, Warady BA, Lum GM, et al. Systemic hypertension in infants with bronchopulmonary dysplasia. *J Pediatr* 1984;104:929.

279. Kwon HW, Kim HS, An HS, et al. Long-term outcomes of pulmonary hypertension in preterm infants with bronchopulmonary dysplasia. *Neonatology*. 2016;110(3):181.

280. Moralıoğlu S, Celayir AC, Bosnalı O, et al. Single center experience in patients with unilateral multicystic dysplastic kidney. *J Pediatr Urol* 2014;10(4):763.

281. Jenkins R, Tackitt S, Gievers L, et al. Phthalate-associated hypertension in premature infants: a prospective mechanistic cohort study. *Pediatr Nephrol* 2019;34(8):1413.

282. Boedy RF, Goldberg AK, Howell CG Jr, et al. Incidence of hypertension in infants on extracorporeal membrane oxygenation. *J Pediatr Surg* 1990;25:258.

283. Cachat F, Van Melle G, McGahren ED, et al. Arterial hypertension after surgical closure of omphalocele and gastroschisis. *Pediatr Nephrol* 2006;21:225.

284. Flynn JT, Tullus K. Severe hypertension in children and adolescents: pathophysiology and treatment. *Pediatric Nephrol* 2009;24:1101.

285. Hammer GB, Lewandowski A, Drover DR. Safety and efficacy of sodium nitroprusside during prolonged infusion in pediatric patients. *Pediatr Crit Care Med* 2015;16(5):397.

286. Gantenbein MH, Bauersfeld U, Baenziger O, et al. Side effects of angiotensin converting enzyme inhibitor (captopril) in newborns and young infants. *J Perinat Med* 2008;36:448.

287. Slaughter JL, Stenger MR, Reagan PB. Variation in the use of diuretic therapy for infants with bronchopulmonary dysplasia. *Pediatrics* 2013;131:716.

288. Stewart A, Brion LP. Routine use of diuretics in very-low birth-weight infants in the absence of supporting evidence. *J Perinatol* 2011;31:633.

289. Blaisdell CJ, Troendle J, Zajicek A, Prematurity and Respiratory Outcomes Program. Acute Responses to Diuretic Therapy in Extremely Low Gestational Age Newborns: Results from the Prematurity and Respiratory Outcomes Program Cohort Study. *J Pediatr* 2018;197:42.

290. Greenberg RG, Gayam S, Savage D, et al.; Best Pharmaceuticals for Children Act—Pediatric Trials Network Steering Committee. Furosemide exposure and prevention of bronchopulmonary dysplasia in premature infants. *J Pediatr* 2019;208:134.

291. Sierra CM, Hernandez EA, Parbuoni KA. Use of arginine hydrochloride in the treatment of metabolic alkalosis or hypochloremia in pediatric patients. *J Pediatr Pharmacol Ther* 2018;23(2):111.

292. Heble DE Jr, Oschman A, Sandritter TL. Comparison of arginine hydrochloride and acetazolamide for the correction of metabolic alkalosis in pediatric patients. *Am J Ther* 2016;23(6):e1469.

293. Hoffman DJ, Gerdes JS, Abbasi S. Pulmonary function and electrolyte balance following spironolactone treatment in preterm infants with chronic lung disease: a double-blind, placebo-controlled, randomized trial. *J Perinatol* 2000;20(1):41.

294. Doggrell SA, Brown L. The spironolactone renaissance. *Expert Opin Investig Drugs* 2001;10:943.

295. Bauer S, Eliakim A, Pomeranz A, et al. Urinary tract infection in very low birth weight preterm infants. *Pediatr Infect Dis J* 2003;22:426.

296. American Academy of Pediatrics Task Force on Circumcision. Circumcision policy statement. *Pediatrics* 2012;130:585.

297. Ellison JS, Dy GW, Fu BC, et al. Neonatal circumcision and urinary tract infections in infants with hydronephrosis. *Pediatrics* 2018;142(1):e20173703.

298. Downey LC, Benjamin Jr DK, Smith PB, et al. Urinary tract infection concordance with positive blood and cerebrospinal fluid cultures in the neonatal intensive care unit. *J Perinatol* 2013;33:302.

299. Tung KT, MacDonald LM, Smith JC. Neonatal systemic candidiasis diagnosed by ultrasound. *Acta Radiol* 1990;31:293.

300. Subcommittee on Urinary Tract Infection, Steering Committee on Quality Improvement and Management; Roberts KB. Urinary tract infection: clinical practice guideline for the diagnosis and management of the initial UTI in febrile infants and children 2 to 24 months. *Pediatrics* 2011;128:595.

301. Levy I, Comarsca J, Davidovits M, et al. Urinary tract infections in preterm infants: the protecting role of breastfeeding. *Pediatr Nephrol* 2009;24:527.

302. Expert Panel on Pediatric Imaging: Karmazyn BK, Alazraki AL, Anupindi SA, et al. ACR appropriateness criteria urinary tract infection-child. *J Am Coll Radiol* 2017;14(5S):S362.

303. Nowell L. Prevalence of renal anomalies after urinary tract infections in hospitalized infants less than 2 months of age. *J Perinatol* 2010;30:281.

304. The RIVUR Trial Investigators. Antimicrobial prophylaxis for children with vesicoureteral reflux. *N Engl J Med* 2014;370(25):2367.

305. Wheeler D, Vimalachandra D, Hodson EM. Antibiotics and surgery for vesicoureteric reflux: a meta-analysis of randomised controlled trials. *Arch Dis Child* 2003;88:688.

306. Upadhyay J, McLorie GA, Bolduc S, et al. Natural history of neonatal reflux associated with prenatal hydronephrosis: long-term results of a prospective study. *J Urol* 2003;169:1837.

307. The online metabolic and molecular bases of inherited disease. In: Valle D, ed. McGraw Hill Medical. Available from: http://ommbid.mhmedical.com/ommbid-index.aspx

308. Mount D, Pollack M. *Molecular and genetic basis of renal disease, a companion to Brenner and Rector's the kidney.* Philadelphia, PA: Saunders, 2008.

309. Sargent JD, Stukel TA, Kresel J, et al. Normal values for random urinary calcium to creatinine ratios in infancy. *J Pediatr* 1993;123(3):393.

310. Schell-Feith EA, Kist-van Holthe JE, van der Heijden AJ. Nephrocalcinosis in preterm neonates. *Pediatr Nephrol* 2010;25(2):221.

311. Lee HS, Sung IK, Kim SJ, et al. Risk factors associated with nephrocalcinosis in preterm infants. *Am J Perinatol* 2014;31(4):279.

312. Giapros V, Tsoni C, Challa A, et al. Renal function and kidney length in preterm infants with nephrocalcinosis: a longitudinal study. *Pediatr Nephrol* 2011;26(10):1873.

313. Lichter-Konecki U, Broman KW, Blau EB, et al. Genetic and physical mapping of the locus for autosomal dominant renal Fanconi syndrome, on chromosome 15q15.3. *Am J Hum Genet* 2001;68(1):264.

314. Klootwijk ED, Reichold M, Helip-Wooley A, et al. Mistargeting of peroxisomal EHHADH and inherited renal Fanconi's syndrome. *N Engl J Med* 2014;370(2):129.

315. Hall AM, Unwin RJ. The not so 'mighty chondrion': emergence of renal diseases due to mitochondrial dysfunction. *Nephron Physiol* 2007;105(1):1.

316. Emma F, Bertini E, Salviati L, et al. Renal involvement in mitochondrial cytopathies. *Pediatr Nephrol* 2012;27(4):539.

317. Hall AM, Bass P, Unwin RJ. Drug-induced renal Fanconi syndrome. *QJM* 2014;107(4):261.

318. Manoli I, Sysol JR, Li L, et al. Targeting proximal tubule mitochondrial dysfunction attenuates the renal disease of methylmalonic acidemia. *Proc Natl Acad Sci U S A* 2013;110(33):13552.

319. Levin B, Snodgrass GJ, Oberholzer VG, et al. Fructosaemia. Observations on seven cases. *Am J Med* 1968;45(6):826.

320. Ezgu F, Senaca S, Gunduz M, et al. Severe renal tubulopathy in a newborn due to BCS1L gene mutation: effects of different treatment modalities on the clinical course. *Gene* 2013;528(2):364.

321. Bockenhauer D, Bokenkamp A, van't Hoff W, et al. Renal phenotype in Lowe syndrome: a selective proximal tubular dysfunction. *Clin J Am Soc Nephrol* 2008;3(5):1430.

322. Dell KM. The spectrum of polycystic kidney disease in children. *Adv Chron Kidney Dis* 2011;18(5):339.

323. Salomon R, Saunier S, Niaudet P. Nephronophthisis. *Pediatr Nephrol* 2009;24(12):2333.

324. Lindstedt E, Lindstedt G. Letter: Tubular proteinuria early in nephronophthisis. *Lancet* 1973;2(7839):1215.

325. Simpson MA, Cross HE, Cross L, et al. Lethal cystic kidney disease in Amish neonates associated with homozygous nonsense mutation of NPHP3. *Am J Kidney Dis* 2009;53:790.

326. Cullinane AR, Straatman-Iwanowska A, Zaucker A, et al. Mutations in VIPAR cause an arthrogryposis, renal dysfunction and cholestasis syndrome phenotype with defects in epithelial polarization. *Nat Genet* 2010;42(4):303.

327. Linshaw MA. Back to basics: congenital nephrogenic diabetes insipidus. *Pediatr Rev* 2007;28(10):372.

328. van Lieburg AF, Knoers VV, Mallmann R, et al. Normal fibrinolytic responses to 1-desamino-8-D-arginine vasopressin in patients with nephrogenic diabetes insipidus caused by mutations in the aquaporin 2 gene. *Nephron* 1996;72(4):544.

329. Fomon SJ, Ziegler EE. Renal solute load and potential renal solute load in infancy. *J Pediatr* 1999;134(1):11.

330. Loffing J. Paradoxical antidiuretic effect of thiazides in diabetes insipidus: another piece in the puzzle. *J Am Soc Nephrol* 2004;15(11):2948.

331. Kleta R, Bockenhauer D. Bartter syndromes and other salt-losing tubulopathies. *Nephron Physiol* 2006;104(2):73.

332. Haque SK, Ariceta G, Batlle D. Proximal renal tubular acidosis: a not so rare disorder of multiple etiologies. *Nephrol Dial Transplant* 2012;27(12):4273.

333. Batlle D, Haque SK. Genetic causes and mechanisms of distal renal tubular acidosis. *Nephrol Dial Transplant* 2012;27(10):3691.

334. Laing CM, Unwin RJ. Renal tubular acidosis. *J Nephrol* 2006;19 (suppl 9): S46.

335. Alper SL. Familial renal tubular acidosis. *J Nephrol* 2010;23(suppl 16): S57.

336. Quigley R. Proximal renal tubular acidosis. *J Nephrol* 2006;19(suppl 9): S41.

337. Chan JC, Scheinman JI, Roth KS. Consultation with the specialist: renal tubular acidosis. *Pediatr Rev* 2001;22(8):277.

338. Sulyok E, Guignard JP. Relationship of urinary anion gap to urinary ammonium excretion in the neonate. *Biol Neonate* 1990;57(2):98.

339. Furgeson SB, Linas S. Mechanisms of type I and type II pseudohypoaldosteronism. *J Am Soc Nephrol* 2010;21(11):1842.

340. Nesbit MA, Hannan FM, Howles SA, et al. Mutations in AP2S1 cause familial hypocalciuric hypercalcemia type 3. *Nat Genet* 2013;45(1):93.

341. Pearce SH, Williamson C, Kifor O, et al. A familial syndrome of hypocalcemia with hypercalciuria due to mutations in the calcium-sensing receptor. *N Engl J Med* 1996;335(15):1115.

342. Malloy PJ, Wang J, Srivastava T, et al. Hereditary 1,25-dihydroxyvitamin D-resistant rickets with alopecia resulting from a novel missense mutation in the DNA-binding domain of the vitamin D receptor. *Mol Genet Metab* 2010;99(1):72.

343. Sabino-Silva R, Mori RC, David-Silva A, et al. The Na(+)/glucose cotransporters: from genes to therapy. *Braz J Med Biol Res* 2010;43(11):1019.

344. Wright EM. I. Glucose galactose malabsorption. *Am J Physiol* 1998;275 (5 Pt 1):G879.

345. Jabbour SA, Hardy E, Sugg J, et al. Dapagliflozin is effective as add-on therapy to sitagliptin with or without metformin: a 24-week, multicenter, randomized, double-blind, placebo-controlled study. *Diabetes Care* 2014;37(3):740.

346. Hinkes BG, et al. Nephrotic syndrome in the first year of life: two thirds of cases are caused by mutations in 4 genes (NPHS1, NPHS2, WT1, and LAMB2). *Pediatrics* 2007;119:2907.

347. Huttunen NP. Congenital nephrotic syndrome of Finnish type: study of 75 patients. *Arch Dis Child* 1976;51:344.

348. Haftel AJ, Eichner J, Haling J, et al. Myoglobinuric renal failure in a newborn infant. *J Pediatr* 1978;93:1015.

39 Structural Abnormalities of the Genitourinary Tract

Irene M. McAleer and Kai-wen Chuang

INTRODUCTION

Anomalies of the genitourinary tract found in the neonatal period make up many pediatric urology problems. Some age-specific problems do not present in early infancy, but many urologic conditions present primarily or specifically in the neonatal period. Antenatal ultrasonography (US) has had a profound effect on the detection, management, and understanding of many conditions of the urinary tract. Genitourinary anomalies account for approximately 50% of all sonographically detected conditions, and hydronephrosis represents about two-thirds of these genitourinary abnormalities (1). Information from antenatal ultrasonography can be further complemented *in utero* with magnetic resonance imaging (MRI), and fetal bladder urine specimen measurements of electrolytes, osmolality, and β_2-microglobulin. *In utero* surgical therapy is also possible, although the benefits from fetal surgery of the urinary tract have not been proven and may have a high complication rate for both fetus and mother (2).

Understanding significant events of embryogenesis of the genitourinary tract is essential to understanding and interpreting findings seen with congenital urologic problems. The ureteral bud arises from the mesonephric duct at 4 to 5 weeks of gestation, the kidney begins to form at 6 weeks, and the bladder develops during the 6th to 7th week. The wolffian duct is incorporated into the bladder (Fig. 39.1). Urine production begins at the 10th week of gestation, but the urinary tract is generally not well imaged until weeks 15 to 16 when the urinary tract is evident on antenatal US (3). Disordered embryogenesis of the ureter or kidney is responsible for a number of anomalies. Most genitourinary anomalies occur sporadically, but some abnormalities are familial or are associated with chromosomal abnormalities. The concept of CAKUT (congenital abnormalities of the kidney and urinary tract) suggests that many seemingly sporadic problems are actually familial (4).

PRENATAL AND POSTNATAL IMAGING

Fetal anomalies of the urinary tract are detected in 1% to 3% of pregnancies (5,6). Urologic diagnostic imaging in the fetus, newborn, and infant has been transformed by the use of US through development as well as after birth.

Many infants with congenital genitourinary conditions have extensive prenatal imaging; so that a presumed diagnosis of urologic conditions, including those incompatible with life, may be determined well before delivery so that families and health professionals can prepare for postnatal management of these varied conditions.

Prenatal Ultrasonography

The advent of high-resolution, real-time US allows antenatal diagnosis of many anomalies of the urinary tract. The hope that antenatal intervention might improve outcome has not been realized. Maternal morbidity with intervention has been reported to be 4% to 5% (7), and there are no clear examples of improvement in fetal outcome with these interventions.

There is no advantage to early delivery for most genitourinary conditions, reinforcing that timing of delivery in fetuses is determined best by obstetric factors rather than fetal concerns (8).

Fetal kidneys, using improved US, can be identified by the end of the first trimester of pregnancy.

Several classification systems developed to standardize interpretation of US findings in prenatal and postnatal studies may help predict improvement or resolution of hydronephrosis and possibly predict adverse outcomes of hydronephrosis, such as febrile urinary tract infection (UTI) or possible surgical intervention. Two systems are commonly used: The Society for Fetal Urology (SFU) Hydronephrosis Grading System and the Urinary Tract Dilation (UTD) Classification System (5,9).

SFU, developed in 1993, grades the severity of the hydronephrosis based on the extent of renal pelvis and calyceal dilatation and parenchymal thinning or atrophy and attempts to standardize the varying terminology used to describe hydronephrosis on US (10). Measuring the anteroposterior renal pelvis diameter (APD) of the renal pelvis has been used to predict the need for postnatal treatment; generally, if APD is greater than 5 mm in the second trimester or 10 mm late in the third, it may indicate obstruction of the renal pelvis. But not all patients with high APDs will have significant hydronephrosis or need surgical treatment.

The UTD, formulated from several medical societies in 2014, classifies US abnormalities by APD, associated renal calyceal dilation, renal parenchymal appearance and thickness, and associated bladder and ureteral abnormalities. This classification system may limit need for voiding cystourethrogram (VCUG) and antibiotic prophylaxis. Higher graded groups, especially if associated with ureteral dilation or bladder abnormalities, benefit most from VCUG, and use of prophylaxis may decrease febrile UTIs (5,11).

While hydronephrosis is fairly common during pregnancy, most patients with prenatal hydronephrosis have mild hydronephrosis postnatally with resolution without intervention usually in early childhood (ages 2 to 3 years). In a recent study, only 8% of patients in an SFU registry required surgical intervention, with 13 of 14 patients having pyeloplasty. Only 15% had vesicoureteral reflux (VUR) on VCUG with only one patient requiring ureteral reimplantation (6).

The newer classification system (UTD) is more complex than the SFU system, but it has more detail for bladder and ureteral abnormalities and is more predictive for febrile UTI in higher grade abnormalities. The UTD system may be helpful in limiting postnatal antibiotic prophylaxis and VCUG.

Renal duplication anomaly, with or without dilation to either moiety, can be detected by prenatal US.

Dilations of the lower pole system usually may be due to ureteropelvic junction obstruction (UPJO) or VUR. Obstruction of the upper pole system are frequently associated with ureteral dilation down to the bladder and may also have a ureterocele or an obstructed ectopic ureter.

Solid intrarenal lesions found on prenatal imaging may represent mesoblastic nephromas, with neuroblastoma seen less frequently.

Ureteral dilation can be massive and may be confused with bowel on sonography; dilated ureters may be distinguished from bowel as a dilated ureter may be followed from the kidney down to the bladder or in the reverse direction and generally do not peristalse. Ureteral walls generally are not as thick as bowel on US, but this is not consistent. Bilateral hydroureter may be associated with bilateral ureterovesical obstruction, high-grade VUR, ectopic ureters, posterior urethral valves (PUVs), obstructing ureterocele, or prune belly syndrome (PBS).

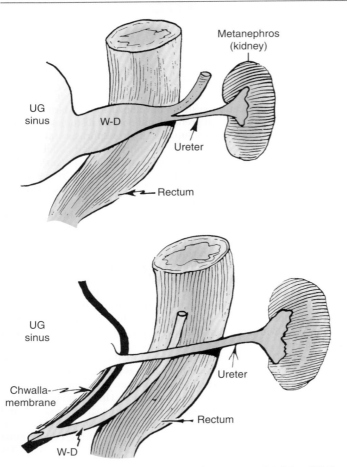

FIGURE 39.1 Incorporation of the wolffian (i.e., mesonephric) duct (W-D) into the UG sinus. (Reprinted from Kelalis PP, King LR, Belman AB, eds. *Clinical pediatric urology*, vol. 1. Philadelphia, PA: WB Saunders, 1976:504. Copyright © 1976 Elsevier. With permission.)

In a male fetus, a thick-walled, enlarged bladder may be secondary to PUVs or PBS, especially if a keyhole posterior urethra is found on US. In females, an enlarged bladder is more likely due to megalocystis–microcolon hypoperistalsis syndrome. Ureteroceles can be identified by US in the bladder. Exstrophy of the bladder may be inferred with no identifiable bladder on serial US or MRI. Following the hypogastric vessels, aorta and branching renal vessels help define which condition may be present but require serial studies to better predict these conditions postnatally (Fig. 39.2A and B).

Conditions associated with hydronephrosis and normal amounts of amniotic fluid usually carry a good prognosis, while those with increased renal echogenicity, cystic changes, and decreased amniotic fluid generally carry a poor prognosis for pulmonary maturation and renal function.

Postnatal Imaging

US and VCUG are not dependent on renal function and are the mainstay of postnatal diagnostic imaging for genitourinary conditions. Renal scintigraphy depends on renal function and may not yield reliable information in the first few weeks of life but may be needed at a relatively young age to determine if there is any renal function in an otherwise grossly abnormal kidney. MRI, magnetic resonance urography (MRU), and computed tomography (CT) imaging may be required if anatomic detail or function of the urinary system is difficult to determine by less-invasive modalities.

ANOMALIES OF THE KIDNEY

Understanding normal embryogenesis is helpful in understanding genitourinary anomalies, and associated problems occurring during fetal development.

Renal Agenesis

Renal agenesis must be considered postnatally when Potter facies (Fig. 39.3) are noted, when there is no urinary output within 24 to 48 hours, or when there is ventilatory failure with hypoplastic lungs on chest radiographs. Postnatally, this diagnosis can be confirmed on US with absence of identifiable kidneys or renal

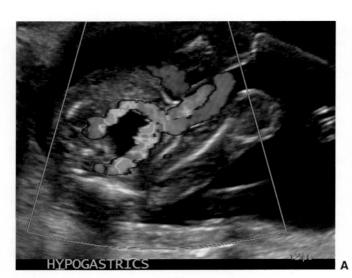

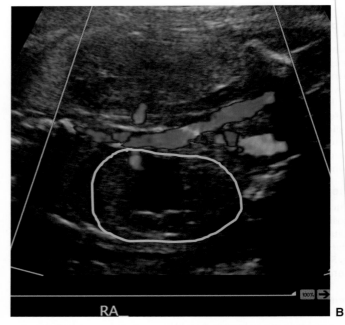

FIGURE 39.2 A: Prenatal ultrasound in an 18-week fetus demonstrating the presence of bladder between the hypogastric vessels. **B:** Same fetus at 22 weeks of gestation with right hydronephrosis (circle) with renal arteries seen with Doppler measurements.

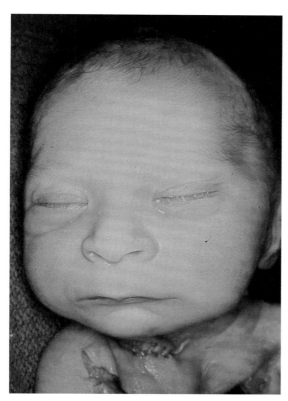

FIGURE 39.3 Potter facies, found in stillborn infant with bilateral renal agenesis, due to compression of fetus from absence of amniotic fluid.

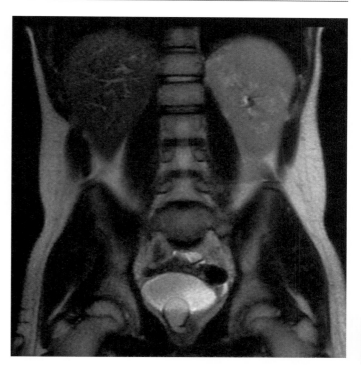

FIGURE 39.4 Renal agenesis on the right with associated seminal vesicle cyst due to abnormal formation of the wolffian duct.

vessels with Doppler, and the absence of urine in the bladder. Renal scintigraphy can be used to prove that there is no identifiable functioning renal tissue; generally, a technetium-99m dimercaptosuccinic acid (DMSA) renal scan is obtained to look for any renal function. When the postnatal diagnosis of bilateral renal agenesis is confirmed, attempts at life support, usually initiated because of respiratory distress, should be abandoned as obtaining any measurable renal function for electrolyte and fluid balance is extremely unlikely and long-term dialysis and renal transplant is very difficult in this group. There have been reports of familial inheritance of bilateral renal agenesis, with up to 3% of siblings of probands having bilateral renal agenesis (12).

Unilateral renal agenesis incidence is roughly 1 in 500 to 1,500 (13). A higher incidence of associated contralateral renal abnormality, either obstructive or reflux-related, is found in these patients when compared to the general population. One-third of patients with a solitary kidney may require surgical intervention on that kidney. Unilateral renal agenesis (Fig. 39.4) may be associated with congenital scoliosis and with vaginal and uterine agenesis in females. It is the most common nonskeletal anomaly seen with imperforate anus. Unilateral renal agenesis is not thought to affect longevity or health as long as the remaining kidney is normal.

Renal and ureteral agenesis with absence of the ipsilateral genital ducts in the male arise if the mesonephros does not develop; if the mesonephric duct develops but the mesonephros does not, there will be renal agenesis with the genital ducts present with a possible blind-ending ureter. In instances with congenital absence of the vas deferens with accompanied renal agenesis, the ipsilateral mesonephric duct does not develop.

Brenner et al. found that most people with unilateral renal agenesis do not develop progressive renal disease. However, long-standing hyperfiltration in people with a solitary kidney from any etiology can cause glomerular hypertension, which may cause progressive glomerular damage with proteinuria and renal insuf-

ficiency (14). Goldfarb et al. (15) reviewed renal function in donor nephrectomy patients and found that renal function was well preserved in most donors over prolonged follow-up averaging 25 years with some increased proteinuria in some donors but with only marginal significance in the group as a whole. Muzaale et al. (16) showed that there was slight increase in the incidence of end-stage renal disease (ESRD) in kidney donors when compared over 15 years to healthy nondonors, but the overall risk of ESRD in donors was only 30.8/10,000.

It is postulated that chronic hypertension and renal disease is associated with low birth weight infants (LBW), primarily due to prematurity and intrauterine growth restriction (IUGR). Because these infants are born before developing a full 36-week complement of nephrons, these infants have lower than expected numbers of nephrons and have associated abnormal renal development and function. These premature LBW or IUGR infants may have a higher risk of developing hypertension and renal disease as adults (17).

Renal Ectopia and Fusion

Failure of renal ascent will result in a pelvic kidney and may be associated with vaginal or vertebral anomalies (18). If the two metanephrogenic masses come into contact with each other in the pelvis, they could fuse forming a pancake or a horseshoe kidney (18) (Fig. 39.5A–C). Horseshoe kidneys are found with increased frequency in girls with Turner syndrome. There can be an increased incidence of UPJO in horseshoe kidneys as the renal pelves do not drain dependently as they would in an otherwise normally placed kidney (18). Some patients with horseshoe kidneys may have increased stone formation, due to relative urinary stasis from nondependent urine drainage.

Embryogenesis of crossed ectopia, with or without fusion, is harder to explain but might result from lateral bending and rotation of the tail bud of the embryo altering the course of renal ascent (19). The left kidney more commonly crosses to the right side than vice versa. (20). There is also an increased incidence of VUR and UPJO in crossed ectopic kidneys (18). Patients with

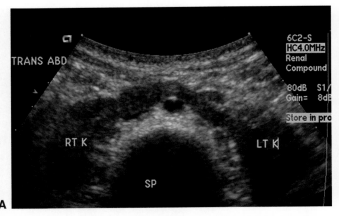

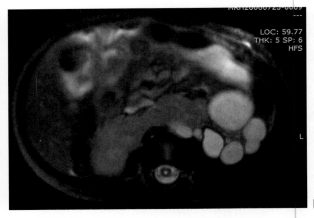

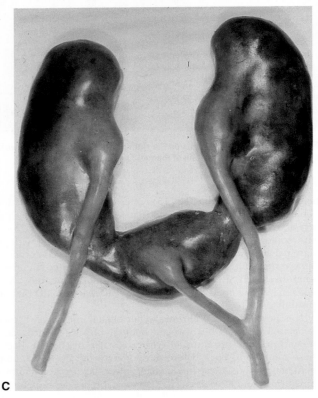

FIGURE 39.5 A: Ultrasound image of horseshoe kidney with isthmus over the spine. **B:** MRI image (T2 image) of horseshoe kidney with multicystic component on the left. **C:** Gross specimen of horseshoe kidney with partial duplication (fused ureters) on the left.

crossed ectopia have an increased incidence of skeletal and cardiac abnormalities (19).

Renal malrotation, or incomplete rotation, occurs when the ascending kidney maintains its early fetal (anteroposterior) orientation with the renal pelvis anteriorly directed. Malrotation is present in fusion anomalies as well as in pelvic and crossed ectopias, but it is also seen in kidneys located in the renal fossa. Incomplete rotation is of no clinical significance but may make interpretation of imaging difficult and should be considered when planning reconstructive procedures. Postnatal MRU may be needed to better define the renal anatomy, particularly if considering surgical reconstruction.

Abnormalities of renal position (i.e., ectopia) are interesting anomalies but are generally not clinically relevant and may be discovered only after renal trauma (i.e., hematuria), a palpable mass, or some associated urologic abnormality. The ectopic kidney may be located in the chest or the pelvis. Thoracic kidneys usually are associated with eventration of the diaphragm and are of no clinical significance except being found on a chest radiograph. Pelvic ectopia is the most common ectopic position and may have associated VUR or UPJO (18). Girls with müllerian

anomalies also have an increased incidence of pelvic kidney compared to the general population. Finding a pelvic kidney in a girl warrants further investigation of the genital tract to uncover associated anomalies.

Supernumerary Kidney

The presence of a supernumerary (i.e., third) renal mass is a very rare anomaly; the clinical significance of this is determined by associated pathologic conditions (21). The supernumerary kidney usually is small and more often caudal than cranial to the normally placed kidney. Many patients and some physicians confuse a supernumerary kidney with duplication of the collecting system and incorrectly refer to ureteral duplication as a third kidney (Fig. 39.6).

Cystic Disease

Renal cystic diseases are a group of disorders frequently presenting in the neonatal period and are increasingly diagnosed with antenatal US. Table 39.1 is a classification that is clinically useful for accurate diagnosis of these conditions for prognosis and for genetic counseling.

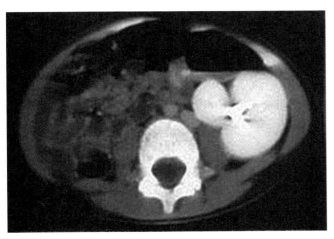

FIGURE 39.6 CT scan of supernumerary kidney on the left (smaller, medial segment). (From Docimo SG, Canning DA, Khoury A, eds. *Clinical pediatric urology.* London: Informa Publishers, 2007:289. Reprinted by permission of Taylor & Francis Ltd, www.tandfonline.com. (Chapter 19, Figure 19.6I))

Autosomal Recessive Polycystic Kidney Disease

Autosomal recessive polycystic kidney disease (ARPCKD) is an inherited disorder whose mode of transmission follows an autosomal recessive pattern. Its reported incidence is between 1 in 6,000 and 1 in 14,000 pregnancies. These kidneys are very large often occupying the entire retroperitoneum (Fig. 39.7A–C). The cysts

TABLE 39.1

Classification of Renal Cystic Disease

Polycystic disease
    Autosomal recessive
    Autosomal dominant

Renal cortical cysts in hereditary syndromes
    Tuberous sclerosis
    von Hippel-Lindau disease
    Meckel syndrome
    Zellweger cerebrohepatorenal syndrome
    Jeune asphyxiating thoracic dysplasia
    Syndromes of multiple malformations that include cortical cysts

Renal medullary cysts
    Familial juvenile nephronophthisis
    Medullary cystic disease
    Renal–retinal dysplasia
    Medullary sponge disease

Renal dysplasia
    Multicystic kidney disease
    Other cystic dysplasias
    Multilocular mesoblastic nephroma

Other cystic diseases
    Simple cysts, single or multiple
    Unilateral segmental cystic disease

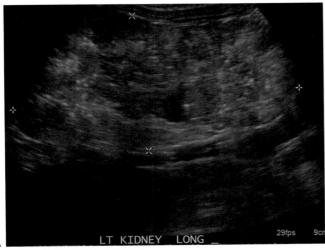

LT KIDNEY LONG   29fps   9cm

A

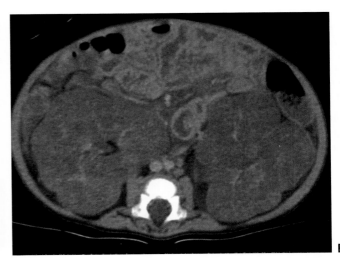

B

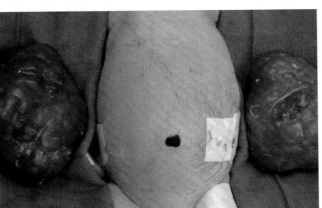

C

FIGURE 39.7 A: Ultrasound image of ARPCK (autosomal recessive polycystic kidney). Note the bright echoes with back shadowing in the kidney from the small cysts. **B:** Noncontrast CT scan of the infant with ARPCK disease showing large striated kidneys filling abdomen. **C:** The infant showing the large kidneys next to the relatively small abdomen after removing both ARPCKs.

are small and are actually enlargements of the collecting ducts. The liver is almost always abnormal. Periportal hepatic fibrosis may be a significant part of this complex. Death, if occurring in the neonatal period, is generally due to either renal or pulmonary failure. Pulmonary failure can be reversed by removing both kidneys so that the lungs can expand. If nephrectomy is done using an extraperitoneal approach, peritoneal dialysis can be used to maintain homeostasis until the child can receive a renal transplant. Those who survive the neonatal period without the need for nephrectomy usually will exhibit decreased renal function and hypertension, but liver failure due to hepatic fibrosis may be the most prominent part of the clinical picture (22). Some of these children may be considered for transplantation of the organs most affected as many survive past infancy with improved medical care. Imaging studies, including antenatal or postnatal US and CT or MRI, usually are diagnostic with very large kidneys demonstrating a sunburst streaking pattern or small echodense or "bright" cysts within the kidneys.

Autosomal Dominant Polycystic Kidney Disease

Autosomal dominant polycystic kidney disease (ADPCKD), inherited in a dominant fashion, is more common than the recessive form. Typically, it presents in adulthood but can be diagnosed at younger ages due to improved imaging techniques. Presenting symptoms with this disorder include hypertension, hematuria, UTI, or renal failure. When this problem is found in childhood, it may present as an abdominal mass or may be found with ultrasound as an antenatal evaluation, screening for polycystic disease, or coincidentally with US being obtained for other reasons. Imaging studies are diagnostic when multiple variably sized cysts are found within one or both kidneys, which may splay or distort the collecting system (Fig. 39.8A and B). A CT or MRI may be confirmatory for the diagnosis, if ADPCKD is suspected, by finding multiple cysts in one or both kidneys that may not be well demonstrated by US only. There may be associated hepatic cysts, but liver failure is not usually found in this disorder. Microdissection studies have shown that the cysts are as a result of abnormal branching of the collecting tubules and cystic dilations of portions of the nephron. Generally, symptomatic renal disease does not develop until middle to late adult life.

Other Cystic Lesions

Tuberous sclerosis can mimic both ARPCKD and ADPCKD where lesions are grossly similar (23) (Fig. 39.9A and B). Microscopically, lesions characteristic of tuberous sclerosis will be seen on biopsy of the affected kidneys. Angiomyolipomas (i.e., renal hamartomas) are the more commonly seen renal lesions in patients with tuberous sclerosis. Usually, there are other family members with this disease and there may be associated skin, brain, and cardiac lesions. Genetic evaluation is warranted in the infant if there is a strong family history.

Multicystic Dysplastic Kidney Disease

Multicystic dysplastic kidney (MCDK) disease, with a frequency of 1 in 1,000 to 4,300 pregnancies (24,25) is the most common form of cystic disease seen in neonates. Originally described in 1836 by Cruveilhier (24) and further defined by Spence, this may be unilateral or bilateral where the entire kidney or part of the kidney is replaced by variably sized cysts. Multicystic kidney disease may be secondary to ureteral obstruction early in gestation or due to disordered induction of the metanephros by a faulty ureteral bud (26).

Grossly, there is no recognizable renal tissue present, but microscopically, there may be dysplastic renal elements in septa between the cysts (Fig. 39.10A–C). Bilateral multicystic kidney disease, like bilateral renal agenesis, is incompatible with life. MCDK is sporadic and is not inherited. Some multicystic kidneys involute, probably by absorption of the cyst fluid. Involution can occur antenatally or in the first few months of life but may take many years to completely resolve. Some cases of presumed renal agenesis may be involuted multicystic kidneys. Multicystic kidneys are generally detected with antenatal US, some diagnosed early in gestation, but some still present during infancy as palpable masses. US will demonstrate multiple, variably sized cysts in a random pattern (Fig. 39.10A and B), with the affected kidney generally without function on renal scan.

Traditionally, nephrectomy was performed for MCDK. Multicystic Kidney Registry collected data on cases followed with observation found that up only to 50% of MCDKs for 3 to 5 years had no change in the multicystic kidney appearance on US although involution may occur (37). The most commonly associated anomalies are contralateral VUR (7% to 26%), contralateral UPJO (1.5% to 5%), and contralateral UVJO (2%) (25).

Currently, pediatric urologists advocate observation because the incidence of sequelae such as infection, pain, hypertension, or malignancy is very low. The major controversy currently is the extent of radiographic study for associated VUR, the duration and

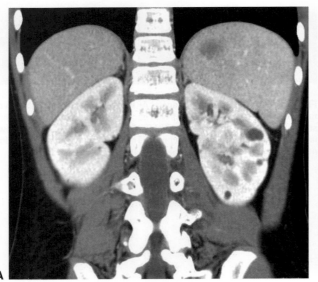
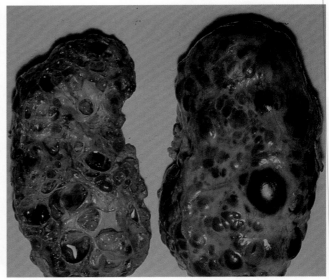

FIGURE 39.8 A: CT scan confirming ADPCK (autosomal dominant polycystic kidney) disease of young child with prior ultrasound demonstrating small cysts in both the kidneys. **B:** Gross specimen of ADPCKs.

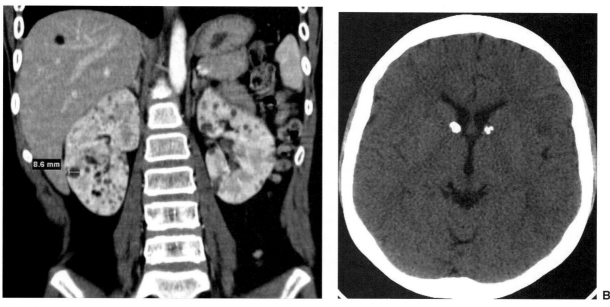

FIGURE 39.9 A: CT scan with contrast in a patient with tuberous sclerosis. Note that the appearance is similar to ADPCK on CT. Angiomyolipomas are not found in this patient. **B:** CT scan of the head demonstrating calcified subependymal nodules lateral to the ventricles. These are found in about 70% of cases.

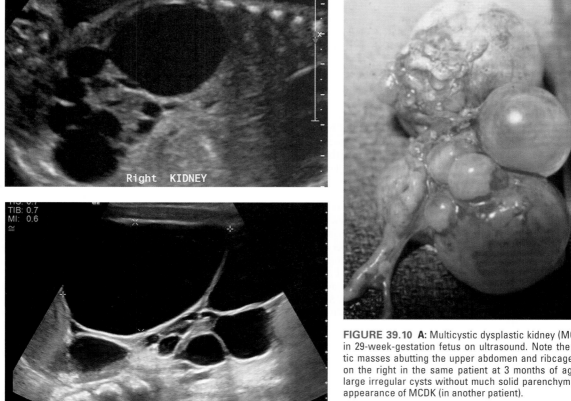

FIGURE 39.10 A: Multicystic dysplastic kidney (MCDK) found in 29-week-gestation fetus on ultrasound. Note the large cystic masses abutting the upper abdomen and ribcage. **B:** MCDK on the right in the same patient at 3 months of age showing large irregular cysts without much solid parenchyma. **C:** Gross appearance of MCDK (in another patient).

THE NEWBORN INFANT

extent of follow-up testing, and use of prophylactic antibiotics to prevent possible febrile UTI.

In a recent meta-analysis, the risk of hypertension in this group was similar to the risk in the general population (26). Additionally, in the same review, the reported risk of Wilms tumor (WT) in MCKD was <1 in 2,000 cases of MCDK and their review of 26 relevant articles comprising over 1,000 patients found no cases of WT.

Since VUR was only found in 21% to 26% in two studies, with low-grade VUR in most cases (only 11% having grade IV reflux) (26), routine VCUG is not indicated unless another indication for VCUG exists (26–28). Other authors reviewed their VUR diagnosis and UTI experience and found that the risk of febrile UTI or need for surgical correction was only 9% of the patients with diagnosed VUR (29).

VCUG should be reserved for patients with potential bladder or ureteral abnormalities, such as contralateral hydroureteronephrosis or those that actually develop signs and symptoms of UTI, particularly a febrile UTI (25). There is also a risk that patients may develop a febrile UTI after invasive VCUG testing, whether or not VUR is found.

Many of these kidneys (60% to 89%) tend to involute generally by 3 to 5 years of age if smaller kidneys at diagnosis (<5 to 6 cm size) (24,25,30). Most children with unilateral MCDK will have compensatory contralateral renal hypertrophy, which is a good prognostic sign for long-term renal health (24,26,29,30).

Duration of follow-up may be up to 3 to 5 years of age with some of follow-up with US imaging done by the patient's primary care provider (PCP) and not necessarily by urology with US done generally every 6 months until age 3 and yearly US up until age 5 years to follow involution for the extremely rare occurrence of malignant transformation. Antibiotic prophylaxis is not indicated for MCDK alone but recommended only if there are associated bladder or contralateral ureteral abnormalities putting the patient at risk for febrile UTIs.

ANOMALIES OF THE URETERS AND BLADDER

Duplication and Triplication of the Ureters

Multiple ureteral buds or premature division of the ureteral bud could produce ureteral duplication or triplication (31). If there are multiple ureteral buds, one bud may meet degenerating rather than normal nephrogenic tissue increasing incidence of renal dysplasia generally in the upper pole of duplicated systems. Duplication of the urinary collecting system is one of the more common abnormalities seen in the urinary tract; its occurrence is about 0.8% (31). Approximately 12% of siblings and parents were affected with ureteral duplication when reviewing family inheritance probands (12). Duplication can be either complete or incomplete. Incomplete duplication is usually of no clinical significance, although there can be ureteroureteral reflux between the two limbs of the partial duplication resulting in dilation of one of the ureters, usually the lower one. Complete duplication occurs once in every 500 cases (31). Complete duplication is usually of no clinical significance but may occasionally have a higher incidence of VUR or obstruction.

VUR probably is more common with ureteral duplication and usually occurs into the lower moiety of the duplicated system (Figs. 39.11A–C and 39.12). Duplication is seen in approximately one in five people with VUR with much higher incidence than the general population. The grade of reflux associated with a complete duplication is usually higher than VUR in a single system. Obstruction is more common if the upper moiety of complete duplication is abnormal. Both obstruction and VUR associated with duplications may present as either mass lesions or urosepsis but are usually first found on antenatal imaging.

If the ureteral bud arises more cranially or caudally than normal, ureteral ectopia, VUR, or paraureteral diverticula might develop (32) (Figs. 39.13A–E and 39.14). Ectopic ureteroceles probably result from abnormalities of the ureteral bud and ureteral ectopia (Fig. 39.15A–C). Simple ureteroceles are thought to be produced by persistence of the Chwalla membrane (the membrane covering the distal end of the ureter during development).

Ureteral obstruction, when present, usually occurs either at the ureteropelvic or at the ureterovesical junction and rarely occurs in the mid ureter. These obstructions usually are intrinsic in nature, and the ureter may have a normal or reduced caliber externally.

Bladder Anomalies

Agenesis of the bladder could result if the allantoic stalk failed to develop (33); or it could occur if there is bilateral failure of ureteral migration resulting in bilateral ureteral ectopia, since ureteral migration is necessary for trigone formation and may also be necessary for enlargement of the allantoic stalk (34). Urachal anomalies occur because of a general mesodermal failure, as in PBS, or because of delayed urachal closure (see Fig. 39.23). Duplications of the bladder and urethra can be associated with duplications of the hindgut and lower spinal cord. It may be that splitting of the hind end of the embryo might be responsible for this anomaly (35).

PUVs probably result from abnormal insertion and persistence of the mesonephric ducts distal to the müllerian tubercle (type I), or from persistence of the cloacal membrane (type III) (36). Type II valves likely are not an obstructing lesion (see Fig. 39.24).

Ureteral Ectopia

Ureteral ectopia exists when the ureter opens in a position other than its normal location at the corner of the trigone. Ectopia may occur in ureters of single or duplex kidneys (Fig. 39.13A–E). The most common form of ureteral ectopia is lateral ureteral ectopia, where the ureteral orifice lies within the bladder lateral to its normal position. This is the etiologic mechanism for primary VUR (see "Vesicoureteral Reflux"). Significant medial or distal ureteral ectopia is less common than lateral ureteral ectopia but may cause variable clinical conditions depending on the location of the ureteral orifice and the gender of the patient. An abnormal proximal budding of the ureteral bud on the mesonephric duct allows the ureteral bud to remain in prolonged contact with the wolffian duct, so that the medially ectopic ureteral orifice may open anywhere along the course of the wolffian duct (Fig. 39.14). In males, this includes the posterior urethra, seminal vesicles, vas deferens, or epididymis. In females, the ectopic ureter may open into the urethra, the uterus, or proximal vagina, or along the course of Gartner duct in the anterolateral wall of the vagina. If a medially ectopic ureter opens within the confines of the bladder, generally, there are no abnormal clinical sequelae. If the ureter opens at the bladder neck location, obstruction of the involved renal unit or VUR may occur.

In females, ectopic ureteral orifices located distal to the internal sphincter mechanism of the bladder neck can cause incontinence (37). Older girls usually present with constant urine leak or dampness and are otherwise asymptomatic with normal voiding patterns but may have a persistent perineal rash. Infant girls may also have a purulent vaginal discharge if the system becomes infected. It is difficult to determine if an ectopically located ureter is causing constant urinary leakage in girls who are not toilet trained. Physical examination suggests the diagnosis if urine can be seen welling up in the vagina or if a spurt of urine is seen coming from an ectopic perineal ureteral orifice. Many ectopic ureters are not diagnosed by physical findings alone. Eighty percent of ectopic ureters arise from the upper pole segment of a

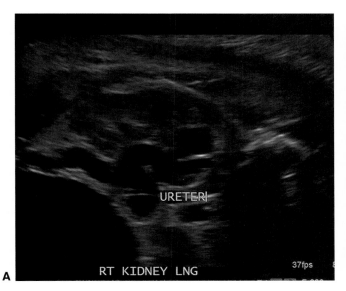

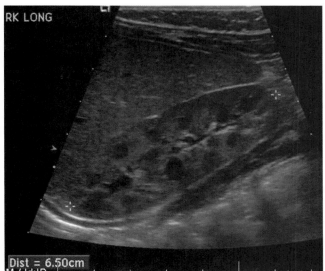

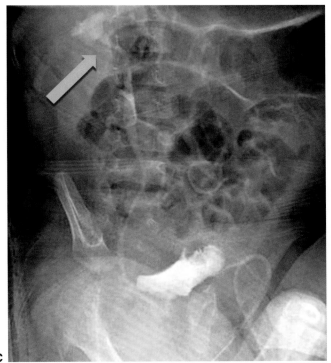

FIGURE 39.11 A: Duplicated collecting system and ureters on the right kidney with possible obstruction of upper system found on fetal ultrasound at 37 weeks of gestation. **B:** Duplicated collecting system on the right in a different patient. Dense band of renal parenchyma separates two slightly dilated renal pelves. **C:** The same patient with upper pole vesicourinary reflux (VUR). Generally, reflux is more common in lower pole duplicated systems. (*Arrow* marks the vesicoureteral reflux to the upper ureter and renal moiety.)

total ureteral duplication. US may suggest a duplicated system with ureteral ectopia, but frequently, CT or MRI may be necessary to define the ectopic ureteral anatomy. An ectopic segment may be visible on CT or MRU even if it functions poorly and an associated dilated ureter may be found and followed to potential area where it terminates. Having a high index of suspicion of possible nonvisible duplication and being aware of radiographic clues, like a "drooping lily" collecting system seen on excretory urography or VUR on VCUG, may lead to the diagnosis. Because an ectopic vaginal ureter may drain a poorly functioning, nonvisualized, single renal unit, congenital absence of one kidney in a girl with incontinence requires a thorough investigation to find a poorly functioning contralateral kidney with an ectopic ureteral orifice. Renal scintigraphy using DMSA may find a functioning renal unit, but MRI may better delineate the anatomic details of a small poorly functioning ectopic kidney.

Treatment of the ectopic ureter depends on the presence or absence of significant function in the involved renal unit. If the ureter drains an otherwise healthy system, ureteral reimplantation into the bladder will correct the problem and preserve maximal renal function. If the ureteral anomaly is associated with a duplex kidney, ipsilateral ureteroureterostomy may be performed whether or not there is good function in both segments of the kidney. Alternatively, excision of the involved segment may be performed if the involved renal unit functions poorly, but generally, this is not needed unless recurrent infection can be localized to the poorly functioning segment. The distal ureteral stump is left undisturbed to avoid or compromise the normal sphincter continence mechanism. Male infants with an ectopic ureter frequently present with antenatal ultrasound findings suggestive of ureteral dilatation, an abdominal mass, UTI, or epididymitis. In boys, an ectopic ureter will arise more frequently from a nonduplicated kid-

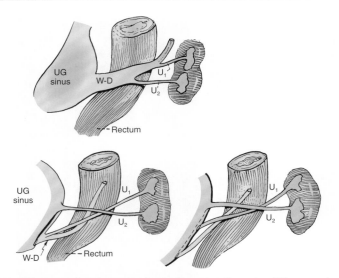

FIGURE 39.12 Development of ectopic ureter. U, ureter; UG, urogenital; W-D, wolffian duct. (Reprinted from Kelalis PP, King LR, Belman AB, eds. *Clinical pediatric urology*, vol. 1. Philadelphia, PA: WB Saunders, 1976:510. Copyright © 1976 Elsevier. With permission.)

ney and may drain into the male genital tract anywhere from the prostatic urethra to the epididymis. Treatment of ectopic ureters in males is similar to that for females.

Ureterocele

A ureterocele is a cystic dilation of the distal submucosal or intravesical portion of a ureter. Ureteroceles account for a broad spectrum of associated pathologic conditions and constitute a complex and confusing group of lower urinary tract anomalies (38).

Ureteroceles in children commonly involve the intravesical end of the upper pole ureter of a duplex kidney (i.e., ectopic ureterocele) but may involve a single-system ureter (i.e., simple ureterocele). Although simple ureteroceles involving a single system are more commonly seen in adults, they are usually not problematic in children. Conversely, ectopic ureteroceles, typically associated with duplication, are more commonly problematic and seen frequently in children. Ureteroceles occur in about 1 in every 4,000 births and generally more common in white ethnic groups. Postmortem occurrence has been recorded as 1 in 500 to 4,000. Ureteroceles are 4 to 6 times more common in females than in males. Orthotopic ureteroceles may represent about 17% to 35% of cases while ectopic ureteroceles occur about 80% in most pediatric series (27). The etiology of ureteroceles is uncertain. Failure

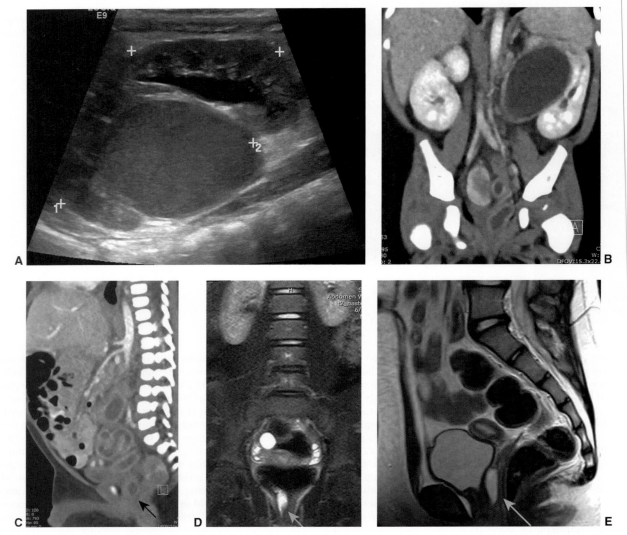

FIGURE 39.13 A: Duplicated collecting system on the left with purulent contents in upper pole and hydronephrosis without infection in lower pole. **B:** CT scan with contrast demonstrating obstructed left upper pole collecting system with ectopic ureter. Note there is a duplication on the right kidney as well. **C:** Ectopic obstructed ureter in the same patient found to be exiting near the prostate (*black arrow*). **D:** MRI study with contrast demonstrating an ectopic duplicated ureter from the right upper pole kidney entering the vagina (see *arrow*). **E:** MRI of the same patient **(D)** on T2-weighted images showing ectopic ureter entering vagina (see *arrow*).

MALE

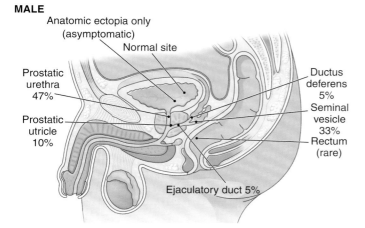

FEMALE

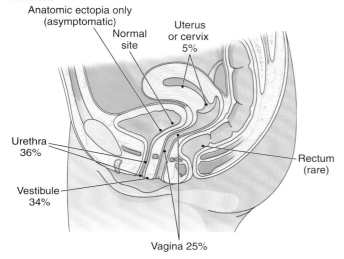

FIGURE 39.14 Sites of ectopic ureteral orifices and their relative frequencies of occurrence in men and women. (Reprinted from Gray SW, Skandalakis JE. *Embryology for surgeons*. Philadelphia, PA: WB Saunders, 1972:536, with permission. Copyright © 1972 Elsevier. With permission.)

of reabsorption of the Chwalla membrane over the ureteral orifice has been proposed as an obstructive etiology. Correct expression of several linking genes, including rearranged in transfection (Ret) and glial-derived neurotrophic factor (GDNF), are needed for ureteral bud and metanephric blastema interaction for normal kidney and ureteral formation. Abnormal interaction will give rise to the many disorders associated with CAKUT. Ureterocele development may be due to abnormal formation of the ureter and possibly include abnormal migration and incorporation of the developing ureter into the cloacal plate through abnormal interactions of multiple genetic, cellular and biochemical factors as yet to be defined (27).

Ureteroceles associated with a single-system ureter (i.e., simple ureteroceles) tend to be intravesical, in the normal position, and are more likely to be found in boys. Intravesical ureteroceles in children may be associated with hydronephrosis of the affected renal unit.

Ureteroceles may be associated with significant abnormalities of the upper and lower urinary tract. Ureteroceles originating from the upper pole ureter of a duplex kidney are frequently associated with secondary pathology, usually hydronephrosis, and impaired function or dysplasia of the upper pole system and

usually with obstruction or reflux in the ipsilateral lower pole system (Fig. 39.15A–C). Contralateral reflux or obstruction also may occur. The pathophysiology of associated findings is easily understood by recognizing that the ureterocele may dissect under the trigonal epithelium and deform the ipsilateral or contralateral ureterovesical junction, resulting in various combinations of VUR or obstruction in any or all of the ureters (28). Ten percent of ureteroceles occur bilaterally (38). A ureterocele prolapsing into the bladder neck or urethra may also block the bladder outlet causing bilateral hydronephrosis and bladder outlet obstruction with urinary retention, infection, and renal dysplasia (Fig. 39.16).

Most ureterocele cases today are diagnosed with antenatal ultrasound, while historically, the most common presentation was an infant with a febrile UTI. If the ureterocele prolapses into the urethra, voiding difficult or azotemia may prompt evaluation. Ureterocele is the most common cause of urinary retention in the female infant. Rarely, a ureterocele will prolapse through the external urethral meatus in a female presenting as an introital mass.

Classically, the diagnosis of a ureterocele is fairly straightforward. Renal and bladder US will show upper tract dilation and the ureterocele wall in the bladder. This can be seen antenatally. VCUG is necessary to establish the presence or absence of associated VUR, potential obstruction of the bladder neck, and bladder wall abnormalities including quality of the detrusor muscle backing the ureterocele. A renal scan can determine if there is reasonable function of the involved upper pole segment and any measurable obstruction of any of the segments, and may be helpful in determining the best surgical approach. If a lower ureteral-only approach is performed, it is not necessary to obtain renal function imaging as it is irrelevant to look for function of the affected segment. If partial nephrectomy is considered due to suspected poor function in the affected segment, a renal scan should be obtained to determine if the segment warrants reconstruction or removal. Many urologists decompress and drain the segment with lower or possibly upper ureteral reconstruction (ureteroureterostomy or ureteropyelostomy) and leave the segment intact as malignant transformation has not generally been reported in these segments.

The age and clinical condition of the patient, the presence or absence of significant function in the involved nephroureteral unit, and the presence of reflux or obstruction in the ipsilateral or contralateral uninvolved ureters all influence the choice of therapy.

With the advent of smaller cystoscopes and small cautery electrodes or endoscopic needles, transurethral incision or puncture of ureteroceles has become more common in infancy and at later presentation as definitive treatment of ureterocele with associated urinary obstruction. Most infants tolerate the procedure well with improved hydronephrosis, but up to 25% of patients can develop VUR to the upper pole moiety subtending the ureterocele (39). Resolution of this new VUR has occurred, but a significant number of children will require further urinary tract reconstruction if they have VUR with recurrent febrile UTIs. Interestingly, most ureterocele patients with single ureteral systems did not require any further surgery. Secondary procedures, including reimplantation, ureterocele reconstruction, and rarely upper pole removal, occurred only with duplicated systems or when associated with ectopic urinary system with ureterocele (39).

Placement of a temporary percutaneous nephrostomy into the involved renal unit may rarely be needed in a critically ill patient.

The best definitive treatment continues to be debated. Many intravesical single-system ureteroceles do not require any surgical treatment.

Treatment options for secondary procedures after ureterocele puncture have included various combinations of partial nephrec-

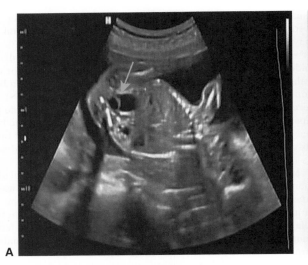

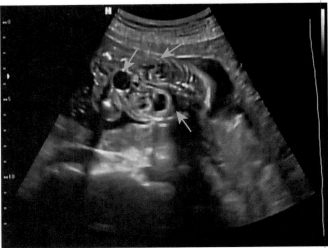

FIGURE 39.15 A: A 22-week fetus with ureterocele seen on ultrasonographic study (see *arrow*). **B:** A 22-week fetus with ureterocele and bilateral duplication with hydronephrosis on both upper and lower poles of the kidneys (see *arrows*). **C:** Postnatal voiding cystourethrogram (VCUG) demonstrating bilateral grade 5 VUR in all four ureters and an ectopic ureterocele that prolapses into the urethra (see *arrows*).

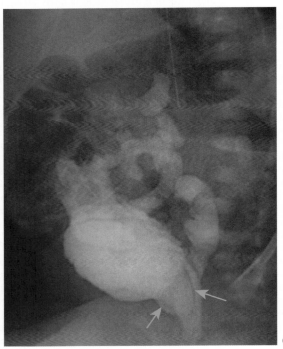

tomy, ureterectomy, marsupialization or excision of the uretero-cele, ureteroneocystostomy, and ureteroureterostomy.

Ureteropelvic Junction Obstruction

Obstruction at the ureteropelvic junction probably is the most common cause of a palpable abdominal mass in the newborn and is the most common cause of antenatal hydronephrosis requiring surgical treatment. This usually is the result of narrowing of the ureter at the junction of the renal pelvis with the ureter. Because the renal pelvis is compliant, there can be a great deal of renal preservation despite massive dilation of the kidney behind the obstruction (Fig. 39.17A–D).

Diagnosis of UPJO can be inferred sonographically where there is a sonolucent central mass within the renal area surrounded by thin renal parenchyma (Fig. 39.17A–D). Grading severity of hydronephrosis and renal parenchymal thickness with either the UTD or SFU grading systems is done to determine if the kidney is likely obstructed and requires surgical repair (Fig. 39.18). VUR

can be excluded from the differential diagnosis using VCUG but is generally not necessary unless there is suspected bladder or distal ureteral pathology. The relative function of the obstructed kidney can be determined by radionuclide scanning or MRU (Fig. 39.17D). Diuretic radionuclide scintigraphy can help esti-mate the relative renal function as well as determine if there is obstruction associated with renal pelvis dilatation. If there is significant dilatation associated with relative obstruction, there will be retention of the radionuclide behind the obstructed ure-teral segment, but if there is no associated obstruction, the diuretic given allows prompt washout of the radionuclide. For valid results, the infant or young patient must be adequately hydrated and have adequate bladder drainage to prevent false interpretation of obstruction due to either relative dehydration or bladder disten-tion (40). In most cases, hydronephrosis in the newborn is phys-iologically insignificant, and will generally stabilize or improve with time without treatment. Obstructive hydronephrosis at the ureteropelvic junction requires repair, generally dismembered pyeloplasty, which may be performed with open or laparoscopic

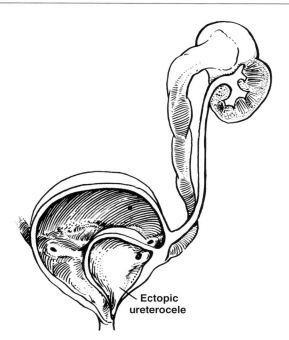

FIGURE 39.16 Ectopic ureterocele. (Reprinted with permission from the Journal of the American College of Surgeons, formerly Surgery Gynecology & Obstetrics, from Malek RS, Kelalis PP, Burke EC, et al. Simple and ectopic ureterocele in infancy and childhood. *Surg Gynecol Obstet* 1972;134:611.)

techniques to improve drainage and occasionally improve renal function. Robotic laparoscopic pyeloplasty is becoming more common but generally is more difficult in smaller patients and is generally not indicated in an infant or young child due to their small size and the relatively longer surgical and anesthesia times required. Some centers are performing more robotic procedures on young patients with improved surgical and anesthesia times obtaining successful results. Despite increased robotic experience in smaller children, open surgical repair is still the mainstay of treatment for UPJO in infancy.

Ureterovesical Obstruction

Obstruction at the ureterovesical junction is not as common as UPJO. Lower ureteral obstruction may present as marked hydroureteronephrosis (i.e., a mass) but may sometimes present as urinary infection or with associated urolithiasis (Fig. 39.19A and B).

As with UPJO, not all hydroureteronephrosis is physiologically significant, and some patients require no treatment. VCUG is recommended in patients with significant hydroureteronephrosis to evaluate for associated VUR or other bladder pathology. Radionuclide scanning with diuretics may help diagnose physiologic obstruction. MRU with intravenous contrast may be necessary to better define the anatomy and possible area of obstruction in cases of lower ureteral obstruction (41). Rarely, an antegrade pyelogram with a pressure perfusion study is necessary to determine if there is a significant narrow segment at the ureterovesical junction. These lesions, if obstructive, may be treated by a variety of procedures including excision of the obstructing segment, tailoring or tapering of the dilated ureter, or reimplantation of the ureter into the bladder. Alternatively, balloon dilation of the obstructed distal ureter with ureteral stenting with one or two stents has been advocated for surgical correction of lower urinary tract obstruction. While long-term results of this technique are not yet fully described, there appears to be some reasonable long-term success, up to 90% in one study (7). At the minimum, there may be enough improvement of the degree of ureteral dilatation by the bladder to allow ureteral reimplantation without tapering, if further definitive surgery is needed later. Temporizing cutaneous ureterostomy may be needed in the infant or neonate if marked obstruction or associated high-grade VUR is present with recurrent febrile UTI. Recently, temporizing ureteral implantation into the bladder bypassing the obstructed area (42) or performing a modified ureteral reimplantation bypassing the obstructed ureteral segment using a long but rolled intravesical neo-ureteral orifice in the bladder (43) have been described. Both of these techniques have the advantage of directly connecting the ureter to the bladder obviating a constantly draining cutaneous ureteral stoma, continuing to allow bladder cycling with some improvement in the degree of hydroureter over time making later reimplantation less likely to require tapering. In the case of the modified ureteral orthotopic reimplantation procedure with the nipple ureteral orifice, some of the patients had no need for further surgery as most of the patients had no obstruction or VUR on long-term follow-up (43).

Vesicoureteral Reflux

VUR is the most common abnormality of the urinary system seen in children; it may occur in 1 of 100 births (44). The actual incidence is unknown, but it is at least as common as cryptorchidism or hypospadias. Genome mapping, performed on families with primary VUR with associated reflux nephropathy, has found an association with a locus on chromosome 1, and may be seen in

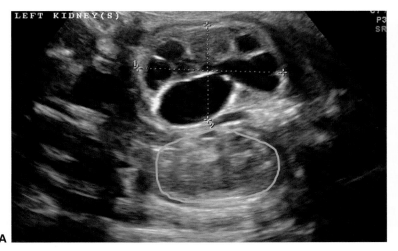
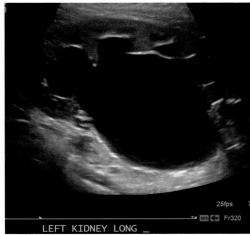

FIGURE 39.17 A: Significant left hydronephrosis found in a 33-week-old fetus with normal right kidney (see marked kidney). **B:** Severe hydronephrosis in the left consistent with UPJO on ultrasound in a child aged 4 months (different patient).

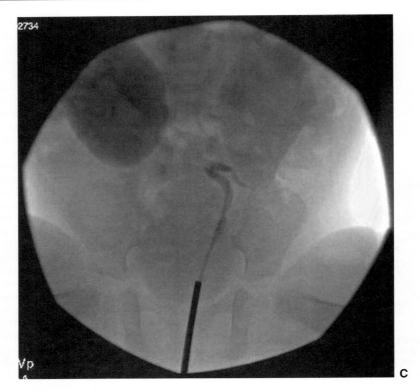

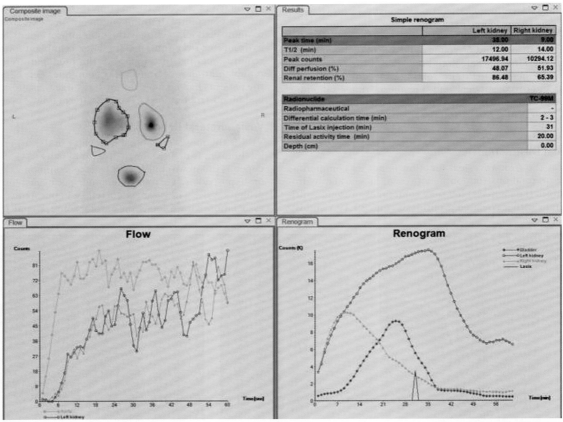

FIGURE 39.17 (*Continued*) **C:** Retrograde pyelography (in same patient) demonstrating narrowed, obstructed UPJ. Retrograde imaging is also important to demonstrate a normal ureter distal to the UPJ. **D:** Renal scan (different patient) demonstrating relative function in both the kidneys and probably obstruction in the left kidney.

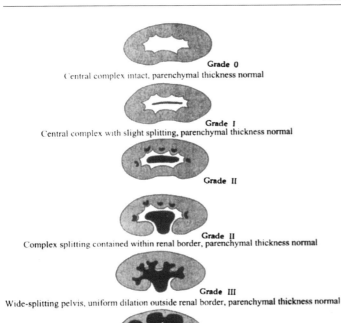

Grade 0
Central complex intact, parenchymal thickness normal

Grade I
Central complex with slight splitting, parenchymal thickness normal

Grade II

Grade II
Complex splitting contained within renal border, parenchymal thickness normal

Grade III
Wide-splitting pelvis, uniform dilation outside renal border, parenchymal thickness normal

Grade IV
Further dilation of renal pelvis and calices, parenchyma thin

FIGURE 39.18 Society for fetal urology (SFU) grading system for ultrasono-graphically detected hydronephrosis. (Reprinted with permission from Baskin LS. Prenatal hydronephrosis. In: Baskin LS, Kogan BA, Duckett JW, eds. *Handbook of pediatric urology*. Philadelphia, PA: Lippincott–Raven, 1997:11. Modified by Curt Powell, MD.)

other families with VUR (45). VUR is known to be a familial problem. When one child in a family is identified as having reflux, as many as 30% to 50% of the siblings of that child may have VUR. The American Urological Association (AUA) previously published

VUR guidelines and found in their meta-analysis that VUR occurs in about 27.4% of siblings and 35.7% in offspring of children with reflux. Previously, all siblings or offspring of children with VUR underwent VCUG screening, but this is now not done unless the child to be screened has had a history of UTI, especially febrile, or an abnormal bladder or ureter on a renal bladder ultrasound, as described in the UTD grading system (46). The normal uretero-vesical junction efficiently allows ureteral urine to drain into the lumen of the bladder and prevents the urine, once in the bladder, from reentering the ureter because of the oblique ureteral course through the bladder wall (**Fig. 39.20**). Additionally, there is maturation of the ureterovesical junction with time and patient growth, as infants typically have a much higher incidence of VUR at diagnosis than do older children.

Reflux is graded on an international scale of 1 to 5 (47). The major significance of this grading system is that with higher grades of reflux, typically grades IV and V, there is an increased likelihood that the reflux will persist despite patient growth and will have a higher risk of associated febrile UTI and reflux nephropathy. Lower grades of reflux are more likely to resolve spontaneously without reflux nephropathy.

Although hydronephrosis suggests an abnormality in the urinary tract, many patients with significant VUR will have a normal US study. The radiologic confirmation of VUR is accomplished by VCUG. VCUG should not be performed while the child is actively infected but may be performed once the urine is sterile and the patient afebrile and under treatment. Because renal scarring occurs easily in the neonate, it is especially important to establish the presence or absence of VUR before discontinuing antibiotics in patients presenting with a febrile UTI.

The AUA VUR task force currently recommends VCUG only in infants with antenatally diagnosed hydronephrosis with high-grade hydronephrosis (SFU grades 3 to 4) or abnormal bladders or hydroureter on ultrasound. If the child later develops a febrile UTI, a VCUG should be obtained at that time (48). Therefore, routine use of VCUG screening in children with antenatal hydrone-phrosis is not indicated thus reducing the number of children with

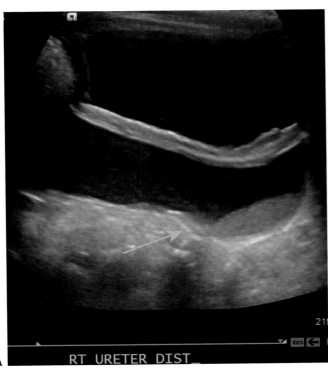

RT URETER DIST

A

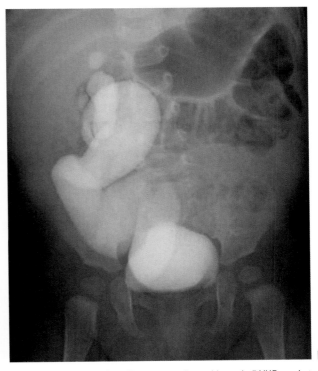

B

FIGURE 39.19 A: Right megaureter with purulent debris layered in the ureter with obstruction (see *arrow*). **B:** The same patient with grade 5 VUR as obstructed refluxing megaureter on the right.

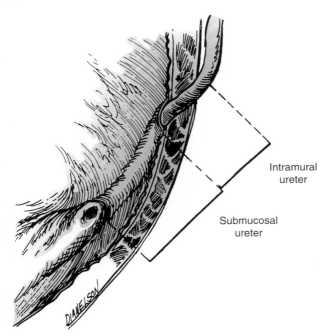

FIGURE 39.20 Normal ureterovesical junction. (Reprinted from Harrison JH, Gittes TA, Stamey AD, et al., eds. *Campbell's urology*, 4th ed. Philadelphia, PA: WB Saunders, 1979:1597. Copyright © 1979 Elsevier. With permission.)

clinically insignificant VUR and sparing infants without reflux from having unnecessary radiation and instrumentation. It is also reasonable to forego routine VCUG in all infants with isolated mild to severe hydronephrosis unless there are other associated findings such as febrile UTI (see below). VCUG should always be obtained in infants or children with recurrent febrile UTIs as this group was found to have higher grades of VUR with VCUG testing and are more prone to UTI-associated renal damage (49,50).

If reflux is demonstrated in the infant, particularly after febrile UTI or with associated bladder or ureteral pathology, the patient should be maintained on low-dose antibacterial therapy until

resolution or decrease in grade of the reflux. The prophylaxis choice is limited in the newborn, but amoxicillin is reasonable until hepatobiliary maturation allows the use of sulfamethoxazole–trimethoprim or nitrofurantoin. A reasonable initial daily suppression dose would be 10 to 25 mg/kg of amoxicillin. If local strains of *Escherichia coli* are resistant to amoxicillin, cefdinir 4 to 5 mg/kg/d and cefixime 5 to 7 mg/kg/d are useful alternatives. With changing VCUG guidelines, many infants will not have a VCUG and will not need prophylaxis. Most infants do not require prophylaxis for lower grades of reflux without associated bladder abnormalities, ureteral dilation, or febrile UTI. It is also more common that uncircumcised males are at higher risk for febrile UTI with or without associated VUR. Several studies have shown an increase in febrile UTI in children with high-grade VUR (grades IV and V), female gender, and significant hydroureteronephrosis and uncircumcised boys regardless of the degree of hydronephrosis (49). The increased risk of febrile UTI in uncircumcised infant boys with tight phimosis, especially with VUR, may be decreased by treating the phimosis with topical steroids (triamcinolone, betamethasone, or hydrocortisone) or circumcision (if family preference) with generally decreased occurrence of febrile UTIs in boys without tight phimosis (51).

Bacterial resistance has increased to amoxicillin and low-dose sulfamethoxazole–trimethoprim. Cephalexin or nitrofurantoin may be used although bacterial resistance to these antibiotics can also occur. Breakthrough infection while the patient is on antibacterial suppression, or poor compliance with prophylaxis use, suggests the need for surgical repair, either with open surgical or with endoscopic techniques.

Studies using DMSA to document pyelonephritis have shown that, even if VUR is present, only some cases of pyelonephritis go on to renal scarring. Additionally, febrile UTIs are fairly uncommon in infants with high grades of isolated hydronephrosis without associated findings of significant hydroureteronephrosis, bladder abnormalities or tight phimosis and, because of this, routine VCUG has not been obtained unless the patient experiences febrile UTIs (50).

Bladder Exstrophy

Exstrophy of the bladder is a rare, but extremely significant, abnormality (Fig. 39.21A and B). It affects roughly 1 child in every 25,000 live births. Exstrophy is not usually associated with other

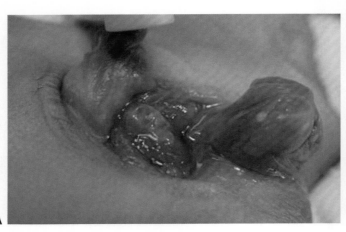
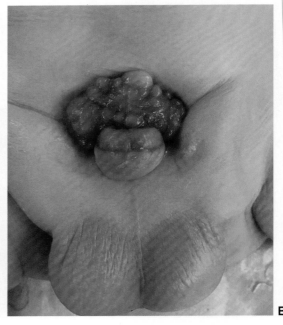

FIGURE 39.21 A: Classic bladder exstrophy in infant male with small bladder defect but adequate split epispadiac penis. **B:** Another male infant with bladder exstrophy and shortened phallus.

organ systems abnormalities except for associated pelvic skeletal anomalies and abnormal external genitalia; the remainder of the urinary tract is generally normal. Functional reconstruction of the exstrophic bladder can be a formidable surgical undertaking, but, in experienced hands, can result in a continent child with a relatively normal upper urinary tract (45). The major factor affecting the success of closure for continence seems to be the presentation size of the exstrophic bladder and, more recently, having reconstruction done in centers where the procedure is more routinely done (52).

The epithelium of the exstrophic bladder is grossly normal at birth but becomes hyperplastic shortly after if the bladder is not closed. It is preferable to protect the exstrophic bladder by leaving the bladder uncovered except for a plastic wrap covering until bladder closure can be accomplished. Gauze or petroleum gauze should not be used, as these can dry the bladder surface and denude the urothelium.

Traditionally, functional closure of exstrophy was a staged procedure. Mitchell advocated bladder closure and epispadias repair as a one-stage procedure, with good initial results that include continence after the single procedure in a significant number of the patients so treated (53). The exstrophic bladder is dissected free from the anterior abdominal wall, closed into a sphere, and dropped back into the pelvis. The abdominal wall is then closed over the bladder. In the infant boy, complete penile disassembly can be done initially creating a hypospadiac penis. Iliac osteotomies are usually performed to facilitate bladder closure. Even though osteotomy can be omitted in newborns, success rates are higher when it is done (54). There is no attempt at the first stage to produce urinary continence, although some children may have reasonable continence after this stage. Generally, after 2 to 3 years, a second-stage procedure may be needed to attempt to achieve urinary control if the patient is incontinent or has a planned staged repair approach. Historically, ureterosigmoidostomy, where the ureters were anastomosed to the sigmoid colon, was used as an alternative to functional closure. Because of associated metabolic abnormalities (e.g., hyperchloremic acidosis) and an increased risk for development of adenocarcinoma of the colon, this procedure is rarely, if ever, performed. It is worth noting that the unclosed exstrophic bladder is also at high risk for development of adenocarcinoma of the bladder in the second or third decade of life. Functional closure seems to obviate this risk. Recently, repair has been delayed until the patient is out of the newborn time period to allow the infant time to get larger and handle lengthy surgical and anesthesia times for exstrophy reconstruction. Additionally, as exstrophy is relatively infrequent, many of these children are best served by being repaired at referral centers where the various surgical subspecialists needed perform exstrophy repair more routinely and obtain more consistent surgical results (52).

Exstrophy of the Cloaca

Cloacal exstrophy is a severe anomaly, previously thought to be incompatible with long-term survival, and still has a high mortality. Its incidence is between 1 in 200,000 to 400,000 live births. Improved survival can be credited to improved neonatal care, nutritional support, and preservation of as much of the intestine as possible. In this anomaly, two halves of the exstrophic bladder are separated by a midline strip of exteriorized cecum (**Fig. 39.22**). The ileum may prolapse through the bowel plate. Additionally, the child has an imperforate anus with almost no colon present distal to the exstrophic bowel plate. The small intestine is often short, and there may be bowel malrotation. The genital tubercle is split and widely separated. It is particularly difficult to produce a functional penis in boys with this anomaly (55). Genetic males with cloacal exstrophy were previously raised as females, but this practice is not currently followed due to gender discordance seen in many older previously gender converted children (56). Cloacal

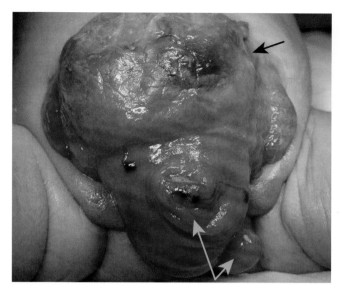

FIGURE 39.22 Severe cloacal exstrophy defect (OEIS) in newborn with large omphalocele with the liver in defect (*black arrow*), split bladder exstrophy plates, very short hind gut, and open ileum in center of the bladder bowel plate (*orange arrows*).

exstrophy children often have spinal dysraphism and may have a neurogenic bladder and bowel. They may also have an associated omphalocele making abdominal wall closure difficult. Because of these associated conditions, OEIS (omphalocele, exstrophy, imperforate anus, and spinal defects) complex has been used to describe this condition (57). A functional anus is almost impossible to produce due to the imperforate anus and the very short colon, so a permanent colostomy, incorporating the exstrophic bowel, is the usual bowel diversion of choice. It is best to preserve as much bowel as possible to improve water reabsorption due to the generally short colon. Permanent ileostomy, used in the past, may lead to problems with dehydration and short gut syndrome. Staged reconstruction when the child is older is generally recommended with bowel preservation, initial colostomy, nutritional support, and delayed reconstruction once patient survival, nutritional status, and bowel function are better determined (58). Bladder closure uniting the two halves of the exstrophic bladder, creating a continent diversion with a catheterizable stoma, utilizing iliac osteotomy before anterior closure, usually will be delayed until the child is 18 to 24 months old or older due to the associated problems with malabsorption due to a short gut where patient may require long-term parenteral nutrition with resultant hepatic compromise. Reconstruction of the external genitalia, if possible, may be performed at the same time (58).

Patent Urachus

The urachus is a tube that connects the urogenital (UG) sinus and the allantois between months 3 and 5 of intrauterine life. The urachus normally regresses to a small-caliber, epithelialized tube and, finally, into a sealed, obliterated cord by term or during the neonatal period. It may remain patent up to the infraumbilical area in premature infants (59). Thirty-two percent of all bladders have tubular remnants of the urachus noted at necropsy. Persistent urachal remnants are quite common and do not require surgical therapy unless symptomatic with umbilical urinary leakage or urachal cyst infections. Significant urachal anomalies are rare but will occur twice as often if present in males as in females.

Complete failure of obliteration of the urachus results in a persistent communication between the bladder and the umbilicus that leaks urine intermittently or continuously. It is the most common

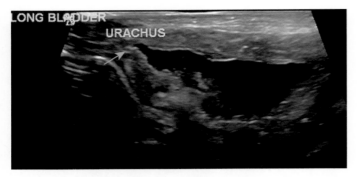

FIGURE 39.23 Patent urachus (*arrow*) demonstrated on ultrasound of the abdomen in a patient with PBS.

urachal anomaly encountered requiring surgical therapy. The etiology of this condition is unknown. It has been suggested that bladder outlet obstruction may be a contributing factor, although the chronology of embryologic events suggests that the urachal lumen obliterates before urethral tubularization. US is easily obtained and the best imaging study to diagnose a persistent tract or cyst up to the umbilicus (**Fig. 39.23**). VCUG will only occasionally demonstrate the communication but may diagnose other associated lower urinary tract anomalies such as obstruction, an abnormal posterior urethra, or VUR. A persistent omphalomesenteric duct must be considered in the differential diagnosis. Umbilical granuloma may also cause a small stain on the diaper or minimal umbilical drainage. Iatrogenic creation of a vesicoumbilical fistula, during an umbilical artery cut down, has also been reported (59). Treatment of a patent urachus involves complete extraperitoneal excision of the urachus with an attached cuff of bladder to completely remove any urachal remnant in the bladder to prevent possible cancer development later in life in residual tissue. Laparoscopic techniques are frequently used to remove the tract and take a bladder cuff while attempting to preserve the umbilicus. Larger urachal cysts may need surgical treatment but many small urachal cysts or urachal remnants are generally incidentally found and do not cause any morbidity and may be observed with serial ultrasound imaging of bladder and lower abdominal regions and, if unchanged over 6 to 12 months' observation, may not warrant further imaging or follow-up unless associated with umbilical infection or enlarging urachal cysts.

Megacystis–Microcolon–Intestinal Hypoperistalsis Syndrome

Megacystis–microcolon–intestinal hypoperistalsis syndrome (MMIHS) was first described in 1976 and is considered rare. The disorder, thought to be an autosomal recessive trait, affects females more than males (4:1 preponderance) and may prove fatal within the first year of life (60). Some long-term survivors do exist using total parenteral nutrition (TPN) or multivisceral transplantation, but these cases are rare (10). In a large review of 72 patients, only 10 survived, with 9 on parenteral nutrition. Most patients die from sepsis, liver failure, short bowel disease, and potential postoperative complications (61). Presentation includes abdominal distention, an abdominal mass (i.e., a distended bladder), and functional intestinal obstruction characterized by bilious vomiting and absent or decreased bowel sounds. The small bowel is short, dilated, and hypoactive and may have associated malrotation and an accompanying microcolon without anatomic obstruction. The abdominal musculature generally is lax. Most of these infants are diagnosed prenatally with ultrasonography demonstrating a large bladder, generally with a thin wall, and bilateral hydroureteronephrosis, with normal or increased amniotic fluid (thought to be as a result of the microcolon). Confirmation with prenatal MRI may be helpful to differentiate this from PBS. The etiology is unknown.

Treatment consists of parenteral alimentation and facilitation of bladder emptying, if the patient cannot void completely, with clean intermittent bladder catheterization (CIC) or urinary diversion by means of a cutaneous vesicostomy, if intermittent catheterization is not anatomically possible or practicable for families. Ochoa urofacial syndrome may also present with megacystis (62).

Posterior Urethral Valves

The most common lesion obstructing the lower urinary tract in a boy is termed PUVs, occurring in 1:5,000 (63) With this high prevalence, it is discouraging that over 50% of the children with PUVs will progress to end-stage renal disease (ESRD) in 10 years (**Fig. 39.24**). The valves are thought to be a diaphragm or membrane that traverses the urethra from a point just distal to the verumontanum in which it connects with urothelial folds and not a "valve" at all (63). Dewan et al. have extensively studied the anatomy of this membrane with videocystourethrography and prefer to classify this anomaly as a congenital posterior urethral membrane (COPUM) because of its variable morphologic expression (64). Embryologically, these membranes may be due to an abnormal anterior insertion and persistence of the distal extent of the wolffian duct or müllerian duct (63). Valves are best considered as a rigid membrane, despite generally having a flimsy appearance, and the vesical neck also is a relatively rigid area. With antegrade urine flow, this membrane obstructs. The urethra dilates proximally and elongates if obstruction is present. The detrusor subsequently

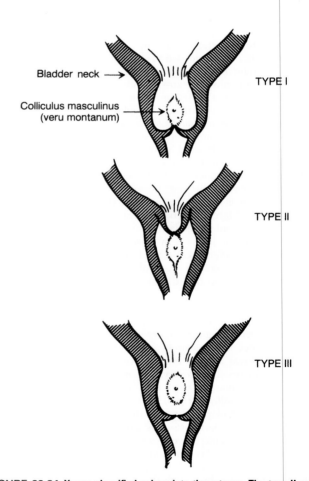

FIGURE 39.24 Young classified valves into three types. The type II valve probably does not exist. (Reprinted from Kelalis PP, King LR, Belman AB, eds. *Clinical pediatric urology*, vol. 1. Philadelphia, PA: WB Saunders, 1976:306. Copyright © 1976 Elsevier. With permission.)

hypertrophies with trabeculation and sacculation, and bladder neck hypertrophy occurs due to increased work of voiding.

VUR may result if there is a primary abnormality of the uretero-vesical junction but usually is secondary to the abnormal development of bladder. Bilateral VUR increases the possibility that renal failure eventually occurs. Hydroureteronephrosis may also develop, with or without reflux. Renal parenchymal damage due to renal dysplasia or interstitial nephritis, with or without pyelonephritis, is concomitant or may be a result of the urethral obstruction. Renal dysplasia, frequently present in infants with PUVs, has been found at as early as 13 to 14 weeks of gestational age in the fetus as found on prenatal US (63) (**Fig. 39.25A**).

In utero intervention, using vesicoamniotic shunts or primary fetal endoscopic ablation of valves, has not improved survival or renal function in these patients; many fetuses expire as a result of premature rupture of membranes or sepsis, and many that survive still develop chronic renal failure and require renal transplantation (2,65). Open fetal surgery, such as vesicostomy, has been generally abandoned as excessively invasive. Percutaneous bladder shunting using a double pigtail catheter is currently the most common fetal procedure currently performed (66). A European randomized controlled trial, PLUTO (percutaneous vesicoamniotic shunting in lower urinary tract obstruction) with the primary outcome of infant survival to 28 days postnatally was abandoned after poor recruitment (31 total recruited of 150 desired), with only 12 live births from each group (16 with prenatal shunting and 15 managed conservatively). Twelve infants survived to 28 days, and only 2 shunted babies survived to 2 years with normal renal function

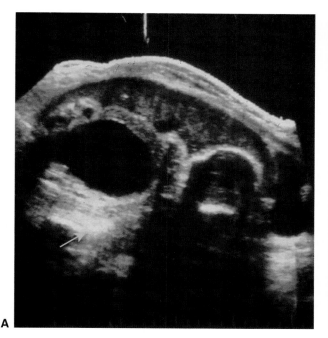

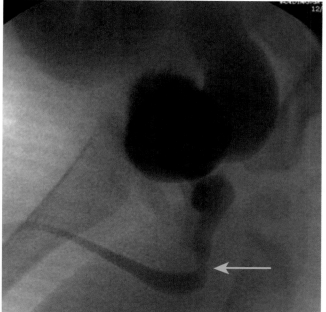

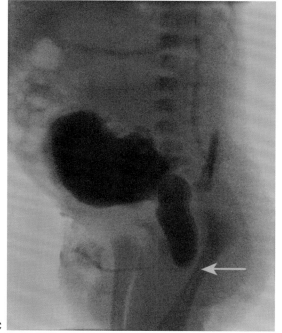

FIGURE 39.25 A: "Keyhole" bladder appearance on prenatal ultrasound indicative of PUV (see *arrow*). **B:** VCUG with PUV (see *arrow*) with grade 5 VUR and small bladder with elongated posterior urethra. **C:** VCUG in another patient with PUV without VUR (see *arrow*). Note the different caliber of the urethra with the same general condition.

(67). Fetal surgical intervention for bladder obstruction currently should be considered experimental and not standard management for presumed congenital bladder outlet conditions (63,66,67).

Some infants with presumed prenatal diagnosis of PUVs with severe oligohydramnios are either born prematurely (<37 weeks gestation) or have LBW <2.5 kg. Some are induced for delivery prematurely due to significant oligohydramnios, severe bilateral hydronephrosis, or IUGR. Although these infants generally had longer hospital stays and a higher rate of vesicostomy (due to small patient size being incompatible for primary valve ablation), they appeared, in one study, to have similar reasonable early renal function outcomes at 2 years of age if their creatinine nadir was 1 mg/dL (68).

Routine use of antenatal US has increased the detection of a thick-walled bladder with a keyhole configuration, with or without hydroureteronephrosis, and oligohydramnios suggestive of PUVs. Hydronephrosis is present in 90% of infants with valves. Interestingly, hydronephrosis found in the 2nd trimester may improve in 80% of PUV cases and up to 40% of infants with PUVs have no evidence of prenatal hydronephrosis, so there should be a high index of suspicion that PUVs may be present and full workup with ultrasonography and VCUG should be obtained after birth (63). Non-renal features of Potter syndrome, due to fetal compression from decreased amniotic fluid, may be seen in some newborns with PUVs, including intrauterine growth deficiency, pulmonary hypoplasia, limb positioning defects (e.g., talipes equinovarus), and characteristic facies. All of the signs and symptoms seen in boys with PUVs are secondary to the obstructive nature of the valves, the effect of intrauterine oligohydramnios, or superimposed urinary infection or azotemia. A palpably enlarged bladder, UTI, ascites, pulmonary difficulties, including isolated pneumothorax, failure to thrive, or gastrointestinal disturbances suggest an investigation for PUVs if not already suspected with prenatal US. A strong urinary stream does not preclude the diagnosis of posterior urethral obstruction. Although fetal urine production may occur at 8 to 10 weeks' gestation, abnormal bladder pressures due to bladder obstruction do not develop until about 13 weeks of gestation with renal damage from obstruction generally seen after about 14 weeks. Critical lung development occurs at about 16 to 25 weeks of gestation, well after renal damage has occurred. Only 14 days of persistent severe oligohydramnios prior to 25 weeks can result in up to 90% fetal mortality (63). Pulmonary hypoplasia at birth presents with respiratory distress, including spontaneous pneumothorax or pneumomediastinum, possibly indicating there may be urethral valves in newborns. Any full-term boy with respiratory distress should be suspect for a renal problem.

Boys presenting with PUVs in infancy have a poorer prognosis than do children who present symptomatically at an older age, especially if serum creatinine levels are higher than 0.8 or 1.0 mg/dL at 1 month after treatment of the valves. On a recent comprehensive study of boys with PUVs, a nadir creatinine of 0.8 to 1.0 mg/dL was the only independent prognostic factor predicting reasonable long-term renal function accounting for other factors such as antenatal diagnosis, ultrasound findings, recurrent UTIs, VUR presence, or need for multiple surgeries (69).

Urinary ascites is a less common presentation for children with PUVs but causes up to one-third of all cases of neonatal ascites (70). Ascites is rarely a result of frank perforation of the urinary tract but is generally due to leakage of urine through renal fornices and transudation of urine across the peritoneal membrane into the peritoneal cavity. The ascitic fluid usually has a chemical content equivalent to that of serum, because the peritoneal membrane has passively dialyzed the urea and creatinine content of urine into the vascular system. These children may not have marked hydronephrosis due to urinary tract decompression by urine leakage. These boys often present as extremely ill infants

but occasionally will initially appear healthy except for abdominal distention. Their prognosis regarding renal preservation often is better than that of the child who does not present with urinary ascites, presumably because the leakage of urine from the distended system protects the upper urinary tract from damage seen with high intraluminal renal pressure. Occasionally, a localized retroperitoneal urinoma will form. The diagnosis of urinary ascites is made clinically and confirmed by ultrasound or a plain radiograph of the abdomen demonstrating bowel displaced to the central abdomen and a ground-glass appearance of the remainder of the abdomen.

Twenty-five to fifty percent of patients with PUVs have VUR at presentation. In one-half of cases, the reflux is bilateral. When there is massive unilateral VUR associated with PUVs, the kidney on the refluxing side often is dysplastic and does not function at presentation or subsequently. This is called VURD (valves, unilateral reflux, and dysplasia) syndrome. VURD syndrome was initially thought to have a protective effect on the nonrefluxing kidney, but long-term follow-up of patients with VURD found that only 25% of the boys between ages 5 and 8 years had normal renal function (71). Marked hydronephrosis without VUR usually carries a better prognosis for long-term renal function than having high-grade bilateral VUR. In refluxing patients with PUVs, VUR may resolve in one-third to one-half of cases once obstruction is relieved.

Obstructive uropathy is suggested on prenatal or postnatal US by finding significant bilateral hydronephrosis with or without hydroureter or a distended, thick-walled bladder. Patients with PUVs often have a dilated and elongated posterior urethra with the thick-walled bladder on US imaging, which has been termed a "keyhole bladder." Perirenal urinoma or ascites can also be detected.

The single most important study in the diagnosis of infravesical obstruction is VCUG. An adequate study requires complete visualization of the urethra from the bladder neck to the meatus and oblique and lateral projections of the urethra during voiding without a catheter in the urethra, because an indwelling catheter may obscure the urethral valves (Fig. 39.25B and C).

PUVs appear as a sharply defined transverse or oblique lucency, with proximal urethral elongation and distention and diminution of flow distal to the valve. The bladder neck may be secondarily thickened and collar-like. The bladder is usually trabeculated with saccules or diverticula, especially paraurethral diverticula (Fig. 39.25B and C). VUR is often present at diagnosis, and refluxing ureters frequently are grossly dilated and tortuous.

Functional renal imaging studies will determine extent of upper tract damage produced by lower tract obstruction. In the newborn or azotemic infant in whom obstruction is suspected, a radionuclide renal scan can provide renal functional information and can often be obtained without the need for sedation. Alternatively, MRU allows estimation of differential renal function and may give better anatomic detail than a radionuclide renal scan and usually does not require a general anesthetic in the newborn (41).

When these infants first present, resuscitative measures may be necessary to treat respiratory distress or associated urinary infection, replace fluid and electrolytes, and, most importantly, drain the urinary tract. A small intraurethral catheter without a balloon (e.g., a feeding tube) will usually suffice to drain the urinary tract. Once the child is stable, either the valves must be primarily resected transurethrally or the urinary tract should be drained for a prolonged period using a cutaneous vesicostomy or, in some cases where there is severe bilateral VUR, with a cutaneous ureterostomy. Many of these infants are anticipated in advance because of antenatal imaging suggestive for PUVs with bladder obstruction; they can be followed closely immediately after birth and may not require resuscitative measures, because the child generally is evaluated almost immediately after birth.

Long-term outlook for infants who present with PUVs is still only fair, because approximately 50% of boys presenting with PUVs eventually progress to renal failure and transplantation despite treatment (72). If serum creatinine is normal at 2 years of age, the prognosis for long-term normal renal function is good but still not perfect (69). In long-term follow-up of 11 to 22 years of children with PUVs, one-third had poor renal function: 10% who survived childhood had died of renal failure, 21% had ESRD or chronic renal failure, and 46% had diurnal enuresis. Diurnal enuresis seen later in life increased the likelihood that there would be progression to renal failure.

Some boys present after infancy without significant prenatal hydronephrosis or oligohydramnios. These boys present with voiding symptoms (50%) or febrile UTIs (28%) in one study. Unfortunately, up to 10% will still develop chronic kidney disease decades later in life, particularly if associated with bilateral hydronephrosis and severe bilateral VUR (73).

Renal Tumors

Fortunately, tumors of the urinary tract are rare in infancy and tend to exhibit a benign behavior. Only 5% of all fetal tumors are found to arise from the kidneys. There are differences in tumors found before birth with fetal imaging and renal tumors diagnosed within the first month of life (74).

Prenatally diagnosed renal tumors may be associated with polyhydramnios (39% in one study) with risk of premature delivery. There may also be associated risk of hemorrhage if the mass rapidly enlarges during pregnancy. These findings may warrant transfer of obstetric care to a specialized center and consideration for cesarean delivery if there is fetal distress and a very large renal tumor with inherent risk of rupture or hemorrhage with a vaginal delivery. Fetal tumors greater than 10 cm are at highest risk for complications, although some centers still maintain close surveillance on these pregnancies and do not routinely deliver these infants prematurely (74).

Although Wilms tumor (WT) is the most frequent renal tumor in childhood, other renal tumors, such as congenital mesoblastic nephroma (CMN) and malignant rhabdoid tumor of the kidney (MRTK), are more common in the fetal and neonatal time periods. Other variants of Wilms tumor can also be seen in the neonatal period including nephroblastomatosis, and benign cystic nephroma. Many of these lesions are found with antenatal US as abnormally large kidneys or kidneys or a large abdominal mass. Previously, they presented in infancy as a palpable flank mass with occasionally associated hypertension. Some of these masses still present this way if there is limited prenatal imaging.

CMNs are generally found to be large, well-circumscribed solid masses, usually replacing a large portion of the kidney, on prenatal US. US shows CMN as generally homogeneous in appearance but occasionally having cystic or calcified components and increased vascularity. These findings make it difficult to differentiate CMN from WT. CMN is the predominant renal tumor diagnosed in the first month of life (54%) but its frequency drops to less than 10% of all renal tumors after age 3 months. After 3 months of age, WT is the more likely seen renal tumor (74). Histologically, CMN is composed largely of mesenchymal stroma with spindle-shaped fibrous or leiomyomatous cells. US demonstrates a solid intrarenal mass. CT will better delineate the mass characteristics and may demonstrate tumor extension outside the renal bed. Although rarely obtained, radionuclide scans will show the mass as nonfunctioning tissue, and MRI or CT will show distortion of the calyceal architecture by the tumor. US and CT will demonstrate the tissue characteristics more clearly than scintigraphy or pyelography. MRI with gadolinium may be necessary to better delineate subtle lesions, determine tumor extensions, and better define the renal vessels and hilum as CMN tumors may extend medially into the perirenal

tissue. Nephrectomy is generally curative with few reports of local recurrence and rare reports of distant metastasis. Metastasis, when it occurs, may be to the brain, lungs, bone, and heart. Up to 7.2% of children had metastasis or recurrent disease in one study, with most of the relapses being found within the first 11 months after surgery and generally determined by US imaging alone (74). Chemotherapy did not prevent recurrence in these patients. Chemotherapy and radiation therapy are not necessary if the entire tumor is removed, which usually requires total nephrectomy due to the absence of a definitive capsule around the tumor.

Nephroblastomatosis can be diffuse or nodular. Diffuse nephroblastomatosis usually presents as marked enlargement of both kidneys. The kidneys are grossly enlarged and have a whitish hue. Biopsy reveals primitive metanephric epithelium resembling tissue seen in Wilms tumor. This lesion usually responds to chemotherapy (i.e., actinomycin D). Nodular renal blastoma consists of microscopic foci of primitive metanephric epithelium and often is an incidental autopsy finding in infants. It is thought that Wilms tumor may arise from foci of nodular renal blastema in some cases.

Benign cystic nephroma can be classified with cystic diseases but belongs with renal tumors because elements of Wilms tumor may be found in the septa between the cysts (74). As with the other tumors, patients with cystic nephroma can present with a palpable mass. US will identify the mass as multiple cysts or as a complex mass (i.e., mixed cystic and solid). Although enucleation of the mass is a theoretical option, nephrectomy is still the treatment of choice. Despite the presence of Wilms tumor elements in the septa, chemotherapy is not necessary for cure.

WT may also be found in the newborn time period with most being of a low stage (stage I or II) although 17% of WT found in the first 7 months in one series presented as stage III disease. It is important to sample at least 7 lymph nodes at time of surgical resection to appropriately stage the tumor as a WT, even when the diagnosis may be CMN based on age of diagnosis. Some infants with WT found to have stage I disease diagnosed less than 2 years old and with a tumor weighing less than 550 g may be treated with surgery and observation only as very low risk WT (VLRWT). Relapse rate was about 15%, and the overall survival was comparable to the group who had planned adjuvant chemotherapy obviating the need for chemotherapy in 85% of this group.

Renal cell carcinoma is extremely rare in the newborn and fetal time periods. MRTK is still very rare and is associated with other tumors including medulloblastoma and neuroectodermal tumors. MRTK presents at a very early age and has a very poor prognosis.

If bilateral renal masses are found in neonatal or fetal US imaging, the diagnosis is almost invariably WT and would be treated with bilateral WT protocol for diagnosis and treatment with adjuvant chemotherapy and renal preserving surgical treatments. Unfortunately, children in this group require more intense surveillance due to finding increased nephrogenic rests and have a poorer 5-year survival in some series (40%) (74).

Renal Vein Thrombosis

Another renal lesion with a definite predilection for the neonatal period is renal vein thrombosis (8). This uncommon problem usually results from hemoconcentration due to dehydration and is often seen in infants of diabetic mothers. It is also seen in infants with cyanotic congenital heart disease, sickle cell disease, perinatal stress, or sepsis. Sludging in the intrarenal venules causes subsequent thrombosis. The thrombus will then propagate centrally. Infants usually present with a palpable mass, hematuria, albuminuria, and thrombocytopenia. When both kidneys are involved, the infant will become uremic. Treatment is supportive and involves correction of the underlying causative problems. Surgery (i.e., nephrectomy) is generally unnecessary if collateral circulation is present allowing renal recovery. Thrombectomy is not helpful since the problem is in the peripheral veins rather than the central veins. Thrombolytic agents developed for clot lysis may be considered for treatment of bilateral renal vein thrombosis but not necessary if the condition is unilateral.

Adrenal Hemorrhage

Hemorrhage in the adrenal gland may occur spontaneously or in association with renal vein thrombosis. Adrenal hemorrhage is more common than renal vein thrombosis. Hemorrhage also occurs following a traumatic delivery, sepsis, large birth weight, or asphyxia. The infant may present with icterus (from absorption of hemoglobin) and an abdominal mass. US will demonstrate a sonolucent or solid mass above the kidney and may be detected with antenatal US as an adrenal mass. It must be followed postnatally to differentiate it from a congenital neuroblastoma or neural crest tumor (CT or MRI may be required to differentiate an adrenal tumor from an adrenal hemorrhage). Resolution of the mass or the rare development of an adrenal pseudocyst will confirm that the mass was due to adrenal hemorrhage. Percutaneous drainage, if necessary, is the preferred mode of treatment of an adrenal pseudocyst, but usually no intervention is needed. Adrenal calcification may be seen several weeks after adrenal hemorrhage. Adrenal hemorrhage can occur bilaterally in 10% of patients with adrenal hemorrhage, but if unilateral, it occurs more commonly on the right side (**Fig. 39.26A and B**).

Abdominal Masses

Finding an abdominal mass is not infrequent in the newborn nursery. Previously, infants in the newborn nursery with abdominal masses arising from the genitourinary tract represented approximately 1 in every 500 admissions, but now most masses are usually diagnosed prior to delivery due to prenatal US imaging. Hydronephrosis and cystic kidneys are the most common lesions in infancy producing abdominal masses, whereas tumors are more common in older children. Postnatally, US is most likely to identify the

TABLE 39.2

Abdominal Masses of Renal Origin

Mass	Texture	Renal Scan	Ultrasonogram
Hydronephrosis	Smooth	Delayed drainage	Sonolucent
Multicystic kidney	Irregular	Nonfunction	Multiple large and small cysts (i.e., cystic dysplasia)
Polycystic kidney	Smooth (recessive); irregular or smooth (dominant)	Delayed function; distortion of collecting system. Multiple large and small cysts (dominant)	Diffuse small cysts (recessive)
Tumor	Smooth	Distortion of collecting system	Solid
Renal vein thrombosis	Smooth	Poor function to nonfunction	Relatively normal renal architecture; enlarged kidney

source of a palpable abdominal mass; occasionally CT or MRI may be required to better delineate some abdominal masses. Physical and radiographic characteristics of the common abdominal masses of renal origin are listed in Table 39.2.

Hematuria

Hematuria in the infant can be a sign of renal vein thrombosis, acute tubular necrosis, renal calculi, urinary infection, or urinary tract obstruction. Hematuria must be confirmed by examination of the urine, both chemically and microscopically. A positive chemical test may reflect hemoglobinuria, rather than hematuria, which implies the presence of cellular elements in the urine. Even more common than the presence of hematuria or hemoglobinuria is

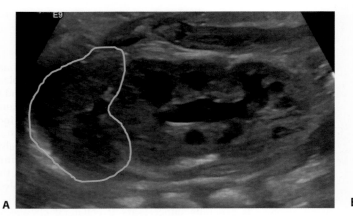

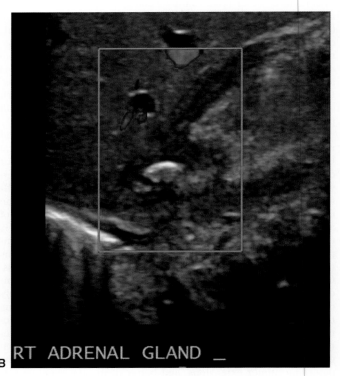

FIGURE 39.26 A: Premature newborn of diabetic mother with bilateral adrenal hemorrhage shortly after birth (adrenal outlined). **B:** The same patient with calcification of right adrenal gland 3 weeks after bilateral adrenal hemorrhage first seen on ultrasound.

finding a red diaper in an infant. Two relatively common causes for red diapers are the presence of urates in the urine, giving a pink hue to the urine, especially in the diaper, and the growth of *Serratia* species on or within a long-standing unchanged urine-soaked diaper. Obviously, these latter two situations are of no clinical consequence but must be separated from true hematuria or hemoglobinuria.

MALE GENITAL ABNORMALITIES AND GENDER AMBIGUITY

Cryptorchidism

Undescended testes are a very common finding in the newborn period, affecting perhaps as many as 1 in every 50 newborn males. Most testes that are undescended at birth will descend during the first 6 to 9 months of life, so that cryptorchidism incidence at 1 year of age is approximately 0.7% to 0.8%, and is exactly the same incidence found in postpubertal males. The newborn examination is important in determining testicular position because the cremasteric reflex then is weak or absent (75). If the testis is well descended in a newborn, it is unlikely that there will be problems with true cryptorchidism later in life. Optimal results from treatment of cryptorchidism are undertaken after the time for testicular descent has passed (i.e., beyond 3 to 6 months of age) and before adverse histologic effects of testicular nondescent are seen (i.e., approximately 1.5 to 2 years of age). Surgical intervention for true cryptorchidism should optimally be before 12 to 18 months of age. Most children now undergo surgical treatment of cryptorchidism between 6 and 9 months of age with good surgical and anesthetic results. Increased mobility of the cord structures is generally seen at this age, even with very high inguinal or abdominal testes, and facilitates placing the testis in the scrotum. But surgical repair should be delayed until the patient is reasonably healthy based on underlying medical or other associated conditions.

Penile Agenesis

Although there are many common penile anomalies, penile agenesis is rare, occurring in 1 in 10 to 30 million live births (Fig. 39.27). Penile agenesis suggests early embryologic failure in the development of the genital tubercle. The urethra usually exits on the perineum or near the anal verge. Previously, these children were raised as females, with castration and reconstruction of the external genitalia performed at an early age (76). With concerns of Y chromosome neurologic imprinting, management of this and other previously sex reassigned conditions continues to be controversial (77).

Penile Duplication

Penile duplication (i.e., true diphallia) is a rare anomaly that may involve duplications of the urethra and bladder (Fig. 39.28) (78). Reconstruction involves complex decisions about functional capability and appearance of the urinary, genital, and gastrointestinal tracts.

Microphallus

The boy born with an abnormally small phallus is therapeutically challenging. Most cases of true microphallus are due to hypogonadism (79) and will respond to testosterone, but occasionally patients with microphallus have end-organ failure or no functioning testosterone receptors, such as 5α-reductase receptors, preventing any response to exogenous testosterone. However, despite the finding of microphallus in the newborn nursery, it is extremely rare to find an adult with a phallus so small that it is incapable of sexual function.

The normal full-term newborn male phallus measures approximately 3 to 3.5 cm in stretched length; microphallus by definition requires a phallus that is less than 2.5 cm in stretched length, excluding ambiguous genitalia or the penis with hypospadias, chordee, or significant penoscrotal webbing or transposition (79). To determine microphallus response to hormonal stimulation, 25 mg of testosterone enanthate is administered intramuscularly every 4 weeks for a total of 75 mg (see Chapter 40). Some response usually is seen after the first dose. Most children will have a relatively normal phallus after the complete stimulation course. If there is no response to testosterone, gender reassignment has been considered in the past, but male gender assignment, due to

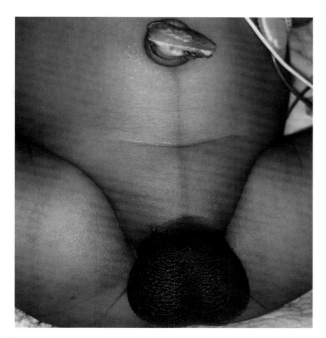

FIGURE 39.27 Penile agenesis.

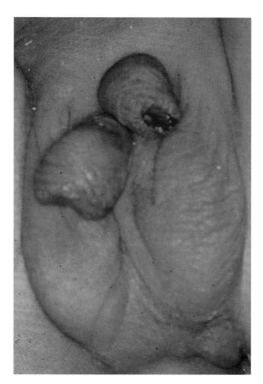

FIGURE 39.28 Penile duplication.

concerns about Y chromosome imprinting, is generally not done for micropenis unless the patient has a different gender preference when they are at an age when they can seriously review available options (77).

Gender Assignment

Gender assignment in the presence of a genital anomaly is an area of significant controversy at present. An optimal multidisciplinary team consensus approach is discussed in detail in Chapter 40. One long-term review of patients with micropenis raised as either male or female, later reassessed when adults found half of the men were dissatisfied with their genitalia but generally satisfied with their gender of rearing, while most raised as female (80%) were dissatisfied with their genitalia requiring surgeries for gender conversion. The neonate should be evaluated for medically treatable conditions, such as congenital adrenal hyperplasia (CAH), and the family counseled as to the conflicts and controversy currently at issue with gender selection.

Hypospadias

Hypospadias, by definition, refers to the abnormal location of the urethral meatus ventral to the normal glanular location (**Fig. 39.29**). The term actually encompasses a complex including chordee (i.e., generally a ventral curvature of the erect penis), abnormal preputial development, or torsion of the penis. Traditionally, hypospadias was categorized by degrees (i.e., first, second, and third). It is more helpful to describe hypospadias based on the urethral meatus location and the presence or absence of chordee (**Fig. 39.29**). Adding a description of foreskin development (complete or incomplete) and accompanying penile torsion will also improve characterizing the child's penile anatomy (**Fig. 39.30A and B**). At times, the hypospadiac meatus can be quite stenotic and very difficult to see, especially in the newborn.

There can be familial occurrence of hypospadias. Male siblings or the monochorionic twin of a child with hypospadias have an increased (14% to 20%) chance of having hypospadias with a similar high association of hypospadias in a child whose father also had hypospadias (80). Hypospadias may be inherited as a multifactorial condition. The historic incidence of hypospadias is 1 in 250 to 300 live births but may be as common as 1 in 125 live male births (81). The apparent incidence of hypospadias, particularly more proximally located hypospadias, may be increasing over the past few decades in the United States and some Scandinavian countries, but it may not have increased occurrence in all countries (82). Studies on *in vitro* fertilization (IVF) with increased incidence of hypospadias have only found an increase (relative risk of 3) in boys conceived with intracytoplasmic sperm injection (ICSI) (82) although progestational agents taken to maintain early pregnancy may also be a risk factor. Maternal exposure to estrogenic compounds such as phytoestrogens thought to increase risk of hypospadias has not been proven in some studies (83). Hypospadias associated with diabetes and gestational diabetes has been studied as other congenital defects are also found in diabetic mothers. However, one study found that increased hypospadias and other malformations were found mostly with preexisting diabetics while gestational diabetes itself did not have an increased risk of malformations (84). There may also be an increased occurrence in twin gestation, particularly in monochorionic twins (80,85,86).

There may be an increased incidence of hypospadias in small for gestational age (SGA) infants with incidence up to 10 times that of the general population (86). SGA infants may occasionally have IUGR, and it is postulated that inadequate human chorionic gonadotropin (HCG) delivery to IUGR fetuses may result in inadequate fetal testosterone production and incomplete virilization during development. This mechanism has not as yet been proven (81).

Children with hypospadias generally do not need to be evaluated for upper urinary tract abnormalities as there is no increased incidence of upper tract abnormalities when compared to the general population. Routine karyotype evaluation of patients with hypospadias and cryptorchidism is not warranted, except where there is a question of ambiguous genitalia especially if accompanied by bilaterally nonpalpable gonads (87). It is reasonable to evaluate the proximal urethra when surgical repair is done in patients with a more proximal hypospadias urethral opening as there may be associated dilation or a prominent utricle increasing the risk for febrile UTI or bladder and urethral emptying difficulties. VCUG may be needed as a newborn if patient does have a febrile UTI or if bladder emptying is at issue, although this is unlikely.

Most patients with hypospadias will have surgical correction of the condition, if needed, in the first year of life, usually after 6 months of age, adjusted for normal term delivery. Circumcision should not be performed in children with hypospadias as the foreskin is generally used for the repair of the hypospadias. Some families may prefer foreskin reconstruction with more distal hypospadias repairs, although this is not always possible if mini-

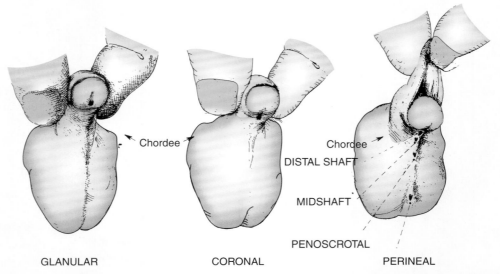

FIGURE 39.29 Classification of hypospadias based on anatomic location of the urethral meatus. The associated chordee is best described in terms of its severity (mild, moderate, or severe). (Reprinted from Kelalis PP, King LR, Belman AB, eds. *Clinical pediatric urology*, vol. 1. Philadelphia, PA: WB Saunders, 1976:577. Copyright © 1976 Elsevier. With permission.)

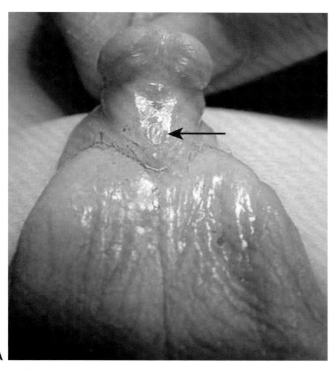 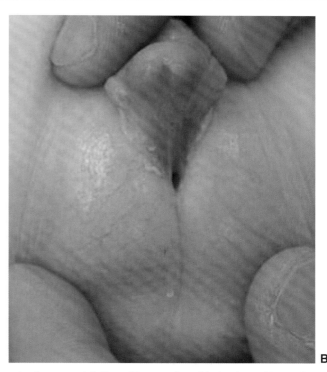

A   **B**

FIGURE 39.30 **A:** Penoscrotal hypospadias with chordee with shallow urethral opening (see *arrow*). **B:** Scrotal hypospadias with chordee and incomplete fore-skin.

mal residual skin is available after the hypospadias repair itself. If there is any question about penile anatomy at birth, circumcision should be delayed until the child can be assessed by a hypospadiologist who can determine whether the foreskin will be necessary for repair or if a repair is even necessary.

Epispadias

Epispadias usually is associated with exstrophy but occasionally appears as an isolated defect (Fig. 39.31). The incidence of isolated epispadias previously reported as 1 in 100,000 live births has now been estimated as occurring in 1 in 40,000 live births (88).

The repair of this condition is fairly complex. The more severe degrees of epispadias are associated with urinary incontinence and are more common than finding epispadias with urinary continence. In incontinent cases, the bladder neck must be reconstructed. Children with epispadias have a relatively short phallus as well as splayed suspensory ligaments making lengthening of the penis difficult despite multiple new techniques of repair. Achieving continence is of paramount importance in these children.

FIGURE 39.31 **Isolated epispadias with wide open bladder neck (*arrow*).**

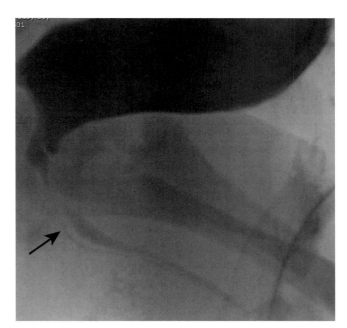

FIGURE 39.32 **Urethral duplication.** Generally, ventral urethra (*arrow*) is the functioning urethra, but in this case, dorsal urethra has wider caliber.

Urethral Duplication

Urethral duplication is an uncommon anomaly presenting as either a partial or complete duplication and is more common in boys. With duplication in boys, the urethras commonly are oriented in an anteroposterior plane, rather than lying side by side (**Fig. 39.32**). The more ventral urethra usually is the functional urethra, and the dorsal urethra often is stenotic and unusable (89). Repairs of these anomalies are tailored to the individual situation. Generally, duplication of the urethra in the female is seen with bladder duplication and is oriented side by side. Urethral duplication in a female with a dorsal urethra and a secondary vaginal urethra is very rare and usually presents with UTIs and the functioning female urethra is the more ventral urethral structure as in males.

Congenital prepubic sinus can occur in males or females as a small orifice located just above the pubis and may be a variant of a duplicated urethra or an exstrophy variant. The tract is usually removed surgically by tracing it down to the bladder or urethra (90).

Ambiguous Genitalia

Ambiguity of the external genitalia, frequently seen in the newborn nursery, often presents a diagnostic and therapeutic dilemma. Gender selection in such cases requires a multidisciplinary team approach, discussed in detail in Chapter 40.

Presence or absence of palpable gonads on physical examination is very helpful. A palpable gonad is most commonly a testis. Bilaterally, palpable gonads strongly suggest that the patient is a genetic male. If there is a unilateral palpable gonad, that too is likely a testis. There could conceivably be a normal testis, a streak gonad, or an ovary on the other side. If no gonads are palpable, the patient could be an XX female, an XY male with abdominal testes or a patient with mixed gonadal dysgenesis, or

ovotesticular disorder of sexual development (DSD), previously termed a true hermaphrodite.

Chromosomal gender is established by karyotype. An XY male who is undervirilized could have Klinefelter syndrome, ovotesticular DSD, 5α-reductase deficiency, hypopituitarism, 17-hydroxylase deficiency, or 3β-hydroxysteroid deficiency.

If the patient is an XX female, ambiguity could be produced by excessive maternal androgens or by adrenogenital syndrome, most commonly caused by a 21-hydroxylase deficiency. XX female must be considered in any phenotypic male patient with nonpalpable gonads, even if the genitalia appear completely masculinized, to avoid an adrenal crisis in a patient with a salt-losing adrenogenital syndrome (**Fig. 39.33A and B**).

Gender assignment should be considered after comprehensive evaluation by endocrinology, including karyotype, and anatomic evaluation, to assure that life-threatening conditions are not likely to occur and to alleviate parental anxiety. A multidisciplinary team will help the parents determine a reasonable gender selection using all information available at the time of review. Elements to consider when determining gender are potential fertility, capacity for future psychosexual function, and the possibility for satisfactory reconstruction. Potential functional reconstruction mandates that an experienced surgeon participate in the discussion regarding gender selection so that parents will understand available surgical options, potential complications or multiplicity of procedures, and lifelong medical treatments that might be required for either gender. Psychological implications of reports of patient dissatisfaction with the chosen gender are typically expressed most strongly in adolescence and adulthood (91). Unfortunately, the choice of possible potential gender is made more difficult with changes in information available as these children age, and potential changes

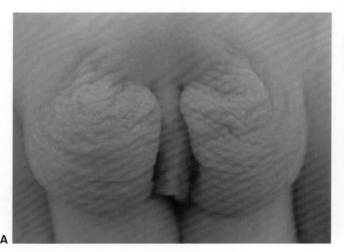

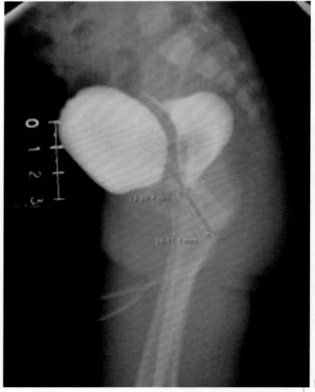

FIGURE 39.33 A: Ambiguous genitalia in a female with congenital adrenal hyperplasia (CAH). Full labioscrotal folds without palpable gonads and prominent phallic structure present in this patient. This patient had low confluence of vagina and urethra. **B:** Genitogram in different female CAH patient where the vagina joins the urethra near bladder neck. (Catheters for the VCUG needed to be placed with cystoscopy and vaginoscopy due to the high confluence.)

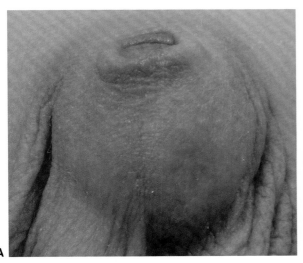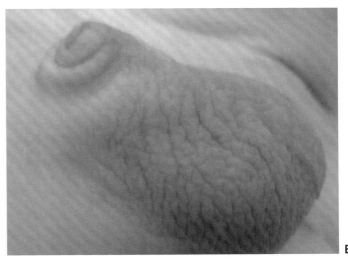

FIGURE 39.34 A: Megaprepuce in young boy. Due to paucity of penile shaft skin, a newborn circumcision should not be attempted as it will cause an entrapment of the penis due to dense scarring requiring further surgical intervention at a later time. **B:** Megaprepuce in a different boy. Note the relative absence of penile shaft skin. Newborn clamp device circumcision should not be done in the patient with similar anatomy.

in patient satisfaction or dissatisfaction with gender initially selected. The neonate should be evaluated for medically treatable or emergent conditions, such as salt wasting associated with conditions such as CAH and counsel the family as to the conflicts and controversy currently at issue with gender assignment.

Development of the Prepuce and Circumcision

The prepuce forms as a roll of epithelium fusing ventrally at the frenulum. Failure of urethral development will interfere with development of the prepuce, so that abnormalities of the prepuce should raise suspicion that other penile abnormalities (e.g., hypospadias, chordee, epispadias, megaprepuce) may be present (Fig. 39.34A and B). As the prepuce covers the glans, its inner epithelial surface fuses with the epithelium of the glans and will not separate from it until later in life. Separation of the inner epithelial layer from the glans occurs when cystic spaces form between these layers that can be filled with desquamated epithelial cells forming white, pearl-like beads (infantile smegma) generally seen through the overlying skin. Occasionally, infantile smegma may become inflamed or infected, although most smegma drains spontaneously without infection.

Because circumcision is common in the United States, the natural history of preputial development is not well understood. Observations in other countries where circumcision is not generally done help with understanding the normal course of preputial separation from the glans. The normal newborn foreskin is not retractable. In a large series from Denmark, the foreskin was not completely retractable in most boys until puberty (92). Phimosis is the inability to retract the foreskin, but this is the normal state from infancy gradually retracting by adolescence. Normal physiologic phimosis allows the foreskin to gradually retract with penile growth, and most children will eventually have retractile skin without infection or voiding difficulty. Forcible retraction of the prepuce produces tearing of the skin at the preputial orifice with resultant scarring that may lead to pathologic phimosis.

Circumcision is performed for a multitude of reasons. Medically, carcinoma of the penis, pathologic phimosis, paraphimosis, some sexually transmitted diseases, and some urinary infections in infancy may be prevented by circumcision. There have been significant benefits with decreased transmission of HIV and HPV in countries where this has significant prevalence and morbidity. Benefits of circumcision are occasionally offset by complications arising from the procedure, just as in any other surgical procedure.

The most common complications seen are hemorrhage and wound infection. Both are relatively uncommon and are usually easily treated. Serious complications including sepsis, necrotizing fasciitis (Fournier gangrene), glans amputation, loss of the entire penis, urethrocutaneous fistulas, bands of scar between the shaft and the glans (Fig. 39.35A–C), denudation of the skin of the entire shaft of the penis, recurrent or pathologic phimosis, and urethral fistulas occur rarely (93). Parents are occasionally very unhappy with the cosmetic appearance of the penis even though there is a good functional result.

Families who do not wish to have their male infant circumcised but whose child is at risk for febrile UTI or if neonatal circumcision cannot be performed can decrease febrile UTI risk by improving tight neonatal phimosis by using topical steroid cream to the tip of the foreskin to help open the preputial skin. Preparations of betamethasone valerate 0.05% or 0.1% twice a day for 6 to 8 weeks, triamcinolone 0.1% four times a day for 6 to 8 weeks, or over-the-counter (OTC) hydrocortisone 1% two to four times a day for 6 to 8 weeks were all found to be quite successful in opening up the foreskin. The skin was not always completely retractile but will generally open enough for less pooling of urine inside the foreskin and less febrile UTIs (51). Adverse reactions were not common in the patients with treatment as prescribed.

Testicular Torsion

Torsion of the testis in the newborn usually presents as a firm, slightly enlarged testis. On presentation, the scrotal skin may be indurated or erythematous, but generally, there is minimal change in the skin. Neonatal torsion seems to be painless on presentation and is likely due to an antenatal event in as many as 72% of the cases (94). Some cases (28%) develop in the postnatal period. Exploration of the twisted testis in the newborn period probably is of limited value, because salvage is unlikely but is warranted if the changes are found shortly after birth and performed expeditiously (<6 hours from the time of change in testicular examination). Salvage with fairly rapid surgical exploration is still unlikely even if performed in less than 6 hours from presentation. Ten percent of neonatal torsions are bilateral, some are asynchronous, and some are intravaginal torsions, as is more common after the neonatal period, rather than the extravaginal torsion seen in newborns. An inguinal approach, in one series, had a salvage rate of about 20% when the torsion had occurred acutely in the neonatal period (95), but this may be an overrepresentation of actual salvage rates in

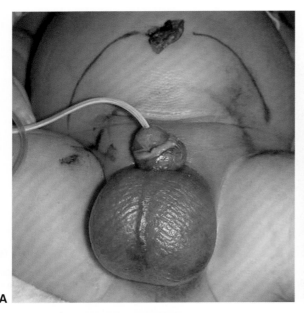

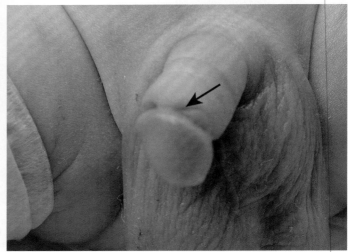

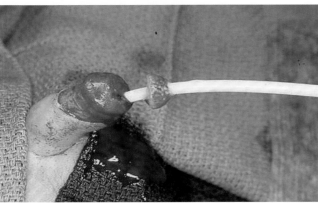

FIGURE 39.35 A: Neonate with necrotizing fasciitis (Fournier gangrene) after a newborn circumcision. Note areas of cellulitic advancement and induration on the scrotum. **B:** Penile skin bridge 1 week after newborn circumcision (see *arrow*). **C:** Partial glans amputation with Mogen clamp neonatal circumcision.

this group. If there is an obviously infarcted testis, contralateral exploration and testicular fixation, when the infant is stable, may prevent later contralateral torsion. Timing for this surgical procedure depends to some extent on the overall health of the infant as well as acuity of testicular or scrotal symptoms with objective physical and/or ultrasonographic findings.

Testicular Tumors

Tumors of the testis occasionally present at birth or in early infancy. These tumors can be evaluated with US to help differentiate them from the more common neonatal torsion, although sometimes, this is difficult. Teratomas of the testis account for 19.7% of cases in the Prepubertal Testicular Tumor Registry, are benign in prepubertal boys, and can usually be treated by testis-sparing tumor excision (96). Gonadal stromal tumors also present in newborns, with Sertoli cell tumors being the most common (96). These tumors appear malignant histologically, but invariably exhibit a benign behavior in infancy, and orchiectomy is curative. Gonadal stromal tumors appearing in later childhood, however, may have malignant behavior.

Yolk sac tumors occur in infancy representing approximately 30% of reported yolk sac tumors of the testis. These malignant tumors are best treated by radical orchiectomy. If there is no evidence of metastatic disease, adjunctive chemotherapy, node dissection, or radiation therapy may be unnecessary. Alpha-fetoprotein (AFP) levels are elevated in patients with yolk sac tumors, but AFP levels are also normally elevated in infancy. Age-adjusted AFP levels should be used to better interpret AFP measurements as a tumor marker in infants (97).

Zinner Syndrome (Congenital Malformation in Males of the Seminal Vesicles with Associated Ipsilateral Renal Agenesis)

Zinner syndrome is an association similar to MRKH in males with unilateral renal agenesis and male genital tract anomalies resulting from faulty development of the distal mesonephric duct. It is generally symptomatic in the second and third decade of life with seminal vesicle dilation or obstruction of the ejaculatory duct. There may be associated infertility in 45% of the patients possibly due to ejaculatory duct obstruction. These are best diagnosed with MRI of the seminal vesicles and ejaculatory ducts but can first be studied with US of abdomen and pelvis (98) (Fig. 39.36A–C).

URINARY TRACT INFECTION

The overall incidence of neonatal UTIs is approximately 1.5 to 5 cases per 1,000 live births. The male-to-female ratio is about 3:1 and 5:1, where later in childhood and in later adult life, there is a female preponderance of patients with UTI. Uncircumcised infant males are more likely to have urinary infections than circumcised males (11,51). The incidence of urinary infection in uncircumcised males approximates 1 per 100. The source of urinary infections can infrequently be hematogenous rather than ascending.

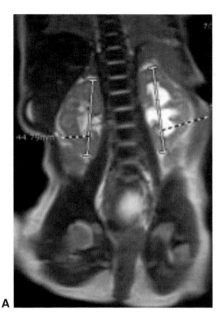
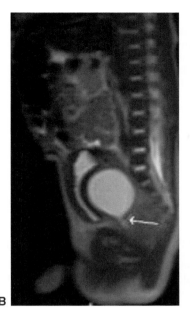
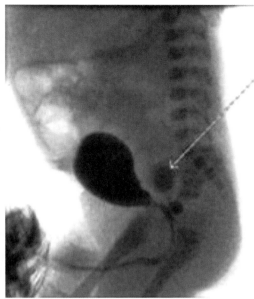

FIGURE 39.36 **A:** Zinner variant with left ectopic obstructed ureter to left seminal vesicle on MRU. **B:** MRU sagittal image of seminal vesicle cyst with left obstructed ureter attached and filling cyst (*arrow* at utricle). **C:** VCUG with prominent utricle and left seminal vesicle cyst filling behind displaced bladder but normal urethra (*arrow* at seminal vesicle cyst).

Any newborn with culture-documented bacteriuria found with bladder catheterization or aspiration should have radiographic evaluation. US is indicated in all children, and VCUG should be obtained, if the US is abnormal or if gross hematuria or fevers are found with the positive urine culture. VUR may be present in approximately half of those evaluated, and obstructive uropathy may also be found. American Academy of Pediatrics' Clinical Practice Guidelines for initial UTI in febrile infants and children for children between 2 and 24 months suggest that no studies are needed until there has been a second documented UTI and these guidelines are used. The guidelines suggest that only a US examination of the urinary tract is necessary. If it is normal, no further imaging is performed. If there is an abnormal ultrasound, or repeated febrile UTI, then a VCUG should be performed (99). Documented febrile UTI in a neonate in most cases still warrants evaluation with US and a VCUG in our opinion.

UROLOGIC ASPECTS OF SPINA BIFIDA

Spina bifida in the United States has a rate of 3.5 per 10,000 births with recent prevalence decreasing by 20% in infants born in non-Hispanic black mothers but remains constant in Hispanic and non-Hispanic white mothers (100,101).

In utero repair of the spinal cord defect, starting in 1997, initially showed slightly decreased need for ventriculoperitoneal shunt (VPS) and some improvement in lower extremity function but without much improved bladder function. The early decreased need for VPS and improved lower extremity function has not persisted over time. To study the effect on bladder function and safety of *in utero* repair of meningomyelocele, the Management of Meningomyelocele Study (MOMS) randomly assigned patients to *in utero* repair versus standard postnatal repair with primary outcomes of survival or need for CIC by 30 months of age. There was a slight advantage in the prenatal surgical group with a smoother bladder at 30 months and with slightly fewer patients starting CIC by 30 months of age (38% of prenatal repaired patients vs. 51% of postnatally repaired patients) and fewer patients with an open bladder neck in the prenatal group than in the postnatal group. There was no significant difference between the groups based on the level

of spinal cord involvement. Ultimately, there was no major difference in overall outcome between the groups except for a speculated potential delay in augmentation cystoplasty in the prenatal group (102).

This study showed that prenatal intervention was not without risks and complications as there was a high risk of premature birth and risks of fetal/neonatal death, intrauterine hemorrhage, and hypovolemia and hypothermia from prenatal surgery itself. Additionally, there are maternal risks and complications from *in utero* surgeries including uterine rupture, sepsis, hemorrhage, and risks for future pregnancies due to uterine scar formation. . Most of these procedures are limited to a few centers that have the most experience and should still be considered experimental and not widespread in application (103).

In 2012, the Centers for Disease Control and Prevention (CDC) met to prospectively develop a protocol for optimal urologic care of spina bifida children from birth through age 5 years. The groups included pediatric urologists, nephrologists, epidemiologists, methodologists, and community advocates (101). Children enrolled underwent frequent US, VCUG and urodynamics (UDS), or videourodynamics (VUDS) at set intervals and yearly creatinine testing. Importantly, infants were initially placed on CIC every 6 hours with decreased frequency once bladder catheterization volumes were less than 30 mL on most catheterizations for 3 consecutive days. Indwelling bladder or Foley catheter drainage was done initially until the family was instructed in CIC. Catheterization frequency decreased as bladder emptying improved and as long as the bladder itself was thought to be hostile if found on VUDS or UDS and VCUG with bladder pressures less and 40 cm H_2O at end filling. Increased CIC frequency every 4 hours at minimum and routine anticholinergic medications was instituted in these patients. This study is still ongoing pending the first 5-year data results. Alternatively, some centers placed infants on routine CIC and anticholinergic treatment and do not take the children off this routine. There is significant controversy as to the best course of management with proactive (ongoing) CIC as compared to reactive CIC (reinstitute CIC if hostile bladder is found on frequent subsequent US, VUDS, or UDS studies). Families can be taught how to informally measure bladder pressures at home by measuring the height of urine in the home intermittent catheter with a ruler on the patient's abdomen. If the measurement is fairly high on the ruler (20 cm or more), this is concerning that the patient's bladder may be becoming more hostile and needs reevaluation and possible change in management (104). Antibiotic prophylaxis use is controversial as well only being used on CDC protocol in patients with grade V VUR or if there was a hostile bladder on testing.

Urinary tract involvement with spina bifida may not be problematic in the newborn period, but these patients should be evaluated shortly after birth, and a urinary tract surveillance program should be instituted. Manual expression of the bladder (Credé maneuver) should not be performed to drain urine from the bladder because it produces very high intravesical pressures causing significant upper tract deterioration, especially if there is associated VUR. CIC is usually recommended to safely and reliably empty the bladder in both male and female infants, but if significant hydronephrosis is present and not improved with CIC and overnight indwelling bladder catheterization or it is difficult or not consistently done by families, temporary cutaneous vesicostomy may be necessary to reliably empty the bladder. Children with spina bifida should, if possible, be managed by a multidisciplinary team that includes neurologists, neurosurgeons, urologists, general pediatrics, nutritionists, and orthopedic surgeons. With this approach, these children have an excellent chance of survival.

Triad Syndrome or Prune Belly Syndrome

Triad syndrome, also known as Eagle-Barrett or PBS, is a spectrum of abnormalities characterized by abdominal wall deficiency, hydronephrosis, and, in males, cryptorchidism. The abdominal wall defect itself gives the patient's characteristic appearance leading to its name. The incidence of this condition is estimated to be 1 per 35,000 to 50,000 live births (105). Males are affected 10 times more frequently than females. Prevalence is generally higher in blacks than whites, and it is more common in children born to younger mothers (105). There is no clear-cut evidence that this is an inherited disorder but there may be an association with Beckwith-Wiedemann syndrome (105). Theories of embryogenesis include obstructive uropathy and mesenchymal dysplasia.

There can be massive hydroureteronephrosis, and the bladder often is very dilated. Because there is prostatic hypoplasia and dilation of the prostatic urethra, antenatal studies may not differentiate these patients from boys with PUVs. The kidneys often are dysplastic determining overall prognosis. Cryptorchidism may be due to bladder distension pushing the testes into the abdomen preventing normal descent. Although some affected children die in infancy, many today survive. Prenatal US may demonstrate a distended bladder, an abnormal prostatic urethra, and possibly hyperechoic or cystic kidneys. Due to the relative absence of abdominal musculature, pulmonary complications, including pulmonary arrest, pulmonary hypoplasia, rib abnormalities, and pneumonia, are common. Associated anomalies are found in up to 65% to 73% of patients with gastrointestinal problems seen in up to 30% and cardiac anomalies in up to 10% of patients. PBS may have a wide spectrum of involvement with high perinatal mortality when severe renal and pulmonary dysplasia and hypoplasia are seen, and some children will have very mild urinary tract abnormalities requiring minimal surgical intervention with fairly efficient voiding and reasonable renal and pulmonary function. Reconstruction of the urinary tract, orchiopexy, and repair of the abdominal wall defect help improve quality of life for these children (**Fig. 39.37A–C**).

UROLOGIC ISSUES WITH ANORECTAL MALFORMATIONS (ARMS)

Development of the lower urinary and gastrointestinal (GI) tract are intimately related, and the urinary tract will be affected in many children with imperforate anus. The higher the lesion, the

greater the chance of urinary involvement with 25% to 50% GU anomalies associated with ARMs (106). All newborns with imperforate anus should be screened for urinary tract abnormalities with US and VCUG because of the close association of the developing lower urinary and GI tracts. VUR has been reported to occur in about 20% to 47% of children with ARMs. These children should be monitored for febrile UTIs because of VUR incidence. Diverting colostomy does not decrease the risk of febrile UTI occurrence. The constellation of other associated anomalies, known as VACTERRL (vertebral, anorectal, cardiac, tracheoesophageal, renal, radial, and limb abnormalities) association is common in many of these children. VACTERRL is a nongenetic and occurs sporadically. As three elements qualify as the association, a third element should be sought if two are present. Lower spine US imaging up to age 3 months should be done to evaluate for possible spinal cord abnormalities.

FEMALE GENITAL ABNORMALITIES

The female reproductive system is formed by the müllerian or paramesonephric ducts. The müllerian system differentiates into a female organ system when müllerian inhibitory substance (MIS) is absent. During the 6th to 8th week of gestation, müllerian ducts will form lateral to the wolffian ducts, cross medially, and fuse in the midline incorporating the UG sinus to form the uterovaginal canal by the 10th week of gestation. The fallopian tubes develop from the lateral ends of the müllerian ducts. The vagina develops from the fused müllerian ducts and the UG sinus. It is believed that the upper four-fifths of the vagina is müllerian derived and the lower fifth is from the UG sinus. Vaginal formation is completed by the 5th month of gestation.

External genitalia differentiates during the 12th to 16th weeks *in utero*. The absence of fetal androgens allows passive development of the genital tubercle into the clitoris, the urethral folds into the labia minora, and the genital swellings into the labia majora.

Vaginal Agenesis

Vaginal agenesis with Mayer-Rokitansky-Küster-Hauser syndrome (MRKH) occurs when the vaginal plate does not canalize. The incidence is reported as 1 in 4,000 to 5,000 live female births. Patients, generally 46XX females, present with primary amenorrhea but have normal secondary female sex features. The ovaries and external genitalia generally are normal, but the vaginal plate is not canalized, and the uterus may be rudimentary. It is common to have associated urinary anomalies; renal anomalies are seen in 34% of the patients (107). Renal agenesis and ectopia are the most common findings. Patients may also have skeletal anomalies, particularly in the spine and ribs. Combinations of these anomalies have been termed as the MURCS (müllerian duct aplasia, renal aplasia, and cervicothoracic somite malformations) association. Surgical correction is individualized based on the location and development of the uterine and vaginal remnants (107).

Hydrocolpos and Hydrometrocolpos

If the vaginal canalization is incomplete, the hymen may be imperforate or a high transverse vaginal septum may be present. The infant may present with hydrocolpos (vaginal distention with secretions stimulated by maternal estrogens) or hydrometrocolpos (distention of the vagina and the uterus also with secretions). Current antenatal US can find this prior to delivery, but many infants still present with an abdominal mass, possible urinary obstruction, and a bulging introital mass. US may demonstrate a fluid-filled or mixed density fluid-filled pelvis mass, and possibly a distended bladder with or without hydroureteronephrosis, or secondary urinary obstruction (**Fig. 39.38**).

Definitive treatment depends on the extent of vaginal canalization; this can be a simple hymenotomy or vaginoplasty or vaginal

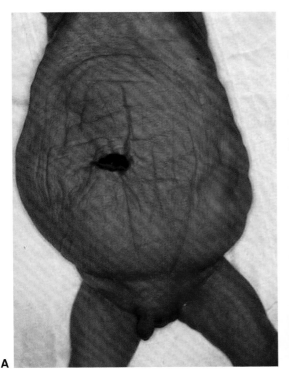
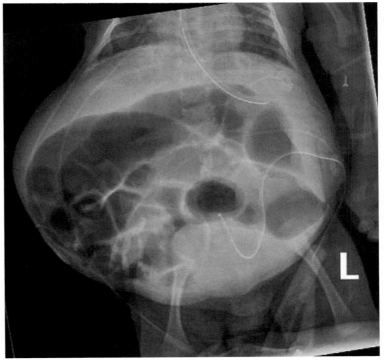
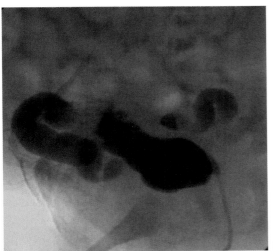

FIGURE 39.37 **A:** PBS with typical abdominal wall appearance due to absent or scant abdominal musculature. **B:** Abdominal x-ray of a baby with PBS with marked distention of the abdomen due to absent abdominal wall. **C:** VCUG on the same PBS patient with patent urachus and high-grade VUR, which is also common in these patients. This patient's prostatic urethra was not well visualized due to catheter in place. This baby also had bilateral dysplastic poorly functioning kidneys.

pull through if the septal defect is high. CT or, preferably MRI with T2-weighted sequences better delineate any vaginal plate, but occasionally, needle aspiration of the fluid with radiographic contrast injection and imaging may be needed to delineate the vaginal plate length.

Duplication or Fusion Anomalies

Duplication of the uterus and vagina occurs if müllerian ducts fusion is incomplete. The child may have two uteri or one or two cervices with either a single vagina or two separate vaginas, with one or both vaginas open to the perineum. These malformations are identified early in life by US but frequently may not present until adolescence. Typical presentation is a menstruating female having cyclic pelvic pain with menses and an enlarging pelvic mass. Treating vaginal duplication usually only requires incising the longitudinal vaginal septum. Successful pregnancies have been reported in some women with duplicated uteri.

Urogenital Sinus (UG) and Cloacal Abnormalities

A common UG sinus is a normal part of development in both sexes. If müllerian duct development arrests during the first trimester, a persistent urovaginal confluence or common UG sinus is found at birth. Depending on the timing of vaginal differentiation, varying locations for the vaginal and urethral junction occur. If the arrest is early, the connection is higher. The anus may be located in a normal location or be more anteriorly placed. These infants have a common introital opening for urethra and vagina and a second opening for the anus. A flush genitogram will delineate the length of the common UG channel and the connection of the urethra and vagina. This is performed by placing a feeding tube or urethral catheter just inside the common opening and injecting contrast material in a retrograde fashion. Surgical reconstruction required is determined by the length of the common channel and the location of the urethral vaginal junction. Corrective surgery can be performed during the first year of life in most

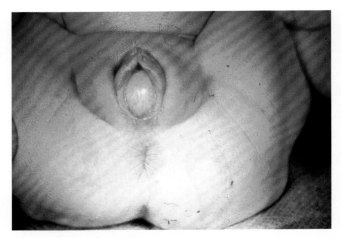

FIGURE 39.38 Bulging imperforate hymen in a newborn infant girl who also had associated hydrocolpos.

cases but is often deferred until the patient weighs about 8 to 10 kg or age 1 to 3 years to allow better convalescence (108). Total or partial UG mobilization has been used to bring a high junction to the perineum, generally without incontinence. More extensive surgery through the rectum may be needed for mobilization of the common sinus if there is high urethra and vagina confluence for better functional and cosmetic results and less urinary incontinence.

Combination of UG sinus and anorectal malformation is termed a cloacal anomaly. This may occur in 1 in 50,000 live births (108). By 4 to 6 weeks of gestation, the uro-rectal septum should divide the common allantoic–hindgut confluence. If this does not occur, a common cloaca will be present at birth. Because of the imperforate anus, these infants have abdominal distention and a single perineal opening. Major pitfalls in newborn management of a cloacal abnormality include failure to recognize and manage hydrocolpos, problems associated with vesicostomy or colostomy, and misdiagnosis of a cloaca (72). Delineating the anatomy in this condition is important for appropriate surgical management, which requires a combined approach with pediatric general surgery and urology input. Infants typically require diverting colostomy as initial treatment. Generally, cystoscopic evaluation should be done at the same time with diverting colostomy and placement of catheters in the vagina and in the bladder done at the same time so radiographic studies can be done to determine important anatomic details for ultimate reconstruction of the anus, vaginal and urethral opening.

Management of associated hydrocolpos is critical using renal and pelvic US to determine associated hydroureteronephrosis. Nephrology consultation is important for management of associated renal disease if bladder outlet obstruction is present with hydrocolpos (72,108).

Typically, intermittent catheterization of the common channel will decompress the vagina or septated vaginas alleviating most urinary obstruction. It is not necessary to drain the bladder itself as the bladder and urethra will usually drain into the common channel and emptying the common channel will ultimately empty the bladder. Rarely, the common channel or urethra may be so stenotic and require either a vesicostomy or a vaginostomy. Successful decompression of the vagina or septated vagina and bladder and improved hydroureteronephrosis may be verified by checking the urinary and vaginal systems with a renal and lower abdomino-pelvic US.

It is better to achieve cloacal emptying with catheterization because a vesicostomy or vaginostomy will cause the bladder and vagina to be fixed higher on the abdomen after surgery causing a higher ultimate cloacal channel length than the original length with higher urethral and vaginal separation requiring more extensive surgery. Additionally, prolapse of the vesicostomy or vaginostomy, if they occur, can be difficult to manage until ultimate reconstruction (108).

These girls may have associated VUR and may have long-term bladder emptying issues from a shortened urethra, incompetent bladder neck or sphincter of the bladder and from associated spinal cord anomalies. These infants should have lower spinal cord US imaging, up until age 3 months, to diagnose spinal anomalies or cord tethering. MRI may be done on the lower spine if ultrasound imaging of the spine is nondiagnostic, if the child older than 3 months, or more comprehensive imaging is needed (108).

Complete reconstruction is generally deferred during infancy and is generally done after 1 year of age or when the patient is about 10 kg as with UG sinus reconstruction. Delaying reconstruction until late childhood or puberty is more difficult, due to scarring from anal pull through and the deeper, less mobile pelvis present in older girls and adolescents (**Fig. 39.39A and B**).

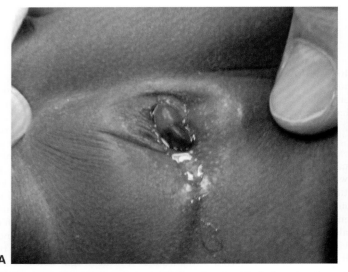
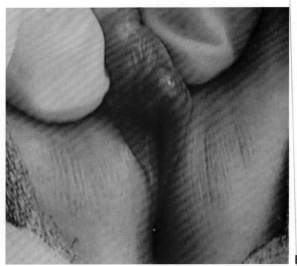

FIGURE 39.39 A: Cloacal abnormality in newborn female with single perineal opening. Note clear urine leaking from single opening. **B:** Infant girl with UG sinus and clitoromegaly but no CAH. The patient has two perineal openings: one for common UG sinus and one for the anus.

Ovarian Cysts

Ovarian cysts develop due to hormonal stimulation and are more commonly seen after puberty. The fetal ovary is stimulated by fetal gonadotropins, maternal estrogens, and placental chorionic gonadotropin and may develop cysts during development and infancy. Ovarian cysts are found more frequently with prenatal US.

Clinically significant ovarian cysts occur in 1/2,500 live births and may be the most common cause of cystic abdominal mass in newborn girls (109).

Vaginal delivery is possible in most cases, with cesarean section being reserved for very large cysts. Recent studies show that most simple cysts less than 5 cm on postnatal US generally will spontaneously resolve and can be followed with serial imaging, with most regressing in the first 3 to 4 months of life. Larger cysts may be followed for involution or can be aspirated for ovary conservation.

Neonatal ovarian torsion is associated with prenatally diagnosed ovarian cyst in up to 91% of patients with most (55%) seen as simple cysts with third trimester US (110).

There is new evidence that up to 92% of torsed neonatal ovaries are found on first postnatal US indicating that most neonatal torsions occurred *in utero*. Additionally, complex ovarian cysts with septa, debris levels, echogenic appearance, or clot may represent neonatal ovarian torsion and may spontaneously resolve (109).

In a recent observational study, 48% resolved spontaneously and those requiring surgery was due to failure of cyst involution or concern for possible interval ovarian torsion and torsion occurred in only 4% overall with around 12% with cysts greater than 5 cm.

Ovarian preservation, including if cysts are complex, may be performed by removing or unroofing the cyst with open or laparoscopic surgery (109). Cysts greater than 5 cm are concerning for possible torsion and loss of the ovary if the vessels are twisted for a prolonged period of time, but most cysts generally involute without surgical treatment.

Occasionally, intestinal obstruction has been noted to occur in newborn girls with ovarian cysts. Generally, these cysts are very large (usually 7 to 10 cm) with associated smaller cysts and bowel obstruction due to inflammatory adhesions from the ovarian torsion. The majority occur within the first 2 days of postnatal life, so there should be a high index of suspicion for intestinal obstruction due to ovarian torsion when large or complex ovarian cysts are present.

Introital Masses

Introital masses generally are seen on the first examination of the infant. The differential diagnosis for introital masses in female infants includes imperforate hymen, prolapsing ureterocele, and Skene or Gartner cysts. Paraurethral cysts (Skene's or Gartner's) present with lateral displacement of the urethral meatus in newborn girls. These cysts involute or rupture spontaneously fairly quickly once maternal estrogen stimulation lessens after birth; surgical treatment is usually unnecessary.

REFERENCES

1. Mandell J, Peters CA, Retik AB. Current concepts in the perinatal diagnosis and management of hydronephrosis. *Urol Clin North Am* 1990;17:247.
2. Fowler SF, Sydorak RM, Albanese CT, et al. Fetal endoscopic surgery: lessons learned and trends reviewed. *J Pediatr Surg* 2002;37(12):1700.
3. Townsend RR, Manlo-Johnson M. Prenatal diagnosis of urinary tract abnormalities with ultrasound: a review. *Scand J Urol Nephrol* 1991;138(suppl):13.
4. Pope JC, Brock JW, Adams MC, et al. How they begin and how they end: classic and new theories for the development and deterioration of congenital anomalies of the kidney and urinary tract CAKUT. *J Am Soc Nephrol* 1999;10(9):2018.
5. Nguyen HT, Benson CB, Bromley B, et al. Multidisciplinary consensus on the classification of prenatal and postnatal urinary tract dilation (UTD classification system). *J Pediatr Urol* 2014;10:982.
6. Zee RS, Herndon CDA, Cooper CS, et al. Time to resolution: a prospective evaluation from the Society for Fetal Urology hydronephrosis registry. *J Pediatr Urol* 2017;13:316e.1.
7. Bujon A, Saldaña L, Caffaratti J. Can endoscopic balloon dilation for primary obstructive megaureter be effective in a long-term follow-up? *J Pediatr Urol* 2015;11:37e1.
8. Belman AB, King LR. The pathology and treatment of renal vein thrombosis in the newborn. *J Urol* 1972;107:852.
9. Maizels M, Reisman ME, Flum ES, et al. Grading nephroureteral dilatation detected in the first year of life: correlation with obstruction. *J Urol* 1992;148:609.
10. Lopez-Munoz E, Hernandez-Zarco A, Polano-Ortiz A, et al. Megacystis-microcolon-intestinal hypoperistalsis syndrome (MMIHS): report of a case with prolonged survival and literature review. *J Pediatr Urol* 2013;9(1):e12.
11. Braga LH, Farrokhyar F, D'Cruz J, et al. Risk factors for febrile urinary tract infection in children with prenatal hydronephrosis: a prospective study. *J Urol* 2015;193:1766.
12. Carter CO. The genetics of urinary tract malformations. *J Genet Hum* 1984;31(1):23.
13. Mackie GG, Stephens FD. Duplex kidneys: a correlation of renal dysplasia with position of the ureteral orifice. *J Urol* 1979;114:274.
14. Brenner BM, Lawler EV, Mackenzie HS. The hyperfiltration theory: a paradigm shift in nephrology. *Kidney Int* 1996;49:1974.
15. Goldfarb DA, Matin SF, Braun WE, et al. Renal outcome 25 years after donor nephrectomy. *J Urol* 2001;166(6):2043.
16. Muzaale AD, Massie AB, Wang M, et al. Risk of end-stage renal disease following live kidney donation. *JAMA* 2014;311(6):579.
17. Luyckx VA, Bertram JF, Brenner BM, et al. Effect of fetal and child health on kidney development and long term risk of hypertension and kidney disease. *Lancet* 2013;382(9888):273.
18. Kelalis PP, Malek RS, Segura JW. Observations on renal ectopia and fusion in children. *J Urol* 1973;110:588.
19. Cook WA, Stephens FD. Fused kidneys: morphologic study and theory of embryogenesis. In: Bergsma D, Duckett JW, eds. *Urinary system malformations in children. Birth defects: original article series*. New York, NY: March of Dimes, 1977:327.
20. McDonald JH, McClellan DS. Crossed renal ectopia. *Am J Urol* 1957;93:995.
21. N'Guessan G, Stephens FD. Supernumerary kidney. *J Urol* 1983;130:649.
22. Blythe H, Ockenden BG. Polycystic disease of kidneys and liver presenting in childhood. *J Med Genet* 1971;8:257.
23. Stapleton FB, Johnson DL, Kaplan GW, et al. The cystic renal lesion in tuberous sclerosis. *J Pediatr* 1980;97:574.
24. Eickmeyer AB, Casanova NF, He C, et al. The natural history of the multicystic dysplastic kidney-Is limited follow-up warranted? *J Pediatr Urol* 2014;10:655.
25. Cardona-Grau D, Kogan BA. Update on multicystic dysplastic kidney. *Curr Urol Rep* 2015;16:67.
26. Cambio AJ, Evans CP, Kurzrock EA. Non-surgical management of multicystic dysplastic kidney. *BJU Int* 2008;101(7):804.
27. Schultz K, Toda LY. Genetic basis of ureterocele. *Curr Genomics* 2016;17:62.
28. Scherz HC, Kaplan GW, Packer MG, et al. Ectopic ureteroceles: surgical management with preservation of continence: review of 60 cases. *J Urol* 1989;142:538.
29. Calaway AC, Whittam B, Syzmanski KM, et al. Multicystic dysplastic kidney: is an initial voiding cystogram necessary? *Can J Urol* 2014;21(5):7510.
30. Gaither TW, Patel A, Patel C, et al. Natural history of contralateral hypertrophy in patients with multicystic dysplastic kidneys. *J Urol* 2017;199:280.
31. Campbell MF. Embryology and anomalies of the urogenital tract. In: Campbell MF, ed. *Clinical pediatric urology*. Philadelphia, PA: WB Saunders, 1951:198.
32. Stephens FD, Lenaghan D. The anatomical basis and dynamics of vesicoureteral reflux. *J Urol* 1962;87:669.
33. Glenn JF. Agenesis of the bladder. *JAMA* 1959;169:2016.
34. Williams DI. The development of the trigone of the bladder. *Br J Urol* 1951;23:123.
35. Satler EJ, Mossman HW. A case of double bladder and double urethra in the female child. *J Urol* 1968;79:274.
36. Stephens FD. *Congenital malformations of the urinary tract*. New York, NY: Praeger, 1983.
37. Brock WA, Kaplan GW. Voiding dysfunction in children. *Curr Probl Pediatr* 1980;2:10.
38. Brock WA, Kaplan GW. Ectopic ureteroceles in children. *J Urol* 1978;119:800.
39. Di Renzo D, Ellsworth PI, Caldamone AA. Transurethral puncture for ureterocele-Which factors dictate outcomes? *J Urol* 2010;184:1620.
40. Conway JJ, Maizels M. The "well-tempered" diuretic renogram: a standard method to examine the asymptomatic neonate with hydronephrosis or hydroureteronephrosis. A report from combined meeting of The Society for Fetal Urology and members of The Pediatric Nuclear Medicine Council—The Society of Nuclear Medicine. *J Nucl Med* 1992;33(11):2047.

THE NEWBORN INFANT

41. Dickerson EC, Dillman JR, Smith EA, et al. Pediatric MR urography: indications, techniques, and approach to review. *Radiographics* 2015;35:1208.

42. Kaefer M, Misseri R, Frank E. Refluxing ureteral reimplantation: a logical method for managing neonatal UVJ obstruction. *J Pediatr Urol* 2014;10:824.

43. Liu W, Du G, Ma R. Modified ureteral orthotopic reimplantation method for managing infant primary obstructive megaureter: a preliminary study. *Int Urol Nephrol* 2016;48:1937.

44. Sargent MA. What is the normal prevalence of vesicoureteral reflux? *Pediatr Radiol* 2000;30(9):587.

45. Feather SA, Malcolm S, Woolf AS, et al. Primary, nonsyndromic vesicoureteric reflux and its nephropathy is genetically heterogeneous, with a locus on chromosome 1. *Am J Hum Genet* 2000;66(4):1420.

46. Vesicoureteral reflux: topic 4—screening of siblings and offspring of patients with vesicoureteral reflux. Management and Screening of Primary Vesicoureteral Reflux in Children: AUA Guidelines, Revised, 2010.

47. Levitt SA, Duckett J, Spitzer A, et al. Medical versus surgical treatment of primary vesicoureteral reflux: report of the International Reflux Study Committee. *Pediatrics* 1981;67:392.

48. Skoog SJ, Peters CA, Arant BS Jr, et al. Pediatric vesicoureteral reflux guidelines panel summary report: clinical practice guidelines for screening siblings of children with vesicoureteral reflux and neonates/infants with prenatal hydronephrosis. *J Urol* 2010;184:1145.

49. Braga LH, Mijovic H, Ferrokhyar F, et al. Antibiotic prophylaxis for urinary tract infection in antenatal hydronephrosis. *Pediatrics* 2013;131(1):e251.

50. Herz D, Merguerian P, McQuiston L. Continuous antibiotic prophylaxis reduces the risk of febrile UTI in children with asymptomatic antenatal hydronephrosis with either ureteral dilation, high-grade vesicoureteral reflux, or ureterovesical junction obstruction. *J Pediatr Urol* 2014;10:650.

51. Chamberlin JD, Dorgalli C, Abdelhalim A, et al. Randomized open-label trial comparing topical prescription triamcinolone to over-the-counter hydrocortisone for the treatment of phimosis. *J Pediatr Urol* 2019;4:1.e1.

52. Borer JG, Vasquez E, Canning DA, et al. An initial report of a novel multi-institutional bladder exstrophy consortium focused on primary surgery and subsequent care. *J Urol* 2014;193:1802.

53. Grady RW, Mitchell ME. Complete primary repair of exstrophy: surgical technique. *Urol Clin North Am* 2000;27(3):569.

54. Scherz HC, Kaplan GW, Sutherland DH, et al. Fascia late and early spica casting as adjuncts in closure of bladder exstrophy. *J Urol* 1990;144:550.

55. Tank ES, Lindenauer SM. Principles of management of exstrophy of the cloaca. *Am J Surg* 1970;119:95.

56. Reiner WG, Kropp BP. A seven year experience of genetic males with severe phallic inadequacy assigned female. *J Urol* 2004;172(6):2395.

57. Phillips TM, Salmasi AH, Stec A, et al. Urological outcomes in the omphalocele exstrophy imperforate anus spinal defects (OEIS) complex: experience with 80 patients. *J Pediatr Urol* 2013;9(3):353.

58. Thomas JC, De Marco RT, Pope JC, et al. First stage approximation of the exstrophic bladder in patients with cloacal exstrophy—should this be the initial surgical approach in all patients? *J Urol* 2007;178:1632.

59. Waffarn F, Devasker UP, Hodgman JE. Vesicoumbilical fistula: a complication of umbilical artery cut-down. *J Pediatr Surg* 1980;15:211.

60. Redman JF, Jimenez JF, Golladay ES, et al. Megacystis microcolon-intestinal hypoperistalsis syndrome: case report and review of the literature. *J Urol* 1984;131:981.

61. Granata C, Puri P. Megacystis-microcolon-intestinal hypoperistalsis syndrome. *J Pediatr Gastroenterol Nutr* 1997;25:12.

62. Ochoa B, Curlin RJ. Urofacial (Ochoa) syndrome. *Am J Med Genet* 1987;27:661.

63. Casella DP, Tomaszewski JJ, Ost MC. Posterior urethral valves: renal failure and prenatal treatment. *Int J Nephrol* 2012;2012:351067.

64. Dewan PA, Keenan RJ, Morris LL, et al. Congenital urethral obstruction: Cobb's collar or prolapsed congenital obstructive posterior urethral membrane (COPUM). *Br J Urol* 1994;73(1):91.

65. McLorie G, Farhat W, Khoury A, et al. Outcome analysis of vesicoamniotic shunting in a comprehensive population. *J Urol* 2001;166(3):1036.

66. Luks FI. New and/or improved aspects of fetal surgery. *Prenat Diagn* 2011;31:232.

67. Morris RK, Malin GL, Quinlan-Jones E, et al. Percutaneous vesicoamniotic shunting versus conservative management for fetal lower urinary tract obstruction (PLUTO): a randomised trial. *Lancet* 2013;382(9903):1496.

68. Sarhan OM. Posterior urethral valves: impact of low birth weight and preterm delivery on final renal outcome. *Arab J Urol* 2017;15:159.

69. Bigutay AN, Roth DR, Gonzales ET Jr, et al. Posterior urethral valves: risk factors for progression to renal failure. *J Pediatr Urol* 2016;12(3):179.e1.

70. Tank ES, Carey TC, Seifert NL. Management of neonatal urinary ascites. *Urology* 1980;16:270.

71. Cuckow PM, Dinneen MD, Risdon RA, et al. Long-term renal function in the posterior urethral valves, unilateral reflux and renal dysplasia syndrome. *J Urol* 1997;158(3 Pt 2):1004.

72. Levitt MA, Peña A. Pitfalls in the management of newborn cloacas. *Pediatr Surg Int* 2005;21:264.

73. Engel DL, Pope JC IV, Adams MC, et al. Risk factors associated with chronic kidney disease in patients with posterior urethral valves without prenatal hydronephrosis. *J Urol* 2011;185:2502.

74. Berger M, von Schweinitz D. Current management of fetal and neonatal renal tumors. *Curr Pediatr Rev* 2015;11:188.

75. Scorer CG, Farrington GH. *Congenital deformities of the testis and epididymis*. London, UK: Butterworths, 1971;4:45.

76. Kessler WO, McLaughlin AP. Agenesis of the penis: embryology and management. *Urology* 1973;1:226.

77. Wisniewski AB, Migeon CJ, Gearhart JP, et al. Congenital micropenis: long-term medical, surgical and psychosexual follow up of individuals raised male or female. *Horm Res* 2001;56:3.

78. Mirshemirani A, Sadeghyian N, Mohajerzadeh L, et al. Diphallus: report on six cases and review of the literature. *Iran J Pediatr* 2010;20(3):353.

79. Lee PA, Mazur T, Danish R, et al. Micropenis: criteria, etiologies, and classification. *Johns Hopkins Med J* 1980;146:156.

80. Clelia T, Stefania M, Rosa S, et al. Hypospadias and associated malformations in twins: a clinical case. *Res J Congenial Dis* 2018;1(1):1.

81. Chen MJ, Macias CG, Gunn SK, et al. Intrauterine growth restriction and hypospadias: is there a connection? *Int J Pediatr Endocrin* 2014;2014(20):1.

82. Anderson B, Mitchell M. Recent advances in hypospadias: current surgical technique and research in incidence and etiology. *Curr Urol Rep* 2001;2(2):122.

83. Carmichael SL, Cogswell ME, Ma C, et al. Hypospadias and maternal intake of phytoestrogens. *Am J Epidemiol* 2013;178(3):434.

84. Aberg A, Westbom L, Källén B. Congenital malformations among infants whose mothers had gestational diabetes or preexisting diabetes. *Early Hum Dev* 2001;61(2):85.

85. Visser R, Burger NC, van Zwet EW, et al. Higher incidence of hypospadias in monochorionic twins. *Twin Res Hum Genet* 2015;18(5):591.

86. Gatti JM, Kirsch AJ, Troyer WA, et al. Increased incidence of hypospadias in small-for-gestational age infants in a neonatal intensive-care unit. *BJU Int* 2001;87:548.

87. McAleer IM, Kaplan GW. Is routine karyotyping necessary in the evaluation of hypospadias and cryptorchidism? *J Urol* 2001;165:2029.

88. Canning DA, Koo HP, Duckett JW. Anomalies of the bladder and cloaca. In: Gillenwater JY, Grayhack JT, Howards SS, et al., eds. *Adult and pediatric urology*, 3rd ed. St. Louis, MO: Mosby-Year Book, 1996:2445.

89. Williams DI, Kenawi MM. Urethral duplications in the male. *Eur Urol* 1975;1:209.

90. Soares-Oliveira M, Juliá V, Garcia Aparicio L, et al. Congenital prepubic sinus. *J Pediatr Surg* 2002;37(8):1225.

91. Migeon CJ, Wisniewski AB, Gearhart JP, et al. Ambiguous genitalia with penoscrotal hypospadias in 46, XY individuals: long-term medical, surgical and psychosexual outcome. *Pediatrics* 2002;110(3):e31.

92. Oster J. Further fate of the foreskin. *Arch Dis Child* 1968;43:200.

93. Kaplan GW. Complications of circumcision. *Urol Clin North Am* 1983;10:543.

94. Das S, Singer A. Controversies in perinatal torsion of the spermatic cord: a review, survey and recommendations. *J Urol* 1990;143:231.

95. Pinto KJ, Noe HN, Jerkins GR. Management of neonatal torsion. *J Urol* 1997;158:1196.

96. Kay R. Prepubertal testicular tumor registry. *Urol Clin North Am* 1993;20:1.

97. Wu JT, Book L, Sudar K. Serum alpha-fetoprotein (AFP) levels in normal infants. *Pediatr Res* 1981;15:50.

98. Mehra S, Ranjan R, Garga UC. Zinner syndrome—a rare developmental anomaly of the mesonephric duct diagnosed on magnetic resonance imaging. *Radiol Case Rep* 2016;11:313.

99. Subcommittee on Urinary Tract Infection, Steering Committee on Quality Improvement and Management; Roberts KB. Urinary tract infection: clinical practice guideline for the diagnosis and management of the initial UTI in febrile infants and children 2 to 24 months. *Pediatrics* 2011;128(3):595.

100. Cardona-Grau D, Chiang G. Evaluation and lifetime management of the urinary tract in patients with myelomeningocele. *Urol Clin Am* 2017;44:391.

101. Routh JC, Cheng EY, Austin JC, et al. Design and methodological considerations of the centers for disease control and prevention urologic and renal protocol for the newborn and young child with spina bifida. *J Urol* 2016;196:1728.

102. Brock JW III, Carr MC, Adzick NS, et al. Bladder function after fetal surgery for myelomeningocele. *Pediatrics* 2015;136(4):e906.

103. Silberberg A, Robetto J, Grillo M. Ethical issues in intrauterine myelomeningocele surgery. *New Bioeth* 2018;24(3):249.

104. Hidas G, Soltani T, Billimek J, et al. Home urodynamic pressures and volume measurement for the neurogenic bladder: initial validation study. *J Urol* 2017;198(6):1424.

105. Tonni G, Alessandro V, Bonasoni MP. Prune-Belly Syndrome: case series and review of the literature regarding early prenatal diagnosis, epidemiology, genetic factors, treatment and prognosis. *Fetal Pediatr Pathol* 2013;32(1):1.

106. Sanchez S, Ricca R, Joyner B, et al. Vesicoureteral reflux and febrile urinary tract infections in anorectal malformations: a retrospective review. *J Pediatr Surg* 2014;49:91.

107. Lopes RI, Tavares A, Srougi M, et al. 27 years of experience with the comprehensive surgical treatment of prune belly syndrome. *J Pediatr Urol* 2016;11:276e1.

108. Shimada K, Hosokawa S, Matsumoto F, et al. Urological management of cloacal anomalies. *Int J Urol* 2001;8:282.

109. Papic JC, Billmire DF, Rescorla FJ, et al. Management of neonatal ovarian cysts and its effect on ovarian preservation. *J Pediatr Surg* 2014;49:990.

110. Kim HS, Yoo SY, Cha MJ, et al. Diagnosis of neonatal ovarian torsion: emphasis on prenatal and postnatal sonographic findings. *J Clin Ultrasound* 2016;44(5):290.

40 Endocrine Disorders

Penny M. Feldman and M. Lee

INTRODUCTION

From the moment of conception, physiologic endocrine processes are actively involved in embryonic and fetal growth and development. Disturbances in these complex hormonal processes can affect the fetus and newborn infant. Clinical disorders of endocrine function in the neonate, therefore, can reflect an altered physiologic state in the fetus, mother, or fetal–maternal unit. Moreover, perturbations of endocrine function at different stages of fetal development may reprogram developmental processes, which may lead to postnatal endocrine disorders and/or increased risk for disease in adolescence or adulthood. Knowledge of the ontogeny of the endocrine glands and their physiologic function during fetal development facilitates understanding disorders of endocrine function in the newborn.

NORMAL SEXUAL DIFFERENTIATION

The normal regulation of sexual differentiation is broadly illustrated in **Figure 40.1**. All embryos are initially undifferentiated, with a bipotential gonad and the anlagen of both male and female reproductive tracts and genitalia (1). Differentiation of the gonads as testes or ovaries dictates the subsequent development of the internal and external genitalia. The gonad forms when germ cells migrate from the dorsal endoderm of the yolk sac to populate the genital ridges. At the 5th to 6th week of gestation, these primitive bipotential gonads consist of both cortical (ovarian) and medullary (testicular) components. The genital ridge is composed of three cell types:

- Primordial germ cells destined to become prespermatogonia in the male or oogonia in the female.
- Epithelial somatic cells support germ cells destined to become Sertoli cells (male) or granulosa cells (female).
- Mesenchymal somatic cells destined to become steroid-producing Leydig cells (male) or theca cells (female).

Figure 40.1 illustrates the genes involved in the differentiation of the genital ridge into a female or male reproductive tract. Wilms tumor suppressor gene (WT1) and steroidogenic factor 1 (SF-1) play a role early on in development of the genital ridge and are critical for gonadal development (2). Mutations in these two genes are clearly associated with gonadal dysgenesis:

- Wilms tumor suppressor gene (WT1) mutations are associated with three related syndromes (WAGR contiguous gene syndrome, Denys-Drash, and Frasier) that affect renal function and gonadal development (3).
- Mutations in the transcription factor, SF-1, cause agenesis of the adrenal glands and gonads (4).

Development of the supporting cells as Sertoli or granulosa cells is critical for shaping the lineage of the germ cells as spermatogonia or oogonia. Sexually dimorphic differentiation of the gonads and reproductive system commences when the testis-determining gene is first expressed. In 1959, Ford and colleagues determined that the Y chromosome was necessary for male development (5); in 1966, the critical region for testis determination was localized to the short arm of the Y chromosome (6), and in 1990, the primary testis-determining gene was identified at Yp11.3 by positional cloning in patients with 46,XX testicular disorders of sex development (DSD) (7). This gene, termed *SRY* (sex-determining region of the Y

chromosome), is a member of the SOX family of transcription factors that contain a high-mobility group (HMG) DNA-binding motif (7). SRY expression at 42 days postconception triggers differentiation of the bipotential gonad as a testis. Reduced SRY expression or an inadequate number of SRY expressing cells can both perturb testicular development. For example, loss-of-function mutations in SRY or a delay in its onset of expression results in 46,XY complete gonadal dysgenesis, while translocation of SRY to the X chromosome or an autosome can cause 46,XX DSD.

SRY and SF-1 work in concert to activate *SOX9* gene expression. SOX9, a presumptive target for SRY, is a related HMG box gene that induces the supporting cells of the gonadal ridge to differentiate as Sertoli cells and helps to suppress development of the müllerian structures and maintenance of wolffian structures (8). Inactivating mutations of SOX9 cause campomelic dysplasia, a syndrome of skeletal anomalies and 46,XY gonadal dysgenesis (9). Mutations affecting genes located downstream of SOX9, SRY, SF-1, and desert hedgehog (DHH) may also disrupt normal testicular determination (**Fig. 40.1**). DMRT$_1$, a critical transcription factor for both Sertoli and germ cell development, is expressed in early gestation by Sertoli cells and later by germ cells. Mutations in this gene cause 46,XY gonadal dysgenesis and 46, XY DSD (8).

Sexually dimorphic differentiation of the wolffian (male anlagen) and müllerian (female anlagen) internal genital tracts depends on the hormonal milieu established by the somatic cells. If SRY is expressed, the primary sex cords develop into testes and the somatic cells differentiate as Sertoli and Leydig cells. SOX9 acts synergistically with WNT1, GATA4, and SF-1 to induce Sertoli cell expression of anti-müllerian hormone (AMH) also known as müllerian-inhibiting substance (MIS), a 140-kDa glycoprotein in the TGF-β family. AMH causes degeneration of the müllerian ducts by inducing apoptotic cell death of the ductal epithelial cells. The Leydig cells secrete testosterone, which stimulates the wolffian ducts to differentiate into the vas deferens, seminal vesicle, and epididymis and virilizes the external genitalia.

Differentiation of the external genitalia requires the further activation of testosterone by 5α-reductase-2 to its more active metabolite, dihydrotestosterone (DHT). DHT stimulates fusion of the urethral folds and the labioscrotal swellings to form the corpus spongiosa and scrotum. DHT also stimulates growth of the genital tubercle and prostate. Sexually dimorphic differentiation of the internal ducts and the external genitalia is complete by 12 weeks of gestation. During the latter part of gestation, the testes descend into the scrotum and the phallus enlarges as testosterone production increases under the stimulus of pituitary gonadotropins.

In addition to the absence of *SRY* gene expression, the expression of β-catenin, follistatin (*Fst*), FOXL2, R-spondin (*RSPO1*), and *WNT4* genes are essential for normal ovarian development. Suppression of the *SOX9* gene by *FOXL2* stimulates ovarian development. *FOXL2* gene mutations are associated with blepharophimosis–ptosis–epicanthus inversus syndrome (BPES), which affects the eyelids and is associated with premature ovarian failure (10). DAX1, a nuclear hormone receptor in the dosage-sensitive sex reversal (DSS) region of the X chromosome, Xp21, represses both SF-1 and SOX9 activity and AMH expression (2). A duplication of either *WNT4* or *DAX-1* genes interferes with normal testicular development to cause a dosage-sensitive form of 46,XY gonadal dysgenesis (4,10). Furthermore, DAX1 mutations cause adrenal hypoplasia congenita (AHC) and hypogonadotropic hypogonadism.

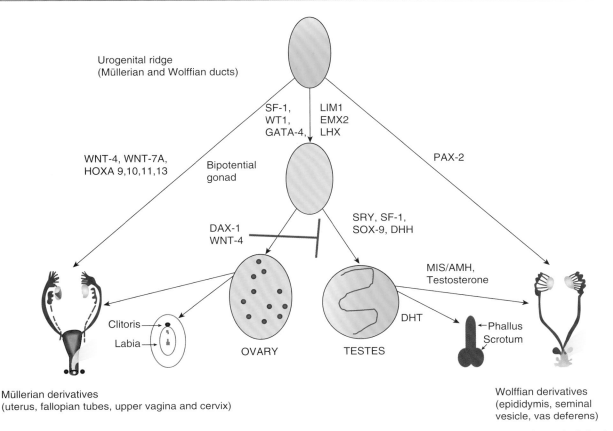

FIGURE 40.1 Schematic of the sex differentiation pathway. The urogenital ridge and gonad are initially undifferentiated. In male embryos, the induction of SRY expression initiates testis determination. The testicular hormones, MIS/AMH, and androgens stimulate male phenotypic development of the internal and external genitalia. In female embryos, the absence of SRY in concert with the expression of DAX1 and WNT-4, which inhibit testicular determination, enables the gonad to develop as an ovary. In the absence of androgens and MIS/AMH, the internal and external genitalia differentiate as female. Note the various genes involved in gonadal differentiation and development of the genital tracts from the müllerian and wolffian derivatives.

The former is life threatening, and early diagnosis in the first few days of life is critical for prompt institution of treatment with corticosteroid and mineralocorticoid replacement therapy (11).

In 46,XX embryos, the primary sex cords form follicles by 10 weeks of gestation and the primordial germ cells differentiate as oogonia. Both X chromosomes are needed for oocyte survival. In the absence of one X chromosome, as in Turner syndrome, the ovaries form initially, but degenerate before birth. In the absence of fetal ovarian secretion of AMH, the müllerian ducts differentiate to form the uterus, fallopian tubes, and upper vagina. The lack of testosterone and DHT production by the fetal ovary leads to degeneration of the wolffian ducts and development of female external genitalia.

DISORDERS OF CHROMOSOMAL SEX

A number of sex chromosome aberrations have been reported (see Chapter 57): some are embryonic lethal (e.g., 45,Y), others cause minimal somatic or hormonal manifestations in the newborn (e.g., 47,XXY and 47,XYY), and a few disrupt gonadal and genital development (45,X/46,XY; 45,X). In contrast to the autosomes, extra genetic material from the X chromosome can be tolerated with minor untoward effects as a result of inactivation of the second and additional X chromosomes. Although ovarian formation and function are intact in patients with X polyploidy, early menopause may occur (12). By contrast, a Y chromosome is generally necessary for testicular development, although rare cases of 46,XX DSD with normal testicular function and male genitalia are reported (13).

The classic sex chromosomal anomalies occur relatively frequently. In the New Haven Study, the frequency of the following karyotypes in newborns were 1/545 males with 47,XXY, 1/728 males with 47,XYY, 1/727 females with 47,XXX, and 1/2,181 females with 45,X karyotype (14). The incidence of 45,X is higher, but this karyotype leads to increased fetal demise and is found in 10% of spontaneous abortions (15). The diagnosis of Turner syndrome, however, is made with greater frequency than the other sex chromosomal aberrations because of mosaicism and the associated somatic abnormalities.

Turner Syndrome

The classic and most common chromosomal abnormality in conceptuses is total loss of one X chromosome. Forty to fifty percent of girls with Turner syndrome have a 45,X karyotype, 15% to 25% are mosaic with 45,X/46,XX, 12% have 45,X/46,XY mixed gonadal dysgenesis, 10% have mosaicism with isochromosome 46,X,i(Xq) or 46 X(idic)(Xp), and 3% are mosaic with a triple X (16). The presence of a mosaic 46,XX cell line has little bearing on stature or somatic abnormalities but does influence gonadal development. A retrospective multicenter Italian Study Group for Turner syndrome found the highest rates of complete pubertal development among girls with mosaicism and a structurally normal second X chromosome or girls with two X chromosomes and structural abnormalities in only one of the X chromosomes (17).

The Turner phenotype in the newborn is secondary to lymphedema of the dorsa of the hands, feet, and neck (pterygium colli). The genetic basis for lymphatic abnormalities is unknown, but studies in adult women suggest that lymphatic aplasia or hypoplasia is the underlying abnormality. The lymphedema frequently resolves by age 2 but can recur or occur later in life. The webbed neck is most often seen as redundant folds of the posterior neck. Many of the somatic defects described in this syndrome become evident with increasing age (15,16). The most common features are triangular facies with low-set ears, high-arched palate, low hairline, shield-like chest with wide spaced and hypoplastic areolae, and cubitus valgus. Skin findings include hemangiomas, cutis laxa, pigmented nevi, dysplastic nails, and tendency to keloid formation. Skeletal abnormalities include "beaking" of the medial tibial condyle, drumstick-shaped distal phalanges, vertebral anomalies, Madelung deformity, and short metacarpals (18). Dermatoglyphic findings include single palmar crease, distal axial triradius, and an increased number of digital ulnar whorls. Growth starts to decline early, and short stature is the most consistent feature in the older child.

Upon diagnosis, screening for associated cardiac and renal defects is imperative. Congenital heart disease occurs in 50% of girls with Turner syndrome with prevalence rates of 15% to 30% for bicuspid aortic valve and 7% to 18% for coarctation of the aorta (16). Atrial septal defect, ventricular septal defect, and partial anomalous pulmonary venous return are also common. Families should be educated about other potential associations, such as recurrent otitis media, increased risk for autoimmune disease, including chronic lymphocytic thyroiditis, celiac disease, diabetes mellitus, sensorineural and conductive hearing loss, metabolic syndrome, liver disease, and idiopathic hypertension. The incidence of intellectual disability is slightly increased with specific X chromosome rearrangements. In most of these girls, cognition is normal with good verbal skills, but some have selective visual–spatial deficits and a nonverbal learning disorder (15,16).

A major concern for girls with Turner syndrome is extreme short stature with a mean adult height of 148 cm. Recombinant growth hormone (GH) increases final height and is approved for treatment of short stature in Turner syndrome. The combination of early use of GH (before 5 years of age) and low-dose estrogen replacement at an appropriate age is thought to have the best outcome in terms of height and psychosexual development (19).

Primary gonadal failure occurs in more than 90% of individuals with Turner syndrome. Women with Turner syndrome, however, have successfully carried offspring to term using donor oocytes, at a rate similar to couples with other causes of infertility (20). Pregnancy complications can result from abnormal uterine development and cardiac abnormalities.

The presence of Y material in the karyotype raises concern for malignant transformation of residual testicular elements. In patients with mosaicism that contain Y material, gonadectomy is recommended to eliminate the risk for gonadoblastoma and to avoid the virilizing effects of hormonally active residual testicular tissue (16).

DISORDERS OF SEXUAL DEVELOPMENT

DSD result when the anatomic development of the external genitalia does not correspond to the chromosomal and gonadal sex. The external genitalia may be truly ambiguous—that is, the sex of the infant cannot be ascertained by physical examination. Alternatively, the phenotype may be normal male or female in morphology, but discordant with the genotype.

These conditions may be secondary to teratogens (radiation, viruses, and drugs), virilizing maternal hormones or genetic defects affecting autosomes, sex chromosomes, or genes involved in fetal gonadal differentiation. Other genetic causes may affect hormonal synthesis or action, timing or regulation of hormone secretion, or receptor binding or signaling. The clinical phenotype of these single gene mutations varies widely, from subtle defects to complete gonadal dysgenesis. Differentiation and development of the

TABLE 40.1

Disorders of Sexual Development (DSD)

DSD	Genotype	Phenotype	Etiology
Complete/ partial gonadal dysgenesis	XY	Female	SRY, SOX9 WT1, SF-1, NR5A1, DHH, DAX-1, WNT4, MAP3K1
46,XX	XX	Variable	SOX9 duplication/ translocation SOX3 duplication/SRY translocation Androgen excess: • CAH: 21-OH def, 11-OH def, 3β-HSD deficiency • Aromatase deficiency, ovarian/adrenal tumor/ exogenous causes
46,XY	XY	Female	SRY deletion; complete/ partial AIS (androgen receptor mutation); Leydig cell hypoplasia, disorder of AMH; DO of AMH and AMR receptor; LH receptor defect; cloacal exstrophy CAH: • Congenital lipoid hyperplasia (StAR) • 17,20 Lyase deficiency • 17α-Hydroxylase deficiency (p450c17) • 17β-Hydroxysteroid deficiency
Ovotesticular	46,XX; 46,XY 45,X/46,XY 46,XX/46,XY	Variable	Mixed gonadal dysgenesis Chimera

internal ducts and external genitalia in these infants depend on the timing and extent of insult to the developing gonad. These are classified as complete/partial gonadal dysgenesis, 46,XX, 46,XY, and ovotesticular DSD (listed in Table 40.1). Aside from autosomal or sex chromosomal anomalies, gene mutations include loss-of-function mutations, gene deletions of SRY, SOX9, NR5A1, WT1, and DHH and gain-of-function mutations of DAX-1 and WNT 4 (21,22).

Complete and Partial Gonadal Dysgenesis

Complete dysgenesis of the genital ridges results in normal female genitalia with no associated somatic findings; thus, the diagnosis may not be clinically evident at birth. Infants with 46,XY complete gonadal dysgenesis, however, may be identified because the genitalia are discordant with the prenatal karyotype. Affected girls tend to be tall with eunuchoid proportions and often present with primary amenorrhea and sexual infantilism. Perrault syndrome is an autosomal recessive form of 46,XX gonadal dysgenesis that is associated with sensory neural deafness and in some individuals with a progressive sensory and motor peripheral neuropathy (23). 46,XY gonadal dysgenesis may be sporadic, but SRY mutations are present in 10% to 20%, and familial forms can vary in inheritance pattern (24,25).

Gain-of-function mutations in the *MAP3K1* gene commonly cause both sporadic and familial partial and complete gonadal dysgenesis. This gene down-regulates downstream factors needed for testicular differentiation and induces the expression of β-catenin and FOXL2 to promote ovarian development (21).

Incomplete loss-of-function of genes essential for testicular differentiation or exposure to teratogens that damage the developing testis causes partial gonadal dysgenesis. If the testicular loss occurs later than 9 to 10 weeks of gestation, regression of the müllerian structures has already been initiated, but midline fusion and development of the external genitalia are affected due to inadequate testosterone. Thus, the external genitalia are severely undervirilized, but the gonads, uterus, and fallopian tubes are absent or rudimentary, and the wolffian structures are incompletely developed.

46,XX DSD

A virilized genotypic (46,XX) female with ovaries is considered to have 46,XX DSD. The female fetus can be virilized by fetal adrenal androgens due to congenital adrenal hyperplasia (CAH) or maternal androgens transferred across the placenta, such as progestational agents used to prevent spontaneous abortion or a rare androgen-producing maternal tumor (26).

Maternal androgen-producing tumors are almost always caused by an ovarian lesion—arrhenoblastomas, Krukenberg tumors, luteomas, or lipoid or stromal cell tumors, although adrenal adenomas are also reported (27). These tumors cause clitoromegaly, acne, deepening of the voice, decreased lactation, and hirsutism in the mothers and are associated with elevated serum androgens and elevated excretion of urinary 17-ketosteroids (28). Fetal exposure to androgens prior to week 12 of gestation results in fusion of the urogenital sinus and genital folds. Exposure to androgens after week 12 of gestation or after birth causes milder manifestations of clitoral enlargement, labial hyperpigmentation, and posterior labial fusion.

In contrast to untreated infants with CAH, infants exposed to maternal androgens through the placenta do not have progressive virilization or continued acceleration of growth and skeletal maturation after birth. No medical intervention is needed as androgens are not elevated. These children will feminize normally at puberty and achieve normal fertility. The enzymatic defects causing virilization due to CAH (21-hydroxylase, 11-hydroxylase, and 3β-hydroxysteroid dehydrogenase defects) are more fully discussed in the section on adrenal disorders.

Aromatase Deficiency

Rare genetic defects in the fetal or placental aromatase gene impair aromatization of maternal and placental androgens to estrogens and cause *in utero* elevations of androgens (29). Both fetal and maternal virilization can occur.

46,XY DSD

A 46,XY male with testes and inadequate virilization is classified as 46,XY DSD. Incomplete masculinization of the male fetus may arise from a myriad of causes that disrupt either androgen action or the response of target tissues to androgens during sexual differentiation. The differential diagnosis of 46,XY DSD is extensive, including enzymatic defects of testosterone synthesis, unresponsiveness to testosterone action (androgen resistance syndromes), hypothalamic or pituitary dysfunction, and vascular or teratogenic insult to the testis. The full details of disorders of testosterone synthesis (17α-hydroxylase/17, 20 lyase, 17β-hydroxysteroid dehydrogenase, steroidogenic acute regulatory protein [StAR], and 3β-hydroxysteroid dehydrogenase deficiencies) including diagnosis and treatment are outlined in the adrenal section.

Syndromes of Androgen Resistance

Androgen resistance is characterized by undervirilized genitalia with normal müllerian duct regression and normal testosterone synthesis (30). The term androgen resistance encompasses androgen receptor or postreceptor defects (androgen insensitivity syndrome [AIS]) and 5α-reductase deficiency in which the conversion of testosterone to its more active metabolite, DHT, is affected.

In both conditions, AMH is produced normally by the fetal testis and causes involution of the müllerian structures. In X-linked AIS, although testosterone is produced, the defect resides in the receptor or its signaling; thus, target tissue is unresponsive. Consequently, all aspects of male development mediated by androgens, including development of the wolffian structures and external genitalia, are affected.

Patients with complete androgen insensitivity syndrome (CAIS) have female external genitalia with a blind vaginal pouch, abdominal or inguinal testes, and no wolffian or müllerian structures. At puberty, peripheral conversion of the high testosterone concentrations to estradiol stimulates breast development and estrogenization of the vaginal mucosa. Most patients have little pubic hair, and some have total absence of sexual hair. In all other respects, including height, habitus, voice, breast development, and gender identity, these individuals are feminine. The diagnosis is made in infancy or childhood as a result of female genitalia that are discrepant with a 46,XY karyotype or when testicular tissue is found during hernia repair. Adolescent patients present with primary amenorrhea. Genetic mutations of the androgen receptor are identified in only two-thirds of individuals with suspected AIS. The gonads in CAIS have a 9% risk for malignant transformation and thus gonadectomy is usually recommended (31). A wide spectrum of phenotypes is observed in individuals with incomplete forms of androgen insensitivity. Partial androgen insensitivity syndrome (PAIS) can range from a female phenotype with clitoromegaly and posterior labial fusion to a male phenotype with oligospermia. Sex assignment may be difficult in patients with PAIS. In some cases, assessment of responsiveness of the phallus to androgens is helpful.

By contrast, in 5α-reductase deficiency, the testosterone produced is sufficient for differentiation of the wolffian structures but is not converted to DHT, which is essential for phallic midline fusion and growth (32). Thus, patients with 5α-reductase deficiency typically have a blind vaginal pouch, a small phallus with chordee, a hooded prepuce, and perineoscrotal hypospadias. At puberty, the rise in testosterone secretion and induction of 5α-reductase and androgen receptor expression in genital tissues enable growth of pubic hair, penile enlargement, and testicular descent. 5α-Reductase deficiency is suspected in 46,XY patients with perineoscrotal hypospadias and an elevated testosterone to DHT ratio of greater than 35 under basal conditions and greater than 74 after human chorionic gonadotropin (hCG) stimulation. The diagnosis is confirmed by genetic testing or finding reduced 5α-reductase activity in genital skin fibroblasts.

Ovotesticular DSD

In ovotesticular DSD, both ovarian and testicular elements are present. Findings may consist of an ovary on one side and a testis on the contralateral side, an ovary or a testis and a contralateral ovotestis, or two ovotestes (33). Although most patients with ovotesticular DSD have genital ambiguity, some have typical female or male external genitalia. The extent of differentiation of the wolffian structures and external genitalia depends on the amount of functioning testicular tissue. The testicular component of the gonad may secrete androgens at puberty to cause unwanted virilization in those reared as female; thus, early gonadectomy may be recommended. Although some patients have sex chromosome abnormalities, 46,XX is the most common karyotype, followed by 46,XY. The pathogenesis of ovotesticular DSD is not well understood but is not consistently associated with alterations in SRY expression. Ovotesticular DSD secondary to 46,XX/46,XY chimerism from *in vitro* fertilization has been reported as well (34).

Other Conditions Involving Genitourinary Development
Hypospadias and Cryptorchidism

Isolated hypospadias occurs in 0.3% to 0.5% of newborn infants, and isolated cryptorchidism is present in approximately 2% to 4%

of full-term and up to 20% to 30% of premature infants. Two percent of boys with cryptorchidism have hypospadias. Generally, neither condition by itself is associated with an endocrine abnormality (35,36). The incidence of DSD, however, is greater if the hypospadias is severe (on the shaft or perineum) and/or if the testes are nonpalpable.

Micropenis

Isolated micropenis with otherwise normally formed genitalia generally is not considered as ambiguous genitalia. This condition is associated with insufficient testosterone secretion during the third trimester. The evaluation of micropenis is discussed under hypopituitarism, the most common treatable cause of this condition.

Evaluation of Disorders of Sexual Development

The evaluation and appropriate sex assignment of a newborn with ambiguous genitalia should be managed expediently by a team of experienced providers comprised of an endocrinologist, urologist, geneticist, psychiatrist or psychologist, pediatrician, and clergy or other support personnel. Parents should be reassured that incomplete or excessive differentiation of the genitals occurred as part of a continuum in the developmental process and that the team will discuss the recommended sex assignment within several days. It is our general philosophy not to discuss pending studies in detail because there are occasions for gender assignment that are inconsistent with either chromosomal or gonadal sex. Presentation of all data available enables a more cohesive explanation. As in any diagnostic problem, the approach to the infant with ambiguous genitalia should begin with a thorough history, careful physical examination, and appropriate laboratory and radiologic testing.

A history of drug ingestion, particularly in the first trimester, or maternal virilization might suggest the cause of 46,XX DSD, whereas first-trimester infections or teratogen exposure might suggest early interference with gonadal development. Unexplained neonatal death or siblings with virilization or precocious puberty is suggestive of CAH, while female relatives with sexual infantilism suggest X-linked causes such as AIS. A family medical history of consanguinity may be helpful when considering disorders with autosomal recessive inheritance.

A thorough physical examination is important, but on no account should a diagnosis be based on physical findings. The presence or absence of palpable gonads helps differentiate the major categories of DSD. In general, gonads lacking testicular elements will not descend below the inguinal region. Thus, a palpable gonad excludes the diagnosis of 46,XX DSD in which both gonads are ovaries by definition. Penile length and diameter are valuable both for prognostic information and as a baseline if treatment is given to enlarge the penis. The urethral opening should be identified, and the existence or absence of a vagina determined. The degree of labial–scrotal fusion and the presence of associated urinary or GI tract anomalies should be assessed.

The physical examination can help direct the laboratory and radiologic investigation. Certain tests are obtained as soon as it is apparent that there is sexual ambiguity, although others may be required at a later stage to make an accurate diagnosis (**Table 40.2**). For example, serum 17-hydroxyprogesterone (17OHP), testosterone, renin, and electrolytes are useful initial screening tests for CAH, but other steroid precursors and genetic studies may help establish the specific diagnosis. 17OHP is normally elevated after birth and should be measured after 36 hours of life. 17OHP should be interpreted based on normative data for gestational age, birth weight, and the infant's postnatal age. In salt-losing CAH, serum electrolytes are usually abnormal by day of life 4, so normal electrolytes in the first couple of days of life are not reassuring. Serum testosterone can be elevated from the gonads or the adrenals and should be interpreted in the context of the examination and other laboratory studies. Measurement of AMH may

TABLE 40.2
Studies to Evaluate Ambiguous Genitalia
Immediate studies
Karyotype
Pelvic ultrasonography
Serum electrolytes
17-Hydroxyprogesterone
17-OH pregnenolone
Testosterone
11-Deoxycortisol
Dihydrotestosterone
Müllerian-inhibiting substance
Follow-up studies
FSH/LH/testosterone at 4–12 wk of age
hCG stimulation testing
Cortrosyn stimulation testing
Genito-urethrogram and other radiologic studies
Exploratory laparotomy and gonadal biopsy
Skin biopsy to evaluate androgen action
Genetic/molecular studies for specific mutations

help determine the presence of testicular tissue (37). It should be stressed that sex assignment does not require that all studies leading to a final diagnosis be completed (e.g., the exact type of CAH may be important for genetic counseling and future prenatal diagnosis, but not necessary for sex assignment). The karyotype can help determine the DSD classification. This, however, should not be used as the primary criteria for sex assignment as other factors such as gonadal function, sensitivity to androgens, future sexual function, and potential for fertility or pregnancy (even if by *in vitro* fertilization) are also critical.

Pelvic ultrasound to evaluate the internal genital structures and gonads should be performed by an experienced radiologist. Ultrasonography may identify nonpalpable gonads and may help distinguish ovarian from testicular tissue (38). The presence of a uterus indicates the absence of AMH, consistent with an early loss of functioning testicular tissue, and usually supports a female sex assignment. Conversely, the absence of müllerian structures implies the presence of functioning testicular tissue at the critical window of 7 to 9 weeks of gestation. This is consistent with SRY expression and suggestive of an XY karyotype, but is not a major determinant of male sex assignment. The karyotype, phallic size and degree of hypospadias, internal genital structures, gonadal pathology, and etiology of the DSD are all part of the equation in gender determination.

To further evaluate the specific etiology of the sexual ambiguity, additional studies may be necessary. The algorithms in **Figures 40.2** and **40.3**, which are based on the initial ultrasound findings, delineate the steps that may be necessary to make a definitive diagnosis. These algorithms include patients with normal male or female phenotypes that are discordant with the genotype. Surgical exploration frequently will be required in cases of ovotesticular DSD or partial gonadal dysgenesis but may be done at a later time. It should be stressed that the final histopathologic diagnosis is not necessary for sex assignment.

After the evaluation is complete, the appropriate sex assignment is determined by a consensus of opinion from the team taking parental input into consideration, especially in cases in which the appropriate sex assignment is uncertain. Gender identity and future sexual function and fertility are key determining factors. The attending physician should discuss the condition fully with the parents, including expectations for future sexual function and fertility and whether any hormonal medications or surgery are recommended.

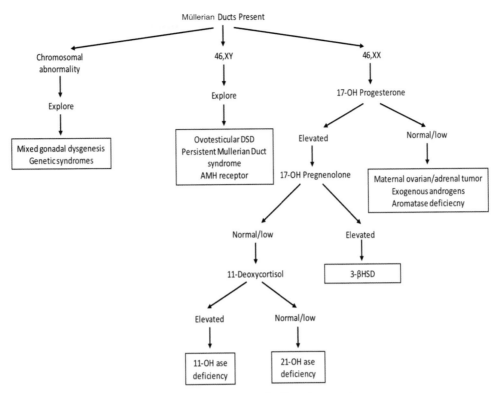

FIGURE 40.2 An algorithm for evaluating in infants with müllerian structures and a discordant genotype.

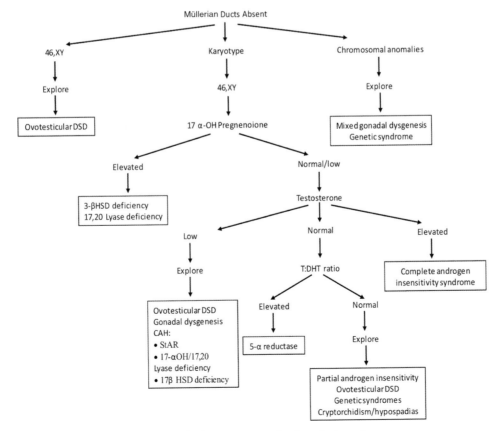

FIGURE 40.3 An algorithm for evaluating in infants without müllerian structures and a discordant genotype.

THE NEWBORN INFANT

Gender assignment for most infants with ambiguous genitalia is straightforward when chromosomal sex and gonadal sex correlate with the internal structures. The external genitalia may require reconstructive surgery to improve function and cosmetic appearance. The timing of surgery has become controversial as a result of heightened concerns regarding the ethics of the parents deciding on surgery for the child, the possibility of gender dysphoria and sex reassignment, and the risk for postsurgical loss of genital sensation. With limited long-term data to support early versus late reconstructive surgery, it may be prudent in many cases to postpone surgery until the family (and child) can fully participate in the decision and gender identity is clear. Hormonal therapy may be required for secondary sexual maturation but is usually not needed during the neonatal period. Rarely, as in cases of PAIS, ovotesticular DSD, or mixed gonadal dysgenesis, gender assignment contrary to chromosomal or gonadal sex is considered. In these cases, careful consideration must be given to the likelihood of gender role and sexual function as an adult (39).

Previously, infants with severe micropenis or agenesis who had functional testes and a 46,XY karyotype were assigned female sex. This practice has since changed, and these infants should generally be assigned male sex because exposure to testosterone *in utero* and other potentially sexually dimorphic differences in the brain influence the programming of gender identity. Furthermore, these individuals have the potential for normal fertility. Recent reports of dissatisfaction with a female sex assignment in some 46,XY individuals with cloacal exstrophy or other nonhormonally mediated causes of aphallia reinforce the need to explore new paradigms for sex assignment that include other factors that affect adult gender identity such as the effect of prenatal hormones on central nervous system (CNS) sex differentiation (39,40).

DISORDERS OF THE HYPOTHALAMUS AND PITUITARY

Development of the Hypothalamic–Pituitary Axis

The hypothalamus arises by proliferation of neuroblasts in the intermediate zone of the diencephalic wall and formation of the supraoptic and periventricular nuclei. **Figure 40.4** illustrates the formation of the anterior and posterior pituitary glands from invaginations of Rathke pouch and the floor of the diencephalon, respectively. Neural fibers migrate from the hypothalamus down to the posterior pituitary to form the neurohypophyseal tract. The hypothalamus regulates the pituitary by secreting both stimulatory and inhibitory hormones. The hypothalamic and pituitary glands are functional after week 12 of gestation. Growth hormone–releasing hormone (GHRH), thyrotropin-releasing hormone (TRH), corticotropin-releasing hormone (CRH), and gonadotropin-releasing hormone (GnRH) stimulate the anterior pituitary

TABLE 40.3

Etiology of Disorders of the Hypothalamic–Pituitary Axis

Malformations
Cleft lip and palate
Optic nerve atrophy
Septo-optic dysplasia
Transsphenoidal encephalocele
Holoprosencephaly
Anencephaly
Trauma associated with delivery (e.g., breech, tight nuchal cord, heart rate decelerations, etc.)
Congenital infection
Rubella
Toxoplasmosis
Tumor
Hypothalamic hamartoblastoma (e.g., Pallister-Hall syndrome)
Rathke pouch cyst
Craniopharyngioma
Glioblastoma
Isolated or combined familial or idiopathic pituitary hormone deficiency
Autosomal recessive or X-linked recessive familial panhypopituitarism

gland to secrete GH, thyroid-stimulating hormone (TSH), adrenocorticotropic hormone (ACTH), and luteinizing hormone (LH) and follicle-stimulating hormone (FSH), respectively. The main inhibitory hormones are somatostatin, which inhibits GH release, and prolactin inhibitory factor, which inhibits prolactin release. The posterior pituitary secretes vasopressin and oxytocin.

Except for the syndrome of inappropriate secretion of antidiuretic hormone (SIADH), most disorders of the hypothalamic–pituitary axis in the newborn period are those of insufficiency related to malformations, trauma, infection, or genetically inherited disorders, as outlined in **Table 40.3**. This differs from older children and adults who may have either functionally active tumors that secrete pituitary hormones or infiltrative disease or tumors that interfere with normal pituitary function.

Disorders of the Anterior Pituitary

Anterior pituitary dysfunction is difficult to detect in the newborn. The predominant features of anterior pituitary insufficiency are hypoglycemia, micropenis, and, occasionally, cholestatic jaundice. The hypoglycemia may be quite severe and comparable to that seen in infants with congenital hyperinsulinism. The infants may even have a brisk glycemic response to glucagon causing further confusion (41). The cholestatic jaundice is initially unconjugated,

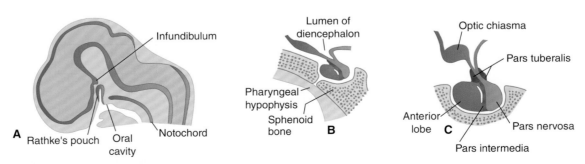

FIGURE 40.4 Schematic drawings illustrating the development of the hypophysis (pituitary gland). A: Midsagittal section through the 6-week-old embryo showing Rathke pouch as a dorsal outpocketing of the oral cavity and the infundibulum as a thickening in the floor of the hypothalamus. **B and C:** Development at 11 and 16 weeks, respectively. The anterior lobe, the pars tuberalis, and the pars intermedia are derived from Rathke pouch. The posterior pituitary gland, neurohypophysis, develops from an invagination from the floor of the diencephalon. (Reprinted with permission from Gould DJ, Fix JD. *BRS neuroanatomy*, 5th ed. Baltimore, MD: Lippincott Williams & Wilkins, 2013:69. (Adapted with permission from Sadler TW. *Langman's medical embryology*, 10th ed. Baltimore, MD: Lippincott Williams & Wilkins, 2006:301.)

TABLE 40.4

Transcription Factors Involved in Cell Differentiation of the Pituitary Gland

Transcription Factor	Mode of Inheritance	Pituitary Hormone Deficiencies	Associated Features
POU1F1 (PIT-1)	AR, AD	TSH, GH, PRL	APH
PROP-1 (Prophet of PIT-1)	AR	GH, TSH, GH, PRL, FSH, LH, and late ACTH deficiency	APH
HESX1	AR, AD	GH, TSH, GH, PRL, FSH, LH, ACTH vasopressin	Septo-optic dysplasia, corpus callosum agenesis
LHX3	AR	GH, TSH, GH, PRL, FSH, LH may develop late-onset ACTH deficiency	Short cervical spine, sensorineural deafness, APH, EPP
LHX4	AD	GH, TSH, FSH, LH, and ACTH	Cerebellar abnormalities, APH, EPP
OTX2	AD	IGHD or GH, TSH, PRL, FSH, and LH	APH, EPP, bilateral anophthalmia, or severe microphthalmia
DAX-1	XL	FSH, LH	Congenital adrenal hypoplasia HH
SOX2	AD	GH, LH, FSH	Anophthalmia, esophageal atresia, sensorineural deafness, genital tract, hypothalamic hamartoma, diplegia
GLI3	AD	Panhypopituitarism	Pallister-Hall syndrome
PITX2	AD	LH, FSH	Rieger syndrome

AD, autosomal dominant; AR, autosomal recessive; XL, X-linked; APH, anterior pituitary hypoplasia; EPP, ectopic posterior pituitary; HH, hypogonadotropic hypogonadism.

then becomes predominantly conjugated, and will often only resolve after hormone replacement. There may be combined deficiency of multiple pituitary hormones or isolated deficiency of a single hormone. At least 30 genes have been reported to cause pituitary hormone deficiencies, some of which are associated with syndromes. Table 40.4 shows the specific patterns of pituitary hormone deficiencies caused by several of these genes. One such gene involves mutations in a homeodomain protein, HESX1, found in some patients with septo-optic dysplasia (SOD), characterized by hypopituitarism, optic nerve hypoplasia, and absent septum pellucidum (42,43). In this disorder, pituitary function can vary from intact to complete panhypopituitarism including diabetes insipidus (DI). SOD is suggested by wandering nystagmus in the newborn, reflective of optic nerve hypoplasia and blindness.

Growth Hormone Deficiency

GH deficiency in the neonate may present with hypoglycemia and/or micropenis. Micropenis is defined as a stretched penile length less than 2.5 cm in the term infant. Congenital deficiency of GH does not cause intrauterine growth restriction and often does not affect linear growth until 6 to 9 months of age. Intrauterine growth is primarily determined by maternal factors, including nutritional status, placental function, and gestational infection or drugs. During early postnatal life, thyroid hormone, insulin, and nutrition are more important growth determinants than is GH. A family history of short stature is pertinent because familial autosomal dominant inheritance of GH deficiency is well recognized.

Gonadotropin Deficiency

Gonadotropin deficiency can occur as either isolated hypogonadotropic hypogonadism or combined multiple pituitary hormone deficiency. Although male infants with combined deficiencies present with micropenis, those with isolated gonadotropin deficiency may not be recognized at birth. The genitalia can be normal male in Kallmann syndrome (hypogonadotropic hypogonadism and anosmia), a syndrome caused by mutations in the KAL gene-encoding anosmin-1. Female infants are asymptomatic at birth and may not be identified until puberty fails to occur. Gonadotropin deficiency is also the cause of micropenis in certain genetic conditions, such as Prader-Willi and CHARGE syndromes.

Adrenocorticotropic Hormone Deficiency

ACTH deficiency rarely presents as an acute adrenal crisis; the cortisol insufficiency is typically mild and may cause hypoglycemia or

hyponatremia without hyperkalemia and, occasionally, prolonged direct hyperbilirubinemia. Isolated ACTH deficiency is extremely rare but has been linked to the CRH gene locus (44). The combination of both GH and ACTH deficiency may cause hypoketotic hypoglycemia of such severity that it is difficult to differentiate from congenital hyperinsulinism (41). ACTH deficiency in the neonate more commonly occurs in association with multiple pituitary hormone deficiencies.

Thyroid-Stimulating Hormone Deficiency

TSH deficiency is essentially asymptomatic in the newborn. On newborn screening (NBS) tests, the serum thyroxine (T_4) concentration is low or low normal with a low, normal, or mildly elevated TSH. A low or low/normal T_4 with a normal TSH may be misinterpreted as the euthyroid sick syndrome (see Disorders of the Thyroid) in a stressed neonate. Furthermore, secondary hypothyroidism may be missed if primary TSH screening is used. TSH deficiency is usually associated with other pituitary deficiencies and rarely occurs in isolation. In an infant with any of the CNS abnormalities outlined in Table 40.3, secondary hypothyroidism should be considered and may be missed with routine newborn screening procedures.

Diagnosis

The diagnosis of hypothalamic and pituitary deficiency may require stimulation testing if random values are nondiagnostic. GH is tonically elevated in the first few days of life; thus, a random GH greater than 10 ng/mL suggests adequate secretion. If a random value is low, confirmatory GH provocative testing is needed. In normal newborn infants, GH values increase to greater than 25 ng/mL with stimulation testing. ACTH deficiency causing adrenal insufficiency is unlikely if a random cortisol is greater than 20 µg/dL, because serum cortisol is low in infants and lacks diurnal variation. In general, ACTH or CRH stimulation testing is necessary to test the hypothalamic–pituitary–adrenal axis. Random sex steroids, FSH, and LH may be diagnostic at 1 to 3 months of age during the minipuberty of infancy when the hypothalamic–pituitary–gonadal axis is transiently active; otherwise, GnRH stimulation testing is needed to assess LH and FSH secretion.

In those infants suspected of anterior pituitary deficiency, ultrasonography through the anterior fontanelle may discern midline malformations of the brain, although magnetic resonance imaging or computed tomography scanning is more sensitive. If SOD is a consideration, ophthalmologic examination should be performed.

THE NEWBORN INFANT

Treatment

Anterior pituitary deficiency may not be detected clinically during the neonatal period if the hypoglycemia, jaundice, and micropenis are mild. Treatment considerations, therefore, are based on the severity of symptoms. The infant with severe hypoglycemia will require immediate GH and glucocorticoid replacement albeit at relatively modest doses. Recombinant GH is injected subcutaneously, at a dose of 0.16 to 0.24 mg/kg/wk. Glucocorticoid replacement with hydrocortisone 8 to 10 mg/m^2/d is often sufficient. This dose should be at least tripled for acute illnesses. Treatment with thyroid hormone replacement therapy can precipitate an adrenal crisis in an individual with hypoadrenalism; therefore, assessment of adrenal function is critical prior to initiating thyroid hormone replacement therapy. If the testes are nonpalpable, AMH determination will ascertain their presence (37). An AMH value in the normal male range for age verifies the presence of testes. In male infants with micropenis, testosterone enanthate or testosterone cypionate at a dose of 25 mg monthly for 3 months can be administered to stimulate penile growth. If the penile response is inadequate, then the 3-month course can be repeated.

Disorders of the Posterior Pituitary

Vasopressin or antidiuretic hormone (ADH) and oxytocin are the two major posterior pituitary endocrine hormones. Oxytocin has no known function in the neonate, although ADH helps to regulate intravascular volume and osmolality. ADH is synthesized in the supraoptic and periventricular nuclei of the hypothalamus by 12 weeks of gestation. It is bound to neurophysin and transported along the neurohypophyseal tract to the posterior pituitary, where it is stored and released as necessary. ADH increases the permeability of the collecting tubules of the kidney to water and urea. Its secretion is stimulated by hyperosmolar states and volume depletion and inhibited by volume overload. The two main disorders of ADH secretion are DI and SIADH.

Diabetes Insipidus

DI in the newborn may result from central ADH insufficiency or renal unresponsiveness to ADH (nephrogenic DI). This section will discuss only central DI.

DI in the neonate may present with failure to thrive, irritability, fever, vomiting, hypernatremia, and a history of polyhydramnios. Polyuria is difficult to appreciate in newborn infants because healthy newborn infants can void up to 20 times a day (45). However, sustained urine output greater than 60% of fluid input and single-void volumes greater than 6 mL/kg suggest DI. In a child with hyperosmolar serum, the diagnosis is confirmed by finding inappropriately dilute urine that becomes more concentrated after vasopressin administration. Failure to respond to vasopressin is suggestive of renal DI. Water deprivation tests should not be done in newborns as acute dehydration and hypernatremia may cause permanent CNS injury. The presence of untreated hypoadrenalism can mask DI because low glucocorticoid deficiency impairs free water excretion possibly by up-regulating aquaporin 2 channels in the kidney. Once glucocorticoid treatment is started, then a diuresis ensues (46).

A list of causes of central DI is given in **Table 40.5**. Secondary DI is more common than primary in the neonatal period and should be strongly suspected in infants with certain malformations.

Treatment

Treatment of DI requires strict management of fluid balance. Infants with DI require enormous quantities of free water; it is not unusual to provide several times the usual maintenance needs as 5% glucose intravenously, while providing nutrition and electrolytes orally. Although a number of different formulations are available, subcutaneous desmopressin, a long-acting analogue

TABLE 40.5

Etiology of Central Diabetes Insipidus

Primary
  Familial
    X-linked recessive
    Autosomal dominant
  Idiopathic
Secondary
  Malformation sequences
    Optic atrophy
    Septo-optic dysplasia
    Holoprosencephaly
  Birth trauma
  Periventricular hemorrhage
  Infection
    Meningitis
    Encephalitis
  Infiltrative disease (in older infants)
    Histiocytosis X
    Granulomatous disease
  Germ cell tumors (in older children)

of vasopressin, elicits the most stable fluid and electrolyte control in infants (47,48). The recommended starting daily dose is 0.01 µg, titrating up to 0.02 to 0.08 µg once to twice daily. The dose and dosing interval must be carefully adjusted in each infant by monitoring fluid intake, urine output, serum electrolytes and osmolality, and state of hydration. Management should include a daily "breakthrough" period of diuresis prior to administering the daily DDAVP dose to avoid fluid overload. Rapid shifts in the serum sodium caused by excessive fluid intake or urine output should be avoided. An alternative approach, which minimizes the risk of water overload, is to use a diluted formula without administering any vasopressin. This treatment is based on the principle that hunger rather than thirst is the driving force behind fluid intake in the neonate. Providing the total daily caloric intake as one-third strength formula will usually result in stable fluid balance. This approach requires 2- to 3-hourly feeds even during the night; thus, sleep may be disrupted. Moreover, the volume of fluid needed can compromise growth in some infants. A third approach is to treat these infants with a low renal solute formula and free water supplementation in conjunction with twice-daily chlorothiazide 5 mg/kg. Through unknown mechanisms, chlorothiazide increases urine osmolality, and this strategy maintains eunatremia (47). For emergency treatment of severe dehydration, intravenous aqueous Pitressin infusion, instead of desmopressin, is recommended as the short half-life of Pitressin allows precise control of fluid balance.

Syndrome of Inappropriate Antidiuretic Hormone Secretion

The secretion of ADH is normally higher in premature infants (49) but can be further increased in sick premature infants for the reasons outlined in **Table 40.6**. A common mechanism in many pathologic cases is intravascular volume depletion, which is detected by stretch receptors in the left atrium. Thus, the elevated ADH levels are appropriate for the volume status, but inappropriate for the osmolar status. SIADH, by definition, occurs in a volume replete or overloaded state when there is dilutional hyponatremia associated with inappropriately concentrated urine with continued sodium loss (urine sodium >20 to 30 mEq/L). This occurs in the absence of volume depletion, renal failure, or adrenal insufficiency. True SIADH is uncommon in neonates (50) and should be differentiated from hyponatremia caused by ADH levels that are appropriately elevated in response to volume depletion.

TABLE 40.6

Causes of Elevated Levels of Antidiuretic Hormone in the Newborn

Birth asphyxia

Acute deterioration of hyaline membrane disease and bronchopulmonary dysplasia

Respiratory syncytial virus infection

Pneumothorax

Pulmonary interstitial emphysema

Artificial ventilation

Acute blood loss

Periventricular hemorrhage

Surgery

Pain

Syndrome of inappropriate ADH secretion

ADH, antidiuretic hormone.

It is vitally important to limit water and sodium intake and prevent hyponatremia in SIADH, but equally important to adequately treat the volume depletion states associated with compensatory increase in ADH secretion.

Hyponatremia occurs more commonly in newborn premature infants who have a higher fractional excretion of sodium than do term infants. The most common nonphysiologic cause of hyponatremia is renal sodium wasting from use of diuretics; other causes include prerenal failure, renal failure, adrenal insufficiency, and SIADH. SIADH is found more frequently in older infants, in conjunction with sepsis and CNS infection, but may occur in critically ill neonates as well. Unlike volume depletion states, SIADH is treated with fluid restriction. The co-occurrence of volume depletion, polyuria, urinary sodium loss, and hyponatremia leads to suspicion of salt wasting.

DISORDERS OF THE ADRENAL GLAND

Development and Function of the Adrenal Gland

The adrenal gland consists of a cortex and medulla, which each function independently and secrete two different classes of hormones. The fetal adrenal cortex is of mesodermal origin, whereas the chromaffin cells of the adrenal medulla are of neuroectodermal origin. Diseases of the adrenal medulla are extremely rare in the neonate; thus, this section will focus on disorders of the adrenal cortex.

The adrenal cortex arises as two large masses on either side of the aorta, at the level of the first thoracic nerve, adjacent to the medullary cells that migrated from the neural crest. Fetal adrenal cortical cells can be identified by 4 weeks of gestation. By 7 weeks of gestation, the medullary cells begin to migrate to the interior of the adrenal cortex. The coelomic epithelium envelopes the cortical cells and remains as an outer shell. The fetal adrenal gland is steroidogenically active and large during gestation, but involutes during the latter half of pregnancy and especially after birth, suggesting a role in the maintenance of pregnancy. The adult adrenal cortex slowly develops from the outer shell, while the fetal zone undergoes involution. *DAX1*, a gene on the X chromosome, is essential for development of the definitive zone of the adrenal cortex (4). Mutations in this gene are responsible for congenital adrenal hypoplasia.

The trophic hormonal control of the fetal adrenal is not clear. In anencephalic fetuses, the fetal adrenal appears to develop normally during the first 12 weeks of gestation, then involutes. In patients with enzymatic defects of cortisol biosynthesis, however, the hyperplasia and increased activity of the adrenal glands

observed during the first 12 weeks of gestation suggest that ACTH must play some role during that time.

The adrenal cortex secretes three main types of steroid hormones:

- Glucocorticoids, of which cortisol (hydrocortisone) is the most important, regulate carbohydrate, protein, and fat metabolism.
- Mineralocorticoids (desoxycorticosterone and aldosterone) maintain salt and water balance by promoting sodium retention in exchange for hydrogen and potassium in the distal convoluted tubules of the kidney.
- Adrenal androgens (dehydroepiandrosterone (DHEA), β4-androstenedione, and 11β-hydroxyandrostenedione) are anabolic steroids that mediate sexual hair growth in girls at puberty. During the neonatal period, adrenal androgens are elevated secondary to the relative deficiency of 3β-hydroxysteroid dehydrogenase in the fetal zone of the fetal adrenal cortex, which is reflected in the higher concentrations of Δ5 steroids (e.g., DHEA, 17-OH pregnenolone), especially in premature infants.

The production of adrenocortical steroids is controlled by a hypothalamic–pituitary–adrenal homeostatic mechanism. Hypothalamic CRH stimulates release of pituitary ACTH, which in turn, stimulates cortisol biosynthesis. Increased levels of cortisol downregulate the axis, probably at the level of the hypothalamus.

Aldosterone secretion is controlled by the renin–angiotensin system rather than ACTH. Acute changes in pressure receptors control the release of renin from the juxtaglomerular cells of the kidney. Circulating renin, in turn, increases angiotensin II, which acts on the zona glomerulosa of the adrenal cortex to stimulate aldosterone secretion and vascular contractility. The increased blood volume and higher pressures within the arterial receptors exert negative feedback inhibition of the renin–angiotensin system. Secondary mechanisms such as a low sodium or high potassium intake also increase aldosterone excretion. ACTH will cause a transient, albeit unsustained, increase in aldosterone excretion, and conversely, aldosterone secretion is diminished in the absence of ACTH. Finally, cortisol itself may have a permissive role in aldosterone action at the tissue level.

Adrenal Insufficiency

During the neonatal period, disorders of the adrenal cortex consist almost entirely of those conditions that cause adrenal insufficiency as opposed to cortisol excess. Cushing syndrome may occur secondary to exogenous steroids such as dexamethasone, but Cushing disease is rare in the infant. Adrenal cortical tumors occur in infants but have not been reported in the neonate. Adrenal insufficiency can result from hypopituitarism, adrenal hemorrhage and other adrenal injury, ACTH receptor abnormalities, inherited degenerative disorders, or inborn errors of adrenal steroid biosynthesis.

Adrenocorticotropic Hormone Insufficiency

In a number of neonatal deaths associated with shock and peripheral vascular collapse in conjunction with severe hyponatremia and hyperkalemia, the adrenal glands were noted to be hypoplastic at autopsy. Because some of these cases were reported in infants with anencephaly or with partial or total pituitary aplasia, the lack of ACTH was thought to be responsible for the failure of development of the definitive zone. The possibility, however, of another critical trophic factor is suggested by finding decreased cortisol production, but normal mineralocorticoid function in patients with congenital hypopituitarism. These patients develop hypoglycemia and failure to thrive, but rarely have hyperkalemia, and can generally maintain water and electrolyte balance and secrete aldosterone in response to sodium deprivation.

Familial glucocorticoid insufficiency (FGD) is an autosomal recessive disorder that can present during the neonatal period or later in childhood with shock, hyperpigmentation, hypoglycemia, and failure to thrive. These patients have cortisol insufficiency and cannot increase serum cortisol or urinary 17-hydroxysteroid excretion in response to ACTH stimulation. They can, however, respond to sodium deprivation with increased aldosterone secretion and conservation of sodium excretion. Some pedigrees have a defect in the ACTH receptor, melanocortin-2 receptor, or the melanocortin 2 receptor accessory protein, causing FGD type 1 and 2, respectively. Partial inactivating mutations in StAR causing nonclassic congenital lipoid adrenal hyperplasia may present with or without a DSD and retain some glucocorticoid and mineralocorticoid capacity leading to misdiagnosis of FGD (51).

Adrenal Gland Injury

Adrenal insufficiency can occur during the newborn period as a result of damage to the relatively large and hyperemic adrenal glands. Trauma in association with a difficult delivery, particularly breech delivery; hemorrhagic diseases; or infectious processes can damage the adrenal glands. Minor hemorrhage or unilateral damage may not cause adrenal insufficiency and may present subsequently as calcification of the adrenal glands detected incidentally on an abdominal radiograph. All patients with shock and hyponatremia should be suspect for adrenal insufficiency. The highly sensitive ACTH immunoradiometric assays can detect elevated levels of plasma ACTH that are diagnostic of primary adrenal insufficiency.

Congenital Adrenal Hyperplasia

CAH is a genetic disorder involving a deficiency of one of several enzymes required for glucocorticoid biosynthesis. Deficient cortisol synthesis secondary to an enzymatic deficiency causes increased ACTH production, which in turn stimulates compensatory hypertrophy of the adrenal cortex and increase in steroidogenesis. This partially compensates for the block in the biosynthetic pathway but also leads to the increased production and accumulation of precursor steroids upstream of the enzymatic defect. Although ACTH chiefly regulates the glucocorticoid pathway, the synthesis of mineralocorticoids and androgens are variably affected depending on the specific enzyme involved.

Synthesis of adrenocortical steroids from cholesterol requires a series of hydroxylations (**Fig. 40.5**) mediated by cytochrome P450 oxidases. The initial step requires that the StAR protein forms contact sites between the outer and inner membranes of the mitochondria to transport cholesterol into the mitochondria and initiate steroidogenesis. Five enzymes are necessary for the synthesis of cortisol: P450scc, P450c17, P450c21, P450c11β, and 3β-hydroxysteroid dehydrogenase (52). The genes for these enzymes have been identified, and genetic defects in any of them can reduce glucocorticoid production and cause CAH. The clinical manifestations of this condition correspond to the particular enzyme affected and are summarized in **Table 40.7**.

Virilization

Virilization of the female is secondary to the elevated adrenal androgens caused by those enzymatic defects subsequent to 17-hydroxylation. In most cases, the labioscrotal folds are partially

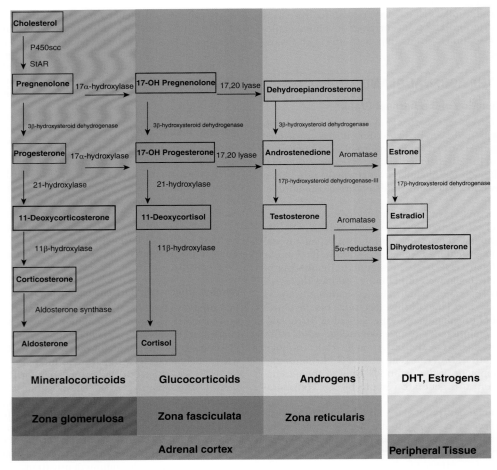

FIGURE 40.5 The biosynthetic pathway of adrenal steroid.

TABLE 40.7

Clinical and Biochemical Findings of the Common Variants of Congenital Adrenal Hyperplasia

Enzyme Deficiency (Classic)	Phenotype		Other Clinical Manifestations	Predominant Steroids
	46,XX	46,XY		
Congenital lipoid adrenal hyperplasia	Female	Female	Salt-wasting crisis	Low level—all steroids No response to ACTH
3β-Hydroxysteroid dehydrogenase deficiency	Virilized	Hypospadias	Salt-wasting crisis	Dehydroepiandrosterone 17-OH pregnenolone Increased Δ^5–Δ^4 ratio of steroids
21-Hydroxylase deficiency	Virilized	Male	Pseudoprecocious puberty in male Late virilization in female Salt-wasting crisis	17-OH progesterone Androstenedione Testosterone
11β-Hydroxylase deficiency	Virilized	Male	Pseudoprecocious puberty in male Hypertension	11-Deoxycortisol 11-Deoxycorticosterone Androstenedione Low renin
17α-Hydroxylase deficiency	Female	Female	Sexual infantilism Hypertension	Corticosterone 11-Deoxycorticosterone Low renin

fused with clitoral enlargement, which may be bound down by chordee. Occasionally, virilization may be so severe that a phallic urethra develops. In male infants, virilization is generally not evident in the neonate; therefore, the diagnosis of milder non–salt-losing forms of this disorder can remain undetected for several years. Boys can present later with secondary sexual changes, increased somatic growth, and well-developed musculature. The classic, and most prevalent virilizing form of CAH, is a defect in cytochrome P450c21 (21-hydroxylase deficiency), accounting for almost 90% of recognized cases (53). Mutations in P450c11 and 3β-hydroxysteroid dehydrogenase also cause female virilization.

Incomplete Masculinization

Failure of complete masculine development occurs in those forms of adrenal hyperplasia in which the androgen pathway is affected. Masculinization in the male, which requires fetal testosterone production, is incomplete, suggesting that the enzymatic defects occur in both the adrenal gland and the testis (54). In defects of 3β-hydroxysteroid dehydrogenase, secreted steroids consist almost entirely of compounds with Δ5-3β-hydroxy configuration (55). Fetal testosterone production by the testis is also impaired, causing incomplete masculinization in the male (56). The elevated Δ5-3β-hydroxyadrenal androgens, especially DHEA, are converted peripherally to active androgens that virilize the female infant. Elevation of serum 17-hydroxypregnenolone is diagnostic of 3β-hydroxysteroid dehydrogenase deficiency, although 17-hydroxyprogesterone concentrations also are markedly elevated (56).

Hypertension

Hyporeninemic hypertension and hypokalemia have been associated with enzymatic blocks of P450c11 β (11-hydroxylase deficiency) and P450c17 (17α-hydroxylase deficiency) resulting in excessive secretion of mineralocorticoids. A defect of cytochrome P450c11β (11-hydroxylase deficiency) causes an accumulation of deoxycorticosterone, a potent mineralocorticoid, and 11-deoxycortisol. The classical form of this disorder also causes virilization in females and pseudoprecocious puberty in males (52). The P450c17 defect (17α-hydroxylase deficiency) blocks 17-hydroxylation of progesterone, interfering with cortisol and androgen biosynthesis and shunting steroid production to the mineralocorticoid pathway (57). In this disorder, genital development in females is unaffected, but males are undervirilized. The hypertension resulting from excess mineralocorticoid production, however, is an inconstant feature, and it is not known if hypertension is present during the newborn period. Whether the hypertension is related to the duration of mineralocorticoid excess, the severity of the defect, or variations in sodium intake, is also unclear.

Salt Loss

Mineralocorticoid insufficiency and sodium loss are seen in the salt-losing form of 21-hydroxylase deficiency and 3β-hydroxysteroid dehydrogenase deficiency. The electrolytes initially are normal, but, within the 1st week of life, serum sodium will slowly decrease with a concomitant rise in serum potassium. These infants may manifest acute adrenal crisis with shock, peripheral collapse, and dehydration, by a week of age.

The underlying metabolic defects for two clinical variants of the 21-hydroxylase enzyme defect are now understood. Bongiovanni and Eberlein postulated that both are the result of the same enzymatic defect (58). In the salt loser, there is almost complete 21-hydroxylase deficiency, whereas in the simple form, there is sufficient 21-hydroxylase activity to permit aldosterone synthesis. A single gene mediates the hydroxylation of both progesterone and 17-hydroxyprogesterone. Different mutations of the P450c21 gene account for the heterogeneity of 21-hydroxylase deficiency disorders, including the nonclassic late-onset variant, although there is phenotypic variability within the same genotype (52,53).

A few instances of aldosterone deficiency caused by a specific defect of 18-dehydrogenase, the last enzymatic process in aldosterone synthesis, have been described (59,60). There is salt and water loss, without the other clinical consequences of CAH. These disorders are secondary to mutations of the P450c11 enzyme.

Congenital pseudohypoaldosteronism (PHA) type 1 is another cause of salt wasting in the neonate and affected infants present with hyponatremia, hyperkalemia, and metabolic acidosis. Elevated renin and aldosterone levels are found in these infants, and the etiology must be distinguished from CAH and transient forms of PHA, such as renal anomalies and urinary tract infections. The autosomal dominant form of type 1 PHA is due to a defect in the mineralocorticoid receptor and is limited to renal aldosterone resistance. This form responds well to salt supplementation, and frequently, by age 3, salt is no longer needed as the diet provides sufficient salt replacement. By contrast, the autosomal recessive form of type 1 PHA is more severe and is caused by a mutation in the epithelial sodium channel, affecting multiple organ systems, including the kidneys, lungs, colon, and salivary and sweat glands. Affected individuals frequently have lower respiratory tract infections and episodes of electrolyte imbalances requiring intensive fluid and electrolyte replacement therapy. Aside from genetic testing, the two types may be readily distinguished by a positive sweat test in the autosomal recessive form of the disorder.

Congenital Lipoid Adrenal Hyperplasia

Previously attributed to a deficiency of 20,22 desmolase (P450scc), the enzyme that mediates the conversion of cholesterol to pregnenolone, this disorder is now recognized as a genetic defect of StAR, a mitochondrial protein that transports cholesterol across the mitochondrial membrane. StAR is needed for acute steroidogenesis; thus, in some individuals, glucocorticoid production is initially preserved, but the accumulation of cholesterol esters causes destruction of the adrenal and adrenal insufficiency at older ages (61). No steroids are produced, and the adrenal glands are markedly enlarged and filled with cholesterol esters. In the classic form, males and females both have female-appearing external genitalia, hyponatremia, hyperkalemia, and dehydration. Males with congenital lipoid adrenal hyperplasia (CLAH) produce adequate AMH *in utero*, causing regression of müllerian structures and formation of wolffian duct derivatives. The accumulation of cholesterol esters damages the fetal Leydig cells, preventing testosterone biosynthesis and virilization, resulting in female external genitalia. Males with nonclassic forms of CLAH have normal male external genitalia. The age at presentation can vary from the newborn period to several months of age and older.

Prenatal Diagnosis and Treatment of Congenital Adrenal Hyperplasia

CAH, 21-hydroxylase deficiency, can be diagnosed prenatally using molecular techniques. Once the diagnosis of 21-hydroxylase deficiency has been established, molecular analysis of the P450c21 gene can be done in the propositus and the parents. Prenatal evaluation and treatment to prevent virilization have been reviewed and are still considered experimental (62). Maternal blood should be tested for fetal Y-chromosome to exclude treating the mother carrying a male, since virilization is not a concern in males. To prevent potential virilization of a female fetus, the mother can be started on dexamethasone, a steroid that crosses the placenta, early in the first trimester to suppress fetal adrenal androgen production. Once the specific gene mutation in an affected family is known, then within 3 weeks genetic analysis of fetal DNA from a maternal blood sample can detect whether the fetus is affected. If the diagnosis is confirmed in a female fetus, dexamethasone treatment is continued to term. Long-term consequences of prenatal steroids remain unknown, and therapy can be associated with cushingoid symptoms in the mother and adrenal suppression in the neonate; thus, prenatal management and therapy should be monitored closely and performed only at centers with expertise (62).

Diagnosis of Adrenal Insufficiency

The diagnosis of acute adrenal insufficiency is difficult to make in the newborn. There must be a high index of suspicion in any acutely ill infant with shock, peripheral collapse, a rapid and weak pulse, poor feeding, failure to thrive, intermittent pyrexia, or even hypoglycemia and convulsions. Hyperpigmentation, especially in the extensor creases and genitalia, is a subtle sign of CAH that is seldom recognized until after diagnosis. Decreased serum sodium and chloride and increased serum potassium levels are suggestive of mineralocorticoid deficiency. Isolated hyponatremia does not exclude glucocorticoid insufficiency and should be viewed as a possible indication of adrenal insufficiency. Certainly, ambiguous external genitalia at birth always should suggest the possibility of CAH.

Serum cortisol levels are low in all newborns, especially in premature infants, and lack diurnal variation; therefore, random cortisol determinations usually are not diagnostic. In clinical situations highly suggestive of adrenal insufficiency, it is recommended that a 1-hour ACTH stimulation test be performed and that pharmacologic doses of glucocorticoids be administered, along with fluid and electrolyte resuscitation, after testing. Plasma concentrations of ACTH are elevated in those infants with primary adrenal insufficiency, including CAH. A plasma sample for ACTH determination should be obtained before ACTH testing.

All 50 states in the United States, 35 countries and regions of 17 additional countries have implemented newborn screening for CAH. 17-hydroxyprogesterone (17-OHP) is elevated at birth and in premature sick infants. Serum values rapidly decrease by the 2nd or 3rd day of life to less than 100 ng/dL (63) but can increase to greater than 200 ng/dL at 1 to 2 months of age in male infants. Newborn values above 1,000 ng/dL are of concern, although 17-hydroxyprogesterone values are higher in stressed newborns, especially preterm sick newborns, in whom it can be greater than 600 ng/dL (64). These values, however, remain significantly lower than those in patients with 21-hydroxylase deficiency, which are often markedly above 2,000 ng/dL. It is important to recognize that elevated serum concentrations of 17-hydroxyprogesterone are not diagnostic of the 21-hydroxylase defect. Serum 17-hydroxyprogesterone can be mildly elevated in the 11-hydroxylase defect and can be markedly elevated in the 3β-hydroxysteroid dehydrogenase defect secondary to peripheral conversion of 17-hydroxypregnenolone to 17-hydroxyprogesterone (56). Serum values of 17-hydroxypregnenolone are especially elevated in the premature infant, and values up to 2,000 ng/dL can be normal (64).

Ideally, the heel stick blood sample should be collected at 48 hours of life, and premature infants should be retested at 2 and 4 weeks of age. Any abnormal NBS should prompt either a repeat NBS filter paper or a serum blood sample obtained for an 8 AM 17OHP to further evaluate for CAH. Delineation of the specific enzyme defect in CAH can be determined with an ACTH stimulation test by measuring serum concentrations of the various steroid precursors (17-OHP, 17-hydroxypregnenolone, dehydroepiandrosterone, androstenedione, cortisol, 11-deoxycorticosterone, and 11-deoxycortisol) at baseline and 60 minutes after administering Cortrosyn 125 µg (see Table 40.7). If results of a repeat NBS or serum 17 OHP are equivocal, then further evaluation with the ACTH stimulation study is recommended as well. NBS results with a high suspicion for CAH should prompt immediate evaluation with blood work for a confirmatory 17 OHP by liquid chromatography–tandem mass spectrometry (LC–MS/MS), electrolytes, and renin followed by prompt initiation of treatment for presumed CAH.

Treatment of Adrenal Insufficiency

The immediate need of a critically ill infant in adrenal crisis is for intravenous fluids. The infant should be given fluid resuscitation, and if possible, obtain blood work for adrenal steroids and ACTH or perform the ACTH stimulation test before administering hydrocortisone. However, if a newborn infant is in shock and in extremis, glucocorticoids should be immediately given as a lifesaving measure. In the usual situation, salt and water alone will relieve the clinical crisis. Intravenous isotonic saline in 5% glucose water should be infused at a rate of 100 to 120 mL/kg during the first 24 hours. If the infant is in severe shock, the use of plasma or 5% albumin, 10 to 20 mL/kg, to restore intravascular volume and cortisol is often necessary. Hydrocortisone sodium succinate, 1.5 to 2 mg/kg, should be given intravenously immediately and continued at a constant infusion of 50 mg/m²/d. Hydrocortisone sodium succinate, 2 mg/kg, can be given intramuscularly if intravenous access is a problem. The infant with severe shock may require a vasopressor, although vasopressor drugs may not be efficacious until hydrocortisone is administered.

Hydrocortisone or cortisone acetate, 10 to 12 mg/m²/d, is the mainstay for long-term treatment of patients with adrenal insufficiency. The newborn with CAH requires 20 to 25 mg/m²/d of hydrocortisone to adequately suppress adrenal androgen production. For acute illness, stress doses of hydrocortisone should be given at triple the maintenance dose. Families are routinely educated to administer both oral and parenteral stress steroids.

Often, a mineralocorticoid is a necessary adjunct for the chronic treatment of adrenal insufficiency. The dose of the oral mineralocorticoid, 9α-fludrocortisone (Florinef), is 0.05 to 0.1 mg/d, which is sufficient for most forms of adrenal insufficiency. In the salt-losing forms of CAH, occasionally higher doses of fludrocortisone are necessary and the addition of supplemental salt 1/4 to 1/2 g four times a day into the infant's formula. Even the compensated (non–salt-losing) variant may benefit from low-dose mineralocorticoid.

Iatrogenic Adrenal Insufficiency

During the neonatal period, pharmacologic doses of glucocorticoids are often needed for adjunctive treatment of a number of diseases and were previously commonly used in the management of bronchopulmonary dysplasia. The dose and duration of glucocorticoid therapy that causes iatrogenic adrenal insufficiency are not known, particularly in infants. High-dose glucocorticoid therapy for a brief duration (<1 week) probably will not cause adrenal insufficiency; therefore, a slow taper is not needed unless the clinical course of the primary condition deteriorates. Treatment longer than 14 days may result in at least transient adrenal insufficiency. After a prolonged course, the dose of glucocorticoids can be decreased by one-half every several days until a physiologic replacement dose (10 mg of hydrocortisone/m²/d orally) is achieved. The dose can then be lowered more gradually, by 20% every 4 or 5 days.

Adrenal function may be suppressed for some time after prolonged pharmacologic glucocorticoid therapy. Again, there are no studies correlating dose, duration of pharmacologic treatment, and time needed for recovery of adrenal function after high-dose glucocorticoid therapy in infants. There are anecdotal reports of adrenal crisis occurring during stress more than 6 months after discontinuation of pharmacologic glucocorticoid therapy. It is possible to evaluate periodically the adrenal response to exogenous ACTH to determine when iatrogenic adrenal insufficiency has resolved; alternatively, pharmacologic doses of glucocorticoids can be used empirically during situations of stress for at least a year after discontinuation of prolonged high-dose glucocorticoid therapy. Hydrocortisone 30 mg/m²/d administer at 6- to 8-hour intervals should be used to cover for the stress of an illness.

DISORDERS OF THE THYROID

Development and Function of the Thyroid

The fetal thyroid begins as a thickening of epithelium at the base of the tongue that migrates down to its location in the neck, leaving the thyroglossal duct as an embryonic remnant. During its caudal migration, the thyroid assumes a more bilobate shape. The developing thyroid concentrates iodide by 12 weeks of gestation and organifies iodide and synthesizes thyroxine (T_4) and triiodothyronine (T_3) by 14 weeks of gestation. Free T_4 and, more so, T_3 can cross the placenta in either direction. It is probable that the gradient is from mother to fetus during the first 12 weeks, then switches from fetus to mother except in the hypothyroid fetus (65,66). There is no placental transfer of maternal or fetal TSH, although thyroid-stimulating immunoglobulins (TSI) and TSH receptor–blocking antibodies (TRAb) will cross the placenta. The hypothalamic–pituitary feedback mechanisms are operative by the latter part of gestation. The hypothalamus secretes a tripeptide, TRH, which stimulates pituitary secretion of TSH. TSH, in turn, stimulates thyroid hormone production by regulating every step of thyroid hormone biosynthesis and release, from iodide accumulation

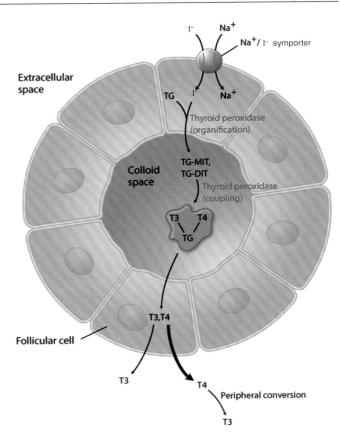

FIGURE 40.6 Thyroid hormone biosynthesis. (Reprinted with permission from Golan DE, Tashjian AH, Armstrong EJ, et al. *Principles of pharmacology*, 3rd ed. Philadelphia, PA: Lippincott Williams & Wilkins, 2011.)

to proteolysis of thyroglobulin. Thyroid hormones exercise negative feedback control of TSH response to TRH at the level of the pituitary and hypothalamus.

The biosynthesis of thyroid hormones is illustrated in **Figure 40.6**. A large percentage of circulating T_3 arises by deiodination of T_4 by deiodinases 1, 2, and 3 (67). Deiodinase 1 (D1) and 2 (D2) are differentially localized in the pituitary and peripheral tissues. At the pituitary level, D2 partially regulates TSH production by modulating T_3 concentrations. Deiodinase 3 (D3) converts T_4 to reverse T_3 and T_2, biologically inactive iodothyronines. Within the thyroid, iodotyrosines and iodothyronines are deiodinated by dehalogenase enzymes and remain within the intrathyroidal iodide pool to be reused. The iodide released from peripheral deiodination enters the circulatory system to be reconcentrated by the thyroid gland or excreted by the kidneys. The iodothyronines are transported in the plasma by proteins. Thyroxine-binding globulin (TBG), an α-globulin, is the major carrier of T_4 and binds T_3 to a lesser extent. Thyroxine also is bound by T_4-binding prealbumin and by albumin. At the cellular level, the unbound free T_3 and T_4 are biologically active. Genetic disorders, acquired conditions, or drugs that quantitatively change the concentration of TBG will alter circulating total T_4 without affecting the free T_4 level, an indicator of the physiologic thyroid status.

Congenital Hypothyroidism

The causes of congenital hypothyroidism are many and include genetic and sporadic disorders of embryogenesis, inborn errors of T_4 biosynthesis, and environmental factors. Table 40.8 lists the incidence of the various causes of permanent and transient congenital hypothyroidism (68–71).

TABLE 40.8

Incidence of Various Forms of Congenital Hypothyroidism

	Incidence
Permanent congenital hypothyroidism	
Congenital thyroid agenesis or dysgenesis	1:4,000
Inborn errors of thyroxine synthesis	1:30,000
TSH resistance	1:50,000
Resistance to thyroid hormone	1:40,000
Hypothalamic–hypopituitary hypothyroidism	1:66,000[a]
Transient congenital hypothyroidism	
[b]Endemic goitrous hypothyroidism	
Maternal transplacental passage of TSH-receptor antibody	1:180,000
Maternal antithyroid drug treatment	1:11,000–1:15,000
Delayed TSH rise	1:250–1:100,000

[a]Hypothalamic–hypopituitary hypothyroidism incidence is based on newborn screening studies so may be underdetected.
[b]Incidence data not available.

Permanent Congenital Hypothyroidism

Agenesis or Dysgenesis of the Thyroid Gland

The most frequent cause of congenital hypothyroidism in the United States is a disorder of embryogenesis, which may result in hypoplasia, athyrosis, or ectopia of the thyroid gland. Thyroid hypoplasia has been reported in children with congenital toxoplasmosis, but *in utero* infectious diseases are rarely a cause of thyroid dysgenesis. Although genetic mutations in thyroid transcription factors (FOXE1, NKX2-1, and PAX-8) have been identified in familial forms of thyroid dysgenesis, more than 95% of cases are sporadic. An ectopic thyroid gland may be located anywhere along its pathway of descent during embryologic development, from the base of the tongue (lingual thyroid) to above its normal location in the neck. Congenital hypothyroidism is also a feature of Townes-Brocks syndrome, DiGeorge syndrome, Johanson-Blizzard syndrome, Williams-Beuren syndrome, Kabuki syndrome, Ohdo syndrome, and genitopatellar syndrome (72).

Inborn Errors of Thyroxine Synthesis

Inherited disorders of T_4 synthesis involve deficiencies in one or more of the enzymes necessary for thyroid hormone production or release, resulting in hypothyroidism (73). A compensatory increase in TSH production produces hyperplasia and enlargement of the thyroid gland, creating the clinical picture of familial goitrous hypothyroidism.

Iodide Transporter Defect

Iodide is transported across the basolateral membrane of the thyroid follicular cell by the sodium–iodide symporter (NIS). In this rare inherited defect of T_4 synthesis, this ability is lost. Several other organs, including the salivary glands, share the ability to concentrate iodide, and this defect can be distinguished from athyrosis because the salivary iodide concentration is low and usually a goiter can be detected by ultrasonography. Radioactive iodine uptake at 24 hours is negligible, and thyroid scans do not detect thyroid tissue. This defect reflects iodine deficiency and can be compensated with high doses of iodide, although treatment with thyroxine is easier and probably more effective.

The chloride/iodide transporter, Pendrin, is present in the inner ear and thyroid gland and transports iodide across the apical membrane of the follicular thyroid cell. Pendred syndrome is associated with sensorineural deafness, goiter, or mild hypothyroidism, and perchlorate discharge is incomplete.

Organification of Peroxidase Defect

DUOX2 is the gene responsible for producing H_2O_2 for organification of iodide. A defect in this gene causes mild–moderate or a transient hypothyroidism and presents with a goiter. The *TPO* gene mediates the organification of the iodide. A defect in the organification of iodide is one of the more frequent disorders of hormonogenesis and usually presents with severe congenital hypothyroidism and a goiter. Monoallelic variants present with a partial iodide organification defect causing mild congenital hypothyroidism. In this defect, the thyroid has an increased uptake of iodide but is unable to oxidize it or combine it with tyrosine or thyronine. In these patients, radioiodine is concentrated in the gland, and when given the anions potassium perchlorate or thiocyanate orally (0.5 to 1 g), it displaces the unorganified iodine, causing rapid discharge of the radioactive iodine from the thyroid gland.

Coupling Defect

Coupling of monoiodotyrosine (MIT) and diiodotyrosine (DIT) into T_4 and T_3 is a complex intermediate step involving several processes and should not be considered a defined single enzymatic deficiency. The inability of the thyroid gland to couple MIT and DIT into T_4 and T_3 leads to the accumulation of large amounts of MIT and DIT in the gland, with small amounts of T_4 and T_3 synthesized and immediately released into the circulation. Radioactive iodine uptake by the thyroid gland is rapid and high. Definitive diagnosis requires thyroid biopsy and chromatographic analysis of the iodotyrosines and iodothyronines with the latter detecting primarily MIT and DIT and only trace quantities of T_4 and T_3.

Dehalogenase Defect

A defect in the *IYD* gene impairs the deiodination of the iodotyrosines and iodothyronines in the thyroid, liver, kidneys, and other organs. The inherited inability of the thyroid to deiodinate MIT and DIT causes leakage of these precursors from the gland and depletion of iodide stores. This loss of iodide causes decreased hormone synthesis, resulting in a compensatory rise in TSH, thyroid hyperplasia, and increased synthesis of MIT, DIT, and iodothyronines. The goitrous hypothyroidism in this defect is not caused by a biosynthetic block but by iodine deficiency, which can be treated with large amounts of iodine. However, thyroid hormone replacement therapy is equally efficacious and easier. Radioactive iodine is rapidly accumulated and turned over. Because this defect is extrathyroidal and intrathyroidal, radioactive MIT and DIT appear unchanged in the urine.

Infants with defects in the sodium–iodide transporter, *DUOX2*, and the *IYD* genes may have normal NBS results and present late, causing neurodevelopmental delays.

Abnormal Thyroglobulin

Thyroglobulin is synthesized exclusively within the thyroid. Defects of thyroglobulin formation include errors of thyroglobulin synthesis and decreased synthesis. Deficient protease activity for thyroglobulin degradation also has been postulated to result in deficiency of thyroid hormone release. These disorders are characterized by abnormal circulating and intrathyroidal iodoproteins. These peptides sometimes have been described as albumin like and have been identified as the iodoalbumin thyroalbumin, in which the major iodinated compounds appear to be monoiodohistidines and diiodohistidines (74,75). The thyroglobulin abnormality is thought to cause iodination of inappropriate proteins, mainly albumin, with a subsequent low yield of T_4. A compensatory increase in TSH secretion causes thyroid hyperplasia and a rapid turnover of T_4 or albumin. Proteolysis of the iodohistidine-rich iodoalbumin results in a high secretion of iodohistidine, which can be detected in the urine.

Thyroid Hormone Receptor Mutations

Refetoff et al. (76) reported a family with deaf–mutism, stippled epiphyses, delayed bone age, and goiter that appeared clinically euthyroid. Serum T_4 was elevated, but thyroid hormone–binding proteins and hormone biosynthesis were normal. This family had the variant of thyroid hormone resistance characterized by generalized tissue unresponsiveness to thyroid hormone. Mutations in the α-and β- isoforms of the thyroid hormone receptor (THR) have been identified. THR-β is present in the liver, kidney, and lung, and affected individuals may present with abnormal NBS studies or later in childhood with a goiter. Affected individuals may have normal or elevated TSH and elevated free T_4 and free T_3 and findings of short stature, attention deficit disorder, and resting tachycardia or be asymptomatic.

THR-α is present in the heart and bone and features include bradycardia, constipation, short stature, delayed bone age, and neurodevelopmental delay. Biochemical findings include an elevated free T_3, low free T_4, and normal TSH. Treatment with thyroid hormone replacement therapy can be difficult in both disorders due to the presence of these mutations in selective organs, in which case treatment could render some organs euthyroid and others hyperthyroid (77).

Thyroid-Stimulating Hormone Receptor (TSHR) Mutations

TSHR mutations cause TSH resistance, and inheritance is autosomal dominant or recessive. The number of affected alleles and type of mutation determine the severity of the condition. TSH in utero stimulates thyroid growth; therefore, severe mutations can result in thyroid hypoplasia with severe biochemical hypothyroidism. Milder mutations may present with mild compensated hyperthyrotropinemia with a normal thyroid gland. Individuals with complete TSH resistance and low free T_4 should be treated with thyroid hormone replacement therapy. Treatment for partial TSH resistance is controversial in those individuals with normal circulating free T_4 because they have normal peripheral sensitivity to the free T_4. Therefore, thyroid hormone replacement therapy could potentially render these individuals hyperthyroid. Long-term follow-up of these patients is essential to determine the need for thyroid hormone replacement therapy (78). Pseudohypoparathyroidism types 1a and 1b also cause TSH resistance due to a G-protein mutation of the TSH receptor and may present in the neonatal period with mild elevations in TSH (79). Patients can be either euthyroid or present with congenital hypothyroidism.

Secondary and Tertiary Hypothyroidism

Central hypothyroidism is caused by failure of the pituitary and hypothalamus to secrete TSH and TRH, respectively. Newborn infants with these disorders may be missed in those NBS programs that rely on primary TSH screening or those directed to primary hypothyroidism, but it will be detected by screening for both low T_4 and elevated TSH levels. All patients with midline abnormalities or suspected pituitary transcription factor mutations (**Tables 40.3 and 40.4**) should be tested for central hypothyroidism with a free T_4 by direct dialysis and an ultrasensitive TSH, because they might be missed by the NBS test. Isolated TSH deficiency is rare, and identification of central hypothyroidism should lead to evaluation of other pituitary function. Reports of autosomal recessive mutations (TSHB and TRHR) and X-linked gene mutations (TBL1X and IGSF1) are other causes of central hypothyroidism (72).

Transient Hypothyroidism

Endemic Goitrous Hypothyroidism

At one time, congenital endemic goitrous hypothyroidism was prevalent worldwide; however, its frequency has markedly declined with the introduction of iodine into various foods, including infant formulas. In 2016, urine iodine levels collected from schoolchildren in 127 countries showed optimal iodine in 102 countries, iodine deficiency in 15 countries, and iodine excess in 10 countries (80). The dietary requirements for iodine vary, but 40 to 100 μg/d is sufficient for most children. In areas with endemic goiters, factors other than iodine, such as enzymatic defects and genetic and dietary factors, probably contribute to goiter formation. Such factors are suggested by the finding that females are more commonly afflicted than males, and not everyone within the endemic area is afflicted despite similar iodine intake. For example, in

the Alps, deaf–mutism is a common finding in association with endemic cretinism, possibly suggesting an associated enzymatic defect of iodine organification. When cretinism occurs in conjunction with endemic goiter, the symptoms are similar to the dysgenetic form of cretinism, except for the presence of a goiter and an elevated radioactive iodine uptake.

Maternal Transplacental Transfer of Thyroid Antibodies

There are two types of thyrotropin receptor antibodies (TRab), stimulating and blocking immunoglobulins. The former binds to the TSH receptor stimulating the production of thyroid hormone (discussed in detail in section on Congenital Thyrotoxicosis), while the latter blocks the production of thyroid hormone causing hypothyroidism. In some cases, the infant may present with primary hypothyroidism followed by hyperthyroidism or hyperthyroidism followed by hypothyroidism due to the presence of both types of antibodies (81). Thyroid antibodies have been detected with increased incidence among mothers of children with hypothyroidism and may cause either transient or persistent congenital hypothyroidism (82). TRAb can be measured in infants and used to guide the duration of treatment. Typically, by 3 to 4 months, these antibodies are no longer present. Most mothers with thyroid antibodies have unaffected children, however, and, conversely, most mothers of children with congenital hypothyroidism do not have thyroid antibodies (83).

Drug-Induced Neonatal Goiter

Many drugs have been demonstrated to be goitrogenic. In the newborn infant, the most commonly implicated drugs are iodides and thiourea derivatives used to treat maternal thyrotoxicosis. These drugs have not only caused goiter in the newborn but are also associated with reports of hypothyroidism (84). Although the correlation between the dose of the drug and the occurrence of goiter is poor, prolonged administration of thiourea drugs to the mother increases the risk of fetal goiter. One recommendation for minimizing this risk is to lower the dose of thiourea drugs during the last trimester and add thyroid hormone concurrently (85). In infants of hyperthyroid mothers, it is necessary to distinguish the drug-induced goiter from the TSI-induced goiter. A low T_4 suggests that the goiter is secondary to the drug, whereas a high T_4 is more compatible with a TSI-induced goiter and maternal antibody–mediated neonatal hyperthyroidism. A mixed picture can also occur with an initially low T_4 that increases within a few days as serum concentrations of the drug decline. The stimulating effects of TSI antibodies, which have a much longer half-life, can manifest as thyrotoxicosis at a few days to a week of age (discussed under congenital thyrotoxicosis). Treatment usually is not necessary for the infant with a drug-induced goiter unless the goiter is asphyxiating or, more rarely, the infant is hypothyroid. Thyroid hormone will cause the goiter to subside.

Treatment with propylthiouracil (PTU) is now restricted to the first trimester of pregnancy because of its association with hepatotoxicity. Methimazole is more teratogenic than PTU and should be avoided in the first trimester. Therefore mothers can be treated with PTU in the first trimester and then switched to methimazole for the remainder of the pregnancy. Concerns have been raised regarding the appropriate use of antithyroid agents in lactating mothers. Carbimazole and methimazole are only transmitted at low levels in breast milk and are safe alternatives for lactating mothers (86,87). Nonetheless, thyroid function should be monitored in the infant.

Delayed TSH Rise in Premature Infants

Woo et al. reported an increased incidence of primary hypothyroidism with a delayed TSH rise in premature infants of very low birth weight (<1,500 g) and extremely low birth weight (<1,000 g). In these infants, the initial NBS was normal, and the increase in TSH was detected at ≥3 weeks of age. These infants no longer needed treatment at 18 months of age, indicating that the hypothyroidism was transient (88). Transient hypothyroidism in these infants may be due to dopamine and/or steroids, which suppress TSH, or iodine exposure during procedures. Screening premature very-low-birth weight infants at 2, 6, and 10 weeks of age or until they reach 1,500 g is recommended.

Symptoms of Hypothyroidism

Symptoms of thyroid agenesis are readily detectable by 6 weeks of age; however, some infants will have clinical manifestations at birth or during the immediate neonatal period (89). Infants with ectopic or residual thyroid tissue or inborn errors of T_4 synthesis often produce enough thyroid hormone to delay the onset of clinical symptoms and are typically asymptomatic when identified by NBS. The signs during the early neonatal period are subtle and include prolonged neonatal jaundice, mottling of the skin, poor suck, poor feeding, lethargy, umbilical hernia, bradycardia, constipation, and intermittent cyanosis. Occasionally, infants with congenital hypothyroidism demonstrate severe respiratory distress. Later, the more classic symptoms of cretinism appear. Progressive myxedema can cause coarsening of the facies with puffy eyelids, flattened nasal bridge, and an enlarged tongue. The cry is hoarse secondary to myxedema of the larynx and epiglottis. Lethargy, hypotonia, constipation, poor feeding, poor weight gain, dry hair, and pallor become more notable with time.

Congenital hypothyroidism is one of the leading causes of preventable intellectual and developmental disabilities worldwide. There is considerable evidence for the essential role of thyroid hormones in the growth and development of the CNS (90). The neurodevelopmental outcome in children with congenital hypothyroidism depends on the severity and duration of the hypothyroidism, age at the time of initiation of therapy, and the dose of thyroid hormone administered. The prognosis appears to be worse if signs of hypothyroidism are clinically evident at diagnosis. Selva et al. performed a randomized study of three different thyroid hormone treatment regimens (37.5 µg daily; 62.5 µg for 3 days and then 37.5 µg or 50 µg daily) showed that free T_4 and T_4 increased into the target range of 10 to 16 µg/dL within 3 days of therapy in the groups treated with 62.5 µg and 50 µg and by 1 week in the group treated with 37.5 µg daily (91). The group treated with 50 µg daily of levothyroxine normalized the TSH by 2 weeks of age. Thirty-one of these children had neurodevelopmental testing at ages <4, 4 to 6,

or >6, which showed that the children started on the higher dose of 50 µg had full-scale IQ scores 11 points higher than those started on the lower dose of 37.5 µg. Regardless of the initial treatment regimen, the subjects with severe congenital hypothyroidism had lower full-scale IQ scores then those with moderate hypothyroidism. Lastly, subjects whose T_4 normalized at 2 weeks and those whose TSH and free T_4 normalized beyond 2 weeks had significantly lower cognitive, attention, and achievement scores (92).

Diagnosis

Thyroid Function Tests

Thyroid function tests in infants are elevated compared to values in older children. Hypothyroidism should not be diagnosed from samples obtained in the immediate postnatal period, less than 48 hours after birth, because of the cold-stimulated surge of TSH and TRH. Maternal estrogen effect accounts for higher TBG concentrations in the neonate. Total T_4 ranges from 7.3 to 22.9 µg/dL during the first month of life, with mean values greater than 10 µg/dL (Table 40.9). Thyroid function tests normally are lower in premature and sick newborns than in healthy term newborn infants (Table 40.9), as a result of lower concentrations of TBG (93,94).

Newborn Screening Program

In view of the desirability for early diagnosis and treatment, NBS programs in the United States test for thyroid dysfunction with a heel-prick blood sample collected on filter paper (95). Only 28.4% of infants born worldwide are screening for congenital hypothyroidism (96). Some screening programs use an initial T_4 screen in which blood samples with a T_4 value below a specified cutoff, such as the 10th percentile, are repeated and a TSH determined on the same sample. If the repeat T_4 is still low (<10 µg/dL) or the TSH elevated, confirmatory tests are requested. Many state screening programs test the TSH level, which will detect primary hypothyroidism, but not central hypothyroidism. The TSH only screen eliminates infants who are premature, euthyroid sick, or have thyroxine-binding protein deficiency. Lastly, some NBS programs run both a T_4 and TSH, which will detect both primary hypothyroidism and central hypothyroidism (95). Following a positive screen, a serum confirmatory sample for free T_4 and TSH should be obtained prior to starting treatment.

TABLE 40.9

Concentrations of Free T_4, T_4, T_3, and TSH in Preterm and Term Infants, in Cord at Birth and Term Infants, in Cord Blood at Birth and at 7, 14, and 28 Days of Age (Mean ± 1 SD)

Gestation (Weeks)	Age of Infant	Free T_4 (ng/dL)	T_4 (µg/dL)	T_3 (ng/dL)	TSH (mU/L)
23–27	Cord	1.28 ± 0.4	5.4 ± 2.0	20 ± 15	6.8 ± 2.9
	7 d	1.47 ± 0.6	4.0 ± 1.8	33 ± 20	3.5 ± 2.6
	14 d	1.45 ± 0.5	4.7 ± 2.6	41 ± 25	3.9 ± 2.7
	28 d	1.5 ± 0.4	6.1 ± 2.3	63 ± 27	3.8± 4.7
28–30	Cord	1.45 ± 0.4	6.3 ± 2.0	29 ± 21	7.0 ± 3.7
	7 d	1.82 ± 0.7	6.3 ±2.1	56 ± 24	3.6 ± 2.5
	14 d	1.65 ± 0.4	6.6 ± 2.3	72 ± 28	4.9 ± 11.2
	28 d	1.71 ± 0.4	7.5 ± 2.3	87 ± 31	3.6 ± 2.5
31–34	Cord	1.49 ± 0.3	7.6 ± 2.3	35 ± 23	7.9 ± 5.2
	7 d	2.14 ± 0.6	9.4 ± 3.4	92 ± 36	3.6 ± 4.8
	14 d	1.98 ± 0.4	9.1 ± 3.6	110 ± 41	3.8 ± 9.3
	28 d	1.88 ± 0.5	8.9 ± 3.0	120 ± 40	3.5 ± 3.4
≥37	Cord	1.41 ± 0.3	9.2 ± 1.9	60 ± 35	6.7 ± 4.8
	7 d	2.70 ± 0.6	12.7 ± 2.9	148 ± 50	2.6 ± 1.8
	14 d	2.03 ± 0.3	10.7 ± 1.4	167 ± 31	2.5 ± 2.0
	28 d	1.65 ± 0.3	9.7 ± 2.2	176 ± 32	1.8 ± 0.9

Data from LaFranchi S. Clinical features and detection of congenital hypothyroidism. In: Post TW, ed. *UpToDate*. Waltham, MA: UpToDate. Accessed October 7, 2019. Copyright © 2019 UpToDate, Inc. For more information visit www.uptodate.com; and Williams FL, Simpson J, Delahunty C, et al. Developmental trends in cord and postpartum serum thyroid hormones in preterm infants. *J Clin Endocrinol Metab* 2004;89:5314.

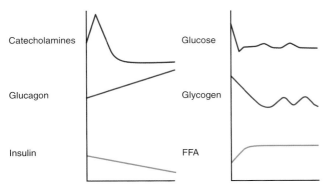

FIGURE 41.1 Levels of hormones and metabolic fuels change after birth. At birth, the counterregulatory hormones (i.e., catecholamines and glucagon) increase greatly, whereas insulin secretion decreases. Neonatal plasma glucose concentrations plummet as a result of cord clamping. The changes in counterregulatory hormones and insulin favor mobilization of glucose and fat and stimulate gluconeogenesis. These changes assure adequate neonatal glucose production. FFA, free fatty acids. (From Kalhan SC, Bier DM, Savin SM, et al. Estimation of glucose turnover and 13C recycling in the human newborn by simultaneous [1-13C]glucose and [6,6-1H2]glucose tracers. *J Clin Endocrinol Metab* 1980;50:456. Reproduced by permission of Oxford University Press.)

The neonatal brain takes up and oxidizes ketone bodies at higher rates than seen in adults, and the neonatal brain uses ketone bodies more efficiently than it does glucose (13).

Glucose levels peak after a feed; any excess glucose available is then stored as glycogen in the liver or, along with fatty acids absorbed after milk feeds, converted to fat for deposition in adipose tissue.

Sometime after each feed, blood glucose level starts to fall and glycogenolysis and gluconeogenesis are again activated to ensure energy availability for organs that are obligate users. Glycogen is an exhaustible source of glucose whose capacity varies according to fetal growth and maturity (14). On average, after approximately 2 hours of fasting, gluconeogenesis must become the major glucose-providing process. Stable isotope turnover studies have shown that neonatal glucose production rates are 4 to 6 mg/kg/min (15). Between feeds, lipolysis and ketogenesis provide alternative fuels to glucose for organs such as the brain, which are not obligate glucose utilizers (16). Indeed, there is evidence that glucose utilization by the neonatal brain is less than in subsequent months, because of utilization of alternative fuels (17). The process of ketogenesis also provides energy and cofactors, which are utilized in gluconeogenesis, again highlighting the importance of fatty fuels.

The control of neonatal metabolism is dependent, first, upon the synthesis of key enzymes, such as hepatic phosphorylase for glycogenolysis, phosphoenolpyruvate carboxykinase (PEPCK) for gluconeogenesis, and carnitine acyltransferases for ketogenesis, and second, upon the induction of enzyme activity by hormonal changes. Glucagon is the major neonatal glucoregulatory hormone (8). The concentration of blood glucagon increases when blood glucose levels fall, and it induces activity of the enzymes of glycogenolysis, gluconeogenesis, and ketogenesis in the liver. The glucoregulatory role of insulin in the neonate is less potent than in the older child and adult (18). In most neonates, insulin does not appear to have a major influence on normal blood glucose homeostasis, but in some extreme cases (see below), high insulin concentrations may result in hypoglycemia. Finally, it is unlikely that other hormones, such as the catecholamines, cortisol, thyroid hormones, and growth hormone, are important regulators in the fast–feed cycle of the healthy neonate, but rare cases of hypopituitarism or cortisol deficiency (see below) may present with neonatal hypoglycemia, which suggests that minimum basal levels are needed to maintain normoglycemia.

Finally, the change from fetal to neonatal metabolism must take into account the important role of gastrointestinal adaptation. The introduction of enteral feeding has been shown to trigger the secretion of gastrointestinal regulatory peptides and hormones, which in turn induce the features of gut adaptation, namely, gut growth, mucosal differentiation, motility, development of digestion and absorption, and even pancreatic hormone responses (19,20).

Differences between Neonatal and Adult Metabolism

The differences between neonatal and adult metabolism are most likely to be evolutionary protective responses. Milk-fed neonates during their normal fast–feed cycle produce and utilize ketone bodies to the extent that is seen in adults only after a prolonged fast. Other fuels such as lactate may also be used in addition to glucose and ketone bodies. Insulin plays a lesser role in neonatal glucoregulation than in the adult, in that its release in response to glucose is blunted and delayed when compared to the adult and that there may be end-organ insensitivities to its action (21). In fact, healthy neonates have insulin–glucose relationships that differ markedly from those of older subjects (22,23). Therefore, when investigating a neonate for possible impaired neonatal glucoregulation, it is essential to have reference data from healthy infants, rather than comparing the neonatal concentrations and interrelationships of fuels and hormones with those of adults. Also, it is inappropriate to consider glucose alone—the availability of alternative fuels must be established.

DISORDERS OF CARBOHYDRATE HOMEOSTASIS

The vast majority of babies are entirely healthy after birth and remain so. For the minority of babies who are born with difficulties or for whom difficulties develop in the hours or days after birth, the etiologies can be described broadly under three headings:

- Intrinsic abnormalities acquired during fetal development
- Intrauterine, intrapartum, or postnatal external insults that directly injure organs and systems
- Failure or delay to make the normal transition from fetal to neonatal life

Taking as an example the cardiovascular system for each of these headings, there may be congenital structural abnormality of the heart acquired during fetal development, there may be myocardial injury and insufficiency arising from a severe hypoxic–ischemic insult, or there may be delayed transition to the normal neonatal circulation with persistent pulmonary hypertension.

With respect to homeostasis of carbohydrate and other metabolic substrates, congenital problems are rare but can cause significant compromise, and severe metabolic disorders arising from external insults are also uncommon. It is the third category (failure or delay to make transition) that is the most common and often significant cause for concern and also for confusion.

Having reviewed, above, the metabolism of the fetus and neonate and the changes that occur at birth in the healthy infant, the three categories of disordered metabolic homeostasis are as follows and in order of increasing occurrence:

- Abnormalities acquired during fetal development—for example, inborn errors of metabolism
- Intrauterine, intrapartum, or postnatal external insults that directly injure organs and systems—for example, hypoxia–ischemia and infection
- Failure or delay in making the normal transition from fetal to neonatal life—for example, following poor control of maternal diabetes mellitus, preterm delivery, or IUGR

THE NEWBORN INFANT

Understanding of disordered metabolic homeostasis must be in the context of a knowledge of normal physiology and normal feeding behavior, in order to understand how these disorders will affect a neonate and to assist formulation of sensible management plans.

NEONATAL HYPOGLYCEMIA

Neonatal hypoglycemia has been recognized for over a century (24–26), although there have been wide swings of opinion regarding the definition of the condition, its clinical significance, and its optimal management (Fig. 41.2). As described above, healthy babies have a number of protective mechanisms to prevent the physiologic postnatal fall in blood glucose from causing harm. However, some babies have absent, delayed, or impaired protective responses and display clinical signs of hypoglycemia. The risk of reduced glucose availability to the brain in such circumstances has been widely acknowledged, and it is a sad fact that babies have come to significant harm (27,28). However, in more recent years, this risk and the increasing practice of defensive medicine have resulted in a swing toward the treatment of large numbers of infants, often unnecessarily, with intravenous glucose, resulting in separation from their mothers and placing at risk the establishment of breast-feeding (29). Therefore, it is important to identify those infants most at risk for the adverse effects of hypoglycemia and determine the most effective and least invasive regimens for prevention of hypoglycemic brain injury (30). To date, no controlled study has addressed either of these issues.

Diagnosis, Definition, and Clinical Significance

Much controversy and confusion have surrounded the definition of hypoglycemia (30,31). In 1988, Koh et al. (32) demonstrated that the "accepted" definition varied widely not only between standard pediatric textbooks but also between neonatologists, with values given ranging from below 1 mmol/L (18 mg/dL) to 4 mmol/L (72 mg/dL). There remain significant variations in definition of hypoglycemia (<2 mmol/L [36 mg/dL] to 4 mmol/L [72 mg/dL]), risk factors for impaired metabolic adaptation, and thresholds for intervention, in contemporary practice (33). Cornblath et al. (30) wrote, "The definition of clinically significant hypoglycemia remains one of the most confused and contentious issues in contemporary neonatology." This continuing controversy regarding the definition and clinical significance of neonatal hypoglycemia arises from a frequent failure to consider the changes of metabolic adaptation in their totality (29,30). Given uncertainties in the evidence base, it is unsurprising that

guidelines for screening, diagnosing, preventing, and treating low glucose concentrations in neonates are varied (34,35). In the UK, a Framework for Practice has recently been published by the British Association for Perinatal Medicine that gives highly practical and family-focused guidance designed to reduce unwanted variation in practices in the identification, management, and admission thresholds of babies admitted to neonatal units for hypoglycemia; and to promote practices that avoid unnecessary separation of mother and baby (36).

The accurate measurement of blood glucose level is essential in the diagnosis of hypoglycemia. In resource-rich settings, the ward-based blood gas biosensor should be considered the reference standard for measuring blood glucose based on accuracy and speed of result. Blood gas analyzers will produce glucose results as a calculated plasma glucose equivalent concentration that should agree with laboratory plasma glucose results in the majority of cases (37), and they can be configured to give a "glucose only" reading on a small volume sample. Central laboratory measurement of glucose from samples sent in fluoride oxalate tubes is inconsistent due to variable inhibition of glycolysis in the first 30 to 90 minutes and variability in time taken to reach the laboratory for processing (38). Processing time may lead to impractical delays in obtaining results and guiding clinical management.

Current cot side technology for measuring blood glucose using reagent strips and glucometers is prone to significant limitations especially in the range of 0 to 2.0 mmol/L (30,39). An International Organisation for Standardisation (ISO) standard for blood glucose meters was implemented in 2016 (ISO:15197:2013). The standard specifies that 95% of measured glucose values shall fall within +/− 0.83 mmol/L of the average measured values of the reference measurement procedure at glucose concentrations less than 5.55 mmol/L. Although handheld glucometers are available that meet this ISO standard, the limits of their accuracy must be understood by the user and in centers where handheld devices are used to screen neonates, low values should be confirmed by accurate measurement to ensure infants are assigned to the appropriate care pathway.

Interesting new techniques for continuous glucose monitoring (CGM) of interstitial glucose levels appear to help target glucose within specific ranges with reduced need for venipuncture and heel pricks in the newborn (39). However, the reliability and calibration of CGM devices has not been fully evaluated, there are no randomized trials showing improved clinical outcomes resulting from their use, there are uncertainties about performance of current technologies in the 0 to 2.0 mmol/L range, and the link between interstitial glucose concentration and cerebral glucose availability is unclear (39,40).

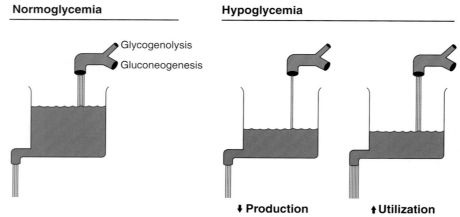

FIGURE 41.2 The rates of glucose production and utilization are represented by the faucet and drain of the sink. The level in the sink is equivalent to plasma or blood glucose concentrations. If production from glycogenolysis and gluconeogenesis is adequate, and use is not excessive, normoglycemia exists and the plasma or blood glucose concentration (i.e., the level in the sink) is normal. Hypoglycemia develops if production is inadequate to meet body needs or if use outstrips production. This results in decreased glucose concentrations (i.e., diminished level in sink). (From Kalhan SC, Bier DM, Savin SM, et al. Estimation of glucose turnover and 13C recycling in the human newborn by simultaneous [1-13C]glucose and [6,6-1H2]glucose tracers. *J Clin Endocrinol Metab* 1980;50:456. Reproduced by permission of Oxford University Press.)

TABLE 41.1

Infants at Risk of Disordered Neonatal Metabolic Adaptation

Preterm (<37 weeks' gestation)

Intrauterine growth restriction (≤2nd centile for gestation age and sex) or clinically wasted

Infants of diabetic mothers

Maternal beta-blocker use in the third trimester and/or at the time of delivery

Unexplained fetal hyperinsulinism causing clinical appearance of macrosomia

Syndrome, for example, Beckwith-Wiedemann

Moderate to severe perinatal hypoxia–ischemia

Infection

Known or family history of pituitary or adrenal insufficiency

Known or family history of inborn error of metabolism

The challenge, in terms of definition, is the description and diagnosis of a pathologic condition, and differentiating this from the changes that are within the physiologic "norm" whereby blood glucose levels fall immediately after birth and then increase, often to lower levels than the normal adult range. The increase in blood glucose levels occurs over the first 2 to 3 postnatal days in healthy, appropriate weight for gestational age (AGA) full-term neonates, sometimes later for those who are breast-fed. These infants have high ketone body levels when blood glucose concentrations are low, and it is likely that this protects them from neurologic sequelae (16,31,41–43). This physiologic pattern in the healthy infant who has no risk factors for impaired metabolic adaptation and has no clinical signs cannot be considered a pathologic condition. Therefore, the definition of the condition we are concerned about is not "a low blood glucose measurement." A more meaningful definition is "a low blood glucose measurement in the absence of protective metabolic responses." The level of blood glucose that may be considered "low" is discussed below.

In the absence of accessible and rapid measurements of levels of alternative fuels in the clinical setting, proxy measures for the presence or absence of protective metabolic responses must be considered. In practical terms, this requires identification of risk factors for impaired or delayed metabolic adaptation (Table 41.1) and/or the recognition of abnormal clinical signs that may arise from hypoglycemia, which is not compensated for by alternative fuel utilization (Table 41.2). Therefore, a full and accurate working definition of the condition, which is referred to in the shorthand

TABLE 41.2

Signs of Clinically Significant Neonatal Hypoglycemia

Perinatal acidosis (cord arterial or infant pH < 7.1 and/or base deficit ≥ −12 mmol/L)

Hypothermia (<36.5°C) not attributed to environmental factors

Suspected/confirmed early-onset sepsis

Cyanosis

Apnea

Altered level of consciousness

Seizures

Hypotonia

Lethargy

High-pitched cry

Abnormal feeding behavior (not waking for feeds, not sucking effectively, appearing unsettled, and demanding very frequent feeds), especially after a period of feeding well

as neonatal hypoglycemia, should be "a persistently low blood glucose level, measured with an accurate device, in a baby at risk of impaired metabolic adaptation but with no abnormal clinical signs," or "a single low blood glucose level in any baby presenting with abnormal clinical signs."

The groups of babies at risk for impaired metabolic adaptation are considered below and in Table 41.1. Signs that may arise from clinically significant hypoglycemia (i.e., a low blood glucose with absent or exhausted metabolic responses) are in Table 41.2. However, no sign is specific to hypoglycemia, and all may arise as the result of coexisting clinical complications, such as perinatal hypoxic–ischemic encephalopathy, or the underlying cause of hypoglycemia (e.g., a metabolic disorder may cause both poor feeding and hypoglycemia).

If early signs of hypoglycemia are not detected and treated, the infant may develop seizures or a reduced level of consciousness. Adverse long-term outcomes have been reported when neurologic signs have been present, although it is difficult to determine the specific impact of hypoglycemia in the presence of preceding or coexisting additional risk factors for brain injury (30,44,45). No study has identified a causal relationship between low blood glucose and brain tissue injury apparent on neuroimaging, but there is evidence from case reports and case series that profound and prolonged hypoglycemia is associated with both transient and permanent structural changes in the brain (46–52). The spectrum of cerebral injury associated with hypoglycemia is wide and includes white matter injury including parenchymal hemorrhage and ischemic stroke, and cortical and deep grey matter injury. Vulnerability of the white matter and cortex of the posterior parietal and occipital lobes has been well reported in human imaging studies, but injury at other sites is also reported, which is consistent with preclinical models of hypoglycemic injury that show a more diffuse neuropathology (**Figs. 41.3 and 41.4**). However, further clinical research is required to differentiate between causal associations and those associations between hypoglycemia and neurologic dysfunction or injury that together may be comorbidities of an underlying condition.

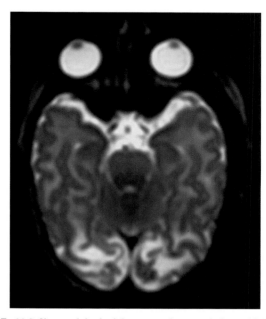

FIGURE 41.3 Neonatal brain injury seen in association with hypoglycemia accompanied by acute neurologic dysfunction. Posterior white matter abnormality in a low transverse plane (T2-weighted MRI scan). There is severe abnormally high signal intensity with loss of gray/white matter differentiation bilaterally in the posterior occipital lobes with bilateral involvement of the visual cortex.

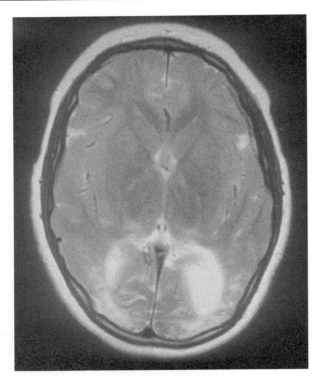

FIGURE 41.4 Imaging in childhood following neonatal hypoglycemia. Atrophy, gliosis, and ulegyria in posterior parietal and occipital regions.

In extreme cases, profound hypoglycemia, usually the result of serious inborn errors of metabolism, may even result in "cot death" or apparent life-threatening events.

No study has yet satisfactorily addressed the duration of absent or reduced availability of metabolic fuels that is sufficient to cause injury to the brain of the human neonate. Studies in neonatal rats have demonstrated that prolonged insulin-induced hypoglycemia, but not starvation-induced hypoglycemia or a short period of hypoglycemia, resulted in neurodegenerative changes (53). A study of rhesus monkeys has shown that a duration of insulin-induced neonatal hypoglycemia (blood glucose <1.5 mmol/L, 27 mg/dL) of 6.5 hours had no demonstrable long-term effects, whereas 10 hours of hypoglycemia was associated with "motivational and adaptability problems" but no motor or cognitive deficit on testing at 8 months of age (54).

Ideally, an evidence-based definition of hypoglycemia should include the blood glucose concentration considered to be the minimum safe level, the duration beyond which the low blood glucose level is considered to be harmful, the presence of clinical signs, the group of infants studied, the consideration of alternative fuel availability, the conditions of sampling, and the assay methods. Most of these criteria have not been adequately addressed by previous studies or publications and, in reality, will vary between babies (31,44,45). This paucity of data has resulted in a pragmatic approach being proposed by groups of clinicians, which is based on thresholds for intervention rather than attempting to define hypoglycemia as a single numerical term (30,36). These groups proposed that regardless of the blood glucose concentration, neurologic signs in association with low blood glucose levels should prompt investigations to establish a firm diagnosis of hypoglycemia and its underlying cause and the institution of urgent treatment. For infants without clinical signs but at risk of neurologic sequelae by virtue of their impaired ability to mobilize alternative fuels at low blood glucose levels (Table 41.1), intervention to raise blood glucose (measured using an accurate device) should be considered if two consecutive blood glucose levels are below 36 mg/dL (2 mmol/L) or a single blood glucose level is below 18 mg/dL (1 mmol/L). A single value below 45 mg/dL (2.5 mmol/L) should prompt intervention in any neonate with abnormal neurologic signs (see **Fig. 41.5A–C**). This approach is supported by a recent RCT that showed that for healthy infants born at 35 weeks of gestation or later with moderate low blood glucose, a threshold of 36 mg/dL (2.0 mmol/L) was noninferior to a threshold of 47 mg/dL (2.6 mmol/L) with respect to psychomotor development at 18 months (55).

To summarize the clinical significance of neonatal hypoglycemia, the likely temporal sequence for the baby is as follows, but the glucose thresholds and time periods for clinical signs and potential injury will vary between babies (29):

Low blood glucose levels are found, but the baby does not have clinical signs or sustain injury because the baby is still able to draw on alternative fuel stores, for example, glycogen and fat. This could be defined as biochemical hypoglycemia with adequate metabolic adaptation.

- If untreated, the baby exhausts alternative fuel stores and develops subtle clinical signs that are not specific to hypoglycemia (e.g., irritability, lethargy, poor feeding), but hypoglycemia is not damaging at this stage. This is the onset of impaired metabolic adaptation.
- If untreated, the baby develops obvious and severe clinical signs (e.g., seizures, coma) but may escape damage if treated very promptly. Metabolic adaptation has failed.
- If not treated sufficiently soon after onset of clinical signs, hypoglycemia becomes damaging and in severe cases results in cardiorespiratory arrest.

Finally, the impact of hypoglycemia and its treatment on the mother and baby must be considered. The early neonatal period is an emotionally sensitive time, and the diagnosis of hypoglycemia may create or add to anxiety for the parents. Treatment of the infant with intravenous glucose involves separation of the baby and mother and may be perceived as invasive or painful. The implications for the establishment of breast-feeding must also not be forgotten, especially as there is evidence that separation disrupts breast-feeding and in turn breast-feeding and avoidance of formula supplementation augments ketogenesis (16,42). Therefore, emphasis should be on the early prevention of hypoglycemia and management strategies that do not involve the separation of mother and baby (56). Parents should be given verbal and written information that describes why their baby is receiving extra support and blood glucose monitoring, how to reduce the likelihood of hypoglycemia, the signs that indicate when a baby is becoming unwell, and how to raise concerns about their baby's well-being or feeding pattern (36).

Mechanisms of Absent, Impaired, or Delayed Metabolic Adaptation in At-Risk Groups

Hypoglycemia may be secondary to increased utilization of glucose, to inadequate supply of glucose, or to a combination of the two (Tables 41.3 and 41.4). As described above, this will reach clinical significance if other aspects of metabolic adaptation are also impaired. Depending on the underlying mechanism, the hypoglycemia may be brief and self-limiting requiring supportive treatment only or, more rarely, may be prolonged and require definitive treatment.

- Dry and place baby skin-to-skin care in a warm, draught free room.

- Put hat on baby, and cover with a warm blanket.

- Encourage and support early breast feeding within the first hour after birth.

- For women who chose to formula feed give 10–15 mL/kg within the first hour after birth.

- Provide verbal and written information to parents that explains how to prevent hypoglycaemia, why their baby needs blood glucose monitoring, lists signs that may indicate hypoglycaemia (see Box 2), and advises parents to inform a member of the healthcare team if they are concerned about their baby's well-being (**Appendix 1**).

Box 1. Infants who require routine blood glucose monitoring

- Intrauterine growth restriction (≤ 2rd centile for gestation age and sex) or clinically wasted

- Infants of diabetic mothers.

- Maternal beta blocker use.

Box 2. Signs that may indicate hypoglycaemia

- Lethargy
- Abnormal feeding behavior especially after a period of feeding well
- High pitched cry
- Altered level of consciousness
- Hypotonia
- Seizures
- Hypothermia (<36.5°C)
- Cyanosis
- Apnoea

Check pre-feed blood glucose level prior to second feed (2–4 hours after birth):
Is the blood glucose level ≥2.0 mmol/L?

YES

NO

See Flowchart B

NO

- Encourage frequent feeding and ensure no longer than 3 hours between feeds.

- Assess the need for helping the mother with: ongoing help with feeding; hand expression; recognition of early feeding cues; and signs of effective attachment and feeding.

- For women who chose to formula feed, give 10–15 ml/kg per feed 3 hourly over the first 24 hours after birth.

- **Check blood glucose level prior to third feed (no longer than 8 hours after birth): Is the blood glucose level ≥2.0 mmol/L?**

YES

- Continue to support responsive breast feeding and ensure that mother understands how to assess effective feeding and knows how to escalate concerns.

- If formula fed give 10–15 mL/kg per feed 3 hourly over the first 24 hours after birth.

- No further blood glucose monitoring required unless there are clinical signs of hypoglycaemia (**Box 2**).

- Observe feeding for 24 hours.

- Complete at least one recorded breastfeeding assessment using local / BFI tool prior to transfer home.

FIGURE 41.5 A: Management of term infants at risk of hypoglycemia.

THE NEWBORN INFANT

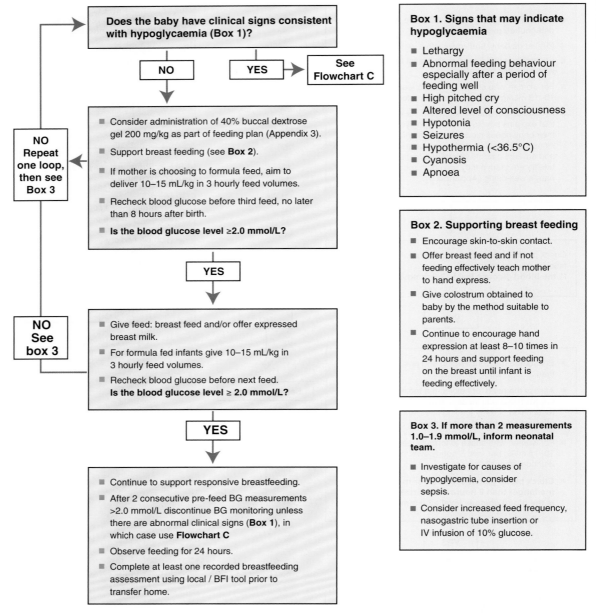

Does the baby have clinical signs consistent with hypoglycaemia (Box 1)?

NO →

YES → **See Flowchart C**

NO Repeat one loop, then see Box 3

- Consider administration of 40% buccal dextrose gel 200 mg/kg as part of feeding plan (Appendix 3).
- Support breast feeding (see **Box 2**).
- If mother is choosing to formula feed, aim to deliver 10–15 mL/kg in 3 hourly feed volumes.
- Recheck blood glucose before third feed, no later than 8 hours after birth.
- **Is the blood glucose level ≥2.0 mmol/L?**

YES

NO See box 3

- Give feed: breast feed and/or offer expressed breast milk.
- For formula fed infants give 10–15 mL/kg in 3 hourly feed volumes.
- Recheck blood glucose before next feed. **Is the blood glucose level ≥ 2.0 mmol/L?**

YES

- Continue to support responsive breastfeeding.
- After 2 consecutive pre-feed BG measurements >2.0 mmol/L discontinue BG monitoring unless there are abnormal clinical signs (**Box 1**), in which case use **Flowchart C**
- Observe feeding for 24 hours.
- Complete at least one recorded breastfeeding assessment using local / BFI tool prior to transfer home.

Box 1. Signs that may indicate hypoglycaemia
- Lethargy
- Abnormal feeding behaviour especially after a period of feeding well
- High pitched cry
- Altered level of consciousness
- Hypotonia
- Seizures
- Hypothermia (<36.5°C)
- Cyanosis
- Apnoea

Box 2. Supporting breast feeding
- Encourage skin-to-skin contact.
- Offer breast feed and if not feeding effectively teach mother to hand express.
- Give colostrum obtained to baby by the method suitable to parents.
- Continue to encourage hand expression at least 8–10 times in 24 hours and support feeding on the breast until infant is feeding effectively.

Box 3. If more than 2 measurements 1.0–1.9 mmol/L, inform neonatal team.
- Investigate for causes of hypoglycemia, consider sepsis.
- Consider increased feed frequency, nasogastric tube insertion or IV infusion of 10% glucose.

FIGURE 41.5 (*Continued*) **B:** Neonates with prefeed blood glucose 18 to 35 mg/dL (1.0 to 1.9 mmol/L) and no abnormal clinical signs.

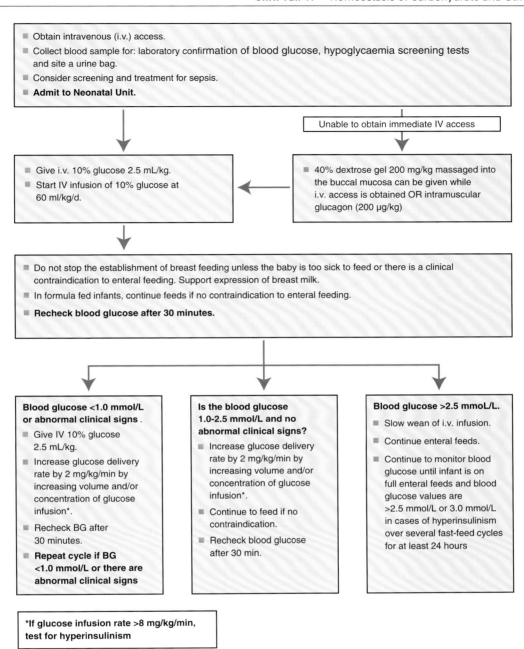

- Obtain intravenous (i.v.) access.
- Collect blood sample for: laboratory confirmation of blood glucose, hypoglycaemia screening tests and site a urine bag.
- Consider screening and treatment for sepsis.
- **Admit to Neonatal Unit.**

Unable to obtain immediate IV access

- Give i.v. 10% glucose 2.5 mL/kg.
- Start IV infusion of 10% glucose at 60 ml/kg/d.

- 40% dextrose gel 200 mg/kg massaged into the buccal mucosa can be given while i.v. access is obtained OR intramuscular glucagon (200 μg/kg)

- Do not stop the establishment of breast feeding unless the baby is too sick to feed or there is a clinical contraindication to enteral feeding. Support expression of breast milk.
- In formula fed infants, continue feeds if no contraindication to enteral feeding.
- **Recheck blood glucose after 30 minutes.**

Blood glucose <1.0 mmol/L or abnormal clinical signs .
- Give IV 10% glucose 2.5 mL/kg.
- Increase glucose delivery rate by 2 mg/kg/min by increasing volume and/or concentration of glucose infusion*.
- Recheck BG after 30 minutes.
- **Repeat cycle if BG <1.0 mmol/L or there are abnormal clinical signs**

Is the blood glucose 1.0-2.5 mmol/L and no abnormal clinical signs?
- Increase glucose delivery rate by 2 mg/kg/min by increasing volume and/or concentration of glucose infusion*.
- Continue to feed if no contraindication.
- Recheck blood glucose after 30 min.

Blood glucose >2.5 mmoL/L.
- Slow wean of i.v. infusion.
- Continue enteral feeds.
- Continue to monitor blood glucose until infant is on full enteral feeds and blood glucose values are >2.5 mmol/L or 3.0 mmol/L in cases of hyperinsulinism over several fast-feed cycles for at least 24 hours

*If glucose infusion rate >8 mg/kg/min, test for hyperinsulinism

FIGURE 41.5 (*Continued*) **C:** Blood glucose less than 18 mg/dL (1.0 mmol/L) and/or clinical signs consistent with hypoglycemia. ((Used with permission by British Association of Perinatal Medicine from Identification and Management of Neonatal Hypoglycaemia in the Full Term Infant: A Framework for Practice. London: British Association of Perinatal Medicine in collaboration with the NHS Improvement Patient Safety Programme 'Avoiding Term Admissions to Neonatal units (Atain); 2017.)

TABLE 41.3
Mechanisms of Hypoglycemia
Reduced production
Reduced availability of gluconeogenic precursors
Reduced activity of enzymes of glycogenolysis or gluconeogenesis
Reduced activity of counterregulatory hormones (glucagon, cortisol, catecholamines)
Increased utilization
Hyperinsulinism
Reduced alternative substrate availability

For some babies, there is a clear single cause of hypoglycemia, for example, the baby born after poor control of maternal diabetes who has fetal and neonatal hyperinsulinism. For others, there may be more than one etiologic mechanism (Table 41.4). For example, neonates who have been subject to IUGR may experience impaired glycogenolysis, secondary to low glycogen stores, and impaired gluconeogenesis, secondary to delayed induction of enzymes. Also, their ability to mount a protective alternative fuel response varies in magnitude and sustainability and cannot be relied upon if blood glucose levels are persistently low (57). In addition to factors arising from intrauterine influences, there is evidence that excessive

TABLE 41.4

Mechanisms of Hypoglycemia in At-Risk Infants

Reduced production

  IUGR

  Preterm delivery

  Perinatal hypoxia–ischemia

  Infection

  Inborn errors of metabolism, for example, glycogen storage disorder

  Endocrine disorders, for example, hypopituitarism, congenital adrenal hyperplasia/hypoplasia

  Maternal beta-blocker medication

Increased utilization

  Hyperinsulinism, for example, after poor control of diabetes in pregnancy, Beckwith-Wiedemann syndrome

  IUGR—to replenish stores

  Reduced availability of alternative substrate, for example, inborn error of fatty acid oxidation

formula milk supplementation may be a cause of the suppressed response, in that ketone body levels are lower in formula-fed infants than in breast-fed infants, and there is a negative relationship between ketone body concentration and daily volume of formula taken (42).

It is important to note that not all IUGR infants will be "small for gestational age," and clinical examination is important for the identification of the "wasted" neonate with disproportionate birth weight and head circumference centiles. Conversely, not all small for gestational age infants will have been subject to placental insufficiency—they may be constitutionally small and will not experience impaired postnatal metabolic adaptation.

Insufficient Supply of Glucose

This is the most common underlying cause of clinically significant neonatal hypoglycemia. In the enterally fed infant, the source of circulating glucose is the absorption and conversion of lactose from milk or, between feeds, from glycogenolysis and gluconeogenesis. Babies receiving intravenous fluids invariably receive glucose as a component of the fluid infusions. If there is insufficient exogenous supply of glucose and the infant fails to switch on glycogenolysis or gluconeogenesis in response to falling blood glucose levels, hypoglycemia will occur. This will be most significant when production of alternative fuels to glucose is also impaired (see above). Three possible mechanisms may cause the failure of glucose production when exogenous supply is too low.

Reduced Availability of Gluconeogenic Precursors

Glycogenolysis and gluconeogenesis may be limited by availability of glycogen, gluconeogenic precursors, or the energy provided by fatty acid oxidation. This may occur after preterm delivery, IUGR, maternal alcohol abuse or perinatal hypoxia–ischemia, or as a consequence of prolonged inadequate intake after birth (58–60).

Reduced Activity of Enzymes of Glycogenolysis, Gluconeogenesis, Lipolysis, and Ketogenesis

Despite normal postnatal endocrine responses, there may be failure of synthesis and activation of the key enzymes described above. This may be the result of a specific inherited metabolic disorder, in which case hypoglycemia is usually severe, and recurrent or persistent, or there may be generalized immaturity of enzymes, as in the preterm infant or following IUGR. Finally, enzyme activity may be suppressed by acquired conditions, such as perinatal bacterial infection or impaired liver function secondary to hypoxia–ischemia. Defective gluconeogenesis may also be the cause of hypoglycemia complicating cases of congenital heart disease and cold injury (61,62).

Impaired Counterregulatory Hormone Response

This will result in failure to activate enzymes of glycogenolysis, gluconeogenesis, lipolysis, and ketogenesis. Hyperinsulinism has a dual mechanism in that glucose utilization is increased (see below) but also counterregulatory hormone release is inhibited. Failure of release of counterregulatory hormones (glucagon, catecholamines) may play a role in hypoglycemia in preterm and IUGR babies, and after maternal medication with beta-blockers in pregnancy (63,64). Finally, there may be rare permanent disorders that result in insufficiency of counterregulatory hormones, for example, low growth hormone and cortisol levels in septo-optic dysplasia and congenital hypopituitarism and low glucocorticoid levels in adrenocortical deficiencies (65–67).

Increased Glucose Utilization

The most common cause of excessive utilization of glucose is neonatal hyperinsulinism. Clinical features are that glucose requirements to maintain normoglycemia are high, in excess of the 8 mg/kg/min, as compared to 4 to 6 mg/kg/min usually required by neonates, and the infant may be macrosomic if hyperinsulinism was of fetal origin. The clinical appearance of macrosomia is of a body size that is large in proportion to head size and must be differentiated from constitutional large size for gestational age, which is not alone a risk factor for hypoglycemia. Hyperinsulinism should be confirmed by the use of a highly specific insulin assay for plasma insulin concentrations and interpretation with reference to normal neonatal insulin–glucose relationships (22,23). Investigation of suspected hyperinsulinism will demonstrate low fatty acid and ketone body concentrations during hypoglycemia, but this feature is not specific to hyperinsulinism as some infants who are not hyperinsulinemic, such as some who are preterm or IUGR, also fail to mount lipolytic and ketogenic responses.

Self-Limiting Hyperinsulinism

Hyperinsulinism may be a temporary phenomenon when the fetus has been rendered hyperglycemic by poorly controlled maternal diabetes, antenatal administration of thiazide diuretics, or the administration of glucose to the mother in labor. It may also occur in infants shortly after abrupt discontinuation of intravenous glucose infusions, after bolus doses of glucose, or if glucose has been infused through an umbilical arterial catheter with the tip placed close to the celiac axis. Rhesus hemolytic disease and perinatal asphyxia have also been associated with transient fetal and neonatal hyperinsulinism, although the etiologic link is not known (68,69).

Iatrogenic or Factitious Hyperinsulinism

Hyperinsulinism may result from erroneous or malicious administration of insulin or from excess glucose infusion or misplaced arterial catheter tip (see above). Although rare, these conditions should be suspected if hypoglycemia is unexpected, profound, or resistant to treatment.

Beckwith-Wiedemann Syndrome

This condition, described independently by Beckwith (70) and Wiedemann (71), is characterized by exomphalos, macroglossia, visceromegaly, earlobe abnormalities, and an increased later incidence of malignancies. Hyperinsulinism is a common but not invariable feature causing high glucose requirements in the early neonatal period and usually resolves sometime after birth. It is likely that the previously reported long-term developmental difficulties were related to undiagnosed and untreated hypoglycemia, and it is anticipated that awareness of the condition and prevention of hypoglycemia should result in improved outcome.

Congenital Hyperinsulinism

Many descriptive terms, such as "nesidioblastosis," "islet-cell dysregulation syndrome," or "persistent hyperinsulinemic hypoglycemia of infancy," have been applied to this condition over the years. Although a rare condition, it is the most common cause of recurrent and persistent hypoglycemia in infancy and childhood (72). It is usually associated with macrosomia and always with extreme hyperinsulinism and high glucose requirements. The condition may be self-limiting in the neonatal period but more often extends beyond this time. As there is no protective ketone body response to hypoglycemia, there are usually neurologic signs, and, untreated, the risk of brain injury is high. Therefore, recognition of hyperinsulinism and early prevention and treatment of hypoglycemia, with referral to a specialist center, are essential to reduce the incidence of permanent neurologic damage, which has been widely reported (72–75).

Currently, histologic classification of congenital hyperinsulinism is into diffuse and focal forms (72). The condition is more often familial than sporadic. Several underlying pathologies have been demonstrated (72). In severe cases of congenital hyperinsulinism, there are mutations in the genes encoding for subunits of the K⁺ATP channel, and the involvement of the pancreas is diffuse. The functional loss of this channel results in dysregulation of calcium fluxes and thus unregulated insulin release. Other forms of hyperinsulinism, which tend to be milder or present later, are linked to defects in genes coding for glutamate dehydrogenase and glucokinase, with activation of these genes in turn affecting the function of the beta cell. The former is the second most common form of congenital hyperinsulinism and is associated with hyperammonemia, so that ammonia levels should always be measured when hyperinsulinemia is suspected. Other mutations are those coding for hepatocyte nuclear factor-4α protein and HADH (a mitochondrial enzyme of fatty acid metabolism). Rarely, an isolated islet-cell adenoma may present with congenital hyperinsulinism (72).

Leucine-Sensitive Hypoglycemia

This was previously described as a distinct entity, but it is more likely that hypoglycemia in response to leucine administration represents underlying hyperinsulinism sensitive to any protein (which may be endogenous as a consequence of catabolism of protein stores or exogenous through parenteral or enteral nutrition) and should be investigated and treated as such (72).

Prevention and Management of Neonatal Hypoglycemia (Table 41.5)

The early identification of at-risk neonates and the understanding of underlying mechanisms of hypoglycemia are important for both diagnosis and treatment. In addition to diagnosing and treating hypoglycemia, the underlying cause must be determined and treated as necessary, for example, to fail to identify and treat bacterial infection may be catastrophic. The underlying cause of hypoglycemia is usually self-evident from the obstetric and perinatal history or clinical examination, but if this is not the case and the hypoglycemia is profound or persistent despite treatment,

TABLE 41.5

Prevention and Management of Neonatal Hypoglycemia

Identify at-risk infants

Clinical monitoring

Glucose monitoring (accurate device)

Adequate energy provision
　Support breast-feeding
　Formula supplementation titrated against clinical condition and blood glucose measurements
　Intravenous glucose if enteral feeds not indicated or tolerated or hypoglycemia resistant to enteral feeds

Investigations and additional treatments if hypoglycemia severe or persistent

further investigations must be performed to identify rare but serious inborn errors of metabolism or hormone deficiencies (see Chapters 40 and 55). As these tests are most informative when carried out at the time of hypoglycemia, it is important to take the necessary blood and urine samples during such episodes and process and store them if necessary out of laboratory working hours. Each unit should devise an appropriate protocol for this, in liaison with local and regional specialized laboratories.

Healthy, Full-Term Appropriate Weight for Gestational Age Babies

As described above, healthy full-term AGA neonates have a physiologic fall in blood glucose concentrations in the first 1 to 2 postnatal days but are protected by the alternative fuels, ketone bodies, and lactate. Thus, it is now generally recognized that for this group, it is not necessary or appropriate to carry out routine blood glucose monitoring, to label low blood glucose as a pathologic entity, or to initiate treatment, which is invasive or which may interfere with the establishment of breast-feeding (30,56,76). Because of the healthy infant's ability to counterregulate, problems with establishment of successful breast-feeding are equally likely to present with excessive weight loss (in excess of 10% birth weight), dehydration, and jaundice as with clinically significant hypoglycemia. Therefore, breast-feeding advice and intervention should not be based on blood glucose levels, but on full assessment of the baby—only proceeding to blood glucose measurement if there are clinical concerns. However, clinicians caring for mothers and babies must be alert to the possibility that other conditions, such as infection or more rarely inborn errors of metabolism, may present with neurologic signs and hypoglycemia. Where appropriate, specific investigations to detect these must be performed.

At-Risk Babies

For practical purposes, the following discussion focuses only on the infants who are at risk of impaired metabolic adaptation and the neurologic sequelae of hypoglycemia (Table 41.1). Early prevention of hypoglycemia is optimal for these infants, so the first step in management must be to identify the risk factors. Although this is easy in some cases (such as the preterm baby), for others, clinical observations are important (e.g., to identify the wasted appearance of the growth-restricted neonate who may not necessarily have a low birth weight).

At-risk infants should have regular, accurate, prefeed blood glucose monitoring. In addition, it is imperative that any infant with neurologic signs, even if not in an at-risk group, has urgent, accurate blood glucose measurement. The monitoring schedule for at-risk infants will vary according to local protocols, but in general, monitoring should be commenced before the second feed (so as to avoid the physiologic nadir in the 1 to 2 hours after birth), and 3 to 4 hourly prefeed monitoring should be continued until the infant has had at least two satisfactory blood levels recorded. Monitoring should be recommended if the infant's clinical condition worsens or energy intake decreases. If monitoring is by reagent strip, low levels must be confirmed by accurate measurement. See **Figure 41.5A** for a suggested care pathway for managing term infants with risk factors for impaired metabolic adaptation.

The importance of early milk feeding has been appreciated for many years (77). Both breast and formula milks provide important gluconeogenic precursors and fatty acids for beta-oxidation. Because milk contains sources of energy other than carbohydrate, it has a higher J/mL content than 10% dextrose. In addition, enteral milk feeding stimulates the secretion of gut hormones, which may facilitate postnatal metabolic adaptation (20). Therefore, all infants who are expected to tolerate enteral feeds should be fed with milk as soon as possible after birth and at frequent intervals thereafter. Babies who are capable of sucking should be offered the breast at each feed (if this is the mother's wish). If it is likely that babies will need complementary or supplementary feeds (by cup, bottle, or gavage), maternal breast milk expression should be encouraged from birth. Women with diabetes but without other complications of pregnancy can begin expressing milk from 36 weeks of gestation if they choose to because this appears to be safe for mother and baby (78). The need for formula supplementation will vary between babies, will diminish with the successful establishment of breast-feeding, and will be guided by the availability of expressed breast milk, regular prefeed blood glucose monitoring, the clinical condition of the baby, and assessment of breast-feeding. In the breast-fed baby, formula intake should be kept to the minimum necessary, so as to enhance breast-feeding and avoid suppression of normal metabolic adaptation (42). Treatment with buccal dextrose gel is a simple and safe treatment to manage hypoglycemia in late preterm and term babies at risk of impaired metabolic adaptation: it is more effective than feeding alone for reversing neonatal hypoglycemia in the first 48 hours after birth, it reduces the incidence of mother–infant separation, and it increases the likelihood of full breast feeding after discharge (79,80). For these reasons, the BAPM Framework recommends its use alongside a feeding plan for babies with risk factors when the BG is 18 to 35 mg/dL (1.0 to 1.9 mmol/L), and there are no abnormal clinical signs.

In the at-risk baby who is establishing oral feeds, there is a potential nadir at which body stores are steadily reducing but milk feeds have not yet started to replenish these stores. Even if the baby is feeding well, this nadir may not occur until at least 48 hours of life. For this reason, vulnerable babies should have regular clinical monitoring for 48 hours and/or until experienced staff are satisfied that feeding is effective.

When it is unlikely that the baby will tolerate full enteral feeds, for example, in the very preterm or sick infant, an intravenous glucose infusion should be commenced as soon as possible after birth. Usually, 10% dextrose at 3 mL/kg/h (5 mg glucose/kg/min) is sufficient to prevent hypoglycemia, but in some cases (such as hyperinsulinism), more is required. If the amount of glucose administered is limited by fluid restriction, more concentrated dextrose solutions should be provided via central venous lines, because these solutions are sclerotic to peripheral veins.

If low blood glucose levels persist or are associated with clinical signs in the milk-fed infant despite the above measures, it may be possible to increase the volume and/or frequency of feeds. If this is not possible, or if the hypoglycemia is resistant to this strategy, intravenous glucose will be required. If the infant is tolerating milk feeds, these should be neither stopped nor reduced. The initial rate of 10% glucose infusion should be 3 mL/kg/h (5 mg/kg/min) but adjusted according to frequent accurate blood glucose measurements. If hypoglycemia persists despite intravenous glucose infusion, it is important to check the infusion site and the infusion apparatus to confirm glucose delivery. All reductions in infusion rate should be gradual, and leaking intravenous cannulae should be promptly resited. Boluses of concentrated glucose solution should be avoided because of the risk of rebound hypoglycemia and cerebral edema (81). If glucose boluses are required (e.g., if there are neurologic signs of hypoglycemia), they should be provided as 10% dextrose (2.5 mL/kg), given slowly, and always followed by an infusion. In cases of hyperinsulinism, intramuscular glucagon will have a temporary glycemic effect if there is delay in siting an intravenous infusion (see below).

Suggested care pathways for managing term infants in the first 48 hours after birth are provided in **Figure 41.5A–C** (36).

Specific Treatments of Neonatal Hypoglycemic Conditions
Hyperinsulinism
It should be stressed again that when hyperinsulinism is not self-limiting and requires or is resistant to very high glucose infusion rates, referral to a specialist center must be made. The treatments outlined below should only be administered in nonspecialist units

on the advice of a specialist center and as a holding measure pending transfer. The risk of precipitating heart failure, especially if there is a coexisting hypertrophic cardiomyopathy, must be considered.

Glucose delivery should be prescribed to maintain blood glucose levels above 3 mmol/L and 54 mg/dL, and early siting of umbilical venous catheter or venous central line is essential to allow adequate delivery rates. If hypoglycemia is resistant to high glucose delivery rates, diazoxide (10 to 20 mg/kg/d) may be effective in suppressing pancreatic insulin release. The effect is optimal if a daily dose of chlorothiazide (7 to 10 mg/kg) is given to potentiate the hyperglycemic effect and prevent the fluid-retentive effect of diazoxide. In cases of persistent hyperinsulinism, response to diazoxide is variable; patients with mutations in the genes coding for HI-GK and HI-GLUD tend to show the best response (72). Some cases of congenital hyperinsulinism respond to the calcium channel blocker, nifedipine (72).

Somatostatin analog (octreotide, Sandostatin, Sandoz Pharmaceuticals) administered intravenously or subcutaneously at a dose of 10 µg/kg/d also suppresses insulin release (75). However, tolerance may develop, and there is concern about possible effects on the secretion of other hormones; for this latter reason, glucagon is administered simultaneously at a dose of 1 µg/kg/h (82).

Glucagon (200 µg/kg bolus i.v. or i.m. or infusion 5 to 10 µg/kg/h) has a temporary glycemic effect via its glycogenolytic action. Given alone, glucagon may be a useful holding measure, for example, when re-siting glucose infusions. However, duration of use is limited because glucagon further stimulates insulin release.

Some cases of neonatal hyperinsulinism, especially those caused by recessive mutations of the genes encoding the SUR1 and Kir6.2 proteins, are unresponsive to medical treatment, and near-total pancreatectomy is required. Referral should be made to specialist surgical centers. In specialist centers, rapid genetic testing allows clinicians to identify those who are likely to have focal disease, and ^{18}F-L-DOPA-PET imaging is then indicated for the preoperative identification and precise anatomical location of focal lesions (72). This is followed by laparoscopic or open targeted focal pancreatectomy.

Adrenocortical Insufficiency
Although parenteral hydrocortisone has been used for many years for the treatment of hypoglycemia of various etiologies, the only specific application of this drug is for rescue and replacement therapy in suspected or proven adrenocortical insufficiency, which is discussed in more detail in Chapter 40.

Inborn Errors of Metabolism
The management of the rare inborn errors of metabolism varies according to diagnosis and is beyond the scope of this chapter. In general, the aim is to provide adequate calories to prevent hypoglycemia and catabolism (see Chapter 55).

NEONATAL HYPERGLYCEMIA

Neonatal hyperglycemia has also been recognized for over a century (83). While "classical" diabetes mellitus may present in the neonatal period (see below), neonatal hyperglycemia is usually self-limiting and like most cases of neonatal hypoglycemia represents the extreme of disturbed neonatal metabolic adaptation. Hyperglycemia is increasingly seen in extremely low–birth-weight infants who are cared for in our neonatal units. As with hypoglycemia, much uncertainty exists regarding definition, clinical significance, and treatment.

Self-Limiting Hyperglycemia
The prevalence of transient hyperglycemia is increasing in parallel with the increased survival of extremely low–birth-weight infants

and the early use of parenteral nutrition solutions and corticosteroid therapy in these babies. Accidental or factitious hyperglycemia must also be considered.

Clinical Significance

It is of the utmost importance to remember that neonatal hyperglycemia may be a sign of a serious underlying disorder, such as infection. However, despite reports of associations between hyperglycemia and adverse outcomes in extremely-low-birth-weight babies, it is still not known whether the high glucose concentrations themselves place the infant at further risk or whether the high blood glucose levels simply reflect the fragile and unstable condition of the babies most at risk of adverse outcome. Unlike adults with insulin deficiency, most hyperglycemic neonates do not develop ketosis or metabolic acidosis (84). There is a risk that at very high blood glucose levels, glycosuria and osmotic diuresis may cause fluid and electrolyte imbalance with dehydration, but in practice, this situation is rare because of the immaturity of the neonatal kidney (84). There is also concern that changes in blood osmolality and fluid shifts may result in cerebral damage. However, cerebral pathology and adverse neurodevelopmental outcome have not been demonstrated to occur as the direct result of hyperglycemia, unless blood glucose levels approximate or exceed 360 mg/dL (20 mmol/L) (85,86).

Definition and Diagnosis

There is no established definition of neonatal hyperglycemia, but the majority of units recently surveyed define hyperglycemia as a blood glucose level above 180 mg/dL (10 mmol/L) (87). However, the upper "safe" limit of blood glucose concentration in the neonate is likely to be above this level.

The use of glucose reagent strips is more useful in the diagnosis of hyperglycemia than for hypoglycemia because the strips are more reliable at high blood glucose levels, and inaccuracies of 8 to 16 mg/dL (0.5 to 1.0 mmol/L) are of less clinical relevance in the context of hyperglycemia. However, clinicians are urged to confirm the diagnosis with a laboratory measurement. It may also be useful to monitor urine for glycosuria, but it should be remembered that neonates, particularly those who are preterm, have a low renal threshold for glucose, and fractional excretion of glucose varies widely, so that glycosuria may be present even in normoglycemia and is independent of circulating blood glucose concentration (84).

Prevalence

Without a clear definition of hyperglycemia, it is difficult to comment on the overall incidence of hyperglycemia. Studies of prevalence vary according to their subjects, with hyperglycemia found most frequently in very-low-birth-weight and preterm infants (88). Small for gestational age infants who are preterm are more at risk for developing hyperglycemia than hypoglycemia when receiving standard intravenous infusions (89).

Mechanisms and At-Risk Groups

The mechanisms underlying neonatal hyperglycemia vary and, as with hypoglycemia, are best understood with reference to the expected metabolic changes at birth. Hyperglycemia may be the result of a high glucose production or infusion rate or a low glucose uptake rate.

Neonatal hyperglycemia is usually secondary to a high rate of appearance of glucose molecules into the blood stream, and it is often seen when glucose infusion rates are high (86,90,91). To maintain control, the infant must be able to adapt to the exogenous administration of glucose by suppressing glucose production by the liver. The ability to glucoregulate in this way has been demonstrated in normoglycemic neonates (92). However, there is evidence from clinical and animal studies that some neonates do not suppress glucose production in response to glucose infusion and/ or increased blood glucose levels (90,93).

The inability to suppress gluconeogenesis may in turn be the result of disordered glucoregulatory hormone control. Although the glucoregulatory role of insulin in the neonate is unclear and may vary between infants, some instances of hyperglycemia result from decreased insulin secretion in immature subjects (94,95). This is analogous to the adult insulin-dependent diabetic. Animal studies have also shown that after chronic hyperglycemia, the fetal pancreas cannot mount an insulin response to a further glucose surge (96). This may be analogous to the condition in preterm babies receiving constant high-rate glucose infusions, whose pancreatic response to hyperglycemia may be "exhausted."

Alternatively, circulating insulin concentrations may be appropriate for the blood glucose concentration, but hyperglycemia may result from end-organ insensitivity to insulin. This is analogous to type II diabetes, which is characterized by insulin resistance. Neonatal insulin resistance has been demonstrated by the persistence of hyperglycemia in the presence of raised insulin concentrations, by the poor hypoglycemic response to large exogenous doses of insulin, and by the high insulin concentrations needed to suppress gluconeogenesis (97,98). Insulin resistance may be secondary to immaturity or down-regulation of peripheral receptors, to the effect of high fatty acid levels resulting from infusion of fat emulsion, or to the peripheral actions of counterregulatory hormones (99).

The excess secretion of counterregulatory hormones, which themselves stimulate glycogenolysis and gluconeogenesis, may in addition block the secretion of insulin and inhibit its peripheral action, thereby contributing to insulin resistance (100). This is the mechanism of hyperglycemia secondary to exogenous corticosteroids, sometimes administered in large doses to neonates with lung disease (101). Aminophylline, used for the prevention of apnea of prematurity, mimics the action of catecholamines and induces glycogenolysis.

These hormonal disturbances may be the consequence of underlying clinical stresses such as infection, respiratory distress, pain, or surgery (102,103).

Prevention and Management

The first step in management, especially in a baby who has previously been normoglycemic, must always be to seek and treat serious underlying disorders. The second step is to prevent the occurrence of high blood glucose concentrations secondary to high glucose infusion rates by instituting careful management of intravenous fluid prescriptions. Clinicians often increase fluid infusion rates to counter renal and extrarenal losses in the immature neonate. It must be recognized that increasing the rate of administration of a glucose solution will result in a proportionate increase in glucose administration. For example, 200 mL/kg/d of 10% dextrose provides 14 mg/kg/min glucose, which is well in excess of the neonate's requirements. Therefore, glucose infusion rates should be calculated, and, if they are found to be excessive (e.g., above 4 to 6 mg/kg/min), more dilute solutions should be used.

Hyperglycemia may occur in some neonates who are clinically stable and who are not receiving excessive glucose intakes. These infants are usually of extremely low birth weight and less than 1 week old. Often, they have received early parenteral nutrition and thus fairly high rates of glucose infusion in combination with amino acids. At the same time, they may have high counterregulatory hormone levels, rendering them "catabolic" with or without peripheral insulin resistance, so that they cannot utilize the infused substrates. The condition is usually self-limiting and may be prevented by the more gradual introduction of parenteral nutrition solutions in those at risk.

As neonatal hyperglycemia is usually self-limiting and not associated with adverse sequelae, attempts to treat the numerical blood glucose value may do more harm than good. There are three strategies for management of hyperglycemia when it occurs in these circumstances.

First, moderate hyperglycemia may be "tolerated" if it does not appear to be causing osmotic diuresis. In most instances, the condition resolves within a few days even if no action is taken.

Second, the rate of glucose infusion may be carefully reduced to the rate at which blood glucose levels become normal and then gradually increased as tolerated. This carries the possible disadvantage of reducing the infant's energy intake, but it is likely that immature infants are unable to effectively utilize all the glucose offered, especially if at a rate in excess of 5 mg/kg/min (93). Accidental hyperglycemia should be prevented by strict attention to stocked glucose solutions, pharmacy TPN production quality control, and glucose infusion devices.

Third, insulin may be administered in order to lower the blood glucose concentration without reducing the glucose infusion rate. If insulin is to be used, the IV tubing should be primed to reduce insulin adsorption to the plastic. Controlled studies of insulin administration to adult intensive care patients on intravenous nutrition have demonstrated that, although there is a short-term improvement in nitrogen balance, there is no advantage in terms of either weight gain or body composition and that a number of patients become hypoglycemic (104). Although there are a number of reports of this practice in the neonatal literature, there is no consistency regarding the clinical situations in which insulin has been given, only short-term outcome measures have been reported, and there are few prospective controlled trials (88,100,105–110). All of these studies reported hypoglycemia in some infants even after the discontinuation of insulin infusion, and some demonstrated progressive tolerance such that increasing insulin doses were required (i.e., the treatment itself may have delayed recovery). Therefore, insulin should not be prescribed without availability of prompt and accurate blood glucose testing. Recent systematic reviews have not supported the strategy of routinely infusing insulin to achieve a specific glucose delivery rate or prevent neonatal hyperglycemia and recommend reserving use of exogenous insulin for infants with severe hyperglycemia (above 220 mg/dL, 14 mmol/L) because the safety of the practice has not yet been determined (108,109). It is not known whether insulin administration promotes linear growth in neonates or merely converts glucose into fat. Epidemiologic studies have suggested that intrauterine nutritional and endocrine status may influence adult metabolism and susceptibility to disease (110). The long-term clinical significance of early high-energy intakes in association with large doses of exogenous insulin in the preterm neonate, and of possible up- or down-regulation of insulin receptors, has not yet been considered. In summary, it is not clear whether insulin therapy confers clinical advantage over expectant management of a condition, which is usually self-limiting.

Finally, the introduction of enteral feeding with small volumes of milk as soon as the infant's gastrointestinal tract will tolerate this may hasten the control of blood glucose homeostasis by inducing surges of gut hormones, which promote insulin secretion (the entero-insular axis) (19).

Neonatal Diabetes Mellitus

This is a rare condition (1:5,000,000 births) presenting in the neonatal period with very high blood glucose levels, low plasma insulin concentrations, dehydration, fever, and failure to thrive despite adequate feeding (111,112). Onset may be after discharge from the neonatal unit or maternity ward. There are a number of identified underlying genetic mechanisms, and small for gestational age babies are most often affected (113,114). In approximately 30% of cases, the condition resolves in the neonatal period, but for others, diabetes mellitus persists (115,116). This condition requires insulin treatment and rehydration in a specialist center or on the advice of specialists.

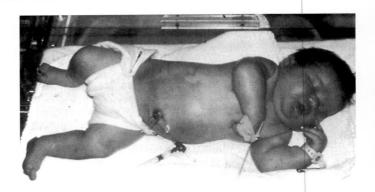

FIGURE 41.6 A macrosomic infant of a diabetic mother (IDM) has head circumference and length that are at the 90th percentile; the IDM's body weight greatly exceeds the 90th percentile. The IDM has considerable fat deposition in the shoulder and intracapsular area.

ADDITIONAL SEQUELAE AFTER DIABETES IN PREGNANCY

The impact of inadequate metabolic control of maternal preexisting or gestational diabetes upon the metabolic homeostasis of the fetus and neonate is described above. There are a number of additional potential adverse outcomes, with the severity and nature of these also reflecting the degree of control of diabetes and periods of vulnerability including the periconceptional period. The affected baby has a characteristic macrosomic appearance (Fig. 41.6).

Some neonatal complications are not specific to diabetes in pregnancy, but relate to being born preterm or by cesarean section. These will be minimized by careful consideration of timing of delivery, maternal steroid administration prior to preterm delivery, and reduced rate of unnecessary cesarean sections. Other complications are secondary to the abnormal metabolic environment of the fetus and ongoing disturbances postnatally and are more specific to diabetes in pregnancy (Table 41.6).

Congenital Anomalies

Despite major improvements in the care of diabetes in pregnancy, there has been little overall change in the incidence of congenital anomalies, which occur with a frequency up to 10 times that observed in the general population (117–119). Congenital anomalies now account for a large proportion of perinatal losses and have replaced RDS as the leading cause of perinatal loss (118–121). Anomalies overrepresented in pregnancies complicated by diabetes are caudal regression syndrome, neural tube defects, holoprosencephaly, vertebral dysplasia, congenital heart disease, ventricular septal defect, transposition of the great vessels, and small left colon syndrome.

TABLE 41.6

Reported Prevalence of Complications after Diabetes in Pregnancy	
Neonatal death	9.3/1,000
Preterm delivery	37%
Congenital anomaly	5.5%
Birth weight >90th centile	52%
Shoulder dystocia	7.9%
Erb palsy	4.5/1,000
Admission neonatal unit	56%

Adapted from Confidential Enquiry into Maternal and Child Health. *Pregnancy in women with type 1 and type 2 diabetes in 2002–2003.* UK: CEMACH, 2005.

The cause of diabetic embryopathy is not fully understood. Genetic factors (diabetes-related genes) are unlikely to play a role, as the incidence of birth defects is not increased in babies of fathers with diabetes (122). It is likely that congenital anomalies are related to the diabetic intrauterine environment during the period of organogenesis, before the seventh week of gestation (123). Possible teratogenic mediators are hyperglycemia hyperketonemia, increased levels of somatomedin-inhibiting factors, decreased myoinositol concentration in the neuroectoderm, and secretion of relaxin, an insulin homologue (123–130). Data from human studies regarding hypoglycemia are reassuring (124).

Macrosomia

Macrosomia is the term for increased body fat and selective organomegaly; the liver and heart are enlarged, but the brain size is not increased relative to gestational age so the head may appear disproportionately small (118,131). The clinical significance of macrosomia is the risk of the complications of delivery of a large infant, such as shoulder dystocia, obstructed labor, perinatal asphyxia, and birth injury (e.g., brachial plexus injury or fractured clavicle or humerus) (118,132,133).

The relationship between overall maternal diabetes control and macrosomia is not universal, in that some infants may be born with macrosomia after a pregnancy in which maternal blood glucose levels were apparently well controlled (134,135). The reason for this may include the fact that glucose level is not the only parameter denoting optimal diabetic control in pregnancy. However, enhanced control of even mild gestational diabetes is associated with reduced fetal overgrowth and risk of should dystocia (136–139).

Parents and health professionals must be prepared for "catch down" in postnatal growth of macrosomic babies, especially when breast-fed. This is a normal and healthy adaptation, and, provided the baby appears to be feeding well and is healthy, there should be no concern if there is an initial period of slow weight gain such that weight crosses down centile lines. Rather, to overfeed the baby and have it remain overweight has long-term health consequences, for example, later risk of cardiovascular disease and diabetes.

Hypertrophic Cardiomyopathy

Some infants of mothers with diabetes manifest generalized myocardial hypertrophy, with a disproportionate thickening of the septum, which may narrow the left ventricular outflow tract, in extreme forms resulting in fetal or neonatal death (135,140–142). However, the condition is usually transient with resolution of the clinical signs in 2 to 4 weeks and of septal hypertrophy within 2 to 12 months (141,143). The majority of the infants need supportive care only. If congestive heart failure develops, propranolol is recommended (143).

Intrauterine Growth Restriction

Impaired fetal growth has been associated with maternal vascular disease leading to placental insufficiency or to overcontrol of diabetes with frequent maternal hypoglycemia (144,145).

Effects of Antenatal and Intrapartum Hypoxia–Ischemia— Stillbirth, Encephalopathy, Hyperviscosity, Polycythemia, and Jaundice

The mechanism for increased risk of fetal hypoxia–ischemia and its sequelae is not fully understood. In addition to stillbirth and hypoxic–ischemic brain injury, there may be polycythemia and hyperviscosity, which in turn lead to sequelae such as hyperbilirubinemia and intravascular thrombosis.

Respiratory Complications

Although the incidence of respiratory distress syndrome was previously reported to be five to six times higher after diabetes in pregnancy than in the normal population, this incidence is falling in line with improved control of diabetes and prevention of preterm delivery (146).

Respiratory problems specific to diabetes may arise from delayed maturation of the pulmonary surfactant system, including surfactant proteins (147–151).

Hypocalcemia and Hypomagnesemia

The incidence and severity of hypocalcemia are related to diabetes control. It is usually associated with hyperphosphatemia and occasionally with hypomagnesemia. The etiology is not entirely clear, but neonatal hypoparathyroidism has been demonstrated and may in part be secondary to maternal renal magnesium loss (152,153).

IATROGENIC COMPLICATIONS

These include preterm delivery or delivery by cesarean section when there is no clear indication, "routine" admission of babies to neonatal units, and "routine" supplementation or replacement of breast-feeds with formula.

Long-Term Outcomes

There are a number of risk factors for adverse neurologic outcomes: placental dysfunction, hypoxia–ischemia, episodes of maternal ketosis or hypoglycemia during pregnancy, and neonatal hypoglycemia (154–156). Some studies report children born to mothers with diabetes are at increased risk for cognitive impairment, inattentiveness, impaired working memory, and altered language development; further research is required to understand whether the relationship is causal and whether increased risk is present if diabetes is well controlled (157–159). The risk of developing obesity is related to maternal diabetes control, birth weight, and weight in infancy (160–163). The risk of insulin-dependent diabetes developing by the age of 20 years in the offspring of women with diabetes is at least seven times that for nondiabetic parents, but only one-third of the risk reported for the offspring of fathers with insulin-dependent diabetes, which is possibly because of a lower rate of dr4 allele transmission from mothers or an effect of programming by the intrauterine environment (157,162,164,165).

Care Delivery

Careful medical and obstetric care to achieve strict glycemic control before and throughout pregnancy, in combination with appropriate neonatal care, greatly reduces the risk of the many complications discussed above. Adequate antenatal screening and assessment should indicate the pregnancies at greatest risk so that an antenatal plan may be made and, at all places of birth, there should be staff trained and competent to recognize and stabilize babies with unexpected complications. All hospitals must have written protocols for the prevention and management of potential neonatal complications, including hypoglycemia, and for admission to the neonatal unit. When there is good preconceptional care and control of diabetes and in the absence of congenital abnormalities, infants may be expected to have an uncomplicated neonatal course and should be managed as any other healthy term baby (166). Therefore, it is important to avoid iatrogenic problems such as needless separation of mothers and babies or practices that impede successful breast-feeding.

SUMMARY

While there is an increasing degree of clarity regarding the pathophysiology of abnormalities of carbohydrate homeostasis and adverse outcomes of a pregnancy affected by diabetes, too many babies still experience these disturbances and their sequelae. Many controversies surrounding the definition, diagnosis, and management of neonatal hypoglycemia and hyperglycemia are still unresolved. A number of key questions remain; examples are given below, but there are many more.

1. What are the long-term effects of moderate hypoglycemia?

   For example, we do not know whether the preterm infant's brain is more or less vulnerable to hypoglycemia than that of the term infant, what duration of hypoglycemia results in permanent disability in different at-risk groups, and whether the effects of hypoglycemia are exacerbated by concurrent complications such as hyperbilirubinemia. We do not know whether impaired neonatal metabolic adaptation predicts future impairment of metabolic responses.

2. Which factors regulate glucose availability and utilization by the brain?

   These may include cerebral blood flow, the ontogeny of glucose transporter proteins, and the role of the astrocyte in neuronal metabolic support.

3. How can brain energy sufficiency best be characterized in the newborn period, and what are the key indicators that are altered when ATP and phosphocreatine are low?

4. How may blood glucose levels be most easily and accurately measured?

   In light of the inadequacy of glucose reagent sticks for the diagnosis and monitoring of hypoglycemia, improved accurate bedside systems should be developed for the measurement of blood glucose concentrations. The ability to measure blood ketone body concentrations in these circumstances would markedly enhance management.

REFERENCES

1. Buchanan TA, Catalano PM. The pathogenesis of GDM: implications for diabetes after pregnancy. *Diabet Rev* 1995;3:584.
2. Hay WW Jr, Sparks JW. Placental, fetal and neonatal carbohydrate metabolism. *Clin Obstet Gynecol* 1985;28:473.
3. Adam PAJ, Raiha N, Rahiala EC, et al. Oxidation of glucose and b hydroxybutyrate by the early human fetal brain. *Acta Paediatr Scand* 1975;64:17.
4. Simmons RA, Flozak A, Ogata ES. The effect of insulin and insulin-like growth factor-I on glucose transport in normal and small for gestational age fetal rats. *Endocrinology* 1993;133:1361.
5. Soothill PW, Nicolaides KH, Campbell S. Prenatal asphyxia, hyperlacticaemia, hypoglycaemia and erythroblastosis in growth retarded fetuses. *BMJ* 1987;294:1051.
6. Miller SL, Huppi PS, Mallard C. The consequences of fetal growth restriction on brain structure and neurodevelopmental outcome. *J Physiol* 2016;594(4):807. doi: 10.1113/JP271402.
7. Obershain SS, Adam PAJ, King KC, et al. Human fetal response to sustained maternal hyperglycemia. *N Engl J Med* 1970;283:566.
8. Sperling MA, Grajwer LA, Leake R, et al. Role of glucagon in perinatal glucose homeostasis. *Metabolism* 1976;25(suppl 1):1385.
9. Sperling MA, Ganguli S, Leslie N, et al. Fetal–perinatal catecholamine secretion: role in perinatal glucose homeostasis. *Am J Physiol* 1984;247:E69.
10. Hägnevik K, Faxelius G, Irestedt L, et al. Catecholamine surge and metabolic adaptation in the newborn after vaginal delivery and caesarean section. *Acta Paediatr Scand* 1984;73:602.
11. Girard JR, Ferre A, Kervran A, et al. Role of the insulin/glucagon ratio in the changes of hepatic metabolism during development of the rat. In: Foa PP, Baja JS, Foa NL, eds. *Glucagon: its role in physiology and clinical medicine.* New York, NY: Springer-Verlag, 1977:563.
12. Medina JM, Fernandez E, Bolaros JP, et al. Fuel supply to the brain during the early postnatal period. In: Cueza JM, Pasaud-Leone AM, Patel MS, eds. *Endocrine development of the fetus and neonate.* New York, NY: Plenum Press, 1990:175.
13. Edmond J, Auestad N, Robbins RA, et al. Ketone body metabolism in the neonate: development and effect of diet. *Fed Proc* 1985;44:2359.
14. Shelley HJ, Neligan GS. Neonatal hypoglycaemia. *Br Med Bull* 1966;22:41.
15. Bougneres PF. Stable isotope tracers and the determination of fuel fluxes in newborn infants. *Biol Neonate* 1987;52(suppl 1):87.
16. Hawdon JM, Ward Platt MP, Aynsley-Green A. Patterns of metabolic adaptation for preterm and term infants in the first neonatal week. *Arch Dis Child* 1992;67:357.
17. Kinnala A, Suhonen-Polvi H, Aarimaa T, et al. Cerebral metabolic rate for glucose during the first six months of life: an FDG positron emission tomography study. *Arch Dis Child* 1996;74:F153.
18. Molsted-Pedersen L. Aspects of carbohydrate metabolism in newborn infants of diabetic mothers. II. Neonatal changes in K values. *Acta Endocrinol* 1972;69:189.
19. Aynsley-Green A. Metabolic and endocrine interrelationships in the human fetus and neonate: an overview of the control of the adaptation to postnatal nutrition. In: Lindblad BA, ed. *Perinatal nutrition.* New York: Academic Press, 1988:162.
20. Lucas A, Aynsley-Green A, Bloom SR. Gut hormones and the first meals. *Clin Sci* 1981;60:419.
21. Johnston V, Frazzini V, Davidheiser S, et al. Insulin receptor number and binding affinity in newborn dogs. *Pediatr Res* 1991;29:611.
22. Hawdon JM, Aynsley-Green A, Alberti KG, et al. The role of pancreatic insulin secretion in neonatal glucoregulation. I. Healthy term and preterm infants. *Arch Dis Child* 1993;68:274.
23. Hawdon JM, Hubbard M, Hales CN, et al. Use of a specific immunoradiometric assay to determine preterm neonatal insulin-glucose relations. *Arch Dis Child* 1995;73:F166.
24. Cobliner S. Blutzuckeruntersuchungen bei Säuglingen. *Z Kinderheilkd* 1911;1:207.
25. Sedgwick JP, Ziegler MR. The nitrogenous and sugar content of the blood of the newborn. *Am J Dis Child* 1920;19:429.
26. Spence JC. Some observations on sugar tolerance, with special reference to variations found at different ages. *Q J Med* 1921;14:314.
27. Cornblath M, Reisner SH. Blood glucose in the neonate, clinical significance. *N Engl J Med* 1965;272:378.
28. Hawdon JM, Beer J, Sharp D, Upton M; NHS Improvement Patient Safety Programme 'Reducing Term Admissions to Neonatal Units'. Neonatal hypoglycaemia: learning from claims. *Arch Dis Child Fetal Neonatal Ed* 2017;102(2):F110. doi: 10.1136/archdischild-2016-310936.
29. Hawdon JM. Hypoglycemia: are evidence based clinical guidelines achievable? *NeoReviews* 2014;15:e91.
30. Cornblath M, Hawdon JM, Williams AF, et al. Controversies regarding definition of neonatal hypoglycemia: suggested operational thresholds. *Pediatrics* 2000;105:1141.
31. Hay WW Jr, Raju TN, Higgins RD, et al. Knowledge gaps and research needs for understanding and treating neonatal hypoglycaemia: workshop report from Eunice Kennedy Shriver National Institute of Child Health and Human Development. *J Pediatr* 2009;155:612.
32. Koh THHG, Eyre JA, Aynsley-Green A. Neonatal hypoglycaemia—the controversy regarding definition. *Arch Dis Child* 1988;63:1386.
33. Dixon KC, Ferris RL, Marikar D, et al. Definition and monitoring of neonatal hypoglycaemia: a nationwide survey of NHS England Neonatal Units. *Arch Dis Child Fetal Neonatal Ed* 2017;102(1):F92. doi: 10.1136/archdischild-2016-311473.
34. Thornton PS, Stanley CA, De Leon DD, et al.; Pediatric Endocrine Society. Recommendations from the Pediatric Endocrine Society for evaluation and management of persistent hypoglycemia in neonates, infants, and children. *J Pediatr* 2015;167(2):238.
35. Adamkin DH; Committee on Fetus and Newborn. Postnatal glucose homeostasis in late-preterm and term infants. *Pediatrics* 2011;127(3):575.
36. British Association of Perinatal Medicine. *Identification and management of neonatal hypoglycaemia in the full term infant*, 2017. Available from: https://www.bapm.org/resources/40-identification-and-management-of-neonatal-hypoglycaemia-in-the-full-term-infant-2017
37. Inoue S, Egi M, Kotani J, Morita K. Accuracy of blood-glucose measurements using glucose meters and arterial blood gas analyzers in critically ill adult patients: systematic review. *Crit Care* 2013;17(2):R48.
38. Joosten KJ, Schellehens AP, Waellens JJ, et al. Erroneous diagnosis 'neonatal hypoglycaemia' due to incorrect preservation of blood samples. *Ned Tijdschr Geneeskd* 1991;135:1691.
39. Woo HC, Tolosa L, El-Metwally D, et al. Glucose monitoring in neonates: need for accurate and non-invasive methods. *Arch Dis Child* 2014;99:F153.
40. Shah R, McKinlay CJD, Harding JE. Neonatal hypoglycemia: continuous glucose monitoring. *Curr Opin Pediatr* 2018; 30(2):204.
41. De Boissieu D, Rocchiccioli F, Kalach N, et al. Ketone body turnover in term and in premature newborns in the first two weeks after birth. *Biol Neonate* 1995;67:84.
42. de Rooy LJ, Hawdon JM. Nutritional factors that affect the postnatal metabolic adaptation of full-term small- and large-for-gestational-age infants. *Pediatrics* 2002;109(3):E42.
43. Thurston JH, Hawhart RE, Schiro JA. β-Hydroxybutyrate reverses insulin-induced hypoglycemic coma in suckling–weanling mice despite low blood and brain glucose levels. *Metab Brain Dis* 1986;1:63.
44. Boluyt N, van Kempen A, Offringa M. Neurodevelopment after neonatal hypoglycaemia: a systematic review and design of optimal future study. *Pediatrics* 2006;117:2231.
45. Rozance PJ, Hay WW. Hypoglycemia in newborn infants: features associated with adverse outcomes. *Biol Neonate* 2006;90:74.
46. Anderson JM, Milner RDG, Strich SJ. Effects of neonatal hypoglycaemia on the nervous system: a pathological study. *J Neurol Neurosurg Psychiatry* 1967;30:295.

47. Auer RN, Siesjo BK. Hypoglycaemia: brain neurochemistry and neuropathology. *Baillieres Clin Endocrinol Metab* 1993;7:611.

48. Barkovich AJ, Ali FA, Rowley HA, et al. Imaging patterns of neonatal hypoglycemia. *AJNR Am J Neuroradiol* 1998;19:523.

49. Kinnala A, Korvenranta H, Parkkola R. Newer techniques to study neonatal hypoglycemia. *Semin Perinatol* 2000;24:116.

50. Murakami Y, Yamashita Y, Matsuishi T, et al. Cranial MRI of neurologically impaired children suffering from neonatal hypoglycaemia. *Pediatr Radiol* 1999;29:23.

51. Burns CM, Rutherford MA, Boardman JP, et al. Patterns of cerebral injury and neurodevelopmental outcomes after symptomatic neonatal hypoglycemia. *Pediatrics* 2008;122:65.

52. Filan PM, Inder TE, Cameron FJ, et al. Neonatal hypoglycemia and occipital cerebral injury. *J Pediatr* 2006;148:552.

53. Zhou D, Qian J, Liu CX, et al. Repetitive and profound insulin-induced hypoglycemia results in brain damage in newborn rats: an approach to establish an animal model of brain injury induced by neonatal hypoglycaemia. *Eur J Pediatr* 2008;167:1169.

54. Schrier AM, Wilhelm PB, Church RM, et al. Neonatal hypoglycaemia in the Rhesus monkey: effect on development and behaviour. *Infant Behav Dev* 1990;13:189.

55. van Kempen AAMW, Eskes PF, Nuytemans DHGM, et al. Lower versus traditional treatment threshold for neonatal hypoglycemia. *N Engl J Med.* 2020;382(6):541. doi: 10.1056/NEJMoa1905593.

56. National Childbirth Trust. Hypoglycaemia of the newborn. *Mod Midwife* 1997;7:31.

57. Hawdon JM, Ward Platt MP. Metabolic adaptation in small for gestational age infants. *Arch Dis Child* 1993;68:262.

58. Ogata ES. Carbohydrate metabolism in the fetus and neonate and altered neonatal glucoregulation. *Pediatr Clin North Am* 1986;33:25.

59. Shelley HJ, Basset JM. Control of carbohydrate metabolism in the fetus and newborn. *Br Med Bull* 1975;31:37.

60. Singh SP, Pullen GL, Snyder AK. Effects of ethanol on fetal fuels and brain growth in rats. *J Lab Clin Med* 1988;112:704.

61. Haymond MW, Strauss AW, Arnold KJ, et al. Glucose homeostasis in children with severe cyanotic congenital heart disease. *J Pediatr* 1979;95:220.

62. Mann TP, Elliot RIK. Neonatal cold injury due to accidental exposure to cold. *Lancet* 1957;i:229.

63. Crooks BN, Deshpande SA, Hall C, et al. Adverse neonatal effects of maternal labetalol treatment. *Arch Dis Child Fetal Neonatal Ed* 1998;79(2):F150.

64. Klarr JM, Bhatt-Mehta V, Donn SM. Neonatal adrenergic blockade following single dose maternal labetalol administration. *Am J Perinatol* 1994;11(2):91.

65. Costello JM, Gluckman PD. Neonatal hypopituitarism: a neurological perspective. *Dev Med Child Neurol* 1988;30:190.

66. Gemelli M, De Luca F, Barberio G. Hypoglycemia and congenital adrenal hyperplasia. *Acta Paediatr Scand* 1979;68:285.

67. Lovinger RD, Kaplan SL, Grumbach MM. Congenital hypopituitarism associated with neonatal hypoglycemia and microphallus. *J Pediatr* 1975;87:1171.

68. Molsted-Pedersen L, Trautner H, Jorgensen KR. Plasma insulin and K values during intravenous glucose tolerance test in newborn infants with erythroblastosis fetalis. *Acta Paediatr Scand* 1973;62:11.

69. Collins JE, Leonard JV. Hyperinsulinism in asphyxiated and small for dates infants with hypoglycaemia. *Lancet* 1984;ii:311.

70. Beckwith JB. Extreme cytomegaly of the adrenal fetal cortex, omphalocele, hyperplasia of kidneys and pancreas and Leydig cell hyperplasia. Another syndrome? Proceedings of the Western Society for Pediatric Research, Los Angeles, CA, November 1963.

71. Wiedemann HR. Complexe malformatif familial avec hernie umbilicale et macroglossie. Un 'syndrome nouveau'? *J Genet Hum* 1964;13:223.

72. Kapoor RR, James C, Hussain K. Advances in the diagnosis and management of hyperinsulinaemic hypoglycaemia. *Nat Clin Pract Endocrinol Metab* 2009;5:101.

73. Meissner T, Brune W, Mayatepak E. Persistent hyperinsulinaemic hypoglycaemia of infancy: therapy, clinical outcome and mutational analysis. *Eur J Pediatr* 1997;156:754.

74. Menni F, de Lonlay P, Sevin C, et al. Neurologic outcomes of 90 neonates and infants with persistent hyperinsulinemic hypoglycemia. *Pediatrics* 2001;107:476.

75. Aynsley-Green A, Hussain K, Hall J, et al. Practical management of hyperinsulinism in infancy. *Arch Dis Child* 2000;82:F98.

76. Eidelman AI. Hypoglycemia and the breastfed neonate. *Pediatr Clin North Am* 2001;48:377.

77. Smallpiece V, Davies PA. Immediate feeding of premature infants with undiluted breast milk. *Lancet* 1964;ii:1419.

78. Forster DA, Moorhead AM, Jacobs SE, et al. Advising women with diabetes in pregnancy to express breastmilk in late pregnancy (Diabetes and Antenatal Milk Expressing [DAME]): a multicentre, unblinded, randomised controlled trial. *Lancet* 2017;389(10085):2204.

79. Harris DL, Weston PJ, Signal M, et al. Dextrose gel for neonatal hypoglycaemia (the Sugar Babies Study): a randomised, double-blind, placebo-controlled trial. *Lancet* 2013;382:2077.

80. Weston PJ, Harris DL, Battin M, Brown J, Hegarty JE, Harding JE. Oral dextrose gel for the treatment of hypoglycaemia in newborn infants. *Cochrane Database Syst Rev* 2016;(5):CD011027.

81. Shah A, Stanhope R, Matthew D. Hazards of pharmacological tests of growth hormone secretion in childhood. *BMJ* 1992;304:173.

82. Hawdon JM, Ward Platt MP, Lamb WH, et al. Tolerance to Sandostatin in neonatal hyperinsulinaemic hypoglycaemia. *Arch Dis Child* 1990;65:411.

83. Kitselle JF. *Kinderh Leipsic* 1852;XVIII:313.

84. Hey E. Hyperglycaemia and the very preterm baby. *Semin Fetal Neonatal Med* 2005;10:3677.

85. Arant BS, Gorsh WM. Effects of acute hyperglycemia on the central nervous system of neonatal puppies. *Pediatr Res* 1978;12:549.

86. Miranda L, Dweck HS. Perinatal glucose homeostasis: the unique character of hyperglycemia and hypoglycemia in infants of very low birth weight. *Clin Perinatol* 1977;4:351.

87. Alsweiler JM, Kuschel CA, Bloomfield FH. Survey of the management of neonatal hyperglycaemia in Australasia. *J Paediatr Child Health* 2007;43:632.

88. Beardsall K, Vanhaesebrouck S, Ogilvy-Stuart A, et al. Early insulin therapy in very-low-birth-weight infants. *N Engl J Med* 2008;359:1873.

89. Chance GW, Bower BD. Hypoglycaemia and temporary hyperglycaemia in infants of low birth weight for maturity. *Arch Dis Child* 1966;41:279.

90. Hawdon JM, Aynsley-Green A, Bartlett K, et al. The role of pancreatic insulin secretion in neonatal glucoregulation. II. Infants with disordered blood glucose homeostasis. *Arch Dis Child* 1993;68:280.

91. Louik C, Mitchell AA, Epstein MF, et al. Risk factors for neonatal hyperglycemia associated with 10% dextrose infusion. *Am J Dis Child* 1985;139:783.

92. Lafeber HN, Sulkers EJ, Chapman TE, et al. Glucose production and oxidation in preterm infants during total parenteral nutrition. *Pediatr Res* 1990;28:153.

93. Van Goudoever JB, Sulkers EJ, Chapman TE. Glucose kinetics and glucoregulatory hormone levels in ventilated preterm infants on the first day of life. *Pediatr Res* 1993;33:583.

94. Milner RDG, Ferguson AW, Naidu SH. Aetiology of transient neonatal diabetes. *Arch Dis Child* 1971;46:724.

95. Zarif M, Pildes RS, Vidyasagar D. Insulin and growth hormone responses in neonatal hyperglycemia. *Diabetes* 1976;25:428.

96. Carver TD, Anderson SM, Aldoretta PA, et al. Glucose suppression of insulin secretion in chronically hyperglycemic fetal sheep. *Pediatr Res* 1995;38:754.

97. Le Dune MA. Insulin studies in temporary neonatal hyperglycaemia. *Arch Dis Child* 1971;46:392.

98. Pollack A, Cowett RM, Schwartz R, et al. Glucose disposal in low birth weight infants during steady state hyperglycemia: effects of exogenous insulin administration. *Pediatrics* 1978;61:546.

99. Yunis KA, Oh W, Kalhan S, et al. Mechanisms of glucose perturbation following intravenous fat infusion in the low birth weight infant. *Pediatr Res* 1989;25:299A.

100. Collins JW Jr, Hoppe M, Brown K, et al. A controlled trial of insulin infusion and parenteral nutrition in extremely low birth weight infants with glucose intolerance. *J Pediatr* 1991;118:921.

101. The Vermont Oxford Network Steroid Study Group. Early postnatal dexamethasone therapy for the prevention of chronic lung disease. *Pediatrics* 2001;108:741.

102. Anand KJS, Hickey PR. Pain and its effects on the human neonate and fetus. *N Engl J Med* 1987;317:1321.

103. Anand KJS, Sipell WG, Schofield N, et al. Does halothane anaesthesia decrease the metabolic and endocrine stress response of newborn infants undergoing surgery? *BMJ* 1988;296:668.

104. Ross RJM, Miell JP, Buchanan CR. Avoiding autocannibalism. *BMJ* 1991;303:1147.

105. Binder ND, Raschko RK, Benda GI, et al. Insulin infusion with parenteral nutrition in extremely low birth weight infants with hyperglycemia. *J Pediatr* 1989;114:273.

106. Ostertag SG, Jovanovic L, Lewis B, et al. Insulin pump therapy in the very low birth weight infant. *Pediatrics* 1986;78:625.

107. Vaucher YE, Watson PD, Morrow G. Continuous insulin infusion in hyperglycemic, very low birth weight infants. *J Pediatr Gastroenterol Nutr* 1982;1:211.

108. Raney M, Donze A, Smith JR. Insulin infusion for the treatment of hyperglycaemia in low birth weight infants: examining the evidence. *Neonatal Netw* 2008;27:127.

109. Sinclair JC, Bottino M, Cowett RM. Interventions for prevention of neonatal hyperglycaemia in very low birth weight infants. *Cochrane Database Syst Rev* 2009;(3):CD007615.

110. Barker DJP. *Fetal and infant origins of adult disease.* London, UK: BMJ; 1992.

THE NEWBORN INFANT

111. Hoffman WH, Knoury C, Byrd HA. Prevalence of permanent congenital diabetes mellitus. *Diabetologia* 1980;19:487.

112. Hutchinson JH, Keay AJ, Kerr MN. Congenital temporary diabetes mellitus. *BMJ* 1962;2:436.

113. Aguilar-Bryan L, Bryan J. Neonatal diabetes mellitus. *Endocr Rev* 2008;29:265.

114. Barbetti F. Diagnosis of neonatal and infancy-onset diabetes. *Endocr Dev* 2007;11:83.

115. Shield JP. Neonatal diabetes: new insights into aetiology and implications. *Horm Res* 2000;53(suppl 1):7.

116. Temple IK, Gardner RJ, Robinson DO, et al. Further evidence for an imprinted gene for neonatal diabetes localised to chromosome 6q22. *Hum Mol Genet* 1996;5(8):1117.

117. Molsted-Pedersen L, Tygstrup I, Pedersen J. Congenital malformations in newborn infants of diabetic women. *Lancet* 1964;i:1124.

118. Confidential Enquiry into Maternal and Child Health. *Pregnancy in women with type 1 and type 2 diabetes in 2002–2003*. London, UK: CEMACH, 2005.

119. Casson IF, Clarke CA, Howard CV, et al. Outcomes of pregnancy in insulin dependent diabetic women: results of a five year population cohort study. *BMJ* 1997;315:275.

120. Confidential Enquiry into Maternal and Child Health. *Diabetes in pregnancy: are we providing the best care? Findings of a national enquiry.* London, UK: CEMACH, 2007.

121. Damm P, Molsted-Pedersen L. Significant decrease in congenital malformations in newborn infants of an unselected population of diabetic mothers. *Am J Obstet Gynecol* 1989;161:1163.

122. Comess LJ, Bennett PH, Man MB, et al. Congenital anomalies and diabetes in the Pima Indians of Arizona. *Diabetes* 1969;18:471.

123. Mills JL, Baker L, Goldman AS. Malformations in infants of diabetic mothers occur before the seventh gestational week. *Diabetes* 1979;28:292.

124. Miodovnik M, Mimouni F, Dignan PSJ, et al. Major malformations in infants of IDDM women. Vasculopathy and early first-trimester poor glycemic control. *Diabetes Care* 1988;11:713.

125. Freinkel N. Diabetic embryopathy and fuel-mediated organ teratogenesis: lessons from animal models. *Horm Metab Res* 1988;20:463.

126. Horton WE Jr, Sadler TW. Effects of maternal diabetes on early embryogenesis: alterations in morphogenesis produced by ketone body, beta-hydroxybutyrate. *Diabetes* 1983;32:610.

127. Sadler TW, Hunter ES II, Wynn RE, et al. Evidence for multifactorial origin of diabetes-induced embryopathies. *Diabetes* 1989;38:70.

128. Sadler TW, Phillips LS, Balkan W, et al. Somatostatin inhibitors from diabetic rat serum after birth and development of mouse embryos in culture. *Diabetes* 1986;35:861.

129. Sussman I, Matschinsky FM. Diabetes affects sorbitol and myo inositol levels of neuroectodermal tissue during embryogenesis in rats. *Diabetes* 1988;37:974.

130. Edwards JRG, Newall DR. Relaxin as an aetiological factor in diabetic embryopathy. *Lancet* 1988;i:1428.

131. Whitelaw A. Subcutaneous fat in newborn infants of diabetic mothers: an indication of quality of diabetic control. *Lancet* 1977;i:15.

132. Acker DB, Sachs BP, Friedman EA. Risk factors for shoulder dystocia. *Obstet Gynecol* 1985;66:762.

133. Mimouni F, Miodovnik M, Siddiqi TA, et al. Perinatal asphyxia in infants of insulin-dependent diabetic mothers. *J Pediatr* 1988;113:415.

134. Bradley RJ, Nicolaides KH, Brudenell JM. Are all infants of diabetic mothers 'macrosomic'? *BMJ* 1988;297:1583.

135. Sardesai MG, Gray AA, McGrath MM, et al. Fatal hypertrophic cardiomyopathy in the fetus of a woman with diabetes. *Obstet Gynecol* 2001;98:925.

136. HAPO Study Cooperative Research Group. Hyperglycemia and adverse pregnancy outcomes. *N Engl J Med* 2008;358:1991.

137. Hod M, Rabinerson D, Kaplan B, et al. Perinatal complications following gestational diabetes mellitus how 'sweet' is ill? *Acta Obstet Gynecol Scand* 1996;75:809.

138. Landon MB, Spong CY, et al. A multicenter, randomized trial of treatment for mild gestational diabetes. *N Engl J Med* 2009;361:1339.

139. Mello G, Parretti E, Mecacci F, et al. What degree of maternal metabolic control in women with type 2 diabetes is associated with normal body size and proportions in full term infants? *Diabetes Care* 2000;23:1494.

140. Mace S, Hirschfeld SS, Riggs T, et al. Echocardiographic abnormalities in infants of diabetic mothers. *J Pediatr* 1979;95:1013.

141. Reller MD, Kaplan S. Hypertrophic cardiomyopathy in infants of diabetic mothers: an update. *Am J Perinatol* 1988;5:353.

142. McMahon JN, Berry PJ, Joffe HS. Fatal hypertrophic cardiomyopathy in an infant of a diabetic mother. *Pediatr Cardiol* 1990;11:211.

143. Way GL, Wolfe RR, Eshaghpour E, et al. The natural history of hypertrophic cardiomyopathy in infants of diabetic mothers. *J Pediatr* 1979; 95:1020.

144. Cordero L, Landon MB. Infant of the diabetic mother. *Clin Perinatol* 1993;20:635.

145. Langer O, Levy J, Brustman C. Glycemic control in gestational diabetes mellitus—how tight is tight enough: small for gestational age versus large for gestational age? *Am J Obstet Gynecol* 1989;161:646.

146. Hanson U, Persson B. Outcome of pregnancies complicated by type I insulin dependent diabetes in Sweden: acute pregnancy complications, neonatal mortality and morbidity. *Am J Perinatol* 1993;10:330.

147. Carlson KS, Smith BT, Post M. Insulin acts on the fibroblast to inhibit glucocorticoid stimulation of lung maturation. *J Appl Physiol* 1984; 57:1577.

148. Gewolb IH. High glucose causes delayed fetal lung maturation in vitro. *Exp Lung Res* 1993;19:619.

149. Nogee L, McMahan M, Whitsett JA. Hyaline membrane disease and surfactant protein, SAP-35, in diabetes in pregnancy. *Am J Perinatol* 1988;5:374.

150. Peterec SM, Nichols KV, Dynia DW, et al. Butyrate modulates surfactant protein mRNA in fetal rat lung by altering mRNA transcription and stability. *Am J Physiol* 1994;267:L9.

151. Smith BT, Giroud CJP, Robert M, et al. Insulin antagonism of cortisol action on lecithin synthesis by cultured fetal lung cells. *J Pediatr* 1975;87:953.

152. Demaini S, Mimouni F, Tsang RC, et al. Impact of metabolic control of diabetes during pregnancy on neonatal hypocalcaemia: a randomized study. *Obstet Gynecol* 1994;83:918.

153. Tsang RC, Kleinman LI, Sutherland JM, et al. Hypocalcemia in infants of diabetic mothers: studies in calcium, phosphorus and magnesium metabolism and parathormone responsiveness. *J Pediatr* 1972;80:384.

154. Haworth JC, McRae KN, Dilling LA. Prognosis of infants of diabetic mothers in relation to neonatal hypoglycaemia. *Dev Med Child Neurol* 1976;18:471.

155. Rizzo TA, Dooley SL, Metzger BE, et al. Prenatal and perinatal influences on long term psychomotor development in offspring of diabetic mothers. *Am J Obstet Gynecol* 1995;173:1753.

156. Stenninger E, Flink R, Eriksson B, et al. Long-term neurological dysfunction and neonatal hypoglycaemia after diabetic pregnancy. *Arch Dis Child* 1998;79:F174.

157. Dionne G, Boivin M, Séguin JR, et al. Gestational diabetes hinders language development in offspring. *Pediatrics* 2008;122:e1073.

158. Bolaños L, Matute E, Ramírez-Dueñas Mde L, et al. Neuropsychological impairment in school-aged children born to mothers with gestational diabetes. *J Child Neurol* 2015;30:1616.

159. Temple RC, Hardiman M, Pellegrini M, et al. Cognitive function in 6- to 12-year-old offspring of women with Type 1 diabetes. *Diabet Med* 2011;28:845.

160. Schwartz R. Hyperinsulinemia and macrosomia. *N Engl J Med* 1990;323:410.

161. Cummins M, Norrish M. Follow-up of children of diabetic mothers. *Arch Dis Child* 1980;55:259.

162. Silverman BL, Rizzo TA, Cho NH, et al. Long term effects of the intrauterine environment. The Northwestern University Diabetes in Pregnancy Center. *Diabetes Care* 1998;21(suppl 2):b142.

163. Vohr BR, Lipsitt LP, Oh W. Somatic growth of children of diabetic mothers with reference to birth size. *J Pediatr* 1980;97:196.

164. Warram JH, Krolewski AS, Gottlieb MS, et al. Differences in risk of insulin dependent diabetes in offspring of diabetic mothers and diabetic fathers. *N Engl J Med* 1984;311:149.

165. Field LL. Insulin-dependent diabetes mellitus: a model for the study of multifactorial disorders. *Am J Hum Genet* 1988;43:793.

166. National Institute for Health and Clinical Excellence. *Diabetes in pregnancy*. London, UK: RCOG, 2008. Available from: http://www.nice.org.uk/Guidance/CG63

Subarna Chakravorty and Irene Roberts

CHANGES IN RED CELL PRODUCTION DURING EMBRYONIC AND FETAL LIFE

Developmental Hematopoiesis

The process that ensures lifelong production of all types of blood cells is known as hematopoiesis. In humans, hematopoiesis begins in the yolk sac at 3 postconceptional weeks (pcw) at which point the majority of cells produced are red blood cells (1,2) (**Fig. 42.1**). Hematopoiesis in the yolk sac is transient and it is not clear that any long-lived stem cells are produced. However, hematopoietic stem cells appear shortly thereafter, by 5 pcw in humans, emerging from a specialized type of endothelium (hemogenic endothelium) that is localized to the ventral wall of the dorsal aorta in a region known as the aorta–gonad–mesonephros (AGM) (3). The AGM is also a transient site of hematopoiesis, serving to initiate the *de novo* generation of lifelong hematopoietic stem cells that then migrate to the fetal liver where they can be found from around 6 pcw (2,4). It is in the fetal liver that hematopoietic stem and progenitor cells begin to rapidly expand and differentiate to produce very large numbers of mature and immature red blood cells (for more detail, see below). The fetal liver remains the main site of hematopoiesis and erythropoiesis throughout fetal life. After birth, the main site of hematopoiesis, at least in term babies, is the bone marrow. However, it is important to note that blood cell production does start in fetal bone marrow much earlier than that (at 11 to 12 pcw), and recent studies show that red blood cell production is fully developed there as early as the second trimester, suggesting that for most of fetal life the circulating red blood cells needed to support the increasing demands of the growing fetus are produced from both the liver and bone marrow. These sequential changes in the sites and regulation of hematopoiesis during development help to explain the natural history of many neonatal hematologic problems, including red cell disorders, such as hemolytic disease of the newborn (HDN).

Erythropoiesis in the Fetus

Erythropoiesis is the process of producing red blood cells from stem or progenitor cells. Except in the yolk sac, where red blood cells develop from transient progenitor cells rather than stem cells, all red cells derive from hematopoietic stem cells through a series of steps (Fig. 42.2) under the control of the hormone erythropoietin (EPO) (5). This is why neonates and children with genetic stem cell defects often develop anemia but also failure of white blood cell and platelet production (see Chapters 43 and 44). When genetic defects occur downstream of the stem cell (in an erythroid progenitor cell, Fig. 42.2), only red cell production is affected (e.g. Diamond-Blackfan Anemia, see below).

Erythropoietin Production in the Fetus and Newborn

During fetal life, EPO is mainly produced in the liver in contrast to adult life when the main source is the kidney (6). Since EPO does not cross the placenta, EPO-mediated regulation of fetal erythropoiesis is predominantly under fetal control, and the only stimulus to EPO production under physiologic conditions is hypoxia with or without anemia (reviewed in Ref. (7)). This explains the high EPO levels in fetuses of mothers with diabetes or hypertension or those with intrauterine growth restriction (IUGR) or cyanotic congenital heart disease (8). EPO is also increased in fetal anemia of any cause, including HDN.

Characteristics of Neonatal Red Blood Cells

The differences in erythropoiesis during fetal development lead to distinct characteristics of red blood cells in term and preterm neonates compared to those in older children. These differences are summarized in **Table 42.1**, and those that are important for our understanding of neonatal anemias are discussed below.

Hemoglobin Synthesis in the Fetus and Newborn

The sequential changes in globin production in humans are well described through work carried out more than two decades ago (1) and have been confirmed in recent studies (2). Erythroblasts and red blood cells in the yolk sac produce mainly epsilon, zeta, and alpha globin that together can combine to produce Hb Gower 1 ($\xi_2 \varepsilon_2$), Hb Gower 2 ($\alpha_2 \varepsilon_2$), and Hb Portland ($\xi_2 \gamma_2$) (**Table 42.2**). Gamma globin chain production begins almost immediately after this so that even in embryonic life a small amount of fetal hemoglobin (HbF; $\alpha_2 \gamma_2$) can be detected. HbF is the predominant hemoglobin until after birth. The fact that the embryo is already so dependent on alpha globin–containing hemoglobins so early during development explains why alpha-thalassemia major (also known as Hb Barts fetalis) causes such severe anemia from early in fetal life (9).

The major hemoglobin synthesized after birth is HbA (adult hemoglobin; $\alpha_2 \beta_2$). Although traces of HbA can normally be detected from as early as 4 pcw, it remains at low levels (10% to 15%) until 30 to 32 weeks pcw. This explains why the diagnosis of some beta globin disorders is very difficult in preterm neonates unless molecular (genetic) tests are used. From 30 pcw onwards, the rate of HbA synthesis increases at the same time as HbF production falls, resulting in an average HbF at term of 70% to 80%, HbA of 25% to 30%, small amounts of HbA₂, and sometimes a trace of Hb Barts (β_4). After birth, HbF falls, to approximately 2% at age 12 months with a corresponding increase in HbA. The molecular control of this change from HbF to HbA is termed globin switching. In recent years, there has been considerable research into the genes involved in globin switching (e.g., *BCL11A*) in order to identify strategies to delay or reverse this physiologic switch after birth and so maintain HbF production for children affected by severe beta globin disorders such as sickle cell disease (SCD) or beta-thalassemia major (10).

The rates of hemoglobin synthesis and of red blood production fall dramatically after birth and remain low for the first 2 weeks of life, probably in response to the sudden increase in tissue oxygenation at birth (11). Although the rates of HbF synthesis fall much more rapidly than do those of HbA, the life span of red cells means that there is little change in HbF over the first 15 days after birth. In preterm babies, who are born with a higher proportion of HbF-containing red blood cells, HbF concentrations may remain at the same level for the first 6 weeks of life before HbA production starts to increase—unless, of course, they are transfused. After this initial period of reduced Hb synthesis, the physiologic resumption of Hb production begins, and by 3 months of age, a healthy infant, whatever the gestation at birth, should be able to produce up to 2 mL of packed RBCs per day (11). Importantly, studies in babies treated with recombinant EPO have calculated that the maximal rate of RBC production is only approximately 1 mL/day in preterm neonates since such babies are unable to maintain their hemoglobin if greater than 1 mL of blood per day is venesected for diagnostic purposes but can do so where sampling losses are less than this (12).

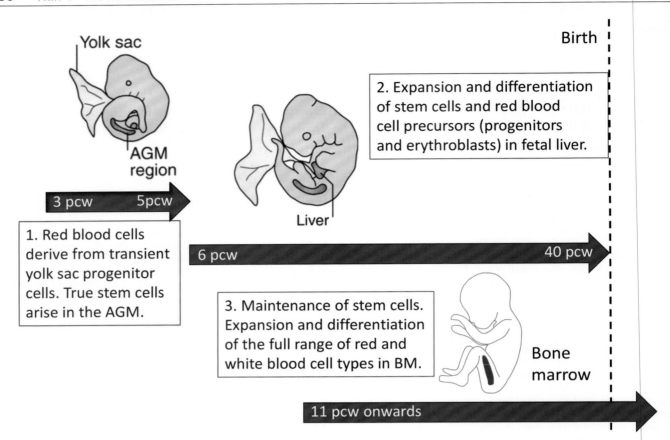

FIGURE 42.1 Human developmental erythropoiesis. Schematic showing the different sites of erythropoiesis during human embryonic and fetal development.

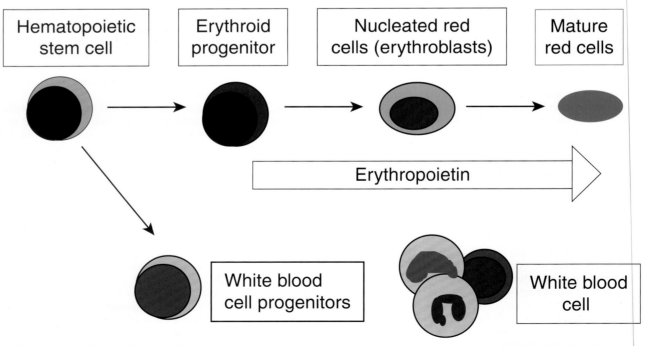

FIGURE 42.2 Development of red blood cells from hematopoietic stem cells. During fetal and postnatal life, all red blood cells originate from erythroid progenitor cells under the influence of the hormone erythropoietin. Erythroid progenitors derive from multipotent hematopoietic stem cells that are tightly regulated by intrinsic and extrinsic mechanisms to ensure controlled production of erythroid progenitors and red blood cells throughout life.

TABLE 42.1

Characteristics of Red Blood Cells in Neonates Compared to Those in Adults

	Preterm Neonate[a]	Term Neonate	Adult
Reduced red cell life span	35–50 d	60–70 d	120 d
Altered red cell metabolism	Susceptible to oxidant damage	Susceptible to oxidant damage	Less susceptible
Higher methemoglobin levels	0.43 g/dL	0.22 g/dL	0.11 g/dL
Hemoglobin and globin chain production	Almost all HbF in the most preterm neonates (85%) Main globin chains produced: alpha gamma beta	Mainly HbF (70%–75%); adult HbA 25%–30% Main globin chains produced: alpha gamma beta delta	HbA 98% HbF < 2% HbA$_2$ 2% Main globin chains produced: alpha beta delta
Erythropoietin			
• Site of production	Liver	Liver	Kidney
• Cause of increase	Increases in response to chronic *in utero* hypoxia (e.g., IUGR, PET) or severe fetal anemia	Increases in response to chronic *in utero* hypoxia (e.g., IUGR, PET) or severe fetal anemia	Increases in response to anemia or chronic hypoxia due to lung or cardiac disease

[a]Less than 37 weeks gestation at birth.

IUGR, intrauterine growth restriction; PET, preeclamptic toxemia.

Red Blood Cell Life Span in the Fetus and Newborn

It has been well recognized from isotope labeling studies that neonatal red cells have a reduced life span compared with adult red cells and that this varies with gestational age. These studies showed that in preterm neonates the red blood cell life span is only 35 to 50 days and this compares with 60 to 70 days for term neonates and 120 days for healthy adults (reviewed in Ref. 11). The reasons

TABLE 42.2

Hemoglobins in the Human Embryo, Fetus, and Neonate

Hemoglobin[a]	Stage of Development	Alpha Cluster (Chromosome 16)	Beta Cluster (Chromosome 11)
Hb Gower 1[b]	Embryo (3–4 pcw)	ξ_2	ε_2
Hb Gower 2	Embryo (4 pcw)	α_2	ε_2
Hb Portland	Embryo (4 pcw)	ξ_2	γ_2
HbF	Embryo/fetus (from 4 pcw)	α_2	γ_2
HbA	Embryo/fetus/ neonate/adult (from 4 pcw)	α_2	β_2
HbA$_2$	Fetus/neonate/ adult (from 30 pcw)	α_2	δ_2

[a]Fetuses with α-thalassemia major, who are unable to synthesize α-globin chains, are only able to synthesize Hb Barts (β$_4$) or, in some cases, Hb Portland.
[b]Hb Gower 1 has also been found as a tetramer containing only epsilon globin chains (ε$_4$).

for reduced red cell life span in neonates are not fully understood but are thought to reflect both biochemical and functional differences in the membrane of neonatal versus adult red blood cells. These differences include increased resistance to osmotic lysis, increased mechanical fragility, increased total lipid content and an altered lipid profile, increased insulin-binding sites, and reduced expression of blood group antigens such as A, B, and I (11).

Altered Red Cell Metabolism in the Fetus and the Newborn

Many studies have demonstrated distinct differences in the glycolytic pathways between neonatal and adult red blood cells. Together, these differences increase the susceptibility of neonatal red blood cells to oxidant-induced damage (13). Overall, glycolysis is impaired and glucose consumption is reduced in normal neonatal red blood cells compared to their adult counterparts. This occurs despite increased activity of the majority of glycolytic pathway enzymes, such as glucose-6-phosphate dehydrogenase (G6PD), pyruvate kinase (PK), and lactate dehydrogenase (LDH), and is believed to be due to reduced phosphofructokinase activity. Neonatal red blood cells also have reduced levels of NADH methemoglobin reductase (about 60% of those in adult red blood cells). This leads to slightly higher methemoglobin levels in neonates compared to those in adults (mean 0.43 g/dL in preterm neonates, 0.22 g/dL in term neonates, and 0.11 g/dL in adults) (11), and neonates are more susceptible to the toxic effects of chemicals (e.g., nitric oxide, local anesthetics) that oxidize hemoglobin to methemoglobin.

NEONATAL ANEMIA

Overview

Anemia is the commonest hematologic abnormality in neonates admitted to neonatal intensive care units, particularly in extremely low birth weight (ELBW) neonates where greater than 90% will receive at least one red cell transfusion during their stay (14). It is important to identify those neonates with pathologic anemia who require specific investigations and more tailored management. However, in the majority of cases, the causes are straightforward, since they reflect a combination of well-recognized physiologic changes and iatrogenic bloodletting. In the neonatal period, the most frequent diseases associated with anemia are immune hemolysis and genetic red cell disorders. The combination of a logical approach and appropriate use of straightforward investigations, as outlined below, reveals the cause in most babies. Treatment options for neonatal anemia remain limited and are based mainly on sensible use of blood transfusion (see below) and prevention of anemia.

Normal Values for Red Blood Cells and Blood Volume

Representative normal values for hemoglobin, hematocrit, mean cell volume (MCV), and reticulocytes for term and preterm babies are shown in Table 42.3. In term babies, as hemoglobin synthesis virtually ceases immediately after birth, reticulocytes fall rapidly and the hemoglobin, hematocrit, and MCV fall gradually over the first few weeks, reaching a mean hemoglobin of 13 to 14 g/dL at 4 weeks of age and 9.5 to 11 g/dL at 7 to 9 weeks of age, with a lower limit of normal for the MCV and mean cell hemoglobin (MCH) of 77 fL and 26 pg, respectively. Similarly, for preterm infants, the hemoglobin, hematocrit, and MCV fall for the first few weeks after birth although this pattern may be difficult to interpret, particularly in ELBW infants, because of the variable clinical course and transfusion requirements of these neonates. However, clinical experience, supported by studies of well preterm infants carried out almost 50 years ago, shows a more rapid and steeper fall in hemoglobin, reaching a mean of 6.5 to 9 g/dL at 4 to 8 weeks' postnatal age after which the reticulocyte count starts to increase (11). Circulating erythroblasts (nucleated red cells), the cells that give rise to mature red cells after enucleation, are

TABLE 42.3

Normal Red Cell Values at Birth in Term and Preterm Neonates

Red Cell Values	Gestational Age at Birth (Weeks)							
	24–25	26–27	28–29	30–31	32–33	34–35	36–37	Term
Hb (g/dL)	**14.5** (11.5–18.5)	**15.5** (11.5–18.5)	**16.0** (12.5–20)	**17.0** (13–20)	**17.0** (13–20)	**17.5** (13.5–21.5)	**18.0** (14–21.5)	**18.5** (14–21.5)
Hct (%)	**43** (30–57)	**45** (30–55)	**47** (38–58)	**50** (40–60)	**50** (40–60)	**51** (40–60)	**52** (42–65)	**54** (43–65)
MCV (fL)	**119** (104–133)	**115** (103–130)	**114** (101–128)	**112** (100–125)	**110** (98–120)	**109** (98–120)	**108** (98–117)	**106** (98–115)
Reticulocytes (%)	**6** (±0.5)	**9.6** (±3.2)	**7.5** (±2.5)	**5.8** (±2.0)	**5** (±1.9)	**3.9** (±1.6)	**4.2** (±1.8)	**3.2** (±1.4)

Values for Hb, Hct, and MCV are mean (5th–95th percentile) and are based on reference ranges in Christensen et al. (15). The reticulocyte data are shown as mean ± SD and are based on our own hospital laboratory data (unpublished).

Reprinted from Christensen R, Henry E, Jopling J, et al. The CBC: reference ranges for neonates. *Sem Perinatol* 2009;33:3. Copyright © 2009 Elsevier. With permission.

present in the peripheral blood of most neonates. Their frequency is higher in preterm neonates than in term neonates (a useful "rule of thumb" is that values of <5 erythroblasts/100 white cells in a term baby and <20 erythroblasts/100 white blood cells in a preterm baby can be considered normal for the first 1 to 2 days of life). The commonest causes of increased numbers of circulating erythroblasts are anemia due to blood loss or hemolysis and acute or chronic hypoxia (e.g., hypoxic ischemic encephalopathy and IUGR, respectively). The blood volume at birth varies not only with gestational age but also with the timing of clamping of the cord (16). In term infants, the average blood volume is 80 mL/kg (range 50 to 100 mL/kg), and in preterm infants, it is higher at 106 mL/kg (range 85 to 143 mL/kg) (17).

Several studies have shown that most term and preterm neonates have adequate stores of iron, folic acid, and vitamin B_{12} at birth. While folic and vitamin B_{12} levels are maintained in term neonates, iron stores will have fallen in the majority of infants by the time they have doubled their birth weight (18). In preterm infants, stores of iron and folic acid are lower and are depleted more quickly, leading to deficiency after 2 to 4 months if the recommended daily intakes are not maintained (reviewed in Ref. 19). A detailed systematic review of randomized trials of enteral iron supplementation in preterm or LBW neonates concluded that supplementation with iron did lead to higher hemoglobin concentrations, although only to a modest extent (0.6 g/dL); iron stores were also improved and the risk of subsequent iron deficiency anemia was reduced confirming the value of supplementation in these neonates (20). However, this review also found that the impact of iron supplementation on neurodevelopmental outcome was unclear.

Definition of Neonatal Anemia

Neonatal anemia is usually defined as a hemoglobin concentration or hematocrit that is 2 standard deviations below the mean or below the 5th percentile, using reference values for term and preterm infants at birth (Table 42.3). Although any term neonate with a hemoglobin of less than 14 g/dL at birth (mean normal value) in a properly taken blood sample could be considered anemic, from a clinical point of view, not every neonate with a hemoglobin concentration at birth of less than 14 g/dL needs detailed further investigation, but thought should be given to the cause (Table 42.4) and appropriate investigations performed. For preterm neonates, the reference ranges for hemoglobin and hematocrit are wider and gestational age at birth must therefore be taken into account. It is also important to consider the possibility of artifactual results, for example due to *in vitro* blood clotting in the sample tube. Where the reduced hemoglobin does not fit the clinical picture, the first step should be to repeat the sample. The site of sampling also influences blood count analyses; for example, the hemoglobin concentration in venous samples is lower than that in heelprick samples collected simultaneously, sometimes by up to 2 to 4 g/dL in the first few hours of life (11). This difference between venous and capillary hemoglobin measurements is less in term than in preterm neonates and falls with increasing postnatal

age, such that by the fifth day of life there is almost no difference in hemoglobin concentration between a well-taken heelprick sample and a venous sample (11).

The Influence of Cord Clamping

The timing of the clamping of the cord and the position of the baby at the time of cord clamping are other major factors determining the hemoglobin concentration at birth (babies held below the placenta receiving more blood). It has been estimated that 25% of the placental blood is transfused within the first 15 seconds and 50% by the end of the first minute (16). Since the placental vessels contain around 100 mL of blood at birth in a term baby, even a short delay has the potential to increase the volume of placental blood transfused by 50 mL. A recent systematic review of delayed (30 seconds or more) versus early clamping of the cord at delivery in preterm infants included 18 randomized studies (21). Overall, the effects on hematocrit and transfusion requirements were modest: the hematocrit increased by 2.7% and the proportion of neonates who were transfused fell by 10%; although, surprisingly, in-hospital mortality was significantly reduced (risk ratio 0.68). At least two of the randomized studies have suggested that neurodevelopmental outcome is improved, and some countries, including the United Kingdom (https://www.resus.org.uk/resuscitation-guidelines/resuscitation-and-support-of-transition-of-babies-at-birth/) and the United States, now recommend delayed cord clamping of at least 30 to 60 seconds for uncompromised preterm and term neonates (https://www.acog.org/clinical/clinical-guidance/committee-opinion/articles/2017/01/delayed-umbilical-cord-clamping-after-birth).

Physiologic Impact of Anemia in the Neonate

The clinical significance of neonatal anemia depends upon not only the hemoglobin concentration but also the ability of the hemoglobin to unload the oxygen it is carrying. This reflects the position of the hemoglobin–oxygen dissociation curve and increases progressively from birth. The two most important factors determining the position of the hemoglobin–oxygen dissociation curve in neonates are the concentration of HbF and the level of 2,3-diphosphoglycerate (2,3-DPG) within the red blood cells: high HbF and low 2,3-DPG both cause the curve to shift to the left, that is, the affinity of hemoglobin for oxygen is increased, so less oxygen is released to the tissues. This is the situation just after birth in both term and preterm babies, when the HbF concentration is above 50%, and may be a significant problem for ELBW (24 to 28 weeks' gestation) neonates where HbF levels are greater than 90% unless they are transfused. Over the first few months of life, as HbF falls and 2,3-DPG levels rise, the hemoglobin–oxygen dissociation curve gradually shifts to the right and oxygen delivery to the tissues increases, to some extent ameliorating the effects of the falling hemoglobin during this time.

Pathogenesis and Causes of Neonatal Anemia

Neonatal anemia has distinct characteristics compared to that in older children. In particular, the results of diagnostic

TABLE 42.4

Principal Mechanisms and Causes of Neonatal Anemia

Mechanism	Principal Causes
Reduced red blood cell production	Parvovirus B19
	Diamond-Blackfan anemia
Increased red cell destruction (hemolysis)	Hemolytic disease of the newborn, e.g., Rh disease
	Red cell membrane disorders, e.g., hereditary spherocytosis
	Red cell enzyme disorders, e.g., G6PD deficiency
	Some hemoglobinopathies (alpha globin disorders)
Blood loss	Fetomaternal
	Twin-to-twin
	Internal hemorrhage, e.g., cephalohematoma

TABLE 42.5

Hematologic Causes of *Hydrops Fetalis*

Red cell aplasia, e.g., parvovirus B19, Diamond-Blackfan anemia

Hemolytic disease of the newborn—mainly due to Rh antibodies (anti-D, anti-C)

Red cell membrane disorders—hydrops is rare except in hereditary stomatocytosis

Red cell enzymopathies, e.g., pyruvate kinase deficiency (rare in G6PD deficiency)

Hemoglobinopathies—alpha-thalassemia major (Hb Bart hydrops fetalis)

Chronic fetal blood loss, e.g., twin-to-twin transfusion

Storage disorders

Hemophagocytic lymphohistiocytosis (HLH)

Malignancies, e.g., transient abnormal myelopoiesis (Down syndrome), congenital acute leukemia in children without Down syndrome

G6PD, glucose-6-phosphate dehydrogenase.

investigations have to be interpreted on the background of the developmental changes affecting the red blood cell membrane and enzymes, as well as the types and rate of hemoglobin production, which vary with gestational and postnatal age. Importantly, anemia in the neonate may be due to pregnancy-related or preexisting disorders in the mother, such as the presence of red blood cell alloantibodies or genetic disorders, and it is important to remember that in many cases evaluating the blood count and blood film of the parents may be the quickest way of identifying the underlying diagnosis in the neonate. Diagnostic tests are also often affected by whether the baby has been transfused, although increasing use of molecular testing for a variety of genetic red cell disorders has much reduced this problem.

The principal causes of neonatal anemia are shown in Table 42.4. In general, anemia can result from one or more of the following mechanisms: reduced red cell production, increased red cell destruction (hemolysis), blood loss, or a combination of these mechanisms, for example, anemia of prematurity.

A Simple Diagnostic Approach to Neonatal Anemia

Clinically, red cell disorders associated with neonatal or fetal anemia usually present in one of three ways: with a low hemoglobin (anemia; see Table 42.4), with jaundice due to hemolysis, or with hydrops. The most common hematologic causes of jaundice and hydrops are shown in **Tables 42.4** and **42.5**, respectively. A diagnostic algorithm to help identify which of these causes is most likely, which can be excluded, and what further investigations are most appropriate, is shown in **Figure 42.3**. This is based on simple observations and simple tests available in almost all hematology

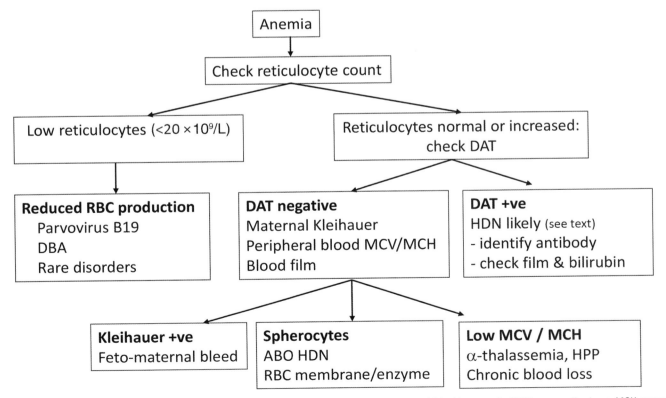

FIGURE 42.3 Diagnostic algorithm for neonatal anemia. DAT, direct antiglobulin test; DBA, Diamond-Blackfan anemia; MCV, mean cell volume; MCH, mean cell hemoglobin; HDN, hemolytic disease of the newborn; HPP, hereditary pyropoikilocytosis.

laboratories. Where in doubt about the best investigations to use and the interpretation of the results, discussion with a hematologist at an early stage may be helpful.

Neonatal Anemia Due to Reduced Red Cell Production
Overview

Anemia due to reduced red cell production is known as red cell aplasia and is not common in the neonatal period. Nevertheless, it is clinically important, because several of the disorders that present in this way are associated with severe, lifelong problems. The full blood count in red cell aplasia is usually normal apart from anemia. Another laboratory clue to the diagnosis of reduced red cell production is the low reticulocyte count ($<20 \times 10^9$/L) and the absence of circulating erythroblasts in the peripheral blood. This is because the normal response to severe anemia in the newborn is to increase the production of new red cells (reticulocytes and erythroblasts), which rapidly appear in the peripheral blood. In addition, the direct antiglobulin test (DAT; Coombs test) is negative as these anemias are not immune.

The most important causes of red cell aplasia are congenital infections (almost all due to parvovirus B19) and the genetic disorder Diamond-Blackfan anemia (DBA). Reduced red cell production may also be part of a general failure of hematopoiesis. In this situation, the white blood cell count and platelet count are also reduced, for example, in congenital leukemias (see Chapter 59) and bone marrow failure syndromes such as Pearson syndrome. Apart from parvovirus B19, other infections that may cause anemia due to reduced red cell production include CMV, toxoplasmosis, congenital syphilis, rubella, and herpes simplex, although the anemia and reticulocytopenia are usually relatively mild (22,23).

Parvovirus B19 and Fetal/Neonatal Anemia

Maternal infection with parvovirus B19 is one of the most common causes of unexplained fetal anemia. The anemia is often very severe and has an *in utero* mortality of almost 10% (24). A diagnosis of fetal parvovirus B19 should be considered in every "unexplained" case of fetal hydrops (Table 42.5) since it has been estimated that parvovirus B19 is responsible for 6% to 7% of cases of nonimmune hydrops (25). Although the anemia is the principal hematologic abnormality in fetal/neonatal parvovirus infection, thrombocytopenia may also occur (22). The reticulocyte count in parvovirus B19 infection is low (usually $<10 \times 10^9$/L) and erythroblasts are absent in the peripheral blood. The diagnosis of parvovirus B19 infection is primarily based on maternal serology together with the demonstration of B19 DNA in the fetus/neonate by dot blot hybridization or polymerase chain reaction (PCR) (22,24). Where results are negative on blood samples but clinical suspicion of parvovirus is high, PCR for B19 should also be carried out on bone marrow (22). Management depends on the severity of the anemia—severe cases diagnosed *in utero* may be treated by intrauterine transfusion (IUT); for those that survive, the majority have no long-term sequelae. However, a small number of neonates with chronic red cell aplasia, with or without evidence of persistent B19 DNA by PCR, have been reported, and for such cases, intravenous immunoglobulin (IVIG) should be given to try and eradicate persistent viral infection (22,26).

Genetic Causes of Failure of Red Cell Production

The most common genetic disorder presenting with red cell aplasia in the newborn is Diamond-Blackfan anemia. Other genetic causes are extremely rare and include congenital dyserythropoietic anemia (CDA) and Pearson syndrome. The other inherited bone marrow failure syndromes, such as Fanconi anemia, rarely present at birth unless there is a family history or the distinctive dysmorphic features lead clinicians to perform specific diagnostic chromosomal breakage investigations.

Diamond-Blackfan Anemia

This disorder, which has an incidence of 5 to 7 cases per million live births, causes congenital red cell aplasia (27). The vast majority of cases are due to heterozygous mutations in one of the ribosomal protein (RP) genes (28). Often, these mutations are *de novo*; indeed, only 20% of cases have a clear family history while 80% are sporadic. Affected children virtually always present in the first year of life; most diagnoses are made around 2 months of age, but 25% of cases present at birth and rare cases present as mid-trimester fetal anemia with or without hydrops (27). DBA usually presents with anemia in an otherwise healthy baby. However, since approximately 40% of infants have associated congenital anomalies, particularly craniofacial dysmorphism, IUGR, neck anomalies (Klippel-Feil syndrome), and thumb malformations (e.g., triphalangeal or bifid thumbs), any infant with these anomalies should be carefully screened for anemia (27). The laboratory features of DBA are normochromic anemia (which may be macrocytic) with reticulocytopenia. Once parvovirus B19 infection has been excluded, neonates with persistent anemia and low reticulocytes should have specific investigations for DBA. These include molecular testing for RP gene mutations (many laboratories now offer next-generation sequencing for DBA diagnosis) and/or a bone marrow examination that will demonstrate the lack of erythroid precursors characteristic of this disease. In case of doubt, or where molecular testing is not available, measurement of red cell adenosine deaminase levels, which are elevated in most affected patients, may be useful (27,29). DBA is almost always a lifelong condition although rare spontaneous remissions later in life are reported. This contrasts transient erythroblastopenia of childhood (TEC), which also causes red cell aplasia in infants and young children but is usually mild and always transient. The only treatment for neonates and infants with DBA is red cell transfusion. After the first year of life, steroids are used as first-line treatment although less than 50% of patients have a lasting response to steroids; the remainder are treated using lifelong red cell transfusion or bone marrow transplantation (27,29).

Congenital Dyserythropoietic Anemia

The CDAs are a rare group of disorders characterized by failure of red cell production due to ineffective erythropoiesis. There are four types of CDA: types I, II, III, and IV depending on the causative gene and characteristic red cell features. Although CDA usually presents during childhood, types I, II, and IV CDA can all present with neonatal anemia and/or hydrops fetalis (30–33). The diagnosis is made using a combination of genetic analysis in tandem with bone marrow examination. Most cases of types I and II disease are caused by mutations in the codanin-1 (*CDAN1*) and *SEC23B* gene, respectively, while type IV disease is caused by mutations in the *GATA1* or *KLF1* genes. In contrast to DBA, the bone marrow has vastly increased numbers of erythroid precursors, but they are grossly abnormal and do not differentiate normally into mature red blood cells. The prognosis of CDA is extremely variable. For transfusion-independent children with CDA, life span is usually normal and quality of life is good. For more severe disease, the treatment options include regular transfusions or bone marrow transplantation.

Pearson Syndrome

This rare disease is caused by mutations in mitochondrial DNA (34). It often presents in neonates who are small for gestational age and thrive poorly in the first few weeks of life (34). The anemia is normocytic and associated thrombocytopenia and neutropenia are common; abnormal leukocyte vacuolation may be seen in the peripheral blood and highly characteristic vacuolation of early erythroid cells on the marrow aspirate should prompt blood to be sent for mitochondrial DNA analysis to establish the diagnosis. The prognosis of Pearson syndrome is very poor: few children survive beyond the second year of life.

Anemia Due to Increased Red Cell Destruction (Hemolytic Anemia)
Overview

Apart from anemia of prematurity, hemolysis is the commonest cause of neonatal anemia. Investigation of the cause of neonatal hemolysis, even if mild and/or transient, is important since this may be the clue to serious disorders later in childhood (e.g., red cell enzymopathies) or to problems that might affect future siblings (e.g., HDN). Diagnostic clues to hemolysis are increased reticulocytes and/or erythroblasts in the peripheral blood, unconjugated hyperbilirubinemia, a positive DAT (if immune), and characteristic changes in the appearance of the red blood cells on a blood film (e.g., hereditary spherocytosis [HS]). The main types of neonatal hemolytic anemia are shown in Table 42.4 and a useful guide to investigations is shown in **Figure 42.3**. Initial investigations of suspected hemolysis should be a full blood count, blood film, and a DAT, which will be positive only in the presence of immune hemolytic anemia, almost always HDN. The main causes of nonimmune hemolysis in neonates are genetic defects affecting the red blood cell membrane, enzymes, or hemoglobins. Congenital and primary infections can also cause neonatal hemolytic anemia including CMV, toxoplasmosis, congenital syphilis, rubella, herpes simplex, and, rarely, malaria. Although it is usually straightforward to distinguish the cause of hemolysis, rarer disorders require specialist investigations (see below) that should be discussed with a hematologist once the basic investigations are to hand.

Immune Hemolytic Anemias, Including HDN

DAT-positive hemolysis is almost always due to HDN caused by transplacental passage of maternal IgG alloantibodies to red cell antigens. Very rarely, maternal autoimmune hemolytic anemia (AIHA) causes a positive DAT in the neonate usually without any clinical evidence of hemolysis or anemia. The principal alloantibodies that cause significant anemia due to HDN are those against Rh antigens (anti-D, anti-C, and anti-E), anti-K, anti-Kidd (J^k), anti-Duffy (F^y), and antibodies of the MNS blood group system, including anti-U. Anti-D remains the most frequent alloantibody to cause significant hemolytic anemia, affecting 1 in 1,200 pregnancies (35). Anti-K antibodies are less common but can cause severe fetal and neonatal anemia since they inhibit erythropoiesis as well as cause hemolysis (36). ABO hemolytic disease occurs only in offspring of women of blood group O and is confined to the 1% of such women who have high-titer IgG antibodies. Although hemolysis due to anti-A is more common (1 in 150 births) than anti-B, HDN due to anti-B is often more severe and may even cause hydrops fetalis (37).

Most babies with HDN present with jaundice and/or anemia, but in severe cases, there may be evidence of extramedullary hematopoiesis, including hepatosplenomegaly and skin lesions due to small foci of erythroid cells producing the clinical appearance of "blueberry muffin baby" (38). In contrast to anti-Rh antibodies, ABO HDN usually causes hyperbilirubinemia without significant neonatal anemia as there are relatively low numbers of group A or B antigenic sites on neonatal red cells, which allows the antibody-coated cells to persist for longer in the circulation (11). Typically, the blood film in HDN shows increased numbers of spherocytes; this is very marked in ABO HDN where it may be the only abnormal feature. In HDN due to Rh disease, there are also large numbers of circulating erythroblasts. The DAT is always positive in Rh HDN and anti-K HDN but may occasionally be negative in ABO HDN (39).

Management of HDN

Management of ABO HDN usually just requires phototherapy; however, close monitoring is essential and exchange transfusion is occasionally required, particularly in cases of ABO HDN due to anti-B antibodies. For HDN due to other alloantibodies, the presence of those antibodies will almost always have been identified antenatally at the time of routine screening. The antenatal management of pregnancies affected by red cell alloimmunization requires cooperation between obstetric, pediatric, and hematology teams

(40). Many countries now have national guidelines for the prevention and management of HDN that are particularly useful as the prevalence of Rh HDN has markedly declined with the widespread introduction of prophylactic antenatal anti-D (41–43). These guidelines recommend that all neonates at risk should have cord blood taken for measurement of hemoglobin, bilirubin, and a DAT. Affected neonates should remain in hospital until hyperbilirubinemia and anemia have been properly managed. Phototherapy should be given from birth to all Rh-alloimmunized infants with hemolysis, as the bilirubin can rise steeply after birth and this expectant approach will prevent the need for exchange transfusion in some infants (44). In HDN due to anti-K, anemia is usually more prominent than jaundice, and minimal phototherapy may be necessary despite severe anemia (40). The indications for exchange transfusion of neonates with HDN recommended by the British Committee for Standards in Haematology (45) are severe anemia (<10 g/dL at birth) and/or severe or rapidly increasing hyperbilirubinemia.

These guidelines also include recommendations about the most appropriate blood products to use for transfusion in this setting. Importantly, irradiated blood must be used for infants who have previously received IUT, to prevent the risk of transfusion-associated graft versus host disease (TA-GvHD) (45). IVIG has been used to reduce the need for exchange transfusion, but the value of this approach remains to be proven in clinical trials (46).

"Late" anemia presents at a few weeks of age in some babies with milder HDN or those who have received intrauterine or exchange transfusion. In these neonates, there is evidence of ongoing hemolysis and the anemia may be aggravated by the normal postnatal suppression of erythropoiesis. Such babies may require top-up red cell transfusion as per conventional guidelines (see Table 42.6). It is important to note that administration of prophylactic antenatal anti-D to Rh D-negative mothers quite commonly causes a weakly positive DAT in the baby at birth. Provided there is a clear history of antenatal prophylaxis and the hemoglobin and blood film are normal, it is not necessary to arrange further investigation and follow-up of such babies. Top-up transfusion for late anemia is rarely needed for neonates with ABO HDN. Folic acid (500 µg/kg/d) should be given to all babies with hemolytic anemia until 3 months of age but is not necessary for babies with ABO HDN who are not anemic. EPO has been used to prevent the need for "top-up" transfusion for late anemia, but there are currently no data from randomized trials to support the routine use of EPO in this setting (47).

TABLE 42.6

Top-Up Red Cell Transfusion for Neonatal Anemia: Indications,^{a} Risks, and Benefits

Indications^a (hemoglobin threshold for transfusion)	0–7 days	10–12 g/dL (oxygen dependent)
		<10 g/dL (oxygen independent)
	8–14 days	9.5–10 g/dL (oxygen dependent)
		<7.5–8.5 g/dL (oxygen independent)
	Day 15 onwards	8.5 g/dL
Benefits	Established: correction of anemia	
	Unclear: improved cardiorespiratory function, weight gain, and neurodevelopmental outcome	
Risks	Established: metabolic complications (e.g., hyperkalemia), transfusion-transmitted infection, e.g., CMV	
	Unclear: NEC, IVH, ROP, BPD	
	Rare: TA-GVHD	
	Unclear in neonates: TRALI, TACO	

^{a}Based on the recommendations of the British Committee for Standards in Hematology (45).

CMV, cytomegalovirus; NEC, necrotizing enterocolitis; IVH, intraventricular hemorrhage; ROP, retinopathy of prematurity; BPD, bronchopulmonary dysplasia; TA-GVHD, transfusion associated graft versus host disease; TRALI, transfusion associated lung injury; TACO, transfusion associated cardiac overload.

From New HV, Berryman J, Bolton-Maggs PHB, et al., on behalf of the British Committee for Standards in Haematology. Guidelines on transfusion for fetuses, neonates and older children. *Br J Haematol* 2016;175:784. Copyright © 2016 John Wiley & Sons Ltd. Reprinted by permission of John Wiley & Sons, Inc.

Neonatal Hemolytic Anemia Due to Red Cell Membrane Disorders

A number of genetic red cell membrane disorders may present in the neonatal period with anemia, the most of which is HS. Most cases present with unexplained hemolysis with jaundice and moderate anemia or the red cell membrane disorder is identified as an incidental finding of abnormal red blood cells on a routine blood film in the absence of jaundice or anemia. Occasionally, however, neonates can present with a severe, transfusion-dependent hemolytic anemia; such cases are nearly always due to the condition hereditary pyropoikilocytosis (HPP), which is described below. The main clues to a diagnosis of a red cell membrane disorder are a family history of anemia or jaundice and an abnormal blood film as these disorders can nearly always be recognized by the characteristic shape of red cells. However, the identification of the exact type of membrane abnormality may require more complex investigations, including molecular diagnosis using a specialized "red cell" gene panel that is unaffected by recent blood transfusion. A brief summary of the three main clinical disorders presenting in neonates is given below; for more detailed information, the reader is referred to comprehensive reviews (48–51).

Hereditary Spherocytosis

The commonest red cell membrane defect, HS, occurs in 1 in 5,000 live births to parents of northern European extraction, but is less frequently seen in other ethnic groups (51). Most forms of HS are autosomal dominant, but recessive forms occur rarely and around 25% of cases are sporadic due to new mutations. HS is caused by mutations in the genes that encode the red cell membrane proteins spectrin, ankyrin, protein 4.1, and protein 3, most commonly mutations in the spectrin gene, SPTA (51). The usual presentation of HS in the neonate is with unconjugated hyperbilirubinemia as most affected neonates are not anemic. A small proportion of neonates have anemia severe enough to require transfusion but this is usually transient and stabilizes to a mild or moderate anemia (8 to 11 g/dL) or even a normal hemoglobin after the first 3 months. The blood film shows increased spherocytes and is identical to that of ABO HDN (the two disorders are distinguishable by the negative DAT in HS). All children with HS should also receive folic acid supplementation (from 500 µg/kg/d in the first 6 months of life and a total daily dose of 2.5 mg from 6 months until 10 years of age of life, increasing to 5 mg daily thereafter). The majority of children will remain well and transfusion independent without additional therapy (49). For those who are more severely affected, splenectomy invariably induces complete remission and may be considered after the age of 6 years (52). Importantly, all patients with HS, including neonates, are at risk of developing severe red cell aplasia if they are infected with parvovirus B19 (49), and all parents of neonates with HS should be advised of this risk.

Hereditary Elliptocytosis and Hereditary Pyropoikilocytosis

Hereditary elliptocytosis (HE) is caused by mutations in the genes for spectrin, ankyrin, or protein 4.1 (51,52). HE is usually autosomal dominant and the most common clinical presentation of the disorder in neonates is as a heterozygote (carrier). HE carriers have increased numbers of elliptocytes on the blood film but they have no clinical manifestations (i.e., no anemia or jaundice) and therefore the diagnosis is made as an incidental finding. No treatment is required and folic acid prophylaxis is unnecessary, as folate deficiency is not a feature of this condition.

By contrast, neonates who are homozygous or compound heterozygotes for HE mutations have severe hemolytic anemia, which starts during the neonatal period (53). This usually manifests as HPP, an uncommon but important condition because it causes severe, transfusion-dependent hemolytic anemia that does not improve with age (53). The diagnosis of HPP should easily be made by examining blood films that show bizarre fragmented red cells and microspherocytes and the full blood count that shows a severe microcytic anemia (MCV usually <60 fL). In addition, one or both parents usually have red cell elliptocytosis. Red cell transfusion is usually necessary until the child is old enough to undergo splenectomy, to which there is an excellent response (53).

Neonatal Hemolysis Due to Red Cell Enzymopathies

G6PD deficiency and PK deficiency are the most common red cell enzymopathies that present in the neonatal period. G6PD deficiency is an extremely common worldwide condition with numbers of affected individuals running into millions, with its epidemiology correlating with malaria. In contrast, PK deficiency is much less common compared to G6PD deficiency, with an estimated incidence of 5:100,000 in Caucasians (50,54). Children with these conditions usually present with unconjugated hyperbilirubinemia; clinically, they are indistinguishable from red cell membrane disorders, although anemia is uncommon in neonates with G6PD deficiency. Unlike with the membrane disorders, there are usually no diagnostic changes on the blood film. Importantly, neonates with PK deficiency can occasionally present with extreme and persistent hyperbilirubinemia leading to hepatic failure, and the absence of changes on the blood film means that the diagnosis may be missed (54).

Glucose-6-Phosphate Dehydrogenase Deficiency

G6PD deficiency is seen in all ethnic groups but has a high prevalence in individuals from central Africa (20%) and the Mediterranean (10%). As the G6PD gene is on the X chromosome, most affected neonates are boys. However, female carriers are sometimes identified through neonatal jaundice screens, and these babies also occasionally develop severe neonatal jaundice (55). In neonatal G6PD deficiency, jaundice usually presents within the first few days of life and is often severe; anemia is unusual and the blood film is completely normal, and thus the diagnosis must be made by assaying G6PD enzyme activity on a peripheral blood sample (55). Mutation analysis of the G6PD gene can also be done in unusual cases—for example, those presenting with severe anemia where there is no evidence of HDN or membranopathy. Some mutations are associated with chronic nonspherocytic hemolytic anemia, and mutation analysis is especially useful in these cases for establishing the diagnosis. It is not clear why some, but not all, G6PD-deficient neonates develop neonatal jaundice (55). In addition, the pathogenesis of the jaundice is also unclear, since most babies with G6PD deficiency have no evidence of hemolysis. Thus, careful management of neonatal hyperbilirubinemia is the principal clinical priority in neonatal G6PD deficiency, particularly where interactions with other risk factors for neonatal hyperbilirubinemia are present, such as Gilbert syndrome or HS, since kernicterus has been reported in this setting (55). Counseling parents of affected babies about which medicines, chemicals, and foods may precipitate hemolysis is also important (see **Table 42.7**), and a suitably designed card or leaflet listing these should be provided to all parents where possible. Fava beans (broad beans) are the most important food item to cause hemolysis in G6PD-deficient individuals and need to be avoided. If exchange transfusion is required for severe hyperbilirubinemia, conventional guidelines for exchange transfusion can be followed (see above and (45)). Additionally, in countries where malaria is endemic, it is important to exclude G6PD deficiency before giving primaquine for malaria eradication due to the high risk of drug-induced hemolysis in affected G6PD-deficient individuals. For the uncommon variants of G6PD deficiency associated with chronic nonspherocytic hemolytic anemia, folic acid supplements should be given (55). However, for the vast majority of patients, there is no chronic hemolysis and no anemia and therefore folic acid supplements are not indicated.

TABLE 42.7

Drugs and Chemicals That May Precipitate Hemolysis in Neonates with G6PD Deficiency[a]

Chemicals	Methylene blue
	Naphthalene (mothballs)
	Fava beans (mother)[b]
Antibiotics	Nitrofurantoin[b]
	Some sulfonamides, e.g., sulfasalazine[b]
	Quinolones (ciprofloxacin[b], nalidixic acid[b])
	Chloramphenicol[a]
	Trimethoprim, Septrin[a,b]
	Isoniazid
Antimalarials	Primaquine[b]
	Chloroquine[a]
	Quinine[a]
Other medication	Rasburicase
	Dapsone[b]
	Aspirin[a,b]

[a]Not absolutely contraindicated but use with caution.
[b]Avoid in breast-feeding mothers.

Pyruvate Kinase Deficiency

PK deficiency is the second most common red cell enzymopathy in neonates. It is autosomal-recessive and clinically heterogeneous, varying from anemia severe enough to cause hydrops fetalis to a mild unconjugated hyperbilirubinemia (54). The majority of cases of PK deficiency are caused by mutations in the *PKLR* gene encoding the PK protein. A very rare cause of PK deficiency is mutations in the gene encoding the erythroid transcription factor Kruppel-like factor 1 (*KLF1*) that can result in reduced PK enzyme levels, aberrant globin gene expression, and chronic hemolytic anemia (56). In severe cases of PK deficiency, the jaundice has a rapid onset within 24 hours of birth and exchange transfusion may be required (54). Enzyme activity assays are cheap, and quick and still frequently used for diagnosis, but often result in aberrant results due to the presence of other confounding features that can affect the results and nonavailability of standardized reagents. Therefore, mutation analysis of the PK gene is increasingly used as the definitive diagnostic tool. This can be done by sequencing the *PKLR* gene through conventional sequencing technology, or part of a targeted next-generation sequencing platform. The blood film is sometimes distinctive but more often shows nonspecific changes of nonspherocytic hemolysis and therefore it is good practice to assay PK in all babies with unexplained hemolysis after the common causes have been excluded. Management in the neonatal period depends on the severity of the jaundice and anemia; some, but not all, children are transfusion dependent and folic acid supplements should be given to prevent deficiency due to chronic hemolysis. Recently, a small molecule allosteric activator of the enzyme resulting in its improved stability in the red blood cell has been tested in Phase 3 studies in PK-deficient adult patients. This molecule has resulted in increased red cell enzyme activity and improvement in baseline hemoglobin (57). However, it is unlikely to be used in neonates until the safety profile is widely understood following long-term studies in children and young adults.

Other Red Cell Enzymopathies Presenting in Neonates

The other red cell enzymopathies are rare. The most important to be aware of in the neonatal period are triosephosphate isomerase (TPI) deficiency and glucose phosphate isomerase (GPI) deficiency, both of which are autosomal recessive (48,50). Both can present with neonatal hemolytic anemia that is often severe, and this may be the only presenting feature at this age. These disorders are important to recognize in the neonatal period because they are both associated with severe neurologic features that may only become apparent 6 to 12 months later. Persistent hemolysis should therefore always be investigated. Diagnosis is mostly done by mutational analysis or enzyme activity analysis including family studies.

Neonatal Hemolysis Due to Hemoglobinopathies

The hemoglobinopathies, with the exception of alpha-thalassemia major, do not usually present in the neonatal period, and symptoms and signs of beta globin hemoglobinopathies (sickle-cell disease and beta-thalassemia major) are especially rare in neonates. HPLC (high-performance liquid chromatography) and other techniques that allow automation and high throughput testing are employed in newborn screening programs in many countries with a high incidence of SCD, including the United Kingdom. The main purpose of identifying SCD in the neonatal period is to initiate penicillin prophylaxis and establish regular specialist medical assessments (58).

Alpha-Thalassemia Major

Alpha-thalassemia major occurs when all four alpha globin genes on chromosome 16 are deleted (59). It predominantly affects families of south-east Asian origin and presents with mid-trimester fetal anemia or hydrops fetalis that is fatal within hours of delivery (occasional babies have lived a few days). Mothers of fetuses with alpha-thalassemia major may also suffer from severe pregnancy-related complications such as preeclampsia (9). The only long-term survivors of alpha-thalassemia major are those who received IUT (9). Prompt prenatal diagnosis and IUT may result in normal growth and development of the affected fetus although there is a high incidence of hypospadias in boys, and other survivors have limb defects and/or severe neurologic problems (9,60). If IUT is delayed until the anemia is severe, neonatal pulmonary hypoplasia is a cause of early mortality. The diagnosis of alpha-thalassemia major should be suspected in any case of severe fetal anemia presenting in the second trimester and any case of hydrops fetalis with severe anemia in which the parents come from south-east Asia (it is also seen occasionally in families who originate from India, the Middle East, or the Mediterranean). The diagnosis of alpha-thalassemia major in babies is confirmed by hemoglobin HPLC or electrophoresis (which shows only Hb Barts and Hb Portland; HbF and HbA are absent) and molecular analysis of the alpha globin gene cluster, which may take several weeks. The blood film, which provides a rapid presumptive diagnosis, shows hypochromic, microcytic red cells with vast numbers of circulating erythroblasts. Checking the blood counts of the parents is also a quick way of identifying whether they are at risk of having a child with alpha-thalassemia major—both parents will be carriers of a chromosome 16 in which both of the two alpha globin genes are deleted and so they will have hypochromic, microcytic red cell indices (MCV usually <74 fL and MCH usually <24 pg). Parental carrier status can be confirmed by molecular diagnosis.

Where IUT has been instituted promptly in the second trimester, neonatal management of alpha-thalassemia major is supportive, including red cell transfusion as required (60). Unfortunately, where the diagnosis and treatment are delayed until after birth, active management has no impact on survival. For surviving neonates, management after the neonatal period is the same as for beta-thalassemia, that is, lifelong red cell transfusions or bone marrow transplantation after the age of 2 years (60). Nevertheless, recent registry data indicate that for many alpha-thalassemia patients rescued by IUT, neurodevelopmental delay and poor growth are common despite long-term postnatal transfusions (9).

Beta-Thalassemias and SCD

Although these disorders are asymptomatic in neonates, if they are identified as a result of neonatal screening programs, specialist advice should be sought as soon as possible. Babies with SCD (homozygous SCD, SC disease, or S-beta-thalassemia) should be started on prophylactic penicillin V (62.5 mg twice daily) (58). Top-up red cell transfusion is not normally necessary for babies with beta-thalassemia major until the age of 4 to 6 months but folic acid supplementation should be given because hemolysis starts even before the need for regular transfusions.

Anemia Due to Blood Loss
Overview
Blood loss causing neonatal anemia may be clinically very obvious, such as rupture of the cord or a large subgaleal hematoma, but more often the blood loss is concealed and easy to miss unless specifically sought (e.g., fetomaternal bleeds). Acute perinatal blood loss leading to severe hypovolemic shock is an underrecognized clinical event, and delay in treatment may occur and may result in death or severe anoxic brain damage leading to neurologic damage (61). The principal causes of neonatal anemia due to blood loss are shown in Table 42.4. In neonates admitted to hospital, the most common cause of anemia is blood loss secondary to iatrogenic bloodletting (see below).

Blood Loss Prior to Birth
Twin-to-Twin Transfusion
Twin-to-twin transfusion occurs in monochorionic twins with monochorial placentas (62). This can be diagnosed early by specific ultrasound techniques (63,64). Bleeding may be acute, particularly during the second stage of labor, or chronic. Chronic twin-to-twin transfusion can cause a marked difference in birth weight between twins, although the majority of twin pairs have a discordance in hemoglobin of less than 5 g/dL (63,64). The most severe cases occur where there has been chronic intertwin transfusion throughout the second and third trimesters of pregnancy (so-called TAPS, twin anemia–polycythemia sequence) (65). The donor (anemic) twin is smaller, pale, and lethargic and may have overt cardiac failure; the recipient (polycythemic) twin is plethoric, with hyperviscosity and hyperbilirubinemia (see below). Twin-to-twin transfusions are now managed by early detection through ultrasound and fetoscopic laser surgery to stop aberrant placental blood flow (64).

Fetomaternal Hemorrhage
Most fetomaternal bleeds occur spontaneously in the third trimester or during labor. Fetomaternal bleeds may also be increased by invasive procedures, such as fetal blood sampling and caesarean section, or occur secondary to trauma, such as traffic accidents or falls (66). The clinical presentation depends on the amount and rate of blood loss. Most episodes involve very small quantities of blood (0.5 mL or less), but acute loss of greater than 20% of the blood volume is an important cause of unexpected intrauterine death, circulatory shock, or hydrops (66). Diagnostic clues to fetomaternal hemorrhage are severe anemia at birth in an otherwise well term baby with no or minimal jaundice. The most useful diagnostic tests are a DAT to exclude immune hemolysis, a reticulocyte count to exclude red cell aplasia, a Kleihauer test on maternal blood to quantitate the number of HbF-containing fetal RBCs in the maternal circulation, and a blood film (67). Accurate quantification of fetal red cells in maternal circulation can be done by flow cytometry, and anti-D dosing in Rh D–negative women can then be accurately calculated (67). Diagnostic difficulties may arise where the baby has bled acutely just prior to delivery. In that situation, the hemoglobin may be normal at delivery but fall rapidly as hemodilution occurs and the blood film may be normal apart from large numbers of erythroblasts.

Where there is chronic blood loss, the baby is often well but may present with cardiac failure; the blood film in this situation is hypochromic/microcytic and the Kleihauer result may be difficult to interpret. In some cases, however, chronic fetomaternal blood loss is followed by an acute bleed, with resultant severe anemia (Hb < 5 g/dL) and a high risk of long-term brain injury (68). Another point of note is that where there is ABO incompatibility between the mother and baby, the fetal cells may be rapidly destroyed within the maternal circulation. Therefore, a high index of suspicion of fetomaternal hemorrhage as a cause of neonatal anemia is needed, in order to perform the Kleihauer test as soon as possible to increase the chance of detecting fetal cells.

Blood Loss at or after Delivery
Blood loss around the time of delivery is usually due to obstetric complications, including placenta previa, placental abruption, incision of the placenta during cesarean section, or umbilical cord trauma and inadequate cord clamping. Blood loss in many of these situations is from the maternal circulation, although the fetus can be subject to hypoxia as a result. Rarely, a vasa previa is present and is inevitably torn when the membranes rupture, leading to severe fetal blood loss. This can easily be missed because the volume of blood is relatively small and it is impossible to distinguish fetal from maternal blood by appearance. The incidence of vasa previa is estimated to be around 1:2,500 and the condition carries a high fetal mortality (69). Although the presence of a vasa previa can be detected antenatally using vaginal ultrasound, this is not routine practice. There is a high risk of vasa previa in cases of *in vitro* fertilization, multiple pregnancies, and morphologically abnormal placentas, all of which can be identified in early gestation (69). Early cesarean section in known cases of vasa previa can prevent catastrophic fetomaternal hemorrhage (69). Internal hemorrhage in the baby, for example, cephalohematoma, pulmonary, or intra-abdominal hemorrhage, is usually associated with traumatic delivery. However, it is important to consider an underlying bleeding diathesis in such babies, particularly hemophilia A or B and vitamin K deficiency. Inherited and acquired coagulation disorders that may present with bleeding at birth or during the neonatal period are discussed in Chapter 44.

Anemia of Prematurity
Overview, Including Pathogenesis
The normal physiologic fall in hemoglobin over the first 4 to 8 weeks of life is greater in preterm compared with term neonates and has been termed "physiologic anemia of prematurity." The pathogenesis is not fully elucidated, but contributory factors include the reduced life span of fetal/neonatal red blood cells, relatively low EPO concentrations, and rapid growth of the baby during this period as well as iatrogenic bloodletting for diagnostic investigations (11). Phlebotomy losses are typically highest in ELBW neonates who have been estimated to lose up to 22 mL/kg per week during the first 6 weeks of life (70). Nutritional deficiency is likely to play only a minor role in modern neonatal practice due to routine, prophylactic supplementation with iron and folic acid (18).

The clinical impact of anemia of prematurity has been the subject of a large number of studies and is only briefly mentioned here. The principal consideration of these studies has been the association between anemia and short- and long-term brain injury, retinopathy of prematurity (ROP), and necrotizing enterocolitis (NEC) (71–74). The relationship between the hemoglobin concentration/hematocrit and state-of-the-art assessment of tissue hypoxia-related damage, as well as the impact of different red cell transfusion strategies and the timing and dose of EPO administration, is described in detail in recent reviews (75–77).

Diagnosis
As mentioned above, the nadir in hemoglobin is 6.5 to 9 g/dL at 4 to 8 weeks of age. The diagnosis is usually straightforward—a well preterm baby has a slowly falling hemoglobin with an unremarkable blood film showing normochromic, normocytic red blood cells, slightly low reticulocytes (20×10^9/L), and no nucleated red cells (erythroblasts). Where active management (red cell

transfusion or EPO therapy) is planned, it is important first to consider other potential causes of anemia using clinical features and a diagnostic algorithm such as shown in **Figure 42.3**.

Management

There are broadly three approaches to managing anemia of prematurity: watchful waiting, top-up red cell transfusion, and/or administration of erythropoiesis-stimulating agents, such as EPO and darbepoietin (77). Whichever option is used, it is important that measures to prevent, or at least minimize the severity and duration of anemia, are taken at the same time. These include limiting iatrogenic blood loss by using blood logs, strict criteria for routine blood tests, and miniaturized assays (78–80); iron supplementation for all preterm neonates (iron 3 mg/kg/d from 4 to 6 weeks of age or iron-fortified formula with 0.5 to 0.9 mg/dL iron); and folate supplementation (50 μg daily or 500 μg once weekly) for all preterm neonates (19). The indications, principles, and hazards of neonatal transfusion are well described in recent reviews (77,81) and are briefly summarized below and in Table 42.6.

Top-Up Red Cell Transfusion for Anemia of Prematurity

The decision to transfuse a neonate with anemia of prematurity differs from transfusion in the setting of pathologic causes of anemia, such as hemolysis, largely because of the differing natural history. Many neonatal hemolytic anemias cause a rapid, precipitous drop in hemoglobin concentration that in most cases occurs within the first 1 to 2 weeks of life and the decision to transfuse in these cases is usually straightforward. By contrast, anemia of prematurity has a slower onset, is always self-limiting, usually has a predictable time course, and can often be ameliorated using simple measures, as discussed above. The decision to transfuse is therefore a much more finely balanced one where most of the benefits are unclear and yet the risks are fairly well defined (see below) (82–84).

At present, the most useful guidance about appropriate indications and thresholds for transfusion comes from consensus guidelines for neonatal transfusion that have been prepared by many national organizations (45,85) (http://www.adhb.govt.nz/newborn/Guidelines/Blood/BloodProducts/RedCellTransfusions.htm) (https://professionaleducation.blood.ca/en/transfusion/guide-clinique/neonatal-and-pediatric-transfusion). These generally recommend a restrictive red cell transfusion threshold, supporting the results of a recent meta-analysis (82). Two large randomized controlled trials of liberal versus restrictive transfusion policies in preterm neonates are due to report in the next few years and should provide the valuable evidence needed: the Effect of Transfusion Thresholds on Neurocognitive Outcome of ELBW infants trial (ETTNO trial; NCT01393496) (86), which completed in October 2018, and the Transfusion of Prematures trial (TOPs trial; NCT01702805), which is due to complete in August 2023. In the meantime, an example of the indications for red cell transfusion in neonates recommended by the British Society for Haematology (45) is shown in Table 42.6, which also summarizes the main risks of transfusion. These include metabolic complications, such as hyperkalemia and hypocalcemia; transmitted-associated infections, such as CMV infection if CMV-unscreened blood products are used; and immunologic complications, such as TA-GvHD, which, though rare in neonates, has a high mortality (77).

To minimize these risks, most countries have changed to using "pedipacks" of up to 6 small volume red cell transfusion bags prepared from a single donor unit. The use of "pedipacks" reduces transfusion exposure for multiply transfused preterm neonates, and although this may mean using older red blood cells, this has not been shown to adversely affect neonatal outcome (45). In the United Kingdom, transfusion of CMV-seronegative blood products is also recommended for all transfusions in neonates up to 44 weeks corrected gestational age. The optimal transfusion volume for top-up transfusions in neonates has not been established but most guidelines currently recommend 10 to 20 mL/kg with higher volumes avoided to minimize volume overload. Although irradiation is not necessary for most neonatal transfusions, red cells for IUT (or for neonates who have received IUT) should always be irradiated to prevent TA-GvHD except in a dire emergency. The most serious hazards of transfusion, such as transfusion-related acute lung injury (TRALI) and transfusion-associated circulatory overload (TACO), are well recognized in adults, but their frequency in neonates is unknown and further studies are needed to properly define these complications in a neonatal setting.

Erythropoiesis-Stimulating Agents to Treat and Prevent Neonatal Anemia

The many controlled trials of erythropoiesis-stimulating agents for prevention of neonatal anemia have recently been the subject of Cochrane systematic reviews (75,76). The only erythropoiesis-stimulating agents currently available for use in neonates are recombinant human EPO and darbepoietin, a reengineered form of EPO with a longer half-life.

Recombinant EPO is biologically effective in that it stimulates erythropoiesis in all, or virtually all, preterm infants and there is no evidence of EPO insensitivity. EPO is also able to reduce red cell transfusion requirements in preterm infants (75). Importantly, the recent Cochrane reviews found that the effects of EPO administration varied depending upon when treatment was started. Early treatment (i.e., before the age of 8 days) reduced not only the number of red blood cell transfusions but also the total transfusion volume and donor exposure (75). In addition, early administration reduced the rate of intraventricular hemorrhage (IVH), periventricular leukomalacia (PVL), and NEC without a significant increase in the rate of ROP. Nevertheless, early administration of EPO is not recommended, mainly because it is not yet clear that the modest reduction in transfusions is clinically meaningful. Indeed, a large randomized study (PENUT; NCT01378273) recently reported no neurodevelopmental benefit for high-dose EPO administered within the first 24 hours of life until 32 postmenstrual weeks (87). The results of late administration are even more disappointing. As Aher and Ohlsson report (76), EPO started between 8 and 28 days, causes a modest reduction in the number of red blood cell transfusions, but has no significant effect on donor exposure and the benefits remain unproven. Despite its marginal role in reducing transfusion requirements, erythropoiesis-stimulating agents may become more important again if worries over the safety of blood transfusion lead to reduced availability and parental acceptance of red blood cell transfusion.

At present, the main therapeutic roles for EPO in neonates are:

- in preventing anemia in infants who have received IUTs for allo-antibody-mediated anemia (47)
- in a nonemergency situation where red blood cell transfusions are against the parents' wishes and are not felt to be absolutely essential to save the life of the baby (e.g., preterm babies of Jehovah's Witnesses) (88).

An effective dose of recombinant EPO in this setting is 100 IU/kg subcutaneous injection 3 times per week starting in the first week of life as the hemoglobin does not start to rise until 10 to 14 days of treatment. Iron supplements should be started as soon as possible, to prevent the rapid development of iron deficiency in EPO-treated infants (the dose may need to be increased up to a maximum of 9 mg/kg if iron deficiency develops on the standard dose) (89).

POLYCYTHEMIA

Overview and Definition

Although a link between polycythemia and reduced blood viscosity and blood flow in neonates has been recognized for 50 years, there is no reliable evidence yet to conclusively define a threshold for clinically significant polycythemia (reviewed in Ref. (90)).

TABLE 42.8

Causes of Neonatal Polycythemia

Chronic intrauterine hypoxia

E.g., IUGR, maternal hypertension/preeclampsia or diabetes

Chromosomal disorders

E.g., trisomy 21, trisomy 18, trisomy 13

Twin-to-twin transfusion (especially TAPS)

Endocrine disorders

E.g., thyrotoxicosis, congenital adrenal hyperplasia

Delayed clamping of the cord

TAPS, twin anemia–polycythemia sequence.

However, since at hematocrits above 0.65, there is an exponential rise in blood viscosity, a reasonable working definition of polycythemia is a central venous hematocrit of greater than 0.65 either in a term or preterm neonate. Nevertheless, even at hematocrits greater than 0.70, only a minority of neonates exhibit clinical signs of hyperviscosity. The clinical manifestations of neonatal polycythemia include lethargy, hypotonia, hyperbilirubinemia, and hypoglycemia (8). In severe cases, the increase in blood viscosity can also cause skin necrosis and ischemia of multiple limbs (91,92). Polycythemia may also be a contributory factor in the pathogenesis of NEC and in thrombotic disorders such as neonatal seizures, stroke, and renal vein thrombosis (93).

Causes of Neonatal Polycythemia

The most common cause of neonatal polycythemia is chronic fetal hypoxia secondary to IUGR, maternal hypertension/preeclampsia, or maternal diabetes (**Table 42.8**), which is self-limiting over the first few weeks of life. Polycythemia may be severe in neonates with Down syndrome (94). This appears to be a direct effect of trisomy 21 stimulating fetal erythropoiesis through a mechanism yet to be explained and is equally common in neonates with or without congenital heart disease. The most severe cases of polycythemia are often in monochorionic twins where there has been chronic intertwin transfusion throughout the second and third trimesters of pregnancy (so-called TAPS) (65).

Treatment

Treatment of neonatal polycythemia is controversial and is probably not necessary in infants with very minor symptoms (e.g., borderline hypoglycemia or poor peripheral perfusion). However, most of the evidence supports active management of infants with a hematocrit greater than 0.65 in association with symptoms or signs indicative of an adverse long-term outcome (e.g., refractory hypoglycemia, neurologic signs) or with disseminated intravascular coagulation (DIC). For these infants, partial exchange transfusion (PET) using a crystalloid solution such as normal saline should be performed to reduce the hematocrit to 0.55 (8). Recipient twins in TAPS appear to be at particular risk of severe complications such as cerebral ischemia, limb ischemia, and skin necrosis, a recent study reporting the need for PET in 13/24 (55%) of recipient twin pairs (65). There is no evidence to support the use of fresh frozen plasma (FFP) or albumin (45) for this procedure, both of which carry the risk of transfusion-transmitted infection.

REFERENCES

1. Huyhn A, Dommergues M, Izac B, et al. Characterization of hematopoietic progenitors from human yolk sacs and embryos. *Blood* 1995;86:4474.
2. Popescu D-M, Botting RA, Stephenson E, et al. Decoding the development of the blood and immune systems during human fetal liver haematopoiesis. *Nature* 2019;574:365.
3. Marshall CJ, Thrasher AJ. The embryonic origins of human haematopoiesis. *Br J Haematol* 2001;112:838.
4. O'Byrne S, Elliott N, Rice S, et al. Discovery of a CD10 negative B-progenitor in human fetal life identifies unique ontogeny-related developmental programs. *Blood* 2019;134:1059.
5. Yan H, Hale J, Jaffray J, et al. Developmental differences between neonatal and adult human erythropoiesis. *Am J Hematol* 2018;93:494.
6. Dame C, Fahnenstich H, Freitag P, et al. Erythropoietin mRNA expression in human and neonatal tissue. *Blood* 1998;92:3218.
7. Teramo KA, Klemetti MM, Widness JA. Robust increases in erythropoietin production by the hypoxic fetus is a response to protect the brain and other organs. *Pediatr Res* 2018;84:807.
8. Watts T, Roberts I. Haematological abnormalities of the growth-restricted infant. *Semin Neonatol* 1999;4:41.
9. Songdej D, Babbs C, Higgs DR; BHFS International Consortium. An international registry of survivors with Hb Bart's hydrops fetalis. *Blood* 2017;129:1251.
10. Vinjamur DS, Bauer DE, Orkin SH. Recent progress in understanding and manipulating haemoglobin switching for the haemoglobinopathies. *Br J Haematol* 2018;180:630.
11. Brugnara C, Platt OS. The neonatal erythrocyte and its disorders. In: Orkin S, et al., eds. *Hematology of infancy and childhood*, 7th ed. Philadelphia, PA: W.B. Saunders, 2009:21.
12. Ohls RK. Erythropoietin in extremely low birthweight infants: blood in versus blood out. *J Pediatr* 2002;141:3.
13. Bracci R, Perrone S, Buonocore G. Oxidant injury in neonatal erythrocytes during the perinatal period. *Acta Paediatr Suppl* 2002;91:130.
14. Von Lindern JS, Lopriore E. Management and prevention of neonatal anemia: current evidence and guidelines. *Expert Rev Hematol* 2014;7:195.
15. Christensen R, Henry E, Jopling J, et al. The CBC: reference ranges for neonates. *Semin Perinatol* 2009;33:3.
16. Linderkamp O, Nelle M, Kraus M, et al. The effect of early and late cord clamping on blood viscosity and other hemorheological parameters in full-term infants. *Acta Paediatr* 1992;81:745.
17. Kiserud T. The fetal circulation. *Prenat Diagn* 2004;24:1049.
18. Rao R, Georgieff MK. Perinatal aspects of iron metabolism. *Acta Paediatr* 2002;91(suppl):124.
19. McCarthy EK, Dempsey EM, Kiely ME. Iron supplementation in preterm and low-birth-weight infants: a systematic review of intervention studies. *Nutr Rev* 2019;77:865.
20. Mills RJ, Davies MW. Enteral iron supplementation in preterm and low birth weight infants. *Cochrane Database Syst Rev* 2012;CD005095.
21. Fogarty M, Osborn DA, Askie L, et al. Delayed vs early umbilical cord clamping for preterm infants: a systematic review and meta-analysis. *Am J Obstet Gynecol* 2018;218:1.
22. Brown K. Haematological consequences of parvovirus B19 infection. *Baillieres Best Pract Res Clin Haematol* 2000;13:245.
23. Ronchi A, Zeray F, Lee LE, et al. Evaluation of clinically asymptomatic high risk infants with congenital cytomegalovirus infection. *J Perinatol* 2020;40:89.
24. Bascietto F, Liberati M, Murgano D, et al. Outcomes associated with fetal Parvovirus B19 infection: a systematic review and meta-analysis. *Ultrasound Obstet Gynecol* 2018;52:569.
25. Bellini C, Donarini G, Paladini D, et al. Etiology of non-immune hydrops fetalis: an update. *Am J Med Genet A* 2014;167A:1082.
26. Lejeune A, Cremer M, von Bernuth H, et al. Persistent pure red cell aplasia in dizygotic twins with persistent congenital parvovirus B19 infection—remission following high dose intravenous immunoglobulin. *Eur J Pediatr* 2014;173:1723.
27. Vlachos A, Ball S, Dahl N, et al. Participants of Sixth Annual Daniella Maria Arturi International Consensus Conference. 2008. Diagnosing and treating Diamond Blackfan anaemia: results of an international clinical consensus conference. *Br J Haematol* 2008;142:859.
28. Ulirsch JC, Verboon JM, Kazerounian S, et al. The genetic landscape of Diamond-Blackfan Anemia. *Am J Hum Genet* 2018;103:930.
29. Bartels M, Bierings M. How I manage children with Diamond-Blackfan Anaemia. *Br J Haematol* 2019;184:123.
30. Fermo E, Bianchi P, Notarangelo LD, et al. CDAII presenting as hydrops foetalis: molecular characterization of two cases. *Blood Cells Mol Dis* 2010;45:20.
31. Liu S, Liu YN, Zhen L, Li DZ. Fetal-onset congenital dyserythropoietic anemia type 1 due to CDAN1 mutations presenting as hydrops fetalis. *Pediatr Hematol Oncol* 2018;35:447.
32. Meznarich JA, Draper L, Christensen RD, et al. Fetal presentation of congenital dyserythropoietic anemia type 1 with novel compound heterozygous CDAN1 mutations. *Blood Cells Mol Dis* 2018;71:63.
33. Ravindranath Y, Johnson RM, Goyette G, et al. KLF1 E325K-associated Congenital Dyserythropoietic Anemia Type IV: insights into the variable clinical severity. *J Pediatr Hematol Oncol* 2018;40:e405.
34. Tadiotto E, Maines E, Degani D, et al. Bone marrow features in Pearson syndrome with neonatal onset: a case report and review of the literature. *Pediatr Blood Cancer* 2018;65. doi: 10.1002/pbc.26939

35. de Haas M, Thurik FF, Koelewijn JM, et al. Hemolytic disease of the fetus and newborn. *Vox Sang* 2015;109:99.
36. Vaughan JL, Manning M, Warwick RM, et al. Inhibition of erythroid progenitor cell growth by anti-Kell (K): a mechanism for fetal anemia in K-immunized pregnancies. *N Engl J Med* 1998;338:798.
37. Ziprin JH, Payne E, Hamidi L, et al. ABO incompatibility due to IgG anti-B antibodies presenting with severe fetal anaemia. *Transfus Med* 2005;15:57.
38. Bowden JB, Hebert AA, Rapini RP. Dermal hematopoiesis in neonates: report of five cases. *J Am Acad Dermatol* 1989;20:1104.
39. Herschel M, Karrison T, Wen M, et al. Isoimmunization is unlikely to be the cause of hemolysis in ABO incompatible but direct antiglobulin test-negative neonates. *Pediatrics* 2002;110:127.
40. Zwiers C, van Kamp I, Oepkes D, et al. Intrauterine transfusion and noninvasive treatment options for hemolytic disease of the newborn—review on current management and outcomes. *Expert Rev Hematol* 2017;10:337.
41. Bennardello F, Coluzzi S, Curciarello G, et al. Recommendations for the prevention and treatment of haemolytic disease of the foetus and newborn. *Blood Transfus* 2015;13:109.
42. White J, Qureshi H, Massey E, et al. Guideline for blood grouping and red cell antibody testing in pregnancy. *Transfus Med* 2016;26:246.
43. Zwiers C, Oepkes D, Lopriore E, et al. The near disappearance of fetal hydrops in relation to current state-of-the-art management of red cell alloimmunization. *Prenat Diagn* 2018;38:943.
44. American Association of Pediatrics Subcommittee on Hyperbilirubinemia: management of hyperbilirubinemia in the newborn infant 35 or more weeks of gestation. *Pediatrics* 2004;114:297.
45. New HV, Berryman J, Bolton-Maggs PHB, et al.; on behalf of the British Committee for Standards in Haematology (2016). Guidelines on transfusion for fetuses, neonates and older children. *Br J Haematol* 2016; 175:784.
46. Zwiers C, Scheffer-Rath ME, Lopriore E, et al. Immunoglobulin for alloimmune hemolytic disease in neonates. *Cochrane Database Syst Rev* 2018;CD003313.
47. Zuppa AA, Alighieri G, Calabrese V, et al. Recombinant human erythropoietin in the prevention of late anemia in intrauterine transfused neonates with Rh-isoimmunization. *J Pediatr Hematol Oncol* 2010;32:e95.
48. Gallagher PG. Diagnosis and management of rare congenital nonimmune hemolytic disease. *Hematology Am Soc Hematol Educ Program* 2015;2015:392.
49. Christensen R, Yaish HM, Gallagher PG. A pediatrician's guide to diagnosing and treating hereditary spherocytosis in neonates. *Pediatrics* 2015;135:1107.
50. Grace RF, Glader B. Red blood cell enzyme disorders. *Pediatr Clin North Am* 2018;65:579.
51. Iolascon A, Andolfini I, Russo R. Advances in understanding the pathogenesis of red cell membrane disorders. *Br J Haematol* 2019;187:13.
52. Iolascon A, Andolfo I, Barcellini W, et al. Working study group on red cells and iron of the EHA. *Haematologica* 2017;102:1304.
53. Niss O, Chonat S, Dagaonkar N, et al. Genotype-phenotype correlations in hereditary elliptocytosis and hereditary pyropoikilocytosis. *Blood Cells Mol Dis* 2016;61:4.
54. Grace RF, Bianchi P, van Beers EJ, et al. Clinical spectrum of pyruvate kinase deficiency: data from the Pyruvate Kinase Deficiency Natural History Study. *Blood* 2018;131:2183.
55. Luzzatto L, Poggi V. Glucose-6-phosphate dehydrogenase deficiency. In: Orkin S, et al., eds. *Hematology of infancy and childhood*, 7th ed. Philadelphia, PA: W.B. Saunders, 2009:883.
56. Viprakasit V, Ekwatanakit S, Riolueang S, et al. Mutations in Kruppel factor-like 1 cause transfusion dependent hemolytic anemia and persistence of embryonic globin expression. *Blood* 2014;123:1586.
57. Grace RF, Rose C, Layton DM, et al. Safety and efficacy of Mitapivat in pyruvate kinase deficiency. *N Engl J Med* 2019;381:933.
58. Shook LM, Ware RE. Sickle cell screening in Europe: the time has come. *Br J Haematol* 2018;183:534.
59. Harteveld CL, Higgs DR. Alpha thalassemia. *Orphanet J Rare Dis* 2010; 5:13.
60. Vichinsky EP. Alpha thalassemia major: new mutations, intrauterine management, and outcomes. *Hematology Am Soc Hematol Educ Program* 2009;2009:35.
61. Loureiro B, Martinez-Biarge M, Foti F, et al. MRI patterns of brain injury and neurodevelopmental outcomes in neonates with severe anemia at birth. *Early Hum Dev* 2017;105:17.
62. Fisk NM, Duncombe DJ, Sullivan MH. The basic and clinical science of twin-to-twin transfusion syndrome. *Placenta* 2009;30:379.
63. Kontopoulos E, Chmait RH, Quintero RA. Twin-to-twin transfusion syndrome: definition, staging and ultrasound assessment. *Twin Res Hum Genet* 2016;19:175.
64. Spruijt MS, Lopriore E, Steggerda S, et al. Twin-to-twin transfusion syndrome in the era of fetoscopic laser surgery: antenatal management, neonatal outcome and beyond. *Expert Rev Hematol* 2020;13:259.
65. Verbeek L, Slaghekke F, Sueters M, et al. Hematological disorders at birth in complicated monochorionic twins. *Exp Rev Hematol* 2017;10:525.
66. Christensen RD, Lambert DK, Baer VL, et al. Severe neonatal anemia from fetomaternal hemorrhage: records from a multihospital healthcare system. *J Perinatol* 2013;33:429.
67. Maier JT, Schalinski E, Schneider W, et al. Fetomaternal hemorrhage (FMH), an update: review of literature and illustrative case. *Arch Gynecol Obstet* 2015;292:595.
68. Troia L, Al-Kouatly HB, McCurdy R, et al. The recurrence risk of fetomaternal hemorrhage. *Fetal Diagn Ther* 2019;45:1.
69. Melcer Y, Maymon R, Jauniaux E. Vasa Previa: prenatal diagnosis and management. *Curr Opin Obstet Gynecol* 2018;30:385.
70. Carroll PD, Widness JA. Nonpharmacological, blood conservation techniques for preventing neonatal anemia—effective and promising strategies for reducing transfusion. *Semin Perinatol* 2012;36:232.
71. Whyte RK, Kirpalani H, Asztalos EV, et al. Neurodevelopmental outcome of extremely low birthweight infants randomly assigned to restrictive or liberal thresholds for blood transfusion. *Pediatrics* 2009;123:207.
72. Patel RM, Knezevic A, Shenvi N, et al. Association of red blood cell transfusion, anemia, and necrotizing enterocolitis in very low-birth-weight infants. *JAMA* 2016;315:889.
73. Lust C, Vesoulis Z, Jackups R Jr, et al. Early red cell transfusion is associated with development of severe retinopathy of prematurity. *J Perinatol* 2019;39:393.
74. Whitehead HV, Vesoulis ZA, Maheshwari A, et al. Progressive anemia of prematurity is associated with a critical increase in cerebral oxygen extraction. *Early Hum Dev* 2019;140:104891.
75. Ohlsson A, Aher SM. Early erythropoiesis-stimulating agents in preterm or low birth weight infants. *Cochrane Database Syst Rev* 2020;2:CD004863.
76. Aher SM, Ohlsson A. Late erythropoiesis-stimulating agents to prevent blood transfusion in preterm or low birth weight infants. *Cochrane Database Syst Rev* 2019;1:CD004868.
77. Saito-Benz M, Flanagan P, Berry MJ. Management of anemia in pre-term infants. *Br J Haematol* 2019;188:354.
78. Lin JC, Strauss RG, Kulhavy JC, et al. Phlebotomy overdraw in the neonatal intensive care nursery. *Pediatrics* 2000;106:E19.
79. Widness JA, Madan A, Grindeanu LA, et al. Reduction in red cell transfusions among preterm infants: results of a randomized trial with an in-line blood gas and chemistry monitor. *Pediatrics* 2005;115:1299.
80. Ballin A, Livshiz V, Mimouni FB, et al. Reducing blood transfusion requirements in preterm infants by a new device: a pilot study. *Acta Paediatr* 2009;98:247.
81. Goel R, Josephson CD. Recent advances in transfusions neonates/infants. *F1000Res* 2018;7:F1000 Faculty Rev-609.
82. Keir A, Pal S, Trivella M, et al. Adverse effects of red blood cell transfusions in neonates: a systematic review and meta-analysis. *Transfusion* 2016;56:2773.
83. Howarth C, Banerjee J, Aladangady N. Red blood cell transfusion in preterm infants: current evidence and controversies. *Neonatology* 2018;114:7.
84. Keir AK, New H, Robitaille N, et al. Approaches to understanding and interpreting the risks of red blood cell transfusion in neonates. *Transfus Med* 2019;29:231.
85. Carson JL, Guyatt G, Heddle NM, et al. Clinical practice guidelines from the AABB: red blood cell transfusion thresholds and storage. *JAMA* 2016;316:2025.
86. Eicher C, Seitz G, Bevot A, et al. Surgical management of extremely low birth weight infants with neonatal bowel perforation: a single center experience and review of the literature. *Neonatology* 2012;101:85.
87. Juul SE, Comstock BA, Wadhawan R, et al. A randomised trial of erythropoietin for neuroprotection in preterm infants. *N Engl J Med* 2020;382:233.
88. Horan M, Stutchfield PR. Severe congenital myotonic dystrophy and severe anaemia of prematurity in an infant of Jehovah's Witness parents. *Dev Med Child Neurol* 2001;43:346.
89. Bechensteen AG, Haga P, Halvorsen S, et al. Erythropoietin, protein, and iron supplementation and the prevention of the anaemia of prematurity. *Arch Dis Child* 1993;69:19.
90. Lucewicz A, Fisher K, Henry A, et al. Review of the correlation between blood flow velocity and polycythemia in the fetus, neonate and adult: appropriate diagnostic levels need to be determined for twin anemia-polycythemia sequence. *Ultrasound Obstet Gynecol* 2016;47:152.
91. Robyr R, Lewi L, Salomon LJ, et al. Prevalence and management of late fetal complications following successful selective laser coagulation of chorionic plate anastomoses in twin-to-twin transfusion syndrome. *Am J Obstet Gynecol* 2006;194:796.
92. Stranak Z, Korcek P, Hympanova L, et al. Prenatally acquired multiple limb ischemia in a very low birthweight monochorionic twin. *Fetal Diagn Ther* 2015;41:237.
93. Kirkham FJ, Zafeiriou D, Howe D, et al. Fetal stroke and cerebrovascular disease: advances in understanding from lenticulostrate venous imaging, alloimmune thrombocytopenia and monochorionic twins. *Eur J Paediatr Neurol* 2018;22:989.
94. Roberts I, Alford K, Hall G, et al. GATA1-mutant clones are frequent and often unsuspected in babies with Down syndrome: identification of a population at risk of leukemia. *Blood* 2013;122:3908.

NEUTROPHILS

Ontogeny and Maturation

Neutrophils often constitute the largest leukocyte subset and participate heavily in the immune response. Mature neutrophils are the last leukocytes to appear in fetal blood and are seen at approximately 16 weeks of gestational age. Granulocyte colony-stimulating factor (G-CSF) levels increase just before birth, which stimulates a rapid increase in neutrophil number (1). The neutrophil life cycle occurs chronologically in three distinct areas: bone marrow, blood, and finally tissues. Granulopoiesis in both term and preterm neonates takes place in the bone marrow, in the form of immature myeloid progenitors: myeloblasts, promyelocytes, and myelocytes (2). These cells constitute the neutrophil proliferative pool (NPP), as they retain the capacity to reproduce. Metamyelocytes develop into band cells and then segmented neutrophils, all of which constitute the neutrophil storage pool (NSP), where proliferation no longer occurs. The NSP is meant to be a readily available source of neutrophils in the face of inflammatory states such as sepsis, which is quickly mobilized in adults. Newborn infants have smaller NSPs, which can be depleted quickly (3). In adult rats, for instance, the NSP contains approximately 6×10^9 cells/kg; a term newborn rat at 21 days' gestation carries an NSP of 1.2×10^9 cells/kg (3). NSP depletion is particularly pronounced in preterm infants (4).

Circulating Neutrophils

The neutrophils in circulation are also conceptually divided into two pools: cells freely traveling in the bloodstream and marginated cells adherent to endothelium. Marginated cells are able to move quickly and transiently into circulation after stressful activities (such as crying or exercise) or administration of sympathomimetic drugs, such as epinephrine or corticosteroids (5,6). Circulating neutrophils, on the other hand, migrate into tissue after a few hours and are more abundant during infection. Normal neutrophil values are difficult to assess in preterm infants, as preterm birth is inherently abnormal and may be influenced by conditions that alter neutrophil counts (e.g., sepsis, preeclampsia). Nevertheless, values from a large database have been helpful in demonstrating typically occurring neutrophil counts in the first 72 hours of life (7). Preterm infants born at less than 28 weeks of gestation frequently have absolute neutrophil counts (ANCs) between 5,000 and 10,000 and gradually peak within that range at 24 to 32 hours of life. The 95th percentile, however, peaks at above 30,000 by 24 hours of life. Older preterm infants born at gestational ages of 28 to 36 weeks have a trajectory similar to that of term infants, peaking at 10 to 12 hours of life and gradually decreasing. Infants at 28 to 36 weeks of gestation peak at a median ANC of approximately 10,000, while infants older than 36 weeks of gestation peak at approximately 15,000 (7). Mode of delivery, sex, and race may impact ANC. Of infants born by cesarean delivery, those born without preceding labor had lower ANCs, and female infants had higher ANCs than did males (8). Neutrophil counts are often lower in infants of African American ancestry, and genetic studies have shown that this difference is particularly notable in a subgroup negative for the Duffy antigen (9).

NEUTROPHIL PATHOLOGY

Neonatal Neutrophilia

Physiologic Neutrophilia

The surge in neutrophil counts in the first week of life can be considered "physiologic," as it is stimulated by cytokines involved in parturition and transition (**Fig. 43.1**). Surges in placental G-CSF and macrophage colony-stimulating factor (M-CSF) have been implicated, with levels peaking the day after birth, still high on days 3 to 5, and returning to baseline by day 14 (10,11). G-CSF participates both in the recruitment of neutrophil progenitors as well as in the terminal differentiation and activation of mature neutrophils.

Nonphysiologic Neutrophilia

Band forms exceeding 20% to 30% of the total neutrophil count should be considered an abnormal increase in neutrophil production (12). Many centers use an "immature:total ratio," often abbreviated as the "I:T ratio," to assist in the diagnosis of sepsis when the clinical scenario is ambiguous. However, the validity of this measurement is controversial as some studies have consistently found neutropenia in septic infants. Additional etiologies of increased production include leukemoid reactions, which describe early transient increases in leukocyte counts to more than 50×10^9/L, associated with accelerated neutrophil production (13). Though some leukemoid reactions are idiopathic, pathogenic causes such as bacterial sepsis or TORCH infections may be implicated. Additionally, such reactions may be seen in Down syndrome. Antenatal betamethasone exposure is a benign etiology of neonatal leukemoid reaction, though it should only be suspected once life-threatening etiologies are excluded (13). Leukemoid reactions are thought to be associated with better survival (14), but also with the later development of bronchopulmonary dysplasia in low birth weight infants (15).

Neonatal Neutropenia

ANCs below 1,000 cells/µL are generally considered clinically significant. When present, neutropenia is most often seen in the first week of life. The neutrophil count should be evaluated along with the full leukocyte count, red blood cells, and platelets, to screen for pancytopenia. Abnormal findings may suggest bone marrow failure, which can eventually lead to biopsy if severe and prolonged (16). More often, neutropenia is isolated. As with all deficiencies, the etiologies of neutropenia can be broadly categorized into those of inadequate production or of excessive usage or destruction. Further workup should be directed by infant and maternal histories, though sepsis should always be considered.

Neutropenia in Infants of Hypertensive Mothers

Early neutropenia is commonly seen in infants born to mothers with hypertension, and is likely due to decreased neutrophil production (17,18). The severity of neutropenia seems to be correlated with the severity of maternal hypertension and also to the degree of growth restriction in the infant. Neutropenia in these infants usually resolves within the first 72 hours and almost always within 1 week. There is conflicting evidence about whether or not these newborns are at greater risk for sepsis before their ANCs normalize (19,20).

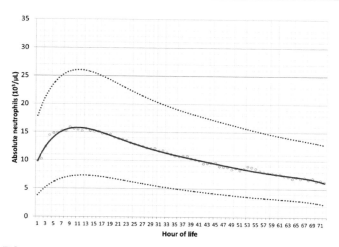

FIGURE 43.1 Neutrophil levels of neonates born at greater than or equal to 36 weeks of gestation during the first 72 hours after birth showing the mean values (*solid blue line*), 5th and 95th percentiles (*dotted red lines*). (Reprinted from Henry E, Christensen RD. Reference intervals in neonatal hematology. *Clin Perinatol* 2015;42:483. Copyright © 2015 Elsevier. With permission.)

Neutropenia of Prematurity

Neutropenia is found commonly in preterm infants in the NICU who are concurrently experiencing anemia of prematurity with active reticulocytosis and are otherwise well. Infants who are born with an extremely low birth weight (ELBW, <1,000 g) are five times more likely to experience neutropenia than babies born weighing greater than 1,000 g (21). However, regardless of absolute size, those who are born small for gestational age have a higher incidence of neutropenia versus those who are born at an appropriate weight for gestational age, 6% versus 1%, respectively (22). It is postulated that the bone marrow commits to erythropoiesis, consuming stem cell progenitors and growth factors and therefore limiting granulopoiesis (23,24). Among those infants with prolonged neutropenia and no identified etiology, the term "idiopathic" neutropenia may be applied and likely reflects diminished production (25).

Immune-Mediated Neutropenia

Alloimmune neutropenia occurs when a sensitized mother produces IgG against paternally acquired antigens on fetal neutrophils (26). IgG antibodies readily cross the placenta, significantly decreasing fetal neutrophil count through pathophysiology that mirrors Rh-hemolytic disease. Neutrophil-specific antibodies will be found in maternal and infant sera; however, the mother's neutrophil count would only be affected if the culpable antibody arises from her own autoimmune neutropenia (27). In such cases, the pathophysiology instead mirrors that of immune thrombocytopenia. Alloimmune neutropenia most frequently involves human neutrophil antigen (HNA)-1a, HNA-1b, or HNA-2a. If an immune-mediated neutropenia is suspected, the mother's neutrophil count, maternal neutrophil antigen typing, and an antineutrophil antibody screen are indicated (28). The disease is typically self-limiting and resolves within 6 to 7 weeks of detachment from the placenta. During this time, neonates are susceptible to infections and should be monitored closely. Most infections are mild and cutaneous, but life-threatening illnesses are also possible (29).

Sepsis

Neutropenia frequently develops in septic infants, as their limited NSPs and NPPs are easily depleted (4,30). This is in contrast to adult sepsis, where both pools are larger and can be replenished quickly. Adult rats exposed to group B streptococci (GBS) responded with a transient decrease in circulating neutrophils

by 33%, followed by profound neutrophilia and an increase in the progenitor pool size. In contrast, neonatal rats infected with GBS depleted 80% of their NSPs and 50% of their NPPs, without increasing production rate (31,32). Once neutrophils are in circulation, there is increased migration into tissues and, in some cases, bone marrow suppression. In addition, classic neutrophil functions such as chemotaxis and phagocytosis may be impaired due to immaturity (30).

Other Causes (Table 43.1)

Inadequate neutrophil production occurs in the setting of several genetic sequences and syndromes, many of which present later in infancy or childhood (e.g., Kostmann syndrome, Shwachman-Diamond syndrome, or cartilage–hair hypoplasia, to name a few). When all hematologic lines are affected, bone marrow suppression may have occurred due to exposure to certain medications or viral infections. Consumptive etiologies of neutropenia are usually related to profound inflammation, such as in necrotizing enterocolitis (NEC). Additionally, donor infants in twin-to-twin transfusion syndrome (TTTS) tend to experience neutropenia (33), as do infants with Rh-hemolytic disease (34). Finally, ANC may be affected by measurement technique, for instance, in cases of pseudoneutropenia due to sample agglutination.

Management of Neutropenia

The management of neutropenia is often directed by its presumed etiology. In cases that are expected to be self-limited, most clinicians opt to wait for resolution. These cases include infants experiencing neutropenia after maternal hypertension, TTTS, or Rh-hemolytic disease (28). Colony-stimulating factors are sometimes considered for infants whose ANC remains low for a prolonged period of time. However, there are conflicting data about their efficacy and risk of mortality secondary to use (35,36).

Recombinant G-CSF stimulates neutrophil production, maturation, and release from the bone marrow and secondarily reduces neutrophil apoptosis (37). G-CSF is the primary endogenous regulator of the circulating neutrophil pool. Granulocyte-macrophage colony-stimulating factor (GM-CSF) generates both granulocyte and macrophage colonies from precursor cells and is an inducible factor present in states of stress and inflammation (38). Rapid recovery of ANC may be seen within 2 days after administration (36). Results of trials employing G-CSF and GM-CSF have been disappointing in terms of preventing sepsis and mortality; however, GM-CSF was shown to be helpful in reducing mortality in infants who were concurrently septic and neutropenic in one cohort (35). Another cohort showed an increased incidence of secondary sepsis and mortality in treated infants; however, the treated group was more ill at baseline as judged by age, weight, and need for cardiopulmonary support (36). Certain subgroups of neutropenic infants may be better selected for this

TABLE 43.1
Causes of Neutropenia

Decreased Production	Increased Consumption or Destruction
Infants of hypertensive mothers	Alloimmune neutropenia
Clinically significant anemia (anemia of prematurity, Rh-hemolytic disease, donors of twin–twin transfusion syndrome)	Bacterial or fungal sepsis
Bone marrow suppression from viral infections (TORCH and others)	Necrotizing enterocolitis
Drug-induced bone marrow suppression	
Genetic syndromes that impair neutrophil precursors or cause bone marrow failure	

drug, such as those with immune-mediated disease. G-CSF has the tendency to down-regulate antigen expression, and newly produced neutrophils may therefore be less susceptible to circulating antibodies (39).

Intravenous immunoglobulin G (IVIG) may be trialed in infants with immune-mediated neutropenia who do not respond to G-CSF alone, to assist with mobilizing neutrophils from the NSP (40). Exchange transfusions and corticosteroid therapy are generally considered ineffective. Immune-mediated neutropenia may recur in following pregnancies, and subsequent siblings should have their ANCs proactively evaluated at birth and at 1 week of age.

Functional Defects of Neutrophils

Qualitatively, cord blood neutrophils of preterm infants are less capable of chemotaxis and chemokinesis than are those of term infants (41). Additionally, exposure to antenatal magnesium sulfate was associated with impaired chemotaxis and random motility of preterm neutrophils, with reduction in functional activity correlating directly with maternal serum magnesium level (42).

Leukocyte Adhesion Deficiency Syndromes

Leukocyte adhesion deficiency syndromes are characterized by the inability of neutrophils and other leukocytes to adequately migrate to a site of inflammation. Migration is completed through rolling, activation, adhesion, and transmigration across a blood vessel, with various proteins necessary for each step. Mutations in any of these proteins, namely integrins, cell adhesion molecules, and chemokines, can be implicated in the inability to form pus at the site of injury. In neonates, the classic first sign of disease is impaired detachment of the dried umbilical cord (43).

MONOCYTES: PHYSIOLOGY AND FUNCTION

Ontogeny and Maturation

Macrophages of monocyte origin are found in the yolk sac as early as 3 to 6 weeks of gestation and are the predominant hematopoietic cell lineage prior to the emergence of erythroid cells. Hematopoiesis moves to the fetal liver at 6 weeks, until the bone marrow takes over during the second trimester (1,44).

Macrophages can be identified by CD11b on the cell surface as early as 12 weeks of gestation. At 15 to 21 weeks of gestation, CD14 begins to appear on monocytes and is expressed at adult levels. Class II major histocompatibility complex (MHC) antigens HLA-DR, HLA-DP, and HLA-DQ show lower expression on neonatal monocytes relative to adult monocytes. Term neonatal monocytes express toll-like receptors (TLR)-2 and -4 at adult levels but show reduced capacity for tumor necrosis factor (TNF) release upon stimulation with TLR agonists. Preterm neonatal monocytes show lower TLR4 expression (30).

The production and differentiation of monocytes as well as their functional activation are attributed to M-CSF. M-CSF is increased in cord blood and continues to rise during the neonatal period (45).

Circulating Monocyte Pool

Evaluation of a cohort of 63,000 neonatal blood counts led to the discovery that absolute monocyte counts (AMCs) rise through the first 2 postnatal weeks (46). Full-term infants tend to display relative physiologic monocytosis throughout the neonatal period. This finding is supported by previous work showing that the concentrations of monocyte precursors rise during this time as well (47). Nonphysiologic explanations for monocytosis during this time have been attributed to prematurity, transfusions of red blood cells or albumin, theophylline therapy, or congenital infections such as candidiasis and syphilis. Early monocytopenia is less frequently encountered than monocytosis and may be found in cases where

all leukocyte lineages are suppressed, for instance, after intrauterine growth restriction (48).

Significant changes in AMC after the first 2 weeks of extrauterine life are likely nonphysiologic. In particular, a connection has been noted between a fall in AMC and NEC, and AMC may emerge as a useful biomarker. In a cohort of infants with feeding intolerance, a drop in AMC of 20% or more carried a sensitivity of 0.70 and specificity of 0.71 in distinguishing NEC from benign symptoms (49). Another cohort showed that the degree of AMC drop correlated with severity of NEC disease (50).

Monocyte Subsets

The circulating monocyte pool is composed of at least two distinct subsets of cells. "Classic" monocytes are CD14+/CD16− and represent the vast majority of blood monocytes in term infants. These monocytes also express C-C chemokine receptor (CCR) 2, as well as CD64 and CD62L. A smaller proportion is composed of "nonclassic" monocytes, characterized as CD14low/CD16+, which lack CCR2. Monocytes that express both CD14 and CD16 demonstrate phagocytic activity upon exposure to lipopolysaccharide (LPS). These cells are capable of producing TNF and interleukin (IL)-1β as part of an inflammatory cascade. Another subset of CD16+ monocytes that express low CD14 (CD14dim/CD16+) is poorly phagocytic and does not produce pro-inflammatory cytokines; these are "resident" monocytes that patrol blood vessels in the steady state and extravasate to tissues once called upon to manage infection or wound healing (51–54).

Immaturity of Neonatal Phagocytosis

Upon injury or bacterial invasion, tissues and organs call upon monocytes by the use of chemoattractants. Once activated, monocytes leave the bloodstream through transendothelial migration to perform a variety of functions at the site of injury, including phagocytosis with a respiratory burst (55). Monocyte chemotaxis to injured tissues is less efficient in neonates than in adults (30).

Once exposed to microbial antigens, monocytes and macrophages are further activated by inflammatory cytokines such as IL-1β, interferon (IFN)-α, and TNF through CD14 and TLR signaling. An oxygen-dependent respiratory burst creates hydroxyl radicals that impart damage to microbial membranes (56). Relative to term monocytes, preterm monocytes may have weaker superoxide production and degranulation in vitro; however, their ability to kill pathogens is probably comparable to adult monocytes. Similarly, TLR expression in term neonatal monocytes approximates that of adult monocytes, but there are functional differences such as sensitivity to TLR ligands (55,57).

Neonates, particularly those born preterm, are at greater risk of sepsis than are older children and adults. Though there are developmental deficiencies throughout the immune system, this increased risk owes partly to the immaturity of neutrophil- and monocyte-derived macrophages (1,30). In order to contribute to immune defense, macrophages must migrate to the site of injury efficiently and in adequate numbers; once present, they must be capable of ingesting and killing microorganisms. Compared to adult neutrophils, neonatal neutrophils showed decreased deformability, adherence, chemotaxis, phagocytosis, aggregation, bacterial killing, and oxidative metabolism. Disparities are also present in neonatal monocytes, but less severe than in neutrophils.

Once presented with a pathogen, leukocytes must be able to respond by up-regulating TLR expression. Monocytes from VLBW infants expressed TLR4 at much lower baseline levels than in mature infants and adults, and also showed decreased production of IL-1β, IL-6, and TNF upon stimulation by LPS. In another cohort, septic neonates were able to increase TLR2 expression on monocytes but not neutrophils and were unable to increase TLR4 expression (1,30,58).

LYMPHOCYTES

Lymphocytes play an important role in battling infections with specificity and building immune memory. There are two primary groups of lymphocytes: T-lymphocytes and B-lymphocytes.

T Lymphocytes

Ontogeny and Maturation

The thymus emerges at approximately 6 weeks of gestation from the third branchial arch. By 9 weeks, the thymic cortex becomes populated with T-cell precursor stem cells, which mature as they migrate inwards to the medulla. During the process of differentiation, these thymocytes undergo genetic rearrangements in order to display a T-cell receptor (TCR) with unique antigen specificity. Prior to differentiation, they are referred to as "double-negative thymocytes," a title they lose upon expression of CD4 and CD8 receptors. Having then earned the title of "double-positive thymocytes," they proceed to lose expression of either CD4 or CD8 to become "single positive." Mature T cells that enter the thymic medulla are single positive. T cells that recognize self-peptides are negatively selected and eliminated during this process (1,59–62).

T-Lymphocyte Subtypes

Broadly, T cells are characterized by their cell surface expression of CD4, CD8, or neither. CD4$^+$ T cells can be further classified as T helper (T_h) cells or T regulatory cells (T_{regs}). CD8$^+$ cells develop into cytotoxic T lymphocytes. Neonates have a high CD4/CD8 ratio owing to higher CD4$^+$ cell counts (63).

Cytotoxic T Lymphocytes

Once activated by antigen recognition, CD8$^+$ cells differentiate into cytotoxic T lymphocytes that effect cell death through the creation of cell membrane pores, using the perforin/granzyme system. They are an important line of defense against intracellular pathogens and play additional roles in graft rejection and tumor surveillance.

Natural Killer T Cells

Natural killer (NK) cells are unique lymphocytes that are part of the innate immune system and therefore do not require priming by prior exposure. They are present in the fetus as early as 9 weeks of gestation (1). NK cells are particularly useful in removing virally infected or malignant cells from circulation, using a perforin system similar to that found in CD8$^+$ cells.

T Helper Cells

T_h cells consist of three distinct subtypes: T_h1, T_h2, and T_h17. T_h1 cells are pro-inflammatory and assist monocyte-derived phagocytes in providing cellular immunity against intracellular pathogens, particularly viruses. T_h2 cells assist B cells and play special roles in defense against helminthic infections as well as allergic reactions through modulation of antibody isotype switching. T_h17 cells enhance neutrophil recruitment to sites of infection and participate in macrophage activation (64). A classic assumption of neonatal T_h cell differentiation is a bias toward T_h2. While most of T-cell development *in utero* is aimed at understanding self-peptides, the exposure to the external environment at birth calls upon T_h cells to start recognizing nonself antigens, and T_h2 cells take a leading role (1). Differentiation and skew of T_h cells begin with the pregnant mother; the degree of maternal T_h2 skew may be predictive of atopic disease in childhood (65).

Regulatory T Cells

Tregs participate in immune response down-regulation by expressing inhibitory cytokines (IL-10, TGF-β) and modulators of cyclic AMP. There have been two Tregs populations identified: those that derive from the thymus (tT_{regs}) and those that develop in the periphery from naïve T cells (pT_{regs}). Though Tregs represent less than 5% of all CD4$^+$ in cord blood at term, they are critical during gestation in promoting self-tolerance. This specific tolerogenic subset constitutes 15% to 20% of all CD4$^+$ cells in the midgestation fetus (66,67). Genetic defects in T_{regs} development may lead to IPEX syndrome (immunodysregulation, polyendocrinopathy, enteropathy), a frequently fatal X-linked disorder characterized by autoimmune symptoms in multiple organs (1).

γδ T Cells

The role of γδ T cells has not yet been fully described. These cells can be detected as early as 6 to 8 weeks in the fetal thymus and liver and constitute approximately 10% of circulating T cells at 16 week of gestation, but only 3% at term. Postnatally, they are found primarily on the skin and mucosal surfaces. They produce pro-inflammatory IFN-γ and TNF and have some cytotoxic capabilities, though diminished in comparison to adults (68,69).

T-Cell Function in Neonates

Despite higher CD4$^+$ counts, cytokine production is overall decreased, particularly of IL-12, IFN-γ, and IL-17. T_{regs} in both term and preterm infants show decreased function as well, particularly in their ability to modulate dendritic cell communication, an important step in T-cell activation (70). Additionally, neonatal T cells show lower expression of CD40 ligand, which binds CD40 cell surface receptor on B cells during immunoglobulin isotype switching (71). Finally, neonatal cytotoxic T cells contain lower levels of perforin and are therefore less capable of cytotoxic pore formation, though some studies have found normal levels by 1 year of age (1,72).

B Lymphocytes

Ontogeny

The pre–B cell can be seen as early as 7 to 8 weeks of gestation in the fetal liver (1,73) and must begin to express surface IgM (sIgM$^+$) before entering the vasculature at approximately 12 weeks of gestation. Cells with other immunoglobulin isotypes (sIgA, sIgG, sIgD) are also seen between 10 and 12 weeks of gestation. The lymph nodes acquire B cells at approximately 16 weeks of gestation. By 22 weeks, the fetal B-cell count is similar to that in adults (73,74). The ratio of B cells to T cells is similar in cord blood and adult blood, though the absolute counts are greater in neonates. B-cell counts continue to rise until 3 to 4 months of age, at which point they gradually decline over the next few years (75). The circulating pool is generally the same in preterm and term infants but may be smaller in those who experienced intrauterine growth restriction (76).

Subtypes

Fetal and neonatal B cells express CD5 and are referred to as B1 cells, differentiating them from the conventional B2 cells seen in adults. Approximately 90% of B cells in cord blood are CD5$^+$, compared to 25% to 35% of adult B cells. The role of these cells has not yet been fully realized, though it is known that they show greater capacity for self-renewal independent of the bone marrow. B1 cells localize to the spleen and peritoneal cavity and have limited immunoglobulin production capabilities, implying that they probably contribute to innate immunity rather than adaptive (74,75,77).

Immunoglobulins

The neonatal antibody response is limited and is usually of the IgM subtype. There is a plethora of IgG antibodies in serum, but the vast majority is acquired transplacentally, starting at 13 weeks of gestation and rising linearly until birth. The majority is transferred in the third trimester, particularly after the 36th week of gestation. Term neonates may have IgG concentrations exceeding their mothers' by 20% to 30% (78). Preterm infants are born with a smaller IgG pool, having not experienced a full third trimester *in utero* (79).

Generally speaking, postnatal age more accurately predicts antibody response than gestational age. Preterm and term infants showed similarly suppressed responses to diphtheria toxoid vaccine in the first 10 days after birth compared with those who were vaccinated at 1 to 2 months of life. Deficiencies in neonatal B-cell function may include a delayed isotype switch or inability to respond to all antigens in a vaccine (80).

Lymphopenia

Lymphopenia refers to patients whose absolute lymphocyte count (ALC) is lower than 1,500 cells/μL blood. In such cases, it is important to evaluate the number of cells in each lymphocyte subset and their relative abundance to each other. Lymphopenia should always raise the question of underlying immunodeficiency, such as severe combined immunodeficiency disorder (SCID), DiGeorge syndrome, ataxia–telangiectasia, hyper-IgM syndrome, or Wiskott-Aldrich syndrome, among others. When triggered by an infection, lymphopenia may be accompanied by neutropenia.

SCID describes a group of syndromes characterized by deficiency or defectiveness in both the B- and T-cell lines. Inheritance is usually recessive and may be autosomal or X-linked. These syndromes are characterized by thymic hypoplasia or aplasia, T-cell cytopenia, along with various degrees of deficiency in the B-cell and NK-cell counts (81). Diagnosis of SCID is often suggested by a low T-cell receptor excision circles (TRECs) count on newborn screening, reflective of low T-cell generation. Preterm infants may have false-positive newborn screen results (82).

DiGeorge syndrome, usually caused by a deletion at chromosome 22q11.2, is characterized by thymic hypoplasia or aplasia in addition to a range of cardiac malformations and characteristic facial features. The parathyroid gland may also be hypoplastic, and the resulting hypocalcemia is often a clue to diagnosis. Patients with hypoplastic thymic glands typically have deficient but not absent T cells, resulting in a sufficient immune response to most insults. DiGeorge syndrome patients with thymic aplasia are more likely to suffer from clinical immunodeficiency (83).

▌DENDRITIC CELLS

DCs (dendritic cells) are uniquely shaped mononuclear cells that are highly specialized to perform antigen presentation, T-cell activation, and other crucial roles in both humoral and adaptive immunity. Visual examination of dendritic cells reveals many lamellipodia, making the cell membranes appear ruffled. The appearance of these cells is similar in neonatal and adult blood, though they are less prevalent in cord blood (0.5% vs. 1% in adult blood).

Ontogeny and Subtypes

Generally, DCs are derived from pluripotent hematopoietic stem cells that proceed along the myeloid or lymphoid differentiation pathways. There are four major subtypes of DCs: myeloid DCs, which present antigens to cytotoxic T cells; plasmacytoid DCs, which localize to lymph nodes and are particularly active during viral infections; CD14+ DCs, which arise from classic monocytes; and organ-specific DCs such as Langerhans cells or microglia. The peripheral blood typically circulates pDCs and mDCs (1,54).

▌EOSINOPHILS

Robust eosinophil counts are frequently noted in neonates, particularly those born preterm. The incidence of eosinophilia was 69% in one cohort of VLBW infants, most commonly in the third week of life. Infants with higher eosinophil counts in the first week of life were more likely to progress to bronchopulmonary dysplasia (84).

Associations have also been drawn between eosinophilia and critical illness, as it was most often noted in those who were intubated, on parenteral nutrition, or receiving blood transfusions (85). The function of these eosinophils in critical illness is unclear; it has been suggested that immaturity of the gastrointestinal and respiratory tracts leads to increased presentation of foreign antigens. Even in well children, eosinophils tend to migrate toward surfaces exposed to the outside world, such as skin and the respiratory tract (86). They are the predominant cell type in erythema toxicum, a benign and common skin rash.

REFERENCES

1. Zhang X, Zhivaki D, Lo-Man R. Unique aspects of the perinatal immune system. *Nat Rev Immunol* 2017;17(8):495.
2. Calhoun DA, Li Y, Braylan RC, et al. Assessment of the contribution of the spleen to granulocytopoiesis and erythropoiesis of the mid-gestation human fetus. *Early Hum Dev* 1996;46(3):217.
3. Erdman SH, Christensen RD, Bradley PP. Supply and release of storage neutrophils. A developmental study. *Biol Neonate* 1982;41:132.
4. Engle WA, McGuire WA, Schreiner RL, et al. Neutrophil storage pool depletion in neonates with sepsis and neutropenia. *J Pediatr* 1988;113(4):747.
5. Steel CM, French EB, Aitchison WRC. Studies on adrenaline-induced leucocytosis in normal man: I. The role of the spleen and of the thoracic duct. *Br J Haematol* 1971;21(4):413.
6. Christensen RD, Rothstein G. Pitfalls in the interpretation of leukocyte counts of newborn infants. *Am J Clin Pathol* 1979;72:608.
7. Henry E, Christensen RD. Reference intervals in neonatal hematology. *Clin Perinatol* 2015;42(3):483.
8. Schmutz N, Henry E, Jopling J, et al. Expected ranges for blood neutrophil concentrations of neonates: the Manroe and Mouzinho charts revisited. *J Perinatol* 2008;28(4):275.
9. Lupton BA, Pendray MR. Regionalized neonatal emergency transport. *Semin Neonatol* 2004;9(2):125.
10. Barak Y, Leibovitz E, Mogilner B, et al. The in vivo effect of recombinant human granulocyte-colony stimulating factor in neutropenic neonates with sepsis. *Eur J Pediatr* 1997;156(8):643.
11. Ishii E, Masuyama T, Yamaguchi H, et al. Production and expression of granulocyte- and macrophage-colony-stimulating factors in newborns: their roles in leukocytosis at birth. *Acta Haematol* 1995;94:23.
12. Akenzua I. Neutrophil and band counts in the diagnosis of neonatal infections. *Pediatrics* 1974;54(1):38.
13. Calhoun DA, Kirk JF, Christensen RD. Incidence, significance, and kinetic mechanism responsible for leukemoid reactions in patients in the neonatal intensive care unit: a prospective evaluation. *J Pediatr* 1996;129(3):7.
14. Rastogi S, Rastogi D, Sundaram R, et al. Leukemoid reaction in extremely low-birth-weight infants. *Am J Perinatol* 1999;16(2):93.
15. Zanardo V, Savio V, Giacomin C, et al. Relationship between neonatal leukemoid reaction and bronchopulmonary dysplasia in low-birth-weight infants: a cross-sectional study. *Am J Perinatol* 2002;19(7):379.
16. Nittala S, Subbarao GC, Maheshwari A. Evaluation of neutropenia and neutrophilia in preterm infants. *J Matern Fetal Neonatal Med* 2012;25 (suppl 5):100.
17. Koenig J, Christensen R. Incidence, neutrophil kinetics, and natural history of neonatal neutropenia associated with maternal hypertension. *N Engl J Med* 1989;321(9):557.
18. Koenig J, Christensen R. The mechanism responsible for diminished neutrophil production in neonates delivered of women with pregnancy-induced hypertension. *Am J Obstet Gynecol* 1991;165(2):467.
19. Doron MW, Makhlouf RA, Katz VL, et al. Increased incidence of sepsis at birth in neutropenic infants of mothers with preeclampsia. *J Pediatr* 1994;125(3):452.
20. Paul DA, Leef KH, Sciscione A, et al. Preeclampsia does not increase the risk for culture proven sepsis in very low birth weight infants. *Am J Perinatol* 1999;16(7):365.
21. Christensen RD, Henry E, Wiedmeier SE, et al. Low blood neutrophil concentrations among extremely low birth weight neonates: data from a multihospital health-care system. *J Perinatol* 2006;26(11):682.
22. Christensen RD, Yoder BA, Baer VL, et al. Early-onset neutropenia in small-for-gestational-age infants. *Pediatrics* 2015;136(5):e1259.
23. Carr R, Modi N, Doré CJ, et al. A randomized, controlled trial of prophylactic granulocyte-macrophage colony-stimulating factor in human newborns less than 32 weeks gestation. *Pediatrics* 1999;103(4):796.
24. Christensen RD, Harper TE, Rothstein G. Granulocyte-macrophage progenitor cells in term and preterm neonates. *J Pediatr* 1986;109(6):1047.
25. Juul S, Calhoun D, Christensen R. "Idiopathic neutropenia" in very low birth weight infants. *Acta Paediatr* 1998;87(9):963.

26. Porcelijn L, de Haas M. Neonatal alloimmune neutropenia. *Transfus Med Hemother* 2018;45(5):311.

27. Kameoka J, Funato T, Miura T, et al. Autoimmune neutropenia in pregnant women causing neonatal neutropenia. *Br J Haematol* 2001;114(1):198.

28. Del Vecchio A, Christensen RD. Neonatal neutropenia: what diagnostic evaluation is needed and when is treatment recommended? *Early Hum Dev* 2012;88:S19.

29. Farruggia P. Immune neutropenias of infancy and childhood. *World J Pediatr* 2016;12(2):142.

30. Levy O. Innate immunity of the newborn: basic mechanisms and clinical correlates. *Nat Rev Immunol* 2007;7(5):379.

31. Christensen RD, Macfarlane JL, Taylor NL, et al. Blood and marrow neutrophils during experimental group B Streptococcal infection: quantification of the stem cell, proliferative, storage and circulating pools. *Pediatr Res* 1982;16(7):549.

32. Christensen RD, Hill HR, Rothstein G. Granulocytic stem cell (CFUc) proliferation in experimental group B Streptococcal sepsis. *Pediatr Res* 1983;17(4):278.

33. Koenig J, Hunter D, Christensen R. Neutropenia in donor (anemic) twins involved in the twin-twin transfusion syndrome. *J Perinatol* 1991;11(4):355.

34. Koenig JM, Christensen RD. Neutropenia and thrombocytopenia in infants with Rh hemolytic disease. *J Pediatr* 1989;114(4):625.

35. Carr R, Modi N, Doré CJ. G-CSF and GM-CSF for treating or preventing neonatal infections. Cochrane Neonatal Group. *Cochrane Database Syst Rev* 2003;(3):CD003066. doi: 10.1002/14651858.CD003066.

36. Lee J, Sauer B, Tuminski W, et al. Effectiveness of granulocyte colony-stimulating factor for hospitalized infants with neutropenia. *Am J Perinatol* 2016;34(5):458.

37. Calhoun DA, Christensen RD. Human developmental biology of granulocyte colony-stimulating factor. *Clin Perinatol* 2000;27(3):559.

38. Burgess A, Metcalf D. The nature and action of granulocyte-macrophage colony stimulating factors. *Blood* 1980;56(6):947.

39. de Haas M, Kerst J, van der Schoot C, et al. Granulocyte colony-stimulating factor administration to healthy volunteers: analysis of the immediate activating effects on circulating neutrophils. *Blood* 1994;84(11):3885.

40. Bux J, Behrens G, Jaeger G, et al. Diagnosis and clinical course of autoimmune neutropenia in infancy: analysis of 240 cases. *Blood* 1998;91(1):181.

41. Birle A, Nebe CT, Hill S, et al. Neutrophil chemotaxis in cord blood of term and preterm neonates is reduced in preterm neonates and influenced by the mode of delivery and anaesthesia. *PLoS One* 2015;10(4):e0120341.

42. Mehta R, Petrova A. Intrapartum magnesium sulfate exposure attenuates neutrophil function in preterm neonates. *Neonatology* 2006;89(2):99.

43. Hanna S, Etzioni A. Leukocyte adhesion deficiencies: leukocyte adhesion deficiencies. *Ann N Y Acad Sci* 2012;1250(1):50.

44. Palis J. Yolk-sac hematopoiesis. The first blood cells of mouse and man. *Exp Hematol* 2001;29(8):927.

45. Park M-Y, Lim B-G, Kim S-Y, et al. GM-CSF promotes the expansion and differentiation of cord blood myeloid-derived suppressor cells, which attenuate xenogeneic graft-vs.-host disease. *Front Immunol* 2019;10:183. Available from: https://www.frontiersin.org/article/10.3389/fimmu.2019.00183/full.

46. Christensen RD, Jensen J, Maheshwari A, et al. Reference ranges for blood concentrations of eosinophils and monocytes during the neonatal period defined from over 63 000 records in a multihospital health-care system. *J Perinatol* 2010;30(8):540.

47. Porcellini A, Manna A, Manna M, et al. Ontogeny of granulocyte-macrophage progenitor cells in the human fetus: development of CFU-Gm in the human fetus. *Int J Cell Cloning* 1983;1(2):92.

48. Wirbelauer J, Thomas W, Rieger L, et al. Intrauterine growth retardation in preterm infants ≤32 weeks of gestation is associated with low white blood cell counts. *Am J Perinatol* 2010;27(10):819.

49. Remon J, Kampanatkosol R, Kaul RR, et al. Acute drop in blood monocyte count differentiates NEC from other causes of feeding intolerance. *J Perinatol* 2014;34(7):549.

50. Desiraju S, Bensadoun J, Bateman D, et al. The role of absolute monocyte counts in predicting severity of necrotizing enterocolitis. *J Perinatol* 2020;40(6):922. Available from: http://www.nature.com/articles/s41372-020-0596-2.

51. de Jong E, Strunk T, Burgner D, et al. The phenotype and function of preterm infant monocytes: implications for susceptibility to infection. *J Leukoc Biol* 2017;102(3):645.

52. Geissmann F, Auffray C, Palframan R, et al. Blood monocytes: distinct subsets, how they relate to dendritic cells, and their possible roles in the regulation of T-cell responses. *Immunol Cell Biol* 2008;86(5):398.

53. Ziegler-Heitbrock L. Blood monocytes and their subsets: established features and open questions. *Front Immunol* 2015;6:423. Available from: http://journal.frontiersin.org/Article/10.3389/fimmu.2015.00423/abstract.

54. Ziegler-Heitbrock L, Ancuta P, Crowe S, et al. Nomenclature of monocytes and dendritic cells in blood. *Blood* 2010;116(16):e74.

55. Tsafaras GP, Ntontsi P, Xanthou G. Advantages and limitations of the neonatal immune system. *Front Pediatr* 2020;8:5.

56. Kuijpers T, Lutter R. Inflammation and repeated infections in CGD: two sides of a coin. *Cell Mol Life Sci* 2012;69(1):7.

57. Levy O, Zarember KA, Roy RM, et al. Selective impairment of TLR-mediated innate immunity in human newborns: neonatal blood plasma reduces monocyte TNF-α induction by bacterial lipopeptides, lipopolysaccharide, and imiquimod, but preserves the response to R-848. *J Immunol* 2004;173(7):4627.

58. Viemann D, Dubbel G, Schleifenbaum S, et al. Expression of Toll-like receptors in neonatal sepsis. *Pediatr Res* 2005;58(4):654.

59. Carlyle JR, Zuniga-Pflucker JC. Lineage commitment and differentiation of T and natural killer lymphocytes in the fetal mouse. *Immunol Rev* 1998;165(1):63.

60. Vacchio M, Ciucci T, Bosselut R. 200 million thymocytes and I: a beginner's survival guide to T cell development. *Methods Mol Biol* 2016;1323:3.

61. Xu X, Zhang S, Li P, et al. Maturation and emigration of single-positive thymocytes. *Clin Dev Immunol* 2013;2013:1.

62. Kumar BV, Connors TJ, Farber DL. Human T cell development, localization, and function throughout life. *Immunity* 2018;48(2):202.

63. Erkeller-Yuksel FM, Deneys V, Yuksel B, et al. Age-related changes in human blood lymphocyte subpopulations. *J Pediatr* 1992;120(2):7.

64. Zhu J, Yamane H, Paul WE. Differentiation of effector CD4 T cell populations. *Annu Rev Immunol* 2010;28(1):445.

65. McFadden JP, Thyssen JP, Basketter DA, et al. T helper cell 2 immune skewing in pregnancy/early life: chemical exposure and the development of atopic disease and allergy. *Br J Dermatol* 2015;172(3):584.

66. Cupedo T, Nagasawa M, Weijer K, et al. Development and activation of regulatory T cells in the human fetus. *Eur J Immunol* 2005;35(2):383.

67. Michaëlsson J, Mold JE, McCune JM, et al. Regulation of T cell responses in the developing human fetus. *J Immunol* 2006;176(10):5741.

68. McVay LD, Carding SR. Extrathymic origin of human gamma delta T cells during fetal development. *J Immunol* 1996;157(7):2873.

69. McVay LD, Jaswal SS, Kennedy C, et al. The generation of human γδ T cell repertoires during fetal development. *J Immunol* 1998;160(12):5851.

70. Rueda CM, Moreno-Fernandez ME, Jackson CM, et al. Neonatal regulatory T cells have reduced capacity to suppress dendritic cell function: cellular immune response. *Eur J Immunol* 2015;45(9):2582.

71. Bishop GA, Hostager BS. B lymphocyte activation by contact-mediated interactions with T lymphocytes. *Curr Opin Immunol* 2001;13(3):278.

72. Toivanen P, Uksila J, Leino A, et al. Development of mitogen responding T cells and natural killer cells in the human fetus. *Immunol Rev* 1981;57(1):89.

73. Gathings WE, Lawton AR, Cooper MD. Immunofluorescent studies of the development of pre-B cells, B lymphocytes and immunoglobulin isotype diversity in humans. *Eur J Immunol* 1977;7(11):804.

74. Hardy RR, Hayakawa K. B cell development pathways. *Annu Rev Immunol* 2001;19(1):595.

75. Paloczi K. Immunophenotypic and functional characterization of human umbilical cord blood mononuclear cells. *Leukemia* 1999;13(S1):S87.

76. Thomas RM, Linch DC. Identification of lymphocyte subsets in the newborn using a variety of monoclonal antibodies. *Arch Dis Child* 1983;58(1):34.

77. Hardy RR, Hayakawa K. Perspectives on fetal derived CD5+ B1 B cells: highlights. *Eur J Immunol* 2015;45(11):2978.

78. Palmeira P, Quinello C, Silveira-Lessa AL, et al. IgG placental transfer in healthy and pathological pregnancies. *Clin Dev Immunol* 2012;2012:1.

79. Ballow M, Cates KL, Rowe JC, et al. Development of the immune system in very low birth weight (less than 1500 g) premature infants: concentrations of plasma immunoglobulins and patterns of infections. *Pediatr Res* 1986;20(9):899.

80. D'Angio C, Maniscalco W, Pichichero M. Immunologic response of extremely premature infants to tetanus, haemophilus influenzae, and polio immunizations. *Pediatrics* 1995;96(1):18.

81. Cirillo E, Giardino G, Gallo V, et al. Severe combined immunodeficiency-an update: severe combined immunodeficiencies. *Ann N Y Acad Sci* 2015;1356(1):90.

82. Blom M, Pico-Knijnenburg I, Sijne-van Veen M, et al. An evaluation of the TREC assay with regard to the integration of SCID screening into the Dutch newborn screening program. *Clin Immunol* 2017;180:106.

83. Kuo CY, Signer R, Saitta SC. Immune and genetic features of the chromosome 22q11.2 deletion (DiGeorge syndrome). *Curr Allergy Asthma Rep* 2018;18(12):75.

84. Yen J-M, Lin C-H, Yang M-M, et al. Eosinophilia in very low birth weight infants. *Pediatr Neonatol* 2010;51(2):116.

85. Bhat AM, Scanlon JW. The pattern of eosinophilia in premature infants. *J Pediatr* 1981;98(4):612.

86. Sullivan SE, Calhoun DA. Eosinophilia in the neonatal intensive care unit. *Clin Perinatol* 2000;27(3):603.

44 Platelets and Disorders of Coagulation

Martha Sola-Visner and Matthew A. Saxonhouse

Bleeding and thrombotic disorders in the neonate may present a diagnostic challenge to the physician. Thrombocytopenia, abnormal levels of coagulation/anticoagulation proteins, and/or acquired risk factors may result in hemorrhagic or thromboembolic (TE) emergencies. The timely diagnosis of a congenital hemorrhagic disorder can potentially avoid significant long-term sequelae, while the lack of standard guidelines addressing the management of neonatal thromboses may leave a neonatologist indecisive on what the optimal treatment strategy should be. In this chapter, neonatal thrombocytopenia and abnormalities of neonatal platelet function will be discussed first, neonatal hemorrhagic disorders with current treatment options second, and neonatal thromboses—including risk factors and common sites of occurrence—third. Finally, suggested evaluation plans for neonates with TE emergencies and the latest treatment recommendations will be outlined.

PLATELETS

Platelet Counts During Development and Incidence of Thrombocytopenia

Thrombocytopenia in neonates (as in adults) has traditionally been defined as a platelet count less than 150×10^9/L and has been classified as mild (100 to 150×10^9/L), moderate (50 to 99 $\times 10^9$/L), and severe ($<50 \times 10^9$/L). The incidence of thrombocytopenia in neonates varies significantly, depending on the population studied. Based on the traditional definitions, large studies in unselected populations established an overall incidence of neonatal thrombocytopenia of 0.7% to 0.9% (1). However, the incidence is much higher among neonates admitted to the NICU, ranging from 18% to 35% (2). The incidence of thrombocytopenia is also inversely correlated to the gestational age, so that the most premature neonates are the most frequently affected. Platelet counts less than 150×10^9/L were found at least once during the hospital stay in 70% of infants with a birth weight less than 1,000 g, and these infants were categorized as being thrombocytopenic (3).

The largest study on neonatal platelet counts conducted to date, which included approximately 47,000 infants delivered between 22 and 42 weeks of gestation (4), showed that platelet counts increased during gestation by approximately 2×10^9/L per week (**Fig. 44.1**). Importantly, the mean platelet count was $\geq 200 \times 10^9$/L (well within the normal adult range) even in the most preterm infants, but the 5th percentile was 104×10^9/L for those ≤ 32 weeks of gestation and 123×10^9/L for late-preterm and term neonates (Fig. 44.1) (4). This study suggested that platelet counts between 100 and 150×10^9/L might be more frequent among otherwise healthy extremely preterm infants than among full-term neonates or older children/adults, and that perhaps different definitions of thrombocytopenia should be applied to neonates at different gestational ages. However, it is important to emphasize that the reference ranges in that study were generated by eliminating the top 5% and the bottom 5% of all available values, rather than by excluding values based on diagnoses. Thus, these should be viewed as "epidemiologic reference ranges" rather than "normal ranges."

Platelet Function and Primary Hemostasis

Studies evaluating various aspects of platelet function (adhesion, aggregation, and activation) have shown that neonatal platelets are hyporesponsive *in vitro* to most agonists, compared with adult platelets (5), and that this hyporeactivity is more pronounced in preterm infants (6). Specifically, platelets from neonatal (full term) cord blood activate and aggregate less than adult platelets in response to traditional platelet agonists such as adenosine diphosphate (ADP), epinephrine, collagen, thrombin, and thromboxane analogs (6,7). More recently, neonatal platelets were also found to exhibit a pronounced hyporesponsiveness to collagen-related peptide (CRP) and to the snake venom toxin rhodocytin, which activate the collagen receptor GPVI and C-type lectin-like receptor 2 (CLEC-2), respectively (8). The same investigators also found developmental differences in platelet *inhibitory* pathways, specifically a hypersensitivity of neonatal platelets to inhibition by prostaglandin E1 (PGE$_1$) of ADP- and collagen-induced platelet aggregation, which might contribute to the hyporeactivity of neonatal platelets (9).

Different mechanisms account for the developmentally unique responses of neonatal platelets to various agents: (a) the hyporesponsiveness to epinephrine is due to fewer α2-adrenergic receptors, the binding sites for epinephrine; (b) the decreased responsiveness to thrombin is related to reduced expression of PAR-1 and PAR-4 in neonatal platelets (10); (c) the decreased response to thromboxane results from reduced signaling downstream from the receptor (5); (d) the reduced responses to collagen and rhodocytin result from mildly reduced expression of GPVI and CLEC-2 combined with a signaling defect evidenced by reduced Syk and PLCγ2 phosphorylation (8); and (e) the hypersensitivity to PGE$_1$ inhibition of platelet aggregation is associated with a functionally increased PGE$_1$–cAMP–PKA axis (9).

Surprisingly, while the hypofunctional *in vitro* platelet phenotype would predict a bleeding tendency, bleeding times (BTs) in healthy term neonates are paradoxically **shorter** than BTs in adults (11). Similarly, studies using the Platelet Function Analyzer (PFA-100, an *in vitro* test of primary hemostasis that measures the time it takes to occlude a small aperture, or closure time [CT]) found that cord blood samples from term neonates exhibited shorter CTs than samples from older children or adults (12). The results of these studies suggest that full-term neonates have enhanced platelet/vessel wall interaction, likely explained by their higher hematocrits, higher mean corpuscular volumes, and higher concentrations of von Willebrand factor (particularly its ultra large multimers). Combined, these factors effectively counteract the intrinsic neonatal platelet hyperreactivity, suggesting that the *in vitro* platelet hyporeactivity of healthy full-term infants should be viewed as an integral part of a well-balanced unique neonatal hemostatic system rather than a developmental deficiency.

These compensatory mechanisms might be less well developed in preterm infants, whose platelets are also more hyporeactive than those of full-term infants, probably leading to a more vulnerable hemostatic system. Specifically, BTs performed on the first day of life were longer in preterm compared with term infants, with neonates less than 33 weeks of gestation exhibiting the longest BTs (13). PFA-100 CTs from nonthrombocytopenic neonates were also inversely correlated to gestational age in both cord blood and neonatal peripheral blood samples obtained on the first day of life (14). However, BTs and CTs in preterm neonates were still near or within the normal range for adults, suggesting that healthy preterm neonates also have adequate primary hemostasis. How disease processes perturb this delicate system and whether these disturbances contribute to bleeding are unanswered questions.

Neonatal platelet function improves significantly and nearly normalizes by 10 to 14 days, even in preterm infants (15). Consistent with this, Del Vecchio et al. found that all infants had shorter

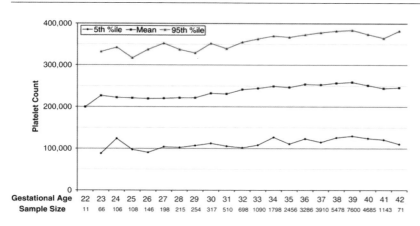

FIGURE 44.1 First recorded platelet counts, obtained in the first 3 days after birth, in neonates born at 22 to 42 weeks of gestation. Mean values are indicated by the *red line*, and the 5th and 95th percentiles are shown in the *blue* and *green lines*, respectively. (Reprinted by permission from Nature: Wiedmeier SE, Henry E, Sola-Visner MC, et al. Platelet reference ranges for neonates, defined using data from over 47,000 patients in a multihospital healthcare system. *J Perinatol* 2009;29:132. Copyright © 2009 Springer Nature.)

BTs by day 10 of life than at birth, and that early gestational age–related differences disappeared by then. Moreover, little or no further shortening occurred between days 10 and 30 (13). While no causal association has been demonstrated, the first 10 days of life also constitute the period of highest bleeding risk in preterm neonates.

NEONATAL THROMBOCYTOPENIA

When evaluating a thrombocytopenic neonate, the most effective first step to narrow the differential diagnosis is by classifying the thrombocytopenia as either **early onset (within the first 72 hours of life)** or **late onset (after 72 hours of life)**, and to determine whether the infant is clinically ill or well.

Early-Onset Thrombocytopenia (Fig. 44.2)

The most frequent cause of early-onset thrombocytopenia in a well-appearing neonate is placental insufficiency, seen in infants born to mothers with pregnancy-induced hypertension/preeclampsia, and in those with intrauterine growth restriction (IUGR). This thrombocytopenia is almost always mild to moderate, presents shortly after birth, and resolves within 7 to 10 days. In a recent large cohort study, approximately one-third of small-for-gestational-age (SGA) infants had thrombocytopenia

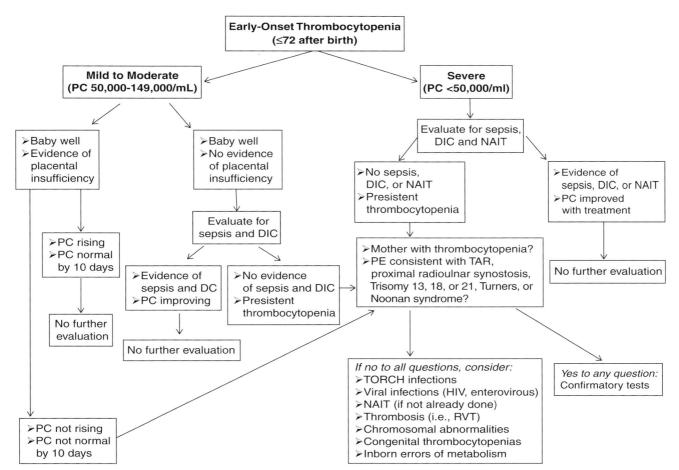

FIGURE 44.2 **Guidelines for the evaluation of neonates with early-onset thrombocytopenia (≤72 hours of life).** PC, platelet count; DIC, disseminated intravascular coagulation; NAIT, neonatal alloimmune thrombocytopenia; RVT, renal vein thrombosis. (Reprinted with permission from Cloherty JP, et al. Neonatal thrombocytopenia. In: Hansen AR, Eichwald EC, Stark AR, et al., eds. *Manual of neonatal care*, 8th ed. Philadelphia, PA: Wolters Kluwer, 2016.)

THE NEWBORN INFANT

(defined as a platelet count $<150 \times 10^9/L$) during the first week of life, compared to only 10% of non-SGA gestational age-matched infants. This type of thrombocytopenia was associated with low mortality (2%), as long as there was no genetic syndrome or congenital infection identified as a cause of the growth restriction (16). If an SGA nondysmorphic infant with mild to moderate thrombocytopenia remains clinically stable and the platelet count normalizes within 10 days, no further evaluation is necessary. However, if the thrombocytopenia becomes severe and/or persists greater than 10 days, further investigation is indicated.

Severe early-onset thrombocytopenia in an otherwise healthy infant should trigger suspicion for an immune-mediated thrombocytopenia, either autoimmune (if the mother is also thrombocytopenic) or alloimmune (if the mother has a normal platelet count). Early-onset thrombocytopenia of any severity in an *ill-appearing* term or preterm neonate should prompt evaluation for sepsis, congenital viral or parasitic infections, or disseminated intravascular coagulation (DIC), most frequently associated with sepsis or birth asphyxia.

In addition, thrombocytopenic neonates should be carefully examined for any radial and thumb abnormalities (suggestive of thrombocytopenia-absent radii syndrome—TAR syndrome, amegakaryocytic thrombocytopenia with radioulnar synostosis, or Fanconi anemia). The inability to rotate the forearm on physical examination, in the presence of severe early-onset thrombocytopenia, suggests the rare diagnosis of congenital amegakaryocytic thrombocytopenia with proximal radioulnar synostosis (ATRUS). Dysmorphic features should warrant investigation for genetic disorders, most commonly trisomy 21, trisomy 18, trisomy 13, Turner syndrome, Noonan syndrome, and Jacobsen syndrome. Hepato- and/or splenomegaly is suggestive of viral infection but can also be seen in hemophagocytic syndrome and liver failure from different etiologies. Other diagnoses, such as renal vein thrombosis, Kasabach-Merritt syndrome, and inborn errors of metabolism (i.e., propionic acidemia and methylmalonic acidemia) should be considered based on specific clinical presentations (i.e., hematuria in renal vein thrombosis, presence of a vascular tumor in Kasabach-Merritt syndrome, metabolic acidosis in propionic acidemia).

Late-Onset Thrombocytopenia (Fig. 44.3)

Thrombocytopenia of any severity presenting after 72 hours of life is most commonly caused by sepsis (bacterial or fungal) or necrotizing enterocolitis (NEC). Affected infants are usually ill appearing and have other signs suggestive of sepsis and/or NEC. However, it is important to note that thrombocytopenia can be the first presenting sign, preceding clinical deterioration.

If bacterial/fungal sepsis and NEC are ruled out, viral infections such as herpes simplex virus, cytomegalovirus (CMV), or enterovirus should be considered. These viral infections are frequently accompanied by abnormal liver enzymes. If the infant has or has recently had a central venous or arterial catheter, thromboses should be part of the differential diagnosis, although they usually only cause thrombocytopenia if the thrombus is enlarging or is infected. Finally, drug-induced thrombocytopenia is rare in neonates, but should be considered if the infant is clinically well, other potential etiologies have been ruled out, and he/she is receiving heparin, antibiotics (penicillins, cephalosporins, metronidazole, vancomycin, or rifampin), indomethacin, famotidine, cimetidine, phenobarbital, or phenytoin, among others.

Novel tools to evaluate platelet production in cases of thrombocytopenia of unclear etiology have been recently developed. Among those, the immature platelet fraction (IPF) can be measured in a standard hematologic cell counter (Sysmex XN Series) as part of the complete cell count. The IPF measures the percentage of newly released platelets (<24 hours) and can be used in a manner similar to the use of reticulocyte counts to evaluate anemia. Thus, an elevated IPF suggests platelet consumption, while a decreased IPF is consistent with a hyporegenerative thrombocytopenia, as

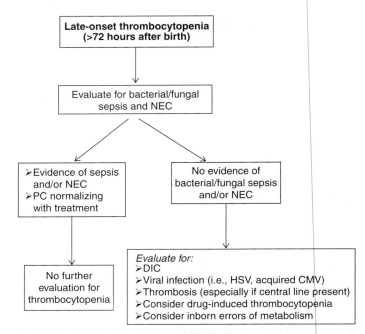

FIGURE 44.3 Guidelines for the evaluation of neonates with late-onset thrombocytopenia (>72 hours of life). PC, platelet count; NEC, necrotizing enterocolitis; HSV, herpes simplex virus; CMV, cytomegalovirus. (Reprinted with permission from Cloherty JP, et al. Neonatal thrombocytopenia. In: Hansen AR, Eichwald EC, Stark AR, et al., eds. *Manual of neonatal care,* 8th ed. Philadelphia, PA: Wolters Kluwer, 2016.)

in bone marrow suppression. Reference intervals for the IPF% (immature platelet fraction percentage) and IPC (immature platelet count; IPF × platelet count) have been evaluated in healthy adult individuals and in full-term umbilical cord blood samples (17), as well as in non-thrombocytopenic NICU patients by Cremer et al. (IPF% = 4.1% ± 1.8%; IPC = 9.5 ± 3.8 × $10^9/L$) (18). Notably, reference ranges for IPF in neonates are slightly higher compared with adults and children, although this is largely driven by preterm neonates (17). In the largest IPF study published to date, MacQueen et al. examined 24,372 platelet counts and IPF percentages from 9,172 term and preterm neonates 0 to 90 days old. Data from nonthrombocytopenic infants in this cohort were used to generate age-specific reference intervals for IPF% and IPCs (Fig. 44.4) (19). As seen in the figure, the IPF at the time of birth was higher in preterm infants, and decreased through gestation until 32 weeks, at which time it stabilized at full-term values

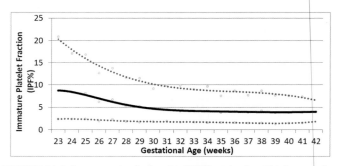

FIGURE 44.4 Immature platelet fraction (IPF%) on the day of birth, according to gestational age. The *lower and upper dashed lines* represent the 5th and 95th percentile reference intervals, and the *solid black line* represents the median. Light circles are the actual medians for 5th, median, and 95th percentile each day. The *dashed* and *solid lines* were generated by smoothing the values in the circles. (Reprinted by permission from Nature: MacQueen BC, Christensen RD, Henry E, et al. The immature platelet fraction: creating neonatal reference intervals and using these to categorize neonatal thrombocytopenias. *J Perinatol* 2017;37:834. Copyright © 2017 Springer Nature.)

TABLE 44.1

Immature Platelet Fraction Values in Neonates with Thrombocytopenia of Different Etiologies

Mechanism of Thrombocytopenia	*N*	IPF%
Hypoproliferative[a]	92	10.4 ± 2.9
Consumptive[b]	98	20.9 ± 7.9
Both	76	17.9 ± 5.9
Indeterminate[c]	14	12.8 ± 8.1

[a]SGA, birth asphyxia, or a syndrome associated with hypoproliferative thrombocytopenia.

[b]Immune-mediated, NEC, sepsis, or DIC.

[c]None of the above diagnoses.

Reprinted by permission from Nature: MacQueen BC, Christensen RD, Henry E, et al. The immature platelet fraction: creating neonatal reference intervals and using these to categorize neonatal thrombocytopenias. *J Perinatol* 2017;37:834. Copyright © 2017 Springer Nature.

(which are similar to adult values). Postnatally, the IPF increased progressively over the first 2 weeks of life and returned to baseline by 1 month in infants of all gestational ages. This study also assessed IPF percentages in neonates with thrombocytopenia and found significantly higher values in neonates with consumptive etiologies compared to those with thrombocytopenia secondary to decreased production (Table 44.1). Thus, when available, the IPF is particularly helpful to guide the diagnostic evaluation of infants with thrombocytopenia of unclear etiology and can help differentiate rare congenital thrombocytopenias (usually low) from NAIT or other consumptive disorders (usually elevated). Recent studies have also shown the usefulness of the IPF to predict platelet recovery in neonates (18,20). In patients with NEC and severe thrombocytopenia, a low IPC has been associated with a poor prognosis and high mortality (21).

IMMUNE THROMBOCYTOPENIA

Immune thrombocytopenia occurs due to the passive transfer of antibodies from the maternal to the fetal circulation. There are two distinct types of immune mediated thrombocytopenia: (a) neonatal alloimmune thrombocytopenia (NAIT) and (b) autoimmune thrombocytopenia.

In NAIT, the antibody is produced in the mother against a specific human platelet antigen (HPA) present in the fetus, but absent in the mother. The antigen is inherited from the father of the fetus. The antigens responsible for NAIT are caused by single-nucleotide polymorphisms on any of the main glycoproteins located on the platelet surface, particularly GPIIb/IIIa. The first platelet antigen was identified in 1959 by von Loghem et al. and was designated Zw-a (later PLA1). The initial nomenclature for these antigens came from the name of the patients, leading to confusion in the field. In 1990, a simplified system for HPA nomenclature was described, in which each antigen was given an HPA number. Antigens were numbered chronologically, according to the date of their initial report. The biallelic antigens were given an alphabetic designation of "a" or "b" in the order of their frequency (higher frequency for "a"). Thus, the Zw-a/PLA1 antigen was named HPA-1, with its two serologic forms designated as HPA-1a for the common form and HPA-1b for the less common form (the latter corresponding to PLA2). Sixteen HPA antigens have been identified so far. The frequency of each antigen varies within ethnic groups: In Caucasians, antibodies to HPA-1a are the major cause of NAIT, followed by HPA-5a and, less frequently, HPA9b, HPA3a and b, and HPA15. Antibodies to HPA-4b are the predominant cause of NAIT in the Japanese population. The anti-HPA antibody produced in the maternal serum crosses the placenta and reaches the fetal circulation, leading to platelet destruction, apoptosis of early

megakaryocyte progenitors (therefore decreased platelet production) (22), and thrombocytopenia.

In autoimmune thrombocytopenia, the antibody is directed against an antigen on the mother's own platelets (autoantibody) as well as on the infant's platelets. The maternal autoantibody also crosses the placenta (both passively and actively transported), resulting in destruction of fetal platelets and thrombocytopenia.

Neonatal Alloimmune Thrombocytopenia

NAIT is the most common underlying cause of early-onset, severe thrombocytopenia, with an incidence among live born neonates of 0.5 to 1.5 per 1,000 births (23). The true incidence of the disease is likely higher, however, since the milder cases might go undetected and the most severe cases lead to intrauterine death. Intrauterine death or intracranial hemorrhage (ICH) may occur as early as at 14 to 16 weeks of gestation, resulting in a relatively high incidence of intrauterine ICH (>10%) (23). The overall incidence of ICH (prenatal and postnatal) is particularly high in this population, affecting up to 20% of infants with NAIT, and potentially leading to lifelong consequences. ICH may occur during the first pregnancy and has a recurrence risk close to 100% in subsequent pregnancies in the absence of prenatal treatment.

NAIT should be considered in any neonate who presents with severe thrombocytopenia at birth or shortly thereafter, particularly in the absence of other risk factors, clinical signs, or abnormalities in the physical exam. In a study of more than 200 neonates with thrombocytopenia, using a platelet count less than $50 \times 10^9/L$ in the first day of life as a screening indicator identified 90% of the patients with NAIT (24). Based on this observation, it is currently recommended that all neonates with platelet counts in this range in the first day of life be screened for NAIT. In addition, the combination of severe neonatal thrombocytopenia with a parenchymal (rather than intraventricular) ICH is highly suggestive of NAIT.

Laboratory Investigation

When NAIT is suspected, blood should be collected from the mother and father and submitted for testing. The initial antigen screening should include HPA 1, 3, and 5. This evaluation should identify approximately 90% of cases of NAIT. However, if the diagnosis is strongly suspected and the initial evaluation is negative, further testing should be undertaken for HPA 9 and 15 (and HPA 4 if the parents are of Asian descent). If positive, these tests will reveal an antibody in the mother's plasma directed against the specific platelet antigen in the father. If blood cannot be collected from the parents in a timely fashion, neonatal serum may be screened for the presence of antiplatelet antibodies. However, a low antibody concentration in the neonate coupled with binding of the antibodies to the infant's platelets can lead to false-negative results. Due to the complexity of testing, evaluations should be performed in an experienced reference laboratory that has a large number of typed controls available for antibody detection and the appropriate DNA-based technology to type multiple antigens. In rare cases, antibodies may be hard to detect in samples drawn at the time of delivery. Therefore, when the clinical diagnosis is most likely NAIT, follow-up serology tests should be performed.

Brain imaging studies (cranial ultrasound) should be performed as soon as NAIT is suspected, *regardless of the presence or absence of neurologic manifestations*, because findings from these studies will dictate the aggressiveness of the treatment regimen for the affected infant and for the mother's future pregnancies. The clinical course of NAIT is short in most cases, often resolving almost entirely within 2 weeks. However, to confirm the diagnosis, it is imperative to follow the platelet count frequently until a normal count is achieved.

THE NEWBORN INFANT

Management

The management of NAIT differs depending on the specific clinical scenario: (a) suspected NAIT (unknown pregnancy); (b) known case of NAIT; and (c) antenatal management of pregnant woman with previous history of NAIT.

Management of the Neonate with Suspected NAIT (Unknown Pregnancy)

Based on recent data demonstrating that a large proportion of *infants with NAIT respond to random donor platelet transfusions, this is now considered the first line of therapy for infants in whom NAIT is suspected* (25). If the patient is clinically stable and does not have an ICH, platelets are usually given when the platelet count is less than 30×10^9/L, although this is arbitrary. In addition to platelets, if the diagnosis of NAIT is confirmed or strongly suspected, intravenous immune globulin (IVIG) (1 g/kg/d for up to 2 consecutive days) may be administered to increase the patient's own platelets and potentially to protect the transfused platelets. Because in NAIT the platelet count usually falls after birth, IVIG may be given when the platelet count is between 30 and 50×10^9/L in a stable neonate, to try to prevent a further drop.

If the patient has evidence of an ICH, the goal is to maintain a platelet count greater than 100×10^9/L. However, this may be challenging in the setting of NAIT. In all of these scenarios, it is important to keep in mind that some infants with NAIT fail to respond to random donor platelets and IVIG. For that reason, the blood bank should be immediately alerted about any infant with suspected NAIT, and arrangements should be made to secure a source of antigen-negative platelets (either from HPA-1b1b and 5a5a donors, which should be compatible in >90% of cases, or from the mother) as soon as possible, so they are available if there is no response to the initial therapies. If maternal platelets are used, they need to be concentrated to decrease the amount of antiplatelet antibodies (present in the mother's plasma) infused into the infant. Platelets can also be washed to eliminate the plasma, although this induces more damage to the platelets than concentrating them. Of note, in some European countries, HPA-1b1b and 5a5a platelets are maintained in the blood bank inventory and are immediately available for use. In those cases, these are preferable to random donor platelets and/or IVIG and should be the first line of therapy.

Management of the Neonate with Known NAIT

When a neonate is born to a mother who had a previous pregnancy affected by confirmed NAIT, genotypically matched platelets (e.g., HPA-1b1b platelets) should be available in the blood bank at the time of delivery and should be the first-line treatment if the infant is thrombocytopenic.

Management of Pregnant Women with Previous History of NAIT

Mothers who delivered an infant with NAIT should be followed in high-risk obstetric clinics during all future pregnancies as the recurrence rate is high, reaching 100% if the father is homozygous for the causative HPA. However, in all cases, fetal genetic testing should be performed. Recently, noninvasive methods have become available through cell-free DNA testing from the mother's plasma. The intensity of prenatal treatment will be based on the severity of the thrombocytopenia and the presence or absence of ICH in the previously affected fetus. This is particularly important to assess the risk of developing an ICH in the current pregnancy and to minimize this risk. Current recommendations involve maternal treatment with IVIG (0.5 to 2 g/kg/wk) ± steroids (0.5 to 1 mg/kg/d prednisone), starting at 12 or at 20 to 26 weeks of gestation, depending on whether the previously affected fetus suffered an ICH, and if so at what time during pregnancy. Most recent studies showed that the combination of IVIG and steroids is the most effective treatment. Regarding mode of delivery, elective cesarean section is recommended in most countries, regardless of ICH status in previous and current fetus, to avoid ICH.

Autoimmune Thrombocytopenia

The diagnosis of neonatal autoimmune thrombocytopenia should be considered in any neonate who has early-onset thrombocytopenia and a maternal history of either immune thrombocytopenic purpura (ITP) or an autoimmune disease (with or without thrombocytopenia). Several large observational studies published in the 1990s concluded that infants born to mothers with ITP have a relatively low but measurable risk of developing severe thrombocytopenia. In one of the earliest studies, Burrows and Kelton found a platelet count less than 50×10^9/L in 10% of infants born to a mother with ITP and a platelet count less than 25×10^9/L in 4.2%. In that study, encompassing 288 infants, no infant suffered an ICH (26). Other studies reported similar incidences of severe thrombocytopenia (defined as a platelet count $<50 \times 10^9$/L) in neonates born to mothers with ITP, ranging from 8.9% to 14.7%, with ICH occurring in 0% to 1.5% of thrombocytopenic infants (27). Unfortunately, the fetal or neonatal platelet count cannot be reliably predicted by maternal platelet count, platelet antibody levels, or history of maternal splenectomy. Neonates born to a mother with history of delivering an infant with thrombocytopenia are usually as affected as the first.

While only a small percentage of neonates are born with severe thrombocytopenia in the setting of maternal ITP, mild to moderate thrombocytopenia is more common and the platelet count typically decreases after birth, reaching a nadir between days 2 and 5. For that reason, the recommendation is to obtain a platelet count immediately after delivery (from the cord or the baby), and to follow platelet counts in all infants with mild or moderate thrombocytopenia. A head ultrasound should be obtained on all infants with a platelet count less than 50×10^9/L at birth. Recommendations from the International Consensus Report on Management of ITP are to treat neonates with either clinical bleeding or a platelet count less than 20×10^9/L with a single dose of IVIG (1 g/kg), which can be repeated if necessary (27). Major bleeding should be treated with random platelet transfusions in addition to IVIG. Severe thrombocytopenia and major hemorrhage secondary to maternal ITP are rare, so evaluation for alloimmune thrombocytopenia or other causes of thrombocytopenia should be considered in those cases (27).

Neonatal thrombocytopenia secondary to maternal ITP can last for weeks to months and requires long-term monitoring and occasionally a second dose of IVIG 4 to 6 weeks after birth. A recent study suggested that antiplatelet antibodies from ITP mothers transferred to the fetus by breast milk are associated with neonatal thrombocytopenia persisting more than 4 months, which disappears following discontinuation of breast-feeding (28).

Maternal Management

Even if the mother has severe ITP, it appears that fetal hemorrhage *in utero* is very rare, compared with the small but definite risk of such hemorrhage in alloimmune thrombocytopenia. Because of that, treatment of ITP during pregnancy and delivery is mostly based on the risk of maternal hemorrhage (27). IVIG given prenatally to the mother with ITP has also not been clearly shown to affect the fetal platelet count. A recent study reported the use of recombinant human thrombopoietin (TPO) to manage ITP during pregnancy. In this study of 31 patients, 74% responded. Furthermore, TPO was well tolerated and no problems were observed in the infants born to treated mothers (29). This paved the way for the use of a new potential therapy to manage ITP during pregnancy.

There is in general little correlation between fetal platelet counts and maternal platelet counts, platelet antibody levels, or history of maternal splenectomy. Attempts to measure the fetal platelet count before delivery are not recommended, due to the risk associated. The only reliable predictive measure of neonatal thrombocytopenia in a mother with ITP has been found to be a history of neonatal thrombocytopenia in previous pregnancy. In regard to the mode of delivery, there is no evidence that cesarean section is safer for the fetus with thrombocytopenia than uncomplicated vaginal delivery. For that reason, the mode of delivery in ITP patients should be determined by purely obstetric indications. However, interventions that increase the risk of bleeding in the fetus should be avoided, such as vacuum extraction or forceps delivery.

CONGENITAL THROMBOCYTOPENIAS

Congenital thrombocytopenias are rare conditions, which most often present at birth and are therefore classified as early-onset thrombocytopenias. This is a heterogeneous group of diseases with variable clinical manifestations. Often, but not always, patients with congenital thrombocytopenia have dysmorphic features and associated abnormalities as part of a genetic syndrome. If a neonate presents with radial abnormalities, the differential diagnosis includes thrombocytopenia-absent radii syndrome (TAR syndrome), amegakaryocytic thrombocytopenia with radioulnar synostosis, and Fanconi anemia. Although thrombocytopenia associated with Fanconi almost always presents later (during childhood), few isolated neonatal cases have been reported (30). In these patients, thumb abnormalities are frequently found, and chromosomal fragility testing is nearly always diagnostic. If the infant has radial abnormalities with normal appearing thumbs, TAR syndrome should be considered. The platelet count is usually less than 50×10^9/L and the white cell count is elevated in greater than 90% of TAR syndrome patients, sometimes exceeding 100×10^9/L and mimicking congenital leukemia. Infants who survive the first year of life generally do well, since the platelet count then spontaneously improves to low–normal levels that are maintained through life (31). The inability to rotate the forearm on physical examination, in the presence of severe early-onset thrombocytopenia, suggests the rare diagnosis of congenital amegakaryocytic thrombocytopenia with proximal radioulnar synostosis (ATRUS). Radiologic examination of the upper extremities in these infants confirms the proximal synostosis of the radial and ulnar bones (32). Most (but not all cases) of ATRUS are associated with Hox-A11 mutations and require bone marrow transplantation. Other genetic disorders associated with early-onset thrombocytopenia include trisomy 21, trisomy 18, trisomy 13, Turner syndrome, Noonan syndrome, and Jacobsen syndrome. Cases of Noonan syndrome presenting with mild dysmorphic features and very severe neonatal thrombocytopenia (mimicking congenital amegakaryocytic thrombocytopenia—CAMT) have been described, so genetic testing should be performed in children who present with a CAMT-like picture and no mutations in the C-mpl gene.

In nonsyndromic cases of congenital thrombocytopenia, there is usually a history of chronic thrombocytopenia in family members. These conditions belong to a heterogeneous group of diseases, and due to diverse clinical manifestations and laboratory findings, the diagnosis is challenging. Often the size of the platelets helps in the differential diagnosis. Myosin heavy chain-9 (MYH-9)-related disorders (May-Hegglin anomaly, Fechtner syndrome, Sebastian syndrome) are inherited in autosomal dominant fashion and present with macrothrombocytopenia. Other congenital thrombocytopenias presenting with large platelets include Bernard-Soulier syndrome (with autosomal recessive inheritance) and X-linked macrothrombocytopenia. Wiskott-Aldrich syndrome, by contrast, should be suspected in male neonates with severe thrombocytopenia and small platelets, particularly if they develop eczema. The diagnosis of congenital amegakaryocytic thrombocytopenia (CAMT) is challenging as it presents with normal sized platelets and may not be diagnosed in the newborn period (when it is usually confused with alloimmune thrombocytopenia) due to

lack of other clinical features. A detailed description of congenital thrombocytopenias and their associated features is provided elsewhere (33). These conditions are often paired with platelet dysfunction as well.

The outcomes for patients with congenital thrombocytopenia are variable depending on the specific disorders. Patients with CAMT often develop bone marrow failure and pancytopenia and require bone marrow transplant. The thrombocytopenia in TAR patients is severe at birth, but improves over time, often reaching platelet counts greater than 100×10^9/L. The hematologic outcome of MYH-9-related disorders is good, although they frequently develop nephritis, hearing loss, and/or cataracts later in life.

MANAGEMENT OF NEONATAL THROMBOCYTOPENIA

Platelet Transfusions in the NICU

Historically, it has been widely accepted that thrombocytopenic preterm neonates should receive platelet transfusions at higher platelet count (PC) thresholds than older children and adults due to their high incidence of spontaneous intracranial bleeding, particularly intraventricular hemorrhage (IVH). Over the last decade, several surveys and observational studies revealed a striking worldwide variability in neonatal platelet transfusion thresholds and an overall more liberal approach to platelet transfusions in U.S. compared to European NICUs (34). This variability was at least in part due to the paucity of high-level evidence in the field. Until recently, there was only one randomized trial of platelet transfusion thresholds in preterm neonates, published 25 years ago (35). That study randomized 152 very low birth weight (VLBW, <1,500 g at birth) neonates to receive platelet transfusions for platelet counts (PCs) less than 150×10^9/L or less than 50×10^9/L in the first week of life and found no differences in the incidence of new IVH or extension of existing IVH (the primary outcome) between the two groups (35). These results likely formed the basis for the use of 50×10^9/L as the most frequent threshold for platelet transfusions in preterm neonates.

The recently published much larger PlaNeT-2 multicenter trial randomized 660 thrombocytopenic neonates with a median gestational age of 26.6 weeks and a median birth weight of 740 g to receive platelet transfusions at PC thresholds of less than 50×10^9/L (<50 group) or less than 25×10^9/L (<25 group). Infants were randomized at any time during their neonatal intensive care unit (NICU) hospitalization when the PC fell below 50×10^9/L, and the primary outcome was a composite of death or new major bleeding within 28 days of randomization (36). Ninety percent of infants in the less than 50 group and 53% in the less than 25 group received at least one platelet transfusion. Unexpectedly, infants in the less than 50 group had a significantly *higher* rate of mortality or major bleeding within 28 days of randomization compared to those in the less than 25 group (26% vs. 19%, respectively; odds ratio 1.57, 95% CI 1.06 to 2.32). In a subgroup analysis, findings were similar for neonates less than 28 weeks of gestation, the group at highest risk of bleeding and death. Among secondary outcomes, infants in the liberally transfused group also had a higher incidence of bronchopulmonary dysplasia. While these findings might have seemed surprising at first, they were in fact consistent with a substantial number of prior observational studies describing a poor association between severity of thrombocytopenia and bleeding risk, a lack of effectiveness of platelet transfusions to prevent bleeding in neonates, and an association between number of platelet transfusions and neonatal mortality and morbidity (37,38).

The results of PlaNeT-2 provided high-level evidence in support of these concepts, although the possibility that the benefits of the lower transfusion threshold would be limited to clinically stable infants with a low risk of bleeding and/or death led to initial skepticism. This question was largely addressed in a follow-up study in which a multivariable logistic regression model was developed (incorporating factors known to influence neonatal bleeding risk and mortality) and used to predict the baseline bleeding/mortality risk of neonates enrolled in PlaNeT-2 (39). Based on their model-predicted baseline risk, 653 neonates in PlaNeT-2 were divided into four quartiles (very low, low, moderate, and high risk), and the absolute risk difference between the less than 50 group and the less than 25 group was assessed within each quartile. Interestingly, the lower transfusion threshold was associated with an absolute risk reduction *in all four groups*, varying from 4.9% in the lowest to 12.3% in the highest risk group. These results suggested that using a lower ($<25 \times 10^9$/L) prophylactic platelet transfusion threshold is beneficial even in high-risk neonates.

While these studies provided strong support for the use of lower platelet transfusion thresholds in nonbleeding preterm infants, some uncertainties remain. First, only 37% of infants in the study were randomized by day of life 5 and 59% by day 10, the period when most clinically significant hemorrhages occur in preterm neonates. While this might have simply reflected the time of onset of thrombocytopenia in the study population, 39% of infants in PlaNeT-2 received one or more platelet transfusions prior to randomization, for unknown reasons and at nonspecified PCs. This raises the question of whether these transfusions were given during the first few days of life, the highest risk period for IVH in preterm neonates. Second, the study required obtaining a head ultrasound within 6 hours of randomization and excluded infants with a significant IVH for 72 hours (after which they could be randomized). Thus, by design, PlaNeT-2 did not assess the effects of a restrictive vs. liberal platelet transfusion threshold on the potential extension of an existing IVH.

In regard to the platelet product that should be transfused, most experts agree that neonates should receive 10 mL/kg of a standard platelet suspension, either a platelet concentrate ("random-donor platelets") or apheresis platelets. Each random-donor platelet unit has approximately 50 mL of volume and contains approximately 10×10^9 platelets per 10 mL. There is no need to pool more than one random-donor unit for a neonatal transfusion, a practice that only increases donor exposures and induces platelet activation without benefit. Two additional important considerations in neonatology are the prevention of transfusion-transmitted CMV infections and graft versus host disease (GVHD). Most blood banks provide either CMV-negative or leuko-reduced products to neonates, both of which significantly reduce (but do not completely eliminate) the risk of transfusion-transmitted CMV. Transfusion of CMV-negative *and* leuko-reduced blood products completely prevents transmission of CMV to VLBW infants (40). GVHD is prevented by irradiating cellular blood products prior to transfusion. Of note, most neonatal cases of GVHD have been reported in neonates with underlying immunodeficiencies, receiving intrauterine or large volume transfusions (i.e., double exchange transfusions), or receiving blood products from a first-degree relative. Thus, these are all absolute indications for irradiating blood products.

PLATELET FUNCTION DISORDERS

Etiology/Pathophysiology

Platelets play a major role in hemostasis, both by supporting the cellular structure for the primary platelet plug, and also by providing a phospholipid surface on which the plasma elements involved in coagulation can bind. Thus, a decrease in the platelet count and/or poor platelet function can result in bleeding symptoms. Platelet function disorders can be broadly categorized as congenital or acquired.

Most platelet function defects seen in the NICU are acquired and can be due to medications, medical conditions, or medical interventions. The list of medications that can affect platelet function is extensive, but the most common medications resulting in platelet dysfunction include aspirin and other nonsteroidal anti-inflammatory drugs (indomethacin and ibuprofen), prostacyclin, certain anticonvulsants (valproic acid in particular), and some antibiotics (beta-lactams). Among the medical disorders associated with platelet dysfunction, the most common and best described is uremia. Although the exact mechanism by which the platelets are affected is not clear, a prevailing theory is that the accumulation of certain substances associated with uremia disrupts the platelet phospholipid surface. Last, certain medical procedures are associated with platelet dysfunction, with the most common being the use of extracorporeal circuits (ECMO and cardiopulmonary bypass). Therapeutic hypothermia, currently standard of care for infants with hypoxic–ischemic encephalopathy, also causes transient platelet dysfunction (41).

Congenital platelet function disorders occur as a result of defects or deficiencies in any of a multitude of components (functional, structural, and regulatory proteins) required for normal platelet function. The most severe platelet function defects, which can present in neonatal life, result from deficiency or absence in the glycoproteins (GP) located on the platelet surface: Bernard-Soulier syndrome, caused by deficiency of GPIb (the vWF receptor), and Glanzmann thrombasthenia, caused by a deficiency of GPIIb/IIIa, the fibrinogen receptor. Both have been reported to present with bleeding in neonatal life, although they most frequently present later in childhood.

Most of the other inherited platelet function defects are mild and very rarely present in the newborn period. Secretory platelet disorders have defective platelet granules and cause mild to moderate bleeding. These include δ-storage pool defects (including the common ADP secretion defect and the less common absence of dense bodies associated with Hermansky-Pudlak syndrome) and α-granules defects (gray platelet syndrome). Over the last decade, the availability of better genetic tools has led to the identification of the genetic causes of many of these platelet functional defects (i.e., mutations in NBEAL2 cause gray platelet syndrome) and of novel mutations associated with platelet dysfunction and bleeding. A thorough review of these disorders is outside of the scope of this chapter, particularly because the degree of bleeding associated with most of these conditions rarely leads to manifestations in the neonatal period.

Clinical Presentation

Patients with platelet function disorders present with bleeding signs similar to thrombocytopenia, including mucocutaneous bleeding (nose, mouth, gastrointestinal tract, genitourinary tract) and bruising. The extent, location, and nature of the bruises are generally related to birth trauma and invasive procedures. Bernard-Soulier syndrome patients present with mild thrombocytopenia, giant platelets on the blood smear (macrothrombocytopenia), and mucosal type bleeding due to platelet dysfunction. Patients with Bernard-Soulier have been reported to present as neonates with gastrointestinal bleeding, bleeding after circumcision, and bleeding after cardiac catheterization in a patient with DiGeorge syndrome. Glanzmann thrombasthenia is a rare autosomal recessive platelet function disorder, caused by a deficiency or abnormality of GPIIb-IIIa expression on the platelet surface. In neonates, the most common manifestations of Glanzmann thrombasthenia are generalized purpura or bleeding after circumcision, although more serious hemorrhages have also been described.

Diagnosis

The diagnosis of platelet function disorders in neonates is problematic, because many of the traditional tests require a large amount of blood (platelet aggregation studies), or lack reference values for neonates. The traditional assay of platelet function is platelet aggregometry. This assay uses a set concentration of platelet-rich plasma and assesses platelet aggregation via light transmission after addition of a variety of platelet agonists (ADP, epinephrine, ristocetin, arachidonic acid, collagen, and thrombin-related activation peptide). Neonates have reduced platelet aggregation compared to older children and adults (based on cord blood values), and therefore, the interpretation of this test in neonates is difficult. The major limitation of platelet aggregometry in neonates has been the large amount of blood required (20 to 30 mL, depending on the platelet count and how many agonists will be tested). Recently, whole blood aggregometry assays have been developed and are becoming increasingly available. These assays require significantly less blood than traditional platelet aggregometry, thus making them accessible to neonates. However, the lack of neonatal reference ranges has hampered the wider use of aggregometry in this age group.

There are two other tests that can screen for platelet function disorders; however, both have significant limitations. The original screening test is the BT, a test that is difficult to perform, particularly in neonates, and is rarely offered clinically. The PFA-100 is a widely used laboratory assay available in most coagulation laboratories and is a useful screening assay to evaluate for disorders of primary hemostasis. Normal ranges for the PFA have been established in cord blood (42) and more recently in neonatal blood (14). The blood volume required for this test is much less than for aggregometry, and thus, it can be used in neonates. Patients with severe platelet function defects such as Bernard-Soulier and Glanzmann thrombasthenia typically have significantly abnormal results. The PFA is also often abnormal in the milder disorders such as the common ADP secretion defects; however, its sensitivity for these disorders is not sufficient to allow such defects to be ruled out if the results are normal. The PFA-100 is also abnormal in patients on aspirin and clopidogrel and ticlopidine (the collagen/ADP cartridge). Neonates on indomethacin, ibuprofen, or certain antibiotics can also have a prolonged PFA-100. The effects of other medications known to affect platelet function are not clear. Thus, the PFA is a useful screen for the platelet function defects. However, it cannot be performed when the patient is on certain medications, and it cannot rule out milder platelet function defects.

More recently, a high-throughput sequencing platform targeting 63 genes relevant for bleeding and platelet disorders was generated, which allows the efficient molecular diagnosis of bleeding and platelet disorders, avoiding the need for multiple sequential tests to narrow the diagnostic possibilities. This DNA-based diagnostic platform will likely become the new approach to patients with suspected inherited platelet function disorders (43).

Treatment

The management of congenital platelet function defects relies on several medications, and platelet transfusions in dire situations when the medications or local measures are ineffective. In acquired conditions, reversal of the condition that led to the platelet dysfunction will reverse the platelet defect, but this is not always possible. In such situations, the approach to management of bleeding is mostly based on platelet transfusions.

Several medications have nonspecific mechanisms whereby they can enhance hemostasis when platelet function is abnormal. These include desmopressin, antifibrinolytic agents, and recombinant activated FVII (rFVIIa). Desmopressin has been demonstrated to improve platelet function in many congenital disorders, in uremia, and during cardiopulmonary bypass. However, desmopressin is generally not used in children less than 2 years of age, because it can lead to vasodilatation and can induce hyponatremic seizures.

Recombinant FVIIa was developed for the management of bleeding in patients with hemophilia and inhibitors; however, it has been shown to also be effective for managing severe bleeding in patients

with severe platelet function defects. It is licensed in Europe for the management of bleeding in patients with Glanzmann thrombasthenia who are refractory to platelet transfusions. The major risk of rFVIIa is the risk of thrombosis. Thus, it is suggested that rFVIIa be used only for patients with severe bleeding in whom standard therapeutic measures have failed. The use of this agent in neonates has been reported, and it appears that neonates are at increased risk for thrombosis compared with older children (44).

For severe bleeding that has not responded to the measures just described, a platelet transfusion should be given in order to provide normally functioning platelets. Although most platelet function defects are mild enough that this will never be required, for the more severe disorders such as Bernard-Soulier and Glanzmann thrombasthenia, a platelet transfusion may be lifesaving. Importantly, however, patients with Bernard-Soulier and Glanzmann thrombasthenia are at risk for alloimmunization, resulting in the formation of antibodies to GPIb and GPIIb/IIIa, respectively. Once these antibodies develop, future platelet transfusions are likely to be ineffective. Thus, it is imperative to withhold platelet transfusions for these patients except in life-threatening hemorrhage, because it may be possible to use this therapy only once in a patient's lifetime. Last, local measures are extremely important in the management of bleeding.

THE NEONATAL HEMOSTATIC SYSTEM

Hemostasis refers to the process in which bleeding is controlled at the site of damaged endothelium. The interaction between endothelium, subendothelium, platelets, circulating cells, and plasma proteins leads to both an immediate localized thrombosis, followed by the development of a confined thrombosis leading to eventual tissue repair. The localized thrombosis leads to the cessation of bleeding, while the thrombus serves as the scaffold for tissue repair and the complete restoration of the endothelial lining (45). Hemostatic processes are regulated by natural anticoagulants containing these processes to the site of injury and preventing these reactions from becoming systemic and pathologic (45).

The neonatal hemostatic system differs from that of adults in regard to platelet function (previously reviewed) and concentrations of procoagulant, anticoagulant, and fibrinolytic proteins (Table 44.2). These differences place a neonate in a "relative" prothrombotic state, but other factors balance the system and prevent a term or "well" premature neonate from experiencing spontaneous thrombosis or hemorrhage.

BLEEDING DISORDERS IN THE NEONATE

When a neonate is either actively bleeding or has suffered a significant hemorrhage, and thrombocytopenia has been excluded, an acquired or inherited coagulation defect must be evaluated for. A detailed family history may assist in establishing such a diagnosis. Laboratory diagnostic criteria that may assist in establishing a diagnosis for the bleeding neonate are presented in Table 44.3.

Laboratory Investigation

Any neonate with a suspected hemorrhagic disorder should have a complete blood count (CBC) and coagulation screen (prothrombin time (PT), activated partial thromboplastin time (APTT) and fibrinogen) performed. Based on these results, more specific testing may then be performed to assist with making the exact diagnosis. How the samples are collected may affect the results. For example, heel stick samples should never be used to confirm thrombocytopenia or a coagulation disorder. Elevated hematocrit levels greater than 55% may result in prolonged diluted coagulation times. When collecting samples from heparinized central catheters, enough blood must be cleared from the line prior to obtaining the sample or heparin should be absorbed from the sample itself (Hepabsorb).

Neonatal Coagulation, Anticoagulation, and Fibrinolytic Protein Levels

	Values Elevated Compared with Adult Values	Values Decreased Compared with Adult Values
Procoagulant	Fibrinogen Factor V[a] Factor VIII VWF	Factors[b] II, VII, IX, X, XI, XII, XIII Prekallikrein High molecular weight kininogen
Anticoagulant	Alpha-2-macroglobulin	Antithrombin III Heparin cofactor II Protein C Protein S
Fibrinolytic	Tissue plasminogen activator Plasminogen activator inhibitor	Plasminogen α-Antiplasmin

[a]Factor V levels are low on day of life 1 but reach adult values within days after birth. (From Will A. Neonatal haemostasis and the management of neonatal thrombosis. *Br J Haematol* 2015;169(3):324. Ref. (46).)

[b]Levels are 50% of adult values. (From Will A. Neonatal haemostasis and the management of neonatal thrombosis. *Br J Haematol* 2015;169(3):324. Ref. (46).)

Adapted from Manco-Johnson M. Controversies in neonatal thrombotic disorders. In: Ohls RY, ed. *Hematology, immunology and infectious disease: neonatology questions and controversies.* Philadelphia, PA: Saunders Elsevier, 2008:59. Copyright © 2008 Elsevier. With permission.

Hemophilia

Hemophilia A (Factor VIII deficiency; 1 per 5,000 males) and hemophilia B (Factor IX deficiency; 1 per 20,000 males), both sex-linked recessive, are the most common congenital bleeding disorders. About one-third of new cases occur in the absence of a family history. The type of mutation and the part of the protein that is affected determine the severity (45). Without Factor VIII or IX, reduced thrombin formation on the surface of activated platelets leads to a thrombus with poor structural integrity and more

Screening Coagulation Parameters for the Bleeding Neonate[a]

Disorder	PT	APTT	Platelets	Fibrinogen
Hemophilia A	Normal	↑↑↑	Normal	Normal
Hemophilia B	Normal	↑↑↑	Normal	Normal
Hemophilia C	Normal	↑↑	Normal	Normal
Factor XIII deficiency	Normal	Normal	Normal	Normal
Factor II, V, and X deficiency	↑↑	↑↑	Normal	Normal
Vitamin K Deficiency Bleeding	↑↑↑	Normal/↑[b]	Normal	Normal
DIC[c]	↑↑↑	↑↑↑	Low	Low
Liver disease[c]	↑↑↑	↑↑↑	Low	Low
vWD	Normal	Normal/↑	Normal	Normal
Hypofibrinogenemia	↑↑↑	↑↑↑	Normal	Low
Dysfibrinogenemia	↑↑↑	↑↑↑	Normal	Normal/Low

[a]A complete blood count and coagulation screening test should be performed for any bleeding infant.

[b]APTT values may be prolonged but not as severe as the elevated PT value.

[c]To differentiate between DIC and liver disease, a factor VIII value should be obtained. Factor VIII values will be normal in infants with liver disease but low in infants with DIC.

PT, prothrombin time(s); APTT, activated partial thromboplastin time(s); DIC, disseminated intravascular coagulation.

susceptible to fibrinolysis, resulting in an increased risk for bleeding. The most common presentation of hemophilia in the neonate is excessive bleeding following surgery or circumcision. The lower the factor level, the greater the risk for more severe early-onset bleeding. The mean age of patients with hemophilia having their first bleed is 28.5 days. Further classifications of hemophilia A and B in neonates are presented in **Table 44.4A**.

When the diagnosis of hemophilia is suspected in a neonate, Factor VIII and IX levels should be immediately obtained. Factor VIII levels are elevated during the neonatal period, so confirmatory testing for hemophilia A should be done at 6 to 12 months of life. Factor IX levels are low at birth, making the diagnosis of mild Hemophilia B difficult. Thus, testing should also be repeated at 6 to 12 months of life.

Treatment with the specific factor should occur in consultation with pediatric hematology. Many neonates do not manifest any bleeding symptoms during the neonatal period and may not require any treatment. Fresh frozen plasma should only be used in the instance of acute hemorrhage when confirmatory testing is not yet available (47).

von Willebrand Disease

von Willebrand Factor (vWF) is the primary plasma protein required for platelet adhesion. It also assists with platelet aggregation and serves as the carrier for Factor VIII (45). Absence, reduction, or abnormal function of vWF result in platelet adhesion and aggregation defects, increasing a neonate's risk for bleeding. However, neonates have higher plasma concentrations of vWF and an increased proportion of high-molecular weight vWF multimers. Therefore, the presentation of von Willebrand disease (vWD) during the neonatal period is very rare.

When a neonate is suspected of having vWD, specialized testing is required. Screening tests (isolated prolonged APTT and/or prolonged epinephrine and ADP CTs measured by the PFA-100) may help support the diagnosis, but further testing would evaluate levels of vWF (vWF antigen assay), platelet-binding function (ristocetin cofactor assay) and Factor VIII–binding function (Factor VIII activity) (48). If confirmed, management depends on the type of vWD and should be in coordination with pediatric hematology (45).

Other Rare Inherited Coagulation Disorders

A complete listing of the other rare coagulation disorders and their treatment, representing 3% to 5% of all coagulation disorders, is presented in Table 44.4A. Deficiencies of fibrinogen and Factors VII and X are the most likely (of the rare disorders) to present during the neonatal period. Factor XIII cross-links fibrin to stabilize thrombi and therefore low levels of Factor XIII will not prolong the PT or APTT. A quantitative assay for Factor XIII is available and should be performed for any neonate with abnormal bleeding that has a normal platelet count, PT, APTT, and fibrinogen level.

Acquired Coagulation Disorders
Vitamin K Deficiency

Vitamin K is an essential cofactor for the γ-carboxylation process of Factors II, VII, IX, and X and proteins C and S (49). Insufficient bacterial colonization of the colon at birth, inadequate dietary intake in solely breast-fed infants, and poor transfer across the placenta place neonates at risk for vitamin K deficiency bleeding (VKDB) formerly known as Hemorrhagic Disease of the Newborn. The different forms and their clinical presentation are displayed in **Table 44.4B**.

Maternal ingestion of certain oral anticoagulants, anticonvulsants, and antituberculosis agents may cause them to cross the placenta and interfere with vitamin K metabolism in the

TABLE 44.4A

Inherited Bleeding Disorders and Their Treatment in Neonates

Disorder	Classification	Treatment	Symptoms
Hemophilia A (FVIII) Hemophilia B (FIX)	Severe (<1%) Moderate (1%–5%) Mild (>40%)	Factor FVIII concentrate Factor FIX concentrate	Bleeding after circumcision and/or blood draws, ICH, extracranial hemorrhage, excessive bruising, muscle hematomas, and bleeding after surgery
Fibrinogen deficiency	Decreased levels (heterozygote): hypofibrinogenemia Absent levels (homozygote): afibrinogenemia Dysfunctional: dysfibrinogenemia	Fibrinogen concentrate FFP or cryoprecipitate if concentrate unavailable	Prolonged bleeding from umbilical stump, bleeding after circumcision, ICH, or mucocutaneous bleeding
Factor II (prothrombin)		Prothrombin concentrate FFP or cryoprecipitate if concentrate unavailable	Mucocutaneous bleeding, ICH, prolonged bleeding from umbilical stump, and bleeding after procedures
Factor V	Commonly associated with congenital anomalies, particularly cardiac defects	Prothrombin complex concentrate (if available) FFP if concentrate unavailable	
Factor VII	Levels do not correlate well with bleeding phenotype	rFVIIa or FFP	
Factor X		rFVIIa or prothrombin complex concentrate (if available)	
Factor XI	Levels do not correlate well with bleeding phenotype	FFP	
Factor XIII		Plasma-derived and recombinant (only for A-subunit deletions) FXIII concentrate Cryoprecipitate if concentrate unavailable	Umbilical cord stump bleeding, ICH, bleeding after procedures

ICH, intracranial hemorrhage.

Reprinted from Saxonhouse MA, Manco-Johnson MJ. The evaluation and management of neonatal coagulation disorders. *Semin Perinatol* 2009;33:52. Copyright © 2009 Elsevier. With permission.

fetus, leading to early VKDB. Classical VKDB is usually due to a physiologic deficiency in vitamin K at birth combined with sole breast milk diet or inadequate feeding. Late VKDB tends to present in either an infant that solely breast-feeds and who

TABLE 44.4B

Acquired Bleeding Disorders and Their Treatment in Neonates

Disorder	Classification	Treatment	Symptoms
DIC		FFP and cryoprecipitate, platelets, heparin	Prolonged bleeding after venipuncture/heel sticks, jaundice, pulmonary hemorrhage
Liver disease		Cryoprecipitate, FFP, prothrombin complex concentrates, platelets, vitamin K, rFVIIa	
Vitamin K deficiency	Early < 24 h Classical 1–7 d	Parenteral vitamin K Prothrombin concentrate for active bleeding	Cephalohematoma, umbilical stump bleeding, ICH GI bleeding, umbilical stump bleeding, mucocutaneous, circumcision, ICH
	Late ≥ 2 wk		ICH, mucocutaneous, GI bleeding

ICH, intracranial hemorrhage; DIC, disseminated intravascular coagulation.

Reprinted from Saxonhouse MA, Manco-Johnson MJ. The evaluation and management of neonatal coagulation disorders. *Semin Perinatol* 2009;33:52. Copyright © 2009 Elsevier. With permission.

received an inadequate dose of vitamin K (none or one oral dose) or has an associated disease process that interferes with the absorption or supply of vitamin K, such as cystic fibrosis, alpha1-antitrypsin deficiency, biliary atresia, hepatitis, or celiac disease (45).

Whenever the diagnosis of VKDB is suspected, a coagulation screening should be performed, which will demonstrate an isolated prolongation of the PT. This can be followed by a prolongation of the APTT, but the prolongation of the PT is usually out of proportion to the elevation of the APTT. If a diagnosis of VKDB is suspected, parenteral treatment (intravenous or intramuscular) with vitamin K should immediately occur. When providing vitamin K IV, the dose should be provided slowly and not more than 1 mg/min. The diagnosis is confirmed by the improvement of the PT and APTT within 2 to 6 hours of the administration of vitamin K. When faced with a neonate with a suspected diagnosis of VKDB and severe hemorrhage, additional therapy with prothrombin complex concentrate (containing all the vitamin K–dependent factors; not available at every institution) aimed at immediate correction of factor deficiencies should occur (45).

The standard of care in the United States is to provide all infants 1.0 mg (0.3 mg/kg for infants <1,000 g and 0.5 mg for infants >1,000 g but <32 weeks of gestation) of intramuscular (IM) vitamin K on the first day of life (50). This dose has been shown to prevent both classical and late VKDB in infants, including in those with cholestatic jaundice (51). The safety of the administration of IM vitamin K has been questioned, but studies have not supported these concerns (52). If a family refuses IM vitamin K, oral dosing may be provided but improper dosing may lead to protection failure from classical and late VKDB. Dosing should be 1 to 2 mg at birth, 1 to 2 mg at 1 to 2 weeks of life, and 1 to 2 mg at 4 weeks of life (53). Dosing regimens for oral vitamin K vary in different countries (see Chapter 18).

Disseminated Intravascular Coagulation

Perinatal and neonatal problems such as birth asphyxia, respiratory failure (respiratory distress syndrome or meconium aspiration syndrome), sepsis, necrotizing enterocolitis, hypothermia, severe placental insufficiency, homozygous deficiency of protein C/S, or thrombosis may lead to the development of DIC. A complex process involving the activation and dysregulation of the coagulation and inflammatory systems, DIC results in massive thrombin generation with widespread fibrin deposition and consumption of coagulation proteins and platelets, ultimately leading to multiorgan damage.

Supporting parameters for making a diagnosis of DIC are presented in Table 44.3. Although supportive care can be provided, the underlying disorder must be treated for the process to subside. Management in the neonate is to support adequate hemostasis and reduce the risk for spontaneous hemorrhage. This is usually achieved with platelet transfusions, FFP, and cryoprecipitate. Another option is to inhibit the activation of the coagulation system using heparin. However, trials in neonates have not been conclusive, and the risk of bleeding may be increased (54).

Liver Disease

Severe, acute liver disease, although rare in neonates, may occur. Birth asphyxia, heart failure, extrahepatic biliary atresia, inborn errors of metabolism, hemophagocytic syndrome, hemochromatosis, and viral hepatitis all may result in acute liver failure in the neonate. Decreased synthesis of coagulation proteins, activation of the coagulation and fibrinolytic systems, poor clearance of activated hemostatic components, loss of coagulation proteins into ascitic fluid, thrombocytopenia, platelet dysfunction, and vitamin K deficiency all may occur and significantly increase a neonate's risk for severe hemorrhage (54). Elevated liver enzymes, direct hyperbilirubinemia, prolongation of the PT and APTT, thrombocytopenia, elevated ammonia levels, decreased fibrinogen levels, and decreased concentrations of Factors VII and V strongly supports the diagnosis of acute liver disease. A normal factor VIII concentration, reflecting extrahepatic synthesis, can help distinguish primary liver disease from DIC (54). Treatment, in addition to treating the underlying cause of liver disease (if able), includes prothrombin complex concentrates (if available) (45), cryoprecipitate (if fibrinogen is low), FFP, recombinant factor VIIa (for bleeding not responsive to platelets and plasma products), platelets, and vitamin K.

▌NEONATAL THROMBOSIS

Incidence/Risk factors

Within the pediatric population, venous thromboembolism (VTE) has an incidence of 0.07 to 0.14/10,000 children, with those less than 1 month of age being most commonly affected (55). Between 1997 and 2018, there was a 13-fold increase in the incidence of neonatal TE, with a greater than 6-fold increase in neonates admitted to the NICU (56). Improving survival rates for the most critically ill and premature neonates (<1,000 g birth weight and <25 to 27 weeks of gestational age), increased utilization of central venous catheters (CVC), and a greater awareness of VTE and its risk factors (**Table 44.5**) have all contributed to this increase (57,58). More than 80% of symptomatic neonatal TE events are associated with the presence of an acquired (maternal, delivery, or neonatal) risk factor (Table 44.5) (58), with the presence of a CVC or arterial catheter being the most common (2.2% to 33.6% incidence) (59). The presence of an umbilical venous catheter (UVC) creates the highest risk for symptomatic VTE in premature neonates (60). Sepsis and congenital heart disease are also significant risk factors for symptomatic VTE in neonates (56).

TABLE 44.5

Acquired Risk Factors for the Development of Neonatal TE

Maternal Risk Factors	Delivery Risk Factors	Neonatal Risk Factors
Infertility	Emergency cesarean section	Central venous/arterial catheters[a]
Oligohydramnios	Fetal heart rate abnormalities	Congenital heart disease
Prothrombotic disorder	Instrumentation	Sepsis/meningitis
Preeclampsia	Meconium-stained fluid	Birth asphyxia
Hypertension		Respiratory distress syndrome
Diabetes		Dehydration
Intrauterine growth restriction		Congenital nephritic/nephrotic syndrome
Chorioamnionitis		Necrotizing enterocolitis
Prolonged rupture of membranes		Polycythemia
Autoimmune disorders		Pulmonary hypertension
		Surgery
		Extracorporeal membrane oxygenation
		Medications (steroids)

[a]Greatest risk factor for thrombosis.

Reprinted from Saxonhouse MA, Manco-Johnson MJ. The evaluation and management of neonatal coagulation disorders. *Semin Perinatol* 2009;33:52. Copyright © 2009 Elsevier. With permission.

Inherited Thrombophilia

The exact role of inherited thrombophilia (IT) in neonatal TE remains poorly defined (58). A recent systematic review found that, while IT may play a role in neonatal TE, clinical risk factors have a bigger influence (61), as demonstrated by CVC-related thromboses in neonates, where only a few cases had an IT associated with them (62). More recent evidence supports that neonatal TE is more influenced by the presence of multiple ITs, or a combination of an IT and clinical risk factors (63). The evaluation for the presence of an IT is appropriate in certain types of neonatal TE, such as those without clinical risk factors or if there is a strong family history. The type of thrombosis, its location, and its severity may also determine the need for an IT evaluation. Due to the large volume of blood required to perform the investigation, a stepwise approach can be used with only certain studies performed during the acute event and most obtained around 3 to 6 months of life (Table 44.6).

The most common IT is the Factor V Leiden (FVL) mutation, with heterozygous mutations affecting about 5% of the Caucasian population. This mutation leads to resistance to activated protein C, resulting in a thrombophilic state. Most people affected by this mutation will not have their first TE event until later in life, but some meta-analyses have found a significant association between FVL mutation and neonatal cerebral sinus venous thrombosis (CSVT) (64).

Prothrombin gene 2021A (PTG) mutation affects approximately 1% to 2% of the Caucasian population and is the second most common IT described in the literature. The mutation results in increasing levels of circulating prothrombin, which increase thrombin concentrations by 15% to 30% and therefore increase TE risk in adults. Reports associating PTG mutations and neonatal TE exist, but these are rare and other studies have not demonstrated a significant association (64).

Both homozygous and heterozygous conditions exist for protein C and protein S deficiencies. If deficient in protein C due to

TABLE 44.6

Evaluation for IT in Neonates[a]

Presence of Other Acquired Risk Factors	No Other Acquired Risk Factors
Antiphospholipid antibody panel, anticardiolipin, and lupus anticoagulant (IgG, IgM)[b]	Antiphospholipid antibody panel, anticardiolipin, and lupus anticoagulant (IgG, IgM)[b]
Protein C activity[c]	Protein C activity[c]
Protein S activity[c]	Protein S activity[c]
Lipoprotein (a) (in Caucasian neonates)[c]	Antithrombin (activity assay)[c]
	Factor V Leiden[d]
Plasminogen level[c] (if considering thrombolytic therapy)	Prothrombin G[d]
	MTHFR mutation[d]
ATIII (activity assay)[c]	PAI-1 4G/5G mutation[d]
Factor V Leiden[d]	Homocysteine[c]
Prothrombin G[d]	Lipoprotein a[c]
	FVIII activity[c]
	FXII activity[c]
	Plasminogen activity[c]
	Heparin cofactor II[c]

If anticoagulation is being administered, then these assays should be obtained 14 to 30 days after discontinuing the anticoagulant.

Lipoprotein (a) levels may need to be repeated at 8 to 12 months of life.

[a]The evaluation presented may be performed in its entirety during the neonatal period or may be performed at 3 to 6 months of age.

[b]May be performed from maternal serum during first few months of life.

[c]Protein-based assays are affected by the acute thrombosis and must be repeated at 3 to 6 months of life, before a definitive diagnosis may be made.

[d]DNA-based assays.

Adapted from Saxonhouse MA, Manco-Johnson MJ. The evaluation and management of neonatal coagulation disorders. *Semin Perinatol* 2009;33:52. Copyright © 2009 Elsevier. With permission.

a heterozygous mutation, FVa and FVIIIa are unable to be inactivated resulting in a 10-fold increased risk for TE. Case reports and case series have suggested that heterozygous protein C deficiency may increase the risk for arterial and venous TE, especially CSVT, in neonates (61). Homozygous mutations resulting in severe protein C deficiency manifests hours after birth with cerebral damage, large vessel thrombosis, and purpura fulminans. Compound heterozygous and homozygous protein S mutations, although rare, also present with purpura fulminans shortly after birth. Newborns affected by purpura fulminans due to either of the mutations have DIC with resulting hemorrhagic complications and large bullous lesions primarily on the extremities, buttock, abdomen, scrotum, and other sites of pressure. Treatment consists of fresh frozen plasma (FFP) at 10 to 20 mL/kg every 12 hours or the use of protein C concentrates until there is resolution of the skin lesions. After the initial treatment, protein C concentrates are safe, efficient, and available for prophylactic use in severe congenital protein C deficiency (65). There are no isolated protein S concentrates available, so treatment involves FFP at 10 to 20 mL/kg every 12 hours until lesions resolve, with potential long-term pharmacologic anticoagulation.

Antithrombin inactivates FIIa (thrombin), FIXa, FXa, FXIa, and FXIIa. Heterozygous antithrombin deficiency has been reported in neonatal arterial and venous TE and in unusual sites such as the coronary arteries, the aorta, and the central nervous system. Homozygous antithrombin deficiency, although rare, has been associated with severe spontaneous neonatal venous and arterial TE (66). Heparin relies on antithrombin as a substrate, so its use for neonates with this deficiency and acute TE is not useful. Plasma-derived concentrates are usually required.

Lipoprotein a (Lp(a)), structurally similar to plasminogen, competes with plasminogen for binding to fibrin. Elevated levels

of Lp(a) can thus reduce fibrinolytic activity significantly enough that TE risk is increased. The true association and risk associated with elevated Lp(a) levels and neonatal TE is not well defined, but it does appear that elevated Lp(a) may play a role in neonatal perinatal arterial ischemic stroke (PAIS) (67).

Clinical Presentations and Locations of Neonatal TE

The various locations of neonatal TE and the recommended imaging modalities to properly diagnose them are presented in Table 44.7. Doppler ultrasonography (US) remains the most widely and safely used modality for neonatal venous and arterial TE, while MRI remains the gold standard for PAIS and CSVT (68).

Arterial TE
Perinatal Arterial Ischemic Stroke

Whether ischemic or hemorrhagic, PAIS occurs from 20 weeks of gestational age to 28 days postnatally. Symptoms, both in term and preterm neonates, consist of acute encephalopathy, seizures, and/or neurologic deficits. Diagnosis is confirmed by MRI demonstrating a parenchymal infarct in the appropriate arterial territory, as cranial ultrasound has been shown to miss as many as 75% of PAIS (69).

The majority of lesions occur in the left hemisphere within the distribution of the middle cerebral artery, with the origin of the left carotid artery from the aorta allowing for a more direct vascular route to the brain as a corridor for cardiac emboli (70). Multifocal cerebral infarctions tend to be embolic in origin. Risk factors implicated in the etiology of PAIS are displayed in Table 44.5. Long-term complications from PAIS include congenital hemiplegic cerebral palsy, seizure disorders, delayed language development, and behavioral disorders (70).

Fetal thrombotic vasculopathy and antiphospholipid antibody syndrome may lead to placental pathology and emboli that break off from the placental circulation and enter the fetal circulation (71).

TABLE 44.7

Locations of Neonatal TE and Recommended Imaging Modalities to Diagnose Them

Vessel	Type of Thromboses (Vessels Potentially Involved)	Imaging Modality
Arterial	Perinatal arterial ischemic stroke (Left middle cerebral artery, anterior cerebral artery, posterior cerebral artery)	Diffusion-weighted MRI/MRA
	Iatrogenic (Abdominal aorta, radial artery, renal artery, mesenteric artery, popliteal artery)	Doppler ultrasound
	Spontaneous (Iliac artery, left pulmonary artery, aortic arch, descending aorta, renal artery)	
Venous	Iatrogenic/spontaneous vessel occlusion (SVC, IVC, hepatic vein, subclavian vein, abdominal veins, peripheral veins)	
	Renal vein	
	Portal venous	
	Cerebral sinovenous (Superior sagittal sinus, transverse sinuses of the superficial venous system, straight sinus of the deep system)	Diffusion-weighted MRI w/venography
	Congenital heart disease related (Right/Left Atria, Right/Left Ventricle, Superior vena cava, Inferior vena cava)	Echocardiography

Adapted from Saxonhouse MA. Management of neonatal thrombosis. *Clin Perinatol* 2012;39:192. Copyright © 2012 Elsevier. With permission.

Iatrogenic/Spontaneous Arterial TE

Arterial catheters (umbilical, peripheral, and femoral), frequently used in the NICU as a means to continuously monitor blood pressure and blood gases, may have significant complications such as infection, limb loss, renal failure, and death (72). In the smallest and most critically ill neonates, umbilical arterial catheters (UACs) are most frequently used. Femoral arterial catheters are used more frequently in neonates with congenital heart disease or those requiring extensive surgery. Suspicion of an arterial TE should be confirmed by Doppler US, but contrast angiography may be required for complicated cases.

Venous TE
Catheter-Related TE

The presence of a CVC represents the greatest risk for neonatal TE. UVCs and peripherally inserted central venous catheters (PCVCs) represent the majority of CVCs placed in neonates. Although vital to improving survival for the smallest and most critically ill neonates, providers must evaluate the risks and benefits every day that a CVC remains in place and removal should occur whenever the risks of a CVC outweigh its benefits. Damage to blood vessel walls during insertion, disrupted blood flow, infusion of substances that damage endothelium, and thrombogenic catheter materials are the main reasons that TE develop (73).

Symptoms such as persistent infection and/or thrombocytopenia, line dysfunction, and bilateral lower limb edema should alert the clinician of a possible UVC-related TE (74). UVCs are typically removed by 7 days, but they should always be removed within 14 days after insertion (75). Symptoms related to either PCVC- or CVC-related TE include unilateral limb swelling/pain/discoloration, superior vena cava syndrome, chylothorax, chylopericardium, intracardiac thrombosis, persistently positive blood cultures, thrombocytopenia, and cardiac failure (60).

Intracardiac TE and TE in Infants with Complex Congenital Heart Disease

Right atrial TE have been associated with endocarditis, pulmonary artery obstruction, ventricular dysfunction, and even death. They may be due to the placement of a CVC, or they may occur before or after repair of a complex congenital heart lesion (76). A recent study demonstrated an incidence of intracardiac TE of 22.5 per 1,000 admissions among infants undergoing palliative cardiac repair (76).

Signs associated with atrial TE include a new onset murmur, sepsis, persistent thrombocytopenia, and cardiac failure.

Renal Vein Thrombosis

The most prevalent non–catheter-related TE during the neonatal period, renal vein thrombosis (RVT), has an incidence of about 0.5 per 1,000 NICU admissions (77). Recent reviews have shown that about 70% of cases are unilateral, with 64% of these involving the left kidney and with a male predominance (78,79). The cardinal signs suggestive of RVT are macroscopic hematuria, a palpable abdominal mass, and thrombocytopenia, with other symptoms including oliguria, proteinuria, acute renal failure, and hypertension. Risk factors are frequently found in RVT cases, with prematurity and perinatal asphyxia being the most common (78). Because of the potential association of an IT and RVT, evaluation for an IT is warranted.

Complications of RVT include adrenal hemorrhage, extension of the clot into the IVC, renal failure, hypertension, and death (79). Survival is currently around 85%. However, renal atrophy did not seem to change regardless of whether supportive care or anticoagulation/fibrinolysis were used, suggesting that many of these events may occur *in utero* and be chronic in nature (78).

Portal Vein Thrombosis

Sepsis/omphalitis and UVC use represent the two major risk factors for portal vein thrombosis (PVT) (80). Diagnosis may be difficult since most cases are clinically silent. Cavernous transformation of the portal vein with subsequent splenomegaly and reversal of portal flow are used to document severity (80). Although spontaneous resolution of asymptomatic PVT in neonates is common, detection of PVT warrants close observation to follow for signs of portal hypertension. This complication may manifest itself up to 10 years after the neonatal period (80).

Cerebral Sinus Venous Thrombosis

A subcategory of perinatal stroke, CSVT symptoms are similar to PAIS (81). Other clinical findings may include anemia and/or thrombocytopenia. Predisposing risk factors are common, with infection, perinatal complications, and IT being the most frequently reported (81). The superficial and lateral sinuses are the most frequently involved vessels, and up to 30% of cases have reported venous infarction with subsequent hemorrhage (70). Intraventricular hemorrhages (especially in term neonates) and hemorrhages within the caudate nucleus and thalamus are associated with thrombosis of the deep cerebral venous sinuses. Therefore, the presence of an intraventricular hemorrhage or thalamic hemorrhage in a term or late preterm infant warrants evaluation for CSVT (82). Diagnosis of CSVT is best made through diffusion MRI with venography (60,74). Mortality rates for neonatal CSVT range from 2% to 24%, with long-term complications consisting of cerebral palsy, epilepsy, and cognitive impairments in 10% to 80% of infants (83).

Management
General Information

The management of neonates with clinically significant TE should occur at a tertiary care center with appropriate pediatric hematology, neonatology, radiology, pharmacology, surgery, and laboratory support (74). Aggressiveness of management depends on type, severity, location, and risk factors. Most cases are managed with either therapeutic anticoagulation or active monitoring for thrombus extension without initial anticoagulation (84). Both short- and long-term complications may develop, and therefore proper follow-up is essential for all neonates evaluated for and/or treated for TE (85).

Arterial TE

In neonates with PAIS, current guidelines recommend anticoagulation only if there is evidence of ongoing cardioembolic sources or recurrence (74,86). Suspicion or confirmation of a TE related to an arterial catheter warrants immediate removal of that catheter (74). Vascular spasm related to arterial catheters in neonates may be alleviated simply by removal of the catheter, but if spasm persists, warming of the contralateral extremity for 15 minutes may resolve symptoms. Further persistence of spasm may require the local application of 2% nitroglycerin ointment at 4 mm/kg with close monitoring of blood pressure (87). Management options for peripheral and femoral arterial catheter-related TE are presented in **Table 44.8**.

Venous TE

When managing neonatal TE associated with CVCs (including UVCs), recommendations are based on whether or not the CVC is still required/vital for care (88). If the CVC is required/vital for care, then the catheter should remain in place during anticoagulation (88). If the CVC is not needed or nonfunctioning, then the catheter should be removed. Delayed removal after 3 to 5 days of anticoagulation is only recommended prior to removing the catheter if the risk for paradoxical emboli is high (88). The majority

TABLE 44.8

Management Options for Peripheral, Femoral, and Umbilical Arterial Catheter-Related TE and Spontaneous TE

Catheter	*Option #1*
Peripheral arterial catheter	Immediate removal of the catheter with no treatment
	Option #2
	If non–limb threatening and mild symptoms after removal, apply topical **2% nitroglycerin ointment at 4 mm/kg**
	Option #3
	If non–limb threatening but concerning symptoms after removal, may start anticoagulation
	Option #4
	If limb threatening symptoms are present after removal, may start rTPA with low-dose UFH
Femoral arterial catheter	*Option # 1*
	If non–limb threatening, start IV UFH until clot resolution but limit treatment to 5–7 d; may convert to LMWH after 48–72 h of UFH treatment and continue until clot resolution
	Option # 2
	If limb or organ threatening, start IV UFH followed by rTPA with UFH within 24–48 h if the thrombus does not improve or symptoms worsen; if rTPA is contraindicated, surgery may be needed
Spontaneous or UAC related	*Option # 1*
	If non–limb or organ threatening, initiate anticoagulation
	Option # 2
	If limb or organ threatening, initiate thrombolytic therapy followed by anticoagulation

UFH, unfractionated heparin; LMWH, low-molecular-weight heparin; rTPA, recombinant tissue plasminogen activator.

Reprinted from Monagle P, Chan AK, Goldenberg NA, et al. Antithrombotic Therapy in neonates and children: Antithrombotic Therapy and Prevention of Thrombosis, 9th ed: American College of Chest Physicians Evidence-Based Clinical Practice Guidelines. *Chest* 2012;141(2 suppl):e737S. Copyright © 2012 The American College of Chest Physicians. With permission.

TABLE 44.9

Management of Renal Vein Thrombosis (RVT), Portal Venous Thrombosis (PVT), and Cerebral Sinus Venous Thrombosis (CSVT)

TE		Clinical Description	Treatment/Monitoring
RVT	Unilateral or bilateral (symptomatic)	Normal renal function	Anticoagulation
		Renal failure	Initial thrombolytic therapy with r-TPA, followed by anticoagulation
PVT		Nonocclusive thrombus and no evidence of portal hypertension	Observation with repeat US in 10 d
		Occlusive thrombus (extension into the IVC, RA, and/or RV)	Anticoagulation *rTPA with UFH may be considered if there is evidence of end-organ compromise*
CSVT		Evidence of CSVT and infant symptomatic	Anticoagulation Repeat MRI and MRV in 6 wk for vessel recanalization. If complete, stop therapy. If not, consider 6 more weeks of treatment

Data from Monagle P, Chan AK, Goldenberg NA, et al. Antithrombotic therapy in neonates and children: Antithrombotic Therapy and Prevention of Thrombosis, 9th ed: American College of Chest Physicians Evidence-Based Clinical Practice Guidelines. *Chest* 2012;141 (2 suppl):e737S; Monagle P, Cuello CA, Augustine C, et al. American Society of Hematology 2018 Guidelines for management of venous thromboembolism: treatment of pediatric venous thromboembolism. *Blood Adv* 2018;2:3292.

Anticoagulation

With baseline antithrombin (AT) levels being lower in neonates compared to children and adults, unfractionated heparin (UFH) treatment in neonates can be challenging. In addition, neonates clear heparin at an increased rate. Thus, neonates frequently require an increase in dosing to attain therapeutic levels (63). Due to the difficulty in obtaining therapeutic heparin levels in neonates, rare cases may require the administration of AT concentrate.

TABLE 44.10

Contraindications for Anticoagulation/Thrombolysis

	Absolute	Relative
Medical conditions	1. CNS surgery or ischemia (including birth asphyxia) within 10 d	1. Platelet count < 50 × 10³/μL (100 × 10³/μL for ill neonates)
	2. Active bleeding	2. Fibrinogen concentration <100 mg/dL
	3. Invasive procedures within 3 d	3. INR > 2
	4. Seizures within 48 h	4. Severe coagulation deficiency
		5. Hypertension

CNS, central nervous system.

Adapted from Manco-Johnson M. Controversies in neonatal thrombotic disorders. In: Ohls RY, ed. *Hematology, immunology and infectious disease: neonatology questions and controversies.* Philadelphia, PA: Saunders Elsevier, 2008:59. Copyright © 2008 Elsevier. With permission.

of neonatal CVC-related TE are treated with anticoagulation, with thrombolytic therapy reserved for life- or limb-threatening cases. Current management options for venous TE in neonates are thrombolysis followed by therapeutic anticoagulation, therapeutic anticoagulation alone, or close observation. A large study in the Netherlands is currently underway determining the best treatment options for neonates with venous TE (89). Thrombolytics and/or anticoagulation should also be used for neonates with infective endocarditis that is resistant to antibiotic therapy alone and should be based on the size and symptoms of the TE (90). RVT, PVT, and CSVT treatment guidelines are provided in **Table 44.9**.

Due to a lack of randomized controlled trials, anticoagulant and thrombolytic dosing regimens for neonates are extrapolated from adult and pediatric data, as well as neonatal case reports and/or series. With the risk of withholding potential life-saving treatment, these trials will likely not be completed within the neonatal TE population (74,91). Therefore, an accurate assessment for serious complications in neonates due to anticoagulant and thrombolytic therapy will never truly be known, especially for premature infants. Before initiating any treatment, absolute and relative contraindications (**Table 44.10**) must be reviewed and family discussions should occur so that the best clinical decision is made.

If AT is provided in neonates, close monitoring of heparin levels is required as supratherapeutic anticoagulant levels may be rapidly obtained, thus increasing the risk of bleeding complications. Therefore, administration of AT concentrate should only occur with pediatric hematology assistance.

Low molecular weight heparin (LMWH) selectively inhibits activated factor X (FXa), with enoxaparin being the LMWH utilized most often (92,93). Compared with UFH, LMWH has fewer bleeding complications, a longer half-life, and a more consistent pharmacokinetic and pharmacodynamic profile (94). LMWH's effectiveness has been demonstrated, with centers reporting either partial or complete resolution of TE events in 59% to 100% of neonates treated (95). Initial dosing guidelines based on gestational age are presented in **Table 44.11**. The challenge with maintaining therapeutic levels in neonates has been demonstrated by a recent review of 240 neonates, in whom the mean maintenance dose of enoxaparin ranged from 1.48 to 2.27 mg/kg every 12 hours for all infants, but was higher for preterm neonates at 1.9 to 2.27 mg/kg every 12 hours (95).

Despite LMWH being the anticoagulant of choice, UFH still has its place in the NICU. UFH has similar activity against both FXa and FIIa, has a much shorter half-life than LMWH, and can be reversed with protamine (63). Therefore, if anticoagulation is necessary in an infant whose risk for bleeding is high, UFH may be the appropriate choice. Initial dosing recommendations based on gestational age are displayed in Table 44.11. Current recommendations are to NOT provide an initial loading dose of UFH to neonates due to an increased bleeding risk (97). Loading doses should be reserved for neonates with significant risk or evidence of thrombus progression. UFH therapy should be limited to short-term use in neonates, with attempts to convert to LMWH if longer anticoagulation is required.

TABLE 44.11
Recommended Dosing for Anticoagulant Therapy in Neonates

Gestational Age[a]	UFH	LMWH
≤32 wk	15 units/kg/h	1.5 mg/kg SQ q12h
>32 wk	28 units/kg/h	2 mg/kg SQ q12h
		Prophylactic dosing
		0.75 mg/kg SQ q12h
		Goal for antifactor Xa level of 0.1–0.3 units/mL

Monitoring for UFH: Maintain anti-Xa UFH assay level of 0.3–0.7 units/mL. Levels should be checked 4–6 h after initiating therapy. If loading dose provided, check level 4–6 h after loading dose provided. If need to make changes in dosing, check levels 4–6 h after each change in infusion rate.

Monitoring for LMWH: Maintain anti-Xa LMWH assay level of 0.5–1.0 units/mL. Check level 4 h after the 2nd or 3rd dose. If therapeutic, repeat level within 24–48 h. If remain therapeutic, then may check weekly (96).

Complete blood count, platelet count, and coagulation screening (including activated partial thromboplastin time, prothrombin time, PT, and fibrinogen) should be performed prior to starting anticoagulation.

Bolus dosing for UFH should be performed only if there is a significant risk or evidence of thrombus progression (97). Otherwise, avoid bolus dosing in neonates. If bolus dosing is recommended: ≤32 weeks 25 units/kg IV over 10 minutes; >32 weeks 50 units/kg IV over 10 minutes.

If infant with renal dysfunction, dosing should be discussed with pharmacist.

Adjustment of dosing based on anti-Xa assay levels are published elsewhere.

[a]Dosing applies also to postconceptional age (GA + weeks of life).

Data from Monagle P, Chan AK, Goldenberg NA, et al. Antithrombotic therapy in neonates and children: Antithrombotic Therapy and Prevention of Thrombosis, 9th ed: American College of Chest Physicians Evidence-Based Clinical Practice Guidelines. *Chest* 2012;141 (2 suppl):e737S; Armstrong-Wells JL, Manco-Johnson MJ. Neonatal thrombosis. In: De Alarcon PW, Werner EJ, Christensen RD, eds. *Neonatal hematology*. New York, NY: Cambridge University Press, 2013:282. Ref. (98).

TABLE 44.12
Neonatal rTPA Dosing/Management Guidelines

Clinical Situation	Recommended Dosing	Appropriate Monitoring
Limb/life-threatening thrombus	0.03 mg/kg/h Infuse UFH at 10 units/kg/h	Dose escalation up to 0.3 mg/kg/h can be considered but must be done slowly with continuing monitoring of the patient. Supplementation with plasminogen (FFP at 10 mL/kg) prior to commencing therapy is recommended to ensure adequate thrombolysis (13)

Dose titrations may be made every 12–24 hours and are as follows: 0.06 mg/kg/h → 0.1 mg/kg/h → 0.2 mg/kg/h → 0.3 mg/kg/h. Max dose is 0.3 mg/kg/h.

- For arterial thrombi, reimage at 6- to 8-hour intervals; for venous thrombi, reimage at 12- to 24-hour intervals.
- If repeat imaging reveals clot lysis <50%, INCREASE infusion to next dosing level and repeat imaging in 12–24 hours.
- If repeat imaging reveals clot lysis 51%–94%, continue same dose of infusion and repeat imaging in 12–24 hours.
- If repeat imaging reveals clot lysis >95%, stop infusion and initiate anticoagulation protocol.
- If no clot dissolution occurring 12–24 hours after starting infusion and/or D-dimers are not increasing, may also give additional 10 mL/kg of FFP to provide plasminogen to increase efficacy of rTPA.
- Attempt to maintain fibrinogen levels >100 mg/dL (provide cryo if <100) and platelet counts >50,000/μL.
- rTPA infusion should not be used for >96 hours unless deemed appropriate by neonatology.

Thrombolysis

Thrombolytic therapy in neonates is mainly used for life- or limb-threatening TE. Recombinant tissue plasminogen activator (rTPA) is the current agent of choice. Data on neonatal use is limited, but case series and cohort studies have reported both safety and efficacy with complete or partial clot lysis in 84% to 94% of cases (99). Due to neonatal plasminogen levels being about 50% of adult levels and with dosing being based on adult data, it is recommended that plasminogen supplementation be provided prior to starting rTPA therapy (74). Dosing recommendations for rTPA as well as proper monitoring guidelines for neonatal use are provided in **Table 44.12**. Once desired effects are achieved from rTPA, therapy should be discontinued and transitioned to therapeutic anticoagulation, preferably LMWH.

Bleeding, particularly ICH, is the major risk associated with rTPA use in neonates. Therefore, other risk factors associated with increasing bleeding risk, such as hypertension, thrombocytopenia, and vitamin K deficiency, should be addressed prior to initiating rTPA therapy in neonates, especially preterm infants.

CONCLUSION

Neonatal bleeding and TE represent significant complications that neonates admitted to the NICU may encounter. With increasing survival of the most critically ill neonates, bleeding and TE events are likely to increase. Neonatologists and hematologists caring for these infants must base their clinical decisions on limited data. Current studies are attempting to determine optimal protocols and care for neonates with symptomatic TE. Despite limited data, the most important goal for anyone caring for neonates with either bleeding or TE emergencies is to treat effectively without causing additional harm. Future studies and improved data registries investigating treatment options for neonatal bleeding and TE will enhance the care provided to these neonates.

REFERENCES

1. Dreyfus M, Kaplan C, Verdy E, et al. Frequency of immune thrombocytopenia in newborns: a prospective study. Immune Thrombocytopenia Working Group. *Blood* 1997;89(12):4402.

2. Castle V, Andrew M, Kelton J, et al. Frequency and mechanism of neonatal thrombocytopenia. *J Pediatr* 1986;108(5 Pt 1):749.

3. Christensen RD, Henry E, Wiedmeier SE, et al. Thrombocytopenia among extremely low birth weight neonates: data from a multihospital healthcare system. *J Perinatol* 2006;26(6):348.

4. Wiedmeier SE, Henry E, Sola-Visner MC, et al. Platelet reference ranges for neonates, defined using data from over 47,000 patients in a multihospital healthcare system. *J Perinatol* 2009;29(2):130.

5. Israels SJ, Odaibo FS, Robertson C, et al. Deficient thromboxane synthesis and response in platelets from premature infants. *Pediatr Res* 1997;41(2):218.

6. Sitaru AG, Holzhauer S, Speer CP, et al. Neonatal platelets from cord blood and peripheral blood. *Platelets* 2005;16(3-4):203.

7. Israels SJ, Rand ML, Michelson AD. Neonatal platelet function. *Semin Thromb Hemost* 2003;29(4):363.

8. Hardy AT, Palma-Barqueros V, Watson SK, et al. Significant hypo-responsiveness to GPVI and CLEC-2 agonists in pre-term and full-term neonatal platelets and following immune thrombocytopenia. *Thromb Haemost* 2018;118(6):1009.

9. Palma-Barqueros V, Torregrosa JM, Caparros-Perez E, et al. Developmental differences in platelet inhibition response to prostaglandin E1. *Neonatology* 2020;117:1.

10. Schlagenhauf A, Schweintzger S, Birner-Gruenberger R, et al. Newborn platelets: lower levels of protease-activated receptors cause hypoaggregability to thrombin. *Platelets* 2010;21(8):641.

11. Andrew M, Paes B, Bowker J, et al. Evaluation of an automated bleeding time device in the newborn. *Am J Hematol* 1990;35(4):275.

12. Israels SJ, Cheang T, McMillan-Ward EM, et al. Evaluation of primary hemostasis in neonates with a new in vitro platelet function analyzer. *J Pediatr* 2001;138(1):116.

13. Del Vecchio A, Latini G, Henry E, et al. Template bleeding times of 240 neonates born at 24 to 41 weeks gestation. *J Perinatol* 2008;6(28):427.

14. Saxonhouse MA, Garner R, Mammel L, et al. Closure times measured by the platelet function analyzer PFA-100 are longer in neonatal blood compared to cord blood samples. *Neonatology* 2010;97(3):242.

15. Bednarek FJ, Bean S, Barnard MR, et al. The platelet hyporeactivity of extremely low birth weight neonates is age-dependent. *Thromb Res* 2009;124(1):42.

16. Christensen RD, Baer VL, Henry E, et al. Thrombocytopenia in small-for-gestational-age infants. *Pediatrics* 2015;136(2):e361.

17. Ko YJ, Kim H, Hur M, et al. Establishment of reference interval for immature platelet fraction. *Int J Lab Hematol* 2013;35(5):528.

18. Cremer M, Weimann A, Schmalisch G, et al. Immature platelet values indicate impaired megakaryopoietic activity in neonatal early-onset thrombocytopenia. *Thromb Haemost* 2010;103(5):1016.

19. MacQueen BC, Christensen RD, Henry E, et al. The immature platelet fraction: creating neonatal reference intervals and using these to categorize neonatal thrombocytopenias. *J Perinatol* 2017;37(7):834.

20. Cremer M, Paetzold J, Schmalisch G, et al. Immature platelet fraction as novel laboratory parameter predicting the course of neonatal thrombocytopenia. *Br J Haematol* 2009;144(4):619.

21. Cremer M, Weimann A, Szekessy D, et al. Low immature platelet fraction suggests decreased megakaryopoiesis in neonates with sepsis or necrotizing enterocolitis. *J Perinatol* 2013;33(8):622.

22. Liu ZJ, Bussel JB, Lakkaraja M, et al. Suppression of in vitro megakaryopoiesis by maternal sera containing anti-HPA-1a antibodies. *Blood* 2015;126(10):1234.

23. Bertrand G, Drame M, Martageix C, et al. Prediction of the fetal status in noninvasive management of alloimmune thrombocytopenia. *Blood* 2011;117(11):3209.

24. Bussel JB, Zacharoulis S, Kramer K, et al. Clinical and diagnostic comparison of neonatal alloimmune thrombocytopenia to non-immune cases of thrombocytopenia. *Pediatr Blood Cancer* 2005;45(2):176.

25. Kiefel V, Bassler D, Kroll H, et al. Antigen-positive platelet transfusion in neonatal alloimmune thrombocytopenia (NAIT). *Blood* 2006;107(9):3761.

26. Burrows RF, Kelton JG. Pregnancy in patients with idiopathic thrombocytopenic purpura: assessing the risks for the infant at delivery. *Obstet Gynecol Surv* 1993;48(12):781.

27. Provan D, Stasi R, Newland AC, et al. International consensus report on the investigation and management of primary immune thrombocytopenia. *Blood* 2010;115(2):168.

28. Hauschner H, Rosenberg N, Seligsohn U, et al. Persistent neonatal thrombocytopenia can be caused by IgA antiplatelet antibodies in breast milk of immune thrombocytopenic mothers. *Blood* 2015;126(5):661.

29. Kong Z, Qin P, Xiao S, et al. A novel recombinant human thrombopoietin therapy for the management of immune thrombocytopenia in pregnancy. *Blood* 2017;130(9):1097.

30. Gershanik JJ, Morgan SK, Akers R. Fanconi's anemia in a neonate. *Acta Paediatr Scand* 1972;61(5):623.

31. Geddis AE. Inherited thrombocytopenia: congenital amegakaryocytic thrombocytopenia and thrombocytopenia with absent radii. *Semin Hematol* 2006;43(3):196.

32. Sola MC, Slayton WB, Rimsza LM, et al. A neonate with severe thrombocytopenia and radio-ulnar synostosis. *J Perinatol* 2004;24(8):528.

33. Smock KJ, Perkins SL. Thrombocytopenia: an update. *Int J Lab Hematol* 2014;36(3):269.

34. Cremer M, Sola-Visner M, Roll S, et al. Platelet transfusions in neonates: practices in the United States vary significantly from those in Austria, Germany, and Switzerland. *Transfusion* 2011;51(12):2634.

35. Andrew M, Vegh P, Caco C, et al. A randomized, controlled trial of platelet transfusions in thrombocytopenic premature infants. *J Pediatr* 1993;123(2):285.

36. Curley A, Stanworth SJ, New H. A randomized trial of neonatal platelet transfusion thresholds. Reply. *N Engl J Med* 2019;380(16):1584.

37. Baer VL, Lambert D, Henry E, et al. Do platelet transfusions in the NICU adversely affect survival? Analysis of 1600 thrombocytopenic neonates in a multihospital healthcare system. *J Perinatol* 2007;12(27):242.

38. Patel RM, Josephson CD, Shenvi N, et al. Platelet transfusions and mortality in necrotizing enterocolitis. *Transfusion* 2019;59(3):981.

39. Fustolo-Gunnink SF, Fijnvandraat K, van Klaveren D, et al. Preterm neonates benefit from low prophylactic platelet transfusion threshold despite varying risk of bleeding or death. *Blood* 2019;134(26):2354.

40. Josephson CD, Caliendo AM, Easley KA, et al. Blood transfusion and breast milk transmission of cytomegalovirus in very-low-birth-weight infants: a prospective cohort study. *JAMA Pediatr* 2014;168(11):1054.

41. Christensen RD, Sheffield MJ, Lambert DK, et al. Effect of therapeutic hypothermia in neonates with hypoxic-ischemic encephalopathy on platelet function. *Neonatology* 2012;101(2):91.

42. Israels SJ. Diagnostic evaluation of platelet function disorders in neonates and children: an update. *Semin Thromb Hemost* 2009;35(2):181.

43. Simeoni I, Stephens JC, Hu F, et al. A high-throughput sequencing test for diagnosing inherited bleeding, thrombotic, and platelet disorders. *Blood* 2016;127(23):2791.

44. Young G, Wicklund B, Neff P, et al. Off-label use of rFVIIa in children with excessive bleeding: a consecutive study of 153 off-label uses in 139 children. *Pediatr Blood Cancer* 2009;53(2):179.

45. Young G. Hemostatic disorders of the newborn. In: Gleason CDS, ed. *Avery's diseases of the newborn*. Philadelphia, PA: Elsevier, 2015.

46. Will A. Neonatal haemostasis and the management of neonatal thrombosis. *Br J Haematol* 2015;169(3):324.

47. Chalmers EA. Neonatal coagulation problems. *Arch Dis Child Fetal Neonatal Ed* 2004;89(6):F475.

48. Ng C, Motto DG, Di Paola J. Diagnostic approach to von Willebrand disease. *Blood* 2015;125(13):2029.

49. Jaffray J, Young G, Ko RH. The bleeding newborn: a review of presentation, diagnosis, and management. *Semin Fetal Neonatal Med* 2016;21(1):44.

50. Saxonhouse MA, Manco-Johnson MJ. The evaluation and management of neonatal coagulation disorders. *Semin Perinatol* 2009;33(1):52.

51. McNinch A, Busfield A, Tripp J. Vitamin K deficiency bleeding in Great Britain and Ireland: British Paediatric Surveillance Unit Surveys, 1993-94 and 2001-02. *Arch Dis Child* 2007;92(9):759.

52. Ross JA, Davies SM. Vitamin K prophylaxis and childhood cancer. *Med Pediatr Oncol* 2000;34(6):434.

53. van Hasselt PM, de Koning TJ, Kvist N, et al. Prevention of vitamin K deficiency bleeding in breastfed infants: lessons from the Dutch and Danish biliary atresia registries. *Pediatrics* 2008;121(4):e857.

54. Albisetti M, Andrew M, Monagle P. Hemostatic abnormalities. In: de Alarcon P, Winter E, eds. *Neonatal hematology*. Cambridge, UK: Cambridge University Press, 2005:310.

55. van Ommen CH, Heijboer H, Buller HR, et al. Venous thromboembolism in childhood: a prospective two-year registry in The Netherlands. *J Pediatr* 2001;139(5):676.

56. Bhat R, Kumar R, Kwon S, et al. Risk factors for neonatal venous and arterial thromboembolism in the neonatal intensive care unit—a case control study. *J Pediatr* 2018;195:28.

57. Uttara N, L H, Roberts C, et al. Risk factors for thrombosis in the neonatal intensive care unit: analysis of large national database. *Annual Meeting of the American Society of Hematology*, 2017.

58. Saracco P, Bagna R, Gentilomo C, et al. Clinical data of neonatal systemic thrombosis. *J Pediatr* 2016;171:60 e61.

59. Park CK, Paes BA, Nagel K, et al. Neonatal central venous catheter thrombosis: diagnosis, management and outcome. *Blood Coagul Fibrinolysis* 2014;25(2):97.

THE NEWBORN INFANT

60. Rajagopal R, Cheah FC, Monagle P. Thromboembolism and anticoagulation management in the preterm infant. *Semin Fetal Neonatal Med* 2016;21(1):50.

61. Klaassen IL, van Ommen CH, Middeldorp S. Manifestations and clinical impact of pediatric inherited thrombophilia. *Blood* 2015;125(7):1073.

62. Demirel G, Oguz SS, Celik IH, et al. Evaluation and treatment of neonatal thrombus formation in 17 patients. *Clin Appl Thromb Hemostasis* 2011;17(6):E46.

63. Saxonhouse MA. Thrombosis in the neonatal intensive care unit. *Clin Perinatol* 2015;42(3):651.

64. Laugesaar R, Kolk A, Tomberg T, et al. Acutely and retrospectively diagnosed perinatal stroke: a population-based study. *Stroke* 2007;38(8):2234.

65. Kroiss S, Albisetti M. Use of human protein C concentrates in the treatment of patients with severe congenital protein C deficiency. *Biologics* 2010;4:51.

66. Swoboda V, Zervan K, Thom K, et al. Homozygous antithrombin deficiency type II causing neonatal thrombosis. *Thromb Res* 2017;158:134.

67. Nowak-Gottl U, Junker R, Hartmeier M, et al. Increased lipoprotein(a) is an important risk factor for venous thromboembolism in childhood. *Circulation* 1999;100(7):743.

68. Pettit J. Assessment of infants with peripherally inserted central catheters: Part 1. Detecting the most frequently occurring complications. *Adv Neonatal Care* 2002;2(6):304.

69. Gacio S, Munoz Giacomelli F, Klein F. Presumed perinatal ischemic stroke: a review. *Arch Argent Pediatr* 2015;113(5):449.

70. Chalmers EA. Perinatal stroke—risk factors and management. *Br J Haematol* 2005;130(3):333.

71. Giacchetti L, De Gaudenzi M, Leoncini A, et al. Neonatal renal and inferior vena cava thrombosis associated with fetal thrombotic vasculopathy: a case report. *J Med Case Rep* 2017;11(1):248.

72. Nouri S, Mahdhaoui N, Beizig S, et al. [Major neonatal aortic thrombosis: a case report]. *Arch Pediatr* 2007;14(9):1097.

73. Bhat R, Monagle P. The preterm infant with thrombosis. *Arch Dis Child Fetal Neonatal Ed* 2012;97(6):F423.

74. Monagle P, Chan AK, Goldenberg NA, et al. Antithrombotic therapy in neonates and children: Antithrombotic Therapy and Prevention of Thrombosis, 9th ed: American College of Chest Physicians Evidence-Based Clinical Practice Guidelines. *Chest* 2012;141(2 suppl):e737S.

75. O'Grady NP, Alexander M, Dellinger EP, et al. Guidelines for the prevention of intravascular catheter-related infections. *Infect Control Hosp Epidemiol* 2002;23(12):759.

76. Ulloa-Ricardez A, Romero-Espinoza L, Estrada-Loza MJ, et al. Risk factors for intracardiac thrombosis in the right atrium and superior vena cava in critically ill neonates who required the installation of a central venous catheter. *Pediatr Neonatol* 2016;57(4):288.

77. Schmidt B, Andrew M. Neonatal thrombosis: report of a prospective Canadian and international registry. *Pediatrics* 1995;96(5 Pt 1):939.

78. Bidadi B, Nageswara Rao AA, Kaur D, et al. Neonatal renal vein thrombosis: role of anticoagulation and thrombolysis—an institutional review. *Pediatr Hematol Oncol* 2016;33(1):59.

79. Lau KK, Stoffman JM, Williams S, et al. Neonatal renal vein thrombosis: review of the English-language literature between 1992 and 2006. *Pediatrics* 2007;120(5):e1278.

80. Williams S, Chan AK. Neonatal portal vein thrombosis: diagnosis and management. *Semin Fetal Neonatal Med* 2011;16(6):329.

81. Wasay M, Dai AI, Ansari M, et al. Cerebral venous sinus thrombosis in children: a multicenter cohort from the United States. *J Child Neurol* 2008;23(1):26.

82. Wu YW, Hamrick SE, Miller SP, et al. Intraventricular hemorrhage in term neonates caused by sinovenous thrombosis. *Ann Neurol* 2003;54(1):123.

83. Berfelo FJ, Kersbergen KJ, van Ommen CH, et al. Neonatal cerebral sinovenous thrombosis from symptom to outcome. *Stroke* 2010;41(7):1382.

84. van Elteren HA, Veldt HS, Te Pas AB, et al. Management and outcome in 32 neonates with thrombotic events. *Int J Pediatr* 2011;2011:217564.

85. Bacciedoni V, Attie M, Donato H; Comite Nacional de Hematología OyMT. Thrombosis in newborn infants. *Arch Argent Pediatr* 2016;114(2):159.

86. van der Aa NE, Benders MJ, Groenendaal F, et al. Neonatal stroke: a review of the current evidence on epidemiology, pathogenesis, diagnostics and therapeutic options. *Acta Paediatr* 2014;103(4):356.

87. Saxonhouse MA. Management of neonatal thrombosis. *Clin Perinatol* 2012;39(1):191.

88. Monagle P, Cuello CA, Augustine C, et al. American Society of Hematology 2018 Guidelines for management of venous thromboembolism: treatment of pediatric venous thromboembolism. *Blood Adv* 2018;2(22):3292.

89. Sol JJ, van de Loo M, Boerma M, et al. NEOnatal Central-venous Line Observational study on Thrombosis (NEOCLOT): evaluation of a national guideline on management of neonatal catheter-related thrombosis. *BMC Pediatr* 2018;18(1):84.

90. Marks KA, Zucker N, Kapelushnik J, et al. Infective endocarditis successfully treated in extremely low birth weight infants with recombinant tissue plasminogen activator. *Pediatrics* 2002;109(1):153.

91. Saxonhouse MA, Tarquinio D, Carney PR, et al. Low-molecular-weight heparin use in a case of noncardiogenic multifocal perinatal thromboembolic stroke. *Adv Hematol* 2009;2009:153643.

92. Young G. Old and new antithrombotic drugs in neonates and infants. *Semin Fetal Neonatal Med* 2011;16(6):349.

93. Chan AK, Monagle P. Updates in thrombosis in pediatrics: where are we after 20 years? *Hematology* 2012;2012:439.

94. Samama MM, Gerotziafas GT. Comparative pharmacokinetics of LMWHs. *Semin Thromb Hemost* 2000;26(suppl 1):31.

95. Malowany JI, Monagle P, Knoppert DC, et al. Enoxaparin for neonatal thrombosis: a call for a higher dose for neonates. *Thromb Res* 2008;122(6):826.

96. Molinari AC, Banov L, Bertamino M, et al. A practical approach to the use of low molecular weight heparins in VTE treatment and prophylaxis in children and newborns. *Pediatr Hematol Oncol* 2015;32(1):1.

97. Bhatt MD, Paes BA, Chan AK. How to use unfractionated heparin to treat neonatal thrombosis in clinical practice. *Blood Coagul Fibrinolysis* 2016;27(6):605.

98. Armstrong-Wells JM-J, M. Neonatal thrombosis. In: De Alarcon PW, Werner EJ, Christensen RD, eds. *Neonatal hematology*. New York, NY: Cambridge University Press, 2013:282.

99. Hartmann J, Hussein A, Trowitzsch E, et al. Treatment of neonatal thrombus formation with recombinant tissue plasminogen activator: six years experience and review of the literature. *Arch Dis Child Fetal Neonatal Ed* 2001;85(1):F18.

Neonatal Hyperbilirubinemia

Vinod K. Bhutani and Ronald J. Wong

INTRODUCTION

Neonatal hyperbilirubinemia occurs in almost all newborns. It is usually reversible, transient, and benign. In some full-term infants, extreme hyperbilirubinemia (EHB) or total serum/plasma bilirubin (TB) greater than 25 mg/dL (428 µmol/L) can develop, and is associated with long-term sequelae. These adverse outcomes can be prevented if the progressive hyperbilirubinemia is managed in a timely manner upon early recognition and diligent monitoring. Hyperbilirubinemia that rapidly progresses or a TB greater than 17 mg/dL (291 µmol/L) is normally due to hemolysis and, in the past, was often because of Rhesus (Rh) disease, ABO blood group isoimmunization, or glucose-6-phosphate dehydrogenase (G6PD) deficiency. In 1953, Hsia et al. (1) were the first to report that cord TB levels in full-term "*ABO-compatible*," full-term "*ABO-incompatible*" infants, and premature infants are essentially the same. However, the average cord TB level of infants with *erythroblastosis fetalis* (a TB level above 5 mg/dL [86 µmol/L] is strongly suggestive of Rh disease) was more than double that of infants without erythroblastosis. They also observed that among normal full-term infants, a rise of TB during the first day of life is indicative of hemolysis. Normally, term infants reach their peak TB levels at about 2 days of life; whereas, in premature infants, the peak occurs later, at about 4 days of life and reach higher levels. In all infants, peak TB levels can be exacerbated by delayed bilirubin elimination processes in the immature newborn liver. Some groups of infants are more vulnerable to bilirubin neurotoxicity because they have poor bilirubin-binding capacity (BBC), concurrent infections, or familial and/or genetic disorders (2). Hyperbilirubinemia is defined as an increase in circulating TB levels and differs from "*jaundice*," which is a yellowing of the skin, mucous membranes, or conjunctiva. Jaundice can be visible during the first 7 days of birth in 84% of all well newborns (3,4). Importantly, the presence or absence of jaundice does not accurately reflect TB levels nor the extent of the hyperbilirubinemia (5). In fact, TB greater than 1.0 mg/dL (17.1 µmol/L) occurs in almost every newborn and is usually benign. Infants with severe hyperbilirubinemia (TB levels >20 mg/dL [342 µmol/L]) are likely to have an increased risk of developing bilirubin neurotoxicity (6). Certain peri- and postnatal conditions can lead to an influx of "*free*" or unbound bilirubin (UB) into the brain, particularly in infants with a disrupted blood–brain barrier (such as in intracranial hemorrhages), asphyxia, acidosis, or hypoalbuminemia (7,8). Thus, bilirubin-induced neurologic dysfunction or BIND may occur at lower TB levels than those observed for term and healthy infants (6,9,10). *In utero*, all unconjugated bilirubin (i.e., fat-soluble and not glucuronidated) is eliminated through the placental circulation such that fetal and maternal bilirubin values are at equilibrium, and unconjugated bilirubin values greater than 2 mg/dL are considered excessive (Table 45.1) (11–14). The immaturity of the fetal liver and its incapacity to conjugate bilirubin via glucuronidation limits the intrauterine elimination of bilirubin, relying solely on the transplacental gradient (15). Certain authors reported that prolonged fetal exposure to elevated unconjugated hyperbilirubinemia could lead to neurologic damage. After birth, hepatic bilirubin conjugating capacity increases exponentially between 6 and 14 weeks of life after placental separation and leads to the natural elimination of bilirubin.

BILIRUBIN METABOLISM

Bilirubin Production (Heme Metabolism)

Heme from circulating hemoglobin (iron protoporphyrin) released by senescing red blood cells (RBCs) is catabolized to equimolar amounts of iron, carbon monoxide (CO) and biliverdin, which is then rapidly converted to bilirubin (16). This process is mediated by the rate-limiting enzyme heme oxygenase (HO) located primarily in the reticuloendothelial system (17). Hemolysis is the destruction of RBCs from circulation before their normal life span of 60 to 90 days in newborn infants. Major causes of hemolysis are discussed below.

Hepatic Uptake of Bilirubin

Unconjugated bilirubin is bound to albumin in the circulation. A primary (high affinity) and a secondary (low-affinity) site for bilirubin exist on each molecule of albumin (2). When the bilirubin-albumin complex reaches the hepatocyte, a proportion is transferred by up to four transport proteins on the plasma membrane. After entry into the hepatocyte, bilirubin is bound principally to ligandin as well as possibly other cytosolic-binding proteins and a network of intracellular microsomal membranes. In this unconjugated form, bilirubin is nonpolar and insoluble and must be converted to polar, water-soluble conjugates (bilirubin mono- and diglucuronides) by the enzyme uridine diphosphoglucuronosyltransferase (UGT1A1) for hepatic excretion. Conjugation in the hepatocytes is mediated by the gene UGT1A1, a specific hepatic isoform of UGT, which encodes the UGT1A1 enzyme. It is located on chromosome 2 at 2q37 and contains 4 common exons and 13 variable exons (18) (**Fig. 45.1**). In addition, an upstream non-coding promoter regulatory region controls gene expression. The UGT1A1 promoter also houses a TATAA box, which is a sequence of thymine (T) and adenine (A) (19). Most conjugation defects arise from mutations of the UGT1A1 exon or its promoter (18,19) (see below).

Biliary and Intestinal Metabolism

Bilirubin is excreted rapidly into the bile canaliculi as conjugated bilirubin after glucuronidation. The process is concentration-gradient dependent and guided by active transport. Hepatocellular injury can disrupt the transport process. Post-intestinal elimination from the biliary system, conjugated bilirubin is not reabsorbed. Colonic bacteria in healthy adults degrades conjugated bilirubin into colorless tetrapyrroles, urobilinogen and stercobilinogens. A significant amount may undergo hydrolysis back to non–water-soluble unconjugated bilirubin that can be re-absorbed back into the circulation—a process called "enterohepatic circulation."

Clinical gastrointestinal (GI) integrity for elimination of conjugated bilirubin and its recirculation can be impacted by prematurity, starvation (decreased enteral intake), decreased GI activity, delayed bacterial colonization of the gut, pyloric stenosis, GI dysmotility or obstruction.

NEONATAL HYPERBILIRUBINEMIA

Neonatal hyperbilirubinemia is a result of decreased bilirubin elimination concurrent with increased bilirubin production rates. In newborns, hepatic conjugation of bilirubin to mono- and diglucuronides is impaired due to low expression of the enzyme UGT1A1

TABLE 45.1

Progression of TB (Postnatal Age: 0 to 96 h) in Infants ≥35 weeks' GA

Postnatal Age (h)	Threshold at TB 95th Percentile Track mg/dL (µmol/L)	Rate of Rise (ROR) mg/dL/h (µmol/L/h)	Predischarge TB ROR (0–60 h) (mg/dL/h) (µmol/L/h)
Cord	≤2.0 (34.2)[a]	<0.20 (3.4)	0.22 (3.8)
24	7.8 (137)	+0.240 (4.1)	
36	11.1 (188)	+0.275 (4.7)	
48	13.2 (222)	+0.175 (3.0)	
60	15.2 (274)	+0.250 (4.3)	
72	15.9 (274)	+0.058 (1.0)	0.03 (0.5)
84	16.7 (274)	+0.067 (1.1)	
96	17.4 (298)	+0.058 (1.0)	

[a]Cord blood values are based on several studies (Data from Carbonell X, Botet F, Figueras J, et al. Prediction of hyperbilirubinaemia in the healthy term newborn. *Acta Paediatr* 2001;90:166; Jones KDJ, Grossman SE, Kumaranayakam D, et al. Umbilical cord bilirubin as a predictor of neonatal jaundice: a retrospective cohort study. *BMC Pediatr* 2017;17:186; Knupfer M, Pulzer F, Gebauer C, et al. Predictive value of umbilical cord blood bilirubin for postnatal hyperbilirubinaemia. *Acta Paediatr* 2005;94:581; Sarici SU, Serdar MA, Korkmaz A, et al. Incidence, course, and prediction of hyperbilirubinemia in near-term and term newborns. *Pediatrics* 2004;113:775). All TB values extrapolated from Bhutani et al. (Bhutani VK, Johnson L, Sivieri EM. Predictive ability of a predischarge hour-specific serum bilirubin for subsequent significant hyperbilirubinemia in healthy term and near-term newborns. *Pediatrics* 1999;103:6.)

TB, total serum/plasma bilirubin; ROR, rate of rise; GA, gestational age.

as well as to the enterohepatic recirculation of bilirubin—all contributing to an infant's circulating bilirubin load (Fig. 45.2). This results in the accumulation of unconjugated bilirubin in neonates. Bilirubin, when not bound to albumin (i.e., UB), can cross the neuronal cell membrane and cause neurotoxicity (see below), which underlies BIND. In addition, infants with hepatic or GI disorders (such as cholestasis), also have impaired bilirubin conjugation, which leads to increased direct bilirubin levels (>1 mg/dL) that can be potentially hepatotoxic (20). Elevated unconjugated bilirubin levels have been reported due to metabolic disorders (detected by routine neonatal metabolic screening) and include hypothyroidism, tyrosinemia, and galactosemia but are rare (21). Table 45.2 lists some proposed biomarkers that can be used to determine risk for developing bilirubin neurotoxicity and the thresholds levels at which to consider initiating interventions.

Hematologic Causes of Increased Bilirubin Production
Rhesus (Rh) Isoimmunization of the Newborn

Rh hemolytic disease is a well-recognized maternal-fetal Rh (D) antigen incompatibility, but is now infrequent due to universal prevention of maternal sensitization in the past 60 years (24,25). *Hydrops fetalis* is a manifestation of severe *in utero* hemolytic disease characterized by progressive anemia, hypoalbuminemia, anasarca (edema), and heart failure. This condition can result in stillbirth or early neonatal death. Survivors rapidly progress to severe hyperbilirubinemia (>20 mg/dL [342 µmol/L]), anemia, and

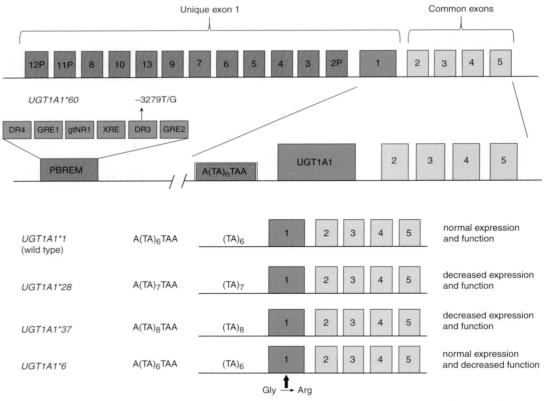

FIGURE 45.1 Schematic of the UG1A1 gene. The uppermost panel represents the entire UGT1A gene complex encompassing: (a) the A1 exon, (b) nine additional exons that encode functional proteins (exons 3–10, 13), (c) three pseudogenes (exons 2P,11Pm12P), and (d) the common domain exon 2–5 sequence shared across all UGT1A transcripts. The UTG1A1 locus and common exons 2–5 are shown in middle panel including the upstream (a) phenobarbital-responsive enhancer module (PBREM) encompassing six nuclear receptor motifs (and hypomorphic variant UGT1A1*60) and (b) TATA box promoter sequences. Lower panels show wild-type UTG1A1*1 and UGT1A1*28, UGT1A1*37, and UGT1A1*6 variant alleles and relevant change in expression function. (Data from Clarke DJ, Moghrabi N, Monaghan G, et al. Genetic defects of the UDP-glucuronosyltransferase-1 (UGT1) gene that cause familial nonhemolytic unconjugated hyperbilirubinemias. *Clin Chim Acta* 1997;166:63; Perera MA, Innocenti F, Ratain MJ. Pharmacogenetic testing for uridine diphosphate glucuronosyltransferase 1A1 polymorphisms. Are we there yet? *Pharmacotherapy* 2008;28:755; Li Y, Buckely D, Wang S, et al. Genetic polymorphisms in the TATA box and upstream phenobarbital-responsive enhancer module of the UGT1A1 promoter have combined effects on UDP-glucuronosyltransferase 1A1 transcription mediated by constitutive androstane receptor, pregnane X receptor, or glucocorticoid receptor in human liver. *Drug Metab Dispos* 2009;37:1978.)

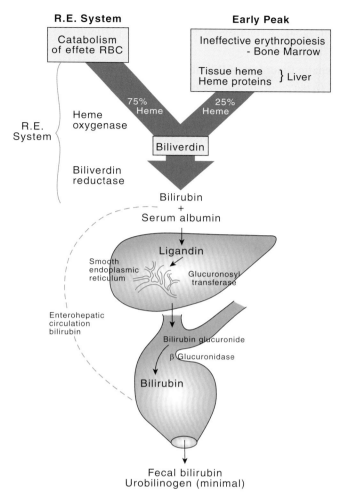

FIGURE 45.2 Neonatal bile pigment metabolism. RBC, red blood cells; RE, reticuloendothelial.

TABLE 45.2

Biomarkers Utilized to Assess Risk of Bilirubin Neurotoxicity and Provide Threshold Limits for Intervention in Preclinical Studies

Proposed Biomarkers	Specific Thresholds	
TB	Consensus values	Adjusted for maturity
TB ROR (22,23)	≥0.2 mg/dL/h	Arithmetically calculated using 2 serial TB measurements (age <60 h)
	≥3.42μmol/L/h	
ETCOc	>2.0 ppm	Hemolysis threshold
COHbc	≥2.5% tHb	Hemolysis threshold
UB	≥10 nmol/L	Phototherapy threshold
	≥18 nmol/L	*Emergency or "crash-cart"* Phototherapy or exchange threshold
BBC	≥45%	Phototherapy threshold
	≥65%	*Emergency or "crash-cart"* Phototherapy or exchange threshold

TB, total serum/plasma bilirubin; ROR, rate of rise; ETCOc, end tidal carbon monoxide, corrected for ambient CO; COHbc, carboxyhemoglobin, corrected for ambient CO; BBC, bilirubin binding capacity; UB, unbound bilirubin; ppm, parts per million; tHb, total hemoglobin.

death due to kernicterus or brain damage. In most high-income countries, Rh disease is rare due to coordinated obstetrical and neonatal care practices of timely exchange blood transfusions, effective phototherapy, and booster RBC transfusions.

ABO Incompatibility and Isoimmunization

ABO hemolytic disease remains one of the important causes of EHB and kernicterus. Mothers of blood type O can be isoimmunized against antigens of fetal blood group A, B, or both. Thus, hemolysis attributed to ABO incompatibility is usually observed in infants with blood groups A or B who are born to group O mothers. The direct antiglobulin test (DAT) detects antibodies which attached to neonatal RBCs as compared with indirect Coombs test that detects circulating IgG antibodies. A positive DAT is the best predictor of hemolysis and hyperbilirubinemia. It has been estimated that ABO-incompatible DAT-positive infants have a two-fold higher chance to develop significant hyperbilirubinemia. Notably, the severity of ABO hemolytic disease varies with the global prevalence of the major blood groups. The clinical diagnosis is dependent on a positive DAT, early onset of jaundice (<36 hours), and supported by the combined presence of reticulocytes (>6%), microspherocytes, or an elevated carboxyhemoglobin (COHbc, >2.5% total hemoglobin) or end-tidal CO (ETCOc, ≥.0 ppm) levels, both corrected for ambient CO. The latter two tests have been shown to be reliable indices of hemolysis (26). ABO incompatibility with hyperbilirubinemia, and a negative DAT generally denotes the absence of hemolysis unless confirmed by an observed increase in bilirubin production rates, such as elevated COHbc and/or ETCOc levels (27,28). The hyperbilirubinemia may also be due to concurrent hemolysis due to G6PD deficiency, Rh disease, minor blood group incompatibilities, or bilirubin elimination disorders, such as Gilbert syndrome. Infants with more mature hepatic elimination usually compensate for increased bilirubin production and often do not sustain hemolytic hyperbilirubinemia. As a policy, the American Academy of Pediatrics (AAP) notes that routine cord blood screening for infants of group O, Rh-positive mothers is an option, but is not required "provided there is appropriate surveillance and risk assessment before discharge and follow-up" (5).

G6PD Deficiency

This is a most common inherited enzymopathy due to major mutations of the X-linked G6PD gene, which results in increased RBC fragility, and hence an increased susceptibility to hemolysis (29,30). It is life-long and can lead to adverse fetal, perinatal, and neonatal outcomes. However, the complex interrelationship between genetic inheritance, the magnitude of G6PD enzyme deficiency (due a particular mutation), and subsequent outcomes are not well known and often leads to confusion in both the provider and family (31). All in all, neonates who are not identified are at risk for developing acute and unpredictable high TB levels and are often re-admitted for EHB post-hospital discharge and bilirubin neurotoxicity can be imminent.

G6PD deficiency can complicate the benign course of the transitional period after birth. This disorder is widespread and the most common genetic condition worldwide (30,32,33). The genetics of G6PD deficiency and its demographic distribution is modulated by migration or community inheritance. "Hot spots" of increased community prevalence can often be identified. Environmental, dietary, or chemical exposures to known "hemolytic triggers" may lead to acute hemolytic crises (34).

The global burden of EHB related to G6PD deficiency is estimated at 1 per 407 live births. G6PD deficiency, by inferential probability, is the major current cause of kernicterus even among facilities that practice TB screening recommended by the AAP (5). Despite this guidance, no changes have been observed in clinical practice nor in the awareness of the impact of infant sex, race, ethnicity, use of phototherapy, or potential health service disparities on this burden. The best mean U.S. incidence of G6PD deficiency is reported to be 3.4%, ranging from 0% to 12.2% (12.2% for African-American males). In 2010, of the 4.3 million live births in the United States, the prevalence ranged from 1.77% to 6.71% with 182,346 babies born at risk for G6PD deficiency (1 per 24 live births). Accurate (phenotypic) and quantitative methods to measure G6PD enzyme activity is needed. Identification of female heterozygotes is the most challenging because it requires both genotypic screening (by polymerase chain reaction [PCR]) and measuring G6PD enzyme activity. Characterization of allele frequencies may generate population-weighted estimates of affected populations (35). This approach leverages a Bayesian geostatistical model that adapts the X-linked inheritance pattern of the G6PD gene to show the development of unpredictable adverse consequences following exposure to aggravating triggers in G6PD-deficient infants. The current recommendation is the avoidance of known environmental triggers that can cause acute hemolysis in these G6PD-deficient infants (36). A dual screening model that utilizes concurrent bilirubin and G6PD enzyme activity measurements (Table 45.3) was proposed when point-of-care technologies become commercially available (34).

Other Causes of Hemolysis

Inherited structural defects of RBC membranes or enzymes are other causes of hemolysis. The type of RBC membrane defect can be diagnosed on peripheral blood smear by examination of RBC shapes. Hereditary spherocytosis is an autosomal dominant-inherited disorder; infants may present with a family history and have no evidence of isoimmunization. Characterized by the presence of elliptocytes, hereditary elliptocytosis can be classified as heterozygous, with pyropoikilocytosis (HPP), spherocytic, South East Asian ovalocytosis, or hereditary stomatocytosis. Presence of chronic hemolysis not manifested in neonatal period are mainly due to hemoglobinopathies such as sickle cell disease and beta-thalassemias. Neonatal hemolysis due to RBC enzymopathy other than G6PD (discussed above), include pyruvate kinase deficiency, an autosomal recessive condition with a defect of the pyruvate kinase (PKLR) gene. Other less common forms of glycolytic enzyme deficiency causing hemolysis include deficiencies in phosphofructokinase, triosephosphate isomerase, hexokinase, and pyrimidine 5' nucleotidase (P5NT).

Hepatic Disorders of Bilirubin Conjugation

- *Crigler-Najjar Syndrome types 1 or 2*, which are autosomal recessive mutations leading to a deficient or absent expression of the UGT1A1 gene, respectively, and diagnosed by liver biopsy
- *Gilbert syndrome (UGT polymorphisms)* is associated with persistent and less severe unconjugated hyperbilirubinemia. This condition may manifest in newborns and children as "breast milk jaundice" or co-inherited with G6PD deficiency.
- *Transient familial neonatal hyperbilirubinemia (Lucey-Driscoll Syndrome)*, which is rare.

Prescription drugs may be eliminated more slowly due to diminished hepatic conjugation (e.g., antibiotics, volatile anesthetics, antivirals (such as atazanavir and indinavir), statins, and antineoplastic agents (such irinotecan and nilotinib).

Combined Conjugated and Unconjugated Hyperbilirubinemia

Co-inheritance of genetic defects in the UGT1A1 gene (such as Gilbert syndrome) with ABO incompatibility, G6PD deficiency, or inherited RBC disorders, etc. underlies the basis for combined conjugated and unconjugated hyperbilirubinemias—combined defects in bilirubin elimination and production. Other conditions of conjugated hyperbilirubinemia with concurrent hemolysis include infections: viral (CMV, herpes, adenovirus, or HIV hepatitis); bacterial (sepsis, urinary tract infections), and protozoal as well as disorders that cause bile duct obstruction (i.e., biliary atresia, perforation of the bile duct, cholelithiasis), hypothyroidism, or septo-optic dysplasia. Other genetic and metabolic diseases to be considered are cystic fibrosis, Alagille syndrome, and alpha-1-antitrypsin deficiency (see Chapter 37 Hepatobiliary Disorders). Metabolic storage disorders in high-risk populations include Gaucher syndrome (glucocerebrosidase deficiency), glycogen storage diseases (Von Gierke, Pompe's, etc.), and Niemann-Pick disease. Drug exposure to high doses or multiple uses of ceftriaxone, methotrexate, erythromycin, or tetracycline can also cause hyperbilirubinemia.

TABLE 45.3

A Proposed Dual Screening Model for Interpretation and Counseling

G6PD Enzyme Activity (*Regardless* of Sex)	Healthy Adult Phenotype	G6PD Enzyme Level (IU/g Hb)	Parental Education	TB Screen (*Regardless* of Sex)		
				Low-Risk Zone	Intermediate Zone	High-Risk Zone
Within Range:	>7–10 IU/g Hb	21.8 ± 2.2	TB FAQs	Use AAP TB Guidelines (2004, 2009)		
Intermediate Range, large variation 10% to <60% activity	Presumes **HEMI**zygote-deficient Male; **HETERO**zygote-deficient **Female** Observed in **MOST** Variants	Variable; hemolysis occurs with stressors/triggers only	G6PD education: safety and follow-up; need for urgent medical attention, drug, chemical and diet modifications (and for lactating mothers)	Assess for hemolysis (may need to track) (*consider ETCOc/COHbc testing*)		
Below Range: <10% activity	**HOMO**zygote-**Deficient Female**	8.5 as a cut-off (range: 2.7 ± 1.1)		Educate alertness for progressive jaundice	For jaundice: start interventions aggressively (within minutes). Clinicians to ensure urgent access to care: i. Access to NICU ii. Access to phototherapy iii. Ability to recognize ABE	

G6PD deficiency defined as <30% of G6PD enzyme activity. IU/g Hb measured at 30°C based on Luzzato L. Recent advances in biological and clinical aspects of paroxysmal nocturnal hemoglobinuria. *Int J Hemato* 2006;84:104; Kaplan M. Neonatal bilirubin production-conjugation imbalance: effect of glucose-6-phosphate dehydrogenase deficiency and borderline prematurity. *Arch Dis Child Fetal Neonatal Ed* 2005;90:F123; and WHO Working Group. Glucose-6-phosphate dehydrogenase deficiency. *Bull World Health Organ* 1989;67:601.

WHO, World Health Organization; G6PD, glucose-6-phosphate dehydrogenase; TB, total serum/plasma bilirubin; Hb, hemoglobin; AAP, American Academy of Pediatrics; ETCOc, end tidal carbon monoxide, corrected for ambient CO; COHbc, carboxyhemoglobin, corrected for ambient CO; ABE, acute bilirubin encephalopathy; NICU, neonatal intensive unit. Crash-cart approach is described in the text.

From WHO Working Group. Glucose-6-phosphate dehydrogenase deficiency. *Bull World Health Organ* 1989;67:601.

BILIRUBIN NEUROTOXICITY

Definition

That bilirubin is neurotoxic was only established in the early 1950s among infants with Rh hemolytic disease. A schematic of a model to illustrate the sequelae following severe hyperbilirubinemia is shown in **Figure 45.3**. Following universal screening for isoimmunization disorders, the incidence of kernicterus is now higher among infants without hemolytic disease. AAP recommends that acute bilirubin encephalopathy (ABE) be used to describe the acute clinical manifestations of bilirubin toxicity that are present in icteric or post-icteric infants. It includes the clinical features associated with ABE to establish a scoring system that can quantify the severity of ABE and its association with developmental outcome. "Kernicterus" or chronic bilirubin encephalopathy (CBE) is a term used for post-icteric, chronic and permanent clinical sequelae of bilirubin toxicity, which manifests a few weeks after acute signs are observed and can still progress until 7 years of age (5). For those infants with high TB levels and no long-term signs of CBE, subtle forms of neurotoxicity may be seen. Recently, the term "syndrome of BIND or bilirubin-induced neurologic dysfunction" has been used to describe a constellation of subtle neurodevelopmental sequelae caused at lower TB levels than those that cause CBE.

Molecular Mechanisms

The pathogenesis of BIND impacts the integrity of plasma, mitochondrial, or endoplasmic reticulum membranes at a molecular level (37), leading to: (a) disruptions of neuronal excitation; (b) failure of mitochondrial energy process; (c) increased oxidative stress; and (d) altered intracellular calcium (iCa^{2+}) concentrations. Increased iCa^{2+} may activate proteolytic enzymes, apoptosis, and/or neuronal necrosis. Activation of microglia and astrocytes and a robust neuroinflammatory response appear to accompany this

injury and may play roles in its evolution and resolution). Brain bilirubin content may affect several of the cytochrome P-450 bilirubin-metabolizing enzymes. These injurious sequences may suggest neuronal cell-specific and region-specific toxicity of bilirubin that are further confounded by regional blood flow (38). Putative bilirubin transporters at the blood–brain (ABCB1) and blood–CSF (ABCC1) barriers also facilitate the clearance of bilirubin from the central nervous system (37).

Isolated Sensorineural Hearing Impairment

Bilirubin-induced toxicity can affect the neuro-auditory pathways. Severe hyperbilirubinemia can manifest as auditory neuropathy spectrum disorder (ANSD) or chronic auditory toxicity with or without reversible ABE. Amin et al. (39) demonstrated the acute auditory neurotoxicity was associated with severe hyperbilirubinemia in infants ≥34 weeks' gestational age (GA). A useful predictor of injury was UB rather than TB levels or bilirubin-albumin molar ratio (BAMR) in term and late preterm infants (40). A more recent study of newborns without kernicterus, possibly with the syndrome of BIND, identified 13% chronic auditory toxicity (odds ratio [OR] = 2.41; 95% confidence interval [CI] = 1.43, 4.07; $p = 0.001$) in 93 newborns with significant hyperbilirubinemia. The receiver operating characteristic curves for UB and TB were reported to be 0.866 and 0.775, respectively, for isolated auditory toxicity ($p = 0.03$) (41).

Structural Neurologic Changes

An infant with ABE (**Fig. 45.4**) and the immediate post-icteric phase after injury are best evidenced by MRI that shows increased T1 signals of globus pallidus and subthalamic nuclei. Subsequently, during infancy between ages 18 months and 3 years, CBE is best diagnosed by bilateral, symmetrical, and heightened T2 signals from the globus pallidus and subthalamic nuclei. Recently, Wisnowski et al. (42) have reported a single case study using

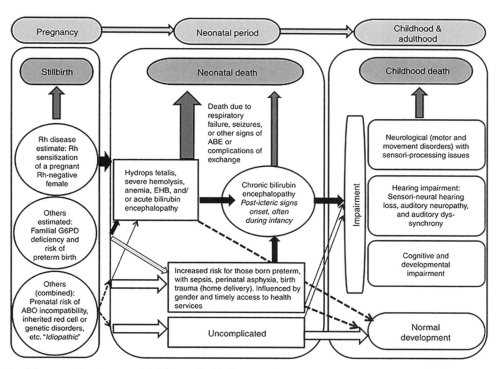

FIGURE 45.3 Schematic of the prenatal and neonatal risk factors for Rh disease and extreme hyperbilirubinemia (EHB) and their impact on stillbirths, neonatal death due to kernicterus, and long-term impairment of kernicterus during childhood. In view of the complex confluence of biologic risk, interaction with other childhood disease, and sociocultural factors, we did not estimate childhood death due to kernicterus. ABE, acute bilirubin encephalopathy. (Reprinted by permission from Nature: Bhutani VK, Zipursky A, Blencowe H, et al. Neonatal hyperbilirubinemia and Rhesus disease of the newborn: incidence and impairment estimates for 2010 at regional and global levels. *Pediatr Res* 2013;74(suppl 1):86. Copyright © 2013 Springer Nature.)

THE NEWBORN INFANT

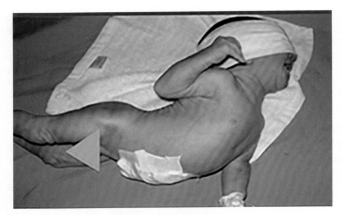

FIGURE 45.4 Photograph of a post-icteric newborn term infant with retrocollis, opisthotonus, and hypertonicity. (Courtesy of Dr. Numan Alhamdani, Children's Hospital. Baghdad, Iraq.)

magnetic resonance spectroscopy that identified a distinct pattern of acute restricted diffusion localized to the dentato-thalamo-cortical pathway during advanced stages of ABE (Fig. **45.5**). Classic brain MRI high intensity signals are reported in T1 images of globus pallidus during ABE (43) and as T2-weighted hyperintense signals as well as fluid-attenuated inversion recovery (FLAIR) images with CBE (44). Similar distinctive MRI findings have been described in preterm infants less than 30 weeks' GA. This constellation of findings is often under-recognized among preterm infants.

Syndrome of Bilirubin-Induced Neurologic Dysfunction

The syndrome of BIND is a spectrum and constellation of subtle neurologic sequelae. Description of specific areas affected include: "basal ganglia, auditory pathways, hippocampus, diencephalon, subthalamic nuclei, midbrain, cerebellum, and the vermis (6,9,10). Pontine nuclei, brainstem nuclei for oculomotor function, respiratory, and neurohumoral and electrolyte control can also be affected" (6,9,10). The subsequent long-term spectrum of neurologic disorders that does develop may occur upon exposure to lower TB levels than has been generally described, especially in

vulnerable infants (10). Subtle neuromotor signs in children have been reported to have objective disturbances of visual processing function (45), sensorineural hearing pathways (46,47), disorders of speech and cognition as well as language processing (48), and movement disorders (49,50). Evidence for associations between bilirubin neurotoxicity (i.e., BIND) and ANSD (39,41,47), or visuo-oculomotor dysfunction (45) is limited and requires further basic science, translational, clinical, and developmental research. Auditory dysfunction is GA-dependent in preterm infants with birthweights (BW) less than 1,500 g and TB levels ($\geq$14 mg/dL [239 μmol/L]), who reportedly may develop hearing deficits (51,52). Duration of bilirubin exposure adds risk (53). For full-term infants, ototoxicity is associated with severe hyperbilirubinemia (54). The bilirubin neurotoxicity is selective to auditory nerve and spiral ganglion, but not to the organ of Corti and thalamocortical auditory pathway (55). Data on the combined impact of prematurity, hemolysis, and severity of hyperbilirubinemia on auditory dysfunction are however still lacking.

Recent data using the swept parameter visual-evoked potential (VEP) to measure visuocortical function in healthy, bilirubin-exposed infants are worrisome. Good et al. (45) compared "steady-state" VEP (sVEP) threshold response amplitudes (contrast, spatial frequency, and vernier offsets) at 12 to 24 weeks' postnatal age in a small cohort of full-term infants with TB levels greater than 10 mg/dL (171 μmol/L) versus matched infants without jaundice. They found that an association between hyperbilirubinemic infants with lower response amplitudes, and worse sVEP thresholds compared with controls for all three measured parameters. The sVEP thresholds for vernier offset sizes appear to correlate with increasing TB levels. The effect of neonatal hyperbilirubinemia on vernier acuity (a surrogate for Snellen or optotype acuity) was found to be dose related. Furthermore, the visuocortical manifestations are diverse lasting beyond the period of hyperbilirubinemia exposure, which suggests a widespread effect.

Effect on Developmental Maturation

Bilirubin can also impair normal developmental maturation and can be further exacerbated by the presence of comorbidities such as: inflammation/sepsis, oxidative stress, prematurity, and genetic factors. These potential risk factors for BIND, most of them

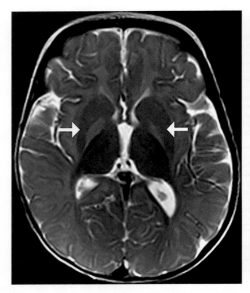
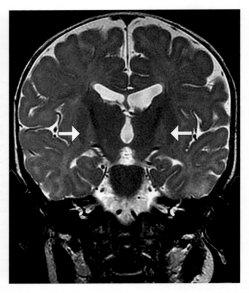

FIGURE 45.5 Axial (left panel) and coronal (right panel) T2-weighted MRI images obtained in a 6-month-old infant with chronic bilirubin encephalopathy (CBE) or kernicterus. This infant had a total serum/plasma bilirubin (TB) of 27.0 mg/dL (462 μmol/L) and dystonia, choreoathetosis, and auditory neuropathy on neurodevelopmental follow-up. Note the high T2-signal in the globus pallidus bilaterally (*arrows*). (Data from Wisnowski JL, Panigrahy A, Painter MP, et al. Magnetic resonance imaging of bilirubin encephalopathy: current limitations and future promise. *Semin Perinatol* 2014;38:422.)

determinants of age-related susceptibilities, may alter individual neurologic outcomes, especially when the developing brain is the most vulnerable (6,9,10). Bilirubin exposure to neurogenic niches, such as microvascular endothelial cells (56), neurons (57), astrocytes (57), glial cells (and their migration) (58), and oligodendrocytes as well as on myelination (59) during preterm and neonatal life retard maturational development.

EVALUATION OF HYPERBILIRUBINEMIA

Clinical Assessment

Visible jaundice can be detected in a neonate by using digital pressure to blanch the skin at the forehead, sternum, iliac crest, patella, or malleolus and assessed along with vital signs—at least at intervals of 8 to 12 hours—and best done in a room under natural light, daylight lamps, or ambient sunlight (5). Placing an infant's leg near the face may help highlight the cephalocaudal progression of jaundice. Visible jaundice on the palms and soles denotes marked jaundice, and that below the elbows and knees also cause concern. The color of jaundice can vary from a lemon yellow to bright orange and sienna. Accurate assessments may be limited by the infant's skin pigmentation, degree of plethora, and previous exposure to sun or phototherapy as well as decreased ambient light. In most light-skinned infants, jaundice progresses cephalocaudally, appearing last on the palms and soles. In darker-skinned neonates, it could appear as a tan. The absence or presence is not predictive of the subsequent development of severe hyperbilirubinemia (TB > 20 mg/dL [342 μmol/L]). In addition, attempts to gauge the skin color to assess TB levels is not recommended and can often lead to errors. However, the onset of jaundice in first 24 to 36 hours of life is considered a sign of an excessive rate of rise (ROR) of TB levels or the presence of ongoing hemolysis (60), and necessitates an immediate measurement of TB levels and further clinical evaluation (Table 45.4).

Routine Laboratory Testing

A seminal postmortem report of infants with kernicterus suggested that the presence of acidosis, perinatal asphyxia, low albumin or disordered BBC predispose newborns to develop kernicterus.

TABLE 45.4

Clinical Evaluation of Infants ≥ 35 Weeks' GA with Hyperbilirubinemia

Postnatal Presentation	Recommended Work-Up
Visible jaundice at age <36 h	Immediate TcB/TB
Visible jaundice excessive for age	TcB/TB
Predischarge TcB/TB (Age: 0–60 h)	Check TB for TcB > 12 mg/dL
	Review history for hemolysis
	Adjust TB for vulnerability
	(GA and other risk factors)
	Assess for hemolysis
	Screen for G6PD deficiency
	(adjust for race/ethnicity)
TB rising rapidly (such as crossing percentiles)	DAT
	Direct fraction of TB
	Consider ETCOc, COHbc, and/or G6PD (quantitative assay)
Consult 2004 AAP guideline	Initiate phototherapy for designated TB threshold

TcB, transcutaneous bilirubin; TB, total serum/plasma bilirubin; GA, gestational age; G6PD, glucose-6-phosphate dehydrogenase; DAT; direct antiglobulin test; ETCOc, end tidal carbon monoxide, corrected for ambient CO; COHbc, carboxyhemoglobin, corrected for ambient CO; AAP, American Academy of Pediatrics.

Kim et al. (61) were unable to identify specific clinical risk factors that are predictive of which infants will develop kernicterus. Clinicians have relied on TB levels, which can be measured either in serum or plasma. In term and late preterm infants, TB levels can be plotted on the hour-specific, percentile-based Bhutani bilirubin nomogram to identify an infant's risk zone status for significant hyperbilirubinemia (until age 7 days) (62) (Fig. 45.6) and recommended to be used in combination with clinical risk factors (4). The nomogram provides an estimate of the magnitude of the hyperbilirubinemia and a projected TB ROR as a function

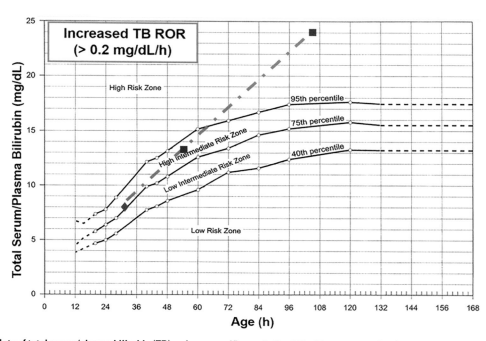

FIGURE 45.6 Serial plots of total serum/plasma bilirubin (TB) on hour-specific predictive bilirubin nomogram for three consecutive TB measurements illustrating the "*crossing of percentiles.*"

TABLE 45.5

Subcohort of Infants (n = 76) with Serial TB/TcB Measurements, Categorized by TB/TcB Percentile Risk < and ≥75th Percentile, and then Stratified by ETCOc < and ≥ 2.0 ppm and by TB ROR

	TB/TcB < 75th Percentile			TB/TcB ≥ 75th Percentile		
	ALL	ETCOc (ppm)		**ALL**	ETCOc (ppm)	
		<2.0	**≥2.0**		**<2.0**	**≥2.0**
n	34	28	6	42	21	21
TB/TcB (mg/dL)	5.28 ± 1.97	5.36 ± 2.05	4.92 ± 1.63	9.53 ± 2.78	9.57 ± 3.33	9.50 ± 2.19
ETCOc (ppm)	**1.72 ± 0.48**	1.56 ± 0.27	2.48 ± 0.52	**2.38 ± 1.89**[a]	1.60 ± 0.25	3.16 ± 2.44
TB ROR (mg/dL/h)	0.011 ± 0.440	0.003 ± 0.485	0.045 ± 0.046	0.172 ± 0.471	0.222 ± 0.643	0.123 ± 0.190
Phototherapy (n)	0	0	0	8	3	5

TB/TcB levels, ETCOc levels, and TB ROR are shown as mean ± SD for each risk category as well as the number of infants that received phototherapy.

[a]$p = 0.050$ using Student unpaired t-tests for values in bold.

From Bhutani VK, Maisels MJ, Schutzman DL, et al. Identification of risk for neonatal hemolysis. *Acta Paediatr* 2018;107:1350. Copyright ©2018 Foundation Acta Pædiatrica. Reprinted by permission of John Wiley & Sons, Inc.

of postnatal age (in hours) as defined for healthy infants (62). As a surrogate, transcutaneous bilirubinometry, a noninvasive measurement of TB levels which uses multiwavelength light, can be used to indirectly quantify circulating TB (63). Transcutaneous bilirubin (TcB) devices have been used as screening tools by providing valid estimates of TB levels (up to 12.5 mg/dL [214 µmol/L]) in neonates less than 14 days of life, although data are limited (64,65). TcB levels, like TB levels, should be based upon an infant's age in hours according to predictive data (66). Normative TcB data of infants in the first week of life do not exist because of variations in clinical practices regarding feeding, the ability to screen and identify hemolytic diseases (increased bilirubin production), and efforts to facilitate bilirubin elimination. The accuracy of TcB devices are affected by infant age, skin thickness, subcutaneous blood flow, and dermal bilirubin kinetics (including skin pigmentation, degree of prematurity, and race). Studies have shown a limited use of TcB as a screening test when TB values are greater than 12 mg/dL (205 µmol/L) (66). However, the accuracy of TcB when plotted as less than 75th percentile for age in hours (based on the bilirubin nomogram) (62) can serve as a useful screening tool or used to monitor TB levels. Because of extensive measurement variations, the mean value of 5 consecutive measurements have been recommended to achieve reasonable equivalency to TB (64). More recently, measurements of ETCOc can serve as an index of bilirubin production rates in conjunction with assessment of TB risk zones as a function of postnatal age can help identify those infants with hemolysis, and therefore at high risk for developing hyperbilirubinemia, but need further validation by multicenter randomized control trials (Table 45.5).

Bilirubin neurotoxicity has been hypothesized to be best predicted by measurements of UB levels. However, development of commercial devices to automate the assay has been challenging (as it is multi-step and labor-intensive) and accurate measurements are confounded by the biologic properties of UB, which is only present in nanomolar concentrations and by the binding characteristics of albumin to bilirubin (67). Historical experiences with UB and bilirubin binding capacity for ABE and BIND are shown in Table 45.6.

Specialized Bilirubin/Albumin Binding (BBC) and UB Testing

The relationship between UB levels, kernicterus, and bilirubin neurotoxicity has yet to be proven. Drugs and chemical agents can alter albumin–bilirubin binding and predispose newborns to develop kernicterus. Thresholds for molecular cellular damage may be resolved by longitudinal clinical studies. BBC is an objective test of bilirubin–albumin binding and possibly predictive of neurotoxicity. The expert opinions that TB levels, by itself, does not reliably predict neurotoxicity or kernicterus has been well

addressed (67,75–78). BBC in preterm and sick infants is highly variable (79,80). Using a protocol device to measure BBC and apparent UB, Lamola et al. (68) have validated that the TB thresholds for phototherapy and exchange transfusion in preterm neonates recommended by Maisels et al. (66) correspond to a 45% and 67% of BBC, respectively (**Fig. 45.7**).

Next-Generation Sequencing

Flow cytometry using eosin-5-maleimide (EMA) uptake can be used to assess RBC membrane integrity. Recently, the use of next-generation sequencing (NGS) has been adapted to characterize inherited RBC defects due to genetic mutations. NGS is a high throughput sensitive assay that utilizes DNA and RNA sequencing techniques to generate large amounts of clinically relevant data. The Christensen team has formulated a panel of 28 genes that are associated with bilirubin production or with defects in hepatocyte bilirubin uptake and its conjugation (81). Using NGS, "*idiopathic*" causes of hyperbilirubinemia due to unknown family histories or inconclusive routine laboratory testing may be identified, such as inherited hemolytic anemias, including RBC membrane defects, RBC enzyme deficiencies, and hemoglobinopathies.

BREAST MILK JAUNDICE MISNOMER

In 1963, Newman and Gross reported five exclusively breast-fed newborns had sustained jaundice as compared with those who were also supplemented with cow's milk (82). Arias et al. (83)

TABLE 45.6

Suggested UB Thresholds for Risk for ABE and BIND

Study (Duration/Exposure Not Measured)	UB (nmol/L)	% Saturation of BBC (Calculated)
Hypothetical model of ABE (68)	20	67
Historical review of ABE (69)	17–23	63–69
Clinical: ABR changes (52,70)	19–33 (median: 23)	66–77 (median: 69)
Transient ABR changes (71,72)	>8.5	>46
Overt BIND (71,72)	>17	>63
Kernicterus present (73)	>27	>73
Kernicterus absent (73)	<13	<57
Kernicterus present (74)	>18	>65
Kernicterus absent (74)	<11	<52

UB, unbound bilirubin; ABE, acute bilirubin encephalopathy; BIND, bilirubin-induced neurologic dysfunction; ABR, auditory brainstem response; BBC, bilirubin binding capacity.

Adapted by permission from Nature: Lamola AA, Bhutani VK, Du L, et al. Neonatal bilirubin binding capacity discerns risk of neurological dysfunction. *Pediatr Res* 2015;77:334. Copyright © 2015 Springer Nature.

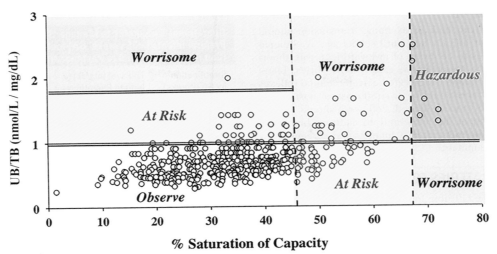

FIGURE 45.7 Distribution of unbound bilirubin (UB)/total serum/plasma bilirubin (TB) as related to bilirubin binding capacity (BBC) in preterm neonates. Quadrants propose intervention options. (Reprinted by permission from Nature: Lamola AA, Bhutani VK, Du L, et al. Neonatal bilirubin binding capacity discerns risk of neurological dysfunction. *Pediatr Res* 2015;77:334. Copyright © 2015 Springer Nature.)

demonstrated a link between decreased UGT1A1 activity and prolonged unconjugated hyperbilirubinemia in seven full-term, breast milk-fed infants. A case report in the *New England Journal of Medicine* first used the label of *"breast milk jaundice"* as a diagnosis (84). A prospective population-based study by Winfield (85) did not confirm these observations. In fact, they showed no incidence of jaundice in cow milk-fed newborns as compared with an incidence of 2.4% of prolonged unconjugated jaundice in those exclusively breast-fed. Gourley et al. (86) subsequently demonstrated that the L-aspartic acid (in cow's milk) enzymatically hydrolyzed casein, which acts as a competitive β-glucuronidase inhibitor to promote bilirubin elimination.

Clinical associations between late prematurity, sustained bruising, unrecognized hemolysis (e.g., G6PD deficiency, ABO incompatibility), Rh disease, hypothyroidism, urosepsis, and certain inborn errors of metabolism with prolonged unconjugated jaundice (persisting >2 weeks) and lasting until 5 and 8 weeks of age has been observed (87). The mean peak TB levels have been reported to be as high as 15.8 ± 4.3 mg/dL (270 ± 74 μmol/L) and in the designated range of 95th and 99th percentile (14.4 mg/dL [246 μmol/L] and 17.2 mg/dL [294 μmol/L], respectively) on the Bhutani nomogram (62). Prolonged unconjugated bilirubin levels have been attributed to UGT genetic mutations. A recent study in Japan performed by Maruo et al. (88) demonstrated a causal relationship in exclusively jaundiced breast-fed infants and homozygosity for *UGT1A1*6*. In fact, TB = 21.8 ± 3.7 mg/dL (373 ± 63 μmol/L) was associated with *UGT1A1*6* and considered *"breast milk jaundice."* Infants of Caucasian backgrounds with Gilbert syndrome exhibit less than 50% of hepatic UGT activity and the presence of an additional TA repeat in the promoter region (19) and co-inheritance with G6PD deficiency (89). In view of the evidence of a link between a spectrum of genetic disorders and prolonged unconjugated hyperbilirubinemia, it is best to retire *"breast milk jaundice"* as a clinical diagnosis (90).

OVERVIEW OF CLINICAL MANAGEMENT

The primary strategy for the clinical management of sick and preterm infants is directed at prevention. Hyperbilirubinemia should be monitored along with other vital signs. TB measurements should be done every 8 to 12 hours and can be decreased to every 12 to 24 hours if the infant is under phototherapy, when TB levels are decreasing, or when the infant is beyond 1 week of age.

Sick and preterm infants may be at increased risk during an acute ROR of TB with concurrent infection or illness, when not fed enterally (NPO), or as a result of a transfusion or acute hemolysis.

Classification of Hyperbilirubinemia
Dependent upon GA

In newborns ≥ 35 weeks' GA:

- Significant hyperbilirubinemia: TB greater than 95th percentile on the bilirubin nomogram (62)
- Severe hyperbilirubinemia: TB at which phototherapy is AAP recommended (5)
- EHB: TB greater than 25 mg/dL (428 μmol/L): a public health index of systems failure for predischarge screening

In newborns less than 35 weeks' GA:

- TB greater than 17 mg/dL (291 μmol/L) at age greater than 96 hours or over the 95th percentile track
- Severe hyperbilirubinemia: TB at which phototherapy is recommended by the AAP (5)
- EHB: TB greater than 25 mg/dL (428 μmol/L) or at which exchange transfusion is recommended by the AAP (5)

Clinical Risk Factors

- TB greater than 75th percentile (≥35 weeks' GA) on the bilirubin nomogram (62)
- Neonatal hemolysis (intravascular or extravascular)
- Male gender
- Asian race
- Prematurity (increases with each early week preterm)
- G6PD deficiency, common in African American, East Asian, Middle Eastern, and Mediterranean populations
- Suboptimal breast milk intake or excessive weight loss of greater than 6% of BW
- Early discharge (before age 72 hours)
- Family history of newborn jaundice (possibly due to inherited disorders)

Post-Icteric Follow-Up

Follow-up is individualized to assess for rebound hyperbilirubinemia and prolonged unconjugated hyperbilirubinemia (TB > 14 mg/dL [239 μmol/L]) and is based on postnatal age, GA, presence of hemolysis, and etiology of the hyperbilirubinemia.

THE NEWBORN INFANT

Developmental Follow-Up

Infants with EHB or who had an exchange transfusion should be followed throughout infancy and until school age. A clinician should instruct families to be aware of awkwardness, gait abnormalities, failure of fine stereognosis, gaze abnormalities, blank stare, poor coordination, and exaggerated extrapyramidal reflexes in the child. These infants could be at subtle risk of post-icteric sequelae during infancy and childhood. Follow-up should include neuroimaging with MRI at discharge and an auditory brainstem response (ABR) measurement during infancy and screening for speech–language development.

TREATMENT STRATEGIES FOR TB REDUCTION

Strategies to reduce the bilirubin load expeditiously are described in the 2004 AAP guideline (5), a recent technical report (91), and an expert review (92). Infants with severe hyperbilirubinemia require immediate and effective phototherapy, and careful evaluation for recognizing the subtle signs of ABE. It is important to be cognizant of non-specific signs of ABE, especially in preterm infants. Severely jaundiced and symptomatic infants should be managed urgently and admitted directly to the NICU.

Promoting Enteral Feeds

The benefits of breast-feeding are well described and valued, and mothers should be encouraged to breast-feed their infants. If breast-feeding is interrupted, mothers should continue to pump and store their breast milk to ensure stimulation for adequate milk production. Breast-feeding should be resumed as soon as possible. The importance of frequent feedings (>8 times per day for the first week) should be emphasized. Lactation consultants and home visits by an expert nurse (after discharge) are helpful. Although any infant who is feeding poorly and with poor weight gain requires increased surveillance for jaundice, late preterm infants (34 to 36 6/7 weeks' GA) are at greater risk of receiving inadequate fluid and nutrition, and thereby require increased surveillance to initiate timely intervention.

Phototherapy

In 1969, the first U.S. national symposium on neonatal hyperbilirubinemia and phototherapy convened by the National Foundation-March of Dimes reported on the effect of light on bilirubin metabolism. The efficacy and mechanisms of phototherapy are well established (91). Extrapolation to moderate and very preterm infants is confounded by their state of maturation (Table 45.7). Clinicians should also be aware of the presence of concurrent diseases, types of light sources and device used, and follow manufacturers' guidelines before initiating phototherapy.

The primary success of phototherapy is in its ability to decrease TB levels and hence bilirubin toxicity (91). Use of exchange transfusion can be prevented with earlier and effective use of phototherapy. Clinician judgment is crucial to safety in deciding when to perform a highly risky exchange transfusion or possible overuse of phototherapy. The absolute indications for commencing an exchange transfusion are listed in Table 45.8. Clinicians are reminded that the margin of safety between risk versus onset of irreversible neurotoxicity is extremely narrow and may be within the limits of TB measurement accuracy (±2 to 3 mg/dL when TB levels are >20 mg/dL [342 μmol/L]).

Photodegradation of Bilirubin

Light absorption by bilirubin takes place in the skin. Nonpolar bilirubin is formed by photoisomerization to excretable polar photoisomers. Other pathways include formation of configurational isomers and structural isomers (i.e., lumirubin) (93,94). Unimpeded isomer excretion help decreases TB. Therapeutic strategies

TABLE 45.7

Operational Thresholds to Manage Hyperbilirubinemia in Preterm Infants (<35 weeks' GA) for the First Week (Can Also Be Adjusted to Postmenstrual Age During Week 2)

Stratification by GA (Weeks)	TB Level (mg/dL) to Initiate Phototherapy	TB Level (mg/dL) to Prepare for Exchange Transfusion
<28	5–6	11–14
28–29	6–8	12–14
30–31	8–10	13–16
32–33	10–12	15–18
≥34	12–14	17–19

These recommendations use the lower range of the listed TB levels for infants at greater risk for bilirubin toxicity, for example: (a) lower GA; (b) serum albumin levels <2.5 g/dL; (c) rapidly TB levels suggestive of hemolytic disease; and (d) if clinically unstable. When a decision is being made about the initiation of phototherapy or exchange transfusion, infants should be considered clinically unstable if they have one or more of the following conditions: (a) blood pH < 7.15; (b) blood culture positive for sepsis in the prior 24 hours; (c) apnea and bradycardia requiring cardiorespiratory resuscitation (bagging and or intubation) during the previous 24 hours; (d) hypotension requiring pressor treatment during the previous 24 hours; and (e) assisted ventilation. (Reprinted by permission from Nature: Maisels MJ, Watchko JF, Bhutani VK, et al. An approach to the management of hyperbilirubinemia in the preterm infant less than 35 weeks of gestation. *J Perinatol* 2012;32:660. Copyright © 2012 Springer Nature.)

GA, gestational age; TB, total serum/plasma bilirubin.

should match bilirubin–albumin absorption to a source of light with a peak emission of about 460 nm (5). The understanding of light and photochemistry that underlies this connection has been well described (91,93–98).

Effective neonatal phototherapy is still the best approach for the treatment of severe hyperbilirubinemia (TB > 20 mg/dL [342 μmol/L]) in term healthy newborns (91). However, it is most important that the device has an effective light footprint (Fig. 45.8). The wavelength range of the emitted light source should overlap the bilirubin action spectrum (91). Light should emit a wavelength range of 450 to 475 nm (blue), the peak absorption spectrum of bilirubin. Broad-band light (such as fluorescent or halogen light) emit harmful ultraviolet (UVA and UVB) radiation and should not be used. The spectral range of effective phototherapy currently recommended by the AAP is 400 to 520 nm, which excludes UV light (5). The efficacy of phototherapy is determined by the light source, the configuration of the device (overhead vs. blanket/wraps), irradiance given, duration of phototherapy, and exposed body surface area (BSA) to an infant (91). For optimal phototherapy (Table 45.9), the light source should: (a) emit light in the blue-to-green range (~460 to 490 nm); (b) produce

TABLE 45.8

Indications for Exchange Transfusion in Infants ≥ 35 weeks' GA

Indications	Clinical Signs	Action
Any neurologic signs[a]	See legend	**IMMEDIATE** intervention
TB > 25 mg/dL in term neonates	Check TB every 2 h for ROR	Escalate care Prepare for exchange transfusion
TB > 20 mg/dL in perterm neonates ≥35 to <38 weeks' GA	Check TB every 2 h for ROR	Escalate care Prepare for exchange transfusion
Sick newborns	See legend Check TB every 2 h for ROR	**IMMEDIATE** intervention Re-evaluate risk vs. benefit of procedure

[a]Lethargy, decreased enteral intake, hypo- or hypertonia, irritability, apnea, seizures, fever, or signs of mild ABE.

TB, total serum/plasma bilirubin; GA, gestational age; ROR, rate of rise; ABE, acute bilirubin encephalopathy.

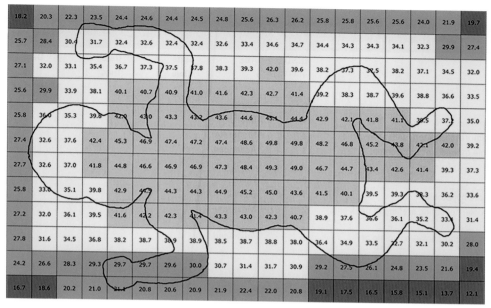

FIGURE 45.8 Irradiance mapping of illuminated footprint with a silhouette of a newborn homunculus. (as described by a methodology described by Vreman HJ, Wong RJ, Murdock JR, Stevenson DK. Standardized bench method for evaluating the efficacy of phototherapy devices. *Acta Paediatr* 2008;97:308 and used by Cline BK, Vreman HJ, Lou HH, Donaldson KM, Bhutani VK. Evaluation of an affordable LED phototherapy device for resource-limited settings. *E-PAS* 2011;2011:4503.) Irradiance ($\mu W/cm^2/nm$) is plotted for square centimeter of the illuminated surface. (From Bhutani VK, Wong RJ. Neonatal phototherapy: choice of device and outcome. *Acta Paediatr* 2012;101:441. Copyright © 2012 The Author(s)/Acta Pædiatrica © 2012 Foundation Acta Pædiatrica. Reprinted by permission of John Wiley & Sons, Inc.)

an irradiance of at least 30 $\mu W/cm^2/nm$ (and confirmed with the appropriate irradiance meter calibrated over the appropriate wavelength range); and (c) illuminate the maximal BSA (80%) of an infant. Photodegradation of bilirubin can occur within 15 to 30 minutes of light exposure. Measured decreases in TB levels can be observed within 4 to 6 hours of light exposure. Misuse, overuse, and/or abuse have been observed with phototherapy. Firstly, accurate measurement of irradiance is a must (95). Secondly, irradiance should be adjusted for use in infants with fragile skin, low antioxidant reserves, and low BBC. Thirdly, intermittent rather than continuous exposure should be considered—"*off*" times used to promote breast-feeding and maternal/infant bonding (99).

Clinicians should not rely on visual brightness, but using recommended light meters to measure irradiance. For the measurement of irradiance, light meters that are supplied by the manufacturer should only be used (91). To achieve maximal irradiance, the light source should be positioned closer to the infant; however, this is not recommended when using devices that incorporate halogen or tungsten lamps as light sources, as they can produce excessive

heat. The irradiance distribution of a device or "*light footprint*" is not uniform, and can be highly variable among phototherapy devices. Therefore, irradiance measurements taken at the center of the footprint may be higher than those taken at the periphery.

For emergency or "*crash-cart*" patient management (outlined in Table 45.10), clinicians need to be prepared for admission who is likely to undergo an exchange transfusion. Emergency

TABLE 45.9

Parameters for TB Reduction in Neonatal Phototherapy

Parameter	GA (weeks)		
	>35	**28–35**	**<28**
Irradiance	25–35	15–25	10–15
Light wavelength (nm)	460	460	460
Body surface area	30% to <80%	30%–80%	<30%

Dosage of phototherapy can be increased in tandem by more extensive body surface exposure and irradiance dose. Irradiance >35 $\mu W/cm^2/nm$ is generally not needed and toxicity for levels >45 $\mu W/cm^2/nm$ have not been reported. Therapy should be prescribed by the parameters rather than the number devices. In larger infants, more than one device maybe necessary for an expanded exposure.

GA, gestational age; TB, total serum/plasma bilirubin.

TABLE 45.10

Steps to Implement a "*Crash-Cart*" Strategy for Urgent TB Reduction

	Step	Double Volume Exchange 160 mL/kg in Term Infants 190 mL/kg in Preterm Infants
1	Infant location	NICU; conduct all procedures with uninterrupted phototherapy
2	Monitor	Cardiorespiratory oxygenation continuously, core temperature, BP
3	BIND score	Clinical progression of BIND before, during and post-exchange
4	Informed consent	Risk/benefit concepts discussed even if it delays procedures
5	Central catheter	Two are optional: umbilical or great vessel. Preferred bore: 5 Fr
6	Cross match blood	For major and minor antibodies; use type O for ABO incompatibility
7	Blood samples	All TB samples to be protected from light exposure
8	Medications	Prepare for medications with appropriate dose and infusions
9	Duration	Within 2 h of NICU admission
10	Technical impediments	A single volume exchange transfusion may be adequate until technical issues are resolved; may need surgical catheterization

NICU, neonatal intensive unit; BP, blood pressure; BIND, bilirubin-induced neurologic dysfunction; TB, total serum/plasma bilirubin.

TABLE 45.11

Clinical BIND Score of Onset, Severity, and Progression of ABE in Infants with Hyperbilirubinemia (TB > 95th Percentile for Age-In-Hours) as Elicited by History and Physical Examination

Clinical Signs	BIND Score	ABE	Date __/__ Time __:__	Date __/__ Time __:__	Date __/__ Time __:__	Date __/__ Time __:__
Mental status						
Normal	0	None				
Sleepy, but arousable; decreased feeding	1	Subtle				
Lethargy, poor suck and/or irritable/jittery with strong suck	2	Moderate				
Semi-coma, apnea, unable to feed, seizures, coma	3	Advanced				
Muscle tone						
Normal	0	None				
Persistent mild to moderate hypotonia	1	Subtle				
Mild to moderate hypertonia, beginning arching of neck and trunk on stimulation	2	Moderate				
Persistent retrocollis and opisthotonos—bicycling or twitching of hands and feet	3	Advanced				
Cry pattern						
Normal	0	None				
High pitched when aroused	1	Subtle				
Shrill, difficult to console	2	Moderate				
Inconsolable crying or cry weak or absent	3	Advanced				
Total BIND score						
Nurse/MD Signature						

Score of 7 to 9 represent advanced ABE: urgent, prompt, and individualized intervention are recommended to prevent further brain damage, minimize severity of sequelae and possibly reverse acute damage.

Score of 4 to 6 represent moderate ABE and is likely to be reversible with urgent and prompt bilirubin reduction strategies.

Score of 1 to 3 are consistent with subtle signs of ABE in infants with hyperbilirubinemia. **An abnormal ABR or "referred" automated ABR** is indicative of likely bilirubin neurotoxicity and would be suggestive of moderate ABE. In infants with these non-specific signs (Scores 1 to 3), a failed ABR hearing screen supports a diagnosis of moderate ABE. Serial ABR may be used as objective measures of progression, stabilization or reversal of acute auditory damage and could interpret effectiveness of bilirubin reduction strategies.

BIND, bilirubin-induced neurologic dysfunction; ABE, acute bilirubin encephalopathy; ABR, auditory brainstem response.

coordination, interventions and close scrutiny of clinical progression relies on the individual and collective responsibilities of the healthcare team, at the bedside as well as within the institution: such as physicians, nurses, patient educators, and even biomedical engineers. These infants are monitored for serial neurologic signs specific to ABE. Progression of increasing BIND scores (Table 45.11) require urgent and immediate interventions with phototherapy and possibly exchange transfusion.

Absolute indications for initiating exchange transfusions are signs of mild to moderate ABE or infants with EHB that is unresponsive to effective phototherapy as well as with documented increasing BIND scores (Table 45.11). Since clinical signs can be subtle or undetectable, monitoring serial BIND scores or assessing population risks for ranges of EHB can inform clinical judgment. With early detection and intervention with effective phototherapy, use of exchange transfusion should be a rarity. Thus far, phototherapy has been considered safe and effective and use of an exchange transfusion reflects a failure in the systems-approach in term neonates.

Side Effects of Phototherapy

Guidelines for standardized phototherapy have eliminated or minimized exposure to mutagenic effects of UV wavelengths (UVA, UVB, and UVC). Reported long-term consequences of prolonged phototherapy exposure has been reported due to the mutagenic action (such as skin cancers) of UV radiation, but only have been theoretical (100), but not proven (101–103). A survey study of phototherapy devices in maternal hospitals affirmed that UV protection is not needed and most of devices are shielded and not contaminated by UV emission. Removal of shields can introduce UV hazards. Operators are unaware of this danger and should be alerted and trained.

Sun as a Light Source

A significant fraction of sunlight is in the UV region, less than 400 nm, and effectively absorbed by various biologic substances. Therefore, unfiltered sunlight should not be used for phototherapy. The safety of direct sunlight and inadvertent exposure to UV lights has been questioned. Recently, the use of window-tinting films, which have the ability to block UVA and infrared (IR) radiation from the sun and to selectively transmit visible light including blue light was evaluated (104). Transmission of therapeutic blue light through films ranged from 24% to 83% compared with unfiltered solar radiation (104). Efficacy of using filtered-sunlight phototherapy has been shown in clinical studies by Slusher et al. (22,105–107).

Pharmacotherapy

Numerous drugs have been proposed to reduce bilirubin load. Most are cathartic in nature and may cause fluid and electrolyte displacements in an infant who may already have intravascular volume depletion, and thus should be used with caution.

Proven concerns of neonatal drug use have already been implemented through public policy. These include compounds that can displace bilirubin from albumin such as sulfa compound and benzyl alcohol, which can lead to increases in UB levels and cause neurotoxicity. Agents that have undergone clinical testing are RhD intravenous immunoglobulin (IVIG) for RhD isoimmunization and use of intravenous gamma globulin for non-RhD isoimmunization. The use of IVIG for minor blood group incompatibilities is unproven. No evidence has been reported for use of albumin. Pharmacotherapy to protect immature neurons has been reported in a piglet model. Derivatives of bovine milk source, enzymatically hydrolyzed and L-aspartic acid to promote bilirubin elimination have also been tested. Competitive inhibitors of HO, such as metalloporphyrins (108,109), have been proposed for use in the prevention of neonatal hyperbilirubinemia (110). Of these, tin mesoporphyrin (SnMP) has been evaluated in FDA-monitored preclinical trials (111). An oral lipid microsphere preparation of zinc protoporphyrin, has been developed and shows promise, but has only been undergoing preclinical testing (112).

INCIDENCE OF EHB AND MORTALITY

Jerold F. Lucey noted in 1982 that the "20 mg/100 mL level" for an exchange transfusion in a full-term infant with hemolytic disease has been effective in avoiding deaths due to kernicterus and brain damage due to bilirubin neurotoxicity. It is not a perfect guideline, but it has been effective. This is amazing because the original studies, judged by modern standards, would not be acceptable today (113). With the absence of a national reporting standards or requirements there are indirect data on the prevalence of EHB, kernicterus, or use of exchange transfusions. In a recent 2012 evidence review, the best estimated reports have been comparisons of these rates between the United States and European nations that have nationalized health systems (114). In a recent U.S. report, Wu et al. (115) performed a retrospective analysis of 525,409 live births from 1995 to 2011 for a single exclusive health care network and found an incidence of TB greater than 30 mg/dL in 8.6 per 100,000 live births ≥ 35 weeks' GA. Brooks et al. (116) reported CBE among live births in California from 1988 to 1997 using Client Development Evaluation Reports from the Department of Developmental Services database. Only 25 cases were found using the strict diagnostic criteria of CBE (or kernicterus), and an incidence of 0.44 per 100,000 live births with a reported mortality rate of 10%. They recognized that even though mortality is an imperfect measure of kernicterus incidence, it can serve as a "rough indicator of incidence" in the United States. Collective reports from the United Kingdom, Denmark, and Canada suggest that the risk increases with the severity of EHB (**Fig. 45.9**).

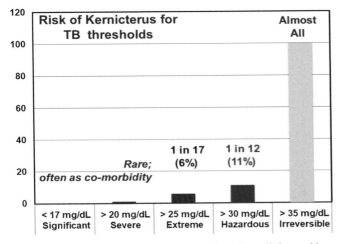

FIGURE 45.9 Population risk of kernicterus using cohort of infants with progressive increments of total serum/plasma bilirubin (TB) reports from United Kingdom, Denmark, and Canada. (Data from Manning D, Todd P, Maxwell M, et al. Prospective surveillance study of severe hyperbilirubinaemia in the newborn in the UK and Ireland. *Arch Dis Child Fetal Neonatal Ed* 2007;92:F342; Sgro M, Campbell DM, Kandasamy S, et al. Incidence of chronic bilirubin encephalopathy in Canada, 2007-2008. *Pediatrics* 2012;130:e886; Donneborg ML, Hansen BM, Vandborg PK, et al. Extreme neonatal hyperbilirubinemia and kernicterus spectrum disorder in Denmark during the years 2000-2015. *J Perinatol* 2020;40:194.)

National Guidelines and Impact on EHB Burden

In 2004, the AAP provided guidelines for the management of hyperbilirubinemia in infants ≥ 35 weeks' GA. Following this guideline, implementation of three systems approaches at national and global levels have resulted in the reduction of TB-related adverse outcomes (117–119). These rely on two advances in maternal care which have had significant impacts on the way in which hyperbilirubinemia is treated and managed. The first is universal screening for maternal blood group and Rh blood type status. The subsequent advent of a global policy of postnatal administration of Rh(D) immunoglobulin to Rh-negative mothers after their first pregnancy dramatically decreased the incidence of Rh alloimmune hemolytic disease in neonates (25). Secondly, introduction of phototherapy as a therapeutic intervention in the United States reduced the use of exchange transfusions. Moreover, it has been shown that concurrent statewide learning collaboratives can impact clinical practice behavior. In the United States, 92.5% of 3,172,762 babies, born from 2007 to 2012, were ≥ 35 weeks' GA. Statewide EHB and exchange transfusion rates decreased from 28.2 to 15.3 and 3.6 to 1.9 per 100,000 live births, respectively (**Fig. 45.10**). From 2007 to 2012, the trends for TB greater than 25 mg/dL (428 μmol/L) rates were −0.92 per 100,000 live births per year (95% CI = −3.71, 1.87; $p = 0.41$; $r^2 = 0.17$). Other regional (**Fig. 45.11**) and statewide implementations of a systems approach to reduce severe hyperbilirubinemia led to a decline in the prevalence of infants with TB greater than 25 mg/dL (428 μmol/L) as well as need for exchange transfusion, and subsequently kernicterus (1 per 61,000 live births in Utah) (120,121).

In Denmark, there were no cases of kernicterus 20 years prior to 1994, and since then sporadic cases have been reported (122). The incidence of EHB among infants ≥35 weeks' GA was 42 per 100,000 live births as reported in a Danish national study from 2000 to 2015 (123). The number of infants with TB ≥ 26.3 mg/dL (450 μmol/L) increased steadily between 2000 and 2007, but decreased between 2005 and 2015. Subtle kernicterus was reported in 1.2 per 100,000 live births mostly associated with blood type ABO-incompatibility.

Estimation of Global Rh Disease Burden

From 184 countries in 2010, an estimated twenty-four million neonates (18% of 134 million live births ≥32 weeks' GA; uncertainty range: 23 to 26 million) were at risk for hyperbilirubinemia-related sequelae (25). Of these, 480,700 (0.36%) had either Rh disease (373,300; uncertainty range: 271,800 to 477,500) or developed EHB from other causes (107,400; uncertainty range: 57,000 to 131,000), with a 24% risk for death (114,100; uncertainty range: 59,700 to 172,000), 13% for kernicterus (75,400), and 11% for stillbirths. Three-quarters of mortality occurred in sub-Saharan Africa and South Asia. Thus, kernicterus with Rh disease ranged from 38, 28, 28, and 25 per 100,000 live births for Eastern Europe/Central Asian, sub-Saharan African, South Asian, and Latin American regions, respectively. More than 83% of survivors with kernicterus had one or more impairments" (**Table 45.12**) (25).

Global Mortality due to Kernicterus

Globally, at least 114,000 neonatal deaths were estimated due to Rh disease and EHB in 2010 (85 per 100,000 live births) (25). The mortality data are disproportionate in high-income countries with 0.1% (n = 94; prevalence 1 per 100,000 live births) as compared with Eastern Europe/Central Asia, Latin America, sub-Saharan Africa, and South Asia, accounting for 6%, 7%, 35%, and 39% of the deaths, respectively (25). Failure to implement national guidelines has led to a re-emergence of kernicterus in the United States (116). Thirty-one infant deaths were reported with clinician documentation from 1979 to 2006. Isolated cases of kernicterus are still being reported and most likely due to G6PD deficiency and other inherited RBC disorders (124).

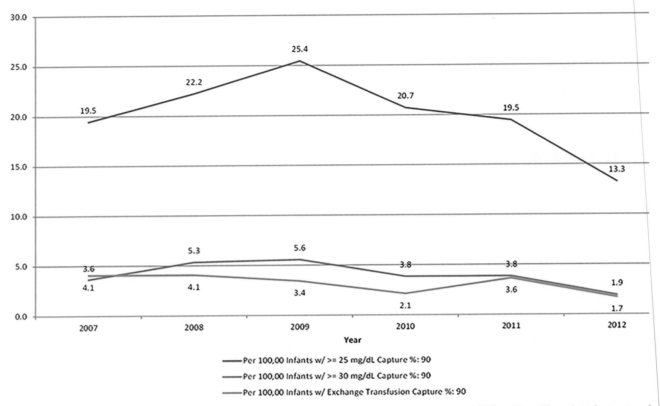

FIGURE 45.10 Serial annual occurrence of extreme hyperbilirubinemia (EHB), total serum/plasma bilirubin (TB) > 30 mg/dL, and exchange transfusion. (Adapted by permission from Nature: Bhutani VK, Meng NF, Knauer Y, et al. Extreme hyperbilirubinemia and rescue exchange transfusion in California from 2007 to 2012. *J Perinatol* 2016;36:853. Copyright © 2016 Springer Nature.)

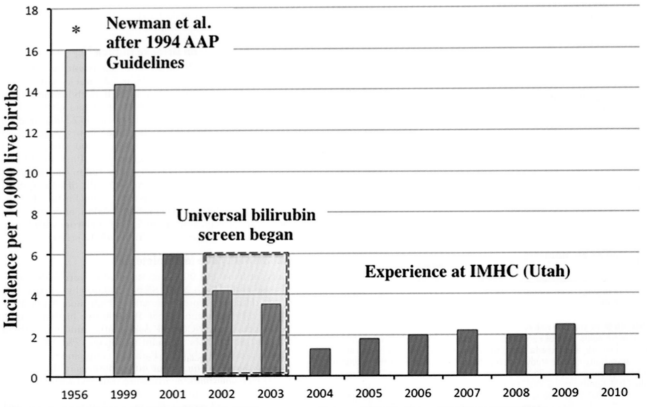

FIGURE 45.11 Serial annual extreme hyperbilirubinemia (EHB) occurrence at Intermountain Healthcare (Utah) from 2004 to 2010.

TABLE 45.12

Annual EHB Global Burden (in Millions)

	Sub-Saharan Africa	Middle East/ North Africa	South Asia	East Asia	Latin America	Europe	North America	Entire World
Need of Rx	5.88	1.13	3.77	2.11	0.24	0.31	0.02	14.11
Unmet need	3.29	0.59	2.36	0.44	–	–	–	6.75
TB > 25 mg/dL	0.80	0.10	0.50	0.10	0.10	0.05	0.10	1.95
TB > 30 mg/dL	0.50	0.10	0.30	0.10	–	–	–	1.00

From a computed model (Reprinted by permission from Nature: Bhutani VK, Zipursky A, Blencowe H, et al. Neonatal hyperbilirubinemia and Rhesus disease of the newborn: incidence and impairment estimates for 2010 at regional and global levels. *Pediatr Res* 2013;74(suppl 1):86. Copyright © 2013 Springer Nature.)

EHB, extreme hyperbilirubinemia; Rx, treatment; TB, total serum/plasma bilirubin.

SUMMARY

Neonatal hyperbilirubinemia is usually benign, but potentially neurotoxic due to a complex multifactorial interaction of the physical, chemical, and photobiologic properties of bilirubin with the existing biology of the neonate (hematologic, genetic, hepatologic, GI, neurologic, and developmental), that can be impacted by nutrition (e.g., breast milk intake) and familial sociocultural beliefs. Currently, a patient safety approach best serves the neonate and family. As clinicians, we should explore novel technologies and advocate to promote and support successful breast-feeding; establish nursery protocols for the early identification and evaluation of hyperbilirubinemia; accurately measure the TB or TcB levels; interpret all TB levels according to the infant's age in hours percentile track to track its ROR. Our purpose is to recognize those infants at risk, who would benefit from closer surveillance and appropriate follow-up. AAP recommends a systems implementation of its guideline (5) and also encourages clinicians to establish office and hospital practices as well as to define replicable universal quality standards that promote earlier use of enteral nutrition and minimalize phototherapy exposure that decreases the use of exchange transfusions, a clinical surrogate measure for kernicterus.

REFERENCES

1. Hsia DY, Jones AR, Allen FH Jr, et al. Studies on erythroblastosis due to ABO incompatibility. *AMA Am J Dis Child* 1953;86:464.
2. Ahlfors CE, Bhutani VK, Wong RJ, et al. Bilirubin binding in jaundiced newborns: from bench to bedside? *Pediatr Res* 2018;84:494.
3. Keren R, Luan X, Friedman S, et al. A comparison of alternative risk-assessment strategies for predicting significant neonatal hyperbilirubinemia in term and near-term infants. *Pediatrics* 2008;121:e170.
4. Bhutani VK, Stark AR, Lazzeroni LC, et al. Predischarge screening for severe neonatal hyperbilirubinemia identifies infants who need phototherapy. *J Pediatr* 2013;162:477.
5. American Academy of Pediatrics. Management of hyperbilirubinemia in the newborn infant 35 or more weeks of gestation. *Pediatrics* 2004;114:297.
6. Johnson L, Bhutani VK. The clinical syndrome of bilirubin-induced neurologic dysfunction. *Semin Perinatol* 2011;35:101.
7. Brodersen R, Cashore WJ, Wennberg RP, et al. Kinetics of bilirubin oxidation with peroxidase, as applied to studies of bilirubin-albumin binding. *Scand J Clin Lab Invest* 1979;39:143.
8. Wennberg RP, Ahlfors CE, Rasmussen LF. The pathochemistry of kernicterus. *Early Hum Dev* 1979;3:353.
9. Bhutani VK, Wong RJ. Bilirubin-induced neurologic dysfunction (BIND). *Semin Fetal Neonatal Med* 2015;20:1.
10. Bhutani VK, Wong RJ. Bilirubin neurotoxicity in preterm infants: risk and prevention. *J Clin Neonatol* 2013;2:61.
11. Carbonell X, Botet F, Figueras J, et al. Prediction of hyperbilirubinaemia in the healthy term newborn. *Acta Paediatr* 2001;90:166.
12. Jones KDJ, Grossman SE, Kumaranayakam D, et al. Umbilical cord bilirubin as a predictor of neonatal jaundice: a retrospective cohort study. *BMC Pediatr* 2017;17:186.
13. Knupfer M, Pulzer F, Gebauer C, et al. Predictive value of umbilical cord blood bilirubin for postnatal hyperbilirubinaemia. *Acta Paediatr* 2005;94:581.
14. Sarici SU, Serdar MA, Korkmaz A, et al. Incidence, course, and prediction of hyperbilirubinemia in near-term and term newborns. *Pediatrics* 2004;113:775.
15. Macias RI, Marin JJ, Serrano MA. Excretion of biliary compounds during intrauterine life. *World J Gastroenterol* 2009;15:817.
16. Tenhunen R, Marver HS, Schmid R. The enzymatic conversion of heme to bilirubin by microsomal heme oxygenase. *Proc Natl Acad Sci U S A* 1968;61:748.
17. Maines MD. The heme oxygenase system: a regulator of second messenger gases. *Annu Rev Pharmacol Toxicol* 1997;37:517.
18. Kaplan M, Hammerman C, Maisels MJ. Bilirubin genetics for the nongeneticist: hereditary defects of neonatal bilirubin conjugation. *Pediatrics* 2003;111:886.
19. Kaplan M, Renbaum P, Vreman HJ, et al. (TA)n UGT 1A1 promoter polymorphism: a crucial factor in the pathophysiology of jaundice in G-6-PD deficient neonates. *Pediatr Res* 2007;61:727.
20. Venigalla S, Gourley GR. Neonatal cholestasis. *Semin Perinatol* 2004;28:348.
21. Newborn Screening. *Program to Enhance the Health & Development of Infants and Children (PEHDIC)*; 2020. Available from: https://www.aap.org/en-us/advocacy-and-policy/aap-health-initiatives/PEHDIC/pages/Newborn-Screening.aspx.
22. Slusher TM, Vreman HJ, Olusanya BO, et al. Safety and efficacy of filtered sunlight in treatment of jaundice in African neonates. *Pediatrics* 2014;133:e1568.
23. Newman TB, Maisels MJ. Response to commentaries re: evaluation and treatment of jaundice in the term newborn: a kinder, gentler approach. *Pediatrics* 1992;89:831.
24. Tovey LA. Haemolytic disease of the newborn—the changing scene. *Br J Obstet Gynaecol* 1986;93:960.
25. Bhutani VK, Zipursky A, Blencowe H, et al. Neonatal hyperbilirubinemia and Rhesus disease of the newborn: incidence and impairment estimates for 2010 at regional and global levels. *Pediatr Res* 2013;74(suppl 1):86.
26. Wong RJ, Bhutani VK, Stevenson DK. The importance of hemolysis and its clinical detection in neonates with hyperbilirubinemia. *Curr Pediatr Rev* 2017;13:193.
27. Herschel M, Karrison T, Wen M, et al. Isoimmunization is unlikely to be the cause of hemolysis in ABO-incompatible but direct antiglobulin test-negative neonates. *Pediatrics* 2002;110:127.
28. Herschel M, Karrison T, Wen M, et al. Evaluation of the direct antiglobulin (Coombs') test for identifying newborns at risk for hemolysis as determined by end-tidal carbon monoxide concentration (ETCOc); and comparison of the Coombs' test with ETCOc for detecting significant jaundice. *J Perinatol* 2002;22:341.
29. Beutler E. Glucose-6-phosphate dehydrogenase deficiency. *Br J Haematol* 1970;18:117.
30. Beutler E. Glucose-6-phosphate dehydrogenase deficiency. *N Engl J Med* 1991;324:169.
31. Lin Z, Fontaine J, Watchko JF. Coexpression of gene polymorphisms involved in bilirubin production and metabolism. *Pediatrics* 2008;122:e156.
32. WHO Working Group. Glucose-6-phosphate dehydrogenase deficiency. *Bull World Health Organ* 1989;67:601.
33. Cappellini MD, Fiorelli G. Glucose-6-phosphate dehydrogenase deficiency. *Lancet* 2008;371:64.
34. Watchko JF, Kaplan M, Stark AR, et al. Should we screen newborns for glucose-6-phosphate dehydrogenase deficiency in the United States? *J Perinatol* 2013;33:499.
35. Howes RE, Piel FB, Patil AP, et al. G6PD deficiency prevalence and estimates of affected populations in malaria endemic countries: a geostatistical model-based map. *PLoS Med* 2012;9:e1001339.
36. Kaplan M, Hammerman C, Bhutani VK. Parental education and the WHO neonatal G-6-PD screening program: a quarter century later. *J Perinatol* 2015;35:779.
37. Watchko JF, Tiribelli C. Bilirubin-induced neurologic damage—mechanisms and management approaches. *N Engl J Med* 2013;369:2021.

THE NEWBORN INFANT

38. Gambaro SE, Robert MC, Tiribelli C, et al. Role of brain cytochrome P450 mono-oxygenases in bilirubin oxidation-specific induction and activity. *Arch Toxicol* 2016;90:279.

39. Amin SB, Wang H, Laroia N, et al. Unbound bilirubin and auditory neuropathy spectrum disorder in late preterm and term infants with severe jaundice. *J Pediatr* 2016;173:84.

40. Amin SB, Saluja S, Saili A, et al. Auditory toxicity in late preterm and term neonates with severe jaundice. *Dev Med Child Neurol* 2017;59:297.

41. Amin SB, Saluja S, Saili A, et al. Chronic auditory toxicity in late preterm and term infants with significant hyperbilirubinemia. *Pediatrics* 2017;140:e20164009.

42. Wisnowski JL, Panigrahy A, Painter MJ, et al. Magnetic resonance imaging abnormalities in advanced acute bilirubin encephalopathy highlight dentato-thalamo-cortical pathways. *J Pediatr* 2016;174:260.

43. Penn AA, Enzmann DR, Hahn JS, et al. Kernicterus in a full term infant. *Pediatrics* 1994;93:1003.

44. Govaert P, Lequin M, Swarte R, et al. Changes in globus pallidus with (pre) term kernicterus. *Pediatrics* 2003;112:1256.

45. Good WV, Hou C. Visuocortical bilirubin-induced neurological dysfunction. *Semin Fetal Neonatal Med* 2015;20:37.

46. Olds C, Oghalai JS. Audiologic impairment associated with bilirubin-induced neurologic damage. *Semin Fetal Neonatal Med* 2015;20:42.

47. Shapiro SM, Popelka GR. Auditory impairment in infants at risk for bilirubin-induced neurologic dysfunction. *Semin Perinatol* 2011;35:162.

48. Wusthoff CJ, Loe IM. Impact of bilirubin-induced neurologic dysfunction on neurodevelopmental outcomes. *Semin Fetal Neonatal Med* 2015;20:52.

49. Rose J, Vassar R. Movement disorders due to bilirubin toxicity. *Semin Fetal Neonatal Med* 2015;20:20.

50. Watchko JF, Painter MJ, Panigrahy A. Are the neuromotor disabilities of bilirubin-induced neurologic dysfunction disorders related to the cerebellum and its connections? *Semin Fetal Neonatal Med* 2015;20:47.

51. de Vries LS, Lary S, Dubowitz LM. Relationship of serum bilirubin levels to ototoxicity and deafness in high-risk low-birth-weight infants. *Pediatrics* 1985;76:351.

52. Nakamura H, Takada S, Shimabuku R, et al. Auditory nerve and brainstem responses in newborn infants with hyperbilirubinemia. *Pediatrics* 1985;75:703.

53. Marlow ES, Hunt LP, Marlow N. Sensorineural hearing loss and prematurity. *Arch Dis Child Fetal Neonatal Ed* 2000;82:F141.

54. Corujo-Santana C, Falcon-Gonzalez JC, Borkoski-Barreiro SA, et al. The relationship between neonatal hyperbilirubinemia and sensorineural hearing loss. *Acta Otorrinolaringol Esp* 2015;66:326.

55. Shapiro SM, Nakamura H. Bilirubin and the auditory system. *J Perinatol* 2001;21(suppl 1):S52.

56. Cardoso FL, Kittel A, Veszelka S, et al. Exposure to lipopolysaccharide and/or unconjugated bilirubin impair the integrity and function of brain microvascular endothelial cells. *PLoS One* 2012;7:e35919.

57. Falcao AS, Silva RF, Vaz AR, et al. Cross-talk between neurons and astrocytes in response to bilirubin: early beneficial effects. *Neurochem Res* 2013;38:644.

58. Brites D. The evolving landscape of neurotoxicity by unconjugated bilirubin: role of glial cells and inflammation. *Front Pharmacol* 2012;3:88.

59. Brites D, Fernandes A. Bilirubin-induced neural impairment: a special focus on myelination, age-related windows of susceptibility and associated co-morbidities. *Semin Fetal Neonatal Med* 2015;20:14.

60. Hsia DY, Allen FH Jr, Diamond LK, et al. Serum bilirubin levels in the newborn infant. *J Pediatr* 1953;42:277.

61. Kim MH, Yoon JJ, Sher J, et al. Lack of predictive indices in kernicterus: a comparison of clinical and pathologic factors in infants with or without kernicterus. *Pediatrics* 1980;66:852.

62. Bhutani VK, Johnson L, Sivieri EM. Predictive ability of a predischarge hour-specific serum bilirubin for subsequent significant hyperbilirubinemia in healthy term and near-term newborns. *Pediatrics* 1999;103:6.

63. Arman D, Topcuoglu S, Gursoy T, et al. The accuracy of transcutaneous bilirubinometry in preterm infants. *J Perinatol* 2020;40:212.

64. Bhutani VK, Gourley GR, Adler S, et al. Noninvasive measurement of total serum bilirubin in a multiracial predischarge newborn population to assess the risk of severe hyperbilirubinemia. *Pediatrics* 2000;106:E17.

65. Rubaltelli FF, Gourley GR, Loskamp N, et al. Transcutaneous bilirubin measurement: a multicenter evaluation of a new device. *Pediatrics* 2001;107:1264.

66. Maisels MJ, Bhutani VK, Bogen D, et al. Hyperbilirubinemia in the newborn infant > or =35 weeks' gestation: an update with clarifications. *Pediatrics* 2009;124:1193.

67. Ahlfors CE. The bilirubin binding panel: a Henderson-Hasselbalch approach to neonatal hyperbilirubinemia. *Pediatrics* 2016;138:e20154378.

68. Lamola AA, Bhutani VK, Du L, et al. Neonatal bilirubin binding capacity discerns risk of neurological dysfunction. *Pediatr Res* 2015;77:334.

69. Ahlfors CE. Unbound bilirubin associated with kernicterus: a historical approach. *J Pediatr* 2000;137:540.

70. Funato M, Tamai H, Shimada S, et al. Vigintiphobia, unbound bilirubin, and auditory brainstem responses. *Pediatrics* 1994;93:50.

71. Amin SB, Ahlfors C, Orlando MS, et al. Bilirubin and serial auditory brainstem responses in premature infants. *Pediatrics* 2001;107:664.

72. Ahlfors CE, Amin SB, Parker AE. Unbound bilirubin predicts abnormal automated auditory brainstem response in a diverse newborn population. *J Perinatol* 2009;29:305.

73. Cashore WJ, Oh W. Unbound bilirubin and kernicterus in low-birth-weight infants. *Pediatrics* 1982;69:481.

74. Ritter DA, Kenny JD, Norton HJ, et al. A prospective study of free bilirubin and other risk factors in the development of kernicterus in premature infants. *Pediatrics* 1982;69:260.

75. Ahlfors CE. Criteria for exchange transfusion in jaundiced newborns. *Pediatrics* 1994;93:488.

76. Wennberg RP, Ahlfors CE, Bhutani VK, et al. Toward understanding kernicterus: a challenge to improve the management of jaundiced newborns. *Pediatrics* 2006;117:474.

77. Ahlfors CE. Predicting bilirubin neurotoxicity in jaundiced newborns. *Curr Opin Pediatr* 2010;22:129.

78. Maisels MJ, Watchko JF, Bhutani VK, et al. An approach to the management of hyperbilirubinemia in the preterm infant less than 35 weeks of gestation. *J Perinatol* 2012;32:660.

79. Cashore WJ, Horwich A, Karotkin EH, et al. Influence of gestational age and clinical status on bilirubin-binding capacity in newborn infants. Sephadex G-25 gel filtration technique. *Am J Dis Child* 1977;131:898.

80. Bender GJ, Cashore WJ, Oh W. Ontogeny of bilirubin-binding capacity and the effect of clinical status in premature infants born at less than 1300 grams. *Pediatrics* 2007;120:1067.

81. Agarwal AM, Nussenzveig RH, Reading NS, et al. Clinical utility of next-generation sequencing in the diagnosis of hereditary haemolytic anaemias. *Br J Haematol* 2016;174:806.

82. Newman AJ, Gross S. Hyperbilirubinemia in breast-fed infants. *Pediatrics* 1963;32:995.

83. Arias IM, Gartner LM, Seifter S, et al. Prolonged neonatal unconjugated hyperbilirubinemia associated with breast feeding and a steroid, pregnane-3(alpha), 20(beta)-diol, in maternal milk that inhibits glucuronide formation *in vitro*. *J Clin Invest* 1964;43:2037.

84. Katz HP, Robinson TA. Breast-milk hyperbilirubinemia: report of a case. *N Engl J Med* 1965;273:546.

85. Winfield CR, MacFaul R. Clinical study of prolonged jaundice in breast- and bottle-fed babies. *Arch Dis Child* 1978;53:506.

86. Gourley GR, Kreamer BL, Cohnen M. Inhibition of beta-glucuronidase by casein hydrolysate formula. *J Pediatr Gastroenterol Nutr* 1997;25:267.

87. Gundur NM, Kumar P, Sundaram V, et al. Natural history and predictive risk factors of prolonged unconjugated jaundice in the newborn. *Pediatr Int* 2010;52:769.

88. Maruo Y, Morioka Y, Fujito H, et al. Bilirubin uridine diphosphate-glucuronosyltransferase variation is a genetic basis of breast milk jaundice. *J Pediatr* 2014;165:36.

89. Agrawal SK, Kumar P, Rathi R, et al. UGT1A1 gene polymorphisms in North Indian neonates presenting with unconjugated hyperbilirubinemia. *Pediatr Res* 2009;65:675.

90. Bhutani VK, Wong RJ. Are genetics disorders masquerading as breast milk jaundice? In: Cabana MD, ed. *Yearbook of neonatal and perinatal medicine*. Philadelphia, PA: Elsevier, 2015:333.

91. Bhutani VK; Committee on Fetus and Newborn. Phototherapy to prevent severe neonatal hyperbilirubinemia in the newborn infant 35 or more weeks of gestation. *Pediatrics* 2011;128:e1046.

92. Maisels MJ, McDonagh AF. Phototherapy for neonatal jaundice. *N Engl J Med* 2008;358:920.

93. McDonagh AF, Lightner DA. Phototherapy and the photobiology of bilirubin. *Semin Liv Dis* 1988;8:272.

94. Lightner DA. *Bilirubin: Jekyll and Hyde pigment of life: pursuit of its structure through two world wars to the new millennium*. Vienna, Austria: Springer-Verlag Wien, 2013.

95. Lamola AA. A pharmacologic view of phototherapy. *Clin Perinatol* 2016;43:259.

96. Turro NJ, Ramamurthy V, Scaiano JC. *Principles of molecular photochemistry: an introduction*. Dulles, VA: University Science Books, 2009.

97. McDonagh AF, Lightner DA. 'Like a shrivelled blood orange'—bilirubin, jaundice, and phototherapy. *Pediatrics* 1985;75:443.

98. Bhutani VK, Konecny CM, Wong RJ. Mechanistic aspects of phototherapy for neonatal hyperbilirubinemia. In: Polin R, Benitz WE, eds. *Fetal and neonatal physiology*, 6th ed. Philadelphia, PA: Elsevier Saunders, 2020.

99. Arnold C, Tyson JE, Pedroza C, et al. Cycled phototherapy for extremely low birth weight infants: a dose-finding clinical trial. *JAMA Pediatr* 2020; in press

100. Matichard E, Le Henanff A, Sanders A, et al. Effect of neonatal phototherapy on melanocytic nevus count in children. *Arch Dermatol* 2006;142:1599.

101. Newman TB, Maisels MJ. Evidence insufficient to recommend mela-noma surveillance following phototherapy for jaundice. *Arch Dermatol* 2007;143:1216; author reply 1216.

102. Lai YC, Yew YW. Neonatal blue light phototherapy and melanocytic nevus count in children: a systematic review and meta-analysis of observational studies. *Pediatr Dermatol* 2016;33:62.

103. Brewster DH, Tucker JS, Fleming M, et al. Risk of skin cancer after neona-tal phototherapy: retrospective cohort study. *Arch Dis Child* 2010;95:826.

104. Vreman HJ, Slusher TM, Wong RJ, et al. Evaluation of window-tinting films for sunlight phototherapy. *J Trop Pediatr* 2013;59:496.

105. Slusher TM, Day LT, Ogundele T, et al. Filtered sunlight, solar powered phototherapy and other strategies for managing neonatal jaundice in low-resource settings. *Early Hum Dev* 2017;114:11.

106. Slusher TM, Olusanya BO, Vreman HJ, et al. A randomized trial of phototherapy with filtered sunlight in African neonates. *N Engl J Med* 2015;373:1115.

107. Slusher TM, Vreman HJ, Brearley AM, et al. Filtered sunlight versus intensive electric powered phototherapy in moderate-to-severe neona-tal hyperbilirubinaemia: a randomised controlled non-inferiority trial. *Lancet Glob Health* 2018;6:e1122.

108. Wong RJ, Bhutani VK, Vreman HJ, et al. Tin mesoporphyrin for the pre-vention of severe neonatal hyperbilirubinemia. *NeoReviews* 2007;8:e77.

109. Schulz S, Wong RJ, Vreman HJ, et al. Metalloporphyrins—an update. *Front Pharmacol* 2012;3:68.

110. Stevenson DK, Rodgers PA, Vreman HJ. The use of metalloporphyrins for the chemoprevention of neonatal jaundice. *Am J Dis Child* 1989;143:353.

111. Bhutani VK, Poland R, Meloy LD, et al. Clinical trial of tin mesoporphyrin to prevent neonatal hyperbilirubinemia. *J Perinatol* 2016;36:533.

112. Fujioka K, Kalish F, Wong RJ, et al. Inhibition of heme oxygenase activ-ity using a microparticle formulation of zinc protoporphyrin in an acute hemolytic newborn mouse model. *Pediatr Res* 2016;79:251.

113. Lucey JF. Bilirubin and brain damage—a real mess. *Pediatrics* 1982;69:381.

114. Knapp AA, Metterville DR, Co JPT, et al. *Evidence review: neonatal hyperbilirubinemia;* 2012. Available from: https://www.hrsa.gov/sites/default/files/hrsa/advisory-committees/heritable-disorders/rusp/previous-nominations/hyperbilirubinemia-evidence-review-report.pdf.

115. Wu YW, Kuzniewicz MW, Wickremasinghe AC, et al. Risk for cere-bral palsy in infants with total serum bilirubin levels at or above the exchange transfusion threshold: a population-based study. *JAMA Pediatr* 2015;169:239.

116. Brooks JC, Fisher-Owens SA, Wu YW, et al. Evidence suggests there was not a "resurgence" of kernicterus in the 1990s. *Pediatrics* 2011;127:672.

117. Bhutani VK, Meng NF, Knauer Y, et al. Extreme hyperbilirubinemia and rescue exchange transfusion in California from 2007 to 2012. *J Perinatol* 2016;36:853.

118. Christensen RD, Baer VL, MacQueen BC, et al. ABO hemolytic disease of the fetus and newborn: thirteen years of data after implementing a universal bilirubin screening and management program. *J Perinatol* 2018;38:517.

119. Mah MP, Clark SL, Akhigbe E, et al. Reduction of severe hyperbilirubi-nemia after institution of predischarge bilirubin screening. *Pediatrics* 2010;125:e1143.

120. Bahr TM, Christensen RD, Agarwal AM, et al. The Neonatal Acute Biliru-bin Encephalopathy Registry (NABER): background, aims, and protocol. *Neonatology* 2019;115:242.

121. Christensen RD, Agarwal AM, George TI, et al. Acute neonatal biliru-bin encephalopathy in the State of Utah 2009-2018. *Blood Cells Mol Dis* 2018;72:10.

122. Ebbesen F. Recurrence of kernicterus in term and near-term infants in Denmark. *Acta Paediatr* 2000;89:1213.

123. Donneborg ML, Hansen BM, Vandborg PK, et al. Extreme neonatal hyper-bilirubinemia and kernicterus spectrum disorder in Denmark during the years 2000-2015. *J Perinatol* 2020;40:194.

124. Christensen RD, Yaish HM. Hemolytic disorders causing severe neonatal hyperbilirubinemia. *Clin Perinatol* 2015;42:515.

THE NEWBORN INFANT

46 Congenital Infections

Swetha G. Pinninti and David W. Kimberlin

INTRODUCTION

The risk of illness due to transmission of infections from pregnant mothers to their infants and from exposures to infections in the first few weeks of life has been recognized for centuries. Advances in diagnostics over the past few decades have enhanced the ability to identify exposures to infectious agents during pregnancy, led to development of screening programs, allowed institution of antimicrobial prophylaxis, and and allowed diagnosis of infection in the newborn. This has been particularly evident in the investigations of the transmission of human immunodeficiency virus (HIV) from mother to infant in which the development of polymerase chain reaction (PCR) testing in the 1990s was necessary to define the risks of transmission and for appropriate diagnosis.

The consequences of infection depend largely on the timing of transmission to the infant (prenatal vs. perinatal vs. postnatal), whether it is a primary maternal infection, the ability to make a quick and accurate diagnosis, rapid institution of appropriate antimicrobial agents, any underlying condition, and the gestational age of the newborn. This chapter will focus on infections acquired in the intrauterine and peripartum period.

Classically, the agents that are most frequently associated with congenital infection have been referred to as the TORCH organisms (toxoplasmosis, other infections, rubella, cytomegalovirus, and herpes). Since the "other" in the mnemonic now stands for a significant number of potential pathogens, it is now considered to be somewhat limited, and a variety of mnemonics have been proposed to help ensure that all potential agents are considered when an infant presents with suspected congenital infection. However, use of maternal identifiable risk factors and knowledge of the local prevalence and incidence of potential infections is a more effective way of developing a diagnostic plan.

It is important for health care providers to consider the possibility of a congenital infection at the time of the initial examination of the infant. Clinical clues as to whether an investigation for congenital infection(s) is warranted and the most likely organisms are listed in Table 46.1. Information concerning the specific agents including the epidemiology, clinical presentation, laboratory diagnosis, and management are detailed below.

VIRAL INFECTIONS

Severe Acute Respiratory Syndrome Coronavirus-2
Epidemiology

Reports of pneumonia caused by a novel coronavirus, severe acute respiratory syndrome coronavirus-2 (SARS-CoV-2), and the infection caused by the virus, referred to as COVID-19, were initially reported from Wuhan, China, in December 2019 (1,2). The World Health Organization (WHO) declared COVID-19 a pandemic on March 11, 2020, and the virus has since been reported from 188 countries/regions across the world, resulting in over 20 million confirmed cases and over 750,000 deaths worldwide, as of August, 2020 (3), contributing to significant morbidity, mortality, and economic losses.

Studies with inclusion of large numbers of children with COVID-19 to date have revealed that the majority of children present with asymptomatic or mild disease (4). A limited number of studies have examined the occurrence of fetal and neonatal infections and documented intrauterine transmission of SARS-CoV-2 (5–10).

In a systematic review, adverse pregnancy outcomes for women with SARS-CoV-2 infection during pregnancy included preterm birth and increased number of perinatal deaths (11,12). Limited reports in the literature have raised concern of possible intrauterine, intrapartum, or peripartum transmission, but the extent and clinical significance of vertical transmission, which appears to be rare, is unclear. In a study of 33 infants born to mothers with COVID-19, 3 babies were positive for SARS-CoV-2 by RT-PCR of nasopharyngeal and anal swabs; all 3 of these infants had pneumonia and required intensive care (13). In more recent studies, four neonates were reported to test positive for SARS-CoV-2 where vertical transmission could not be excluded, and one neonate was described with neurologic manifestations after transplacental transmission (14,15). Overall, the likelihood of intrauterine transmission of SARS-CoV-2 seems low but needs further confirmation.

Pathophysiology and Clinical Presentation

The incubation period for COVID-19 is estimated to be 14 days with a median of 4 to 5 days (5,16). Cardiac, hematologic, thromboembolic, and neurologic complications, particularly in critically ill patients, have been reported (17–19). Transmission of SARS-CoV-2 to neonates is thought to occur primarily through respiratory droplets during the postnatal period when neonates are exposed to mothers or other caregivers with SARS-CoV-2 infection.

Clinical presentation in the newborn period has varied in reports across the world, including complete lack of symptoms (20), fever and lethargy (13) or fever and feeding difficulty (21), perioral cyanosis and subsequent hypoxia requiring high flow nasal cannula (22), late-onset neonatal sepsis, and respiratory distress syndrome (13). Current evidence suggests that SARS-CoV-2 infections in neonates are uncommon (23). When neonates do become infected, the majority have either asymptomatic infections or mild disease.

The pediatric cohort described by Dong et al. included 376 children in the less than 1 year age group (4). A majority (336, 89.4%) had mild to moderate symptoms or were asymptomatic. A more recent pediatric case series of 130 children from Italy found that infants less than 6 months old were at increased risk of critical disease compared with older children, though no deaths occurred (24). Typical laboratory findings in children with COVID-19 have included mild abnormalities in white blood cell count (decreased lymphocyte counts), mildly elevated inflammatory markers, and mildly elevated liver enzymes. Radiologic findings in children with COVID-19 include unilateral or bilateral infiltrates on chest radiograph or CT, and ground-glass opacities on CT.

Diagnosis and Follow-Up

Diagnosis is confirmed by testing for SARS-CoV-2 RNA by reverse transcription polymerase chain reaction (RT-PCR). Detection of SARS-CoV-2 RNA is by collecting nasopharynx, oropharynx, or nasal swab samples (25,26). Serologic testing is not recommended at this time to diagnose acute infection in neonates. The optimal timing of testing of newborns is currently unknown. Early testing potentially can produce false positives (if the neonate's nares, nasopharynx, and/or oropharynx are contaminated by SARS-CoV-2 RNA from maternal fluids) or false negatives (in situations where SARS-CoV-2 RNA may not yet be detectable immediately after exposure following birth).

TABLE 46.1

Common Signs Associated with Congenital Infections

Sign	Chagas	CMV	HSV	LCMV	Malaria	Parvovirus B19	Rubella	Syphilis	Toxoplasma	TB	VZV	ZIKV
Microcephaly		X	X	X			X		X		X	X
Hydrocephalus		X		X				X	X			
IC calcifications		X	X	X			X		X		X	
Chorioretinitis		X	X	X			X		X		X	
Cataracts			X	X			X				X	
SNHL		X	X	X			X	X				X
Cardiac involvement	X					X	X					
Hepatosplenomegaly	X	X		X	X		X	X	X	X		
IUGR	X	X			X		X	X	X		X	X
Limb abnormalities												
Rash/skin lesions		X	X				X	X		X	X	X
Radiographic long-bone abnormalities			X					X			X	
Neonatal jaundice	X	X			X		X	X	X			
Anemia	X					X	X	X	X	X		
Thrombocytopenia		X		X	X	X	X	X				X
Neutropenia/lymphopenia		X				X		X				X

CMV, cytomegalovirus; HSV, herpes simplex virus; LCMV, lymphocytic choriomeningitis virus; TB, tuberculosis; VZV, varicella-zoster virus; ZIKV, Zika virus; IC, intracranial; SNHL, sensorineural hearing loss; IUGR, intrauterine growth retardation.

The current recommendation is for both symptomatic and asymptomatic neonates born to mothers with suspected or confirmed COVID-19, regardless of mother's symptoms, to be tested by PCR at approximately 24 hours of age. If initial test results are negative, testing should be repeated at 48 hours of age. Measures to minimize postnatal transmission include maternal masking and practicing hand hygiene during all contact with their neonates. While SARS-CoV-2 RNA has been detected in breast milk, transmission through breast milk has not been definitively proven at this time. Taking into consideration the long-term benefits of breast-feeding, mothers are encouraged to either breast-feed or express and feed with proper precautions as outlined (27).

Treatment

There are currently no specific approved drugs for the treatment of COVID-19 in neonates and children, and treatment remains largely supportive, including management of complications. Multiple trials at various stages are currently under way to test the efficacy of different treatment modalities (antivirals, immunomodulators, convalescent plasma). To date, remdesivir and dexamethasone have shown clinical benefit in trials in adults (28,29). Remdesivir is now being studied in children, including term and preterm neonates (ClinicalTrials.gov Identifier: NCT04431453).

Cytomegalovirus

Epidemiology

Cytomegalovirus (CMV) is an enveloped double-stranded DNA member of the Herpesviridae family. Hundreds of thousands of children are born all over the world each year with congenital cytomegalovirus infection (cCMV), contributing significantly to hearing loss and developmental disabilities. In the United States, Western Europe, Australia, and Canada, cCMV occurs in approximately 5 to 7 per 1,000 live births (30). However, in populous regions of the world like Latin America, Africa, and most countries in Asia, cCMV rates are much higher at 10 to 30 per 1,000 live births (31–33).

Rates of cCMV in the population are determined heavily by the maternal CMV seroprevalence rates, with higher rates of cCMV being observed in populations with high maternal CMV seroprevalence. Unlike other congenital infections like rubella, where primary infections during pregnancy are responsible for vertically transmitted infections, cCMV can occur in children born to mothers infected with CMV prior to pregnancy (nonprimary infection). Systematic reviews and modeling data have suggested that a majority of infants with cCMV are currently born to mothers with nonprimary infections, due to either reactivation of previously acquired virus or reinfection with a new viral strain.

cCMV-associated hearing loss is the most common cause of nongenetic hearing loss as an etiology of permanent hearing loss during childhood (34,35). In addition, cCMV-associated developmental disabilities are more common than other well-recognized diseases like Down syndrome, fetal alcohol syndrome, and spina bifida (36). Despite the frequency of cCMV sequelae, there are significant awareness and knowledge gaps among pregnant women and health care providers (37).

Pathophysiology and Clinical Presentation

CMV acquisition during pregnancy in seronegative and seropositive women is through contact with children shedding the virus or through sexual activity. Primary infections during pregnancy are associated with higher risk of in utero transmission at 30% to 35%, while for nonprimary infections, the transmission rate is estimated to be lower at 1.1% to 1.7% (38). While the rate of maternal-to-fetal transmission increases with increase in gestational age (third trimester > second trimester > first trimester), the severity of infection is higher when infection occurs in the early stages of pregnancy (39,40). Congenital CMV is a multisystem disease with predilection for reticuloendothelial system and the central nervous system. The majority of children with cCMV (85% to 90%) do not have clinical findings at birth (asymptomatic infection), and the remaining 10% to 15% are born with clinical abnormalities at birth of varying severity (41) and categorized as symptomatic infection (42–44). Physical signs in the newborn period occurring in greater than 50% of symptomatic cCMV babies are petechial rash, jaundice, hepatosplenomegaly, and neurologic abnormalities such as microcephaly and lethargy. The intracranial calcifications seen in congenital CMV infections tend to be periventricular in location as is seen in **Figure 46.1**. Other neurologic abnormalities may include intraventricular hemorrhages, periventricular necrosis, cerebral hypoplasia, periventricular leukomalacia, hydrocephalus,

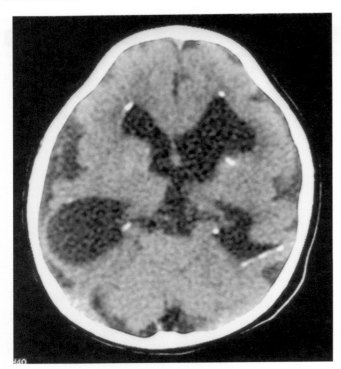

FIGURE 46.1 Computerized axial tomogram of a microcephalic 3-month-old boy with symptomatic congenital CMV following primary maternal gestational CMV infection. Shown are subependymal periventricular calcifications, enlarged ventricles and CSF spaces, and loss of periventricular and subcortical white matter volume.

and porencephalic cysts. Chorioretinitis and/or optic atrophy are evident on ophthalmologic examination in 10% of symptomatic infants. About half of symptomatic infants are small for gestational age, and one-third are born prematurely. Laboratory findings observed in greater than 50% of symptomatic newborns include conjugated hyperbilirubinemia, thrombocytopenia, and elevations of hepatic transaminases (43).

Approximately 40% to 60% of symptomatic infants and 10% to 15% of asymptomatic newborns will develop long-term sequelae related to cCMV, with sensorineural hearing loss (SNHL) being the most common and to a lesser extent, particularly in the asymptomatic group, cognitive impairment, chorioretinitis, and cerebral palsy. SNHL may be present at birth (early-onset), or in 33% to 50% can occur later in the first few years of life (late-onset) (45). About 50% with symptomatic and asymptomatic infection will have worsening SNHL in the first few years (progressive SNHL), and hearing can fluctuate over time (46).

Diagnosis

Routine antenatal screening for CMV during pregnancy is not recommended at this time. Diagnosis of acute CMV infection in the pregnant woman is performed by documentation of seroconversion during pregnancy, rising IgG titers, and/or the presence of IgM antibodies with a low IgG avidity response.

In pregnant women with documented primary infection, options for prenatal diagnosis with invasive (amniocentesis/cordocentesis) and noninvasive (ultrasound) techniques are available for prenatal diagnosis of cCMV. Detection of the virus by PCR in high titers in the amniotic fluid is associated with higher incidence of fetal infection likely resulting in symptomatic infants at birth (47). While the sensitivity of ultrasound to detect fetuses with cCMV is low, it is useful for detecting and monitoring fetal abnormalities suggestive of cCMV. Normal ultrasound examinations in a documented cases

of fetal cCMV have been shown to be associated with a low risk of severe symptomatic infection.

Both symptomatic and asymptomatic newborns with cCMV shed large amounts of virus in saliva and urine, making either of these specimens ideal for the diagnosis. It is imperative that the specimens be collected in the first 2 to 3 weeks of life to distinguish congenital from postnatally acquired CMV.

Detection of infectious virus or viral antigens in urine or saliva have long been the gold standard for identification of infants with cCMV (48,49). Sensitivities for PCR detection of CMV DNA are similar with both specimen types (99.7% agreement) (50). PCR assays from these samples have been shown to be superior to culture methods (51) and have the advantages of being less expensive with rapid turnaround times with no requirement for maintaining tissue culture facilities. While use of dry blood spot (DBS) samples collected for metabolic and genetic screening programs is promising as a screening specimen to identify newborns with cCMV, DBS PCR currently is not utilized due to low sensitivity of the assay (52).

Treatment and Management

Due to lack of data supporting the use of CMV-specific hyperimmune globulin (HIG) (53) and antiviral therapy (54) to prevent maternal-to-fetal transmission of CMV, the mainstay of interventions to prevent maternal infections during pregnancy and cCMV has focused on CMV awareness and behavioral interventions to minimize exposure to the virus (55).

For treatment of symptomatic cCMV, 6 months of valganciclovir therapy has been shown to be more beneficial for hearing loss and neurodevelopmental outcomes (56–58). Benefit of antiviral therapy is currently unknown in infants with isolated SNHL and asymptomatic cCMV, and antiviral therapy in these populations is not recommended at this time. For infants undergoing treatment, close monitoring for neutropenia (absolute neutrophil count weekly for 6 weeks and then monthly for the duration of treatment) and hepatic involvement (transaminases levels monthly for the duration of treatment) is recommended. There is no evidence for monitoring CMV viral loads levels to determine duration of treatment or efficacy.

Long-term audiologic follow-up with testing at 6-month intervals for the first 3 years and annually through adolescence with appropriate intervention (speech, hearing aids, and cochlear implants) when needed is strongly recommended. Ophthalmologic examinations with required follow-up and developmental assessments are recommended on a case-by-case basis (56).

Herpes Simplex Virus
Epidemiology

Herpes simplex viruses (HSV-1 and HSV-2) are large, enveloped viruses that are members of the *Herpesviridae* family. They consist of a double-stranded DNA core with glycoproteins on the surface that are responsible for attachment to cells and evoking immune responses.

Seroprevalence rates of HSV-1 and -2 vary significantly depending on age, sex, race, and geographic distribution. Among pregnant women, seroprevalence rates are estimated to be 20% to 30%. A majority of genital infections caused by HSV-1 or -2 are asymptomatic (*clinically inapparent*). The risk of transmission of HSV to the neonate remains significantly higher with primary maternal infections acquired closer to the time of delivery compared with recurrent infections (50% to 60% with primary infections vs. <3% for recurrent infections).

Infections with HSV are classified as first-episode primary (acquisition of either HSV-1 or HSV-2 in a person without prior infection with either), first-episode nonprimary (e.g., acquisition of HSV-2 in a person previously infected with HSV-1, or vice versa), or recurrent (reactivation of a latent HSV-1 infection or a latent HSV-2 infection).

HSV infection of the neonate is uncommon with varying rates across the world due to differing birth rates and HSV seroprevalence. Both HSV-1 and HSV-2 have been recognized to cause neonatal herpes infection. The overall global rate of neonatal HSV, based on seroprevalence, birth rates, and infections in pregnancy, is estimated to be 10 per 100,000 live births, with a best estimate of 14,000 cases annually (59,60).

Pathogenesis and Clinical Presentation

The major risk factors for HSV transmission to the neonate are type of maternal infection (61) (first-episode primary > first-episode nonprimary > recurrent), maternal HSV serostatus, mode of delivery (vaginal > C-section), duration of rupture of membranes (62), and disruption of cutaneous barrier (use of fetal scalp electrodes and other instrumentation). Fetal/newborn acquisition of HSV can occur in utero (5%), in the peripartum period (85%), or in the postnatal period (10%).

In utero infection with HSV is a rare entity but is unlikely to be missed because of presentation at birth and extent of involvement. It occurs in approximately 1 in 300,000 deliveries (63) with affected infants presenting with a triad of clinical findings (64,65): cutaneous (scarring, rash, aplasia cutis, hyperpigmentation, or hypopigmentation); ophthalmologic (microphthalmia, chorioretinitis, optic atrophy); and neurologic (intracranial calcifications, microcephaly, encephalomalacia).

Peri- and postpartum HSV acquired by the neonate present as (a) SEM disease (skin, eye, and/or mouth), (b) CNS disease (central nervous system), and/or (c) disseminated disease.

In infants with SEM disease, infection is confined to the skin, eye, and/or mouth of newborns without any involvement of CNS or visceral organs. Infants with SEM disease present at 10 to 12 days of life and 80% of these infants have a vesicular rash on physical examination (66) (Fig. 61.25A and B). Almost one-third of cases of neonatal herpes disease present as encephalitis and are categorized as CNS disease, with or without skin involvement. Neonates usually present at 16 to 19 days of life with focal/generalized seizures, lethargy, irritability, poor feeding, temperature instability, and bulging fontanel. Newborns with disseminated disease present around days 10 to 12 of life with respiratory and hepatic failure with disseminated intravascular coagulation (DIC). Disease involves multiple organs, including CNS, lungs, liver, adrenal, skin, eye, and/or mouth. Two-thirds of infants with disseminated disease have concurrent encephalitis, and approximately 40% of infants never develop a vesicular rash during the entire illness. Death from disseminated disease is usually due to severe coagulopathy and extensive hepatic and pulmonary involvement.

Diagnosis

Culture of the virus from skin and mucosal sites will confirm neonatal infection, as does detection of HSV DNA by PCR at these sites as well as the blood and CSF. The application of PCR to CSF samples has revolutionized the diagnosis of CNS neonatal herpes disease with overall high sensitivities and specificities (67,68). In comparison, blood PCR has been evaluated to a lesser extent and appears to be a powerful tool in the diagnosis of neonatal HSV infections (69,70). Serologic studies are not helpful for the diagnosis of neonatal HSV infection.

The following specimens should be obtained from a newborn before initiating antiviral therapy: (a) swab for viral culture/PCR from the base of vesicles or suspicious skin or mucous membrane lesions; (b) swab of mouth, conjunctiva, nasopharynx, and rectum (surface cultures) for viral culture/PCR; (c) CSF for indices and HSV DNA PCR; (d) whole blood for HSV DNA PCR; and (e) blood to determine alanine aminotransferase (ALT) level.

Treatment and Management

All neonates with HSV disease should receive parenteral acyclovir at 60 mg/kg/d divided every 8 hours (71). Duration of treatment is 14 days for infants with SEM disease and 21 days for CNS and disseminated disease presentations. All neonates with CNS involvement should have repeat CSF PCR near the end of 21 days of treatment to document a negative CSF PCR result. In those rare neonates with positive CSF PCR at the end of therapy, antiviral therapy should be continued until PCR negativity is achieved. Serial measurement of blood DNA PCR for assessing response to therapy is not recommended at this time. Neutropenia is an anticipated side effect with acyclovir and should be monitored for closely. After completion of 2 to 3 weeks of treatment, neonatal HSV patients then should receive oral acyclovir at 300 mg/m^2/dose, three times a day for 6 months for improved long-term developmental outcomes (72).

Guidance has been developed to address the management of asymptomatic infants born to mothers with suspected or proven genital HSV lesions (73,74). The management of asymptomatic infants born to mothers with known HSV lesions depends upon whether the mother has a primary infection, maternal treatment, and lesions at delivery. All infants must be monitored for signs of infection; parents must be counseled about clinical signs that should trigger an investigation.

- Asymptomatic term infants born to mothers with recurrent HSV but no lesions at delivery are monitored clinically. If symptoms or signs concerning for neonatal HSV occur, the neonate should be thoroughly evaluated for HSV infection and started on intravenous (IV) acyclovir as outlined above pending results.
- Asymptomatic infants born to mothers with HSV lesions and known recurrent HSV disease should be screened for HSV colonization by viral culture or PCR testing of mucosal surfaces at 24 hours of age. If HSV is detected, the infant should be evaluated for HSV disease and treated with IV acyclovir (60 mg/kg/d) for 10 days provided the CSF studies are normal.
- Asymptomatic infants born to mothers with lesions present at delivery, and no previous history of HSV infection should be screened for HSV colonization by PCR testing of mucosal surfaces at 24 hours of age, and for HSV infection by blood PCR testing, blood ALT determination, and lumbar puncture for CSF cell count, chemistries, and HSV PCR. Maternal lesions should be tested for HSV by culture and/or PCR at the time of labor, and if possible, maternal serologic studies should be obtained to try to determine if they have IgG antibodies directed against the HSV strain type that is recovered. While investigations are ongoing, the infant should be treated with IV acyclovir (60 mg/kg/d). The duration of acyclovir depends on the results of investigations. Management of the neonate then depends on the results of these assessments:
  - If the mother is found to have a primary infection and the infant remains well, treatment should be continued as preemptive therapy for 10 days.
  - If the mother's type-specific serologic investigations are not available and the infant remains well, treatment should be continued as preemptive therapy for 10 days.
  - If the mother is confirmed to have recurrent disease based on the comparison of her virologic and serologic testing, and if the infant's surface swabs are positive, treatment should be continued as preemptive therapy for 10 days.
  - If the mother is confirmed to have recurrent disease based on the comparison of her virologic and serologic testing, and if the infant's surface swabs are negative, the acyclovir can be discontinued when these results become available.
  - In all of these scenarios, if the neonate's evaluation reveals HSV disease, then the duration of therapy should be 14 days (for SEM disease) to 21 days (for CNS or disseminated disease).

Human Immunodeficiency Virus
Epidemiology

Human immunodeficiency viruses (types HIV-1 and HIV-2) are RNA viruses that belong to family Retroviridae, with humans as the only reservoir. There are two distinct species of the virus identified (HIV-1 and HIV-2). Both are responsible for infection but are characterized by distinct transmission patterns, demographics, and rate of disease progression. Both viruses are responsible for a chronic fatal infection in the absence of treatment. HIV-1 is more frequently responsible for pediatric HIV, while HIV-2 is closely related to simian immunodeficiency virus (SIV) with lower documented rates of mother-to-child transmission (MTCT) and a protracted disease course. In 1983, HIV was identified as the causative agent of a newly identified entity termed human acquired immunodeficiency syndrome (AIDS). Per the WHO estimates, there were an estimated 38.0 million people living with HIV at the end of 2019, with over two-thirds of all people living with HIV living in the WHO African Region (25.7 million). While HIV continues to be a major global public health issue, WHO estimates between 2000 and 2019, new HIV infections fell by 39% and HIV-related deaths fell by 51%, with 15.3 million lives saved due to antiretroviral therapy (ART) due to increasing access to effective HIV diagnosis, treatment, and prevention strategies. HIV infection has now become a manageable chronic health condition, enabling people living with HIV to lead long and healthy lives.

Well-established modes of transmission of HIV include (a) sexual contact (orogenital, vaginal, or anal); (b) mucous membrane exposure—blood or body fluids; (c) MTCT—in utero, perinatal, and postnatal (through breast-feeding); and (d) contact with contaminated blood—transfusion or percutaneous exposure. This section will focus on characteristics of MTCT.

Rates of pediatric HIV due to MTCT have drastically decreased in the last two decades in countries that have developed and implemented HIV antenatal testing programs and instituted antiretroviral (ARV) prophylaxis during the antepartum, intrapartum, and postpartum periods, including increasing use of cesarean section for delivery and complete avoidance of breast-feeding. However, in resource-limited settings, postnatal HIV transmission through breast-feeding is the most common mode of MTCT due to lack of safe alternatives to breast milk.

Pathophysiology and Clinical Presentation

Retroviruses carry a viral reverse transcriptase (RT) enzyme that converts the single-stranded viral RNA genome into a double-stranded DNA copy, termed a provirus, that integrates into the host cell genome. HIV affects almost all immune cell types with the gp120 component of the HIV virion binding to the CD4+ T cells. Host expression of chemokine receptors such as CXCR4 and CCR5 promote viral binding to the host cell membranes and entry into cells. Mechanisms of immune dysfunction, particularly in instances of perinatal transmission, where very high viral load levels are observed, include T-cell (lymphopenia), B-cell (hypergammaglobulinemia), and NK-cell functions. Additionally, monocytes and macrophages serve as reservoirs for HIV. In children, HIV infection is staged based on age-specific CD4+ T-lymphocyte count or T-lymphocyte percentage.

HIV staging based on age-specific CD4+ T-lymphocyte count (75):
Stage 1:

- ≥1,500 cells/μL (≥34%) for children less than 1 year
- ≥1,000 cells/μL (≥30%) for children 1 to 5 years
- ≥500 cells/μL (≥26%) for 6 years to adult

Stage 2:

- 750 to 1,499 cells/μL (26% to 33%) for children less than 1 year
- 500 to 999 cells/μL (22% to 29%) for children 1 to 5 years
- 200 to 499 cells/μL (14% to 25%) for 6 years to adult

Stage 3:

- Less than 750 cells/μL (<26%) for children less than 1 year
- Less than 500 cells/μL (<22%) for children 1 to 5 years
- Less than 200 cells/μL (<14%) for 6 years to adult

Acute retroviral syndrome, characterized by nonspecific symptoms such as fever, malaise, lymphadenopathy, and skin rash, is more frequently seen in adolescents and adults than in infants with MTCT. Manifestations of untreated pediatric HIV infection include nonspecific presentations such as unexplained fevers, generalized lymphadenopathy, hepatomegaly, splenomegaly, failure to thrive, persistent or recurrent oral and diaper candidiasis, recurrent diarrhea, and other opportunistic viral, fungal, and parasitic infections (OIs) (76). The introduction of combination antiretroviral therapeutic regimens (cART) has dramatically improved the clinical outcome and hospitalization rates of children with HIV. Without cART, the prognosis for survival is poor for untreated infants who acquire HIV infection through MTCT and have high viral load levels (>100,000 copies/mL) and severe suppression of CD4+ T-lymphocyte counts. Besides OIs, malignant neoplasms and HIV encephalopathy are more common among children with untreated HIV infection.

Diagnosis

Schedules for testing of HIV-exposed infants vary by nation. The following are recommendations followed in the United States.

Diagnosis of HIV in children less than 18 months is performed by the following methodologies:

1. *Serologic assays*: Due to the presence of maternal passively acquired antibodies, serologic assays are not ideal for the diagnosis of HIV in children less than 24 months.
2. *Nucleic acid amplification assays*: The preferred test for diagnosis in children less than 2 years is by HIV DNA or RNA PCR. HIV DNA PCR assay detects cell-associated integrated HIV DNA with a sensitivity of 100% by 3 months of age. RNA assays also can be used to diagnose infection in HIV-exposed infants, particularly as a supplemental test for an infant with positive DNA PCR assay results. Diagnostic testing is recommended at 14 to 21 days of age and, if results are negative, again at 1 to 2 months of age and at 4 to 6 months of age. An infant is considered infected if two samples from two different time points test positive by DNA or RNA PCR assay.

In HIV-exposed children younger than 18 months who are not breast-fed, a *presumptive exclusion of HIV* infection is based on the following criteria in the absence of other laboratory or clinical evidence of HIV:

- Two negative HIV DNA or RNA assays, from separate specimens, obtained at 2 weeks of age or older, with at least one obtained at 4 weeks of age or older; OR
- One negative HIV DNA or RNA virologic test result from a specimen obtained at 8 weeks of age or older; OR
- One negative HIV antibody test result obtained at 6 months of age or older.

In HIV-exposed children younger than 12 months who are not breast-feeding with negative HIV virologic test results without other virologic or clinical evidence of HIV, *definitive exclusion* of HIV is based on the following:

- At least 2 negative HIV DNA or RNA assays, from separate specimens, both obtained at 1 month of age or older with at least one obtained at 4 months of age or older; OR
- At least 2 negative HIV antibody test results from separate specimens obtained at 6 months of age or older

Treatment and Management

With early diagnosis of HIV infection in pregnant women, infants, and children, and with the initiation of appropriate treatment (cART), the occurrence of AIDS-defining illnesses is rare among children in industrialized countries.

Without cART initiation, infants who acquire HIV by MTCT develop AIDS-defining conditions during the first 6 months of life due to high viral load and suppression of CD4+ T-lymphocytes.

MTCT Prevention Strategies

The three interventions widely utilized in the United States are: (a) ARV prophylaxis; (b) cesarean delivery at 38 completed weeks of gestation, before labor and before rupture of membranes; and (c) avoidance of breast-feeding. However, as outlined previously, in resource-limited countries where complete avoidance of breast-feeding may not be safe or available, exclusive breast-feeding is favored because it is associated with a lower risk of postnatal HIV transmission or infant morbidity/mortality compared with mixed breast-feeding and formula feeding. The WHO in 2010 strongly recommended that HIV-infected mothers exclusively breast-feed for the first 6 months of life where there are no safe alternatives available. The recommendation for breast-feeding infants is to receive daily nevirapine prophylaxis until 1 week after breast milk consumption stops, and for their mothers to receive ARV (consisting of an effective cART regimen) indefinitely.

Maternal ARV Therapy and MTCT Prophylaxis

Due to variations in treatment approaches across nations, the reader is referred to resources such as http://aidsinfo.nih.gov for detailed recommendations on use of ARVs in HIV-infected pregnant women. The primary goal of treatment during pregnancy is virologic suppression during pregnancy and following delivery for the prevention of MTCT.

Several of the approaches to prevent MTCT are highlighted as follows (77):

- HIV-infected women with HIV RNA ≥1,000 copies/mL (or unknown HIV RNA) near delivery should receive IV zidovudine during labor, regardless of antepartum regimen or mode of delivery.
- For women in labor with undocumented HIV infection status, a rapid HIV test should be performed as soon as possible.
- For an HIV-infected woman, routine oral ARVs should be continued on schedule.
- Procedures that compromise the integrity of fetal skin during labor and delivery should be avoided.
- Newborn infants should begin ARV prophylaxis as soon as possible after birth, preferably within 12 hours. In the United States, neonatal prophylaxis generally consists of zidovudine for 6 weeks.
- For infants born to mothers who did not receive any ARVs before the onset of labor, neonatal postexposure prophylaxis with a two- or three-drug ARV regimen is recommended.
- In instances with maternal HIV RNA ≥ 1,000 copies/mL (or unknown HIV RNA) near delivery, three doses of oral nevirapine are indicated for the infant within the first week of life, in addition to oral zidovudine. Detailed guidance is available regarding infant ARV prophylaxis regimens.

For infants with documented HIV infection, cART should be provided as soon as possible after diagnosis with goals for treatment being: (a) suppression of viral replication; (b) restoration and preservation of immune function; (c) reduction of HIV-associated morbidity and mortality; and (d) maintenance of normal growth and development.

Parvovirus B19
Epidemiology

Human Parvovirus B19 is a small, nonenveloped, single-stranded DNA virus, responsible for causing fifth disease or erythema infectiosum. Viral spread is predominantly through contact with respiratory secretions. The incubation period is 4 to 21 days with a majority of infections occurring in the winter months. Seroprevalence studies of pregnant women have revealed varying seroprevalence rates of 30% to 80%, depending on country of residence, socioeconomic status, and exposure to young children (78,79).

Pathophysiology and Clinical Presentation

Erythema infectiosum is a syndrome usually seen in children associated with a characteristic immune-mediated "slapped cheek" rash (80). The rash is lacy or reticulated, spreads to the trunk and extremities, and may last up to 2 weeks. It may be more pronounced with exposure to sunlight, temperature changes, or emotional stress. Some adults will have an influenza-like illness, with an associated immune-mediated symmetrical arthritis frequently involving the hands but may also involve the wrists, ankles, and knees. Most infected adults have a subclinical presentation. The virus causes a lytic infection in human erythroid progenitor cells due to tropism for erythrocyte P antigen (globoside).

The estimated risk of hydrops fetalis when a mother acquires Parvovirus B19 in pregnancy is around 2%. Suppression of fetal bone marrow leads to chronic anemia and congestive heart failure. The primary outcome is fetal loss if the infection occurs in the first 20 to 22 weeks of gestation. While a number of other congenital abnormalities have been reported among infants with Parvovirus B19 infection, causation has not been established.

Diagnosis

The diagnosis of infection is made clinically with the appearance of the characteristic rash in children and adults. The presence of Parvovirus B19–specific IgM antibody is the usual method of diagnosing new or recent infection. Parvovirus B19 can also be detected in blood samples using PCR but may persist for several months complicating the diagnosis of acute infections. Pregnant women who seroconvert during pregnancy should be monitored closely. If there is a suspicion for hydrops fetalis, diagnosis of fetal infection can be made by a combination of fetal blood tests for Parvovirus B19 IgM antibody and Parvovirus B19 DNA PCR testing of amniotic fluid. Diagnosis of infection in the infant is made primarily by the detection of Parvovirus B19–specific antibody or the presence of Parvovirus B19 DNA in blood or tissues (81).

Treatment and Management

There is no specific treatment for Parvovirus B19 infections. Despite one published report of successful treatment with IVIG, no large scale studies have been performed and IVIG is not recommended therapy (82). Management of hydrops fetalis in the postnatal period is supportive and involves partial exchange transfusions or simple transfusions of packed red cells until the hemoglobin is stabilized. In general, there are no long-term sequelae for those infants who recover, although there have been recent reports of adverse neurodevelopmental outcome. Children with congenital infection are not at risk of chronic infection.

Rubella Virus
Epidemiology

Rubella (German measles, third disease) is caused by the rubella virus, which is an enveloped, single positive-stranded RNA virus. Transmission occurs exclusively across the placenta, depending on the trimester of pregnancy. Prior to institution of universally funded immunization programs, major rubella epidemics occurred about every 5 to 10 years (83). In 1966, rubella became a notifiable disease and with the licensure of the rubella vaccine in 1969 in the United States, the effect of the immunization program on congenital rubella syndrome (CRS) risk is well documented (84,85). The incidence of CRS is an estimate, which in countries with an immunization program is believed to be approximately 0.4 per 100,000 live births. Primary infection during pregnancy, particularly in the first trimester, is a major risk factor for congenital infection (86,87).

Pathophysiology and Clinical Presentation

After maternal infection, the virus initially multiplies in cells of the nasopharynx followed by a period of systemic viremia and shedding from the throat during which the placenta and fetus are infected. Pathogenesis involves placental vascular endothelial cell necrosis leading to small vessel thrombosis, hypoxic tissue damage, and virus-infected emboli.

Congenital rubella infection may present with a wide variety of clinical findings at birth or the infant may appear normal at birth and develop symptoms over time (83,88). The initial characterization of CRS as the triad of heart defects, cataract, and hearing defects in association with maternal rubella infection in the first trimester of pregnancy has expanded considerably over time. The most common abnormalities in decreasing order of frequency are as follows: SNHL > mental retardation > cardiac malformations > ocular defects.

Hearing loss is the most common specific congenital defect and is usually bilateral. It may be present at birth or it may develop over time and be progressive. Heart defects are seen more commonly in infants infected in the first trimester. Patent ductus arteriosus is found in 30% of affected infants and which may be associated with other cardiac defects, most commonly pulmonary valvular or artery stenosis. Cataract is found in 35% of infants and additionally, retinopathy in 35% to 60%. It is often unilateral and has a distinctive "salt and pepper" appearance. Intrauterine growth restriction is present in 50% to 85% of infants. Approximately 20% of infants will have a transient meningoencephalitis, which may manifest with bulging anterior fontanelle, hypotonia, irritability, and seizures. CSF findings show a mononuclear pleocytosis, increased protein content, and rubella virus isolation in 30% of affected infants. Some infants will present with microcephaly and/or intracranial calcifications and/or a large anterior fontanelle. Approximately 5% will develop an interstitial pneumonia that is thought to be immune mediated. In approximately 5%, blueberry muffin spots may be transiently seen and some children will have chronic rashes from which rubella virus can be isolated. More than 50% of symptomatic infants will have hepatosplenomegaly at birth that resolves over several weeks. Obstructive jaundice occurs in about 5% of infants. In infants with severe disease, thrombocytopenic purpura occurs at birth in 5% to 10% of infants, with transient anemia that may be hemolytic in nature.

Diagnosis

The presence of rubella-specific IgM antibodies in a sample collected within 1 month of a rash suggestive of rubella illness is diagnostic of acute infection. Additionally, viral detection using RNA PCR techniques can be done from maternal nasopharyngeal swabs, and the virus is reliably detected from these specimens up to 7 days after the appearance of the rash (89).

The diagnosis of congenital rubella involves both serologic testing and virus isolation (90). It is possible to attempt diagnosis of congenital infection by sampling fetal cord blood prenatally or in the postnatal period for rubella-specific IgM antibodies. PCR is the preferred method of testing for the virus and can be performed on fetal and placental tissues, amniotic fluid, chorionic villus samples, and fetal blood (89–91). The diagnosis of CRS is based on a combination of laboratory and clinical findings. Infants require a thorough evaluation including an echocardiogram, neurologic imaging, and ophthalmologic and audiologic assessment. Infants should have a complete blood count (CBC), hepatic function tests, and radiographs of the long bones.

Infants with clinical abnormal findings consistent with rubella from whom the virus has been detected by PCR or has been isolated and/or has a positive rubella-specific IgM titer and/or has

persistence of rubella-specific IgG antibody titers are considered to have confirmed CRS. Infants who do not have any congenital defects but who have laboratory evidence of congenital infection are considered to have congenital rubella infection. Infants with two or more of the eye, cardiac, or hearing clinical manifestations consistent with CRS with or without other commonly described abnormalities but without complete laboratory confirmation are classified as having a CRS compatible condition.

Treatment and Management

There is no specific antiviral treatment for rubella infections. Management of infected individuals is supportive with close long-term monitoring of children diagnosed with CRS or CRS-compatible disease.

Prevention of infection via immunization programs to ensure that the incidence of rubella is low and that pregnant women are not susceptible to rubella is the hallmark of the strategy to combat congenital rubella (92). Immunization with rubella vaccine during pregnancy is contraindicated. Susceptible pregnant women should avoid contact with children with CRS or congenital rubella infection for the first year of the infant's life.

Varicella–Zoster Virus

Epidemiology

Varicella–zoster virus (VZV) is an enveloped double-stranded DNA virus in the *Herpesviridae* family and causes a primary infection varicella (chickenpox) and a distinctive illness associated with reactivation—herpes zoster (shingles). Prior to 1995, it was estimated that 95% of pregnant women were immune to varicella. With the introduction of the varicella vaccine for children, the incidence of disease has dropped dramatically in jurisdictions that have universal childhood immunization programs that include varicella vaccine (93). While the risk of exposure to varicella is low, immunization coverage has not been universally high, and since women from tropical countries are less likely to be immunized or exposed to the virus, varicella remains a concern.

Pathophysiology and Clinical Presentation

Transmission of the virus occurs through exposure to infected respiratory secretions or direct contact with zoster lesions. The incubation period ranges from 10 to 21 days after exposure to respiratory droplets. Individuals are most infectious on the day immediately before and the day the rash develops. Overall, congenital varicella syndrome is rare with an estimated risk less than 0.5% of maternal infections acquired before 12 weeks of gestation, 2% if the mother acquired varicella between 13 and 20 weeks of gestation, and 1% if she acquired it after that period (94,95). Approximately 25% of newborns whose mothers contracted varicella in the last 3 weeks of gestation will have clinical infection. The risk of congenital varicella syndrome with exposure of pregnant woman to zoster is negligible.

The congenital abnormalities associated with gestational varicella are primarily cutaneous, musculoskeletal, neurologic, and ocular (94,95). The most common skin abnormalities are cicatricial lesions. Cutaneous scars are found on hypoplastic limbs or trunk (see **Fig. 46.2**). Limb abnormalities include hypoplasia, atrophy, and/or paresis. Limb hypoplasia is usually unilateral and involves lower extremities. The pathophysiology of the limb abnormalities is thought to be the consequence of a neuropathy resulting from damage to the dorsal ganglia and anterior columns of the spinal cord. CNS findings more commonly include microcephaly, cortical and cerebral atrophy, psychomotor retardation, seizures, and focal brain calcifications. Unilateral or bilateral ocular abnormalities are common including optic nerve atrophy, cataracts, chorioretinitis, microphthalmos, and/or nystagmus.

Perinatal infection is a major concern if the mother develops clinical varicella between 5 days before or 2 days after the infant's

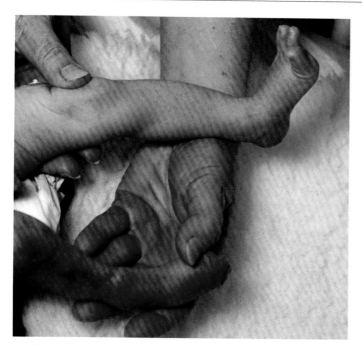

FIGURE 46.2 Limb atrophy and cicatricial skin scarring in an infant with congenital varicella syndrome. (Reprinted with permission from Knipe DM, Howley PM, eds. *Fields virology*, 6th ed. Philadelphia, PA: Lippincott Williams & Wilkins, 2013.)

birth (96). The incubation period for neonatal development of varicella is between 5 and 10 days after delivery. Illness may vary from very mild with only a few cutaneous lesions to severe and life threatening with fever, hemorrhagic rash, and wide spread systemic involvement. Infants can develop pneumonia, hepatitis, and meningoencephalitis. The mortality rate is high at 30% with death usually resulting from pulmonary involvement.

Diagnosis

Prenatal diagnosis of congenital varicella syndrome is made by a combination of ultrasonogram appearance of findings suggestive of congenital abnormalities and detection of VZV DNA by PCR from fetal blood or amniotic fluid. The VZV PCR can be done between 17 and 21 weeks of gestation and is very sensitive. A detailed anatomic ultrasound investigation should be done at a minimum of 5 weeks after the maternal infection to detect any abnormalities. A negative VZV PCR and a normal result of the ultrasound examination indicate that congenital VZV infection or congenital varicella syndrome is unlikely. A positive DNA PCR is suggestive of a high risk of congenital varicella syndrome. Postnatal diagnosis of congenital varicella syndrome depends on the history of maternal disease during pregnancy, physical examination compatible with congenital varicella syndrome, and laboratory confirmation by detection of VZV DNA from blood, VZV-specific IgM antibodies in the infant's blood obtained shortly after birth or the persistence of VZV-specific IgG beyond 7 months of age.

The diagnosis of varicella in the newborn is made by isolation from the lesions of VZV by culture or the detection of the VZV antigen by direct fluorescent antibody or DNA by PCR testing. VZV grows slowly in culture, and so culture is not useful for rapid diagnosis. VZV PCR testing of CSF is currently the most common method to detect CNS infection.

Treatment and Management

Treatment considerations of varicella have evolved over the past decade (92). Oral acyclovir is recommended for individuals at risk for moderate to severe disease. Children receiving treatment

with oral acyclovir will have a shortened course of illness and period of infectivity. Pregnant women with varicella pneumonia or other varicella-related complications need admission to hospital and treatment with IV acyclovir (10 mg/kg every 8 hours). There have not been any controlled studies addressing the treatment of uncomplicated varicella in pregnancy. Many experts would recommend treatment in pregnant women with uncomplicated varicella with oral valacyclovir. Whether treatment reduces the risk or the severity of congenital varicella syndrome is unknown. There are no antiviral treatment recommendations for children born with congenital varicella syndrome.

Varicella vaccine is contraindicated in pregnancy, but it can be safely used in the postpartum period in nonimmune mothers. For instances of nonimmune pregnant women known or suspected to be exposed to VZV, varicella-zoster immune globulin administration can prevent or lessen the severity of infection when administered within 10 days of exposure. The current formulation in the United States and Canada is VariZIG, and the adult dose is 625 units, given IM. If VariZIG or a similar product is not available, IVIG at a dose of 400 mg/kg has been used. Whether the use of either of these products will prevent congenital varicella syndrome is unknown.

Zika Virus

Epidemiology

Zika virus (ZIKV) is an RNA virus that belongs to *Flaviviridae* and transmitted predominantly by mosquitoes, particularly *Aedes aegypti*. ZIKV was first isolated in the rhesus monkey in 1947 in Uganda and in 1952 from humans in Nigeria. The first reported outbreak of ZIKV was documented initially in 2007 on Yap island in Micronesia (97) and later from French Polynesia in 2013 (98). Most recently, the largest outbreak that highlighted maternal–fetal and sexual transmission with ZIKV was reported from Brazil, starting in 2014 (99).

Pathophysiology and Clinical Presentation

While the primary mode of transmission is through mosquito bites, the importance of sexual transmission and maternal–fetal transmission cannot be overstated. The clinical presentations of ZIKV infections during pregnancy are not significantly different from nonpregnant individuals. Symptoms are usually self-limited and include a descending maculopapular pruritic rash, fever, arthralgias, conjunctivitis, and headache and overlaps significantly with clinical presentations from other arboviral infections like dengue and chikungunya. Infections are symptomatic in approximately 20% of infected pregnant women (97,98). However, the consequences of infection during pregnancy may have devastating effects on the fetus. Data are limited regarding absolute risks of maternal–fetal transmission with infections during pregnancy. Adverse fetal outcomes have been documented regardless of the trimester of documented infection, with worse outcomes associated with earlier gestation infections (55% in first trimester vs. 52% in second trimester vs. 29% in third trimester) (100).

Infection in the infant is likely a spectrum from mild symptoms to findings of severe congenital ZIKV infection. Ultrasound findings in the fetus concerning for congenital ZIKV infection predominantly involve the central nervous system including cerebral atrophy, ventriculomegaly, cerebellar hypoplasia, and arthrogryposis. Findings reported frequently in infants born to pregnant women exposed to ZIKV are microcephaly, redundant scalp skin, overlapping sutures, and skull collapse (101). Congenital arthrogryposis has frequently been reported in these infants and is unique in ZIKV infections when compared with other congenital infections (102). Eye involvement is frequent and includes chorioretinal atrophy, pigmented retinopathy, macular atrophy, and microphthalmia (103). Auditory involvement presents as SNHL. Postnatal imaging of brain and spinal cord shows varying involvement with findings of cortical thinning, lissencephaly, cerebellar hypoplasia, and subcortical and brainstem calcifications (104,105).

Based on histopathologic studies of fetuses, newborns, and animal models, the underlying pathogenesis is likely a combination of virus-induced destruction of neural cells and host-mediated inflammation.

Diagnosis

Serologic testing for ZIKV infections is complicated by cross-reactivity with other flaviviruses, particularly dengue, chikungunya, and yellow fever vaccine recipients in endemic countries. IgG testing with plaque reduction assays might be necessary to differentiate between these infections but are laborious. In non-endemic areas, ZIKV-specific IgM testing has high specificity. Diagnosis is currently achieved by detection of viral RNA in body fluids (serum, urine, CSF) or tissues (106). Clinical guidelines have been issued by the CDC for the care of pregnant women and newborns exposed or infected with ZIKV (http://www.cdc.gov/zika/hc-providers/index.html).

Treatment and Management

Many individuals with ZIKV will likely be asymptomatic or have mild nonspecific symptoms. There are currently no effective antiviral treatments for congenital ZIKV infection or vaccine for prevention. Close long-term follow up for neurodevelopmental, visual, and audiologic outcomes should be undertaken pending further recommendations.

Syphilis

Epidemiology

Treponema pallidum (TP), a spirochete, is the causative agent of syphilis. It is a Gram-negative spirochete that primarily infects humans but can cause disease in other primates, pigs, and rabbits in the laboratory setting. It does not grow on conventional media, and the disease lacks an animal model to study the pathogenesis of congenital syphilis. Syphilis is a sexually transmitted disease, and congenital syphilis results primarily from transplacental transmission from an infected mother to her infant. The prevalence of syphilis among adult childbearing populations varies considerably. Worldwide, syphilis is suspected to complicate the lives of 36 million people (2008 WHO report). The risk of congenital syphilis is dependent upon the prevalence of syphilis in the local adult populations, the stage of maternal disease, maternal coinfection with HIV, and, to a great extent, the effectiveness of maternal prenatal screening and treatment programs (107,108). Syphilis can be transmitted throughout gestation, but the risk of transmission increases as gestation progresses. Transmission occurs between 60% and 100% of pregnancies when mothers have primary or early secondary syphilis. Mothers in the latent and late–latent stages transmit in 40% and 8% of pregnancies, respectively. In the past decade, the rate of congenital syphilis in the United States has varied from 8 to 11 cases per 100,000 live births (107).

Pathophysiology and Clinical Presentation

Once the spirochete crosses the placental barrier, it widely disseminates throughout the fetus (109). The manifestations of congenital syphilis are a result of the host responses to *T. pallidum* (110,111). Regardless of the organ system involved, the pathologic appearance of infected tissue shows perivascular infiltration by lymphocytes, plasma cells, and histiocytes producing obliterative endarteritis and extensive fibrosis. Placentas in pregnancies complicated by syphilis tend to be relatively large with focal villitis and, in those infants who are symptomatic at birth, a necrotizing funisitis (112). Approximately 60% of affected infants will develop some clinical manifestation of congenital syphilis by 3 months of life. The development of "snuffles," a thick purulent nasal discharge that is highly infectious and teeming with spirochetes, along with palmar and plantar bullae (also highly infectious) and splenomegaly is a highly suggestive clinical presentation of congenital syphilis and usually is seen beginning around the third week of life. Osteochondritis and periostitis may be seen in the long bones or in the ribs. This may be present at birth in an otherwise asymptomatic infant. In some instances, this may result in fracture, and the infant will decline to move the affected limb (pseudoparalysis of Parrot).

Other signs are less specific and include fever, lymphadenopathy, pneumonitis, irritability, meningitis, hepatosplenomegaly, hepatitis, jaundice, pancreatitis, glomerulonephritis or nephrotic syndrome, hemolytic anemia, DIC, thrombocytopenia, and failure to thrive. Pneumonia due to syphilis classically shows complete opacification of both lung fields if not treated (pneumonia alba). The hemolytic anemia may be associated with cryoglobulinemia, immune complex formation, and macroglobulinemia and be refractory to treatment and last for months. The hepatosplenomegaly is caused by extramedullary hematopoiesis and inflammation. The associated jaundice is caused by hemolysis and/or hepatitis. Some children may have fulminant sepsis-like presentations with hypoglycemia, lactic acidosis, encephalopathy, and DIC in association with hepatic failure. Hepatic abnormalities may persist for up to a year after treatment. Premature infants are more likely to develop severe early disease than are term infants. However, signs may not develop until puberty in some infected children. These late signs include alterations of the permanent teeth (Hutchinson teeth—peg-shaped and notched upper central incisors; mulberry molars—multicuspid first molars), interstitial keratitis, secondary glaucoma, eighth nerve deafness, saddle nose deformity due to scarring by syphilitic rhinitis, cranial nerve palsies, developmental delay, hydrocephalus, epilepsy, optic nerve atrophy, frontal bossing, saber shins (anterior bowing of the mid tibia), and Clutton joints (synovial effusions of the knees).

Diagnosis

T. pallidum can be detected with immunohistochemical stains or PCR performed directly from the placental tissue. However, diagnosis is usually made via serologic testing, and management decisions are based on maternal treatment history and the infant's initial evaluations.

An infant is diagnosed with congenital syphilis in the presence of physical, laboratory, or radiographic signs of syphilis (confirmed/highly probably congenital syphilis) or the child was born to a mother with untreated, inadequately treated or suboptimally treated syphilis (presumed congenital syphilis) (92). Laboratory diagnosis requires demonstration of *T. pallidum* by dark field microscopy, fluorescent antibody stains, or other specific stains in infant or placental tissues but is not readily available (113). Alternatively, if antibody testing of the infant's serum (not cord blood) shows a fourfold higher titer than a simultaneously tested maternal sample by either rapid plasma reagin (RPR) or venereal disease research laboratory (VDRL) measurements, then the diagnosis is likely.

In addition to serologic testing, infants who are suspected as having congenital syphilis need to be assessed with long-bone radiographs, CSF examination, CBC, and liver enzyme determinations. The criteria used to diagnose congenital neurosyphilis include CSF mononuclear pleocytosis ($\geq$25 cells/mm^3), elevated protein concentration (>150 mg/dL in term infants and >170 mg/dL in premature infants), and a reactive CSF VDRL (114). The elevated CSF WBC has a sensitivity of 38% and a specificity of 88%. The elevated CSF protein has a sensitivity of 56% and a specificity of 78%. The CSF VDRL has a sensitivity of 54% and a specificity of 90%.

Screening serologic testing for syphilis traditionally used RPR and VDRL as the initial test, and the diagnosis of positive syphilis serology was then confirmed using specific treponemal antigen testing (the most usual one used being the TP passive particle agglutination assay—TPPA). However, this sequence of laboratory tests has changed in many laboratories in recent years for screening for syphilis. The development of more automated treponemal-specific testing has led to their use first followed by using the RPR and VDRL for confirmation (115–117). The VDRL and RPR tests are still used to evaluate response to therapy and are the tests that should be used to determine whether the infant requires investigation and treatment for congenital syphilis and for follow-up monitoring the infant's status.

Management and Treatment

Management and treatment algorithms are based on a combination of the results of syphilis investigation of the mother, treatment she has received, syphilis testing of the infant, and results of hematologic, CSF studies, hepatic function studies, and radiologic evaluation of the infant (92). All infants born to mothers with reactive RPR/VDRL and positive specific treponemal antibody tests should have a complete physical examination and a VDRL or RPR test to compare titers with that of the mother. All infants should have follow-up titers done until either they are negative or they have reached a serofast state. The management plans are based on the results of testing and treatment records of the mother and the physical examination of the infant (92).

- No treatment is needed for the infant only in the situation where the mother has received adequate treatment with penicillin *before* pregnancy with a demonstrated low stable titer (serofast) of VDRL ≤ 1:2 or RPR ≤ 1:4, and the infant's physical examination is normal.
- Recommendation for the infant to be given benzathine penicillin G, 50,000 units/kg IM as a single dose in the following circumstances:
  ◦ The mother has received adequate treatment with penicillin before pregnancy with a demonstrated low stable titer (serofast) of VDRL ≤ 1:2 or RPR ≤ 1:4, and the infant's physical examination is normal, but there are concerns that the infant will not return for follow-up.
  ◦ The mother has received adequate treatment with penicillin *during* pregnancy more than 4 weeks prior to delivery and demonstrated a reduction of the VDRL or RPR ≤ 1:4; the infant's VDRL or RPR is the *same or less* than fourfold higher than the maternal titer, and the infant's physical examination is normal.
- Infant to receive treatment for congenital syphilis, which is aqueous penicillin G, 50,000 units/kg IV every 12 hours if 1 week of age or younger and every 8 hours if older than 7 days in circumstances as outlined below. Alternatively, procaine penicillin G 50,000 units/kg IM daily × 10 days. Even if a single day of therapy is missed, the entire course should be restarted.
  ◦ Mother has received adequate treatment with penicillin during pregnancy more than 4 weeks prior to delivery, but the infant's VDRL or RPR is *fourfold or more higher* than the maternal titer or the infant's physical examination is *abnormal*.
  ◦ Mother received adequate treatment but *within* 4 weeks of delivery.
  ◦ Mother did *not* receive treatment.
  ◦ Maternal treatment was *not documented*.
  ◦ Maternal treatment course involved *a nonpenicillin drug* was used.
  ◦ There is maternal evidence or relapse or reinfection with *similar or increase in maternal VDRL/RPR*.

Tuberculosis

Epidemiology

Mycobacterium tuberculosis, the causative agent of tuberculosis, is an acid-fast staining aerobic bacteria (AFB) found worldwide and is one of the top ten causes of death worldwide, based on the 2019 WHO global Tuberculosis report. In 2018, an estimated 10 million were newly diagnosed with Tuberculosis, including 1.1 million children, with 1.5 million deaths. People with HIV accounted for 9% of all new cases of TB. Drug-resistant TB is an emerging issue, and in 2018, globally, approximately half a million people contracted rifampicin-resistant Tb (RR-TB), and of these, 78% had multidrug-resistant TB (MDR-TB) with very low treatment success rates. The prevalence and incidence of tuberculosis in pregnancy and incidence of congenital tuberculosis remain largely unknown.

Pathophysiology and Clinical Presentation

The pathophysiology of tuberculosis in pregnancy is similar to that of the nonpregnant women (118). Pregnant women are no more likely to contract tuberculosis or reactivate latent disease than nonpregnant women. The usual route of infection is by inhalation of the bacteria with deposition in the lung. After initial replication in the lung and spread to the regional lymph nodes via infected macrophages, the bacteria disseminate to the rest of the body. After 1 to 3 months, the body can mount a cell-mediated immune response and control the infection, at which point the tuberculin skin test becomes positive. The affected regions in the lung are essentially walled off by deposition of fibrin and calcium, but viable *M. tuberculosis* bacteria remain and the individual is considered to have latent tuberculosis (LTBI), with the likelihood of subsequent reactivation in immune-compromised conditions. Congenital tuberculosis occurs through two mechanisms (119): a primary mechanism of bacteremia and infection of the placenta, leading to formation of primary complexes in the fetal lungs or liver and by a second mechanism of aspiration or ingestion of contaminated amniotic fluid resulting in primary complex formation in the lung or gastrointestinal tract, respectively. Frequently, the mode of transmission cannot be determined. Overall, congenital tuberculosis is rare.

Maternal primary infection with *M. tuberculosis* is frequently asymptomatic or mild and unrecognized (120). Reactivated maternal disease may only present with weight loss, cough, and fatigue. Over time, fever and night sweats occur in approximately 50%, chest pain in 30%, dyspnea in 30%, and hemoptysis in 25%. Chest radiographs are helpful in the diagnosis as most patients will have abnormalities and are appropriate to perform in pregnant women as part of the investigation for potential tuberculosis.

Congenital tuberculosis can present at birth or in the first few weeks of life and should be differentiated from postnatally acquired infection (119). The clinical signs are related to the location and the size of the granulomatous lesions. Approximately 75% will have hepatomegaly in association with liver function abnormalities. A primary complex in the liver or caseating hepatic granuloma is diagnostic of congenital tuberculosis. Around 70% will have respiratory symptoms, most with an abnormal chest radiograph with infiltrates and 50% with a miliary pattern of disease. Occasionally, an infant will have a rapidly progressive pulmonary illness with the development of cavitary lesions. Other nonspecific findings include fever in approximately 50%, lymphadenopathy in approximately 40%, abdominal distention in 25%, and lethargy in 20%. Other abnormalities that occur less frequently are ear discharge, papular skin rash, apnea, vomiting, jaundice, seizures, cyanosis, and petechiae.

Diagnosis

The diagnosis of tuberculosis in pregnancy is based on clinical sus-picion of symptoms and a history of either direct exposure or resi-dence in an area of high tuberculosis prevalence (121). Pregnant women who are HIV seropositive are at high risk for TB and should be tested for tuberculosis. Similarly, pregnant women diagnosed with tuberculosis should be offered HIV testing. General screening for tuberculosis in low prevalence areas is not indicated. Testing should be performed in women who are symptomatic, and tuber-culosis is in the differential diagnosis.

Diagnosis for LTBI in pregnancy includes a chest radiograph with appropriate shielding of the fetus along with either tuberculin skin testing (TST) or interferon gamma release assays (IGRAs) (122).

Neither the TST nor the IGRAs have been systematically studied for the diagnosis of congenital tuberculosis. For children exposed to tuberculosis in the perinatal period, the TST does not reliably become positive for a few months. For suspected congen-ital tuberculosis and for the diagnosis of clinically symptomatic tuberculosis in pregnant women, bacterial cultures are preferred. Cultures of tissues including the placenta once delivered, fluid, or drainage from suspected infected sites should be tested for acid fast bacilli (AFB) by stains and cultures and molecular methods. For pulmonary tuberculosis in pregnant women, serial sputum samples should be used. For infants, tracheal aspirates and gas-tric washings are necessary for isolation of bacteria. Blood cul-tures collected in tubes designed for mycobacterial isolation may be helpful in some cases. Rapid probes can now be used to confirm the diagnosis on specimen samples, which are positive on staining and on cultures when growth is detected (123).

Treatment and Management

Asymptomatic pregnant women diagnosed with LTBI may be offered therapy during pregnancy depending upon the risk assess-ment of likelihood of progression to active disease (121). Treat-ment approach to women with uncomplicated active tuberculosis in pregnancy is similar to nonpregnant women with the use of iso-niazid, rifampin, and ethambutol as first-line drugs. In the situa-tion where there may be drug-resistant tuberculosis or the mother is coinfected with HIV, alternative regimens may be used, and their care is usually done in conjunction with an expert in tuber-culosis and/or HIV care. While there are no evidence-based treat-ment guidelines for the treatment of congenital tuberculosis, the same general principles used for treatment of postnatal infection are used in consultation with an expert in tuberculosis. Prognosis is better with early effective treatment, and it is acceptable to initi-ate treatment while awaiting confirmation if the diagnosis is highly suspected and the infant is clinically ill.

The usual medications used are as follows:

- Isoniazid syrup (10 mg/mL) at a dose of a single dose of 10 to 15 mg/kg/d if used as daily dosing or 20 to 30 mg/kg/dose if used twice weekly.
- Rifampin (syrup derived from 150 mg capsules) at a single dose of 10 to 20 mg/kg/d given either daily or twice a week.
- Pyrazinamide (provided in 500 mg tablets) at a single dose of 30 to 40 mg/kg/d if given daily and 50 mg/kg/dose if given weekly.
- Streptomycin 20 mg/kg IM given daily or 50 mg/kg IM given twice a week OR ethambutol (provided in 100 mg tablets) at a single dose of 20 mg/kg/d if given daily or 50 mg/kg/dose if given twice a week.
- The anticipated treatment duration is 9 to 12 months, although shorter courses are under consideration.

Other Viruses of Importance

Epstein-Barr virus (EBV) is an enveloped double-stranded DNA virus in the *Herpesviridae* family. Infections can occur during pregnancy but are rare as most women of child-bearing age are seropositive. The majority of primary infections among mothers are asymptomatic, but some have a mononucleosis like illness. There is no evidence to date that maternal primary EBV infection causes birth defects or illness in the infant.

Human herpes virus 6 (HHV-6) and *Human herpes virus 7* (HHV-7) are enveloped double-stranded DNA herpes viruses that belong to *Herpesviridae* family that are commonly associated with roseola infantum in infants among other viral syndromes. Most women of childbearing age show serologic evidence of previous infection with HHV-6 and HHV-7, and primary infection by either virus in pregnancy is rare (124). Congenital infection with HHV-6 occurs in approximately 1% of newborn infants, as determined by the presence of HHV-6 DNA in cord blood. Most congenital infec-tions appear to result from the germ line passage of maternal or paternal chromosomally integrated HHV-6 (ciHHV-6), a unique mechanism of transmission of human viral congenital infection. Transplacental HHV-6 infection also may occur from reinfection or reactivation of maternal HHV-6 infection or from reactivated maternal ciHHV-6 (125). Risk of HHV-7 transmission is largely unknown. *Human herpes virus 8* (HHV-8) is associated with Kaposi sarcoma, multicentric Castleman disease, and one type of non-Hodgkin lymphoma. Seroprevalence among pregnant women in North America varies from 0% to 20% but may be as high as 50% in women in areas of Africa. At this time, transmission to the fetus is known to occur, with unclear clinical relevance (126).

Lymphocytic choriomeningitis virus (LCMV) is an RNA virus in the *Arenaviridae* family and found in rodents such as mice and hamsters. Rodents excrete the virus in nasal secretions, saliva, milk, urine, semen, and feces and transmit the virus transplacen-tally. Humans acquire the infection by inhaling aerosolized virus or by contact with contaminated fomites. LCMV infections are asymptomatic in about a third of cases with half of those infected developing aseptic meningitis or meningoencephalitis.

Congenital infections are well documented (127). Early tri-mester infections result in spontaneous abortions and infections in later part of pregnancy lead to symptomatic infants present-ing with eye findings like chorioretinitis or chorioretinal scars, optic atrophy, nystagmus, conjunctivitis, esotropia, microphthal-mos, and cataract. Infants may be either microcephalic or mac-rocephalic and have hydrocephalus or intracranial calcifications. Hearing loss, hepatosplenomegaly, and thrombocytopenia have been documented. The majority will develop long-term disabili-ties. Due to a significant overlap with symptoms with congenital CMV infection, in situations where CMV is suspected but testing is negative, LCMV testing should be pursued.

Diagnosis is by detection of virus by RT-PCR from serum and CSF. Treatment is supportive without definitive antiviral treat-ment. Prevention involves counseling pregnant women to avoid areas of exposure to rodent excretions. Pet hamsters and mice are potential sources, and pregnant women should refrain from han-dling the animals or cleaning their cages.

Enteroviruses and Parechoviruses are small RNA nonen-veloped viruses grouped together in family Picornaviridae (*pico* means small). Enteroviruses as a group are among the most com-mon etiologic agents of human disease with an estimated 10 to 15 million symptomatic infections in the United States each year (128). An estimated 10% of these infections occur in neonates in the first 29 days of life.

MTCT is most likely by perinatal exposure and less likely by transplacental or ascending infection. In more than 60% of infected infants, there is maternal report of a febrile illness dur-ing the last week of pregnancy. Maternal illness may be asymp-tomatic, an undifferentiated febrile illness, or an illness with fever and any of the following: diarrhea, vomiting, rash, petechia, pur-pura, herpangina, aseptic meningitis, encephalitis, paralysis, acute hemorrhagic conjunctivitis, pleurodynia, or myopericarditis. Clin-ical illness in the infant depends in part on the viral type and on the gestational age of the infant, with premature infants having a worse outcome. Some serotypes may cause febrile illnesses associated with nonspecific rashes or self-limited meningitis. Group B Coxsackie virus serotypes 2 to 5 and Echovirus 11 are the types that are more frequently associated with the development of overwhelming systemic illness in the neonatal period. Most infants become symptomatic between 3 and 7 days of age. Early signs of illness are usually mild and may include listlessness, poor feeding, or some respiratory distress. Severe disease in infants manifests as either myocarditis or fulminant hepatitis and associated with a poor prognosis (128).

Clinical presentations of parechoviral infections are indistinguishable from those of other enteroviruses. Classic clinical presentation involves fever with a sepsis-like presentation and a maculopapular rash. CNS and hepatic involvement are not uncommon with clinical presentations of aseptic meningitis and mild transaminitis. Rarely, hepatic necrosis has been reported in newborns.

Diagnosis is by detection of virus by either culture or PCR methodologies from multiple sites like CSF, respiratory tract, serum or urine. In general, serologic testing is not used for the diagnosis of enteroviral disease as the assays are strain specific.

Treatment is supportive. There is currently no specific antiviral therapy available, although the experimental drug pleconaril has demonstrated benefit in treatment of neonatal enteroviral sepsis (129). IVIG has been used anecdotally, without any direct evidence of benefit based on trials (130). Infants with suspected or known enterovirus infections need to be placed on contact precautions. In situations where more than one infant is affected in a nursery, cohorting of infected infants is appropriate. There is currently no enteroviral or parechoviral vaccine.

PARASITIC INFECTIONS

Toxoplasmosis

Epidemiology

Toxoplasmosis is caused by the protozoan *Toxoplasma gondii*, an obligate intracellular parasite (131). It is a zoonotic disease in that part of the complex life cycle of the pathogen involves infection in animals. Susceptible cats acquire *T. gondii* through either ingesting oocysts or parasite-infested tissues of other animals. Humans acquire *T. gondii* primarily through ingestion of oocyst-contaminated water, soil, dust, contact with cat litter, consumption of cyst-containing raw or undercooked beef, pork, mutton, lamb, chicken, or contaminated raw eggs (132). Accidental contamination of laboratory workers has been reported. In addition, transmission has occurred through transfusion of infected blood, blood products, and organ transplants. However, the main route of human-to-human transmission is via the transplacental route.

The percent of women of childbearing age with antibodies to *T. gondii* varies considerably worldwide from 0% to 90% (133). Women from lower socioeconomic circumstances or who work in soil-related professions have a higher likelihood of being seropositive. Specific risks for acquisition of *T. gondii* in pregnancy include consumption of cured pork, raw meat (including tasting while preparing foods), eating unwashed raw vegetables or fruits, infrequent washing of hands or kitchen utensils after preparation of raw meat before handling another food items, contact with soil, and the cleaning of cat litter boxes (134). The actual incidence of congenital toxoplasmosis is unknown with surveys showing varying rates ranging from 0 to 10 per 1,000 live births, with a lower incidence reported in North America compared with regions in Europe (135).

Pathophysiology and Clinical Presentation

In pregnant women, the infection is asymptomatic in 80% to 90% with lymphadenopathy in the head and neck the most common clinical finding when symptomatic (136). An estimated 1% to 5% of acute infectious mononucleosis is attributed to toxoplasmo-

sis. Rare clinical presentations in pregnant women may include hepatitis, pneumonia, myocarditis, encephalitis, or deafness. Ocular involvement usually presents as chorioretinitis or retinochoroidal scars. Fulminant disease is common in immunosuppressed patients such as pregnant women with advanced HIV infection (AIDS).

T. gondii causes transplacental infection in the fetus in about 1% if the infection occurred in the months immediately preceding the pregnancy, 10% to 25% of untreated pregnancies with acute infection in the first trimester, 20% to 54% in the second trimester, and 65% to 70% in the third trimester (137,138). At least two-thirds of infants with congenital toxoplasmosis are asymptomatic at birth (139,140). On careful evaluation, however, one-third of these infants will have some abnormality attributable to the infection such as an abnormal cerebrospinal fluid (CSF) examination with pleocytosis and/or elevated protein (20%), chorioretinitis (15%), or intracranial calcifications (10%). Over time, untreated infants will begin to show manifestations of the disease.

Symptomatic congenital toxoplasmosis can be mild, moderate, or severe at birth (141) and can involve multiple organ systems or present as an isolated abnormality, specifically hydrocephalus, hepatosplenomegaly, or prolonged hyperbilirubinemia. Between 25% and 50% of symptomatic infants are born prematurely. Approximately 10% of affected infants have severe disease at birth, of whom 10% die; the remainder generally have major neurologic abnormalities including mental retardation, seizures, spasticity, and visual defects. Systemic manifestations of congenital toxoplasmosis include fever, jaundice, anemia, hepatomegaly, splenomegaly, and/or chorioretinitis.

Neurologic abnormalities include encephalitis, seizures, hydrocephalus, and/or intracranial calcifications with frequent CNS involvement. Occasionally, hydrocephalus is the only manifestation of congenital toxoplasmosis. It may present at birth or later and be static or progressive, requiring shunt placement. Diffuse intracranial calcifications occur in 10% to 20% of infants but are found in up to 70% of those with symptomatic disease at birth as is seen in **Figure 46.3**. Although they may increase in number and

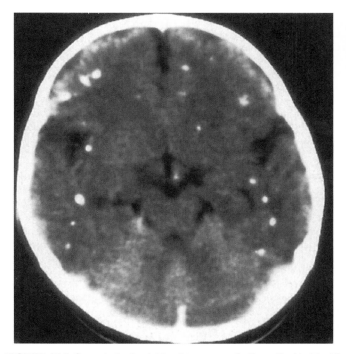

FIGURE 46.3 Computerized axial head tomogram of a 5-month-old girl with congenital toxoplasmosis. Notice the diffuse parenchymal calcifications and the prominent subarachnoid space bilaterally.

THE NEWBORN INFANT

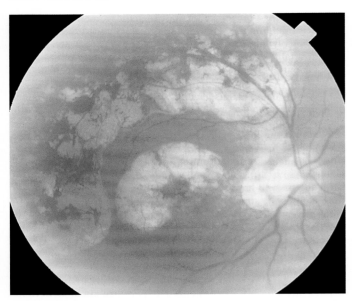

FIGURE 46.4 Multiple chorioretinal scars in a patient with a history of congenital toxoplasmosis. ((Reprinted with permission from Gold DH, Weingeist TA. *Color atlas of the eye in systemic disease.* Baltimore, MD: Lippincott Williams & Wilkins, 2001.)

size in some untreated infants, with treatment, 75% will decrease or totally resolve within a year.

Ocular toxoplasmosis can have a multitude of clinical presentations, including chorioretinitis, chorioretinal scars, iritis, leukocoria, microphthalmia, nystagmus, optic atrophy, optic coloboma, retinal folds and traction detachments, granulomas in the posterior pole, strabismus, microcornea, and/or cataracts (142) (see **Fig. 46.4**). Chorioretinal scars are the most common finding and are usually located peripherally. Macular scars are seen in up to 75% and may be bilateral in one-quarter of cases leading to markedly decreased visual acuity.

Unfortunately, most infants with severe symptomatic congenital toxoplasmosis who survive will have significant sequelae despite therapy. This frequently involves developmental delay and blindness. Those who are born with a subclinical infection and are not treated will invariably develop eye disease by 10 to 20 years of age, and approximately 50% will go on to develop neurologic sequelae. Children born with subclinical infection who receive treatment have a better long-term prognosis, with 75% with some evidence of retinal disease of varying severity. Both untreated and treated infants can have recurrences of ocular toxoplasmosis, but recurrences are less frequent among treated infants (40% to 60% compared to 76% to 82%) (142).

Diagnosis

Acute toxoplasmosis in an adult is not likely to be diagnosed clinically. Acute symptomatic infections are usually investigated as part of work up for infectious mononucleosis with negative testing for EBV and a clinical suspicion for toxoplasmosis. Serologic diagnosis of a recent infection in a pregnant woman and congenital infection in an "at-risk" infant is important to make but can be complicated due to the nature of the immune response to this pathogen and the sensitivity/specificity of the antibody testing (143).

Toxoplasma-specific IgM antibodies can be measured by IFA, ELISA, or IgM immunosorbent agglutination assay (IgM-ISAGA). False-positive IgM-IFA or IgM-ELISA can occur in the presence of rheumatoid factor or other lipid factors in the blood that are extracted along with the parasite lipids during testing. Alterations in the ELISA testing by using a double sandwich technique (DS-IgM-ELISA) can correct this. Toxoplasma-specific IgM antibodies

can be detected 1 to 2 weeks after acute infection. They also can be detected for several years after infection if the IgM-ISAGA or DS-IgM-ELISA methods are used. Therefore, the detection of Toxoplasma-specific IgM antibodies in a single sample from an adult is not necessarily proof of a recent infection. Specificity testing can be helpful as highly specific IgM antibodies coupled with high titers of IgG antibodies (1:1,000 or higher) as measured by either the Sabin-dye test or IFA indicate a recent infection. Low specific IgM titers measured by DS-IgM-ELISA or IgM-ISAGA are generally more often found in individuals whose infection occurred several months previously. IgM-IFA tests are less sensitive and are positive in 60% to 70% of adults with acute infection and only 25% to 50% of infants with congenital toxoplasmosis. Toxoplasma IgG antibodies as measured by the dye test, IFA, or ELISA usually appear early in an acute infection and peak at around 2 months and then fall gradually but remain detectable for years afterward. By contrast, Toxoplasma IgG titers measured by indirect hemagglutination assays are not detectable for several months after infection. A high IgG titer is suggestive of a recent infection but again is not necessarily proof of it. Avidity testing can be done to try to determine whether the infection is recent, and low avidity is seen in acute infections, and high avidity is seen in chronic ones. Anti–Toxoplasma IgA antibodies against one of the surface proteins of the tachyzoites are present in almost all acute infections and disappear after approximately 6 months to a year. They are rarely seen in patients with chronic infections. Similarly, specific IgE antibodies appear with acute infection and disappear over the next 4 to 8 months.

The determination of an acute infection during pregnancy is complex (144).

- A recent *T. gondii* infection can be diagnosed in an immune competent pregnant woman if seroconversion is detected. The timing of the infection can be narrowed down to the time period between the negative specimen and the one in which antibodies were detected.
  - If the initial specimen was collected immediately prior to pregnancy or in early gestation, then the diagnosis of toxoplasmosis in pregnancy can be reasonably established.
  - If there is a longer time period between testing, the nature of the antibodies would need to be further characterized to determine whether the fetus is at risk for toxoplasmosis (see below).
- Alternatively, if the initial specimen collected from a pregnant woman is positive, the determination of a fourfold rise or greater in antibody titers in a repeat serum sample collected 3 to 6 weeks later is needed to establish the diagnosis of toxoplasmosis.
- For an immune competent pregnant woman with no preceding serologic studies whose initial antibody titers are positive and stable on repeat testing, further studies of the nature of the antibody response is also necessary to determine whether the fetus is at risk.
  - Absence of IgM antibodies and a negative rheumatoid factor test would rule out a recent infection and the fetus would not be considered to be at risk.
  - Positive IgM titers with high IgG titers of low avidity would indicate a recent infection, and the fetus would be considered at risk. Further testing for the presence of IgA or IgE titers will provide data regarding the timing of infection to determine if the fetus is at risk.
- An immunocompromised pregnant woman in whom toxoplasmosis is suspected may not develop a serologic response, and tests for detection of the parasite in body fluids or tissues would be needed.

Specific diagnosis of intrauterine infection with *T. gondii* can be done with amniocentesis or ultrasound-guided cordocentesis (145). When available, samples can be sent for parasite isolation using tissue cultures or injection into mice, which is the most sensitive method to determine fetal infection (approximately 80%).

Fetal blood that is documented to be free of maternal blood contamination can be assayed for Toxoplasma-specific IgM or IgA antibodies, but the sensitivity is low (approximately 20% to 50%). Congenitally infected fetuses may have high levels of total IgM and gamma-glutamyltransferase, and these results have been used along with results from abnormalities on fetal ultrasound to provide a tentative diagnosis of congenital infection when serology or culture studies are not available. Studies using PCR detection of *T. gondii* DNA in amniotic fluid have shown promise with high sensitivity (up to 98%) and specificity (90%) in some research laboratories (138,146,147). However, PCR testing is not standardized across laboratories, leading to interlaboratory variability. PCR test results do have the advantage of a shorter turn-around time (few days vs. weeks for culture).

The laboratory diagnosis of congenital toxoplasmosis in the infant also is not straightforward. At birth, Toxoplasma-specific IgM antibodies can be detected in only 25% of congenitally infected infants with the use of the IFA method, and therefore, other testing methods are recommended. IgM antibodies are detectable in at least 75% of congenitally infected infants with use of the DS-IgG-ELISA or the ISAGA assays. Congenitally infected infants who are IgM antibody positive may remain so for up to a year after birth. Maternally transmitted IgG antibody titers drop by 50% each month and, depending upon the maternal titer, may persist for at least a year after birth. Measuring infant's IgG titers over time is another method to determine whether an infant has congenital toxoplasmosis. If the titers do not decline as expected, congenital toxoplasmosis should be suspected. Finally, most congenitally infected infants produce specific IgA titers, and many produce IgE-specific antibodies. These tests can additionally be useful in unclear cases. For infants with CNS disease, determining if there has been intrathecal production of specific IgG and/or IgA antibodies may be helpful.

In summary, infants born to mothers suspected to have had toxoplasmosis within 6 months of becoming pregnant or based on clinical examination should be investigated for congenital toxoplasmosis (92):

- Infants should have IgM tests for *T. gondii*-specific IgM antibodies using DS-IgG-ELISA or the ISAGA
  ◦ Immediately after birth
  ◦ One month after birth if the initial IgM tests are negative
- Infants should have IgG *T. gondii*–specific antibody titers obtained
  ◦ Immediately after birth
  ◦ If IgM testing is negative, IgG testing should be repeated at 6 weeks and 3 months of age to determine if the titers are declining as expected.

Treatment and Management

Treatment of acute toxoplasmosis is not usually undertaken except during pregnancy or an immunocompromised state. For pregnant women who elect to continue their pregnancy, treatment with spiramycin is strongly recommended (137,144,148). Spiramycin is a macrolide antibiotic that is active against *T. gondii* and can cross the placenta and enter the cord blood. Side effects are primarily maternal nausea, vomiting, and diarrhea. It is designated as a class C drug in pregnancy and is licensed for use in Canada and Europe in pregnancy and is available for special access in the United States. The recommended dose is 1 g three times daily. While it is thought to reduce the risk of intrauterine infection to the fetus, it does not seem to affect the course of infection once established.

In instances of established fetal infection, a combination of pyrimethamine and sulfadiazine is recommended. Pyrimethamine is an antimalarial drug and is a folic acid antagonist with a long half-life and achieves high tissue concentrations, particularly in brain. Side effects include bone marrow suppression resulting in

anemia, granulocytopenia, thrombocytopenia, and pancytopenia, which on occasion is severe. Other side effects include a bad after taste, headache, and gastrointestinal upset. The drug is known to be teratogenic in animals and so should be avoided in the first 5 months of pregnancy. Sulfadiazine acts synergistically with pyrimethamine against *T. gondii* and is also a folic acid antagonist. Major side effects include bone marrow suppression with patients frequently reporting rashes, crystalluria, hematuria, and reversible renal failure.

Despite the lack of randomized controlled trials to guide therapy, treatment protocols have been developed for congenitally infected infants that show effectiveness when compared to historical outcomes (139,149,150). The treatment of symptomatic infants during the first 12 months of life usually involves the use of pyrimethamine, sulfadiazine, and folinic acid (151). Infants with chorioretinitis or CSF protein elevations (≥ 1 g/dL) also generally receive prednisone or methylprednisolone to reduce the inflammatory response while on treatment. Weekly CBC monitoring is recommended during the first 6 months of therapy and every other week thereafter while on pyrimethamine. The dose of folinic acid can be increased if neutropenia develops and pyrimethamine held if severe neutropenia develops. For infants who develop an allergy to sulfadiazine, clindamycin at a dosage of 20 to 30 mg/kg/d can be substituted. The usual presentation of allergy to sulfadiazine is skin rash, such as hives or allergic dermatitis. Renal and hepatic function should be tested at the beginning of therapy and monitored every few months while on therapy.

Additionally, infants determined to have congenital toxoplasmosis who are otherwise asymptomatic on physical examination at birth should also be treated. The recommended treatment involves an initial 6-week course of pyrimethamine, sulfadiazine, and folinic acid in the same doses used for symptomatic infants. They then continue with alternating courses of spiramycin for 6 weeks and pyrimethamine, sulfadiazine, and folinic acid for 4 weeks to complete a 1-year course of therapy. Monitoring for drug adverse effects while on pyrimethamine is similar to that described above.

For asymptomatic infants born to mothers with documented gestational toxoplasmosis for whom the suspected diagnosis of congenital toxoplasmosis is not yet confirmed, initial treatment with pyrimethamine, sulfadiazine, and folinic acid can be started while awaiting definitive study results. If the diagnosis is confirmed, then the treatment for asymptomatic congenital toxoplasmosis should be instituted. For healthy infants born to mothers with suspected but not confirmed gestational toxoplasmosis, spiramycin can be started while awaiting definitive test results. All infants with congenital toxoplasmosis who survive will need close follow-up in childhood for developmental disabilities and lifelong for ocular disease regardless of initial presentation.

Prevention Strategies

There is no effective vaccine against *T. gondii*. Prevention of congenital toxoplasmosis involves educating pregnant women on avoiding contact with the parasite. While indoor cats fed dried, cooked, or canned food have a low risk of becoming infected with *T. gondii*, contact with cat feces should be avoided. Disposable gloves should be used when cleaning cat litter and ideally avoided completely by pregnant women. Gardening is another risk activity for inadvertent contact with cat feces, so gloves should be worn and strict attention paid to hand hygiene. Children's sand boxes should be covered to avoid inadvertent contact with cat feces. Meat should be cooked appropriately. Women should avoid touching their eyes and mouth when handling raw meat and should wash their hands immediately afterward. Care should be taken to clean kitchen surfaces after preparation of meat-containing dishes. Fruits and vegetables may be contaminated with oocysts and so should be peeled and/or washed before being consumed. Secondary prevention includes identification and treatment of women who become infected immediately before or during pregnancy. Presently, only a few regions with high prevalence rates of toxoplasmosis, such as France, have a routine screening program in pregnancy.

Malaria

Epidemiology

Malaria in humans is caused by five different strains of protozoan parasites of genus *Plasmodium*: *P. falciparum*, *P. ovale*, *P. vivax*, *P. malariae*, and *P. knowlesi*. They are transmitted frequently by the bite of an infected anopheles mosquito and occasionally by blood transfusion, organ transplantation, and from mother to fetus leading to congenital infection. Malaria is a major international public health problem with an estimated 228 million cases worldwide and approximately 405,000 deaths in 2018, based on the 2019 WHO World Malaria Report. Of these, 11 million pregnant women are estimated to be exposed to malaria, predominantly from West Africa, leading to a substantial proportion of newborns with low birth weight and severe anemia. Transmission rates vary depending on geographic area, weather conditions, and mosquito vector density. The malaria parasites have a complex life cycle involving developmental stages in both the anopheles mosquito vector and the human host. *P. falciparum* is the species most associated with poor prognosis, followed by *P. vivax*.

Pathophysiology and Clinical Presentation

The degree of illness associated with malaria is based on the degree of parasitemia during the erythrocyte phase, parasite species, previous immunity to the parasite, and the status of the immune system in general. Pregnant women in general and women with HIV in particular are at a greater risk for severe disease, compared to nonpregnant women (152). Placental malaria occurs in approximately 40% of affected primigravida pregnancies (range 16% to 63%) compared with 20% of multigravidas (range 12% to 33%).

The symptoms of malaria in the pregnant woman are similar to those of the nonpregnant adult (153). Almost all nonimmune individuals will present with fever that is periodic suggestive of the cyclical release of parasites from the infected erythrocytes into the blood. Frequently, the patient has chills, sweats, headaches, myalgias, fatigue, nausea, abdominal pain, vomiting, diarrhea, and/or cough in association with the fever spikes. Pregnant women are more likely to have severe hypoglycemia (58%) compared with nonpregnant women (8%). In cases of severe malaria, there is significant anemia, jaundice, and sequestration of erythrocytes in the brain (cerebral malaria) and kidney (black water fever), leading to death. In the context of congenital transmission, maternal infection can result in low birth weight (10% to 20%) or fetal loss (6% to 8%).

Congenital infection can occur with all malaria species, but infections with *P. falciparum* and *P. vivax* have been described the most. For mothers who are partially immune, the actual risk of transmission to the fetus is low (0.1% to 1.5%) but may be as high as 10% for previously nonimmune mothers. In endemic areas, distinguishing congenital infection from mosquito-borne disease is not always possible. Infants with congenital malaria generally present in the first 2 months of age with irritability, fever, anemia, thrombocytopenia, hyperbilirubinemia, splenomegaly, hepatomegaly, feeding difficulties with vomiting, and/or diarrhea. Infants with congenital *P. vivax* malaria may present at several months of age.

Diagnosis

The clinical diagnosis of malaria and of congenital malaria is based on the presence of maternal or infant symptoms, maternal present or past residence or visit to an endemic area, and clinical suspicion of disease based on unexplained maternal anemia and/or thrombocytopenia. The standard method of determining if malarial parasites are present, their speciation, and the degree of parasitemia is by examination of Giemsa-stained thick and thin blood smears and rapid diagnostics assays (154–156).

Infants born to mothers who were successfully treated for malaria do not need to be routinely screened at birth but should be tested if they develop signs compatible with disease. However, asymptomatic infants born to mothers with suspected or diagnosed malaria who were not successfully treated should be tested as soon as possible after birth. In all cases where malaria is suspected, the placenta should be submitted for examination for malarial parasites.

Treatment and Management

Treatment choices of malaria in pregnancy depend on the suspected or identified species, the degree of parasitemia if *P. falciparum* is suspected, and the clinical illness (92,157). Despite lack of large studies to determine the side effect profile of medications during pregnancy, due to the potential severity of disease and risk of maternal and fetal mortality, treatment with antimalarial medications is not withheld during pregnancy. In general, pregnant woman with malaria residing in nonendemic regions should be managed in consultation with an infectious disease or travel medicine specialist. Treatment protocols vary over time as resistance patterns change. The CDC Web site is a reference source most commonly used to help guide therapy based on prevalence of various malarial species and the antimalarial resistance patterns in the regions (http://www.cdc.gov/malaria). Pregnant women with severe disease due to *P. falciparum* are usually treated with therapy that may include clindamycin with either artesunate or quinine. Quinine is associated with hypoglycemia, which can adversely affect the fetus. Chloroquine can be used for chloroquine-sensitive malarial strains. The use of doxycycline and primaquine is generally contraindicated in pregnancy and while breast-feeding.

There are limited clinical studies to guide therapy (157), and the choice of treatment regimen is dependent on the malarial species. One suggested treatment guideline is as follows, but treatment of an infant with congenital malaria is best done in consultation with an expert in infectious diseases:

- Mild infections or parasitemia with chloroquine-sensitive *P. vivax*, *P. ovale*, *P. malariae*, or *P. falciparum*:
  - Chloroquine orally 10 mg/kg for the first dose, followed by a second dose of 5 mg/kg after 6 hours then 5 mg/kg once a day for the next 2 days.
  - Primaquine is not needed for additional treatment as there is no tissue phase in congenital malaria.
- Severe infection or infections with chloroquine-resistant *P. falciparum*
  - Quinine IV in 5% dextrose with the first dose being 20 mg/kg given over 4 hours in an ICU setting followed by 10 kg/kg every 8 hours IV until the medication can be given orally to complete a 7-day course, plus
  - Clindamycin 10 mg/kg as a first dose then 5 mg/kg/dose given three times per day for 7 days of treatment, also given IV until medication can be given orally.

Supportive therapy includes hydration and monitoring for hypoglycemia.

Preventive strategies include travel deferral by pregnant women to areas in which malaria is endemic. If travel is necessary, measures should be taken to reduce exposure to mosquitoes, along with use of insect repellent and malaria chemoprophylaxis. Pregnant women should be advised to seek medical care if signs or symptoms compatible with malaria develop. Women should also be advised to report the details of any travel to a malarial area (both travel prior to and during the pregnancy) when presenting for delivery.

Chagas Disease

Epidemiology

Trypanosoma cruzi is a hemoflagellate protozoan parasite that is transmitted to humans via the bite of hemipteran insects (primarily *Triatoma infestans* and *Panstrongylus megistus* in South America and *Rhodnius prolixus* and *Triatoma dimidiata* in Central America and Mexico) in endemic regions, causing an illness called Chagas disease (158). Transmission is predominantly vector borne but can also be transmitted congenitally and by blood transfusion or organ transplant from an infected donor.

It is estimated that there are between 6 and 7 million people infected worldwide in the Americas and that approximately 12,000 people die each year of the infection in this region. With immigration, Chagas disease is now diagnosed worldwide. Approximately 15,000 cases of congenital Chagas disease are diagnosed per year in Latin America, 63 to 315 cases per year in the United States, and 20 to 200 cases per year in Europe (159–161).

Pathophysiology and Clinical Presentation

T. cruzi is found in high concentration in the feces of infected insects. The insect defecates on the skin during or after a blood meal, and the parasite enters via the wound. Transit is also possible via intact conjunctiva or mucosa.

Chagas disease is divided into two phases—acute and chronic. The acute phase lasts 8 to 12 weeks with detectable parasitemia by microscopy. Most individuals are asymptomatic or have nonspecific symptoms in association with fever. Rarely, swelling at the site of the inoculation, called chagoma, is appreciated, usually on the face or extremities. If the inoculation occurs via the conjunctiva, there may be a unilateral swelling of the upper and lower eyelid called Romaña sign.

In 20% to 30% of patients, the chronic phase begins after the parasitemia falls below the level detectable by light microscopy. This phase can be indeterminate, without any signs or symptoms, or can have clinical manifestations of the disease with cardiac and/or gastrointestinal involvement. However, individuals in the chronic phase still serve as reservoirs for the insect vectors, and pregnant women can transmit the parasite transplacentally (161). Moreover, individuals in this phase can develop reactivation of disease, which is a return to acute phase with detectable parasitemia and dissemination, seen in transplant recipients on immunosuppressive therapy or HIV/AIDS patients with low CD4 counts.

Approximately 1% to 5% of infants born to infected mothers have acute *T. cruzi* infection. Transmission occurs predominantly during second and third trimesters. While the risk factors responsible for transmission remain largely unknown, factors that likely influence congenital transmission are level of parasitemia (high parasite load > low parasitemia), maternal infection status (acute > reactivated infection), and maternal HIV infection. While a majority (60% to 90%) of infected infants are asymptomatic at birth, 10% to 40% of infected infants present with nonspecific symptoms such as prematurity, low Apgar scores at birth, low birth weight, hepatosplenomegaly, anemia, or jaundice, with severe infection with meningoencephalitis, myocarditis, cardiomegaly, arrhythmias, hydrops fetalis, megaesophagus, megacolon, and/or respiratory failure. Untreated infants who survive the acute infection have the same 20% to 30% lifetime risk of cardiac and gastrointestinal disease as do individuals who acquired the parasite at an older age.

Diagnosis

The diagnosis of chronic Chagas disease in the pregnant woman is by serologic testing for *T. cruzi* antibodies, followed by confirmation from reference laboratory testing. Diagnosis of acute Chagas disease is by either demonstration of the parasite in the blood smears or PCR testing, if available (161).

Diagnosis of congenital Chagas disease involves detecting the parasite in centrifuged cord blood or neonatal blood samples. The sensitivity of detection of a single sample is approximately 50%; therefore, multiple repeat samples are recommended. PCR testing is more sensitive and recommended where available. In instances where testing at birth is negative, retesting at 4 to 6 weeks with similar methodologies is recommended. Infants suspected to be infected with negative testing at these intervals are recommended to undergo serology-based testing at greater than 9 months of age. All positive tests require additional testing for confirmation of Chagas disease.

Treatment and Management

All cases of congenital Chagas disease should receive treatment as soon as the diagnosis is confirmed with either with benznidazole at a dose of 10 mg/kg/d divided bid for 60 days or with nifurtimox 15 to 20 mg/kg/d divided three to four times per day for 90 days (161,162). Treatment in infancy and early childhood is thought to reduce the risk of chronic infection and therefore the risk of late manifestations of the disease. Treatment should be deferred during pregnancy and breast-feeding.

REFERENCES

1. Zhu N, et al. A novel coronavirus from patients with pneumonia in China, 2019. *N Engl J Med* 2020;382:727.
2. Wu Z, McGoogan JM. Characteristics of and important lessons from the coronavirus disease 2019 (COVID-19) outbreak in China: summary of a report of 72314 cases from the Chinese Center for Disease Control and Prevention. *JAMA* 2020;323(13):1239.
3. World Health Organization. 2020. Available from: https://covid19.who.int
4. Dong Y, et al. Epidemiology of COVID-19 among children in China. *Pediatrics* 2020;145(6):e20200702.
5. Guan WJ, et al. Clinical characteristics of coronavirus disease 2019 in China. *N Engl J Med* 2020;382:1708.
6. Schwartz DA, et al. Spectrum of neonatal COVID-19 in Iran: 19 infants with SARS-CoV-2 perinatal infections with varying test results, clinical findings and outcomes. *J Matern Fetal Neonatal Med* 2020;12:1. doi:10.10 80/14767058.2020.1797672.
7. Juan J, et al. Effect of coronavirus disease 2019 (COVID-19) on maternal, perinatal and neonatal outcome: systematic review. *Ultrasound Obstet Gynecol* 2020;56:15.
8. Yang H, Hu B, Zhan S, et al. Effects of SARS-CoV-2 infection on pregnant women and their infants: a retrospective study in Wuhan, China. *Arch Pathol Lab Med* 2020;144(10):1217.
9. Yang Z, Liu Y. Vertical transmission of severe acute respiratory syndrome coronavirus 2: a systematic review. *Am J Perinatol* 2020;37:1055.
10. Yan J, et al. Coronavirus disease 2019 in pregnant women: a report based on 116 cases. *Am J Obstet Gynecol* 2020;223:111.e111.
11. Alzamora MC, et al. Severe COVID-19 during pregnancy and possible vertical transmission. *Am J Perinatol* 2020;37:861.
12. Huntley BJF, et al. Rates of maternal and perinatal mortality and vertical transmission in pregnancies complicated by severe acute respiratory syndrome coronavirus 2 (SARS-Co-V-2) infection: a systematic review. *Obstet Gynecol* 2020;136:303.
13. Zeng L, et al. Neonatal early-onset infection with SARS-CoV-2 in 33 neonates born to mothers with COVID-19 in Wuhan, China. *JAMA Pediatr* 2020;174(7):722.
14. Zimmermann P, Curtis N. COVID-19 in children, pregnancy and neonates: a review of epidemiologic and clinical features. *Pediatr Infect Dis J* 2020;39:469.
15. Vivanti AJ, et al. Transplacental transmission of SARS-CoV-2 infection. *Nat Commun* 2020;11:3572.
16. Li Q, et al. Early transmission dynamics in Wuhan, China, of novel coronavirus-infected pneumonia. *N Engl J Med* 2020;382:1199.
17. Liu PP, Blet A, Smyth D, et al. The science underlying COVID-19: implications for the cardiovascular system. *Circulation* 2020;142:68.
18. Whittaker A, Anson M, Harky A. Neurological manifestations of COVID-19: a systematic review and current update. *Acta Neurol Scand* 2020;142:14.
19. Su H, et al. Renal histopathological analysis of 26 postmortem findings of patients with COVID-19 in China. *Kidney Int* 2020;98:219.
20. Mithal LB, Machut KZ, Muller WJ, et al. SARS-CoV-2 infection in infants less than 90 days old. *J Pediatr* 2020;224:150.
21. Feld L, et al. A case series of the 2019 novel coronavirus (SARS-CoV-2) in 3 febrile infants in New York. *Pediatrics* 2020;146(1):e20201056.

22. Sinelli M, et al. Early neonatal SARS-CoV-2 infection manifesting with hypoxemia requiring respiratory support. *Pediatrics* 2020;146(1):e20201121.

23. CDC COVID-19 Response Team. Coronavirus Disease 2019 in Children—United States, February 12-April 2, 2020. *MMWR Morb Mortal Wkly Rep* 2020;69(14):422. doi: 10.15585/mmwr.mm6914e4.

24. Parri N, et al. Characteristic of COVID-19 infection in pediatric patients: early findings from two Italian Pediatric Research Networks. *Eur J Pediatr* 2020;179:1315.

25. Centers for Disease Control and Prevention. *Interim guidelines for collecting, handling, and testing clinical specimens from persons for coronavirus disease 2019 (COVID-19)*. Atlanta, GA: US centers for Disease Control and Prevention (CDC), 2020. Available from: https://www.cdc.gov/coronavirus/2019-ncov/lab/guidelines-clinical-specimens.html.

26. Pinninti S, et al. Comparing nasopharyngeal and mid-turbinate nasal swab testing for the identification of SARS-CoV-2. *Clin Infect Dis* 2020:ciaa882. doi: 10.1093/cid/ciaa882.

27. Kimberlin DW, Puopolo KM. Breastmilk and COVID-19: what do we know? *Clin Infect Dis* 2020:ciaa800. doi: 10.1093/cid/ciaa800.

28. Beigel JH, et al. Remdesivir for the treatment of Covid-19—preliminary report. *N Engl J Med* 2020;383(10):993.

29. RECOVERY Collaborative Group; Horby P, et al. Dexamethasone in hospitalized patients with Covid-19—preliminary report. *N Engl J Med* 2020;NEJMoa2021436. doi: 10.1056/NEJMoa2021436.

30. Dollard SC, Grosse SD, Ross DS. New estimates of the prevalence of neurological and sensory sequelae and mortality associated with congenital cytomegalovirus infection. *Rev Med Virol* 2007;17:355.

31. Dar L, et al. Congenital cytomegalovirus infection in a highly seropositive semi-urban population in India. *Pediatr Infect Dis J* 2008;27:841.

32. Noyola DE, et al. Congenital cytomegalovirus infection in San Luis Potosi, Mexico. *Pediatr Infect Dis J* 2003;22:89.

33. Manicklal S, Emery VC, Lazzarotto T, et al. The "silent" global burden of congenital cytomegalovirus. *Clin Microbiol Rev* 2013;26:86.

34. Fowler KB, Boppana SB. Congenital cytomegalovirus (CMV) infection and hearing deficit. *J Clin Virol* 2006;35:226.

35. Morton CC, Nance WE. Newborn hearing screening—a silent revolution. *N Engl J Med* 2006;354:2151.

36. Cannon MJ. Congenital cytomegalovirus (CMV) epidemiology and awareness. *J Clin Virol* 2009;46(suppl 4):S6.

37. Binda S, et al. What people know about congenital CMV: an analysis of a large heterogeneous population through a web-based survey. *BMC Infect Dis* 2016;16:513.

38. Kenneson A, Cannon MJ. Review and meta-analysis of the epidemiology of congenital cytomegalovirus (CMV) infection. *Rev Med Virol* 2007;17:253.

39. Enders G, Daiminger A, Bäder U, et al. Intrauterine transmission and clinical outcome of 248 pregnancies with primary cytomegalovirus infection in relation to gestational age. *J Clin Virol* 2011;52:244.

40. Pass RF, Fowler KB, Boppana SB, et al. Congenital cytomegalovirus infection following first trimester maternal infection: symptoms at birth and outcome. *J Clin Virol* 2006;35:216.

41. Dreher AM, et al. Spectrum of disease and outcome in children with symptomatic congenital cytomegalovirus infection. *J Pediatr* 2014;164:855.

42. Britt WJ. Chapter 24: Cytomegalovirus. In: Remington JS, Klein JO, Wilson CB, et al., eds. *Infectious diseases of the fetus and newborn infant*. Philadelphia, PA: Elsevier Saunders, 2011:706.

43. Boppana SB, Pass RF, Britt WJ, et al. Symptomatic congenital cytomegalovirus infection: neonatal morbidity and mortality. *Pediatr Infect Dis J* 1992;11:93.

44. Townsend CL, et al. Long-term outcomes of congenital cytomegalovirus infection in Sweden and the United Kingdom. *Clin Infect Dis* 2013;56:1232.

45. Fowler KB, Dahle AJ, Boppana SB, et al. Newborn hearing screening: will children with hearing loss caused by congenital cytomegalovirus infection be missed? *J Pediatr* 1999;135:60.

46. Dahle AJ, et al. Longitudinal investigation of hearing disorders in children with congenital cytomegalovirus. *J Am Acad Audiol* 2000;11:283.

47. Revello MG, Zavattoni M, Furione M, et al. Quantification of human cytomegalovirus DNA in amniotic fluid of mothers of congenitally infected fetuses. *J Clin Microbiol* 1999;37:3350.

48. Boppana SB, Smith R, Stagno S, et al. Evaluation of a microtiter plate fluorescent antibody assay for rapid detection of human cytomegalovirus infections. *J Clin Microbiol* 1992;30:721.

49. Balcarek KB, Warren W, Smith RJ, et al. Neonatal screening for congenital cytomegalovirus infection by detection of virus in saliva. *J Infect Dis* 1993;167:1433.

50. Yamamoto AY, et al. Is saliva as reliable as urine for detection of cytomegalovirus DNA for neonatal screening of congenital CMV infection? *J Clin Virol* 2006;36:228.

51. Pinninti SG, et al. Comparison of saliva PCR assay versus rapid culture for detection of congenital cytomegalovirus infection. *Pediatr Infect Dis J* 2015;34:536.

52. Boppana SB, et al. Dried blood spot real-time polymerase chain reaction assays to screen newborns for congenital cytomegalovirus infection. *JAMA* 2010;303:1375.

53. Revello MG, et al. A randomized trial of hyperimmune globulin to prevent congenital cytomegalovirus. *N Engl J Med* 2014;370:1316.

54. Leruez-Ville M, et al. In utero treatment of congenital cytomegalovirus infection with valacyclovir in a multicenter, open-label, phase II study. *Am J Obstet Gynecol* 2016;215:462.e461.

55. Price SM, et al. Educating women about congenital cytomegalovirus: assessment of health education materials through a web-based survey. *BMC Womens Health* 2014;14:144.

56. Rawlinson WD, et al. Congenital cytomegalovirus infection in pregnancy and the neonate: consensus recommendations for prevention, diagnosis, and therapy. *Lancet Infect Dis* 2017;17:e177.

57. Kimberlin DW, et al. Valganciclovir for symptomatic congenital cytomegalovirus disease. *N Engl J Med* 2015;372:933.

58. Oliver SE, et al. Neurodevelopmental outcomes following ganciclovir therapy in symptomatic congenital cytomegalovirus infections involving the central nervous system. *J Clin Virol* 2009;46(suppl 4):S22.

59. Looker KJ, et al. First estimates of the global and regional incidence of neonatal herpes infection. *Lancet Glob Health* 2017;5:e300.

60. Kimberlin DW. Why neonatal herpes matters. *Lancet Glob Health* 2017;5:e234.

61. Brown ZA, et al. Effect of serologic status and cesarean delivery on transmission rates of herpes simplex virus from mother to infant. *JAMA* 2003;289:203.

62. Nahmias AJ, et al. Perinatal risk associated with maternal genital herpes simplex virus infection. *Am J Obstet Gynecol* 1971;110:825.

63. Baldwin S, Whitley RJ. Intrauterine herpes simplex virus infection. *Teratology* 1989;39:1.

64. Hutto C, et al. Intrauterine herpes simplex virus infections. *J Pediatr* 1987;110:97.

65. Pinninti SG, et al. Neonatal herpes disease following maternal antenatal antiviral suppressive therapy: a multicenter case series. *J Pediatr* 2012;161:134, e133.

66. Kimberlin DW, et al. Natural history of neonatal herpes simplex virus infections in the acyclovir era. *Pediatrics* 2001;108:223.

67. Kimberlin DW, et al. Application of the polymerase chain reaction to the diagnosis and management of neonatal herpes simplex virus disease. National Institute of Allergy and Infectious Diseases Collaborative Antiviral Study Group. *J Infect Dis* 1996;174:1162.

68. Malm G, Forsgren M. Neonatal herpes simplex virus infections: HSV DNA in cerebrospinal fluid and serum. *Arch Dis Child Fetal Neonatal Ed* 1999;81:F24.

69. Diamond C, Mohan K, Hobson A, et al. Viremia in neonatal herpes simplex virus infections. *Pediatr Infect Dis J* 1999;18:487.

70. Samies N, Jariwala R, Boppana S, et al. Utility of surface and blood polymerase chain reaction assays in identifying infants with neonatal herpes simplex virus infection. *Pediatr Infect Dis J* 2019;38:1138.

71. Kimberlin DW, et al. Safety and efficacy of high-dose intravenous acyclovir in the management of neonatal herpes simplex virus infections. *Pediatrics* 2001;108:230.

72. Kimberlin DW, et al. Oral acyclovir suppression and neurodevelopment after neonatal herpes. *N Engl J Med* 2011;365:1284.

73. Kimberlin DW. When should you initiate acyclovir therapy in a neonate? *J Pediatr* 2008;153:155.

74. Kimberlin DW, Baley J; Committee on Infectious Diseases, Committee on Fetus and Newborn. Guidance on management of asymptomatic neonates born to women with active genital herpes lesions. *Pediatrics* 2013;131:383.

75. Centers for Disease Control and Prevention (CDC). Revised surveillance case definition for HIV infection—United States, 2014. *MMWR Recomm Rep* 2014;63:1.

76. Mofenson LM, et al. Guidelines for the prevention and treatment of opportunistic infections among HIV-exposed and HIV-infected children: recommendations from CDC, the National Institutes of Health, the HIV Medicine Association of the Infectious Diseases Society of America, the Pediatric Infectious Diseases Society, and the American Academy of Pediatrics. *MMWR Recomm Rep* 2009;58:1.

77. Panel on Treatment of Pregnant Women with HIV Infection and Prevention of Perinatal Transmission. Recommendations for the Use of Antiretroviral Drugs in Pregnant Women with HIV Infection and Interventions to Reduce Perinatal HIV Transmission in the United States. Available from: https://clinicalinfo.hiv.gov/sites/default/files/inline-files/PerinatalGL.pdf. Accessed 1/12/21.

78. Valeur-Jensen AK, et al. Risk factors for parvovirus B19 infection in pregnancy. *JAMA* 1999;281:1099.

79. Harger JH, Adler SP, Koch WC, et al. Prospective evaluation of 618 pregnant women exposed to parvovirus B19: risks and symptoms. *Obstet Gynecol* 1998;91:413.

80. Young NS, Brown KE. Parvovirus B19. *N Engl J Med* 2004;350:586.

81. Yamakawa Y, Oka H, Hori S, et al. Detection of human parvovirus B19 DNA by nested polymerase chain reaction. *Obstet Gynecol* 1995;86:126.

82. Selbing A, Josefsson A, Dahle LO, et al. Parvovirus B19 infection during pregnancy treated with high-dose intravenous gammaglobulin. *Lancet* 1995;345:660.

83. Reef SF, et al. Preparing for elimination of congenital Rubella syndrome (CRS): summary of a workshop on CRS elimination in the United States. *Clin Infect Dis* 2000;31:85.

84. Centers for Disease Control and Prevention (CDC). Elimination of rubella and congenital rubella syndrome—United States, 1969-2004. *MMWR Morb Mortal Wkly Rep* 2005;54:279.

85. Centers for Disease Control and Prevention (CDC). Progress toward elimination of measles and prevention of congenital rubella infection—European region, 1990-2004. *MMWR Morb Mortal Wkly Rep* 2005;54:175.

86. Miller E, Cradock-Watson JE, Pollock TM. Consequences of confirmed maternal rubella at successive stages of pregnancy. *Lancet* 1982;2:781.

87. Munro ND, Sheppard S, Smithells RW, et al. Temporal relations between maternal rubella and congenital defects. *Lancet* 1987;2:201.

88. Webster WS. Teratogen update: congenital rubella. *Teratology* 1998;58:13.

89. Bosma TJ, Corbett KM, O'Shea S, et al. PCR for detection of rubella virus RNA in clinical samples. *J Clin Microbiol* 1995;33:1075.

90. Bosma TJ, et al. Use of PCR for prenatal and postnatal diagnosis of congenital rubella. *J Clin Microbiol* 1995;33:2881.

91. Tanemura M, Suzumori K, Yagami Y, et al. Diagnosis of fetal rubella infection with reverse transcription and nested polymerase chain reaction: a study of 34 cases diagnosed in fetuses. *Am J Obstet Gynecol* 1996;174:578.

92. Kimberlin D, Brady M, Jackson MA, et al. Red book. In: Kimberlin D, ed. *Herpes simplex*. Itasca, IL: American Academy of Pediatrics, 2018.

93. Marin M, et al. Varicella among adults: data from an active surveillance project, 1995-2005. *J Infect Dis* 2008;197(suppl 2):S94.

94. Enders G, Miller E, Cradock-Watson J, et al. Consequences of varicella and herpes zoster in pregnancy: prospective study of 1739 cases. *Lancet* 1994;343:1548.

95. Pastuszak AL, et al. Outcome after maternal varicella infection in the first 20 weeks of pregnancy. *N Engl J Med* 1994;330:901.

96. Meyers JD. Congenital varicella in term infants: risk reconsidered. *J Infect Dis* 1974;129:215.

97. Duffy MR, et al. Zika virus outbreak on Yap Island, Federated States of Micronesia. *N Engl J Med* 2009;360:2536.

98. Musso D, et al. Zika virus in French Polynesia 2013-14: anatomy of a completed outbreak. *Lancet Infect Dis* 2018;18:e172.

99. Brasil P, et al. Zika virus outbreak in Rio de Janeiro, Brazil: clinical characterization, epidemiological and virological aspects. *PLoS Negl Trop Dis* 2016;10:e0004636.

100. Brasil P, et al. Zika virus infection in pregnant women in Rio de Janeiro. *N Engl J Med* 2016;375:2321.

101. Mlakar J, et al. Zika virus associated with microcephaly. *N Engl J Med* 2016;374:951.

102. van der Linden V, et al. Congenital Zika syndrome with arthrogryposis: retrospective case series study. *BMJ* 2016;354:i3899.

103. Ventura CV, Ventura Filho MC, Ventura LO. Ocular manifestations and visual outcome in children with congenital Zika syndrome. *Top Magn Reson Imaging* 2019;28:23.

104. Chimelli L, et al. Persistence of Zika virus after birth: clinical, virological, neuroimaging, and neuropathological documentation in a 5-month infant with congenital Zika syndrome. *J Neuropathol Exp Neurol* 2018;77:193.

105. Britt WJ. Adverse outcomes of pregnancy-associated Zika virus infection. *Semin Perinatol* 2018;42:155.

106. Munoz-Jordan JL. Diagnosis of Zika virus infections: challenges and opportunities. *J Infect Dis* 2017;216:S951.

107. Bowen V, Su J, Torrone E, et al. Increase in incidence of congenital syphilis—United States, 2012-2014. *MMWR Morb Mortal Wkly Rep* 2015;64:1241.

108. Centers for Disease Control and Prevention (CDC). Congenital syphilis—United States, 2003-2008. *MMWR Morb Mortal Wkly Rep* 2010;59:413.

109. Obladen M. Curse on two generations: a history of congenital syphilis. *Neonatology* 2013;103:274.

110. Lago EG, Vaccari A, Fiori RM. Clinical features and follow-up of congenital syphilis. *Sex Transm Dis* 2013;40:85.

111. Arrieta AC, Singh J. Congenital syphilis. *N Engl J Med* 2019;381:2157.

112. Sheffield JS, et al. Placental histopathology of congenital syphilis. *Obstet Gynecol* 2002;100:126.

113. Workowski KA. Centers for Disease Control and Prevention sexually transmitted diseases treatment guidelines. *Clin Infect Dis* 2015;61(suppl 8):S759.

114. Michelow IC, et al. Central nervous system infection in congenital syphilis. *N Engl J Med* 2002;346:1792.

115. Centers for Disease Control and Prevention (CDC). Discordant results from reverse sequence syphilis screening—five laboratories, United States, 2006-2010. *MMWR Morb Mortal Wkly Rep* 2011;60:133.

116. Pillay A. Centers for Disease Control and Prevention Syphilis Summit—diagnostics and laboratory issues. *Sex Transm Dis* 2018;45:S13.

117. Peng J, et al. Analysis of 2 reverse syphilis testing algorithms in diagnosis of syphilis: a large-cohort prospective study. *Clin Infect Dis* 2018;67:947.

118. Loto OM, Awowole I. Tuberculosis in pregnancy: a review. *J Pregnancy* 2012;2012:379271.

119. Cantwell MF, et al. Brief report: congenital tuberculosis. *N Engl J Med* 1994;330:1051.

120. Kothari A, Mahadevan N, Girling J. Tuberculosis and pregnancy—results of a study in a high prevalence area in London. *Eur J Obstet Gynecol Reprod Biol* 2006;126:48.

121. Lewinsohn DM, et al. Official American Thoracic Society/Infectious Diseases Society of America/Centers for Disease Control and Prevention clinical practice guidelines: diagnosis of tuberculosis in adults and children. *Clin Infect Dis* 2017;64:e1.

122. Malhamé I, Cormier M, Sugarman J, et al. Latent tuberculosis in pregnancy: a systematic review. *PLoS One* 2016;11:e0154825.

123. Walzl G, et al. Tuberculosis: advances and challenges in development of new diagnostics and biomarkers. *Lancet Infect Dis* 2018;18:e199.

124. Okuno T, et al. Human herpesviruses 6 and 7 in cervixes of pregnant women. *J Clin Microbiol* 1995;33:1968.

125. Adams O, Krempe C, Kögler G, et al. Congenital infections with human herpesvirus 6. *J Infect Dis* 1998;178:544.

126. Brayfield BP, et al. Postnatal human herpesvirus 8 and human immunodeficiency virus type 1 infection in mothers and infants from Zambia. *J Infect Dis* 2003;187:559.

127. Barton LL, Mets MB. Congenital lymphocytic choriomeningitis virus infection: decade of rediscovery. *Clin Infect Dis* 2001;33:370.

128. Tebruegge M, Curtis N. Enterovirus infections in neonates. *Semin Fetal Neonatal Med* 2009;14:222.

129. Abzug MJ, et al. A randomized, double-blind, placebo-controlled trial of pleconaril for the treatment of neonates with enterovirus sepsis. *J Pediatr Infect Dis Soc* 2016;5:53.

130. Johnston JM, Overall JC. Intravenous immunoglobulin in disseminated neonatal echovirus 11 infection. *Pediatr Infect Dis J* 1989;8:254.

131. Dubey JP, Jones JL. Toxoplasma gondii infection in humans and animals in the United States. *Int J Parasitol* 2008;38:1257.

132. Hill DE, Dubey JP. Toxoplasma gondii prevalence in farm animals in the United States. *Int J Parasitol* 2013;43:107.

133. Berger F, Goulet V, Le Strat Y, et al. Toxoplasmosis among pregnant women in France: risk factors and change of prevalence between 1995 and 2003. *Rev Epidemiol Sante Publique* 2009;57:241.

134. Cook AJ, et al. Sources of toxoplasma infection in pregnant women: European multicentre case-control study. European Research Network on Congenital Toxoplasmosis. *BMJ* 2000;321:142.

135. Varella IS, et al. Prevalence of acute toxoplasmosis infection among 41,112 pregnant women and the mother-to-child transmission rate in a public hospital in South Brazil. *Mem Inst Oswaldo Cruz* 2009;104:383.

136. Montoya JG, Liesenfeld O. Toxoplasmosis. *Lancet* 2004;363:1965.

137. Montoya JG, Remington JS. Management of Toxoplasma gondii infection during pregnancy. *Clin Infect Dis* 2008;47:554.

138. Wallon M, et al. Congenital toxoplasma infection: monthly prenatal screening decreases transmission rate and improves clinical outcome at age 3 years. *Clin Infect Dis* 2013;56:1223.

139. Sever JL, et al. Toxoplasmosis: maternal and pediatric findings in 23,000 pregnancies. *Pediatrics* 1988;82:181.

140. Guerina NG. Congenital infection with Toxoplasma gondii. *Pediatr Ann* 1994;23:138, 147.

141. McLeod R, et al. Severe sulfadiazine hypersensitivity in a child with reactivated congenital toxoplasmic chorioretinitis. *Pediatr Infect Dis J* 2006;25:270.

142. Phan L, et al. Longitudinal study of new eye lesions in children with toxoplasmosis who were not treated during the first year of life. *Am J Ophthalmol* 2008;146:375.

143. McAuley J, et al. Early and longitudinal evaluations of treated infants and children and untreated historical patients with congenital toxoplasmosis: the Chicago Collaborative Treatment Trial. *Clin Infect Dis* 1994;18:38.

144. Foulon W, et al. Prenatal diagnosis of congenital toxoplasmosis: a multicenter evaluation of different diagnostic parameters. *Am J Obstet Gynecol* 1999;181:843.

145. Boyer KM. Diagnostic testing for congenital toxoplasmosis. *Pediatr Infect Dis J* 2001;20:59.

146. Romand S, et al. Usefulness of quantitative polymerase chain reaction in amniotic fluid as early prognostic marker of fetal infection with Toxoplasma gondii. *Am J Obstet Gynecol* 2004;190:797.

147. Thalib L, et al. Prediction of congenital toxoplasmosis by polymerase chain reaction analysis of amniotic fluid. *BJOG* 2005;112:567.

148. Gilbert RE, et al. Effect of prenatal treatment on mother to child transmission of Toxoplasma gondii: retrospective cohort study of 554 mother-child pairs in Lyon, France. *Int J Epidemiol* 2001;30:1303.

149. Koppe JG, Loewer-Sieger DH, de Roever-Bonnet H. Results of 20-year follow-up of congenital toxoplasmosis. *Lancet* 1986;1:254.

150. McLeod R, et al. Outcome of treatment for congenital toxoplasmosis, 1981-2004: the National Collaborative Chicago-Based, Congenital Toxoplasmosis Study. *Clin Infect Dis* 2006;42:1383.

151. Maldonado YA, Read JS; Committee on Infectious Diseases. Diagnosis, treatment, and prevention of congenital toxoplasmosis in the United States. *Pediatrics* 2017;139:e20163860.

152. Ezeoke U, et al. Prevalence of malaria in HIV positive and HIV negative pregnant women attending antenatal clinics in south eastern Nigeria. *Malawi Med J* 2018;30:256.

153. Bauserman M, et al. An overview of malaria in pregnancy. *Semin Perinatol* 2019;43:282.

154. Visser T, et al. Rapid diagnostic tests for malaria. *Bull World Health Organ* 2015;93:862.

155. Prestel C, Tan KR, Abanyie F, et al. Malaria diagnostic practices in U.S. Laboratories in 2017. *J Clin Microbiol* 2018;56:e00461-18.

156. Amir A, Cheong FW, De Silva JR, et al. Diagnostic tools in childhood malaria. *Parasit Vectors* 2018;11:53.

157. Coll O, et al. Treatment and prevention of malaria in pregnancy and newborn. *J Perinat Med* 2008;36:15.

158. Bern C. Chagas' disease. *N Engl J Med* 2015;373:1882.

159. Rassi A, Marin-Neto JA. Chagas disease. *Lancet* 2010;375:1388.

160. Bern C, Montgomery SP. An estimate of the burden of Chagas disease in the United States. *Clin Infect Dis* 2009;49:e52.

161. Cevallos AM, Hernández R. Chagas' disease: pregnancy and congenital transmission. *Biomed Res Int* 2014;2014:401864.

162. Carlier Y, et al. Congenital Chagas disease: updated recommendations for prevention, diagnosis, treatment, and follow-up of newborns and siblings, girls, women of childbearing age, and pregnant women. *PLoS Negl Trop Dis* 2019;13:e0007694.

47 Evaluation and Management of Infection in the Newborn

Miren B. Dhudasia, Dustin D. Flannery, and Karen M. Puopolo

INTRODUCTION

Infection is one of the most common causes of neonatal mortality. Deaths in the first month after birth account for nearly half of the estimated 2 to 2.5 million early childhood deaths that occur worldwide (1). The overwhelming majority occur in low- and middle-income countries (LMIC) in Asia and Africa, but infants particularly those born preterm, in high-income countries (HIC) such as the United States may also succumb to infection, particularly those born preterm. It is therefore imperative to identify neonates at risk for infection in a timely manner and intervene with antimicrobial and other supportive care to prevent both mortality and complications of infection. This chapter will review the epidemiology, microbiology, approach to risk assessment, and empiric therapy for early and late-onset bacteremia and meningitis, as well as site-specific bacterial infection including urinary tract infection (UTI), omphalitis, neonatal tetanus, and ophthalmia neonatorum (conjunctivitis).

EARLY-ONSET SEPSIS

Definitions

Early-onset sepsis (EOS) is defined as invasive microbial infection that occurs within the first 3 to 7 days after birth. Among infants born at term gestation (≥37 weeks' gestation) in HIC, EOS is a very low-incidence but still potentially fatal complication of birth. Among preterm, particularly low-gestation, very low birth weight (VLBW, birth weight <1,500 g) and extremely low birth weight (ELBW, birth weight <1,000 g) infants, EOS is more common and a significant contributor to morbidity and mortality in both HIC and LMIC. Among continuously hospitalized, primarily preterm infants, EOS diagnosis is limited to infection occurring ≤72 hours after birth. Among term infants, EOS diagnosis is most commonly made at less than 48 hours after birth; for example, 95% of EOS caused by group B *Streptococcus* (GBS) in the United States (U.S.) occurs less than 48 hours of age (2). Although less common, otherwise healthy infants may be discharged from the birth hospital and develop EOS up to 7 days of age. Bacteria are the primary cause of EOS; fungal species are occasionally isolated, primarily among very preterm infants (3–5).

EOS is further defined in most countries as isolation of a pathogenic species from a blood or cerebrospinal fluid (CSF) culture, but clinical criteria are frequently used in LMIC without consistent access to laboratory facilities. In all settings, the nonspecific nature of signs of infection in the newborn present difficulties to caregivers that must distinguish such signs from the normal process of physiologic transition after birth, from the instability inherent to prematurely born infants, and from noninfectious causes of instability after birth, including hypoxic–ischemic injury.

Epidemiology

The incidence of EOS is inversely related to gestational age at birth and varies widely by country. Active national surveillance conducted by the U.S. Centers for Disease Control and Prevention (CDC) demonstrates that overall U.S. incidence has been constant from 2005 to 2015 at approximately 0.7 to 0.8 cases/1,000 live births (3). Among infants born ≥37 weeks of gestation, the incidence is approximately 0.5 cases/1,000 live births (3,4). The overall incidence reported in other HIC countries such as the United Kingdom, Australia, Italy, and France is similar (Table 47.1). In contrast, the incidence of EOS among LMIC is variable but overall higher, ranging widely depending on study population and definition used to identify EOS (Table 47.1). Studies limited to preterm populations find rates of EOS markedly higher that those observed in term infants. Prospective surveillance among centers participating in the U.S. Neonatal Research Network from 2015 to 2017 found an incidence of 18.5 cases/1,000 live births occurring at 22 to 28 weeks' gestation and 6.2/1,000 among those born at 29 to 33 weeks' gestation (4). As assessed by birth weight, the study observed an incidence of 13.9 cases/1,000 live birth among VLBW infants, consistent with prior NRN reports over the prior 20 years that ranged from 11 to 19 cases/1,000 live births (27,28).

Pathophysiology

The pathogenesis of EOS begins with invasion of the intra-amniotic compartment with bacterial species from maternal genitourinary and gastrointestinal tracts. In areas of poor hygiene, nosocomial and environmental sources of bacteria can also be a source of ascending colonization and infection from the maternal genitourinary tract. The pathologic processes of EOS were described in seminal papers by Bernirscke and Blanc who described the "amniotic infection syndrome" as the cause of congenital bacterial sepsis and pneumonia, contrasting this entity to the transplacental, hematogenous origin of congenital viral infection (29,30). Rarely, pathogenic bacteria infecting the maternal bloodstream may cause EOS via transplacental route. *Listeria monocytogenes* is a foodborne pathogen with placental tropism that can cause fetal infection via the maternal bloodstream.

Several characteristics of neonatal physiology contribute to vulnerability of the newborn, and particularly the preterm newborn, to EOS. Labor, particularly after rupture of membranes (ROM), provides the opportunity for fetal exposure to maternal bacterial flora. Although labor and ROM begin the normally physiologic process of developing the newborn microbiome, it also provides opportunity for colonization and bacterial replication in amniotic fluid, fetal skin, and fetal membranes. Transition from fetal colonization to invasive infection via skin and membranous surfaces then occurs, either *in utero* or after birth. Fetal infection may also occur *in utero* by aspiration of infected amniotic fluid. This pathogenesis primarily proceeds during labor, and is promoted by membrane rupture, but rarely can occur before the onset of labor (31,32). Characteristics of preterm infants provide increased vulnerability to infection. Preterm skin is characterized by immature stratum corneum, providing an incomplete barrier to microbial invasion (33). Surfactant deficiency characteristic of the immature lung contributes to the susceptibility of the preterm fetus to invasive infection, as surfactant proteins A and D are members of the collectin family of host defense proteins with roles in binding and opsonization of bacterial pathogens such as GBS (34). Relative deficiencies in mucosal antimicrobial proteins and peptides may also contribute to the vulnerability of the preterm infant to infection (35,36). Finally, transplacental antibody transfer is evident as early as 22 weeks' gestation but does not reach levels greater than 50% of maternal levels until after 30 weeks' gestation (37). Active transport mechanisms active at the end of the third trimester result in cord blood antibody levels that may exceed maternal levels. Effective immune response to the majority of organisms causing EOS require opsonic antibody in combination with neutrophil- and complement-mediated defense mechanisms, and antibody deficiency contributes to preterm vulnerability to EOS.

TABLE 47.1

International Incidence and Microbiology of Early-Onset Sepsis among All Live Births

References	Years Included	Country/Region	Population (Live Births, n)	Definition of EOS	Incidence (Cases/1,000)	Predominant Organisms
United States and Europe						
Schrag et al. (3)	2005–2014	U.S. (surveillance in four states)	All GA (n~2,000,000)	Bacteria isolated from blood or cerebrospinal fluid <72 hours of age	0.74	GBS > E. coli
Stoll et al. (4)	2015–2017	U.S. (18 high-risk birth centers)	All GA (n = 217,480)	Bacteria isolated from blood or cerebrospinal fluid <72 hours of age and antibiotics for ≥5 days or until death	1.08	E. coli > GBS
Berardi et al. (6)	2009–2012	Italy (Emilia-Romagna)	All GA (n = 146,682)	Bacteria isolated from blood or cerebrospinal fluid <72 hours of age	0.60	GBS > E. coli
Kuhn et al. (7)	2004–2005	France (Alsace)	All GA (n = 20,131)	Bacteria isolated from blood or cerebrospinal fluid <72 hours of age and antibiotics for ≥5 days or until death	1.19	GBS > E. coli
Morris et al. (8)	Prior to 2020	England and Wales	GA ≥34 weeks' gestation (n = 142,333)	Bacteria isolated from blood or cerebrospinal fluid <72 hours of age and antibiotics for ≥5 days or until death	0.5	GBS in 88%
Braye et al. (9)	2006–2016	Australia (New South Wales)	All GA (n = 93,584)	Bacteria isolated from blood or cerebrospinal fluid <72 hours of age	0.7	GBS (term) E. coli (preterm)
Asia						
Gao et al. (10)	2012–2016	China (Guangzhou)	All GA (n = 91,215)	Bacteria isolated from blood or cerebrospinal fluid <72 hours of age and clinical diagnosis of sepsis	0.8	GBS > E. coli
Shim et al. (11)	1996–2005	South Korea (Seoul)	All GA (n = 13,742)	Bacteria isolated from blood or cerebrospinal fluid ≤4 days of age and clinical diagnosis of sepsis	0.6	No dominant species
Lim et al. (12)	2005–2009	Taiwan (Taoyuan City)	VLBW infants (n = 1042)	Bacteria isolated from blood or cerebrospinal fluid <72 hours of age and clinical diagnosis of sepsis	9.6 per 1,000 VLBW	E. coli
Tran et al. (13)	2010–2011	Vietnam	All GA (admitted to neonatal unit) (n = 2,555)	Bacteria isolated from blood or cerebrospinal fluid <72 hours of age	8.0	CONS S. aureus
Turner et al. (14)	2009–2012	Thailand and Myanmar border region	All GA[a] (n = 4,173)	Clinical sepsis[b]	44.8 (clinical EOS)	N/A
Investigators of the Delhi Neonatal Infection Study (DeNIS) Collaboration (15)	2011–2014	India (Delhi)	All GA (n = 88,636 births) (n = 13,530 NICU admits)	Bacteria isolated from blood or cerebrospinal fluid <72 hours of age	6.5 (all births) 42.8 (NICU admits)	Acinetobacter CONS Klebsiella
Swarnkar and Swarnkar (16)	2008–2010	India (Maharashtra)	All GA (n = 3,574)	Bacteria isolated from blood or cerebrospinal fluid <48 hours of age in setting of clinical sepsis	20.1 (clinical) 10.4 (culture-confirmed)	Klebsiella
Middle East						
Shehab El-Din (17)	2011–2012	Egypt (Mansoura)	All GA (in NICU) (n = 344)	Egyptian Neonatal Network (EGNN) guidelines[c]	142 (per 1,000 NICU admissions)	CONS Acinetobacter E. coli
Chan et al. (18)	2011	Bangladesh (Dhaka)	GA ≥30 wk (n = 600)[d]	Bacteria isolated from blood culture or clinical signs in first 7 days of life	128.3	N/A
Akbarian-Rad et al. (19)	2000–2019	Iran	All GA (in hospital) (n = 14,683)	Bacteria isolated from blood <3 days age	Pooled prevalence 11.0%	Enterobacter Klebsiella
Glikman et al. (20)	2010–2015	Israel	All GA (n = 180,000)	Bacteria isolated from blood or cerebrospinal fluid <72 hours of age (preterm) and <7 days (term)	0.6	E. coli GBS Eco preterm
Zareifar et al. (21)	2007–2009	Iran (Shiraz)	All GA (screened for G6PD deficiency) (n = 150,996)	Bacteria isolated from blood <72 hours of age	0.7	N/A

TABLE 47.1

International Incidence and Microbiology of Early-Onset Sepsis among All Live Births (Continued)

References	Years Included	Country/Region	Population (Live Births, n)	Definition of EOS	Incidence (Cases/1,000)	Predominant Organisms
Afsharpaiman et al. (22)	2003–2006	Tehran, Iran	All GA (n = 19,573)	Bacteria isolated from blood <72 hours of age with clinical illness	2.2	*Enterobacter*
Africa						
Velaphi et al. (23)	2013–2014	South Africa (Soweto)	All GA[e] (n = 31,359)	Bacteria isolated from blood or cerebrospinal fluid <72 hours of age	3.2	GBS (by culture) *Ureaplasma* (by molecular assay)
Olorukooba et al. (24)	2017–2018	Nigeria (Zaria)	All GA (admitted to special care unit) (n = 465)	Bacteria isolated from blood or <72 hours of age with clinical illness	200 per 1,000 admissions	*E. coli*
Kayom et al. (25)	2012	Uganda (Kampala)	All GA[f] (n = 317)	Clinical definition (IMNCI criteria)[g]	63.1	N/A
Pérez et al. (26)	2013–2014	Mexico (Guadalajara)	All GA (n = 14,207)	Bacteria isolated from blood or CSF cultures <72 hours of age	4.7	N/A

[a]Infants excluded if they had severe congenital anomaly or prior treatment with antibiotics ≤6 days of age.

[b]Infant <7 days of age with fever (>38°C or >37.5°C × 2) or at least two clinical signs (poor perfusion, respiratory distress, persisting glucose imbalance, abdominal distension, bilious aspirates, or blood in the stool).

[c]Egyptian Neonatal Network (EGNN) guidelines—presence of at least 3 out 4 of the following: risk factors of sepsis (e.g., prematurity, chorioamnionitis); two or more clinical signs of sepsis (poor reflexes, lethargy, respiratory distress, bradycardia, apnea, convulsions, abdominal distension, and bleeding); abnormal hemogram and positive CRP and positive culture.

[d]Women who presented with fetal distress, obstructed labor, hemorrhage, or severe preeclampsia were excluded to facilitate their need for urgent care. Women who used antibiotics or steroids within 2 weeks of labor were also excluded from the study. Newborns were excluded if they were born with birth injuries or surgical conditions. Clinical signs of sepsis were defined as the presence of convulsion, severe chest indrawing, fever >37.5°C, hypothermia <35.5°C, movement only with simulation, history of poor feeding, or fast breathing >60 breaths/minute confirmed twice.

[e]Newborns excluded were those with major congenital anomalies; with care directed for anticipated demise; born to mothers <18 years of age; or born between 3:00 PM Friday to midnight Saturday (due to inability to enroll).

[f]Congenital malformation and or ELBW (birth weight <1,000 g) excluded.

[g]IMNCI criteria: temperature >37.5°C or felt hot to touch, convulsions (by history), fast breathing (>60 breaths/minute), severe chest in drawing, nasal flaring, grunting, bulging fontanelle, pus draining from ear, umbilical redness extending to the skin, feels cold (by history), many or severe skin pustules, difficult to wake up, cannot be calmed within 1 hour, less than normal movement, not able to feed by bottle or breast.

Once infected, the quality of the fetal and neonatal immune responses determines whether infection leads to the development of the systemic immune response syndrome (SIRS) that is the hallmark of severe EOS (35,36). Adaptive immune responses are not present at birth, leaving the newborn dependent on innate immune responses and maternally derived humoral immunity. Pattern recognition through innate immune cell surface molecules such as toll-like receptors (TLR) on monocytes and macrophages initiate the neonatal innate immune response. Gram-positive pathogens primarily signal by lipoteichoic acid stimulation of TL2-mediated pathways, and Gram-negative bacteria primarily signal by lipopolysaccharide (endotoxin) stimulation of TL4-mediated pathways (35,36). Intracellular signaling and activation of gene expression results in a release of a variety of proinflammatory molecules, including cytokines, chemokines, complement proteins, and coagulant proteins. These molecules function in host defense by activating endothelial responses, recruiting neutrophils, and activating complement. Anti-inflammatory counter-regulatory responses are also activated; the complex balance of these responses contributes to the overall severity of SIRS. Circulating bacteria also prompt additional innate responses such as the production of acute phase reactants, including procalcitonin and C-reactive protein (CRP) (35,36,38).

Clinical Features

The signs and symptoms of EOS among newborns are nonspecific, often similar to the transitional instability that may occur among term infants, and especially difficult to distinguish from the cardiorespiratory immaturity commonly displayed among preterm infants (4,27,39–42). A very small proportion of term infants with confirmed bacteremia may remain asymptomatic of infection but in many term and preterm infants, EOS can progress to severe septic shock (42,43). Vital sign instability is often present, including tachycardia, tachypnea, and temperature instability. Respiratory signs may range from mild tachypnea with or without a requirement for supplemental oxygen to profound respiratory failure due to pneumonitis, primary or secondary surfactant deficiency, and/or pulmonary hypertension with persistent fetal circulation. Persistent pulmonary hypertension is characteristic of neonatal sepsis and may be worsened by specific bacterial toxins such as the phospholipid components of the GBS cell membrane (44). Cardiovascular systemic symptoms range from poor perfusion and metabolic acidosis to hypotension and cardiac dysfunction. Cardiovascular instability can result from the production of vasoactive substances in activated endothelium, classically with peripheral vasodilation, decreased vascular resistance and hypotension, or so-called warm shock. Neonates may also present with so-called cold shock characterized by cardiac dysfunction and variable degrees of blood pressure instability. Severe sepsis may be complicated by hypoxic–ischemic encephalopathy with or without meningitis. Septic shock may evolve to multisystem organ failure with oliguria, liver dysfunction including coagulopathy, bone marrow suppression with leukopenia, neutropenia, and thrombocytopenia. Disseminated intravascular coagulation can result from the overproduction of coagulant protein production and endothelial activation and damage. Ultimately the combination of hypotension, hypoxia, and endothelial and microangiopathic injury may result in irreversible multisystem organ failure and death.

Approximately 50% to 70% of infants with EOS will present with signs of illness at the time of birth in HIC such as the United States, and approximately 90% will present by 24 hours of age (41,43). However, a small proportion of term infants can present after 24 hours of age, particularly those ultimately determined to be infected with GBS, despite negative maternal antenatal screening results and no significant intrapartum risk factors for EOS (41). Such cases may represent infants born to mothers who screened falsely negative for GBS or whose colonization status changed during the period between screening and delivery. In LMIC, EOS may present more frequently up to 3 to 7 days of age among infants in the community.

Risk factors

Factors that promote or reflect intra-amniotic infection (IAI) may be used to assess risk of EOS (45–49). Preterm birth and low birth weight are strong risk factors for infection: IAI is a significant cause of preterm birth itself in addition to the immune vulnerability of the preterm infant. At the other end of the gestational age spectrum, postterm infants born after 41 weeks of completed gestation are also at slightly higher (approximately 1.6-fold) risk of EOS compared to those born 37 to 40 weeks of gestation (49). The etiology of increased risk associated with postterm birth is unclear, but changes in the integrity of the amniotic membranes and cervical mucosa as well as placental senescence may contribute to decreased barrier defenses to infection.

Multiple intrapartum characteristics are also predictive of EOS in both HIC and LMIC settings. Duration of ROM is a risk factor for EOS among term and late preterm infants, as longer ROM promotes ascending colonization and infection of the uterine and fetal compartments. Preterm, prelabor rupture of membranes (PPROM) is associated with increased risk of EOS among preterm infants, but the exact relationship between duration of PPROM and infection is modified by the administration of latency antibiotics and obstetric management. Signs of maternal IAI (previously referred to as clinical chorioamnionitis) are strong predictors of neonatal infection. These signs include maternal intrapartum fever, maternal tachycardia, and uterine tenderness, all of which are reasonably sensitive but lack specificity for predicting EOS. The American College of Obstetrics and Gynecology (ACOG) provides guidance for the definitive and suspected diagnosis of maternal IAI (50). The diagnosis of IAI is confirmed by amniotic fluid culture, Gram stain and/or biochemical analysis consistent with infection, as well as by placental histopathology consistent with infection and inflammation. Amniotic fluid–based diagnostic information is usually obtained when assessing a pregnant woman who presents with preterm labor and is less relevant to women laboring at term for whom definitive evidence of IAI is more often obtained by placental histopathology. Suspected IAI is diagnosed in the laboring woman when maternal intrapartum temperature ≥39.0°C occurs alone, or maternal temperature in the 38.0°C to 38.9°C range occurs as well as when maternal leukocytosis, purulent cervical drainage, or fetal tachycardia is present. Isolated maternal fever is defined as the occurrence of maternal intrapartum temperature ≥39.0°C alone, or persistent maternal temperature in the 38.0°C to 38.9°C range without additional clinical risk factors. The administration of maternal intrapartum antibiotics for confirmed or suspected IAI as well as for isolated intrapartum maternal fever can decrease the risk of both serious maternal infectious complications as well as the risk of neonatal EOS.

Maternal vaginal–rectal colonization GBS is a predictor for GBS-specific EOS in populations where this organism is prevalent (see *Microbiology*). Vertical transmission of GBS from mother to fetus and newborn is almost exclusively the source of neonatal early-onset GBS disease, in contrast to late-onset neonatal GBS disease, which may be due to either vertical or horizontal maternal transmission or horizontal transmission from nonmaternal caregivers and household sources. The risk posed by maternal GBS colonization is significantly reduced by administration of intrapartum antibiotic prophylaxis (IAP) to laboring GBS-colonized mothers (51). IAP can temporarily reduce maternal and fetal colonization with GBS and reduce the risk of progression to invasive GBS infection. Widespread implementation of recommended practices for maternal antenatal culture-based screening for GBS colonization and appropriate administration of IAP has been associated with a nearly 10-fold decline in the incidence of GBS-specific EOS in the United States (52). This approach is not universally accepted. The U.K. National Health Service does not recommend antenatal GBS screening but recommends use of IAP if specific risk factors are identified during labor (53). In contrast, GBS screening using intrapartum nucleic acid amplification testing and use of IAP to prevent GBS disease was recommended by a European consensus conference of perinatal experts (54). Nonetheless, as seen in Table 47.1, the relative importance of this organism varies across different settings.

Obstetric practices such as the frequency of vaginal examinations during labor and the use of invasive fetal monitoring have been associated with increased risk of EOS in some observational studies (47,55). These findings are confounded by their associations with other factors such as length of labor and ROM and preterm delivery and may be related to introduction of nosocomial pathogens in settings with poor hygiene at delivery.

Microbiology

The organisms causing EOS across international settings are shown in Table 47.1. In the United States and other HIC, Gram-positive organisms, primarily GBS, predominate. Fungal infections are reported but are uncommon, constituting approximately 2% of all infections in U.S. surveillance and occurring exclusively among preterm infants. Despite use of targeted IAP, GBS is the most common organism isolated in U.S. EOS case infants born ≥37 weeks' gestation, whereas *Escherichia coli* is the predominant organism isolated among those born ≤36 weeks' gestation. The differential between these two most common causes of EOS is greater with decreasing gestational age: among those born at 22 to 28 weeks' gestation, the rate of *E. coli* disease is 120-fold higher than among those born at ≥37 weeks' gestation (12 cases/1,000 among low-gestation vs. 0.10 cases/1,000 among term infants). Gram-negative organisms predominate in India and other Asian countries, with *Klebsiella*, *Acinetobacter*, and *E. coli* most commonly isolated.

Although GBS are predominantly identified in HIC, the role of this pathogen in neonatal sepsis may be underestimated in LMIC where clinical (rather than culture-based) approaches are taken to identify infection. An international meta-analysis estimated that worldwide in 2015, over 300,000 cases of early- and late-onset GBS disease occurred, accounting for approximately 90,000 neonatal deaths and greater than 50,000 fetal deaths or stillbirths (56). GBS are found as colonizing species in approximately 18% of pregnant women worldwide, with significant regional variation (11% to 35%) (57). Of the 10 immunologically distinct GBS serotypes, types I to V predominate, and type III accounts for approximately 25% of most neonatal disease. Serotype distribution also varies regionally, however, and the less common types VI to IX are found predominantly in Asian countries. Unlike *E. coli*, GBS are not considered a normal and necessary constituent of the maternal gastrointestinal and genitourinary flora, and thus, efforts are ongoing to develop effective multivalent GBS vaccines. Such vaccines could reduce the international burden of perinatal GBS disease, with potential positive impacts on maternal, fetal, and neonatal infection as well as on preterm birth (58).

Risk Assessment

Different approaches may be taken to determine the risk that an individual infant is at enough risk of EOS to administer empiric antibiotic therapies and pursue diagnostic testing. In both LMIC and HIC, clinical illness prompts concern for EOS among newborns of all gestational ages. In HIC, the presence of specific risk factors has been used to assess risk of EOS at birth among well-appearing infants, with the rationale that infants may be identified in early, presymptomatic or minimally symptomatic stages of infection and administered antibiotics to prevent progression into severe sepsis syndrome. The efficacy of this rationale is not clear, but bacteremia is documented to occur in initially well-appearing newborns in the United States where this approach to EOS risk assessment is routinely taken, albeit at very low rates approaching 1 in 10,000 live births (42).

Table 47.2 summarizes representative international approaches to EOS risk assessment. The American Academy of Pediatrics (AAP) provides guidance for term and preterm infants separately (59,60). The rationale for this approach is that among term infants (defined as those born ≥35 0/7 weeks' gestation), the pathogenesis of EOS most commonly develops during the course of labor, and

TABLE 47.2

EOS Risk Assessment among Infants Born ≥35 0/7 Weeks' Gestation

Source	Approach/Population	Factors Considered	Recommendations
AAP 2018/2019	Categorical Infants ≥35 0/7 gestation	1. Signs of newborn clinical illness (defined by clinician) 2. Maternal intrapartum temperature ≥38°C 3. Inadequate GBS intrapartum antibiotic prophylaxis (when indicated)	Blood cultures and antibiotics for indications (1) and (2) Clinical observation for (3) Alternative: Blood cultures and antibiotics for indications (1) only Clinical observation for (2) and (3)
AAP 2018/2019	Neonatal Early-Onset Sepsis Calculator[a] Infants ≥35 0/7 gestation	1. GA at birth 2. Highest maternal intrapartum temperature 3. Duration of ROM 4. Maternal GBS status 5. Type and duration of intrapartum antibiotic 6. Infant clinical status over the first 6–12 hours of age (clinical issues defined by calculator)	Calculator makes recommendations for laboratory evaluation, blood cultures and antibiotics based on risk estimates
AAP 2018/2019	Delivery characteristics ≤34 6/7 gestation	Reason for preterm birth 1. Concern for intra-amniotic infection 2. Preterm labor 3. Preterm, prelabor rupture of membranes 4. Maternal health indications (non–infection related) 5. Fetal status (non–infection related)	Blood cultures and antibiotics indicated for (1–3) Blood cultures and antibiotics NOT recommended for infants born for (4, 5) if born by cesarean section in absence of labor and with ROM at delivery Blood cultures and antibiotics indicated for (4, 5) if born with induced labor or attempts to induce labor (with vaginal or cesarean delivery) if newborn has respiratory or cardiorespiratory instability
WHO/YIP	All gestational ages (primary for evaluation in community setting)	1. Not feeding well or 2. Convulsions or 3. Fast breathing (60 breaths/min or more) or 4. Severe chest indrawing 5. Fever (≥37.5°C) 6. Hypothermia (<35.5°C) 7. Movement only when stimulated or no movement at all	Administer antibiotics (give first dose intramuscular if evaluated in community) Refer for hospital admission
NICE (United Kingdom)	All gestational ages	1. Red flags: a. Maternal antibiotic treatment for confirmed or suspected invasive bacterial infection 24 h before; during labor; or 24 h after delivery (excluding GBS IAP) b. Suspected or confirmed infection in another baby in the case of a multiple pregnancy c. Respiratory distress starting >4 hours age d. Seizures e. Mechanical ventilation in term infant f. Signs of shock 2. Risk factors: a. Mother GBS positive b. Invasive GBS infection in a prior infant c. Prelabor rupture of membranes d. Spontaneous preterm birth e. ROM > 18 h in preterm birth f. Intrapartum fever >38°C, or confirmed or suspected chorioamnionitis 3. Clinical indicators[b]	Laboratory evaluation, blood cultures and antibiotics for infants with • Any red flag • Two or more "non–red flag" risk factors or clinical indicators Antibiotics should not be delayed pending test results.

[a]Neonatal Early-Onset Sepsis Calculator found at: https://neonatalsepsiscalculator.kaiserpermanente.org/.

[b]Clinical indicators include the following: Altered behavior or responsiveness; altered muscle tone; feeding refusal; vomiting, excessive gastric aspirates or abdominal distension; bradycardia or tachycardia; signs of respiratory distress; hypoxia; jaundice within 24 hours of birth; apnea; signs of neonatal encephalopathy; need for cardiopulmonary resuscitation; need for mechanical ventilation in a preterm baby; persistent pulmonary hypertension; temperature <36°C or >38°C; unexplained excessive bleeding, thrombocytopenia, or abnormal coagulation (INR >2.0); oliguria persisting beyond 24 hours after birth; hypoglycemia or hyperglycemia; metabolic acidosis (base deficit ≥ 10); local signs of infection.

EOS, early-onset sepsis; GBS, Group B *Streptococcus*; IAP, intrapartum antibiotic prophylaxis; ROM, rupture of membranes.

THE NEWBORN INFANT

the overall incidence of EOS among such infants (approximately 1/2,000 live births) is low. Therefore, the goal of risk assessment is to determine which newborns are at *high* enough risk to *warrant* EOS evaluation and empiric antibiotic therapy. In contrast, the majority of infants born preterm are born due to spontaneous preterm labor with or without preterm ROM, meaning that infection may be both a cause and a complication of preterm birth. Further, the baseline risk is as high as 1/50 live births for infants born less than 29 weeks' gestation in HIC—meaning that the goal of EOS risk assessment among preterm infants is to determine which infants are at *low* enough risk to be *spared* initiation of empiric antibiotics.

AAP recommends use of categorical or multivariate approaches to risk assessment among term infants. The categorical approach uses dichotomous cutoff values for risk factors, assigning risk on the basis of the presence or absence of specific risk factors and recommends that laboratory evaluation and empiric therapy be administered when the risk factor is present. This approach was recommended in U.S. GBS perinatal prevention guidance from 1996 to 2010, and widely applied to the evaluation of newborns for all microbial causes of EOS. The categorical approach to EOS risk assessment was not prospectively evaluated prior to recommendation, but retrospective studies among infants born ≥35 to 36 weeks' gestation demonstrate that implementation results in 5% to 12% of infants treated with empiric antibiotics (42,61,62). Alternatively, centers may choose to administer empiric antibiotics only to those infants who are clinically ill at birth. Other infants flagged as at risk for EOS can undergo serial, structured physical assessments for 24 to 36 hours after birth and empiric therapies administered if signs of illness develop. A single center in the United States has reported on use of this approach among infants born to mothers diagnosed with chorioamnionitis and reports significantly decreased overall rates of empiric antibiotic use (61).

Multivariate prediction models have been developed that utilize specific risk factors for EOS and account for use of intrapartum antibiotics as well as the evolving clinical condition of the newborn over the first 6 to 12 hours after birth (41,49). These models provide estimated risk of EOS for the individual infant and have been formulated as a Web-based "*Neonatal Early-Onset Sepsis Calculator*" (https://neonatalsepsiscalculator.kaiserpermanente.org). Prospective implementation studies in large birth cohorts demonstrate that this approach can reduce the rate of EOS evaluation and empiric antibiotic administration without safety concerns (42,62). Depending on the thresholds used for specific clinical actions, empiric antibiotic rates of 2.6% to 3.7% have been reported among infants born ≥35 to 36 weeks' gestational age using the sepsis risk calculator. Multiple studies across the United States, United Kingdom, and Europe have validated use of the sepsis calculator and a recent meta-analysis concluded that its use is associated with overall reductions in empiric antibiotic use among term infants without safety concerns. Given that the sepsis calculator was developed in the United States and reflects both obstetric practice common in HIC and universal use of antenatal GBS screening, some concerns remain regarding use of this tool in LMIC.

The comparatively high rate of EOS among preterm infants compared to term infants and the high rates of sepsis-associated mortality among preterm infants has resulted in near-universal use of empiric antibiotic administration among these infants. In a study of over 40,000 preterm infants cared for in 297 centers across the United States from 2009 to 2015, 78.6% of VLBW and 87% of ELBW infants were treated with empiric antibiotics for risk of EOS. Prolonged administration of antibiotics for proven or presumed infection occurred in 20% to 40% of VLBW and ELBW infants, respectively, rates that are roughly 10-fold higher than the incidence of EOS in this population. AAP management guidance now recommends that clinicians focus on delivery characteristics

of preterm infants to identify those that are low risk for EOS and may be spared antibiotic initiation. This guidance is based on evidence from studies that demonstrate the markedly lower risk of EOS among preterm infants born for maternal health indications (primarily preeclampsia) or fetal indications (primarily growth restriction) when there is no additional concern for IAI. When such infants are born by cesarean section in the absence of labor or attempts to induce labor, with ROM at delivery, they are not subject to factors that promote the pathogenesis of EOS and are very low to no risk of EOS, regardless of their clinical condition at birth (63,64). While a very preterm infant born to a woman with clinical concern for IAI, with evidence of histologic chorioamnionitis on placental pathology, may have a risk of EOS as high as 1/20, the risk among infants born by cesarean section, without labor or ROM prior to delivery, for maternal preeclampsia may be close to zero (64). One center reported on the impact of using this approach to EOS risk assessment in a study of VLBW infants admitted to the NICU over an 11-year period with declines in overall antibiotic use without safety concerns (65).

The U.K. National Health Service provides extensive guidance for the use of risk factors and clinical findings to determine which newborns are at highest risk for EOS and should be administered empiric therapies. The National Institute for Health and Care Excellence (NICE) guidelines consider many of the same factors considered by the AAP guidance and apply to both term and preterm infants. Because many of the clinical indicators are nonspecific, the NICE guidelines have been associated with relatively high rates of empiric antibiotic therapies compared to the incidence of culture-confirmed EOS in the United Kingdom (66).

In LMIC, EOS risk assessment often occurs in the community setting due to home birth and/or rapid maternal hospital discharge after birth. In such settings, the goal of neonatal evaluation is to rapidly identify infants at risk for EOS, administer initial antibiotic therapy, and refer for hospitalization. The Young Infants Clinical Signs Study sought to determine if the WHO Integrated Management of Illness approach to clinical assessment could be utilized in infants less than 7 days of age. The study enrolled over 3,000 infants in the first week of age and established the utility of seven signs (Table 47.2) to identify infants with severe illness who would derive benefit from initiation of antibiotic therapy in the community and referral for hospitalization (67).

Diagnostic Evaluation for Early-Onset Infection

The diagnosis of EOS is optimally made by culture of a pathogenic species from blood and/or CSF, prior to administration of empiric antibiotics. If not done with the initial evaluation, CSF analysis and culture should be performed when bacteremia is identified. Urine culture is not indicated for EOS diagnosis, and culture of tracheal or gastric secretions or skin surfaces will not distinguish colonization from infection. When clinical criteria are used in LMIC settings, particularly when used in community setting remote from advanced medical care, antibiotics may be administered intramuscularly prior to any diagnostic evaluation. In such settings, markers of inflammation and/or molecular methods may be used in place of culture-based methods in both clinical care and in formal studies to assess the presence of bacterial or viral infection.

Blood cultures

Appropriate blood culture technique can minimize concerns around the sensitivity of blood culture to detect bacteremia. Standard pediatric blood culture bottles should be inoculated with a minimum of 1 mL of blood to optimize organism recovery. The use of both aerobic and anaerobic culture bottles can optimize isolation of strict anaerobic species, particularly among preterm infants. One site that routinely obtained both aerobic and anaerobic cultures among VLBW reported that 17% of isolates were strict anaerobes, primarily *Bacteroides* species (63). Obtaining two blood cultures may optimize recovery of potentially low-level bacteremias. Modern blood culture systems use automated, continuous detection technologies with identification of a positive culture within 24 hours for most clinically relevant bacterial pathogens. Time-to-positivity data for neonatal EOS cultures collected from multiple sites over a 20-year period found that the median TTP was 21.0 hours (IQR, 17.1 to 25.3 hours) with 68% of bacterial pathogens isolated by 24 hours, 94% by 36 hours, and 97% by 48 hours' incubation. In this study, neither gestational age (term vs. preterm) or organism Gram stain (gram positive vs. gram negative) nor the administration of maternal intrapartum antibiotics significantly impacted TTP (67).

Cerebrospinal Fluid Culture and Analysis

Although meningitis is most often a metastatic complication of bacteremia, meningitis can very rarely occur in isolation. CDC active surveillance identified 1,277 cases of GBS EOS occurring in the United States from 2005 to 2016; CSF was the only source of bacterial isolation in 11 (0.1%) of cases. Overall rates of culture-confirmed early-onset meningitis range from 0.01 to 0.03 cases/1,000 live births among infants in HIC, although the incidence may be 10-fold higher when assessed by CSF cell counts, and as high as 0.8 cases/1,000 live birth among infants born in LMIC. Lumbar puncture is often deferred as part of the initial evaluation for EOS if the newborn is physiologically unstable. Evidence supports deferring lumbar puncture and CSF culture when EOS evaluation is being performed on the basis of risk factors for an initially well-appearing infant, with later CSF examination in the rare cases of confirmed bacteremia. In contrast, lumbar puncture for CSF culture and analysis is considered to the standard of care for evaluation of the febrile infant 8 to 90 days of age.

Ideally, when indicated, lumbar puncture and CSF cell count, protein and glucose measurement, and culture should be done prior to initiation of empiric antibiotic therapy at high risk for meningitis. CSF can be rapidly sterilized with parenteral antibiotic administrations, and determination of normative values for CSF is challenging (68). Values can vary by gestational age at birth and by postnatal age at the time of lumbar puncture, resulting in wide ranges of potential "normal values." Among term-born infants from 0 to 90 days of age, mean values for CSF WBC range from 3 to 20 cells per high-power field in the majority of studies, with reported upper limits as high as 130 (69). Mean and median values for studies performed in preterm infants generally fall in the 2 to 30 range. Normative CSF protein levels are reported for both term and preterm in 30 to 100 mg/dL range, with upper limits as high as 150 to 200. In contrast, CSF glucose normative values are reported more consistently in the 40 to 60 mg/dL in nearly all studies of both term and preterm infants. Lumbar punctures present a variety of technical difficulties that can result in peripheral blood contamination of the CSF sample. Although a number of algorithms are used to interpret the "bloody tap" CSF, a large study evaluating such approaches demonstrated that none resulted in a reliable estimation of true pleocytosis—emphasizing the importance of obtaining CSF for culture prior to antibiotic administration in high-risk infants (70).

Complete Blood Count

Multiple studies have evaluated the efficacy and utility of the complete blood count (CBC) for EOS diagnosis using test characteristics such as sensitivity, specificity, and positive and negative predictive value. These test characteristics are impacted by the incidence of disease; because of the relatively low incidence of EOS, the optimal test characteristic for evaluation of laboratory test performance is the likelihood ratio (LR). The test is also impacted by a variety of factors other than infection: gestational age at birth, sex, *in utero* growth restriction, mode of delivery,

time (in hours) after birth, maternal pregnancy complications such as preeclampsia and diabetes all can impact some component of the CBC. Two large studies addressed the performance of the white blood cell (WBC) count, immature/total neutrophil ratio (I/T), and absolute neutrophil count (ANC) in predicting culture-confirmed EOS using large multicenter data sets (38,71). Both studies found that values obtained at less than 1 hour age were associated with low LRs, meaning that the results did not significantly modify the prior probability of EOS. Values obtained greater than 4 hours of age were more predictive; extreme values (total WBC count <5,000/μL; I/T >0.3; ANC <2,000/μL in one study and WBC count <1,000/μL; ANC <1,000/μL; and I/T>0.5 in the other) were associated with the highest LRs but very low sensitivities. WBC count greater than 20,000/μL and platelet counts were not associated with EOS in either study. The I/T squared (I/T divided by the ANC) performs better than any of the more traditional tests and is independent of age in hours but also had modest sensitivity and specificity. Overall, no component of the CBC has adequate sensitivity to be used alone as a screen to make decisions regarding antibiotic initiation for EOS.

Inflammatory Biomarkers

Measurements of CRP and procalcitonin have been studied for use in determining risk of EOS, both as single screening values and as serial assessments (38). CRP is an acute-phase reactant synthesized by the liver in response to interleukin-6 release from immune cells. CRP levels do rise during bacterial infection, but CRP will also rise in the setting of common perinatal noninfectious conditions. Elevated CRP has been associated with respiratory conditions including transient tachypnea of the newborn and meconium aspiration, and with birth-associated tissue damage such as bruising and cephalohematoma, as well as with iatrogenic tissue damage such as with placement of chest tube for pneumothorax (71). The sensitivity of CRP at the time of EOS evaluation is particularly poor; in one series of 1,002 EOS evaluations, CRP levels performed at the time of sepsis evaluation had a 35% sensitivity for EOS, with a positive predictive value (PPV) of 6.7% and a positive LR of 3.5. In this study, three serial CRP obtained over the 48 hours after EOS evaluation together had increased sensitivity for EOS, but the PPV (5.2%) and LR (3) declined (72). We recently evaluated 4,201 infants of all gestational ages who had CRP performed at the time of blood culture for EOS evaluation at our local institutions. Abnormal CRP levels at the time of EOS evaluation occurred in only 42% of culture-confirmed cases of EOS and also were found in 10% of newborns with sterile cultures. The PPV for CRP at EOS evaluation in this study was 2.3%, with a positive LR of 4. The poor performance of CRP at the time of EOS evaluation means that this laboratory test should not be used alone to determine empiric antibiotic therapy for EOS, particularly among the lowest risk term infants for whom an LR 3–4 will not substantially increase the estimated risk of infection. Nonetheless, serial normal CRP levels over the 36 to 48 hours after birth are associated with the absence of EOS and may be of use in LMIC where blood culture is not readily available. PCT, an inflammatory mediator that is produced both by the liver and directly by WBCs, rises in response to bacterial infection faster than does CRP. However, PCT rises normally in the hours after birth, and like CRP, PCT levels also rise in response to noninfectious conditions. Specific normative ranges by age in hours as well as by gestational age at birth are needed to optimally interpret PCT, limiting its use for evaluating risk of EOS as a single measurement at birth (38). Interleukin-6 itself and other cytokines such as soluble interleukin-2 receptor, interleukin-8, and tumor necrosis factor as well as inflammatory cell adhesion molecules have been studied as predictive markers of EOS. None have demonstrated sufficient sensitivity and specificity, and none are widely available for clinical use.

Molecular Methods

Advanced molecular-based methods for identification of infectious organisms are emerging, including polymerase chain reaction and microarray techniques. Use of such techniques, if available, can add to the use of blood culture to identify the organisms causing EOS. Such techniques do not distinguish live bacteria from traces of bacterial nucleic acid, however, and may identify organisms of uncertain clinical impact. In a large prospective study conducted in South Africa, use of a molecular assay identified five times as many organisms in blood than culture, with *Ureaplasma* the most common isolates (23).

Imaging Studies

Chest radiographs should be obtained in the diagnostic evaluation when respiratory signs are present. Radiographs may aid in distinguishing lung immaturity, pneumonia, and retained fetal lung fluid, although the radiographic abnormalities associated with each can overlap in the newborn period. The typical diffuse ground-glass opacities found with surfactant deficiency may also be present with pneumonitis, and the patchy opacities of retained lung fluid may mimic infectious infiltrates.

Empiric Therapy

Empiric therapy for EOS should target the most common microbial isolates identified in local surveillance studies. In the United States, United Kingdom, and Europe, where GBS and *E. coli* predominate, an aminopenicillin and aminoglycoside are commonly used in combination as empiric therapy. Increasing resistance among Gram-negative organisms is a challenge in both HIC and LMIC settings. Resistance to both ampicillin and gentamicin was reported in 10% of EOS cases caused by *E. coli* in U.S. reports from 2009 to 2017 (73). Despite the prevalence of gram-negative infections in LMIC, the WHO recommends intramuscular ampicillin and gentamicin as first-line antibiotics for clinical neonatal sepsis prior to hospital admission (74). Definitive therapy should be targeted to the identified organism in culture-confirmed cases, and the duration of therapy should be tailored to the clinical response and extent of infection: EOS complicated by meningitis will require longer therapy. There is no current evidence to support the use of adjunctive therapies such as granulocyte-stimulation factors or intravenous immunoglobulin (IVIG) in EOS. An international study that randomized 3,493 infants (95 with EOS) to two infusions of IVIG or placebo observed no difference in the combined outcome of death or disability at 2 years of age (75). Supportive therapies should be targeted to organ dysfunction, with the use as needed of supplemental oxygen, mechanical ventilation, inhaled nitric oxide, intravenous volume, vasoactive pressors, blood product transfusion, and intravenous nutrition to optimize oxygenation, maintain blood pressure and end-organ perfusion, minimize bleeding and thrombosis, and reverse acid/base, glucose, and electrolyte imbalance. Infants of adequate birth weight and gestational age may require extracorporeal membrane oxygenation support (as available), if conventional intensive care fails to provide adequate cardiopulmonary support.

▌LATE-ONSET SEPSIS

Definitions

There are important differences in the epidemiology, microbiology, evaluation, and management of continuously hospitalized, primarily preterm infants with suspected infection in the first weeks after birth, as compared to previously healthy newborns who present from the community with suspected serious bacterial infection (SBI) up to 3 months of age. The evaluation of hospitalized infants for late-onset, nosocomial infection is covered in Chapter 22. The following section will address the evaluation of previously healthy term and late preterm infants presenting from the community for suspected SBI from 8 to 89 days of age.

Epidemiology

While viral infections accounts for most febrile episodes among infants less than 90 days of age, the risk of SBI is substantial. The incidence of SBI in febrile otherwise healthy infants less than 90 days of age in the United States is approximately 5% to 11% when defined as bacteremia, bacterial meningitis, or UTI (76,77). Risk of SBI is higher in infants less than 1 month of age (and particularly among those <21 days of age), higher in those presenting to an emergency department, and lower in infants with confirmed viral infection and in those presenting to an outpatient clinic (76,78–80). SBI prevalence is lower in infants with a reported history of fever who are afebrile at evaluation, compared with those who remain febrile at emergency department visit (81). UTI is the most common type of SBI among these infants, occurring in approximately 10% to 15% of evaluations among infants less than 90 days of age (78). UTI usually occurs alone but can occur concomitantly with bacteremia and/or meningitis (82,83). Bacteremia is less common, identified in 3% to 7% of infants less than 29 days of age and 1% to 2% of febrile infants 29 to 60 days of age, while bacterial meningitis is identified in 1% to 2% of infants less than 29 days of age and 0.2% to 0.4% of those ages 29 to 60 days (78,82,83). Depending on age, up to 20% of bacteremic infants may also have meningitis. The ANISA study prospectively evaluated the incidence of infection among 63,114 infants born in communities in Bangladesh, India, and Pakistan from 2011 to 2014 (84). Using the WHO/YIP clinical criteria for possible SBI (**Table 47.2**), the overall infection rate from birth to 59 days of age was 9.5% (84).

Microbiology

The bacterial microbiology of SBI infants less than 3 months of age continues to evolve, with recent reports in the United States establishing *E. coli* as the most commonly identified organism (79,82,85). GBS remains a common cause, and although the incidence of GBS in the first week after birth has declined significantly since the introduction of IAP for colonized women, late-onset GBS disease incidence remains unchanged in the United States at 0.2 to 0.3 cases per 1,000 live births (2,86). *Listeria monocytogenes*, a classic cause of neonatal infection, is relatively rare now in HIC, possibly related to advances in food safety (82). Other reported Gram-positive pathogens include *Streptococcus viridans*, *Staphylococcus aureus*, *Enterococcus* species, as well as *Streptococcus pneumoniae*, which is more common in older infants (76,82,83). Other reported gram-negative organisms include *Klebsiella* species and *Salmonella*; *Neisseria meningitidis* may present in infants with an underlying immune disorder such as complement deficiency or asplenia (76,83).

Viral infections are the underlying cause of most febrile illnesses among infants less than 90 days of age. Respiratory syncytial virus (RSV), influenza virus, enterovirus, parechovirus, adenovirus, rhinovirus, parainfluenza virus, and rotavirus are common etiologies (78,87). Parechovirus type 3 and enteroviruses may cause sepsis-like illness that is particularly difficult to distinguish from SBI and may be associated with aseptic meningitis (88–91). One study used molecular methods to identify parechovirus in 9.5% of 1,475 febrile infants less than 60 days of age (89). Diagnosis of a viral infection decreases the risk of SBI, but coinfection is possible. In a multicenter study of 2,945 febrile infants less than 60 days who were tested for at least one viral pathogen, the incidence of UTI was 2.8% and of bacteremia was 0.8% among virus-positive infants, whereas UTI was identified in 10.7% and bacteremia in 2.9% among virus-negative infants (80). Rhinovirus diagnosis by molecular methods can be particularly problematic, as infants may have PCR-detectable virus for weeks after initial infection and this diagnosis may therefore not lower the risk of SBI (78).

Herpes simplex virus (HSV) is an uncommon but life-threatening viral cause of febrile illness among young infants (111). HSV infection occurs at a rate of 4 to 5 cases per 10,000 live births in a large U.S. study (92). Unlike other viral causes of fever in the young infant, HSV infection must be treated with antiviral medications to mitigate severe morbidity and mortality. Clinicians should consider this pathogen among febrile infants with lesions suggestive of HSV, in those with evidence of CSF pleocytosis, in those with unexplained transaminitis, and/or in those infants with severe clinical presentation (93,94) (see Chapter 46).

Diagnostic Evaluation

Routine evaluation of well-appearing febrile infants less than 90 days of age starts with a thorough history and physical examination in both HIC and LMIC. Sick contacts and immunization history, respiratory signs associated with viral infection, as well as focal infection sources such as otitis media or skin and soft tissue infections may help to narrow the differential diagnosis. In LMIC, the WHO/YIP signs are useful in identifying infants who require empiric therapy and referral to higher levels of care, coupled with diagnostic cultures and laboratory tests when available.

Blood Culture, Urinalysis and Urine Culture, CSF Analysis and Culture

Diagnostic culture-based evaluation includes blood, urine, and CSF culture. Urine specimens should be obtained by catheterization (or less commonly, sterile bladder aspiration) to avoid contamination (90). Lumbar puncture is generally recommended in febrile infants less than 1 month of age given the relatively higher risk of among febrile but well-appearing infants less than 21 days of age (91). In contrast, the incidence of meningitis is significantly lower among otherwise well-appearing infants 29 to 90 days of age; among these infants, the value of routine lumbar puncture is an area of debate and site-specific practice variation persists (85,95–99). Normative values for CSF analysis are discussed in the section above on EOS. Most blood and CSF cultures for bacterial pathogens turn positive within 24 hours among febrile infants with SBI (100).

Urinalysis may indicate the presence of UTI, and different indices (WBC per high power field, nitrite, leukocyte esterase) are used in common risk algorithms (Table 47.3). Abnormal urinalysis is highly correlated with culture-confirmed UTI among febrile infants less than 60 days of age (105). UTI is diagnosed by growth of a pathogenic species at a colony count of $\geq$50,000 species from a catheter specimen and $\geq$10,000 species from a bladder aspirate specimen; variably, UTI may be diagnosed by $\geq$100,000 species from a urine bag specimen if the same species is isolated from a blood culture.

Complete Blood Count and Inflammatory Markers

Additional diagnostic tests with utility in the evaluation of suspected SBI include the CBC and ANC, CRP, and procalcitonin. In contrast to the use of these tests in evaluation of EOS, each has clinical utility in the evaluation of the febrile infant for SBI when combined with other components of the evaluation (76,85,106). Multiple studies have demonstrated that clinical appearance alone is not a sensitive indicator of SBI in febrile infants (107). Different approaches have been proposed and evaluated (Table 47.3) with

TABLE 47.3

Evaluation of Outpatient Febrile Infant

Criteria (References)	Age	Exclusion Criteria	Low-Risk for SBI Criteria	Management Goal	% SBI	Outcome or Statistics
Boston (101)	28–89 d	• Ill-appearing • Vaccines <48 h prior • Antibiotics <48 h prior • Concern for site-specific infection	• WBC <20,000 • CSF <10 • No leukocyte esterase on urinalysis	Outpatient management with IM ceftriaxone	27/503 (5.4%)	95% managed entirely as outpatient
Philadelphia (102)	29–56 d	• Infant observation score >10 • Concern for site-specific infection • Bloody CSF	• WBC <15,000 • WBC <10 and few bacteria on urinalysis • CSF WBC<8 • Chest film without focal infiltrate	Outpatient management without antibiotics	Low risk: 1/287 (0.4%) Not low risk: 64/460 (13.9%)	SBI prediction: Sensitivity: 98% Specificity: 42% Positive LR: 1.7 Negative LR: 0.05
Rochester (103)	≤60 d	• Ill-appearing • Birth ≤36 weeks' gestation • Perinatal antibiotics • Recent antibiotics • Unexplained hyperbilirubinemia • Hospitalized at birth longer than mother • Underlying health issues	• WBC 5–15,000 • ANC ≤1,500 • WBC <10 on urinalysis • WBC <5 in stool[a]	Rule development for potential management without antibiotics	Low risk: 5/437 (1.1%) Not low-risk: 61/494 (12.3%)	Negative predictive value of low-risk criteria for SBI: 99%
Clinical prediction rule (104)	≤60 d	• Ill-appearing • Antibiotics <48 h prior • Birth ≤36 weeks' gestation • Preexisting medical conditions (including immunodeficiency) • Indwelling devices • Concern for site-specific infection	Leukocyte esterase, nitrite or WBC >5 on urinalysis ANC >4,090 PCT ≥1.7 ng/mL	Rule development: Secondary analysis of RNA microarray study	Low risk: 1/522 (0.2%) Not low risk: 81/386 (21%)	SBI prediction: Sensitivity: 97.7% Specificity: 60.0% Positive LR: 2.44 Negative LR: 0.04

[a]Stool analysis performed if infant had history of diarrhea.

ANC, absolute neutrophil count; CSF, cerebrospinal fluid; IM, intramuscular; LR, likelihood ratio; WBC, white blood count; PCT, procalcitonin. Units: Peripheral blood WBC expressed as count per 10^9 cells/L; ANC expressed as count per 10^6 cells/L; CSF cell counts expressed as count per high-power field or cubic millimeter; urine and stool WBC as count per high-power field.

THE NEWBORN INFANT

the goal of decreasing the proportion of otherwise well-appearing febrile infants that are hospitalized and/or treated with empiric antibiotics. The Boston, Philadelphia, and Rochester risk stratification criteria utilize routine testing components, yet each algorithm has notable differences (Table 47.3). The Philadelphia and Rochester criteria were developed for infants under 60 days of age while the Boston criteria were developed for infants under 90 days. Research continues into new prediction rules and tools; one recent approach proposes the use of urinalysis, ANC, and procalcitonin (Table 47.3) to identify otherwise well-appearing infants who can be spared empiric antibiotics.

Viral Testing

HSV testing should be performed in febrile newborns less than 1 month of age and in infants with vesicular skin lesions, CSF pleocytosis, or seizures (76,94,103). Testing should include HSV PCR-based testing of blood, CSF and mucosal surfaces (eyes, nasopharynx, mouth, rectum), and any skin lesions. Chest radiograph and respiratory viral testing for RSV, influenza, and other respiratory viruses including SARS-CoV-2 (individually or as part of a "respiratory panel") may be indicated in febrile infants with respiratory distress to modify SBI risk as well as to evaluate for evidence of viral and bacterial pneumonia (76). PCR-based testing is available to identify enteroviruses and parechoviruses in both blood and CSF; one study identified parechovirus in 9.5% of 1,475 febrile infants less than 60 days of age (89). Routine use of enteroviral testing has been shown to reduce hospitalization and antibiotic use and duration of hospitalization among febrile infants (90,91).

Empiric Treatment

Empiric antimicrobial coverage for infants with suspected SBI presenting from the community should target the most likely infecting pathogens. For infants 8 to 28 days of age who are not critically ill and in whom meningitis is not overtly suspected, ampicillin and ceftazidime are the recommended combination, while ceftriaxone is the recommended empiric monotherapy for infants for infants aged 29 to 90 days in the United States (83,86). For all infants between 8 and 90 days of age who are critically ill or with concern for meningitis (i.e., bulging fontanelle, seizure, CSF pleocytosis), the addition of vancomycin should be considered given the potential for infection with beta-lactam–resistant S. pneumoniae (86). Given the evolving threat of antimicrobial resistance, regional infection epidemiology and local antibiograms should be taken into account when choosing appropriate empirical therapies (76). Empiric acyclovir should be included for infants undergoing evaluation for HSV (94). The WHO recommends use of oral amoxicillin and intramuscular gentamicin for community treatment of infants with clinical signs of possible SBI before referral to tertiary care centers (74).

SITE-SPECIFIC INFECTION

Omphalitis

Omphalitis is characterized by signs of infection in the periumbilical region, including periumbilical cellulitis and purulent discharge from the umbilical stump. This infection can be caused by the same organisms as those that cause EOS, as well as by environmental contamination of the cord. Omphalitis may progress to severe cellulitis and invasive abdominal wall and peritoneal infection, with progression to involve the abdominal blood vessels and liver in the most severe cases. Severe omphalitis is rare in HIC, and clean, dry cord care is the standard recommendation. In LMIC setting with poor sanitation, the WHO recommends the application of 4% chlorhexidine daily for the first week after birth to prevent cord infection (74). Systemic antibiotics are recommended for treatment of omphalitis after obtaining blood and pus samples for culture.

Neonatal Tetanus

Neonatal tetanus infection is caused by the anaerobic bacterium *Clostridium tetani*. The clinical syndrome is caused by a neurotoxin elaborated by this bacterium that binds to presynaptic motor neurons and results in loss of inhibitory action on motor and autonomic responses (108). Neonatal infection can occur by colonization and infection of the umbilical cord stump, often resulting from unsanitary childbirth and/or cord care practices. The clinical syndrome begins with poor newborn feeding and untreated, proceeds over several days to muscle spasms, seizures, and death. Treatment consists of intensive care support with mechanical ventilation and sedation; specific treatment includes administration of tetanus toxoid and penicillin G. *Clostridia* species are found in soil and can be normal constituents of the intestinal microbiome, and are therefore a common exposure in LMIC with poor sanitation. Maternal tetanus vaccination can prevent neonatal tetanus by transplacental transfer of vaccine-induced antibody to tetanus toxoid. The WHO Maternal and Neonatal Tetanus Elimination initiative has aimed to eliminate neonatal tetanus in LMIC with maternal vaccination. WHO estimated that 787,000 deaths due to neonatal tetanus occurred worldwide in 1988; although not eliminated, it was estimated that by 2018, deaths due to neonatal tetanus had declined to 25,000 (109). The condition is almost entirely eliminated in the United States where the ACOG recommends routine TdaP vaccination during each pregnancy (110). Notably, infants surviving neonatal tetanus infection do not develop immunity and require standard childhood vaccination for tetanus.

Neonatal Conjunctivitis (*Ophthalmia Neonatorum*)

Both viral and bacterial organisms may cause infection and inflammation of the neonatal conjunctivae in the first month after birth. Common bacterial causes include *Neisseria gonorrhoeae* and *Chlamydia trachomatis*, as well as staphylococci and all organisms causing EOS. HSV may also cause conjunctivitis as part of skin, mouth, and eye infection (94). Routine birth eye prophylaxis with erythromycin ophthalmic ointment is standard care in the United States to prevent neonatal conjunctivitis. In LMIC, the WHO recommends one of the following for routine eye prophylaxis at birth: tetracycline hydrochloride 1% eye ointment; erythromycin 0.5% eye ointment; povidone–iodine 2.5% solution (water-based); silver nitrate 1% solution; or chloramphenicol 1% eye ointment (74). Eye prophylaxis, however, will not prevent chlamydial conjunctivitis. Screening pregnant women for gonococcal and chlamydia infection, administering treatment, and ensuring negative test of cure during pregnancy is an important component of preventing neonatal conjunctivitis.

Neonatal conjunctivitis is characterized by conjunctival injection, swollen eyelids, and purulent exudate. Treatment of clinical conjunctivitis is targeted to the most common etiologies. Exudate from neonatal conjunctivitis should be submitted for bacterial culture and additionally tested for gonococcus, chlamydia, and HSV (if indicated) using molecular methods. Gonococcal disease is treated with ceftriaxone and chlamydial disease with erythromycin; in neither condition is topical treatment alone adequate or necessary (108). Infants with gonococcal conjunctivitis should additionally be evaluated for invasive infection. Chlamydial disease may be complicated by pneumonitis. Other bacterial infections may be treated topically with appropriate agents if nonsevere, but severe cases require evaluation for invasive infection and parenteral antibiotic therapy. Infants born to women with untreated gonococcal infection at delivery should receive parenteral ceftriaxone or other appropriate cephalosporin therapy, but prophylactic systemic treatment for infants born to mothers with chlamydial infection at delivery is not indicated.

REFERENCES

1. Newborns: improving survival and well being. Available from: https://www.who.int/news-room/fact-sheets/detail/newborns-reducing-mortality. Accessed October 20, 2020.
2. Nanduri SA, Petit S, Smelser C, et al. Epidemiology of invasive early-onset and late-onset group B streptococcal disease in the United States, 2006 to 2015: multistate laboratory and population-based surveillance. *JAMA Pediatr* 2019;173:224.
3. Schrag SJ, Farley MM, Petit S, et al. Epidemiology of invasive early-onset neonatal sepsis, 2005 to 2014. *Pediatrics* 2016;138:e20162013.
4. Stoll BJ, Puopolo KM, Hansen NI, et al. Early-onset neonatal sepsis 2015 to 2017, the rise of *Escherichia coli*, and the need for novel prevention strategies. *JAMA Pediatr* 2020;174:e200593.
5. Polewiartek LB, Smith PB, Benjamin DK, et al. Early-onset sepsis in term infants admitted to neonatal intensive care units (2011-2016). *J Perinatol* 2021;41:157.
6. Berardi A, Baroni L, Bacchi Reggiani ML, et al. The burden of early-onset sepsis in Emilia-Romagna (Italy): a 4-year, population-based study. *J Matern Fetal Neonatal Med* 2016;29:3126.
7. Kuhn P, Dheu C, Bolender C, et al. Incidence and distribution of pathogens in early-onset neonatal sepsis in the era of antenatal antibiotics. *Paediatr Perinat Epidemiol* 2010;24:479.
8. Morris R, Jones S, Banerjee S, et al. Comparison of the management recommendations of the Kaiser Permanente neonatal early-onset sepsis risk calculator (SRC) with NICE guideline CG149 in infants ≥34 weeks' gestation who developed early-onset sepsis. *Arch Dis Child Fetal Neonatal Ed* 2020;105:581.
9. Braye K, Foureur M, de Waal K, et al. Epidemiology of neonatal early-onset sepsis in a geographically diverse Australian health district 2006-2016. *PLoS One* 2019;14:e0214298.
10. Gao K, Fu J, Guan X, et al. Incidence, bacterial profiles, and antimicrobial resistance of culture-proven neonatal sepsis in South China. *Infect Drug Resist* 2019;12:3797.
11. Shim GH, Kim SD, Kim HS, et al. Trends in epidemiology of neonatal sepsis in a tertiary center in Korea: a 26-year longitudinal analysis, 1980-2005. *J Korean Med Sci* 2011;26:284.
12. Lim WH, Lien R, Huang YC, et al. Prevalence and pathogen distribution of neonatal sepsis among very-low-birth-weight infants. *Pediatr Neonatol* 2012;53:228.
13. Tran HT, Doyle LW, Lee KJ, et al. A high burden of late-onset sepsis among newborns admitted to the largest neonatal unit in central Vietnam. *J Perinatol* 2015;35:846.
14. Turner C, Turner P, Hoogenboom G, et al. A three-year descriptive study of early onset neonatal sepsis in a refugee population on the Thailand Myanmar border. *BMC Infect Dis* 2013;13:601.
15. Investigators of the Delhi Neonatal Infection Study (DeNIS) Collaboration. Characterisation and antimicrobial resistance of sepsis pathogens in neonates born in tertiary care centres in Delhi, India: a cohort study. *Lancet Glob Health* 2016;4:e752.
16. Swarnkar K, Swarnkar M. A study of early onset neonatal sepsis with special reference to sepsis screening parameters in a tertiary care centre of rural India. *Internet J Infect Dis* 2012;10:1.
17. Shehab El-Din EM, El-Sokkary MM, Bassiouny MR, et al. Epidemiology of neonatal sepsis and implicated pathogens: a study from Egypt. *Biomed Res Int* 2015;2015:509484.
18. Chan GJ, Baqui AH, Modak JK, et al. Early-onset neonatal sepsis in Dhaka, Bangladesh: risk associated with maternal bacterial colonisation and chorioamnionitis. *Trop Med Int Health* 2013;18:1057.
19. Akbarian-Rad Z, Riahi SM, Abdollahi A, et al. Neonatal sepsis in Iran: a systematic review and meta-analysis on national prevalence and causative pathogens. *PLoS One* 2020;15:e0227570.
20. Glikman D, Curiel N, Glatman-Freedman A, et al. Nationwide epidemiology of early-onset sepsis in Israel 2010-2015, time to re-evaluate empiric treatment. *Acta Paediatr* 2019;108:2192.
21. Zareifar S, Pishva N, Farahmandfar M, et al. Prevalence of G6PD Deficiency in Neonatal Sepsis in Iran. *Iran J Pediatr* 2014;24:115.
22. Afsharpaiman S, Torkaman M, Saburi A, et al. Trends in incidence of neonatal sepsis and antibiotic susceptibility of causative agents in two neonatal intensive care units in Tehran, I.R Iran. *J Clin Neonatol* 2012;1:124.
23. Velaphi SC, Westercamp M, Moleleki M, et al. Surveillance for incidence onset and etiology of early-onset neonatal sepsis in Soweto, South Africa. *PLoS One* 2019;14:e0214077.
24. Olorukooba AA, Ifusemu WR, Ibrahim MS, et al. Prevalence and factors associated with neonatal sepsis in a Tertiary Hospital, North West Nigeria. *Niger Med J* 2020;61:60.
25. Kayom VO, Mugalu J, Kakuru A, et al. Burden and factors associated with clinical neonatal sepsis in urban Uganda: a community cohort study. *BMC Pediatr* 2018;18:355.
26. Pérez RO, Lona JC, Quiles M, et al. Sepsis neonatal temprana, incidencia y factores de riesgo asociados en un hospital público del occidente de México [Early neonatal sepsis, incidence and associated risk factors in a public hospital in western Mexico]. *Rev Chilena Infectol* 2015;32:387.
27. Stoll BJ, Hansen NI, Sánchez PJ, et al. Early onset neonatal sepsis: the burden of group B Streptococcal and *E. coli* disease continues. *Pediatrics* 2011;127:817.
28. Stoll BJ, Hansen NI, Higgins RD, et al. Very low birth weight preterm infants with early onset neonatal sepsis: the predominance of gram-negative infections continues in the National Institute of Child Health and Human Development Neonatal Research Network, 2002-2003. *Pediatr Infect Dis J* 2005;24:635.
29. Benirschke, K. Routes and types of infection in the fetus and the newborn. *Am J Dis Child* 1960;99:714.
30. Blanc, WA. Pathways of fetal and early neonatal infection. Viral placentitis, bacterial and fungal chorioamnionitis. *J Pediatr* 1961;59:473.
31. Goldenberg RL, McClure EM, Saleem S, Reddy UM. Infection-related stillbirths. *Lancet* 2010;375:1482.
32. Gibbs RS, Roberts DJ. Case records of the Massachusetts General Hospital. Case 27-2007. A 30-year-old pregnant woman with intrauterine fetal death. *N Engl J Med* 2007;357:918.
33. Kusari A, Han AM, Virgen CA, et al. Evidence-based skin care in preterm infants. *Pediatr Dermatol* 2019;36(1):16.
34. Griese M. Pulmonary surfactant in health and human lung diseases: state of the art. *Eur Respir J* 1999;13:1455.
35. Cuenca AG, Wynn JL, Moldawer LL, et al. Role of innate immunity in neonatal infection. *Am J Perinatol* 2013;30:105.
36. Wynn JL, Levy O. Role of innate host defenses in susceptibility to early-onset neonatal sepsis. *Clin Perinatol* 2010;37:307.
37. Fouda GG, Martinez DR, Swamy GK, et al. The impact of IgG transplacental transfer on early life immunity. *Immunohorizons* 2018;2:14.
38. Benitz WE. Adjunct laboratory tests in the diagnosis of early-onset neonatal sepsis. *Clin Perinatol* 2010;37:421.
39. Wynn JL, Wong HR. Pathophysiology and treatment of septic shock in neonates. *Clin Perinatol* 2010;37:439.
40. Wynn J, Cornell TT, Wong HR, et al. The host response to sepsis and developmental impact. *Pediatrics* 2010;125:1031.
41. Escobar GJ, Puopolo KM, Wi S, et al. Stratification of risk of early-onset sepsis in newborns ≥ 34 weeks' gestation. *Pediatrics* 2014;133:30.
42. Kuzniewicz MW, Puopolo KM, Fischer A, et al. A quantitative, risk-based approach to the management of neonatal early-onset sepsis. *JAMA Pediatr* 2017;171:365.
43. Wortham JM, Hansen NI, Schrag SJ, et al. Chorioamnionitis and culture-confirmed, early-onset neonatal infections. *Pediatrics* 2016;137:e20152323.
44. Curtis J, Kim G, Wehr NB, et al. Group B streptococcal phospholipid causes pulmonary hypertension. *Proc Natl Acad Sci U S A* 2003;100:5087.
45. Benitz WE, Gould JB, Druzin ML. Risk factors for early-onset group B streptococcal sepsis: estimation of odds ratios by critical literature review. *Pediatrics* 1999;103:e77.
46. Escobar GJ, Li DK, Armstrong MA, et al. Neonatal sepsis workups in infants ≥2000 grams at birth: a population-based study. *Pediatrics* 2000;106:256.
47. Dutta S, Reddy R, Sheikh S, et al. Intrapartum antibiotics and risk factors for early onset sepsis. *Arch Dis Child Fetal Neonatal Ed* 2010;95:F99.
48. Mukhopadhyay S, Puopolo KM. Risk assessment in neonatal early onset sepsis. *Semin Perinatol* 2012;36:408.
49. Puopolo KM, Draper D, Wi S, et al. Estimating the probability of neonatal early-onset infection on the basis of maternal risk factors. *Pediatrics* 201;128:e1155.
50. Committee on Obstetric Practice. Committee opinion No. 712: intrapartum management of intraamniotic infection. *Obstet Gynecol* 2017;130:e95.
51. Boyer KM, Gotoff SP. Prevention of early-onset neonatal group B streptococcal disease with selective intrapartum chemoprophylaxis. *N Engl J Med* 1986;314:1665.
52. Verani JR, McGee L, Schrag SJ; Division of Bacterial Diseases, National Center for Immunization and Respiratory Diseases, Centers for Disease Control and Prevention (CDC). Prevention of perinatal group B streptococcal disease—revised guidelines from CDC, 2010. *MMWR Recomm Rep* 2010;59:1.
53. UK National Screening Committee. Universal antenatal culture-based screening for maternal Group B Streptococcus (GBS) carriage to prevent early-onset GBS disease. Available from: https://legacyscreening.phe.org.uk/groupbstreptococcus. Accessed October 20, 2020.
54. Di Renzo GC, Melin P, Berardi A, et al. Intrapartum GBS screening and antibiotic prophylaxis: a European consensus conference. *J Matern Fetal Neonatal Med* 2015;28:766.
55. Schuchat A, Zywicki SS, Dinsmoor MJ, et al. Risk factors and opportunities for prevention of early-onset neonatal sepsis: a multicenter case-control study. *Pediatrics* 2000;105:21.
56. Seale AC, Bianchi-Jassir F, Russell NJ, et al. Estimates of the burden of group B streptococcal disease worldwide for pregnant women, stillbirths, and children. *Clin Infect Dis* 2017;65:S200.
57. Russell NJ, Seale AC, O'Driscoll M, et al.; GBS Maternal Colonization Investigator Group. Maternal colonization with group B streptococcus and serotype distribution worldwide: systematic review and meta-analyses. *Clin Infect Dis* 2017;65:S100.

THE NEWBORN INFANT

58. Bianchi-Jassir F, Paul P, To KN, et al. Systematic review of Group B Streptococcal capsular types, sequence types and surface proteins as potential
vaccine candidates. *Vaccine* 2020;38:6682.

59. Puopolo KM, Benitz WE, Zaoutis TE; Committee on Fetus and Newborn,
Committee on Infectious Diseases. Management of neonates born at ≥35
0/7 weeks' gestation with suspected or proven early-onset bacterial sepsis.
Pediatrics 2018;142:e20182894.

60. Puopolo KM, Benitz WE, Zaoutis TE; Committee on Fetus and Newborn,
Committee on Infectious Diseases. Management of neonates born at ≤34
6/7 weeks' gestation with suspected or proven early-onset bacterial sepsis.
Pediatrics 2018;142:e20182896.

61. Joshi NS, Gupta A, Allan JM, et al. Clinical monitoring of well-
appearing infants born to mothers with chorioamnionitis. *Pediatrics*
2018;141:e20172056.

62. Dhudasia MB, Mukhopadhyay S, Puopolo KM. Implementation of the sepsis risk calculator at an academic birth hospital. *Hosp Pediatr* 2018;8:243.

63. Mukhopadhyay S, Puopolo KM. Clinical and microbiologic characteristics
of early-onset sepsis among very low birth weight infants: opportunities for
antibiotic stewardship. *Pediatr Infect Dis J* 2017;36:477.

64. Puopolo KM, Mukhopadhyay S, Hansen NI, et al. Identification of
extremely premature infants at low risk for early-onset sepsis. *Pediatrics*
2017;140:e20170925.

65. Garber SJ, Dhudasia MB, Flannery DD, et al. Delivery-based criteria for
empiric antibiotic administration among preterm infants. *J Perinatol*
2021;41:255.

66. Neonatal infection (early onset): antibiotics for prevention and treatment.
Available from: https://www.nice.org.uk/guidance/cg149. Accessed October 20, 2020.

67. Kuzniewicz MW, Mukhopadhyay S, Li S, et al. Time to positivity of neonatal blood cultures for early-onset sepsis. *Pediatr Infect Dis J* 2020;39:634.

68. Aleem S, Greenberg RG. When to Include a lumbar puncture in the evaluation for neonatal sepsis. *NeoReviews* 2019;20:e124.

69. Srinivasan L, Harris MC, Shah SS. Lumbar puncture in the neonate:
challenges in decision making and interpretation. *Semin Perinatol*
2012;36:445.

70. Greenberg RG, Smith PB, Cotten CM, et al. Traumatic lumbar punctures
in neonates: test performance of the cerebrospinal fluid white blood cell
count. *Pediatr Infect Dis J* 2008;27:1047.

71. Pourcyrous M, Bada HS, Korones SB, et al. Significance of serial C-reactive protein responses in neonatal infection and other disorders. *Pediatrics* 1993;92:431.

72. Benitz WE, Han MY, Madan A, et al. Serial serum C-reactive protein levels
in the diagnosis of neonatal infection. *Pediatrics* 1998;102:E41.

73. Flannery DD, Akinboyo IC, Mukhopadhyay S, et al. Antibiotic susceptibility of *Escherichia coli* among infants admitted to neonatal intensive care
units across the U.S. from 2009 to 2017. *JAMA Pediatr* 2021;175:168.

74. WHO recommendations on newborn health. Updated May 2017. Available from: https://apps.who.int/iris/bitstream/handle/10665/259269/WHO-
MCA-17.07-eng.pdf?sequence=1. Accessed October 20, 2020.

75. INIS Collaborative Group; Brocklehurst P, Farrell B, King A, et al. Treatment of neonatal sepsis with intravenous immune globulin. *N Engl J Med*
2011;365:1201.

76. Biondi EA, Byington CL. Evaluation and management of febrile, well-
appearing young infants. *Infect Dis Clin North Am* 2015;29:575.

77. Nigrovic LE, Mahajan PV, Blumberg SM, et al. The Yale observation scale
score and the risk of serious bacterial infections in febrile infants. *Pediatrics* 2017;140:e20170695.

78. Biondi EA, Lee B, Ralston SL, et al. Prevalence of bacteremia and bacterial meningitis in febrile neonates and infants in the second month of life:
a systematic review and meta-analysis. *JAMA Netw Open* 2019;2:e190874.

79. Powell EC, Mahajan PV, Roosevelt G, et al. Epidemiology of bacteremia in
febrile infants aged 60 days and younger. *Ann Emerg Med* 2018;71:211.

80. Mahajan P, Browne LR, Levine DA, et al. Risk of bacterial coinfections in
febrile infants 60 days old and younger with documented viral infections.
J Pediatr 2018;203:86.

81. Ramgopal S, Janofsky S, Zuckerbraun NS, et al. Risk of serious bacterial
infection in infants aged ≤60 days presenting to emergency departments
with a history of fever only. *J Pediatr* 2019;204:191.

82. Mischler M, Ryan MS, Leyenaar JK, et al. Epidemiology of bacteremia in previously healthy febrile infants: a follow-up study. *Hosp Pediatr* 2015;5:293.

83. Woll C, Neuman MI, Pruitt CM, et al. Epidemiology and etiology of invasive
bacterial infection in infants ≤60 days old treated in emergency departments. *J Pediatr* 2018;200:210.

84. Saha SK, Schrag SJ, El Arifeen S, et al. Causes and incidence of community-acquired serious infections among young children in south Asia
(ANISA): an observational cohort study. *Lancet* 2018;392:145.

85. Dorney K, Bachur RG. Febrile infant update. *Curr Opin Pediatr*
2017;29:280.

86. Puopolo KM, Lynfield R, Cummings JJ; Committee on Fetus and Newborn; Committee on Infectious Diseases. Management of infants at risk
for group B streptococcal disease. *Pediatrics* 2019;144:e20191881.

87. Tomatis Souverbielle C, Wang H, Feister J, et al. Year-round, routine testing of multiple body site specimens for human parechovirus in young
febrile infants. *J Pediatr* 2021;229:216.

88. Olijve L, Jennings L, Walls T. Human parechovirus: an increasingly recognized cause of sepsis-like illness in young infants. *Clin Microbiol Rev*
2017;31:e00047.

89. Souverbielle CT, Wang H, Feister J, et al. Year-round, routine testing of multiple body site specimens for human parechovirus in young
febrile infants. *J Pediatr* 2020;S0022-3476(20)31266-X. Online ahead of
print.

90. Paioni P, Barbey F, Relly C, et al. Impact of rapid enterovirus polymerase
chain reaction testing on management of febrile young infants < 90 days
of age with aseptic meningitis. *BMC Pediatr* 2020;20:166.

91. Wallace SS, Lopez MA, Caviness AC. Impact of enterovirus testing on
resource use in febrile young infants: a systematic review. *Hosp Pediatr*
2017;7:96.

92. Mahant S, Hall M, Schondelmeyer AC, et al. Neonatal herpes simplex
virus infection among medicaid-enrolled children: 2009-2015. *Pediatrics*
2019;143:e20183233.

93. Kimberlin DW. When should you initiate acyclovir therapy in a neonate?
J Pediatr 2008;153:155.

94. Kabani N, Kimberlin DW. Neonatal herpes simplex virus infection. *NeoReviews* 2018;19:e89.

95. Martinez E, Mintegi S, Vilar B, et al. Prevalence and predictors of bacterial
meningitis in young infants with fever without a source. *Pediatr Infect
Dis J* 2015;34:494.

96. Scarfone R, Murray A, Gala P, et al. Lumbar puncture for all febrile infants
29-56 days old: a retrospective cohort reassessment study. *J Pediatr*
2017;187:200.

97. Mintegi S, Benito J, Astobiza E, Well appearing young infants with fever
without known source in the emergency department: are lumbar punctures always necessary? *Eur J Emerg Med* 2010;17:167.

98. Aronson PL, Thurm C, Alpern ER, et al. Variation in care of the febrile
young infant <90 days in US pediatric emergency departments. *Pediatrics* 2014;134:667.

99. Rogers AJ, Kuppermann N, Anders J, et al. Practice variation in the evaluation and disposition of febrile infants ≤60 days of age. *J Emerg Med*
2019;56:583.

100. Alpern ER, Kuppermann N, Blumberg S, et al. Time to positive blood and
cerebrospinal fluid cultures in febrile infants ≤60 days of age. *Hosp Pediatr* 2020;10:719.

101. Baskin MN, O'Rourke EJ, Fleisher GR. Outpatient treatment of febrile
infants 28 to 89 days of age with intramuscular administration of ceftriaxone. *J Pediatr* 1992;120:22.

102. Baker MD, Bell LM, Avner JR. Outpatient management without antibiotics of fever in selected infants. *N Engl J Med* 1993;329:1437.

103. Jaskiewicz JA, McCarthy CA, Richardson AC, et al. Febrile infants at low
risk for serious bacterial infection—an appraisal of the Rochester criteria and implications for management. Febrile Infant Collaborative Study
Group Pediatrics. *Pediatrics* 1994;94:390.

104. Kuppermann N, Dayan PS, Levine DA, et al. A clinical prediction rule to
identify febrile infants 60 days and younger at low risk for serious bacterial infections. *JAMA Pediatr* 2019;173:342.

105. Tzimenatos L, Mahajan P, Dayan PS, et al. Accuracy of the urinalysis for
urinary tract infections in febrile infants 60 days and younger. *Pediatrics*
2018;141:e20173068.

106. Milcent K, Faesch S, Gras-Le Guen C, et al. Use of procalcitonin assays to
predict serious bacterial infection in young febrile infants. *JAMA Pediatr*
2016;170:62.

107. Pantell RH, Newman TB, Bernzweig J, et al. Management and outcomes of
care of fever in early infancy. *JAMA* 2004;291:1203.

108. American Academy of Pediatrics. Tetanus (Lockjaw). In: Kimberlin DW,
Brady MT, Jackson MA, et al., eds. Red Book: 2018 *Report of the Com-
mittee on Infectious Diseases.* 31st ed. Itasca, IL: American Academy of
Pediatrics, 2018:793.

109. Maternal and Neonatal Tetanus Elimination (MNTE). Available from:
https://www.who.int/immunization/diseases/MNTE_initiative/en/.
Accessed October 20, 2020.

110. Committee on Obstetric Practice, Immunization and Emerging Infections Expert Work Group. Committee opinion no. 718: update on immunization and pregnancy: tetanus, diphtheria, and pertussis vaccination.
Obstet Gynecol 2017;130:e153.

111. Caviness AC, Demmler GJ, Almendarez Y, et al. The prevalence of neonatal herpes simplex virus infection compared with serious bacterial illness
in hospitalized neonates. *J Pediatr* 2008;153:164.

48 Immunology

Kristin Scheible

INTRODUCTION

The immune system is diverse and flexible, and its primary role is to protect against pathogen invasion. In the fetus and neonate, however, it also plays an important role in organ development (1,2). The human immune system is organized by solid organs (thymus, spleen, lymph nodes), soluble (complement, antimicrobial peptides, immunoglobulin), and cellular (myeloid and lymphoid) components and begins to develop in the early first trimester of gestation. Immune functions during early embryogenesis primarily support organ development, including brain, lung, gut, and secondary lymphoid organs (3–7). Toward the end of pregnancy, the immune system acquires specialized functions to enable coordinated protection and regulation during the postnatal period of rapid microbial colonization and exposure to novel infections (8).

Newborns experience more frequent and more severe infections compared to older pediatric patients. In the healthy full term, susceptibility can be attributed to physiologic immaturity of the (naive) adaptive immune system that will eventually acquire protective antigen-specific memory. The premature infant, however, is in a relatively immunodeficient state due to additional factors such as lack of maternal antibody transfer, disrupted physical barriers between a newborn's internal and external environment (central lines, endotracheal tubes), and exposure to immunosuppressive medications such as steroids (**Fig. 48.1**). Even nonsteroidal anti-inflammatories, which are commonly used for IVH prophylaxis, for ductal closure, and as antipyretics, may play a role in altering vaccine- or infection-induced cytokine responses and mucosal immunity (9–13). Developmentally determined differential immunity affects responses to natural infections as well as vaccines administered in the first year and may also increase risk for immune dysregulation in preterm infants (14–18). For these reasons, primary immunodeficiencies (PID) can be difficult to distinguish from other causes of infection in newborns, particularly in preterms. Although the most severe PID phenotypes and genotypes are rare, it is essential that providers caring for newborns recognize concerning signs and initiate time-critical evaluation and therapies, as PID survival improves with earlier treatment. PID should be considered in any infant with recurrent, severe, or opportunistic infections, deep tissue infections, failure to thrive, chronic, immune dysregulation, or chronic diarrhea, when out of proportion to expected course for a given gestational age (**Fig. 48.2**).

There are over 300 known PID, and these disorders can affect cellular components, soluble mediators, and solid organs of the immune system (19). Clinical and laboratory features have been used in the past to organize diagnostics and treatment strategies, and these strategies are increasingly being replaced by more targeted treatments tailored to diagnostics determined by genetic sequencing (19–24). Given the breadth of PID phenotypes and genotypes, this chapter will focus on those immunodeficiencies more commonly encountered in the newborn period, with an emphasis on aspects of fetal and neonatal immune development that can mimic PID.

SOLID ORGAN DEVELOPMENT AND DISORDERS

Congenital Athymia and Thymic Hypoplasia

The thymus is an anterior mediastinal structure originating from the bilateral 3rd and 4th pharyngeal pouches that develops during the 7th week of gestation. T-cell precursors can be found in the thymus by 8 weeks, and thymic function, as measured by recent thymic emigrant (RTE) T cells in the peripheral blood, can be detected as early as 23 weeks' gestation (25). In addition to T cells, natural killer cells and T regulatory cells also mature in the thymus. T-cell lineages are severely diminished in conditions associated with congenital athymia or thymic hypoplasia (**Table 48.1**). Acquired thymic dysfunction and acute thymic involution can also be seen in preterm and full-term newborns exposed to hypoxic stress, acidosis, severe infection, or exogenous steroids and should also be considered in cases of apparent thymic insufficiency (26–29).

Prior to genetic studies, conditions with congenital heart disease, thymic, and parathyroid hypoplasia/aplasia were collectively referred to as DiGeorge syndrome, based on their shared clinical phenotype. 22q11.2 deletion is now found in over 85% of patients with DiGeorge (30), and the majority (90% to 95%) are de novo mutations. The 22q11.2DS clinical phenotype is due to interrupted migration of structures derived from the rostral neural crest (31). Eighty-five percent of patients with DiGeorge have hypoparathyroid/parathyroid aplasia, which causes a profound hypocalcemia. In addition to thymus and parathyroid gland, 22q11 deletion can, but does not always, involve other neural crest–derived midline structures, including cardiac (interrupted aortic arch, truncus arteriosus, tetralogy of Fallot) and craniofacial (laryngomalacia, palatal or lip cleft, hypertelorism, broad nasal bridge, hearing loss). Patients with 22q11.2 are at increased risk for neuropsychiatric complications, including intellectual disabilities and schizophrenia (32).

22q11 deletion was previously diagnosed by fluorescence *in situ* hybridization (FISH) targeting the deleted *N25* and *TUPLE* genes. Sequencing methods are now favored due to their more complete coverage of affected regions proximal or distal to those targeted by FISH, including the regions containing low copy repeats (LCR22B-D) associated with the familial forms of 22q11.2 syndromes (31,32). The clinical phenotype of complete DiGeorge overlaps with severe combined immunodeficiency (SCID), due to the severely diminished or absence of peripheral T cells. Death is nearly universal by 2 years of age without intervention. However, even in the apparent absence of thymus in the expected anatomic location, ectopic rests of functional thymic tissue can deposit along its migratory track, and severity of infectious complications from DiGeorge correlate with the amount of residual functional thymic tissue. Patients with Down syndrome also display diminished thymic function, and there is overlap in thymus histopathology between patients with Down syndrome and DiGeorge, including poor corticomedullary differentiation and epithelial dysfunction marked by decreased AIRE (autoimmune regulator) expression. Complete DiGeorge, the most extreme phenotype where there is total absence of thymic function, is only found in 1% of patients, but 30% of patients with 22q11 deletions will have mild–moderate lymphopenia (31,33–35).

Treatment for DiGeorge involves a multidisciplinary approach, and prevention of immune-related complications depends on the degree of immunosuppression. Antibiotic prophylaxis, immunoglobulin replacement, and calcium supplementation may be needed, as well as surgery to address hearing loss and palate and cardiac abnormalities. Live vaccines are strictly avoided. Outcomes following hematopoietic cell transplant are not as favorable in comparison to SCID, because progenitor cells still require a thymus to fully mature. Whole blood from an HLA-matched sibling

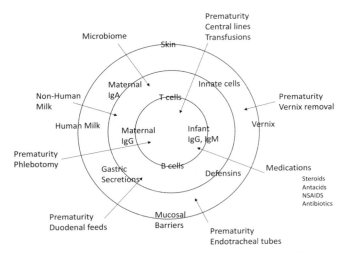

FIGURE 48.1 Immunodeficiency secondary to breeches of natural immunity in the newborn.

TABLE 48.1

Disorders of Thymic Development

Disorder	Gene	Features
CHARGE	*CHD7, SEMA3E*	Coloboma, cardiac anomalies, choanal atresia, genitourinary anomalies, ear anomalies
DiGeorge	Chromosome 22q11.2	Facial dysmorphisms, conotruncal anomalies, hypoparathyroidism
TBX1 deficiency	*TBX1*	Renal disease, deafness

can provide mature T cells, however, which may be beneficial in the setting of life-threatening infection (36). Thymus transplant for complete DiGeorge is currently under investigation, and early trials suggest that there may be survival advantage compared to hematopoietic cell transplant (37–40).

CHARGE syndrome is another known syndrome with thymic hypoplasia and is defined by a constellation of symptoms: Coloboma

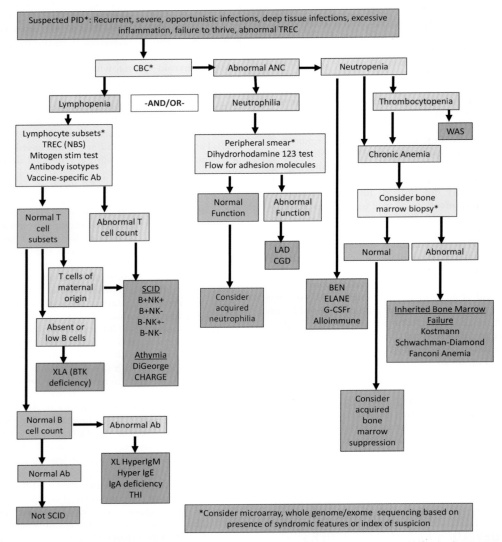

FIGURE 48.2 Algorithm for initial PID evaluation. PID, primary immune deficiency; CBC, complete blood count; ANC, absolute neutrophil count; TREC, T-cell receptor excision circle; Ab, antibody, XLA, X-linked agammaglobulinemia; THI, transient hypogammaglobulinemia of infancy; LAD, leukocyte adhesion defect; CGD, chronic granulomatous disease; BEN, benign ethnic neutropenia; NBS, newborn screen; WAS, Wiskott-Aldrich syndrome.

of the eye, *H*eart defects, *A*tresia of the choanae, *R*etardation of growth, *G*enitourinary abnormalities, and *E*ar abnormalities. De novo mutations in the CHD7 gene are found in 90% of children meeting diagnostic criteria (41). In a meta-analysis of studies describing clinical phenotype of patients with CHARGE, 80% of patients had low or absent T cells and 61% had hypogammaglobulinemia. Ninety-five percent of patients with T-cell lymphopenia had thymic aplasia or hypoplasia. Abnormalities of B and NK cells were rare (42). Treatment for CHARGE-associated immunodeficiency parallels DiGeorge, in that it is dependent on severity of lymphopenia and is focused on prophylaxis against opportunistic infection. Patients with SCID-like phenotype may be candidates for immune replacement therapy (19).

Asplenia and Hyposplenia

The spleen buds off from the dorsal mesogastrium by 5 weeks, and hilar vessels appear by 8 weeks. Hematopoietic cells populate the spleen at 7 to 8 weeks, and their secretion of Lymphotoxin-alpha stimulates the development of splenic functional compartments. Red pulp develops first, followed by white pulp in the late second trimester. The marginal zone defines the interface between the red and white pulp and is not fully developed until 1 to 2 years of age. The spleen is organized to facilitate antigen presentation between professional antigen-presenting cells (APC) and T and B cells, which triggers the generation of cellular and humoral memory (43–45). Marginal zone B cells and macrophages are specialized cell populations that recognize polysaccharides contained in the cell wall of encapsulated bacteria such as *Streptococcus pneumoniae*, *Haemophilus influenza b*, *Neisseria meningitides*, *Staphylococcus aureus*, *Salmonella*, *Klebsiella*, and *Escherichia coli* (46). Two opsonins, tuftsin and properdin, are produced in the spleen, and lower levels can be a harbinger of diminished splenic function (47). Due to the multiple spleen-dependent mechanisms central to clearing encapsulated bacteria in the bloodstream, neonates respond poorly to encapsulated bacteria in part due to the structural immaturity of the spleen.

Asplenia or hyposplenia has a 60% male predominance and can be found in isolation as an autosomal dominant condition or as part of one of several syndromes associated with isomerism (Table 48.2). Suspicion for asplenia or hyposplenia should be raised in newborns with abnormal visceral situs, high fraction of Howell-Jolly bodies on complete blood counts, persistent thrombocytosis, or recurrent, severe infections from encapsulated bacteria. Patients with hyposplenia/asplenia should undergo genetic evaluation and anatomic screening by ultrasound to assess for associated cardiac or other visceral anomalies. The presence of polysplenia in patients with left-sided isomerism on imaging studies does not exclude functional hyposplenia. To assess for functional hyposplenia in high-risk patients, a pitted erythrocyte count, which contain perimembranous vacuoles of accumulated waste visible by microscopy, greater than 4% is concerning. If the spleen is unable to be identified on abdominal ultrasound, or if the splenic function is uncertain, ^{99m}Tc-labelled, heat-altered, autologous erythrocyte scintigraphy can be considered for more definitive functional testing (47–49).

Management of asplenia focuses on prophylaxis against encapsulated organisms. Conjugate vaccines, which recruit T helper cells to promote B-cell maturation and antibody class switching, are recommended for asplenic patients, as T-independent B-cell responses are impaired. Conjugate pneumococcal PCV13 and Hib vaccines are given at 2, 4, 6, and 12 months. Quadrivalent meningococcal conjugate vaccine MCV4 (Menveo) is also added to the 2-, 4-, 6-, and 12-month infant series. PPV23, the pneumococcal polysaccharide vaccine, is administered after 24 months, even in asplenic infants who were fully vaccinated with PCV13. Yearly influenza vaccine starting at 6 months is recommended, and all household contacts are encouraged to receive the complete age-appropriate series of vaccinations (50). Antibiotic prophylaxis with oral amoxicillin, preferably with clavulanate until 3 months if tolerated, or penicillin VK should be initiated upon diagnosis (49,50).

▌IMMUNE CELL DEVELOPMENT AND DISORDERS

Developmental Hematopoiesis

Hematopoiesis begins with hematopoietic stem cells (HSCs) and is the process from which all lineages of circulating cells arise, including both myeloid and lymphoid immune cells. HSCs are a self-renewing, pluripotent cell population found in the human embryo as early as day 25, and their presence continues through adulthood (6). The fate of an HSC is determined by sequentially restricted expression of lineage-specific molecular signals, and gene mutations leading to interruptions in these signals are associated with loss of function or number of their dependent cell populations (Fig. 48.2), and the evaluation of PID can therefore be informed by specific features of a patient's immune cell distribution (Fig. 48.3). The earliest erythroid and myeloid progenitor populations are derived from *primitive hematopoiesis* occurring in the yolk sac (2 to 6 weeks' gestation) and are the only monocyte progenitors capable of forming microglia. Next, *definitive hematopoiesis I* happens in the aorta–gonad–mesonephros and liver (5 to 22 weeks' gestation), forming erythroid, myeloid, and select lymphoid populations. Finally, *definitive hematopoiesis II* begins in the bone marrow (11 weeks' gestation–adulthood), and these progenitors differentiate into the fully diverse, mature pool of circulating myeloid and lymphoid cells. Whether or not there are functional immune consequences in premature newborns resulting from the relative admixture of immune cells derived from *definitive hematopoiesis I and II* has not been fully explored, but likely contributes to immunoinsufficiency during the newborn period.

Inherited Bone Marrow Failure Syndromes

Inherited bone marrow failure (IBMF) syndromes are characterized by loss of one or more hematopoietic cell lines and cause primary immunodeficiency when leukocyte cell lineages are affected (Table 48.3). Defects underlying IBMF affect mechanisms common to many critical cell cycle processes, including DNA repair, telomere maintenance, or ribosomal biosynthesis, and therefore often manifest multiorgan involvement beyond the hematopoietic system. IBMF presentation in the newborn can be indolent, and sometimes, disease discovered only after a first acute severe infection and progressive or persistent hematologic abnormalities are identified. IBMF syndromes are rare, and their recognition is confounded by the far more prevalent causes of bone marrow suppression and cytopenias in the newborn, including sepsis, congenital infections (TORCHS), intrauterine growth restriction, and preeclampsia (51–54).

TABLE 48.2
Disorders of Spleen Development

Syndrome	Gene (Inheritance)	Features
Isolated congenital asplenia	*RPSA* (AD)	Isolated
Ivemark syndrome	Unknown	Right-sided isomerism, heterotaxy
Stomorken syndrome	*STIM1* (AD)	Myopathy, thrombocytopenia, ichthyosis
Polysplenia syndrome	Multiple	Left-sided isomerism, heterotaxy

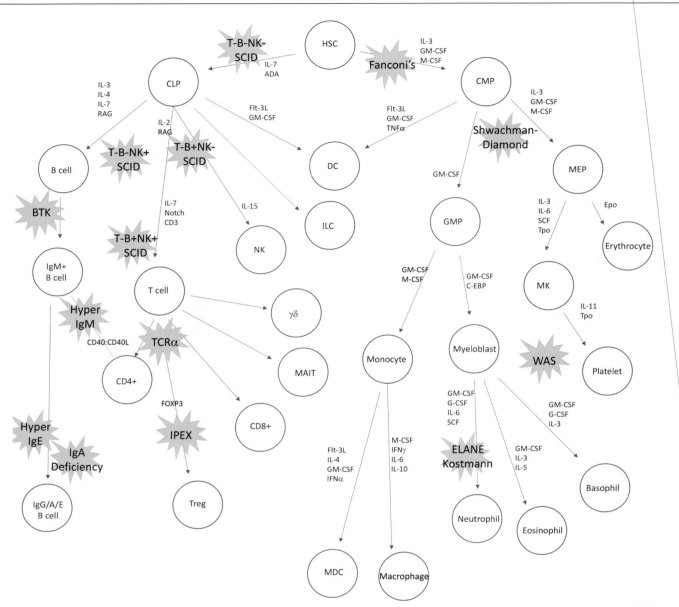

FIGURE 48.3 Immune cell ontogeny and related PID. HSC, hematopoietic stem cell; CMP, common myeloid progenitor; MEP, myeloerythroid progenitor; GMP, granulocyte myeloid progenitor; MK, megakaryocyte; MDC, myeloid dendritic cell; CLP, common lymphoid progenitor; DC, dendritic cell; ILC, innate lymphoid cell; NK, natural killer cell; MAIT, mucosal-associated invariant T cell; Treg, T regulatory cell. (Image courtesy of Dr. Kristin Scheible.)

Fanconi Anemia

Fanconi anemia (FA) is usually an autosomal recessive and less often an X-linked disorder affecting DNA repair genes (55). Bone marrow failure rarely presents in the newborn period, though FA can present in the newborn period when associated with common nonhematologic findings, including short stature, upper limb abnormalities, microcephaly, triangular facies, and renal anomalies. Diagnosis of FA should be considered in patients with VACTERL-H (VACTERL with hydrocephalus) as there is considerable phenotypic overlap (56,57). Patients with FA are treated with granulocyte colony-stimulating factor (G-CSF), often in combination with androgens and erythropoietin in order to improve blood counts. HSCT is considered definitive treatment, though transplant has not been proven to reduce the risk of FA-associated malignancy (58).

Shwachman-Diamond Syndrome

Shwachman-Diamond syndrome (SDS) is an AR IBMF disorder associated with mutations in the SDBS gene in greater than 90% of patients. SDBS mutations affect ribosome biogenesis, a critical

pathway in protein synthesis for all cells. SDS can present early in life, most often with exocrine pancreatic insufficiency or systemic features including failure to thrive, skin rashes, palatal defects, metaphyseal dysostosis, and syndactyly (57,59). Immunodeficiency is generally less severe than other PID and is associated with neutropenia and impaired neutrophil chemotaxis (60). The CBC in SDS is distinct from other IBMF syndromes in that the B-cell counts are usually normal to elevated, and the bone marrow response will show an appropriate reticulocyte count. Treatment should include G-CSF to address the neutropenia and fat-soluble vitamin supplementation to compensate for poor fat absorption. HSCT has been successful in treating patients with severe, progressive pancytopenia (61).

Congenital Neutropenias and Disorders of Neutrophil Function

Mature, circulating neutrophils are activated through a range of environmental sensing mechanisms and are typically the first to localize to sites of acute infection and injury. Under normal conditions,

TABLE 48.3

Select PID Associated with Neutropenia with or without Bone Marrow Failure

Syndrome	Features	Gene Defect (Inheritance)	Treatment
Congenital neutropenia secondary to ELANE mutations	**Most frequent primary neutropenia**, congenital, chronic or cyclic neutropenia recurrent, severe infections	ELANE mutations (AR)	G-CSF, bactrim
Kostmann syndrome	Severe, chronic neutropenia Neurologic disease Monocytosis, eosinophilia Arrest of neutrophils at promyelocytes, cognitive delay, and epilepsy	HAX1 gene (AR)	G-CSF, bactrim, BMT
Autoimmune primitive neutropenia	**Most frequent chronic neutropenia in children**, late arrest of neutrophils, macrophagia of intramedullary PMNs	(Auto-antibody against FcRgIIIb)	Conservative
Fanconi anemia	Pancytopenia Short limbs, upper limb anomalies, microcephaly, renal anomalies	DNA repair genes (AR, XL)	G-CSF Androgens HSCT
Shwachman-Diamond syndrome	Intermittent neutropenia Pancytopenia Exocrine pancreas insufficiency Narrow thorax, respiratory distress Neurologic disease	SDBS (AR)	G-CSF Bactrim Erythropoietin Growth hormone ADEK vitamins
Cartilage hair hypoplasia	Short-limbed dwarfism, fine hair, lymphopenia	RMRP	Bactrim
Wiskott-Aldrich syndrome	Eczema, thrombocytopenia	WAS (XL)	IVIG Bactrim HSCT
Chédiak-Higashi syndrome	Oculocutaneous albinism, bleeding	LYST (AR)	Bactrim HSCT

neutrophils develop in the bone marrow in response to G-CSF and other cytokines, and are then released into circulation as mature polymorphonuclear cells (PMN cells). Inflammatory states, both sterile and infectious, can trigger release of immature neutrophil precursors. Neutrophils peak in the newborn by 12 hours of age and contract to steady-state levels after 72 hours. Egress from the circulation into tissue follows a series of receptor-regulated steps, from endothelial attachment, rolling, and arrest to crawling and transmigration. Once localized, neutrophils phagocytose and destroy pathogen through ROS production, and release of antimicrobial peptide-decorated neutrophil extracellular traps (NETs).

An absolute neutrophil count (ANC) below 1,000/µL is a generally accepted threshold for defining neutropenia, and ANC below 500/µL is associated with a significant risk for infection if persistent (62). Sepsis, maternal hypertension, twin–twin transfusion, alloimmunization, and hemolytic disease are the most frequent causes of neutropenia. Small for gestational age (SGA) infants are more likely to experience neutropenia, and counter to earlier studies, the association appears to be independent of either maternal hypertension or preeclampsia (63). Inflammatory states can suppress neutrophil function (chemotaxis, phagocytosis, and oxidative burst) in adults, though the extent to which sepsis impairs neutrophils in neonates is not well studied (64,65). Maturation of neutrophil function continues through gestation for each of these functions (66,67), and neutrophil impairments can therefore be a consequence of either developmental physiology (e.g., extreme prematurity), perinatal exposures, or from an inherited neutrophil disorder. Neutrophils in premature infants, for example, have impaired NET-related antimicrobial function, and in full terms, dysregulated NET function may contribute to illness severity during sepsis (68,69). The above etiologies are the most common causes of transient neutropenia in the newborn, and improvement can be expected within 1 to

2 weeks following birth or with resolution of the inflammatory state (66). Another reversible neutropenia that can persist to 3 to 6 months is alloimmune neutropenia, which can be diagnosed based on identification of serum human neutrophil antigen (HNA)-reactive antibodies in the mother (70).

Perinatal causes of neutropenia usually resolve within a week, whereas primary congenital neutropenias are distinguished by severe (<500/µL) and *persistently* diminished ANC in the absence of infection or other secondary cause (71). While there is significant overlap in phenotype between congenital neutropenias and IBMF, IBMF can be distinguished by more than one cell lineage being affected. Persistent neutropenia in an otherwise well-appearing infant should raise concern for a congenital syndrome affecting neutrophil maturation. Of the dozens of inherited neutropenic syndromes, relatively few present in the newborn period, but when they do occur, can associate with severe infections or inflammatory conditions such as necrotizing enterocolitis. Treatment for the majority of congenital neutropenias, with the exception of those due to G-CSF receptor defects, targets stimulating neutrophil maturation using high-dose G-CSF (70).

Benign ethnic neutropenia (BEN) is the most frequent form of chronic neutropenia. BEN is found in individuals of African descent and is defined based on a lower neutrophil count relative to normal ranges established in populations predominantly of European descent, but normal neutrophil maturation and function (72). Many single-nucleotide polymorphisms predict lower neutrophil count in patients with BEN, and population-based cohort studies have linked BEN to a Duffy null allele, rs2814778 (73). The Duffy null allele may be more frequent in individuals of African descent as it confers protection against *Plasmodium vivax* malaria infection (74). As the name suggests, BEN is benign, and treatment is not indicated.

THE NEWBORN INFANT

The most common inherited form of isolated congenital neutropenia, representing 40% to 55% of infants with congenital neutropenia, is caused by mutations in the genes encoding ELANE (neutrophil elastase). ELANE mutations are inherited in an autosomal dominant fashion and cause arrest of neutrophil development at the promyelocyte stage. ELANE mutations present either as cyclic, oscillating in a 21-day cycle, or persistent, severe congenital phenotypes, and serial neutrophil counts are needed to distinguish between these patterns. The severe congenital phenotype is associated with systemic and deep tissue bacterial and fungal infections, and there are no known extrahematopoietic manifestations. In a series of G-CSF untreated patients, mouth ulcers occurred in 80% and pneumonia was documented in 49% (75).

The most common congenital neutropenia *with extrahematopoietic findings* is Kostmann syndrome. Kostmann syndrome is an autosomal recessive form of neutropenia caused by mutations in the *HAX-1* gene, which encodes for the protein HS-1-associated protein X. HAX-1 plays a role in maintaining mitochondrial membrane potential and cell survival, and mutations result in early-stage maturational arrest of neutrophils (76,77). Kostmann syndrome is a severe form of congenital neutropenia and is characterized by neurologic sequelae including developmental delay and epilepsy (78). Severe congenital neutropenia due to ELANE-related and HAX-1 mutations are associated with acute leukemia, and because the risk is increased in patients requiring high-dose G-CSF exposure to maintain neutrophil counts, these patients may benefit from early HSCT (79).

Disorders of neutrophil function (**Table 48.4**) should be suspected in cases of recurrent serious bacterial infections and are differentiated from other phagocyte-related PID in the presence of neutrophilia and absence of purulence. Leukocyte adhesion deficiencies (LAD1 to LAD3) are due to defects in neutrophil chemotaxis and adhesion; cells are able to mature and proliferate but are unable to localize to sites of inflammation. LAD-associated infections of the skin and mucosa include *S. aureus*, Gram-negative bacteria, and Candida species. Newborns can have delayed cord separation, but LAD1 will usually have an associated omphalitis. Autosomal recessive LAD1 caused by diminished leukocyte integrin CD18 expression is the most common form and can be diagnosed by low CD18 expression assessed by flow cytometry (80–84). Treatment involves prompt use of antibiotics and surgical wound debridement, and HSCT is curative (85–87).

Chronic granulomatous disease (CGD) is a PID that presents in early life with failure to thrive, recurrent respiratory tract infections, lymphadenitis, visceral abscesses, and granulomatous lesions infected with *S. aureus*, *Burkholderia cepacia*, *Serratia marcescens*, *Nocardia*, and *Aspergillus* spp. CGD is most often inherited in males in an X-linked pattern (XL-CGD) and is linked to mutations in the *CYBB* gene. More recently, autosomal recessive

(AR-CDG) forms of CGD have been found associated with other loci related to the NADPH oxidase system. Formation of characteristic granulomas is secondary to defects in the bactericidal oxidative burst that normally follows phagocytosis of bacteria. Persistence of intracellular bacterial antigen leads to formation of granulomas in an effort to contain spread of infection (88). Confirmatory testing for CGD includes flow cytometric analysis of the neutrophil oxidative burst using dihydrorhodamine 123 (DHR) (88). Genetic sequencing is indicated, especially in females with suspected CGD. TMP/SMX and antifungal prophylaxis should be initiated upon diagnosis, and HSCT has been successful at achieving long-term survival (89–91).

T-Cell Deficiencies

SCID is a heterogeneous set of conditions that affect lymphoid cells. Impaired CD3+ T-cell development is a shared feature among all SCID conditions, but because of the mutual dependence of lymphoid cells on T-cell help, as well as their common molecular determinants for differentiation, B and natural killer (NK) cells are also either directly or indirectly affected. The majority of infants with SCID do not typically present immediately at birth, as placentally transferred maternal antibody affords transient protection. By 6 months of age, however, maternal antibody wanes significantly, and most SCID-affected infants will show signs within this time such as recurrent severe or opportunistic infections, growth failure, chronic diarrhea, or chronic candidiasis (22). With the exception of X-linked interleukin-2 receptor gamma (IL2rγ) disorder, the more common SCID diseases are inherited in an autosomal recessive pattern. Continued advances in genetic sequencing-based diagnostics have led the Errors of Immunity Committee's (previously International Union of Immunologic Societies) PID Expert Committee to regularly revise classification schemes for SCID and other PID (21). SCID can be organized into four broad groups based on lymphoid lineages affected (B+/NK+, B+/NK−, B−/NK+, and B−/NK−), and more than one lineage is affected when there are shared molecular determinants for differentiation (Table 48.5). As with other PID, SCID can be further divided into syndromic or nonsyndromic groups, and associated examination findings can be helpful for targeting evaluation and additional screening based on a narrowed diagnosis.

Concern for SCID should be raised in an infant presenting with two or more of several criteria: chronic diarrhea, failure to thrive, abnormal newborn screen, abnormal lymphocyte counts, family history of SCID, family history of pediatric deaths from opportunistic infection, atypical frequency, severity or location of infection, or physical stigmata consistent with immunodeficiency syndrome. SCID is a medical emergency and should prompt *immediate* consultation and referral to a regional immunodeficiency specialist. Diagnostic measures to evaluate for SCID include tests

TABLE 48.4

Leukocyte Function Defects

Function	Disorder (Gene/Inheritance)	Presentation	Diagnosis	Management
Adhesion	Leukocyte adhesion deficiency (Types I-III) (CD18/AR)	Neutrophilia, delayed cord separation, omphalitis, gingivitis, peritonitis, absence of abscess formation or pus accumulation	Low CD18 and CD11b	Oral hygiene, antibiotics HSCT
Respiratory burst	Chronic granulomatous disease (*CYBB*/XL, AR)	Recurrent pneumonia, abscesses, Aspergillus infection	Abnormal oxidative burst activity	Antimicrobial prophylaxis, HSCT
	Myeloperoxidase deficiency (compound heterozygous)	May be asymptomatic, *Candida albicans* infections	Normal burst, absent MPO staining	Treatment of infections
Antigen presentation	MHC II (AR)	Hypogammaglobulinemia, CD4 lymphopenia, severe, recurrent infections (SCID phenotype)	Absent MHC II on B cells	Avoid live vaccines, HSCT
	MHC I (unknown)	Necrotizing granulomatous skin lesions, frequent respiratory infections, bronchiectasis	Absent MHC I on cells	Avoid live vaccines HSCT

TABLE 48.5

Severe Combined Immunodeficiencies (SCID)

Cell Type (All T− or T Low)	Gene Defect (Inheritance)	Cell Activity Impaired	Management
B+NK+	IL7rα and IL7rγ (X-linked)	T-cell maturation, survival, and differentiation	Isolation
			Avoid live vaccines
			Bactrim
			IVIG
			HSCT
	CD3-complex defects (AR)	T-cell signaling and T-cell regulation	
	PTPRC (CD45) (AR)	T-cell receptor signaling regulation	
	CORO1A (variable)	T-cell thymic egress and actin dynamics, calcium release	
B+NK−	IL2RG (X-linked)	IL-2cγr-mediated T and NK survival (shared receptor for IL-2, IL-4, IL-7, IL-9, IL-15, and IL-21), antibody maturation in B cells	
	JAK3 (AR)	IL-2cγr signal transduction (see above)	
B−NK−	ADA (AR)	Purine salvage/clearance (purines are toxic to lymphocytes), induce apoptosis	
	AK2 (reticular dysgenesis) (AR)	Regulation of adenosine diphosphate (accumulation causes apoptosis in myeloid and lymphoid precursors)	
B+NK+	RAG1 (Omenn) (AR)	V(D)J recombination	
	RAG2 (Omenn) (AR)	V(D)J recombination	
	DCLRE1C (Artemis)	V(D)J recombination, double-strand DNA repair	

for both cellular and humoral immunity and should be pursued aggressively in parallel. A complete blood count and enumeration of lymphocyte subsets by flow cytometry (CD45RA+ naive and CD45RO+ memory CD4+ and CD8+ T cells, CD19+ B-cell subsets, CD56+ NK cells) are first steps. B-cell function is assessed by measuring IgG, IgA, and IgM antibody isotype levels, though newborns with SCID may still have low or normal IgG antibody levels due to transplacental maternal IgG antibody, and should be interpreted with caution, and in tandem with neonatal-derived IgM and IgA levels. Once lymphopenia is confirmed, maternal chimerism can be tested in females by comparing buccal tissue and whole-blood variable tandem repeats, and in males using whole blood FISH for XX/XY chimeric genotype. T-cell function is evaluated by *in vitro* mitogen stimulation test, and in an infant who is old enough to have received vaccinations, antigen-specific antibody levels can be helpful in assessing both T helper and B-cell function. Genetic diagnosis is recommended using either whole-genome sequencing or sequencing panels designed to test for an array of SCID and CID, but treatment should not be delayed while awaiting results (92,93).

Early diagnosis and initiation of treatment prior to the first infectious complication dramatically increases survival from 40% to 90%, prompting routine newborn screening for SCID (94). Typical SCID is defined as <300 T cells/mm³, and an *in vitro* mitogen stimulation response of <10%. Since the advent of newborn screening, the reported incidence of SCID increased from 1 in 100,000 to 1 in 58,000 (95), indicating that nearly half of SCID-positive patients were previously undiagnosed. Newborn screening programs quantify blood T-cell excision circle (TREC) concentrations, which are enriched in RTE T cells; threshold counts of less than 200 to 300 TRECs/mL should prompt further testing. Though suggestive of perturbed immune homeostasis, a low (nonzero) TREC count is not specific for SCID, but an undetectable level should always prompt further investigation (95). Peripheral lymphocyte counts may appear normal on the complete blood count of a newborn with SCID, as transplacentally acquired maternal T cells can engraft in an infant without responsive autologous T cells. Maternal cells, however, are low in TRECs, and therefore will not affect NBS results (96). TRECs increase linearly with advancing gestational age, and premature or low–birth-weight infants have a higher false-positive rate compared to full-term infants.

Detectable, but below SCID-positive threshold, TRECs level in a premature infant warrants repeat NBS but may not require investigation for PID unless other stigmata are present (97). One caveat is that persistently low TREC or low T-cell count that does not meet typical SCID criteria may be a sign of "leaky SCID," a less severe SCID phenotype that often presents later in life.

Antimicrobial prophylaxis beginning at 1 month is critical to avoid infection-associated mortality and to maximize survival with the definitive treatment for SCID, HLA-matched sibling donor hematopoietic stem cell transplant (HSCT). Prophylaxis regimens are designed against *Pneumocystis*, bacterial and fungal infections (TMP-SMX, IVIG, and fluconazole, respectively). Infants should be screened for CMV, EBV, adenovirus, HHV6, HSV, HIV-1, and hepatitis. As with many PID, live vaccines are absolutely contraindicated, palivizumab should be given during RSV season. Live vaccines are contraindicated in patients with SCID, and the benefits of inactivated vaccine will depend on the residual function of intact immune cells. Pneumococcal and *Hib* vaccines are generally recommended. Healthy household contacts (HHC) should not receive live oral polio vaccine due to the high risk of viral shedding, but all other vaccines, including MMR, are indicated in HHC given their low risk for viral shedding (98). Breast-feeding is usually discouraged until maternal CMV-seronegative status is confirmed, and risk for CMV transmission through breast milk with either new or reactivated maternal infection should be discussed (93).

Early HSCT (transplant at <3.5 months), or therapy initiated before the onset of infections (if >3.5 months), is associated with >90% long-term survival (99). More recently, gene therapy for adenosine deaminase deficiency (ADA) and X-linked (IL2rγ) SCID has achieved long-term stable engraftment, though some patients succumbed to leukemic transformation (100). Enzyme replacement therapy with polyethylene glycol-adenosine deaminase (PEG-ADA) for ADA SCID is recommended as a bridge to transplant (101).

Isolated B-Cell Deficiencies

B cells, which are identified by their CD19 expression, in the newborn are predominantly naive in both the preterm and full-term infant and acquire the ability to secrete antibody following postnatal antigen exposure. Overall, B-cell numbers rapidly spike in the first 6 months, then gradually decline through adolescence (102). The central mechanism by which B cells protect is through secretion of antibodies, which is the soluble form of B-cell receptor (BCR). Antibodies are secreted by plasma cells (PC) that arise from mature, naive B cells following binding of the cell-bound BCR with its cognate (receptor-specific) antigen. B cells from newborns display differential maturation and class switching function, and assessment of both B-cell number and function should be done using age-adjusted normative values. A small fraction of a more "primitive" B-cell phenotype derived during early fetal hematopoiesis, termed B-1 B cells, is able to secrete IgM spontaneously without prior antigen exposure, and based on animal studies, these cells are thought to serve a more innate-like function against encapsulated bacteria (103). Whether or not B-1 B cells can compensate for other functional immune deficiencies in newborns is unknown. B-cell function during fetal development and in premature infants is poorly understood. B-cell and antibody maturation is highly dependent on appropriate costimulation by other cells, and these highly regulated interactions are orchestrated within specific secondary lymphoid organs that continue to develop postnatally, and these multiple factors likely converge to dampen normal B-cell responses in early life (104,105).

B-cell deficiencies (Table 48.6), when caused by shared molecular defects limiting both T- and B-cell lymphocyte differentiation, fall within the B-T-SCID category (RAG1, RAG2, artemis, ADA, and reticular dysgenesis, among others). B-cell defects with normal T-cell numbers can be grouped based on the types of antibody isotypes that are affected in a given disorder, and range phenotypically from absence of all antibody classes (agammaglobulinemia, CD19+ B cells <2%) to single isolated isotype deficiencies (age-dependent ranges). B-cell deficiencies typically present with recurrent bacterial respiratory tract infections, particularly otitis media and pneumonia in infants. *S. pneumoniae* and *H. influenzae* are the most common organisms associated with B-cell disorders. Susceptibility to infection with encapsulated bacteria, such as *Streptococcus* and *Haemophilus* species, is physiologic in neonates secondary to their normally low abundance of marginal zone B cells, which specialize in recognizing bacterial cell polysaccharides (46,106). However, B-cell deficiency should still be considered in those infants who present with more frequent or severe sinopulmonary infections, or those with additional systemic findings such as failure to thrive.

Bruton tyrosine kinase, or BTK deficiency (also known as X-linked Agammaglobulinemia, XLA), accounts for 85% of agammaglobulinemias. XLA is caused by the arrest of B cell differentiation at the pre-B-cell stage, resulting in low to absent circulating B cells. Neutrophil maturation is also dependent on BTK signaling activity, and XLA can therefore be associated with severe neutropenia (70). Disease severity varies based on a given *BTK* gene mutation and its impact on function and level of BTK protein (107). Autosomal recessive clinical variant localizing to other (non-BTK) genes regulating B-cell maturation can be considered in males who present with XLA phenotype but have normal BTK sequencing, as well as in females with low B cells and clinical phenotype consistent with XLA (107).

Maternal IgG is the only antibody isotype that is licensed to cross into the fetal compartment and is actively transported by FcγR across the placenta during the third trimester. An infant's maternal IgG level reaches a nadir between 3 and 6 months, and this nadir is accompanied by rising levels of endogenous IgG. Persistently low IgG and IgA beyond 6 to 12 months without an associated immunodeficiency syndrome is rare, and when present is termed transient hypogammaglobulinemia of infancy (THI). THI can present similarly to other PID affecting B cells, including an increased susceptibility to infection with encapsulated bacteria and diminished antibody responses to vaccines. Patients with THI, however, have normal B-cell numbers and IgM, and antibody levels recover spontaneously by 4 years of age, though there are reports that recovery is over decades for some patients (108,109). Conservative management is usually indicated, but IVIG may be beneficial in cases of severe, life-threatening, or recurrent infections (110).

Specific defects isolated to B-cell antibody class switching can result in single isotype deficits, as in selective IgA deficiency, or accumulation of isotypes that are unable to mature, as in X-linked hyper IgM. Selective IgA deficiency (SIgAD) is the most common PID and is defined as a decreased or absent IgA level in association with normal IgG and IgM antibody levels. Although infants presenting with recurrent respiratory infections can be found to have low serum IgA, diagnosis of SIgAD cannot be considered until after 4 years of age due to physiologically (normal) low IgA levels expected during earlier immune development, as well as falsely reassuring IgA levels from maternal breast milk–derived IgA. As with other PID, SIgAD is most often associated with recurrent sinopulmonary infections, but infections are usually less severe than those seen with more global B-cell disorders. Multiple distinct genetic pathways are involved in SIgAD, but the shared endpoint of these pathways is impaired maturation of B cells into IgA-secreting plasma cells (111,112).

Unlike SIgAD, X-linked hyperimmunoglobulin IgM (HIGM) usually presents in infancy and has clinical features similar to other

TABLE 48.6

B-Cell Deficiencies

Disorder	Gene Defect (Inheritance)	Associated Features	Management	Vaccines
Transient hypogammaglobulinemia of infancy	None	Exaggerated physiologic nadir beyond 6 months (excellent prognosis)	Conservative IVIG (as needed)	Yes, all
X-linked agammaglobulinemia	*BTK* deficiency (XL, AR)	Failure of B cell Low–absent B cells	IVIG	Avoid live vaccines
X-linked Hyper IgM	*TNFSF5, TNFRSF5* (XL)	Absence of CD40L on T cells causes failure of antibody class switching neutropenia, poor prognosis	IVIG HSCT	Avoid live vaccines
IgA deficiency	Unknown gene (AD)	Impaired class switching isolated to IgA isotype (**most common PID**, good prognosis)	Symptomatic, **avoid IVIG** (host anti-IgA antibodies can react against donor IgA)	Yes, all
Hyper IgE (AD)	STAT3 (AD) and DOCK8 (AR)	Signaling defect causes dysregulated cytokine production with secondary preference for IgE class switching dermatitis, course facial features, and craniosynostosis	Skin care, bactrim, immunomodulators (IFN-γ, IVIG) Consider HSCT	Yes

B-cell deficiencies, including with severe upper and lower respiratory tract infections, opportunistic infections, and also neutropenia and chronic anemia. Cholangitis is common over time without treatment and is linked to worse outcomes (113). HIGM is caused by mutations in TNF superfamily 5 or TNF receptor superfamily 5 (*TNFSF5* and *TNFRSF5*, respectively), genes encoding receptor surface protein CD40, and its ligand CD40L. CD40 is constitutively expressed on B cells, neutrophils, and monocytes, and CD40L is expressed on activated T cells, and their engagement provides costimulatory signals necessary for antibody maturation and class switching; arrest of antibody maturation results in normal or elevated serum levels of IgM isotype, and low or absent IgG and IgA. There is some disagreement in the literature regarding the level of expression and activity of CD40:CD40L coreceptors in the newborn, though more recent evidence suggests that both preterm and full-term infants likely have diminished CD40:CD40L function (105,114–116). PCP prophylaxis is indicated, and G-CSF can be used in cases with severe, prolonged neutropenia. Recommended treatment for both CD40 and CD40L deficiency is HSCT. HSCT for HIGM is recommended and has shown benefit for 20-year survival and long-term quality of life measures (113,117).

Hyper IgE syndrome (HIgES or Job syndrome) is a rare immune disorder caused most commonly by autosomal dominant (AD) *STAT3* or autosomal recessive (AR) *DOCK8* genetic mutations, leading to an exaggerated immediate hypersensitivity, impaired Th17 function, and dysregulation of cytokine responses (118). Clinical manifestations include a classic triad of recurrent staphylococcal abscesses, recurrent respiratory infections, and high serum IgE. Over 80% of patients with HIgES will present within 1 month with elevated serum IgE and a distinctive exudative maculopapular rash that begins on the face (119). Systemic manifestations of disease include bronchiectasis, bone fragility, hyperextensible joints, and delayed shedding of primary teeth. The autosomal dominant form is also associated with characteristic course, asymmetric facial features, and sometimes craniosynostosis. Allergen-specific reactions are not typical of AD HIgES but appear to be common in AR forms (120,121). Initial treatment for HIgES focuses on prevention of infectious complications using prophylactic antibiotics and antifungals, and counseling regarding prevention of pathologic fractures. IVIG, monoclonal antibody against IgE, or IFN-γ treatment may be helpful in some cases, and HSCT is considered beneficial in some AR (*DOCK8*) cases (122).

INFLAMMATORY AND AUTOIMMUNE DISORDERS IN THE NEWBORN

The normal developing immune system is biased toward tolerance, due to sudden, countless environmental exposures to which the newborn needs to adapt at birth. Fetal-derived immune cells, however, display inflammatory properties that may increase susceptibility to acute and chronic activation, such as necrotizing enterocolitis and bronchopulmonary dysplasia. Clinicians should be vigilant in their consideration of primary inflammatory disorders presenting during infancy, however, in order to prevent sequelae by initiating early evaluation and treatment.

Immune dysregulation, polyendocrinopathy, enteropathy, X-linked syndrome (IPEX) is a rare PID that classically affects the forkhead box protein 3 (*FOXP3*) gene expression, the master transcription factor necessary for regulatory Treg development. Loss of Treg function in affected males causes excessive, uncontrolled effector T-cell proliferation, resulting in an early, progressive multiorgan autoimmune phenotype. Patients most often present in infancy with enteropathy, dermatitis, diabetes, hypoparathyroidism, thyroiditis, and other autoimmune phenomena. Sequencing has revealed a number of genes that associate with an IPEX-like clinical phenotype, but without involvement of the X-linked *FOXP3*

locus. Initial evaluation begins with enumeration of FOXP3-expressing T cells by flow cytometry, but this should be followed by genetic testing due to the IPEX-like syndromes that may have normal FOXP3 expression patterns. Initial treatment includes immunosuppression with systemic steroids, calcineurin inhibitor or MTOR inhibitor, and early HSCT should be considered (123–126).

Hemophagocytic lymphohistiocytosis (HLH) is characterized by dysregulated activation of cytotoxic T cells (CTL) and NK cells and frequently presents in the newborn period. HLH can be primary (familial) or secondary to infection (acquired) and presents clinically in the newborn with progressive pancytopenia, hepatic failure, coagulopathy, and a dramatically elevated serum ferritin (>500 ng/mL). Defective trafficking and degranulation of perforin-containing vesicles in CTL and NK cells results in poorly controlled infection, persistence of antigen, and ultimately cytokine storm that is fatal if left untreated (127–130). Primary disease involves one of several predisposing genetic mutations governing CTL degranulation and can present in association with physical examination findings when part of a syndrome. Primary HLH with syndromic features include Chediak-Higashi (*LYST*), Griscelli (*SH2D1A*), and Hermansky-Pudlak (*AP3B1*) syndromes, all of which are associated with partial albinism (129,131). Epstein-Barr virus triggers HLH in males with X-linked proliferative disease (XLP), which is caused by mutations in the *SH201A* gene encoding for T and NK cell receptor signaling. Secondary forms of HLH can occur in newborns exposed perinatally by intracellular bacterial or viral infections such as enteroviruses and adenovirus (132–134). Initial treatment of primary HLH targets suppression of T-cell proliferation and activation using a combination of dexamethasone and etoposide, and in some cases refractory to initial suppression, cyclosporin, and antithymocyte globulin (ATG), early HSCT is indicated prior to onset of multiorgan failure. Secondary HLH management is not standardized, but trial of steroids followed by biologics may be beneficial (128,135).

DISORDERS OF SECRETED IMMUNE MEDIATORS

Soluble components of the immune system play critical roles in neutralizing bacteria and viruses, in intercellular communication of changes to homeostasis, and in the initiation and regulation of immune responses. Key soluble factors include complement and antimicrobial proteins and peptides (APP). Little is known about the normal activity of APP across the lifespan, but they serve as first-line nonspecific defense against the most common novel pathogens that a neonate will encounter, making them uniquely suited to protect the naive newborn against a diversity of invasive infections. With the exception of cathelicidins and lactoferrin, which are both elevated in breast milk and vernix, full-term newborn APP levels are mostly comparable to adult levels. Premature infants, however, are deficient in many of these bacterial neutralizing proteins, which may contribute to their age-related susceptibility to infection (136).

Complement

Complement is produced in the liver and is activated through multiple mechanisms, and together, the components and their activity serve as a chemical bridge between nonimmune cells, innate immunity, and adaptive immunity (137,138). The classical pathway is activated through circulating antibody and antigen complexes, the lectin pathway through lectin, bacterial carbohydrate, and IgA binding, and the alternative pathway has low-level spontaneous hydrolysis of C3. With the exception of Factor D in the alternative pathway which is elevated in full terms, components of all three pathways are diminished relative to adults. Terminal component C9 is neurotoxic, and levels are significantly diminished in the newborn. There is inconsistency between studies comparing preterm to full-term complement levels, which may be an artifact

TABLE 48.7

Sentinel Infections Associated with PID

Infection	Disorder
Nocardia, Aspergillus spp., and *Burkholderia cepacia* pneumonia	Chronic granulomatous disease
Recurrent *Neisseria* spp.	Terminal complement deficiency
Escherichia coli bacteremia	Galactosemia
Pneumocystis carinii	T-lymphocyte deficiency
Recurrent *Streptococcus pneumonia* bacteremia	Asplenia, B-cell deficiencies, complement deficiencies
CMV, HSV	Hyper IgE, SCID, HIV
Gingivostomatitis	Neutrophil abnormalities

of the difficulty in accurately measuring the individual components in older studies. The complement system is assessed using the CH50 test, which measures the lysis activity of serial dilutions of human sera against sheep erythrocytes (139–141). Complement system function overlaps with antibody, and not surprisingly, clinical presentation of primary deficiencies overlap with antibody and B-cell disorders, including recurrent bacterial infections with encapsulated bacteria (especially *Pneumococcus*), autoimmunity, and angioedema. Diagnosis is made following detection of below age-appropriate levels of individual complement (19,21,142).

SUMMARY

The fetal and newborn immune system is in a state of continued development and is uniquely suited to prevent immunopathology while transitioning to an *ex utero* environment. Many of the features of the developing immune system also place them at risk for recurrent, severe infections, and their clinical susceptibility can mimic many PID. Evaluation for PID should be pursued without delay in those infants with infections that exceed the frequency and severity seen at similar gestational ages, especially when accompanied by opportunistic infections, failure to thrive, abnormal immune cell distribution, or stigmata consistent with known PID. Molecular diagnosis can be pursued in parallel with quantification and functional immunity evaluation targeted based on the combination of features present.

REFERENCES

1. Godinho-Silva C, Cardoso F, Veiga-Fernandes H. Neuro-immune cell units: a new paradigm in physiology. *Annu Rev Immunol* 2019;37:19. doi: 10.1146/annurev-immunol-042718-041812.
2. Stras SF, Werner L, Toothaker JM, et al. Maturation of the human intestinal immune system occurs early in fetal development. *Dev Cell* 2019;51(3):357. doi: 10.1016/j.devcel.2019.09.008.
3. Heinig K, Sage F, Robin C, et al. Development and trafficking function of haematopoietic stem cells and myeloid cells during fetal ontogeny. *Cardiovasc Res* 2015;107(3):352. doi: 10.1093/cvr/cvv146.
4. Kollmann TR, Kampmann B, Mazmanian SK, et al. Protecting the newborn and young infant from infectious diseases: lessons from immune ontogeny. *Immunity* 2017;46(3):350. doi: 10.1016/j.immuni.2017.03.009.
5. Mold JE, Venkatasubrahmanyam S, Burt TD, et al. Fetal and adult hematopoietic stem cells give rise to distinct T cell lineages in humans. *Science* 2010;330(6011):1695. doi: 10.1126/science.1196509.
6. Pahal GS, Jauniaux E, Kinnon C, et al. Normal development of human fetal hematopoiesis between eight and seventeen weeks' gestation. *Am J Obstet Gynecol* 2000;183(4):1029. doi: 10.1067/mob.2000.106976.
7. Tavian M, Peault B. Embryonic development of the human hematopoietic system. *Int J Dev Biol* 2005;49(2-3):243. doi: 10.1387/ijdb.041957mt.
8. Krow-Lucal ER, McCune JM. Distinct functional programs in fetal T and myeloid lineages. *Front Immunol* 2014;5:314. doi: 10.3389/fimmu.2014.00314.
9. Demirel G, Celik IH, Canpolat FE, et al. The effects of ibuprofen on sepsis parameters in preterm neonates. *Early Hum Dev* 2012;88(4):195. doi: 10.1016/j.earlhumdev.2011.07.021.
10. Falup-Pecurariu O, Man SC, Neamtu ML, et al. Effects of prophylactic ibuprofen and paracetamol administration on the immunogenicity and reactogenicity of the 10-valent pneumococcal non-typeable *Haemophilus influenzae* protein D conjugated vaccine (PHiD-CV) co-administered with DTPa-combined vaccines in children: an open-label, randomized, controlled, non-inferiority trial. *Hum Vaccin Immunother* 2017;13(3):649. doi: 10.1080/21645515.2016.1223001.
11. Langhendries JP, Allegaert K, Van Den Anker JN, et al. Possible effects of repeated exposure to ibuprofen and acetaminophen on the intestinal immune response in young infants. *Med Hypotheses* 2016;87:90. doi: 10.1016/j.mehy.2015.11.012.
12. Sirota L, Shacham D, Punsky I, et al. Ibuprofen affects pro- and anti-inflammatory cytokine production by mononuclear cells of preterm newborns. *Biol Neonate* 2001;79(2):103. doi: 10.1159/000047075.
13. Theisen E, McDougal CE, Nakanishi M, et al. Cyclooxygenase-1 and -2 play contrasting roles in Listeria-stimulated immunity. *J Immunol* 2018;200(11):3729. doi: 10.4049/jimmunol.1700701.
14. Das A, Rouault-Pierre K, Kamdar S, et al. Adaptive from innate: human IFN-gamma(+)CD4(+) T cells can arise directly from CXCL8-producing recent thymic emigrants in babies and adults. *J Immunol* 2017;199(5):1696. doi: 10.4049/jimmunol.1700551.
15. Gibbons D, Fleming P, Virasami A, et al. Interleukin-8 (CXCL8) production is a signatory T cell effector function of human newborn infants. *Nat Med* 2014;20(10):1206. doi: 10.1038/nm.3670.
16. Olin A, Henckel E, Chen Y, et al. Stereotypic immune system development in newborn children. *Cell* 2018;174(5):1277. doi: 10.1016/j.cell.2018.06.045.
17. Scheible KM, Emo J, Laniewski N, et al. T cell developmental arrest in former premature infants increases risk of respiratory morbidity later in infancy. *JCI Insight* 2018;3(4). doi: 10.1172/jci.insight.96724.
18. Scheible KM, Emo J, Yang H, et al. Developmentally determined reduction in CD31 during gestation is associated with CD8+ T cell effector differentiation in preterm infants. *Clin Immunol* 2015;161(2):65. doi: 10.1016/j.clim.2015.07.003.
19. Bonilla FA, Khan DA, Ballas ZK, et al.; Joint Task Force on Practice Parameters, representing the American Academy of Allergy, Asthma & Immunology; the American College of Allergy, Asthma & Immunology; and the Joint Council of Allergy, Asthma & Immunology. Practice parameter for the diagnosis and management of primary immunodeficiency. *J Allergy Clin Immunol* 2015;136(5):1186, e1. doi: 10.1016/j.jaci.2015.04.049.
20. Rivers L, Gaspar HB. Severe combined immunodeficiency: recent developments and guidance on clinical management. *Arch Dis Child* 2015;100(7):667. doi: 10.1136/archdischild-2014-306425.
21. Bousfiha A, Jeddane L, Picard C, et al. The 2017 IUIS phenotypic classification for primary immunodeficiencies. *J Clin Immunol* 2018;38(1):129. doi: 10.1007/s10875-017-0465-8.
22. Aluri J, Desai M, Gupta M, et al. Clinical, immunological, and molecular findings in 57 patients with severe combined immunodeficiency (SCID) from India. *Front Immunol* 2019;10:23. doi: 10.3389/fimmu.2019.00023.
23. Picard C, Al-Herz W, Bousfiha A, et al. Primary immunodeficiency diseases: an update on the classification from the International Union of Immunological Societies Expert Committee for primary immunodeficiency 2015. *J Clin Immunol* 2015;35(8):696. doi: 10.1007/s10875-015-0201-1.
24. Gratzinger D, Jaffe ES, Chadburn A, et al. Primary/congenital immunodeficiency: 2015 SH/EAHP Workshop Report-Part 5. *Am J Clin Pathol* 2017;147(2):204. doi: 10.1093/ajcp/aqw215.
25. Farley AM, Morris LX, Vroegindeweij E, et al. Dynamics of thymus organogenesis and colonization in early human development. *Development* 2013;140(9):2015. doi: 10.1242/dev.087320.
26. Dooley J, Liston A. Molecular control over thymic involution: from cytokines and microRNA to aging and adipose tissue. *Eur J Immunol* 2012;42(5):1073. doi: 10.1002/eji.201142305.
27. Glavina-Durdov M, Springer O, Capkun V, et al. The grade of acute thymus involution in neonates correlates with the duration of acute illness and with the percentage of lymphocytes in peripheral blood smear. Pathological study. *Biol Neonate* 2003;83(4):229. doi: 10.1159/000069481.
28. Toti P, De Felice C, Stumpo M, et al. Acute thymic involution in fetuses and neonates with chorioamnionitis. *Hum Pathol* 2000;31(9):1121. doi: 10.1053/hupa.2000.16676.
29. Varas A, Jimenez E, Sacedon R, et al. Analysis of the human neonatal thymus: evidence for a transient thymic involution. *J Immunol* 2000;164(12):6260. doi: 10.4049/jimmunol.164.12.6260.
30. Driscoll DA, Salvin J, Sellinger B, et al. Prevalence of 22q11 microdeletions in DiGeorge and velocardiofacial syndromes: implications for genetic counselling and prenatal diagnosis. *J Med Genet* 1993;30(10):813. doi: 10.1136/jmg.30.10.813.
31. McDonald-McGinn DM, Sullivan KE, Marino B, et al. 22q11.2 deletion syndrome. *Nat Rev Dis Primers* 2015;1:15071. doi: 10.1038/nrdp.2015.71.
32. Michaelovsky E, Frisch A, Carmel M, et al. Genotype-phenotype correlation in 22q11.2 deletion syndrome. *BMC Med Genet* 2012;13:122. doi: 10.1186/1471-2350-13-122.

33. Marcovecchio GE, Bortolomai I, Ferrua F, et al. Thymic epithelium abnormalities in DiGeorge and Down syndrome patients contribute to dysregulation in T cell development. *Front Immunol* 2019;10:447. doi: 10.3389/fimmu.2019.00447.

34. Pierdominici M, Marziali M, Giovannetti A, et al. T cell receptor repertoire and function in patients with DiGeorge syndrome and velocardiofacial syndrome. *Clin Exp Immunol* 2000;121(1):127. doi: 10.1046/j.1365-2249.2000.01247.x.

35. Davies EG. Immunodeficiency in DiGeorge syndrome and options for treating cases with complete athymia. *Front Immunol* 2013;4:322. doi: 10.3389/fimmu.2013.00322.

36. Ip W, Zhan H, Gilmour KC, et al. 22q11.2 deletion syndrome with life-threatening adenovirus infection. *J Pediatr* 2013;163(3):908. doi: 10.1016/j.jpeds.2013.03.070.

37. Markert ML, Devlin BH, Chinn IK, et al. Factors affecting success of thymus transplantation for complete DiGeorge anomaly. *Am J Transplant* 2008;8(8):1729. doi: 10.1111/j.1600-6143.2008.02301.x.

38. Markert ML, Devlin BH, Chinn IK, et al. Thymus transplantation in complete DiGeorge anomaly. *Immunol Res* 2009;44(1-3):61. doi: 10.1007/s12026-008-8082-5.

39. Lee JH, Markert ML, Hornik CP, et al. Clinical course and outcome predictors of critically ill infants with complete DiGeorge anomaly following thymus transplantation. *Pediatr Crit Care Med* 2014;15(7):e321. doi: 10.1097/PCC.0000000000000219.

40. Davies EG, Cheung M, Gilmour K, et al. Thymus transplantation for complete DiGeorge syndrome: European experience. *J Allergy Clin Immunol* 2017;140(6):1660. doi: 10.1016/j.jaci.2017.03.020.

41. Verloes A. Updated diagnostic criteria for CHARGE syndrome: a proposal. *Am J Med Genet A* 2005;133A(3):306. doi: 10.1002/ajmg.a.30559.

42. Wong MT, Scholvinck EH, Lambeck AJ, et al. CHARGE syndrome: a review of the immunological aspects. *Eur J Hum Genet* 2015;23(11):1451. doi: 10.1038/ejhg.2015.7.

43. Endo A, Ueno S, Yamada S, et al. Morphogenesis of the spleen during the human embryonic period. *Anat Rec* 2015;298(5):820. doi: 10.1002/ar.23099.

44. Mebius RE, Kraal G. Structure and function of the spleen. *Nat Rev Immunol* 2005;5(8):606. doi: 10.1038/nri1669.

45. Vellguth S, von Gaudecker B, Muller-Hermelink HK. The development of the human spleen. Ultrastructural studies in fetuses from the 14th to 24th week of gestation. *Cell Tissue Res* 1985;242(3):579.

46. Martin F, Kearney JF. Marginal-zone B cells. *Nat Rev Immunol* 2002;2(5):323. doi: 10.1038/nri799.

47. de Porto AP, Lammers AJ, Bennink RJ, et al. Assessment of splenic function. *Eur J Clin Microbiol Infect Dis* 2010;29(12):1465. doi: 10.1007/s10096-010-1049-1.

48. William BM, Corazza GR. Hyposplenism: a comprehensive review. Part I: basic concepts and causes. *Hematology* 2007;12(1):1. doi: 10.1080/10245330600938422.

49. William BM, Thawani N, Sae-Tia S, et al. Hyposplenism: a comprehensive review. Part II: clinical manifestations, diagnosis, and management. *Hematology* 2007;12(2):89. doi: 10.1080/10245330600938463.

50. Salvadori MI, Price VE; Canadian Paediatric Society, Infectious Diseases and Immunization Committee. Preventing and treating infections in children with asplenia or hyposplenia. *Paediatr Child Health* 2014;19(5):271.

51. Marchant EA, Kan B, Sharma AA, et al. Attenuated innate immune defenses in very premature neonates during the neonatal period. *Pediatr Res* 2015;78(5):492. doi: 10.1038/pr.2015.132.

52. Melvan JN, Bagby GJ, Welsh DA, et al. Neonatal sepsis and neutrophil insufficiencies. *Int Rev Immunol* 2010;29(3):315. doi: 10.3109/08830181003792803.

53. Mouna K, Doddagowda SM, Junjegowda K, et al. Changes in haematological parameters in newborns born to preeclamptic mothers—a case control study in a rural hospital. *J Clin Diagn Res* 2017;11(7):EC26. doi: 10.7860/JCDR/2017/29137.10303.

54. Lewin S, Bussel JB. Review of fetal and neonatal immune cytopenias. *Clin Adv Hematol Oncol* 2015;13(1):35.

55. Wegman-Ostrosky T, Savage SA. The genomics of inherited bone marrow failure: from mechanism to the clinic. *Br J Haematol* 2017;177(4):526. doi: 10.1111/bjh.14535.

56. Dokal I, Vulliamy T. Inherited bone marrow failure syndromes. *Haematologica* 2010;95(8):1236. doi: 10.3324/haematol.2010.025619.

57. Khincha PP, Savage SA. Neonatal manifestations of inherited bone marrow failure syndromes. *Semin Fetal Neonatal Med* 2016;21(1):57. doi: 10.1016/j.siny.2015.12.003.

58. Dietz AC, Savage SA, Vlachos A, et al. Late effects screening guidelines after hematopoietic cell transplantation for inherited bone marrow failure syndromes: consensus statement from the Second Pediatric Blood and Marrow Transplant Consortium International Conference on Late Effects After Pediatric HCT. *Biol Blood Marrow Transplant* 2017;23(9):1422. doi: 10.1016/j.bbmt.2017.05.022.

59. Alter BP. Diagnosis, genetics, and management of inherited bone marrow failure syndromes. *Hematology Am Soc Hematol Educ Program* 2007;2007:29. doi: 10.1182/asheducation-2007.1.29.

60. Giri N, Alter BP, Penrose K, et al. Immune status of patients with inherited bone marrow failure syndromes. *Am J Hematol* 2015;90(8):702. doi: 10.1002/ajh.24046.

61. Alter BP. Inherited bone marrow failure syndromes: considerations pre- and posttransplant. *Blood* 2017;130(21):2257. doi: 10.1182/blood-2017-05-781799.

62. Maheshwari A. Neutropenia in the newborn. *Curr Opin Hematol* 2014;21(1):43. doi: 10.1097/MOH.0000000000000010.

63. Christensen RD, Yoder BA, Baer VL, et al. Early-onset neutropenia in small-for-gestational-age infants. *Pediatrics* 2015;136(5):e1259. doi: 10.1542/peds.2015-1638.

64. Hibbert JE, Currie A, Strunk T. Sepsis-induced immunosuppression in neonates. *Front Pediatr* 2018;6:357. doi: 10.3389/fped.2018.00357.

65. Kan B, Razzaghian HR, Lavoie PM. An immunological perspective on neonatal sepsis. *Trends Mol Med* 2016;22(4):290. doi: 10.1016/j.molmed.2016.02.001.

66. Lawrence SM, Corriden R, Nizet V. Age-appropriate functions and dysfunctions of the neonatal neutrophil. *Front Pediatr* 2017;5:23. doi: 10.3389/fped.2017.00023.

67. Sacchi F, Rondini G, Mingrat G, et al. Different maturation of neutrophil chemotaxis in term and preterm newborn infants. *J Pediatr* 1982;101(2):273. doi: 10.1016/s0022-3476(82)80139-x.

68. Colon DF, Wanderley CW, Franchin M, et al. Neutrophil extracellular traps (NETs) exacerbate severity of infant sepsis. *Crit Care* 2019;23(1):113. doi: 10.1186/s13054-019-2407-8.

69. Yost CC, Cody MJ, Harris ES, et al. Impaired neutrophil extracellular trap (NET) formation: a novel innate immune deficiency of human neonates. *Blood* 2009;113(25):6419. doi: 10.1182/blood-2008-07-171629.

70. Donadieu J, Fenneteau O, Beaupain B, et al. Congenital neutropenia: diagnosis, molecular bases and patient management. *Orphanet J Rare Dis* 2011;6:26. doi: 10.1186/1750-1172-6-26.

71. Del Vecchio A, Christensen RD. Neonatal neutropenia: what diagnostic evaluation is needed and when is treatment recommended? *Early Hum Dev* 2012;88(suppl 2):S19. doi: 10.1016/S0378-3782(12)70007-5.

72. Hsieh MM, Everhart JE, Byrd-Holt DD, et al. Prevalence of neutropenia in the U.S. population: age, sex, smoking status, and ethnic differences. *Ann Intern Med* 2007;146(7):486. doi: 10.7326/0003-4819-146-7-200704030-00004.

73. Reich D, Nalls MA, Kao WH, et al. Reduced neutrophil count in people of African descent is due to a regulatory variant in the Duffy antigen receptor for chemokines gene. *PLoS Genet* 2009;5(1):e1000360. doi: 10.1371/journal.pgen.1000360.

74. Miller LH, Mason SJ, Clyde DF, et al. The resistance factor to *Plasmodium vivax* in blacks. The Duffy-blood-group genotype, FyFy. *N Engl J Med* 1976;295(6):302. doi: 10.1056/NEJM197608052950602.

75. Makaryan V, Zeidler C, Bolyard AA, et al. The diversity of mutations and clinical outcomes for ELANE-associated neutropenia. *Curr Opin Hematol* 2015;22(1):3. doi: 10.1097/MOH.0000000000000105.

76. Klein C, Grudzien M, Appaswamy G, et al. HAX1 deficiency causes autosomal recessive severe congenital neutropenia (Kostmann disease). *Nat Genet* 2007;39(1):86. doi: 10.1038/ng1940.

77. Welte K, Zeidler C, Dale DC. Severe congenital neutropenia. *Semin Hematol* 2006;43(3):189. doi: 10.1053/j.seminhematol.2006.04.004.

78. Roques G, Munzer M, Barthez MA, et al. Neurological findings and genetic alterations in patients with Kostmann syndrome and HAX1 mutations. *Pediatr Blood Cancer* 2014;61(6):1041. doi: 10.1002/pbc.24964.

79. Rotulo GA, Beaupain B, Rialland F, et al. HSCT may lower leukemia risk in ELANE neutropenia: a before-after study from the French Severe Congenital Neutropenia Registry. *Bone Marrow Transplant* 2020;55(8):1614. doi: 10.1038/s41409-020-0800-1.

80. Bunting M, Harris ES, McIntyre TM, et al. Leukocyte adhesion deficiency syndromes: adhesion and tethering defects involving beta 2 integrins and selectin ligands. *Curr Opin Hematol* 2002;9(1):30. doi: 10.1097/00062752-200201000-00006.

81. Etzioni A. Genetic etiologies of leukocyte adhesion defects. *Curr Opin Immunol* 2009;21(5):481. doi: 10.1016/j.coi.2009.07.005.

82. Mortaz E, Alipoor SD, Adcock IM, et al. Update on neutrophil function in severe inflammation. *Front Immunol* 2018;9:2171. doi: 10.3389/fimmu.2018.02171.

83. Moutsopoulos NM, Konkel J, Sarmadi M, et al. Defective neutrophil recruitment in leukocyte adhesion deficiency type I disease causes local IL-17-driven inflammatory bone loss. *Sci Transl Med* 2014;6(229):229ra40. doi: 10.1126/scitranslmed.3007696.

84. Schmidt S, Moser M, Sperandio M. The molecular basis of leukocyte recruitment and its deficiencies. *Mol Immunol* 2013;55(1):49. doi: 10.1016/j.molimm.2012.11.006.

85. Horikoshi Y, Umeda K, Imai K, et al. Allogeneic hematopoietic stem cell transplantation for leukocyte adhesion deficiency. *J Pediatr Hematol Oncol* 2018;40(2):137. doi: 10.1097/MPH.0000000000001028.

86. Al-Dhekri H, Al-Mousa H, Ayas M, et al. Allogeneic hematopoietic stem cell transplantation in leukocyte adhesion deficiency type 1: a single center experience. *Biol Blood Marrow Transplant* 2011;17(8):1245. doi: 10.1016/j.bbmt.2010.12.714.

87. Qasim W, Cavazzana-Calvo M, Davies EG, et al. Allogeneic hematopoietic stem-cell transplantation for leukocyte adhesion deficiency. *Pediatrics* 2009;123(3):836. doi: 10.1542/peds.2008-1191.

88. Song E, Jaishankar GB, Saleh H, et al. Chronic granulomatous disease: a review of the infectious and inflammatory complications. *Clin Mol Allergy* 2011;9(1):10. doi: 10.1186/1476-7961-9-10.

89. Connelly JA, Marsh R, Parikh S, et al. Allogeneic hematopoietic cell transplantation for chronic granulomatous disease: controversies and state of the art. *J Pediatr Infect Dis Soc* 2018;7(suppl_1):S31. doi: 10.1093/jpids/piy015.

90. Kato K, Kojima Y, Kobayashi C, et al. Successful allogeneic hematopoietic stem cell transplantation for chronic granulomatous disease with inflammatory complications and severe infection. *Int J Hematol* 2011;94(5):479. doi: 10.1007/s12185-011-0932-6.

91. Seger RA, Gungor T, Belohradsky BH, et al. Treatment of chronic granulomatous disease with myeloablative conditioning and an unmodified hempoietic allograft: a survey of the European experience, 1985-2000. *Blood* 2002;100(13):4344. doi: 10.1182/blood-2002-02-0583.

92. Kelly BT, Tam JS, Verbsky JW, et al. Screening for severe combined immunodeficiency in neonates. *Clin Epidemiol* 2013;5:363. doi: 10.2147/CLEP.S48890.

93. Thakar MS, Hintermeyer MK, Gries MG, et al. A practical approach to newborn screening for severe combined immunodeficiency using the T cell receptor excision circle assay. *Front Immunol* 2017;8:1470. doi: 10.3389/fimmu.2017.01470.

94. Brown L, Xu-Bayford J, Allwood Z, et al. Neonatal diagnosis of severe combined immunodeficiency leads to significantly improved survival outcome: the case for newborn screening. *Blood* 2011;117(11):3243. doi: 10.1182/blood-2010-08-300384.

95. Kwan A, Abraham RS, Currier R, et al. Newborn screening for severe combined immunodeficiency in 11 screening programs in the United States. *JAMA* 2014;312(7):729. doi: 10.1001/jama.2014.9132.

96. Muller SM, Ege M, Pottharst A, et al. Transplacentally acquired maternal T lymphocytes in severe combined immunodeficiency: a study of 121 patients. *Blood* 2001;98(6):1847. doi: 10.1182/blood.v98.6.1847.

97. van der Spek J, Groenwold RH, van der Burg M, et al. TREC based newborn screening for severe combined immunodeficiency disease: a systematic review. *J Clin Immunol* 2015;35(4):416. doi: 10.1007/s10875-015-0152-6.

98. Medical Advisory Committee of the Immune Deficiency Foundation; Shearer WT, Fleisher TA, Buckley RH, et al. Recommendations for live viral and bacterial vaccines in immunodeficient patients and their close contacts. *J Allergy Clin Immunol* 2014;133(4):961. doi: 10.1016/j.jaci.2013.11.043.

99. Pai SY, Logan BR, Griffith LM, et al. Transplantation outcomes for severe combined immunodeficiency, 2000-2009. *N Engl J Med* 2014;371(5):434. doi: 10.1056/NEJMoa1401177.

100. Kuo CY, Kohn DB. Gene therapy for the treatment of primary immune deficiencies. *Curr Allergy Asthma Rep* 2016;16(5):39. doi: 10.1007/s11882-016-0615-8.

101. Kohn DB, Hershfield MS, Puck JM, et al. Consensus approach for the management of severe combined immune deficiency caused by adenosine deaminase deficiency. *J Allergy Clin Immunol* 2019;143(3):852. doi: 10.1016/j.jaci.2018.08.024.

102. Blanco E, Perez-Andres M, Arriba-Mendez S, et al.; EuroFlow PID Group. Age-associated distribution of normal B-cell and plasma cell subsets in peripheral blood. *J Allergy Clin Immunol* 2018;141(6):2208. doi: 10.1016/j.jaci.2018.02.017.

103. Montecino-Rodriguez E, Dorshkind K. B-1 B cell development in the fetus and adult. *Immunity* 2012;36(1):13. doi: 10.1016/j.immuni.2011.11.017.

104. Pihlgren M, Friedli M, Tougne C, et al. Reduced ability of neonatal and early-life bone marrow stromal cells to support plasmablast survival. *J Immunol* 2006;176(1):165. doi: 10.4049/jimmunol.176.1.165.

105. Kaur K, Chowdhury S, Greenspan NS, et al. Decreased expression of tumor necrosis factor family receptors involved in humoral immune responses in preterm neonates. *Blood* 2007;110(8):2948. doi: 10.1182/blood-2007-01-069245.

106. Glaesener S, Jaenke C, Habener A, et al. Decreased production of class-switched antibodies in neonatal B cells is associated with increased expression of miR-181b. *PLoS One* 2018;13(2):e0192230. doi: 10.1371/journal.pone.0192230.

107. Lee PP, Chen TX, Jiang LP, et al. Clinical characteristics and genotype-phenotype correlation in 62 patients with X-linked agammaglobulinemia. *J Clin Immunol* 2010;30(1):121. doi: 10.1007/s10875-009-9341-5.

108. Ameratunga R, Ahn Y, Steele R, et al. Transient hypogammaglobulinaemia of infancy: many patients recover in adolescence and adulthood. *Clin Exp Immunol* 2019;198(2):224. doi: 10.1111/cei.13345.

109. Moschese V, Cavaliere FM, Graziani S, et al. Decreased IgM, IgA, and IgG response to pneumococcal vaccine in children with transient hypogammaglobulinemia of infancy. *J Allergy Clin Immunol* 2016;137(2):617. doi: 10.1016/j.jaci.2015.06.014.

110. Memmedova L, Azarsiz E, Edeer Karaca N, et al. Does intravenous immunoglobulin therapy prolong immunodeficiency in transient hypogammaglobulinemia of infancy? *Pediatr Rep* 2013;5(3):e14. doi: 10.4081/pr.2013.e14.

111. Abolhassani H, Aghamohammadi A, Hammarstrom L. Monogenic mutations associated with IgA deficiency. *Expert Rev Clin Immunol* 2016;12(12):1321. doi: 10.1080/1744666X.2016.1198696.

112. Yazdani R, Azizi G, Abolhassani H, et al. Selective IgA deficiency: epidemiology, pathogenesis, clinical phenotype, diagnosis, prognosis and management. *Scand J Immunol* 2017;85(1):3. doi: 10.1111/sji.12499.

113. de la Morena MT, Leonard D, Torgerson TR, et al. Long-term outcomes of 176 patients with X-linked hyper-IgM syndrome treated with or without hematopoietic cell transplantation. *J Allergy Clin Immunol* 2017;139(4):1282. doi: 10.1016/j.jaci.2016.07.039.

114. Nonoyama S, Penix LA, Edwards CP, et al. Diminished expression of CD40 ligand by activated neonatal T cells. *J Clin Invest* 1995;95(1):66. doi: 10.1172/JCI117677.

115. Splawski JB, Nishioka J, Nishioka Y, et al. CD40 ligand is expressed and functional on activated neonatal T cells. *J Immunol* 1996;156(1):119.

116. Han P, McDonald T, Hodge G. Potential immaturity of the T-cell and antigen-presenting cell interaction in cord blood with particular emphasis on the CD40-CD40 ligand costimulatory pathway. *Immunology* 2004;113(1):26. doi: 10.1111/j.1365-2567.2004.01933.x.

117. Mitsui-Sekinaka K, Imai K, Sato H, et al. Clinical features and hematopoietic stem cell transplantations for CD40 ligand deficiency in Japan. *J Allergy Clin Immunol* 2015;136(4):1018. doi: 10.1016/j.jaci.2015.02.020.

118. Schimke LF, Sawalle-Belohradsky J, Roesler J, et al. Diagnostic approach to the hyper-IgE syndromes: immunologic and clinical key findings to differentiate hyper-IgE syndromes from atopic dermatitis. *J Allergy Clin Immunol* 2010;126(3):611. doi: 10.1016/j.jaci.2010.06.029.

119. Eberting CL, Davis J, Puck JM, et al. Dermatitis and the newborn rash of hyper-IgE syndrome. *Arch Dermatol* 2004;140(9):1119. doi: 10.1001/archderm.140.9.1119.

120. Happel CS, Stone KD, Freeman AF, et al. Food allergies can persist after myeloablative hematopoietic stem cell transplantation in dedicator of cytokinesis 8-deficient patients. *J Allergy Clin Immunol* 2016;137(6):1895. doi: 10.1016/j.jaci.2015.11.017.

121. Siegel AM, Stone KD, Cruse G, et al. Diminished allergic disease in patients with STAT3 mutations reveals a role for STAT3 signaling in mast cell degranulation. *J Allergy Clin Immunol* 2013;132(6):1388. doi: 10.1016/j.jaci.2013.08.045.

122. Freeman AF, Holland SM. The hyper-IgE syndromes. *Immunol Allergy Clin North Am* 2008;28(2):277, viii. doi: 10.1016/j.iac.2008.01.005.

123. Barzaghi F, Amaya Hernandez LC, Neven B, et al.; Primary Immune Deficiency Treatment Consortium (PIDTC) and the Inborn Errors Working Party (IEWP) of the European Society for Blood and Marrow Transplantation (EBMT). Long-term follow-up of IPEX syndrome patients after different therapeutic strategies: an international multicenter retrospective study. *J Allergy Clin Immunol* 2018;141(3):103. doi: 10.1016/j.jaci.2017.10.041.

124. d'Hennezel E, Bin Dhuban K, Torgerson T, et al. The immunogenetics of immune dysregulation, polyendocrinopathy, enteropathy, X linked (IPEX) syndrome. *J Med Genet* 2012;49(5):291. doi: 10.1136/jmedgenet-2012-100759.

125. Gambineri E, Ciullini Mannurita S, Hagin D, et al. Clinical, immunological, and molecular heterogeneity of 173 patients with the phenotype of immune dysregulation, polyendocrinopathy, enteropathy, X-linked (IPEX) syndrome. *Front Immunol* 2018;9:2411. doi: 10.3389/fimmu.2018.02411.

126. Wildin RS, Smyk-Pearson S, Filipovich AH. Clinical and molecular features of the immunodysregulation, polyendocrinopathy, enteropathy, X linked (IPEX) syndrome. *J Med Genet* 2002;39(8):537. doi: 10.1136/jmg.39.8.537.

127. Abdullatif H, Mohsen N, El-Sayed R, et al. Haemophagocytic lymphohistiocytosis presenting as neonatal liver failure: a case series. *Arab J Gastroenterol* 2016;17(2):105. doi: 10.1016/j.ajg.2016.06.002.

128. Chandrakasan S, Filipovich AH. Hemophagocytic lymphohistiocytosis: advances in pathophysiology, diagnosis, and treatment. *J Pediatr* 2013;163(5):1253. doi: 10.1016/j.jpeds.2013.06.053.

129. Gurgey A, Unal S, Okur H, et al. Neonatal primary hemophagocytic lymphohistiocytosis in Turkish children. *J Pediatr Hematol Oncol* 2008;30(12):871. doi: 10.1097/MPH.0b013e31818a9577.

130. Isaacs H Jr. Fetal and neonatal histiocytoses. *Pediatr Blood Cancer* 2006;47(2):123. doi: 10.1002/pbc.20725.

131. Whaley BF. Familial hemophagocytic lymphohistiocytosis in the neonate. *Adv Neonatal Care* 2011;11(2):101. doi: 10.1097/ANC.0b013e318210d02c.
132. Censoplano N, Gorga S, Waldeck K, et al. Neonatal adenovirus infection complicated by hemophagocytic lymphohistiocytosis syndrome. *Pediatrics* 2018;141(suppl 5):S475. doi: 10.1542/peds.2017-2061.
133. Edner J, Rudd E, Zheng C, et al. Severe bacteria-associated hemophagocytic lymphohistiocytosis in an extremely premature infant. *Acta Paediatr* 2007;96(11):1703. doi: 10.1111/j.1651-2227.2007.00505.x.
134. Fukazawa M, Hoshina T, Nanishi E, et al. Neonatal hemophagocytic lymphohistiocytosis associated with a vertical transmission of coxsackievirus B1. *J Infect Chemother* 2013;19(6):1210. doi: 10.1007/s10156-013-0629-2.
135. Stephan JL, Kone-Paut I, Galambrun C, et al. Reactive haemophagocytic syndrome in children with inflammatory disorders. A retrospective study of 24 patients. *Rheumatology (Oxford)* 2001;40(11):1285. doi: 10.1093/rheumatology/40.11.1285.
136. Battersby AJ, Khara J, Wright VJ, et al. Antimicrobial proteins and peptides in early life: ontogeny and translational opportunities. *Front Immunol* 2016;7:309. doi: 10.3389/fimmu.2016.00309.
137. Carroll MC. The complement system in regulation of adaptive immunity. *Nat Immunol* 2004;5(10):981. doi: 10.1038/ni1113.
138. Carroll MC. The complement system in B cell regulation. *Mol Immunol* 2004;41(2-3):141. doi: 10.1016/j.molimm.2004.03.017.
139. Grumach AS, Ceccon ME, Rutz R, et al. Complement profile in neonates of different gestational ages. *Scand J Immunol* 2014;79(4):276. doi: 10.1111/sji.12154.
140. McGreal EP, Hearne K, Spiller OB. Off to a slow start: under-development of the complement system in term newborns is more substantial following premature birth. *Immunobiology* 2012;217(2):176. doi: 10.1016/j.imbio.2011.07.027.
141. Wolach B, Dolfin T, Regev R, et al. The development of the complement system after 28 weeks' gestation. *Acta Paediatr* 1997;86(5):523.
142. Turvey SE, Bonilla FA, Junker AK. Primary immunodeficiency diseases: a practical guide for clinicians. *Postgrad Med J* 2009;85(1010):660. doi: 10.1136/pgmj.2009.080630.

THE NEWBORN INFANT

49 Brain Injury at Term

Andrew Whitelaw and Marianne Thoresen

NEONATAL ENCEPHALOPATHY

Encephalopathy means a clinically apparent disturbance in brain function. In the context of a newborn infant at term, this means that tone, activity, and responsiveness of the infant are abnormal. The infant may have become very hypotonic with marked head lag or very hypertonic. Spontaneous activity may be markedly reduced or increased with tremors and/or clonic movements. Responsiveness to stimuli is generally reduced or even absent, but in mild encephalopathy, increased irritability and tremors on touch or noise indicate abnormally increased responsiveness. A detailed description of the neurologic examination is in Chapter 17. We have based our own neurologic examination on the work of Dubowitz (1). Clinical seizures are not an essential criterion but, if present, they do indicate encephalopathy. The term, encephalopathy, is used particularly when an infant develops new signs or deteriorates neurologically.

Neonatal encephalopathy is used to describe any such state in the first 28 days, but, in practice, the first 7 days. Initially, the clinician can recognize the disturbance in brain function by observation and examination, but causation requires investigation of the differential diagnosis (Table 49.1).

Encephalopathy after Birth Asphyxia

Birth asphyxia means a critical shortage of oxygen during labor and delivery sufficient to produce a lactic acidosis at birth and delayed onset of respiration.

Lactic Acidosis

Initially hypoxia–ischemia results in cells switching energy production from aerobic metabolism in mitochondria to anaerobic glycolysis in cytoplasm. Glycolysis produces less than 10% of the energy in the form of adenosine triphosphate (ATP) per gram of glucose than does aerobic metabolism (oxidative phosphorylation). Thus, essential functions can be maintained only for a time during severe hypoxia or hypoxia–ischemia but at the cost of rapid consumption of glucose and buildup of lactic acid.

Reduced placental gas exchange results in lower PaO_2 and higher $PaCO_2$, leading to increases in hydrogen ion concentration and so lowers pH. Bicarbonate (HCO_3^-) is the most important immediate buffer in blood, and if $PaCO_2$ increases, HCO_3^- buffers H^+ and HCO_3^- is reduced. At pH 7.4 and $PaCO_2$ 5.3 kPa (40 mm Hg), bicarbonate is 24 mmol/L. If HCO_3^- has been reduced to 8 mmol/L, 16 mmol has been used to buffer H^+, and we say that base deficit is 16 mmol/L, that is, we lack 16 mmol/L of HCO_3^- in order to restore pH back to 7.4. This is called base excess when using negative values. A smaller additional part of base deficit is accounted for by phosphate and proteins.

Base excess (or the opposite, base deficit) is not directly measured by a blood gas machine but is calculated using formulae and constants including temperature, hemoglobin, pH, bicarbonate, and $PaCO_2$. A number of assumptions are used to calculate base deficit, which may not apply precisely in particular circumstances. Lactate, on the other hand, is directly measured in modern blood gas machines. A lactate concentration over 10 mmol/L in cord blood has been taken as more indicative of intrapartum hypoxia than base excess or pH (2).

It is sometimes the case that umbilical cord compression before delivery followed by early cord clamping with the blood sample then being drawn from the placental side of the clamp rather than the baby side of the clamp can result in the cord venous blood gas result being relatively normal despite the baby being in poor condition (3). The real acidotic state of the fetus may then be revealed by a blood sample drawn directly from the infant a few minutes after birth.

Criteria for "Birth Asphyxia"

"Poor condition at birth" involves the five items of the Apgar score, heart rate, respiration, tone, responsiveness, and color. An Apgar score of 6 or less for more than 5 minutes indicates a poor response to initial resuscitation.

The conventional criteria for "birth asphyxia" involve low Apgar score, low pH, and/or increased base deficit. In a much cited article on the link between birth asphyxia and subsequent cerebral palsy, an Apgar score of 6 or less for more than 5 minutes and a base deficit of greater than 12 mmol/L or pH below 7.0 were chosen as criteria for significant asphyxia (4). These thresholds for base deficit and pH have been adopted by the American College of Obstetrics & Gynecology (5). Birth asphyxia does not, per definition, mean that the brain has been acutely injured. A low Apgar score with normal pH and base deficit in umbilical cord (and very early neonatal) blood suggests that the low Apgar score is not due to recent hypoxia in the last hour before delivery and may be due to another cause such as infection, prepartum brain injury, congenital anomaly, or maternal medication.

Hypoxic–Ischemic Encephalopathy

The term hypoxic–ischemic encephalopathy (HIE) is used when encephalopathy follows delivery with persistently low Apgar scores, a significant metabolic (lactic) acidosis, and no evidence of other causes of encephalopathy. In some centers, clinical signs of encephalopathy are taken as sufficient diagnostic criteria, but in many centers including ours, electroencephalography (EEG) is used as confirmation. Modern amplitude-integrated EEG (aEEG) equipment is sufficiently user friendly that a busy neonatologist or neonatal nurse can apply electrodes and can initiate useful aEEG recordings with acceptable impedance within a few minutes, particularly if needle electrodes are used in emergency settings. It is important that all infants of 36 or more weeks' gestation with significant birth asphyxia are urgently assessed neurologically because a provisional diagnosis of HIE now means that the infant should receive therapeutic hypothermia as soon as possible.

Pathophysiology of HIE

Animal models of HIE have been important in understanding processes and interventions. Dr Ronald Myers pioneered such studies in pregnant monkeys in the late 1960s and distinguished between acute total asphyxia and prolonged partial asphyxia (6).

The acute total asphyxia model involved opening the uterus just before term, clamping the umbilical cord, and preventing the fetal monkey from breathing. Blood pressure briefly rose and then rapidly decreased as did pH which was below 7.0 after 10 minutes. Base deficit typically reached 16 mmol/L by 12 minutes. If cord clamping lasted less than 10 minutes, the fetus could be resuscitated without neuropathologic injury. If cord clamping lasted between 10 and 25 minutes, the fetus could be resuscitated but with neuropathology in the spinal cord, brain stem, and thalamus. If cord clamping continued beyond 25 minutes, the fetal monkey could not be resuscitated.

TABLE 49.1

Differential Diagnosis of Neonatal Encephalopathy

Severe hypoxia during labor and delivery

Perinatal stroke, that is, infarction, focal ischemia in the territory of a blood vessel

Severe infection especially meningitis or encephalitis (discussed in Chapters 22 and 46)

Hypoglycemia (discussed in Chapter 41)

Severe unconjugated hyperbilirubinemia (discussed in Chapter 45)

Severe hypocalcemia, hypomagnesemia, hyponatremia

Trauma to the brain, for example, subdural hematoma (discussed in Chapter 53)

Spontaneous hemorrhage in or around the brain, including hemorrhagic infarction and subgaleal hemorrhage

Acute hydrocephalus (discussed Chapter 53)

Various malformations of the brain including holoprosencephaly and migration disorders

Various genetic conditions including some metabolic diseases, especially hyperammonemia, nonketotic hyperglycinemia, pyridoxine dependence, and molybdenum cofactor deficiency (discussed in Chapter 55)

Very early presentation of epilepsy syndromes such as Ohtahara (discussed in Chapter 51)

Prolonged partial asphyxia was produced by inducing hypotension by halothane anesthesia to the pregnant monkey, by intravenous infusion of oxytocin producing prolonged frequent uterine contractions, or by constricting the maternal abdominal aorta. If this was maintained for 2 to 4 hours, the fetal monkey could be resuscitated but usually developed extensor posture and seizures. Neuropathology showed a completely different pattern, there being widespread injury in the cerebral hemispheres, particularly frontally and occipitally, the watershed areas between two main cerebral arteries, and not in the brain stem and spinal cord. Basal ganglia injury was only seen in fetal monkeys who had experienced prolonged partial asphyxia and then acute total asphyxia (6).

In a global hypoxic–ischemic newborn pig model, reducing blood oxygen saturation to around 30% for 45 minutes combined with halothane-induced moderate hypotension resulted in encephalopathy with posthypoxic seizures and widespread neuropathology in basal ganglia, thalamus, cortex, hippocampus, and cerebellum (7).

Uterine Contractions and Fetal Hypoxia

During labor, every uterine contraction compresses the uterine arteries bringing oxygenated blood from the mother's circulation to the placental bed. Normally the human fetus tolerates this because the uterine contractions are short enough and the relaxation periods are long enough to avoid critical fetal hypoxia. Overstimulation with continuous infusion of oxytocin may however contribute to such short relaxation between contractions that critical fetal hypoxia can result.

In human obstetrics, examples of "sentinel events" corresponding to acute total asphyxia are umbilical cord prolapse, uterine rupture, shoulder dystocia, and placental abruption. Typically, prolonged partial asphyxia corresponds to the postmature fetus (>42 weeks) in labor with an aging placenta or an intrauterine growth–restricted fetus in labor with placental insufficiency. In practice, there are likely to be many fetuses without a sentinel event, who are subjected to considerably longer than 25 minutes of partial hypoxia but then more severe hypoxia that comes progressively worse until it is "total" (8).

Posthypoxic Cell Death and Secondary Energy Failure

An important realization in the 1980s was that processes continued to injure and kill brain cells for hours and days after oxygenation

and circulation had been restored. These processes include free radical injury, calcium entry, excitotoxicity from extracellular glutamate, inflammation, and apoptosis. Magnetic resonance spectroscopy showed that the energy status of the brain (ATP levels) in the newborn pig reversible carotid occlusion model returned to prehypoxic levels after cerebral perfusion and overall homeostasis was restored but then declined after about 24 hours (9). This was described as "secondary energy failure." These insights provided a window of opportunity, and models of neonatal hypoxic–ischemic brain injury then enabled testing of therapies.

A further advance in understanding was the discovery that inflammation increased vulnerability to hypoxia–ischemia. Hypoxia–ischemia, which was not sufficiently severe to cause permanent brain injury on its own, when sensitized with mild preinsult inflammation such as that produced by lipopolysaccharide resulted in extensive injury (10).

Clinical Signs of HIE

After resuscitation, the neonatologist must look for abnormal neurologic signs to see if encephalopathy develops. The pattern of clinical signs allows the neonatologist to grade the severity of encephalopathy. This was first systematized by Sarnat and Sarnat (11) and modified by Levene (12). This is summarized in Table 49.2. The Sarnat grading concerns patterns, and it is not necessary to have all the features listed to allocate a grade. For example, some infants with grade 3 encephalopathy do not have clinical seizures but they are completely unresponsive, hypotonic, and require ventilation. Not all infants with grade 2 encephalopathy have clinical seizures. Some will show hypotonia but others show pathologically increased trunk tone with neck extensor hypertonia, hands held in a fist, legs adducted, and exaggerated knee and ankle tendon reflexes (Fig. 49.1).

Since moderate and severe grades of HIE have a poor prognosis and mild encephalopathy does not, two combinations of signs have been used as diagnostic criteria for moderate/severe HIE in trials (Table 49.3) (13,14). The Thompson neonatal encephalopathy score was developed in South Africa and has been used in many hospitals as an alternative to aEEG. A Thompson score of 7 or more correlates well with moderate or severely abnormal aEEG (15).

Following resuscitation, encephalopathy develops with signs changing over time. Initially, some severely injured infants with respiratory drive hyperventilate because of lactic acidosis.

TABLE 49.2

Grade of Neonatal Encephalopathy

Grade 1 (Mild <24 h)	Grade 2 (Moderate)	Grade 3 (Severe)
No seizures	Clinical seizures	Persistent seizures
Mild alterations in tone	Marked abnormalities of tone	Severe hypotonia
Suck intact	Weak suck	Absent suck
Exaggerated Moro	Moro incomplete	Moro absent
Pupils react normal	Pupils constricted	Deviated, dilated, or nonreactive
Hyperalert	Reduced responsiveness to sound, light, and touch	Unresponsive
Jittery, tremor on handling	Reduced activity	No activity
	Distal flexion, proximal extension	Extended
		Impaired breathing

Modified from Sarnat HB, Sarnat MS. Neonatal encephalopathy following fetal distress. A clinical and electroencephalographic study. *Arch Neurol* 1976;33:696; Levene MI, Sands C, Grindulis H, et al. Comparison of two methods of predicting outcome in perinatal asphyxia. *Lancet* 1986;8472:67.

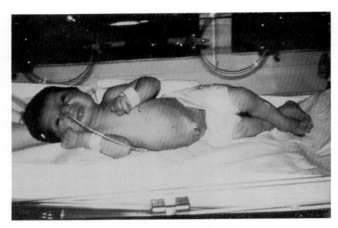

FIGURE 49.1 Infant with grade II HIE pathologically increased trunk tone, neck extensor hypertonia, hands held in a fist, and legs adducted.

The majority have not demonstrated clinical seizures within the first 6 hours but the majority have by 24 hours. When aEEG is applied early, nonclinical seizures are shown in 50% of infants before 6 hours of age (16). Some infants show grade 2 encephalopathy signs and then improve, reaching normality within 3 to 5 days. Others will first be in grade 2 and then worsen to grade 3 without ever normalizing. It is the worst grade of HIE over several days, not the best grade, which is important prognostically. Thus, clinical observation in the first 6 hours may not give a true picture of the severity.

TABLE 49.3

Combinations of Signs Used as Criteria for Moderate or Severe HIE

1. Reduced responsiveness with hypotonia or incomplete reflexes (including weak suck) or clinical seizures (13)
2. At least three signs from the following categories:
   Reduced responsiveness
   Reduced activity
   Abnormal posture
   Abnormal tone
   Incomplete reflexes
   Abnormal pupil response, heart rate, or respiration (14)

Investigations to Support a Diagnosis of HIE
Electroencephalography

The need for rapid confirmation of encephalopathy has been greatly helped by the use of aEEG. In addition to being relatively straightforward to apply, the display shows, in a compressed form (6 cm corresponds to 1 hour), the voltage range (amplitude) and pattern of aEEG over several hours on the screen. The awake full-term infant has continuous EEG activity with the lower voltage margin being well over 10 µV (Fig. 49.2) and also displaying sleep–wake cycling (17). The mildest response to a hypoxic insult is for the EEG to change from being continuous to being discontinuous, that is, having periods where the aEEG is less active and the lower margin amplitude reduces for some seconds below 5 µV and then

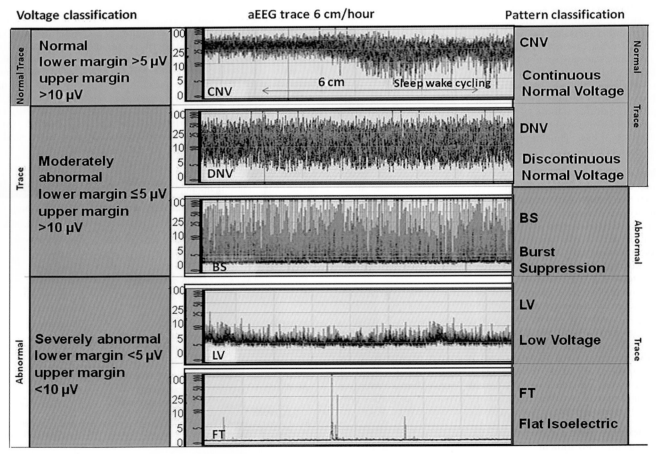

FIGURE 49.2 Amplitude-integrated EEG classification. Continuous EEG; discontinuous normal voltage; burst suppression; low voltage; and flat trace.

reverts to the previous normal amplitude. This is called "discontinuous normal voltage" (DNV). If the injury is more severe, the aEEG reduces to a low-voltage background with periodic brief bursts of normal amplitude for 1 to 2 seconds with longer periods (over 20 seconds of very low voltage background in between). This is "burst suppression." If the disturbance is even more severe, there are no bursts, only continuous low-voltage activity. If the disturbance is worse still, there is no electrical activity at all (flat trace).

Amplitude-integrated EEG is valuable because it provides an objective record which can be reviewed by an expert if there is doubt in a way that is impossible with neurologic examination unless it is videoed. Amplitude-integrated EEG can be set up within 10 minutes by a nurse or neonatologist in a critically ill infant using as few as three thin 27-G needle electrodes or using skin electrodes. Our experience with courses is that neonatal staff can be trained to obtain interpretable recordings and to recognize the vast majority of clinically important neonatal abnormalities (and artifacts) within 1 day (18). It is important that all recordings are reviewed within 24 hours by a neurophysiologist or neonatologist with in-depth experience of the subject. The compressed recordings and "raw EEG" can be viewed by video or Internet link or scanned and then sent to an expert anywhere in the world. A neonatal chest or abdominal radiograph is often taken as an emergency and interpreted immediately by the neonatologist on the spot but is then reviewed within 24 hours by a radiologist who writes a definitive report that may differ from the original interpretation. A similar system of review of aEEG is important as quality control.

Animal modeling of hypoxia–ischemia shows that during severe hypoxia–ischemia, the EEG becomes a flat trace or very low voltage. After reoxygenation, the amplitude of the EEG gradually increases over time, the speed of normalizing being inversely proportional to the severity of the brain injury on subsequent neuropathologic grading (7,19).

If one waits long enough in some cases, the EEG will show continuous normal amplitude activity even in the presence of severe brain injury and subsequent cerebral palsy. Continuous aEEG during the first 72 to 96 hours is valuable in confirming not only encephalopathy but also the time it takes for the trace to recover to at least a normal voltage pattern and the occurrence of and drug responses to seizures (16–18).

Clinical Chemistry and Multi-Organ Injury

Elevated creatinine, liver enzymes, cardiac troponins-T or -I, and prolonged coagulation times and thrombocytopenia indicate multi-organ dysfunction, which provides evidence of total body hypoxia.

Cranial ultrasound should be done on admission as it may show evidence of antenatal injury or anomaly, for example, dilated ventricles, hemorrhage, or corpus callosum (CC) agenesis. Relatively severe cases of HIE often show echodensity in thalami/basal ganglia, but apparently normal anatomy on cranial ultrasound on days 1 to 2 does not exclude encephalopathy. Scanning on day 3 and at 1 week can show an evolving pattern of injury consistent with HIE, and this may be useful in settings without access to magnetic resonance imaging (MRI).

Cerebral MRI taken 5 to 14 days after birth is valuable in confirming HIE and in excluding congenital anomalies and prenatal developmental disturbances. In HIE following acute total asphyxia, MRI typically shows abnormal signal in the basal ganglia and thalamus and absence of myelin signal in the posterior limb of the internal capsule (PLIC) (**Fig. 49.3**). The brain stem and rolandic cortex may also show abnormal signal (20–22). Following a more prolonged period of hypoxia, there is typically abnormal signal in the watershed areas (frontal and occipital cortex and subcortical white matter) (**Fig. 49.4**). In severe cases, both distributions of brain injury may be seen in the same child.

Prediction of Outcome in Birth Asphyxia and HIE
Grade of Encephalopathy

In the original study by Sarnat and Sarnat (11), well before the era of therapeutic hypothermia, infants with grade 2 encephalopathy who normalized within 5 days had normal developmental outcome, whereas those who had not normalized by 7 days died or were neurodevelopmentally abnormal, typically with cerebral palsy. Overall, grade 2 HIE has been associated with later disability in 20% to 40% and grade 3 HIE with a very high rate of death or disability. The figures vary widely probably reflecting different definitions of HIE grades and different thresholds for withdrawing life support.

Lactic Dehydrogenase

Lactic dehydrogenase (LDH) sampled within 6 hours of birth as well as at 72 hours gives prognostic information. In one study, all infants with HIE and LDH values less than 2,085 U/L survived without disability, whereas those who died or were disabled had median LDH value 3,555 U/L (inter quartile range 3,003 to 8,705) (23).

Doppler Cerebral Blood Flow Velocity

While ultrasound images are being obtained, pulsed Doppler can be used to measure Pourcelot resistance index (systolic velocity minus diastolic velocity)/systolic velocity on the anterior cerebral artery. After about 24 hours of HIE, there is pathologic cerebral vasodilatation with, paradoxically, the highest cerebral blood flow being found in the most severely injured infants. This cerebral vasodilatation may be reflected in a cerebral resistance index below 0.55. This was found to have a positive predictive value for death or disability of 84% (24).

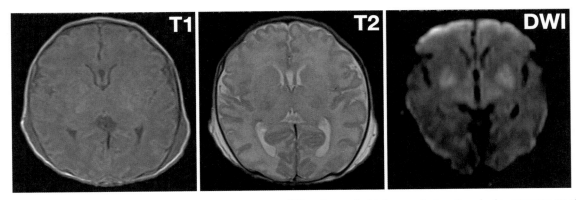

FIGURE 49.3 MRI from a term male infant, intubated and ventilated for severe HIE, and treated with therapeutic hypothermia. Appearances are of a symmetrical abnormality affecting the deep gray structures and the perirolandic gray and white matter. T2 hyperintensity, reduction in gray–white differentiation and diffusion restriction. These are features of profound hypoxic–ischemic injury. (Case courtesy of Dr Jeremy Jones, Radiopaedia.org, **rID**: 73220.)

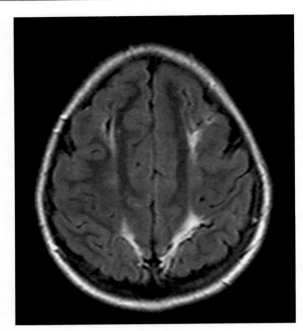

FIGURE 49.4 MRI T1 axial image showing abnormal (*white*) signal in frontal and occipital areas (watershed brain injury).

Electroencephalography

Van Rooij (25) showed that aEEG at 6 hours was predictive of outcome. If the trace shows very low voltage or a flat trace at 6 hours, only 5 out of 65 had normal outcome, but if EEG had normalized by 24 hours, then 5 out of 6 had normal outcome. If there was burst suppression at 6 hours, 6 out of 28 had normal outcome or mild disability later and all of these had achieved normal aEEG by 24 hours. All of those who still had burst suppression at 24 hours had poor outcome. Examining the aEEG over several days gives additional information in that time to restoration of normal voltage amplitude and time to regain sleep–wake cycling are also prognostic (19).

The usefulness of aEEG at 6 and 24 hours has been further confirmed in a meta-analysis of prognostic tests (26).

In a study using continuous EEG in 47 infants with HIE, the presence of seizures *per se* was not associated with abnormal outcome ($p = 0.126$). However, the odds of an abnormal outcome increased over ninefold if a neonate had a total seizure burden of more than 40 minutes and eightfold if a neonate had a maximum hourly seizure burden of more than 13 minutes per hour (27).

Neuroimaging

Cerebral ultrasound and CT scan may show changes in relatively severe cases but, in our experience, do not provide sufficient detail on injured areas to be useful for prognosis in a clinical setting. On conventional MRI, abnormal signal in the basal ganglia and thalamus is highly predictive of subsequent cerebral palsy as is absence of myelin signal in the PLIC. The severity of basal ganglia lesions is useful in predicting the severity of subsequent motor impairment. In a large study of 175 infants with HIE and basal ganglia lesions, the predictive accuracy of severe BGT lesions for severe motor impairment was 0.89 (21). Abnormal PLIC signal intensity predicted the inability to walk independently by 2 years (sensitivity 0.92, specificity 0.77, positive predictive value 0.88, negative predictive value 0.85). Brainstem injury was the only factor with an independent association with death.

Abnormal signal in the cortex and white matter, in the absence of basal ganglia and thalamic abnormality, is not so predictive of cerebral palsy (only 5 out of 84), but severe changes were associated with cognitive impairment, epilepsy, and visual impairment, and there were a variety of behavioral and communication problems (22).

Diffusion-weighted imaging, when added to T1 and T2 imaging, can give early confirmation of injury in centrum semiovale, CC, anterior and posterior limbs of the internal capsule, external capsules, fornix, cingulum, cerebral peduncles, optic radiations, and inferior longitudinal fasciculus that correlates with later neurologic development (28). MR spectroscopy (MRS) can measure *in vivo* the relative concentrations of chemical substances in tissue. Some researchers have reported that thalamic/basal ganglia Lac/NAA on 1H MRS at 3T at 4 to 14 days accurately predicted neurodevelopmental outcome in infants with HIE (29,30). However, other authors have come to different conclusions and pointed out the lack of consistency between different MRS software and equipment (31–33). The complexity of acquiring and interpreting MRS means this promising technology requires further evaluation before introduction into standard clinical pathways. Hypothermia has changed early prognostic indicators (Table 49.4).

Other Conditions That Can Mimic HIE

Not every infant born with low Apgar scores has suffered critical hypoxia, and a number of long-standing disorders of the nervous system can present with a hypotonic infant who does not breathe. This is especially true of congenital myotonic dystrophy and congenital muscular dystrophies and myopathies. Molybdenum cofactor deficiency and isolated sulfite oxidase deficiency can give seizures of prenatal onset so that the infant is observed to have seizures very soon after birth (35). High-dose magnesium, benzodiazepine, or opiate therapy to the mother may produce low Apgar scores and a hypotonic, poorly responsive infant but without a severe metabolic acidosis, burst suppression, or seizures. Intrapartum infection, if established hours before birth, may result in a floppy infant with delayed respiration. Rarely, severe birth trauma can injure the brain to such an extent that there is delayed onset of respiration.

If there is a consistent sequence of obstetric sentinel event, fetal distress, low Apgar score for more than 5 minutes, marked lactic acidosis, clinical encephalopathy, low voltage or burst suppression EEG, multiorgan dysfunction, and initial cranial ultrasound showing normal anatomy, then the diagnosis of HIE is not in doubt. In the cases where important pieces of the HIE jigsaw are missing, other investigations need to be considered with MR imaging, ammonia, uric acid, amino acids, urine sulfite reaction and S-sulfo-L-cysteine, and organic acids.

Evidence Base for Therapeutic Hypothermia

For many decades, the one aspect of neonatal care on which all nurses and neonatologists were agreed was that it was harmful to let a sick baby get cold. However, it had been known for decades that being cooled during hypoxia protected the brain. This had made possible some early open heart surgery. The demonstration of a lengthy posthypoxic or reperfusion cascade of molecular and cellular processes ending in cell death raised the question of whether hypothermia after (rather than during) hypoxia might reduce brain injury.

First Laboratory Evidence of Hypothermia's Benefit

The first convincing demonstration in a newborn animal model was in the newborn pig and published in 1995. Bilateral carotid artery temporary occlusion produced, on MRS, severe depletion of energy nucleotides that returned to normal for some hours and then declined in irreversible secondary energy failure. Posthypoxic cooling to 35°C prevented secondary energy failure (36). More research in rats (37), sheep (38), and pigs (39) showed that cooling by 2 to 6 degrees for 6 to 72 hours reduced neuropathologic injury, long-term neurobehavioral deficits (40), cerebral edema, excitotoxic amino acids and free radical indicators (41), inflammation (42), and apoptosis (43). Furthermore, no adverse effects of cooling were identified. Being cooled is stressful, and there is extensive evidence that prolonged stress and elevated corticosteroid has a negative effect on the brain. When newborn pigs were anesthetized during posthypoxic hypothermia, brain injury was reduced but, when no anesthesia or sedation was given, plasma cortisol concentrations were increased approximately three times and cooling was not neuroprotective (44).

Hypothermia was also found to be not protective in the presence of inflammation (lipopolysaccharide given a few hours before hypoxia–ischemia) (45). Although neuroprotection had been obtained after 6 to 24 hours of hypothermia, Davidson (46) showed that better protection was obtained with 72 hours cooling than with 48 hours cooling.

Pilot Clinical Trials

Evidence from three species of newborn animal made it ethical to start clinical trials in 1997–1998 (47). Because there was still concern that cooling might have harmful effects, the brain was cooled more than the rest of the body using a cooling cap, thereby lowering rectal temperature to 34.5°C. Blood pressure rose during active cooling and could fall significantly during rapid warming (48). Heart rate fell by an average of 14 beats/°C, and rates of 70 to 80 per minute were tolerated without evidence of inadequate perfusion.

Large Randomized Trials

The first large multicenter randomized trial (CoolCap) of selective head cooling for 72 hours enrolled infants of 36 or more weeks' gestation with asphyxia, signs of encephalopathy, and abnormal aEEG (13). This trial showed a reduction in death or disability at 18 months in the infants who had less severe EEG changes at enrollment. The next trial was conducted by the US National Institute of Child Health and Development Network and used cooling of the whole body at 33.5°C (14), showing significant reduction in death or disability. The TOBY (Total Body Hypothermia) trial cooled the whole infant body to 33.5°C for 72 hours, and this, the largest trial, showed a significant increase in survival without neurologic impairment (49). All three of these early trials followed up infants and have evidence that the protection at 18 months lasts into the school years. A meta-analysis of hypothermia trials in intensive care settings has confirmed that hypothermia reduced both disability and mortality (50) (Table 49.5).

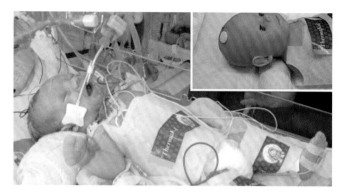

FIGURE 49.5 A term ventilated baby being cooled to 33.5°C rectal temperature for 72 hours using a wrap around body and legs circulated with water. The temperature is servocontrolled to the preset temperature. The picture of a doll in the upper right corner shows the insulation pillow made from six layers of "bubblewrap," which also positions the head in neutral extension in the midline.

Practical Aspects of Therapeutic Hypothermia (51)

1. Cooling is most effective the earlier it is applied. In animals, most benefit has been lost by 5.5 hours delay, and there was no benefit by 8.5 hours. A study in Bristol showed better neurodevelopmental outcome when cooling had been started before 3 hours than when started between 3 and 6 hours. There must be no delay in identifying candidates. If a term infant still needs resuscitation at 10 minutes, turn the overhead heater off to avoid hyperthermia, and check the cord blood or neonatal acid–base analysis while resuscitation continues. The infant will start to cool passively, and it is essential that the core temperature is monitored rectally (6 cm in) or via the esophagus, while the infant is being moved to the neonatal intensive care unit.

2. Allow passive hypothermia to occur by not actively rewarming the child. Target temperature for initial passive hypothermia is suggested to be 34°C to 35°C (to avoid accidental overcooling during transport to NICU). The sicker the infant, the faster the temperature will fall passively. If the infant fulfils asphyxia criteria and shows neurologic criteria, this will be enough evidence in many centers to cool at 33.5°C for 72 hours but we strongly recommend the use of aEEG to confirm encephalopathy and assess severity.

3. If the infant has to be transported to a tertiary center for therapeutic cooling, core temperature must be monitored continuously during transport and cooling/warming adjusted. For short periods, low-tech cooling techniques can be used within a transport incubator. We initially used surgical gloves filled with cold water and applied around the axilla, groin, and trunk. Do not use ice or anything colder than 10°C as this is painful.

Figure 49.5 shows an infant with HIE being cooled with a water-filled wrap around the trunk and thighs. This is connected to a servo system which automatically adjusts the temperature of the water to maintain rectal temperature at 33.5°C. The original selective head cooling system "CoolCap" is no longer in production but some are still in use.

TABLE 49.5

Meta-Analysis of 10 Randomized Trials of Hypothermia for Term Infants with HIE				
	n	Relative Risk	Risk Difference	NNT
Death or major disability	1,344	0.75 (0.68–0.83)	−0.15 (−0.20 to −0.10)	7 (5–10)
Mortality	1,468	0.75 (0.64–0.88)	−0.09 (−0.13 to −0.04)	11 (8–25)
Major disability	917	0.77 (0.63–0.94)	−0.13 (−0.19 to −0.07)	8 (5–14)

NNT, number needed to treat.

From Jacobs SE, Berg M, Hunt R, et al. Cooling for newborns with hypoxic ischaemic encephalopathy. *Cochrane Database Syst Rev* 2013;1:CD003311. Ref. (50).

TABLE 49.6

General Support for Infants with HIE

- Monitor arterial blood pressure and assess hypotension with echocardiography to guide volume replacement or choice of inotrope.
- Maintain oxygen saturation 93%–98% or PaO_2 60–100 mm Hg (8–13 kPa).
- $PaCO_2$ 45–58 mm Hg (6–8 kPa) if blood analyzed at 37°C.
- Monitor Na, K, Ca, and Mg. Correct hypocalcemia and hypomagnesemia as they may contribute to seizures.
- Monitor and maintain a safe blood glucose (45–140 mg/dL [2.5–8 mmol/L]).

It is recommended that the infant head should be uncovered to allow heat loss and placed on a pillow made by six layers of bubblewrap to insulate from any heating under the head (52). It is also recommended to keep the head in midline as head rotation may impede venous drainage. It is important to protect the skin at pressure points by periodic adjustment of posture. We have seen one infant with extensive skin necrosis following an adrenaline infusion and lying supine, not changing position on a cold mattress for 72 hours.

It is essential that the rectal (or esophageal probe) does not slide out as it will then register a temperature lower than the true core temperature, resulting in overheating.

4. In addition to requiring monitoring of seizures and anticonvulsant therapy, infants with HIE usually have multisystem dysfunctions affecting circulation, respiration, metabolism, kidney function, and blood components, which require interventions (Table 49.6).

5. The intestines of any infant with HIE will have been subjected to hypoxia–ischemia, and it has been common practice to withhold enteral feeding during hypothermia but some infants can safely tolerate minimal enteral feeding. In a retrospective study of 52 Swedish infants judged to be stable with HIE, 91% received enteral feeding with breast milk (53). The enteral feeds started at a median of 24 hours with 1 to 2 mL/kg boluses every 3 hours and stopped if gastric residuals were large, bilious, or blood stained and increased if feeds were tolerated The authors point out that enteral feeding can stimulate gut function even in small amounts and hypothermia protects the gut and liver after ischemia. They concluded that minimal enteral feeding was feasible with no significant complications.

Stress and Sedation

In the neonatal pig model, therapeutic hypothermia after hypoxia/ischemia did not protect the brain if there was no anesthesia (44) or sedation but gave good protection if anesthesia was used (39). Plasma cortisol concentrations were approximately three times higher during hypothermia without anesthesia than with anesthesia. Combining these findings with the extensive information on the adverse effect of prolonged stress on the brain, we conclude that infants being cooled should be assessed for signs of stress/pain, and unless the infant is already comatose, we use a continuous infusion of morphine, starting at 20 µg/kg/h and then titrating to the infant's need aimed at the lowest effective dose (51).

Drug metabolism is slowed during hypothermia (54). If continuous infusions of drugs or repeated doses are used, drug accumulation will occur more readily than at normal temperature. This means that continuous infusions of drugs such as benzodiazepines and opiates need to be carefully assessed to avoid misinterpreting a drug-induced coma as brain death.

Blood gas and pH measurements change with temperature, and the blood gas machine has to have the current body temperature

entered at the time the blood sample was taken. Analyzed at 33.5°C, a blood sample shows higher pH, lower $PaCO_2$, and lower PaO_2 than the same sample analyzed at 37°C. Hypocapnia stimulates cerebral vasoconstriction and must be avoided.

Although initial cooling can be rapid, rewarming must be carried out no faster than 0.5°C per hour. Rapid rewarming can precipitate hypotension and seizures.

Initiating Cooling after 6 Hours?

Although the large randomized trials mostly used 6 hours as a time limit for initiation of hypothermia, hypothermia should be started as soon as the need is recognized: "Time is brain" (55). The evidence from fetal sheep is that protection is reduced as time passes until about 5.5 hours with no protection after 8.5 hours (38). A multicenter randomized clinical trial investigating hypothermia starting at a median of 16 (6–23,56) hours after birth found death or moderate/severe disability in 24.4% of cooled infants and 27.9% of noncooled infants ($p = 0.23$), which is not significant protection if conventional trial statistical analysis is used. The authors claimed that Bayesian analysis showed benefit; however, reanalysis disputed this (56,57).

How Deep Should the Temperature Drop?

In 7-day-old rat pups, cooled to 33.5°C, 32°C, 30°C, 26°C, or 18°C for 5 hours after hypoxia–ischemia, there was no additional protection with temperatures below 33.5°C (58). Similarly, in newborn pigs, whole body hypothermia with a reduction in body temperature of 3.5°C or 5°C was associated with significant (and similar) neuroprotection, but a reduction of 8°C resulted in loss of neuroprotection after global cerebral ischemia (59). A multicenter randomized clinical trial found that cooling infants with moderate or severe HIE to 32°C instead of 33.5°C did not confer any further reduction in mortality or moderate or severe disability at 18 months (60).

Cooling for Longer

Given the evidence in sheep that cooling for 72 hours gives better neuroprotection than cooling for 48 hours, it was natural to consider whether cooling for longer than 72 hours would increase protection. However, hypothermia started at 3 hours and continued for 5 days instead of 3 days gave no further improvement in electrophysiologic recovery or neuropathology (61). A multicenter randomized clinical trial comparing 120 and 72 hours of hypothermia found no improvement in mortality or moderate/severe disability after cooling for 120 hours (60).

Hypothermia for "HIE" outside Trial Criteria

The large randomized clinical trials have confined recruitment to term infants with moderate or severe HIE after birth asphyxia. There is a good case for therapeutic hypothermia for HIE after postnatal collapse as the posthypoxia encephalopathy is essentially the same. The timing of postnatal collapse can be determined accurately, and thus, ideally, hypothermia can be started very early with maximum effect (62).

A number of centers have extended treatment criteria to include term infants assessed as having mild HIE. The criteria for mild HIE as described by Sarnat (11) and others are quite subtle and subjective particularly distinguishing between "mild altered tone" and normal variation in tone and between "hyperalert" and normal alertness. "Jitteriness" and tremor on handling can also be normal. When does this become excessive? Another characteristic of mild HIE in Sarnat's paper was normalization within 48 hours but that can only be determined in retrospect. In Sarnat's original paper, infants with mild HIE all recovered. More recent reports of prognosis and treatment of mild HIE have varied in diagnostic criteria (63). There are, as yet, no published randomized trials of hypothermia with neurodevelopmental outcome for mild HIE.

TABLE 49.7

Clinical Trials of Treatments Added to Hypothermia for HIE

- Allopurinol (65)
- Erythropoietin (66–68)
- Melatonin (69,70)
- Xenon (71–73)

Therapeutic hypothermia should not be considered as a benign treatment that can be added "just in case," particularly if transport by ambulance or aircraft, mechanical ventilation, and sedation for 72 hours are involved.

Infants at 34 and 35 weeks' gestation with birth asphyxia may behave very similarly to term infants with HIE and with similar sequelae. Late preterm infants have been cooled in a number of centers, apparently without adverse consequences. Despite the absence of randomized trial evidence on safety or efficacy, we do not think it is wrong to cool infants of 34 and 35 weeks' gestation who meet all the other criteria for therapeutic hypothermia (64). Conversely, it is also reasonable to specify 36 weeks as the minimum age for cooling because that was the minimum gestation in most major trials.

Infants below 34 weeks' gestation, especially those below 30 weeks, must be considered as different from the term infant with HIE. The pattern of brain injury is very different (intraventricular hemorrhage and periventricular leukomalacia), pulmonary and cardiovascular derangement is a much bigger problem, organ function and metabolism are less mature, and bleeding is much more common. Thus, we advise against therapeutic hypothermia in infants below 34 weeks' gestation (64).

Despite therapeutic cooling, 30% to 40% of infants with HIE still die or are disabled, and Table 49.7 shows interventions in addition to hypothermia that are being currently investigated in clinical trials for HIE (65–73). At the present time, none of these can be recommended as standard of care (Table 49.7). The role of hypothermia for neuroprotection in HIE in low and middle income settings is currently uncertain and requires further research.

PERINATAL STROKE

The term perinatal stroke refers to acute onset of neurologic signs in the first 7 days attributable to focal brain infarction or hemorrhage and typically presents with seizures (74). "Presumed perinatal stroke" refers to infants who present later in childhood usually with cerebral palsy or seizures and in whom neuroimaging indicates infarction probably of perinatal origin. This chapter deals with stroke in term infants and does not include germinal matrix/intraventricular hemorrhage in preterm infants.

Perinatal Arterial Ischemic Stroke

This typically occurs in the territory of the middle cerebral artery (or branches of it), and the left side is more commonly affected than the right (Fig 49.6). The presentation is usually seizure activity in the early postnatal period (74). The seizures are usually focal, sometimes just one limb, and respond quickly to conventional anticonvulsant therapy (unlike HIE). Despite the location of the infarct involving a motor area, physical examination reveals no sign of hemiplegia. At this age, the necessary myelination and connectivity have not yet developed. This amazes adult neurologists when faced with the neonatal imaging.

Perinatal arterial ischemic stroke (PAIS) often presents in a term infant aged about 24 hours who is on the postnatal ward and where there has been no prolonged resuscitation but, in many cases, risk factors can be identified. Seizures can be difficult to distinguish from the variety of neonatal movements, and

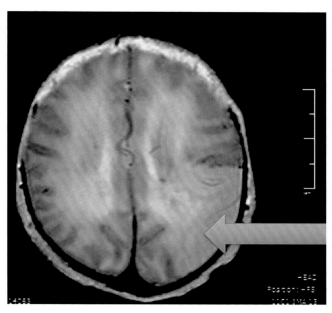

FIGURE 49.6 Stroke. MRI T2 axial image showing abnormal signal in the left parietal area (*arrowed*).

this probably explains why some cases only come to light many months later when the child shows hemiplegia or other signs and is then imaged (presumed perinatal stroke).

PAIS occurs in 1 in 3,500 newborns (75). The risk factors for PAIS are listed in Table 49.8 (76,77). Diagnosis is by urgent MR imaging including MR angiography and MR venography. Routine testing for thrombophilia is not recommended.

Mechanisms

The epidemiology strongly suggests that the origin of most perinatal arterial stroke is in labor and delivery and not in the postnatal period. Thus, seizures present many hours (perhaps even a day or two) after the causative injury. It is postulated that thrombi form in the placenta as a result of sluggish flow and then travel via umbilical vein, right atrium, foramen ovale, left atrium, and aorta

TABLE 49.8

Perinatal Factors Associated with Neonatal Arterial Stroke

Fetal heart rate abnormality

Emergency cesarean section

Chorioamnionitis

Prolonged rupture of membranes

Prolonged second stage of labor

Vacuum extraction

Cord abnormality

Preeclampsia

Intrauterine growth restriction

Low 5-min Apgar score

Coagulation abnormalities

Mutation of the gene COL4A1

Congenital heart disease

Extracorporeal membrane oxygenation

From Lee J, Croen LA, Backstrand KH, et al. Maternal and infant characteristics associated with perinatal arterial stroke in the infant. *JAMA* 2005;293(6):723. Ref. (76); Wu YW, March WM, Croen LA, et al. Perinatal stroke in children with motor impairment: a population-based study. *Pediatrics* 2004;114(3):612. Ref. (77).

to the left carotid artery (74). Sluggish or slow cardiac output, polycythemia, inflammation, and local pressure on the side of the head may also contribute to the final result being ischemia in the territory of the middle cerebral artery. Congenital heart disease with right to left shunting provides a route for placental and endocardial thrombi to embolize to the aorta and carotid artery. Furthermore, postnatal interventions such as balloon septostomy, cardio-pulmonary bypass, and surgery can introduce thrombi (and also air) into the circulation. Extracorporeal membrane oxygenation (ECMO) can also give rise to emboli and subsequent infarction (78). The brain is further at risk because these infants have often been hypoxemic in order to meet the criteria for ECMO.

Prevention

No interventions have been shown to reduce or prevent perinatal stroke. Minimizing the risk factors is part of good antenatal and intrapartum care.

Management

Seizures should be controlled. Oxygen saturation and blood glucose should be maintained and dehydration or anemia corrected. Antiplatelet therapy, anticoagulation, and thrombolytic therapy are not recommended. Theoretically, hypothermia should help in stroke. Much of the preclinical research showing that posthypoxic hypothermia reduced brain injury was carried out on the Rice-Vanucci model in the rat pup (40). This is, in fact, a stroke model rather than a global hypoxic–ischemic model. On that basis, it is very likely that therapeutic hypothermia would reduce injury in perinatal stroke. The problem is the frequent delay of 12 to 24 hours, often longer, between the onset of ischemia (probably late in labor/delivery) and diagnosis of stroke by recognition of seizure and then MR imaging. All the animal evidence suggests that delay would be too late for hypothermia to be protective and therefore hypothermia cannot be recommended.

Prognosis

Only a proportion of infants with PAIS develop neurodevelopmental impairments later. In a Swiss study of 100 full-term neonates with symptomatic PAIS, 39% were diagnosed with cerebral palsy and 31% with cognitive impairment by the age of 2 years (79). Lesion topography is an important determinant of cerebral palsy in PAIS with concomitant involvement of cerebral cortex, posterior limb of internal capsule, and basal ganglia/thalamus being closely associated with hemiplegia (80). The larger the infarct, the more likely are later impairments in cognition, speech, attention, and executive function and epilepsy (81). Recurrence risk after noncardiac perinatal arterial stroke is very low, presumably because the mechanisms are linked to labor and delivery. Thus long-term therapy with antiplatelet or anticoagulant therapy is not indicated.

Physical Therapy

The vast majority of arterial stroke is unilateral with resulting cerebral palsy being hemiplegic. Eliasson (82) conducted a randomized trial comparing constraint-induced movement therapy (CIMP) with baby massage starting at 5 to 6 months in infants showing asymmetric hand function. CIMP involves preventing the use of the (normal) limb, thus encouraging use of the impaired limb on the opposite side. At 18 months of age, function of the affected hand was significantly better in the CIMP group.

Cerebral Sinovenous Thrombosis

This presents with seizures, lethargy, and has risk factors similar to arterial stroke with dehydration and meningitis in addition (74). The venous obstruction often results in secondary hemorrhage, which may enter a lateral ventricle (**Fig. 49.7**).

Thrombophilia investigations are not recommended.

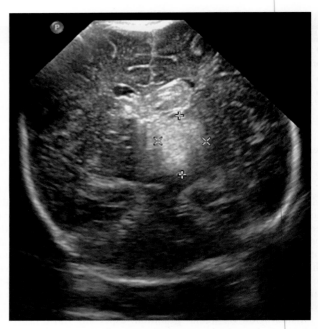

FIGURE 49.7 Cerebral sinovenous thrombosis and intraventricular hemorrhage. Ultrasound coronal view showing echodensity (*white*) in the basal ganglia/thalamus and within the lateral ventricle.

Prognosis

Fitzgerald (83) described 42 neonates with cerebral sinovenous thrombosis (CSVT). Forty-one survived and 59% had cerebral palsy, 67% cognitive impairment, and 41% epilepsy. Recurrence of neonatal CSVT has not been described.

Management

Controlling seizures and correcting dehydration are important. There is a significant risk of the thrombus propagating with worsening outcome, and this is the basis for anticoagulant therapy. Moharir (84) treated 29 of 83 CSVT neonates with heparin or warfarin. Of those receiving anticoagulation, only 4% showed propagation of thrombus compared to 28% of those not anticoagulated. Of those who had a preexisting hemorrhage and received anticoagulation, secondary hemorrhage occurred in 14% but without worsening of outcome.

Kersbergen (85) described 10 neonates with unilateral thalamic hemorrhage and CSVT who were treated with low-molecular-weight heparin. No side effects were observed and repeat MRI at 3 to 7 months showed recanalization in all cases. Thus, despite the absence of a randomized trial, the evidence is that anticoagulation is safe and useful in confirmed CSVT, even in the presence of hemorrhage, although this is not an official recommendation by the American Heart Association (74).

Neonatal Hemorrhagic Stroke

Nontraumatic spontaneous hemorrhagic stroke is rare in term neonates, probably one in more than 10,000. The main risk factors are severe thrombocytopenia (e.g., neonatal alloimmune thrombocytopenia) and coagulopathy either inherited or from vitamin K deficiency, see Chapters 42 and 44. Congenital vascular malformation is an extremely rare cause of hemorrhagic stroke at term and would be suggested by cardiac failure or a cranial bruit.

▌ HYPOGLYCEMIC BRAIN INJURY

Diagnosis and management of hypoglycemia are fully covered in Chapter 41.

Like oxygen, glucose is a fundamental source of energy for neurons. However, newborn infants are able to use alternative fuels such as fatty acids, lactate, and ketone bodies to achieve cerebral energy sufficiency in the hours after birth immediately after placental glucose supply has ceased, but this depends on the capacity to mobilize and use alternative substrates.

The definition of neonatal hypoglycemia is controversial (see Chapter 41), and there are still variations in practice with clinicians using values ranging between <2 mmol/L [36 mg/dL] and <4 mmol/L [72 mg/dL]) (86). Although the concentration of blood glucose that is associated with brain injury is uncertain, there is consensus that values less than 18 mg/dL (1.0 mmol/L) that are prolonged and associated with acute neurologic dysfunction present the greatest risk, and that values greater than 18 mg/dL (1.0 mmol/L) that are transient and are not associated with abnormal clinical signs in an infant who is establishing feeding successfully, are not known to lead to brain injury. This gives rise to the pragmatic "operational threshold" approach to interventions, which states that for infants without clinical signs but at risk of neurologic sequelae by virtue of their impaired ability to mobilize alternative fuels at low blood glucose levels (i.e., IUGR, maternal diabetes, exposure to beta-blockers), clinicians should intervene to raise blood glucose if two consecutive blood glucose levels are below 36 mg/dL (2 mmol/L) or a single blood glucose level is below 18 mg/dL (1 mmol/L).

Intrapartum hypoxia–ischemia disturbs the typical metabolic transition and increases the likelihood of low blood glucose concentrations through several mechanisms. There is prolonged duration of anaerobic glycolysis, evidenced by increased lactate, a fall in pH, and a decrease in high-energy phosphates: two molecules of ATP are generated per molecule of glucose by anaerobic glycolysis, whereas 38 molecules are generated under oxidative conditions. This substrate expensive process leads to a rapid depletion of glycogen stores. Seizures consume cerebral energy, thereby increasing glucose utilization. In addition to depleted stores and increased CNS utilization, an infant with HIE may have increased peripheral glucose utilization, which may be compounded by transient hyperinsulinism, reduced availability of gluconeogenic precursors, and impaired counterregulatory hormone and enzyme responses that compromise the mobilization and uptake of alternative cerebral fuels. The liver is responsible for gluconeogenesis and the production of alternative fuels; so reduced perfusion and impairment of liver function has direct effects on substrate supply. Exogenous glucose supply is usually limited because this group of infants is often managed with fluid volume restriction, and because enteral feeding with breast milk, which promotes ketogenesis, may be delayed.

The brain has altered vulnerability to hypoglycemia under conditions of hypoxia–ischemia in experimental models, and clinical studies suggest a potentiating relationship between hypoxia–ischemia and early postnatal low blood glucose concentration. Therefore in HIE, blood glucose concentrations that would not normally be considered damagingly low, for example, 36 to 45 mg/dL (2.0 to 2.5 mmol/L) may worsen the severity of the injury. It has been recommended to maintain blood glucose in the range 45 to 144 mg/dL (2.5 to 8 mmol/L) in HIE. There are no randomized trials of treatment of hypoglycemic brain injury.

In situations where hypoglycemia arises due to impaired metabolic adaptation in an infant with a previously intact nervous system (e.g., due to mechanisms of reduced gluconeogenesis, reduced availability of gluconeogenic precursors, reduced activity of enzymes of glycogenolysis or gluconeogenesis, reduced activity of counterregulatory hormones, increased glucose utilization, hyperinsulinism) after a few hours, the infant becomes jittery and less responsive. We have observed that infants of normal birth weight may develop serious hypoglycemia if they are deprived of calories for long enough (e.g., 48+ hours), sometimes without problems with breastfeeding being recognized (87,88). The initially mild neurologic change may progress to hypotonia, and irregular respiration and then seizures. The neurologic sequence can be likened to hypoxia/ischemia but taking longer.

The initial phase is asymptomatic hypoglycemia during which alternative fuels maintain the energy status, followed by a phase of mild/moderate neurologic signs during which there is reversible energy depletion, followed by a phase of critical energy failure with severe neurologic disturbance, usually involving seizures and usually irreversible.

In our experience, hypoglycemia needs to have lasted for at least 6 hours and sometimes 8 hours or longer, before seizures occur, with blood glucose being below 18 mg/dL (1.0 mmol/L). In these circumstances, administration of intravenous glucose normalizes blood glucose but does not normalize neurologic status, nor control seizures. Once the prolonged hypoglycemia has produced critical energy failure in the brain severe enough to cause seizures, a sequence of damaging processes similar to posthypoxia continues for hours after correction of glucose.

As in HIE, infants with prolonged neurologic abnormality after hypoglycemia have poor prognosis with cognitive impairment and epilepsy and spastic cerebral palsy in the worst cases. The typical MRI changes associated with low blood glucose are in the white matter and cortex of occipital and parietal regions, but changes can be more widespread to include white matter injury including parenchymal hemorrhage and ischemic stroke (89).

BILIRUBIN AND BRAIN INJURY

Chapter 45 deals with diagnosis and management of hyperbilirubinemia.

Unconjugated bilirubin, in sufficient concentrations, can injure the cell membranes of neurons, enter, and then injure mitochondria, endoplasmic reticulum, and nucleus, leading to neuronal death. The term "kernicterus" originally came from postmortem neuropathology and referred to yellow staining of specific nuclei, but the term has come to be used to describe the clinical manifestations (Fig. 49.8).

Acute bilirubin encephalopathy (kernicterus) is characterized initially by lethargy, hypotonia, and poor sucking (90). This is followed by increased extensor tone with arching backward (opisthotonus), high pitched cry, and reduced level of consciousness.

Chronic bilirubin encephalopathy typically consists of extrapyramidal movements, failure of upward gaze, and sensorineural hearing impairment and may not be apparent until well after 1 year. Cognitive function may be relatively preserved but difficult to test because of the motor and hearing impairment.

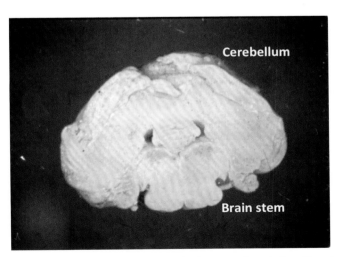

FIGURE 49.8 Kernicterus. Postmortem brain stem and cerebellum. There is *yellow* (bilirubin) staining in nuclei in the brain stem.

The nucleus referred to in the term "kernicterus" is the globus pallidus, and localized injury can be demonstrated on imaging but MRI is not as useful prognostically as it is in HIE. Careful serial neurologic examination (including hearing) is probably more meaningful in individual infants. There are no randomized trials of treatment of bilirubin encephalopathy. The emphasis must be on prediction of hyperbilirubinemia and control of bilirubin levels.

REFERENCES

1. Dubowitz LM, Dubowitz V, Palmer P, et al. A new approach to the neurological assessment of the preterm and full-term newborn infant. *Brain Dev* 1980;2:3.
2. Wiberg N, Källén K, Herbst A, et al. Relation between umbilical cord blood pH, base deficit, lactate, 5-minute Apgar score and development of hypoxic ischemic encephalopathy. *Acta Obstet Gynecol Scand* 2010;89(10):1263.
3. Pomerance JJ. Comment on "Intrapartum intrauterine fetal demise with normal umbilical cord blood gas values at birth". *Case Rep Obstet Gynecol* 2015;2015. Article ID 191426. doi: 10.1155/2015/191426
4. MacLennan A. A template for defining a causal relation between acute intrapartum events and cerebral palsy: international consensus statement. *BMJ* 1999;319:1054.
5. American College of Obstetricians and Gynecologists Task Force on Neonatal Encephalopathy. *Obstet Gynecol* 2014;123:896.
6. Myers RE. Two patterns of perinatal brain damage and their conditions of occurrence. *Am J Obstet Gynecol* 1972;112:246.
7. Thoresen M, Haaland K, Løberg EM, et al. A piglet survival model of post-hypoxic encephalopathy. *Pediatr Res* 1996;40:738.
8. Martinez-Biarge M, Diez-Sebastian J, Wusthoff CJ, et al. Antepartum and intrapartum factors preceding neonatal hypoxic-ischemic encephalopathy. *Pediatrics* 2013;132(4):e952.
9. Hope PL, Costello AM, Cady EB, et al. Cerebral energy metabolism studied with phosphorus NMR spectroscopy in normal and birth-asphyxiated infants. *Lancet* 1984;8399:366.
10. Eklind S, Mallard C, Leverin AL, et al. Bacterial endotoxin sensitizes the immature brain to hypoxic–ischaemic injury. *Eur J Neurosci* 2001;13(6):1101.
11. Sarnat HB, Sarnat MS. Neonatal encephalopathy following fetal distress. A clinical and electroencephalographic study. *Arch Neurol* 1976;33:696.
12. Levene MI, Sands C, Grindulis H, et al. Comparison of two methods of predicting outcome in perinatal asphyxia. *Lancet* 1986;8472:67.
13. Gluckman PD, Wyatt JS, Azzopardi D, et al. Selective head cooling with mild systemic hypothermia after neonatal encephalopathy: multicentre randomized trial. *Lancet* 2005;365:663.
14. Shankaran S, Laptook AR, Ehrenkranz RA, et al. Whole-body hypothermia for neonates with hypoxic-ischemic encephalopathy. *N Engl J Med* 2005;353:1574.
15. Horn AR, Swingler GH, Myer L, et al. Early clinical signs in neonates with hypoxic ischemic encephalopathy predict an abnormal amplitude-integrated electroencephalogram at age 6 hours. *BMC Pediatr* 2013;13:52. doi: 10.1186/1471-2431-13-52
16. Liu X, Jary S, Cowan F, et al. Reduced infancy and childhood epilepsy following hypothermia-treated neonatal encephalopathy. *Epilepsia* 2017;58:1902.
17. Toet MC, Hellström-Westas L, Groenendaal F, et al. Amplitude integrated EEG 3 and 6 hours after birth in full term neonates with hypoxic-ischaemic encephalopathy. *Arch Dis Child Fetal Neonatal Ed* 1999;81(1):F19.
18. Whitelaw A, White RD. Training neonatal staff in recording and reporting continuous electroencephalography. *Clin Perinatol* 2006;33(3):667.
19. Thoresen M, Hellström-Westas L, Liu X, et al. Effect of hypothermia on amplitude-integrated electroencephalogram in infants with asphyxia. *Pediatrics* 2010;126(1):e131.
20. Okereafor A, Allsop J, Counsell SJ, et al. Patterns of brain injury in neonates exposed to perinatal sentinel events. *Pediatrics* 2008;121:906.
21. Martinez-Biarge M, Diez-Sebastian J, Kapellou O, et al. Predicting motor outcome and death in term hypoxic-ischemic encephalopathy. *Neurology* 2011;76:2055.
22. Martinez-Biarge M, Bregant T, Wusthoff CJ, et al. White matter and cortical injury in hypoxic-ischemic encephalopathy: antecedent factors and 2-year outcome. *J Pediatr* 2012;161:799.
23. Thoresen M, Liu X, Jary S, et al. Lactate dehydrogenase in hypothermia-treated newborn infants with hypoxic-ischaemic encephalopathy. *Acta Paediatr* 2012;101:1038.
24. Archer LN, Levene MI, Evans DH. Cerebral artery Doppler ultrasonography for prediction of outcome after perinatal asphyxia. *Lancet* 1986;2(8516):1116.
25. Van Rooij LG, Toet MC, Osredkar D, et al. Recovery of amplitude integrated electroencephalographic background patterns within 24 hours of perinatal asphyxia. *Arch Dis Child Fetal Neonatal Ed* 2005;90:F245.
26. van Laerhoven H, de Haan TR, Offringa M, et al. Prognostic tests in term neonates with hypoxic-ischemic encephalopathy: a systematic review. *Pediatrics* 2013;131:88.
27. Kharoshankaya L, Stevenson NJ, Livingstone V, et al. Seizure burden and neurodevelopmental outcome in neonates with hypoxic-ischemic encephalopathy. *Dev Med Child Neurol* 2016;58(12):1242.
28. Tusor N, Wusthoff C, Smee N, et al. Prediction of neurodevelopmental outcome after hypoxic-ischemic encephalopathy treated with hypothermia by diffusion tensor imaging analyzed using tract-based spatial statistics. *Pediatr Res* 2012;72(1):63.
29. Lally PJ, Montaldo P, Oliveira V, et al. Magnetic resonance spectroscopy assessment of brain injury after moderate hypothermia in neonatal encephalopathy: a prospective multicentre cohort study. *Lancet Neurol* 2019;18(1):35.
30. Mitra S, Kendall GS, Bainbridge A, et al. Proton magnetic resonance spectroscopy lactate/N-acetylaspartate within 2 weeks of birth accurately predicts 2-year motor, cognitive and language outcomes in neonatal encephalopathy after therapeutic hypothermia. *Arch Dis Child Fetal Neonatal Ed* 2019;104(4):F424. doi: 10.1136/archdischild-2018-315478.
31. Walløe L. Pitfalls in using neonatal brain NAA to predict infant development. *Lancet Neurol* 2019;18(5):423. doi: 10.1016/S1474-4422(19)30111-5
32. Barta H, Jermendy A, Kolossvary M, et al. Prognostic value of early, conventional proton magnetic resonance spectroscopy in cooled asphyxiated infants. *BMC Pediatr* 2018;18(1):302. doi: 10.1186/s12887-018-1269-6
33. Moss HG, Jenkins DD, Yazdani M, et al. Identifying the translational complexity of magnetic resonance spectroscopy in neonates and infants. *NMR Biomed* 2019;32(6):e4089. doi: 10.1002/nbm.4089
34. Thoresen M. Patient selection and prognostication with hypothermia treatment. *Semin Fetal Neonatal Med.* 2010 Oct;15(5):247.
35. Hobson EE, Thomas S, Crofton PM, et al. Isolated sulphite oxidase deficiency mimics the features of hypoxic ischaemic encephalopathy. *Eur J Pediatr* 2005;164:655.
36. Thoresen M, Penrice J, Lorek A, et al. Mild hypothermia after severe transient hypoxia-ischemia ameliorates delayed cerebral energy failure in the newborn piglet. *Pediatr Res* 1995;37:667.
37. Thoresen M, Bågenholm R, Løberg EM, et al. Posthypoxic cooling of neonatal rats provides protection against brain injury. *Arch Dis Child Fetal Neonatal Ed* 1996;74(1):F3.
38. Gunn AJ, Gunn TR, de Haan HH, et al. Dramatic neuronal rescue with prolonged selective head cooling after ischemia in fetal lambs. *J Clin Invest* 1997;99(2):248.
39. Tooley JR, Satas S, Porter H, et al. Head cooling with mild systemic hypothermia in anesthetized piglets is neuroprotective. *Ann Neurol* 2003;53(1):65.
40. Bona E, Hagberg H, Løberg EM, et al. Protective effects of moderate hypothermia after neonatal hypoxia-ischemia: short- and long-term outcome. *Pediatr Res* 1998;43(6):738.
41. Thoresen M, Satas S, Puka-Sundvall M, et al. Post-hypoxic hypothermia reduces cerebrocortical release of NO and excitotoxins. *Neuroreport* 1997;8(15):3359.
42. Yuan X, Ghosh N, McFadden B, et al. Hypothermia modulates cytokine responses after neonatal rat hypoxic-ischemic injury and reduces brain damage. *ASN Neuro* 2014;6(6):1759091414558418.
43. Thornton C, Rousset CI, Kichev A, et al. Molecular mechanisms of neonatal brain injury. *Neurol Res Int* 2012;2012:506320.
44. Thoresen M, Satas S, Løberg EM, et al. Twenty-four hours of mild hypothermia in unsedated newborn pigs starting after a severe global hypoxic-ischemic insult is not neuroprotective. *Pediatr Res* 2001;50:405.
45. Osredkar D, Thoresen M, Maes E, et al. Hypothermia is not neuroprotective after infection-sensitized neonatal hypoxic-ischemic brain injury. *Resuscitation* 2014;85(4):567.
46. Davidson JO, Draghi V, Whitham S, et al. How long is sufficient for optimal neuroprotection with cerebral cooling after ischemia in fetal sheep? *J Cereb Blood Flow Metab* 2018;38(6):1047.
47. Gunn AJ, Gluckman PD, Gunn TR. Selective head cooling in newborn infants after perinatal asphyxia: a safety study. *Pediatrics* 1998;102 (4 Pt 1):885.
48. Thoresen M, Whitelaw A. Cardiovascular changes during mild therapeutic hypothermia and rewarming in infants with hypoxic-ischemic encephalopathy. *Pediatrics* 2000;106:92.
49. Azzopardi DV, Strohm B, Edwards AD, et al. Moderate hypothermia to treat perinatal asphyxial encephalopathy. *N Engl J Med* 2009;361:1349.
50. Jacobs SE, Berg M, Hunt R, et al. Cooling for newborns with hypoxic ischaemic encephalopathy. *Cochrane Database Syst Rev* 2013;1:CD003311.
51. Thoresen M. Hypothermia after perinatal asphyxia: selection for treatment and cooling protocol. *J Pediatr* 2011;158(2 suppl):e45.

THE NEWBORN INFANT

52. Liu X, Chakkarapani E, Hoque N, et al. Environmental cooling of the newborn pig brain during whole-body cooling. *Acta Paediatr* 2011;100(1):29.

53. Thyagarajan B, Tillqvist E, Baral V, et al. Minimal enteral nutrition during neonatal hypothermia treatment for perinatal hypoxic-ischaemic encephalopathy is safe and feasible. *Acta Paediatr* 2015;104(2):146.

54. Frymoyer A, Bonifacio SL, Drover DR, et al. Decreased morphine clearance in neonates with hypoxic ischemic encephalopathy receiving hypothermia. *J Clin Pharmacol* 2017;57(1):64.

55. Thoresen M, Tooley J, Liu X, et al. Time is brain: starting therapeutic hypothermia within three hours after birth improves motor outcome in asphyxiated newborns. *Neonatology* 2013;104(3):228.

56. Laptook AR, Shankaran S, Tyson JE, et al. Effect of therapeutic hypothermia initiated after 6 hours of age on death or disability among newborns with hypoxic-ischemic encephalopathy: a randomized clinical trial. *JAMA* 2017;318(16):1550.

57. Walløe L, Hjort NL, Thoresen M. Major concerns about late hypothermia study. *Acta Paediatr* 2019;108(4):588.

58. Wood T, Osredkar D, Puchades M, et al. Treatment temperature and insult severity influence the neuroprotective effects of therapeutic hypothermia. *Sci Rep* 2016;6:23430.

59. Alonso-Alconada D, Broad KD, Bainbridge A, et al. Brain cell death is reduced with cooling by 3.5°C to 5°C but increased with cooling by 8.5°C in a piglet asphyxia model. *Stroke* 2015;46(1):275.

60. Shankaran S, Laptook AR, Pappas A, et al. Effect of depth and duration of cooling on death or disability at age 18 months among neonates with hypoxic-ischemic encephalopathy: a randomized clinical trial. *JAMA* 2017;318(1):57.

61. Davidson JO, Wassink G, Yuill CA, et al. How long is too long for cerebral cooling after ischemia in fetal sheep? *J Cereb Blood Flow Metab* 2015;35(5):751.

62. Thoresen M. Who should we cool after perinatal asphyxia? *Semin Fetal Neonatal Med* 2015;20(2):751.

63. El-Dib M, Inder TE, Chalak LF, et al. Should therapeutic hypothermia be offered to babies with mild neonatal encephalopathy in the first 6 h after birth? *Pediatr Res* 2019;85(4):442.

64. Smit E, Liu X, Jary S, et al. Cooling neonates who do not fulfil the standard cooling criteria—short- and long-term outcomes. *Acta Paediatr* 2015;104(2):138.

65. Kaandorp JJ, van Bel F, Veen S, et al. Long-term neuroprotective effects of allopurinol after moderate perinatal asphyxia: follow-up of two randomised controlled trials. *Arch Dis Child Fetal Neonatal Ed* 2012;97(3):F162.

66. Malla RR, Asimi R, Teli MA, et al. Erythropoietin monotherapy in perinatal asphyxia with moderate to severe encephalopathy: a randomized placebo-controlled trial. *J Perinatol* 2017;37(5):596.

67. Garg B, Sharma D, Bansal A. Systematic review seeking erythropoietin role for neuroprotection in neonates with hypoxic ischemic encephalopathy: presently where do we stand. *J Matern Fetal Neonatal Med* 2018;31(23):3214.

68. Zhu C, Kang W, Xu F, et al. Erythropoietin improved neurologic outcomes in newborns with hypoxic-ischemic encephalopathy. *Pediatrics* 2009;124(2):e218.

69. Aly H, Elmahdy H, El-Dib M, et al. Melatonin use for neuroprotection in perinatal asphyxia: a randomized controlled pilot study. *J Perinatol* 2015;35(3):186.

70. Robertson NJ, Martinello K, Lingam I, et al. Melatonin as an adjunct to therapeutic hypothermia in a piglet model of neonatal encephalopathy: a translational study. *Neurobiol Dis* 2019;121:240.

71. Chakkarapani E, Dingley J, Liu X, et al. Xenon enhances hypothermic neuroprotection in asphyxiated newborn pigs. *Ann Neurol* 2010;68(3):330.

72. Dingley J, Tooley J, Liu X, et al. Xenon ventilation during therapeutic hypothermia in neonatal encephalopathy: a feasibility study. *Pediatrics* 2014;133(5):809.

73. Azzopardi D, Robertson NJ, Bainbridge A, et al. Moderate hypothermia within 6 h of birth plus inhaled xenon versus moderate hypothermia alone after birth asphyxia (TOBY-Xe): a proof-of-concept, open-label, randomised controlled trial. *Lancet Neurol* 2016;15(2):145.

74. Ferriero DM, Fullerton HJ, Bernard TJ, et al. Management of stroke in neonates and children: a scientific statement from the American Heart Association/American Stroke Association. *Stroke* 2019;50(3):e51.

75. Agrawal N, Johnston SC, Wu YW, et al. Imaging data reveal a higher pediatric stroke incidence than prior US estimates. *Stroke* 2009;40(11):3415.

76. Lee J, Croen LA, Backstrand KH, et al. Maternal and infant characteristics associated with perinatal arterial stroke in the infant. *JAMA* 2005;293(6):723.

77. Wu YW, March WM, Croen LA, et al. Perinatal stroke in children with motor impairment: a population-based study. *Pediatrics* 2004;114(3):612.

78. Wien MA, Whitehead MT, Bulas D, et al. Patterns of brain injury in newborns treated with extracorporeal membrane oxygenation. *AJNR Am J Neuroradiol* 2017;38(4):820.

79. Grunt S, Mazenauer L, Buerki SE, et al. Incidence and outcomes of symptomatic neonatal arterial ischemic stroke. *Pediatrics* 2015;135(5):e1220.

80. Boardman JP, Ganesan V, Rutherford MA, et al. Magnetic resonance image correlates of hemiparesis after neonatal and childhood middle cerebral artery stroke. *Pediatrics* 2005;115(2):321.

81. Bosenbark DD, Krivitzky L, Ichord R, et al. Clinical predictors of attention and executive functioning outcomes in children after perinatal arterial ischemic stroke. *Pediatr Neurol* 2017;69:79.

82. Eliasson AC, Nordstrand L, Ek L, et al. The effectiveness of Baby-CIMT in infants younger than 12 months with clinical signs of unilateral-cerebral palsy; an explorative study with randomized design. *Res Dev Disabil* 2018;72:191.

83. Fitzgerald KC, Williams LS, Garg BP, et al. Cerebral sinovenous thrombosis in the neonate. *Arch Neurol* 2006;63(3):405.

84. Moharir MD, Shroff M, Stephens D, et al. Anticoagulants in pediatric cerebral sinovenous thrombosis: a safety and outcome study. *Ann Neurol* 2010;67(5):590.

85. Kersbergen KJ, de Vries LS, van Straaten HL, et al. Anticoagulation therapy and imaging in neonates with a unilateral thalamic hemorrhage due to cerebral sinovenous thrombosis. *Stroke* 2009;40(8):2754.

86. Dixon KC, Ferris RL, Marikar D, et al. Definition and monitoring of neonatal hypoglycaemia: a nationwide survey of NHS England Neonatal Units. *Arch Dis Child Fetal Neonatal Ed* 2017;102(1):F92.

87. Perlman JM, Volpe JJ. Glucose. In: Volpe JJ, Inder T, Barras B, et al., eds. *Volpe's neurology of the newborn*, 6th ed. Philadelphia, PA: Elsevier, 2017:701.

88. Dyer C. NHS failed to communicate feeding advice to refugee mother, court rules. *BMJ* 2018;361:k1711. doi: 10.1136/bmj.k1711

89. Boardman JP, Wusthoff CJ, Cowan FM. Hypoglycaemia and neonatal brain injury. *Arch Dis Child Educ Pract Ed* 2013;98(1):2.

90. Perlman JM, Volpe JJ. Bilirubin. In: Volpe JJ, Inder T, Barras B, et al., eds. *Volpe's neurology of the newborn*, 6th ed. Philadelphia, PA: Elsevier, 2018:730.

50 Brain Development and Injury in Preterm Infants

David Edwards, Serena J. Counsell, and Pierre Gressens

INTRODUCTION

Premature birth is a worldwide problem, estimated to be annually responsible for 77 million lost disability-adjusted life years, 3.1% of the global total (1). The rates of impairment and disability among survivors are improving but remain significant, particularly for nonmotor problems.

Data from the population-based Epipage studies show that with modern intensive care, the overall rate of cerebral palsy at 24 to 26, 27 to 31, and 32 to 34 weeks of gestation is 7% (95% confidence intervals 5% to 10%), 4% (3% to 5%), and 1% (0.5% to 12%), respectively. Survival without neuromotor or sensory disabilities among live births increased between 1997 and 2011 from 45% (39% to 52%) to 62% (57% to 67%) at 25 to 26 weeks of gestation (2). Emerging data from low- and middle-income countries seem broadly comparable: the rate of cerebral palsy in preterm infants in Vietnam is 7% (3).

However, a high proportion of preterm infants have non-motor problems: in the Epipage studies, the percentage of children below threshold on a well-accepted measure of functional development at 24 to 26, 27 to 31, and 32 to 34 weeks of gestation were 50% (44% to 56%), 41% (38% to 43%), and 36% (32% to 40%), respectively (2). Cognitive, socialization, educational, sexual, and behavioral problems are apparent in up to half of preterm infants (4–7). Neuropsychiatric disorders develop as the children grow older: autistic spectrum disorder, attention deficit disorders, schizophrenia, and other mental health problems are more common, and preterm infants are approximately 7 times more likely to be diagnosed with bipolar disease (8).

It is increasingly clear that the adverse cerebral sequelae of preterm birth leading to these varied problems arise from a combination of brain injury and dysmaturation. The increasingly high survival rates for preterm infants means that understanding the nature of these abnormalities relies heavily on noninvasive investigation, particularly neuroimaging. This chapter will describe relevant features of brain development and review what is known about preterm cerebral lesions and dysmaturation, mechanisms of injury, clinical assessment, and strategies to reduce adverse outcomes.

BRAIN DEVELOPMENT

Between 23 and 44 weeks of gestation, the brain grows from a smooth lissencephalic organ resembling a coffee bean to the familiar, much larger, walnut-like structure with complex gyrification (Fig. 50.1) (9,10). Cortical sulcation develops from around 14 weeks of gestation: the medial surface folds before the lateral surface, and morphologic differentiation of sulci begins in the central region and progresses in an occipitorostral direction (Fig. 50.2) (11). This rapid cortical growth is matched by concomitant increase in connections within and between brain regions, and cerebellar development is particularly rapid from 24 to 40 weeks of gestation with an exponential growth in foliation. The program that determines early brain growth is largely genetic, but other influences play a role, for example, gyrification appears to be influenced by the mechanical tension between brain regions created by early axonal connections (12). These developments require a complex choreography of cellular elements, which has been comprehensively reviewed in the context of preterm birth by Volpe (4), and are summarized below.

Neuronal Development

Neurogenesis

The central nervous system is initially derived from the embryonic neural tube, formed in approximately the 3rd to 4th weeks of gestation. In the most rostral section of the neural tube, two vesicles are formed: the telencephalon, which gives rise to the cerebral cortex, and the diencephalon, which gives rise to deep structures including the thalamus and hypothalamus.

The growing cortex is initially composed of a single layer of radially oriented proliferating neuroepithelial cells lining the walls of the lateral ventricles, known as the ventricular zone. This early proliferation gives rise to neurons, and also to radial glia that grow to span the width of the cerebrum from the ventricular zone to the pial surface and form tracks that guide the movement of postmitotic neurons from their point of creation in the ventricular zone to the cortex. Around the 7th gestational week, a second zone of proliferation develops, the internal subventricular zone, derived from precursors in the ventricular zone. The cells of the internal subventricular zone do not adopt a radial configuration. More recently, a third proliferative zone has been identified in the developing neocortex: the external subventricular zone, which appears around the 11th gestational week.

Brain development involves overproduction of neurons and connections, followed by elimination of unnecessary elements. Some 15% to 20% of all neurons produced die through apoptosis, around 70% these between 28 and 41 weeks of gestation, with electrical activity and synaptic stimulation appearing to be important survival factors. In rodents, substances that block electrical activity (such as anticonvulsants and anesthetics) during brain development lead to widespread cell death.

Neural Migration

Neurons migrate from their origin in the proliferative zone to their eventual position, with the fate of individual differentiating neuroblasts dependent upon their position in proliferative zones, their exposure to chemical attractant and repellent cues in the surrounding tissue, and whether or not they form functional connections. Neurons form the cortex from the inside out: the first wave of postmitotic neurons migrate orthogonally from the ventricular/subventricular zones along radial glia to form the preplate; later cohorts migrate through the preplate to create the cortical plate, splitting preplate into layer one above and subplate beneath (Fig. 50.3). Younger-born neurons migrate past previously formed layers toward the pial surface and form progressively layers six to two. A large proportion of neurons, which later give rise to the GABAergic interneuron population, adopt a different migration pattern by first moving tangentially from the ganglionic eminence toward targets in the cortex and thalamus.

Neuronal migration reaches its peak between 12 and 20 weeks of gestation and is mostly complete by 26 to 29 weeks, although late migrating GABAergic neurons arrive in cortex in the third trimester and form a substantial proportion of the population of cortical inhibitory neurons.

Axon Formation

Axonal bundles that will later develop into major white matter pathways appear as early as 8 weeks of gestation. Specialized growth cones at the end of the axon interact with guidance cues in the extracellular environment to navigate the growing axon

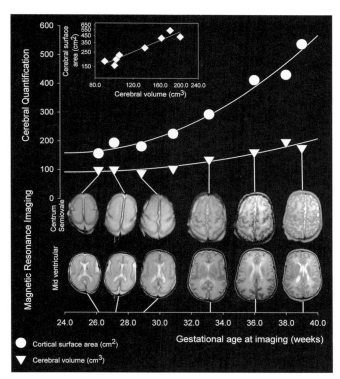

FIGURE 50.1 Growth of cerebral volume and cortical surface area in one preterm infant. (From Kapellou O, Counsell SJ, Kennea N, et al. Abnormal cortical development after premature birth shown by altered allometric scaling of brain growth. *PLoS Med* 2006;3(8):e265. Copyright © 2006 Kapellou et al.)

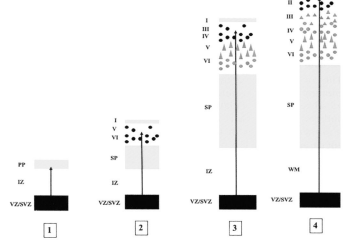

FIGURE 50.3 Schematic representation of neocortical neurogenesis and neural migration. VZ/SVZ, ventricular/subventricular zones where neurogenesis is taking place; IZ, intermediate zone (prospective white matter—WM); PP, preplate; SP, subplate; I, cortical layer I or molecular layer; II to VI, cortical layers II to VI. *Arrows* and *blue circles* indicate migrating neurons, while *red circles* (granular neurons) and *triangles* (pyramidal neurons) represent postmigratory neurons. (Credit of Dr. Pierre Gressens.)

front to its correct position. Guidance cues can either be substrate bound or diffusible and include semaphorins, netrins, and ephrins, which act as chemoattractants or repellents for specific axonal subtypes. Interaction of these guidance cues and growth cone receptors facilitates or inhibits axonal growth and directs the axon to its correct target.

Cortical Subplate

The cortical subplate is an important transient structure situated below the developing cortex in regions destined to become white matter in the mature brain. The subplate reaches its greatest extent at around 20 weeks of gestational age and persists until around term. It serves as a "waiting station" for neuronal afferents from the thalamus, basal forebrain, and brainstem on their way to the cortex. These afferents synapse transiently with subplate neurons, which themselves connect with and mediate functional maturation of the cortex. Afferent neurons then disconnect from the subplate and make permanent connections with targets in the

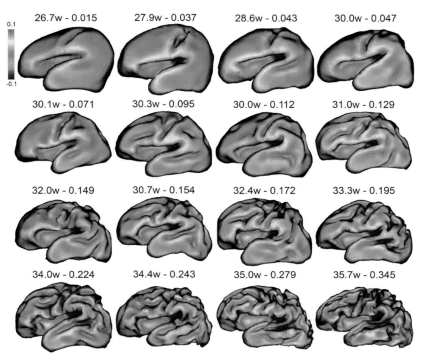

FIGURE 50.2 Inner cortical surface reconstructions: examples of the 3D interface between the developing cortex and white matter zone for newborns of different gestational age (in weeks, left numbers) and SI (right numbers). The colors outline the surface curvature. The surfaces are not displayed with the same spatial scale. (From Dubois J, Benders M, Cachia A, et al. Mapping the early cortical folding process in the preterm newborn brain. *Cereb Cortex* 2008;18:1444. Copyright © The Author 2007. Reproduced by permission of Oxford University Press.)

cortex. If afferents do not make these transient subplate synapses, they will often fail to connect to the correct cortical targets and there is disruption to normal cortical development. Disturbance of this process offers one potential mechanism for cerebral dysmaturation in preterm infants.

Cortical Maturation

The cortical plate develops into distinct layers beginning in sensorimotor cortex at around 25 weeks of gestation, and by 32 weeks, mostly cortex has six layers, each with distinct arrays of cell types and connections. Cells that are vertically adjacent are organized into radial columns that have distinct connections and histologic appearances, which form the basis of the cortical atlases defined by Brodman and Von Economo.

Interneuron formation, elaboration of dendritic trees, and axonal outgrowth cause the marked increase in cortical surface area and the number and complexity of gyri. Dendritic development is especially rapid and correlates with electrical activity, depending on afferent input from thalamic, commissural, and corticocortical fibers. Thalamocortical axons are developing rapidly from around 26 weeks, and this development correlates with electroencephalographic maturation.

At this stage of development, GABAergic interneurons, which are inhibitory in mature brain, are paradoxically stimulatory. Activation of chloride-permeable GABA-a receptors, which in the mature brain is inhibitory, leads to neuronal excitation due to simultaneous expression of the Na^+ K^+ $2Cl^-$ cotransporter (NKCC1), which causes intracellular chloride accumulation, elevated chloride levels, and a depolarized equilibrium potential. GABA becomes inhibitory as net outward neuronal transport of Cl^- develops during maturation. This maturational sequence has implications to the generation and therapeutic intervention of neonatal seizures.

Proliferation of cells of the external granular layer of the cerebellum allows the external layer to expand horizontally to create a 30-fold increase in surface area. The cerebellum is particularly rich in glucocorticoid receptors which may affect its vulnerability to stress.

Synaptic Development

Like neurogenesis, synaptic development proceeds by production of excess elements followed by pruning. Synaptogenesis appears to proceed in five main phases: (a) around 6 to 8 weeks, synaptogenesis is limited to deep structures; (b) around 12 to 17 weeks, a relatively small number of synapses are produced in the cortex; (c) from around mid-pregnancy to 8 months after birth, synaptogenesis grows dramatically, with many thousands estimated to be formed each minute; (d) synapse production continues until puberty; and (e) in adulthood, synaptogenesis may be masked by loss of synapses related to aging. Experimentally, the two initial phases are not influenced by the deprivation of sensory stimuli, the third phase is partly dependent on sensory input, whereas the fourth phase is strongly influenced by sensory stimuli and experience.

Synapse production is largely genetically controlled, and it appears that during the course of evolution, a moderate increase in the number of genes involved in synaptogenesis has led to a richer substrate upon which environmental factors and experience can act, to result in a more complex network. Both synaptogenesis and synaptic pruning normally requires the participation of microglial cells.

Neuroglia

Astrocytes

Astrocytes are involved in axonal guidance, the growth and survival of neurons via trophic factor production, synapse formation and maintenance, the transfer of metabolites between blood vessels and neurons, the establishment of templates for certain brain structures, myelination, and maintenance of the blood–brain barrier. Neonatal astrocytes are of two origins: at the end of neuronal migration, radial glia are transformed into astrocytes populating deep cortical layers and white matter, while in superficial cortical layers, astrocytes are derived principally from glial precursors that migrated from the subventricular zone. Astrocytic proliferation probably starts at around 24 weeks of gestation, with a peak at around 26 to 28 weeks and may be largely complete by the end of a normal pregnancy, presenting another vulnerability for infants born preterm.

Oligodendrocytes

Oligodendrocytes are the cells responsible for myelination, which begins before term and is largely but not entirely complete by 2 to 3 years of age. Primary sensory functions such as olfactory auditory pathways and primary sensorimotor cortex are the first structures to be myelinated, while projection and heteromodal association cortex, in particular the prefrontal structures, myelinate later.

Oligodendrocytes mature through four stages: (a) during the third trimester and early postnatal period bipolar, mitotically active oligodendrocyte precursors arise in the subventricular zone; (b) differentiation into multipolar preoligodendrocytes takes place during migration through white matter; (c) multipolar immature oligodendrocytes surround axons preparatory to myelination; and (d) mature oligodendrocytes mediate myelination.

Preoligodendrocytes, the predominant variety in the preterm brain, are highly vulnerable to oxidative stress, excitotoxic injury, and hypoxic–ischemic insults, and their maturation and function are disrupted by neuroinflammation. Attenuated oligodendrocyte maturation appears to play a critical role in the adverse effects of preterm birth.

Microglia

Microglia have an important role in normal synapse formation, synapse pruning, and neurite remodeling and are also central to controlling and mediating neuroinflammation in response to central or peripheral inflammatory stimuli. They constitute 5% to 15% of the total number of brain cells and are derived from precursors that arise from the yolk sac early during development and invade the developing brain. Although sometimes called "the brain's macrophages," they are a separate cell lineage, with different embryologic origins, cell surface markers, and functions.

During the first trimester, microglia have an amoeboid morphology that progressively evolves into a mature phenotype consisting of a small cell body and long processes. In mid pregnancy, microglial populations are principally detected in white matter bundles, such as the internal and external capsules, the corpus callosum, and the intersections of axonal fiber bundles. High microglial density correlates with high risk for white matter lesions, and microglia are thought to play an important role in the genesis of lesions: inflammation induces microglial activation, and microglia control the functions of blood-derived macrophages trafficking to the brain, although it remains to be understood fully how this influences brain injury and development.

PRETERM BRAIN DAMAGE

Clinical Associations of Adverse Outcomes

The neurologic risks associated with prematurity begin before delivery. Placental dysfunction and abruption, oligohydramnios, preeclampsia, chorioamnionitis, maternal stress, and substance abuse all increase risks to fetal brain development, and intrauterine growth retardation is independently associated with worse outcomes in preterm infants (13,14).

However, there is a strong relationship between adverse neurologic outcome and younger age at birth (5), at least in part because extreme prematurity increases the prevalence of comorbidities associated with brain injury, although it is not clear if this is a causal relationship or due to shared vulnerabilities (15). Respiratory disease, particularly bronchopulmonary dysplasia, is strongly associated with adverse neurocognitive outcome (15). Inflammatory conditions including necrotizing enterocolitis and infection are associated with brain injury (16,17). Circulatory instability is linked to periventricular hemorrhage and periventricular leukomalacia (PVL): hypoxia–ischemia may initiate cerebral injury, as possibly may chronic hypoxia, although the evidence for this is less strong (18). Inflammation and hypoxia–ischemia together have a synergistic effect so that insults that individually are too small to induce significant damage can combine to cause significant injury (19). It is likely that nutrition is important, but strong evidence of a role for specific nutrients is sparse (20). Infants probably have individual levels of intrinsic genetic vulnerability, which predispose or protect them from injury (21,22), and current evidence would support a "multiple hit" model in which multiple environmental, clinical, and genetic elements combine together (23).

Iatrogenic risk factors for cerebral injury include birth outside a hospital with a neonatal intensive care unit and the ex utero transfer of infants between hospitals (24). Care pathways probably have wider, less well-documented effects, as there are significant differences between geographical regions that are not accounted for by maternal or infant characteristics (25). Hypoglycemia is thought to be a risk to brain development, but this is poorly understood, and the critical lower level where brain risks become significant is hard to define (26,27). Blood gas measurements outside the normal range are also believed to carry a significant risk to brain development, although it is difficult to separate these factors from other manifestations of clinical instability (28). Despite the incomplete evidence base, good clinical practice emphasizes maintaining physiologic stability.

Cerebral Damage and Dysmaturation

In many cases, the neuropathologic mechanism for the neurologic, cognitive, and psychiatric problems associated with prematurity is unclear, and only a small proportion of infants show clear evidence of destructive brain lesions. It is emerging that in addition to recognizable cerebral damage, adverse outcomes are associated with abnormal brain maturation, and persistent abnormalities of growth and development can be detected in gray and white matter throughout the cerebrum and cerebellum, with some predilection for particular regions but wide variations between individuals (4).

However, some cerebral lesions, including periventricular haemorrhage and PVL, have been extensively described and studied by neuropathology and neuroimaging.

Periventricular Hemorrhage

This was first noted postmortem in the early 20th century, and systematically characterized in the 1920s. Influential studies that defined the neuropathology and hypothesized mechanisms were codified by Wigglesworth and Pape and formed the basis for much early thinking about preterm brain injury (29). The advent of three-dimensional neuroimaging defined the clinical associations and prevalence of hemorrhage, and characterized the developmental consequences in survivors. In 1978, using the newly developed CT scanner, Papile and colleagues produced a simple classification of hemorrhage into four grades (Table 50.1) (see Chapter 21) (30). This formed the basis for clinical classifications, which became widely used after the discovery of transfontanellar ultrasonography by Reynolds (31) and Cooke (32) in 1979.

Ultrasound detects hemorrhage with high levels of accuracy, and it became clear that hemorrhage occurs around the time of birth, so that new lesions appearing after the first week are

TABLE 50.1

Classification of Periventricular Hemorrhage

	Papile (30)	Volpe (34)
Grade 1	Subependymal hemorrhage	Germinal matrix hemorrhage with no or minimal intraventricular hemorrhage (<10% of ventricular area in parasagittal view)
Grade 2	Intraventricular hemorrhage without ventricular dilatation	Intraventricular hemorrhage (10%–50% of ventricular area in parasagittal view)
Grade 3	Intraventricular hemorrhage with ventricular dilation	Intraventricular hemorrhage (>50% of ventricular area in parasagittal view: usually distends lateral ventricle)
Grade 4	Intraventricular hemorrhage with parenchymal hemorrhage	Not graded: separate notation for hemorrhagic parenchymal infarction

Several different systems have been developed to classify periventricular hemorrhage, and the use of different definitions contributes to the variance in the literature on the outcome of particular lesions. The earliest was by Papile, based on CT scan appearance, and this remains the simplest. Volpe revised the classification based on neuropathologic considerations.

Grade 1: Defined by Papile as subependymal hemorrhage, this is confined to the subependymal in the region of the germinal matrix and is often called "germinal matrix hemorrhage." Classically detected by ultrasound in the thalamocaudate notch, MRI shows that it can occur anywhere along the germinal matrix. Volpe includes small amounts of ventricular blood in this grade. In practice, many neonatologists follow Papile.

Grade 2: Papile and Volpe definitions are largely compatible. Blood in the ventricles can sometimes be difficult to distinguish from choroid plexus on ultrasound examination.

Grade 3: Defined by Papile as "intraventricular hemorrhage with ventricular dilation"; there is some disagreement about whether the distention has to be by blood or can be by CSF. Volpe does not require ventricular distention, just a significant quantity of blood in the ventricle. Many clinicians would classify any large hemorrhage with ventricles distended by blood or CSF as grade 3.

Grade 4: Defined by Papile as "intraventricular hemorrhage with parenchymal hemorrhage"; Volpe separates hemorrhagic parenchymal infarction, with or without blood in the ventricles, as a separate entity but in practice there is consistency.

uncommon. Hemorrhage, particularly grade 4, which is a hemorrhagic parenchymal infarction due to venous infarction (33) caused by obstructed venous outflow, is associated with disrupted hemodynamics: impaired cerebral autoregulation; abnormal blood flow related for example to hypercarbia; increased cerebral venous pressure, classically linked to pneumothorax or right ventricular overload; and hypotension followed by volume loading. In general, circulatory instability before, during or after delivery seems to predispose to periventricular hemorrhage. Hemorrhagic lesions are characteristically thought to be focal, with the remainder of the brain relatively unaffected (34).

Severe hemorrhages are uncommon: population-based data from the Epipage studies suggests that hemorrhagic parenchymal infarction occurs in 4% (95% confidence limits 3 to 4); grade 3 in 3% (3 to 4); grade 2 in 12% (11 to 13); and grade 1 in 17% (15 to 18) (13). While the global incidence is hard to ascertain, a study of 1760 infants in China reported an incidence of 17% for all periventricular hemorrhages (35) and a similar value was reported from the United Arab Emirates, including 2% hemorrhagic parenchymal infarction (36).

Periventricular Leukomalacia

Periventricular leukomalacia, "softening of the white matter" associated with cystic destructive lesions, was classically described by Banker and Larroche in 1962 as a form of "anoxic encephalopathy" in infants born between 26 and 40 weeks of gestation with a variety of clinical problems not confined to prematurity but including congenital heart disease and erythroblastosis fetalis (37). They described focal periventricular necroses with loss of all cellular elements and diffuse axonal injury thought to be due to global hypoxic–ischemic damage to the immature brain. In contradistinction to hemorrhagic parenchymal infarction, PVL is regarded as an arterial infarction and usually involves large volumes of brain tissue.

Classical cystic PVL is only rarely detected and can sometimes be difficult to confirm using only cerebral ultrasound, but if seen, it is characteristically around 2 weeks following a period of severe hypoperfusion or hypoxia when the focal cysts give evidence of global cerebral injury. In the Epipage studies, cystic PVL occurs in fewer than 5% of infants, and the incidence is no higher in unselected groups studied with magnetic resonance imaging (MRI) (13,38).

Lenticulostriate Vasculopathy

Hyperechogenic blood vessels are sometimes detected forming a trident shape in the thalamus and basal ganglia. In term infants, these lesions raise the suspicion of congenital infection, but in the preterm infant, the cause is usually unknown. In the large prospective ePrime study, they were detected in 143 of 510 infants at term-corrected age and had no association with adverse outcome.

Punctate Lesions

The advent of MRI for extremely preterm infants allowed investigators to detect further types of brain lesion not seen on ultrasound (39). Small focal changes, "punctate lesions," can be detected immediately after delivery and in a proportion of cases persist until term. They can be single or multiple, and isolated punctate lesions are typically associated with higher gestational age and birth weight, and less severe chronic lung disease. In one study, 24% of infants had punctate lesions at term, predominantly in the centrum semiovale and corona radiata. The pathology of these lesions is unclear, but it is likely that they are small focal regions of cell death and neuroinflammation. Punctate lesions probably represent part of a more widespread abnormality, as they are associated with reduced thalamic volume and diffuse microstructural changes in white matter (**Fig. 50.4**) (punctate lesions) (40,41).

Cerebellar Lesions

MRI also showed that cerebellar lesions are common and include hemorrhage, infarction and reduced growth; this is a poorly understood and probably underrecognized problem. Small studies have shown adverse outcome in a high proportion of infants, but interpretation is complex because cerebellar damage is often associated with supratentorial lesions (42).

Diffuse White Matter Abnormalities and the Encephalopathy of Prematurity

The abnormality most frequently detected by MRI in preterm infants is diffuse and widespread abnormality in white matter without cystic change, seen in up to 80% of preterm infants at term-corrected age, although with extreme variation in the location and severity between individuals (**Fig. 50.5**) (40). Diffuse white matter disease is often associated with corpus callosal thinning, ventriculomegaly, and reduced cortical and thalamic growth. It is possible that these diffuse lesions are the mild end of a spectrum of a single pathologic process that includes PVL and punctate lesions; however, this remains unproven (43).

A significant overall finding from the totality of neuroimaging and postmortem neuropathologic studies is that focal lesions are relatively rare and do not explain the prevalence or variety of adverse long-term adverse outcomes; however, abnormalities of growth, development, and maturation are common. To encompass both injury and abnormal development, Volpe introduced the descriptive term *"Encephalopathy of Prematurity"* (44) including the spectrum of cystic PVL; small focal lesions; nonclastic diffuse white matter abnormalities; abnormal cortical and deep gray matter; and reduced brain growth.

The mechanism appears to be fundamentally inflammatory, initiated by local or systemic infection, hypoxia–ischemia or biotrauma. Activation of microglia diverts them from their normal homeostatic role and induces production of pro-inflammatory cytokines and reactive oxygen species, and probably also

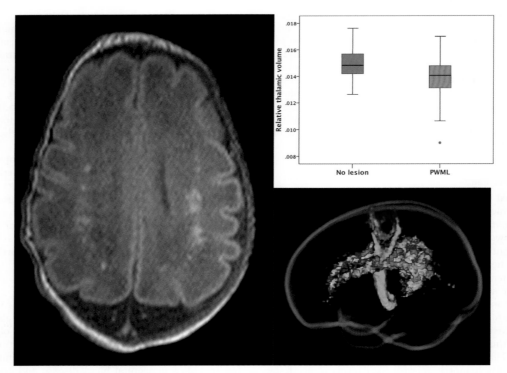

FIGURE 50.4 Punctate lesions in preterm brain (left) are associated with reduced growth in the thalamus (right upper). The distribution of punctate lesions in 131 infants, shown in relation to white matter tracts traversing the internal capsule (*blue*) rendered in a transparent brain image (*right lower*). PWML, punctate white matter lesion. (From Tusor N, Benders MJ, Counsell SJ, et al. Punctate white matter lesions associated with altered brain development and adverse motor outcome in preterm infants. *Sci Rep* 2017;7:13250. http://creativecommons.org/licenses/by/4.0/.)

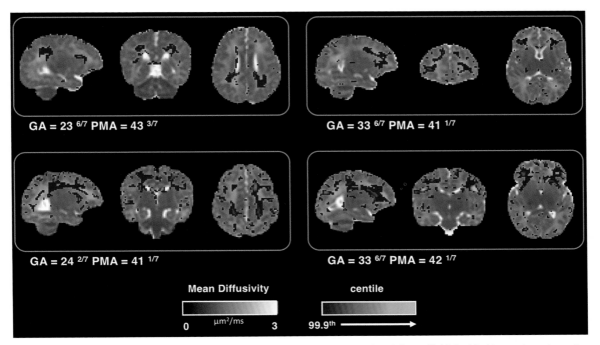

FIGURE 50.5 dMRI images showing mean diffusivity, a measure of tissue microstructure, in four infants. Highlighted in *blue* are the regions where each preterm infant had significantly abnormal mean diffusivity (>99.9 centile). These examples demonstrate the high levels of heterogeneity in white matter abnormalities following preterm birth. GA, gestational age at birth; PMA, postmenstrual age at scan (in weeks + days). (Credit: Dr Ralica Dimitrova and the Developing Human Connectome Project.)

recruitment of circulating phagocytes into the brain. Activated microglia lose their normal functions in synapse development, function, and plasticity, with potentially detrimental effects on neuronal differentiation and connectivity (45).

Microglial activation can also induce oligodendrocyte precursor death or dysmaturation, leading to deficient myelination. In animal models, moderate systemic inflammation causes a blockade to maturation of oligodendrocyte precursors beyond the precursor stage, while severe systemic inflammation, protracted hypoxia, or hypoxic–ischemic insult lead to a combination of oligodendrocyte precursor death and maturation blockade. However, it would appear that maturational blockade rather than death is a key feature of diffuse white matter injury. In most rodent models, oligodendrocyte precursor maturation does finally catch up (at a time-point equivalent to young adulthood or late puberty), allowing normal myelination; however, behavioral impairments persist. This is consistent with imaging and behavioral outcomes in humans after preterm birth. These multiple deleterious effects mean that microglial activation has emerged as a key hallmark of encephalopathy of prematurity (45).

During the preterm period, interneurons are actively migrating to the cortex where they play a key role in the balance between excitation and inhibition. Postmortem and experimental studies suggest specific deficits in cortical interneurons: parvalbumin interneurons are instrumental for neuronal circuit plasticity, and recent studies suggest that this specific subset of interneurons is decreased in the cortex of preterm infants; these data suggest one potential mechanism for the reduced cortical growth associated with preterm birth (46).

Evolution of Cerebral Abnormalities

Germinal matrix (grade 1) hemorrhages usually resolve to form subependymal pseudocysts by term-corrected age, and intraventricular blood is slowly cleared by the endogenous fibrinolytic system.

Parenchymal hemorrhagic infarction resolves to form porencephalic cysts that are frequently in communication with the lateral ventricles. Residual blood clot and cerebral debris can cause posthemorrhagic hydrocephalus, which appears to increase the injury to the brain (47). A large retrospective study found that hydrocephalus developed in 28% of grade 4 and 25% of grade 3 hemorrhages, 38% of whom were treated with ventriculoperitoneal shunts (45). The optimal timing for intervention is unclear, although many clinicians would aim to reduce cerebrospinal fluid volumes by spinal or ventricular tap (often utilizing a neurosurgically placed reservoir to avoid repeated ventricular puncture) when the Ventricular Index (the width of the lateral ventricles measured at the level of the foramen of Munro) is size greater than the 97th centile (see Chapter 21). However, there is no good evidence that repeated tapping reduces the need for ventriculoperitoneal shunts or improves outcome (48). Attempts to improve outcomes using fibrinolysis have to date produced equivocal results (49).

In cystic PVL, the cavitating lesions disappear over the course of a few weeks due to growth of adjacent brain tissue; unfortunately, this does not imply resolution of associated functional deficits and "disappearing" cystic PVL retains a poor prognosis. Some punctate lesions disappear; the functional relevance of this is not known.

The plasticity of the developing brain significantly modifies outcomes after preterm brain injury. The location of critical functions within the cortex is known to change following injury: after injury involving primary sensorimotor cortex sensory and motor functions have been detected by functional MRI (fMRI) in distant cortical regions, together with appropriate white matter connections (50). Varying plasticity is probably one of the factors that reduce the precision of perinatal neuroimaging as a guide to neurodevelopment (44).

Long after insults to the immature brain, there may be persisting injury processes in addition to developmental disruption. The mechanisms are poorly understood but probably include persistent inflammation, reduced growth, abnormal dopamine synthesis, altered epigenetics, and impaired endogenous repair. These factors may predispose to the development of later cognitive dysfunction and sensitization to further injury (45,51).

CLINICAL ASSESSMENT OF PERINATAL BRAIN INJURY

Ultrasound and MRI abnormalities are associated with a variety of adverse outcomes at a group level, and these data have been valuable in understanding the pathogenesis of preterm brain injury. They also offer the clinician a valuable guide in the case of severe focal brain damage, particularly hemorrhage. However, as a diagnostic tool for routinely assigning individual prognosis, imaging is often imprecise and clinical judgment is needed to make the best use of the information.

Cranial Ultrasound

Cranial ultrasonography is the workhorse for clinical assessment of preterm brain injury and is an excellent tool for detecting periventricular hemorrhage. Hemorrhages are usually classified into four grades based on the original work of Papile et al. (30), although the growth of slightly different classifications can lead to some confusion (see Table 50.1). Although much less sensitive at detecting PVL, arterial stroke, or other lesions, ultrasound can still sometimes provide useful information.

Many studies have reported the relationship between ultrasound appearances and neurodevelopmental outcomes, although rather fewer have examined cognitive abilities. Most report outcomes at around 2 years of age when ascertainment of long-term problems may not be completely precise. Studies can be combined through a meta-analysis, although inconsistent classification, the low incidence of high-grade lesions, and heterogeneity in the study cohorts as well as changes in practice over time means that results can only be approximate (52). Nevertheless, the results are broadly consistent across studies.

Prediction of Cerebral Palsy and Motor Impairment

Normal scan: A series of studies over a 30-year period have shown that a normal ultrasound scan provides considerable confidence that an infant will have normal neuromotor development; the predictive accuracy is high and confidence limits narrow. Meta-analysis showed that the pooled probability of *not* having cerebral palsy is 94% (95% CI 92% to 96%).

Grades 1 or 2 intraventricular hemorrhage: Meta-analysis showed a pooled probability of abnormal neuromotor development of 9% (4 to 22%).

Grade 3 intraventricular hemorrhage: Meta-analysis showed a pooled probability of abnormal motor development of 26% (13% to 45%), but with wide confidence intervals.

Grade 4 intraventricular hemorrhage (hemorrhagic parenchymal infarction): Meta-analysis showed that the chance of abnormal motor outcome was 53%, (29% to 75%). The high level of uncertainty may reflect many factors including the highly variable nature of these lesions and neuroplasticity, but also the relative rarity of this lesion in published studies. There have been attempts to refine the prognosis by considering the location of the lesions: meta-analysis of these small studies suggests that the probability of abnormal neuromotor development with anterior lesions is 32% (16% to 53%) and in posterior lesions 48% (24% to 73%); however, the confidence limits remain very wide. Bilateral lesions have much worse prognosis than unilateral lesions (53).

Cystic periventricular leukomalacia (PVL): Meta-analysis showed that the chance of motor impairment was 74% (42% to 92%) but with considerable uncertainty in the individual case. The large ELGANS study reported the prognostic value of "echolucent" lesions, which likely include both PVL and hemorrhagic parenchymal infarction as 61%. There is some evidence from a large retrospective study that sensitivity is improved by repeated scanning early and late in the perinatal period (54).

Ventricular dilatation and posthemorrhagic hydrocephalus: Meta-analysis is unreliable due to inconsistent classification, but the ELGANS study reported positive predictive values of 55% for motor impairment (55), and in the untreated patients in the Drift study of irrigation and fibrinolysis, 69% (50% to 83%) had adverse motor outcomes (49).

Cerebellar hemorrhage: Cerebellar hemorrhages are not commonly reported. They are often detected in association with supratentorial lesions, although they can rarely occur in isolation. One study found that they predicted psychomotor and cognitive impairment, but with wide confidence intervals: positive predictive value of 72% (41 to 92).

Combining lesions: The ePrime study examined the overall prognostic value of combining: grade 3 to 4 periventricular hemorrhage; PVL; porencephalic cysts; and/or ventricular size ≥4 mm above the 97th centile for age. The positive predictive value for motor impairment was 47.6% (25.7% to 70.2%) (38).

Prediction of Cognitive Impairment

Cranial ultrasound is not an accurate tool for predicting cognitive outcomes. Meta-analysis showed that the probability of a normal cognitive outcome with a normal ultrasound scan is 82% (79% to 85%). In the ELGANS study, the positive predictive value of echolucent lesions or ventriculomegaly for the Bayley Mental Development Index (MDI) was 45% (55), and in the ePrime study, the positive predictive value for the Bayley III Cognitive Domain was 67% (43% to 85%) and for the Language Domain it was 52% (30% to 74%) (38).

Magnetic Resonance Imaging

MRI has significantly better anatomical definition than ultrasonography. T1- and T2-weighted MRI detects lesions not seen on cranial ultrasound, in particular diffuse nonfocal changes, and allows precise morphometric measurements of brain size and structure.

White matter abnormalities: MRI detects diffuse changes in the white matter in the majority of preterm infants. However, the relationship between MRI findings and the encephalopathy of prematurity is complex. Diffuse excessive high signal on T2-weighted imaging (DEHSI) is seen in up to 80% of infants less than 33 weeks, and there is a relationship between diffuse white matter changes and adverse outcomes. However, taken as a single radiologic sign, DEHSI is poorly predictive of neurologic outcome in individuals (56), and composite scoring systems that grade a range of abnormalities in white and/or gray matter are often used in prognostication in preference to commenting on specific lesions. The most commonly used system was published by Woodward et al in which white matter abnormality is assessed through the nature and extent of T1 and T2 signal abnormality; periventricular white matter volume; cystic changes; ventricular dilatation; and thinning of the corpus callosum. Gray matter abnormality is assessed for the presence of gray matter cortical signal abnormality, the quality of gyral maturation, and the size of the subarachnoid space (57).

Van Hoof et al. presented a meta-analysis of this approach to predict a number of important outcomes, and while the number and size of the individual studies were small, this analysis provides a useful overview. Pooled sensitivity and specificity values for prediction of cerebral palsy were 77% (53% to 91%) and 79% (51% to 93%), respectively. For prediction of motor function, the values were 72% (52% to 86%) and 62% (29% to 87%), respectively. Prognostic accuracy for visual and/or hearing problems, neurocognitive, and/or behavioral function was very poor.

Punctate lesions: The ePrime study reported on the prognostic value of punctate lesions in white matter. Punctate lesions predicted unfavorable motor outcome with sensitivity 71% (43% to 88%) and specificity 72% (69% to 77%), but the positive predictive value for individuals is low 0.09% (0.04% to 0.15%) (41).

Cerebellar lesions: The same study detected small cerebellar hemorrhages in 112/506 of the infants, often associated with abnormalities elsewhere in the brain, and none of these infants had a Gross Motor Function Classification System score greater than 2. Seven infants had isolated large cerebellar hemorrhage, six of these had normal neurodevelopment at 20 months, and one had abnormal cognitive and language scores. In smaller studies, cerebellar lesions have been associated with worse cognitive outcomes, but it can be difficult to determine the role of associated supratentorial lesions (42).

Neuroimaging in Clinical Practice

Cranial ultrasound is a valuable tool in routine clinical practice, giving useful if not completely precise information about the risk of neuromotor impairment in infants with hemorrhage or PVL and allowing the need for intervention in posthemorrhagic hydrocephalus to be judged. A normal ultrasound scan is reassuring.

It has been suggested that MRI might be superior to ultrasound in defining prognosis. To assess the relative value of routine MRI and ultrasound in predicting neurocognitive outcomes, the large ePrime study prospectively compared routine T1- and T2-weighted MRI with ultrasound for the prediction of neurodevelopmental prognosis (38) (Table 50.2). It found that MRI was only slightly more predictive of motor impairments than ultrasound, and the differences did not translate to major improvements in predictive power or clinical utility. The ability of both ultrasound and MRI to predict cognitive outcomes is poor. The performance of MRI was not due to the scoring system used: an unpublished secondary analysis of the trial was unable to find a better scoring system.

Routine T1- and T2-weighted MRI thus adds little to ultrasound but may be warranted in specific cases, for example, where there is disagreement about a significant abnormality on ultrasound, if a congenital anomaly is suspected, or if neurosurgical intervention is being considered. MRI may also add information in specific cases with ultrasound detected lesions. For example, if a localised parenchymal infarction is detected on ultrasound there is around a 50% chance of later cerebral palsy; MRI may detect other lesions, for example associated PVL or abnormalities of the internal capsule ipsilateral to the infarct, which would increase the likelihood of later problems.

Assessment of the Encephalopathy of Prematurity Using Neuroimaging

The limitations of conventional T1- and T2-weighted MRI and ultrasound have led to the use of more advanced imaging modalities such as volumetric MRI, diffusion MRI (dMRI), and fMRI. Although not yet able accurately to predict outcomes for individual infants, these techniques are providing significant insights into the nature of the encephalopathy of prematurity. Common messages from a wide range of studies are that brain growth and maturation is profoundly affected by preterm birth; that the distribution of lesions is heterogeneous; and that abnormalities detected at term are associated with long-term risks and impairments.

Brain Growth

MRI measurement of brain volumes show that brain growth trajectories are slower in preterm infants than in healthy fetuses, and at term-equivalent age, brain volume is reduced in preterm infants compared to term-born infants (58,59). This reduction in brain volume is probably not inevitable, as growth appears to be preserved in infants who escape adverse events such as intrauterine growth restriction, infection, surgery, and chronic lung disease (60). However, on average, total brain volume, deep gray matter volume, and cerebellar volume are reduced, and this is associated with impaired neurodevelopment: for example, impaired fine motor function at 6 years is associated with reduced cerebellar, brain stem, and precentral gyrus volume (61).

In addition to diminished total and regional brain volumes, preterm infants have impaired cortical growth with reduced cortical surface area (9). The rate of growth of cortical surface area is less in those infants born at lower gestational ages or with multiple clinical problems and is related to subsequent adverse neurodevelopmental outcome (10).

Reduced brain volumes in survivors of preterm birth persist into adulthood (62). However, the long-term effect of prematurity on brain growth is complex, with subcortical and medial temporal regions showing reduced gray matter volume, and parts of frontal and lateral parietotemporal cortices demonstrating increased gray matter volume compared to term-born controls, perhaps suggesting resilience to the adverse consequences of preterm birth in these gray matter regions, as lateral parietotemporal gray matter volume correlated with full-scale IQ in the very preterm group; it has also been suggested that preterm birth may lead to more rapid brain ageing (63).

Intensive care practices can influence brain growth, and more frequent procedural pain has been associated with smaller thalamic volumes (64). Better nutrition is associated with improved brain development and early childhood outcome (65–67).

White Matter Microstructural Development

dMRI provides quantitative tools to study microstructural changes associated with brain maturation and injury in preterm infants. Commonly used dMRI methods include diffusion tensor imaging (DTI), which measures fractional anisotropy (FA, a measure of the directional dependence of water molecular motion that increases as nerve tracts become established), and mean diffusivity (MD, representing overall water molecular motion, which decreases as cell and neurite density increase). These and other DTI metrics are relatively nonspecific and reflect many underlying parameters of brain tissue, which has led to the development of biophysical models, such as NODDI, that aim to provide greater specificity by separating the influence of neurite density and orientation from each other and to provide distinct indices such as an orientation dispersion index that captures the degree of dispersion of axonal or dendrite orientations (e.g., through fanning, bending, crossing), and a neurite density index. (68)

The perinatal period is characterized by increasing FA and decreasing MD in the white matter associated with normal axonal growth and myelination. This follows a heterogeneous spatiotemporal pattern, with different fasciculi maturing at different times and different rates in a posterior-to-anterior and a central-to-peripheral direction of maturation (69). Early myelinating structures such as the posterior limb of the internal capsule demonstrate higher FA and lower MD from around 30 weeks of GA. By contrast, MD in some association tracts can remain relatively high up to term-equivalent age. Complimentary analyses using the NODDI model show that neurite density increases in the white matter with increasing maturation, with the highest neurite density values observed at term in primary motor and somatosensory tracts and lower values in association fibers (70).

These complex microstructural developments are disrupted by preterm birth. Compared to term-born infants, preterm infants at term-equivalent age display significantly lower FA and higher MD in the white matter in the absence of abnormalities visible on conventional MRI; infants who are most immature at birth display lowest FA at term, most likely due to the increased rate of adverse clinical events in the most preterm infants (23). As with reduced growth in brain volume, abnormal white matter microstructure appears not to be an inevitable consequence of premature extrauterine life but is associated with multiple comorbidities (23,71). Chronic lung disease and the need for prolonged respiratory support are associated with decreases in FA, suggestive of diffuse white matter damage. Postnatal infection is associated with elevated MD values and reduced FA, independent of extreme prematurity and common neonatal comorbidities. Other risk factors include fetal growth restriction, longer duration of total parenteral nutrition, surgery for necrotizing enterocolitis, chorioamnionitis, pain, stress, and illness severity (23,72). Adverse effects on white matter can begin before birth: prenatal exposure to selective serotonin reuptake inhibitors (SSRIs) or maternal stress appears to be associated with altered brain development in preterm infants (73,74).

TABLE 50.2

Comparison of Cranial Ultrasound and MRI for Predicting Neurodevelopmental Outcomes at Term-Corrected Age[a]

Outcome	MRI (n = 480) Normal versus Moderate or Severe Changes Using Woodward Score					Ultrasound (n = 484) Normal versus PVH grade 3–4, PVL, Porencephalic Cysts, and/or Ventricular Dilation					
	Sensitivity (95% CI)	Specificity (95% CI)	PPV (95% CI)	NPV (95% CI)	MRI Prognosis AUROC (95% CI)	Sensitivity (95% CI)	Specificity (95% CI)	PPV (95% CI)	NPV (95% CI)	Ultrasound Prognosis AUROC (95% CI)	P Value
Gross motor function classification score grade 2–5											
	60.6 (42.1–77.1)	88.4 (85.0–91.2)	27.8 (17.9–39.6)	96.8 (94.6–98.3)	0.74 (0.66–0.83)	29.4 (15.1–47.5)	97.6 (95.7–98.8)	47.6 (25.7–70.2)	94.8 (92.4–96.7)	0.64 (0.56–0.72)	0.01
Bayley scales of infant development III											
Motor domain score <85	38.9 (27.6–51.1)	89.2 (85.8–92.1)	38.9 (27.6–51.1)	89.2 (85.8–92.1)	0.64 (0.58–0.70)	16.4 (8.8–27.0)	97.8 (95.9–99.0)	57.1 (34.0–78.2)	86.8 (83.4–89.8)	0.57 (0.53–0.62)	0.008
Cognitive domain score <85	27.9 (19.8–37.2)	88.9 (85.2–91.9)	43.1 (31.4–55.3)	80.4 (76.2–84.1)	0.58 (0.54–0.63)	12.5 (7.0–20.1)	98.1 (96.2–99.2)	66.7 (43.0–85.4)	78.8 (74.8–82.5)	0.55 (0.52–0.59)	0.13
Language domain score <85	19.9 (14.3–26.6)	87.8 (83.6–91.3)	48.6 (36.7–60.7)	65.4 (60.6–70.1)	0.54 (0.50–0.57)	6.2 (3.1–10.8)	96.7 (94.1–98.4)	52.4 (29.8–74.3)	63.9 (59.4–68.3)	0.51 (0.49–0.54)	0.14

[a]Prediction of motor and cognitive outcomes at 20 months of age by cranial ultrasound and MRI in the ePrime Study. Both imaging modalities were quite specific but less sensitive and confidence limits for positive predictive frequently crossed 50%. MRI was statistically more accurate, with a higher area under the receiver operator characteristics curve, but this did not provide any clinically meaningful increase in predictive power.

PVH, periventricular hemorrhage; PVL, periventricular leukomalacia; ventricular dilation, ventricular size ≥4 mm above the 97th centile for age; CI, confidence intervals; PPV, positive predictive value; NPV, negative predictive value; AUROC, area under the receiver operator characteristics curve; MRI, magnetic resonance imaging.

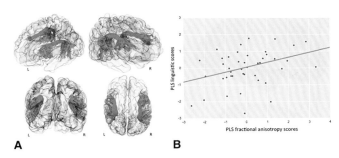

FIGURE 50.6 Linguistic performance at 2 years associated with fractional anisotropy of the left and right arcuate fasciculus at term-equivalent age, independent of degree of prematurity. A: Visualization of an infant brain and the reconstructed arcuate fasciculi from left-frontal, right-frontal, frontal, and top views. The tracts are colored by direction: *green* for anteroposterior; *red* for left-right; *blue* for superoinferior. **B:** Relation between linguistic performance at 20 months and fractional anisotropy using cross-validated partial-least-square regression. (From Salvan P, Tournier JD, Batalle D, et al. Language ability in preterm children is associated with arcuate fasciculi microstructure at term. *Hum Brain Mapp* 2017;38:3836. Copyright © 2017 The Authors Human Brain Mapping Published by Wiley Periodicals, Inc. Reprinted by permission of John Wiley & Sons, Inc.)

Neurodevelopmental outcome is correlated to FA values in a number of white matter tracts including cingulum, fornix, anterior commissure, corpus callosum, and right uncinate fasciculus (75). Widespread disruptions to thalamocortical connectivity are evident in preterm infants a term-equivalent age, with highly significant differences being observed in the frontal lobe, the supplementary motor and premotor regions, and in the medial occipital lobe. These neural systems subserve executive, coordination, and sensory functions, and impaired thalamocortical connectivity in the neonatal period is associated with cognitive performance at 2 years (76).

dMRI also allows the mapping of white matter tracts by detecting the motion of water molecules along nerve fibers, and *dMRI tractography* defines specific white matter tracts, connections, and structure–function relationships. For example, **Figure 50.6** shows the relation between language ability in early childhood is associated with FA values in the arcuate fasciculus at term-equivalent age (77).

These microstructural alterations are persistent (78). In childhood and adolescence, poorer cognitive and motor abilities are associated with reduced white matter FA. Executive function in adolescents born preterm is associated with white matter microstructure in the inferior-occipital fasciculi, and structural connectivity alterations in the limbic system are associated with impaired memory function.

Cortical Microstructural Development

Cortical maturation can also be observed by MRI. Unlike the changes observed in white matter, until around 38 weeks of gestational age, cortical gray matter maturation is characterized by decreasing MD and FA, reflecting increased interneuron development and dendritic arborization (79,80). These changes in cortical microstructure demonstrate regional specificity, developing first in primary sensory cortex, with association heteromodal cortex in parietal and frontal lobe lagging behind then developing rapidly (80). dMRI changes are mirrored by an increase in cortical lipid content measured by T1/T2-weighted MRI, which is principally due to cortical myelination (**Fig. 50.7**) (81). Again, prematurity is associated with disruption to this process of cortical maturation (80,81).

Neural Systems and the Connectomes

The brain is a complex system with emergent properties. Networks of connectivity emerge at many levels as cellular components mature, and it is now normal (if complicated) to speak of the brain's *connectome* meaning the totality of intracerebral connections (82). This is observed at different scales, from electron microscopy of individual synapses to MRI of millimeter-scale

fiber tracts (83). New forms of connectivity are being discovered, creating multiple connectomes: following Hebb dictum that "neurons that fire together wire together" correlated activation in *resting-state networks* has been studied as a form of functional connectome (84).

dMRI and fMRI provide the data for network-based analyses of these various connectomes based on graph theoretical approaches that summarize network topology with parameters that capture the network characteristics, including global network features such as global efficiency and characteristic path length, which assess the ease of connection between regions, and characterization of network hubs and core or peripheral connections. Such approaches shift attention from pinpointing focal damage or specific regions toward a more holistic view, where alterations in separate but functionally related regions give rise to behavioral dysfunction. There is increasing evidence that the perinatal development of both specific tracts serving particular neurocognitive functions and overall connectome architectures underpin normal cerebral functioning in childhood and adolescence (84).

Structural Connectivity

The rapid development of white matter tracts during the preterm period forms an increasingly complex network of structural connections (84). The evolution of this structural connectome is beginning to be defined: the large-scale architecture develops rapidly, and by term-corrected age, the network has many of the characteristics of the adult connectome, including a "rich club" network structure with a small number of highly interconnected nodes that form a rapid communication spine into which other brain regions feed. Preterm infants show deficits in a wide variety of these structures that are associated with neurocognitive deficits (85,86) that persist into childhood and beyond (87,88).

Functional Connectivity

Regional cerebral activity can be mapped using fMRI. Increased neuronal activity leads to local increases in blood flow, providing more oxygen than is needed so that local tissue oxygenation increases; this can be detected using the blood oxygen level–dependent MRI signal (BOLD) (89). BOLD has been used to map both the cerebral response to stimulation and spontaneous brain activity associated with movement or EEG changes (90). By recording spontaneous fluctuations that reflect specific infra-slow neurophysiologic processes (91) and defining regions with coordinated activity, fMRI captures resting-state networks of correlated activation that form a connectome of brain regions that function together. These regions map precisely onto known functional regions, such as the visual system or thalamic nuclei, and appear to be a resilient infrastructure for cortical function, still largely present in altered states such as sleep.

This intrinsic functional architecture is already rich and complex even from birth. Resting-state networks develop rapidly in the last trimester with primary cortex maturing earlier than association cortex (**Fig. 50.8**) (92). By term, a good facsimile of the adult functional networks corresponding to primary sensorimotor, visual, and auditory cortices is instantiated, while the networks involving association cortex appear relatively fragmented and undergoing continuing maturation.

While the development of these resting-state networks appears to be intrinsically programmed to arise at specific postmenstrual ages, more detailed analyses of large-scale datasets have shown that preterm birth significantly affects the establishment of functional connections (**Fig. 50.9**).

Neuroprotection

Neuroprotection of the preterm brain is a health care priority both in terms of suffering and economy. It would appear that brain injury is not inevitable and that well-organized perinatal care

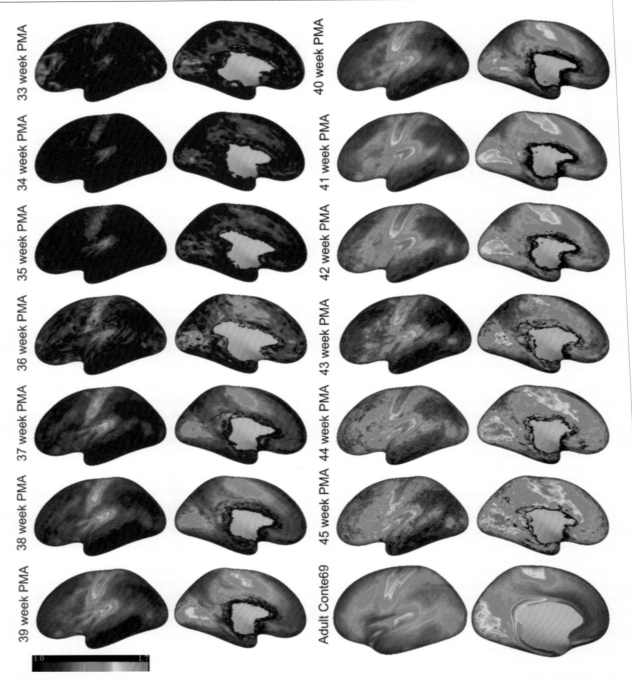

FIGURE 50.7 Growth of cortical myelination, visualized as increasing cortical lipid content using T1/T2 MRI. (Courtesy of Bozek J, Bastiani M, Makropoulos A, et al. In Vivo Cortical Myelination of the Neonatal Brain in the Developing Human Connectome Project 22nd Annual Meeting of the Organization for Human Brain Mapping. Geneva, Switzerland, 2016; Data from Bozek J, Makropoulos A, Schuh A, et al. Construction of a neonatal cortical surface atlas using Multimodal Surface Matching in the Developing Human Connectome Project. *Neuroimage* 2018;179:11. Copyright © 2018 Elsevier. With permission.)

and the avoidance of major comorbidities will allow good brain development (24,60,71) Developing specific therapies is challenging; however, optimal antenatal and neonatal care and repurposing existing drugs have significant potential to improve neurocognitive outcomes.

Corticosteroids

Antenatal corticosteroid administration in high-income settings reduces the incidence of periventricular hemorrhage of any grade and a wide range of the adverse clinical conditions associated with encephalopathy of prematurity. Meta-analysis shows that treated infants have less developmental delay in early childhood, but the data were inconclusive about the effect on cerebral palsy (93). Despite previous evidence that dexamethasone was more beneficial than betamethasone, recent analyses reported that both drugs increased intact survival (94). Antenatal steroids are now known to improve outcomes in low and middle income settings as well as developed health economies (95).

Postnatal corticosteroid administration has been linked to adverse neurodevelopmental outcomes and is generally used only with considerable caution. However, a recent meta-analysis did not find a conclusive association (96), and there is now interest in the possibility that prophylactic low-dose hydrocortisone may improve outcomes (97).

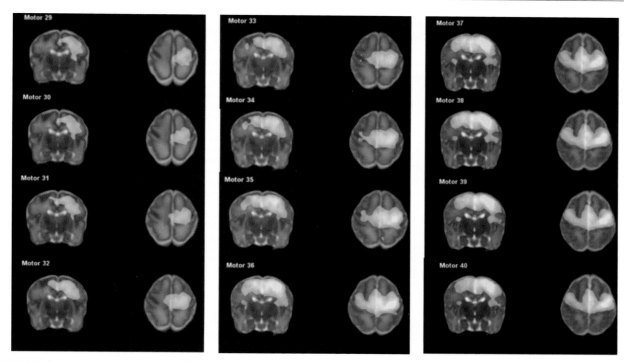

FIGURE 50.8 Axial and transverse resting-state functional magnetic resonance images of the right motor cortex from 29 to 40 weeks of gestational age. At 29 weeks, the activity is clearly unilateral. Correlated activity ('functional connectivity') with the left side of the brain develops over the next few weeks, so that by term age, the right and left brain are in functional connection. (Adapted from Doria V, Beckmann CF, Arichi T, et al. Emergence of resting-state networks in the preterm human brain. *Proc Natl Acad Sci U S A* 2010;107:20015. With permission.)

Antenatal Magnesium Sulfate

Maternal administration of magnesium sulfate is a proven therapy for eclampsia and preeclampsia, and a recent analysis shows that given prior to preterm birth, it reduces the combined risk of fetal/infant death or motor deficits (98) probably by preventing mitochondrial dysfunction. The effect size is modest, but given the high prevalence of prematurity, widespread adoption worldwide of this relatively inexpensive treatment could have a major impact.

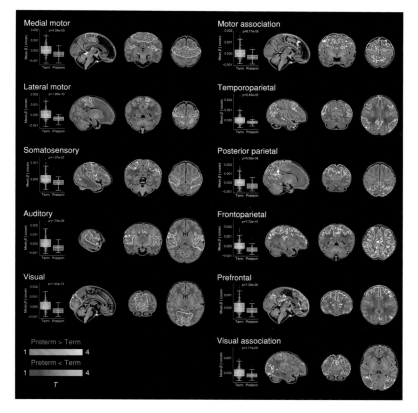

FIGURE 50.9 Reduced functional connectivity in preterm infants at term showing brain regions with reduced (*blue*) or increased (*red-yellow*) functional connectivity in preterm-born infants. *White lines* represent the outlines of the resting-state network in normal term infants. *Boxplots* show group differences in core network strength, taking account of age at scan, sex, and motion. Most networks show reduced network connectivity in preterm infants. (Reprinted from Eyre M, Fitzgibbon SP, Ciarrusta J, et al. The Developing Human Connectome Project: typical and disrupted perinatal functional connectivity. *Brain* 2021:awab118.)

THE NEWBORN INFANT

Maternal Milk

Predominant breast milk feeding in the first 28 days of life was associated with a greater deep nuclear gray matter volume at term-equivalent age and better IQ, academic achievement, working memory, and motor function at 7 years of age, demonstrating that this relatively easy to implement therapy, with no adverse effect, is a key step toward protecting the brain of preterm infants (65,66).

Caffeine

A large randomized trial has shown that caffeine significantly reduced motor deficits in preterm infants without impacting negatively on their cognitive outcome at 11 years of age (99). Through its effects on adenosine receptors, caffeine has potentially multiple impacts on the developing brain of a preterm infant. Increasing the dose of caffeine might increase the neuroprotective effects and further randomized controlled trials seem warranted.

Early Developmental Interventions

It is well established that adverse family and social conditions are associated with worse cognitive development in children (100). Developmental intervention programs initiated soon after discharge from hospital have a positive influence on cognitive and motor outcomes in preterm infants, with cognitive benefits persisting into preschool age (101). Further research is needed to determine which early developmental interventions are most effective and to determine the longer-term effects of these programs.

However, there is less evidence that developmental care during hospital admission has benefits, and an early enthusiasm generated by an initial small trial has not been sustained in later studies (102).

Erythropoietin

Erythropoietin has been used safely for decades in preterm infants to reduce the risk of transfusions. Erythropoietin also has neuroprotective effects in animal models, and there was optimism that it might have useful clinical effects. However, although a randomized controlled trial with erythropoietin given after preterm birth found a decrease in brain lesions on MRI, there was no benefit in neurodevelopment and a recent large trial has confirmed no benefit in 2-year outcomes (103). It is possible that 2-year neurodevelopment is not an optimal outcome measure, and long-term follow-up will be valuable.

Other Interventions

A review of the Cochrane Library (www.cochranelibrary.com) will show that a large number of interventions have been studied without convincing evidence of neurodevelopmental benefit being found, including thyroid hormone administration, manipulation of oxygen saturation, prophylactic intravenous indomethacin, and supplementation of vitamin A or vitamin E. Delayed cord clamping probably increases survival and reduces the incidence of all grades of IVH in high-income settings but was not associated with a reduction in grade 3 to 4 IVH, and the effect on neurodevelopmental outcomes remains unclear (104).

REFERENCES

1. Blencowe H, Lee AC, Cousens S, et al. Preterm birth-associated neurodevelopmental impairment estimates at regional and global levels for 2010. *Pediatr Res* 2013;74(suppl 1):17.
2. Pierrat V, Marchand-Martin L, Arnaud C, et al. Neurodevelopmental outcome at 2 years for preterm children born at 22 to 34 weeks' gestation in France in 2011: EPIPAGE-2 cohort study. *BMJ* 2017;358:j3448.
3. Do CHT, Kruse AY, Wills B, et al. Neurodevelopment at 2 years corrected age among Vietnamese preterm infants. *Arch Dis Child* 2020;105(2):134.
4. Volpe JJ. Dysmaturation of premature brain: importance, cellular mechanisms, and potential interventions. *Pediatr Neurol* 2019;95:42.

5. MacKay DF, Smith GC, Dobbie R, et al. Gestational age at delivery and special educational need: retrospective cohort study of 407,503 schoolchildren. *PLoS Med* 2010;7(6):e1000289.
6. Twilhaar ES, de Kieviet JF, Aarnoudse-Moens CS, et al. Academic performance of children born preterm: a meta-analysis and meta-regression. *Arch Dis Child Fetal Neonatal Ed* 2018;103(4):F322.
7. Twilhaar ES, Wade RM, de Kieviet JF, et al. Cognitive outcomes of children born extremely or very preterm since the 1990s and associated risk factors: a meta-analysis and meta-regression. *JAMA Pediatr* 2018;172(4):361.
8. Nosarti C, Reichenberg A, Murray RM, et al. Preterm birth and psychiatric disorders in young adult life. *Arch Gen Psychiatry* 2012;69(6):E1.
9. Ajayi-Obe M, Saeed N, Cowan FM, et al. Reduced development of cerebral cortex in extremely preterm infants. *Lancet* 2000;356(9236):1162.
10. Rathbone R, Counsell SJ, Kapellou O, et al. Perinatal cortical growth and childhood neurocognitive abilities. *Neurology* 2011;77(16):1510.
11. Dubois J, Benders M, Cachia A, et al. Mapping the early cortical folding process in the preterm newborn brain. *Cereb Cortex* 2008;18(6):1444.
12. Van Essen DC. A tension-based theory of morphogenesis and compact wiring in the central nervous system. *Nature* 1997;385(6614):313.
13. Chevallier M, Debillon T, Pierrat V, et al. Leading causes of preterm delivery as risk factors for intraventricular hemorrhage in very preterm infants: results of the EPIPAGE 2 cohort study. *Am J Obstet Gynecol* 2017;216(5):518.e1.
14. Korzeniewski SJ, Allred EN, Joseph RM, et al. Neurodevelopment at age 10 years of children born <28 weeks with fetal growth restriction. *Pediatrics* 2017;140(5):e20170697.
15. Laughon M, O'Shea MT, Allred EN, et al. Chronic lung disease and developmental delay at 2 years of age in children born before 28 weeks' gestation. *Pediatrics* 2009;124(2):637.
16. Leviton A, Joseph RM, Allred EN, et al. The risk of neurodevelopmental disorders at age 10 years associated with blood concentrations of interleukins 4 and 10 during the first postnatal month of children born extremely preterm. *Cytokine* 2018;110:181.
17. Stoll BJ, Hansen NI, Adams-Chapman I, et al. Neurodevelopmental and growth impairment among extremely low-birth-weight infants with neonatal infection. *JAMA* 2004;292(19):2357.
18. Gilles F, Gressens P, Dammann O, et al. Hypoxia-ischemia is not an antecedent of most preterm brain damage: the illusion of validity. *Dev Med Child Neurol* 2018;60(2):120.
19. Eklind S, Mallard C, Leverin AL, et al. Bacterial endotoxin sensitizes the immature brain to hypoxic—ischaemic injury. *Eur J Neurosci* 2001;13(6):1101.
20. Cormack BE, Harding JE, Miller SP, et al. The influence of early nutrition on brain growth and neurodevelopment in extremely preterm babies: a narrative review. *Nutrients* 2019;11(9):2029.
21. Krishnan ML, Wang Z, Aljabar P, et al. Machine learning shows association between genetic variability in PPARG and cerebral connectivity in preterm infants. *Proc Natl Acad Sci U S A* 2017;114(52):13744.
22. Cullen H, Krishnan ML, Selzam S, et al. Polygenic risk for neuropsychiatric disease and vulnerability to abnormal deep grey matter development. *Sci Rep* 2019;9(1):1976.
23. Barnett ML, Tusor N, Ball G, et al. Exploring the multiple-hit hypothesis of preterm white matter damage using diffusion MRI. *Neuroimage Clin* 2018;17:596.
24. Helenius K, Longford N, Lehtonen L, et al. Association of early postnatal transfer and birth outside a tertiary hospital with mortality and severe brain injury in extremely preterm infants: observational cohort study with propensity score matching. *BMJ* 2019;367:l5678.
25. Edstedt Bonamy AK, Zeitlin J, Piedvache A, et al. Wide variation in severe neonatal morbidity among very preterm infants in European regions. *Arch Dis Child Fetal Neonatal Ed* 2019;104(1):F36.
26. van Kempen A, Eskes PF, Nuytemans D, et al. Lower versus traditional treatment threshold for neonatal hypoglycemia. *N Engl J Med* 2020;382(6):534.
27. Goode RH, Rettiganti M, Li J, et al. Developmental outcomes of preterm infants with neonatal hypoglycemia. *Pediatrics* 2016;138(6):e20161424.
28. Leviton A, Allred E, Kuban KC, et al. Early blood gas abnormalities and the preterm brain. *Am J Epidemiol* 2010;172(8):907.
29. Wigglesworth JS, Pape KE. An integrated model for haemorrhagic and ischaemic lesions in the newborn brain. *Early Hum Dev* 1978;2(2):179.
30. Papile LA, Burstein J, Burstein R, et al. Incidence and evolution of subependymal and intraventricular hemorrhage: a study of infants with birth weights less than 1,500 gm. *J Pediatr* 1978;92(4):529.
31. Lipscombe AP, Blackwell RJ, Reynolds EO, et al. Ultrasound scanning of brain through anterior fontanelle of newborn infants. *Lancet* 1979;2(8132):39.
32. Cooke RW. Ultrasound examination of neonatal heads. *Lancet* 1979; 2(8132):38.
33. Gould SJ, Howard S, Hope PL, et al. Periventricular intraparenchymal cerebral haemorrhage in preterm infants: the role of venous infarction. *J Pathol* 1987;151(3):197.

34. Inder T, Perlman J, Volpe JJ. Preterm intraventricular hemorrhage/post-hemorrhagic hydrocephalus. In: Volpe JJ, Darras BT, Du Plessis AJ, et al., eds. *Volpe's neurology of the newborn*, 6th ed. Elsevier, 2018:637.

35. Kong X, Xu F, Wu R, et al. Neonatal mortality and morbidity among infants between 24 to 31 complete weeks: a multicenter survey in China from 2013 to 2014. *BMC Pediatr* 2016;16(1):174.

36. Chedid F, Shanteer S, Haddad H, et al. Short-term outcome of very low birth weight infants in a developing country: comparison with the Vermont Oxford Network. *J Trop Pediatr* 2009;55(1):15.

37. Banker BQ, Larroche JC. Periventricular leukomalacia of infancy. A form of neonatal anoxic encephalopathy. *Arch Neurol* 1962;7:386.

38. Edwards AD, Redshaw ME, Kennea N, et al. Effect of MRI on preterm infants and their families: a randomised trial with nested diagnostic and economic evaluation. *Arch Dis Child Fetal Neonatal Ed* 2018;103(1):F15.

39. Battin M, Maalouf EF, Counsell SJ, et al. Magnetic resonance imaging of the brain of premature infants. *Lancet* 1997;349(9067):1741.

40. Dyet LE, Kennea N, Counsell SJ, et al. Natural history of brain lesions in extremely preterm infants studied with serial magnetic resonance imaging from birth and neurodevelopmental assessment. *Pediatrics* 2006;118(2):536.

41. Tusor N, Benders MJ, Counsell SJ, et al. Punctate white matter lesions associated with altered brain development and adverse motor outcome in preterm infants. *Sci Rep* 2017;7(1):13250.

42. Limperopoulos C, Chilingaryan G, Sullivan N, et al. Injury to the premature cerebellum: outcome is related to remote cortical development. *Cereb Cortex* 2014;24(3):728.

43. Volpe JJ. Confusions in nomenclature: "Periventricular Leukomalacia" and "White Matter Injury"-identical, distinct, or overlapping? *Pediatr Neurol* 2017;73:3.

44. Volpe JJ. Brain injury in premature infants: a complex amalgam of destructive and developmental disturbances. *Lancet Neurol* 2009;8(1):110.

45. Hagberg H, Mallard C, Ferriero DM, et al. The role of inflammation in perinatal brain injury. *Nat Rev Neurol* 2015;11(4):192.

46. Stolp HB, Fleiss B, Arai Y, et al. Interneuron development is disrupted in preterm brains with diffuse white matter injury: observations in mouse and human. *Front Physiol* 2019;10:955.

47. Isaacs AM, Smyser CD, Lean RE, et al. MR diffusion changes in the perimeter of the lateral ventricles demonstrate periventricular injury in post-hemorrhagic hydrocephalus of prematurity. *Neuroimage Clin* 2019;24:102031.

48. Whitelaw A, Lee-Kelland R. Repeated lumbar or ventricular punctures in newborns with intraventricular haemorrhage. *Cochrane Database Syst Rev* 2017;4:CD000216.

49. Whitelaw A, Jary S, Kmita G, et al. Randomized trial of drainage, irrigation and fibrinolytic therapy for premature infants with posthemorrhagic ventricular dilatation: developmental outcome at 2 years. *Pediatrics* 2010;125(4):e852.

50. Arichi T, Counsell SJ, Allievi AG, et al. The effects of hemorrhagic parenchymal infarction on the establishment of sensori-motor structural and functional connectivity in early infancy. *Neuroradiology* 2014;56(11):985.

51. Froudist-Walsh S, Bloomfield MA, Veronese M, et al. The effect of perinatal brain injury on dopaminergic function and hippocampal volume in adult life. *Elife* 2017;6:e29088.

52. Nongena P, Ederies A, Azzopardi DV, et al. Confidence in the prediction of neurodevelopmental outcome by cranial ultrasound and MRI in preterm infants. *Arch Dis Child Fetal Neonatal Ed* 2010;95(6):F388.

53. Maitre NL, Marshall DD, Price WA, et al. Neurodevelopmental outcome of infants with unilateral or bilateral periventricular hemorrhagic infarction. *Pediatrics* 2009;124(6):e1153.

54. Sarkar S, Shankaran S, Laptook AR, et al. Screening cranial imaging at multiple time points improves cystic periventricular leukomalacia detection. *Am J Perinatol* 2015;32(10):973.

55. O'Shea TM, Kuban KC, Allred EN, et al. Neonatal cranial ultrasound lesions and developmental delays at 2 years of age among extremely low gestational age children. *Pediatrics* 2008;122(3):e662.

56. Murner-Lavanchy IM, Kidokoro H, Thompson DK, et al. Thirteen-year outcomes in very preterm children associated with diffuse excessive high signal intensity on neonatal magnetic resonance imaging. *J Pediatr* 2019;206:66.

57. Woodward LJ, Anderson PJ, Austin NC, et al. Neonatal MRI to predict neurodevelopmental outcomes in preterm infants. *N Engl J Med* 2006;355(7):685.

58. Kapellou O, Counsell SJ, Kennea N, et al. Abnormal cortical development after premature birth shown by altered allometric scaling of brain growth. *PLoS Med* 2006;3(8):e265.

59. Bouyssi-Kobar M, du Plessis AJ, McCarter R, et al. Third trimester brain growth in preterm infants compared with in utero healthy fetuses. *Pediatrics* 2016;138(5):e20161640.

60. Boardman JP, Counsell SJ, Rueckert D, et al. Early growth in brain volume is preserved in the majority of preterm infants. *Ann Neurol* 2007;62(2):185.

61. Bolk J, Farooqi A, Hafstrom M, et al. Developmental coordination disorder and its association with developmental comorbidities at 6.5 years in apparently healthy children born extremely preterm. *JAMA Pediatr* 2018;172(8):765.

62. Nosarti C, Giouroukou E, Healy E, et al. Grey and white matter distribution in very preterm adolescents mediates neurodevelopmental outcome. *Brain* 2008;131(Pt 1):205.

63. Karolis VR, Froudist-Walsh S, Kroll J, et al. Volumetric grey matter alterations in adolescents and adults born very preterm suggest accelerated brain maturation. *Neuroimage* 2017;163:379.

64. Duerden EG, Grunau RE, Guo T, et al. Early procedural pain is associated with regionally-specific alterations in thalamic development in preterm neonates. *J Neurosci* 2018;38(4):878.

65. Belfort MB, Anderson PJ, Nowak VA, et al. Breast milk feeding, brain development, and neurocognitive outcomes: a 7-year longitudinal study in infants born at less than 30 weeks' gestation. *J Pediatr* 2016;177:133.

66. Blesa M, Sullivan G, Anblagan D, et al. Early breast milk exposure modifies brain connectivity in preterm infants. *Neuroimage* 2019;184:431.

67. Coviello C, Keunen K, Kersbergen KJ, et al. Effects of early nutrition and growth on brain volumes, white matter microstructure, and neurodevelopmental outcome in preterm newborns. *Pediatr Res* 2018;83(1–1):102.

68. Zhang H, Schneider T, Wheeler-Kingshott CA, et al. NODDI: practical in vivo neurite orientation dispersion and density imaging of the human brain. *Neuroimage* 2012;61(4):1000.

69. Dubois J, Dehaene-Lambertz G, Perrin M, et al. Asynchrony of the early maturation of white matter bundles in healthy infants: quantitative landmarks revealed noninvasively by diffusion tensor imaging. *Hum Brain Mapp* 2008;29(1):14.

70. Batalle D, O'Muircheartaigh J, Makropoulos A, et al. Different patterns of cortical maturation before and after 38 weeks gestational age demonstrated by diffusion MRI in vivo. *Neuroimage* 2019;185:764.

71. Bonifacio SL, Glass HC, Chau V, et al. Extreme premature birth is not associated with impaired development of brain microstructure. *J Pediatr* 2010;157(5):726.

72. Chau V, Brant R, Poskitt KJ, et al. Postnatal infection is associated with widespread abnormalities of brain development in premature newborns. *Pediatr Res* 2012;71(3):274.

73. Lautarescu A, Pecheva D, Nosarti C, et al. Maternal prenatal stress is associated with altered uncinate fasciculus microstructure in premature neonates. *Biol Psychiatry* 2020;87:559.

74. Podrebarac SK, Duerden EG, Chau V, et al. Antenatal exposure to antidepressants is associated with altered brain development in very preterm-born neonates. *Neuroscience* 2017;342:252.

75. Counsell SJ, Edwards AD, Chew AT, et al. Specific relations between neurodevelopmental abilities and white matter microstructure in children born preterm. *Brain* 2008;131(Pt 12):3201.

76. Ball G, Pazderova L, Chew A, et al. Thalamocortical connectivity predicts cognition in children born preterm. *Cereb Cortex* 2015;25(11):4310.

77. Salvan P, Tournier JD, Batalle D, et al. Language ability in preterm children is associated with arcuate fasciculi microstructure at term. *Hum Brain Mapp* 2017;38(8):3836.

78. Skranes J, Evensen KI, Lohaugen GC, et al. Abnormal cerebral MRI findings and neuroimpairments in very low birth weight (VLBW) adolescents. *Eur J Paediatr Neurol* 2008;12(4):273.

79. McKinstry RC, Mathur A, Miller JH, et al. Radial organization of developing preterm human cerebral cortex revealed by non-invasive water diffusion anisotropy MRI. *Cereb Cortex* 2002;12(12):1237.

80. Ball G, Srinivasan L, Aljabar P, et al. Development of cortical microstructure in the preterm human brain. *Proc Natl Acad Sci U S A* 2013;110(23):9541.

81. Bozek J, Makropoulos A, Schuh A, et al. Construction of a neonatal cortical surface atlas using multimodal surface matching in the developing human connectome project. *Neuroimage* 2018;179:11.

82. Hagmann P, Grant PE, Fair DA. MR connectomics: a conceptual framework for studying the developing brain. *Front Syst Neurosci* 2012;6:43.

83. Swanson LW, Lichtman JW. From cajal to connectome and beyond. *Annu Rev Neurosci* 2016;39:197.

84. Smyser CD, Wheelock MD, Limbrick DD Jr, et al. Neonatal brain injury and aberrant connectivity. *Neuroimage* 2019;185:609.

85. Ball G, Boardman JP. The influence of preterm birth on the developing thalamocortical connectome. *Cortex* 2013;49(6):1711.

86. Ball G, Aljabar P, Zebari S, et al. Rich-club organization of the newborn human brain. *Proc Natl Acad Sci U S A* 2014;111(20):7456.

87. Pandit AS, Robinson E, Aljabar P, et al. Whole-brain mapping of structural connectivity in infants reveals altered connection strength associated with growth and preterm birth. *Cereb Cortex* 2014;24(9):2324.

88. Froudist-Walsh S, Karolis V, Caldinelli C, et al. Very early brain damage leads to remodeling of the working memory system in adulthood: a combined fMRI/tractography study. *J Neurosci* 2015;35(48):15787.

89. Biswal B, Yetkin FZ, Haughton VM, et al. Functional connectivity in the motor cortex of resting human brain using echo-planar MRI. *Magn Reson Med* 1995;34(4):537.

90. Arichi T, Whitehead K, Barone G, et al. Localization of spontaneous bursting neuronal activity in the preterm human brain with simultaneous EEG-fMRI. *Elife* 2017;6:e27814.

91. Mitra A, Kraft A, Wright P, et al. Spontaneous infra-slow brain activity has unique spatiotemporal dynamics and laminar structure. *Neuron* 2018;98(2):297.

92. Doria V, Beckmann CF, Arichi T, et al. Emergence of resting state networks in the preterm human brain. *Proc Natl Acad Sci U S A* 2010;107(46):20015.

93. Roberts D, Brown J, Medley N, et al. Antenatal corticosteroids for accelerating fetal lung maturation for women at risk of preterm birth. *Cochrane Database Syst Rev* 2017;3:CD004454.

94. Crowther CA, Ashwood P, Andersen C, et al. Maternal intramuscular dexamethasone versus betamethasone before preterm birth (ASTEROID): a multicentre, double-blind, randomised controlled trial. *Lancet Child Adolesc Health* 2019;3(11):769.

95. WHO ACTION Trials Collaborators. Antenatal dexamethasone for early preterm birth in low-resource countries. *N Engl J Med* 2020;383(26):2514.

96. Doyle LW, Cheong JL, Ehrenkranz RA, et al. Late (>7 days) systemic postnatal corticosteroids for prevention of bronchopulmonary dysplasia in preterm infants. *Cochrane Database Syst Rev* 2017;10:CD001145.

97. Baud O, Trousson C, Biran V, et al. Two-year neurodevelopmental outcomes of extremely preterm infants treated with early hydrocortisone: treatment effect according to gestational age at birth. *Arch Dis Child Fetal Neonatal Ed* 2019;104(1):F30.

98. Shepherd E, Salam RA, Middleton P, et al. Antenatal and intrapartum interventions for preventing cerebral palsy: an overview of Cochrane systematic reviews. *Cochrane Database Syst Rev* 2017;8:CD012077.

99. Murner-Lavanchy IM, Doyle LW, Schmidt B, et al. Neurobehavioral outcomes 11 years after neonatal caffeine therapy for apnea of prematurity. *Pediatrics* 2018;141(5):e20174047.

100. Ene D, Der G, Fletcher-Watson S, et al. Associations of socioeconomic deprivation and preterm birth with speech, language, and communication concerns among children aged 27 to 30 months. *JAMA Netw Open* 2019;2(9):e1911027.

101. Spittle A, Orton J, Anderson PJ, et al. Early developmental intervention programmes provided post hospital discharge to prevent motor and cognitive impairment in preterm infants. *Cochrane Database Syst Rev* 2015;(11):CD005495.

102. Symington A, Pinelli J. Developmental care for promoting development and preventing morbidity in preterm infants. *Cochrane Database Syst Rev* 2006;(2):CD001814.

103. Juul SE, Comstock BA, Wadhawan R, et al. A randomized trial of erythropoietin for neuroprotection in preterm infants. *N Engl J Med* 2020;382(3):233.

104. Rabe H, Gyte GM, Diaz-Rossello JL, et al. Effect of timing of umbilical cord clamping and other strategies to influence placental transfusion at preterm birth on maternal and infant outcomes. *Cochrane Database Syst Rev* 2019;9:CD003248.

51 Neonatal Seizures

Amanda G. Sandoval Karamian and Courtney J. Wusthoff

INTRODUCTION

Seizures are among the most common neurologic problems during the neonatal period, affecting an estimated 1 to 5 per 1,000 live births (1,2). Studies examining the prevalence of neonatal seizures have been primarily in high-income countries, with incidence and prevalence of neonatal seizures in low- and middle-income countries not well characterized (2). Risk factors for neonatal seizures include maternal, intrapartum, and infant factors (3). Maternal age greater than 40 years, nulliparity, and gestational diabetes have been associated with increased risk of neonatal seizures. Intrapartum fetal distress, placental abruption, cord prolapse, uterine rupture, and chorioamnionitis are also associated with neonatal seizures, likely related to associated brain injury. Infant risk factors include low-birth weight, lower gestational age in preterm infants, and birth post-term after 42 weeks (3,4).

With the growing emphasis on newborn neuroprotection and increasingly available EEG technology, neonatal seizures are an area of intense research and clinical focus. This chapter will discuss neonatal seizures, including pathophysiology, common etiologies, approach to diagnosis and evaluation, treatment, and related prognosis.

PATHOPHYSIOLOGY

Seizures are abnormal, uncontrolled, rhythmic electrical activity in the brain, propagated in the setting of disrupted circuit physiology. Neonates have increased susceptibility to seizures as compared to older children and adults. This is at least in part because immature neurons in the neonatal brain have increased excitatory and decreased inhibitory activity in comparison with neurons at later stages of development. One contributing mechanism is the difference in ion gradients seen in immature as compared to mature neurons. Immature neurons have high intracellular chloride levels. As a result, when GABA transmission triggers opening of chloride channels, there is a unique depolarizing, or excitatory, effect. This is in contrast to the chloride channel's typical hyperpolarizing, or inhibitory, effect in mature neurons. In addition to creating a lower seizure threshold in neonates, these transient gradient properties also may render GABAergic antiseizure medications (ASMs) (such as phenobarbital) less effective. This is again due to depolarization rather than the expected hyperpolarization of the neuron with GABA-triggered opening of the postsynaptic chloride channel (5). While this is not the only mechanism underlying the relatively hyperexcitable state of the neonatal brain, it does illustrate how unique neonatal physiology increases the risk for seizures at this developmental stage.

In addition to having a relatively excitatory state, the newborn brain also undergoes rapidly evolving structural connectivity. This incomplete connectivity may alter how neonatal seizures propagate through the brain and change their clinical manifestations. For example, focal seizures beginning outside of the motor cortex may remain focal and in neonates are less likely to spread to adjacent brain regions. If they do not spread to motor cortex, seizures may not generate an outward motor sign. Thus, even while a focal electrographic seizure is ongoing within the brain, it may remain subclinical, with no outward motor signs to reflect the abnormal brain activity. Neonatal seizures are most often focal or multifocal in onset; seizures which begin simultaneously across the whole brain (primary generalized seizures) are exceedingly rare in this age group.

DIAGNOSIS

Clinical Presentation

Neonatal seizures vary in presentation, ranging from easily recognizable stereotyped movements to subclinical seizures with no outward signs. The clinical appearance of neonatal seizures is most often subtle, with electrographic seizures having no associated clinical correlate 80% to 90% of the time, and clinical seizures becoming subclinical electrographic seizures in up to 58% of neonates after treatment with ASMs (6–8). Bedside clinical observation for detection and diagnosis of neonatal seizures has been shown to be incorrect even by experienced clinicians, with clinical identification of seizures only 27% to 50% accurate (9,10). Jitteriness, shivering, benign myoclonus, excessive startle, and clonus are all nonepileptic paroxysmal phenomena in neonates that may be confused with true seizures (11). Care must be taken to avoid conflating mimics with true seizures; one study reported high rates of overdiagnosis, with 73% of documented clinical "seizures" having no correlating ictal activity present on EEG, meaning these events were not actually seizures (9).

Unlike in older children and adults, neonatal seizures tend to remain focal electrographically and with limited outward signs clinically. Studies of electrographic seizures in neonates have demonstrated that electrographic onset of neonatal seizures is nearly always focal (12,13). The "generalized tonic–clonic seizure" is exceedingly rare in neonates. This is, in part, due to the immature connections within the neonatal brain limiting the generalization and propagation of seizures. Until recently, the International League Against Epilepsy's (ILAE) classification of neonatal seizures has been included in the same system as that for older children and adults (14,15). Because the unique features of neonatal seizures do not fit this framework easily, a proposed modification specific to neonatal seizures is currently underway. While this modification is eagerly awaited, neonatal seizures are described in this chapter according to the most recent 2017 ILAE Guidelines. The majority of neonatal seizures are focal or multifocal in onset, with categories relevant for neonates as per the 2017 ILAE guidelines shown in **Figure 51.1**.

By the 2017 ILAE guidelines, neonatal seizures are broadly categorized into motor onset and nonmotor onset, though the majority of neonatal seizures have no clinical correlate. Motor automatisms can include cycling movements of the legs, swimming movements of the arms, or oral-motor movements such as lip-smacking (16). Clonic seizures are rhythmic jerks of the face, arms, legs, or trunk, which can occur at single or multiple (multifocal) sites, and can shift from one site to another (17). Clonic jerks are characterized by rapid contraction and slow relaxation and are not suppressible with touch. Epileptic spasms typically manifest as sudden, bilateral, or rarely asymmetric flexion or extension of the neck, trunk, and/or extremities associated with a brief loss of consciousness. These are less frequently observed in the neonatal period, though can be seen in infancy (18). Myoclonic seizures are rapid, isolated jerks which can be irregular (17). They are typically brief and isolated as compared to the longer sustained rhythmicity of clonic jerks. Tonic seizures are a sustained muscle contraction and posture in either flexion or extension which can affect the limbs, trunk, head/neck, or eyes (17). In the nonmotor category of seizures, autonomic changes can be the only outward sign of seizure, with paroxysmal apnea, pallor, flushing, tearing,

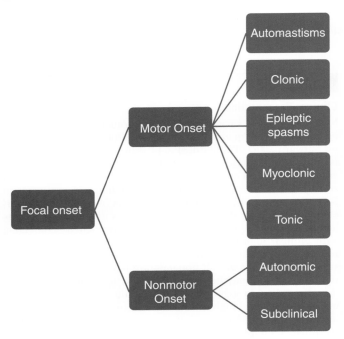

FIGURE 51.1 Neonatal seizure classification. (Adapted from Fisher RS, Cross JH, French JA, et al. Operational classification of seizure types by the International league against epilepsy: position paper of the ILAE Commission for classification and terminology. *Epilepsia* 2017;58(4):522.)

and tachycardia or elevated blood pressures all possible indicators of seizure (16). Apnea may be the only outward clinical sign of seizure; in a term newborn, unexplained apnea should be investigated as possible seizure if no other cause is apparent. Other isolated paroxysmal vital sign changes, particularly bradycardia

or blood pressure changes, are rarely seizures; however, seizure is more likely when these are in combination or associated with other clinical signs such as changes in tone or eye movements (19). Seizures are difficult to distinguish from other nonepileptic paroxysmal events in the neonatal period based on clinical appearance alone (9). Because most neonatal seizures are acute symptomatic seizures of an underlying process, clinical presentation of seizures is often accompanied by encephalopathy, poor feeding, or other symptoms of illness.

Diagnostic Monitoring

Neonatal seizures with outward observable signs are described as "clinical seizures." When clinical seizures are confirmed to have electrographic correlate on EEG, they are described as "electroclinical seizures." However, the majority of neonatal seizures are subclinical, or "electrographic-only", and have no clear associated clinical correlate. Subclinical seizures are identifiable only by EEG (8). Because of this, and because mimics can be difficult to distinguish from true electroclinical seizures, continuous video EEG (cEEG) monitoring is the gold standard for evaluation of suspected neonatal seizures. The World Health Organization (WHO) recommends EEG confirmation of all clinical neonatal seizures where this technology is available (2).

The American Clinical Neurophysiology Society (ACNS) recommends long-term, conventional EEG monitoring in neonates to definitively diagnose suspected clinical seizures and for detection of subclinical seizures in high-risk groups (16). With cEEG, 10 to 13 electrodes are applied by a neurodiagnostic technologist, with locations according to the International 10 to 20 system modified for neonates. In most cases, concurrent video is recorded. Electrical activity of the brain is recorded; a neurophysiologist reviews the recording for identification of electrographic and electroclinical seizures. Continuous video EEG allows the neurophysiologist to correlate clinical events with ictal changes on EEG; this is important as bedside clinical identification of seizures is often inaccurate (9,10). **Figure 51.2** shows an example of neonatal seizure

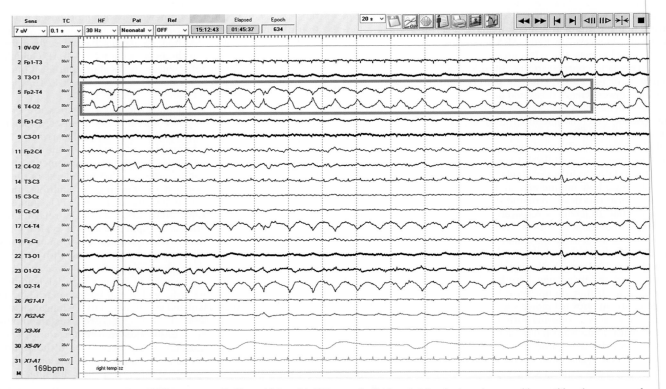

FIGURE 51.2 Neonatal conventional EEG montage at 7 μV sensitivity with 16.5 seconds displayed. A focal seizure is seen with repetitive sharp waves of approximately 1.5 Hz frequency maximal in the right temporal region at T4, outlined in *green*. The seizure segment shown is 15 seconds in duration.

on neonatal montage of cEEG. Rather than obtain a routine (also called "spot") EEG for just 30 to 60 minutes, ACNS guidelines recommend monitoring neonates at high risk for seizures for a minimum of 24 hours, given seizures may occur outside a 30 to 60 minute recording. For example, seizures occur at any point within 6 hours of birth in more than half of neonates with hypoxic–ischemic encephalopathy (HIE). Similarly, seizures occur at a mean of 21 hours postoperatively with a wide range in newborns undergoing cardiac surgery (16,20,21). Monitoring should continue for at least 24 hours, or until 24 hours of seizure freedom (16). Neonates, both term and preterm, considered at high risk for seizures warrant long-term EEG monitoring for definitive diagnosis. Conditions conferring increased risk for seizures in which cEEG monitoring should be considered include neonatal encephalopathy, HIE, significant respiratory conditions that may compromise cerebral oxygenation, ECMO, congenital heart defects requiring surgery with cardiopulmonary bypass, CNS infection, CNS trauma, CNS hemorrhage, inborn errors of metabolism, perinatal stroke, venous sinus thrombosis, high-grade IVH in premature neonates, and brain structural abnormalities (16). Automated seizure detection software is emerging technology that can complement cEEG; however, its use in neonates is not well established and is not yet of sufficient validity to recommend for widespread use in the detection of neonatal seizures (22,23).

Where conventional EEG monitoring is not available, amplitude-integrated EEG (aEEG) can serve as a useful screening tool. aEEG is a form of digital trending that modifies the raw EEG recording by filtering frequencies, displaying EEG amplitude on a semilogarithmic scale, and showing trends over time in a time-compressed format (16). With aEEG, a limited number (2 to 5) of electrodes are placed by a nurse or other NICU team member; the modified EEG tracing is interpreted at the bedside by NICU providers. **Figure 51.3** shows an example of neonatal seizures on aEEG. aEEG is superior to detection of seizures solely by clinical observation, though it has limitations as compared to full array EEG monitoring (16). The key advantage of aEEG is relative ease of use, with application and interpretation possible by trained neonatal staff in the absence of neurodiagnostic technologists and neurophysiologists. The sensitivity and specificity of aEEG for seizure detection are highly dependent on the user's level of expertise in interpretation. Sensitivity of seizure detection ranges from 27% to 90% with reported specificities ranging from 39% to 97% (16,24–26). While aEEG is a useful tool, it is most powerful in combination with conventional EEG for confirmation of seizures. This allows the benefit of real-time monitoring at the bedside, with expert confirmation of suspected seizures using full-array conventional EEG. To use both tools in combination requires a full set of cEEG electrodes placed for interpretation by neurophysiologists, with equipment displaying limited channel aEEG at the bedside for interpretation by NICU providers. NICU providers can then communicate any concerns regarding suspicious aEEG changes to the neurophysiologist for confirmation on cEEG.

All neonatal seizures should be confirmed with EEG wherever possible, as per WHO Guidelines. At the same time, in settings where cEEG and aEEG are unavailable, seizures can be monitored clinically via abnormal movements and changes in vital signs (see section on Clinical Presentation above).

Causes of Neonatal Seizures

There are many underlying etiologies for neonatal seizures. The majority (80% to 85%) of neonatal seizures are acute symptomatic, meaning that the seizures are symptomatic of an underlying acute brain injury (3,27,28). A minority of neonatal seizures are due to neonatal-onset epilepsy, such as those due to a genetic etiology or a CNS malformation (28,29).

A number of causes may underlie acute symptomatic seizures (see Table 51.1). For term neonates, HIE is the most common underlying etiology, present in about 40% of neonates with seizures (3,27,28). Ischemic infarction, or stroke, is the second most common cause of neonatal seizures, accounting for 15% to 20% of cases (3,28). Intracranial hemorrhage follows at 10% to 15% in term neonates; in preterm newborns, this is the most common cause of seizures, due to the higher incidence of intraventricular hemorrhage (3,28). Other acute symptomatic causes include intracranial infections such as meningitis and encephalitis and electrolyte and metabolic derangements such as hypoglycemia, hypo- or hypernatremia, hypocalcemia, and hypomagnesemia (30).

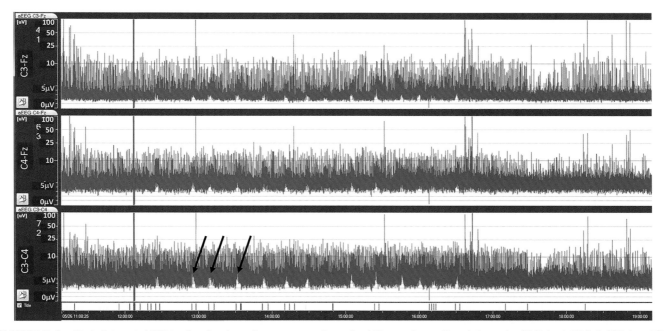

FIGURE 51.3 **Amplitude-integrated EEG tracing showing a time-compressed sample of 8 hours of recording of electrodes C3-Fz (top), C4-Fz (middle), and C3-C4 (bottom).** Background shows amplitude suppression with baseline less than 5 μV and intermittent areas of baseline amplitude elevation, representing seizure (examples marked by *black arrows*).

TABLE 51.1
Causes of Neonatal Seizures

Acute symptomatic	Hypoxic–ischemic brain injury	Hypoxic–ischemic encephalopathy
	Vascular	Ischemic infarction/stroke
		Cerebral venous sinus thrombosis
	Intracranial hemorrhage	Intraventricular hemorrhage
		Intraparenchymal hemorrhage (including cerebellar hemorrhage)
		Subdural hemorrhage
		Subarachnoid hemorrhage
	Central nervous system infection	Meningitis
		Encephalitis
	Toxic/metabolic etiologies	Hypoglycemia
		Hyper- or hyponatremia
		Hypocalcemia
		Hypomagnesemia
		Hyperbilirubinemia
		Neonatal abstinence syndrome
Neonatal-onset epilepsy	Metabolic disorders	Inborn errors of metabolism (organic acid and amino acid synthesis disorders)
	Developmental abnormalities of the brain	Brain malformations
	Epilepsy syndromes	Genetic epilepsy (including benign familial neonatal convulsions)
		Vitamin-responsive epilepsy (including pyridoxine deficiency, biotinidase deficiency)
		Early Infantile Epileptic Encephalopathy (EIEE)
		Early Myoclonic Encephalopathy (EME)

Reprinted with permission from Whitelaw A, Osredkar D, Thoresen M. Neurological & Neuromuscular Disorders. In: MacDonald M, Seshia M, eds. *Avery's neonatology: pathophysiology and management of the newborn*, 7th ed. Philadelphia, PA: Wolters Kluwer, 2016:994.

Less commonly, in about 15% to 20% of cases, seizures in the neonatal period are the beginning of neonatal-onset epilepsy. These are most often due to a chronic cause such as an underlying inborn error of metabolism, brain malformation, or genetic abnormalities. These etiologies cause a small but important minority of seizures presenting in the neonatal period.

Onset of neonatal seizures is typically within the first week after birth, dependent upon the underlying etiology (3). Seizure onset within the first 24 hours is common in HIE (31). Similarly, seizures from stroke typically begin in the first few days after delivery (29,32). CNS infections may cause seizures that do not begin until after the first few days after birth, whereas seizures related to an underlying metabolic disorder may present at any time within the first few weeks (32).

Etiologic Evaluation

Prompt recognition and diagnosis of neonatal seizures is imperative both for identifying the etiology and to facilitate treatment. In any case of suspected neonatal seizures, the patient should be assessed for reversible causes, including hypocalcemia, hypoglycemia, hypomagnesemia, and hypo- or hypernatremia. An indirect bilirubin level should be obtained to assess for possible bilirubin encephalopathy. Neonates with seizures should also be evaluated for systemic and central nervous system infections, with initiation of antimicrobial therapy when indicated.

Concurrent with the initial rapid assessment for potential reversible causes of neonatal seizures, the history can provide important clues toward etiology. Prenatal history should include medication and substance exposures, maternal diabetes, any evidence and timing of maternal infection, and quality of fetal movements during pregnancy and prior to delivery. Birth history should include evidence of fetal distress, need for resuscitation in the delivery room, blood gas or other evidence of acidosis, vitamin K administration, and condition at birth. Family history of seizures, epilepsies, genetic conditions, bleeding disorders, or early childhood deaths should be obtained. Physical examination should take note of head circumference, dysmorphic features and/or other congenital anomalies, neurocutaneous stigmata, and particular attention to the neurologic examination for signs of lethargy, feeding difficulty, or encephalopathy.

Neuroimaging should be obtained urgently, with head ultrasound typically the most readily available modality. Head ultrasound can reveal the presence of hemorrhage, certain brain malformations, and, in some cases, evidence of ischemia. Though the image resolution of ultrasound is limited, it requires no radiation exposure, is inexpensive, and widely available. Head ultrasound is a highly useful immediate study, with magnetic resonance imaging (MRI) the definitive imaging modality in the evaluation of neonatal seizures, to be obtained as soon as possible (30,33). The high image quality of MRI allows for identification of more subtle findings, including those associated with HIE, stroke, intracranial hemorrhage, CNS infections, and brain malformations. MRI involves no radiation exposure. In active neonates, sedation is sometimes required to minimize patient movement for optimal image quality; however, encephalopathic or ill neonates often do not require sedation. Computed tomography (CT) scans are not recommended in neonates due to the resulting radiation exposure and limited resolution of images (30). CT may be used, however, in rare situations, for example, when ultrasound reveals a large intracranial hemorrhage requiring potential neurosurgical intervention, and MRI is unavailable, though head ultrasound may also be used as a modality of urgent neuroimaging and might be more readily available.

If history and neuroimaging do not reveal the etiology of neonatal seizures, additional metabolic and/or genetic testing is warranted. As guided by the clinical presentation, this may include screening serum labs for inborn errors of metabolism, CSF studies for specific metabolic and genetic disorders, and/or urine studies in combination with serum and CSF testing to assess for vitamin-responsive epilepsies (see Table 51.2). Testing for neonatal-onset genetic epilepsies should also be considered, with gene panels often useful. As genetic testing methods and availability continue to improve, more expanded testing such as rapid whole-genome sequencing may allow quick identification of genetic epilepsy etiologies for timely targeted intervention. In a sample of 38 critically ill children, 45% had a molecular diagnosis made by rapid whole-genome sequencing, which led to a change in management in 24% of those with a genetic diagnosis identified (35). This is particularly relevant for neonates, as a high proportion of neonatal-onset epilepsy may be due to genetic causes. In a large sample of neonates with seizures, a genetic etiology was identified in 59% of neonates with epilepsy who had testing performed (36).

Neonatal-onset genetic epilepsies vary widely in presentation. The most common genetic cause of neonatal seizures is mutation in *KCNQ2*, a potassium channel gene. Mutations in *KCNQ2* can cause a phenotypic spectrum of neonatal-onset epilepsies. Benign Familial Neonatal Epilepsy is characterized by seizures within the first week of life that typically resolve later in infancy. However, *KCNQ2* mutations can also cause a neonatal epileptic encephalopathy (EIEE) with refractory seizures that is associated with poor neurodevelopmental outcomes (37,38). Early diagnosis of *KCNQ2*-related epilepsy has important implications

TABLE 51.2

Investigations to Consider for Neonatal Seizures

Initial evaluations	Serum	Electrolytes, including sodium, magnesium, calcium, glucose
		Indirect bilirubin
		CBC with differential
		CRP
		Blood cultures
	Urine	Urinalysis, urine culture
	CSF	Consider lumbar puncture to assess for infection
	Neuroimaging	Head ultrasound
		MRI brain
Additional evaluations to consider when clinically indicated	Serum	Screen for inborn errors of metabolism: Ammonia, lactate, pyruvate, acyl carnitine profile, free and total carnitine, serum amino acids
		Genetic testing (including epilepsy gene panels)
		Testing for vitamin-responsive epilepsies (34): pipecolic acid, alpha-aminoadipic semialdehyde (AASA)
	Urine	Screen for organic acidemias: urine organic acids
		Testing for vitamin-responsive epilepsies (34): vanillactic acid, AASA, reducing substances
	CSF	CSF glucose level (paired with serum glucose)
		Testing for vitamin-responsive epilepsies (34): AASA, neurotransmitter metabolites

for treatment because this form of epilepsy responds well to sodium channel blocking ASMs, such as oxcarbazepine. A growing number of other genetic etiologies have been identified as causative for early-onset epileptic encephalopathies. These are largely characterized by refractory seizures with high risk of mortality or poor neurodevelopmental outcomes (39). Early infantile epileptic encephalopathy (EIEE), or Ohtahara syndrome, is characterized by refractory seizures, encephalopathy, and burst suppression on EEG. Early myoclonic encephalopathy (EME) is characterized by myoclonic seizures and often is associated with encephalopathy between seizures (40). In addition to genetic etiologies, brain malformations and inborn errors of metabolism are also causative of neonatal-onset epilepsies.

TREATMENT

Goals of Treatment

The goals of treatment should be made explicit for each individual patient. Most often, the goal of treatment is to stop all seizures, both clinical and electrographic. Though there is no evidence from high-quality randomized controlled trials with long-term follow-up data to demonstrate seizure treatment improves outcomes, mounting evidence supports neonatal seizures as a potentially modifiable risk factor for adverse outcomes. Among neonates with known brain injury, seizures are associated with worse neurodevelopmental outcomes as compared to brain injury without seizures (28,41). Similarly, seizures in themselves have been shown

to cause neuronal apoptosis in animal studies (42,43). There appears to further be a dose–response effect: in humans, higher seizure burden and presence of status epilepticus increases the risk of poor outcomes (43–45). Therefore, treatment with the goal of complete cessation of seizures is advised when possible for both term and preterm neonates. In those cases where complete resolution of seizures is not possible, such as neonatal-onset epilepsies, an appropriate treatment goal may be reduction of seizures as much as possible without excessive adverse effects of medication. Though more evidence is needed to understand the independent impact of ASMs on neurodevelopmental outcomes, current guidelines recommend seizure control with ASM therapy when possible (2). In cases of comfort care, it may be appropriate to only treat clinical seizures, and forego evaluation for and treatment of subclinical seizures. Implementation of a neonatal neurocritical care service, including prolonged cEEG monitoring and seizure management guidelines, has been shown to be beneficial for the management of neonatal seizures by allowing decreased use of phenobarbital via more precise seizure recognition and treatment (46).

Immediate Treatment

For neonates having seizures, initial management is to stabilize the patient: secure and maintain the airway, assess and confirm appropriate breathing and ventilation, and confirm or provide adequate circulation. The neonate should be rapidly assessed for reversible causes of seizures, with any derangements in electrolytes or glucose corrected. If indicated, treatment of infection should be initiated. Concurrently, EEG monitoring should be initiated for confirmation of the seizure diagnosis. With confirmation of seizures on EEG or with high clinical suspicion of seizures, ASM treatment should begin.

Antiseizure Medications

Phenobarbital is the first-line agent for the treatment of neonatal seizures, as recommended by current WHO guidelines (2). If seizures continue despite adequate loading doses of phenobarbital, a second-line agent should be given. Second-line agents include benzodiazepines, phenytoin, and lidocaine, with no clear evidence for the use of one agent over another (2). There are no specific guidelines for third-line treatment beyond the agents above, though levetiracetam is increasingly popular as a second- and/or third-line treatment (47). Table 51.3 summarizes loading doses, maintenance doses, and drug levels for ASMs. If seizures are refractory to multiple ASMs, trials of pyridoxine, pyridoxal 5′-phosphate (PLP), and folinic acid should be given to assess for possible vitamin-responsive epileptic encephalopathies (34).

Phenobarbital

Phenobarbital is one of the oldest ASMs used for neonatal seizure treatment and remains first-line therapy (2). It is a barbiturate that enhances inhibitory neurotransmission as a gamma-aminobutyric acid type A (GABA-A) receptor agonist (48). For decades, there has been only one published randomized trial assessing the efficacy of phenobarbital, conducted by Painter and colleagues (49). This compared phenobarbital to phenytoin, using the end point of 80% seizure reduction in 59 neonates. With phenobarbital, only 43% of neonates had this degree of improvement in seizure burden (49). Other small retrospective and prospective studies have reported seizure control rates ranging from 43% to 63% (48,50,51). The NeoLEV2 trial recently demonstrated a higher rate of seizure control following phenobarbital, with seizure resolution on EEG reported in 80% of subjects randomized to phenobarbital loading doses after onset of seizures on EEG, further supporting the use of phenobarbital as first-line therapy for neonatal seizures caused by various etiologies (52). Phenobarbital has several important adverse effects to consider, most commonly sedation

THE NEWBORN INFANT

TABLE 51.3

Antiseizure Medication Treatment Doses and Drug Monitoring Levels

ASM	Loading Dose	Maintenance Dose	Goal Serum Level
Phenobarbital	20 mg/kg IV Additional 10 mg/kg doses up to 40 mg/kg total	5 mg/kg/d divided in 1–2 doses	Goal 20–40 µg/mL 1–2 h after loading dose
Phenytoin/fosphenytoin	15–20 mg PE/kg IV Additional 10 mg PE/kg one time	3–5 mg/kg/d divided in 2–4 doses	Goal level 10–20 µg/mL total or 1–2 µg/mL free phenytoin 1 h after loading dose
Midazolam	0.05 mg/kg IV over 10 min	Continuous infusion of 0.15 mg/kg/h, increase stepwise by 0.05 mg/kg/h, typical maximum 0.5 mg/kg/h or as limited by side effects	No established drug levels for monitoring
Lorazepam	0.05–0.1 mg/kg over 2–5 min Repeat doses up to total dose of 0.15 mg/kg	—	
Clonazepam	0.01 mg/kg IV	0.01 mg/kg/dose for 3–5 doses	
Levetiracetam	40–80 mg/kg IV	30–60 mg/kg/d divided in 2 doses	No established drug levels for monitoring
Topiramate	5–10 mg/kg enteral	1–5 mg/kg/d	5–20 µg/mL for adults Goal level for neonates not established

PE, phenytoin equivalents.

and respiratory depression. This risk is increased at serum levels greater than 50 µg/mL (50,53). Animal studies have demonstrated neuronal apoptosis with early and prolonged phenobarbital use, raising concern for risk to neurodevelopmental outcomes if administered chronically. This potential risk supports the importance of only using this ASM for definite seizures (42,48).

Phenytoin

Phenytoin, and the prodrug fosphenytoin, is a commonly used second-line agent for neonatal seizure treatment. Phenytoin decreases excitatory neurotransmission at the glutamatergic synapse by inhibiting voltage-gated sodium channels (48). This mechanism of action differs from phenobarbital or benzodiazepines, justifying phenytoin as a reasonable choice for polypharmacy in seizures not responsive to phenobarbital. In the Painter trial, 45% of neonates showed improvement in seizure burden with phenytoin (49). No other randomized trial has evaluated phenytoin for the treatment of neonatal seizures. A challenge with phenytoin use is that neonates rapidly metabolize phenytoin through hepatic clearance, requiring frequent dosing to maintain therapeutic levels, up to four times daily. Phenytoin has several notable adverse effects, including hepatotoxicity, arrhythmias, hypotension, and soft tissue injury from extravasation. Infusion-related side effects are less frequent, though still possible, with fosphenytoin use (30,54–56). Phenytoin should not be given concurrently with lidocaine, as these drugs together have a higher risk for cardiac complications.

Similar to phenobarbital, phenytoin has been shown to cause neuronal apoptosis in animal studies, though without similar findings in humans (42).

Lidocaine

Lidocaine is another second-line agent for treatment of neonatal seizures, also with a mechanism of decreasing excitatory neurotransmission at the glutamatergic synapse through action on sodium channels (48). Reported response rates vary, with seizure control reported to range from 53% to 76% (57–60). Lidocaine is given as a continuous infusion, with suggested dosing regimens in Table 51.4. The dosing is adjusted for preterm neonates and infants undergoing therapeutic hypothermia due to decreased clearance. The most significant adverse effects of lidocaine are cardiac toxicity; neonates require continuous cardiac monitoring throughout infusion due to the risk for arrhythmias (2,60–64). Similarly, with ongoing infusion, there is accumulation of a toxic metabolite, limiting lidocaine use to 24 to 48 hours maximum duration. At high concentrations, lidocaine has proconvulsant activity; however, this does not occur at doses used for neonatal seizure treatment (60). Lidocaine should not be used in conjunction with phenytoin, due to the increased risk of adverse effects.

Benzodiazepines

Midazolam, lorazepam, and clonazepam are also recommended as second-line agents for treatment of neonatal seizures (2). This

TABLE 51.4

Lidocaine Dosing, General (61), and Stratified by Birth Weight (62) and Hypothermia Status (63)

	Loading Dose	First Infusion		Second Infusion		Third Infusion	
		mg/kg/h	h	mg/kg/h	h	mg/kg/h	h
General dosing	2 mg/kg IV over 10 min	6	6	4	12	2	12
Birth weights 0.8–1.5 kg		5	4	2.5	6	1.25	12
Birth weights 1.6–2.5 kg		6	4	3	6	1.5	12
Birth weights 2.6–4.5 kg		7	4	3.5	6	1.75	12
Hypothermia, birth weights 2.0–2.5 kg		6	3.5	3	12	1.5	12
Hypothermia, birth weights 2.5–4.5 kg		7	3.5	3.5	12	1.75	12

class of drugs increases inhibitory neurotransmission by modulating the GABA-A receptor chloride channel (48). Limited, small case series and prospective studies report variable response to benzodiazepines for neonatal seizures (57,58,65–68). Potential adverse effects of benzodiazepines include sedation, respiratory depression, and hypotension (48,50,51).

Levetiracetam

While levetiracetam is not specifically included in the WHO Guidelines as a recommended AED for neonatal seizures, it is increasingly popular in clinical use (47,69). The postulated mechanism of action is through decreasing excitatory neurotransmission at the glutamatergic synapse by inhibition of calcium channels and synaptic vesicle protein 2A (64). Small retrospective and prospective studies report variable efficacy, with seizure control rates ranging from 35% to 82% (48,70,71). However, the randomized NEOLEV2 trial found seizure control rates of only 28% to 36% with levetiracetam, dependent on dose (52). The side effect profile of levetiracetam is favorable, with no relevant drug–drug interactions, no need for drug level monitoring, and many study populations reporting no acute adverse effects (47,51,69–71).

Topiramate

Topiramate is less frequently used in neonates because it requires enteral administration. It is not included in current WHO Guidelines for neonatal seizure treatment, lacking data supporting use for this age group (50,51). Small case series and retrospective studies have demonstrated variable efficacy. A recent randomized trial of topiramate therapy versus placebo in combination with therapeutic hypothermia for HIE showed no significant difference in seizure burden between the topiramate and placebo groups (72–74). There is no intravenous form of topiramate, which limits its use for acute seizure control (75). One small case series described 4 preterm neonates who developed necrotizing enterocolitis after receiving topiramate; this risk has not been fully defined (76). Otherwise, adverse effects have not been well described from existing case series of topiramate in neonates, though it is known to commonly cause metabolic acidosis in other age groups (75).

Vitamins

In cases where seizures continue despite treatment with adequate doses of multiple ASMs, vitamin-responsive epilepsies should be considered. These are the class of metabolic and genetic disorders manifesting as seizures that respond to specific vitamin supplementation. Pyridoxine-dependent epilepsy is caused by alpha-aminoadipic semialdehyde (AASA) dehydrogenase (antiquin) deficiency due to *ALDH7A1* mutations. It may be empirically diagnosed by a trial of high-dose pyridoxine (34). While on EEG monitoring, an initial load of 100 mg pyridoxine IV should be given, with assessment for electrographic response. This can be repeated every 10 minutes up to a total dose of 500 mg (34). This should only be attempted under hospital conditions with cardiorespiratory monitoring, as resulting bradycardia has been reported. Of note, not every patient will have an immediate response to IV pyridoxine on EEG or clinically. In suspected cases, maintenance therapy with IV or oral pyridoxine 15 to 18 mg/kg/d divided twice daily should be continued until results of confirmatory tests are obtained, or until an alternate etiology is identified (34). PLP-dependent seizures, caused by pyridox(am)ine 5′-phosphate oxidase (PNPO) deficiency, may similarly be diagnosed by response to an empiric PLP trial or by genetic testing for mutations in the *PNPO* gene. Enteral PLP is given at a dose of 30 mg/kg/d divided three to four times daily, with observation for response. Folinic acid–responsive seizures are allelic with pyridoxine-dependent seizures and may similarly respond to administration of folinic acid, with 3 to 5 mg/kg/d given maintenance therapy.

Duration of Therapy

In neonates who achieve seizure control on a single ASM, WHO Guidelines recommend discontinuation without tapering of the medication prior to hospital discharge (2). This reflects that the majority of neonatal seizures are acutely symptomatic, with risk for ongoing seizures significantly decreased outside of the period of acute illness. If more than one ASM is required for seizure control, medications can be discontinued one by one (2). Earlier discontinuation of ASMs has become more common due to the largely unknown neurodevelopmental consequences of ASMs and concerns for adverse effects with prolonged use (77). In cases of neonatal-onset epilepsy, however, long-term ASM therapy likely will be required for seizure control. Each case of neonatal seizures must be evaluated individually when deciding the appropriate interval to discontinue therapy, with WHO Guidelines as a framework.

▌ PROGNOSIS

Overview and Risk Factors

Neonates with seizures have an increased risk of mortality and neurodevelopmental problems, including epilepsy, cerebral palsy, developmental delays, and intellectual disability (78). The prognosis for neonates with seizures is highly dependent on the etiology of the seizures. Neonates with reversible causes typically have more favorable outcomes than those with genetic or structural etiologies or those with severe brain injuries. Across the continuum of seizure etiologies, several risk factors have been correlated with worse outcomes. Higher seizure burden and status epilepticus are correlated with worse neurodevelopmental outcomes (79–81). In HIE, this effect is seen independent of severity of injury on MRI (4,82). In a study of 47 neonates with HIE, there was a nine-fold increased odds of abnormal neurodevelopmental outcome in those with total seizure burden greater than 40 minutes (81).

Mortality

In a recent large prospective cohort study of neonates with seizures, 17% died or were transferred to hospice care, with mortality rates significantly higher for preterm as compared to term infants (28). Additional studies have reported mortality rates ranging from 7% to 30% for infants with neonatal seizures (29,78,79,83).

Morbidity—Neurodevelopmental Outcomes
Epilepsy

The majority of seizures in the neonatal period are acute symptomatic seizures of an underlying inciting factor and therefore are not considered epilepsy. Following this acute period, however, 34% of patients develop postneonatal epilepsy, with higher risk in preterm infants (78). The median age of onset of epilepsy following neonatal seizures is 9 months, with a wide range (78). Neonates with genetic and metabolic etiologies, or structural brain malformations, are considered to have neonatal-onset epilepsy with ongoing high risk for seizures expected to continue beyond the neonatal period.

Cerebral Palsy

Cerebral palsy, a static disorder of motor function caused by nonprogressive brain injury, occurs in 25% to 45% of survivors of neonatal seizures (78,84). This is also dependent on the etiology of neonatal seizures, with cerebral palsy most common in neonates with seizures due to brain injury. Higher risk of cerebral palsy is also seen in preterm infants following neonatal seizures, due to the common underlying etiologies of intraventricular hemorrhage and ischemic injury in this age group (78).

Developmental Delay/Intellectual Disability

Neonatal seizures are also associated with later global developmental delays and intellectual disability. In a population-based study with a 10-year follow-up of subjects with neonatal seizures, 25% developed intellectual disability, with an additional 27% having learning disabilities (78). Rates of intellectual disability were higher in preterm as compared with term infants (78). As above, the etiology significantly impacts these risks.

CONCLUSIONS

Neonatal seizures are common, with many underlying etiologies. As the majority of neonatal seizures are reflective of an acute brain injury, prompt assessment for reversible causes with appropriate intervention is imperative. The clinical appearance of seizures in neonates is often subtle or subclinical, requiring continuous EEG monitoring for accurate diagnosis. Given this need for EEG monitoring and skilled interpretation, an area requiring further exploration is how to leverage advances in teleneurology and remote EEG review to create an efficient pooled resource for neonatal neurology. Currently for one region, a center can review EEG for multiple hospitals; this can be adapted for countries or larger regions where experts are less available. Current guidelines recommend treatment of neonatal seizures to decrease seizure burden because untreated seizures are associated with poorer neurodevelopmental outcomes, though further research in this area is needed. Phenobarbital is the first-line agent recommended for the treatment of neonatal seizures, supported by recent efficacy data. Research into additional treatments for neonatal seizures is required, as data have demonstrated only partial responses with current treatment options. Overall, neonates with seizures are at increased risk of mortality and poor neurodevelopmental outcomes including future epilepsy, cerebral palsy, and intellectual disability and require special attention for early intervention and rehabilitation services.

REFERENCES

1. Abend NS, Jensen FE, Inder TE, et al. Chapter 12—neonatal seizures. In: Volpe JJ, Inder TE, Darras BT, et al., eds. *Volpe's neurology of the newborn*, 6th ed. Philadelphia, PA: Elsevier, 2018:275. doi: 10.1016/B978-0-323-42876-7.00012-0
2. Di Giorgio R, ed. *Guidelines on neonatal seizures.* Geneva, Switzerland: World Health Organization, 2011. Available from: http://www.ncbi.nlm.nih.gov/books/NBK304092/. Accessed February 26, 2019.
3. Vasudevan C, Levene M. Epidemiology and aetiology of neonatal seizures. *Semin Fetal Neonatal Med* 2013;18(4):185. doi: 10.1016/j.siny.2013.05.008
4. Glass HC, Glidden D, Jeremy RJ, et al. Clinical neonatal seizures are independently associated with outcome in infants at risk for hypoxic-ischemic brain injury. *J Pediatr* 2009;155(3):318. doi: 10.1016/j.jpeds.2009.03.040
5. Booth D, Evans DJ. Anticonvulsants for neonates with seizures. *Cochrane Database Syst Rev* 2004;(4):CD004218. doi: 10.1002/14651858.CD004218.pub2
6. Scher MS, Alvin J, Gaus L, et al. Uncoupling of EEG-clinical neonatal seizures after antiepileptic drug use. *Pediatr Neurol* 2003;28(4):277.
7. Shellhaas RA. Continuous long-term electroencephalography: the gold standard for neonatal seizure diagnosis. *Semin Fetal Neonatal Med* 2015;20(3):149. doi: 10.1016/j.siny.2015.01.005
8. Abend NS, Wusthoff CJ. Neonatal seizures and status epilepticus. *J Clin Neurophysiol* 2012;29(5):441. doi: 10.1097/WNP.0b013e31826bd90d
9. Murray DM, Boylan GB, Ali I, et al. Defining the gap between electrographic seizure burden, clinical expression and staff recognition of neonatal seizures. *Arch Dis Child Fetal Neonatal Ed* 2008;93(3):F187. doi: 10.1136/adc.2005.086314
10. Malone A, Ryan CA, Fitzgerald A, et al. Interobserver agreement in neonatal seizure identification. *Epilepsia* 2009;50(9):2097. doi: 10.1111/j.1528-1167.2009.02132.x
11. Loman AMW, ter Horst HJ, Lambrechtsen FACP, et al. Neonatal seizures: aetiology by means of a standardized work-up. *Eur J Paediatr Neurol* 2014;18(3):360. doi: 10.1016/j.ejpn.2014.01.014
12. Shellhaas RA, Clancy RR. Characterization of neonatal seizures by conventional EEG and single-channel EEG. *Clin Neurophysiol* 2007;118(10):2156. doi: 10.1016/j.clinph.2007.06.061
13. Clancy RR. The contribution of EEG to the understanding of neonatal seizures. *Epilepsia* 1996;37(suppl 1):S52. doi: 10.1111/j.1528-1157.1996.tb06022.x
14. Berg AT, Berkovic SF, Brodie MJ, et al. Revised terminology and concepts for organization of seizures and epilepsies: report of the ILAE Commission on Classification and Terminology, 2005–2009. *Epilepsia* 2010;51(4):676. doi: 10.1111/j.1528-1167.2010.02522.x
15. Fisher RS, Cross JH, French JA, et al. Operational classification of seizure types by the International League Against Epilepsy: Position Paper of the ILAE Commission for Classification and Terminology. *Epilepsia* 2017;58(4):522. doi: 10.1111/epi.13670
16. Shellhaas RA, Chang T, Tsuchida T, et al. The American Clinical Neurophysiology Society's Guideline on continuous electroencephalography monitoring in neonates. *J Clin Neurophysiol* 2011;28(6):611. doi: 10.1097/WNP.0b013e31823e96d7
17. Whitelaw A, Osredkar D, Thoresen M. Chapter 46—Neurological & neuromuscular disorders. In: MacDonald M, Seshia M, eds. *Avery's neonatology: pathophysiology and management of the newborn*, 7th ed. Philadelphia, PA: Lippincott Williams & Wilkins, 2016:994.
18. Hancock EC, Osborne JP, Edwards SW. Treatment of infantile spasms. *Cochrane Database Syst Rev* 2013;(6):CD001770. doi: 10.1002/14651858.CD001770.pub3
19. Dang LT, Shellhaas RA. Diagnostic yield of continuous video electroencephalography for paroxysmal vital sign changes in pediatric patients. *Epilepsia* 2016;57(2):272. doi: 10.1111/epi.13276
20. Gluckman PD, Wyatt JS, Azzopardi D, et al. Selective head cooling with mild systemic hypothermia after neonatal encephalopathy: multicentre randomised trial. *Lancet* 2005;365(9460):663. doi: 10.1016/S0140-6736(05)17946-X
21. Clancy RR, Sharif U, Ichord R, et al. Electrographic neonatal seizures after infant heart surgery. *Epilepsia* 2005;46(1):84. doi: 10.1111/j.0013-9580.2005.22504.x
22. Din F, Lalgudi Ganesan S, Akiyama T, et al. Seizure detection algorithms in critically ill children: a comparative evaluation. *Crit Care Med* 2020;48(4):545. doi: 10.1097/CCM.0000000000004180
23. Ansari AH, Cherian PJ, Caicedo A, et al. Neonatal seizure detection using deep convolutional neural networks. *Int J Neural Syst* 2019;29(04):1850011. doi: 10.1142/S0129065718500119
24. Rennie JM, Chorley G, Boylan GB, et al. Non-expert use of the cerebral function monitor for neonatal seizure detection. *Arch Dis Child Fetal Neonatal Ed* 2004;89(1):F37.
25. Shellhaas RA, Soaita AI, Clancy RR. Sensitivity of amplitude-integrated electroencephalography for neonatal seizure detection. *Pediatrics* 2007;120(4):770. doi: 10.1542/peds.2007-0514
26. Frenkel N, Friger M, Meledin I, et al. Neonatal seizure recognition—comparative study of continuous-amplitude integrated EEG versus short conventional EEG recordings. *Clin Neurophysiol* 2011;122(6):1091. doi: 10.1016/j.clinph.2010.09.028
27. Weeke LC, Groenendaal F, Toet MC, et al. The aetiology of neonatal seizures and the diagnostic contribution of neonatal cerebral magnetic resonance imaging. *Dev Med Child Neurol* 2015;57(3):248. doi: 10.1111/dmcn.12629
28. Glass HC, Shellhaas RA, Wusthoff CJ, et al. Contemporary profile of seizures in neonates: a prospective cohort study. *J Pediatr* 2016;174:98. doi: 10.1016/j.jpeds.2016.03.035
29. Tekgul H, Gauvreau K, Soul J, et al. The current etiologic profile and neurodevelopmental outcome of seizures in term newborn infants. *Pediatrics* 2006;117(4):1270. doi: 10.1542/peds.2005-1178
30. Glass HC. Neonatal seizures: advances in mechanisms and management. *Clin Perinatol* 2014;41(1):177. doi: 10.1016/j.clp.2013.10.004
31. Wusthoff CJ, Dlugos DJ, Gutierrez-Colina A, et al. Electrographic seizures during therapeutic hypothermia for neonatal hypoxic-ischemic encephalopathy. *J Child Neurol* 2011;26(6):724. doi: 10.1177/0883073810390036
32. Calciolari G, Perlman JM, Volpe JJ. Seizures in the neonatal intensive care unit of the 1980s. Types, etiologies, timing. *Clin Pediatr (Phila)* 1988;27(3):119. doi: 10.1177/000992288802700301
33. Wilmshurst JM, Gaillard WD, Vinayan KP, et al. Summary of recommendations for the management of infantile seizures: Task Force Report for the ILAE Commission of Pediatrics. *Epilepsia* 2015;56(8):1185. doi: 10.1111/epi.13057
34. Gospe SM. Neonatal vitamin-responsive epileptic encephalopathies. *Chang Gung Med J* 2010;33(1):1.
35. Sanford EF, Clark MM, Farnaes L, et al. Rapid whole genome sequencing has clinical utility in children in the PICU. *Pediatr Crit Care Med* 2019;20(11):1007. doi: 10.1097/PCC.0000000000002056
36. Shellhaas RA, Wusthoff CJ, Tsuchida TN, et al. Profile of neonatal epilepsies: Characteristics of a prospective US cohort. *Neurology* 2017;89(9):893. doi: 10.1212/WNL.0000000000004284
37. Goto A, Ishii A, Shibata M, et al. Characteristics of KCNQ2 variants causing either benign neonatal epilepsy or developmental and epileptic encephalopathy. *Epilepsia* 2019;60(9):1870. doi: 10.1111/epi.16314
38. Kato M, Yamagata T, Kubota M, et al. Clinical spectrum of early onset epileptic encephalopathies caused by KCNQ2 mutation. *Epilepsia* 2013;54(7):1282. doi: 10.1111/epi.12200

39. Beal JC, Cherian K, Moshe SL. Early-onset epileptic encephalopathies: Ohtahara syndrome and early myoclonic encephalopathy. *Pediatr Neurol* 2012;47(5):317. doi: 10.1016/j.pediatrneurol.2012.06.002

40. Olson HE, Kelly M, LaCoursiere CM, et al. Genetics and genotype-phenotype correlations in early onset epileptic encephalopathy with burst suppression. *Ann Neurol* 2017;81(3):419. doi: 10.1002/ana.24883

41. van Rooij LGM, Toet MC, van Huffelen AC, et al. Effect of treatment of subclinical neonatal seizures detected with aEEG: randomized, controlled trial. *Pediatrics* 2010;125(2):e358. doi: 10.1542/peds.2009-0136

42. Kaushal S, Tamer Z, Opoku F, et al. Anticonvulsant drug-induced cell death in the developing white matter of the rodent brain. *Epilepsia* 2016;57(5):727. doi: 10.1111/epi.13365

43. Kang SK, Kadam SD. Neonatal seizures: impact on neurodevelopmental outcomes. *Front Pediatr* 2015;3:101. doi: 10.3389/fped.2015.00101

44. Miller SP, Weiss J, Barnwell A, et al. Seizure-associated brain injury in term newborns with perinatal asphyxia. *Neurology* 2002;58(4):542. doi: 10.1212/wnl.58.4.542

45. van Rooij LGM, de Vries LS, Handryastuti S, et al. Neurodevelopmental outcome in term infants with status epilepticus detected with amplitude-integrated electroencephalography. *Pediatrics* 2007;120(2):e354. doi: 10.1542/peds.2006-3007

46. Wietstock SO, Bonifacio SL, McCulloch CE, et al. Neonatal neurocritical care service is associated with decreased administration of seizure medication. *J Child Neurol* 2015;30(9):1135. doi: 10.1177/0883073814553799

47. Shoemaker MT, Rotenberg JS. Levetiracetam for the treatment of neonatal seizures. *J Child Neurol* 2007;22(1):95. doi: 10.1177/0883073807299973

48. Donovan MD, Griffin BT, Kharoshankaya L, et al. Pharmacotherapy for neonatal seizures: current knowledge and future perspectives. *Drugs* 2016;76(6):647. doi: 10.1007/s40265-016-0554-7

49. Painter MJ, Scher MS, Stein AD, et al. Phenobarbital compared with phenytoin for the treatment of neonatal seizures. *N Engl J Med* 1999;341(7):485. doi: 10.1056/NEJM199908123410704

50. van Rooij LGM, van den Broek MPH, Rademaker CMA, et al. Clinical management of seizures in newborns : diagnosis and treatment. *Paediatr Drugs* 2013;15(1):9. doi: 10.1007/s40272-012-0005-1

51. Slaughter LA, Patel AD, Slaughter JL. Pharmacological treatment of neonatal seizures: a systematic review. *J Child Neurol* 2013;28(3):351. doi: 10.1177/0883073812470734

52. Sharpe C, Reiner GE, Davis SL, et al. Levetiracetam versus phenobarbital for neonatal seizures: a randomized controlled trial. *Pediatrics* 145(6):e20193182. doi: 10.1542/peds.2019-3182

53. Patsalos PN, Berry DJ, Bourgeois BFD, et al. Antiepileptic drugs—best practice guidelines for therapeutic drug monitoring: a position paper by the subcommission on therapeutic drug monitoring, ILAE Commission on Therapeutic Strategies. *Epilepsia* 2008;49(7):1239. doi: 10.1111/j.1528-1167.2008.01561.x

54. Appleton RE, Gill A. Adverse events associated with intravenous phenytoin in children: a prospective study. *Seizure* 2003;12(6):369.

55. Sharief N, Goonasekera C. Soft tissue injury associated with intravenous phenytoin in a neonate. *Acta Paediatr* 1994;83(11):1218. doi: 10.1111/j.1651-2227.1994.tb18288.x

56. Mueller EW, Boucher BA. Fosphenytoin: current place in therapy. *J Pediatr Pharmacol Ther* 2004;9(4):265. doi: 10.5863/1551-6776-9.4.265

57. Boylan GB, Rennie JM, Chorley G, et al. Second-line anticonvulsant treatment of neonatal seizures: a video-EEG monitoring study. *Neurology* 2004;62(3):486. doi: 10.1212/01.wnl.0000106944.59990.e6

58. Shany E, Benzaqen O, Watemberg N. Comparison of continuous drip of midazolam or lidocaine in the treatment of intractable neonatal seizures. *J Child Neurol* 2007;22(3):255. doi: 10.1177/0883073807299858

59. Lundqvist M, Ågren J, Hellström-Westas L, et al. Efficacy and safety of lidocaine for treatment of neonatal seizures. *Acta Paediatr* 2013;102(9):863. doi: 10.1111/apa.12311

60. Malingré MM, Van Rooij LGM, Rademaker CMA, et al. Development of an optimal lidocaine infusion strategy for neonatal seizures. *Eur J Pediatr* 2006;165(9):598. doi: 10.1007/s00431-006-0136-x

61. Weeke LC, Schalkwijk S, Toet MC, et al. Lidocaine-associated cardiac events in newborns with seizures: incidence, symptoms and contributing factors. *Neonatology* 2015;108(2):130. doi: 10.1159/000430767

62. van den Broek MPH, Huitema ADR, van Hasselt JGC, et al. Lidocaine (lignocaine) dosing regimen based upon a population pharmacokinetic model for preterm and term neonates with seizures. *Clin Pharmacokinet* 2011;50(7):461. doi: 10.2165/11589160-000000000-00000

63. van den Broek MPH, Rademaker CMA, van Straaten HLM, et al. Anticonvulsant treatment of asphyxiated newborns under hypothermia with lidocaine: efficacy, safety and dosing. *Arch Dis Child Fetal Neonatal Ed* 2013;98(4):F341. doi: 10.1136/archdischild-2012-302678

64. Tulloch JK, Carr RR, Ensom MHH. A systematic review of the pharmacokinetics of antiepileptic drugs in neonates with refractory seizures. *J Pediatr Pharmacol Ther* 2012;17(1):31. doi: 10.5863/1551-6776-17.1.31

65. van Leuven K, Groenendaal F, Toet MC, et al. Midazolam and amplitude-integrated EEG in asphyxiated full-term neonates. *Acta Paediatr* 2004;93(9):1221.

66. Sirsi D, Nangia S, LaMothe J, et al. Successful management of refractory neonatal seizures with midazolam. *J Child Neurol* 2008;23(6):706. doi: 10.1177/0883073807313041

67. Deshmukh A, Wittert W, Schnitzler E, et al. Lorazepam in the treatment of refractory neonatal seizures. A pilot study. *Am J Dis Child* 1986;140(10):1042. doi: 10.1001/archpedi.1986.02140240088032

68. Maytal J, Novak GP, King KC. Lorazepam in the treatment of refractory neonatal seizures. *J Child Neurol* 1991;6(4):319. doi: 10.1177/088307389100600406

69. Mruk AL, Garlitz KL, Leung NR. Levetiracetam in neonatal seizures: a review. *J Pediatr Pharmacol Ther* 2015;20(2):76. doi: 10.5863/1551-6776-20.2.76

70. Abend NS, Gutierrez-Colina AM, Monk HM, et al. Levetiracetam for treatment of neonatal seizures. *J Child Neurol* 2011;26(4):465. doi: 10.1177/0883073810384263

71. Khan O, Chang E, Cipriani C, et al. Use of intravenous levetiracetam for management of acute seizures in neonates. *Pediatr Neurol* 2011;44(4):265. doi: 10.1016/j.pediatrneurol.2010.11.005

72. Glass HC, Poulin C, Shevell MI. Topiramate for the treatment of neonatal seizures. *Pediatr Neurol* 2011;44(6):439. doi: 10.1016/j.pediatrneurol.2011.01.006

73. Riesgo R, Winckler MI, Ohlweiler L, et al. Treatment of refractory neonatal seizures with topiramate. *Neuropediatrics* 2012;43(6):353. doi: 10.1055/s-0032-1327771

74. Nuñez-Ramiro A, Benavente-Fernández I, Valverde E, et al. Topiramate plus cooling for hypoxic-ischemic encephalopathy: a randomized, controlled, multicenter, double-blinded trial. *Neonatology* 2019;116(1):76. doi: 10.1159/000499084

75. Silverstein FS, Ferriero DM. Off-label use of antiepileptic drugs for the treatment of neonatal seizures. *Pediatr Neurol* 2008;39(2):77. doi: 10.1016/j.pediatrneurol.2008.04.008

76. Courchia B, Kurtom W, Pensirikul A, et al. Topiramate for Seizures in preterm infants and the development of necrotizing enterocolitis. *Pediatrics* 2018;142(1):e20173971. doi: 10.1542/peds.2017-3971

77. Shellhaas RA, Chang T, Wusthoff CJ, et al. Treatment duration after acute symptomatic seizures in neonates: a multicenter cohort study. *J Pediatr* 2017;181:298. doi: 10.1016/j.jpeds.2016.10.039

78. Ronen GM, Buckley D, Penney S, et al. Long-term prognosis in children with neonatal seizures: a population-based study. *Neurology* 2007;69(19):1816. doi: 10.1212/01.wnl.0000279335.85797.2c

79. Pisani F, Spagnoli C. Neonatal seizures: a review of outcomes and outcome predictors. *Neuropediatrics* 2016;47(1):12. doi: 10.1055/s-0035-1567873

80. Glass HC, Hong KJ, Rogers EE, et al. Risk factors for epilepsy in children with neonatal encephalopathy. *Pediatr Res* 2011;70(5):535. doi: 10.1203/PDR.0b013e31822f24c7

81. Kharoshankaya L, Stevenson NJ, Livingstone V, et al. Seizure burden and neurodevelopmental outcome in neonates with hypoxic-ischemic encephalopathy. *Dev Med Child Neurol* 2016;58(12):1242. doi: 10.1111/dmcn.13215

82. Shah DK, Wusthoff CJ, Clarke P, et al. Electrographic seizures are associated with brain injury in newborns undergoing therapeutic hypothermia. *Arch Dis Child Fetal Neonatal Ed* 2014;99(3):F219. doi: 10.1136/archdischild-2013-305206

83. Garfinkle J, Shevell MI. Prognostic factors and development of a scoring system for outcome of neonatal seizures in term infants. *Eur J Paediatr Neurol* 2011;15(3):222. doi: 10.1016/j.ejpn.2010.11.002

84. Uria-Avellanal C, Marlow N, Rennie JM. Outcome following neonatal seizures. *Semin Fetal Neonatal Med* 2013;18(4):224. doi: 10.1016/j.siny.2013.01.002

52 Neuromuscular Disorders

Eugenio Mercuri and Marika Pane

The field of neuromuscular disorders has dramatically changed over the last two decades. The advent of next-generation sequencing (NGS) has simplified the diagnostic process by identifying an underlying genetic defect in most cases (1–4); over 200 loci responsible for neuromuscular disorders have been identified. This has resulted in new approaches to classification based on phenotype–genotype correlations, with a subsequent improvement in standards of care. Most importantly, a better understanding of the mechanisms underlying individual disorders or groups of disorders has, in some cases, led the development of specific therapeutic approaches with exciting translational research work, especially in the field of genetic therapy.

In this chapter, we will review the current state of knowledge of neuromuscular disorders with neonatal onset, including primary muscle disorders, such as muscular dystrophies and congenital myopathies, and motor neuron disorders; we provide clinical and pathologic details for each form. When available, we will also provide an update on care recommendations and review the most significant therapeutic advances for neonatal-onset neuromuscular diseases. The final part of the chapter will summarize suggestions to be considered in the differential diagnosis of neonates with hypotonia in whom a neuromuscular disorder is suspected.

WHEN TO SUSPECT A NEUROMUSCULAR DISEASES IN THE NEONATE

Hypotonia is the most typical and common symptom of neuromuscular disease in the newborn infant, but it can also be a sign of many nonneuromuscular disorders, and in some cases, the differential diagnosis can be quite difficult. A detailed clinical examination and a good clinical and obstetric history often provide a foundation to distinguish infants with peripheral involvement from those with central nervous system (CNS) involvement, and in some cases, clinical assessment provides important clues for a more specific diagnosis.

Weakness is one of the key signs to detect neuromuscular disorders (5,6). Weakness can be detected by looking for antigravity movements, as weak infants are unable or have severe difficulties in performing antigravity movements, even in response to stimulation. Other clinical signs highly suggestive of neuromuscular disorders include contractures that can be generalized or in a pattern (arthrogryposis), feeding difficulties, reduced fetal movements, and polyhydramnios, which suggest weakness with onset *in utero* (6).

Weakness in the respiratory musculature is an important sign because some neuromuscular disorders, such as some of the congenital muscular dystrophies (CMDs) or congenital myopathies, may show diaphragmatic weakness with paradoxical movement of the abdominal muscles, while others, like spinal muscular atrophy (SMA), show intercostal weakness with an abdominal breathing pattern. More details on clinical signs will be provided when discussing the individual neuromuscular forms, and the reader is also referred to Chapter 17 "Physical Assessment and Classification."

The chances of detecting a neuromuscular disorder further increase if serum creatine kinase (CK) level is increased, although a normal CK level does not exclude the possibility of a neuromuscular disorder, as the enzyme levels are normal or only mildly elevated in congenital myopathies and spinal muscular atrophies, for example. Muscle biopsy has been, until recently, the next step in investigation. The advent of NGS technologies, however, now offers the possibility to achieve a genetic diagnosis, although the technique identifies many DNA variations with unpredictable meaning. In this situation, muscle biopsy is often still required.

MUSCULAR DYSTROPHIES

Muscular dystrophies share a severe disruption of the muscle cells, with a typical "dystrophic pattern" on muscle biopsy. CMDs and congenital myotonic dystrophy are the most common forms of dystrophies with neonatal onset, while other dystrophies, such as Duchenne, Becker, or limb–girdle muscular dystrophies, that are overall more frequent in the pediatric population, are with very rare exceptions, generally not clinically symptomatic in the first year.

Congenital Muscular Dystrophies

Although by definition all the genetically inherited disorders should be considered as congenital, in clinical practice, the term "congenital" is generally applied to the forms with overt clinical signs in the neonatal period or during the first months after birth. The CMD include a heterogeneous group of disorders sharing some features, namely dystrophic changes on muscle biopsy; weakness, usually from birth, or within 6 months; and often contractures (7–9).

A recent nationwide population study reported that, in Italy, the prevalence of CMD is of 0.563 per 100,000 (10). Over the years, the classification of CMD has become increasingly complicated due to the ever-growing number of genes and proteins identified. Mutations in more than 20 genes have been reported (11,12). In the last few years, CMDs have been classified according to combined clinical, genetic, and pathologic approaches (7). Table 52.1 provides a complete list of the CMD types, including protein and gene defects.

As a group, the CMDs share some clinical signs. Generalized weakness, hypotonia, and contractures are usually present at birth. Facial weakness is frequently present but generally is not as striking as in congenital myotonic dystrophy. Respiratory and swallowing involvement is also frequent at birth. In dystroglycanopathies, clinical signs of CNS involvement may predominate. From a practical point of view, for the clinician, it is useful to separate forms with CNS involvement from those in which CNS involvement is absent or rare.

A comprehensive review of all the CMD forms is beyond the scope of this chapter; here, we describe the forms associated with alpha-dystroglycan (α-DG) deficiency and brain involvement and those with merosin deficiency, which often present in the neonatal period.

Forms of Congenital Muscular Dystrophy with Structural Brain Changes and Eye Involvement

The major recent contribution to our understanding of new forms of CMD comes from the identification of a family of genes involved in the glycosylation of α-DG. Under the term of "dystroglycanopathies," we include a clinically and genetically heterogeneous group of muscle disorders, which have hypoglycosylated α-DG on muscle biopsy (7,12,13).

Some clinical features, such as predominant involvement of the upper limbs compared to lower limbs and markedly elevated CK, are common. Brain and eye involvement are also frequent but are not invariably found in all forms. While the early studies mainly focused on distinct known phenotypes, namely muscle–eye–brain disease (MEB), Walker-Warburg syndrome (WWS), and Fukuyama muscular dystrophy (FCMD), it has become increasingly obvious

TABLE 52.1

Types of Congenital Muscular Dystrophy by Biochemical Defect, Protein, Gene, Chromosome Location, and Phenotype

Biochemical Defect	Protein	Gene	Chromosome Location	CMD Disease Phenotype(s)
Extracellular matrix proteins	Laminin α2 chain of merosin	LAMA2	6q22-23	Primary merosin deficiency
	Collagen type VI, subunit alpha 1/2/3	COL6A1	21q22.3	Ullrich CMD
		COL6A2	2q37	
		COL6A3		
External sarcolemmal proteins	Integrin a7	ITGA7	12q13	Integrin a7-related CMD
	Integrin a9	ITGA9	3p23-21	Integrin a9-related CMD
Dystroglycan and glycosyltransferase enzymes	Protein-1-O-mannosyl-transferase 1	POMT1	9q34.1	Walker-Warburg syndrome, MEB, CMD with cerebellar involvement, CMD with mental retardation and microcephaly, CMD with no mental retardation
	Protein-O-mannosyltransferase 2	POMT2	14q24.3	Walker-Warburg syndrome, MEB, CMD with cerebellar involvement, CMD with mental retardation and microcephaly
	Protein-O-linked mannose beta1,2-N-aminyltransferase 1	POMGnT1	1q32-34	Walker-Warburg syndrome, MEB, CMD with cerebellar involvement
	Fukutin-related protein	FKRP	19q13.3	Walker-Warburg syndrome, MEB, CMD with cerebellar involvement, CMD with mental retardation and microcephaly, CMD with no mental retardation
	Fukutin	FCMD	9q31	Fukuyama CMD, CMD with mental retardation, CMD with no mental retardation
	Like-glycosyltransferase	LARGE	22q12.3-13.1	Walker-Warburg syndrome, MEB, white matter changes
	Dolichyl-phosphate mannosyltransferase polypeptide 2/3	DPM2/DPM3	1q12-q21	CMD with mental retardation and severe epilepsy
	Isoprenoid synthase domain	ISPD	7p21.2	WWS
	O-mannose β-1,4-N-acetylglucosaminyltransferase	GTDC2	3p22.1	WWS
	Beta-1,3-N-acetylgalactosaminyltransferase 2	B3GALNT2	11q13.2	WWS, MEB
	GDP-mannose pyrophosphorylase	GMPPB		CMD with mental retardation and severe epilepsy
	Beta-dystroglycan	DAG1	3p21	Primary dystroglycanopathy
	Protein O-mannose kinase	SGK196	8p11.21	MEB
		—	1q42	MDC1B
Endoplasmic reticulum protein	Selenoprotein N1	SEPN1	1p35-36	CMD with spinal rigidity (RSMD1)
Nuclear envelope proteins	Nesprin 1	SYNE1	6q25	CMD with adducted thumbs
	Lamin A	LMNA	1q21.2	Congenital laminopathy
Mitochondrial membrane protein	Choline kinase	CHKB	22q13	Mitochondrial CMD (CMDmt)

CMD, congenital muscular dystrophy; MEB, muscle–eye–brain disease; WWS, Walker-Warburg syndrome; MDC1B, muscular dystrophy, congenital, 1B; RSMD1, rigid spine with muscular dystrophy type 1.

that the spectrum of CNS involvement is much more complex (7,12). New OMIM entries have been created subdividing this group into three broad phenotypic subgroups.

Type A includes the phenotypes with cortical involvement and the most severe phenotypes: WWS, WWS-like, MEB, and FCMD-like.

WWS is the most severe phenotype, with severe neonatal-onset weakness, hypotonia, CNS involvement, and ocular abnormalities ranging from severe myopia to retinal dysgenesis, microphthalmia, or anterior chamber malformations (14). Type II lissencephaly with the typical polymicrogyric cobblestone cortex, severe and diffuse white matter abnormalities, and cerebellar and brainstem hypoplasia or dysplasia are typical features of WWS (14).

MEB also presents with severe neonatal-onset weakness and hypotonia, CNS involvement, and ocular abnormalities, but brain involvement is less severe (15). Brain MRI shows extensive abnor-

malities of neuronal migration, such as pachygyria and polymicrogyria and often brainstem and cerebellar hypoplasia and periventricular white matter changes (16).

Type B includes cases of CMD with posterior fossa abnormalities or normal MRI, and patients may or may not have intellectual disability. Cerebellar dysplasia/hypoplasia is frequent; there are a number of cases with neonatal onset of weakness and hypotonia, and cerebellar cysts (17) and/or hypoplasia (16,18,19) who also develop cognitive impairment.

There is also a type C including the limb–girdle muscular dystrophy (LGMD) forms, but these will not be discussed in this chapter as they have onset well beyond the neonatal period.

As a rule of thumb, whenever there are structural brain abnormalities, especially if associated with eye abnormalities and clinical signs of weakness, it is useful to measure CK levels because so far, with very few exceptions, all reported cases have increased CK levels (>5 times the normal levels). The diagnostic process originally included a muscle biopsy and the search for mutations in the different genes. This was not straightforward as there are many genes currently associated with these forms of CMD. Mutations in individual genes have been associated with different phenotypes, and conversely, the same phenotype has been reported in association with many, if not all, known genes (15,20). This suggests that the identity of the defective gene cannot be predicted from the clinical phenotype. The new NGS techniques have now simplified this diagnostic process (21) because they can identify possible mutations in the known genes.

Merosin-Negative Congenital Muscular Dystrophy

This form classified as merosin-deficient congenital muscular dystrophy type 1A (MDC1A) is an autosomal recessive form due to mutations in the *LAMA2* gene on chromosome 6, encoding merosin (laminin α2), an extracellular matrix protein (22).

Children with merosin deficiency are usually symptomatic at birth, or in the first few weeks of life, with hypotonia, muscle weakness, weak cry, and, in 10% to 30% of cases, contractures (23). Weakness often affects upper limbs more than lower limbs. CK levels in these children are always grossly elevated. In the past, muscle biopsy was invariably performed and showed a classical dystrophic picture with reduction or absence of laminin α2 chain (merosin) on immunofluorescence. The diagnosis of merosin-deficient CMD is now more often genetically confirmed by studying the laminin α2 chain (*LAMA2*) gene, mapped to chromosome 6q22-23 either in isolation or as part of an NGS panel (24).

Affected children show severe motor delay and never acquire independent ambulation (9,23).

Brain MRI shows diffuse white matter changes on MRI, which are a typical feature of merosin-deficient CMD (25). These changes only become evident around 6 months and are not obvious on conventional imaging performed in the first months of life (26). Other patterns of brain lesions, such as cerebellar hypoplasia and/or cortical dysplasia, can be observed in a small proportion of these patients (25).

Congenital Myotonic Dystrophy

Congenital myotonic dystrophy is the congenital form of myotonic dystrophy type 1 (DM1) (27), a genetic disease caused by expansion of a CTG trinucleotide repeat in the noncoding region of the dystrophia myotonica gene (DM1 protein kinase, *DMPK*) (28). Its incidence is approximately 2.1/100,000 (1/47,619) live births (29).

The neonatal form of myotonic muscular dystrophy differs from the adult form both clinically and pathologically. Infants with congenital myotonic dystrophy are often born following a pregnancy complicated by polyhydramnios and reduced fetal movements. At birth, clinical signs include weakness, hypotonia, and often severe contractures affecting feet (bilateral equinovarus talipes deformity), knees, and hips, which may be dislocated. Marked difficulty in sucking and swallowing are often present in association with striking facial weakness, with a triangular-shaped open mouth.

There is also often respiratory muscle weakness, and ventilation is often required at least in the first weeks of life. Severe neonatal feeding difficulties are present, and nasogastric/jejunal tube feeding may be required for several months even in infants who breathe spontaneously.

Both respiratory and feeding difficulties may improve over the first months of life, and gastrostomy feeding is rarely needed. The duration and severity of respiratory involvement is one of the most important determinants of the long-term survival of these infants. During the first year of life, there is a 30% mortality for those infants ventilated for more than 3 months (29,30). It is important to remember that many of the signs invariably present or frequently found in the adult form, such as clinically evident myotonia or cardiologic and ocular abnormalities, are not always present in the neonatal period.

Congenital myotonic dystrophy is one of the most frequent causes of neonatal-onset muscle disorders. Therefore, in an infant with clinical signs that are consistent with this diagnosis, signs of the disease should be investigated in the mother, who is often affected. A detailed pedigree and the examination of the mother are generally strongly indicative of the diagnosis because although myotonic dystrophy is an autosomal dominant trait, the mother is the transmitting parent in most cases. Facial weakness, percussion myotonia of the tongue, and myotonic discharge on the EMG can generally be found in the mothers. Clinical myotonia of the hands or eye opening is often present and will further support the diagnosis, which should be confirmed by molecular genetic testing.

Other Forms of Muscular Dystrophies

In the most common forms of muscular dystrophies occurring in pediatric population, such as Duchenne or limb–girdle muscular dystrophies, the onset of clinical signs is generally well beyond the first year of age. However, Ullrich CMD and CMD related to mutations in the lamin A/C (*LMNA*) gene can present in the neonatal period.

Ullrich CMD is due to deficiency of collagen type VI (31) and is characterized by marked distal laxity, contractures of the proximal joints, skin changes, and normal intelligence (32,33). The onset is generally in the first years, but patients at the severe end of the clinical spectrum may have a neonatal onset with weakness, contractures, and hypotonia, often associated with torticollis and hip dysplasia (33). Serum CK is often normal or only mildly elevated (34). Marked deficiency or absence of collagen VI on skin or muscle fibers is a clear marker of Ullrich CMD (35). The diagnosis should be confirmed by genetic analysis looking for mutations in the collagen VI genes: *COL6A1* and *COL6A2* on chromosome 21q22 or *COL6A3* on chromosome 2q37 (33,36).

A dominantly inherited form of CMD due to mutations in the *LMNA* gene can have a very early presentation with reduced fetal movements, severe hypotonia, and weakness at birth with marked involvement of the neck muscles (37,38).

CONGENITAL MYOPATHIES

The term congenital myopathies includes a group of genetically inherited primary myopathies characterized by "nondystrophic" changes on muscle biopsies (for a review, see Sewry et al. (39)). Unlike muscular dystrophies, congenital myopathies generally have better preservation of muscle fiber architecture and less severe changes such as fiber-type disproportion. The point prevalence is approximately 1:26,000, with core myopathies the most common histopathologic subtype and ryanodine receptor 1 (*RYR1*)-related myopathies the most prevalent genetic subtype (40).

Clinically, they tend to be relatively nonprogressive, although respiratory muscle weakness may affect prognosis. Although congenital myopathies are reported to have a relatively benign, nonprogressive course, this is not always the case in the neonatal-onset forms.

This group of disorders is clinically, biochemically, and genetically very heterogeneous. Until recently, the classification of congenital myopathies was mainly based on histopathologic findings that separated forms with rods from those with cores (41). With the classical approach, the most frequent forms of congenital myopathies with neonatal onset are nemaline myopathy, CNMs, core myopathies (central core disease [CCD] and multiminicore myopathy), and congenital fiber–type disproportion (42).

The advent of molecular genetics techniques with NGS has enabled better definition of the spectrum of these disorders. It has become increasingly apparent that there is great heterogeneity even within specific morphologic subtypes, and as for CMDs, the boundaries between conditions are often indistinct. Mutations in the same gene can give rise to diverse clinical and histopathologic phenotypes, and conversely, the same phenotype can arise from mutations in a variety of genes (21,39). For example, the same clinical and pathologic phenotype, such as nemaline myopathy, can be associated with different genes, and an individual gene can be associated with multiple phenotypes, such as CCD or nemaline myopathy. Because of this heterogeneity and overlap, the clinical and pathologic diagnosis should be confirmed by genetic testing.

From a clinical point of view, there are features that raise suspicion of a diagnosis of congenital myopathy. In the forms with neonatal onset, clinical signs consist of floppiness associated with contractures and weakness and often also affecting the facial muscles. In nemaline myopathy, minicore disease, and myotubular myopathy, there is a tendency to develop progressive respiratory failure, probably related to diaphragmatic involvement. Unlike in muscular dystrophies, the serum CK levels are frequently normal or only mildly elevated. Muscle biopsy is often performed to obtain information on the possible structural changes, but there is an increasing number of etiologies that can be confirmed by genetic analysis (NGS) without performing biopsy. Table 52.2 shows a summary of the conditions that have been recognized to date. The names generally reflect the underlying structural change.

TABLE 52.2
Congenital Myopathies, Inheritance Pattern, and Genetic Basis

Myopathy Subtype	Inheritance Pattern	Gene	Chromosome Location
Nemaline myopathy	AD, AR	ACTA1	1q42.1
	AR	CFL2	14q13.1
	AD	KBTBD13	15q22.31
	AR	KLHL40	3p33.1
	AR	KLHL41	2q31.1
	AR	NEB	2q23.3
	AR	RYR1	19q13.2
	AR	TNNT1	19q13.42
	AD	TPM2	9p13.3
	AD, AR	TPM3	1q21.3
Central core/ multiminicore disease	AR	RYR1	19q13.2
	AR	SEPN1	1p36.11
	AD	MYH7	14q11.2
Centronuclear myopathy	AR	BIN1	2q14.3
	AD	CCDC78	16p13.3
	AD	DNM2	19p13.2
	XL	MTM1	Xq28
	AD	MYF6	12q21.31
	AR	RYR1	19q13.2
	AR	TTN	2q31.2
	AR	SPEG	2q35
	AR	NEB	2q23.3
	AD, AR	RYR1	19q13.2
	AD	TPM2	9p13.3
Congenital fiber–type disproportion	AD	ACTA1	1q42.1
	AD	MYH7	14q11.2
	AR	RYR1	19q13.2
	AR	SEPN1	1p36.11
	AD	TPM2	9p13.3
	AD	TPM3	1q21.3

ACTA1, skeletal muscle α-actin; *CFL2*, Cofilin 2; *KBTBD13*, Kelch repeat and BTB domain-containing 13; *KLHL40*, Kelch-like family member 40; *NEB*, nebulin; *RYR1*, ryanodine receptor 1; *TNNT1*, troponin T; *TPM3*, tropomyosin 3; *SEPN1*, selenoprotein N; *MYH7*, myosin heavy chain 7; *BIN1*, bridging integrator 1; *CCDC78*, coiled-coil domain-containing 78; *DNM2*, Dynamin 2; *MTM1*, myotubularin 1; *MYF6*, myogenic factor 6; *TTN*, Titin; *SPEG*, striated muscle enriched protein kinase; *TPM2*, tropomyosin 2.

Nemaline Myopathy

This condition takes the name from the rods observed on muscle biopsy resembling thread-like structures (Greek: *nema*—thread). The classification of nemaline myopathy is based on age of onset and severity of motor and respiratory involvement. In the neonatal period, we identify severe congenital, intermediate congenital and typical congenital; childhood-onset; and adult-onset forms (43–45). There are two main modalities of presentation. In the "typical" congenital form, infants show hypotonia, general weakness predominantly affecting axial muscles and the face, which is typically elongated, with tented upper lip, and high-arched palate. There are bulbar and feeding difficulties, requiring frequent suctioning, tube feeding, and gastrostomy. In the severe form, there is also often a history of polyhydramnios, and at birth, infants present with arthrogryposis, severe weakness with complete immobility, respiratory failure, and severe feeding difficulties. The intermediate are cases in between the "classical" variant and this severe form.

The prognosis is highly variable. Although some infants will not survive the first weeks or months due to respiratory insufficiency, several patients, including some with severe floppiness and lack of spontaneous respiration at birth, will survive, and some will have little residual disability. Of note, the prognosis or degree of respiratory muscle involvement does not always reflect the severity of skeletal muscle weakness (43,45).

The serum CK level is normal or only slightly elevated. Mutations in nine different genes have been identified: α-tropomyosin slow (*TPM3*), nebulin (*NEB*), skeletal muscle α-actin (*ACTA1*), β-tropomyosin (*TPM2*), Kelch repeat and BTB domain-containing 13 (*KBTBD13*), Cofilin 2 (*CFL2*), Kelch-like family member 40 (*KLHL40*), Kelch-like family member 41 (KLHL41), and troponin T (TNNT1) (41,42). In the neonatal forms, *de novo* dominant mutations in the *ACTA1* gene account for a significant proportion of the severe form; mutations in *NEB* and *TPM3* have also been frequently reported.

Central Core Disease

Core myopathies are a heterogeneous group of disorders characterized by the presence of areas devoid of oxidative staining, which may appear as "central cores" or multiple smaller "minicores" (41,42,46,47). This group of disorders usually have onset in infancy or childhood, and only in some cases is there neonatal onset with severe neonatal weakness, arthrogryposis, and respiratory failure often requiring respiratory support (42,48,49).

Mutations in the ryanodine receptor 1 gene (*RYR1*) are the most frequent in this group and have often been found in the neonatal cases (42,48).

Centronuclear (Myotubular) Myopathy

The term CNMs derives from the numerous centrally placed (centronuclear) nuclei with a surrounding central zone devoid of oxidative enzyme activity seen on muscle biopsy. The disease has been also known as myotubular myopathy as the muscle fibers with central nuclei resemble myotubes seen during fetal muscle development.

There are three clinical and genetic subtypes but only the severe X-linked type presents in the neonatal period. The other two forms, a less severe infantile type and the mild juvenile or adult type, have later onset and a different modality of inheritance (42,50,51). The severe neonatal form is characterized by male infants presenting with polyhydramnios, reduced fetal movements, and after birth, marked hypotonia, a variable degree of external ophthalmoplegia, respiratory failure, dysphagia, and often undescended testes (42,50–52).

Until recently, the diagnosis was based on muscle biopsy, which shows typical centronuclear features, but now, as for the other congenital myopathies, diagnosis can be made directly by genetic

THE NEWBORN INFANT

testing (53) for mutations in the myotubularin gene (*MTM1*) (42), which is generally responsible for the X-linked form of the disease.

The disease was often considered to be fatal, with the exception of a few cases with a "mild" phenotype with only slightly delayed milestones and no need for ventilatory support beyond the newborn period (54,55). However, the advent of a gene replacement therapy AT132, using an AAV8 vector to deliver a functional copy of the *MTM1* gene, appears to be extremely promising for improving function and survival.

SPINAL MUSCULAR ATROPHY

The term "spinal muscular atrophy" includes a group of disorders characterized by a progressive degenerative disease of spinal and brainstem motoneurons (56). The most frequent forms of motor neuron involvement in infancy are related to mutations in the *SMN* gene on chromosome 5. This includes a wide range of clinical forms ranging from the severe neonatal forms to those that present in adulthood with mild signs. Classically, SMA has been subdivided into three main types (57), taking into account the age of onset and the maximum functional ability achieved:

Type 1. Severe. Unable to sit unsupported, with onset at birth or in the first months

Type 2. Intermediate. Able to sit unsupported. Unable to stand or walk unaided

Type 3. Mild. Able to stand and walk

In the severe spinal muscular atrophy, also called Werdnig-Hoffmann Disease or type 1 SMA, the onset is generally within the first 6 months. The clinical features in type 1 SMA are very typical and consist of a combination of hypotonia and severe weaknesses with almost complete absence of movements in both axial and limb muscles, but sparing the facial muscles. There is a typical posture with the arms held internally rotated in a "jug-handle" position by the side of the body and hands facing outward, which is associated with absent tendon reflexes, a bell-shaped chest, and a diaphragmatic breathing pattern. Classically, bulbar weakness with difficulty in sucking and swallowing and an associated accumulation of mucus in the pharynx are constant features and may occur at presentation or later during the first year. These are consistent features and are strongly suggestive of the diagnosis on initial assessment of the infant.

Recent natural history studies have shown that type 1 SMA is heterogeneous, and there have been attempts to identify clinical subgroups (58–61). Dubowitz proposed a decimal classification (62) identifying as type 1.5 the most common presentation described above in infants who at diagnosis have no feeding and swallowing or respiratory involvement. Some infants may have a milder phenotype, type 1.9, achieving some head control and having a less severe respiratory involvement (type 1.9) but still not achieving the ability to sit independently. At the other end of the spectrum are infants with early severe respiratory and bulbar difficulties and severe weakness from birth, with an overtly poor prognosis for survival (type 1.1). Contractures are generally not observed in type 1 SMA, and the very few cases with prenatal onset with reduced fetal movements, multiple contractures, severe respiratory failure at birth, and short survival time are labeled as SMA 0 (63).

With genetic testing now readily available and providing reliable results in approximately 95% of cases, the diagnosis is easily achieved by identifying deletions in the SMN gene (64).

The management of type 1 SMA has changed dramatically over the last decade because of improved care recommendations and the availability of new therapies. The median age of survival in infants with SMA 1 is reported to be around 9 months with only 8% surviving by 20 months (60). Recent standards of care recommendations highlight the importance of noninvasive ventilatory support, of feeding and nutritional management (64,65), also providing recommendations for other aspects related to acute care, physiotherapy and posturing, orthopedic involvement, and medications.

The most exciting results, however, come from recent clinical trials. Several therapeutic approaches have been used in the last few years that target restoration of production of full-length SMN protein that is missing in SMA as a result of the mutation in the *SMN1*. These include gene replacement therapy and molecular therapies acting at mRNA level.

A phase 1 clinical trial used gene replacement therapy to assess safety and efficacy of a single-dose intravenous administration of self-complementary adeno-associated viral vectors (scAAV)—SMN delivering the *SMN1* gene in type 1 SMA infants (66). The long-term results showed that all the treated patients are not only still alive well beyond 20 months of age but also had a rapid increase on the CHOP INTEND scale following gene delivery, with most patients achieving the ability to sit unsupported, which is classically never achieved in type 1 SMA. Preliminary results of two larger trials (STRIVE US and STRIVE EU) appear to confirm the results of the first study.

Other approaches aimed at restoring the production of full-length SMN protein use a different target than *SMN1* gene. In SMA patients, mutations in the *SMN1* gene are only partly compensated by the activity of a second neighboring centromeric gene, *SMN2*. *SMN2* gene is intact in all patients but contains a C-to-T variation in exon 7 that leads to production of only a very small part of full-length protein, while the majority of the protein produced is unstable and cannot substitute for mutant *SMN1*. Various therapeutic approaches have targeted the possibility of increasing exon 7 inclusion in the majority of *SMN2* at mRNA level and thereby increase the production of fully functional SMN protein (67,68).

Nusinersen, an antisense oligonucleotide, was the first drug to complete pivotal studies in both type 1 and late-onset SMA (69,70) with results leading to the worldwide approval and commercialization of the drug. In type 1 SMA, a large randomized double-blind sham-controlled clinical trial (ENDEAR) in type 1 infants under 7 months of age (69), there was a significant difference in survival and motor function between the two groups. Those receiving the sham procedure had no improvement in milestones on the Hammersmith Infant Neurological Examination (HINE), while over 50% of those treated with nusinersen had a motor-milestone response. Better results were observed in younger infants and in those with shorter disease duration. The results of the study have recently been confirmed by real-world data (71). The need for early initiation of treatment is further confirmed by the dramatic improvement observed in the results of the phase 2, open-label, single-arm NURTURE study using nusinersen in presymptomatic SMA patients (72). Most of these patients achieved motor milestones such as sitting or walking at the time these are achieved by their peers.

Small molecules, such as risdiplam, have also just completed phase 2/3 clinical trials with similarly encouraging results. All studies strongly indicate that the need for early diagnosis as the response to treatment was significantly better in those treated soon after onset of clinical signs and markedly better in those identified presymptomatically. This highlights the need to raise more awareness among neonatologists to promote early diagnosis and referral for type 1 infants and to promote neonatal screening that is increasingly available in many countries.

CONGENITAL AND NEONATAL MYASTHENIA

Transient Neonatal Myasthenia Gravis

Neonatal myasthenia gravis is a transient disorder that may occur in newborns born to myasthenic mothers. It is due to the transfer of acetylcholine receptor (ACHR) antibodies across the placenta (73).

Within a few days, but often within a few hours from birth, there are feeding difficulties and often inability to handle pharyngeal secretions, generalized weakness and poor respiratory effort. The severity of signs of neonatal myasthenia is not always related to the severity or duration of maternal disease (74). Ventilatory support and feeding by gavage may be needed during this period. In symptomatic infants, neostigmine (or pyridostigmine) should be given orally or by nasogastric tube until the infant is no longer symptomatic. Recovery is anticipated by 2 to 4 months in most infants.

Congenital Myasthenic Syndromes

Congenital myasthenic syndromes (CMS) are a heterogeneous group of inherited disorders characterized by neuromuscular transmission dysfunction. They are not related to maternal myasthenia but have a very heterogeneous genetic background caused by multiple mechanisms (75–79). Over 30 CSM disease genes have been identified in the last few years (76,78–80).

In the neonatal period, CMS presents with signs of fatigable weakness affecting especially the ocular and other cranial muscles, sometimes occurring with swallowing difficulties and apnea. These features raise suspicion of CMS, especially in the presence of a positive family history.

While a positive family history can help to target specific genes, when this is not present, NGS or other genetic techniques should be used to identify the specific gene defect. Diagnostic accuracy is important because there are specific therapeutic approaches for some forms of CMS (76,79,80).

CONCLUSIONS

Recent advances in diagnostic and therapeutic strategies for neuromuscular disorders should be considered by clinicians faced with managing the "floppy infant." This is particularly true for disorders for which therapeutic options are available, such as myasthenia and, more recently, SMA and myotubular myopathy. It is also important for the other forms of neuromuscular disease that present in the neonatal period, because early and accurate diagnosis enhances genetic counseling and may help the clinician to provide high-quality prognostic information to families about likely progress of their child's disease.

REFERENCES

1. Savarese M, Di Fruscio G, Tasca G, et al. Next generation sequencing on patients with LGMD and nonspecific myopathies: findings associated with ANO5 mutations. *Neuromuscul Disord* 2015;25(7):533.
2. Savarese M, Di Fruscio G, Torella A, et al. The genetic basis of undiagnosed muscular dystrophies and myopathies: results from 504 patients. *Neurology* 2016;87(1):71.
3. Cummings BB, Marshall JL, Tukiainen T, et al. Improving genetic diagnosis in Mendelian disease with transcriptome sequencing. *Sci Transl Med* 2017;9(386):eaal5209.
4. Ghaoui R, Cooper ST, Lek M, et al. Use of whole-exome sequencing for diagnosis of limb-girdle muscular dystrophy: outcomes and lessons learned. *JAMA Neurol* 2015;72(12):1424.
5. Dubowitz V. The floppy infant—a practical approach to classification. *Dev Med Child Neurol* 1968;10(6):706.
6. Vasta I, Kinali M, Messina S, et al. Can clinical signs identify newborns with neuromuscular disorders? *J Pediatr* 2005;146(1):73.
7. Mercuri E, Muntoni F. The ever-expanding spectrum of congenital muscular dystrophies. *Ann Neurol* 2012;72(1):9.
8. Dubowitz V. 22nd ENMC sponsored workshop on congenital muscular dystrophy held in Baarn, The Netherlands, 14–16 May 1993. *Neuromuscul Disord* 1994;4(1):75.
9. Philpot J, Sewry C, Pennock J, et al. Clinical phenotype in congenital muscular dystrophy: correlation with expression of merosin in skeletal muscle. *Neuromuscul Disord* 1995;5(4):301.
10. Graziano A, Bianco F, D'Amico A, et al. Prevalence of congenital muscular dystrophy in Italy: a population study. *Neurology* 2015;84(9):904.
11. Sframeli M, Sarkozy A, Bertoli M, et al. Congenital muscular dystrophies in the UK population: clinical and molecular spectrum of a large cohort diagnosed over a 12-year period. *Neuromuscul Disord* 2017;27(9):793.
12. Bonnemann CG, Wang CH, Quijano-Roy S, et al. Diagnostic approach to the congenital muscular dystrophies. *Neuromuscul Disord* 2014;24(4):289.
13. Godfrey C, Foley AR, Clement E, et al. Dystroglycanopathies: coming into focus. *Curr Opin Genet Dev* 2011;21(3):278.
14. Dobyns WB, Pagon RA, Armstrong D, et al. Diagnostic criteria for Walker-Warburg syndrome. *Am J Med Genet* 1989;32(2):195.
15. Godfrey C, Clement E, Mein R, et al. Refining genotype phenotype correlations in muscular dystrophies with defective glycosylation of dystroglycan. *Brain* 2007;130(Pt 10):2725.
16. Clement E, Mercuri E, Godfrey C, et al. Brain involvement in muscular dystrophies with defective dystroglycan glycosylation. *Ann Neurol* 2008;64(5):573.
17. Topaloglu H, Brockington M, Yuva Y, et al. FKRP gene mutations cause congenital muscular dystrophy, mental retardation, and cerebellar cysts. *Neurology* 2003;60(6):988.
18. Godfrey C, Escolar D, Brockington M, et al. Fukutin gene mutations in steroid-responsive limb girdle muscular dystrophy. *Ann Neurol* 2006;60(5):603.
19. Mercuri E, Brockington M, Straub V, et al. Phenotypic spectrum associated with mutations in the fukutin-related protein gene. *Ann Neurol* 2003;53(4):537.
20. Mercuri E, Messina S, Bruno C, et al. Congenital muscular dystrophies with defective glycosylation of dystroglycan: a population study. *Neurology* 2009;72(21):1802.
21. O'Grady GL, Lek M, Lamande SR, et al. Diagnosis and etiology of congenital muscular dystrophy: we are halfway there. *Ann Neurol* 2016;80(1):101.
22. Tome FM, Evangelista T, Leclere A, et al. Congenital muscular dystrophy with merosin deficiency. *C R Acad Sci III* 1994;317(4):351.
23. Geranmayeh F, Clement E, Feng LH, et al. Genotype-phenotype correlation in a large population of muscular dystrophy patients with LAMA2 mutations. *Neuromuscul Disord* 2010;20(4):241.
24. Hillaire D, Leclere A, Faure S, et al. Localization of merosin-negative congenital muscular dystrophy to chromosome 6q2 by homozygosity mapping. *Hum Mol Genet* 1994;3(9):1657.
25. Philpot J, Cowan F, Pennock J, et al. Merosin-deficient congenital muscular dystrophy: the spectrum of brain involvement on magnetic resonance imaging. *Neuromuscul Disord* 1999;9(2):81.
26. Mercuri E, Pennock J, Goodwin F, et al. Sequential study of central and peripheral nervous system involvement in an infant with merosin-deficient congenital muscular dystrophy. *Neuromuscul Disord* 1996;6(6):425.
27. Vanier TM. Dystrophia myotonica in childhood. *Br Med J* 1960;2(5208):1284.
28. Buxton J, Shelbourne P, Davies J, et al. Detection of an unstable fragment of DNA specific to individuals with myotonic dystrophy. *Nature* 1992;355(6360):547.
29. Campbell C, Levin S, Siu VM, et al. Congenital myotonic dystrophy: Canadian population-based surveillance study. *J Pediatr* 2013;163(1):120.e1-3.
30. Johnson NE, Butterfield R, Berggren K, et al. Disease burden and functional outcomes in congenital myotonic dystrophy: a cross-sectional study. *Neurology* 2016;87(2):160.
31. Camacho Vanegas O, Bertini E, Zhang RZ, et al. Ullrich scleroatonic muscular dystrophy is caused by recessive mutations in collagen type VI. *Proc Natl Acad Sci U S A* 2001;98(13):7516.
32. Mercuri E, Yuva Y, Brown SC, et al. Collagen VI involvement in Ullrich syndrome: a clinical, genetic, and immunohistochemical study. *Neurology* 2002;58(9):1354.
33. Nadeau A, Kinali M, Main M, et al. Natural history of Ullrich congenital muscular dystrophy. *Neurology* 2009;73(1):25.
34. Foley AR, Quijano-Roy S, Collins J, et al. Natural history of pulmonary function in collagen VI-related myopathies. *Brain* 2013;136(Pt 12):3625.
35. Sabatelli P, Gara SK, Grumati P, et al. Expression of the collagen VI alpha5 and alpha6 chains in normal human skin and in skin of patients with collagen VI-related myopathies. *J Invest Dermatol* 2011;131(1):99.
36. Yonekawa T, Nishino I. Ullrich congenital muscular dystrophy: clinicopathological features, natural history and pathomechanism(s). *J Neurol Neurosurg Psychiatry* 2015;86(3):280.
37. Mercuri E, Poppe M, Quinlivan R, et al. Extreme variability of phenotype in patients with an identical missense mutation in the lamin A/C gene: from congenital onset with severe phenotype to milder classic Emery-Dreifuss variant. *Arch Neurol* 2004;61(5):690.
38. Quijano-Roy S, Mbieleu B, Bonnemann CG, et al. De novo LMNA mutations cause a new form of congenital muscular dystrophy. *Ann Neurol* 2008;64(2):177.
39. Sewry CA, Jimenez-Mallebrera C, Muntoni F. Congenital myopathies. *Curr Opin Neurol* 2008;21(5):569.
40. Amburgey K, McNamara N, Bennett LR, et al. Prevalence of congenital myopathies in a representative pediatric United States population. *Ann Neurol* 2011;70(4):662.
41. North KN, Wang CH, Clarke N, et al. Approach to the diagnosis of congenital myopathies. *Neuromuscul Disord* 2014;24(2):97.
42. Maggi L, Scoto M, Cirak S, et al. Congenital myopathies—clinical features and frequency of individual subtypes diagnosed over a 5-year period in the United Kingdom. *Neuromuscul Disord* 2013;23(3):195.

43. Wallgren-Pettersson C, Laing NG. 138th ENMC Workshop: nemaline myopathy, 20–22 May 2005, Naarden, The Netherlands. *Neuromuscul Disord* 2006;16(1):54.

44. North KN, Laing NG, Wallgren-Pettersson C. Nemaline myopathy: current concepts. The ENMC International Consortium and Nemaline Myopathy. *J Med Genet* 1997;34(9):705.

45. Laing NG, Wallgren-Pettersson C. 161st ENMC International Workshop on nemaline myopathy and related disorders, Newcastle upon Tyne, 2008. *Neuromuscul Disord* 2009;19(4):300.

46. Ferreiro A, Monnier N, Romero NB, et al. A recessive form of central core disease, transiently presenting as multi-minicore disease, is associated with a homozygous mutation in the ryanodine receptor type 1 gene. *Ann Neurol* 2002;51(6):750.

47. Ferreiro A, Quijano-Roy S, Pichereau C, et al. Mutations of the selenoprotein N gene, which is implicated in rigid spine muscular dystrophy, cause the classical phenotype of multiminicore disease: reassessing the nosology of early-onset myopathies. *Am J Hum Genet* 2002;71(4):739.

48. Jungbluth H. Central core disease. *Orphanet J Rare Dis* 2007;2:25.

49. Klein A, Lillis S, Munteanu I, et al. Clinical and genetic findings in a large cohort of patients with ryanodine receptor 1 gene-associated myopathies. *Hum Mutat* 2012;33(6):981.

50. Jungbluth H, Wallgren-Pettersson C, Laporte J. Centronuclear (myotubular) myopathy. *Orphanet J Rare Dis* 2008;3:26.

51. Romero NB, Bitoun M. Centronuclear myopathies. *Semin Pediatr Neurol* 2011;18(4):250.

52. Heckmatt JZ, Sewry CA, Hodes D, et al. Congenital centronuclear (myotubular) myopathy. A clinical, pathological and genetic study in eight children. *Brain* 1985;108(Pt 4):941.

53. North KN. Clinical approach to the diagnosis of congenital myopathies. *Semin Pediatr Neurol* 2011;18(4):216.

54. Barth PG, Dubowitz V. X-linked myotubular myopathy—a long-term follow-up study. *Eur J Paediatr Neurol* 1998;2(1):49.

55. Pierson CR, Agrawal PB, Blasko J, et al. Myofiber size correlates with MTM1 mutation type and outcome in X-linked myotubular myopathy. *Neuromuscul Disord* 2007;17(7):562.

56. D'Amico A, Mercuri E, Tiziano FD, et al. Spinal muscular atrophy. *Orphanet J Rare Dis* 2011;6:71.

57. Mercuri E, Bertini E, Iannaccone ST. Childhood spinal muscular atrophy: controversies and challenges. *Lancet Neurol* 2012;11(5):443.

58. De Sanctis R, Coratti G, Pasternak A, et al. Developmental milestones in type I spinal muscular atrophy. *Neuromuscul Disord* 2016;26(11):754.

59. De Sanctis R, Pane M, Coratti G, et al. Clinical phenotypes and trajectories of disease progression in type 1 spinal muscular atrophy. *Neuromuscul Disord* 2018;28(1):24.

60. Finkel RS, McDermott MP, Kaufmann P, et al. Observational study of spinal muscular atrophy type I and implications for clinical trials. *Neurology* 2014;83(9):810.

61. Kolb SJ, Coffey CS, Yankey JW, et al. Baseline results of the NeuroNEXT spinal muscular atrophy infant biomarker study. *Ann Clin Transl Neurol* 2016;3(2):132.

62. Dubowitz V. Chaos in the classification of SMA: a possible resolution. *Neuromuscul Disord* 1995;5(1):3.

63. MacLeod MJ, Taylor JE, Lunt PW, et al. Prenatal onset spinal muscular atrophy. *Eur J Paediatr Neurol* 1999;3(2):65.

64. Mercuri E, Finkel RS, Muntoni F, et al. Diagnosis and management of spinal muscular atrophy: part 1: recommendations for diagnosis, rehabilitation, orthopedic and nutritional care. *Neuromuscul Disord* 2018;28(2):103.

65. Finkel RS, Mercuri E, Meyer OH, et al. Diagnosis and management of spinal muscular atrophy: part 2: pulmonary and acute care; medications, supplements and immunizations; other organ systems; and ethics. *Neuromuscul Disord* 2018;28(3):197.

66. Mendell JR, Al-Zaidy S, Shell R, et al. Single-dose gene-replacement therapy for spinal muscular atrophy. *N Engl J Med* 2017;377(18):1713.

67. Hua Y, Sahashi K, Rigo F, et al. Peripheral SMN restoration is essential for long-term rescue of a severe spinal muscular atrophy mouse model. *Nature* 2011;478(7367):123.

68. Porensky PN, Mitrpant C, McGovern VL, et al. A single administration of morpholino antisense oligomer rescues spinal muscular atrophy in mouse. *Hum Mol Genet* 2012;21(7):1625.

69. Finkel RS, Mercuri E, Darras BT, et al. Nusinersen versus Sham control in infantile-onset spinal muscular atrophy. *N Engl J Med* 2017;377(18):1723.

70. Mercuri E, Darras BT, Chiriboga CA, et al. Nusinersen versus Sham control in later-onset spinal muscular atrophy. *N Engl J Med* 2018;378(7):625.

71. Pane M, Coratti G, Sansone VA, et al. Nusinersen in type 1 spinal muscular atrophy: twelve-month real-world data. *Ann Neurol* 2019;86(3):443.

72. De Vivo DC, Bertini E, Swoboda KJ, et al. Nusinersen initiated in infants during the presymptomatic stage of spinal muscular atrophy: interim efficacy and safety results from the Phase 2 NURTURE study. *Neuromuscul Disord* 2019;29(11):842.

73. Djelmis J, Sostarko M, Mayer D, et al. Myasthenia gravis in pregnancy: report on 69 cases. *Eur J Obstet Gynecol Reprod Biol* 2002;104(1):21.

74. D'Amico A, Bertini E, Bianco F, et al. Fetal acetylcholine receptor inactivation syndrome and maternal myasthenia gravis: a case report. *Neuromuscul Disord* 2012;22(6):546.

75. McMacken G, Whittaker RG, Evangelista T, et al. Congenital myasthenic syndrome with episodic apnoea: clinical, neurophysiological and genetic features in the long-term follow-up of 19 patients. *J Neurol* 2018;265(1):194.

76. Nicole S, Azuma Y, Bauche S, et al. Congenital myasthenic syndromes or inherited disorders of neuromuscular transmission: recent discoveries and open questions. *J Neuromuscul Dis* 2017;4(4):269.

77. Natera-de Benito D, Topf A, Vilchez JJ, et al. Molecular characterization of congenital myasthenic syndromes in Spain. *Neuromuscul Disord* 2017;27(12):1087.

78. McMacken G, Abicht A, Evangelista T, et al. The increasing genetic and phenotypical diversity of congenital myasthenic syndromes. *Neuropediatrics* 2017;48(4):294.

79. Souza PV, Batistella GN, Lino VC, et al. Clinical and genetic basis of congenital myasthenic syndromes. *Arq Neuropsiquiatr* 2016;74(9):750.

80. Beeson D. Congenital myasthenic syndromes: recent advances. *Curr Opin Neurol* 2016;29(5):565.

53 Neurosurgery

Kristian Aquilina

Treatment of structural and functional abnormalities of the neonatal central nervous system (CNS) provides unique challenges to both the neurosurgeon and neonatologist caring for the infant. Considerations of several interrelated pathophysiologic processes can provide an understanding of the nature of the abnormality and goal of treatment. This understanding forms the basis for a successful interdisciplinary team approach to the management of these infants.

THE PATHOPHYSIOLOGY OF NEONATAL NEUROSURGERY

Almost all neurosurgical interventions in the neonate can be discussed in terms of four categories of technical intervention: (a) drainage or diversion of fluids, (b) closure of openings (including neural tube defects), (c) removal of tissue (including neoplasms and anomalous masses), and (d) opening of fusions (such as craniosynostoses). In the management of many newborn patients, two or more of these interventions may be necessary. Some neonatal nervous system problems, such as some vascular disorders, do not yet have a workable neurosurgical intervention. Parallel developments in interventional radiology have, however, mitigated this problem to a large extent.

When applying these interventions to neonatal care, their use must be guided by pathophysiologic mechanisms unique to the neonate, such as (a) the biomechanics of neonatal brain tissue and a distensible skull, (b) recognized and unrecognized congenital anomalies (microscopic and macroscopic), and (c) the plasticity of neonatal CNS tissue and its effects on response to injury. Recent advances in antenatal diagnosis allow unprecedented opportunity to manage these processes even before birth. Frequently, solutions to a neonatal neurosurgical problem must address combinations, or complex interactions, of these pathophysiologic mechanisms.

The biomechanical nature of neonatal brain tissue and a distensible skull accounts for one of the best-known cardinal signs of neurosurgical difficulty in the neonate, namely abnormal head growth. The prodigious ability of the skull to grow and sutures to widen can allow some of the most severe cases of hydrocephalus to result in relatively mild pressure effects, even when the need for cerebrospinal fluid (CSF) shunting is clear. These same considerations in the type and nature of response of the tissues to abnormal fluid buildup can result in dramatic craniocephalic disproportion once the pressure is relieved. The change in brain and skull biomechanics over time adds particular challenge to management of these problems.

Obvious congenital anomalies, especially those involving open neural-tube defects and exposed CNS tissue, may require urgent neurosurgical intervention. A complicating aspect is the potential occurrence of concurrent microscopic abnormalities, such as widespread synaptic miswiring. In many cases, neurologic deficits may be present in a patient with macroscopic structural abnormalities, but major neurologic disability may come from less obvious problems with tissue development, currently not treatable by neurosurgical means. Diffusion tractography has identified multiple white matter abnormalities in association with open myelomeningocele and Chiari II.

The details of the plasticity and vulnerability of the neonatal CNS is discussed in Chapters 49 and 50. It is well known that the ability to recover function after CNS injury is age dependent and seems to be better in younger individuals. Interaction between the age-dependent variables of CNS plasticity, recoverability, and vulnerability make the task of estimating prognosis after an injury or neurosurgical intervention extremely difficult.

Antenatal diagnosis has changed many aspects of neurosurgical conditions. Obstetric management may be altered, for example, by site and mode of delivery, if there is a known neural-tube defect. Antenatal surgery for open myelomeningocele has been investigated in a randomized control trial. In addition, the psychological issues around the time of neurosurgical therapy for the newborn are altered, as the child's family now has the opportunity to meet the neurosurgeon prenatally and fully discuss and decide upon any contemplated care plan before birth.

FLUID COLLECTIONS AND THEIR MANAGEMENT

Disorders of Cerebrospinal Fluid Accumulation

The most common neurosurgical consultation for newborn patients is to evaluate and treat enlargement of the ventricular system. The survival and outcomes of progressively more premature neonates continue to improve, and intraventricular hemorrhage, and subsequent hydrocephalus of prematurity, remains a frequent neurosurgical issue (1). The clinical signs of progressive enlargement of the ventricular system include excessive increase in the head circumference (HC), fullness in the anterior fontanelle (especially when the patient is upright when the venous and fontanelle pressures should be low), episodic apnea and bradycardia, general lethargy, and abnormalities of ocular movement, especially restricted upward gaze. Many of these findings are nonspecific and can be seen with hydrocephalus of any etiology. At a practical level, the most important distinction is between progressive and static abnormalities in ventricular volume. This is relatively easy to determine with serial clinical and ultrasound examinations (Fig. 53.1). Resistive index (RI) measurements add a physiologic dimension to the anatomic images gathered by ultrasonography (2). The presence of dramatic changes in the Doppler-measured flow signals in the anterior cerebral artery with gentle, brief compression of the anterior fontanelle correlates extremely well with the intracranial pressure by measurement and the probability of eventual need for a ventriculoperitoneal (VP) shunt (2).

The majority of hydrocephalus seen in neonates is associated with, and traditionally thought to result from, abnormal resorption of CSF; other causes of hydrocephalus, including those associated with neural tube defects, aqueduct stenosis, or CSF-secreting tumors, are relatively rare (Fig. 53.2). After intraventricular hemorrhage (IVH) (Fig. 53.1), partial occlusion of the normal resorptive pathways of CSF through the arachnoid villi, as well as scarring in the basal cisterns, leads to communicating hydrocephalus (3–5). However, despite traditional teaching, the neonatal sagittal sinus does not contain arachnoid granulations and therefore dysfunction of the minor pathways of CSF absorption must be particularly relevant (6). Elegant studies in small and large animals, including nonhuman primates, have demonstrated bulk flow from the intraventricular CSF to the subfrontal subarachnoid space and on to the cribriform plate, lymphatics in the nasal mucosa, and subsequently large lymphatic channels in the neck (7). An extensive network of lymphatic vessels has also been identified in and around the meninges; these have been shown to mediate transport of fluid from the brain interstitial space and subarachnoid

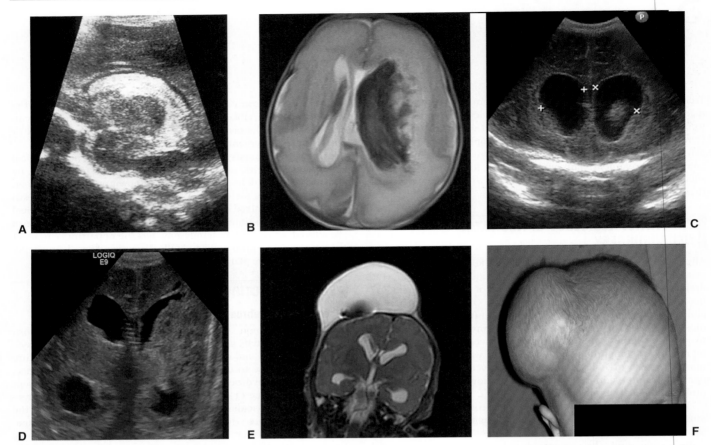

FIGURE 53.1 Intraventricular hemorrhage of prematurity. A: Transfontanelle sagittal ultrasound image in a preterm neonate at 28 weeks' gestational age. Extensive intraventricular hemorrhage is evident throughout the left lateral ventricle, also seen as a hypointense area on the axial T2-weighted MR image in **(B)**. Posthemorrhagic ventricular dilatation is evident on the axial ultrasound image in **(C)**. In **(D)** the catheter of a ventriculosubgaleal shunt can be seen in the larger lateral ventricle, adjacent to the septum pellucidum; this has been effective at reducing the degree of ventricular. A coronal T2-weighted MRI scan in **(E)** shows similarly decompressed ventricles and a large subgaleal collection; this is visible clinically in **(F)**. This child underwent conversion of the VSG shunt to a VP shunt at term equivalent and a body weight of 2 kg.

space into extracranial lymphatics (8). Aquaporin 4 also mediates the flow of CSF through perivascular spaces into interstitial brain fluid, eventually draining into parenchymal veins (9).

Implantation of a VP shunt is the primary treatment for hydrocephalus in the neonate; other treatment options include endoscopic third ventriculostomy (ETV) and choroid plexus coagulation, but their role in the management of overt neonatal hydrocephalus is uncertain. Once a shunt is implanted, it becomes the principal conduit through which CSF flows out of the ventricles. The subarachnoid space does not develop to the same extent as in non-shunted neonates, and there is a tendency to microcephaly. Chronic shunt overdrainage in an infant may cause slit ventricle syndrome later in childhood, where the ventricles are small and brain compliance is reduced. Recurrent obstruction of the ventricular catheter, due to coaptation of the ependymal surfaces on the catheter, in the presence of poor compliance, leads to acute and symptomatic elevation in intracranial pressure (10,11). These children have frequent shunt revisions, emphasizing the importance of selecting a valve that reduces overdrainage (12). Incorporation of an antisiphon device, reducing gravity-dependent overdrainage, has been shown to reduce the incidence of shunt malfunction (13).

In clinical practice, it is difficult to determine whether a shunt continues to be required in a growing child. Absence of shunt flow in an asymptomatic child is difficult to establish, although recent evaluation of a device able to detect temperature difference of the skin along the distal shunt tubing has been promising (14). An ice

cube is placed on the skin along the palpable tubing, and a temperature drop distally along the tube is a good indicator of CSF flow (14). An alternative involves externalization of the distal catheter, with gradual raising of the drainage chamber and occlusion over 2 to 3 days. If this is tolerated, it is possible that the child is shunt independent, although flow through an established subcutaneous tract still cannot be excluded.

One of the problems with assessing growth of ventricular size in the neonate is the possibility that enlargement of the ventricles may at least partially reflect loss of tissue in the brain, rather than increase in pressure. This can become a difficult problem, as prolonged hydrocephalus itself certainly can cause loss of tissue bulk (15), and the value of shunt placement may be more difficult to determine when the tissue loss is not obviously the result of high pressure. The specific loss of myelin or white matter, called periventricular leukomalacia, is discussed in Chapter 50. The relationship between periventricular leukomalacia and hydrocephalus is of particular concern in neurosurgical decision-making. When a preterm infant, especially one who has sustained an intracranial hemorrhage, shows lateral ventricular enlargement, it is difficult to determine to what extent this is a result of impaired CSF flow or absorption, versus diffuse white matter damage or inadequate density of axons. In general, the absence of macrocephaly is an indicator of brain atrophy. An MRI scan showing transependymal CSF flow on T2-weighted images, effacement of the cortical sulci, distension of the recesses of the third ventricle, and inferior displacement of the third ventricular floor are indicators of hydrocephalus.

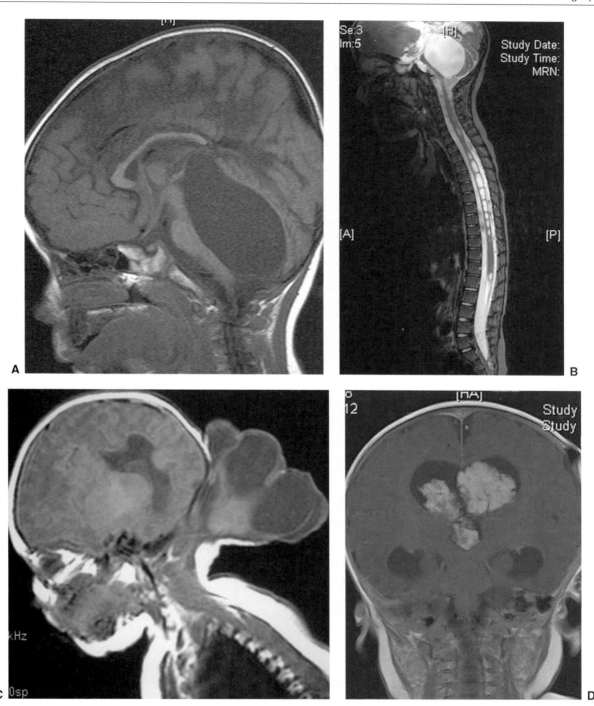

FIGURE 53.2 Hydrocephalus. A: Mid-sagittal T1-weighted MR scan showing a trapped fourth ventricle in a 1-year-old child with a supratentorial ventriculoperitoneal shunt for posthemorrhagic hydrocephalus. **B:** A sagittal T2-weighted MR scan of the same child demonstrating an associated syrinx. Both the trapped fourth ventricle and the syrinx were effectively treated by an additional shunt catheter placed in the fourth ventricle. **C:** Mid-sagittal T1 MR scan showing a large occipital encephalocele that also contained brainstem; debulking of the encephalocele led to hydrocephalus. **D:** Postcontrast coronal MR image showing multiple choroid plexus papillomata involving the lateral and third ventricles with hydrocephalus secondary to increased CSF production.

Regular measurement of occipitofrontal circumference (OFC) with reference to established centile charts is crucial (16). In general, an OFC growth of less than 1 cm/wk is acceptable, whereas growth of more than 1.5 cm/wk is considered excessive. Head growth must be interpreted in the context of overall somatic growth measured by weight and length. Babies can demonstrate brain catch-up growth, but it is suspicious if the rate of OFC growth is plotted at the high end of the normal range while the weight and length remain rela-

tively unchanged. Because major intervention decisions are based on the intrinsically imprecise measurement of OFC, any effort to improve its precision is worthwhile. Minimizing the number of care providers obtaining the measurement and overtly standardizing the measurement site and technique improves accuracy. The effect of interpreter variability can be reduced by comparing the OFC to the previous day and also to 1 week earlier to calculate average daily growth by dividing by seven. Using a correct and accurate growth curve is also important (17). In achondroplasia, OFC growth is different, and a specific HC centile chart for this condition has been developed (18).

The increasing availability of detailed antenatal imaging with ultrasound and fetal MRI has allowed earlier diagnosis of congenital hydrocephalus, providing an opportunity to manage such pregnancies prospectively. Fetal ventriculomegaly is defined as an atrial width of over 10 mm; this same value applies throughout pregnancy (19). Ventriculomegaly is present in 2 per 1,000 live born babies (19). For isolated mild fetal ventriculomegaly (10 to 15 mm) diagnosed after 24 weeks' gestation, the risk of moderate to severe neurodevelopmental delay is only 4%; 83% show normal development and 8% minor delay (20). Severe ventriculomegaly (>15 mm) is often associated with other neurologic abnormalities, which then primarily influence prognosis. A meta-analysis including 110 fetuses with prenatal diagnosis of isolated severe ventriculomegaly demonstrated that more than one-third survived without disability (21). In a recent large series, fetal hydrocephalus due to intracranial hemorrhage or associated with corpus callosum agenesis, atresia of the foramen of Monro or arachnoid cyst had a good prognosis; those associated with holoprosencephaly, encephalocele, or virus infection demonstrated poorer outcomes (22). Outcomes in fetuses with isolated unilateral ventriculomegaly are significantly better, with a prevalence of abnormal neurologic development of only 7% in a large meta-analysis (23). Cavalheiro et al. have described the intrauterine management of fetal hydrocephalus, involving endoscopic insertion of a ventriculo-amniotic curled catheter; this is only suitable for progressive hydrocephalus, unrelated to brain atrophy, in the absence of congenital infection, additional malformations, or abnormal karyotype, as confirmed by cordocentesis, and is ideally considered between 24 and 32 weeks' gestation (24).

Benign external hydrocephalus is characterized by a rapid increase in HC. In an epidemiologic study on 176 children with BEH, 86.4% were boys (25). Although the HC was nearly normal at birth, an abnormally high value was always reached by the age of 7 months, at a mean of 3.4 months. Imaging shows enlargement of the subarachnoid spaces with slightly enlarged or normal sized ventricles. There is at least one close relative with macrocephaly in up to 90%. HC growth stabilizes by 18 months and then continues to follow a higher centile parallel to the 98th. This condition probably represents delayed maturation of CSF absorption capacity, and CSF diversion is not required (26). Up to half of the children eventually have an HC at or above the 97th centile (25). In macrocephalic children, it is important to exclude glutaric aciduria type I, which, if identified early, can be treated with dietary and metabolic measures, reducing the risk of significant neurologic morbidity (27).

Treatment of Neonatal Hydrocephalus

Due to the disadvantages and complications of VP shunting, the decision to place a shunt must be made only after all nonsurgical options have failed. The fact that CSF resorption may change with time, and indeed may improve, provides a rationale for conservatism. As a patient grows and the dynamic relationship between CSF production and resorption changes, the need and indications for diversion of CSF may change over the child's lifetime.

Children born with hydrocephalus due to nonhemorrhagic causes, such as aqueductal stenosis, posterior fossa cysts, holoprosencephaly, or hydranencephaly, can be shunted within 1 to 2 days of birth, pending evaluation of general medical status. Affected infants are usually born at or near term. At a pre-operative body weight of approximately 1,500 to 2,000 g peritoneal drainage of ventricular CSF is generally well-supported (28). There are ethical issues that should be raised before placing a VP shunt in a child suffering from hydrocephalus with significantly reduced brain function from either an *in utero* event or developmental anomaly. Frank discussion with the child's parents regarding prognosis is critical. Shunting for affected children without other life-threatening anomalies is certainly reasonable for the purposes of controlling head size in the growing infant. With maximal interventive therapy, most of these children are expected to live beyond a few weeks, and such day-to-day issues as whether the child's head will fit in an infant car seat, as well as the risk of skin pressure and breakdown related to the large head, need to be considered. Shunting at birth is a relatively low-risk method of preventing massive head enlargement and allowing other factors aside from congenital hydrocephalus to determine the child's outcome (29). Despite the progress in endoscopic techniques and the establishment of ETV for CSF diversion in obstructive hydrocephalus, its efficacy in neonates remains controversial. A large Canadian review of 368 children who underwent ETV in nine centers showed that the 5-year success rate for ETV in children under 1 month of age was only 28% (30). The International Infant Hydrocephalus Study allowed a direct comparison between ETV and VP shunt in infants under 24 months of age with symptomatic triventricular hydrocephalus due to aqueduct stenosis (31). One hundred and fifty-eight patients were recruited between 2004 and 2013 in 27 neurosurgical centers; 115 and 43 infants underwent ETV and VP shunt, respectively. Only 32.9% were randomized, with the rest treated according to parental preference. At 6 months, the success rate of ETV versus shunt was 66% versus 88%, but those under 6 months of age did relatively worse with ETV (58.6% success rate at 6 months' follow-up) (31). Evaluation of health status and quality of life measures at 5 years did not demonstrate a significant difference between the two groups (31).

The addition of choroid plexus coagulation (CPC) to ETV in infants was investigated in a large infant population in Uganda and subsequently in a prospective study through the Hydrocephalus Research Network (HCRN) in the United States (32,33). In the former study, 266 children underwent ETV and CPC, and were compared to 284 who underwent ETV alone (32). In children under 1 year of age, combined ETV and CPC had a superior success rate of 66%, compared to 47% for ETV alone; the combined procedure led to best outcomes in infants with myelomeningocele and non-postinfectious hydrocephalus. In the HCRN prospective study, 118 infants, with a median corrected age of 1.3 months, underwent ETV with CPC; the principal causes of hydrocephalus were myelomeningocele, IVH of prematurity, and aqueduct stenosis. The 6-month success rate was 36%. Infants were matched to others who underwent ETV only or insertion of a VP shunt; outcomes of combined ETV–CPC were similar to ETV alone, but clearly inferior to VP shunt (33). At age over 1 year, higher extent of CPC, smaller ventricles, and clear basal cisterns without scarring were associated with better CPC outcomes (33,34). A further prospective study by the HCRN analyzed 191 children who underwent primary ETV and CPC (35). Infants under 6 months of age constituted 79% of the cohort. At 6 months, ETV with CPC was successful in 48% of the cohort; age under 1 month and PHH were the only two independent predictors of failure (35).

Nearly all acquired hydrocephalus in the premature infant in high income countries is posthemorrhagic (Fig. 53.1). Although the incidence of IVH declined from about 50% to 20% in the late 1980s, it has remained stable in recent decades; its incidence in very premature infants weighing 500 to 750 g remains about 40% (1). The germinal matrix is still abundant up to 32 weeks' gestation; it contains fragile and unsupported arterioles and capillaries, with poor autoregulatory control and pressure-passive circulation, and is therefore susceptible to hemorrhage with changes in blood pressure or respiratory distress (3). The highest risk for bleeding is in the first 48 hours after birth large hemorrhages rupture through the ependyma and cause IVH, with subsequent hydrocephalus. Brain injury in the developing brain is related to increased intracranial pressure, distension of periventricular white matter, disturbance of neuronal generation and migration from the subventricular zone, and the pro-inflammatory effects of intraventricular blood; cell-free intraventricular hemoglobin and methemoglobin induce the expression of pro-inflammatory cytokines and free radicals, and transforming growth factor beta released from platelets has a role in promoting fibrosis in the subarachnoid space (4,36–38). At the time when ventricular dilatation first appears, these infants have usually not achieved adequate body weight for safe placement of permanent VP shunts, and the final determination of lifelong hydrocephalus has not been made. Serial lumbar punctures are, initially, the best way to reduce ventricular size and intracranial pressure. As the cranial sutures are open, the risk of coning after LP is extremely rare in this situation. Up to 10 mL/kg of CSF may be removed at one time. As these neonates often have a combination of communicating and obstructive hydrocephalus, LPs often soon become ineffective. Obstruction of CSF pathways at the spinal level may also occur (10). Direct ventricular puncture through the anterior fontanelle is not ideal and parenchymal needle tracks appear on ultrasound examination after multiple aspirations. In the Ventriculomegaly trial, the risk of ventriculitis and repeated LPs was 7% (39). In practice, once two LPs or one ventricular tap have been unsuccessful at controlling ventriculomegaly, insertion of a ventricular subgaleal (VSG) shunt or ventricular access device (VAD) would be recommended (40). Acetazolamide and furosemide were investigated in the International PHVD Drug Trial Group study in a randomized trial in 1998 (41). The trial was discontinued prematurely by the data monitoring committee as it became clear that the treatment group fared worse. This was likely related to $PaCO_2$ elevation in ventilator-dependent neonates with immature renal function.

An additional approach that has been tried for posthemorrhagic hydrocephalus (PHH) is the introduction of fibrinolytic therapy directly into the ventricular system. Enzymes such as streptokinase, urokinase, and tissue plasminogen activator all have been proposed and tested with variable success. Some centers have suggested that the risk of VP shunts can be reduced using this technique (42). Others have been unable to show a decrease in the need for VP shunting with this maneuver (43,44). It is possible that the trials that found no helpful effect from fibrinolytic therapy had less favorable results because of patient selection, with a trend toward enrolling the most severe and potentially intractable cases.

Drainage, irrigation, and fibrinolysis therapy (DRIFT) developed out of an attempt to reduce intracranial pressure and wash out toxic cytokines from the ventricular system as early as possible (45). This involves insertion of right frontal and left occipital external ventricular catheters. Tissue plasminogen activator is injected and, 8 hours later, irrigation with artificial CSF is commenced under intracranial pressure monitoring. The drainage fluid clears from dark and thick to straw colored CSF within about 72 hours. A phase I study enrolled 24 infants with ventriculomegaly (97th centile + 4 mm) (45). Mortality, disability, and shunt dependence (74%) was lower than historical controls. Seventy infants, between 24 and 34 weeks' gestation, were subsequently randomized in a multicenter trial to DRIFT or standard treatment (46). Although shunt insertion rates were not different, a follow-up study at 2 years demonstrated that severe cognitive disability was significantly reduced in the DRIFT group (47). Seventy-one percent of infants who had received standard treatment were severely disabled or dead, compared to 54% in the DRIFT group. Thirty-one percent of infants surviving DRIFT had severe cognitive disability, compared to 59% in the standard treatment group.

A 10-year follow-up of the DRIFT study evaluated 52 of the original 77 randomized children (48). Twenty-eight children had received DRIFT and 24 had standard treatment. After correction for gender, birth weight, and grade of IVH, DRIFT children had a cognitive quotient advantage of 23.5 points ($p = 0.009$); the binary outcome, alive without severe cognitive disability, showed an adjusted odds ratio of 10 for improved cognition with DRIFT. The

number needed to treat was three. Reduction for special education suggested that this treatment could also be cost-effective (48).

DRIFT is a demanding procedure, requiring significant expertise in neonatal intensive care units. A similar approach involves endoscopic lavage of the intraventricular hematoma, aiming to clear the hemorrhagic CSF and remove solid clot from the ventricular system and aqueduct within a single neurosurgical procedure (49,50). An endoscopic septostomy ensures access to both sides of the ventricular system. An initial study reported on a comparison between 19 neonates with PHH who underwent endoscopic lavage with 10 neonates treated conventionally with temporizing procedures (49). Median gestational age at first intervention was 32 weeks. In the lavage group, only 58% required a VP shunt, compared to 100% in the group treated conventionally. In addition, the lavage group required fewer procedures overall, had fewer infections, and demonstrated a lower incidence of supratentorial multiloculated hydrocephalus (49). An extended case series from two centers subsequently reported on 56 neonates, median age of 31 weeks' gestation and weight of 1,523 g, where after lavage only 57% required a VP shunt (50). Neonates underwent insertion of an external ventricular drain or a VAD after endoscopy, allowing ongoing removal of CSF and blood products from the ventricles as determined by regular ultrasound assessment; this may have been relevant to the low requirement for a VP shunt (50). A prospective randomized trial (ENLIVEN—Endoscopic Lavage after Intraventricular Hemorrhage in Neonates) to directly compare endoscopic lavage plus VSG shunt with conventional therapy using a VSG shunt alone is currently recruiting in the author's institution and hopes to report by 2022.

Persisting increase in ventricular size in the preterm post-IVH neonate, still too small to allow implantation of a VP shunt, is managed by insertion of a VAD or a VSG shunt, allowing intermittent or continuous CSF drainage from the ventricles (Fig. 53.3). A VAD provides a safe route for repeated aspiration of ventricular CSF, with low reported infection rates (51,52). Insertion, through the frontal corner of the anterior fontanelle, can be safely performed in neonates under 800 g. In a large series of 325 preterm infants with grade III to IV IVH studied over a 10-year period, 65 infants underwent insertion of a VAD. There were four infections during the course of treatment and three had to be revised due to malfunction (51). Revision and infection rates were similar in a Dutch study on 76 preterm infants over a 12-year period (52). Tapping frequency is determined by regular measurements of the ventricular index. VSG shunts are also used as temporizing devices prior to placement of a VP shunt. The device, as well as

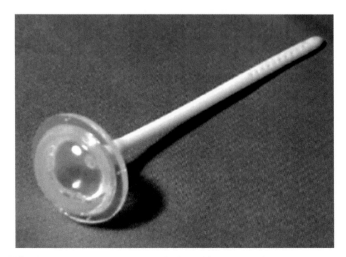

FIGURE 53.3 Ventricular access device with 40-mm catheter. Implantation allows easy percutaneous access to ventricular fluid.

THE NEWBORN INFANT

the surgical implantation technique, is very similar to the VAD. The ventricular catheter is connected to a reservoir with a side arm. This can either be left open into the subgaleal space or 10 cm of shunt tubing may be attached to it and coiled within the subgaleal pocket, fashioned by blunt dissection between the pericranium and galeal aponeurosis. The major advantage is that the subgaleal pocket may allow some resorption of CSF and can absorb fluid pulsations. Infants with VSG shunts typically require far less frequent taps and sometimes no taps at all (39). If necessary, the reservoir or subcutaneous fluid collection can be tapped, just like a VAD. The indications for tapping VSG shunt devices are the same as for VADs, and the follow-up assessment for both involves regular, at least twice weekly, sonographic assessment of ventricular size. In the large St Louis series, there was no difference between VADs and VSGs in terms of infection, need for revision, shunt insertion rate (66.7% for VSG shunts vs. 75.4% for VADs), shunt infection, and revision rate or mortality rate (51). Similarly, a large HCRN review evaluated 145 preterm neonates in six centers in the United States, where a standard management protocol was followed (53). Thirty-six underwent a VSG shunt and 66 a VAD; infection rates were 14% and 17%, respectively. 180-Day conversion rates to a VP shunt were also similar at 63.5% and 74%, respectively (53).

Traditionally, decisions to drain CSF were taken on the basis of signs and symptoms of raised intracranial pressure. These included a tense anterior fontanelle, rapidly increasing OFC, splaying of cranial sutures as well as episodes of bradycardia and apnea. The current trend is to intervene earlier on the basis of serial ventricular measurements on ultrasound. The ventricular index, defined as the distance between the lateral ventricular wall and the falx on coronal ultrasonography through the anterior fontanelle, is the most commonly used measurement of ventricular size (54). In the preterm neonate, its correlation with HC is poor (55). The broadly accepted action point is a ventricular index 4 mm above the 97th centile. Physiologically, earlier drainage may maintain a lower intracranial pressure over a longer period of time and may reduce white matter stretch and injury. The use of near-infrared spectroscopy, Doppler, and EEG have demonstrated that cerebral perfusion and oxygenation in neonates are reduced with progressive ventriculomegaly and improve with CSF drainage (56,57). In a survey of 37 neonatal intensive care units in Europe, 72% started therapy to drain CSF once the ventricular index crossed 4 mm over the 97th centile; 25%, however, intervened earlier, when the 97th centile was crossed (58). A recent study compared two populations of neonates from two centers—one center consistently used an early approach, with CSF drainage at a ventricular index at p97 + 4 mm; the second center only instituted CSF drainage for symptomatic raised intracranial pressure (59). Most of the infants in the second group underwent insertion of a VP shunt as a primary CSF diversion procedure. The overall rate of VP shunt placement was 20% in the early approach group and 92% in the late approach group. In addition, the majority of survivors within the first group (55 from 62) had cognitive and motor outcome scores within the normal range, whereas 14 of 27 in the late approach group had moderately to severe abnormal outcomes. Although the populations were different, with a higher proportion of infants in the late approach group having grade IV IVH, this study suggests that earlier treatment may be beneficial if the complications related to the interventions are low and the rates of intervention are equivalent (59).

In a Dutch study, early intervention resulted in a lower shunt requirement rate than intervention at the 4 mm + 97th centile, and the incidence of moderate or severe disability was higher in the group where intervention was late (60). The authors went on to explore this further in a prospective randomized study (ELVIS—Early vs Late Intervention Study) that recruited 126 preterm infants with PHH, following grade III or IV IVH, under 34 weeks' gestation from 14 neonatal intensive care units in six countries (61). Neonates were randomized to treatment at low threshold (ventricular index > p97 or anterior horn width > 6 mm) or high threshold (ventricular index >p97 + 4 mm or anterior horn width >10 mm). A VAD was inserted if three consecutive lumbar punctures failed to reduce ventricular size. The rate of shunt insertion was very low, and similar in both groups at 19% and 23% in the low- and high-threshold neonates, respectively; infants treated at the lower threshold required more shunt revisions and underwent more invasive procedures than those treated at the higher threshold. At 24 months corrected age, the composite adverse outcome (death or cerebral palsy or Bayley composite cognitive/motor scores <-2 standard deviations) did not differ significantly between groups, but in post hoc analyses, earlier intervention was associated with a lower odds of death or severe neurodevelopmental disability (61).

In three recent large single-center studies, the rate of shunt implantation for neonates with ventricular dilatation following grades III to IV IVH have varied between 16% and 75% (51,62,63). The decision to insert a VP shunt should not be taken too early. Shunts in this population have a higher rate of failure and infection (12,64). It is ideal to wait at least until about term, when the body weight is at least 2 kg. This reduces the risk of infection and skin ulceration over the shunt. CSF protein should be lower than 1.5 g/L, and repeated cultures should be confirmed negative. At this stage, tapping is discontinued. If the OFC increases by at least 2 mm daily for several days, and ultrasonography confirms this to be related to an increase in the ventricular index, then insertion of a shunt is indicated. The contraindications to implantation of a permanent VP shunt are similar to those in older children: evidence of CSF infection, significantly elevated CSF protein, presence of a high-CSF red blood cell count that may mechanically obstruct the shunt, peritoneal inflammation, or infection such as necrotizing enterocolitis. These problems necessitate a delay in implantation. CSF glucose is sometimes quite low (<20 mg/dL) in neonates with PHH in the absence of infection. The significance of this finding is unclear, and there is not an increase in shunt infection in these patients. Similarly, patients with IVH, whether adult or neonatal, can manifest fever perhaps from the presence of blood in the CSF. The exact cause of this increased temperature in the neonate is unclear; without positive bacteriologic data, it is unlikely to be infection. Therefore, in the absence of positive culture data, shunt placement should not be delayed.

The neurodevelopmental outcome of IVH and PHVD is closely related to the severity of the hemorrhage and the extent of parenchymal infarction (4). Early mortality rates of up to 50% have been described in very premature infants with large hemorrhages with a birth weight under 750 g (4). In a cohort of 75 children with large intraparenchymal echodensities, 87% demonstrated major motor deficit and 68% had cognitive function below 80% of normal (65). On the basis of MRI-based cortical volumetric studies, even uncomplicated IVH is associated with reduced cortical grey matter at near-term age (66). In addition to major motor and cognitive deficits, these children often demonstrate fine motor coordination difficulties, cortical visual impairment, anxiety, and attention deficit hyperactivity disorder (67). IVH and PHH are also both associated with slow cerebellar growth and reduced cerebellar volume at birth; this may be related to diaschisis after parenchymal brain injury and leads to difficulties with mobility, balance, and language development (68).

A large study involving follow-up of over 6,000 very low birth weight infants across multiple centers demonstrated that children with severe IVH who also have a shunt have a cerebral palsy rate of up to 90% (69). If there are no persistent echolucencies on ultrasonography, up to 40% of infants with IVH will develop cerebral palsy and up to 25% will have multiple disabilities (39,41). A logistic regression analysis of factors affecting school performance at 14 years of age in a cohort of 278 preterm infants showed that peri- or intraventricular hemorrhage was the primary risk factor for special education (70).

Complications of Ventriculoperitoneal Shunting

Many problems related to CSF diversion can be managed with simple surgical techniques. For example, since shunts tend to obstruct with very high protein concentrations, an externally draining system or a ventricular catheter with a tapping reservoir is initially placed (Fig. 53.2). At a later time, it is revised into a VP shunt if the infant requires permanent diversion (29). Another potential problem is patients outgrowing their shunts. Initial placement of longer tubing eliminates the need to periodically lengthen the peritoneal catheter because of growth. Catheters up to 90 cm in length are well tolerated, even by neonates. Prospective studies have not shown any increase in complications, even with tubing up to 120 cm in length (71). Therefore, many centers now place a long catheter into the peritoneum, even in a neonate.

Shunt infection and malfunction are the most serious complications of VP shunting at any age. Neonates are at particularly high risk of these complications because of their relatively thin skin, nutritional difficulties causing delayed wound healing, and the tendency for CSF to be proteinaceous. Plastic hardware items such as shunts are particularly susceptible to infection, because a small pathogen inoculation, even with a relatively nonpathogenic bacterium, can avoid normal immune surveillance. In several series, the rate of infection correlated significantly with patient's age and often with little else (72). Intravenous antibiotic prophylaxis is generally used to cover a 24-hour period around shunt implantation. Impregnation of shunt tubing with antibiotics, typically clindamycin and rifampicin, reduces the incidence of shunt infections in the first 6 months after implantation. In a study evaluating shunt infection rates 18 months before and after the introduction of antibiotic impregnated catheters, shunt infections dropped from 12% with standard catheters to 1.4% with newer catheters (73). In a later larger study from the same institution, the introduction of antibiotic-impregnated catheters reduced shunt infection in high-risk situations, such as in premature infants with hydrocephalus, shunt implantation after CSF infection, and conversion of external drains to shunts (74). A meta-analysis of 5,613 reported adult and pediatric cases confirmed reduction of shunt infection with these catheters without an increased incidence of antibiotic-resistant microorganisms (75). In the United Kingdom, a recent randomized controlled trial involving 3,505 patients of all ages demonstrated a significantly lower shunt infection rate with catheters impregnated with rifampicin and clindamycin, at 2%, compared to nonimpregnated (6%) and silver impregnated (6%) catheters (76).

Another complication of VP shunting sometimes seen in infants, although rarely seen in older individuals, is injury to bowel or other abdominal viscera (77). A relatively frequent difficulty in this population is the development of peritoneal adhesions following surgery for necrotizing enterocolitis. In these infants, the pleural cavity is still too small to permit satisfactory CSF drainage and a ventriculoatrial shunt is preferable when peritoneal absorption fails.

Especially with very large ventricles, rapid decompression of the ventricular system can cause bleeding into the subdural space, ventricles, or parenchyma of the brain. For this reason, only moderate amounts of CSF are typically removed at the time of surgery, and patients are kept flat for the immediate postoperative period, with elevation of the head titrated gradually based on assessment of the anterior fontanelle. The head can be raised as long as there is no extreme concavity of the anterior fontanelle. Other authors have suggested the use of high-pressure valves or valves incorporating anti-siphon devices when the ventricles are large (78).

Programmable valves allow an additional degree of freedom in the management of pediatric hydrocephalus, enabling gradual stepwise change in shunt opening pressure without the need to surgically revise the valve. The disadvantages of programmable valves include higher cost, the possibility of the settings changing with exposure to the strong magnetic field of an MRI scanner, and their reduced tolerance to high protein or debris in the CSF. The development of low-profile reliable anti-siphon services, as well as flow-controlled valves, allow safer shunting of large ventricles, reducing the risk of subdural collections and slit ventricle syndrome.

Asymmetry in the size of the lateral ventricles occurs frequently. Spontaneous resolution of ventricular asymmetry sometimes occurs and therefore, in the absence of an associated asymmetric physical examination, ventricular asymmetry can generally be tolerated with close observation. Endoscopic septostomy is a useful technique to allow interventricular communication. Alternatively, image-guided insertion of a ventricular catheter across the septum pellucidum is an effective way of draining both sides (79). Endoscopic foraminal dilatation may be valuable in unilateral hydrocephalus due to stenosis of the foramen of Monro. Endoscopy is also useful when multiple ventricular loculations occur after IVH or ventriculitis and may facilitate simple control of hydrocephalus by the minimal number of ventricular catheters. A trapped or encysted fourth ventricle, rarely associated with syringomyelia due to disruption of CSF flow at the obex (Fig. 53.3), may require a separate catheter. This must be connected above the valve of the shunt draining the supratentorial ventricles.

Intracranial Cystic Spaces in the Neonate

Interhemispheric, temporal fossa, posterior fossa, and other arachnoid cysts may be found incidentally or may present with macrocephaly or hydrocephalus (Fig. 53.4). They may also be identified on routine antenatal imaging. In general, arachnoid cysts identified incidentally are followed up. Those causing symptomatic mass effect or accelerated head growth need intervention, and may be fenestrated, endoscopically or by open microsurgical technique, into the basal cisterns or ventricle. Direct shunting of the cyst is preferably avoided if at all possible.

Dilation of the isolated fourth ventricle is a particularly difficult surgical problem, both because the posterior fossa is a more technically difficult area into which to place a catheter that will continue to work over a long period of time, and because the neurologic risks of even transient catheter failure are high, resulting in brainstem symptoms such as apnea and bradycardia. The risks of fourth ventricular cysts and specific placement of shunts into the cysts to drain them have been documented in several reports (80). In principle, fourth ventricular catheters are best placed using image guidance and should be connected above the valve of a coexisting supratentorial shunt. Severe fourth ventricular entrapment may also cause syringomyelia, which should improve once CSF drainage from the ventricle is secured.

MANAGEMENT OF THE INFANT WITH AN OPEN DEFECT OF THE NEURAL AXIS

Abnormal developmental folding of the neural tube and anterior neuropore can result in a wide spectrum of abnormalities. Although the average prevalence of neural tube defects (NTD) worldwide is estimated at one case per 1,000 births, geographical variation is high, with some regions in China reporting a prevalence that is 20 times higher than in Europe or the United States (81). On the basis of prevalence surveys in the United Kingdom in the 1960s, the heritability of NTDs has been estimated at 60 to 70%; fewer than 10% occur as part of a syndrome (81). For a particular woman, the empirical risk for a second offspring with NTD is 3%, rising to 10% after two affected pregnancies. Beyond genetic factors, folate

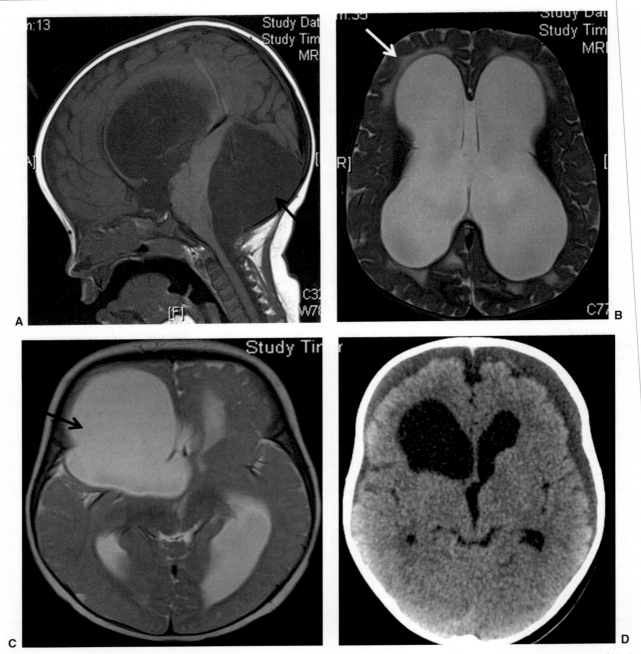

FIGURE 53.4 Intracranial cysts in the neonate. A: T1-weighted MR mid-sagittal image showing a large posterior fossa arachnoid cyst in a neonate (*black arrow*). Brainstem distortion and aqueduct obstruction caused obstructive hydrocephalus, best seen on axial T2-weighted MR image **(B)**; the *white arrow* points to extensive frontal subependymal CSF flow. Open fenestration of the cyst into the spinal and basal cisterns treated both the cyst and the hydrocephalus. **C:** Large right frontal extraventricular arachnoid cyst (*black arrow*), causing displacement of the ventricular system and hydrocephalus. **D:** CT scan demonstrating restoration of normal ventricular size following endoscopic fenestration of the cyst into the basal cisterns.

deficiency is the best known factor affecting NTD risk (81). The most benign presentation is spina bifida occulta, a bifid spinal arch seen in up to 30% of the general population with no neurologic sequelae. The most severe presentation is anencephaly or craniospinal rachischisis, representing complete absence of neuraltube closure.

The general guideline is to defer urgent repair of these defects if they are small and truly skin covered, that is, lipomyelomeningocele. Open defects, such as myelomeningocele, or defects that leak CSF or interfere with airway patency, such as large nasofrontal encephaloceles, require repair within a few days of birth. Infants

with enlarging lesions such as occipital encephaloceles are often managed most safely with close observation until they achieve adequate weight to minimize surgical risks.

Neurosurgeons frequently are called upon to evaluate a variety of midline "lumps, bumps, and dimples" along the neural axis from nose to coccyx. These lesions often represent myelodysplasia that will require repair. However, in the stable newborn, evaluation and treatment can be deferred until after 3 months of age when surgical intervention is medically safer. Even MRI evaluation can be deferred until that time to obtain a technically superior and dedicated study. Head and spine ultrasound are useful in the neonatal period for screening these lesions, but a high false-negative rate has been noted. The MRI scan remains the gold standard for preoperative planning of these occult lesions.

Myelomeningocele

Antenatal diagnosis has markedly changed the management of patients with myelomeningoceles. The majority of patients with this deformity are diagnosed prenatally on the basis of an ultrasound study, elevated maternal serum alpha-fetoprotein, and an antenatal MRI scan (82,83). Ultrasonography shows an irregular contour of the fetal back, as well as the "lemon sign," referring to the concave shape of the frontal calvarium, and the "banana sign," related to the appearance of the posterior convexity of the cerebellum in the presence of a Chiari II malformation. Delivery of patients with myelomeningocele by cesarean section prior to labor may improve the functional outcome relative to the anatomic level of the myelomeningocele (84). The optimal obstetric mode of delivery of a fetus with myelomeningocele is however indeterminate in the literature (85). Unless rapidly progressive ventriculomegaly is present, there is no indication for a preterm delivery.

Postnatal surgery for repair of a myelomeningocele has been well described (86). The goal of surgery is to reconstruct the terminal end of the neuraxis and approximate the topologic relationships that would have occurred if closure of the neural tube had been complete. The neural placode itself is usually visible beneath translucent abnormal tissue, representing arachnoid, stretching from the edge of the skin defect inward to the small island of pink tissue, which represents the termination of the spinal cord. It is flat and has a groove down the middle (**Fig. 53.5**). On surgical dissection, nerve roots projecting ventrally, through the remnants of the sacrum and lumbar bony elements, and laterally, out into the soft tissue and skin, can be identified. The placode tissue tends to dry out before closure, and dressing with sterile gauze kept continuously moist with sterile saline is crucial. Prophylaxis with broad-spectrum antibiotics is administered until the skin defect is closed. Closure within 72 hours of birth is recommended, decreasing the risk of infection and potentially improving neurologic outcome. In a large retrospective review infants undergoing closure within 72 hours showed better bladder stability on urodynamic evaluation than those closed later (87).

Once in the operating room, the patient is handled and managed so as to avoid any further trauma to the placode. The patient is usually intubated in the lateral or supine position, with padding very carefully arranged to avoid any pressure on the meningocele sac or placode.

The dissection begins with a circumferential division of the abnormal, thinly epithelialized translucent tissue, which joins the placode to the surrounding skin. It is important that any residual dermal elements that may end up inside the dura are removed. Such elements can subsequently grow to form intradural dermoid cysts with potential for chronic inflammation and further cord tethering. The tissue of the placode itself is trimmed. Magnification with loupes or operating microscope is extremely helpful in preserving all of the neural tissue but removing any possible dermal remnant. The placode can then be rolled into a tubular structure if its shape permits, anchoring pia to pia using fine sutures. It is important at this stage of the procedure to examine both above and below the placode for other intraspinal pathology, such as a fatty filum or diastematomyelia. Sometimes removal of one lumbar lamina above the area of exposure is necessary to permit full exploration.

Serial cranial ultrasonography is important after myelomeningocele closure as many of these neonates develop hydrocephalus. Progressive ventriculomegaly or symptoms and signs of raised intracranial pressure require insertion of a VP shunt. Similarly, neonates who develop an acute neurologic change, such as stridor, apnea, or swallowing difficulties also need prompt CSF diversion (88). Shunts in this population have a high revision and infection rate (89). Neurologically stable neonates, with stable ventriculomegaly, may be watched carefully and thereby avoid a VP shunt. In many of these infants, head growth will slow and start to follow their centile (88). About 10% of neonates with spina bifida have overt hydrocephalus at birth; insertion of a VP shunt at the same time as myelomeningocele closure is often undertaken in this select group. This may be associated with an increased risk of CSF infection. Overall shunt implantation rates in the spina bifida population have varied from 90% in historical controls to 52% with a conservative watch and wait policy (85).

It is hypothesized that chronic leakage of CSF through the open posterior neuropore into the amniotic fluid reduces expansion of the rhombencephalic vesicle, causing a small posterior fossa and ectopia of the caudal fourth ventricle, brainstem, and

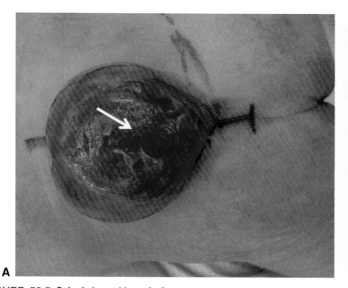
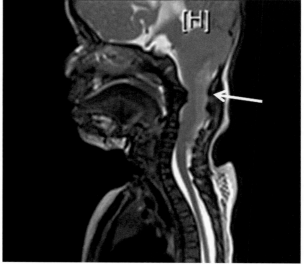

FIGURE 53.5 Spinal dysraphism. A: Preoperative photograph of lumbosacral myelomeningocele; the *white arrow* points to the midline of the placode. **B:** A mid-sagittal T2-weighted MR scan demonstrating the small posterior fossa and Chiari II malformation (*white arrow*).

cerebellar tonsils into the cervical spine, known as the Chiari II malformation. The principal symptoms related to this malformation include central apnea, stridor, vocal cord palsy, and, in older neonates, swallowing difficulties and recurrent chest infections. Hydrocephalus worsens these symptoms by increasing pressure on the brainstem within a crowded posterior fossa. In the first instance, the management of these symptoms involves confirmation of effective CSF diversion (Fig. 53.5B). The role of posterior fossa and cervical spine decompression is unclear; despite effective decompression, neurologic status may still not improve. Such symptoms may be related to abnormal brainstem nuclei organization, rather than simple mechanical brainstem compression (90). It is reasonable to consider decompression if the neonate is normal at birth but then develops acute symptoms despite effective CSF diversion (91).

In view of the associated complications related to open myelomeningocele, care for such neonates is ideally provided by a multidisciplinary team involving specialists from neurosurgery, orthopedics, urology, neurology, and, at a later stage, rehabilitation.

Reliable early diagnosis of myelomeningocele within the second trimester, an improved understanding of the progressive chemical and mechanical injury to the exposed placode during pregnancy, as demonstrated in animal models, and the impact of the small posterior fossa on hydrocephalus and brainstem function stimulated research into prenatal repair. The randomized Management of Myelomeningocele Study (MOMS) recruited patients from three centers and reported in 2011 (92). The study was terminated after recruitment of 187 out of a planned 200 patients due to the benefits in the prenatal surgery arm. The 12-month outcomes for 158 randomized patients are described. *In utero* surgery was undertaken before 26 weeks' gestation. The rate of shunt placement at 12 months was 40% in the prenatal surgery group and 82% in the postnatal surgery group. At 1 year of age, the proportions of infants who had no evidence of hindbrain herniation were 36% and 4%, respectively; brainstem kinking and syringomyelia were also less prevalent in the prenatal group. Infants in the prenatal surgery group were more likely to have a level of function that was two or more levels better than expected from the anatomical level and were better able to walk without orthotics or devices. Pregnancy complications were more common in the prenatal surgery group; the average gestational age at birth for the prenatal group was 34.1 weeks and for the postnatal group was 37.3 weeks. Thirteen percent of neonates in the prenatal group were delivered before 30 weeks and one-fifth had evidence of respiratory distress syndrome at birth (92). A second analysis of the MOMS cohort at 30 months confirmed that prenatal repair improves motor development and reduces the rate of VP shunt requirement (93).

Several neurosurgical units currently offer prenatal myelomeningocele closure, and experience in the technique has grown significantly over the last 8 years. A dedicated team including fetal, obstetric, and neurosurgical expertise is required; extensive preoperative counseling and postnatal care are also essential. In one of the largest post-MOMS published series, 101 mothers underwent intrauterine closure, and similar results to the MOMS trial were obtained (94). The mean gestational age at the time of surgery was 23.3 weeks, and 54% of babies were born at 35 weeks or later. Premature rupture of membranes, oligohydramnios, and maternal transfusion were less common than in the MOMS trial. Seventy-one percent of infants demonstrated no evidence of hindbrain herniation postnatally (94). Some of the pre-MOMS neonates who had undergone fetal closure are now in early adolescence. A recent review of 42 children showed nearly 80% were community ambulators, and only 14% were wheelchair bound at 10 years; 25% had normal bladder function (95). Long-term evaluation of the MOMS and subsequent neonates is eagerly awaited.

Endoscopic fetal closure has the potential to reduce uterine scarring and risk of prematurity. Initial fetoscopic procedures, using an onlay synthetic patch to protect the exposed defect from the amniotic fluid, with subsequent formal skin closure at birth, were not as successful. Progress is being made, however, and early reports of multilayered closure through the endoscopic route are demonstrating a low rate of prematurity and equivalent improvement in hindbrain herniation and the need for CSF diversion (96).

Spinal Dysraphism Other Than Myelomeningocele

Although myelomeningocele is the easiest spinal cord defect to identify, the diagnosis of tethered cord syndrome, spinal lipomas, or other related closed malformations can be made in the newborn period. In general, patients who have hemangiomas, hairy patches, fatty lumps, or deep sinus tracts in the area of the lumbosacral spine deserve investigation within the first few months of life. Spinal ultrasound can be an excellent screening test for determining the level of the conus medullaris, as well as the respiratory excursions of the nerve roots. Ultrasound is also useful in cases of dimples without any other associated findings. As mentioned previously, in the absence of a truly open defect or draining sinus that increases the risk of meningitis or other infection, there is no urgent need to surgically correct these deformities (Fig. 53.6). To diminish the risk of surgical complication, elective repair of tethered spinal cords is typically delayed until the patient is at least 3 months old. Urodynamic evaluation with electromyographic studies of sphincter function can be useful in comparing the preoperative to postoperative bladder functions in precontinent children. An MRI is extremely useful, preferably obtained at several months of age, shortly before surgery, when the characteristics of the tissue allow better anatomic definition of structures.

Encephaloceles

The cranial analogue of the open myelomeningocele is the meningocele or encephalocele (Fig. 53.7). It is part of a spectrum of abnormalities thought to arise from disordered closure of the anterior neuropore. This spectrum spans from cranial dermal sinuses, through cranial meningoceles, to encephaloceles, where meninges and variable amount of brain parenchyma herniates through a cranial defect (88). Again, the availability of ultrasound and MRI scanning antenatally has allowed improvements in the planning and advice given to prospective parents of babies with these problems. As with open myelomeningocele defects, open cranial defects require acute closure, generally within 24 hours of birth, to minimize the risk of meningitis. Closed lesions can be managed in a variety of ways. If the lesion is large or enlarging, or could potentially cause airway obstruction, early repair is required. As with occult spinal dysraphic states, repair of small lesions can be deferred until radiologic imaging quality is maximized and surgical risks are minimized. Vertex encephaloceles are often associated with venous anomalies, such as a vertical straight sinus or a superior sagittal sinus fenestrated or bifurcated at the vertex; radiologic investigations are important to allow safe surgery (97).

The surgical repair of an encephalocele is analogous to myelomeningocele repair. The encephalocele sac is entered and explored for neural tissue. Generally, extracranial tissue is truncated and discarded because it is nonfunctional. The remainder of the repair is devoted to reconstructing a barrier between brain and subcutaneous tissue by repairing the dural lining and forming a reinforced barrier to CSF leakage through the skin.

The normal skin around the margin of the encephalocele is inspected and trimmed to yield a skin edge that eventually can be closed. There is typically a defect in the cranium as well as in the normal dura. As with myelomeningoceles, there is usually a gradual change from normal tissue to abnormal scar tissue around the edges of the lesion. If the encephalocele is large, it is often

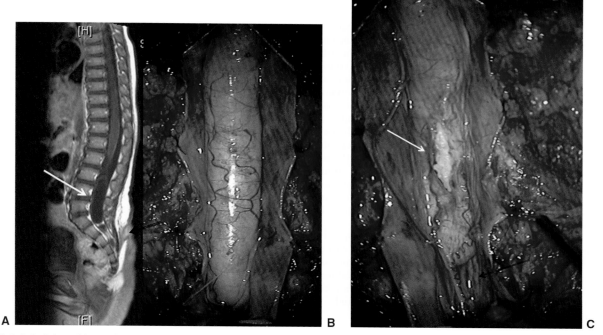

FIGURE 53.6 Spinal dermoid cyst. A: Mid-sagittal postcontrast T1 weighted MR image showing a dermoid cyst (*white arrow*) below the conus. A dermal sinus tract is also visible. **B:** Preoperative photograph showing the dura opened at the midline; the dermoid cyst is visible within the dural sac, and extrudes white keratin when opened **(C)**.

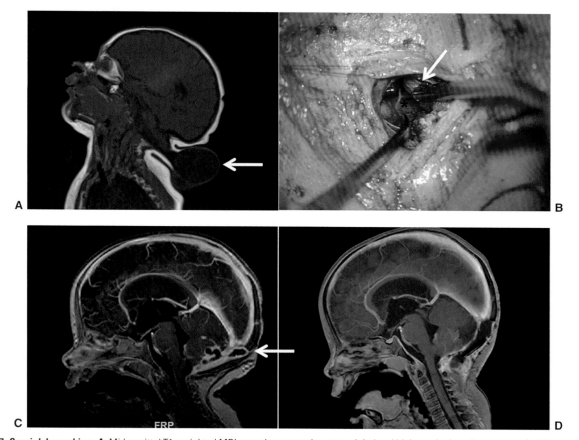

FIGURE 53.7 Cranial dysraphism. A: Mid-sagittal T1-weighted MRI scan demonstrating an occipital and high cervical sac in a neonate (*white arrow*). **B:** An intra-operative photomicrograph, in which the sac has been opened and its CSF has been drained. The cerebellar tonsil on the right has been lightly retracted (*white arrow*) to expose the lower brainstem and upper cervical spine. This represents a Chiari III malformation, a rare anomaly where a high cervical or low occipital neural tube defect may contain cerebellum, brainstem, fourth ventricle, or even occipital lobe. **C:** A postcontrast mid-sagittal MR scan of an occipital dermoid sinus tract. This neonate presented at 4 weeks with symptoms of meningitis. A small closed dimple was evident in the midline at the posterior occipital protuber-ance (*white arrow*). The tract was explored surgically and led through a bone defect to an infected dermoid cyst within the cerebellar vermis. **D:** A postoperative T1-weighted MRI scan with gadolinium confirming resection of the lesion. (Figures **(A)** and **(B)** were kindly provided by Mr. Dominic Thompson.)

essentially pedunculated glial material, and it becomes necessary to amputate the excess neural tissue to allow possibility of closure. The edges of relatively normal dura are identified and then either closed primarily or with a patched graft, which can be taken from pericranium in some cases, or commercially available dural substitute materials can be used. After a watertight seal is created, the scalp over the dural closure is approximated. In some cases, relaxing incisions or rotational flaps have to be made to allow for a satisfactory closure. Postoperatively, the patient must be carefully observed for the development of symptomatic hydrocephalus, which may have been masked by a gradual leakage of fluid out of the encephalocele. Some encephalocele patients require shunts, but most do not. Frontal encephaloceles, commoner in Asia, may project into the cribriform plate and naso-ethmoidal cavities and may require more complex surgical procedures in conjunction with maxillofacial and plastic surgeons.

Outcome in encephaloceles is related to anatomical site, volume of neural contents, and the presence of coexisting malformations (88). More rostral encephaloceles carry a better prognosis. Hydrocephalus and seizures are commoner in those located more occipitally. Herniation of posterior fossa structures and brainstem is a poor prognostic marker. The presence of an associated congenital anomaly adversely affects prognosis (88).

REMOVAL OF EXCESS INTRACRANIAL MASS

An increase in the contents of the cranial vault can be due to sources other than CSF accumulation. Head trauma and congenital CNS tumors are pathophysiologic categories that cause an increase in intracranial contents that are amenable to neurosurgical intervention. Regardless of the etiology, excess intracranial mass may not present with neurologic symptoms because of the distensibility of the neonatal skull. The fontanelle provides the capacity for constant monitoring of intracranial pressure.

Head Trauma in the Neonate

Mechanical injury to the CNS or peripheral nervous system in the neonate generally is a result of conditions immediately surrounding birth itself. These injuries are dramatically less frequent than they were only a decade or two ago, largely because of improvements in monitoring and imaging that have improved the overall level of obstetric care. The true incidence of head trauma is unknown because clinically insignificant injuries are rarely diagnosed. Among diagnosed cases of neonatal head trauma, 1 in 20 is fatal. Isolated spinal cord or brainstem injury has been observed in 3% to 10% of neonatal autopsies (98).

Extracranial injuries resulting in blood collections in the neonate can be important because of the low circulating blood volume and relatively large capacity for sequestration of blood in infants of this size. An important example is subgaleal hemorrhage, where dramatic blood loss can occur because blood collects below the galea and is therefore not bounded by suture lines. Occasionally, these require aspiration of unclotted blood. Coagulopathies and thrombocytopenia should be excluded.

Cephalohematoma is the collection of blood below the pericranium of the outer surface of the skull. It does not cross suture lines, is unilateral, and is almost always over parietal areas. These clots resolve spontaneously over time. Because these hemorrhages are generally self-limited, the clots are usually not aspirated to avoid the risk of introducing infection. Neurosurgical intervention is largely limited to the occasional cephalohematoma that calcifies and causes an obvious cosmetic deformity.

In the majority of cephalohematomas, there is probably an underlying skull fracture that is never formally diagnosed and reduces spontaneously. These minimally depressed, "ping pong" fractures generally involve the parietal bones. If they do not reduce spontaneously, they can either be elevated by limited and careful digital manipulation or can be surgically reduced with a very simple procedure in which an instrument is passed through a small hole adjacent to the fracture to raise it back into place.

Leptomeningeal cysts, also called growing skull fractures, are rare consequences of a skull fracture in which a dural tear has also occurred. The dural tear accommodates herniated cerebral tissue and grows over several months. Treatment involves dural reconstruction with a patch of autologous pericranium, covered by a split calvarial graft (99). Although they only rarely require surgical exploration or treatment, the full range of intracranial injuries can occur in the neonate: epidural, subdural, subarachnoid, and parenchymal hemorrhages. An important sign frequently seen on scans is the accumulation of blood within the leaves of the tentorium, which may mimic a tentorial subdural hematoma. It is important to identify this condition because it may look quite dramatic on computed tomographic scan, but surgical exploration can lead to disastrous, uncontrolled bleeding, essentially from the communication of this intradural space with the sinuses. The distensibility of the head and the open sutures and fontanelle provides the neurosurgeon with unique, direct access to the intracranial space. The newborn's cranium allows for percutaneous aspiration of subdural hematoma or intraparenchymal clot (112).

Spinal Cord Injury

Ligaments are generally lax in the pediatric patient, and in the newborn particularly. However, it is possible to stretch the spinal cord beyond its elastic capacity to the point of injury. Though some patients recover with no observable abnormalities, others will suffer permanent nerve damage that can cause neurologic syndromes with pathophysiologic correlation with the involved nerves. High cervical injury will result in quadriplegia. An extensive lesion of the lower cervical cord would be expected to cause partial dysfunction in the upper extremities, impaired diaphragmatic movement, and paraplegia. The presence or absence of Horner syndrome (failure of sympathetic innervation to the pupil and face on one side) can be an important clue to the structural integrity of the roots emerging from the cervical spinal cord.

Congenital Tumors of the Central Nervous System

There are several types of congenital CNS tumors (**Fig. 53.8**), all of which are rare. In view of their large size, significant mass effect, and vascularity, in the context of a small child with low total blood volume, these tumors present a formidable surgical challenge. Their biologic behavior depends primarily on their histology and biologic behavior (100). Important types of tumors include choroid plexus papillomas, teratomas, and anaplastic lesions such as astrocytomas, glioblastomas, and primary neuroblastomas (101). In a recent single-institution retrospective review on infants presenting with intracranial tumors in the first 3 months of life, the most common histopathologic subtypes were gliomas and embryonal tumors (101). Thirteen of 27 were supratentorial and 14 were infratentorial. Treatment involved a combination of surgery, chemotherapy, and deferred radiotherapy. At a median follow-up of 2.1 years, 44% of patients had died; infants with gliomas were much more likely to survive than those with embryonal tumors. In a separate study, the authors report on 13 infants who underwent neoadjuvant chemotherapy prior to definitive surgical resection (102). This was effective at reducing tumor vascularity and increasing the chance of obtaining gross total tumor resection at a later stage.

In a recently published series of brain tumors presenting under the age of 1 year, from Great Ormond Street Hospital, London, from a total of 98 children, survival was 93% at 1 month, 64% at 1 year, 44% at 5 years, and 28% at 10 years (103). The commonest tumors were choroid plexus papilloma, PNET, and atypical teratoid rhabdoid tumors (ATRT). Low-grade gliomas and choroid plexus

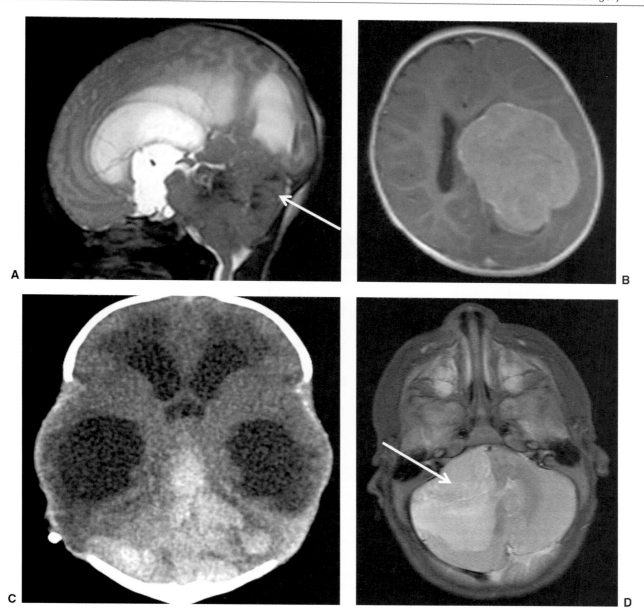

FIGURE 53.8 Neonatal brain tumors. Congenital tumors are rare, and a diagnosis during the neonatal period is unusual. **A:** Mid-sagittal T2-weigthed MR scan showing large posterior fossa atypical teratoid rhabdoid tumor (ATRT) in a term newborn (*white arrow*). **B:** Postcontrast axial MR image showing a large left hemispheric choroid plexus carcinoma. In **(C)**, a newborn presented at 2 days of age with acute neurologic and respiratory deterioration related to acute hemorrhage within a large previously undiagnosed posterior fossa tumor; acute obstructive hydrocephalus is also evident. **D:** A 1-week-old baby presenting with irritability and vomiting was found to have a large right posterior fossa lesion (*white arrow*); histopathology showed an embryonic tumor with multilayered rosettes (ETMR).

tumors had the best prognosis and GBM/PNET the worst. Seventy-seven percent of children reaching school age were in mainstream education. Endovascular embolization (**Fig. 53.9**), staged surgery, and preoperative chemotherapy were important preoperative components of the management strategy (103).

OPENING PREMATURE FUSIONS IN THE NEONATE

Craniofacial Anomalies

With the exception of severe synostosis of all of the sutures, treatment of craniosynostosis is aimed at allowing development of a more cosmetically acceptable spherically shaped skull. It has minimal or no effect on ultimate neurologic outcome. Generally, the earlier synostosis is treated, the less severe is the surgery. The

most common isolated synostosis is sagittal synostosis, which produces a long, narrow cranium, often with a ridge and characteristic lack of movement in the sagittal suture on physical examination. A variety of procedures have been proposed for this condition, but a wide sagittal craniectomy is favored, within the first few months of life. The rounding effect of brain growth is usually adequate for restoring excellent contours. The use of spring-assisted cranioplasty, in which skull incisions free the involved suture and two metallic springs are then inserted to promote cranial reshaping, has become more prevalent (104). New endoscopic techniques have also been used for sagittal and coronal craniosynostoses, reducing blood loss and achieving equivalent long-term results (105). For more complex deformities, particularly the syndromic categories of Crouzon, Apert, and Pfeiffer syndromes, all of which

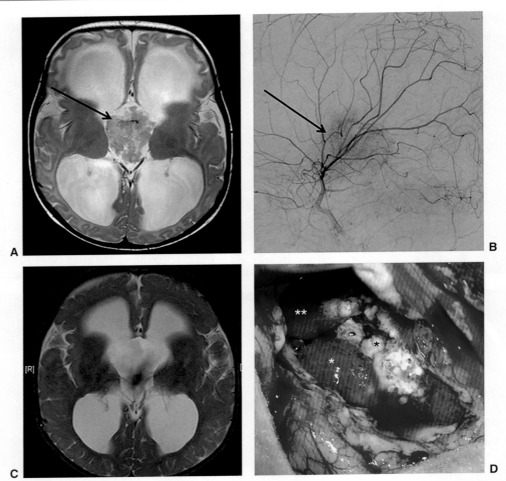

FIGURE 53.9 Choroid plexus tumors. A: T2-weighted axial MR image of a choroid plexus papilloma in the third ventricle presenting with acute hydrocephalus. **B:** Angiography demonstrated a vascular blush (*black arrow*); the lesion was embolized endovascularly. **C:** Postoperative T2-weighted axial MR image after resection of the tumor. Spontaneous improvement in hydrocephalus had been noted after embolization. **D:** An operative photomicrograph of a large choroid plexus papilloma in the lateral ventricle, approached through the cerebral cortex; the blue tumor component (*white asterisk*) is embolized tumor; the red component (*double asterisk*) was not embolized; the white component (*black asterisk*) was coagulated during the resection.

have associated abnormalities of the extremities and other congenital defects, treatment of the brachycephaly is usually deferred for several months beyond the neonatal period so that a more definitive and planned craniofacial approach can be taken, if necessary, with frontal advancement and orbital reshaping.

Treatment of the kleeblattschädel, or cloverleaf deformity, when all sutures are congenitally closed, is the only craniosynostotic syndrome requiring treatment in the neonatal period. Such multisuture synostosis requires early craniectomy, with total calvarial remodeling and expansion. It generally requires one or more frontal advancements, starting several months later, to achieve an acceptable cranial shape. Ventriculomegaly and hydrocephalus with raised intracranial pressure may also occur in the context of multisutural craniosynostosis and early treatment with a VP shunt may be indicated.

CEREBROVASCULAR ANOMALIES OF THE NEWBORN

A wide range of neurovascular pathology has been described in the neonate. The most distinct neonatal neurovascular anomaly is the vein of Galen aneurysmal malformation (VGAM) (**Fig. 53.10**). Arteriovenous malformations, arteriovenous fistulas (dural and pial), as well as cavernous malformations, are also described (106,107).

These lesions can be classified according to the morphology of the channels comprised (e.g., venous vs. arteriovenous), flow characteristics (low vs. high), and location (galenic, parenchymal, pial, or dural). For high-flow lesions, the flow itself becomes the major symptom, with systemic signs of high-output cardiac state and, in severe cases, cardiac failure with multiple organ dysfunction. Smaller lesions with lower flow may present as macrocephaly and hydrocephalus related to the increased venous pressure and subsequent reduction in CSF absorption (105). In addition, as a result of progressive veno-occlusive disease, progressive cerebral atrophy, and intracranial calcification may develop.

VGAMs represent shunting of arterial blood into an ectatic median prosencephalic vein of Markowski. VGAMs are believed to occur between 6 and 11 weeks of gestation as a result of arterial communications, predominantly from the choroidal arteries and the developing anterior cerebral arteries, with the median prosencephalic vein. The proximal part of the median prosencephalic vein normally involutes as the maturing arterial network of the cortex drains into its distal part becoming the vein of Galen. Persisting shunting of arterial inflow throughout its length leads to ectasia and development of VGAM (108). There are two types of VGAMs—the mural type has one or more direct arterial connections into the wall of median prosencephalic vein; in the choroidal type, multiple choroidal feeders form a nidal network that drains into the median prosencephalic vein. In neonates, VGAMs often present with cardiac failure due to the high flow, low resis-

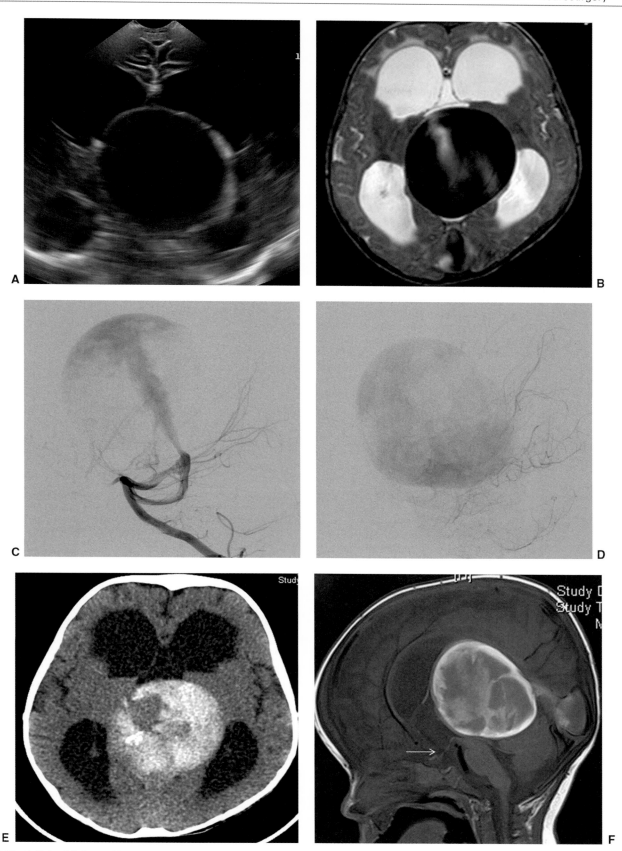

THE NEWBORN INFANT

FIGURE 53.10 Vein of Galen malformation, identified in a newborn presenting with macrocephaly and heart failure, on axial transfontanelle ultrasound (**A**), T2-weighted MRI (**B**) and angiography (**C, D**). Endovascular transarterial embolization led to progressive thrombosis of the sac, demonstrated on CT scan (**E**). The size of the sac caused aqueduct obstruction with hydrocephalus; an endoscopic third ventriculostomy (*white arrow*) on the mid-sagittal postcontrast MR scan in (**F**), reduced the progressive increase in head circumference.

tance arteriovenous connections within the malformation. This may be associated with pulmonary hypertension and myocardial ischemia, particularly if there is also a patent ductus arteriosus (108). Presentation with heart failure and suprasystemic pulmonary hypertension predict poor survival (109).

In neonates, the goal of treatment is stepwise, partial embolization to restore hemodynamic balance. Endovascular embolization can be accomplished by either a transarterial or transvenous route. Although the transarterial modality is preferred by many endovascular centers, a transvenous approach involving access to the venous drainage by transtorcular, transfemoral, or transjugular catheterization can result in subtotal occlusion of the venous drainage, thereby reducing the shunt volume and cardiac failure. Ultimate cure by thrombosis can potentially be seen in either type of therapy. In cases of severe cardiac failure, however, the cardiac prognosis is poor enough that the outcome is guarded. In the largest reported series of 233 patients, the overall mortality was 10.6% but 52% in neonates (110). Seventy-four percent of surviving patients were neurologically normal during a median follow-up of 4.4 years. Longer follow-up, however, has shown that long-term outcome is less favorable than short-term reports suggest; in one recent study that evaluated children aged between 6 and 11 years, 14 of 33 survivors had a poor neurodevelopmental outcome (109). Even those with a good outcome, able to attend normal school, had developed neuropsychological disorders. Complete obliteration of the VGAM was not necessary to achieve a good clinical result. The value of managing these rare and complex lesions within an experienced multidisciplinary team cannot be overstated. Antenatal diagnosis makes such coordinated postnatal evaluation considerably more feasible.

PROGNOSIS AND LONG-TERM OUTLOOK FOR THE NEUROSURGICAL NEONATE

An understanding of the long-term prognosis for any particular type of abnormality is crucial for planning and evaluating therapeutic strategies and for counseling parents. Unfortunately, these weighty decisions must be based on general guidelines that are often not predictive for an individual baby. du Plessis and Volpe have outlined a rational sequence of considerations to use when discussing prognosis in these cases (111). They emphasize the importance of establishing the etiology of a disease process as the most important predictor. Thus, a particular degree of ventriculomegaly may be associated with a significantly worse cognitive prognosis in Dandy-Walker malformation or aqueductal stenosis than in myelomeningocele or communicating PHH. Such differences can be understood on the basis of major contributions from associated cerebral dysgenesis, earlier called the microanatomic malformations or "wiring" abnormalities. In addition, hydrocephalus resulting from infection will depend, to a very large degree, on the nature of the infection at the cellular level. This will be more predictive of developmental outcome than the degree of secondary ventriculomegaly. From the neurosurgical point of view, it is important to separate the portion of projected disability that is based on hydrodynamic or other neurosurgically solvable problems from that which is intrinsic to the neurons themselves and not remediable by the neurosurgeon. In counseling parents, this distinction should be made quite explicitly, and it should be stated that the disease process involves at least two types of processes: those that can be treated with neurosurgical intervention such as a shunt and those that the intervention will not alter. This enables the neurosurgeon to say, for example, that a shunt may be absolutely necessary to treat a particular infant's condition, but that it may not be sufficient to correct the overall neurologic problem. In effect, this defers part of the issue of prognosis back to the medical and neurologic teams, while enforcing the importance of the proposed neurosurgical intervention. Nevertheless, the general

implications of recent literature on the outcome of patients with common neurosurgical conditions should be well understood by neurosurgeons and other clinicians involved at the time of this family counseling.

REFERENCES

1. Wilson-Costello D, Friedman H, Minich N, et al. Improved survival rates with increased neurodevelopmental disability for extremely low birth weight infants in the 1990s. *Pediatrics* 2005;115(4):997.
2. Taylor GA, Madsen JR. Neonatal hydrocephalus: hemodynamic response to fontanelle compression—correlation with intracranial pressure and need for shunt placement. *Radiology* 1996;201(3):685.
3. Ballabh P. Intraventricular hemorrhage in premature infants: mechanism of disease. *Pediatr Res* 2010;67(1):1.
4. Volpe JJ. Brain injury in premature infants: a complex amalgam of destructive and developmental disturbances. *Lancet Neurol* 2009;8(1):110.
5. Larroche JC. Post-haemorrhagic hydrocephalus in infancy. Anatomical study. *Biol Neonate* 1972;20(3):287.
6. Oi S, Di Rocco C. Proposal of "evolution theory in cerebrospinal fluid dynamics" and minor pathway hydrocephalus in developing immature brain. *Childs Nerv Syst* 2006;22(7):662.
7. Johnston M, Zakharov A, Koh L, et al. Subarachnoid injection of Microfil reveals connections between cerebrospinal fluid and nasal lymphatics in the non-human primate. *Neuropathol Appl Neurobiol* 2005;31(6):632.
8. Tamura R, Yoshida K, Toda M. Current understanding of lymphatic vessels in the central nervous system. *Neurosurg Rev* 2020;43(4):1055.
9. Jessen NA, Munk ASF, Lundgaard I, et al. The glymphatic system: a beginner's guide. *Neurochem Res* 2015;40(12):2583.
10. Rudas G, Almássy Z, Varga E, et al. Alterations in spinal fluid drainage in infants with hydrocephalus. *Pediatr Radiol* 1997;27(7):580.
11. Bruce DA, Weprin B. The slit ventricle syndrome. *Neurosurg Clin N Am* 2001;12(4):709, viii.
12. Drake JM, Kestle JR, Milner R, et al. Randomized trial of cerebrospinal fluid shunt valve design in pediatric hydrocephalus. *Neurosurgery* 1998;43(2):294, discussion 303.
13. Koueik J, Kraemer MR, Hsu D, et al. A 12-year single-center retrospective analysis of antisiphon devices to prevent proximal ventricular shunt obstruction for hydrocephalus. *J Neurosurg Pediatr* 2019;1–10.
14. Madsen JR, Abazi GS, Fleming L, et al. Evaluation of the ShuntCheck noninvasive thermal technique for shunt flow detection in hydrocephalic patients. *Neurosurgery* 2011;68(1):198, discussion 205.
15. McAllister JP, Chovan P. Neonatal hydrocephalus. Mechanisms and consequences. *Neurosurg Clin N Am* 1998;9(1):73.
16. Gross SJ, Eckerman CO. Normative early head growth in very-low-birth-weight infants. *J Pediatr* 1983;103(6):946.
17. Sherry B, Mei Z, Grummer-Strawn L, et al. Evaluation of and recommendations for growth references for very low birth weight. *Pediatrics* 2003;111(4 Pt 1):750.
18. Rekate HL. Pathogenesis of hydrocephalus in achondroplastic dwarfs: a review and presentation of a case followed for 22 years. *Childs Nerv Syst* 2019;35(8):1295.
19. McKechnie L, Vasudevan C, Levene M. Neonatal outcome of congenital ventriculomegaly. *Semin Fetal Neonatal Med* 2012;17(5):301.
20. Laskin MD, Kingdom J, Toi A, et al. Perinatal and neurodevelopmental outcome with isolated fetal ventriculomegaly: a systematic review. *J Matern Fetal Neonatal Med.* 2005;18(5):289.
21. Carta S, Kaelin Agten A, Belcaro C, et al. Outcome of fetuses with prenatal diagnosis of isolated severe bilateral ventriculomegaly: systematic review and meta-analysis. *Ultrasound Obstet Gynecol* 2018;52(2):165.
22. Yamasaki M, Nonaka M, Bamba Y, et al. Diagnosis, treatment, and long-term outcomes of fetal hydrocephalus. *Semin Fetal Neonatal Med* 2012;17(6):330.
23. Scala C, Familiari A, Pinas A, et al. Perinatal and long-term outcomes in fetuses diagnosed with isolated unilateral ventriculomegaly: systematic review and meta-analysis. *Ultrasound Obstet Gynecol* 2017;49(4):450.
24. Cavalheiro S, da Costa MDS, Mendonça JN, et al. Antenatal management of fetal neurosurgical diseases. *Childs Nerv Syst* 2017;33(7):1125.
25. Zahl SM, Egge A, Helseth E, et al. Clinical, radiological, and demographic details of benign external hydrocephalus: a population-based study. *Pediatr Neurol* 2019;96:53.
26. Zahl SM, Egge A, Helseth E, et al. Benign external hydrocephalus: a review, with emphasis on management. *Neurosurg Rev* 2011;34(4):417.
27. Kölker S, Christensen E, Leonard JV, et al. Diagnosis and management of glutaric aciduria type I—revised recommendations. *J Inherit Metab Dis* 2011;34(3):677.
28. Gurtner P, Bass T, Gudeman SK, et al. Surgical management of posthemorrhagic hydrocephalus in 22 low-birth-weight infants. *Childs Nerv Syst.* 1992;8(4):198.

29. Frim DM, Scott RM, Madsen JR. Surgical management of neonatal hydrocephalus. *Neurosurg Clin N Am* 1998;9(1):105.

30. Drake JM; Canadian Pediatric Neurosurgery Study Group. Endoscopic third ventriculostomy in pediatric patients: the Canadian experience. *Neurosurgery* 2007;60(5):881, discussion 881.

31. Kulkarni AV, Sgouros S, Constantini S; IIHS Investigators. International Infant Hydrocephalus Study: initial results of a prospective, multicenter comparison of endoscopic third ventriculostomy (ETV) and shunt for infant hydrocephalus. *Childs Nerv Syst* 2016;32(6):1039.

32. Warf BC. Comparison of endoscopic third ventriculostomy alone and combined with choroid plexus cauterization in infants younger than 1 year of age: a prospective study in 550 African children. *J Neurosurg* 2005;103(6 suppl):475.

33. Kulkarni AV, Riva-Cambrin J, Rozzelle CJ, et al. Endoscopic third ventriculostomy and choroid plexus cauterization in infant hydrocephalus: a prospective study by the Hydrocephalus Clinical Research Network. *J Neurosurg Pediatr* 2018;21(3):214.

34. Warf BC, Campbell JW, Riddle E. Initial experience with combined endoscopic third ventriculostomy and choroid plexus cauterization for posthemorrhagic hydrocephalus of prematurity: the importance of prepontine cistern status and the predictive value of FIESTA MRI imaging. *Childs Nerv Syst* 2011;27(7):1063.

35. Riva-Cambrin J, Kestle JRW, Rozzelle CJ, et al. Predictors of success for combined endoscopic third ventriculostomy and choroid plexus cauterization in a North American setting: a Hydrocephalus Clinical Research Network study. *J Neurosurg Pediatr* 2019;1–11.

36. Gram M, Sveinsdottir S, Ruscher K, et al. Hemoglobin induces inflammation after preterm intraventricular hemorrhage by methemoglobin formation. *J Neuroinflammation* 2013;10:100.

37. Wu Y, Song J, Wang Y, et al. The potential role of ferroptosis in neonatal brain injury. *Front Neurosci* 2019;13:115.

38. Whitelaw A, Cherian S, Thoresen M, et al. Posthaemorrhagic ventricular dilatation: new mechanisms and new treatment. *Acta Paediatr Suppl* 2004;93(444):11.

39. Randomised trial of early tapping in neonatal posthaemorrhagic ventricular dilatation: results at 30 months. Ventriculomegaly Trial Group. *Arch Dis Child Fetal Neonatal Ed* 1994;70(2):F129.

40. Whitelaw A, Aquilina K. Management of posthaemorrhagic ventricular dilatation. *Arch Dis Child Fetal Neonatal Ed* 2012;97(3):F229.

41. Kennedy CR, Ayers S, Campbell MJ, et al. Randomized, controlled trial of acetazolamide and furosemide in posthemorrhagic ventricular dilation in infancy: follow-up at 1 year. *Pediatrics* 2001;108(3):597.

42. Hudgins RJ, Boydston WR, Hudgins PA, et al. Treatment of intraventricular hemorrhage in the premature infant with urokinase. A preliminary report. *Pediatr Neurosurg* 1994;20(3):190.

43. Hansen AR, Volpe JJ, Goumnerova LC, et al. Intraventricular urokinase for the treatment of posthemorrhagic hydrocephalus. *Pediatr Neurol* 1997;17(3):213.

44. Luciano R, Velardi F, Romagnoli C, et al. Failure of fibrinolytic endoventricular treatment to prevent neonatal post-haemorrhagic hydrocephalus. A case-control trial. *Childs Nerv Syst* 1997;13(2):73.

45. Whitelaw A, Pople I, Cherian S, et al. Phase 1 trial of prevention of hydrocephalus after intraventricular hemorrhage in newborn infants by drainage, irrigation, and fibrinolytic therapy. *Pediatrics* 2003;111(4 Pt 1):759.

46. Whitelaw A, Evans D, Carter M, et al. Randomized clinical trial of prevention of hydrocephalus after intraventricular hemorrhage in preterm infants: brain-washing versus tapping fluid. *Pediatrics* 2007;119(5):e1071.

47. Whitelaw A, Jary S, Kmita G, et al. Randomized trial of drainage, irrigation and fibrinolytic therapy for premature infants with posthemorrhagic ventricular dilatation: developmental outcome at 2 years. *Pediatrics* 2010;125(4):e852.

48. Luyt K, Jary S, Lea C, et al. Ten-year follow-up of a randomised trial of drainage, irrigation and fibrinolytic therapy (DRIFT) in infants with posthaemorrhagic ventricular dilatation. *Health Technol Assess* 2019;23(4):1.

49. Schulz M, Bührer C, Pohl-Schickinger A, et al. Neuroendoscopic lavage for the treatment of intraventricular hemorrhage and hydrocephalus in neonates. *J Neurosurg Pediatr* 2014;13(6):626.

50. d'Arcangues C, Schulz M, Bührer C, et al. Extended experience with neuroendoscopic lavage for posthemorrhagic hydrocephalus in neonates. *World Neurosurg* 2018;116:e217.

51. Limbrick DD, Mathur A, Johnston JM, et al. Neurosurgical treatment of progressive posthemorrhagic ventricular dilation in preterm infants: a 10-year single-institution study. *J Neurosurg Pediatr* 2010;6(3):224.

52. Brouwer AJ, Groenendaal F, van den Hoogen A, et al. Incidence of infections of ventricular reservoirs in the treatment of post-haemorrhagic ventricular dilatation: a retrospective study (1992-2003). *Arch Dis Child Fetal Neonatal Ed* 2007;92(1):F41.

53. Wellons JC, Shannon CN, Holubkov R, et al. Shunting outcomes in posthemorrhagic hydrocephalus: results of a Hydrocephalus Clinical Research Network prospective cohort study. *J Neurosurg Pediatr* 2017;20(1):19.

54. Levene MI. Measurement of the growth of the lateral ventricles in preterm infants with real-time ultrasound. *Arch Dis Child* 1981;56(12):900.

55. Ingram M-CE, Huguenard AL, Miller BA, et al. Poor correlation between head circumference and cranial ultrasound findings in premature infants with intraventricular hemorrhage. *J Neurosurg Pediatr* 2014;14(2):184.

56. Norooz F, Urlesberger B, Giordano V, et al. Decompressing posthaemorrhagic ventricular dilatation significantly improves regional cerebral oxygen saturation in preterm infants. *Acta Paediatr* 2015;104(7):663.

57. Olischar M, Klebermass K, Hengl B, et al. Cerebrospinal fluid drainage in posthaemorrhagic ventricular dilatation leads to improvement in amplitude-integrated electroencephalographic activity. *Acta Paediatr* 2009;98(6):1002.

58. Brouwer AJ, Brouwer MJ, Groenendaal F, et al. European perspective on the diagnosis and treatment of posthaemorrhagic ventricular dilatation. *Arch Dis Child Fetal Neonatal Ed* 2012;97(1):F50.

59. Leijser LM, Miller SP, van Wezel-Meijler G, et al. Posthemorrhagic ventricular dilatation in preterm infants: when best to intervene? *Neurology* 2018;90(8):e698.

60. de Vries LS, Liem KD, van Dijk K, et al. Early versus late treatment of posthaemorrhagic ventricular dilatation: results of a retrospective study from five neonatal intensive care units in The Netherlands. *Acta Paediatr* 2002;91(2):212.

61. Cizmeci MN, Groenendaal F, Liem KD, van Haastert IC, Benavente-Fernández I, van Straaten HLM, Steggerda S, Smit BJ, Whitelaw A, Woerdeman P, Heep A, de Vries LS; ELVIS study group. Randomized Controlled Early versus Late Ventricular Intervention Study in Posthemorrhagic Ventricular Dilatation: Outcome at 2 Years. J Pediatr 2020;Aug 12:S0022-3476(20)30996-3.doi: 10.1016/j.jpeds.2020.08.014. Epub ahead of print. PMID: 32800815.

62. Alan N, Manjila S, Minich N, et al. Reduced ventricular shunt rate in very preterm infants with severe intraventricular hemorrhage: an institutional experience. *J Neurosurg Pediatr* 2012;10(5):357.

63. Brouwer AJ, Groenendaal F, Han KS, et al. Treatment of neonatal progressive ventricular dilatation: a single-centre experience. *J Matern Fetal Neonatal Med* 2015;28(suppl 1):2273.

64. Pople IK, Bayston R, Hayward RD. Infection of cerebrospinal fluid shunts in infants: a study of etiological factors. *J Neurosurg* 1992;77(1):29.

65. Guzzetta F, Mercuri E, Spanò M. Mechanisms and evolution of the brain damage in neonatal post-hemorrhagic hydrocephalus. *Childs Nerv Syst* 1995;11(5):293.

66. Vasileiadis GT, Gelman N, Han VKM, et al. Uncomplicated intraventricular hemorrhage is followed by reduced cortical volume at near-term age. *Pediatrics* 2004;114(3):e367.

67. Dorner RA, Burton VJ, Allen MC, et al. Preterm neuroimaging and neurodevelopmental outcome: a focus on intraventricular hemorrhage, posthemorrhagic hydrocephalus, and associated brain injury. *J Perinatol* 2018;38(11):1431.

68. Tam EWY, Rosenbluth G, Rogers EE, et al. Cerebellar hemorrhage on magnetic resonance imaging in preterm newborns associated with abnormal neurologic outcome. *J Pediatr* 2011;158(2):245.

69. Adams-Chapman I, Hansen NI, Stoll BJ, et al; NICHD Research Network. Neurodevelopmental outcome of extremely low birth weight infants with posthemorrhagic hydrocephalus requiring shunt insertion. *Pediatrics* 2008;121(5):e1167.

70. van de Bor M, Ouden den L. School performance in adolescents with and without periventricular-intraventricular hemorrhage in the neonatal period. *Semin Perinatol* 2004;28(4):295.

71. Couldwell WT, LeMay DR, McComb JG. Experience with use of extended length peritoneal shunt catheters. *J Neurosurg* 1996;85(3):425.

72. Dallacasa P, Dappozzo A, Galassi E, et al. Cerebrospinal fluid shunt infections in infants. *Childs Nerv Syst* 1995;11(11):643, discussion 649.

73. Sciubba DM, Stuart RM, McGirt MJ, et al. Effect of antibiotic-impregnated shunt catheters in decreasing the incidence of shunt infection in the treatment of hydrocephalus. *J Neurosurg* 2005;103(2 suppl):131.

74. Parker SL, Attenello FJ, Sciubba DM, et al. Comparison of shunt infection incidence in high-risk subgroups receiving antibiotic-impregnated versus standard shunts. *Childs Nerv Syst* 2009;25(1):77, discussion 85.

75. Copp AJ, Adzick NS, Chitty LS, et al. Spina bifida. *Nat Rev Dis Primers* 2015;1:15007.

76. Mallucci CL, Jenkinson MD, Conroy EJ, et al. Antibiotic or silver versus standard ventriculoperitoneal shunts (BASICS): a multicentre, single-blinded, randomised trial and economic evaluation. *Lancet* 2019;394(10208):1530.

77. Alonso-Vanegas M, Alvarez JL, Delgado L, et al. Gastric perforation due to ventriculo-peritoneal shunt. *Pediatr Neurosurg* 1994;21(3):192.

78. Bass T, White LE, Wood RD, et al. Rapid decompression of congenital hydrocephalus associated with parenchymal hemorrhage. *J Neuroimaging* 1995;5(4):249.

79. Steinbok P, Poskitt KJ, Cochrane DD, et al. Prevention of postshunting ventricular asymmetry by transseptal placement of ventricular catheters. A randomized study. *Pediatr Neurosurg* 1994;21(1):59, discussion 65.

80. Rademaker KJ, Govaert P, Vandertop WP, et al. Rapidly progressive enlargement of the fourth ventricle in the preterm infant with post-haemorrhagic ventricular dilatation. *Acta Paediatr* 1995;84(10):1193.

81. Parker SL, Anderson WN, Lilienfeld S, et al. Cerebrospinal shunt infection in patients receiving antibiotic-impregnated versus standard shunts. *J Neurosurg Pediatr* 2011;8(3):259.

82. Levine D, Barnes PD, Madsen JR, et al. Fetal central nervous system anomalies: MR imaging augments sonographic diagnosis. *Radiology* 1997;204(3):635.

83. Madsen J, Estroff J, Levine D. Prenatal neurosurgical diagnosis and counseling. *Neurosurg Clin N Am* 1998;9(1):49.

84. Luthy DA, Wardinsky T, Shurtleff DB, et al. Cesarean section before the onset of labor and subsequent motor function in infants with meningomyelocele diagnosed antenatally. *N Engl J Med* 1991;324(10):662.

85. Bowman DG. Neurosurgical management of spina bifida: research issues. *Dev Disabil Res Rev* 2010;16(1):82.

86. McLone DG. Care of the neonate with a myelomeningocele. *Neurosurg Clin N Am* 1998;9(1):111.

87. Tarcan T, Onol FF, Ilker Y, et al. The timing of primary neurosurgical repair significantly affects neurogenic bladder prognosis in children with myelomeningocele. *J Urol* 2006;176(3):1161.

88. Thompson DNP. Postnatal management and outcome for neural tube defects including spina bifida and encephalocoeles. *Prenat Diagn* 2009;29(4):412.

89. Bowman RM, McLone DG, Grant JA, et al. Spina bifida outcome: a 25-year prospective. *Pediatr Neurosurg* 2001;34(3):114.

90. Fujii M, Tomita T, McLone DG, et al. Natural course of brainstem auditory evoked potentials in infants less than 6 months old with asymptomatic meningomyelocele. *Pediatr Neurosurg* 1996;25(5):227.

91. McLone DG, Dias MS. The Chiari II malformation: cause and impact. *Childs Nerv Syst* 2003;19(7-8):540.

92. Adzick NS, Thom EA, Spong CY, et al. A randomized trial of prenatal versus postnatal repair of myelomeningocele. *N Engl J Med* 2011;364(11):993.

93. Farmer DL, Thom EA, Brock JW, et al. The Management of Myelomeningocele Study: full cohort 30-month pediatric outcomes. *Am J Obstet Gynecol* 2018;218(2):256.e1.

94. Moldenhauer JS, Soni S, Rintoul NE, et al. Fetal myelomeningocele repair: the post-MOMS experience at the Children's Hospital of Philadelphia. *Fetal Diagn Ther* 2015;37(3):235.

95. Danzer E, Thomas NH, Thomas A, et al. Long-term neurofunctional outcome, executive functioning, and behavioral adaptive skills following fetal myelomeningocele surgery. *Am J Obstet Gynecol* 2016;214(2):269.e1.

96. Belfort MA, Whitehead WE, Shamshirsaz AA, et al. Fetoscopic open neural tube defect repair: development and refinement of a two-port, carbon dioxide insufflation technique. *Obstet Gynecol* 2017;129(4):734.

97. Gao Z, Massimi L, Rogerio S, et al. Vertex cephaloceles: a review. *Childs Nerv Syst* 2014;30(1):65.

98. Morota N, Sakamoto K, Kobayashi N. Traumatic cervical syringomyelia related to birth injury. *Childs Nerv Syst* 1992;8(4):234.

99. Tamada I, Ihara S, Hasegawa Y, et al. Surgical treatment of growing skull fracture: technical aspects of cranial bone reconstruction. *J Craniofac Surg* 2019;30(1):61.

100. Fort DW, Rushing EJ. Congenital central nervous system tumors. *J Child Neurol* 1997;12(3):157.

101. Qaddoumi I, Carey SS, Conklin H, et al. Characterization, treatment, and outcome of intracranial neoplasms in the first 120 days of life. *J Child Neurol* 2011;26(8):988.

102. Van Poppel M, Klimo P, DeWire M, et al. Resection of infantile brain tumors after neoadjuvant chemotherapy: the St. Jude experience. *J Neurosurg Pediatr* 2011;8(3):251.

103. Toescu SM, James G, Phipps K, et al. Intracranial neoplasms in the first year of life: results of a third cohort of patients from a single institution. *Neurosurgery* 2019;84(3):636.

104. Borghi A, Schievano S, Rodriguez Florez N, et al. Assessment of spring cranioplasty biomechanics in sagittal craniosynostosis patients. *J Neurosurg Pediatr* 2017;20(5):400.

105. Jimenez DF, McGinity MJ, Barone CM. Endoscopy-assisted early correction of single-suture metopic craniosynostosis: a 19-year experience. *J Neurosurg Pediatr* 2018;23(1):61.

106. Zuccaro G, Argañaraz R, Villasante F, et al. Neurosurgical vascular malformations in children under 1 year of age. *Childs Nerv Syst* 2010;26(10):1381.

107. Burrows PE, Robertson RL. Neonatal central nervous system vascular disorders. *Neurosurg Clin N Am* 1998;9(1):155.

108. Recinos PF, Rahmathulla G, Pearl M, et al. Vein of Galen malformations: epidemiology, clinical presentations, management. *Neurosurg Clin N Am* 2012;23(1):165.

109. Taffin H, Maurey H, Ozanne A, et al. Long-term outcome of vein of Galen malformation. *Dev Med Child Neurol* 2020;62(6):729.

110. Lasjaunias PL, Chng SM, Sachet M, et al. The management of vein of Galen aneurysmal malformations. *Neurosurgery* 2006;59(5 suppl 3):S184, discussion S3.

111. du Plessis A, Volpe JJ. Prognosis for development in the newborn requiring neurosurgical intervention. *Neurosurg Clin N Am* 1998;9(1):187.

112. Macdonald RL, Hoffman HJ, Kestle JR, et al. Needle aspiration of acute subdural hematomas in infancy. *Pediatr Neurosurg* 1994;20(1):73, discussion 77.

54 Neonatal Abstinence Syndrome

Hendrée E. Jones, Gerri R. Baer, and Jonathan M. Davis

A HISTORY OF OPIOID USE IN WOMEN

Early History and Opioid Definition

Humans have used opium since the earliest times known to humankind as recorded in medical documents written in 2100 BC. Communities in Greece, Cyprus, and Egypt also had knowledge of the opium poppy (1). Physicians from many cultures around the world mixed opium with other substances in search of a treatment for all diseases including alleviating pain for women for gynecologic problems and during and after childbirth. Opioids are now generally defined as substances binding to opioid receptors of delta, kappa, and mu. Different opioids have variable receptor-binding affinity and may stimulate or block the receptors (agonist or antagonist, respectively) (2). While nociception and analgesia are established domains of the mu receptor, the functions of the delta and kappa receptors are less well articulated. In the early 1800s, morphine, a mu-receptor (μ) agonist, was isolated from opium allowing for a safer and more consistent effect (1). The development of more pure forms of opioids ushered in an era of recreational opioid use in addition to medical use.

Opioid Use Varies around the World

The United Nations report on pain reliever use shows that the United States uses more opioid pain medicine than any other country (3). In fact, the United States uses 50% more opioids than Germany, the next highest using country (which may be related to the size of the population). Global opioid use is also high in Canada, Australia, and parts of Europe. In contrast, many other countries have very limited access to opioids to treat pain. While opioids can improve the quality of life through pain control, they can also cause significant harm through fatal overdose and addiction. For example, the United States constitutes 4% of the world population, yet has 27% of the world's drug overdose deaths. Overdose deaths and addiction have been directly linked to prescription opioids in the United States with 75% of those who began their opioid misuse reporting that they started with a prescription opioid. That trajectory shifted in the past decade with heroin increasing as the primary opioid of misuse (4).

Opioid Use or Misuse and its Relationship to Neonatal Opioid Withdrawal

While the prevalence of opioid use around the world among women of childbearing age continues to increase, it is critical to examine the different types of use and the extent of the problems encountered (5). For example, substance use of all types, including opioids, occurs on a continuum that encompasses no, occasional, and regular use. Opioid use that occurs after adverse consequences in life domains leads to a diagnosis of opioid use disorder (OUD) that is graded as mild, moderate, or severe according to the Diagnostic and Statistical Manual, Fifth Edition (DSM-5) criteria. For women who continue to use opioids without a prescription after pregnancy awareness, such behavior indicates that they have at least a mild OUD that merits intervention. Consistent with the general population, the prevalence of OUD at delivery has significantly increased from 1.5 per 1,000 in 1999 to 6.5 per 1,000 delivery hospitalizations in 2014 (6). However, the proportion of women who deliver: (a) while taking opioid agonist medications for OUD, (b) with active yet untreated OUD, or (c) while taking opioids that were prescribed for treatment of chronic pain are unknown. Such data are needed because management of the mother who

has taken opioids during pregnancy and her neonate, who may have postnatal opioid withdrawal (e.g., neonatal abstinence syndrome—NAS), both require individualized approaches within the bounds of standard medical care.

DEFINING NEONATAL ABSTINENCE SYNDROME

Early History of Neonatal Withdrawal from Opioids

Given that men and women have been using opioids for centuries, it is not surprising that women may use opioids for a variety of reasons after becoming pregnant. When neonates are delivered and the umbilical cord is cut, drug supply is terminated abruptly and signs of withdrawal can then occur. The first documented case of neonatal opioid withdrawal was in 1875 in Germany (7) and then in the United States in 1892 (8). The term "congenital morphinism" was coined, and later "infant addiction" and "congenital neonatal addiction" were used to describe neonatal opioid withdrawal (9,10). Early cases were often fatal due to the lack of effective treatments used to alleviate withdrawal (e.g., breast-feeding only, opium smoke exposure, etc.) (11). The term "Neonatal Abstinence Syndrome" (NAS) emerged in 1975 to describe withdrawal from opioids as well as substances such as alcohol, tobacco, and other psychotropic medications (12,13). Similar to opioid withdrawal in adults, opioid withdrawal in the neonate is characterized by gastrointestinal distress (e.g., loose stools, vomiting) and autonomic dysfunction (e.g., irritability, tremors, hypertonicity, difficulty sleeping, temperature dysregulation, sneezing etc.). The neonate with untreated opioid withdrawal differs from an adult due to the potential impact of withdrawal on growth and development. Untreated withdrawal can lead to feeding problems (e.g., uncoordinated suck–swallow reflexes, not latching, etc.), increased caloric needs, and loss of fluids due to diarrhea and vomiting. These problems may lead to dehydration, suboptimal growth and development, and impaired maternal–infant attachment.

Neonatal Opioid Withdrawal Syndrome—A Subset of Neonatal Abstinence Syndrome

NAS is a nonspecific term that could refer to neonatal withdrawal from a variety of psychotropic substances. To more clearly link the postnatal withdrawal to prenatal opioid exposure, government agencies (e.g., U.S. Department of Health and Human Services) have suggested the more specific term neonatal opioid withdrawal syndrome (NOWS). "NOWS" highlights opioids as the driving factor in the signs of withdrawal. The term "NAS" continues to be used in the literature to reflect common polysubstance exposure, as withdrawal signs are likely opioid related but may be altered by other nonopioid substances (prescribed or illicit) (14).

Pathophysiology of Opioid Withdrawal

Maternal opioids easily pass through the placenta and enter the fetal circulation. At birth the maternal supply of opioids to the neonate ceases and physical withdrawal can then occur. NAS occurs on a continuum and may depend on the bioavailability and pharmacokinetic profile of the opioid (and/or other substances) and the ability of the drug(s) to cross the fetal blood–brain barrier (15). The cellular and molecular mechanisms that correlate with the physiology and clinical signs of withdrawal (including from opioids) have yet to be fully elucidated. Additional challenges to understanding NAS involve the rapid developmental and maturational changes that occur in the fetal and postnatal periods. Further adding to the complexity is that opioids act largely through opioid receptors, which are primarily distributed across the central and peripheral nervous systems and the gastrointestinal tract. While the affinity and density of mu-receptors in the neonatal brain are comparable to adults, this may not be true for kappa and delta receptors (16). A reduced number of opioid receptors that are in a chronically stimulated state increase overall activity leading to increased adenyl cyclase activity and cellular ionic imbalance. Ultimately, these changes result in the increased production of various neurotransmitters through a cascade of enzymatic activities (e.g., increased noradrenaline, acetylcholine, corticotrophin; decreased serotonin, dopamine) (17) that may help frame the signs of withdrawal as a stress response (18). NAS can be seen as early as 24 to 48 hours after birth and as long as 120 to 240 hours after birth (depending on fetal exposure) (18). Observation for up to 5 days prior to discharge in most neonates will be adequate to allow time for significant signs of withdrawal to appear (19).

TOOLS TO IDENTIFY AND ASSESS NAS

Screening for Maternal Opioid Use

Pregnancy represents a unique opportunity to provide medical care to both the mother and fetus. Pregnant women may be taking opioids prescribed therapeutically or may have an active OUD. Although universal screening for an OUD using standard verbal instruments is recommended for all pregnant women, studies have suggested that many health care providers do not routinely perform these assessments (20). If an OUD is suspected and with the mother's consent, urine toxicology testing may provide important information about what drugs the fetus has been exposed to. However, this testing is not sufficient to diagnose an OUD. When the neonate is born, samples of urine, meconium, or umbilical

cord can be sent for testing using immunoassays and/or liquid chromatography time-of-flight mass spectrometry (21,22). These testing approaches have been studied, but research has been complicated by (a) small sample size, (b) differences in drug deposition and accumulation, (c) inconsistent limits of detection, (d) inconsistent testing panels of drugs and their metabolites, (e) difficulties collecting meconium, and (f) differences in assay methods.

In the past, neonatal urine was routinely collected to test for the presence of various licit and illicit substances. However, it is now recognized that the first void may be difficult to obtain and typically reflects drug exposure within days of delivery, with low sensitivity for more distant exposures (21). Although meconium drug screening is now considered the "gold standard," some have suggested that umbilical cord tissue may have higher sensitivity to detect both recent and more remote antenatal opioid exposures. Colby and associates tested meconium and umbilical cord tissue from 501 neonates born to mothers with substance use disorders (23). Although the overall agreement between umbilical cord and meconium ranged from 80% to 100%, paired results often demonstrated significant discordance. The sensitivity for detecting opioids in umbilical cord tissue ranged from 53% for most opioids to 75% for methadone. In another study, five individual opioids were able to be detected in meconium (24). For three of the five opioids, the concentration of drug measured in meconium did not correlate well with qualitative detection in umbilical cord. These data suggest that there are different sensitivities of drug detection in umbilical cord tissue and meconium. For opioids, meconium appears to provide greater sensitivity and is likely to remain the specimen of choice since sensitivity is usually of greatest importance.

Clinical Signs of Withdrawal

Table 54.1 summarizes the various scoring tools that exist to quantify the signs and severity of withdrawal in NAS. These tools

TABLE 54.1

Measures that Assess NAS

Name of NAS Assessment	Number of Items	Comments
Finnegan Neonatal Abstinence Scoring Tool (FNAST) (13)	21	• Developed as a research tool by Loretta Finnegan in 1975 • Comprehensive training needed • Frequent booster trainings can reduce variability. • FNAST (with many modifications) remains the predominant approach used worldwide, likely because of its comprehensive nature.
Simplified Finnegan Neonatal Abstinence Scoring Tool (sFNAST) (25)	10	• More rapid and objective assessment of neonates • Pearson's correlation between the sFNAST and the FNAST was 0.914. • Optimal treatment cutoff values for the sFNAST were 6 and 10 to predict FNAST scores ≥8 and ≥12, respectively. • Excellent specificity and negative predictive value for identifying infants with FNAST scores ≥8 and ≥12 (typically when neonates receive pharmacologic treatment)
MOTHER NAS scale (MNS) Short Form (26)	5	• The AUC of the five-item MNS was 0.90, which was close to the AUC of 0.94 for the 19-item MNS.
Lipsitz Tool (also known as Neonatal Drug Withdrawal Scoring System) (27)	11	• Less comprehensive than the FNAST and not routinely used
The Neonatal Withdrawal Inventory (28)	11	• Simplified scoring system with better interrater reliability than the FNAST • Interrater reliability (range, 0.89–0.98) was superior to the FNAST (range, 0.70–0.88). • Allows for accurate assessment within 10 min under blinded conditions
The Neonatal Narcotic Withdrawal Index (NNWI) (29)	7	• This scoring system results in fewer neonates requiring pharmacotherapy and shorter length of treatment compared with neonates with similar exposures who were not assessed with the NNWI.
Eat, Sleep, and Console (ESC) (30)	3	• Approach that focuses on three central signs of withdrawal that impact important physiologic functions, that is, eating, sleeping, and ability to be consoled • Fewer neonates receive pharmacologic treatment compared to other approaches. • Widespread applicability and impact on short- and longer-term outcomes being investigated

were primarily designed to evaluate term neonates in relation to maternal opioid exposure (31,32). However, available tools can be complicated to use, have high interrater variability, and require significant training (initial and ongoing) to improve accuracy and reduce subjectivity. Only a few are in widespread use today.

Several studies report the FNAST may be streamlined without loss of accuracy (25). For example, Devlin and associates demonstrated that 8 (sleeps <3 hours after feeding, any tremors, increased muscle tone, fever ≥37.2°C, respiratory rate greater than 60 per minute, excessive sucking, poor feeding, regurgitation) of 21 items were independently associated ($p < 0.05$) with pharmacologic therapy, with area under the curve = 0.86 (95% CI: 0.79, 0.93) (33). Thresholds of 4 and 5 for the simplified scale yielded the closest agreement with FNAST thresholds of 8 and 12 (weighted κ = 0.55, 95% CI: 0.48 to 0.61). These 8 signs of withdrawal appear sufficient to assess whether a neonate meets criteria for pharmacologic therapy. Of note, 7 of the 8 items in the Devlin et al. scale were also reported in the sFNAST study (33).

A five-item MOTHER NAS scale (tremors while undisturbed, increased muscle tone, excoriation, tachypnea, excessive irritability) has similar items and also appears sufficient for determining the use of pharmacologic treatment for NAS (26). A focus on these signs could simplify and significantly enhance the clinical utility of the FNAST.

The NICU Network Neurobehavioral Scale (NNNS) has demonstrated significant neurobehavioral differences between neonates prenatally exposed to methadone who did or did not require pharmacotherapy to treat NAS (34,35). The NNNS has not been used to assess NAS treatment, yet it may capture additional signs not included in the FNAST and may serve as a clinical tool to examine neurobehavioral outcomes of opioid-exposed neonates (36).

Other efforts to assess neonates for NAS have included (a) measurement of skin conductance (37,38), (b) larger pupillary diameters in neonates needing pharmacotherapy (39), and (c) alterations in sleep state with increased wakeful periods in neonates with NAS compared to healthy control neonates (40). Future studies aim to develop an objective and simple assessment tool that can be uniformly applied to all prenatally opioid-exposed neonates to more accurately and efficiently define the need for pharmacologic treatment and the response.

INCIDENCE AND SEVERITY OF NAS

As the rates of opioid use increased in the United States and Canada, so did the rates of NAS. Between 2000 and 2014, the incidence of NAS rose from 1.2 to 8.0 per 1,000 hospital births in the United States (41), and between 2003 and 2016 NAS rates increased from 0.99 to 5.94 per 1,000 live births in Ontario, Canada (42). For both countries, there are differences in NAS incidence by geography, with rural populations having higher rates of NAS compared to high-density urban population areas.

NAS Severity Occurs on a Continuum

Similar to acute withdrawal in adults, withdrawal in neonates occurs along a continuum. Many neonates with regular prenatal opioid exposure will demonstrate signs of NAS after birth. However, there are numerous factors that appear to modify the expression, timing, and intensity of NAS including the timing and duration of prenatal opioid use, types of opioids used (e.g., prescription opioids, illicit opioids), cigarette smoking, polysubstance use (e.g., other illicit substances and/or psychotropic medications), sex of the child, and birth weight (19).

The short-term use of prescription opioids during pregnancy without additional risk factors was found to be associated with a lower risk of NAS compared to longer-term opioid use (defined as >30 days), especially when the additional risk factors described above are present (e.g., absolute risk of NAS 5.9 per 1,000 births

vs. 220 per 1,000 births, respectively) (43). This finding may be reassuring both to women taking opioids for a limited time during pregnancy and their physicians prescribing the opioids. Furthermore, the absolute dose of opioid agonist medications (methadone or buprenorphine) has not been found to significantly and consistently be related to measures of NAS severity (44–47).

Other Substance Exposure and Withdrawal

Substances such as alcohol, cannabis, and/or stimulants (cocaine and methamphetamines) have not been found to produce a specific withdrawal syndrome. However, simultaneous exposure to cocaine and heroin is associated with more severe NAS (48) compared to cocaine and methadone, which has been found to have more variable effects (18,49,50). Among neonates exposed to prenatal buprenorphine, polysubstance exposure is a strong predictor of NAS severity (51). Furthermore, fetal exposure to selective serotonin reuptake inhibitors (SSRIs), benzodiazepines, and tobacco influences the severity of NAS. When SSRIs are taken by pregnant women receiving either methadone or buprenorphine for their OUD, higher peak NAS scores and doses of morphine needed to treat NAS have been noted (19,52). Despite higher scores and need for more pharmacologic treatment, SSRI use does not appear to correlate with the duration of treatment for neonates prenatally exposed to methadone or buprenorphine (50,53).

Benzodiazepine use (prescribed and/or misused) in pregnant women receiving methadone or buprenorphine is also associated with increased use and duration of pharmacologic treatment for NAS, longer hospital stay, and more adjunct medication use relative to neonates without this exposure (54,55). More recently, it has been noted that prescribed and nonprescribed gabapentin use is increasing among individuals who take opioids. In two of three studies, gabapentin appears to alter NAS expression of the neonates. (54,56) Gabapentin administered to neonates with or without an opioid agonist may help alleviate clinical signs of NAS when more standard treatments are not effective. For neonates prenatally exposed to prescription opioids, prenatal exposure to two or more psychotropic medications was associated with a twofold increased risk of NAS (57).

One of the most common substances used in conjunction with opioids is tobacco. Cigarette smoking among women receiving methadone or buprenorphine for OUD adversely affects the total amount of medication required to treat NAS and length of treatment (58). The impact of smoking on NAS outcomes is clearly associated with the number of cigarettes smoked daily. Thus, smoking cessation/reduction/intervention programs may be highly beneficial for pregnant women with OUD, and their infants.

Other Factors Related to NAS Expression

Male sex has been associated with a higher risk and severity of NAS in some studies, but this association is inconsistent (59,60). Higher birth weight has been a predictor of requiring medication to treat NAS (19,50,61). Although this finding correlates with gestational age at delivery, women should not be delivered early to reduce the risk of NAS.

There are nonpharmacologic actions that caregivers and clinicians can take to influence NAS expression. These supports are aimed at enhancing neonatal regulation of the central and autonomic nervous systems so that NAS does not impair feeding, sleeping, and the neonate's ability to be alert and communicate cues to caregivers. Such actions and environmental supports can greatly reduce the use of pharmacologic treatment of NAS as well as shorten the length of hospital stay (14).

The Genetics and Epigenetics of NAS

Significant variability has been observed in the expression of NAS in neonates exposed to opioids and other psychotropic drugs in utero. Associated genetic and/or epigenetic factors involved in maternal, fetal, and placental drug metabolism and opioid receptor expression may play a significant role. Rapidly improving "chip" and sequencing technology has increased the possibilities of discovering genomic variants that could better explain the development and severity of NAS and facilitate new therapeutic strategies (62). Previous studies in neonates with antenatal opioid exposure have found an association (in both mothers and their neonates) of specific single nucleotide polymorphisms (SNPs) in the *OPRM1, COMT, and PNOC* genes associated with a shorter length of hospital stay and less need for treatment (63,64). A single base pair change leading to a single amino acid substitution can affect the protein/receptor significantly (changing the dynamics of endogenous and exogenous opioid binding and metabolism). Epigenetic regulation of these same genes (methylation) also appears to contribute to disease severity, potentially by silencing important regulatory elements (65). Some of these findings have been subsequently validated in independent cohorts (66). Ongoing and future studies must include much larger cohorts with comprehensive clinical and demographic data linked to genetic/epigenetic information to establish predictive models and a better understanding of the pharmacogenomics of NAS.

TREATMENT APPROACHES FOR NAS

The general principles of treatment include monitoring neonates for signs of NAS, optimizing nonpharmacologic care, treating with medication(s) when needed, and systematically tapering medications as signs resolve. The specifics of treatment protocols may vary across clinicians, medical centers, regions, and countries, and there is no consensus to guide the optimal threshold for medication, pharmacologic regimen, or tapering protocols. Quality improvement efforts with standardization of care pathways appear to reduce the length of pharmacologic treatment (67).

Nonpharmacologic Treatment for NAS

Once an in utero exposure has been identified, the first course of action is to optimize nonpharmacologic care to reduce any emerging signs of NAS. However, there are no broadly accepted standardized approaches to effective nonpharmacologic care (68). Table 54.2 provides commonly used nonpharmacologic interventions (69). Opioid-exposed neonates who are managed successfully with nonpharmacologic measures should be monitored in the hospital for 5 to 7 days prior to discharge (70).

Pharmacologic Treatment for NAS
Opioid Agonists

If nonpharmacologic approaches alone fail to adequately control the signs of NAS, then medication is required. Appropriate medication treatment approaches are designed to promote growth and development, treat physiologic effects of withdrawal, and allow for mother–infant bonding. The foundation of pharmacologic treatment for NAS is treatment with an opioid, typically morphine or methadone. Some clinicians are using sublingual buprenorphine, but the existing formulation contains 30% alcohol, which may be harmful to neonates. Opioid agonist medications have been

TABLE 54.2	
Nonpharmacologic Approaches to Reduce Signs of NAS	
Observation	**Nonpharmacologic Response**
Prenatal exposure to opioids is known	• Keep room quiet and dim. • Mother and child room together • Skin-to-skin contact • Encourage breast-feeding in mothers without active illicit drug use and HIV infection. • Tube feeding, intravenous fluids, and electrolyte replacement may be needed. • In-hospital monitoring of neonates with opioid exposure for 5–7 d prior to discharge.
Hyper- or hyporesponsive neonates to sensory stimulation and regulatory issues	• Handling of infant should be soft and slow. • Specific holding/containing techniques • Newborn's hands against his/her chest in a supine or side position, providing firm but gentle pressure to the trunk or head • Swaddling may help to better tolerate stimulation. • Look for self-soothing abilities, such as bringing the hands to the mouth or self-clinging. • Education on supporting child and not discouraging the neonate's self-soothing behaviors • Consider using a pacifier for organizing a dysregulated infant and preventing disorganization during activity.
Behavioral states, transitions between states and duration in states	• Environment should be tailored to helping the neonate achieve quiet alert or restful sleep states. • Only wake a neonate who is sleeping if feeding is needed. • Slow arousal, keeping the environment minimally stimulating, and using gentle handling before feeding, bathing, or changing • A pacifier, gentle and slow vertical rocking, and containing the arms can facilitate eye contact and interaction. • Using black and white objects or determining which colors or visual stimuli are comfortable may prevent overstimulation.
Motor and tone control	• Gentle handling • Positioning • Nonnutritive sucking and swaddling • Simulating the fetal position • Slow vertical rocking may help with relaxation. • If neonates are hyperthermic, may just need a blanket across the chest to contain the arms • Helping the neonate to keep the head still to facilitate the insertion of a pacifier or breast nipple • Frequent burping during feeds and rubbing the back instead of patting
Autonomic signs of stress	• Teach staff and caregivers to monitor for signs of stress (e.g., hiccups, color change, spitting up, bowel sounds, sneezing, back arching). • If signs of stress are noted, modify care. • Teach caregivers to avoid vigorous stimulation. • Provide small and frequent feedings with gentle handling.

shown to be effective in numerous clinical trials and retrospective examinations in controlling signs of NAS (14). Once medication is initiated, the dose may be titrated up until signs are minimal. If nonpharmacologic measures and opioid substitution are not adequate to manage the signs of NAS, an adjunct medication may be added (e.g., phenobarbital, clonidine). Following a period of clinical stability, medication doses are carefully and gradually reduced and then discontinued. Table 54.3 summarizes the medications to treat NAS and includes both opioid agonists and nonopioids. Diluted tincture of opium is no longer recommended.

TABLE 54.3
Types of Medications Used to Treat NAS

Type of Medication	Pharmacology	Dosing for NAS	Key Research Support
Opioids			
Morphine	• Natural μ-receptor agonist • Oral bioavailability 40%–50% • Undergoes first-pass hepatic metabolism by the cytochrome P-450 system • Half-life 6–9 h in term neonates, 2–4 h in older infants and children • Metabolized by glucuronidation and demethylation • Glucuronidation results in active metabolites including morphine-3 glucuronide (M3G) and morphine-6 glucuronide (M6G). • ~5% demethylated and eliminated via the gastrointestinal tract • Most metabolites are water soluble and excreted by the kidney. • Developmental trajectory of glucuronidation changes over the first few weeks of life	• No universal regimen (32) • **Weight-based dosing:** Initiate 0.02–0.06 mg/kg/dose given every 3–4 h, can increase by 0.05 mg/kg/dose to a maximum of 0.2 mg/kg/dose—literature references give maximum daily dose of 1.3 mg/kg/d • **Sign-based dosing:** uses fixed doses based upon severity of signs (31) • Standard neonatal morphine solution (NMS) concentration is 0.4 mg/mL.	• Weight-based more common; assumes that patient weight is the primary source of variability • A hybrid dosing regimen combining the two approaches has been used in the setting of a clinical trial comparing methadone and morphine (71).
Methadone (30)	• Synthetic complete μ-receptor agonist and N-methyl-D-aspartate (NMDA) receptor antagonist • Lipophilic with high bioavailability (>90% in most patients) • Plasma half-life 16–25 h • Metabolized in the liver by demethylation and cytochrome P-450 cyclization	• Suggested initial dose 0.05–0.1 mg/kg/dose every 6–24 h followed by a detailed escalation and tapering regimen • Maximum recommended dose 1 mg/kg/d	• Several studies have demonstrated a shorter length of stay in neonates treated with methadone (71–73). • In all published reports, safety appears to be similar between methadone and other opioids in an inpatient setting.
Buprenorphine (74)	• Semisynthetic partial μ-receptor agonist; κ-receptor antagonist • Half-life in neonates is ~11 h. • Metabolized by CYP3A4/5 and to a lesser extent fetal CYP3A7	• Suggested initial dose 4–5 μg/kg/dose every 8 h, may be increased to total 60 μg/kg/d (72) • There is no age-appropriate formulation currently marketed. • The formulation used in referenced clinical studies contains 30% ethanol and can be stored at room temperature for ≥30 d.	• Small RCTs and observational studies suggest decreased length of treatment using buprenorphine (vs. morphine or methadone) (75,76). • *Maternal* use of buprenorphine has a favorable profile relative to methadone for MAT, with a lower incidence and severity of withdrawal in neonates with NAS (77).
Nonopioid medications			
Clonidine (74)	• α-2-adrenergic agonist, affecting central presynaptic receptors • Inhibits norepinephrine release and down-regulates sympathetic tone • Elimination half-life 48–72 h in neonates and clearance increases markedly in the second week of life. • Oral bioavailability of clonidine is ~90%. • Metabolized by CYP enzymes, primarily CYP2D6	• Typically used as adjunctive therapy • Suggested initial dose: 0.5–1 μg/kg, followed by 0.5–1.25 μg/kg/dose every 4–6 h	• A placebo-controlled RCT of clonidine given in parallel to morphine (in the form of diluted tincture of opium) was associated with lower doses of morphine and had a significantly shorter duration of treatment compared with morphine alone (78). • A pilot study of clonidine vs. morphine as primary therapy for NAS demonstrated significantly shorter duration of treatment with clonidine (79).
Phenobarbital (also known as phenobarbitone) (74)	• GABA_A receptor agonist • Half-life in neonates ranges from 67 to 115 h.	• Most commonly used adjunctive therapy • Suggested loading dose 16 mg/kg on day 1, followed by 1–4 mg/kg every 12 h	• More global sedative effect and is less specific to opioid-driven signs than clonidine • It may provide additional benefit in cases where the fetus has been exposed to both opioids and other psychotropic medications. • Long-term studies raise concerns of adverse neurodevelopmental outcomes.

THE NEWBORN INFANT

Nonopioid Medications

Although small studies have examined nonopioid medications such as clonidine or phenobarbital as a primary treatment of NAS, these medications are typically used as adjunctive treatment when the opioid did not adequately reduce NAS severity. Such combination drug treatment with an opioid may be synergistic, resulting in enhanced efficacy. The opioid is often weaned first followed by tapering of the adjunct medication in an inpatient or outpatient setting. Completion of adjunctive pharmacologic therapy as an outpatient may be associated with a shorter hospitalization, but longer total duration of therapy (80). However, shorter hospital stays may not be the best outcomes to assess the adequacy of treatment. In a population-based observation of 532 infants treated with phenobarbital in the state of Tennessee, outpatient treatment was associated with higher number of emergency department visits over the first 6 months of life (81). Though not statistically significant, the point estimate odds ratio for an emergency visit at 6 weeks, or any hospitalization at 6 or 24 weeks was approximately 1.5 times higher for outpatient compared to inpatient treatment. This phased medication approach is more common for phenobarbital than clonidine. Another strategy is initiating treatment with both an opioid and clonidine therapy, which may reduce the total duration of pharmacologic treatment. The optimal protocol for NAS management with adjunctive medications has not been clearly defined.

CHOOSING AN NAS MEDICATION REGIMEN

Two recent systematic reviews/meta-analyses compared various pharmacotherapies to treat NAS (75,82). In both meta-analyses, length of treatment for the opioid agonists was shortest with buprenorphine, followed by methadone and morphine. However, buprenorphine was associated with an increased need for adjunct treatment and methadone was associated with the lowest use of adjunct medications. The authors of both publications acknowledged significant limitations and suggested further controlled studies (75,82). A new multisite clinical trial using an alcohol-free formulation of sublingual buprenorphine is being planned to confirm these initial findings.

A treatment protocol should define the specific medication(s) to be used, initial dose, dose escalation, maximum dose, adjunctive medications, weaning rate, cessation dose, and duration of observation once the opioid is discontinued. Important differences between protocols may include the approach to nonpharmacologic measures, NAS assessment tool, NAS severity score cut points used to initiate and modify pharmacologic treatment, as well as the choice, dose, titration, and weaning of any adjunctive therapy. Future studies may use pharmacometric modeling to measure drug exposure along with covariates of NAS severity. This may result in a medication regimen that will link drug(s) and dose to desired control of NAS. Ultimately, the answer to "what is the best opioid for NAS" may be rephrased to "which opioid is best for which type of neonate with NAS?"

LONG-TERM FOLLOW-UP FOR CHILDREN WITH NAS

Although exposure to opioids and other drugs during the antenatal and postnatal periods may increase the risk of developing longer-term medical (e.g., hepatitis C, HIV) and neurodevelopmental abnormalities, it is difficult to differentiate the primary impact of the drug exposure from other associated medical, genetic, and/or environmental influences. Sequelae of intrauterine exposures and postnatal conditions may not be apparent in the neonatal period but may be recognizable as children develop and reach preschool and school age. This suggests that key knowledge gaps exist regarding longer-term neurocognitive and mental health outcomes. Jones and colleagues reviewed multiple long-term follow-up studies of neonates with NAS and found many of the studies to have significant limitations including (a) not adequately describing

antenatal/postnatal drug exposure (single or multiple drugs with the potential for drug–drug interactions); (b) using large datasets with a coded diagnosis of NAS that may be inaccurate and subject to excessive variability; (c) not describing if prenatal toxicology testing was performed to confirm opioid exposure during pregnancy (especially in the third trimester); (d) not using well-defined or matched comparison groups; (e) using very large population-based datasets where many variables may be statistically significant, but not clinically relevant; and (f) recognition that children who had NAS can be influenced by multiple factors that may be impossible to control for in a single follow-up study (83). All of these factors need to be considered when examining existing follow-low literature.

In a follow-up to the MOTHER study, Kaltenbach and colleagues followed 96 infants to 36 months of age (84). They found no differences in outcomes between infants born to mothers who had received antenatal methadone or buprenorphine. Although a separate control group of unexposed infants was not included, infants in the MOTHER study appeared to have developed normally over this time period. Czynski and associates studied 99 infants who had been randomized to receive either methadone or morphine for NAS at approximately 18 months of age (85). In primary prespecified analyses, no significant differences were found between treatment groups on the NNNS, Bayley-III, or Child Behavior Checklist (CBCL). However, in post-hoc analyses, neonates receiving adjunctive phenobarbital had lower Bayley-III scores and more behavior problems on the CBCL. In adjusted analyses, internalizing and total behavior problems were associated with the need for phenobarbital, maternal psychological distress, and infant medical problems. Externalizing problems were associated with maternal psychological distress and continued maternal substance use. Although these data suggest that neurodevelopmental outcomes may be associated with receiving phenobarbital, it is unclear whether the outcomes are related to increased severity of NAS or a more direct effect of the drug. Other factors that impact the outcomes are the overall health of the child and the postnatal caregiving environment.

Three major analyses of the literature regarding long-term follow-up of opioid-exposed infants have recently been conducted. A meta-analysis of 26 studies by Yeoh and associates found that antenatal opioid exposure was associated with adverse cognitive, mental, and physical/motor performance as early as 6 months and persisting through adolescence (86). An expert panel convened by the Substance Abuse and Mental Health Services Administration (SAMHSA) affirmed that despite a limited number of high-quality longitudinal follow-up studies, there may be an association between antenatal opioid exposure and adverse neurocognitive, behavioral, and developmental outcomes in children (87). A literature review performed to inform the research agenda for the Environmental Influences on Child Health Outcomes (ECHO) consortium found equivocal results (88). While some studies did not find a difference in cognitive outcomes between opioid exposed and nonexposed infants, others did document significant differences in IQ, language, neurodevelopmental, and behavioral performance as well as issues with executive functioning. However, many of these differences disappeared when controlling for important confounders associated with environmental variables.

Finally, investigators have performed neuroimaging of opioid-exposed neonates in order to identify any potential structural abnormalities present at the time of birth. Merhar and colleagues studied 20 term neonates with prenatal opioid exposure and 20 term controls at 4 to 8 weeks of age (89). They found that 40% of the opioid-exposed neonates had punctate white matter lesions or white matter signal abnormalities compared to none of the controls. Monnelly and associates performed diffusion MRI around the time of birth on 20 methadone-exposed neonates and compared them to 20 controls (90). They found that prenatal methadone exposure was associated with microstructural alterations in major white matter tracts in these high-risk neonates. While the investigators could not directly attribute the white matter alterations to exposure to methadone (since exposure to multiple antenatal psychotropic drugs was common), these results do reinforce the need to conduct future longitudinal studies with larger sample sizes and more diverse populations. The only way to better delineate key structure function relationships is to perform serial MRIs (pre- and postnatal) and neurodevelopmental testing while adjusting for important prenatal and postnatal drug exposures and other environmental influences.

Neonates with prenatal opioid exposure may be at risk of developing eye abnormalities including delayed visual development, abnormal visual evoked potentials, strabismus, nystagmus, and reduced visual acuity, suggesting the need for careful ophthalmologic follow-up (91). For individual clinicians, data on long-term outcomes may be difficult to assess and provide limited guidance on creating a personalized and optimal treatment approach for neonates with NAS. However, these data do support the need for (a) better understanding the influence of genetics and epigenetics, polysubstance use, and psychosocial and environmental factors on childhood outcomes and (b) providing psychosocial support for these children and their families (including early intervention) to optimize longer-term outcome.

SUMMARY

Opioid use and misuse have been a part of human life for thousands of years. The rise in opioid use and problems with use shows a geographic diversity, with the United States having the greatest rates of use while African countries have the lowest reported use. In North America, Australia, and Europe, there has been an unprecedented focus on women who have an OUD and become pregnant. The greatest focus has been on NAS that may develop after birth. It is clear from the data presented that identification, assessment, and treatment of NAS need further examination. Given the repeated findings regarding prenatal polysubstance exposure as a potent predictor of NAS severity, interventions that reduce maternal polysubstance use during medication-assisted treatment for OUD may be beneficial. An objective measure of NAS derived from a rigorous psychometric and/or biomarker approach is needed in addition to research that focuses on evaluation of the effectiveness and safety of pharmacologic and nonpharmacologic treatment protocols. More effective ways for engaging parents in treatment and identifying interventions that improve rates of parents maintaining custody may help prevent maternal substance use relapse and improve child outcomes in the short- and longer term life trajectories.

REFERENCES

1. Norn S, Kruse PR, Kruse E. History of opium poppy and morphine. *Can Medicinhist Arbog* 2005;33:171.
2. Trescot AM, Datta S, Lee M, et al. Opioid pharmacology. *Pain Physician* 2008;11(2 suppl):S133.
3. *Narcotic drugs—technical report. Estimated world requirements for 2019—statistics for 2017.* New York, NY: United Nations Publications, 2019. Available from: https://www.incb.org/incb/en/narcotic-drugs/Technical_Reports/2018/narcotic-drugs-technical-report-2018.html. Accessed October 25, 2019.
4. Cicero TJ, Ellis MS, Surratt HL, et al. The changing face of heroin use in the United States: a retrospective analysis of the past 50 years. *JAMA Psychiat* 2014;71(7):821.
5. GBD 2016 Alcohol and Drug Use Collaborators. The global burden of disease attributable to alcohol and drug use in 195 countries and territories, 1990-2016: a systematic analysis for the global burden of disease study 2016. *Lancet Psychiatry* 2018;5(12):987.
6. Haight SC, Ko JY, Tong VT, et al. Opioid use disorder documented at delivery hospitalization—United States, 1999-2014. *MMWR Morb Mortal Wkly Rep* 2018;67(31):845.
7. Die morphinkrankheit der neugeborenen morphinistischer mutter [The morphine disease of the newborn in morphine-using mothers]. *Monatsscr Kinderh* 1934;60:182.
8. Happel JJ. Morphinism in its relation to the sexual functions and appetite and its effect on the off-spring of the users of the drug. *Med Surg Rep* 1892;68:403.
9. Pettey GE. Congenital morphinism, with report of cases: general treatment of morphinism. *South Med J* 1912;65:95.
10. Rosenthal T, Patrick SW, Krug DC. Congenital neonatal narcotics addiction: a natural history. *Am J Public Health Nations Health* 1964;54:1252.
11. Goodfriend MJ, Shey IA, Klein MD. The effects of maternal narcotic addiction on the newborn. *Am J Obstet Gynecol* 1956;71(1):29.
12. Desmond MM, Wilson GS. Neonatal abstinence syndrome: recognition and diagnosis. *Addict Dis* 1975;2(1-2):113.
13. Finnegan LP, Connaughton JFJ, Kron RE, et al. Neonatal abstinence syndrome: assessment and management. *Addict Dis* 1975;2(1-2):141.
14. Jones HE, Kraft WK. Analgesia, opioids, and other drug use during pregnancy and neonatal abstinence syndrome. *Clin Perinatol* 2019;46(2):349.
15. Scott CS, Riggs KW, Ling EW, et al. Morphine pharmacokinetics and pain assessment in premature newborns. *J Pediatr* 1999;135(4):423.
16. Barr GA, McPhie-Lalmansingh A, Perez J, et al. Changing mechanisms of opiate tolerance and withdrawal in early development: animal models of the human experience. *ILAR J* 2011;52(3):329.
17. Rehni AK, Jaggi AS, Singh N. Opioid withdrawal syndrome: emerging concepts and novel therapeutic targets. *CNS Neurol Disord Drug Targets* 2013;12(1):112.
18. Kocherlakota P. Neonatal abstinence syndrome. *Pediatrics* 2014;134(2):e547.
19. Kaltenbach K, Holbrook AM, Coyle MG, et al. Predicting treatment for neonatal abstinence syndrome in infants born to women maintained on opioid agonist medication. *Addiction* 2012;107(suppl 1):45.
20. Nikoo N, Nikoo M, Song M, et al. Effectiveness of prenatal screening for substance use: critical consciousness, a promising curriculum for compassionate screening. *Ment Health Fam Med* 2017;13:401.
21. Colby JM, Cotten S. Facing challenges in neonatal drug testing: how laboratory stewardship enhances care for a vulnerable population. 2018. Available from: https://www.aacc.org/cln/articles/2018/march/facing-challenges-in-neonatal-drug-testing. Accessed October 25, 2019.
22. Marin SJ, Metcalf A, Krasowski MD, et al. Detection of neonatal drug exposure using umbilical cord tissue and liquid chromatography time-of-flight mass spectrometry. *Ther Drug Monit* 2014;36(1):119.
23. Colby JM, Adams BC, Morad A, et al. Umbilical cord tissue and meconium may not be equivalent for confirming in utero substance exposure. *J Pediatr* 2019;205:277.
24. Colby JM. Comparison of umbilical cord tissue and meconium for the confirmation of in utero drug exposure. *Clin Biochem* 2017;50(13-14):784.
25. Gomez Pomar E, Finnegan LP, Devlin L, et al. Simplification of the Finnegan Neonatal Abstinence Scoring System: retrospective study of two institutions in the USA. *BMJ Open* 2017;7(9):e016176.
26. Jones HE, Seashore C, Johnson E, et al. Measurement of neonatal abstinence syndrome: evaluation of short forms. *J Opioid Manag* 2016;12(1):19.
27. Lipsitz PJ. A proposed narcotic withdrawal score for use with newborn infants. A pragmatic evaluation of its efficacy. *Clin Pediatr (Phila)* 1975;14(6):592.
28. Zahorodny W, Rom C, Whitney W, et al. The neonatal withdrawal inventory: a simplified score of newborn withdrawal. *J Dev Behav Pediatr* 1998;19(2):89.
29. Green M, Suffet F. The neonatal narcotic withdrawal index: a device for the improvement of care in the abstinence syndrome. *Am J Drug Alcohol Abuse* 1981;8(2):203.
30. Grossman MR, Lipshaw MJ, Osborn RR, et al. A novel approach to assessing infants with neonatal abstinence syndrome. *Hosp Pediatr* 2018;8(1):1.
31. Jansson LM, Velez M, Harrow C. The opioid-exposed newborn: assessment and pharmacologic management. *J Opioid Manag* 2009;5(1):47.
32. Raffaeli G, Cavallaro G, Allegaert K, et al. Neonatal abstinence syndrome: update on diagnostic and therapeutic strategies. *Pharmacotherapy* 2017;37(7):814.
33. Devlin LA, Breeze JL, Terrin N, et al. A simplified Finnegan Scoring System to assess the need for treatment in neonatal abstinence syndrome. *JAMA Netw Open* 2020;3(4):e202275.
34. Lester BM, Tronick EZ, Brazelton TB. The Neonatal Intensive Care Unit Network Neurobehavioral Scale procedures. *Pediatrics* 2004;113(3 Pt 2):641.
35. Velez ML, Jansson LM, Schroeder J, et al. Prenatal methadone exposure and neonatal neurobehavioral functioning. *Pediatr Res* 2009;66(6):704.
36. Velez ML, McConnell K, Spencer N, et al. Prenatal buprenorphine exposure and neonatal neurobehavioral functioning. *Early Hum Dev* 2018;117:7.
37. Oji-Mmuo CN, Michael EJ, McLatchy J, et al. Skin conductance at baseline and postheel lance reflects sympathetic activation in neonatal opiate withdrawal. *Acta Paediatr* 2016;105(3):e99.
38. Schubach NE, Mehler K, Roth B, et al. Skin conductance in neonates suffering from abstinence syndrome and unexposed newborns. *Eur J Pediatr* 2016;175(6):859.

39. Heil SH, Gaalema DE, Johnston AM, et al. Infant pupillary response to methadone administration during treatment for neonatal abstinence syndrome: a feasibility study. *Drug Alcohol Depend* 2012;126(1-2):268.

40. O'Brien CM, Jeffery HE. Sleep deprivation, disorganization and fragmentation during opiate withdrawal in newborns. *J Paediatr Child Health* 2002;38(1):66.

41. Winkelman TNA, Villapiano N, Kozhimannil KB, et al. Incidence and costs of neonatal abstinence syndrome among infants with medicaid: 2004-2014. *Pediatrics* 2018;141(4):e20173520.

42. Dawson E, Lew J, Mauer-Vakil D, et al. A longitudinal analysis of temporal and spatial incidence of neonatal abstinence syndrome in Ontario: 2003-2016. *J Opioid Manag* 2019;15(3):205.

43. Desai RJ, Huybrechts KF, Hernandez-Diaz S, et al. Exposure to prescription opioid analgesics in utero and risk of neonatal abstinence syndrome: population based cohort study. *BMJ* 2015;350:h2102.

44. Jansson LM, Velez ML, McConnell K, et al. Maternal buprenorphine treatment during pregnancy and maternal physiology. *Drug Alcohol Depend* 2019;201:38.

45. Jones HE, Dengler E, Garrison A, et al. Neonatal outcomes and their relationship to maternal buprenorphine dose during pregnancy. *Drug Alcohol Depend* 2014;134:414.

46. Jones HE, Jansson LM, O'Grady KE, et al. The relationship between maternal methadone dose at delivery and neonatal outcome: methodological and design considerations. *Neurotoxicol Teratol* 2013;39:110.

47. Wong J, Saver B, Scanlan JM. Does maternal buprenorphine dose affect severity or incidence of neonatal abstinence syndrome? *J Addict Med* 2018;12(6):435.

48. Fulroth R, Phillips B, Durand DJ. Perinatal outcome of infants exposed to cocaine and/or heroin in utero. *Am J Dis Child* 1989;143(8):905.

49. Mayes LC, Carroll KM. Neonatal withdrawal syndrome in infants exposed to cocaine and methadone. *Subst Use Misuse* 1996;31(2):241.

50. Seligman NS, Salva N, Hayes EJ, et al. Predicting length of treatment for neonatal abstinence syndrome in methadone-exposed neonates. *Am J Obstet Gynecol* 2008;199(4):396, e391.

51. Jansson LM, Velez ML, McConnell K, et al. Maternal buprenorphine treatment and infant outcome. *Drug Alcohol Depend* 2017;180:56.

52. Jansson LM, Dipietro JA, Elko A, et al. Infant autonomic functioning and neonatal abstinence syndrome. *Drug Alcohol Depend* 2010;109(1-3):198.

53. Dryden C, Young D, Hepburn M, et al. Maternal methadone use in pregnancy: factors associated with the development of neonatal abstinence syndrome and implications for healthcare resources. *BJOG* 2009;116(5):665.

54. Wachman EM, Warden AH, Thomas Z, et al. Impact of psychiatric medication co-exposure on Neonatal Abstinence Syndrome severity. *Drug Alcohol Depend* 2018;192:45.

55. Sanlorenzo LA, Cooper WO, Dudley JA, et al. Increased severity of neonatal abstinence syndrome associated with concomitant antenatal opioid and benzodiazepine exposure. *Hosp Pediatr* 2019;9(8):569.

56. Loudin S, Murray S, Prunty L, et al. An atypical withdrawal syndrome in neonates prenatally exposed to gabapentin and opioids. *J Pediatr* 2017;181:286.

57. Huybrechts KF, Bateman BT, Desai RJ, et al. Risk of neonatal drug withdrawal after intrauterine co-exposure to opioids and psychotropic medications: cohort study. *BMJ* 2017;358:j3326.

58. Jones HE, Heil SH, Tuten M, et al. Cigarette smoking in opioid-dependent pregnant women: neonatal and maternal outcomes. *Drug Alcohol Depend* 2013;131(3):271.

59. Unger A, Jagsch R, Bawert A, et al. Are male neonates more vulnerable to neonatal abstinence syndrome than female neonates? *Gend Med* 2011;8(6):355.

60. Charles MK, Cooper WO, Jansson LM, et al. Male sex associated with increased risk of neonatal abstinence syndrome. *Hosp Pediatr* 2017;7(6):328.

61. Dysart K, Hsieh HC, Kaltenbach K, et al. Sequela of preterm versus term infants born to mothers on a methadone maintenance program: differential course of neonatal abstinence syndrome. *J Perinat Med* 2007;35(4):344.

62. Cole FS, Wegner DJ, Davis JM. The genomics of neonatal abstinence syndrome. *Front Pediatr* 2017;5:176.

63. Wachman EM, Hayes MJ, Brown MS, et al. Association of OPRM1 and COMT single-nucleotide polymorphisms with hospital length of stay and treatment of neonatal abstinence syndrome. *JAMA* 2013;309(17):1821.

64. Wachman EM, Hayes MJ, Sherva R, et al. Association of maternal and infant variants in PNOC and COMT genes with neonatal abstinence syndrome severity. *Am J Addict* 2017;26(1):42.

65. Wachman EM, Hayes MJ, Lester BM, et al. Epigenetic variation in the mu-opioid receptor gene in infants with neonatal abstinence syndrome. *J Pediatr* 2014;165(3):472.

66. Wachman EM, Hayes MJ, Shrestha H, et al. Epigenetic variation in OPRM1 gene in opioid-exposed mother-infant dyads. *Genes Brain Behav* 2018;17(7):e12476.

67. Walsh MC, Crowley M, Wexelblatt S, et al. Ohio Perinatal Quality Collaborative improves care of neonatal narcotic abstinence syndrome. *Pediatrics* 2018;141(4):e20170900.

68. Coyle MG, Brogly SB, Ahmed MS, et al. Neonatal abstinence syndrome. *Nat Rev Dis Primers* 2018;4(1):47.

69. Velez M, Jansson LM. The opioid dependent mother and newborn dyad: non-pharmacologic care. *J Addict Med* 2008;2(3):113.

70. Hudak ML, Tan RC; Committee on Drugs; Committee on Fetus and Newborn; American Academy of Pediatrics. Clinical report. Neonatal drug withdrawal. *Pediatrics* 2012;129(2):e540.

71. Davis JM, Shenberger J, Terrin N, et al. Comparison of safety and efficacy of methadone vs morphine for treatment of neonatal abstinence syndrome: a randomized clinical trial. *JAMA Pediatr* 2018;172(8):741.

72. Brown MS, Hayes MJ, Thornton LM. Methadone versus morphine for treatment of neonatal abstinence syndrome: a prospective randomized clinical trial. *J Perinatol* 2015;35(4):278.

73. Burke S, Beckwith AM. Morphine versus methadone treatment for neonatal withdrawal and impact on early infant development. *Glob Pediatr Health* 2017;4:2333794x17721128.

74. NeoFax. IBM Watson Health, 2019. Available from: https://www.ibm.com/products/micromedex-neofax-pediatrics/details. Accessed October 28, 2019.

75. Lee JJ, Chen J, Eisler L, et al. Comparative effectiveness of opioid replacement agents for neonatal opioid withdrawal syndrome: a systematic review and meta-analysis. *J Perinatol* 2019;39(11):1535.

76. Kraft WK, Adeniyi-Jones SC, Chervoneva I, et al. Buprenorphine for the treatment of the neonatal abstinence syndrome. *N Engl J Med* 2017;376(24):2341.

77. Jones HE, Kaltenbach K, Heil SH, et al. Neonatal abstinence syndrome after methadone or buprenorphine exposure. *N Engl J Med* 2010;363(24):2320.

78. Agthe AG, Kim GR, Mathias KB, et al. Clonidine as an adjunct therapy to opioids for neonatal abstinence syndrome: a randomized, controlled trial. *Pediatrics* 2009;123(5):e849.

79. Bada HS, Sithisarn T, Gibson J, et al. Morphine versus clonidine for neonatal abstinence syndrome. *Pediatrics* 2015;135(2):e383.

80. Murphy-Oikonen J, McQueen K. Outpatient pharmacologic weaning for neonatal abstinence syndrome: a systematic review. *Prim Health Care Res Dev* 2018;20:1.

81. Maalouf FI, Cooper WO, Slaughter JC, et al. Outpatient pharmacotherapy for Neonatal Abstinence Syndrome. *J Pediatr* 2018;199:151.

82. Disher T, Gullickson C, Singh B, et al. Pharmacological treatments for neonatal abstinence syndrome: a systematic review and network meta-analysis. *JAMA Pediatr* 2019;173(3):234.

83. Jones HE, Kaltenbach K, Benjamin T, et al. Prenatal opioid exposure, neonatal abstinence syndrome/neonatal opioid withdrawal syndrome, and later child development research: shortcomings and solutions. *J Addict Med* 2019;13(2):90.

84. Kaltenbach K, O'Grady KE, Heil SH, et al. Prenatal exposure to methadone or buprenorphine: early childhood developmental outcomes. *Drug Alcohol Depend* 2018;185:40.

85. Czynski AJ, Davis JM, Dansereau LM, et al. Neurodevelopmental outcomes of neonates randomized to morphine or methadone for treatment of neonatal abstinence syndrome. *J Pediatr* 2020;219:146.

86. Yeoh SL, Eastwood J, Wright IM, et al. Cognitive and motor outcomes of children with prenatal opioid exposure: a systematic review and meta-analysis. *JAMA Netw Open* 2019;2(7):e197025.

87. Larson JJ, Graham DL, Singer LT, et al. Cognitive and behavioral impact on children exposed to opioids during pregnancy. *Pediatrics* 2019;144(2):e20190514.

88. Conradt E, Flannery T, Aschner JL, et al. Prenatal opioid exposure: neurodevelopmental consequences and future research priorities. *Pediatrics* 2019;144(3):e20190128.

89. Merhar SL, Parikh NA, Braimah A, et al. White matter injury and structural anomalies in infants with prenatal opioid exposure. *AJNR Am J Neuroradiol* 2019;40(12):2161.

90. Monnelly VJ, Anblagan D, Quigley A, et al. Prenatal methadone exposure is associated with altered neonatal brain development. *Neuroimage Clin* 2017;18:9.

91. McGlone L, Hamilton R, McCulloch DL, et al. Visual outcome in infants born to drug-misusing mothers prescribed methadone in pregnancy. *Br J Ophthalmol* 2014;98(2):238.

55 Inherited Metabolic Disorders

Barbara K. Burton

INTRODUCTION

Major advances in the recognition and treatment of inborn errors of metabolism have made it more essential than ever that the neonatologist be familiar with the clinical presentation of these disorders. Many of the diseases in this group are associated with symptoms in the neonatal period, and many affected infants find their way into neonatal intensive care units. The likelihood of establishing a diagnosis often is directly related to the level of awareness of the neonatologist responsible for the infant's care. Although many of the individual inborn errors of metabolism occur infrequently, collectively, they are not rare. There is no doubt that a significant number of children with these disorders are undiagnosed. Every geneticist has had the experience of diagnosing an inborn error of metabolism in a child and discovering that the parents have had one or more other children who died in early infancy of vague or undetermined causes. In such cases, it is reasonable to assume that the other children were similarly affected but undiagnosed. Autopsy findings in such cases are often nonspecific and unrevealing unless specific biochemical studies are done (see later for a list of samples to obtain from a dying child with a suspected IEM). Infection often is suspected as the cause of death, and sepsis is a common accompaniment of inherited metabolic disorders.

The significance of the precise diagnosis of metabolic disease cannot be overemphasized. Increasingly, these disorders are lending themselves to successful medical management. If treatment means the prevention of significant mental retardation or death, even when the numbers are small, the diagnosis is clearly worth pursuing. However, the success of most treatment regimens depends on the earliest possible institution of therapy, stressing the importance of early clinical diagnosis. Even when no effective therapy exists or an infant cannot be salvaged, diagnosis is critical for purposes of genetic counseling.

Inborn errors of metabolism are all genetically transmitted, typically in an autosomal recessive or X-linked recessive fashion, and there is usually a substantial risk of recurrence. Prenatal diagnosis is available for many conditions in this group. Awareness of the diagnosis before birth of an at-risk infant can lead to earlier therapy and an improved prognosis.

This chapter defines the constellation of findings in the newborn that should alert the clinician to the possibility of inherited metabolic disease. The discussion is confined to the disorders for which manifestations are observed in the first few months of life and does not include the many disorders (e.g., most lysosomal storage diseases such as Fabry disease or type 1 Gaucher disease) that typically present in later infancy or childhood. The laboratory tools used to evaluate infants suspected of having inherited metabolic disease are discussed. Treatment of important groups of metabolic disorders is addressed, focusing on the stabilization and acute management of patients with these conditions. Although newborn screening panels have been expanded to include many more inborn errors of metabolism than was the case only a decade ago, many infants become symptomatic and may die before the results of newborn screening tests are available. Therefore, there is still a role for astute clinical diagnosis of these disorders.

CLINICAL MANIFESTATIONS OF INBORN ERRORS OF METABOLISM

Acute Metabolic Encephalopathy

Several groups of inherited metabolic disorders, most notably the organic acidemias (such as methylmalonic acidemia, propionic acidemia, or isovaleric acidemia), urea cycle defects (such as ornithine transcarbamylase [OTC] deficiency or citrullinemia), and certain disorders of amino acid metabolism (such as maple syrup urine disease or nonketotic hyperglycinemia), typically present with acute life-threatening symptoms in the neonatal period. Affected infants are typically full term and usually appear normal at birth. The interval between birth and clinical symptoms ranges from hours to weeks. The initial findings are usually those of lethargy and poor feeding, as seen in almost any sick infant. Although sepsis is often the first consideration in infants who present in this way, these symptoms in a full-term infant with no specific risk factors strongly suggest a metabolic disorder. Infants with inborn errors of metabolism may rather quickly become debilitated and septic; therefore, it is important that the presence of sepsis not preclude consideration of other possibilities. The lethargy associated with these conditions is an early symptom of a metabolic encephalopathy that may progress to coma. Other signs of central nervous system (CNS) dysfunction, such as seizures and abnormal muscle tone, may also exist. Evidence of cerebral edema may be observed, and intracranial hemorrhage occasionally occurs (1).

An infant with an inborn error of metabolism who presents more abruptly or in whom the lethargy and poor feeding go unnoticed may first come to attention because of apnea or respiratory distress. The apnea is typically central in origin and a symptom of the metabolic encephalopathy, but tachypnea may be a symptom of an underlying metabolic acidosis, as occurs in the organic acidemias (such as methylmalonic and propionic acidemia). Infants with urea cycle defects (such as OTC deficiency and citrullinemia) and evolving hyperammonemic coma initially exhibit central hyperventilation, which leads to respiratory alkalosis. Indeed, the finding of respiratory alkalosis in an infant with lethargy is virtually pathognomonic of hyperammonemic encephalopathy.

Vomiting is a striking feature of many of the inborn errors of metabolism associated with protein intolerance, although it is less common in the newborn than in the older infant. If persistent vomiting occurs in the neonatal period, it usually signals significant underlying disease. Inborn errors of metabolism should always be considered in the differential diagnosis. It is common for an infant to be diagnosed as having a metabolic disorder after having undergone surgery for suspected pyloric stenosis (2). Formula intolerance frequently is suspected, and many affected infants have numerous formula changes before a diagnosis finally is established.

The basic laboratory studies that should be obtained for an infant who has acute life-threatening symptoms consistent with an inborn error of metabolism are listed in Table 55.1.

Hyperammonemia

Among the most important laboratory findings associated with inborn errors of metabolism presenting with an acute encephalopathy is hyperammonemia. A plasma ammonia level should be

TABLE 55.1

Laboratory Studies for an Infant Suspected of Having an Inborn Error of Metabolism

Complete blood count with differential

Urinalysis

Blood gases

Electrolytes

Blood glucose

Plasma ammonia

Urine reducing substances

Urine or serum ketones

Plasma and urine amino acids, quantitative

Urine organic acids

Plasma lactate

obtained for any infant with unexplained vomiting, lethargy, or other evidence of an encephalopathy. Significant hyperammonemia is observed in a limited number of conditions. Inborn errors of metabolism, including urea cycle defects (especially OTC deficiency and citrullinemia) and many of the organic acidemias (especially propionic acidemia), are at the top of the list. It can also be seen in the severe form of several long chain fatty acid oxidation disorders such as carnitine palmitoyltranferase II (CPTII) deficiency. Also in the differential diagnosis is a condition referred to as transient hyperammonemia of the newborn (THAN), although this is very uncommon (3). Ammonia levels in all of these conditions may exceed 1,000 µmol/L. The finding of marked hyperammonemia provides an important clue to diagnosis and indicates the need for urgent treatment to reduce the ammonia level. The

degree of neurologic impairment and developmental delay subsequently observed in infants and children with urea cycle disorders depends on many factors, but an important one is the duration of the neonatal hyperammonemic coma (4).

A flowchart for the differentiation of conditions producing significant hyperammonemia in the newborn is shown in **Figure 55.1**. The timing of the onset of symptoms may provide an important clue. Infants with urea cycle defects typically do not become symptomatic until after 24 hours of age. Patients with some of the organic acidemias, such as glutaric acidemia type II, or with pyruvate carboxylase deficiency may exhibit symptomatic hyperammonemia during the first 24 hours. Symptoms in the first 24 hours are characteristic of the aforementioned THAN, a condition that is poorly understood but apparently not genetically determined. The typical patient with this disorder is a large premature infant (mean gestational age of 36 weeks) who has symptomatic pulmonary disease, often from birth, and severe hyperammonemia. Survivors do not have recurrent episodes of hyperammonemia and may or may not exhibit neurologic sequelae, depending on the extent of the neonatal insult. There are some affected infants who survive with normal intelligence despite extraordinarily high ammonia levels (3). The disorder has become extremely rare in recent years for unknown reasons.

Infants who develop severe hyperammonemia after 24 hours of age usually have a urea cycle defect or an organic acidemia; infants with organic acidemias typically exhibit a metabolic acidosis and ketonuria as well. Urine organic acids should always be obtained, regardless of whether or not acidosis is present. Metabolic acidosis is not a feature of the urea cycle defects unless shock is a complicating feature. Plasma amino acid analysis is helpful in the differentiation of the specific defects in this group. Characteristic amino acid abnormalities provide a definitive diagnosis of citrullinemia

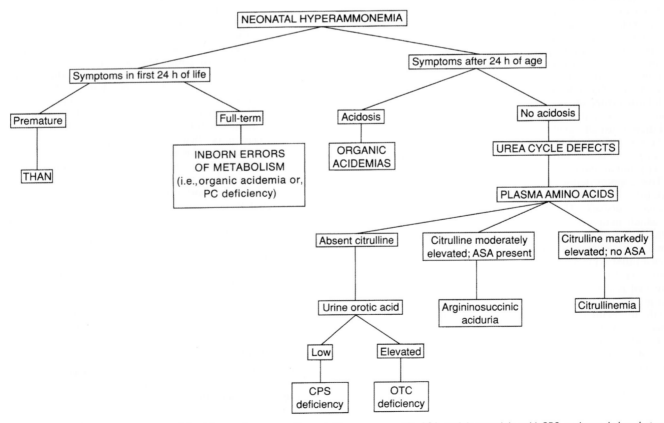

FIGURE 55.1 Differentiating between conditions that produce severe neonatal hyperammonemia. ASA, argininosuccinic acid; CPS, carbamoyl phosphate synthetase; OTC, ornithine transcarbamylase; PC, pyruvate carboxylase; THAN, transient hyperammonemia of the newborn.

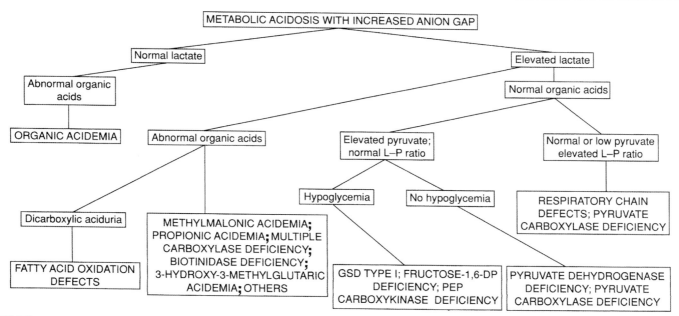

FIGURE 55.2 Evaluating metabolic acidosis in the young infant. Fructose-1,6-DP, fructose-1,6-bisphosphatase; GSD, glycogen storage disease; L/P, lactate/pyruvate; PEP, phosphoenolpyruvate.

and argininosuccinic aciduria. Although no diagnostic amino acid elevations are observed in carbamoyl phosphate synthetase deficiency or OTC deficiency, a low or undetectable level of plasma citrulline is observed in both of these conditions. This finding is helpful in differentiating these two conditions from THAN, in which the plasma citrulline level is normal. Carbamoyl phosphate synthetase deficiency and OTC deficiency may be differentiated by measuring urine orotic acid, which is low in the former and elevated in the latter. The pattern of inheritance of the two may also help to differentiate them; OTC deficiency, an X-linked disorder, rarely produces severe hyperammonemia in a female infant, whereas carbamoyl phosphate synthetase deficiency, an autosomal recessive disorder, occurs with equal frequency in the two sexes.

Although the clinical and laboratory evaluation outlined should lead to a specific tentative diagnosis for virtually all patients, molecular testing to identify the causative gene mutation or mutations may be indicated for confirmation of the diagnoses of carbamoyl phosphate synthetase and OTC deficiencies, because these diagnoses dictate rigid lifelong therapy or consideration of hepatic transplantation. Acute treatment should be based on the presumptive diagnosis.

Less significant elevations of plasma ammonia than those associated with inborn errors of metabolism and THAN can be observed in a variety of other conditions associated with liver dysfunction, including sepsis, generalized herpes simplex infection, and perinatal asphyxia. Liver function studies should be obtained in evaluating the significance of moderate elevations of plasma ammonia. However, even in cases of severe hepatic necrosis, it is rare for ammonia levels to exceed 500 μmol/L (5). Mild transient hyperammonemia with ammonia levels as high as twice normal is relatively common in the newborn, especially in the premature infant, and is usually asymptomatic. It appears to be of no clinical significance, and there are no long-term neurologic sequelae (6).

Metabolic Acidosis

The second important laboratory feature of many of the inborn errors of metabolism during acute episodes of illness is metabolic acidosis with an increased anion gap, readily demonstrable

by measurement of arterial blood gases or serum electrolytes and bicarbonate (7). A flowchart for the evaluation of infants with this finding is shown in **Figure 55.2**. An increased anion gap (>16) is observed in many inborn errors of metabolism and in most other conditions producing metabolic acidosis in the neonate. The differential diagnosis of metabolic acidosis with a normal anion gap essentially is limited to two conditions, diarrhea and renal tubular acidosis. Among the inborn errors, the largest group typically associated with overwhelming metabolic acidosis in infancy is the group of organic acidemias, including methylmalonic acidemia, propionic acidemia, and isovaleric acidemia, among others.

In addition to specific organic acid intermediates, plasma lactate often is elevated in organic acidemias as a result of secondary interference with coenzyme A (CoA) metabolism. Neutropenia and thrombocytopenia commonly are observed and further underscore the clinical similarity of these disorders to neonatal sepsis. Hyperammonemia, sometimes as dramatic as that associated with urea cycle defects, is seen commonly but not uniformly in critically ill neonates with organic acidemias.

Inborn Errors Masquerading as Other Diseases

The metabolic acidosis associated with organic acidemias and certain other inborn errors of metabolism may have significant adverse impact on many different organ systems, which may lead to the erroneous diagnosis of a wide variety of seemingly unrelated disorders. I had the experience of caring for an infant with isovaleric acidemia who presented at 10 days of age with respiratory distress, severe metabolic acidosis, a dilated heart, and poor cardiac output. The infant was suspected of having the hypoplastic left heart syndrome or other severe congenital heart disease. Cardiac catheterization was performed, even though members of the nursing staff had observed that the infant had a strong unpleasant odor, reminiscent of sweaty feet. Personnel in the catheterization laboratory also noticed that the blood had a strong peculiar odor, but it was not until 18 hours later, long after significant heart disease had been ruled out, that the diagnosis of metabolic disease was first considered. Despite attempts at therapy with dialysis and other measures, the child succumbed to the disease. In this case, the metabolic acidosis associated with isovaleric acidemia led to poor function of the myocardium and not the reverse.

THE NEWBORN INFANT

Another child subsequently found to have methylmalonic acidemia was admitted through the emergency room with severe metabolic acidosis and a tight, distended abdomen with evidence of multiple air–fluid levels on x-ray films. The history revealed that the child had fed poorly since birth and had repeated episodes of vomiting despite several formula changes. Intestinal obstruction was suspected, and the child was taken to the operating room, in which most of the small intestine was found to be infarcted, presumably secondary to the acidosis and poor tissue perfusion. No anatomic abnormalities were found. Postoperatively, metabolic disease was considered, and the diagnosis of a vitamin B_{12}–responsive form of methylmalonic acidemia was made. The infant died of complications of the disease even though the early diagnosis and treatment of this disorder, before the terminal episode, should have been associated with a good prognosis.

Defects in pyruvate metabolism or in the respiratory chain may lead to primary lactic acidosis presenting as severe metabolic acidosis in infancy (8,9). Unlike most of the other conditions presenting acutely in the newborn, the clinical features of these disorders are unrelated to protein intake. Disorders in this group should be considered in patients with lactic acidosis who have normal or nondiagnostic urine organic acids. Differentiation of the various disorders in this group can be facilitated by measuring plasma pyruvate and calculating the lactate to pyruvate ratio. A normal ratio (<25) suggests a defect in pyruvate dehydrogenase (PDH) or in gluconeogenesis, and an elevated ratio (>25) suggests pyruvate carboxylase deficiency or a mitochondrial respiratory chain defect.

Alternate Presentations

Not all infants with life-threatening metabolic disease have metabolic acidosis or hyperammonemia. For example, patients with nonketotic hyperglycinemia typically present in the neonatal period with evidence of severe and progressive CNS dysfunction but do not exhibit metabolic acidosis or hyperammonemia (10). Even patients with galactosemia may present with symptoms of acute CNS toxicity, which may progress to cerebral edema, when galactose-1-phosphate levels rise precipitously. Therefore, a series of laboratory studies designed to screen for inborn errors of metabolism should be obtained for any infant with clinical findings suggesting an inborn error of metabolism, even if metabolic acidosis and hyperammonemia are not present. These studies are listed in Table 55.1. Most are self-explanatory. Although not available in many hospital laboratories, amino acid and organic acid analysis can be obtained in any part of the country through reference laboratories or through referral of samples to medical center genetics units. It is important to insist that any reference laboratory used for this purpose provide prompt test results and reference ranges and provide interpretation of abnormal results.

Urine testing for reducing substances can be performed using Benedict reagent (Clinitest tablets, Miles, Elkhart, IN). If the result is positive, the urine should be tested for glucose by dipstick. A nonglucose reducing substance in the urine is probably galactose, but there are other possibilities (Table 55.2).

Several disorders associated with an acute metabolic encephalopathy in the neonate deserve special mention because they typically are not associated with hyperammonemia or metabolic acidosis.

Nonketotic Hyperglycinemia

This condition typically results in severe and progressive CNS dysfunction, including obtundation, seizures, and altered muscle tone. Routine laboratory studies all yield normal findings. The first diagnostic clue is usually the finding of elevated glycine on plasma amino acid analysis. The diagnosis is confirmed by measurement of cerebrospinal fluid (CSF) glycine and demonstration of an elevated CSF to plasma glycine ratio. Although therapy of infants with nonketotic hyperglycinemia has been attempted with dietary protein restriction, sodium benzoate, dextromethorphan, and a variety of other drugs, the results have been disappointing. Essentially all infants with this disorder die or exhibit significant neurologic impairment.

Molybdenum Cofactor Deficiency

A second disorder that produces a progressive encephalopathy with no clues on routine laboratory studies is molybdenum cofactor deficiency. The neurologic findings in the affected infant are virtually indistinguishable from those associated with hypoxic–ischemic encephalopathy. Surviving infants exhibit similar neurologic sequelae including cerebral palsy, mental retardation, and seizures. The diagnosis may be suggested by the finding of hypouricemia or, beyond the neonatal period, by ectopia lentis noted on ophthalmologic examination. If it is suspected, urine should be screened for the presence of sulfites, a finding attributable to a deficiency of the enzyme sulfite oxidase, which accompanies the disorder. Other less common metabolic causes of neonatal metabolic encephalopathy include defects in purine and pyrimidine metabolism and neurotransmitter disorders.

A summary of the inborn errors of metabolism most likely to be associated with an acute encephalopathy in the newborn are summarized in Table 55.3. The typical laboratory findings in each condition or group of conditions also are listed.

TABLE 55.2

Disorders Associated with Nonglucose Reducing Substances in Urine

Disorder	Compound
Galactosemia	Galactose
Hereditary fructose intolerance	Fructose
Hereditary tyrosinemia	p-Hydroxyphenylpyruvic acid
Galactokinase deficiency	Galactose
Essential fructosuria	Fructose
Pentosuria	Xylulose
Severe liver disease with secondary galactose intolerance	Galactose

TABLE 55.3

Major Inborn Errors of Metabolism Presenting in the Neonate as an Acute Encephalopathy

Disorders	Characteristic Laboratory Findings
Organic acidemias (includes MMA, PA, IVA, MCD and many less common conditions)	Metabolic acidosis with increased anion gap; elevated plasma and urine ketones; variably elevated plasma ammonia and lactate; abnormal urine organic acids
Urea cycle defects	Respiratory alkalosis, no metabolic acidosis; markedly elevated plasma ammonia; elevated urine orotic acid in OTCD; abnormal plasma amino acids
Maple syrup urine disease	Metabolic acidosis with increased anion gap; elevated plasma and urine ketones; abnormal plasma amino acids
Nonketotic hyperglycinemia	No acid–base or electrolyte abnormalities; normal ammonia; abnormal plasma amino acids
Molybdenum cofactor deficiency	No acid–base or electrolyte abnormalities; normal ammonia; normal amino and organic acids; low serum uric acid; elevated sulfites in urine

IVA, isovaleric acidemia; MCD, multiple carboxylase deficiency; MMA, methylmalonic acidemia; OTCD, ornithine transcarbamylase deficiency; PA, propionic acidemia.

EMERGENCY TREATMENT OF THE INFANT WITH AN ACUTE METABOLIC ENCEPHALOPATHY

When an inborn error of metabolism, such as an organic acidemia or urea cycle defect, is suspected in a critically ill infant, immediate treatment should be initiated even if a definitive diagnosis may not yet be established. Within 48 to 72 hours, the results of amino acid and organic acid analyses should be available, allowing diagnostic confirmation in most cases. Appropriate and aggressive treatment before the confirmation of a diagnosis may be lifesaving and may avert or reduce the neurologic sequelae of some of these disorders. The immediate treatment of infants with disorders in this group has two primary goals. The first is the removal of accumulated metabolites, such as organic acid intermediates or ammonia. At the first suspicion of a disorder associated with protein intolerance, protein intake in the form of breast milk, infant formula, or hyperalimentation should be discontinued immediately. In critically ill infants with hyperammonemia, arrangements should be made for hemodialysis or continuous renal replacement therapy (11). Although peritoneal dialysis, continuous arteriovenous hemoperfusion, and exchange transfusion all have been used in the past to lower plasma ammonia levels, all are substantially less effective than hemodialysis (12). In infants who are comatose, ventilator dependent, or exhibit evidence of cerebral edema, dialysis should be instituted immediately without waiting to see if there is a response to dietary manipulation, medication, or other less aggressive therapy. Maximal supportive care should be provided simultaneously. In patients suspected of having a urea cycle defect because of significant hyperammonemia without acidosis, an infusion of 6 mL/kg of 10% arginine hydrochloride (HCl) (0.6 g/kg) can be given intravenously over 90 minutes. In patients with citrullinemia and argininosuccinic aciduria, this often results in a precipitous drop in the plasma ammonia level. An intravenous arginine preparation is commercially available and should be readily accessible from any hospital pharmacy.

If an organic acidemia is suspected, vitamin B_{12} (1 mg) should be given intramuscularly in case the patient has a vitamin B_{12}–responsive form of methylmalonic acidemia. Biotin (10 mg) should be given orally or by nasogastric tube, because some patients with multiple carboxylase deficiency are biotin responsive. If acidosis exists, intravenous bicarbonate should be administered liberally. Calculations of bicarbonate requirements appropriate for the treatment of other conditions rarely are adequate in these disorders because of ongoing production of organic acids or lactate. The acid–base status should be monitored frequently, with therapy adjusted accordingly.

While there is debate about the role of bicarbonate therapy in infants whose acidosis is secondary to impaired tissue perfusion, there is no such debate in inborn errors of metabolism. In these cases, primary acid excess is the primary pathology and abnormal circulatory function is a secondary side effect, whereas in shock, circulatory dysfunction is the primary pathology and acidosis is the side effect. Therefore, in inborn errors of metabolism, bicarbonate therapy is clearly and urgently indicated.

After removing toxic metabolites, the second major goal of therapy in infants with inborn errors of metabolism should be to prevent catabolism. Ten percent glucose should be liberally administered intravenously with higher concentrations given if the patient has central access. Intravenous lipids can be given to infants with urea cycle defects and other disorders in which dietary fat plays no role. Protein should not be withheld indefinitely. If clinical improvement is observed and a final diagnosis has not been established, some amino acid intake should be provided after 2 to 3 days of complete protein restriction. Essential amino acids or intact protein can be provided orally or intravenously at an initial dose of 0.5 g protein/kg body weight/24 hours. This should

be increased incrementally to 1.0 g/kg/24 hours (over 2 to 3 days) and held at that level until the diagnostic evaluation is complete, and plans can be made for definitive long-term therapy. Therapy should be planned in conjunction with a geneticist or specialist in metabolic disease. Until then, supplemental calories and nutrients can be provided orally using protein-free diet powder (Pro-Phree, Ross Laboratories; PFD-1, Mead Johnson Nutritionals).

The chronic therapy of urea cycle defects and most of the organic acidemias involves restriction of dietary protein. Depending on the specific diagnosis, this may be accomplished by simple restriction of intact protein intake in breast milk or standard infant formula or by use of special formulas designed for individual inborn errors of metabolism. Formulas have been developed for many of the more common metabolic disorders and are commercially available. These specialized formulas typically have reduced amounts of one or several specific amino acids. Dietary treatment alone may be effective in management of some patients with organic acidemias and in several disorders of amino acid metabolism, such as maple syrup urine disease.

In several of the vitamin-responsive disorders, such as methylmalonic acidemia, multiple carboxylase deficiency, and homocystinuria; dietary protein restriction may be combined with specific cofactor therapy. In the organic acidemias and certain other disorders, L-carnitine, usually beginning with a dose of 100 mg/kg/d, may be given. Acyl-CoAs accumulating in these disorders combine with carnitine to produce acylcarnitines that are water soluble and excreted in the urine. Without treatment, many patients with these disorders develop a secondary carnitine deficiency. Treatment with exogenous carnitine prevents the development of symptoms of carnitine deficiency and provides a measure of protection against recurrent episodes of metabolic decompensation by providing an augmented mechanism for excretion of accumulated metabolites.

Patients with urea cycle defects require supplementation with oral arginine or, in some cases, citrulline, which is converted to arginine in the body. In normal persons, adequate amounts of arginine are synthesized via the urea cycle. Patients with a defect in urea synthesis have deficient arginine production and must depend on dietary supplementation. In the case of carbamoyl phosphate synthetase, OTC deficiency, and some cases of the more distal disorders, drug therapy also is required. These disorders were formerly almost uniformly lethal in the neonatal period. The development of novel drugs that provide an alternate pathway for waste nitrogen excretion has allowed survival of many affected infants (13). Sodium benzoate and sodium phenylacetate were the agents originally used, but these have been replaced largely for oral use by sodium phenylbutyrate and, more recently, by glycerol phenylbutyrate.

Despite rigorous therapy and intensive surveillance, patients with urea cycle defects remain at risk for intercurrent episodes of hyperammonemia, which may result in death or neurologic sequelae. The risk appears to be greatest for patients with neonatal-onset carbamoyl phosphate synthetase and OTC deficiency. Liver transplantation should be considered seriously for patients with these disorders, once they are stabilized.

HYPOGLYCEMIA

Hypoglycemia and its associated symptoms occasionally may be seen in infants with disorders of protein intolerance, but it more commonly is seen in disorders of carbohydrate metabolism or of fatty acid oxidation.

Disorders of Carbohydrate Metabolism

Among the best-known inborn errors of metabolism associated with hypoglycemia are the glycogen storage diseases, of which types I (von Gierke disease) and III (Cori disease or debrancher deficiency) are the most likely to be associated with manifestations in the neonatal period. The hypoglycemia in these disorders is related to the inability of the liver to release glucose from glycogen, and it is most profound during periods of fasting. Hypoglycemia, hepatomegaly, and lactic acidosis are prominent features of these disorders, but, in the neonate, hypoglycemia may be the only finding. Hypoglycemia is not a feature of glycogen storage disease type II (Pompe disease) because cytoplasmic glycogen metabolism and release are normal in this disorder, in which glycogen accumulates within lysosomes as a result of the deficiency of the lysosomal enzyme α-1,4-glucosidase. The clinical manifestations of this disorder include macroglossia, hypotonia, cardiomyopathy with congestive heart failure, and hepatomegaly. Hypertrophic cardiomyopathy is the most striking finding and is essentially always present in the neonatal period. Congestive heart failure has been the cause of death in most cases in the past, but enzyme replacement therapy (with synthetic acid alpha glucosidase) is now commercially available and, when administered early in the course of the disease, can be lifesaving. Pompe disease is now on the recommended uniform screening panel (RUSP) in the United States, and newborn screening for this disorder is being widely implemented.

A disorder that presents clinically with findings virtually indistinguishable from the hepatic glycogen storage diseases types I and III is fructose-1,6-bisphosphatase deficiency, a disorder of gluconeogenesis. Several other disorders of gluconeogenesis have been described. The basic immediate treatment of all of these disorders is frequent feedings and glucose administration. The definitive diagnosis of most of these disorders can be established by molecular genetic testing.

Fatty Acid Oxidation Defects

A number of inherited defects in fatty acid oxidation have been identified in infants presenting with hypoglycemia. Although many of the disorders in this group typically present after 2 months of age, neonatal manifestations may be observed. These disorders are important because of their apparent frequency and because of the variability of the initial presentation. Affected infants have an impaired capacity to use stored fat for fuel during periods of fasting and readily deplete their glycogen stores. Despite the development of hypoglycemia, acetyl-CoA production is diminished, and ketone production is impaired. The hypoglycemia occurring in these conditions typically is characterized as nonketotic, although small amounts of ketones may be produced. Hypoglycemia may occur as an isolated finding or may be accompanied by many of the other biochemical derangements typically associated with Reye syndrome, such as hyperammonemia, metabolic acidosis, and elevated transaminases. Hepatomegaly may or may not be present. Any infant presenting with findings suggesting Reye syndrome should be evaluated for fatty acid oxidation defects. As the incidence of true Reye syndrome has decreased, most children presenting at any age with this constellation of findings have an inherited metabolic disorder.

The most common of the fatty acid oxidation defects is medium-chain acyl-CoA dehydrogenase deficiency, which is estimated to occur in 1 of 15,000 births, an incidence similar to that observed for phenylketonuria (PKU) (14,15). It is among the most common inborn errors of metabolism. In addition to presenting as nonketotic hypoglycemia or a Reye-like syndrome, it may present as sudden death or an acute life-threatening event. Microvesicular fat in the liver or muscle of any infant who dies unexpectedly should strongly suggest the possibility of this or a related disorder of fatty acid oxidation. Very-long-chain fatty acyl-CoA dehydrogenase deficiency is associated with similar clinical findings, although there may be evidence of a significant cardiomyopathy. Infants with this defect may present with cardiac arrhythmias or unexplained cardiac arrest. Defects in the carnitine cycle or in

carnitine uptake also may lead to a profound defect in fatty acid oxidation and result in sudden neonatal death.

The accumulation of fatty acyl-CoAs in patients with fatty acid oxidation defects leads to a secondary carnitine deficiency, probably as a result of excretion of excess acylcarnitine in the urine (16,17). Urine organic acid analysis and measurement of serum carnitine and analysis of the plasma acylcarnitine profile are the most helpful laboratory studies in the initial screening for defects in fatty acid oxidation. These studies are sufficient to establish the diagnosis of medium-chain acyl-CoA dehydrogenase deficiency, which is associated with the presence of a characteristic metabolite, octanoylcarnitine, on the acylcarnitine profile. Enzymatic assays or molecular testing may be necessary for the definitive diagnosis of some of the fatty acid oxidation defects. As is true for the defects in carbohydrate metabolism leading to hypoglycemia, treatment of the fatty acid oxidation defects involves avoidance of fasting and provision of adequate glucose. Supplemental L-carnitine therapy at a dose of 50 to 100 mg/kg/d may be recommended. With appropriate therapy, patients with medium-chain acyl-CoA dehydrogenase deficiency appear to have an excellent prognosis. The prognosis for the other fatty acid oxidation defects is more variable. All states in the United States now screen infants for fatty acid oxidation disorders with an acylcarnitine profile, but, as is true for some of the other inborn errors of metabolism, they may become symptomatic before the results of the screening tests become available.

Congenital Disorders of Glycosylation

Another group of disorders that may present with hypoglycemia in the neonate is the group of congenital disorders of glycosylation (the process by which cells build glycoproteins). This is a very heterogeneous and large group of conditions, which affect multiple organ systems. A common method of screening involves isoelectric focusing of serum transferrin with demonstration of underglycosylation (18).

▮ JAUNDICE AND LIVER DYSFUNCTION

Jaundice or other evidence of liver dysfunction may be the presenting finding in a number of inherited metabolic disorders in the neonatal period (19). These are listed in Table 55.4, along with the laboratory studies useful in diagnosis. For most of the inborn errors of metabolism associated with jaundice, the elevated serum bilirubin is of the direct-reacting type. This generalization does not include those inborn errors of erythrocyte metabolism, such as glucose-6-phosphate dehydrogenase deficiency or pyruvate kinase deficiency, which occasionally are responsible for hemolytic disease in the newborn.

Galactosemia

The best-known metabolic disease associated with jaundice is galactosemia, in which the deficiency of the enzyme galactose-1-phosphate uridylyl transferase results in an accumulation of galactose-1-phosphate and other metabolites, such as galactitol, which are thought to have a direct toxic effect on the liver and on other organs. Jaundice and liver dysfunction in this disorder are progressive and usually appear at the end of the first or during the second week of life, with vomiting, diarrhea, poor weight gain, and eventual cataract formation if the infant is receiving breast milk or a galactose-containing formula. Hypoglycemia may be observed. The disease may present initially with indirect hyperbilirubinemia resulting from hemolysis secondary to high levels of galactose-1-phosphate in erythrocytes. Alternatively, the effects of acute galactose toxicity on the brain rarely may cause the CNS symptoms to predominate, and, in some cases, *Escherichia coli* sepsis is the presenting problem.

TABLE 55.4

Inborn Errors of Metabolism Associated with Neonatal Liver Disease and Laboratory Studies Useful in Diagnosis

Disorder	Laboratory Studies
Galactosemia	Urine reducing substances; red blood cell galactose-1-phosphate uridyl transferase
Hereditary tyrosinemia	Plasma quantitative amino acids; urine succinylacetone
α_1-Antitrypsin deficiency	Quantitative serum α_1-antitrypsin; protease inhibitor (Pi) typing
Neonatal hemochromatosis	Serum ferritin; liver biopsy; buccal biopsy
Zellweger spectrum disorder	Plasma very-long-chain fatty acids
Niemann-Pick disease type C	Skin biopsy for fibroblast culture; filipin staining of cultured cells; molecular testing on peripheral blood
Glycogen storage disease type IV (brancher deficiency)	Liver biopsy for histology and biochemical analysis or skin biopsy with assay of branching enzyme in cultured fibroblasts; molecular testing on peripheral blood
Congenital disorders of glycosylation	Transferrin isoelectric focusing N- or O-glycan analysis in blood and/or urine
Mitochondrial DNA depletion syndromes	Plasma lactic acid; molecular testing on peripheral blood

If galactosemia is suspected, the urine should be tested simultaneously with Benedict reagent and with a glucose oxidase method. The glucose oxidase method is specific for glucose, and Benedict reagent can detect any reducing substance. A negative dipstick for glucose with a positive Benedict reaction means that a nonglucose reducing substance is present. With appropriate clinical findings, this is most likely to be galactose. Paper or thin-layer chromatography can be used to identify positively the reducing substance. If a child with galactosemia has been on intravenous fluids and has not recently been receiving galactose in the diet, galactose may not be present in the urine.

If the diagnosis of galactosemia is suspected, whether or not reducing substances are found in the urine, galactose-containing feedings should be discontinued immediately and replaced by soy formula or other lactose-free formula, pending the results of appropriate enzyme assays on erythrocytes to confirm the diagnosis. Untreated galactosemics, if they survive the neonatal period, have persistent liver disease, cataracts, and severe mental retardation. Many affected infants die of E. coli sepsis in the neonatal period, and the early onset of sepsis may alter the presentation of the disorder (20).

Treatment of the disorder by maintenance of strict dietary restriction of galactose, if started early, results in complete reversal of liver disease and enables many affected individuals to develop normal or near-normal intelligence. Unfortunately, there continues to be an increased incidence of intellectual disability even among treated patients, and many have speech disorders or learning disabilities. Additionally, there are some late sequelae of the disorder that appear to be unaffected by current therapy. These include premature ovarian failure in females and a late-onset neurologic syndrome involving ataxia and tremors in both sexes (21,22). All states in the United States have newborn screening programs for galactosemia, but clinical manifestations of the disorder often appear before the results of screening studies are available; therefore, it is critical that physicians remain alert to this possibility.

Hereditary Fructose Intolerance

Another inborn error of metabolism that rarely presents in the newborn period with jaundice, hepatomegaly, and the presence of reducing substances in the urine is hereditary fructose intolerance, which is characterized by episodes of profound hypoglycemia, vomiting, and metabolic acidosis. This disorder is seen uncommonly in the neonate, because most newborns are not exposed immediately to a fructose-containing diet unless they have been given a soy formula with sucrose as the carbohydrate source. In the uncommon event that an infant who has been receiving fructose should present with these findings, this diagnosis should be considered. Analysis of the urine reveals the presence of a nonglucose reducing substance that can be demonstrated by chromatography to be fructose. Treatment involves elimination of fructose from the diet and results in complete resolution of all clinical signs and symptoms. Confirmation of the diagnosis is by assay of the deficient enzyme fructose-1-phosphate aldolase in liver tissue, but this rarely is necessary.

α_1-Antitrypsin Deficiency

α_1-Antitrypsin deficiency, a puzzling disorder that is among the most common of all inherited metabolic diseases, also may present with neonatal jaundice (23). The clinical manifestations of this disorder may be identical to those of traditional neonatal or giant cell hepatitis, and a determination of serum α_1-antitrypsin should be a part of the initial evaluation of all children presenting with this syndrome. Infants with deficient levels of α_1-antitrypsin on quantitative analysis should have protease inhibitor typing performed to confirm the diagnosis. There is no specific treatment for the liver disease associated with α_1-antitrypsin deficiency, but approximately one-half of all affected infants eventually exhibit complete resolution of the liver dysfunction. Others may progress to end-stage disease and require liver transplantation. A history of chronic pulmonary disease in adult family members may be obtained.

Hereditary Tyrosinemia

Hereditary tyrosinemia (tyrosinemia type I) is another disorder that presents with liver disease, typically including a severe coagulopathy, in early infancy. The biochemical hallmarks of this disorder include marked elevations of plasma tyrosine and methionine and generalized aminoaciduria with a disproportionate increase in the excretion of tyrosine. However, these findings are relatively nonspecific and may be observed as a secondary phenomenon in other forms of liver disease. Hereditary tyrosinemia once was among the most difficult of inborn errors of metabolism to diagnose clinically. The finding of succinylacetone in the urine of patients with this disease has led to a helpful diagnostic test for the disorder (24). It also has become possible to establish the diagnosis definitively by demonstrating a deficiency of the enzyme fumarylacetoacetate fumarylhydrolase in lymphocytes and cultured skin fibroblasts of affected individuals (25). Plasma tyrosine is measured in newborn screening programs but has a low sensitivity for the detection of hereditary tyrosinemia since tyrosine levels are rarely significantly elevated at 24 hours of age. Plasma succinylacetone is being developed as a newborn screening marker and may turn out to be a much more sensitive tool for the detection of the disorder.

Neonatal Hemochromatosis/Gestational Alloimmune Liver Disease

Neonatal hemochromatosis, now regarded as an alloimmune disorder, is the most common cause of acute liver failure in the neonate. The condition is now understood to be caused by maternal production of IgG antibodies that are directed against fetal hepatocytes. Its fulminating course distinguishes it from many of the other metabolic disorders associated with neonatal liver disease. In addition to being associated with severe liver failure from birth, the disorder is characterized by distinctive hepatic morphology and hepatic and extrahepatic parenchymal iron deposition. Serum ferritin and iron typically are elevated, whereas total transferrin is low, but these findings are not diagnostic. Abdominal MRI can be helpful at times. The definitive diagnosis is established by liver biopsy or autopsy. If liver biopsy is contraindicated because of a secondary coagulopathy, biopsy of the salivary glands or buccal mucosa is a useful alternative. Many affected infants succumb to the disorder during the early weeks of life. Treatment with antioxidants and chelation therapy has now successfully been replaced by exchange transfusions and intravenous immunoglobulin substitution. Antenatal treatment with intravenous immunoglobulins has been shown to prevent recurrence of the disorder in subsequent pregnancies such that making the diagnosis, even postmortem, is vital for management of subsequent pregnancies (26).

Other Causes

Less common metabolic causes of neonatal liver dysfunction include Niemann-Pick disease type C and glycogen storage disease type IV. Infants with Niemann-Pick disease type C exhibit cholestatic jaundice, which often resolves by several months to several years of age. They then may be clinically normal for a period of months to years before developing findings of a degenerative neurologic disorder. A subset of infants with Niemann-Pick disease type C have neonatal liver disease progressing to liver failure making them candidates for liver transplantation. Infants with glycogen storage disease type IV accumulate an abnormal form of glycogen in the liver as a result of a deficiency of the glycogen branching enzyme. This leads to progressive cirrhosis and generalized hepatic dysfunction. Hypoglycemia is not a prominent feature, as it is in some other forms of glycogen storage disease.

Zellweger spectrum disorder, formerly referred to as the cerebrohepatorenal syndrome, is another cause of neonatal jaundice and hepatic dysfunction, but it usually is recognizable clinically because of the associated hypotonia and dysmorphic features. It is the prototype of the peroxisome assembly disorders and is associated with generalized peroxisomal dysfunction.

In contrast to disorders in which there is an elevation of the direct-reacting bilirubin, a persistent elevation of indirect bilirubin beyond the limits of physiologic jaundice, without evidence of hemolysis, suggests the diagnosis of the Crigler-Najjar syndrome. The hyperbilirubinemia in this disorder is related to a partial or complete deficiency of glucuronyl transferase, the liver enzyme responsible for the normal conjugation of bilirubin to bilirubin diglucuronide. There is no effective long-term therapy for all patients with this disorder, but the standard modalities of phototherapy and exchange transfusion may prevent the development of kernicterus in the neonatal period (27,28). Hepatic transplantation has been performed successfully in patients with this disorder. Patients with a partial deficiency of the enzyme may respond to phenobarbital therapy (29).

FINDINGS SUGGESTIVE OF A STORAGE DISEASE

Many of the well-known lipid storage diseases typically do not present in the neonatal period. Among those that occasionally may be associated with hepatosplenomegaly in the neonatal period are GM$_1$ gangliosidosis type I, Gaucher disease, Niemann-Pick disease, and Wolman disease. The glycogen storage diseases that are associated with hepatomegaly in the newborn have previously been discussed in reference to hypoglycemia. Infants with the most common mucopolysaccharidoses, such as the Hurler and Hunter syndromes, uncommonly exhibit clinical abnormalities in the first month of life. Newborns with the typical features of these syndromes, such as coarse facial features, hepatosplenomegaly, skeletal abnormalities, and hernias, are more likely to have GM$_1$ gangliosidosis or a mucolipidosis, such as I-cell disease. Beta-glucuronidase deficiency, also classified as mucopolysaccharidosis type VII, may present in the neonatal period with features virtually indistinguishable clinically from those seen later in the Hurler and Hunter syndromes. An infantile form of sialidosis (i.e., neuraminidase deficiency) typically is associated with findings at birth. The clinical manifestations of several of these conditions may be so severe in utero that fetal hydrops develops. Certainly, a storage disorder should be considered in the differential diagnosis of nonimmune fetal hydrops, particularly if organomegaly is present (30).

If one of these disorders is suspected, urine screening tests for mucopolysaccharides (glycosaminoglycans) and oligosaccharides should be performed. These can be helpful diagnostically, but negative results do not rule out the possibility of a storage disorder. False-positive mucopolysaccharide spot tests are commonly observed in neonates. The definitive diagnosis of most disorders of lipid or mucopolysaccharide metabolism is made by appropriate biochemical studies or molecular studies on leukocytes or cultured skin fibroblasts. A number of laboratories offer lysosomal enzyme screening panels for this indication.

ABNORMAL ODOR

Abnormal body or urinary odor, more commonly observed by nurses or mothers rather than physicians, is an important but often overlooked clue to the diagnosis of several of the inborn errors of metabolism and may be the most specific clinical finding in these patients. It is best described for PKU, for which the urine was found to have a peculiar musty odor years before the biochemical basis of the disease was understood. In the era of newborn screening, the abnormal odor of PKU is essentially never observed. In the acutely ill neonate with an abnormal odor, isovaleric acidemia, glutaric acidemia type II, and maple syrup urine disease are the most likely entities to be encountered. In maple syrup urine disease, the urine has a distinctive sweet odor, said to be reminiscent of maple syrup or burnt sugar. The odor associated with isovaleric acidemia and glutaric acidemia type II is pungent and unpleasant and similar to that of sweaty feet or pungent cheese.

DYSMORPHIC FEATURES

There formerly appeared to be a clear distinction between inborn errors of metabolism and dysmorphic syndromes, both of which may be inherited in a similar fashion. Infants with inherited metabolic disease were thought to be phenotypically normal at birth, with no evidence of major or minor structural anomalies. It is becoming increasingly apparent that inherited metabolic disorders may be associated with consistent patterns of birth defects, suggesting that metabolic derangements in utero may disrupt the normal process of fetal development.

Peroxisomal Disorders

This phenomenon is illustrated clearly by the group of disorders associated with multiple defects in peroxisomal enzymes, including those involved in fatty acid oxidation and plasmalogen synthesis (29,31). These include Zellweger spectrum disorder, neonatal adrenoleukodystrophy, and several variant conditions, all of which are associated with congenital hypotonia and dysmorphic features, such as epicanthal folds, Brushfield spots, large fontanels, simian creases, and renal cysts.

Glutaric Acidemia

Patients with the most severe form of glutaric acidemia type II, one of the organic acidemias, have a characteristic phenotype, including a high forehead, hypertelorism, low-set ears, abdominal wall defects, palpably enlarged kidneys, hypospadias, and rocker bottom feet (32,33). An energy-deficient mechanism, referred to as fuel-mediated teratogenesis, similar to that postulated for maternal diabetes mellitus, has been suggested to explain these findings. Several of the other organic acidemias, such as mevalonic aciduria and 3-hydroxyisobutyric aciduria, have also been associated with multiple dysmorphic features.

Pyruvate Dehydrogenase Deficiency

Some infants with pyruvate dehydrogenase (PDH) deficiency have dysmorphic facial features resembling those observed in the fetal alcohol syndrome (FAS) (34). The specific findings observed include a narrow forehead with frontal bossing, a broad nasal bridge, short nose with anteverted nostrils, and a long philtrum. The resemblance to FAS has been explained by suggesting that there is a common mechanism in the two disorders, involving a deficiency of PDH activity. It has been postulated that, in FAS, acetaldehyde from the maternal circulation inhibits fetal PDH, which leads to malformations.

Smith-Lemli-Opitz Syndrome

The Smith-Lemli-Opitz syndrome, an autosomal recessive disorder of cholesterol biosynthesis, is an autosomal recessive disorder associated with a wide range of malformations, including dysmorphic facies, cleft palate, congenital heart disease, hypospadias, polydactyly, and 2–3 syndactyly of the feet. Recent observations have revealed that this disorder is an inborn error of cholesterol biosynthesis. Affected infants have decreased levels of plasma cholesterol accompanied by markedly elevated levels of the cholesterol precursor 7-dehydrocholesterol (35).

ISOLATED MALFORMATIONS

Isolated malformations may be even more commonly associated with inherited metabolic disorders than are specific malformation patterns. Patients with nonketotic hyperglycinemia frequently have agenesis of the corpus callosum and may have gyral malformations related to defects in neuronal migration as well (36). Patients with PDH deficiency also may exhibit agenesis of the corpus callosum (37). It is not uncommon for patients with almost any of the inborn errors of metabolism to exhibit one or more dysmorphic features or anomalies that are nonspecific. The observation of dysmorphic features in an infant in no way should preclude consideration of an inherited metabolic disorder. In selected circumstances, it may heighten the clinical suspicion.

ABNORMAL EYE FINDINGS

Abnormal eye findings typically are associated with many of the inborn errors of metabolism, although they are not always found at the time of initial presentation. Cataracts classically are associated with galactosemia and other disorders of galactose metabolism but also are observed in disorders such as Zellweger syndrome and Lowe syndrome. Dislocated lenses, seen in homocystinuria, molybdenum cofactor deficiency, and sulfite oxidase deficiency, may be found as early as the first month of life and are an important clue to diagnosis. Retinal degenerative changes are typical of the peroxisomal disorders, including Zellweger syndrome and neonatal adrenoleukodystrophy, and are observed in several other conditions. Other abnormalities that may be associated with inborn errors of metabolism include corneal clouding and congenital glaucoma. A careful eye examination, preferably by an ophthalmologist, should be performed whenever an inherited metabolic disorder is suspected. A summary of some of the inherited metabolic disorders associated with specific ocular abnormalities is shown in Table 55.5.

TABLE 55.5

Eye Abnormalities Associated with Inborn Errors of Metabolism

Eye Finding	Associated Disorders
Cataracts	Galactosemia
	Homocystinuria
	Lowe syndrome
	Zellweger syndrome
	Rhizomelic chondrodysplasia punctata
	Sengers syndrome
	Hypophosphatasia
Ectopia lentis	Homocystinuria
	Molybdenum cofactor deficiency
	Sulfite oxidase deficiency
Cherry red spot	Niemann-Pick disease types A and B
	Gaucher disease type II
	GM_2 gangliosidosis (Tay-Sachs; Sandhoff)
	Sialidosis type II
	Farber disease
Corneal clouding	Mucopolysaccharidoses
	Mucolipidoses
	Lowe syndrome
	Homocystinuria
Pigmentary retinopathy	Zellweger syndrome
	Neonatal adrenoleukodystrophy
	Long-chain 3-hydroxyacyl-CoA dehydrogenase deficiency

SAMPLES TO OBTAIN FROM A DYING CHILD WITH A SUSPECTED INBORN ERROR OF METABOLISM

If death appears imminent in a child suspected of having an inborn error of metabolism, it is important to obtain the appropriate samples for postmortem analysis. This is critical for resolution of the cause of death and is essential for subsequent genetic counseling and prenatal diagnosis. The following samples should be collected and stored: urine, frozen; plasma, separated from whole blood and frozen; and whole blood from which DNA can be extracted. If an autopsy is performed, a sample of unfixed liver tissue should be obtained as soon as possible after death and frozen at $-20°C$ for subsequent biochemical studies. Additional tissue should be preserved for electron microscopy. If consent for autopsy is denied, consent for a postmortem needle biopsy of the liver should be requested if it is appropriate given the symptoms. The liver tissue should be frozen in total or in part if histologic studies appear to be indicated. As soon as possible after death, the case should be reviewed with a metabolic specialist and plans made for the transport of samples to the appropriate laboratory.

NEWBORN SCREENING FOR INHERITED METABOLIC DISORDERS

All 50 states and the District of Columbia in the United States and many other countries have newborn screening programs in place for genetic disorders. While there were once significant state-to-state differences in the disorders that were included, with the establishment of a federal advisory committee within the Department of Health and Human Services that has developed a core panel of disorders, which are recommended for inclusion in newborn screening panels by the states ("the recommended uniform screening panel or RUSP"), these differences have now largely been eliminated. However, there are still significant differences in how newborn screening is implemented by each state health department, and new disorders may be added by individual states without the recommendation of the federal advisory committee. The disorders that were included on the RUSP as of 2019 are listed in Table 55.6. A mechanism exists for the nomination of new disorders to the RUSP. Nominations can be submitted by any interested individual, group, or organization. In general, requirements for addition to a disorder to the RUSP include evidence that a disorder is medically significant, the availability of a screening test that is appropriate for analysis of large numbers of samples in a short period of time, the availability of treatment for the disorder,

TABLE 55.6

Disorders on the Recommended Uniform Screening Panel

Amino acid disorders	Phenylketonuria
	Maple syrup urine disease
	Homocystinuria
	Hereditary tyrosinemia (tyrosinemia type I)
Urea cycle disorders	Citrullinemia
	Argininosuccinic aciduria
Organic acid disorders	Methylmalonic acidemia
	Methylmalonic acidemia (cobalamin disorders)
	Proprionic acidemia
	Isovaleric acidemia
	3-Methylcrotonyl-CoA carboxylase deficiency
	Holocarboxylase synthase deficiency
	Biotinidase deficiency
	3-Hydroxy-3-methylglutaric aciduria
	β-Ketothiolase deficiency
	Glutaric acidemia type I
Fatty acid oxidation disorders	Medium-chain acyl-CoA dehydrogenase deficiency
	Very long-chain acyl-CoA dehydrogenase deficiency
	Long-chain hydroxyl acyl-CoA dehydrogenase deficiency
	Trifunctional protein deficiency
	Carnitine uptake defect
Lysosomal disorders	Pompe disease (glycogen storage disease type I)
	Mucopolysaccharidosis type 1
Endocrine disorders	Congenital hypothyroidism
	Congenital adrenal hyperplasia
Other	Galactosemia
	Severe combined immunodeficiency disease
	X-linked adrenoleukodystrophy
	Cystic fibrosis
	Critical congenital heart disease
	Hearing loss
	Spinal muscular atrophy
Hematologic disorders	S, S disease
	S, C disease
	S, β-Thalassemia

and evidence that treatment prior to the time of clinical diagnosis improves the outcome.

Positive newborn screening tests are common among sick or premature hospitalized neonates and are often not a reflection of true disease. For some analytes, positive test results may be more common in premature infants because of immaturity of metabolic pathways. Abnormal amino acid levels, often not suggestive of a single specific diagnosis, are common among infants receiving total parenteral nutrition. Physicians should become familiar with the recommendations for follow-up of abnormal screening test results in their practice areas. In many cases, sending a repeat filter paper sample may be appropriate. However, if a specific diagnosis is suggested by the test result particularly one with urgent implications for treatment (such as galactosemia, maple syrup urine disease, or a urea cycle disorder), definitive diagnostic testing should be pursued. In some cases, presumptive treatment should be initiated. For example, if the newborn screening test result suggests a high risk of galactosemia, galactose should be eliminated from feedings until diagnostic test results are available. The American College of Medical Genetics and Genomics provides fact sheets regarding each of the newborn screening disorders and diagnostic algorithms on its website www.acmg.net.

MATERNAL METABOLIC DISORDERS

With advances in therapy for inborn errors of metabolism, it is now common for patients with many of these disorders to reach adult life with normal or near-normal intelligence and the desire to have families of their own. This has led to serious concerns about the potential adverse effects of maternal metabolic derangements on fetal growth and development. The real potential for adverse consequences is illustrated by the experience that has accumulated with maternal PKU. In the past, patients with PKU were severely intellectually disabled and were unlikely to reproduce. This changed completely with the initiation of newborn screening programs and early dietary management. Dietary therapy was once maintained until 5 to 6 years of age and then discontinued. Treatment for PKU is now recommended for life, because it has been demonstrated that some patients exhibit neurologic deterioration and loss of intelligence quotient (IQ) points after discontinuation of the diet and because chronically elevated blood phenylalanine levels are associated with adverse neurocognitive and psychiatric symptoms. Nonetheless, many patients with PKU who are now adults have been off the diet for years, have high phenylalanine levels, and are resistant to treatment. In addition, many adults on continuous treatment have poorly controlled blood phenylalanine levels due to difficulties in adhering to the very restrictive low phenylalanine diet. After women with PKU began reproducing, it became clear that the maternal metabolic environment in this condition had extremely harmful effects on fetal development. A spectrum of findings referred to as "maternal PKU syndrome" is observed in a large percentage of infants exposed to high phenylalanine levels *in utero*, while most of these infants do not themselves have PKU (38,39). Typical findings include microcephaly, developmental disabilities, growth restriction, and congenital heart defects. Altered facial features, similar to those observed in FAS, may be observed.

There is evidence that dietary treatment of pregnant women before conception and throughout pregnancy, with careful control of phenylalanine levels, reduces the risk to the fetus (40). This may be a difficult goal to achieve, however, in all cases because the phenylalanine-restricted diet is an onerous one to patients who have ever been on a normal diet, and some adult patients, despite early therapy, may have borderline intellectual functioning. There has been no evidence for an increased risk of birth defects or any other problems in infants born to fathers with PKU.

Pregnancies have been reported in mothers with a variety of other inherited metabolic disorders, including several forms of glycogen storage disease, propionic acidemia, isovaleric acidemia, homocystinuria, hereditary orotic aciduria, and several others, with no adverse outcomes clearly attributable to the maternal disorder. The collaborative experience with many disorders, however, is limited to single cases or small numbers of patients. It is probable that other maternal metabolic disorders will be identified that adversely affect fetal development.

REFERENCES

1. Fischer AQ, Challa VR, Burton BK, et al. Cerebellar hemorrhage complicating isovaleric acidemia: a case report. *Neurology* 1981;31(6):746.
2. Nyhan WL. Patterns of clinical expression and genetic variation in the inborn errors of metabolism. In: Nyhan WL, ed. *Heritable disorders of amino acid metabolism*. New York, NY: John Wiley and Sons, 1974.
3. Ballard RA, Vinocur B, Reynolds JW, et al. Transient hyperammonemia of the preterm infant. *N Engl J Med* 1978;299:920.
4. Msall M, Batshaw ML, Suss R, et al. Neurologic outcome in children with inborn errors of urea synthesis. *N Engl J Med* 1984;310:1500.
5. Goldberg RN, Cabal LA, Sinatra FR, et al. Hyperammonemia associated with perinatal asphyxia. *Pediatrics* 1979;64(3):336.
6. Batshaw ML, Wachtel RC, Cohen L, et al. Neurologic outcome in premature infants with transient asymptomatic hyperammonemia. *J Pediatr* 1986;108(2):271.
7. Schillaci L-AP, DeBrosse SD, McCandless SE. Inborn errors of metabolism with acidosis. Organic acidemias and defects of pyruvate and ketone body metabolism. *Pediatr Clin North Am* 2018;65:209.
8. Robinson BH, Taylor J, Sherwood WG. The genetic heterogeneity of lactic acidosis: occurrence of recognizable inborn errors of metabolism in a pediatric population with lactic acidosis. *Pediatr Res* 1980;14:956.
9. Robinson BH, Glerum DM, Chow W, et al. The use of skin fibroblast cultures in the detection of respiratory chain defects in patients with lactic acidemia. *Pediatr Res* 1990;28:549.
10. Dalla Bernardina B, Aicardi J, Goutieres F, et al. Glycine encephalopathy. *Neuropadiatrie* 1979;10:209.
11. Hanudel M, Avasare S, Tsai E, et al. A biphasic dialytic strategy for the treatment of neonatal hyperammonemia. *Pediatr Nephrol* 2014;29(2):315.
12. Wiegand C, Thompson T, Bock GH, et al. The management of life-threatening hyperammonemia: a comparison of several therapeutic modalities. *J Pediatr* 1980;96:142.
13. Enns GM, Berry SA, Berry GT, et al. Survival after treatment with phenylacetate and benzoate for urea-cycle disorders. *N Engl J Med* 2007;356:2282.
14. Matsubara Y, Narisawa K, Tada K, et al. Prevalence of K329E mutation in medium-chain acyl-CoA dehydrogenase gene determined from Guthrie cards. *Lancet* 1991;1:552.
15. Ziadeh R. Medium chain acyl-CoA dehydrogenase deficiency in Pennsylvania: neonatal screening shows high incidence and unexpected mutation frequencies. *Pediatr Res* 1995;37:675.
16. Stanley CA, Hale DE, Coates PM, et al. Medium chain acyl-CoA dehydrogenase deficiency in children with non-ketotic hypoglycemia and low carnitine levels. *Pediatr Res* 1983;17:877.
17. Engel AG, Rebouche CJ. Carnitine metabolism and inborn errors. *J Inherit Metab Dis* 1984;1(suppl 7):38.
18. Woods AG, Woods CW, Snow TM. Congenital disorders of glycosylation. *Adv Neonatal Care* 2012;12:90.
19. Ferreira CR, Cassiman D and Blau N. Clinical and biochemical footprints of inherited metabolic diseases. II. Metabolic liver diseases. *Mol Genet Metab* 2019;127:117.
20. Levy HL, Sepe SJ, Shih VE, et al. Sepsis due to *Escherichia coli* in neonates with galactosemia. *N Engl J Med* 1977;297:823.
21. Kaufman FR, Kogut MD, Donnell GN, et al. Hypergonadotropic hypogonadism in female patients with galactosemia. *N Engl J Med* 1981;304:994.
22. Friedman JH, Levy HL, Boustany RM. Late onset of distinct neurologic syndromes in galactosemic siblings. *Neurology* 1989;39:741.
23. Cutz E, Cox DW. Alpha1-antitrypsin deficiency: the spectrum of pathology and pathophysiology. *Perspect Pediatr Pathol* 1979;5:1.
24. Lindbland B, Lindstedt S, Stein G. On the enzymic defects in hereditary tyrosinemia. *Proc Natl Acad Sci U S A* 1977;74:4641.
25. Kvittingen EA, Halvorsen S, Jellum E. Deficient fumarylacetoacetate fumarylhydrolase activity in lymphocytes and fibroblasts from patients with hereditary tyrosinemia. *Pediatr Res* 1983;14:541.
26. Lopriore E, Mearin ML, Oeples D, et al. Neonatal hemochromatosis: management, outcome, and prevention. *Prenat Diagn* 2013;33:1221.
27. Karon M, Imach D, Schwartz A. Effective phototherapy in congenital non-obstructive non-hemolytic jaundice. *N Engl J Med* 1970;282:377.
28. Gorodischer R, Levy G, Krasner J, et al. Congenital non-obstructive non-hemolytic jaundice: effect of phototherapy. *N Engl J Med* 1970;282:375.
29. Schutgens RB, Heymans HS, Wanders RJ, et al. Peroxisomal disorders: a newly recognized group of genetic diseases. *Eur J Pediatr* 1986;144:430.
30. Holtz M, Montaño AM, Sly WS. Association between mucopolysaccharidosis type VII and hydrops fetalis. *Ultrasound Obstet Gynecol* 2020;55(3):416. doi: 10.1002/uog.20371.
31. Wilson GN, Holmes RD, Hajra AK. Peroxisomal disorders: clinical commentary and future prospects. *Am J Med Genet* 1988;30:771.
32. Sweetman L, Nyhan WL, Trauner DA, et al. Glutaric aciduria type II. *J Pediatr* 1980;96:1020.
33. Chalmers RA, Tracy BM, King GS, et al. The prenatal diagnosis of glutaric acidemia type II using quantitative gas chromatography–mass spectroscopy. *J Inherit Metab Dis* 1985;2:145.
34. Robinson BH, McMillan H, Petrova-Benedict R, et al. Variable clinical presentation in patients with defective E component of pyruvate dehydrogenase complex. A review of 30 cases with a defect in the E component of the complex. *J Pediatr* 1987;111:525.
35. Opitz JM, de la Cruz F. Cholesterol metabolism in the RSH/Smith–Lemli–Opitz syndrome: summary of an NICHD conference. *Am J Med Genet* 1994;50:326.
36. Dobyns WB. Agenesis of the corpus callosum and gyral malformations are frequent manifestations of nonketotic hyperglycinemia. *Neurology* 1989;39:817.
37. Wick H, Schweizer KK, Baumgartner R. Thiamine dependency in a patient with congenital lactic acidemia due to pyruvate dehydrogenase deficiency. *Agents Actions* 1977;7:405.
38. Lenke RR, Levy HL. Maternal phenylketonuria and hyperphenylalaninemia. An international survey of untreated and treated pregnancies. *N Engl J Med* 1980;303:1202.
39. Levy HL, Waisbren SE. Effects of untreated maternal phenylketonuria and hyperphenylalaninemia on the fetus. *N Engl J Med* 1983;309:1269.
40. Koch R, Friedman E, Azen C, et al. The International Collaborative Study of Maternal Phenylketonuria: status report 1998. *Eur J Pediatr* 2000;159(suppl 2):S156.

56 Genetics and Genomics

Margo Sheck Breilyn and Bruce D. Gelb

INTRODUCTION

Genetic disorders and congenital birth defects are a major cause of morbidity and mortality in high-resource countries and impact approximately 6% of births in the United States (1). Arriving at a diagnosis in these patients requires an understanding of the strengths and limitations of the available genetic testing technologies. This chapter reviews the types of human genetic variation and the technologies that can detect them. Specimen collection and types of results are also briefly reviewed.

OVERVIEW OF THE HUMAN GENOME

The human genome comprises the complete set of genetic material contained in the nuclear and mitochondrial genomes. The nuclear genome consists of approximately 3.2×10^9 nucleotides of DNA and encodes approximately 20,000 genes. This large dataset is packaged into 24 chromosomes, including 22 autosomes and 2 sex chromosomes (X and Y). At least one full copy of the human genome is found in every normal nucleated cell in the human body. Somatic cells are *diploid*, meaning they have two copies of each autosome plus two sex chromosomes (46, XY or 46, XX), while gametes are *haploid* with 23 chromosomes per cell. The genomic sequence is subdivided into protein coding portions (*exons*), genetic material separating the exons (*introns*), and other noncoding sequences including promoters, enhancers, and other intergenic sequences. An *exome* is defined as the entire collection of exonic sequences and the flanking intron boundaries and accounts for only 1.5% of the genome.

The mitochondrial genome is a circular DNA molecule that is 16,562 nucleotides in length. It encodes 37 genes that are important for mitochondrial structure and function (2). The remaining proteins required for mitochondrial function are nuclearly encoded.

The basic unit of DNA is a base pair (bp). Multiplying by a factor of 1,000, 1×10^3 bp is a kilobase (kb), 1×10^6 bp is a megabase (Mb), and 1×10^9 bp is a gigabase (Gb). The full length of the genome is 3.2 Gb (the human genome). Although highly variable, the median length of a protein-coding gene is estimated at 26 kb (3). Chromosomes range in size from 25 Mb to nearly 250 Mb (4) (**Fig. 56.1**).

HUMAN GENETIC VARIATION

"Normal" Genetic Variation

The Human Genome Project was an international collaboration to decode the nucleotide sequence of the human nuclear genome. As a result of this project, a reference human genome was released in 2004 (5). Although this reference was initially felt to be representative of most healthy individuals, further sequencing efforts revealed genetic variation in the absence of disease. The 1,000 Genomes Project involved sequencing the genomes of more than 2,500 healthy individuals from 26 populations. The data revealed a broad spectrum of variation in these populations, with over 88 million total variants (6). This project supported the idea that the reference genome does not incorporate the full spectrum of "normal" variation in healthy individuals and that variation from the reference, therefore, does not always confer disease. This principle is important to interpreting sequencing variants in patients.

Variation at the Genomic and Chromosomal Levels

Human genetic variation can be grouped based on the size of the change. Beginning with the largest variants, *polyploidy* is a defect at the genomic scale. Defined as an aberrant multiple of the complete set of the haploid genome, polyploidy may be seen in products of conception (e.g., 72, XXX). *Aneuploidy* is a comparable defect at the chromosomal scale. This involves an abnormal number of a single or select set of chromosomes. Aneuploidy affects up to 5% of all recognized pregnancies and 1 in 160 live births (7). Trisomies occur when there are three copies of a representative chromosome. Trisomies observed in live births are trisomy 13, 18, 21, X, and Y. *Monosomy*, or reduction to a single copy of a representative chromosome, is generally not compatible with life with the notable exception of monosomy X (45, X, or Turner syndrome).

Uniparental disomy (UPD) can also be considered a variant at the chromosomal scale. It is observed when the total number of chromosomes is normal, but rather than biparental inheritance, both copies of a chromosome were inherited from the same parent. This is clinically relevant when the chromosome is *imprinted*, meaning there is parent-of-origin-specific gene expression, or as an unusual mechanism for autosomal recessive conditions (inheritance of two copies of a pathogenic allele from one parent). Imprinting conditions with UPD as an underlying mechanism include Prader Willi and Angelman syndromes.

Variation at the Subchromosomal Level

Variation at the subchromosomal scale includes alterations in the copy number of a chromosomal segment and structural rearrangements. These are observed with a frequency of 1 in 375 newborns (7). Structurally abnormal chromosomes include translocations, inversions, and supernumerary chromosomes (marker and ring chromosomes). The addition and deletion of subchromosomal genetic material can be subdivided based on size. Copy number variants (CNVs) are the largest alterations in this category and involve the addition or deletion of 1 kb to greater than 1 Mb. Indels are small insertions and deletions that involve a single nucleotide or up to 1 kb. Examples of syndromes caused by CNVs include DiGeorge syndrome (22q11.2 deletion), Cri du chat syndrome (5p deletion), and Williams syndrome (7q11.23 deletion).

Repeat expansion disorders are a unique mechanism of nucleotide addition. Nucleotide repeats (e.g., CGGCGGCGG...) are a normal occurrence within the genome but may become unstable and expand between generations. Disease is observed when the number of repeats expands beyond some gene-specific threshold. Repeat expansion disorders include fragile X syndrome, Friedrich ataxia, and myotonic dystrophy, among others.

Variation at the Nucleotide Level

The smallest scale of genetic variation is at the bp level and includes alteration of a nucleotide relative to the reference sequence. Alterations of a nucleotide sequence may result in a change in the encoded amino acid (missense variant), or terminate translation by coding for a stop codon (nonsense variant). Alternatively, the coding sequence may remain unchanged (silent variant). An alternative sequence of a gene at a specific locus is referred to as an *allele*. Nucleotide substitutions are a common mechanism of genetic disease and account for approximately 80% of disease-causing variants. Sickle cell disease, for example, is caused by the replacement of an adenine with a thymine in the β-globin gene (G*A*G → G*T*G), which results in a change from glutamic acid to

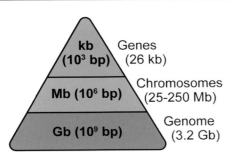

FIGURE 56.1 Units in genetics and genomics. The basic unit of DNA is a base pair (bp). Genes are on the kilobase scale (kb), chromosomes are on the megabase scale (Mb), and the genome in its entirety is on the gigabase scale (Gb).

valine in the sixth amino acid of the protein (p.Glu6Val). If both copies of a patient's β-globin genes have this change, they will manifest with sickle cell disease (8). This illustrates the potential for genetic changes at the smallest scale to result in systemic disease.

Mosaicism

Mosaicism is an important concept in human genetic variation. This occurs when there are two or more distinct cell populations in an individual or tissue, arising from the same zygote. Chromosomal abnormalities, for example, may be mosaic and result in an attenuated phenotype. An example of chromosomal mosaicism is trisomy 21, whereby an individual has cells lines with both a normal karyotype and trisomy 21 karyotype (46, XY/47, XY+21).

MITOCHONDRIAL GENOME

Alterations of the mitochondrial genome constitute a distinct category of genetic variation. There are 80 to 2,000 mitochondria per cell, each maternally inherited and independently replicating. Like the nuclear genome, the mitochondrial genome is susceptible to deletions, duplications, and point alterations. Phenotypes resulting from mitochondrial genomic alterations depend upon the fraction of abnormal mitochondria in any given cell. This variability is referred to as *heteroplasmy*.

The mitochondrial genome encodes just a small proportion of the proteins necessary for mitochondrial integrity and function. The majority of these proteins are nuclearly encoded. As such, while mitochondrial disease may result from variation in the mitochondrial genome, the majority result from nuclear variation (9). Leigh syndrome, for example, is a mitochondrial disease characterized by progressive neurologic decline and characteristic symmetric T2 hyperintensities on MRI. This prototypical mitochondrial disease has been attributed to variants in more than 50 nuclear genes and 14 mitochondrial genes. Such genetic heterogeneity is characteristic of many mitochondrial diseases, often spanning both the mitochondrial and nuclear genomes.

SPECIMEN COLLECTION

Genetic testing is most commonly performed on whole blood. Saliva, dried blood spots, and urine can also be used. Tubes with EDTA are preferred for specimens for DNA analysis, with best results when samples are refrigerated at 4°C and processed within 9 days (10). Some testing laboratories also permit blood samples to be collected in citric acetate or potassium oxalate/sodium fluoride tubes. Tubes with sodium heparin are required for karyotype and fluorescence *in situ* hybridization (FISH) tests as those typically require living white blood cells to be grown in culture. Skin biopsy may be considered for fibroblast culture. This should be collected under sterile conditions to avoid culture contamination. Fibroblasts are favored for long-term cell culture and are sometimes useful in the postmortem setting for this reason.

TECHNOLOGIES

Detection of Aneuploidies and Copy Number Variants
Karyotype

A karyotype is a photomicrograph of condensed chromosomes organized by number. Preparation involves cell culture, arrest in metaphase, and then staining. Giemsa staining, or "G staining," is most commonly used and results in a characteristic staining pattern of dark and light bands. The pattern of bands can be used to identify chromosomes and their structure. Loss of a band or bands corresponds to loss of the sequences and genes within it. Karyotyping is the gold standard for detecting structural and numerical chromosomal changes. The ability to detect deletions or duplications is limited by resolution. Standard karyotyping has a resolution of 5 to 10 Mb. High-resolution karyotypes, obtained during prometaphase, have a resolution of 2 to 3 Mb and, therefore, can detect smaller deletions and duplications.

Fluorescence *In Situ* Hybridization

Fluorescence *in situ* hybridization, abbreviated FISH, is used to rapidly identify the copy number of a specific chromosome or subchromosomal segment. FISH involves hybridization of a fluorescently labeled DNA probe, followed by fluorescent microscopy to visualize the copy number for the tagged region(s). Compared to karyotyping, FISH offers faster return of results because it can be performed without cell culture. It is useful in neonates for rapid identification of aneuploidies and common microdeletion syndromes, such as 22q11.2 deletion syndrome. However, it is only informative for the regions specific to the ordered DNA probes, typically chromosomes 18, 13, 21, X and Y, and 22q11.2. Structural abnormalities are not detected and low-level mosaicism may be missed. For these reasons, FISH should be ordered as a complement to karyotype (11).

Chromosomal Microarray

Chromosomal microarray (CMA) offers high-resolution detection of CNVs on a genome-wide scale. This technology involves comparison of a patient's genomic DNA to a reference genome. There are two major platforms used in CMA analysis, comparative genome hybridization (CGH), and single-nucleotide polymorphism (SNP) analysis. In CGH, labeled control and sample DNAs are hybridized to probes spaced throughout the genome, which are on the microarray, and the relative hybridization is compared. An excess or reduction of hybridization of the patient sample relative to the reference genome represents a duplication or deletion, respectively. Microarrays have the advantage of identifying CNVs that are too small to be visualized on karyotyping. SNP arrays incorporate the relative representation of single-nucleotide variants seen in the healthy population (referred to as single-nucleotide polymorphisms or SNPs). The addition of SNP analysis allows identification of uniparental disomy and areas of homozygosity reflective of a common ancestor. The resolution of a microarray depends on the number and distribution of probes and varies by the commercial platform. Typically, resolution is at least 250 kb (7). Since this test reflects gene dosage but not position, balanced structural rearrangements cannot be detected with CMAs.

A comparison of the technologies used to detect aneuploidies and CNVs can be seen in Table 56.1.

Detection of Trinucleotide Repeat Disorders
Southern Blotting and PCR

Accurate sizing of a repeat is important for prognostic purposes in many triplet repeat disorders. Quantification of moderate length expansions can be performed by PCR, but for longer expansions as is seen in myotonic dystrophy and fragile X syndrome, Southern blotting, or long-range PCR methods are required (12).

TABLE 56.1

Comparison of Technologies for Detection of Aneuploidies (e.g., Trisomy 21) and Copy Number Variants (e.g., DiGeorge Syndrome)		
Technology	Major Advantage	Limitations
Karyotype	Allows visualization of balanced and imbalanced structural rearrangements	Will miss small copy number variants that could be detected on CMA
FISH	Fast turnaround time (generally 2–3 d)	Highly targeted—only informative with regard to the FISH probes used
CMA	Able to detect smaller CNVs than karyotype	Does not detect balanced rearrangements

FISH, fluorescence *in situ* hybridization (FISH); CMA, chromosomal microarray; CNV, copy number variants.

Detection of Base Pair Substitutions

Technologies

There are two types of sequencing technologies that are in practice today: Sanger sequencing and next-generation sequencing (NGS). Sanger sequencing involves controlled termination of DNA synthesis by incorporation of dideoxy-NTPs (ddNTPs). DNA fragments are sorted by size using capillary gel electrophoresis, and sequencing is performed by detecting the fluorescent emission of the ddNTP. This technology is costly and time consuming. NGS is a newer technology that allows for massively parallel sequencing reactions. There are a variety of NGS platforms; however, these follow a common general approach that involves (a) fragmentation of DNA (referred to as library prep), followed by (b) simultaneous amplification and sequencing of the fragments, and (c) assembly into continuous sequence using computer-based algorithms. The advent of NGS dramatically reduced per bp costs and increased sequencing capacity. NGS, as currently implemented clinically, is not as effective at sequencing repetitive regions as Sanger sequencing. Both technologies are still employed today, with Sanger sequencing often used for

validation of NGS findings (13). Sequencing technologies continue to advance. Real-time single molecule sequencing is currently in development and may allow for point-of-care genetic testing (14). If successful, such sequencing will enable reads through repetitive regions and other areas of the human genome not currently interpretable with NGS.

In addition to the above sequencing technologies, targeted genotyping can be performed using hybridization or amplification techniques. These methods include allele-specific polymerase chain reaction (PCR) and allele-specific hybridization. Targeted genotyping provides a yes/no answer regarding the presence of a *specific* nucleotide sequence, or allele, at a given locus. This may be used, for example, to detect variants in cystic fibrosis known to be common in a population. However, this testing does not cover the remaining coding sequence or alleles not tested for (15).

Nucleotide analysis can be subdivided based on the breadth of coverage. Targeted approaches include panel testing and genotyping, as compared to the untargeted approaches of whole exome sequencing. These technologies are represented graphically in **Figure 56.2** and are further discussed below.

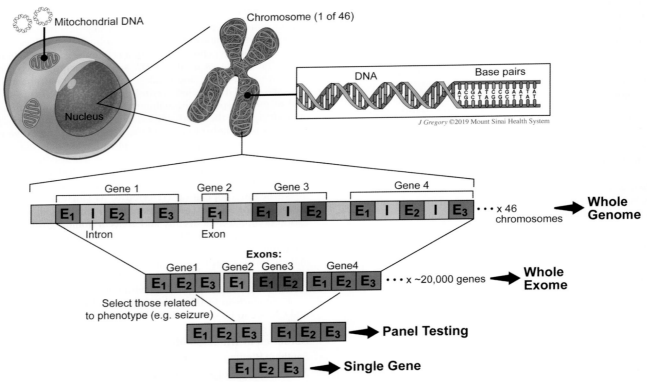

FIGURE 56.2 Detection of base pair substitutions at the whole genome, whole exome, or gene level. A graphic representation of the relative breadth of coverage of whole genome sequencing (WGS), whole exome sequencing (WES), panel testing, and single gene testing. Both WGS and WES involve sequencing of all genes associated with human disease. In WES, both the exonic (labeled *E1, E2, E3,* etc.) and intronic material (labeled *I*) of these genes are sequenced. By contrast, WES is restricted primarily to the exons. Panel testing also involves sequencing of exons and narrows the scope of genes to those associated with a phenotype. (Illustration by Jill Gregory. Used with permission from © Mount Sinai Health System.)

Panel Testing

Panel testing refers to analysis of the nucleotide sequence of a single gene or set of genes associated with a phenotype. Common indications for panel testing in neonatology include seizures disorders and surfactant deficiency.

When the phenotype is well delineated and there is a finite list of causative genes, a panel may be an appropriate first-tier test. However, panels can vary considerably between clinical laboratories. The technology used to analyze these genes may be a targeted genotyping approach versus full sequencing of the exons and selected intronic regions. The latter approach is more common but not exclusively applied. Additionally, the genes selected for inclusion on a panel often vary between labs.

Panels can be a more cost- and time-effective approach but will fail to detect causal variants in genes not covered. Furthermore, if targeted genotyping was used, the result is informative only with respect to the tested allele. For those genes that are sequenced, shorter read lengths in panel testing allows for higher coverage and, therefore, greater sensitivity. Providers should be careful to seek appropriate genetic expertise of both the test methods and the genes included when ordering a panel and interpreting the results.

Whole Exome and Whole Genome Sequencing

Whole exome and whole genome sequencing (WES and WGS, respectively) are untargeted approaches to genetic testing. WES involves fragmenting the genomic DNA, capturing fragments containing exons, and then sequencing those. This process enriches the exome from 2% of the starting DNA to greater than 65% of the sequencing reads. Sequencing read depth, however, varies from one exon to another, depending on the efficiency of the capture. This creates challenges when attempting to "call" (detect) CNVs from these data. WGS, by contrast, uses all of the DNA fragments, which results in more even read depths and more reliable detection of CNVs. The relative ability to detect aneuploidy, CNVs, indels, and SNVs via WES or WGS, as compared to karyotype, CMA, and FISH is shown in **Figure 56.3**.

WES and WGS have the advantage of being untargeted approaches in which the coding regions of all genes are surveyed. As these approaches become increasingly affordable and efficient, WES and WGS will likely replace panel testing as a first-tier test in intensive care settings. As per base sequencing costs continue to fall, WGS is likely to dominate. In addition to providing more information, the costs of generating the required libraries for WGS are less expensive than for WES.

The impact of WES and WGS for critically ill neonates with respect to diagnostic yield, actionability of positive results, and economic utility are currently under study. Studies published so far are indicating that the yield of WES and WGS is in the 30% to 50% range when critically ill newborns and young infants deemed likely to have genetic disorders are studied (16,17). Notably, yield is higher when parent-affected child trios are studied (17). Turnaround times for WES of under 2 weeks and, for rapid WGS, less than 3 days have been achieved. The genetic diagnoses achieved with WES or WGS impact medical management in roughly 50% of cases. While these outcomes are encouraging, they have all been achieved under the auspices of research protocols and the rates cited are undoubtedly sensitive to case selection.

Gene-Level Deletion and Duplication Testing

For many genetic conditions, disruption of gene function may be due to a single-nucleotide variant, a gene level deletion, or a combination of both. When not included in the order, deletion and duplication analysis should therefore be ordered concurrently with sequencing for conditions associated with high occurrence of deletion or duplication as the underlying mechanism. Gene-level deletion and duplication analysis is commonly detected by high-resolution microarray, multiplex ligation-dependent probe amplification (MLPA), or quantitative PCR.

Future Directions

Sequencing technologies continue to advance. Real-time single molecule sequencing is currently in development and may allow for point-of-care genetic testing (3). If successful, such sequencing will enable reads through repetitive regions and other areas of the human genome not currently interpretable with NGS.

█ MITOCHONDRIAL SEQUENCING

As mentioned above, the mitochondrial genome is distinct from the nuclear genome. If a defect of the mitochondrial genome is suspected, mitochondrial sequencing must be ordered separately. This can be added to clinical WES or WGS. However, consistent with the predominance of nuclear-encoded proteins necessary for mitochondrial functioning, the majority of mitochondrial diseases actually result from nuclear mutations (9). A complete evaluation for genetic etiologies of mitochondrial diseases should include both nuclear and mitochondrial sequencing.

█ TYPES OF RESULTS

Genetic testing has the potential to yield a variety of unexpected results. It is essential that ordering providers understand the types of possible results and incorporate this information into pretest counseling with patients and their families. Ideally, consent is obtained from a physician, genetic counselor, or other health care provider familiar with genetic testing.

Genetic Variation Type	Testing Technology				
	Karyotype	CMA*	FISH**	WES	WGS
Aneuploidy	●	●	●		●
Copy number variant:					
1×10^6 base pairs (large)	●	●	●		●
1×10^5 base pairs (medium)		●	●		●
1×10^4 base pairs (small)		●			●
Indels				●	●
Single nucleotide variant				●	●

*Imbalanced variations only; **Specific to probe target

FIGURE 56.3 Resolution of commonly employed testing technologies. A tabular representation of the ability of karyotype, chromosomal microarray (CMA), fluorescence *in situ* hybridization (FISH), whole exome sequencing (WES), and whole genome sequencing (WGS) to detect aneuploidy, copy number variants, insertions and deletions (indels), and single-nucleotide variants. A colored dot indicates the ability of the corresponding testing technology (columns) to detect a given type of variation (rows). For example, while karyotype can detect large copy number variants, it will miss medium and small copy number variants seen by CMA.

Variant Interpretation (for CMA and Sequencing)

The American College of Medical Genetics and Genomics (ACMG) and the Association for Molecular Pathology have created guidelines for categorizing genetic variants detected with NGS and CMA into five categories: pathogenic, likely pathogenic, uncertain significance, likely benign, and benign. Allocation to these categories is based on the ACMG guidelines, which incorporate evidence from population, computational, functional, and segregation data (18). A pathogenic variant is a change in the genetic material known to cause disease and indicates a definitively positive result. A likely pathogenic variant is a change for which the overall supporting evidence is less conclusive than for a pathogenic variant but still sufficient to conclude that the variant is likely disease causing. Conversely, a benign variant is one with sufficient evident to conclude definitively that it is not associated with human disease. A likely benign variant is one with less definitive evidence that it is not associated with human disease but enough evidence to deem that likely. Typically, benign and likely benign variants are not reported. A variant of uncertain clinical significance, which will be reported, is one without clear evidence of its pathogenicity or lack thereof. Periodic reanalysis is recommended since variant interpretation is based on present knowledge and can change with time.

Parental samples can be useful in clarifying the pathogenicity of a variant. For variants in genes associated with dominant diseases, observation of the variant in a healthy parent reduces the likelihood of pathogenicity. Alternatively, if the change is new in the patient (*de novo*), this supports pathogenicity (there are only approximately 1.5 *de novo* variants per exome). Parental samples can also be useful in the study of variants in genes with autosomal recessive inheritance, whereby demonstrating that both parents carry one of the variants supports that the variants are in trans (on opposite chromosomes). Parental samples are therefore recommended to be included, when possible, for variant interpretation as part of WES or WGS (referred to as a "trio") and for larger panels (18).

Secondary Findings (for WES/WGS)

WES and WGS have the potential to reveal variation in genes that are unrelated to the indication for testing but are medically actionable, for example a pathogenic variant in *BRCA1* or *BRCA2*, which confer cancer risk in adults. To guide clinical laboratories on return of such results, the ACMG has published a list of genes for which it recommends reporting known pathogenic or expected pathogenic variants regardless of the indication for testing, referred to as "secondary findings." This list currently has 59 genes but is curated and updated over time. Patients can opt out of receiving secondary findings, and discussion of the risks and benefits of receiving secondary findings is an important component of pretest counseling (19).

Misattributed Parentage (for WES/WGS)

Misattributed parentage can be detected on genetic testing when biologic relatives undergo testing, for example, family-based whole exome or whole genome sequencing. The American Society of Human Genetics recommends that parents be informed about the possibility of detecting misattributed parentage during pretest counseling (20).

CONCLUSION

Genetic testing technologies have rapidly advanced over recent years. This has made clinical WES and WGS increasingly accessible for neonatal care. In the years ahead, we can safely anticipate further reductions in cost, improvements in variant annotation, and increasing application of these technologies for routine care.

REFERENCES

1. March of Dimes Foundation Data Book for Policy Makers. *Maternal, infant, and child health in the United States*, 2016. Available from: https://www.marchofdimes.org/March-of-Dimes-2016-Databook.pdf.
2. Anderson S, Bankier AT, Barrell BG, et al. Sequence and organization of the human mitochondrial genome. *Nature* 1981;290(5806):457.
3. Piovesan A, Caracausi M, Antonaros F, et al. GeneBase 1.1: a tool to summarize data from NCBI gene datasets and its application to an update of human gene statistics. *Database (Oxford)* 2016;2016:baw153.
4. Chromosome map. In: *Genes and disease*. Bethesda, MD: National Center for Biotechnology Information, 1998. Available from: https://www.ncbi.nlm.nih.gov/books/NBK22266/
5. International Human Genome Sequencing Consortium. Finishing the euchromatic sequence of the human genome. *Nature* 2004;431(7011):931.
6. Genomes Project C, Auton A, Brooks LD, et al. A global reference for human genetic variation. *Nature* 2015;526(7571):68.
7. Nussbaum RL, McInnes RR, Willard HF. *Thompson & Thompson genetics in medicine e-book.* Elsevier Health Sciences, Philadelphia, PA: 2015.
8. Nussbaum RL, McInnes RR, Willard HF, et al. *Thompson & Thompson genetics in medicine,* 7th ed. Philadelphia, PA: Saunders/Elsevier, 2007.
9. Calvo SE, Mootha VK. The mitochondrial proteome and human disease. *Annu Rev Genomics Hum Genet* 2010;11:25.
10. Permenter J, Ishwar A, Rounsavall A, et al. Quantitative analysis of genomic DNA degradation in whole blood under various storage conditions for molecular diagnostic testing. *Mol Cell Probes* 2015;29(6):449.
11. Test, Technology Transfer Committee ACoMGRPBMDUS. Technical and clinical assessment of fluorescence in situ hybridization: an ACMG/ASHG position statement. I. Technical considerations. Test and Technology Transfer Committee. *Genet Med* 2000;2(6):356.
12. Budworth H, McMurray CT. A brief history of triplet repeat diseases. *Methods Mol Biol* 2013;1010:3.
13. Grody WW, Thompson BH, Hudgins L. Whole-exome/genome sequencing and genomics. *Pediatrics* 2013;132(suppl 3):S211.
14. Goodwin S, McPherson JD, McCombie WR. Coming of age: ten years of next-generation sequencing technologies. *Nat Rev Genet* 2016;17(6):333.
15. Beauchamp KA, Muzzey D, Wong KK, et al. Systematic design and comparison of expanded carrier screening panels. *Genet Med* 2018;20(1):55.
16. Petrikin JE, Cakici JA, Clark MM, et al. The NSIGHT1-randomized controlled trial: rapid whole-genome sequencing for accelerated etiologic diagnosis in critically ill infants. *NPJ Genom Med* 2018;3:6.
17. Meng L, Pammi M, Saronwala A, et al. Use of exome sequencing for infants in intensive care units: ascertainment of severe single-gene disorders and effect on medical management. *JAMA Pediatr* 2017;171(12):e173438.
18. Richards S, Aziz N, Bale S, et al. Standards and guidelines for the interpretation of sequence variants: a joint consensus recommendation of the American College of Medical Genetics and Genomics and the Association for Molecular Pathology. *Genet Med* 2015;17(5):405.
19. Kalia SS, Adelman K, Bale SJ, et al. Recommendations for reporting of secondary findings in clinical exome and genome sequencing, 2016 update (ACMG SF v2.0): a policy statement of the American College of Medical Genetics and Genomics. *Genet Med* 2017;19(2):249.
20. Botkin JR, Belmont JW, Berg JS, et al. Points to consider: ethical, legal, and psychosocial implications of genetic testing in children and adolescents. *Am J Hum Genet* 2015;97(1):6.

57 Congenital Anomalies and Genetic Disease

Tara L. Wenger and Elizabeth J. Bhoj

Congenital anomalies and suspected genetic disease are common among infants admitted to neonatal intensive care units (NICUs). For the vast majority of these infants, the specific diagnosis is not known at the time of their admission, which can pose challenges for admitting providers seeking out information about their underlying disease processes. While some genetic syndromes can be readily recognized on physical examination by most neonatal providers (e.g., achondroplasia, Cornelia de Lange syndrome, trisomy 13, trisomy 18, trisomy 21, Turner syndrome), the vast majority of genetic syndromes cannot. Moreover, most infants with congenital anomalies will not have an underlying monogenic disorder. This chapter will provide a framework for providers to evaluate infants with congenital anomalies and suspected genetic disease (**Fig. 57.1**), to aid in initial evaluation and categorization of the suspected underlying differences.

APPROACH TO HISTORY TAKING FOR NEONATES WITH CONGENITAL ANOMALIES

A complete family history is essential for the proper evaluation of an infant with congenital anomalies. However, there are several barriers that can pose an obstacle for obtaining this information:

- **Parents not at bedside.** After a neonate with congenital anomalies has been born, the neonate is often transferred to a children's hospital for management. In many cases, this is not the same hospital where the mother has delivered. There is typically a delay in the ability of parents to be present at the bedside of a neonate who has been admitted to an NICU. Additionally, there may be visiting restrictions that limit a parent's ability to stay with the infant and/or limited space and privacy.
- **Parents not aware of details of family history.** Parents will often describe the time their child spends in an NICU as being some of the most stressful times in their lives. In addition to the postpartum hormonal changes and sleep deprivation experienced by all new parents, parents of children with congenital anomalies also experience distress related to separation from their child, anxiety regarding management of medical challenges facing their child, fear of the unknown long-term prognosis, and often profound loss and grief. Individuals in crisis have difficulty remembering complete details of medical history of family members. Additionally, different family communication styles and openness about medical issues can affect the amount of information an individual knows about his or her history. It is not uncommon for parents to provide a family history to the best of their knowledge, only to return a few days later with significant details they were previously unaware of.
- **Assumption that medical record contains complete information.** Neonates who were not expected to be born with congenital anomalies will often be admitted urgently to the NICU. The nature of the admission often emphasizes medical stabilization and transport to a facility that can provide proper monitoring and definitive treatment. In the setting of a rushed transfer, it is common for incomplete family history to be documented. In the Electronic Health Record, this may look like a family history with an extremely focused or incomplete history obtained from charts or a terrified parent (e.g., "Family history: no cleft palate"). When subsequent providers care for the child, this abbreviated history is often copied forward, with an assumption that a complete family history was elicited and this is the only piece of relevant information. A provider evaluating an infant with congenital anomalies should always obtain a complete pedigree and should not assume a complete family history was elicited unless it is specifically stated and pedigree is documented. Even in this case, it is essential to review the pedigree or history with family when the child is stabilized to ensure it is complete and appropriate.

Several techniques can be used to increase the chance of obtaining a proper and complete medical history:

- **Give parents time to obtain necessary portions of history**. At the time of initial consultation, a preliminary history should be obtained, and a follow-up time should be arranged to speak again after they have had a chance to elicit more information from family members. It is important to speak with each parent, because they may not have a full picture of the medical issues in their partner's history. Parents should be reassured that it is normal that they may not have all of the information or find it difficult to remember all of the details when they are adjusting to the birth of a child with congenital anomalies. Ask each parent to speak with family members to ask about birth defects, losses, major medical issues, types of cancer and age at time of cancer diagnosis, causes of death for deceased family members and neurocognitive development. Agree on a time to follow up to review the information they are able to obtain. Some parents will be able to provide this information later the same day, while it may take others more time to gather this information from family members. Many parents will find that when they reach out to family members with these specific questions, they will learn that there are medical issues they were not told about. It is helpful if they can emphasize to their family members that understanding a complete family history may help the neonatologists better care for their infant. For parents that are unable to be at the bedside, a phone call can be scheduled to review what they were able to find in their family history. When information regarding paternal identity or paternal family history is not possible to obtain (e.g., no contact with father or paternal relatives; father deported; paternal identity unknown), providers should keep an open mind about the possibility of disease that typically runs in families.
- **For donor-conceived children, reach out to reproductive clinics.** For children who are donor conceived, parents should be encouraged to reach out to the reproductive clinic or clinics through which they obtained donor gametes. Family history should be recorded for donors, but they also will want to track any birth defects in children conceived via that donor (1). They may have information that was not available at the time of conception about the health outcomes of genetic siblings of the child.
- **Ask parents to bring photographs**. It is also helpful to ask parents to bring with them baby pictures of themselves and of siblings, as well as any family member who has birth defects that are similar to the affected infant. Parents who have donor-conceived children will often have a baby photograph of the donor or may have photographs of genetic siblings they have connected with through the Donor Sibling Registry or their specific

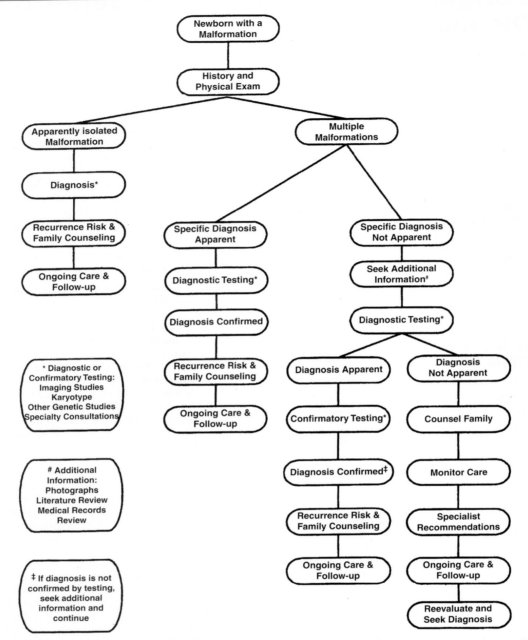

FIGURE 57.1 Integrated approach to management. (Modified from Hall JG. When a child is born with congenital abnormalities. *Contemp Pediatr* 1988;78. With permission.)

agency. Photographs of these children are also helpful. While speaking with a family, it may be helpful to suggest that parents access photographs on social media platforms and/or text family members of interest for photographs. If there is a specific structure of interest, many patients will be willing to ask for specific photographs to be texted to them from family members of interest (e.g., ask them to have family members text a photo of their ears). If there have been infants or children who have passed away, or were stillbirths, it is worth asking if there are photographs of these children. Due to the growth of organizations such as "Now I Lay Me Down to Sleep," many families have professional photographs of children who have passed away. Many choose to share these photographs on social media and may be accessed by a relative during a family history, and others may be willing to share photographs individually with their family members.

- **Schedule a time to follow up to review new information.** Providers should always reconnect with parents of affected children at a later date to find out if parents have learned any new information about family history, or if they have learned that any information they had provided was inaccurate.
- **Empower parents to text relatives for clarifications during family history.** When parents are at the bedside and an initial pedigree is obtained, parents should be empowered and encouraged to text family members for clarification of specific issues during the consultation visit. Though it can add a few minutes to the consultation, this is an efficient way to clarify medical information and may save time in the long run. Social norms in many regions would prohibit parents from taking out their cell phone during a visit with a physician, but they will do so if encouraged that it is acceptable by the provider.

Family History

The following components of family history should be elicited for all patients:

- **Prior losses**. Parents should be specifically asked how many pregnancies they have had together and with other partners. Gestational age at the time of the losses as well as any abnormalities on ultrasound, prenatal screening, or genetic testing on products of conception should be recorded.
- **Birth defects**. Any individuals in the family with structural anomalies should be noted in the pedigree, even beyond the immediate family members. It can be helpful to ask if any family members had surgery as infants or were followed by any specialists as children. The description of what the birth defects were felt to be due to should be recorded, but unless there is definitive testing, the provider should keep an open mind. It is common for parents and providers to want to ascribe a "reason" for a birth defect, and some of these turn out to be false (e.g., attributing a birth defect to an exposure to a teratogen during pregnancy).
- **Cancer**. Type of cancer and age of diagnosis should be recorded for each affected individual. Many people may not mention cancers in adult family members when they are focusing on the reason for congenital anomalies. However, many cancer predisposition syndromes have congenital anomalies as a presenting feature (e.g., thumb anomalies in Fanconi anemia, craniosynostosis in Baller-Gerold syndrome, cleft lip and palate in Gorlin syndrome). Additionally, some genes that predispose to cancer in the heterozygous state can cause multiple congenital anomalies in the homozygous state (e.g., a patient with one pathogenic variant in *BRCA2* will have an increased risk for breast and ovarian cancer, but if a child has a pathogenic variant on both copies of *BRCA2*, they will manifest Fanconi anemia). If a relative who had cancer is available, it is helpful to do a quick dysmorphology examination to look for minor anomalies that would suggest a cancer predisposition syndrome that could explain the birth defects in the infant (2).
- **Genetic conditions in family members**. Diagnosed or suspected genetic conditions in family members, including independent review of genetic test reports of affected family members. When considering different genetic diagnoses, it is helpful to explore the penetrance, inheritance pattern, and spectrum of features that can be seen in each condition of interest. Variably penetrant conditions may apparently "skip" individuals who are affected (e.g., Van der Woude syndrome). X-linked conditions may be present in a maternal uncle with a mildly affected mother (e.g., Aarskog syndrome). Caution should be taken to rule out X-linked conditions in families with few male family members. Some conditions may have similar features in all affected individuals (e.g., achondroplasia), while others can manifest differently (e.g., an infant with 22q11.2 deletion syndrome may have congenital heart disease and hypocalcemia, while his affected parent had learning issues and hypothyroidism). Autosomal dominant conditions in each parent can result in a more severe or qualitatively different phenotype when the child inherits the allele with the pathogenic variant from both parents (e.g., double dominance in achondroplasia, which is lethal). Approximately 5% of individuals with suspected genetic disease will have a dual diagnosis, which is important to keep in mind when there are features that cannot be attributed to a single genetic cause (3). With the advent of direct-to-consumer genetic testing, there have been many instances of families who were told they had a particular genetic condition, but evaluation by a licensed geneticist confirms that the variant represented a benign change. Variant reclassification has also resulted in individuals erroneously being told they did or did not harbor a particular genetic disease. Additionally, laboratories that perform genetic testing but do not have the rigorous controls of laboratories that specialize in genetic testing will sometimes report

generic text related to cytogenetic changes on a particular chromosomal band. Individual mapping of the breakpoints sometimes reveals that the text given for these cytogenetic reports was erroneous and does not apply to the individual. *Copies of the genetic testing reports should be obtained for all family members who have had genetic testing for direct review.*
- **Ethnicity**. It is important to determine ethnicity, as well as to assess the likelihood of consanguinity. Some genetic conditions have a higher likelihood of occurring in particular ethnic groups (e.g., Ellis–van Creveld in Pennsylvania Dutch, *TBCK*-related disorder in Puerto Rican population). Although families may not believe they are consanguineous, families from the same geographic regions can sometimes have a higher risk for recessive conditions. Patients with known consanguinity will often have stretches of lack of heterozygosity (LOH) on SNP array. Knowledge of the conditions of interest and ethnic background can facilitate diagnosis. It is also helpful to be aware of cultural beliefs regarding genetic testing within specific populations.

Pregnancy History

There are several facets of prenatal history that are important to explore for children born with congenital anomalies. As discussed above, there are many prenatal exposures that cause structural and developmental defects in newborns (4). One of the most common teratogens is ethanol, which leads to fetal alcohol spectrum and syndrome (FAS). FAS is extremely variable and does not correlate well with the amount of alcohol consumed. It can cause neurologic and facial differences in a typical pattern, including a smooth long philtrum and thin upper lip (5). For more detail, please refer to Chapter 14.

History of Infertility

Couples with a history of infertility are at increased risk of having a child with congenital anomalies, even when they conceive spontaneously. The reasons for this are unclear and may be a combination of increased risk of genetic disease, as well as decreased egg or sperm quality. It is important to elicit whether they believe they may have had multiple early losses (a.k.a. chemical pregnancies) or that they never became pregnant. Depending on the reason for infertility, there are different types of assisted reproductive technologies that can be used to assist in conception. These different methods harbor variable risks for specific types of genetic disease and rate of birth defects (6). Patients who have conceived with the use of ovarian hyperstimulation (e.g., Clomid, letrozole), either alone or during *in vitro* fertilization, are at increased risk of methylation defects including Beckwith-Wiedemann syndrome (BWS). The risk of having a child with BWS is approximately 18 times the background population risk after ovarian hyperstimulation, though fortunately the risk appears to be limited to the mechanism of hypomethylation at DMR2, the lowest risk group for BWS-associated malignancies (7). It is important to remember that any child conceived via IVF with or without egg donation would have been conceived with the use of ovarian hyperstimulation medications. *In vitro* fertilization is associated with a small increased risk of birth defects. Children conceived via IVF with intracytoplasmic sperm injection have the highest risk of birth defects, although the overall risk is still low (8). Children conceived via IVF also have a higher risk of macrosomia. Interestingly, despite larger birth weights in IVF-conceived children in general, children who are carried by a woman who is not genetically related to the embryo (i.e., egg donation, embryo donation, surrogacy) have a higher risk of placental disorders and low-birth-weight infants (9). Children who have been conceived via IVF may have undergone preimplantation genetic screening (PGS) or preimplantation genetic diagnosis (PGD). The specific laboratory tests performed utilizing PGS and PGD vary depending on laboratory, so it is important to obtain the reports to determine exactly what testing was completed.

Both PGS and PGD are performed on a small blastocyst biopsy, and therefore, mosaic disorders cannot be ruled out. Most PGS will evaluate for chromosomal number and sometimes presence of microdeletions. Sequencing is not routinely performed unless targeted to a specific familial variant in PGD.

Travel History

Travel history to Zika virus–endemic areas should be elicited for both the mother and the father. Zika virus can cause birth defect with infection from early in pregnancy through the third trimester (for more information see Chapter 46: Congenital Infections). Therefore, travel of a mother *or father* to a Zika endemic region in the 6 months prior to conception through the remainder of the pregnancy should be recorded. If there has been travel to a Zika endemic region, history of viral symptoms and their timing should be recorded, though it does not rule out infection if a mother cannot recall having viral symptoms (10).

Immunization History

Waning immunity to vaccines in adulthood and suboptimal immunization rates in childhood over the past couple of decades leave some women vulnerable to birth defects associated with vaccine-preventable illnesses. Infection with rubella during pregnancy is associated with cataracts, blindness, microcephaly, and severe intellectual disability in affected children. Varicella and measles infections during pregnancy can also affect the fetus, leaving it vulnerable to intellectual disability, deafness, and blindness (for more information see Chapter 46: Congenital Infections) It is estimated that there are significantly more women entering childbearing years who are not immune to rubella. This is anticipated to result in a rise in congenital rubella syndrome, a vaccine-preventable blindness-intellectual disability syndrome. Also, depending on the age of the patient, they may or may not have received varicella vaccine.

Maternal Medical History

It is extremely important to obtain a full medical history from the birth mother of the child, which may be in addition to the "genetic" mother of the child if there was an egg/embryo donation or a gestational carrier was used. Vital points include if the mother had diabetes, risks for nutritional deficiency, maternal infections, hypertension, autoimmune issues, metabolic disorder, or uterine anomalies.

Maternal Diabetes

Maternal diabetes has been known for decades to cause not just glucose imbalance in neonates but congenital malformations as well. There is an imperfect but significant increase in risk for mothers with preexisting diabetes (as opposed to gestational diabetes) and those who are insulin dependent. It is helpful to know average glucose or hemoglobin A1C levels during different stages of pregnancy to help determine risk. In a recent study of nearly 300,000 births the most common defects associated with maternal diabetes were neural tube defects (9%), congenital heart defects (4%), renal agenesis or dysgenesis (6%), and vertebral anomalies (4%) (11).

Nutritional Deficiencies

Nutritional deficiencies in the mother can pose significant risk to the developing infant. Those mothers at risk include those with eating disorders, both restrictive and purging disorders, severe hyperemesis, restricted access to food due to local conditions, or bariatric surgery (which is underreported to medical professionals). There are many macro- and micronutrients that are vital for normal fetal development, but folate is the best studied. Women who are deprived of folate during pregnancy have higher risk of neural tube defects. With fortification of foods the rates of neural tube defect (NTD) have dropped worldwide, but women are still recommended

to take folic acid 4 mg/day if they are at high risk or 0.4 mg/day if at lower risk (12). Lack of additional nutrients that can lead to suboptimal neonatal health include iodine, vitamin K, zinc, magnesium, vitamin A, vitamin B6, vitamin B12, and vitamin C (13).

Maternal Infections

Maternal infections are also capable of causing malformations, neurologic compromise, and other medical issues in the neonate (for more information see Chapter 46: Congenital Infections.) The "TORCH" (T)oxoplasmosis, (O)ther agents, (R)ubella, (C)ytomegalovirus, and (H)erpes simplex are the most commonly tested for. "Other" agents can include syphilis, varicella–zoster, and parvovirus B19. The majority of these infections can cause mild or even unrecognized symptoms in the mothers but have severe consequences for the fetus. An emerging risk is congenital infection with Zika virus. The most notable feature is microcephaly and neurologic complications, which can include vision and hearing impairment, seizures, contractures, and feeding difficulty (12). There is also a small risk of various birth defects and neurologic impairment with any maternal fever, and it is important to note the timing, duration, and degree of fever.

Hypertension

Hypertension (preexisting as well as gestational hypertension) is increasingly diagnosed in pregnant women and can have negative consequences for their infants. Multiple studies have linked maternal hypertension with IUGR and congenital heart defects. (14)

Autoimmune Disorders

Autoimmune disorders are of particular concern, because of several mechanisms. Many drugs used to treat autoimmune disorders have been shown to lead to nutritional deficiencies as above. During gestation, the developing infant may have experienced placental vascular disruptions as many autoimmune conditions are associated with hypercoagulable states. In addition, certain conditions may lead to the neonate having organ-specific symptoms, such as cardiac arrhythmias, or myasthenia gravis from maternal antibodies (15).

Metabolic Disorders

Metabolic disorders such as phenylketonuria (PKU) in a pregnant mother may lead to birth defects because of exposure of the fetus to teratogenic substances. Infants born to mothers with untreated PKU are exposed to toxic levels of the amino acid phenylalanine, which causes microcephaly, congenital heart disease, dysmorphic facial features, and developmental delays (16).

Maternal Medical Conditions Treated with Teratogenic Medications

Maternal medical conditions that are typically treated with teratogenic medications should be specifically questioned, as many mothers may not think of a well-controlled medical condition as being an active issue (Table 57.1). It is also important to check for well-controlled maternal conditions where the treatment may be associated with teratogenic medications. Some conditions to especially ask about should include seizures/epilepsy, bipolar and other psychiatric disorders, acne, malignancy, and autoimmune conditions. Many of these conditions may not cause a risk to the pregnancy directly (e.g., maternal seizures) but the mother may have been on a teratogenic medication during early gestation. Obstetricians may recommend that a woman stop taking a teratogenic medication when they learn she is pregnant, but it may have already resulted in a birth defect before it was stopped. Therefore, it is imperative to question what medications they stopped taking when they learned they were pregnant, and how far along they were at the time. There are some medications that are mildly teratogenic that are often continued during pregnancy because the risk of maternal relapse is of greater risk to the fetus. It is also

TABLE 57.1		
Selected Teratogens and Their Effects		
Teratogen	**Anomalies**	**Comments**
Phenytoin (Dilantin)	Growth deficiency Wide anterior fontanelle Hypertelorism Cleft lip and palate Hypoplastic distal phalanges Small nails	Similar facial features seen with exposure to carbamazepine, valproate, mysoline, phenobarbital Full spectrum in 10%; milder effects in one-third
Warfarin (Coumadin)	Nasal hypoplasia Stippled epiphyses Short fingers Seizures	Critical period between 6 and 9 weeks of gestation. One-third of exposed fetuses are affected.
Retinoic acid (Accutane)	Microtia or anotia Hypertelorism Micrognathia Conotruncal cardiac defects Hydrocephalus Microcephaly Cortical, cerebellar dysplasia	If exposed more than 15 days after conception, one-third have embryopathy.
Rubella	Growth deficiency Microcephaly Deafness Cataracts Microphthalmia Chorioretinitis Cardiac septal defects Patent ductus arteriosus Peripheral pulmonic stenosis	Fifty percent chance of effects if exposed in the first trimester, but risk extends into the second trimester. May have late, persistent infectious sequelae, for example, diabetes mellitus.
Varicella	Developmental delay Seizures Cortical atrophy/microcephaly Growth deficiency Limb hypoplasia/club foot Cutaneous scars	One to two percent with effects when exposed between 8 and 20 weeks of gestation; wide spectrum of severity
Maternal phenylketonuria	Developmental delay (73%–92%) Hypertonia Low birth weight (52%) Microcephaly (73%) Cardiac defects (15%) Spontaneous abortion (30%)	Even when "on diet," phenylalanine levels may rise above 4–10 mg/dL, the apparent threshold for fetal effects. Percentages cited here are for levels >16 mg/dL. Normal is <2 mg/dL.

important to ask if any medications are currently being taken and which will be reinitiated after delivery, to make sure that they are compatible with breast-feeding. The Drugs and Lactation Database (LactMed) can be a helpful resource (www.ncbi.nlm.nih.gov/books/NBK501922) (17).

Multiple Gestation Pregnancy

Multiple gestation pregnancy increases the risk of all congenital malformations, which is higher for monochorionic than dichorionic (18). The hypothesized mechanisms for these vary. For example, some kinds of craniosynostosis are hypothesized to result from mechanical compression of the developing skull. Others such as BWS can occur due to a disruption of methylation patterns in monozygotic twins. Twins are also at a higher risk of various deformation anomalies and sequences.

Uterine Anomalies

Another risk for deformation in neonates is maternal uterine anomalies, such as fibroids or bicornuate uterus, which can decrease fetal movement and restrict growth in unusual patterns (19).

Screening during Pregnancy

As mentioned previously, it is important to get pregnancy records when possible to see what screening tests were performed during the pregnancy. It is important to distinguish between screening tests, which can only be used to modify risk assessment, and diagnostic testing that gives a more definitive direct result. Examples of screening during pregnancy include testing for diabetes and hypertension, and any disease-specific screening for preexisting conditions.

Sequential Screening versus Noninvasive Prenatal Screening (For additional information refer to Chapter 10: Prenatal diagnosis and Management)

Women will usually be offered screening for a selection of genetic disorders, especially trisomies. Traditionally, sequential screening was performed, which first involves a nuchal translucency measurement by ultrasound at 11 to 13 weeks as well as measurements of pregnancy-associated plasma protein-A (PAPP-A), and human chorionic gonadotropin (hCG) in the mother's blood. This information is combined with the age of the mother (or the egg donor) to stratify the risk that the fetus carries an abnormality. The second part of the sequential screen measures hCG again, as well as inhibin-A, unconjugated estradiol (uE3), and alpha-fetoprotein (AFP). All of this information is used to calculate a risk for trisomy 21 or trisomy 18. Now many women are choosing to have cell-free fetal DNA sequencing, or noninvasive prenatal testing/screening (NIPT/NIPS). This is one blood draw performed during the first trimester that captures some of the extracellular placental DNA that is found in the maternal blood. There is a variety of conditions that can be tested for, but most laboratories include at least trisomies 13, 18, and 21 and sex chromosome abnormalities. It is also possible to screen for any chromosome anomaly, including microdeletions and duplications, including those for cri-du-chat, 22q11.2 deletion syndrome, and Williams syndrome. Again, NIPT/NIPS is only a screening test that can modify risk but can never completely rule in or rule out a diagnosis.

Diagnostic Genetic Testing

For diagnostic testing a chorionic villus sample (CVS) can be performed as early as 10 weeks, in which a small portion of the developing placenta is removed for direct testing. This testing can be sequencing for a known familial variant or include varied testing such as a karyotype, SNP array, or even exome sequencing. It is important to note that it is the placental DNA being tested, so cases of mosaicism may be difficult to interpret with just CVS. An amniocentesis obtains DNA from cells shed directly from the fetus and is the gold standard for a sample for pregnancy testing. Any test can be performed on samples from amniocentesis, so it is important to clarify what testing was performed as a result of the procedure, not just that the procedure was performed. Due to the issues of mosaicism it can be important to follow a prenatal karyotype with a postnatal karyotype as well. In addition, there may be limited reporting of some variants in the results on SNP arrays and other tests performed in the prenatal setting, so it can be important to contact the laboratory directly if other information exists and was not reported. As with all genetic testing, it is vitally important to directly view the original test results, as they are often misrepresented by both medical professionals in the official records and verbal histories from families.

Anatomy Scan

Many women will also have ultrasound imagining during pregnancy, including an anatomy scan to identify any fetal issues around 18 to 20 weeks. There is a high level of variability of detail and skill in different centers, and some women may only have a superficial test to determine the sex without further detail. It is not at all uncommon for even major malformations to be missed on prenatal ultrasound. Specifically, the findings associated with achondroplasia are often only evident several weeks after traditional anatomy scans, and therefore lead to an initial diagnosis only after birth. If an abnormality was found on a screening anatomy screen, then further testing may have been recommended, such as a cardiac or brain MRI. These results are very helpful if the postnatal imaging has yet to be performed but should never take the place of a traditional echocardiogram or brain MRI on the neonate. In addition, infants that were found to be in an unusual (including breech) position on ultrasound may have resulting deformation. An abnormal head shape with a flattened top and prominent occipital shelf from prolonged breech positioning is the most common example.

Preconception Genetic Testing

In addition, the parents may have had screening to see if they are carriers of any recessive genetic conditions, such as cystic fibrosis, fragile X syndrome, or ethnicity specific testing such as sickle cell disease or common Ashkenazi Jewish diseases. Some couples of Ashkenazi heritage may have participated in programs where they are not aware of their own carrier status but have been told that there are no tested conditions where both parents are carriers. It is important to remember that some carrier screening programs only test for common variants and do not completely rule the disease out in the neonate.

Birth History

It is important to gather details of the birth, including the method of delivery (C-section or vaginal), how long the labor lasted (which can cause deformations if prolonged), and if there were any complications such as meconium or hypoxia. It is also important to note any medications that the infant may have been exposed to during the birth, both illicit and as part of the hospital stay. Some medications may mimic neurologic injury or hypotonia and are important to be aware of before genetic testing is sent. It is also important to note if the birth was performed at home and what type of clinician attended the birth. Vacuum- or forceps-assisted deliveries may cause temporary head shape deformities. "Ping pong" skull fractures in the infant can result from strong external pressure, including from maternal pelvic bones, but seldom lead to lasting sequelae.

EVALUATION OF THE NEONATE WITH CONGENITAL ANOMALIES

Infants with Apparently Isolated Anomalies

Some infants will have apparently isolated anomalies, which still need to be carefully considered. It is useful to think of three categories of congenital differences. A major anomaly is an anatomic abnormality severe enough to reduce normal life expectancy or compromise normal function. A minor anomaly is a structural alteration that either requires no treatment or can be corrected in a straightforward manner, with no permanent consequences, and present in less than 4% of the normal population. A minor variant is a physical feature, often familial, that is present in only a small proportion (1% to 5%) of normal individuals. Many infants will have at least one minor anomaly at birth, and even some major isolated anomalies are common in specific ethnic backgrounds, such as polydactyly and umbilical hernias in African American infants. However, even one anomaly should prompt a thorough evaluation for other major or minor malformations, especially facial dysmorphology. If dysmorphic features are present, it is more likely that other anomalies have not presented themselves yet, and additional imaging may be warranted. Typically, a major clue to evaluating an isolated anomaly is the course of the patient's development, which will not be evident in the neonate. However certain neonatal tasks can be helpful to use as proxies for more advanced developmental milestones. Feeding is one that requires many systems; therefore, feeding assessment can be helpful in identifying malformations of airway, tone of airway, neurologic status, aspiration, and fatigue (as with congenital heart disease). Some anomalies are common in an isolated state, while others are less likely to occur in the absence of a genetic syndrome (Table 57.2). Note that the severity of the defect is not necessarily the most important factor and many of these defects will not cause a major functional consequence.

TABLE 57.2

Example of Birth Defects that Are More Likely to be Truly Isolated versus Those That Occur in Setting of a Genetic Syndrome

System	Birth Defects More Likely to be Isolated	Birth Defects More Likely to be Associated with Syndrome
Craniofacial	Microtia Sagittal craniosynostosis Unilateral cleft lip and palate	Ear asymmetry without microtia Coronal or multisuture craniosynostosis Cleft palate with micrognathia
Cardiac	VSD, ASD, TGA	TOF with PA, coarctation, cardiomyopathy, cardiac masses
Hearing	Conductive hearing loss due to fluid or bony atresia with microtia	Sensorineural hearing loss Absent semicircular canals
Limb	Postaxial polydactyly Transverse limb defect Ectrodactyly Asymmetry due to limb hypoplasia	Preaxial polydactyly Radial ray defect Polysyndactyly Asymmetry due to limb overgrowth
Abdominal	Gastroschisis	Omphalocele
Genitourinary	Pelviectasis Bladder exstrophy in infant of diabetic mother	Polycystic kidneys Uterine didelphys
Skin	Circumscribed vascular malformations with normal surrounding tissue Isolated hemangioma	Vascular malformations that invade surrounding tissue/organs Hemangioma in the V1 distribution of facial nerve Pigmentary differences along lines of Blaschko Cutis aplasia
Ophthalmologic	Microphthalmia/anophthalmia in setting of transverse facial cleft/amniotic banding that disrupts orbit Strabismus	Colobomas, cataracts, microphthalmia/anophthalmia, epibulbar dermoid, heterochromia, posterior embryotoxon, abnormalities of optic nerve, cherry-red spot
Spine	Spina bifida	Extra or missing vertebral body

Infants with Multiple Anomalies

The evaluation of the infant with multiple anomalies may feel overwhelming given that there are more than 10,000 possible etiologies, and that there is often phenotypic variability even within conditions. To provide a framework for these conditions, it is often helpful to work within the larger categories of disorders (Table 57.3). One useful classification system for congenital anomalies is the overreaching etiology of the anomalies. These etiologies can be divided into deformation, disruption, malformation, and dysplasia.

- **Deformations** result from unusual external pressures on an otherwise normal tissue, such as talipes from uterine malformations or fetal positioning, or an infant with breech presentation having a head that is flattened on the top with a prominent occipital shelf (which has developed while constrained by the maternal diaphragm).
- **Disruptions** are caused by destruction of normal structures, and can be caused by vascular insults, infections, teratogens, and other causes. Recognizable disruptions from amniotic bands can cause limb anomalies or facial clefting depending on the position of the band in utero.
- **Dysplasia** is similar and results when the underlying structure of the tissue is compromised at the cellular level. Most disorders of connective tissue, such as osteogenesis imperfecta or achondroplasia, are dysplasias.
- **Malformation** is caused when one or more tissues did not form correctly and can be the result of either a genetic or environmental effect.

TABLE 57.3

Definitions of Major Concepts in Medical Genetics

Major anomaly	An anatomic abnormality severe enough to reduce normal life expectancy or compromise normal function, for example, NTD, cleft lip
Minor anomaly	A structural alteration that either requires no treatment or can be corrected in a straightforward manner, with no permanent consequences, and present in <4% of the normal population, for example, preauricular skin tag, small ventricular septal defect
Minor variant	A physical feature, often familial, that is present in only a small proportion (1%–5%) of normal individuals, for example, single palmar crease of the palm, epicanthal folds
Malformation	A morphologic defect of an organ, part of an organ, or region due to an *intrinsically abnormal developmental process*, for example, microphthalmia, ectrodactyly
Deformation	An abnormal form, shape, or position of a part of the body caused by *unusual mechanical forces on normal tissue*, for example, club foot, plagiocephaly
Disruption	A morphologic defect due to extrinsic interference with a normal developmental process resulting in *breakdown of normal tissue*, for example, amniotic band sequence, fetal alcohol syndrome
Sequence	Several anomalies that occur due to a cascade of events, caused by a single initiating event or anomaly, for example, Potter sequence, Pierre Robin sequence
Developmental field defect	A set of morphologic defects that share a common or contiguous region during embryogenesis, for example, hemifacial microsomia
Syndrome	A recognizable pattern of anomalies that "run together," for example, Down syndrome, SLOS, CHARGE syndrome (*C*oloboma, *H*eart disease, *A*tresia choanae, *R*etarded growth and development and/or CNS anomalies, *G*enital hypoplasia, and *E*ar anomalies or deafness)

- **Vascular malformations/masses** do not fit within one of these categories but can arise as a discrete mass or can be diffusely infiltrated into the surrounding tissue (e.g., beard distribution lymphatic malformation.

When a child has multiple major and/or minor anomalies, it is important to attempt to define the relationship of the anomalies to one another. It is invaluable for the primary neonatology team to try to determine which anomalies could be related to one another (e.g., U-shaped cleft palate and micrognathia in Robin sequence) and which are physiologically unrelated anomalies (e.g., vertebral anomaly and congenital heart disease in VACTERL). The major categories of relationships between multiple malformations include the following:

An **association** is when a set of anomalies tend to occur together, but the etiology that connects the differences remains unknown. Examples include VACTERL and most forms of craniofacial microsomia.

A **sequence** refers to a set of malformations that all result from a single initial malformation. For example, in Pierre Robin sequence, microretrognathia leads to failure of descent of the fetal tongue, which obstructs the closure of the palatal shelves resulting in a U-shaped cleft palate and airway obstruction. The unique malformations are microretrognathia and a U-shaped cleft palate, along with resultant glossoptosis and airway obstruction. However, these are not unique features but rather stem from a single initial abnormality.

A **syndrome** refers to a set of differences that occur and are due to the same underlying cause. A syndrome may result from a genetic abnormality or from an environmental exposure (e.g., fetal alcohol syndrome; fetal hydantoin syndrome).

If an infant with a suspected genetic condition dies before discharge, it can be helpful to encourage the family to allow for an autopsy. If there are religious or cultural beliefs prohibiting a complete autopsy, it is well worth the time to discuss additional options, such as a partial or "virtual" autopsy, which usually involves postmortem advanced imaging (20). Blood and tissue samples can also be collected and saved for future genetic analysis, especially if additional affected children are born later. It can be valuable to emphasize to families that an autopsy or DNA banking may allow for a definitive genetic diagnosis, which can lead to more appropriate recurrence risk counseling, or even open the possibility of PGD in future pregnancies.

SELECTED CONDITIONS THAT PRESENT IN THE NEWBORN

Chromosomal Abnormalities

Chromosome abnormalities can be caused by either the addition or loss of an entire chromosome (such as trisomy 21), the deletion or duplication of just a small critical region of a chromosome (such as 22q11.2 deletion syndrome), or a translocation between two chromosomes. Of the three tests usually used to identify these differences, the first is a karyotype, which can show large chromosome copy number changes and also the position of the chromosomes. These location data are important to identify the mechanism of chromosome changes, and also the major way to identify balanced chromosomal translocations. The second is fluorescent in situ hybridization (FISH), in which colored probes to specific regions bind and identify exact chromosome regions. The third and most common is a single nucleotide polymorphism (SNP) chromosomal microarray, which gives more detailed copy number variation data, and also can show LOH through the SNP sequencing. With the advent of next generation sequencing, there is also usually a copy number analysis performed on sequencing data, such as exome and genome sequencing. In addition, long-range sequencing can often identify complex chromosome

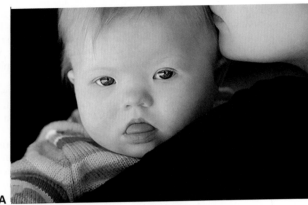
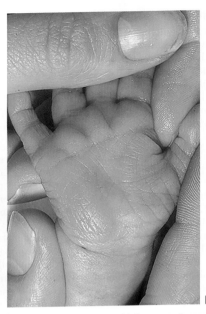

FIGURE 57.2 A: Typical facies in an infant with Down syndrome. **B:** Single palmar crease, a typical feature in an infant with Down syndrome. Reprinted with permission from Ricci S. *Essentials of maternity, newborn, and women's health*, 5th ed. Philadelphia, PA: Wolters Kluwer Health, 2020. Figure 10.18.)

rearrangements that are difficult to otherwise uncover. Instances where one test is superior when concerned about specific conditions will be detailed below, but in general, an SNP microarray is the first-tier test for a neonate with an undiagnosed suspected chromosomal condition.

Trisomy 21

Trisomy 21, also called Down syndrome, is one of the most common and recognizable genetic conditions. The risk of trisomy 21 due to a free-standing copy of chromosome due to a maternal meiosis error is increased with advanced maternal age. However, women of any age can give birth to an infant with trisomy 21. Prevalence differs across populations but is between 1:319 to 1:1,000 live births (21). Due to the high uptake of prenatal screening for Down syndrome, there is usually at least a concern for the diagnosis before an affected infant is even born. However, many families choose to skip screening, and as no screening is perfect there are still many infants born with Down syndrome without prior information. There is a recognizable facial gestalt including upslanting palpebral fissure, but prematurity and other factors may complicate clinical diagnosis (**Fig. 57.2A and B**). The Atlas of Human Malformation Syndromes is a valuable resource to see clinical photographs of patients from diverse backgrounds, including those with a diagnosis of trisomy 21 (research.nhgri.nih.gov/atlas/condition/trisomy-21). Tables **57.4 and 57.5** list the major and minor anomalies, respectively, that have been observed in children with Down syndrome. Vital studies before discharge include an echocardiogram as 50% of infants will have cardiac issues, feeding evaluation, red reflex examination for cataracts, newborn hearing screen, complete blood count for hematologic abnormalities (including both true leukemia and leukemoid reactions), and screening for hypothyroidism. Also important to remember are careful examination and history for signs and symptoms of Hirschsprung disease or renal anomalies. Every child with Down syndrome should have a karyotype (not microarray) to evaluate for a "free" chromosome 21 or a robertsonian translocation. The recurrence risk for a family with certain robertsonian translocations can be as high as greater than 99%, so this is a step that

should not be overlooked, even if the clinical diagnosis has been made. With appropriate surgical and medical management, the life expectancy for individuals with Down syndrome is in the 60s, with 78% of infants without congenital heart disease surviving to their first birthday, and 96% of patients without congenital heart disease reaching the same milestone (22). Early-onset Alzheimer disease becomes the major medical concern for individuals with Down syndrome when they reach middle age. There are many wonderful support groups for families with a new diagnosis of Down syndrome, including some who will have an experienced parent meet with the family in the hospital before discharge.

Trisomy 18

Trisomy 18 (or Edwards syndrome) is the second most common autosomal trisomy and has higher rates of morbidity and mortality than does Down syndrome. Families make many different choices about the direction of care for infants with trisomy 18, so it is very important to make an accurate diagnosis quickly. Despite the

TABLE 57.4		
Major Anomalies at Birth in Down Syndrome		
Cardiac: all types		40%
Atrioventricular canal	16%–20%	
Ventricular septal defect	16%	
Patent ductus arteriosus	3%–5%	
Atrial septal defect	4%–10%	
Gastrointestinal: all types		10%–18%
Duodenal stenosis/atresia	3%–5%	
Imperforate anus	2%	
Other	6%	
Hematologic: leukemoid reaction		Common
Hypothyroidism (congenital)		1%

Adapted from Jones KL, Jones MC, Del Campo M. *Smith's recognizable patterns of human malformation*, 7th ed. Philadelphia, PA: Elsevier Saunders, 2013; and Curry CJ. Chapter 43—autosomal trisomies. In: Rimoin D, Pyeritz R, Korf B, eds. *Emery and Rimoin's principles and practice of medical genetics*. Philadelphia, PA: Academic Press, 2013.

TABLE 57.5

Minor Anomalies in Down Syndrome	
Microbrachycephaly	75%
Upslanting palpebral fissures[a]	80%
Epicanthal folds	59%
Speckling of the iris (Brushfield spots)[b]	56%
Flat facial profile[a]	90%
Low nasal bridge	68%
Small ears[b]	100%
Mildly dysplastic ears[a]	50%
Short neck	61%
Excess skin at the nape of the neck[a,b]	80%
Protruding tongue	47%
Narrow palate	76%
Open mouth	58%
Short hands and fingers	
Clinodactyly (curving) of the fifth finger[a]	60%
Single transverse palmar crease[a]	45%
Wide gap between the first and second toes[b]	68%
Poor Moro reflex[a]	85%
Hyperflexibility of joints[a]	80%
Hypotonia[a]	80%

[a]Cardinal features.

[b]Features with superior discriminative efficacy and power.

generally poor prognosis, there has been increasing consensus that the diagnosis does not necessarily preclude interventions, including cardiac surgery etc. With intensive care, about 50% of affected infants will survive for at least a week, and between 5% and 10% will survive more than a year (23). There can be improved prognosis for patients with mosaic trisomy 18, which can be hard to distinguish without genetic testing. Facial features suggestive of the diagnosis including small and narrow palpebral fissures, small mouth, and prominent occiput; they also have increased rates of omphalocele, club feet, hypoplastic nails, "rocker bottom" feet, and clenched fists with overriding fingers (**Fig. 57.3A and B**). Clinically, the infants often present with severe neurologic and cardiac problems and often require aggressive management from birth to

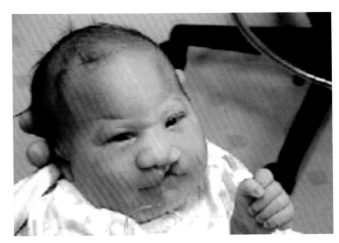

FIGURE 57.4 Typical facies including facial clefting in an infant with trisomy 13. (Reprinted with permission from Baum VC, O'Flaherty JE. *Anesthesia for genetic, metabolic, and dysmorphic syndromes of childhood*, 3rd ed. Philadelphia, PA: Wolters Kluwer, 2015. Figure 19.8.)

maintain their cardiorespiratory status. Involvement with a palliative care team as early as possible is often helpful to families in determining the direction of care.

Trisomy 13

Trisomy 13 (also known as Patau syndrome) is the third autosomal trisomy that is compatible with postnatal life. It also has a very high rate of morbidity and mortality, so a prompt diagnosis is essential for families for planning the direction of care. Again, like trisomy 21 and 18, it is essential that a karyotype (not microarray) is performed to determine if there is a "free" chromosome 13 or if the trisomy is the result of a robertsonian translocation. There may be an indication from prenatal screening that a fetus is at risk for trisomy 13, or in many cases there is no unifying prenatal diagnosis but multiple anomalies seen on ultrasound. Facial features in the disorder include scalp skin defects (cutis aplasia), hypotelorism (close-set eyes), prominent nasal bridge, and cleft lip and/or palate. Addition findings include rocker bottom feet, congenital heart defects, hypoplastic nipples, polydactyly, and severe neurologic deficits. **Figure 57.4** shows a neonate with trisomy 13.

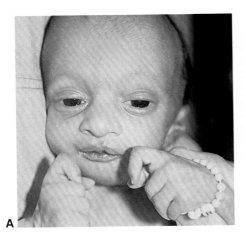 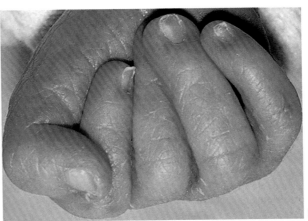

FIGURE 57.3 A: Typical facies in an infant with trisomy 18. **B:** Clenched and overlapping fingers, a typical feature in an infant with trisomy 18. (Reprinted with permission from Kyle, T, Carman S. *Essentials of pediatric nursing*, 4th ed. Philadelphia, PA: Wolters Kluwer, 2020. Figure 27.9.)

THE NEWBORN INFANT

Abnormalities in Sex Chromosomes

Turner Syndrome

While the loss of any autosome is not compatible with life, the complete or partial loss of one of the sex chromosomes (leaving at least a single X chromosome behind) causes 45 X, or Turner syndrome. The other sex chromosome anomalies do not typically cause medical issues that would arise in the neonatal period. As with other chromosomal anomalies there are multiple specific chromosome differences that can cause Turner syndrome, making a karyotype essential for both prognostication and recurrence risk. For example, if there is even a low percent mosaicism for a Y chromosome then there is a risk of gonadal malignancy. There is a limited correlation with specific X chromosome differences and cognitive outcomes (24). Some sex chromosome differences are identified by cfDNA screening, but not all, so it can be helpful while waiting for definitive testing to obtain original results of the testing to see if a normal complement of sex chromosomes was predicted. The physical features of Turner syndrome can be quite variable, especially in cases of mosaic chromosomal differences. Classic physical examination findings include a wide webbed neck, broad chest and widely spaced nipples, and transient edema of the tops of the hands and feet. Further investigation should include echocardiogram for cardiac anomalies (classically aortic coarctation), renal bladder ultrasound, and pelvic ultrasound. If there is a mosaic 46XY/45X karyotype there may be male gonad tissue with a risk for malignant transformation that should be referred for possible surgical removal. There can be many psychosocial issues for parents of children with sex chromosome differences, and in addition to the medical needs of the infant, the social and emotional issues of the parents should also be addressed.

Chromosomal Deletion Syndromes

22q Deletion Syndrome

The most common microdeletion in humans is 22q11.2 deletion syndrome (22q11.2 DS), which encompasses approximately 40 genes on chromosome 22. It has a similar prevalence to trisomy 21. Previously, 22q11.2 DS has also been called DiGeorge syndrome, velocardiofacial syndrome, and conotruncal anomaly face syndrome, among other names, before the molecular diagnosis was established. Approximately 90% are de novo, with the remainder inherited from an affected parent. Children with 22q11.2 DS can often be recognized because of subtle dysmorphic features, including hooded lids, a tubular nose, and overfolded helices. Congenital heart disease is found in approximately 30% of patients and often triggers testing during pregnancy or shortly after birth. Patients without congenital heart disease are often not diagnosed until much older. Other medical problems common in 22q11.2 DS are cervical spine anomalies, hypocalcemia associated with hypoparathyroidism, hypothyroidism, renal anomalies, submucous cleft palate, and velopharyngeal insufficiency. Most have developmental delay, with notable delay in expressive language. Though many have a diagnosis of autism, they typically fail to meet strict diagnostic criteria. Approximately half have attention deficit/hyperactivity disorder, and 25% will go on to develop schizophrenia as adults. It is critical to reach a diagnosis as early as possible, as children need to undergo screening for medical conditions associated with 22q11.2 DS and should be enrolled in Early Intervention Services.

5p Minus (Cri-du-chat) Syndrome

One of the most recognizable chromosome deletion syndromes is 5p minus, or cri-du-chat syndrome (due to the distinctive "cat-like" high-pitched cry.) The syndrome is sometimes detected prenatally if cfDNA analysis includes microdeletion syndromes, or if an SNP microarray is performed on amniocytes after anomalies are identified by prenatal ultrasound. However, most affected infants are born with either no prenatal diagnosis or only nonspecific findings found on ultrasound. Therefore, the physical examination can be vital for making the diagnosis;

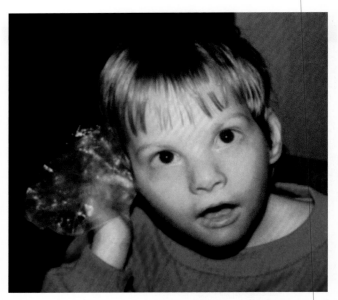

FIGURE 57.5 Typical facies in a young child with cri-du-chat syndrome. (Reprinted by permission from Springer: Schaaf C, Zschocke J. Angeborene Fehlbildungs syndrome. In: *Basiswissen Humangenetik*. Springer-Lehrbuch. Berlin, Heidelberg: Springer, 2013;190. Copyright © 2013 Springer-Verlag Berlin Heidelberg. https://doi.org/10.1007/978-3-642-28907-1_19.)

major features include microcephaly, hypertelorism (wide-spaced eyes) with epicanthi, low-set posteriorly rotated ears, cleft lip/palate, and micrognathia (**Fig. 57.5**). Further investigation may reveal congenital heart defects, urogenital anomalies, and megacolon. There is usually significant developmental delay, but an exact delineation of the deletion size can be helpful for prognosis.

Single-Gene Disorders

Achondroplasia

Achondroplasia is arguable the most recognizable genetic condition, although it is often missed prenatally because the limb differences become most prominent during the late second and third trimester after the traditional screening ultrasound at 20 weeks of gestation. Therefore, it is not uncommon to make a diagnosis in the delivery room or just after to unprepared families. It is an autosomal dominant condition, although the majority of cases are *de novo* without a family history. The children have a distinctive set of findings including rhizomelic (involving proximal more than distal bones) shortening of the arms and legs, disproportionately macrocephaly with a large forehead, and "trident" hands where the fingers are more splayed than typical (**Fig. 57.6**). Importantly, unless there is an untreated neurosurgical issue, the cognition is normal, although some motor delays are expected due to physical differences. Neurosurgical emergencies can arise due to the abnormal anatomy of the head and spine, especially cervicomedullary compression, which rarely can arise in the neonatal period. Although there are many forms of dwarfism, which are often lumped together, achondroplasia is a specific distinct entity caused by activating variants in the gene *FGFR3*, and nearly all patients have the same exact variant, which simplifies testing. Syndromes with activating variants (also called gain-of-function) are often found only in "hotspots" where the specific variant allows for constitutive activation of the resulting protein.

Treacher Collins Syndrome

Treacher Collins Syndrome has a distinctive but variable set of facial differences that are often identified prenatally but are more diagnostic after birth. The most notable features are often small

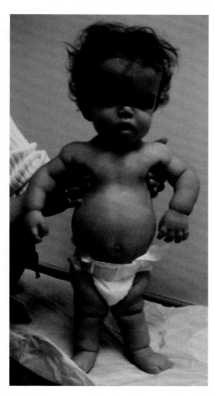

FIGURE 57.6 Typical stature and physical features in an infant with achondroplasia. (Courtesy of Paul S. Matz, MD.)

or absent ears (including the auditory canal), wide mouths with lateral clefts, and cleft palates. Other features include downslanting palpebral fissures with notched lower eyelids, zygomatic arch hypoplasia, ear tags/pits, and micrognathia (**Fig. 57.7**). Unless there is hypoxic brain injury due to the anatomic differences, cognition is expected to be unaffected. Hearing loss is very common and should be followed closely. This is an autosomal dominant

condition and can be either *de novo* or inherited. There is striking phenotypic variability even within families, which can lead a very mildly affected parent to have a child who is not viable due to being very severely affected. Patients most often have pathogenic variants in the gene *TCOF1*, with less than 10% in either *POLR1C* or *POLR1D*. Occasionally a clinical diagnosis will be made with negative molecular testing.

Apert, Beare-Stevenson, Crouzon, Pfeiffer, and Saethre-Chotzen Syndromes

There are a few craniosynostosis syndromes that are usually readily identifiable after birth, including Apert (**Fig. 57.8**), Beare-Stevenson, Crouzon, Pfeiffer, and Saethre-Chotzen syndromes. Each of these syndromes is associated with multisuture craniosynostosis and multilevel airway obstruction. Though the coronal sutures are the most commonly involved sutures, each of these syndromes can have involvement of multiple sutures. The head shape for each child will depend on which sutures fused prematurely, and the timing of their closure. Head shapes in these conditions can vary from normal to cloverleaf skull. There is typically midface retrusion and prognathism. Crouzon, Pfeiffer, and Saethre-Chotzen syndromes can be challenging to distinguish without molecular testing. Multilevel airway obstruction ranges from mild to severe, and some children will require tracheostomy. Apert and Beare-Stevenson syndromes are readily identifiable at birth, due to the presence of unique features (i.e., polysyndactyly and synonychia in Apert syndrome; cutis gyrate in Beare-Stevenson). Patients with these syndromes should be evaluated in a craniofacial center with experience in the treatment of children with tracheal anomalies and multisuture craniosynostosis. Neurologic outcomes are better in children who have early surgery to address cephalocranial disproportion. Genetic testing typically involves a panel that includes *FGFR1*, *FGFR2*, *FGFR3*, and *TWIST1* and sometimes includes additional genes.

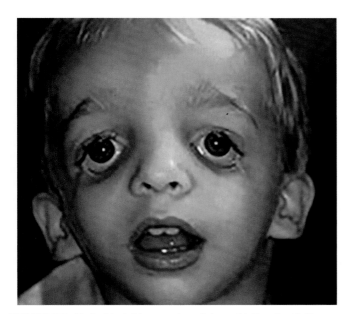

FIGURE 57.7 Typical facial features in an infant with Treacher Collins syndrome. (Reprinted with permission from Gold DH, Weingeist TA. *Color atlas of the eye in systemic disease.* Baltimore, MD: Lippincott Williams & Wilkins, 2001.)

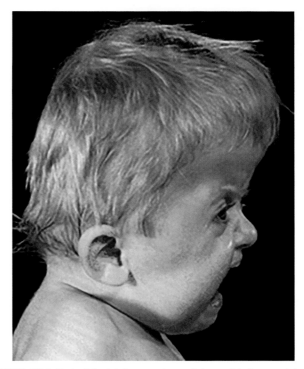

FIGURE 57.8 Typical facial features in an infant with Apert syndrome. (From Chung KC, van Aalst J. *Operative Techniques in Craniofacial Surgery.* Philadelphia, PA: Wolters Kluwer, 2019.)

Disorders in Imprinting/Methylation

Prader-Willi/Angelman Syndrome

Prader-Willi and Angelman syndrome are both caused by variations in the imprinted region on chromosome 15. While Angelman syndrome does not cause symptoms until 6 to 12 months of age, Prader-Willi is characterized by infantile hypotonia (which can be severe enough to confuse with spinal muscular atrophy), poor feeding, and failure to thrive. They can also have fair skin for their family, genital hypoplasia, small hands and feet, and mildly dysmorphic features including a narrow forehead, almond-shaped eyes, and a triangular mouth. It is important to remember that neither a SNP array nor exome sequencing will pick up some cases of these syndromes, and methylation testing of the affected region of chromosome 15 is the gold standard for diagnosis.

Beckwith-Wiedemann Syndrome

BWS is a genetic condition caused by multiple types of perturbations of the imprinted locus on chromosome 11p. It can sometimes be predicted prenatally due to classic findings on prenatal ultrasounds, including overgrowth (including hemihypertrophy), omphalocele, macroglossia, and placental abnormalities. On postnatal examination it is also important to note horizontal ear lobe creases and posterior ear pits, and glabellar nevus flammeus, which can lead to the diagnosis (**Fig. 57.9**). When considering the diagnosis it is important to be alert for hypoglycemia (usually with hyperinsulinemia), and the increased risk for specific malignancies, including Wilms tumor, hepatoblastoma, and adrenal cortical tumors. Due to the complicated molecular aberrations that can cause BWS, it is usually best to send a panel of testing that will look for abnormal methylation patterns in the region, as well as paternal uniparental disomy or other chromosomal differences, and

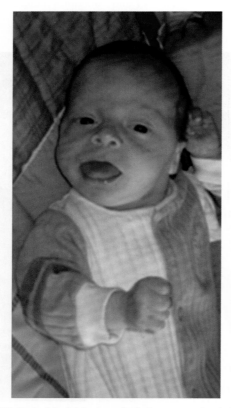

FIGURE 57.9 Typical facial features including macroglossia in an infant with Beckwith-Wiedemann syndrome.

TABLE 57.6

Multifactorial Disorders and Their Recurrence Risks	
Disorder	**Empiric Recurrence Risk**
Cleft lip with or without cleft palate	4%–5%
Cleft palate	2%–6%
Ventricular septal defect	3%–4%
Pyloric stenosis	3%
Hirschsprung anomaly	3%–5%
Clubfoot	2%–8%
Congenital hip dysplasia	3%–4%
Neural tube defects	3%–5%
Atrial septal defect (secundum)	2%–3%

pathogenic variants in the *CDKN1C* gene. Once the exact molecular mechanism has been established, recurrence risk can be calculated, but in many cases a clinical diagnosis can be made without abnormal genetic testing. These cases may be due to mosaicism, but still require tumor screening as recommended by expert guidelines.

Multifactorial Disorders

As discussed above, the vast majority of major and minor anomalies in newborns are not caused by single-gene or chromosome disorders, but by a combination of multiple gene and environmental effects. When a certain threshold has been reached for all these risk factors, then the disorder or malformation manifests. The most common multifactorial disorders and their recurrence risks are in Table 57.6.

Incomplete closure of the neural tube in the first month of pregnancy leads to a range of disorders under the umbrella term NTDs. These can be as mild as spina bifida occulta (as evidenced by a spinal dimple) to complete anencephaly, which is incompatible with life. The vast majority of cases of NTD are caused by a combination of environmental and genetic effects, including many teratogens. Unlike most birth defects, there is an effective prevention for NTD: pre- and early postconception folic acid. Studies have demonstrated up to 80% decrease in NTD after food fortification programs (25). It is important to recognize that many women taking folic acid also give birth to children with NTD, and because of the high level of public literacy surrounding folic acid and NTD, there is a higher level of guilt/shame for women who give birth to children with this particular defect and it should be taken into consideration during family counseling.

Inborn Errors of Metabolism with Dysmorphology

There are multiple categories of inborn errors of metabolism that can cause dysmorphology in the neonate. One of the most groups is those that affect cholesterol disorders, specifically Smith-Lemli-Opitz (SLO) and Antley-Bixler type 1 syndromes. SLO is an autosomal recessive disorder caused by a deficiency of the enzyme 7-dehydrocholesterol (7-DHC) reductase. On examination it can be recognized by facial features that include a narrow forehead, epicanthal folds, ptosis, short mandible, short nose, anteverted nares, and low-set ears (Fig. 57.10A and B). Other anomalies can include cleft palate, cardiac defects, undeveloped male genitalia, and postaxial polydactyly; 2 to 3 syndactyly of the toes is especially characteristic. Antley-Bixler type 1 syndrome is an autosomal recessive disorder associated with mutations in the POR gene encoding cytochrome P450 oxidoreductase. Anomalies include severe radiohumeral synostosis and craniosynostosis, with facial features that include midface hypoplasia and choanal stenosis. Affected patients can also have joint contractures and congenital anomalies of the genitourinary system. Peroxisomal disorders, including Zellweger syndrome and rhizomelic chondrodysplasia

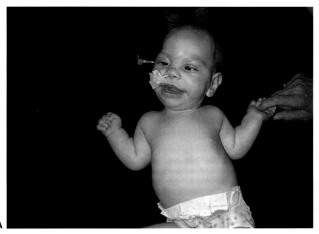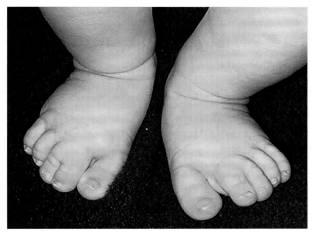

FIGURE 57.10 A: Facial features of an infant with Smith-Lemli-Opitz syndrome. **B:** 2–3 toe syndactyly in an infant with Smith-Lemli-Opitz Syndrome. (Reprinted by permission from Springer: Schaaf CP. Angeborene Fehlbildungssyndrome. In: *Basiswissen Humangenetik.* Springer-Lehrbuch. Berlin, Heidelberg; Springer, 2018:249. Copyright © 2018 Springer-Verlag GmbH Deutschland. https://doi.org/10.1007/978-3-662-56147-8_19.)

punctate, can be identified in the newborn period due to their dysmorphic features. Zellweger and related disorders can cause abnormally large fontanelles, epicanthi, high broad forehead, and a flat nasal bridge. Rhizomelic chondrodysplasia punctata will demonstrate a characteristic rhizomelic shortening of the limbs and epiphyseal stippling on radiographs. Additional biochemical disorders with congenital anomalies include pyruvate dehydrogenase deficiency (dysmorphic facial features and brain malformations), multiple acyl-CoA dehydrogenase deficiency (macrocephaly, hypospadias, dysmorphic facial features, and rocker bottom feet), lysosomal storage disorders (fetal hydrops), and congenital disorders of glycosylation (abnormal fat distribution).

CONCLUSION

Consultation with a clinical geneticist is an important part of the evaluation of an infant with congenital anomalies. Due to a widespread shortage of clinical geneticists, many NICUs will not have a geneticist readily available. A through history and evaluation will help the neonatal providers determine whether a child with congenital anomalies needs to be transferred to a hospital with geneticists available, or whether this can wait until after discharge. In addition to helping the neonatal team understand the nature of the child's differences, a thorough history and evaluation as discussed in this chapter may aid a neonatologist in reaching a diagnosis or determining the urgency of a genetics consultation if possible. Categorization of anomalies and suspected underlying etiologies will also aid in choice of initial genetic tests and discussions with families of infants with congenital anomalies (Table 57.7).

TABLE 57.7

Online Diagnostic Decision Support Sites	
OMIM	www.omim.org/
GeneReviews	www.genetests.org/
GeneMatcher	https://genematcher.org
Atlas of Human Malformation Syndromes in Diverse Populations	research.nhgri.nih.gov/atlas
Simulconsult	www.simulconsult.com/
POSSUM	www.possum.net.au/ (subscription required)

ACKNOWLEDGMENT

The authors gratefully acknowledge the contributions of Dr. Scott D. McLean who wrote this chapter in the 7th edition and compiled Tables 57.1, 57.3, 57.4, 57.5, and 57.6.

REFERENCES

1. Isley L, Falk RE, Shamonki J, et al. Management of the risks for inherited disease in donor-conceived offspring. *Fertil Steril* 2016;106(6):1479.
2. Kwiatkowski F, Perthus I, Uhrhammer N, et al. Association between hereditary predisposition to common cancers and congenital multimalformations. *Congenit Anom (Kyoto)* 2020;60(1):22.
3. Posey JE, Harel T, Liu P, et al. Resolution of disease phenotypes resulting from multilocus genomic variation. *N Engl J Med* 2017;376(1):21.
4. Rasmussen SA. Human teratogens update 2011: can we ensure safety during pregnancy? *Birth Defects Res A Clin Mol Teratol* 2012;94(3):123.
5. Goh PK, Doyle LR, Glass L, et al. A decision tree to identify children affected by prenatal alcohol exposure. *J Pediatr* 2016;177:121.
6. Hoorsan H, Mirmiran P, Chaichian S, et al. Congenital malformations in infants of mothers undergoing assisted reproductive technologies: a systematic review and meta-analysis study. *J Prev Med Public Health* 2017;50(6):347.
7. Kalish JM, Doros L, Helman LJ, et al. Surveillance recommendations for children with overgrowth syndromes and predisposition to wilms tumors and hepatoblastoma. *Clin Cancer Res* 2017;23(13):e115.
8. Zhao J, Yan Y, Huang X, et al. Do the children born after assisted reproductive technology have an increased risk of birth defects? A systematic review and meta-analysis. *J Matern Fetal Neonatal Med* 2020;33(2):322.
9. Mascarenhas M, Sunkara SK, Antonisamy B, et al. Higher risk of preterm birth and low birth weight following oocyte donation: a systematic review and meta-analysis. *Eur J Obstet Gynecol Reprod Biol* 2017;218:60.
10. Krauer F, Riesen M, Reveiz L, et al. Zika virus infection as a cause of congenital brain abnormalities and Guillain-Barre syndrome: systematic review. *PLoS Med* 2017;14(1):e1002203.
11. Nasri HZ, Houde Ng K, Westgate MN, et al. Malformations among infants of mothers with insulin-dependent diabetes: is there a recognizable pattern of abnormalities? *Birth Defects Res* 2018;110(2):108.
12. De-Regil LM, Pena-Rosas JP, Fernandez-Gaxiola AC, et al. Effects and safety of periconceptional oral folate supplementation for preventing birth defects. *Cochrane Database Syst Rev* 2015;(12):CD007950.
13. Morrison JL, Regnault TR. Nutrition in pregnancy: optimising maternal diet and fetal adaptations to altered nutrient supply. *Nutrients* 2016;8(6):342.
14. Ramakrishnan A, Lee LJ, Mitchell LE, et al. Maternal hypertension during pregnancy and the risk of congenital heart defects in offspring: a systematic review and meta-analysis. *Pediatr Cardiol* 2015;36(7):1442.
15. Wainwright B, Bhan R, Trad C, et al. Autoimmune-mediated congenital heart block. *Best Pract Res Clin Obstet Gynaecol* 2020;64:41.

THE NEWBORN INFANT

16. Prick BW, Hop WC, Duvekot JJ. Maternal phenylketonuria and hyperphenyl-alaninemia in pregnancy: pregnancy complications and neonatal sequelae in untreated and treated pregnancies. *Am J Clin Nutr* 2012;95(2):374.

17. Anderson PO. LactMed update—an introduction. *Breastfeed Med* 2016;11(2):54.

18. Yu Y, Cozen W, Hwang AE, et al. Birth anomalies in monozygotic and dizygotic twins: results from the California twin registry. *J Epidemiol* 2019;29(1):18.

19. Martinez-Frias ML, Bermejo E, Rodriguez-Pinilla E, et al. Congenital anomalies in the offspring of mothers with a bicornuate uterus. *Pediatrics* 1998;101(4):E10.

20. Filograna L, Pugliese L, Muto M, et al. A practical guide to virtual autopsy: why, when and how. *Semin Ultrasound CT MR* 2019;40(1):56.

21. Asim A, Kumar A, Muthuswamy S, et al. Down syndrome: an insight of the disease. *J Biomed Sci* 2015;22:41.

22. Skotko BG, Davidson EJ, Weintraub GS. Contributions of a specialty clinic for children and adolescents with Down syndrome. *Am J Med Genet A* 2013;161A(3):430.

23. Cereda A, Carey JC. The trisomy 18 syndrome. *Orphanet J Rare Dis* 2012;7:81.

24. Viuff M, Skakkebaek A, Nielsen MM, et al. Epigenetics and genomics in Turner syndrome. *Am J Med Genet C Semin Med Genet* 2019;181(1):68.

25. Imbard A, Benoist JF, Blom HJ. Neural tube defects, folic acid and methylation. *Int J Environ Res Public Health* 2013;10(9):4352.

58 Eye Disorders

Stacy L. Pineles and Sherwin J. Isenberg

INTRODUCTION

The eye is possibly the fastest developing organ in the body. As soon as 4 to 6 months after birth, some ocular functions are permanently set and if impaired, cannot be fully restored to normalcy. The neonate with a serious ophthalmic disorder may be compared to a time bomb. It is not adequate to simply reverse or cure the immediate problem, since amblyopia may remain. The treatment must be conducted rapidly and effectively, and treatment for amblyopia must be commenced. Thus, the neonatologist has some responsibility to recognize ocular abnormalities and enable early treatment.

GENERAL CONSIDERATIONS

Amblyopia

Amblyopia can be defined as a reduction in vision in the absence of, or beyond that explained by, an apparent organic cause. Amblyopia can be classified as follows: deprivational, strabismic, or refractive. The form of amblyopia that is most feared in infants is deprivation amblyopia. It usually arises before 3 months of age. The cause is blockage of all images from reaching the retina. It may be unilateral or bilateral and may be caused by anything that obstructs the visual axis, such as a cataract, corneal opacity, or severe eyelid ptosis. There is considerable urgency in reversing this form of amblyopia because good vision can only be attained if the visual axis is cleared within the first 3 to 6 months after birth. This timetable coincides with the "critical period" of ocular development in humans (1). Thus, for example, if a significant unilateral congenital cataract is discovered after 6 months of age, one would not expect excellent visual recovery, even after surgery and optical (usually contact lens or intraocular lens) therapy.

Strabismic amblyopia results from a child preferring one eye when the visual axes are misaligned. Reversal, generally with occlusion of the preferred eye, can usually only be achieved before age 7 to 9 years; the earlier treatment begins, the better. Refractive amblyopia generally results from significant inequality of the refractive errors in each eye. This form of amblyopia also should be reversed by 7 to 9 years of age, with treatment usually consisting of spectacles (or contact lenses) and, often, occlusion or penalization of the sound eye. Either of these two forms of amblyopia can begin within the first few postnatal months.

Growth and Development of the Eye

At birth, the sagittal (axial) diameter of the eye is 16 mm in full-term neonates (2). It is less in preterm infants at birth. Ultrasonography can be utilized to determine precisely the size of the entire eye. In the first year, this dimension grows 3.8 mm, with half the expected lifetime increase achieved by 12 months of age. With this information, one can appreciate the early anatomic maturity of the eye.

The corneal diameter is often used as an indicator of the size of the entire eye. At term, the corneal diameter averages 10.0 mm. Microcornea (<9 mm) or megalocornea (>11 mm) (Fig. 58.1) suggests a similar abnormality in size of the entire globe, which should lead to an appropriate workup (see following). The tactile corneal reflex is absent in 90% of infants at birth but develops in all by 3 months of age (3).

Three developmental markers exist in the preterm eye that can help the neonatologist define a neonate's postconceptional age. The tunica vasculosa lentis is a temporary plexus of vessels, which is visible prior to 32 to 34 weeks postconception, crossing the pupil anterior to the lens. The lens surface is covered by these vessels at 27 to 28 weeks postconception, at which time they begin to regress (4). Except for a few vessels at the lens periphery, they should be fully regressed by 34 weeks (Fig. 58.2).

The status of the pupil follows a relatively predictable developmental pattern (Fig. 58.3) (5). At 26 to 31 weeks postconception, the pupillary diameter in relative darkness is quite large (up to 5.0 mm), and the pupil does not respond to light. By 31 weeks, the pupil diameter has decreased to a stable size of 3.5 mm, and the pupil begins to react to light. The light reaction increases in magnitude until reaching stability at term.

The appearance of the macula in the retina is easily appreciated with the ophthalmoscope after the pupil is dilated. The examiner can assess the infant's postconceptional age by observing the development of three landmarks in the macula: pigmentation, annular reflex, and foveola (Table 58.1) (6). With these three anatomic findings, a neonate's postconceptional age can be estimated from 27 weeks postconception to term.

EXAMINATION TECHNIQUES

Visual Acuity

In the neonatal period, there is seldom a reason to even attempt to determine the infant's visual acuity. In the first 2 months after birth, the visual acuity is no better than 20/400 because of immaturity of the retina. The retinal periphery, however, can be stimulated with horizontal optokinetic targets to produce nystagmus. This will prove that the infant is developing some vision. Vertical nystagmus responses develop later. Laboratory techniques can be utilized, if necessary, to more precisely determine the visual acuity. These techniques include preferential forced looking, pattern electroretinograms, and visual-evoked potential. A blink response to light confirms the presence of light perception.

Anterior Segment

The anterior segment can be examined using a strong penlight, with magnification as provided with loupes. Alternatively, a direct ophthalmoscope with a setting of about +5 can be utilized. The examiner should observe the eyelids, conjunctiva, cornea, iris, and lens. The corneal diameter can be measured. As described previously, the pupil diameter initially should be observed with a dim light, followed by evaluation of the reactivity to a bright light.

Posterior Segment

Prior to examining the vitreous and retina, it is usually necessary to dilate the pupil. The choice of dilating agents is important because retinal examinations often are indicated in low-weight preterm infants to rule out retinopathy of prematurity (ROP). Sympathomimetic eye drops can raise a low-weight neonate's blood pressure (7), whereas anticholinergic eye drops that are thought to be of low concentration can significantly increase gastric acid (8). A safe and effective combination mydriatic eye drop, which is commercially available, is 1.0% phenylephrine/0.2% cyclopentolate. One drop should be applied to both eyes and then repeated 5 to 10 minutes later. A third set occasionally may be required if the iris is darkly pigmented.

Although the eyelids can be held open by an assistant if the examination will be brief, usually an eyelid speculum specifically designed for neonatal use is utilized after application of an anesthetic eye drop. When the examiner is manipulating the eye,

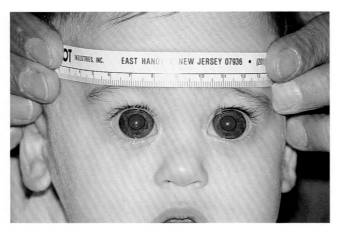

FIGURE 58.1 Megalocornea. Notice the corneal clarity as revealed by the red reflex. The ruler on the forehead allows the corneal diameter to be measured without an examination under anesthesia. (Reprinted with permission from Tasman W, Jaeger E. *The Wills Eye Hospital Atlas of clinical ophthalmology*, 2nd ed. Philadelphia, PA: Lippincott Williams & Wilkins, 2001.)

infants have been shown to display an oculocardiac reflex, defined as any dysrhythmia or a bradycardia of 10% or more, in as many as 31% of cases (9). Therefore, the assistant should monitor the baby, as well as the eye, as the retinal examination progresses. During the retinal examination, the cornea tends to become dry and opacify somewhat because of the heat of the light, exposure, evaporation, and reduced tear production especially in preterm infants (10). Thus, while ensuring the stability of the speculum, the assistant also will need to lubricate the cornea. A number of nonpharmacologic (sucrose, nonnutritive sucking, swaddling) and pharmacologic (topical anesthesia) approaches can be used to reduce the stress experienced by neonates during a retinal examination (11). There is also evidence that sensitivity to light following pupillary dilatation contributes to the stress of a retinal examination in the newborn, with some authors recommending the use of eye shields for 4 hours after the examination (12).

CONGENITAL ANOMALIES

Ocular Size and Shape
Enlarged Eyes

An enlarged eye is suspected when the corneal diameter exceeds 11.0 mm in a term newborn. For confirmation, an A-scan (short for amplitude scan) ultrasound can be obtained easily to measure

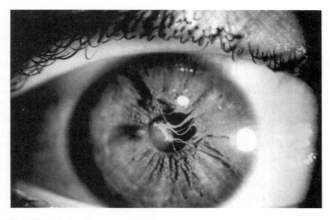

FIGURE 58.2 Persistent pupillary membranes, remaining from tunica vasculosa lentis vessels, are the most common embryonic remnants found in adults.

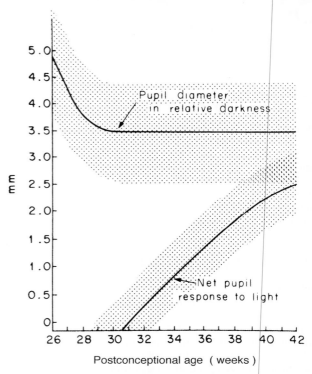

FIGURE 58.3 Diameter of the pupil (mean ± standard deviation) in term and preterm neonates in relative darkness (<10 feet-c) and after light stimulation (600 feet-c). (Reprinted from Isenberg SJ. Examination methods. In: Isenberg SJ, ed. *The eye in infancy*, 2nd ed. St. Louis, MO: Mosby-Year Book, 1994:47. Copyright © 1994 Elsevier. With permission.)

the ocular axial length, which is normally 16 mm at birth (2). If the eye is enlarged, infantile glaucoma caused by an elevated intraocular pressure should be suspected immediately. Infantile glaucoma also often will present with tearing, squinting, photosensitivity, and a cloudy cornea (**Fig. 58.4**). The cornea often is found to have horizontal lines called Haab striae, which result from a disruption of the Descemet membrane. The optic nerve is noted to have an enlarged cup on fundus examination. To differentiate the tearing of glaucoma from that of the much more common nasolacrimal duct obstruction, the examiner should look at, or into, the nostrils. If tears emanate from the nostrils, the nasolacrimal apparatus is patent and glaucoma is possible. If no tears are found in the nostril, a nasolacrimal duct obstruction is more likely.

The treatment of glaucoma is fairly urgent because uncontrolled infantile glaucoma will cause opacification of the cornea, enlargement of the eye, creation of significant myopia, and damage to the optic nerve. If unilateral, the myopia engendered can cause amblyopia, even if the cornea is fairly clear. The corneal opacification can cause deprivation amblyopia.

The infant must be examined while under anesthesia to confirm the diagnosis. After confirmation, the treatment is surgical.

TABLE 58.1	
Development of the Macula	
Observations in the Macula	**Postconceptional Age (wk)**
No pigmentation exists	31.5 ± 1.5
Dark red pigmentation appears	34.8 ± 1.0
Part of the annular reflex is evident	34.7 ± 2.4
Annular reflex is complete	36.3 ± 2.2
Foveolar pit is difficult to appreciate	37.6 ± 3.3
Foveolar light reflex is easily observed	41.7 ± 4.0

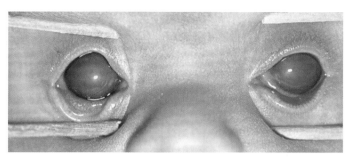

FIGURE 58.4 This cornea is diffusely opacified and enlarged from infantile glaucoma.

The ophthalmologist must open the trabecular meshwork filtration system either internally (goniotomy) or externally (trabeculotomy). If those approaches fail, the ophthalmologist may create an external filtration area (trabeculectomy) or implant an artificial drainage device. Medical management with topical application of agents to reduce aqueous humor secretion (beta-blockers, carbonic anhydrase inhibitors) or increase aqueous humor drainage (prostaglandin analogues) has very limited efficacy in management of glaucoma but may be indicated as an interim treatment while awaiting surgery, or as an adjunct to maximize intraocular pressure reduction postoperatively (13).

Infantile glaucoma has been associated with other ocular problems, such as aniridia; goniodysgeneses (or mesodermal dysgeneses), which include Axenfeld and Rieger syndromes; and persistent fetal vasculature (see below) and following cataract surgery. It has been associated with a number of systemic disorders and syndromes, including Sturge-Weber, neurofibromatosis, Marfan, Pierre Robin, homocystinuria, Lowe, rubella, Rubinstein-Taybi, and chromosomal abnormalities.

The cornea also may be enlarged on a structural basis without glaucoma. However, in this case, the rest of the eye has a normal shape, as can be demonstrated by ultrasonographic examination and a normal intraocular pressure. Megalocornea is uncommon and usually has an X-linked inheritance pattern.

Small Eyes

A small eye will present with a corneal diameter less than 9 mm in a term birth. Confirmation of an axial length less than the normal 16 mm, as shown by ultrasound, is desirable. Microphthalmos can range from an eye that is slightly smaller than normal but other-

wise intact to an eye that is so small that it cannot be found on routine examination (anophthalmos). In cases of anophthalmos, a small, often cystic, eye sometimes can be demonstrated by MRI, CT, or ultrasound. It may be associated with Klinefelter syndrome or trisomy 13.

There are two, not infrequent, ophthalmic disorders associated with microphthalmos. A coloboma is a developmental gap generally located inferiorly in the eye. It can be recognized externally as an inferior notch in the pupil caused by missing iris tissue ("keyhole pupil"), which by itself does not affect vision. More ominously, the defect also can include the optic nerve, macula, and other parts of the retina, which can result in severe visual impairment (Fig. 58.5). Ophthalmologists are now recognizing the frequent combination of systemic findings associated with CHARGE syndrome, consisting of coloboma (C), heart defects (H), atresia choanae (A), retarded growth and development (R), genital hypoplasia (G), and ear anomalies and deafness (E). Facial palsy also is common. At least four of these findings must be present to make the diagnosis.

A second ophthalmic disorder commonly associated with microphthalmos is persistent fetal vasculature, previously known as persistent hyperplastic primary vitreous (14). This disorder often is associated with microphthalmos and hypoplasia of the fovea, as it represents an arrest of ocular development. Many of the sequelae result from abnormal vessels in the vitreous, anterior lens, and equator, causing persistent pupillary membranes, pigmented star-shaped structures on the anterior lens capsule, fibrovascular remnants on the optic nerve (Bergmeister papilla), and nonattachment of the retina. Serious secondary events can ensue, including cataract, glaucoma, lens subluxation, corneal opacities, intraocular hemorrhages, retinal detachments, and chronic inflammation. Because some of these manifestations are treatable, the neonatologist should seek an ophthalmic consultation for any infant with a small eye.

Eyelid Abnormalities

Congenital eyelid ptosis is readily apparent to the parents and all who observe a baby. An early referral to an ophthalmologist should be made. Appropriate timing of surgical correction is important. If the ptosis threatens the infant's vision, it should be corrected early—even within the first few postnatal months. The vision can be threatened in two ways. If the ptosis is total or near total, the visual axis will be obstructed and the child may develop

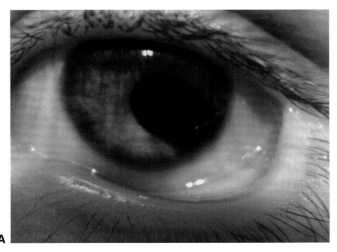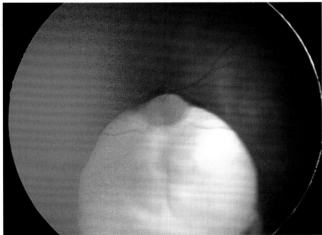

FIGURE 58.5 A: The inferior iris defect, which resembles a keyhole, does not by itself affect vision. **B:** In this coloboma of the posterior pole of the fundus, the optic nerve is seen at the *top*. A defect as large as this will compromise vision, especially if fibers to the macula are deficient.

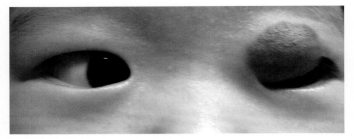

FIGURE 58.6 A hemangioma of the eyelid may not affect vision, even if it is large.

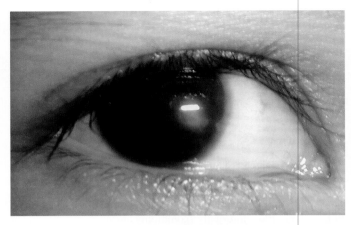

FIGURE 58.7 In this unilateral case of Peters anomaly, the cornea is opaque centrally and clear peripherally. (Courtesy of Dr. Federico Velez.)

deprivation amblyopia. This is unusual because ptosis is seldom total, which allows the child, once head control is established, to elevate the chin to see under the ptotic eyelid. A more likely mechanism of potential visual loss is by an astigmatism induced by the ptotic eyelid applying subtle pressure to the cornea. This unilateral astigmatism can cause refractive amblyopia, even in a young infant. If vision is not threatened, surgery can be deferred until 4 or 5 years of age.

A number of eyelid tumors can present at birth. Most frequent is the capillary hemangioma (Fig. 58.6), which generally continues to grow after birth. The skin overlying the mass can be dimpled and red, resembling a strawberry, or it can assume a diffuse purple color if the lesion is deeper. The lesion does not transilluminate and feels spongy. Left untreated, most of these tumors will spontaneously involute after 1 to 4 years of age. Treatment is indicated if vision is threatened by obstruction of the visual axis or induction of astigmatism, as noted previously. Systemic beta-blockers have become accepted first-line therapy for infantile hemangioma (15). Dramatic responses have been seen in children even after a few days of oral propranolol treatment. However, the use of propranolol requires monitoring for systemic side effects such as bradycardia, hypoglycemia, and respiratory distress. Therefore, the risks and benefits of all treatment options must be weighed and individualized for each patient. Injection of a combination of corticosteroids directly into the tumor or by systemic corticosteroids may also be considered. One other treatment option that can be effective in the more superficial tumors is the topical application of timolol drops or gel to the skin overlying the mass. Lymphangiomata and dermoid cysts of the eyelid also can present at birth and surgical treatment may be required in certain cases.

Corneal Opacities

A number of congenital anomalies can cause corneal opacities at birth. Congenital glaucoma and persistent fetal vasculature have been discussed and must always be ruled out; however, other diagnoses also should be considered.

Birth trauma, usually induced by a forceps placed at or near the eye during delivery, can cause opacities of the cornea. These opacities usually clear within a few days but may leave corneal scars. The corneal damage can leave scarring in the visual axis or induce significant refractive error, which can result in poor vision.

Sclerocornea is a nonprogressive, usually bilateral, anomaly in which the cornea is replaced by opaque sclera-like tissue. Central or total sclerocornea usually is devastating to a child's vision.

Dermoid tumors of the cornea may affect vision similarly if located centrally. A peripheral corneal tumor can affect vision by inducing refractive error. The tumor may be isolated or part of Goldenhar syndrome.

Peters anomaly, characterized by a central corneal opacity and variable iris–corneal or lens–corneal adhesions, is uncommon but a frequent reason for corneal transplant in infants (Fig. 58.7). The periphery of the cornea usually is normal. It has been associated

with fetal alcohol syndrome. Corneal surgery during infancy often is reserved for bilateral cases because the prognosis for good vision following even initially successful corneal transplantation is guarded. In unilateral cases, poor vision is almost inevitable because of amblyopia in the affected eye. The amblyopia may result from a number of causes, including a possible graft rejection, significant refractive errors, recurrent opacities, and secondary glaucoma.

Aniridia

Aniridia, in which much or even the entire iris visible to the examiner is missing, can be compatible with good vision (Fig. 58.8). However, vision can be quite compromised by other ocular associations, including cataracts, peripheral corneal opacities, foveal hypoplasia, glaucoma, and nystagmus. If the vision is quite reduced in infancy, nystagmus usually is found, especially in bilateral cases.

These children must be followed closely because some of the problems, such as glaucoma and central corneal pannus, may arise later in childhood. The glaucoma is particularly difficult to treat because it often is refractory to medical management. Surgical treatment of the glaucoma can induce a cataract because there may be no iris to protect the lens during and after the operation.

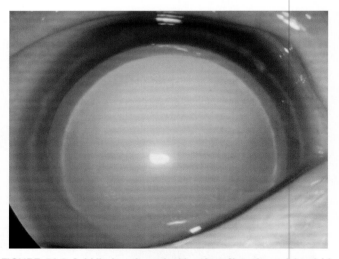

FIGURE 58.8 Aniridia in a 6-month-old patient. Note the peripheral iris rim and the clear view of the lens equator. (Reprinted with permission from Allingham RR, Damji KF, Freedman SF, et al. *Shields textbook of anatomy*, 6th ed. Philadelphia, PA: Wolters Kluwer, 2010.)

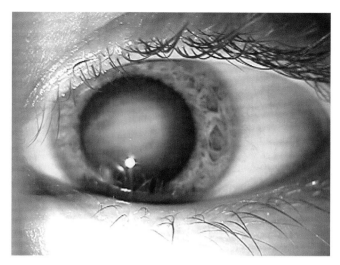

FIGURE 58.9 Congenital cataract. Congenital nuclear cataract: large central nuclear opacity. This cataract is visually significant and requires surgical removal. (Reproduced with permission from Nelson LB. *Pediatric ophthalmology*, 2nd ed. Philadelphia, PA: Wolters Kluwer, 2018.)

Wilms tumor has been reported to occur in up to one-third of all sporadic aniridia cases. Therefore, periodic abdominal ultrasonography of children with aniridia is justified. An 11p deletion has been associated with the complex of aniridia, ambiguous genitalia, and mental retardation. Wilms tumor also may occur with this deletion.

Cataracts

Lens opacities in infants may be isolated or associated with a systemic condition. The morphology of infantile cataracts often is distinctive, which differentiates the infantile from other forms of cataract (Fig. 58.9). The location of the opacity within the baby's lens permits a classification of polar, zonular (or lamellar), nuclear, sutural, or total cataract.

About 25% of infantile cataracts are hereditary, especially if bilateral. Therefore, in the workup of infantile cataracts, it is important to examine the parents and siblings. If an asymptomatic cataract that resembles an infantile cataract is found in a family member, the etiology is attributed to heredity, and an extensive workup can be avoided. The most frequent mode of inheritance is autosomal dominant with variable expressivity but almost complete penetrance.

Metabolic problems have been noted to cause cataracts in infants. Among these are hypoglycemia, mannosidosis, hypoparathyroidism, maternal diabetes, and galactosemia. Galactosemia, inherited as an autosomal recessive trait, should be diagnosed on most neonatal blood spot screening protocols. But a child with a galactosemia cataract may still present to the pediatrician if he or she was not screened for congenital disorders or has the galactokinase deficiency type, which usually presents after 5 months of age. The cataract resembles a typical oil droplet. Early intervention with a lactose-free diet may reduce the lens level of dulcitol and reverse some or all of the lens opacity. Medications, such as corticosteroids, may cause cataracts but seldom in neonates.

A number of systemic conditions are associated with cataracts. In congenital rubella, cataracts are characteristically total or near-total opacities in a smaller-than-normal lens. In addition, the eye in rubella often is small, has abnormalities of the retinal pigment epithelium (noted as "salt and pepper" changes), and may be glaucomatous. Live rubella virus can survive in the lens for years. Therefore, at surgery, care should be taken with the lens aspirates, especially if personnel in the operating room may be

pregnant. Cataracts have been described in other congenital infections, including herpes simplex and varicella.

The presence of a cataract should initiate an appropriate workup with the many causes and associations in mind. The list of other conditions associated with infantile cataract is very long and has been discussed elsewhere (16). To rule out familial cataract, both a family history, including any consanguinity, and an examination of the lenses of the parents and siblings should be undertaken. The history should include questions regarding low-birth weight, ROP, hypoglycemia, serum calcium abnormalities, syndromes, or any systemic disorders. A maternal history of infections while pregnant, diabetes, drug ingestion, and toxin exposure should be sought. Laboratory evaluation should include serum for glucose, blood urea nitrogen, calcium, phosphorus, galactose, and "TORCH" titers (toxoplasmosis, rubella, cytomegalovirus, varicella, and herpes simplex). Lymphocytic choriomeningitis virus may also be responsible for some cataracts in families exposed to rodents (17). Urine should be sent for amino acid levels and hematuria. Other tests should be ordered as indicated by the nonocular findings.

An ophthalmologist should judge if the cataracts are vision threatening. If so and if the child is less than about 4 months old in unilateral cases or 4 to 6 months old in bilateral cases, surgery is urgent to avoid legal blindness from deprivation amblyopia (the definition of legally blind in the USA is a visual acuity of 20/200 or worse in the best seeing eye). Cataract surgery is typically deferred until after 4 weeks in unilateral cases and after 6 to 8 weeks in bilateral cases due to the increased risk of aphakic glaucoma in cases where surgery is initiated before 4 weeks of life. The surgeon will remove the cataract using an intraocular suction-cutting device (lensectomy) and remove the anterior vitreous (vitrectomy) to avoid the postoperative development of posterior opacified membranes. It should be emphasized that many of the techniques used for cataract surgery in adults are not applicable to children. Compared with adults, a baby's sclera is more elastic, which can allow an eye to collapse during surgery; the lens itself is softer; the lens capsule is stiffer; and the vitreous is more solid. For these reasons, special training and experience are desirable prior to operating on the cataracts of babies.

The end of the surgery is far from the end of the infant's visual rehabilitation. An optical device must be used to provide focus after loss of the lens. Spectacles could work, but few infants will keep spectacles in place while in the crib or toddling later. The current method of choice to rehabilitate infant's eyes after cataract surgery is contact lenses. The parents are taught to insert the lens in the morning and remove it in the evening. Certain types of contact lenses may be left in overnight, but some ophthalmologists avoid them because of the increased risk of ocular infection. With contact lenses, the eye doctor can easily change the power as the eye grows and the hyperopic prescription decreases.

Intraocular lenses, as commonly utilized in adults, have been assessed for use in babies. Current intraocular lenses have one fixed power (focal length), which the surgeon must choose at the time of surgery. The refractive power of the baby's eye will decrease up to 8 diopters by 12 months of age and decrease even more later (18). Thus, a lens properly powered for a 1-month-old infant will make the baby highly myopic by 1 year of age. Conversely, a lens placed in an infant's eye with a power appropriate for later in life will leave him quite hyperopic in infancy, when good focus is crucial to developing vision and avoiding amblyopia. For these reasons and because of the concern of leaving a "plastic" lens in an eye for perhaps more than 80 years, intraocular lenses generally were generally not used by ophthalmologists in infants under 6 months, unless under a special protocol. The Infant Aphakia Treatment Study randomized infants between 1 and 6 months of age to cataract extraction with or without an intraocular lens placement (19). The 1- and 5-year outcomes revealed a higher number of immediate and late complications in the patients with intraocular lens placement; however, visual outcomes between the groups at 4.5 years of age were similar amongst groups (20,21). In low- and middle-income countries where no alternative exists, intraocular lenses may be utilized in infants.

In all unilateral cases and some bilateral cases, optical rehabilitation must be accompanied by occlusion of the better seeing eye to reverse amblyopia. Whether to occlude many hours a day to best improve visual acuity or fewer hours to maximize binocularity is a controversial subject (22).

Optic Nerve Hypoplasia

Optic nerve hypoplasia is a frequent cause of unsuspected visual loss. It results in a diminished number of axons in the optic nerve. The number can be low enough to cause legal or complete blindness or sufficiently reduced vision to cause peripheral field loss with normal visual acuity. The appearance of the nerve can vary from a subtle reduction in size in one segment to a grossly small nerve surrounded by a pigment ring and yellow halo known as the "double ring sign" (Fig. 58.10). If bilateral and vision reducing, this entity often will cause nystagmus in infancy. If unilateral and vision reducing, it may present as a unilateral strabismus in the first 5 years of life. The diagnosis can be made with the direct ophthalmoscope by comparing features of the two optic nerves or with other instruments.

Although this disorder is associated with a number of other entities, two deserve the special interest of neonatologists. Fetal alcohol syndrome appears to be a major cause of optic nerve hypoplasia. In Scandinavia, optic nerve hypoplasia was found to occur in almost half the cases of fetal alcohol syndrome (23). It may be the most frequently encountered ocular teratogenic event.

Another association with optic nerve hypoplasia is commonly known as septooptic dysplasia or de Morsier syndrome, in which the child has a number of midline central nervous disorders, such as absence of the septum pellucidum, agenesis of the corpus callosum, and dysplasia of the third ventricle. Hypopituitarism, most commonly evident by short stature, occurs frequently. Hypothyroidism, neonatal hypoglycemia, sexual infantilism or precocity, hypoadrenalism, hyperprolactinemia, and diabetes insipidus also have been reported. This diagnosis, suggested by the presence of optic nerve hypoplasia, can lead to early treatment to modify these endocrinopathies. Therefore, all infants with optic nerve hypoplasia should have neuroimaging to look for abnormalities of the septum pellucidum, corpus callosum, and third ventricle as well as an endocrinologic evaluation (see also Chapter 40). Endocrine abnormalities are especially likely if the posterior pituitary is ectopic or bright on MRI or the infundibulum is absent (24).

Strabismus

In the first few months after birth, infants may display a variable intermittent exotropia (outward deviation of the eyes). This divergence decreases with time, as visual acuity and binocularity develop, until the eyes are generally straight by 3 to 6 months of age. Even infants who develop infantile esotropia (inward deviation of the eyes) are initially exotropic after birth (25). Unless the eye position is constantly abnormal in the first 3 postnatal months, observation is appropriate until the baby is 4 months old. Babies with small or variable angles of esotropia may spontaneously improve. A constant unilateral strabismus may suggest an examination for the strabismus and the presence of amblyopia, possibly caused by an organic lesion such as retinoblastoma. Neonatologists and pediatricians should examine the posterior fundus of any child with unilateral constant strabismus to rule out a retinoblastoma because an early diagnosis can be life saving.

ACQUIRED DISORDERS

Infections

Ophthalmia Neonatorum

This infection arises in the first postnatal month by microorganisms entering the eye during the birth process. The most feared infection is caused by *Neisseria gonorrhoeae*. In the 19th century, neonatal gonococcal conjunctivitis was the major cause of blindness in European children. An extremely marked inflammation characterized by eyelid swelling, conjunctival edema, and copious amounts of purulent discharge usually arises at postnatal days 4 to 6 (Fig. 58.11). Left untreated, the cornea can be perforated within days, which can lead to loss of the eye or corneal scarring and possible blindness in milder cases. The majority of cases are bilateral. As the incidence of adult gonococcal infections has increased in recent decades, so has the incidence of neonatal gonococcal conjunctivitis. Treatment is with ceftriaxone 50 mg/kg intravenously or intramuscularly with proper toilet for the eye to prevent conjunctival membranes. Prophylaxis of ophthalmia neonatorum is discussed below.

Chlamydia trachomatis infection is the most common form of ophthalmia neonatorum today, occurring in up to 1% of births in developed countries. The infection produces a mild and chronic conjunctivitis, with pseudomembrane formation and corneal scarring. The signs first appear between 4 and 12 days of age. After a few months, follicles appear in the conjunctiva. Because these infants also can develop pneumonitis, systemic treatment is necessary with erythromycin (usually as an oral syrup), as well as ocular treatment with erythromycin or sulfacetamide ointment.

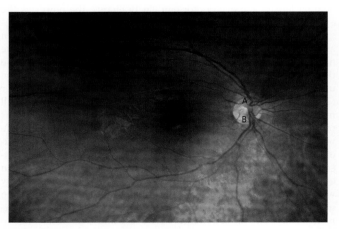

FIGURE 58.10 The diagnosis of optic nerve hypoplasia, although not extremely small, is revealed by the rings of white representing sclera and pigmentation representing retinal pigment epithelium.

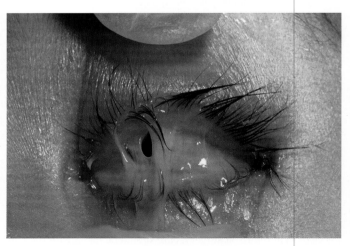

FIGURE 58.11 Gonococcal ophthalmia neonatorum.

Other organisms, such as *Staphylococcus* and *Streptococcus*, also can cause ophthalmia neonatorum. The onset of infection usually is later—often after 1 week of age. Some of these organisms may be acquired postnatally. Treatment is with a broad-spectrum ocular antibiotic ointment, such as sulfacetamide or polymyxin B–bacitracin combination.

Chemical conjunctivitis must always be ruled out. This is a non-infectious inflammation caused by the toxic effects of some prophylactic eye medications on the sensitive conjunctiva of newborns. The inflammation almost always is gone by 24 to 48 hours after birth. It is especially frequent after application of silver nitrate to the eyes.

Prophylaxis against ophthalmia neonatorum began in 1881 by Credé in Leipzig, Germany. Using 2% silver nitrate solution placed in the eyes at birth, he reduced the incidence of ophthalmia neonatorum in his hospital from 10% to 0.3%. Silver nitrate is no longer manufactured in the United States and most other countries. Tetracycline ointment can be useful but has lost popularity because of the frequency of tetracycline-resistant gonococci. Erythromycin ointment may be used, but it is better at reducing than eliminating organisms (26). A new prophylactic agent, povidone–iodine 2.5% ophthalmic solution, has proven to be very effective and inexpensive in a large clinical trial in Kenya when compared with silver nitrate and erythromycin (27). It now is being used in many low- and middle-income countries and may become the medication of choice for ophthalmia neonatorum prophylaxis.

In 2019, the United States Preventive Services Task Force (USPSTF) reaffirmed its recommendation for prophylaxis against gonococcal ophthalmia neonatorum in all newborns, with topical erythromycin ointment being the most widely used agent nationally. However, prophylaxis is no longer recommended in Canada or the United Kingdom.

Workup for a neonate with an inflamed eye includes a history obtained from each parent about genital discharge, genital vesicles, and a history of any sexually transmitted diseases. Laboratory analysis includes conjunctival scrapings for Gram and Giemsa stains. *Chlamydia* is assessed by nucleic acid amplification test (NAAT), culture, or direct fluorescent antibody assay. Cultures could be sent using Thayer-Martin and blood agar media. More specific tests can be ordered if herpes or other organisms are considered.

Nasolacrimal Obstructions

The distal end of the nasolacrimal duct frequently is imperforate at birth. Subsequent infection of the nasolacrimal sac is evidenced by a purulent discharge from the puncta and tearing in the presence of a relatively white eye. In most cases, the infection is alleviated by spontaneously opening of the occluded duct by 7 months of age (28). The opening may occur spontaneously or be induced by conservative treatment, which consists of digital massage over the duct followed by application of an antibiotic eye drop if a discharge is observed. Ointments may only further occlude the duct.

When the symptoms persist beyond 6 to 7 months of age, a probing of the duct usually is indicated (Fig. 58.12). The success rate of a probing procedure is greater than 90%. For persistent obstruction, the probing can be repeated, the turbinate bone can be infractured, or the entire nasolacrimal system can be intubated with silicone tubing. The tubes are removed in 3 to 6 months. A new and quite successful method of treating cases that fail an initial simple probing is to dilate the nasolacrimal duct with a balloon catheter (29). Nasolacrimal duct obstruction has also been associated with an increased risk of anisometropic amblyopia (30) and so children with nasolacrimal duct obstruction should have a comprehensive eye examination in the ensuing years after treatment.

Systemic Infections

Rubella

Ocular manifestations of congenital rubella syndrome include pigmentary retinopathy, cataracts, glaucoma, shallowing of the anterior

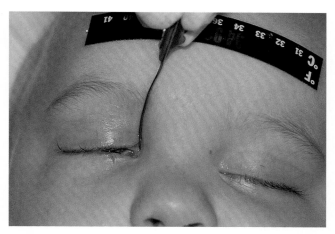

FIGURE 58.12 Nasolacrimal duct probing. The probe is directed inferiorly, laterally, and posteriorly through the nasolacrimal duct. (Reprinted with permission from Chern KC, Saidel MA. *Ophthalmology review manual*, 2nd ed. Philadelphia, PA: Lippincott Williams & Wilkins, 2012.)

chamber, anterior uveitis, microphthalmos, and corneal clouding with or without glaucoma. About half of all children with rubella will have ocular symptoms, which are bilateral in 70% of cases.

Rubella retinopathy, characterized by pigmentary changes secondary to damage to the retinal pigment epithelium, may be the most common ocular manifestation. The appearance has led to the term "salt and pepper" retinopathy. It usually is concentrated in the posterior pole and can be seen with the direct ophthalmoscope if the media are clear. Visual acuity is seldom affected by the retinal involvement alone.

Cataracts occur in 30% to 75% of cases (Fig. 58.13). The morphology of the cataract is fairly typical, being either a total opacification or dense nuclear opacities. About half of the cataracts develop and worsen after birth. The surgeon must obsessively remove all the lens protein and much of the capsule. Residual lens particles in rubella can cause a severe inflammation that itself can lead to blindness.

Cytomegalovirus

The cytomegalovirus reaches the eye hematogenously. It essentially affects only the retina and choroid. The retinopathy presents

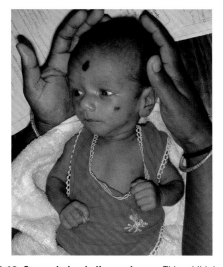

FIGURE 58.13 Congenital rubella syndrome. This child has congenital rubella syndrome. Although full term, the baby is small for his gestational age. There is leukocoria due to a cataract in the left eye. (Reprinted with permission from Garg SJ. *Uveitis*. Philadelphia, PA: Wolters Kluwer, 2018.)

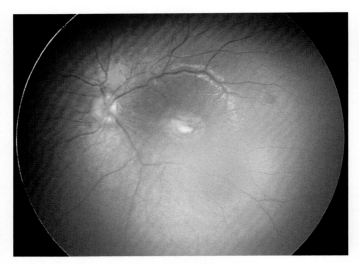

FIGURE 58.14 A large chorioretinal scar has destroyed the fovea in this child with toxoplasmosis. (Courtesy of Dr. Irena Tsui.)

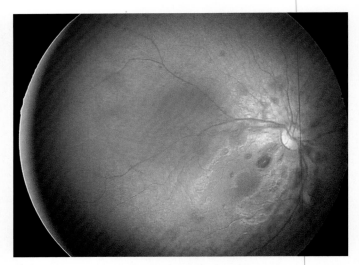

FIGURE 58.15 Retinal hemorrhages in an infant 1 day after birth. (Courtesy of Dr. Irena Tsui.)

as patches of retinal whitening, generally in the periphery. The borders of the lesions are indistinct, and retinal hemorrhages with vascular sheathing may be found. The retinopathy occurs in about 5% of infected infants either at birth or later.

Toxoplasmosis

Seventy-five percent of all patients with congenital toxoplasmosis will have ocular involvement. In 10%, the ocular lesions will be present with no evidence of infection in other organs. *Toxoplasma gondii* causes a focally destructive retinal lesion, with severe inflammation that also affects the choroid. The overlying vitreous becomes hazy with inflammatory cells and exudate. The infection often is unappreciated when it is acute but is recognized later as a discrete yellow-white atrophic scar with hyperpigmented borders and smaller satellite scars (**Fig. 58.14**). Involvement of the macula (in approximately 46% of cases) will reduce vision and may cause a secondary strabismus (31). This is the single major cause of pediatric blindness in some areas of South America and other regions of the world. Peripheral retinal lesions are generally asymptomatic. Although lesions may look quiescent, live organisms may survive within them for years. This is probably a common cause of recurrent inflammation in children and adults.

Local treatment with subconjunctival corticosteroid injections usually is reserved for severely inflamed eyes in conjunction with systemic therapy, as with pyrimethamine and sulfonamides (32). Treatment may not prevent late recurrence.

▎TRAUMA

Birth Trauma

Any portion of the eye or adnexa can be injured in the birth process, and some degree of ocular injury is seen in up to 50% of difficult deliveries. The eyelids may be swollen and ecchymotic. Rarely, the eyelids may be everted totally, with the conjunctiva exposed to the environment. If everted, the exposed surfaces should be kept moist with lubricants until reversion is achieved spontaneously or with manual or surgical measures.

The eyeball may be subluxated, usually by delivery forceps. Orbital fractures and hemorrhages have been reported. The conjunctiva may have hemorrhages in at least 13% of births.

A cloudy cornea may result from forceps injury. It almost always is unilateral. Glaucoma, which also presents with a cloudy cornea, must be ruled out (see "Enlarged Eyes" section). Following birth, the cornea trauma often is accompanied by eyelid edema

and ecchymosis, as well as conjunctival hemorrhage. Corneal examination may reveal linear opacities, usually oriented vertically, caused by Descemet membrane rupture. Although the overall corneal opacity usually clears within 2 weeks, healing of the Descemet membrane rupture can create a severe astigmatism or myopia, which can lead to amblyopia and strabismus.

A hyphema (hemorrhage within the anterior chamber) may result from forceps delivery, especially if residual fetal vessels are present. These hyphemas clear in a few weeks with no specific treatment. Vitreous hemorrhages, however, can cause amblyopia and severe myopia, especially if they persist for more than 3 weeks. They have been associated with protein C deficiency. Vitrectomy ultimately may be necessary if the hemorrhage does not spontaneously clear. Compression of the head in the course of a vaginal delivery often results in retinal hemorrhages (**Fig. 58.15**). The incidence has been reported to be 40% within 1 hour of birth, which decreases to 11% by 72 hours (33). Even extensive hemorrhage will resorb within 6 weeks after birth. Rarely, hemorrhages in the fovea resorb slower, resulting in amblyopia in a normal-appearing eye.

Nonaccidental Trauma

Amniocentesis has been reported to damage eyes, usually in the midtrimester of pregnancy. Although most cases have resulted in blindness with frequent loss of the eye, early repair may salvage vision (34). The presence of segmental edema of the conjunctiva or corneal edema in a neonate should raise the possibility of an amniocentesis injury.

Child abuse often will affect the eye. There are many possible ocular effects of abuse, but intraocular hemorrhage is the most specific sign. Buys and colleagues (35) reported no retinal hemorrhages in a series of 75 children with documented accidental head trauma; however, their nonaccidental trauma cases all had retinal hemorrhages. Thus, any case of suspected child abuse, unexplained coma, seizure, intracranial hemorrhage, or injury should have an ophthalmology consultation (36).

In addition, maternal substance abuse during pregnancy may affect ocular development. The most frequent teratogenic effect is probably optic nerve hypoplasia in fetal alcohol syndrome, as described previously. Cocaine abuse has been noted to affect the eye by inducing hypervascularization of the iris (37). The dilated and tortuous vessels, which run from the pupil to the periphery, usually are gone 1 week after birth. If these vessels are noted shortly after birth, a toxicology screen, which includes cocaine, is indicated.

PHOTOTHERAPY FOR HYPERBILIRUBINEMIA

Light has the ability to photooxidize bilirubin from the skin and subcutaneous tissue. Although useful to reduce hyperbilirubinemia, animal studies have shown that very intense light damages the outer retinal layers irreversibly. In human infants, however, there has been little evidence of long-term damage from these lights (38). Nonetheless, it is prudent to occlude both eyes with an opaque mask or eye patches during this therapy. To prevent the possibility of amblyopia, both eyes should be occluded equally and securely.

RETINOPATHY OF PREMATURITY

In high-income countries, ROP is one of the major causes of blindness in infants. This disorder of abnormal vascularization of the retina, formerly called retrolental fibroplasia, tends to occur in low-weight neonates often exposed to large amounts of oxygen. The more premature the child, the more likely is the disease. Of infants with a birth weight under 1 kg, 82% will develop ROP, with 9.3% progressing to vision-threatening sequelae (39). Of infants with a birth weight between 1 and 1.5 kg, 47% will develop ROP and 2% will be in danger of losing vision.

Risk Factors

Infants who develop ROP often have other morbidities of the very preterm infant, as well as a complicated hospital course. This makes clinical correlations between ROP and other clinical entities difficult to interpret. Nonetheless, measures have been taken to prevent ROP. Oxygen use has long been minimized as hyperoxemia has been conclusively shown cause ROP (40). However, studies showing that lower target oxygen saturations for the first 6 to 8 weeks of life are associated with lower rates of ROP, also suggested increased mortality (41). Other studies have evaluated oxygen targets after 32 weeks of gestational age and have shown that higher oxygen levels may be better tolerated during this time period (41).

The Neonatal Oxygenation Prospective Meta-analysis (NeO-ProM) was a 15-year-long collaboration (initiated in 2003) to address optimal oxygen targeting in preterm infants. This group of investigators carried out five separate but similar randomized clinical trials, prospectively planning to share outcome data. A total of 4,965 infants were randomized to higher (90% to 95%) or lower (85% to 89%) oxygen saturations in the newborn period. Despite some debate over study performance and reliability of the oxygen saturation algorithm used (42), a consensus towards targeting saturations of 90% to 95% is now emerging (43). Infants in the lower saturation group did have lower rates of ROP requiring treatment (10.9% vs. 14.9%) but also had higher rates of death (19.9% vs. 17.7%) and severe necrotizing enterocolitis (9.2% vs. 6.9%) (44).

Low gestational age and low birth weight for gestational age are each independent major risk factors for ROP. In addition, poor postnatal weight gain and low serum IGF-1 concentrations are also associated with increased rates of ROP (45). IGF-1 may contribute to the suppression of vascular growth in ROP patients, and low values are also highly associated with poor postnatal weight gain in preterm children.

There is great interest in predictive models to identify high-risk infants to reduce the burden of unnecessary screening examinations. In addition to gestational age and birth weight, various models have incorporated variables such as oxygen use, postnatal weight gain, serum IGF-1 and IGFBP3 levels, and other medical conditions. Although some models have resulted in decreased screening burden as part of a research protocol, they have not yet been widely adopted in clinical practice (46,47).

Pathogenesis

The pathogenesis of ROP is thought to begin from a combination of prematurity, supplemental oxygen, and other possible factors causing vasoconstriction of immature retinal vessels. Premature deliveries combined with supplemental oxygen therapy lead to a relative retinal hyperoxia in the extrauterine environment. This relative hyperoxia leads to suppression of hypoxia-inducible factor and vascular endothelial growth factor (VEGF), leading to a cessation of retinal vascular development and vasoconstriction. This vasoconstriction interrupts the normal developmental migration of the blood vessels from the optic nerve peripherally to the ora serrata. Vascular closure may cause localized ischemia. In addition, further retinal growth and high metabolic demands then cause upregulation of VEGF and other growth factors from the avascular immature retina, leading to abnormal vessel development. Endothelial proliferation adjacent to the vessels extends within the retina and into the vitreous. Fibrous and glial tissue grows, producing hemorrhage, traction, and retinal detachment.

Examination

The decision of which babies to screen is somewhat controversial. Some nurseries desire an examination of any infant with a birth weight below 1,250 g, whereas others use a weight as high as 1,600 g. A University of Pittsburgh study found that above a birth weight of 1,500 g, ROP developed only in infants exposed to at least 6 weeks of continuous oxygen (47). The American Academy of Pediatrics (AAP) published updated recommendations in 2018; these recommendations state that infants with birth weight less than 1,500 g or gestational age of 30 weeks or less, and selected infants with birth weight between 1,500 and 2,000 g or gestational age greater than 30 weeks with an unstable clinical course should have retinal screening performed (48). Similar guidelines with slight variation in gestational and birth weight criteria are in place internationally.

The examination should be performed as soon as the media are clear enough to permit ophthalmoscopy, and the neonate can tolerate the "trauma" of a retinal examination. The use of proper dilating eye drops and soothing techniques was discussed previously. A number of centers advise the first examination be performed 6 weeks after birth. Because vision-threatening ROP has been shown to arise at 33 to 41 weeks postconception, it would be wise to time the first examination at approximately 31 to 32 weeks, if possible. Larger preterm newborns may need their first examination sooner after birth than do smaller ones. The AAP recommendations suggest a screening examination at 31 weeks for babies born at 27 weeks or earlier and an examination at 4 weeks of chronologic age for infants born at 28 weeks or later (48). See Table 58.2.

TABLE 58.2

AAP Recommendation of Age at First ROP Screening

Gestational Age at Birth (wk)	Age at Initial Examination (wk)	
	Postmenstrual	Chronologic
22[a]	31	9
23[a]	31	8
24	31	7
25	31	6
26	31	5
27	31	4
28	32	4
29	33	4
30	34	4
Older gestational age, high-risk factors[b]	—	4

Shown is a schedule for detecting prethreshold ROP with 99% confidence, usually before any required treatment.

—, not applicable.

[a]This guideline should be considered tentative rather than evidence based for infants with a gestational age of 22 to 23 weeks because of the small number of survivors in these postmenstrual age categories.

[b]Consider timing on the basis of the severity of comorbidities.

TABLE 58.3

Stages of Retinopathy of Prematurity

Stage	Character
1	Demarcation line
2	Ridge
3	Extraretinal fibrovascular proliferation
4A	Partial retinal detachment, macula still attached
4B	Partial retinal detachment, macula detached
5	Total retinal detachment
Plus	Dilation and tortuosity of posterior retinal vessels

Subsequent examinations should be conducted as indicated by the findings of the first examination. If no ROP is found, but the retina is still being vascularized, the examination should be repeated every 1 to 2 weeks. If ROP is found, the examinations should be repeated weekly. If "plus disease" (tortuosity and dilation of the blood vessels in the posterior pole of the fundus) is noted, the disease may be progressing faster, justifying a repeat evaluation in 3 to 4 days. The examinations are continued until the retinal vascularization has reached zone III (see following), the threshold for treatment (see following) is achieved, or the disease has definitely regressed. There are some rare cases in which regression was followed by reactivation.

Recently, telemedicine has been utilized as an important screening tool in the management of ROP. Wide-angle digital retinal photography has been used to detect "plus disease" as well as posterior ROP. Telemedicine allows expansion of ROP screening and education to underserved areas throughout the world (49).

Classification

The internationally established classification of acute ROP is meant to characterize accurately the extent of the disorder in a particular eye. Three dimensions or criteria are used—stage, location (anterior to posterior), and extent.

The staging scheme is presented in Table 58.3. In stage 1, the normal progression of vascularization of the retina toward the periphery is halted at a thin demarcation line found by an abrupt change in color of the retina. The line divides the vascularized from the nonvascularized retina. Importantly, the vessels mul-

tibranch or arcade at the line. The latter appearance differentiates early ROP from normal vascularization because in the normal state, the advancing vessels usually bifurcate and do not break into an arcade. In stage 2, the demarcation line extends up out of the retinal plane toward the vitreous. This ridge may change color from white or tan to red. In stage 3, extraretinal fibrovascular tissue grows either on the top of the ridge, yielding a ragged appearance, or just posterior. As it grows, it reaches into the vitreous (Fig. 58.16). Stage 4 is reached when the retina begins to detach from traction exerted by the extraretinal fibrovascular tissue condensing (analogous to a purse string) or, less commonly, from serous fluid elevating the retina. The macula still is spared from detachment in stage 4A, and the visual prognosis is still hopeful. The visual prognosis decreases markedly in stage 4B as the macula detaches. In stage 5, the retinal detachment is total and shaped like a funnel or tulip.

In describing the stage, one also should indicate if "plus disease" is present. "Plus disease" is the presence of tortuosity and dilation of the blood vessels in the posterior pole of the fundus. These posterior vascular changes usually indicate that an arteriovenous shunt is occurring in the extraretinal fibrovascular tissue on top of the ridge. "Plus disease" is a worse prognostic sign and may indicate that the disease is progressing faster.

The location is described in zones (Fig. 58.17). Zone I, the most posterior, is a circle centered on the optic nerve, with a radius twice the distance from the optic nerve to the fovea. Zone II extends from the edge of zone I all the way to the ora serrata on the nasal side and, on the temporal side, to the anatomic equator. This leaves zone III, which is a peripheral crescent on the temporal side. ROP in zone I is potentially the most dangerous, whereas disease in zone III is seldom of any concern. The circumferential extent of the disease is noted in clock hours, with an entire eye composed of 12 clock hours. One clock hour equals 30 degrees.

This classification pertains to the acute changes of ROP. There also are cicatricial changes that should be considered. Classification of the cicatricial changes is not yet universally accepted. Usually these changes arise in eyes that have reached acute stage 3 but did not progress to a significant retinal detachment. In these eyes, the vessels are drawn to the lateral side by cicatrization distorting the optic nerve and dragging the fovea laterally (Fig. 58.18). A retinal fold may form. These developments often reduce vision significantly.

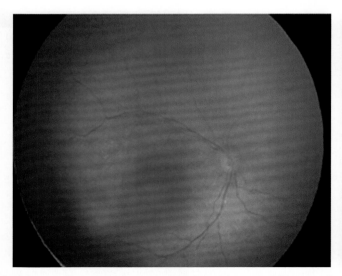
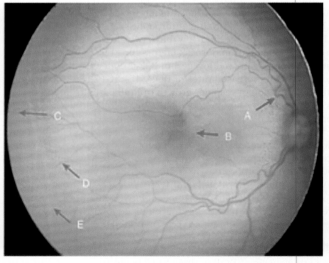

FIGURE 58.16 Retinal telephotoscreening of the right eye for ROP taking place in the NICU using the RetCam. Left: normal retina; right: stage 3 ROP in zone 2 with plus disease (pretreatment). **A:** Increased tortuosity and dilatation of retinal vessels at the optic disc. **B:** Fovea. **C:** Avascular peripheral retina. **D:** Increased vascular branching posterior to the ridge. **E:** Stage 3 ROP at the demarcation line between the vascular and avascular retina. (Courtesy of Dr. Ian Clark.)

Right eye

Left eye

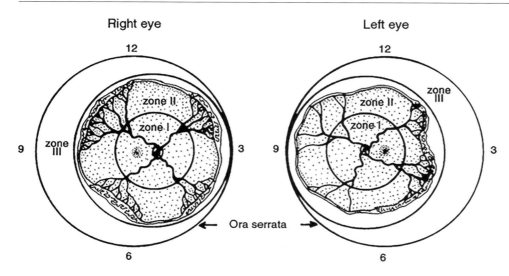

FIGURE 58.17 Schematic representation of the retinas divided into three zones, with the relevant anatomic landmarks. (Reprinted with permission from Hartnett ME. *Pediatric retina,* 2nd ed. Philadelphia, PA: Wolters Kluwer, 2013.)

Treatment

Many eyes that develop ROP will improve without treatment to the point that few or no remnants of the disorder are evident later. The point at which the prognosis for regression is below 50% is considered the threshold level for treatment. The multicenter trial of cryotherapy defined the threshold level as stage 3 in five adjacent or eight cumulative clock hours in combination with "plus disease" (50,51). This definition has proven appropriate for disease in zone II. Recent studies have suggested that treatment should be indicated for any stage ROP with "plus disease" in zone I, zone I stage 3 disease without "plus disease," or zone II stage 2 or 3 with "plus disease" (48).

Currently, cryotherapy has been replaced for most applications by the use of lasers, which usually are mounted on an indirect ophthalmoscope worn on the head of the surgeon (47). Laser surgery can be performed in the nursery with mild sedation and only topical anesthesia because it probably causes less pain than does cryotherapy.

The rationale behind this treatment is to ablate the peripheral avascular retina for 360 degrees in the affected eye(s). This approach has been shown in numerous studies to improve diabetic retinopathy, presumably by reducing or eliminating the signal from the ischemic or avascular tissue to the retina to produce neovascular vessels.

The long-term beneficial effects demonstrated by both cryotherapy and laser therapy have been evaluated in large multicenter trials. The frequency of the potentially blinding ROP sequelae of retinal detachment and retinal fold was reduced by half after cryotherapy (52), with the benefit of laser therapy presumed to be similar. At about 6 years of age, poor visual acuity (20/200 or worse) was found in 62% of untreated eyes compared with 47% of cryotreated eyes (53). Using laser treatment and current recommendations for earlier treatment, the rate of poor visual acuity was decreased to 25% of eyes at 6 years (54). Despite the destruction of parts of the peripheral retina by cryotherapy and laser therapy, long-term follow-up has found only a 6-degree loss of peripheral visual field (55). Whether their infant is treated with laser or cryotherapy, the parents must be informed that although the treatment will reduce the possibility of blindness, blindness may still result despite treatment. Too often, parents assume that, with treatment, blindness definitely will be avoided.

Recently published studies have indicated that anti-VEGF treatments may also be useful for the treatment of ROP (56). The medication is injected through the sclera near the cornea into the vitreous humor. Studies have shown that regression is usually induced by one injection into the affected eye. There are concerns about the possibility of systemic side effects and that recurrence can arise up to nearly a year after birth, necessitating many repeat examinations. Currently, AAP recommendations state that this therapy may be considered for patients with severe ROP (zone I, stage 3+). However, the use of these agents is not currently approved by the U.S. Food and Drug Administration for the treatment of ROP; therefore, a detailed informed consent process is required, and full disclosure of the lack of long-term data regarding dosage, timing, visual outcomes, and other long-term effects must be performed (48).

If retinal detachment occurs, all is not lost. Modern vitreoretinal surgery can reattach a detached retina with ROP more than 30% of the time. Once the macula detaches, however, the visual prognosis decreases markedly, even if the retina is reattached successfully. For stage 4A, visual acuity results as good as 20/20 have been reported with the macula still attached. Stage 4B results have been in the 20/80 to 20/200 range. With a total detachment (stage 5), the results decrease considerably to the 20/600 to 20/1,600 range or even lower (57). This low level of vision may allow the child to ambulate independently and certainly is better than the blindness that would occur without surgery.

Long-Term Problems

Aside from the problems of poor vision from a detached retina or retinal folds, there are other sequelae that can arise in the eyes

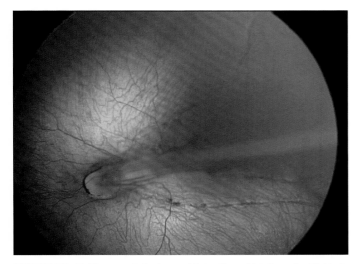

FIGURE 58.18 The macula is dragged laterally amidst the retinal folds in cicatricial retinopathy of prematurity.

of infants with regressed ROP. Even with an attached retina and intact macula, children with regressed ROP have been shown to be more susceptible to a number of visual disorders, including myopia, amblyopia, strabismus, and nystagmus. Children who develop cicatricial retinal changes, even with good vision, are at risk for future retinal problems, including detachment. Therefore, these children should be examined at least annually throughout their life, or at least until they are mature and literate enough to rule out amblyopia and strabismus.

COMMON DIFFERENTIAL DIAGNOSTIC PROBLEMS

Leukocoria

When faced with an infant with a white pupil or unusual retinal light reflex, the neonatologist or pediatrician should consider the differential diagnosis and begin a workup (**Fig. 58.19**). The first obligation is to rule out the potentially fatal retinoblastoma, even in a neonate (**Fig. 58.20**). The most common lesions that may, to some extent, simulate a retinoblastoma by presenting with leukocoria in infancy include cataract, persistent fetal vasculature, Coats disease, large retinal coloboma, and retinal detachment resulting from ROP. Toxocariasis is not a disease of infants. Coats disease is caused by anomalous telangiectatic retinal vessels that cause massive exudation and retinal detachment. It is important to realize that behind an opaque cataract can lie other problems, such as retinal detachment or a mass.

The history should reveal the presence of prematurity, oxygen use, illnesses during pregnancy (such as rubella, toxoplasmosis, and cytomegalovirus), possible child abuse, or traumatic birth. The nonocular history may help. Deafness suggests the possibility of rubella or Norrie disease (cataract with retinal detachment). Toxoplasmosis or tuberous sclerosis may present with seizures. Incontinentia pigmenti or tuberous sclerosis may have skin lesions. Bilateral leukocoria would favor the diagnoses of ROP, Norrie disease, child abuse, and retinal dysplasias. Unilateral leukocoria is more consistent with Coats disease, persistent fetal vasculature, and intraocular foreign body. Although Norrie and Coats diseases are more common in males, incontinentia pigmenti is more frequent in females.

The examination may actually begin with the eyes of the parents. Parents have been found to have an asymptomatic congenital cataract, regressed retinoblastoma, unappreciated coloboma, and findings of familial exudative retinopathy, which closely resembles ROP. Any of these findings in a parent, who usually cooperates better in the examination, generally establishes the diagnosis for the baby. Examination of the child may reveal microphthalmos, which is consistent with coloboma or persistent fetal vasculature. The level of the opacity may be evident with a light or portable slit lamp. If there is a defect in the inferior iris, coloboma should be considered. Lens opacity, of course, constitutes a cataract, but additional examinations, perhaps with ultrasound or radiologic tests, may reveal pathology in the vitreous or retina. A detailed

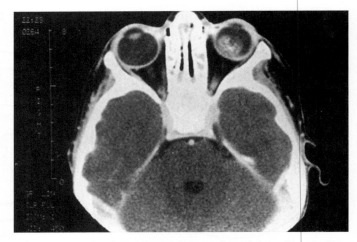

FIGURE 58.20 A calcified intraocular mass in an infant with retinoblastoma.

retinal examination is crucial if the media are sufficiently clear, to diagnose many entities that present with leukocoria.

Cloudy Cornea

Profound amblyopia will result from an opacified cornea, especially if it is unilateral. Although some opacities clear with time, others remain. The history, associated findings, and examination will clarify the prognosis.

The history should include illnesses during pregnancy to rule out rubella, syphilis, and herpes, which can cause keratitis. Delivery by forceps of a large neonate suggests birth trauma (**Fig. 58.21**). Conjunctival hemorrhages suggest a traumatic etiology. The presence of conjunctival inflammation implies infection or pupillary block glaucoma as an etiology.

Systemic physical abnormalities may imply an etiology as an umbilical hernia suggests glaucoma associated with Rieger syndrome. Glaucoma also is suggested by a history of photosensitivity and tearing. Family history is important. On examination, the eyelids may reveal evidence of phakomatoses as the angiomatosis of Sturge-Weber syndrome or a neurofibroma.

Most important is the corneal examination. The corneal diameter should be measured as accurately as possible. An enlarged cornea strongly indicates glaucoma, whereas a small opacified cornea may result from sclerocornea, microphthalmos, trisomy 13,

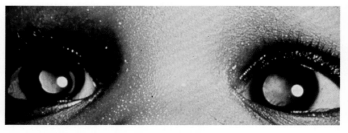

FIGURE 58.19 Bilateral leukocoria was found in this neonate. A family history of Norrie disease simplified the diagnosis.

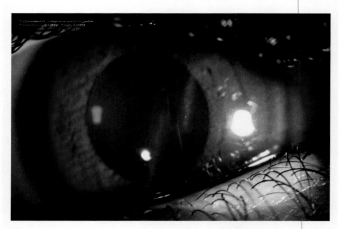

FIGURE 58.21 Cloudy cornea after forceps delivery. (Courtesy of Ms. Cynthia VandenHoven, BAA, CRA, FOPS and the Hospital for Sick Children, Toronto, Canada.)

or rubella. Striae in the cornea are often helpful. Horizontally oriented striae are compatible with glaucoma, whereas vertical or oblique ones often result from birth trauma. A mass overlying the cornea may be a dermoid tumor.

Measurement of the intraocular pressure in these cases often is imperative to rule in glaucoma. Examination of the iris may reveal adhesions to the cornea. This can result from trauma or may indicate a mesodermal dysgenesis syndrome. This syndrome encompasses a number of developmental disorders, such as Peters anomaly—the most frequent reason to perform corneal transplants in infants. A cataractous lens behind an opacified cornea may be caused by rubella, birth trauma, Lowe syndrome, or mesodermal dysgenesis. If the eye and intraocular pressure are otherwise normal, the opacified cornea may result from a hereditary corneal dystrophy.

REFERENCES

1. Rakic P. Development of visual centers in the primate brain depends on binocular competition before birth. *Science* 1981;214:928.
2. Isenberg SJ, Neumann D, Cheong PY, et al. Growth of the internal and external eye in term and preterm infants. *Ophthalmology* 1995;102:827.
3. Snir M, Axer-Siegel R, Bourla D, et al. Tactile corneal reflex development in full-term babies. *Ophthalmology* 2002;109:526.
4. Hittner HM, Hirsch NJ, Rudolph AJ. Assessment of gestational age by examination of the anterior vascular capsule of the lens. *J Pediatr* 1977;91:455.
5. Isenberg SJ. Clinical application of the pupil examination in neonates. *J Pediatr* 1991;118:650.
6. Isenberg SJ. Macular development in the premature infant. *Am J Ophthalmol* 1986;101:74.
7. Isenberg SJ, Everett S. Cardiovascular effect of mydriatics in low-birth-weight infants. *J Pediatr* 1984;105:111.
8. Isenberg SJ, Abrams C, Hyman PE. Effect of cyclopentolate eyedrops on gastric secretory function in pre-term infants. *Ophthalmology* 1985;92:698.
9. Clarke WN, Hodges E, Noel LP, et al. The oculocardiac reflex during ophthalmoscopy in premature infants. *Am J Ophthalmol* 1985;99:649.
10. Isenberg SJ, Apt L, McCarty JA, et al. Development of tearing in preterm and term neonates. *Arch Ophthalmol* 1998;116:773.
11. Francis K. What is best practice for providing pain relief during retinopathy of prematurity eye examinations? *Adv Neonatal Care* 2016;16:220.
12. Szigiato AA, Speckert M, Zielonka J, et al. Effect of eye masks on neonatal stress following dilated retinal examination: the MASK-ROP randomized clinical trial. *JAMA Ophthalmol* 2019;137(11):1265.
13. Yu Chan JY, Choy BN, Ng AL, et al. Review on the management of primary congenital glaucoma. *J Curr Glaucoma Pract* 2015;9:92.
14. Goldberg MF. Persistent fetal vasculature (PFV): an integrated interpretation of signs and symptoms associated with persistent hyperplastic primary vitreous (PHPV). LIV Edward Jackson Memorial Lecture. *Am J Ophthalmol* 1997;124:587.
15. Yang H, Hu DL, Shu Q, et al. Efficacy and adverse effects of oral propranolol in infantile hemangioma: a meta-analysis of comparative studies. *World J Pediatr* 2019;15:546.
16. Hiles DA, Kilty LA. Disorders of the lens. In: Isenberg SJ, ed. *The eye in infancy*, 2nd ed. St. Louis, MO: Mosby-Year Book, 1994:336.
17. Barton LL, Mets MB, Beauchamp CL. Lymphocytic choriomeningitis virus: emerging fetal teratogen. *Am J Obstet Gynecol* 2002;187:1715.
18. Neumann D, Weissman BA, Isenberg SJ, et al. The effectiveness of daily wear contact lenses for the correction of infantile aphakia. *Arch Ophthalmol* 1993;111:927.
19. Plager DA, Lynn MJ, Buckley EG, et al.; Infant Aphakia Treatment Study. Complications, adverse events, and additional intraocular surgery 1 year after cataract surgery in the Infant Aphakia Treatment Study. *Ophthalmology* 2011;118:2330.
20. Plager DA, Lynn MJ, Buckley EG, Wilson E, Lamber SR; Infant Aphakia Treatment Study Group. Complications in the first 5 years following cataract surgery in infants with and without intraocular lens implantation in the Infant Aphakia Treatment Study. *Am J Ophthalmol* 2014;158(5):892.
21. The Infant Aphakia Treatment Study Group; Lambert SR, Lynn MJ, Hartmann EE, et al. Comparison of contact lens and intraocular lens correction of monocular aphakia during infancy. A randomized clinical trial of HOTV optotype acuity at age 4.5 years and clinical findings at age 5 years. *JAMA Ophthalmol* 2014;132(6):676.
22. Wright KW. Pediatric cataracts. *Curr Opin Ophthalmol* 1997;8:50.
23. Stromland K. Ocular abnormalities in the fetal alcohol syndrome. *Acta Ophthalmol Suppl* 1985;171:1.
24. Phillips PH, Spear C, Brodsky MC. Magnetic resonance diagnosis of congenital hypopituitarism in children with optic nerve hypoplasia. *J AAPOS* 2001;5:275.
25. Birch E, Stager D, Wright K, et al.; for the Pediatric Eye Disease Investigator Group. The natural history of infantile esotropia during the first six months of life. *J AAPOS* 1998;2:325.
26. Hammerschlag MR, Cummings C, Roblin PM, Williams TH, Delke I. Efficacy of neonatal ocular prophylaxis for the prevention of chlamydial and gonococcal conjunctivitis. *N Engl J Med* 1989;320(12):769.
27. Isenberg SJ, Apt L, Wood M. A clinical trial of povidone-iodine as prophylaxis against ophthalmia neonatorum. *N Engl J Med* 1995;332:562.
28. Petersen RA, Robb RM. The natural course of congenital obstruction of the nasolacrimal duct. *J Pediatr Ophthalmol Strabismus* 1978;15:246.
29. Lueder GT. Balloon catheter dilation for treatment of persistent nasolacrimal duct obstruction. *Am J Ophthalmol* 2002;133:337.
30. Matta NS, Silbert DI. High prevalence of amblyopia risk factors in preverbal children with nasolacrimal duct obstruction. *J AAPOS* 2011;15:350.
31. Hogan MJ, Kimura SJ, O'Connor GR. Ocular toxoplasmosis. *Arch Ophthalmol* 1964;72:592.
32. Engstrom RE Jr, Holland GN, Nussenblatt RB, et al. Current practices in the management of ocular toxoplasmosis. *Am J Ophthalmol* 1991;111:601.
33. Jain IS, Singh YP, Grupta SL, et al. Ocular hazards during birth. *J Pediatr Ophthalmol Strabismus* 1980;17:14.
34. Naylor G, Roper JP, Willshaw HE. Ophthalmic complications of amniocentesis. *Eye* 1990;4:845.
35. Buys YM, Levin AV, Enzenauer RW, et al. Retinal findings after head trauma in infants and young children. *Ophthalmology* 1992;99:1718.
36. Christian CW, Levin AV. AAP Council on Child Abuse and Neglect, AAP Section on Ophthalmology, American Association of Certified Orthoptists, American Association for Pediatric Ophthalmology and Strabismus, American Academy of Ophthalmology. The Eye Examination in the Evaluation of Child Abuse. *Pediatrics* 2018;142(2):e20181411.
37. Isenberg SJ, Spierer A, Inkelis SH. Ocular signs of cocaine intoxication in neonates. *Am J Ophthalmol* 1987;103:211.
38. Kalina RE, Forrest GL. Ocular hazards of phototherapy for hyperbilirubinemia. *J Pediatr Ophthalmol* 1971;8:116.
39. Palmer EA, Flynn JT, Hardy RJ; for the Cryotherapy for Retinopathy of Prematurity Cooperative Group. Incidence and early course of retinopathy of prematurity. *Ophthalmology* 1991;98:1628.
40. Flynn JT, Bancalari E, Snyder ES, et al. A cohort study of transcutaneous oxygen tension and the incidence and severity of retinopathy of prematurity. *N Engl J Med* 1992;326:1050.
41. Hellstrom A, Smith LEH, Dammann O. Retinopathy of prematurity. *Lancet* 2013;382:1445.
42. Schmidt B, Whyte RK. Oxygen saturation target ranges and alarm settings in the NICU: what have we learnt from the neonatal oxygenation prospective meta-analysis (NeOProM)? *Semin Fetal Neonatal Med* 2020;25:101080.
43. Darlow BA, Husain S. Primary prevention of ROP and the oxygen saturation monitoring trials. *Semin Perinatol* 2019;43:333.
44. Askie LM, Darlow BA, Finer N. Association between oxygen saturation targeting and death or disability in extremely preterm infants in the neonatal oxygenation prospective meta-analysis collaboration. *JAMA* 2018;319:2190.
45. Phelps DL. Vitamin E and retinopathy of prematurity. In: Silverman WA, Flynn JT, eds. *Contemporary issues in fetal and neonatal medicine 2: retinopathy of prematurity*. Boston, MA: Blackwell, 1985:181.
46. Kim SJ, Port AD, Swan R, Campbell JP, Chan RVP, Chiang MF. Retinopathy of prematurity: a review of risk factors and their clinical significance. *Surv Ophthalmol* 2018;63(5):618.
47. Brown DR, Biglan AW, Stretavsky MAM. Screening criteria for the detection of retinopathy of prematurity in patients in a neonatal intensive care unit. *J Pediatr Ophthalmol Strabismus* 1987;24:212.
48. Fierson WM; American Academy of Pediatrics Section on Ophthalmology; American Academy of Ophthalmology; American Association for Pediatric Ophthalmology and Strabismus; American Association of Certified Orthoptists. Screening examination of premature infants for retinopathy of prematurity. *Pediatrics* 2018;142(6):e20183061.
49. Weaver DT. Telemedicine for retinopathy of prematurity. *Curr Opin Ophthalmol* 2013;24:425.
50. Cryotherapy for Retinopathy of Prematurity Cooperative Group. Multicenter trial of cryotherapy for retinopathy of prematurity: preliminary results. *Arch Ophthalmol* 1988;106:471.
51. Hunter DG, Repka MX. Diode laser photocoagulation for threshold retinopathy of prematurity. A randomized study. *Ophthalmology* 1993;100:238.
52. Cryotherapy for Retinopathy of Prematurity Cooperative Group. Multicenter trial of cryotherapy for retinopathy of prematurity. One-year outcome—structure and function. *Arch Ophthalmol* 1990;108:1408.

53. Cryotherapy for Retinopathy of Prematurity Cooperative Group. Multicenter trial of cryotherapy for retinopathy of prematurity: Snellen acuity and structural outcome at 5½ years after randomization. *Arch Ophthalmol* 1996;114:417.

54. Early Treatment for Retinopathy of Prematurity Cooperative Group; Good WV, Hardy RJ, Dobson V, et al. Final visual acuity results in the early treatment for retinopathy of prematurity study. *Arch Ophthalmol* 2010;128:663.

55. Quinn GR, Dobson V, Hardy RJ, et al.; for the CRYO-Retinopathy of Prematurity Cooperative Group. Visual fields measured with double-arc perimetry in eyes with threshold retinopathy of prematurity from the cryotherapy for retinopathy of prematurity trial. *Ophthalmology* 1996; 103:1432.

56. Mintz-Hittner HA, Kennedy KA, Chuang AZ; BEAT-ROP Cooperative Group. Efficacy of intravitreal bevacizumab for stage 3+ retinopathy of prematurity. *N Engl J Med* 2011;17:603.

57. Maguire AM, Trese MT. Visual results of lens-sparing vitreoretinal surgery in infants. *J Pediatr Ophthalmol Strabismus* 1993;30:28.

59 Oncology

Lauren H. Boal and Howard J. Weinstein

INTRODUCTION

Although neoplasia in infancy is quite rare, it presents important and unique biologic, diagnostic, and therapeutic problems. Many tumors in early life are composed of persistent embryonal or fetal tissues, suggesting a failure of proper maturation or cytodifferentiation during intrauterine or early postnatal life. This failure of proper maturation of fetal tissue at times may be difficult to distinguish from neoplasia. Spontaneous regression and cytodifferentiation also occur most frequently in tumors of early life. Additionally, a large number of neoplasms of early life are associated with growth disturbances and congenital anomalies. The unique physiology of the developing neonate provides the clinician with special problems in terms of therapeutic interventions and their long-term sequelae, including secondary malignancies.

EPIDEMIOLOGY

From the data in the Third National Cancer Survey (1969–1971), Bader and Miller (1) reported that, in the United States, the annual incidence of malignant neoplasms in infants younger than 1 year of age was 183.4 per 1 million live births and within the first 28 days of life was 36.5 per 1 million live births. They further estimated that approximately 653 infants per year in the United States are diagnosed with cancer and that about 130 (20%) of these patients are neonates. In a later study from Denmark, the incidence of neonatal cancer was calculated to be in a similar range, with values of 1.88 to 2.98 cases per 100,000 births (2). In contrast, the annual incidence of cancer in the United States for persons under the age of 20 years is approximately 15 per 100,000. Approximately one-half of the neonatal malignancies are noted on the first day of life, and there does not appear to be any gender bias.

Further, the distribution of the types of malignancies found in infants younger than 1 year of age differs from that found in later childhood. For example, neuroblastoma is the most common malignancy in infants under 1 year of age and accounts for about 50% of malignancies in the neonatal period; it is followed by leukemia, renal tumors, sarcomas, central nervous system (CNS) tumors, and hepatic malignancy (3). However, when one considers the total spectrum of neoplastic disorders of infancy, teratomas are usually reported as the most frequently encountered neoplasm, followed by hemangiomas, lymphangiomas, and small nevi lesions. In children younger than 15 years of age, leukemia is the most common malignancy (about 30%), followed by CNS tumors, lymphoma, neuroblastoma, sarcoma, and renal tumors. Thus, the incidence and types of neoplastic disorders of infancy contrast greatly compared to later childhood and define the neonatal period as epidemiologically distinct.

ORIGINS AND CAUSES OF NEONATAL CANCER

Developmental Growth Disturbances, Genetic Aberrations, and Cancer Pathogenesis

Naturally occurring DNA sequences homologous to transforming viral oncogenes exist in normal, untransformed cells of all metazoa. Such DNA sequences, termed cellular oncogenes, control growth, development, and differentiation of normal cells in precise temporal and tissue-specific patterns. Because of their expression and critical role during normal development, inherited or acquired mutations affecting cellular oncogene expression and/or function can lead to a variety of developmental abnormalities and congenital defects, such as hemihypertrophy syndromes and hamartomas. Additionally, the persistent expression beyond birth of certain growth-related oncogenes may play a role in such proliferative states as the transient myeloproliferative disorder (TMD) associated with Down syndrome and stage MS neuroblastoma found in infants, both of which are characterized by subsequent, spontaneous regression.

Inherited syndromes usually occur as a result of chromosomal aneuploidy, deletions, translocations, increased fragility, or altered epigenetic imprinting. An example of aneuploidy is Down syndrome (trisomy 21), in which the frequency of acute leukemia is approximately 15 times the normal. Additionally, an increased incidence of solid tumors has been reported for persons with trisomies 8, 9, 13, and 18 (4). Deletion of part of the long arm of chromosome 13 is associated with psychomotor retardation, microcephaly, cardiac and skeletal defects, and the early development of retinoblastoma. The deletion of the short arm of chromosome 11 results in mental retardation, microcephaly, aniridia, ear and genital anomalies, and an increased incidence of Wilms tumor (WAGR syndrome). These syndromes provided support for the assignment of a retinoblastoma-associated locus to chromosome 13q14 and a Wilms tumor–associated locus to 11p13 followed by identification of the retinoblastoma (RB) and the Wilms tumor genes (WT1). These mutant genes are usually heterozygous in germ-line DNA and homozygous in tumors, thus resulting in the loss of heterozygosity characteristic of tumor suppressor genes. WAGR syndrome results from loss of several genes from the 11p13 region. Deletion of one copy of PAX 6 is responsible for aniridia, and loss of one WT1 allele results in genitourinary anomalies. Homozygosity at the Wilms tumor locus on chromosome 11 has also been found in embryonal rhabdomyosarcomas (RMS) and hepatoblastomas, suggesting a common pathogenesis for these embryonal tumors. The specific loss of constitutional heterozygosity and its relationship to oncogenesis has been confirmed in studies of transgenic mice that lack a functional tumor suppressor gene, p53. The inherited human counterpart, termed Li-Fraumeni syndrome in humans, is characterized by a higher incidence of embryopathy and an increased incidence of malignancies including bone and soft tissue sarcomas, breast cancer, adrenocortical and brain tumors, leukemias, and choroid plexus carcinomas (CPC).

A number of inherited syndromes, including Bloom syndrome, Fanconi anemia, ataxia–telangiectasia, xeroderma pigmentosum, and Werner syndrome, are characterized by developmental abnormalities and increased incidence of various types of cancer (5). Many of these syndromes are known to be caused by defects in genes encoding key proteins involved in DNA recombination and repair, such as in Fanconi anemia or Bloom syndrome or excision repair enzymes associated with xeroderma pigmentosum. It is of note that when these defective genes are inherited through the germ line, patients show both developmental abnormalities and an increased incidence of cancer, thus linking genes leading to developmental defects to cancer predisposition.

Malformations and malformation syndromes without obvious cytogenetic abnormalities include hemihypertrophy and Beckwith-Wiedemann syndrome (BWS), which consists of mental retardation, gigantism, macroglossia, omphalocele, and organomegaly as well as being associated with the development of Wilms tumor, hepatoblastoma, and adrenocortical carcinoma. BWS, which occurs in approximately 1 in 13,000 births, is usually sporadic, although an autosomal dominant inheritance pattern with incomplete penetrance has also been proposed. Patients with BWS have an approximately 7.5% to 10% risk of developing a tumor.

Hamartomas are pathologically benign proliferations of cells in their normal anatomic location. Hamartomas in which malignant neoplasms arise include congenital melanotic nevi, which can progress to melanoma, and familial polyposis, which may evolve into colonic carcinoma. Examples of malignancies developing from persistent fetal rests include craniopharyngioma, which arises from tissue derived embryologically from the Rathke pouch, and neuroblastoma arising from persistent adrenal neuroblasts.

These predisposing conditions share at least one common element: an inherited or developmental disturbance of cellular growth and/or cell survival, which may be linked to the molecular pathways regulating these genetically determined cellular responses. The identification of these different classes of genes helps to define the molecular links between conditions of abnormal development (i.e., teratogenesis) and neoplastic transformation.

Prenatal Exposure to Maternal Genotoxins

There are relatively few reports and/or studies of outcome in infants born to mothers undergoing chemotherapy and/or radiation therapy for cancer. The risk of developmental problems increases with decreased gestational age at the time of maternal exposure. Termination of a pregnancy is commonly recommended when significant numbers and doses of anticancer drugs are used during the first trimester because of an increased risk of major birth defects and spontaneous abortions. Outcomes for infants whose mothers are treated during the second and third trimesters are significantly better, although reports have shown some risk of low birth weight, intrauterine growth restriction, and stillbirths (6,7).

Some prenatal drug exposures may lead to increased risk of cancer in offspring. For example, prenatal exposure to diethylstilbestrol has been closely linked to the development of clear cell adenocarcinoma of the vagina, Dilantin exposure with neuroblastoma, nitrosourea compounds with CNS tumors, and topoisomerase II inhibitors (epipodophyllotoxins, flavonoids, catechins, caffeine) with leukemia associated with mixed lineage leukemia (MLL) gene rearrangements. Significant use of alcohol and tobacco/marijuana and exposure to pesticides have been reported to be associated with an increased risk of congenital leukemia, although this association remains controversial (8). Radiation therapy or significant exposures to radiation through diagnostic testing such as computed tomography (CT) scanning are usually avoided whenever possible in pregnant mothers because of concerns of potential morbidity and cancer risk to the developing fetus.

Exposure to Maternal Malignancy

In addition to the susceptibility of the fetus to adverse effects of chemotherapy during pregnancy, there is also the very rare possibility that the maternal cancer will metastasize to the placenta and fetus. The types of tumors transmitted from the mother to the placenta or fetus are quite varied, with melanoma most commonly cited and anecdotal cases of lymphoma and leukemia. The evaluation of infants born to mothers with cancer has not been clearly established, in part because of the rarity of such events. However, close follow-up is recommended during the first year of life, including physical exams, blood studies such as complete blood count (CBC) and liver function tests, and scans only when clinically indicated. The frequency of transfer of a maternal cancer to an infant appears to be higher when the infant suffers from immunodeficiency. Careful examination of the placenta is an important component of this evaluation.

SPECIFIC TUMORS AFFECTING NEONATES

Tumors of Neuroepithelial Origin

Neuroectodermal cells of the neural tube differentiate to neuroblasts, which can then develop into several key cell lineages and subtypes, including nervous system tissue and melanocytes; free spongioblasts, which become either astrocytes or oligodendroglia cells; and ependymal spongioblasts, which become ependymal cells. Neoplasia may arise in any of these primitive neuroectodermal cellular compartments, giving rise to a group of morphologically similar tumors involving central and peripheral sites of the nervous system. Neonatal tumors originating from neuroectodermal cells include neuroblastoma, retinoblastoma, peripheral nerve tumors (i.e., neuroepithelioma), medulloblastoma, choroid plexus papilloma (CPP), ependymoblastoma, and melanotic neuroectodermal tumors. These tumors show varying degrees of cellular differentiation, have similar histologic features (e.g., small, primitive cells with rosettes or pseudorosettes), and tend to spread along cerebrospinal fluid pathways. The most common and clinically important are discussed in more detail.

Neuroblastoma

Neuroblastoma is the most common malignant tumor in neonates. It originates from neural crest cells that normally give rise to the adrenal medulla and sympathetic ganglia. Observation of patients with close family members with neuroblastoma suggested that some cases are hereditary and led to the identification of germline mutations, particularly in ALK and PHOX2B, in familial neuroblastoma (9). In such cases, the tumors are usually diagnosed at an earlier age and often characterized by having multifocal primary tumors (10). In a review of fetal and neonatal neuroblastoma, 50% of patients were diagnosed through prenatal ultrasound typically with the finding of an adrenal mass that can be a combination of solid and cystic tissue (11).

Although at least half of infants with neuroblastoma present with an abdominal mass from tumors arising in the adrenal medulla or retroperitoneal sympathetic ganglia, neuroblastoma may arise anywhere along the sympathetic nervous system and/or present with disseminated disease. In adrenal neuroblastoma, an abdominal ultrasound or CT scan demonstrates displacement of the kidney without distortion of the calyceal system. The neoplasm also may originate in the posterior mediastinum, neck, or pelvis. Cervical sympathetic ganglion involvement may result in Horner syndrome; mediastinal tumors may cause respiratory distress; paravertebral tumors tend to grow through the intervertebral foramina and cause symptoms of spinal cord compression; and presacral neuroblastomas may mimic presacral teratomas. Two unusual presentations of neuroblastoma are intractable diarrhea secondary to release of vasoactive intestinal peptide, and the paraneoplastic syndrome of opsoclonus, myoclonus, and truncal ataxia. The diarrhea secondary to vasoactive intestinal peptide abates after removal of the neuroblastoma while, in contrast, opsoclonus–myoclonus often persists despite treatment.

Metastatic lesions are common presenting findings of neuroblastoma in the neonatal period. The primary tumor often cannot be found in infants younger than 6 months of age. These infants present with bluish, subcutaneous nodules and extensive hepatomegaly. The liver may be studded with tumor nodules and be so large that it causes respiratory distress secondary to abdominal distention. Clumps of tumor cells often are found in the bone marrow aspirates. Metastases to bones, skull, and orbit, which present as periorbital ecchymoses, are, however, rare in the neonate. The unique metastatic pattern to liver, bone marrow, and skin in infants is classified as stage MS neuroblastoma according to the recently established International Neuroblastoma Risk Group Staging System (INRGSS) (12).

The differential diagnosis for neuroblastoma is limited. The subcutaneous nodules appear similar to those found in congenital leukemia cutis and several congenital infections. The leukoerythroblastosis secondary to bone marrow metastases from neuroblastoma also is observed with congenital infection, severe hemolytic disease, and leukemia. More than 90% of children with neuroblastoma will have elevated urinary excretion of catecholamine metabolites, vanillylmandelic acid or homovanillic acid, or both. The diagnosis of neuroblastoma is typically made by biopsy of the primary tumor or metastatic lesions. The most histologically primitive lesion is neuroblastoma without differentiation and is composed of small, round cells with scant cytoplasm. The ganglioneuroma, its benign counterpart, is composed of large, mature ganglion cells. Ganglioneuroblastoma has components of both. In the absence of a tissue specimen, the findings of elevated urinary catecholamines and tumor pseudorosettes in a bone marrow specimen can be sufficient to make a definitive diagnosis.

The prognosis for children with neuroblastoma is correlated to the age of the child at diagnosis, histology, tumor biology (chromosomal changes), and the extent of disease. In neonatal neuroblastoma, patients diagnosed on prenatal ultrasound have a higher survival rate than do those diagnosed in the neonatal period (11). Infants with stage MS frequently have spontaneous regression of disease and may undergo maturation into mature ganglioneuroma without need for surgical or chemotherapeutic interventions. The incidence of spontaneous regression of neuroblastoma may be more common than is clinically evident. Primitive sympathetic neuroblasts, which are derived from neural crest ectoderm, migrate in early embryonic life into the adrenal primordium, in which they arrange themselves in nodules before differentiation into adrenomedullary tissue. These nodules are present in all fetal adrenal glands at 14 to 18 weeks of gestation. Beckwith and Perrin (13) detected the presence of microscopic clusters of neuroblastoma cells (i.e., neuroblastoma in situ) in the adrenal glands in a number of autopsies from infants younger than age 3 months who had no clinical evidence of tumor. They estimated that neuroblastoma in situ occurs in 1 of 250 stillborn infants and infants younger than 3 months of age. However, clinically detectable neuroblastoma is noted in only 1 of 10,000 live births. Also pertinent to these observations are the results from neonatal catecholamine screening programs, which resulted in an increased incidence of early-stage neuroblastoma that, most likely, would not have presented as clinically detectable disease (14,15).

The treatment for neuroblastoma depends on the stage of the disease and biologic factors such as histology, MYCN amplification, and DNA ploidy. An infant with stage MS disease with favorable biologic features is usually observed for a period of weeks to months before treatment is initiated because of the reasonable likelihood of spontaneous regression. However, respiratory difficulties, blood vessel (usually vena cava) obstruction, and gastrointestinal compression secondary to rapid tumor expansion often require treatment. Chemotherapy is usually the first line of treatment (10,16). About 8% to 10% of patients with stage MS disease have MYCN amplification and are then recommended to receive treatment according to high-risk regimens.

Complete surgical removal of neuroblastoma is usually accomplished in infants with stage L1 or L2 disease, especially for patients in the perinatal group who mostly have localized adrenal tumors with favorable biology. Postoperative treatment is not generally indicated for these patients, and their long-term survival is excellent (12). Similarly, many infants with remaining gross residual tumor after surgery may not require further therapy (17). Chemotherapy is used for infants with localized or stage M disease and can be combined with immune/cytokine treatment, radiation, and autologous transplantation based on biologic risk factors combined with age and extent of disease (18). Active chemotherapeutic agents against neuroblastoma include alkylating compounds (e.g., cisplatin, temozolomide, cyclophosphamide, dacarbazine), vincristine, and doxorubicin. Outcomes for infants with intermediate-risk neuroblastoma have a greater than 90% overall survival, while those with MYCN amplification have an approximately 50% overall survival, suggesting that the biology plays a more significant role in prognosis than does age alone (19).

Retinoblastoma

Retinoblastoma is a congenital malignant tumor arising from the nuclear layer of the retina and is the most common ocular tumor of childhood. The median age at presentation is 18 months and 14 months for bilateral cases, but a small percentage of infants are diagnosed during the first few months of life. Prenatal diagnosis by sonography has been observed. Approximately 10% of children with retinoblastoma have a family history of the disease while about 20% with bilateral or multifocal unilateral tumors have a positive family history (20). These two groups can transmit the disease to their offspring in an autosomal dominant fashion through mutations in the retinoblastoma (RB) gene located on chromosome 13q14. Retinoblastoma has also been associated with chromosome 13 deletion mosaicism. If an asymptomatic child is at an elevated risk of retinoblastoma due to family history of retinoblastoma, an experienced ophthalmologist should perform regular dilated funduscopic exams up to 7 years of age (21).

The most common initial signs of retinoblastoma include an abnormal white pupil (i.e., leukocoria), known as a cat's-eye reflex and a squint or strabismus. Other potential diagnoses that can resemble retinoblastoma include granulomatosis uveitis, congenital defects, and severe retrolental fibroplasia. Once the diagnosis of retinoblastoma is suspected, both eyes should be examined with the infant under general anesthesia (22). A bone marrow aspiration and spinal tap for malignant cells are performed for staging when metastatic disease is suspected secondary to optic nerve extension or extensive choroidal invasion. A staging system for retinoblastoma is based on the size, location, number of tumors in each eye, and distant hematogenous metastases. Vitreous seeding, tumors extending anteriorly to the ora serrata, tumors invading over one-half of the retina, residual orbital disease, and optic nerve or distant metastases are all adverse prognostic features.

Retinoblastoma is curable in most patients when diagnosed early; vision often need not be sacrificed even when bilateral disease is present, and targeted local therapies are becoming increasingly common to avoid the morbidity of enucleation and/or irradiation (23–25). Children with very advanced and metastatic disease require aggressive chemotherapy regimens.

Brain Tumors and Other Neuroectodermal Tumors

Intracranial tumors presenting in the first year of life are uncommon. Brain tumors in children in this age group tend to be very large and supratentorial, in contrast to those of older children, which are usually infratentorial. In infants, the most common presenting symptom is macrocranium, with a bulging fontanelle secondary to either hydrocephalus or tumor volume. Seizures, vomiting, failure to thrive, abnormal eye movement, irritability, and hemorrhage also are frequent.

Treatment of infants with brain tumors historically included surgical removal or biopsy followed by radiotherapy. Operative mortality was high, and few infants survived for longer than 1 year. In these few, brain radiotherapy resulted in severe intellectual and psychomotor retardation (26). In attempts to avoid the adverse effects of radiotherapy on the developing brain, subsequent therapeutic approaches have typically used surgery followed by preradiation chemotherapy or intensive chemotherapy without radiation (27).

THE NEWBORN INFANT

Teratomas have been reported to represent the single most frequent intracranial tumors in neonates (28). The histologic diagnoses of the neuroectodermal tumors are similar to those of tumors in later childhood, with gliomas accounting for most. Aggressive embryonal tumors are also found including medulloblastoma, supratentorial primitive neuroectodermal tumor (PNET), and atypical teratoid/rhabdoid tumor (ATRT).

Choroid plexus tumors represent 10% to 20% of brain tumors in the neonatal period, most commonly seen in the lateral ventricle. Choroid plexus papilloma (CPP) is a benign tumor with high survival rates with gross total resection alone. Choroid plexus carcinoma (CPC) is less commonly seen in the neonatal period, and has a poorer prognosis typically including invasion of adjacent brain parenchyma and subsequent brain edema (29). More than half of CPC have TP53 mutations, and germ-line TP53 mutations have also been seen in patients with CPC. Therapy includes surgical resection and chemotherapy, with radiation remaining controversial due to patient age (30).

Desmoplastic infantile gangliogliomas are rare, massive, cystic tumors that usually occur supratentorially in the neonatal period (31). They present most commonly with signs of increased intracranial pressure, including seizures. Therapy has included surgery and chemotherapy. For patients who have a complete surgical resection, additional therapy may not be required. Prognosis may be better than that observed with other tumors, such as high-grade astrocytoma. In contrast, pineoblastomas are malignant tumors with an extremely poor outcome, even when treated with surgery, chemotherapy, and radiation therapy. Part of the reason for the poor outcome in these infants may be the propensity of pineoblastoma to involve the leptomeninges and extraneural spread.

ATRTs of the CNS, although rare, are usually large and aggressive and have historically had very poor outcomes with the use of conventional therapies used in children with brain tumors. More aggressive, multidisciplinary approaches have started to show some improvement in patients with this type of brain tumor, although median survival is still estimated to be less than 2 years (32). These tumors all share the inactivation of the *SNF5/INI1* gene, which encodes for a key developmental chromatin remodeling factor (33).

Congenital/Neonatal Leukemia

Leukemia in the newborn is extremely rare with approximately five cases reported per million live births (34). The kinetics of leukemic cell growth and the estimated leukemic cell burden at the time of diagnosis make it reasonable to assume that clinically detectable leukemia during the first 4 weeks of life originated *in utero* (35,36). Backtracking this process through molecular studies indicates a prenatal initiation of the common subtypes of acute lymphoblastic leukemia (ALL with KMT2A and ETV6-RUNx1 fusions) and some acute myeloid leukemias, in children diagnosed as neonates, during infancy, or even later in life.

An increasing number of germ-line mutations have been identified in children that predispose to leukemia. However, these mutations are seen in a small percentage of children with acute leukemia. Interestingly, the concordance of leukemia in identical twins is not due to a genetic predisposition but to placental transfer (twin–twin transmission) of a preleukemia clone (35,36). If leukemia develops in one of a set of identical twins before 6 years of age, the risk of disease in the other twin is nearly 100%. Leukemia usually develops in the other twin within weeks to months of the first case (35,36). For fraternal twins and siblings, the risk of development of leukemia is two to four times higher than in the general population. Down syndrome is associated with an estimated 20-fold increased risk of leukemia. Other syndromes carrying an increased risk for leukemia include neurofibromatosis 1, Bloom syndrome, Fanconi anemia, congenital neutropenia, and ataxia–telangiectasia.

More than 95% of the childhood leukemias, including congenital leukemia, are classified as acute, because they are characterized by a predominance of immature lymphoid or myeloid precursors that replace the normal bone marrow. The proportion of cases of ALL to acute myelogenous leukemia (AML) is approximately four to one in children, but AML is more common in neonates (34). Lymphoblasts from most children with congenital/neonatal ALL are of B lineage, lack CD10, often express both lymphoid and myeloid cell surface antigens, and have KMT2A rearrangements. These infants have a higher incidence of CNS leukemia at diagnosis, a higher leukocyte count, increased frequency of hepatosplenomegaly, and a poor prognosis (37). The most common subtype of AML in neonates and children less than 2 years of age is acute monoblastic/monocytic leukemia (M5), which accounts for only 20% of AML in older children. This subtype is commonly associated with t(9;11) or a KMT2A (MLL) rearrangement (38).

Cutaneous manifestations are the most frequent clinical findings noted in congenital or neonatal AML. In addition to petechiae and purpura, leukemic skin nodules (i.e., leukemia cutis) have been observed in approximately 50% of cases. These skin nodules may vary in size from a few millimeters to a few centimeters, are bluish to slate gray in color, may appear in all sites, and are palpated as firm tumors of the deep skin (Fig. 59.1). Neonatal leukemia cutis may undergo a spontaneous, temporary regression, but tends to recur in a more generalized form within a few weeks to months. Hepatosplenomegaly is common, but lymphadenopathy is not. Respiratory distress, secondary to leukostasis within the pulmonary vasculature, may complicate the clinical course. Other

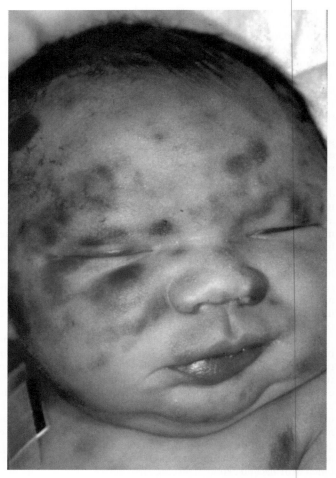

FIGURE 59.1 Congenital acute monocytic leukemia with skin nodules.

nonspecific symptoms of neonatal leukemia include lethargy, pallor, poor feeding, and umbilical, gastrointestinal, or genitourinary bleeding. The diagnosis of leukemia is confirmed by microscopic examination of a bone marrow aspirate obtained from the posterior iliac crest with concomitant immunophenotyping and cytogenetic and molecular analyses.

Several illnesses in the newborn may present with clinical and laboratory features that are suggestive of congenital leukemia. The newborn bone marrow response to infection, hypoxemia, or severe hemolysis is often associated with a leukemoid reaction. One may see an increase in nucleated red blood cells and immature myeloid cells in the peripheral blood. In addition, several congenital viral infections are associated with a rash that may mimic leukemia cutis. A bone marrow aspirate or skin biopsy will clarify the diagnosis.

The transient myeloproliferative syndrome or transient abnormal myelopoiesis (TAM) in infants with Down syndrome or mosaic Down syndrome shares many clinical features and hematologic findings with congenital AML (39). This syndrome usually presents during the first few days to weeks of life. Peripheral leukocyte counts can range from normal to greater than 50,000, and the bone marrow may contain greater than 30% blasts. Hepatosplenomegaly and thrombocytopenia are also common findings. The blood counts and clinical manifestations in approximately 80% of these neonates return to normal within in 1 to 4 months after diagnosis, with only supportive therapy. However, up to 10% of these children may die of cardiac, pulmonary, or liver disease or sepsis before resolution of their transient myeloproliferative syndrome. Treatment with chemotherapy is only recommended for a small subgroup of these infants. Chemotherapy should be withheld in all neonates with suspected AML until cytogenetic results are available because TAM has been observed in phenotypically normal infants who have trisomy 21 mosaicism. These neonates are also likely to have spontaneous regression. The leukemic blasts in this syndrome are of the megakaryocytic lineage and have a GATA1 mutation (38,39). GATA1 is a key transcription factor that regulates megakaryopoiesis and erythropoiesis. Interestingly, approximately 30% of neonates who have spontaneous resolution of TAM will develop AML within the next 3 years (40). Treatment with chemotherapy in that setting is very effective with a high likelihood of achieving long-term survival. There have also been reports of spontaneous remissions of congenital AML in neonates with a translocation t(8;16)(p11;p13) suggesting that some cases can be initially conservatively managed with observation and/or supportive care (41).

It is recommended that all other children with congenital/neonatal AML be treated with chemotherapy. The prognosis for neonates with AML has improved over the past few decades, but intensive chemotherapy in this age group is often associated with life-threatening complications. If possible, these neonates should be treated on a clinical research trial (42).

Neoplasms of the Kidney
Mesoblastic Nephroma

Most abdominal masses presenting in infancy are renal in origin, and most can be accounted for by cystic disease of the kidney and congenital malformations of the urinary tract leading to hydronephrosis. Although neoplasms of the kidney are rare in infancy, they do occur and have important prognostic implications, making it mandatory that they be included in the evaluation of abdominal masses.

The most common renal tumor found in infants is mesoblastic nephroma, which accounts for nearly 80% of renal tumors in the neonatal period (43). It also has been called fetal renal hamartoma, mesenchymal hamartoma of infancy, and leiomyomatous hamartoma. Mesoblastic nephroma commonly presents as an asymptomatic, enlarging abdominal mass during the first few months of life

but may be associated with severe hypertension. It is not associated with congenital anomalies and has no race predilection. Of note is the more frequent occurrence of polyhydramnios and premature labor in women whose infants have mesoblastic nephroma. The differential diagnosis includes renal cystic disease, congenital malformations of the urinary tract resulting in hydronephrosis, and Wilms tumor. The chromosomal translocation resulting in a fusion protein, ETV6-NTRK3, has been reported in both mesoblastic nephroma and infantile fibrosarcoma (44).

Most patients with mesoblastic nephroma are cured by surgical excision without adjuvant chemotherapy or radiotherapy (45). The addition of chemotherapy has resulted in increased morbidity and, in some instances, fatal complications. In rare cases, such as older infants presenting with metastatic disease or when there is tumor rupture and spillage, chemotherapeutic intervention with regimens containing actinomycin D, vincristine, cyclophosphamide, and sometimes doxorubicin have been effectively used. Similar regimens have been used for recurrences.

Persistent Renal Blastema, Nephroblastomatosis, and Wilms Tumor

The adult or metanephric kidney arises from a complex, inductive interaction between the evaginating uteric bud and its bifurcations with the metanephric, mesodermally derived blastema. By 36 weeks of gestation, normal nephrogenesis is usually complete, with no residual metanephric blastema. When these metanephric blastemal elements persist, they usually are characterized by microscopic clusters of primitive blastema and occasionally some tubular differentiation (i.e., persistent metanephric blastema). If these fetal rests proliferate, they may develop along several different histologic pathways, each of which has particular relevance to the evolution of Wilms tumor. Nephroblastomatosis represents the persistence and growth of metanephric blastema beyond the cessation of nephrogenesis. Nephroblastomatosis may be histologically multifocal or diffuse.

Multifocal nephroblastomatosis refers to the widespread proliferation of blastemal cells, most prominently in the subcapsular cortex and along the penetrating columns of Bertin. Nephromegaly is not always evident. Unlike mesoblastic nephroma, multifocal nephroblastomatosis is associated with congenital malformation syndromes and chromosomal abnormalities. Within the category of multifocal nephroblastomatosis, there are several characteristic lesions. When persistent blastemas proliferate in small 100- to 300-mm foci separated by normal renal parenchyma, they are referred to as nodular renal blastema. These lesions may regress or evolve into what has been called sclerosing metanephric hamartoma and/or into Wilms tumorlets, which are 0.3 to 3.5 cm in diameter, noninfiltrating, often multiple, neoplastic tumors separated by normal renal parenchyma. They usually consist of blastema with a monomorphous epithelial pattern of differentiation. Although they resemble true Wilms tumor, they are distinguishable by their smaller size and their noninfiltrating behavior.

Although diffuse nephroblastomatosis is quite rare, it is more commonly observed in infants and young children. The blastemal proliferation may be pan-nephric or superficial, with the latter lesion encasing a normal cortex and medulla. Diffuse nephroblastomatosis presents as bilateral, palpable nephromegaly in association with congenital malformations. Radiographic examination reveals distortion and elongation of the calyceal system without obstruction. On gross inspection, there is an exaggerated pattern of fetal lobulation of the enlarged kidneys.

That these various histologic patterns are related to one another and to the evolution of frank Wilms tumor has been strongly suggested by case studies and by epidemiologic and pathologic correlations. In about one-third of cases of Wilms tumor, there is suggestive pathologic evidence for the association of nodular renal blastema, nephroblastomatosis, and Wilms tumorlets; in bilateral Wilms tumor, this association is nearly always present. Several overgrowth syndromes have been associated with these abnormalities and the development of Wilms tumor (46).

Management of nephroblastomatosis involves renal tissue–preserving surgery and sometimes chemotherapy, depending on the extent of disease. Radiation therapy is not very effective. If only one kidney is involved, surgical resection is sufficient, but exploration and biopsy of the contralateral kidney are important. When both kidneys are extensively involved, nephroblastomatosis usually will respond to combination chemotherapy used in Wilms tumor (i.e., vincristine and actinomycin). The goal of such treatment is to cause regression of the nephroblastomatosis or push its development into an end-stage hamartoma. The duration of treatment is based on clinical response. Close follow-up with both radiographic and second-look operations is important in that patients may still progress to the development of true Wilms tumor despite therapy.

True Wilms tumor rarely is seen in the neonatal period (43). It generally presents as an asymptomatic abdominal mass that does not cross the midline, but, occasionally, the mass is large enough to cause dystocia at the time of delivery. It is rarely associated with gross hematuria, hypertension, or polycythemia secondary to increased erythropoietin levels. Congenital abnormalities occur in 12% to 15% of cases, and the most frequent include hemihypertrophy, BWS, aniridia, and genitourinary anomalies including WAGR syndrome (Wilms tumor, aniridia, genitourinary malformations, and mental retardation). Additionally, the Wilms tumor–aniridia syndrome is associated with a deletion of part of the short arm of chromosome 11. CT scan, as well as magnetic resonance imaging (MRI) and renal ultrasonography, can help define the extent of the tumor. Infants with hemihypertrophy and Beckwith-Wiedemann should have abdominal ultrasounds performed every 3 to 6 months up to 6 years of age for early detection of both Wilms tumor and hepatoblastoma.

Classic Wilms tumor consists of neoplastic blastemal elements with epithelial and stromal components. In the neonate, Wilms tumor is predominantly epithelial and localized, displaying little invasiveness or metastatic potential. The primary prognostic variables in the neonatal period include histology, extent of disease, and age. The management of a patient with Wilms tumor depends primarily on staging. In the neonate, most patients will be classified as stage I, in that the tumors usually are relatively small (i.e., <550 g), localized, noninvasive, and completely resectable. At the time of surgery, a frozen section diagnosis can be helpful in ascertaining whether or not nephroblastomatosis is also present. If nephroblastomatosis is present, wedge biopsy of the contralateral kidney may be also helpful. The management of bilateral Wilms tumor must often be individualized, with the intent of trying to spare as much normal renal parenchyma as possible (47,48). Careful follow-up in such cases is critical.

For patients with stage I disease, 18 weeks of combination chemotherapy with vincristine and actinomycin without the use of radiation therapy is recommended. Disease-free, long-term survival is greater than 90% (45). For advanced stages and for tumors with anaplastic histology, more aggressive therapy, including radiation and intensive chemotherapy, is recommended.

Renal Neoplasms Not Associated with Wilms Tumor

Malignant rhabdoid tumor of the kidney, which represents about 2% of primary renal malignancies during childhood and for which the mean age at diagnosis is 13 months, was first described as a rhabdomyosarcomatoid variant of Wilms tumor. Malignant rhabdoid tumors may also arise in the liver, chest wall, or paravertebral area. There is an association with posterior fossa brain tumors and a predilection for metastasizing to the brain (49). Prognosis depends on stage and ranges from about 15% for advanced-stage disease to 40% to 50% for early-stage disease.

Clear cell sarcoma of the kidney, also originally described as a Wilms tumor variant, is considered a separate entity. It represents about 2% to 5% of all childhood malignant tumors of the kidney and is rarely seen in the neonatal period or in infants. Age at presentation is similar to that in Wilms tumor. Clear cell renal sarcoma demonstrates a predilection to metastasize to bone and carries a poor prognosis when metastatic, but recent studies have demonstrated improved survival for advanced stage III and IV disease (50).

Tumors of Germ Cell Origin

Germ cell tumors are derived from the stem cells of the embryo that ultimately are determined to differentiate into spermatocytes or ova. Such cells are developmentally multipotent and, therefore, are capable of giving rise to tumors containing any fetal, embryonal, or adult tissue. Additionally, their spatial distribution and migration pattern during embryogenesis help explain the various anatomic sites in which such tumors may develop. For example, human primordial germ cells can be recognized first in the 4-week embryo as large cells embedded in a restricted area of the yolk sac. During the 5th week of gestation, the germ cells migrate from the yolk sac to the hindgut wall and along the mesentery to the gonadal ridge, in which they encounter the gonadal anlage. From there, they descend into the pelvis or scrotal sac. During their migration from the yolk sac to the definitive gonad, germ cells may be left behind or they may migrate too far along the dorsal wall of the embryo near the midline. Thus, aside from the gonads, germ cell–derived tumors quite commonly arise in locations at or near the midline, anywhere from the sacrum to the head. Depending on their viability, embryonic stage, and anatomic location, they may differentiate along a variety of different cell lineages.

The malignant germ cell tumors include germinoma, embryonal carcinoma, yolk sac tumor, and choriocarcinoma. These tumors are very rare in the neonate except for yolk sac tumors that may appear as a component of a sacrococcygeal teratoma. The rare case of choriocarcinoma detected in neonates represents metastasis from a maternal or placental gestational trophoblastic primary tumor. Patients usually present with pallor, hepatomegaly, and a history of gastrointestinal bleeding with hemoptysis or hematuria. There may be endocrinologic manifestations, with breast enlargement and pubic hair. Chest radiographs may reveal pulmonary metastases; human chorionic gonadotropin levels most often are elevated. Such gestational-related choriocarcinomas are particularly responsive to treatment with methotrexate.

Teratomas

Sacrococcygeal teratomas are the most common germ cell tumor of childhood with about 67% diagnosed by the age of 1 year. They arise from the embryonal compartment, and are the most recognized neoplasm of neonates. These tumors occur at a rate of 1 in 25,000 to 1 in 40,000 live births and display a significant gender predilection, with females being affected more than 75% of the time (51). These neoplasms contain cellular or tissue derivatives of more than one of the three primary embryonal germ layers and are foreign to the anatomic region in which they arise. The name teratoma is derived from the Greek teratos, which literally means monster, plus the ending "-oma," which is used to denote a neoplasm. This name derived from cases in which these tumors contained tissue elements so well organized they resembled a deformed fetus. About 15% to 20% of these tumors have a malignant yolk sac component. However, pure sacrococcygeal yolk sac tumors are not usually seen in neonates and peak at the age of 6 to 12 months.

In neonates and infants, teratomas primarily occur as extragonadal masses located along the midline axis; about 40% to 50% occur in the sacrococcygeal region, with head and neck, brain, mediastinum, retroperitoneum, abdomen, spinal cord, and other soft tissue locations accounting for 1% to 5% each (51). Gonadal teratomas occur more frequently after puberty, particularly in the ovary. About 80% to 90% of early childhood teratomas are benign; malignant teratomas usually are characterized histologically by areas containing embryonal carcinoma or endodermal sinus/yolk sac tumor. Such malignant lesions most often arise in the sacrococcygeal region.

Clinically, these tumors usually present as a mass protruding between the coccyx and the rectum (**Fig. 59.2**). They nearly always arise from the tip of the coccyx and vary greatly in the amount of their internal versus external tissue extensions. Some lesions can be diagnosed only by rectal examination; however, this examination should be done with extreme care in the neonate to avoid any traumatic damage. The differential diagnosis of a sacrococcygeal teratoma includes meningomyelocele, rectal abscess, pilonidal cyst, bladder neck obstruction, rectal prolapse, duplications of the rectum, imperforate anus, dermoid cyst, angioma, lymphangioma, lipoma, neurogenic tumors of the pelvis and perineum, giant cell tumor of the sacrum, and soft tissue sarcoma.

Benign teratomas usually will produce no functional problems other than obstruction, whereas the presence of bowel or bladder dysfunction suggests a malignant lesion. Evidence for venous or lymphatic obstruction or lower leg paralysis is found more commonly in malignant tumors. Approximately 15% of patients with sacrococcygeal teratomas have associated congenital anomalies, including imperforate anus, sacral bone defects, genitourinary abnormalities such as duplication of the uterus or vagina, and occasionally spina bifida and meningomyelocele. Radiographic evaluation of the spine can be informative in that meningomyeloceles are associated with characteristic vertebral abnormalities. Abdominal and pelvic ultrasonography along with CT or MRI scanning is useful in assessing the internal extension of the mass. Barium enema may help distinguish between a bowel duplication and displacement caused by a tumor mass. Chest radiographs or CT is used to access mediastinal or pulmonary involvement. Serum AFP and human chorionic gonadotropin levels may be elevated in those teratomas with mixed cellular elements.

The prognosis for a patient with a sacrococcygeal teratoma depends primarily on whether the lesion is benign or malignant (52). The management of a patient with a benign sacrococcygeal teratoma is primarily surgical and includes removal of the coccyx, the site in which the tumor arises. Leaving the coccyx is associated with a 10% to 40% incidence of recurrence within 3 years,

about 40% to 50% of which are malignant (53). For patients with malignant teratomas, chemotherapy regimens that include bleomycin, etoposide, and cisplatin have resulted in overall survivals of just over 92% (54). After surgical resection, neonates with mature or immature teratomas should be followed with intermittent serum AFP determinations.

Primary Hepatic Neoplasms

The differential diagnosis of hepatomegaly or a liver mass in infants is extensive and includes nonneoplastic lesions and a variety of benign and malignant tumors. Infantile hemangioma is the most common benign tumor of the liver in infancy. Hepatoblastoma is the most common malignant liver tumor in children. However, hepatomegaly associated with malignant disease in neonates and infants may be secondary to leukemia or disseminated neuroblastoma rather than a primary hepatic malignancy.

Hepatoblastoma occurs primarily but not exclusively in children younger than age 3 years, with a mean age of 18 months; it can also occur in neonates. There have been anecdotal reports of patients with hepatoblastoma associated with the maternal use of oral contraceptives or with the fetal alcohol syndrome (55,56). Low birth weight also has been associated with the development of hepatoblastoma (57). Familial cases of hepatoblastoma have been documented, suggesting an environmental or genetic contribution in some instances (58). Hepatoblastoma has been associated with a variety of congenital anomalies, most notably hemihypertrophy, renal abnormalities, macroglossia, Meckel diverticulum, tetralogy of Fallot, diaphragmatic hernia, talipes equinovarus, and digital clubbing. Wilms tumor and adrenal cortical neoplasms also have been found in patients with hepatoblastoma (58,59).

Hepatoblastoma presents in most cases with an asymptomatic right upper quadrant or epigastric mass. In approximately 25% of patients, there also will be associated poor feeding, weight loss, pallor, and pain. Less common are vomiting and jaundice. Diarrhea, fever, and precocious puberty are rare. Laboratory studies may show a mild anemia and thrombocytosis. Increased levels of liver enzyme transaminases and alkaline phosphatase are variable, but mild elevation of bilirubin may be present in up to 15% of cases. AFP is elevated manifold in nearly 70% of patients (60). Although not specific for hepatoblastoma, this protein marker, with a half-life of 4 to 6 days, is useful in the diagnostic workup, assessment of the response to therapy, and detection of tumor recurrence. It should be noted, however, that not all recurring metastatic lesions are positive for AFP, even though the primary tumor was positive. All values for AFP should be compared to age-matched values, because levels normally are elevated in the neonatal period and normalize to adult values for up to 9 months (61).

Abdominal radiographs show enlargement of the liver, with right lobe involvement being more common. Areas of calcification occur in up to 20% of cases. Chest radiographs or CT may reveal pulmonary metastases, present in about 10% of cases at diagnosis. Abdominal CT or MRI scanning can help assess tumor size and surgical resectability.

The prognosis for patients with hepatoblastoma appears to depend primarily on the lesion's surgical resectability, on histology, and whether it is metastatic (62). Complete surgical excision is possible in about 40% to 75% of patients, although perioperative mortality has been reported as high as 10% to 25%. Pretreatment extent of tumor (PRETEXT) staging has been widely adopted as a risk stratification system. Local and metastatic recurrences after surgical resection usually appear within 36 months; recurrences can occur as late as 8 years after surgery.

The histopathology of hepatoblastoma can be viewed as occurring in two major patterns. The first is the pure fetal epithelial type that is associated with an improved outcome. The second type, composed of both epithelial and mesenchymal elements, usually is referred to as a mixed hepatoblastoma and has been associated

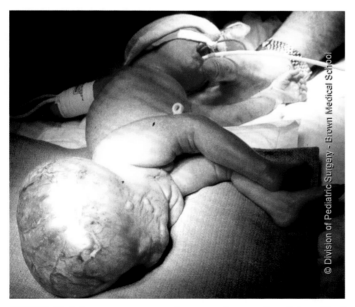

FIGURE 59.2 Large sacrococcygeal teratoma in a newborn infant. (Used by permission, Division of Pediatric Surgery, Alpert Medical School of Brown University.)

with a poorer prognosis. Additionally, some hepatoblastomas may have anaplastic or sarcomatous elements that portend a poor prognosis.

Although some reports have demonstrated that approximately 30% to 60% of patients can be cured with only complete surgical resection for localized disease, others have shown that adjuvant chemotherapy after tumor resection significantly reduces the risk of development of distant metastases. For those children with unresectable primary tumors, combination chemotherapy is usually successful in reducing tumor size to allow resection (63,64). Most chemotherapy regimens are cisplatin based with survival rates of greater than 90% for patients with stages I and II and about 75% for more advanced stages. For situations in which the tumor cannot be resected, even after cytoreductive therapy, liver transplantation has been used (65,66).

Soft Tissue Sarcomas

Soft tissue tumors represent a diverse group of neoplasms, all of which share a common cellular origin from mesenchymal elements. In the infant, soft tissue sarcomas are rare and include congenital infantile fibrosarcoma (CIF), rhabdomyosarcoma (RMS), non-RMS soft tissue sarcomas, and the malignant rhabdoid tumor (see section on "Neoplasms of the Kidney"). Ewing sarcoma is very rare in neonates and infants.

Although RMS accounts for about one-half of soft tissue sarcomas in children it is extraordinarily rare in the neonate (67). It may present at a variety of anatomical sites, including orbit, nasopharynx, sinuses, trunk, or extremity. As a genitourinary tract tumor presentation, the tumor usually arises from the bladder, prostate, vagina, or as a paratesticular mass. At the time of diagnosis, about 15% to 25% of patients have evident metastatic disease, usually to lung, lymph nodes, liver, bone marrow, and bone.

After appropriate assessment of the primary tumor and possible metastatic sites, surgery should be planned if it will not result in greatly impaired function or cosmesis (68). Adjuvant chemotherapy with regimens usually containing vincristine, actinomycin D, anthracyclines, and cyclophosphamide is always given and significantly increases disease-free and overall survival rates. Radiation therapy is given if there is residual microscopic or gross residual disease after surgery. However, radiation therapy carries both acute and long-term side effects in neonates and infants. Unlike neuroblastoma, the prognosis for children less than 1 year of age with RMS is not favorable (68).

CIF is a cellular, mitotically active neoplasm with a paradoxically limited metastatic potential in most children in contrast to fibrosarcomas in older children. CIF is a locally aggressive tumor that rarely metastasizes and commonly arises in the extremities, retroperitoneum, and head or neck. Complete surgical resection is curative in more than 90% of cases. Local recurrences occur in approximately 20% to 40% of cases. For tumors that are not amenable to surgical resection because of size, location, or both, combination chemotherapy may be effective in shrinking the tumor and facilitating a surgical resection. Infantile fibrosarcomas and mesoblastic nephromas are characterized by a translocation resulting in an ETV6-NTRK3 fusion protein (42). Recent studies have demonstrated high response rates in children with CIF who have been treated with larotrectinib, a pan TRK inhibitor (69).

Other fibroblastic proliferative disorders may also be seen in the infant and newborn. Digital fibromas most commonly occur as a soft tissue mass on the medial side of digits and usually exclude the thumbs and great toes. As with fibrosarcoma, surgical resection can be curative, although recurrence rates may be as high as 75% to 90%.

Congenital (i.e., infantile) fibromatosis may occur as solitary or multiple soft tissue lesions. The solitary lesions occur nearly anywhere on the body. An autosomal dominant presentation has been associated with mutations of PDGFRB and NOTCH3 (70). When present as multiple lesions, they can involve subcutaneous tissue, muscle, and bones; in some cases, there may be significant morbidity and mortality from visceral organ involvement. These disorders are pathologically benign in appearance. Curative treatment of solitary lesions is complete resection. Spontaneous regression can occur. Visceral involvement is associated with a poorer prognosis. Chemotherapy, including vincristine, actinomycin D, and cyclophosphamide along with other agents, has been reported to induce excellent responses in infants with unresectable fibromatosis and improves prognosis (71). Gain-of-function PDGFRB mutations in the majority of patients with multifocal infantile myofibromatosis are facilitating diagnosis and treatment with targeted therapies (72).

Vascular Neoplasms and Malformations

Hemangiomas are the most common tumors found in infancy and childhood (73). Most commonly, they appear during late fetal or early neonatal life and more frequently affect girls. Skin is the most frequent site of involvement, although they may arise in any organ and often occur in multiple locations. They are soft, compressible, bright red to blue lesions. They range in size from a few millimeters to quite large where they can involve large areas of the skin or internal organs. Several inherited syndromes associated with vascular tumors have been linked to specific gene defects; in addition, somatic mutations in key regulatory genes have been reported in different vascular abnormalities (73,74).

Their natural course is characterized by rapid growth for the first 4 to 6 months of life, followed by stabilization and then gradual involution over several years. They should be distinguished from vascular malformations such as arteriovenous fistulas, which represent anomalous vascular development and do not demonstrate endothelial cell proliferation. Vascular malformations commonly present at birth and increase in size along with the patient, without the usual phase of involution. Lymphangiomas also represent malformations and may be seen in conjunction with blood vessel malformations (75).

The clinical complications that arise from hemangiomas are usually secondary to their size, site of origin, and physiology. They may compromise vision by encroaching on the eye, cause respiratory distress by impinging on the trachea, lead to severe and even fatal congestive heart failure when they are very large, produce gastrointestinal or CNS hemorrhage, or cause a consumptive coagulopathy with thrombocytopenia. Kaposiform hemangioendotheliomas are vascular tumors that are responsible for most cases of Kasabach-Merritt syndrome. MRI is a quite useful imaging modality for vascular tumors.

The first principle of treatment should be to do no harm, because most hemangiomas will eventually spontaneously regress. Nevertheless, when they are the cause of significant morbidity, intervention may be necessary. Several treatment approaches can be effective depending on individual patient circumstances. Radiotherapy is usually avoided because of poor response but also resulting adverse side effects, such as cutaneous scarring, dermatitis, growth disturbances, and secondary malignancies. Surgery may be difficult for large lesions and may result in unsightly scarring. For large lesions of the liver, hepatic artery ligation and embolization occasionally have been successful in controlling high-output cardiac failure, but liver necrosis, renal failure, and other embolic complications may result. Laser therapy also has been used. Hemangiomas usually respond to corticosteroids. However, propranolol has been successfully used and is now the treatment of choice (76,77).

Malignant tumors arising from vascular endothelium, such as hemangioendothelioma, hemangiopericytoma, and angiosarcoma, are extremely rare but have been reported in infants (67).

Histiocytoses

The histiocytoses represent a heterogeneous group of disorders primarily involving bone marrow–derived antigen-presenting cells (78). These disorders are typically classified as (a) dendritic cell disorders, including Langerhans cell histiocytosis (LCH), juvenile xanthogranulomatous disease (JXG), and Erdheim-Chester disease (ECD); (b) macrophage-related disorders including hemophagocytic lymphohistiocytosis (HLH) and Rosai-Dorfman disease (RDD); and (c) malignant histiocytic disorders, including histiocytic sarcomas. While LCH, ECD, or RDD can occur together in the same patient, ECD and RDD are not usually observed in infants.

LCH includes disorders historically referred to as eosinophilic granuloma, Hand-Christian-Schüller disease, and Abt-Letterer-Siwe disease. The diagnosis is made by biopsy that shows characteristic pathologic changes that typically include a histologically mixed, reactive infiltrate of cells including eosinophils, neutrophils, lymphocytes, multinucleated giant cells, and histiocytes. The lesional histiocytes usually express CD1a, CD205 (langerin), and S100 antigens. Several studies have demonstrated that LCH is a clonal neoplastic disorder with 50% to 60% of cases associated with activating mutations of *BRAF* or members of the RAS/RAF/ERK pathway (79). Congenital cases observed with such mutations and a high level of concordance in identical twins suggest germline inheritance as well as sharing of placental circulation of the neoplastic cells that have acquired a somatic mutation (80).

Disseminated involvement of LCH is usually clinical fulminant and most commonly presents within the first year of life and occasionally in neonates. Infants often present with scaly, seborrheic, eczematoid, or maculopapular rashes involving the scalp, face, ear canals, abdomen, axilla, anus, and groin (**Fig. 59.3**). Hepatosplenomegaly is common, and there may be signs of hepatic dysfunction with hypoproteinemia and coagulopathy. Draining ears, lymphadenopathy, cough, and tachypnea are common. These infants are commonly irritable and fail to thrive, secondary either to chronic disease and liver dysfunction or to malabsorption as a result of gastrointestinal infiltration. Lytic bone lesions often are often present.

The prognosis for systemic disease involving liver, spleen, and bone marrow along with dysfunction is poor despite combination chemotherapy, especially for those patients who show a poor response to initial therapy. Treatment is usually based on international Histiocyte Society study regimens that use vinblastine and corticosteroids (81,82). Clofarabine has recently been successfully used to treat refractory disease (83). Drugs that selectively target the RAS/RAF/ERK pathway for patients whose LCH has relevant mutations are associated with high response rates (84). Long-term

sequelae are common, with sclerosing cholangitis, pulmonary fibrosis, and neurodegenerative disease of the CNS the most severe; thus, infants treated for LCH should have close and long-term follow-up (85,86). Importantly, about 50% of infants with only skin involvement may show spontaneous remissions over several weeks to months; such infants should be closely followed without treatment (87–89). Congenital self-healing histiocytosis is also referred to as self-healing reticulohistiocytosis or Hashimoto-Pritzker disease. The disease is really a self-resolving form of LCH that usually is evident at birth or during the neonatal period as cutaneous, reddish-brown papules that can sometimes ulcerate. Spontaneous regression usually occurs over the first 3 months of life, and therapeutic interventions are not necessary. Because the disease in some patients will progress to a disseminated involvement, close follow-up is important.

JXG most commonly presents with single or multiple cutaneous nodules that are yellowish-brown to red, firm, and raised. In infants, JXG also can present in a disseminated form referred to as xanthoma disseminatum. The average age of onset is approximately 2 years. The disease is histologically characterized, like ECD, by lipid-laden histiocytes that show variable expression of S100 and some multinucleated giant cells.

JXG usually remains limited in extent and frequently undergoes spontaneous remission, especially in neonates and infants (90). Even the disseminated form of JXG, which can involve multiple organs, can undergo spontaneous remission. Excision of local lesions can be curative, and chemotherapy, such as vinblastine plus prednisone, can be effective, albeit not necessarily able to eradicate the disease, in nonregressive, disseminated disease. ECD occurs primarily in older adults and, although it has some histologic similarities to JXG, it is also associated with a different clinical pattern of organ involvement and a high frequency of *BRAF* mutations (91).

The HLH disorders are characterized by systemic and excessive production of inflammatory cytokines that lead to macrophage activation, hemophagocytosis, hepatosplenomegaly, fever, hypotension, renal failure, pulmonary insufficiency with capillary leak, lymphadenopathy, pancytopenia, coagulopathy, and CNS involvement with seizures and sometimes obtundation (91). HLH can be inherited as an autosomal recessive disease due to mutation of a variety of genes important for cytolytic granule formation and function of cytolytic T lymphocytes and natural killer (NK) cells. Some forms of HLH are also X-linked and involve lymphocyte activation and survival pathways. The inherited forms are associated with parental consanguinity and more commonly present during infancy and very early childhood, often initiated by a viral infection (92). HLH can also occur as an acquired disease

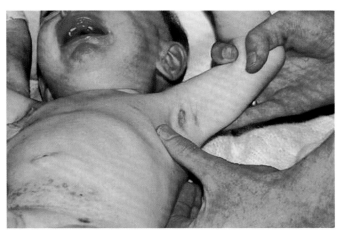
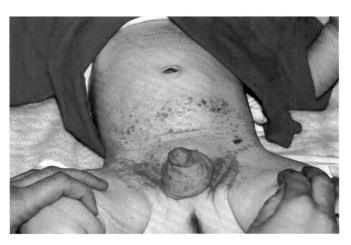

FIGURE 59.3 Skin presentations of infant LCH.

THE NEWBORN INFANT

usually related to certain viral infections such as CMV and EBV, but also to a variety of other causes including immunodeficiency syndromes as well as concomitant malignancy.

Specific diagnostic criteria have been developed for HLH. The presence of 5 out of 8 of the following criteria is necessary: fever, splenomegaly, cytopenias (greater than two affected lineages), hypertriglyceridemia and/or hypofibrinogenemia, bone marrow hemophagocytosis, low or absent NK cell activity, high ferritin (>500 mg/mL), and elevated soluble CD25 (IL-2 receptor, >2,400 units/mL). Evidence of loss-of-function mutations of any of the genes that have been linked to HLH is also diagnostic (91,93).

Recognition and rapid initiation of treatment for infants with HLH are critical. International trials have established the use of immunochemotherapy approaches that include high-dose dexamethasone and etoposide along with cyclosporine (94). Antithymocyte globulin (ATG) or anti-CD52 (campath) has also been used, and in some instances, anti-IL6 (tocilizumab). The only curative therapy for the inherited forms of HLH is hematopoietic stem cell transplantation, with approximately 70% survival, although adverse long-term sequelae are common.

RDD, sometimes referred to as sinus histiocytosis with massive lymphadenopathy (SHML), is a rare macrophage-related disorder, characterized by the accumulation of macrophages that express CD14, CD68, CD163, variable expression of S100, and fascin (95,96). The presence of emperipolesis, the engulfment of intact cells into the cytoplasm of another cell, is a distinct feature of RDD. The disease, which usually occurs during the first two decades of life, can affect persons of any age. Signs and symptoms include fever, fatigue, and weight loss, along with skin nodules and infiltration into lymph nodes, parotid, and salivary glands as well as any other organ, including the CNS. While the disease is usually self-limited, systemic therapy with chemotherapy may sometimes be warranted by significant clinical problems. In such cases, treatment with vinblastine plus prednisone, cladribine, clofarabine, or oral 6-mercaptopurine and methotrexate has shown efficacy in small numbers of patients.

Malignant histiocytic sarcomas can be of histiocytic or dendritic cell lineages. Pathology is characterized by large, noncohesive cells with pleomorphic nuclei and prominent nucleoli; hemophagocytosis may be present along with multinucleated giant cells. They rarely occur in very young children. Presentation may be a solitary mass at any anatomic site or may be as disseminated disease. A complete surgical excision for localized disease can be curative, but chemotherapy based on lymphoma-directed regimens and sometimes radiation may be necessary (95,96). Histiocytic sarcomas may harbor mutations in the mitogen-activated protein kinase (MAPK) pathway and respond to trametinib, a MAPK kinase inhibitor of MEK1 and 2 (97).

THERAPEUTIC ISSUES AND LATE EFFECTS OF THERAPY

The issues surrounding the treatment of cancer in infants and young children are unique. Because of their very young age, the balance between therapy and long-term side effects becomes especially important. A close collaboration and coordination by subspecialists and primary care physicians are critical.

Surgical management must consider the distinctive aspects of neonatal biology. Some tumors, such as hemangiomas and stage MS neuroblastoma, frequently involute or regress on their own, obviating surgical intervention. With other tumors, such as localized neuroblastomas, a complete resection may be unnecessary, whereas in cases of hepatoblastoma, a complete resection is more critical.

The detrimental effects of irradiation to infants are profoundly demonstrated in the treatment of patients with brain tumors, resulting in a high incidence and degree of physical and neurocognitive deficits. Skeletal growth also may be severely affected, with deformities of limbs and scoliosis. Liver, lung, and kidney are major organs whose short- and long-term function can be compromised. Additionally, the late appearance of second tumors may be significantly increased as a result of the mutagenic effects of irradiation.

The use of chemotherapy in the newborn is complicated by unique differences in absorption, distribution, metabolism, and excretion of such drugs (26,98). Additionally, these characteristics are constantly changing, as the infant undergoes rapid developmental changes. There are special considerations concerning drug absorption, distribution, metabolism, and elimination. Absorption through the gastrointestinal tract is slower in neonates, averaging about 6 to 8 hours. There are also decreased levels of key gastrointestinal enzymes, especially for infants under 4 months of age. The distribution of drugs in neonates and infants is also altered in part because of the high body water content (approximately 75% of total body weight and 40% is extracellular), thus impacting on the distribution of water-soluble drugs; such unique physiology suggests that water-soluble drugs be dosed based on body surface area rather than weight. Neonatal and infant drug metabolism is also decreased, in part due to reduced levels of various drug-metabolizing enzymes, such as those of the liver p450 pathway and reduced biliary excretion. Drugs such as cyclophosphamide, anthracyclines, and vincristine may thus result in prolonged exposures and increased toxicity. Elimination of drugs, particularly renal excretion, in neonates and infants is also slowed due to their reduced glomerular filtration rate, which does not reach adult levels until after 3 to 5 months of age. In addition, urine pH is lower in neonates and infants, thus requiring special consideration for drugs like methotrexate that are preferentially excreted at a higher pH.

Importantly, some of the signs and symptoms of drug toxicity may be subtle in infants and reflect the often more limited behavioral repertoire. For instance, neurotoxicity from vincristine may be reflected by irritability and hoarseness of crying. Survivors of the successful treatment of malignancy in infancy should be followed closely for long-term sequelae.

REFERENCES

1. Bader JL, Miller RW. US cancer incidence and mortality in the first year of life. *Am J Dis Child* 1979;133(2):157.
2. Borch K, et al. Neonatal cancer in Denmark 1943–1985. *Ugeskr Laeger* 1994;156(2):176.
3. Vasilatou-Kosmidis H. Cancer in neonates and infants. *Med Pediatr Oncol* 2003;41(1):7.
4. Plon SE, Malkin D. Childhood cancer and heredity. In: Pizzo PA, Poplack DG, eds. *Principles and practice of pediatric oncology*, 7th ed. Philadelphia, PA: Wolters Kluwer, 2016:13.
5. Aplan PD, Shern JE, Khan J. Molecular and genetic basis of childhood cancer. In: Pizzo PA, Poplack DG, eds. *Principles and practice of pediatric oncology*, 7th ed. Philadelphia, PA: Wolters Kluwer, 2016:32.
6. Abdel-Hady el-S, et al. Cancer during pregnancy: perinatal outcome after in utero exposure to chemotherapy. *Arch Gynecol Obstet* 2012;286(2):283.
7. Milojkovic D, Apperley JF. How I treat leukemia during pregnancy. *Blood* 2014;123(7):974.
8. Infante-Rivard C, et al. Childhood acute lymphoblastic leukemia associated with parental alcohol consumption and polymorphisms of carcinogen-metabolizing genes. *Epidemiology* 2002;13(3):277.
9. Mosse YP, et al. Identification of ALK as a major familial neuroblastoma predisposition gene. *Nature* 2008;455(7215):930.
10. Fisher JP, Tweddle DA. Neonatal neuroblastoma. *Semin Fetal Neonatal Med* 2012;17(4):207.
11. Isaacs H. Fetal and neonatal neuroblastoma: retrospective review of 271 cases. *Fetal Pediatr Pathol* 2007;26:177.
12. Monclair T, Brodeur GM, Ambros PF, et al. The International Neuroblastoma Risk Group (INRG) staging system: an INRG Task Force report. *J Clin Oncol* 2009;27(2):298.
13. Beckwith JB, Perrin EV. In situ neuroblastomas: a contribution to the natural history of neural crest tumors. *Am J Pathol* 1963;43:1089.
14. Woods WG. Screening for neuroblastoma: the final chapters. *J Pediatr Hematol Oncol* 2003;25(1):3.
15. Tsubono Y, Hisamichi S. A halt to neuroblastoma screening in Japan. *N Engl J Med* 2004;350(19):2010.

16. Twist CJ, Naranjo A, Schmidt ML, et al. Defining risk factors for chemotherapeutic intervention in infants with stage 4S neuroblastoma: a report from Children's Oncology Group Study ANBL0531. *J Clin Oncol* 2019;37(2):115.
17. Strother DR, et al. Outcome after surgery alone or with restricted use of chemotherapy for patients with low-risk neuroblastoma: results of Children's Oncology Group study P9641. *J Clin Oncol* 2012;30(15):1842.
18. Rubie H, et al. Excellent outcome with reduced treatment in infants with nonmetastatic and unresectable neuroblastoma without MYCN amplification: results of the prospective INES 99.1. *J Clin Oncol* 2011;29(4):449.
19. Davidoff AM. Neuroblastoma. *Semin Pediatr Surg* 2012;21(1):2.
20. Field M, Shanley S, Kirk J. Inherited cancer susceptibility syndromes in paediatric practice. *J Paediatr Child Health* 2007;43(4):219.
21. Skalet AH, Gombos DS, Gallie BL, et al. Screening children at risk for retinoblastoma: consensus report from the American Association of Ophthalmic Oncologists and Pathologists. *Ophthalmology* 2018;125:453.
22. Carr N, Foster P. Examination of the newborn: the key skills. Part 1. The eye. *Pract Midwife* 2014;17(1):26.
23. Chantada GL, et al. Impact of chemoreduction for conservative therapy for retinoblastoma in Argentina. *Pediatr Blood Cancer* 2014;61(5):821.
24. Manjandavida FP, et al. Management and outcome of retinoblastoma with vitreous seeds. *Ophthalmology* 2014;121(2):517.
25. Ortiz MV, Dunkel IJ. Retinoblastoma. *J Child Neurol* 2016;31(2):227.
26. Dunham C, Pillai S, Steinbok P. Infant brain tumors: a neuropathologic population-based institutional reappraisal. *Hum Pathol* 2012;43(10):1668.
27. Venkatramani R, et al. Outcome of infants and young children with newly diagnosed ependymoma treated on the "Head Start" III prospective clinical trial. *J Neurooncol* 2013;113(2):285.
28. Orbach D, et al. Neonatal cancer. *Lancet Oncol* 2013;14(13):e609.
29. Dash C, Moorthy S, Garg K, et al. Management of choroid plexus tumors in infants and young children up to 4 years of age: an institutional experience. *World Neurosurg* 2019;121:e237.
30. Merino DM, Shlien A, Villani A, et al. Molecular characterization of choroid plexus tumors reveals novel clinically relevant subgroups. *Clin Cancer Res* 2015;21:184.
31. Friedrich C, et al. Treatment of young children with CNS-primitive neuroectodermal tumors/pineoblastomas in the prospective multicenter trial HIT 2000 using different chemotherapy regimens and radiotherapy. *Neuro Oncol* 2013;15(2):224.
32. Chi SN, et al. Intensive multimodality treatment for children with newly diagnosed CNS atypical teratoid rhabdoid tumor. *J Clin Oncol* 2009;27(3):385.
33. Kreiger PA, et al. Loss of INI1 expression defines a unique subset of pediatric undifferentiated soft tissue sarcomas. *Mod Pathol* 2009;22(1):142.
34. Vormoor J, Chintagumpala M. Leukaemia & cancer in neonates. *Semin Fetal Neonatal Med* 2012;17(4):183.
35. Wiemels J, Kang M, Greaves M. Backtracking of leukemic clones to birth. *Methods Mol Biol* 2009;538:7.
36. Ford AM, Greaves M. ETV6-RUNX1 acute lymphoblastic leukemia in identical twins. *Adv Exp Med Biol* 2017;962:217.
37. Guest E, Stam R. Updates in the biology and therapy of infant acute lymphoblastic leukemia. *Curr Opin Pediatr* 2017;29:20.
38. Creutzig U, Zimmermann M, Reinhardt D, et al. Changes in cytogenetics and molecular genetics in acute myeloid leukemia from childhood to adult age groups. *Cancer* 2016;122(24):3821.
39. Massey GV, Zipursky A, Chang MN, et al. A prospective study of the natural history of transient leukemia in neonates with Down syndrome: Children's Oncology Group (COG) study POG 9481. *Blood* 2006;107(12):4406
40. Nikolaev SI, et al. Exome sequencing identifies putative drivers of progression of transient myeloproliferative disorder to AMKL in infants with Down syndrome. *Blood* 2013;122(4).
41. Daifu T, Kato I, Kozuki K, et al. The clinical utility of genetic testing for t(8;16)(p11;p13) in congenital acute myeloid leukemia. *J Pediatr Hematol Oncol* 2014;36:325.
42. Burnett AK, et al. Optimization of chemotherapy for younger patients with acute myeloid leukemia: results of the medical research council AML15 trial. *J Clin Oncol* 2013;31(27):3360.
43. Lamb M, Aldrink J, O'Brien S, et al. Renal tumors in children younger than 12 months of age: a 65 year single institution review. *J Pediatr Hematol Oncol* 2017;39(2):103.
44. Church A, Calicchio M, Skalova N, et al. Recurrent EML4-NTRK3 fusions in infantile fibrosarcoma and congenital mesoblastic nephroma suggest a revised testing strategy. *Mod Pathol* 2018;31(3):463.
45. Berger M, von Schweinitz D. Current management of fetal and neonatal renal tumors. *Curr Pediatr Rev* 2015;11(3):188.
46. Neylon OM, Werther GA, Sabin MA. Overgrowth syndromes. *Curr Opin Pediatr* 2012;24(4):505.
47. Hamilton TE, et al. The management of synchronous bilateral Wilms tumor: a report from the National Wilms Tumor Study Group. *Ann Surg* 2011;253(5):1004.
48. Sudour H, et al. Bilateral Wilms tumors (WT) treated with the SIOP 93 protocol in France: epidemiological survey and patient outcome. *Pediatr Blood Cancer* 2012;59(1):57.
49. Wagner L, Hill D, Fuller C, et al. Treatment of metastatic rhabdoid tumor of the kidney. *J Pediatr Hematol Oncol* 2002;24:385.
50. Seibel NL, et al. Effect of duration of treatment on treatment outcome for patients with clear-cell sarcoma of the kidney: a report from the National Wilms' Tumor Study Group. *J Clin Oncol* 2004;22(3):468.
51. Barksdale EM Jr, Obokhare I. Teratomas in infants and children. *Curr Opin Pediatr* 2009;21(3):344.
52. Mann JR, et al. Mature and immature extracranial teratomas in children: the UK Children's Cancer Study Group experience. *J Clin Oncol* 2008;26(21):3590.
53. Gabra HO, et al. Sacrococcygeal teratoma—a 25-year experience in a UK regional center. *J Pediatr Surg* 2006;41(9):1513.
54. Frazier A, Hale J, Rodriguez-Galindo C, et al. Revised risk classification for pediatric extracranial germ cell tumors based on 25 years of clinical trial data from the United Kingdom and United States. *J Clin Oncol* 2015;33:195
55. Khan A, et al. Hepatoblastoma in child with fetal alcohol syndrome. *Lancet* 1979;1(8131):1403.
56. Otten J, et al. Hepatoblastoma in an infant after contraceptive intake during pregnancy. *N Engl J Med* 1977;297(4):222.
57. McLaughlin CC, et al. Maternal and infant birth characteristics and hepatoblastoma. *Am J Epidemiol* 2006;163(9):818.
58. Spector LG, Birch J. The epidemiology of hepatoblastoma. *Pediatr Blood Cancer* 2012;59(5):776.
59. Trobaugh-Lotrario AD, Venkatramani R, Feusner JH. Hepatoblastoma in children with Beckwith-Wiedemann syndrome: does it warrant different treatment? *J Pediatr Hematol Oncol* 2014;36(5):369.
60. Murray MJ, Nicholson JC. alpha-Fetoprotein. *Arch Dis Child Educ Pract Ed* 2011;96(4):141.
61. Blohm ME, et al. Alpha 1-fetoprotein (AFP) reference values in infants up to 2 years of age. *Pediatr Hematol Oncol* 1998;15(2):135.
62. Trobaugh-Lotrario AD, et al. Outcomes for patients with congenital hepatoblastoma. *Pediatr Blood Cancer* 2013;60(11):1817.
63. Czauderna P, et al. Guidelines for surgical treatment of hepatoblastoma in the modern era—recommendations from the Childhood Liver Tumour Strategy Group of the International Society of Paediatric Oncology (SIOPEL). *Eur J Cancer* 2005;41(7):1031.
64. Roebuck DJ, et al. 2005 PRETEXT: a revised staging system for primary malignant liver tumours of childhood developed by the SIOPEL group. *Pediatr Radiol* 2007;37(2):123 [quiz 249].
65. Meyers RL, et al. Hepatoblastoma state of the art: pre-treatment extent of disease, surgical resection guidelines and the role of liver transplantation. *Curr Opin Pediatr* 2014;26(1):29.
66. Ravaioli M, et al. Liver transplantation for hepatic tumors: a systematic review. *World J Gastroenterol* 2014;20(18):5345.
67. Ferrari A, et al. Neonatal soft tissue sarcomas. *Semin Fetal Neonatal Med* 2012;17(4):231.
68. Joshi D, Anderson J, Paidas C, et al. Age is an independent prognostic factor in rhabdomyosarcoma: a report from the Soft tissue sarcoma committee of the Children's Oncology Group. *Pediatr Blood Cancer* 2004;42:64.
69. Drilon A, Laetsch T, Kummar S, et al. Efficacy of larotrectinib in TRK-fusion-positive cancers in adults and children. *N Engl J Med* 2018:378:731.
70. Lee JW. Mutations in PDGFRB and NOTCH3 are the first genetic causes identified for autosomal dominant infantile myofibromatosis. *Clin Genet* 2013;84(4):340.
71. Wu SY, et al. Chemotherapy for generalized infantile myofibromatosis with visceral involvement. *J Pediatr Hematol Oncol* 2015;37(5):402.
72. Mudry P, Slaby O, Neradil J, et al. Case report: rapid and durable response to PDGFR targeted therapy in a child with refractory infantile myofibromatoisis and a heterozygous germline mutation of the PDGFRB gene. *BMC Cancer* 2017;17(1): 119.
73. Hook KP. Cutaneous vascular anomalies in the neonatal period. *Semin Perinatol* 2013;37(1):40.
74. Kirkorian A, Grossberg A, Puttgen K. Genetic basis for vascular anomalies. *Semin Cutan Med Surg* 2016;35(3):128
75. Blei F. Congenital lymphatic malformations. *Ann N Y Acad Sci* 2008;1131:185.
76. Leaute-Labreze L, Dumas del la Rogue, Hubich T, et al. Propranolol for severe hemangiomas of infancy. *N Engl J Med* 2008;358:2649.
77. Hong SY, Tammareddi N, Walvekar R, et al. Successful discontinuation of propranolol for infantile hemangiomas of the head and neck at 12 months of age. *Int J Pediatr Otorhinolaryngol* 2013;77(7):1994
78. Janka GE, Lehmberg K. Hemophagocytic syndromes—an update. *Blood Rev* 2014;28(4):135.
79. Berres ML, et al. BRAF-V600E expression in precursor versus differentiated dendritic cells defines clinically distinct LCH risk groups. *J Exp Med* 2014;211(4):669.

80. Bates SV, et al. BRAF V600E-positive multisite Langerhans cell histiocytosis in a preterm neonate. *AJP Rep* 2013;3(2):63.

81. Badalian-Very G, et al. Pathogenesis of Langerhans cell histiocytosis. *Annu Rev Pathol* 2013;8:1.

82. Gadner H, et al. Therapy prolongation improves outcome in multisystem Langerhans cell histiocytosis. *Blood* 2013;121(25):5006.

83. Simko SJ, et al. Clofarabine salvage therapy in refractory multifocal histiocytic disorders, including Langerhans cell histiocytosis, juvenile xanthogranuloma and Rosai-Dorfman disease. *Pediatr Blood Cancer* 2014;61(3):479.

84. Kolenova A, Schwentner R, Jug G, et al. Targeted inhibition of the MAPK pathway: emerging salvage option for progressive life threatening multisystem LCH. *Blood Adv* 2017;1:352.

85. Nanduri VR, et al. Long term morbidity and health related quality of life after multi-system Langerhans cell histiocytosis. *Eur J Cancer* 2006;42(15):2563.

86. Mittheisz E, et al. Central nervous system-related permanent consequences in patients with Langerhans cell histiocytosis. *Pediatr Blood Cancer* 2007;48(1):50.

87. Lau L, et al. Cutaneous Langerhans cell histiocytosis in children under one year. *Pediatr Blood Cancer* 2006;46(1):66.

88. Battistella M, et al. Neonatal and early infantile cutaneous Langerhans cell histiocytosis: comparison of self-regressive and non-self-regressive forms. *Arch Dermatol* 2010;146(2):149.

89. Kansal R, et al. Identification of the V600D mutation in Exon 15 of the BRAF oncogene in congenital, benign Langerhans cell histiocytosis. *Genes Chromosomes Cancer* 2013;52(1):99.

90. Oza V, Stringer T, Campbell C, et al. Congenital type juvenile xanthogranuloma: a case series and literature review. *Pediatr Dermatol* 2018;35(5):582.

91. Henter JI, et al. HLH-2004: diagnostic and therapeutic guidelines for hemophagocytic lymphohistiocytosis. *Pediatr Blood Cancer* 2007;48(2):124.

92. Heeg M, Amman S, Klemann C, et al. Is an infectious trigger always required for primary hemophagocytic lymphohistiocytosis? Lessons from in utero and neonatal disease. *Pediatr Blood Cancer* 2018;65(11):e27344.

93. Sepulveda F, de Saint Basile G. Hemophagocytic syndrome: primary forms and predisposing conditions—review. *Curr Opin Immunol* 2017;49:20.

94. Ehl S, Astigarraga I, von Bahr Greenwood, et al. Recommendations for the use of etoposide based therapy and bone marrow transplantation for the treatment of HLH: consensus statements by the HLH Steering Committee of the Histiocyte Society. *J Allergy Clin Immunol Pract* 2018;6(5):1508.

95. Vaiselbuh SR, et al. Updates on histiocytic disorders. *Pediatr Blood Cancer* 2014;61(7):1329.

96. Weitzman S, Jaffe R. Uncommon histiocytic disorders: the non-Langerhans cell histiocytoses. *Pediatr Blood Cancer* 2005;45(3):256.

97. Gounder M, Solit D, Tap W. Trametinib in histiocytic sarcoma with an activating MAP2K1(MEK1) mutation. *N Engl J Med* 2018;378(20):1945.

98. Veal GJ, Boddy AV. Chemotherapy in newborns and preterm babies. *Semin Fetal Neonatal Med* 2012;17(4):243.

Orthopedics

Deborah M. Eastwood

INTRODUCTION

Assessment of the musculoskeletal system (MSK) is an essential part of neonatal evaluation. Normal variations in contour, size, and range of movement may be influenced by factors such as ethnicity and the position *in utero*, but these should be distinguished from the potentially more significant congenital or acquired problems. Certain conditions respond well to early, appropriate treatment within the neonatal period, while for other abnormalities, there is no "quick and easy fix" no matter how much the parents and clinicians may wish there was. In essence, the aim of the neonatal assessment is to distinguish between these two.

HISTORY

No examination, not even that of a neonate, should take place before a history has been taken. The history may be short, but it can include important information relating to family history and the pregnancy. The parents may already be aware that their child has a "problem" as many skeletal abnormalities, generalized and focal, can be identified on antenatal ultrasound scans. It is important to know what counseling they have received and what information they have been given. Similarly, it is always important to ask about the family history, for example, of developmental dysplasia of the hip (DDH) or indeed syndromes with a genetic cause. Please remember that the parents in the room may not be those with the genetic input. A history of reduced fetal movements may also be relevant.

GENERAL EXAMINATION

Good observational skills are the hallmark of a good clinician. Every doctor should develop a routine for a general screening examination of a newborn so that he/she is confident that a complete examination has been performed. This routine must be flexible to adapt to the infant's behavior and to the signs identified/elicited. The orthopedic tried and tested adage is **"Look, Feel, Move"** starting generally and then focusing on individual parts of the MSK system. Please remember that sometimes the subtle signs are more relevant to neonatal management than are the obvious abnormalities. The purpose of the examination is to identify the pathologic "something" from the physiologic "nothing" of concern.

First and foremost, you should look for normality and symmetry of appearance and movement both in prone and in supine. Certain neonatal reflexes are, by definition, asymmetrical, but overall movements left and right, upper and lower limbs should be the same. Skin creases are normal; their absence can be concerning (**Fig. 60.1**). Dimples may be considered cute, but on the front of the tibia, for example, they suggest a significant underlying bony abnormality. The cutaneous stigmata of underlying conditions such as the café au lait marks associated with neurofibromatosis must be documented. A limb that seems to lie in an abnormal position may still show good movement out of/away from that position, and it is important to recognize the difference between a postural flexible deformity and a structural one that is fixed. A simple syndactyly may be just that or may be associated with other more significant failures of normal development. Obvious major abnormalities such as absence of part of a limb or lack of movement in an arm or legs will direct the subsequent examination but not at the expense of a full assessment.

Once you start examining the infants by touching them, it is important to judge their response to this stimulus. Is their response "expected" or not? While it is important to identify MSK problems, they are often interlinked with problems in the peripheral and/or central neurologic systems. General features such as warmth, swelling, and tenderness are also important findings.

As you observe the active movements of the child, passive range of movements can be examined while remembering that the neonate differs from the child in its joint ranges. The infant is born with a flexion deformity at hip, knee, and elbow exacerbated perhaps by the "molded baby syndrome (MBS)."

INVESTIGATION

The mainstays of orthopedic investigations in the neonatal period are plain radiographs (including a full skeletal survey for dysplasia if indicated), ultrasound scans, and rarely an MRI scan that can often be done under "feed and wrap" sedation.

It is not within the scope of this chapter to discuss all the MSK abnormalities that can be identified in the neonate, but the aim is to help the reader feel confident in diagnosing the common and/or important generalized and focal conditions.

GENERAL CONGENITAL CONDITIONS

The Molded Baby Syndrome

Babies may be subjected to significant molding pressures while *in utero* resulting in postural abnormalities, which are obvious at birth in an estimated 10% of infants (1). The MBS consists of a variety of signs not all of which are present in every case (**Table 60.1**).

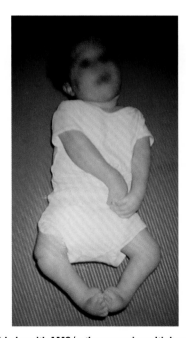

FIGURE 60.1 A baby with AMC (arthrogryposis multiplex congenita) affecting all four limbs.

TABLE 60.1

Main Clinical Features of the Molded Baby Syndrome

- Plagiocephaly
- Torticollis
- Adduction contracture of the hip
- Foot deformities
  - Postural club foot, metatarsus adductus
- Pelvic obliquity, spinal curvature

A careful examination will exclude more significant structural abnormalities, and identify postural problems which will improve with time and some stretching exercises. The asymmetric hip movements are important to note: the *adduction contracture* of MBS may seem exactly the same as the *limited abduction*, which is present in DDH.

Amniotic Band Syndrome

The exact cause of this syndrome is unclear, although the popular theory remains that if the inner layer of the amniotic sac ruptures, the fetus is exposed to strands of fibrous tissue, which, once floating in the amniotic fluid, may then wrap around a developing limb or digit constricting it as it grows (2). An alternative theory suggests that the constriction band is secondary to an underlying localized area of poor blood flow. The clinical picture is very variable ranging from ring-like constrictions around the limb to partial amputation of digits, and or/tissue linking digits together (**Fig. 60.2**). Rarely, at birth, the limb distal to a circumferential constriction may appear ischemic, and urgent surgical release or indeed amputation is required (**Fig. 60.3A and B**). More commonly, any surgical treatment required to improve function or cosmesis takes place later in childhood.

Arthrogryposis Multiplex Congenita

By definition, this condition is associated with multiple (two or more) stiff joints present from birth with legs more often affected than arms. Most cases occur randomly, and over 400 different conditions have been associated with isolated or multiple joint contractures (3). The most severe form of the condition is amyloplasia,

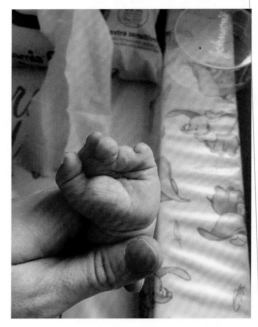

FIGURE 60.2 Picture of a left hand where most of the digits are missing secondary to an amniotic band syndrome.

while in distal arthrogryposis, as its name implies, problems are more limited to the distal joints of upper and lower limbs. Distal arthrogryposis may be associated with a genetic disorder. There may be non-MSK-associated conditions present too.

While the exact cause(s) of AMC are not known, it is associated with decreased fetal movements. The joints form at 5 to 6 weeks of embryologic life, and they need movement in order to develop normally. In the absence of intrauterine movement (due to any cause), connective tissue forms further limiting joint motion. The muscles are poorly developed. The joints have never moved, and the overlying soft tissues confirm this with a noticeable absence of the normal skin creases. The limbs are often described as tubular and featureless (Fig. 60.1).

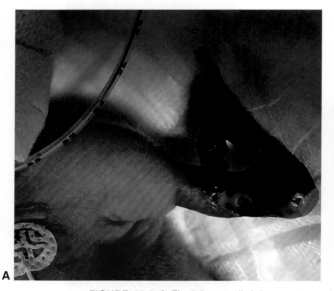

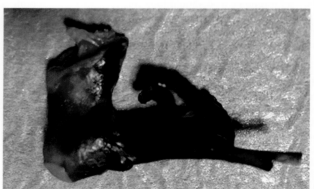

FIGURE 60.3 A: The left upper limb in neonate aged 2 days who was born with an ischemic limb. **B:** The necrotic portion was removed in the NICU as the child was already intubated.

Some limited improvement in joint contractures may occur in response to physiotherapy stretching exercises started soon after birth, but joint movement will never be normal. The associated clubfoot (CTEV: congenital talipes equinovarus) or vertical talus (CVT: congenital vertical talus) deformities may respond to a more formal Ponseti program (*see CTEV section*). Dislocated hips do not respond well to conservative treatment, and surgical management may be considered. A holistic approach to care is essential with sensible long-term goals identified and planned for from an early age.

Skeletal Dysplasias

The majority of skeletal dysplasias are associated with short stature and hence may have been identified on an antenatal scan. They are a heterogeneous group of genetic disorders characterized by abnormalities in the growth of both bone and cartilage leading to abnormal shapes and sizes of bones and joints, particularly in the limbs and the spine (4). The head size may be relatively large. Most often these conditions are associated with joint contractures and stiffness, but in some conditions, joint laxity is evident. The molecular basis of many of these conditions has now been established, which may lead to new avenues of prevention and treatment. Perhaps, the two most common dysplasias are achondroplasia and osteogenesis imperfecta.

Achondroplasia

Achondroplasia is an autosomal dominant condition, which usually presents as a *de novo* mutation (5). The physical appearance is considered characteristic in the child, but many features may be

TABLE 60.2
Main Clinical Features of Achondroplasia in the Neonate

- Macrocephaly with frontal bossing, a large anterior fontanelle, and a flattened midface and nasal bridge
- Disproportionate short stature
  - Short limbs, particularly proximally (rhizomelic)
  - Spine length normal (thoracolumbar kyphosis later)
  - Small chest
- Bowed legs
- Joint laxity (apart from the elbows where there is a fixed flexion)
- Hypotonia
- Short fingers and a trident hand

difficult to detect in the newborn. A skeletal survey should confirm the diagnosis. No specific orthopedic problems exist at this stage; referral for a spinal opinion and general genetic and clinical advice will be required (Table 60.2).

Osteogenesis Imperfecta

Osteogenesis imperfecta (OGI) is an umbrella term for a group of genetic conditions characterized by inadequate production and/or poorly functioning collagen (6). Bones may fracture easily, in response to minimal force, but bone healing is unaffected. The neonate with a severe form of the condition may present with multiple fractures that occurred *in utero* and/or during delivery (Fig. 60.4A and B). Alternatively fractures may occur as a result of normal handling in the neonatal period and beyond (Fig. 60.4C).

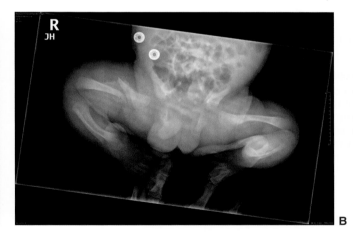
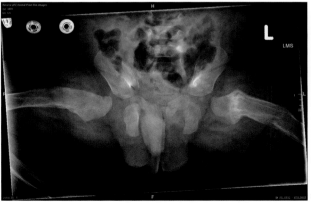

FIGURE 60.4 **A:** Right femoral shaft fracture on day of birth with minimal trauma. The child was subsequently diagnosed with OGI. **B:** Same fracture on day 14: note the significant amount of callus (new bone formation) despite the separation of one part of the bone from the other. **C:** Same child age 4 months. The right femoral fracture has already remodeled well, but there is now evidence of two healed left-sided fractures too, which may have occurred within the neonatal period.

Blue sclerae and a characteristic facies are present in some cases but not obvious in other children.

Fractured limbs require minimal splintage, but the child may require very gentle handling at least until a diagnosis is established.

Overgrowth Syndromes

Growth is usually proportionate and symmetrical so that localized overgrowths of all tissue types may be very obvious. Presentation is very variable depending on the tissues involved ranging from a localized vascular malformation to an isolated macrodactyly or lipomatous swelling, but the overgrowth can be quite dramatic. Treatment in the neonatal period is rarely required, although some high-flow vascular malformations can lead to signs of cardiac failure. Accurate diagnosis is essential, and multidisciplinary follow-up should take place.

LOCALIZED CONGENITAL ABNORMALITIES OF THE THORACOLUMBAR SPINE

Myelomeningocele

The most urgent and most serious spinal abnormality is a neural tube defect (NTD) (see also Chapter 53) manifesting as a myelomeningocele: in high-income countries, these have usually been diagnosed in the antenatal period with plans in place for surgical closure within a few days of birth (**Fig. 60.5**). However, any stigmata of a NTD such as a sacral pit or hairy patch should raise concerns, particularly if associated with abnormal muscle tone or function. A change in function and/or conscious level following closure of the lesion demands exclusion of a secondary hydrocephalus. The associated hip, knee, and foot deformities may require early conservative treatment as part of a multidisciplinary plan.

In general, the overall mortality, morbidity, and disability correlate well with the level of the defect, the presence of an associated hydrocephalus, and a significant kyphotic deformity.

Caudal Regression Syndrome or Sacral Agenesis

In this rare condition, the development of the caudal (lower) part of the body is deficient. The lumbar vertebrae, sacrum, and corresponding sections of the spinal cord may be absent or poorly formed with limbs that may show a flaccid paralysis and/or fixed deformity. In less severe cases, the foot deformities may respond to physiotherapy. Associated abnormalities of the genitourinary and GIT systems are common.

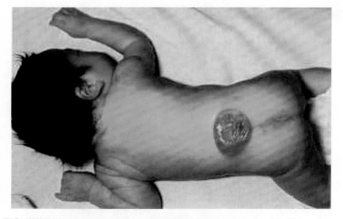

FIGURE 60.5 A neonate with a closed myelomeningocele of the lower lumbar spine.

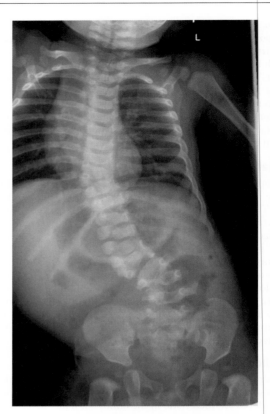

FIGURE 60.6 An x-ray of the spine showing abnormal shapes to the bony vertebrae at several levels: these represent hemivertebrae and may lead to severe deformity over time and with growth.

Other Congenital Anomalies of the Thoracolumbar Spine

In the absence of an NTD or an obvious skeletal dysplasia, it is unusual to see anything but a straight and mobile thoracolumbar spine with the infant held in your hand in the prone position. Therefore, any suggestion of significantly reduced movement (in the neck for example) or significant curvature in either the AP/coronal (for scoliosis) or lateral/sagittal (for kyphosis) planes mandates further assessment. The imaging method of choice is often a plain x-ray (**Fig. 60.6**), and despite the cartilaginous nature of much of the infant skeleton, hemivertebrae can be identified. In experienced hands, ultrasound scanning is both an accurate and cost-effective examination for evaluating the bony and soft tissue components of the infant spine (7).

Congenital spinal deformities have a high incidence of associated cardiac and genitourinary problems, which will require assessment. A documented spinal abnormality requires referral to a spinal team, but no treatment is required in the neonatal period.

LOCALIZED CONGENITAL ABNORMALITIES OF THE CERVICAL SPINE

Torticollis

A head held in the "cock robin" (tilted) position is frequently due to tightness in the sternocleidomastoid muscle (SCM), which limits *rotation toward* and *lateral flexion away* from the lesion. The etiology is unclear, but the two most popular theories relate to intrauterine molding and minor trauma during delivery. The head tilt and "tumor" in the SCM may not be apparent until a few days after birth. See also Chapter 59.

Other Congenital Anomalies of the Cervical Spine

As with the thoracolumbar spine, failures of formation or segmentation do occur as in the Klippel-Feil syndrome where the neck is short and stiff. The stiffness and asymmetric movements may mimic a torticollis, but a plain radiograph will confirm the diagnosis.

CONGENITAL ABNORMALITIES OF THE LIMBS

Missing Parts/Amputations

One to two percent of newborns will have a congenital defect, and 10% of those affect the upper limb. The embryonic development of the limb buds is now more fully understood as is the influence of genetic mutations on this process. Congenital limb malformations may be classified in several ways; perhaps the easiest to recognize is a *transverse deficiency* where the limb has developed essentially normally up to a particular point but beyond this point, there may be nothing more than digital remnants. When "parts are missing," it is still important to examine the whole limb according to the look, feel, and move principle. Joints proximal to the "amputation" should move well. An x-ray does help define the skeletal problem, and an USS may identify cartilaginous anlages of other as yet unossified bones and possibly tendons/muscles (Fig. 60.7) (Table 60.3). No treatment other than explanation, reassurance, and advice to encourage normal infant development is required. Referral to a rehabilitation service, particularly for those with a lower limb amputation, is recommended. The distal limb amputations/partial amputations may be associated with the ABS.

Cleft Hands and Feet

Ectrodactyly or failure of formation of the central rays affects hands more commonly than feet. It can be an autosomal dominant condition, but severity is very variable. It is usually bilateral and may be associated with other abnormalities. The function is often surprisingly good. Treatment in infancy is rarely required.

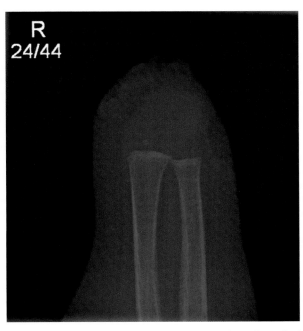

FIGURE 60.7 Failure of formation of the right hand. AP radiograph shows the radius and ulnar and a soft tissue "paddle hand" with rudimentary digits present.

TABLE 60.3

Examination of a Limb with a Part Missing

- Are there cartilaginous "bones" within the paddle hand for example?
- Is there active and/or passive movement where you expect the joints to be?
- Are the proximal joints normal?

Limb Deformity

In a *longitudinal deficiency*, there is a reduction or absence of bone and soft tissue elements in the long axis of the limb often associated with significant deformity of the limb. There may be normal skeletal elements both distal and proximal to the affected area, but often the whole limb will show subtle abnormalities particularly with growth. Missing toes or rays of the hand/foot suggest that there is a more widespread underlying deficiency (Figs. 60.8 to 60.10). Previously, these conditions had descriptive names such as radial or ulna club hand or fibula or tibial hemimelia.

Tibial Bowing

Of the uncommon conditions, tibial bowing or deformity is quite common, and the type of deformity gives a good clue as to the underlying abnormality. The deformity is always defined in terms of where the apex of the deformity is clinically (and indeed radiographically). The anterolateral bow may present with deformity or a "fracture" but without pain and true swelling. Splintage is rarely necessary unless perhaps the child

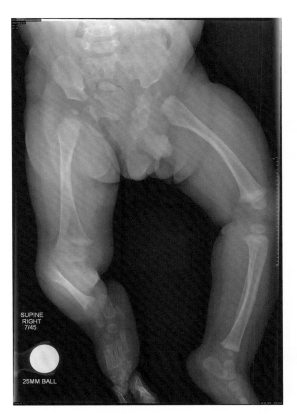

FIGURE 60.8 Tibial amelia. AP radiograph of a neonatal limb showing only one bone in the lower leg with five metatarsals. The single bone is often considered to be the tibia, but it is too lateral and not articulating with the distal femur—thus, it is the fibula.

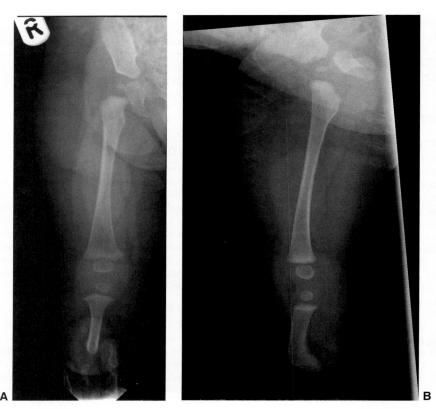

FIGURE 60.9 A: AP radiograph of a longitudinal deficiency. **B:** Lateral radiographs of a longitudinal deficiency. The apex of the deformity is anteromedial, and the underlying abnormality is fibula hemimelia. There is no fibula present.

appears distressed particularly if there is a pseudarthrosis of both the tibia and the fibula. The anteromedial bow (**Fig. 60.11**) is in effect a manifestation of the longitudinal deficiency mentioned above (**Table 60.4**).

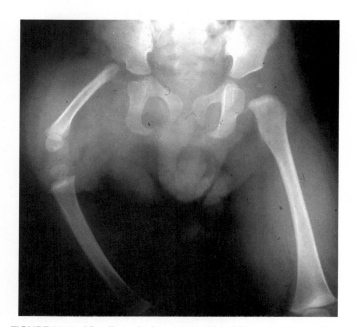

FIGURE 60.10 AP radiograph of a neonate with a right proximal femoral focal deficiency demonstrating abnormal formation of the femur and no hip joint.

The posteromedial bow often presents with the top (dorsal surface) of the foot touching the anterior surface of the tibia (**Fig. 60.12**). There is a lump palpable posteriorly. Physiotherapy stretches are the mainstay of treatment. This condition improves significantly over time and may even resolve completely. It is the least serious of the three types of tibial bow.

Hyperextended Knee

A hyperextended knee may present as an isolated finding, for example, in association with an extended breech position or as part of a generalized neuromuscular disorder such as spina bifida or AMC. Clinically, the leg lies in external rotation, and the hyperextension may appear as a valgus knee. The femoral condyles are prominent posteriorly. Many hyperextended knees do respond to stretching exercises alone or combined with serial casting, but it is essential to ensure the limb is held in neutral rotation (patella facing forward) before the stretching commences (8). Some do not respond, particularly if the knee is dislocated, and there is significant contracture of the quadriceps with anterior subluxation of the hamstring tendons (**Fig. 60.13A and B**). Surgical intervention may be required within the first year of life. The subluxed knee usually reduces with casting, but a dislocated knee may require open reduction.

Important Common Conditions of the Lower Limb

The following two conditions are relatively common with an incidence around 1 to 2/1,000 live births. Both need to be detected promptly as early treatment results in a significantly improved long-term outcome. One condition is obvious, and the other has to be looked for.

THE NEWBORN INFANT

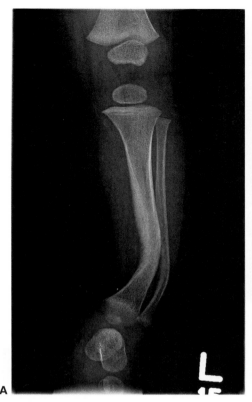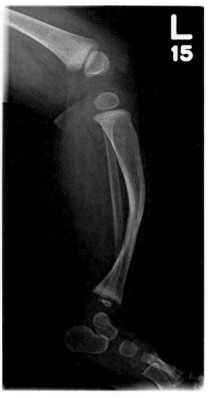

FIGURE 60.11 A: AP radiograph in an 8-month-old child showing an apex anterolateral bow consistent with "congenital pseudarthrosis of the tibia CPT," but in this case, the tibia has yet to break. **B:** Lateral radiograph of the same child showing the apex anterolateral bow.

Developmental Dysplasia of the Hip

DDH describes a spectrum of hip pathology, present in the neonate, that ranges from dysplasia perhaps seen only on an ultrasound scan, through clinical hip instability and subluxation to a frank dislocation, which may or may not be reducible. Etiologic factors include *in utero* mechanical forces and the influence of maternal hormones on the tissues of both herself and the infant (9). A delay in diagnosis and treatment has a profound effect on outcome, and the results of treatment initiated under the age of 6 weeks are better than those where treatment commences at a later stage; hence the emphasis on surveillance programs and selective or universal ultrasound screening programs. Clinical suspicion should be high

in all female, firstborn babies, especially those with a positive family history and/or a breech position in the last trimester of pregnancy. The left hip is more frequently affected in unilateral cases, but DDH may be bilateral.

The examination of a newborn's hip should seek to answer three questions, which determine whether further investigation is required. Guidelines vary from one country to another (Table 60.5).

The findings are often more subtle in the newborn compared to the infant, and limited hip abduction in flexion may only be noticed "in passing" as the hip goes into full abduction with spontaneous reduction of the femoral head. The static images

TABLE 60.4

Where is the Apex?

		Look for	Outcome
Anteromedial (Fig. 60.9)	Congenital pseudarthrosis (tibia may not yet be broken)	Neurofibromatosis	Usually requires surgical management
Anterolateral (Fig. 60.11)	Longitudinal deficiency	Skin dimples	Usually requires surgical management
	Fibula hemimelia	Short leg	
		Foot deformity	
Posteromedial (Fig. 60.12)		May be confused with a positional calcaneovalgus foot deformity	May require surgical management of residual deformity and LLD
Posterolateral (never seen)			

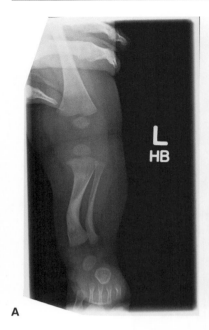
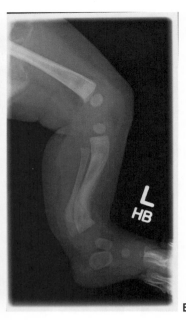

FIGURE 60.12 A: AP radiograph of an apex posteromedial tibial bow. **B:** Lateral radiograph of a posteromedial tibial bow.

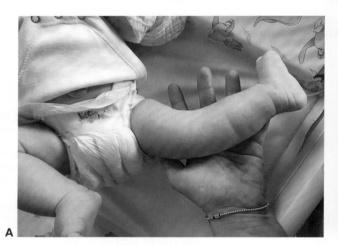
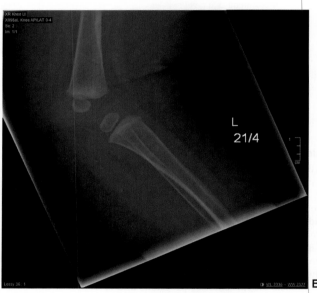

FIGURE 60.13 A: Clinical photograph of a child with a hyperextended knee. On examination, the femoral condyles are easily palpable posteriorly, suggesting the knee is dislocated. **B:** Lateral radiograph of a lower limb showing dislocation of the knee. (Tibia has moved forward on the femur.)

TABLE 60.5

Questions to be Asked during the Clinical Examination of a Neonatal Hip

1. Is the hip dislocated at rest?
   - If so, is it reducible?
     - If so, this is an Ortolani positive hip.
   - If not, this is an irreducible Ortolani negative hip.
2. If the hip is not dislocated, is it dislocatable?
   - If so, the hip is a Barlow positive hip.
3. If the hip is neither dislocated, nor dislocatable, is it therefore clinically normal?
   - Does it require further investigation?

With a history of risk factors, an USS is indicated (10).

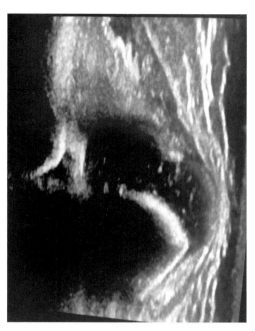

FIGURE 60.14 An ultrasound scan showing a reasonably formed acetabulum, but the femoral head is not in contact with the acetabulum, and therefore, the hip is dislocated.

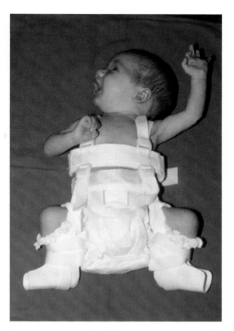

FIGURE 60.15 A neonate in a Pavlik harness as treatment for its left-sided DDH. Note the presence of the Moro reflex.

from a hip ultrasound are used to define the anatomy of the hip and quantify the dysplasia (Fig. 60.14). The dynamic scan is performed as the examiner provokes instability by performing a Barlow test (applying downward pressure to the flexed and adducted hip).

There is clinical equipoise among the profession as to when treatment should be started given that many cases of hip instability improve spontaneously over the first few weeks of life (11). A safe practice would be to ensure that investigations were performed by 2 to 4 weeks and that review by the treating physician was between 2 and 6 weeks. The Barlow positive hip simply needs to be held safely in joint. For the dislocated hip, the femoral head reduces with the hip flexed past 90 degrees and in comfortable abduction: as the flexed thigh abducts, the dislocated femoral head can be lifted into the acetabulum manually (Ortolani maneuver) or it will relocate spontaneously. Treatment with a Pavlik harness involves full time wear for a period of 6 to 12 weeks dependent on the pathology being treated and the response of the hip to the harness treatment (Fig. 60.15). Follow-up will then continue until normal development has been documented.

CTEV

Congenital talipes equinovarus (the club foot, CTEV) is the most common significant foot abnormality (Fig. 60.16). In high-income countries, the diagnosis has often been made on the antenatal scans with high sensitivity and positive predictive values, but the scans are unable to comment on the severity of the deformity, that is, how fixed or flexible it is. Bilateral cases are more often associated with other abnormalities.

The classic clubfoot is a developmental anomaly of the entire foot. The foot points "down and in" and described in terms of equinus and varus of the hindfoot, adduction of the forefoot, and apparent cavus. The talonavicular joint is subluxed, and the talar head palpable dorsolaterally. Treatment of the foot with a fixed deformity is by the Ponseti method, a structured process where the four elements of the deformity are corrected in a sequential manner by serial manipulations and casting performed weekly (12).

A tenotomy of the Achilles tendon, done under local anesthetic in the clinic room, is required in around 80% to 90% of cases after a mean of five casts. Surgery should be avoidable in greater than 90% of idiopathic CTEV. Ponseti casting usually starts within the neonatal period (Fig. 60.17). Idiopathic deformities respond better than do nonidiopathic deformities (Fig. 60.18).

There is a positional/postural form of CTEV which by definition is much more flexible and can be fully corrected with gentle pressure by the examiners hand.

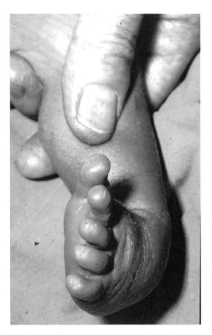

FIGURE 60.16 A foot with the signs of an idiopathic club foot deformity (CTEV: congenital talipes equino varus).

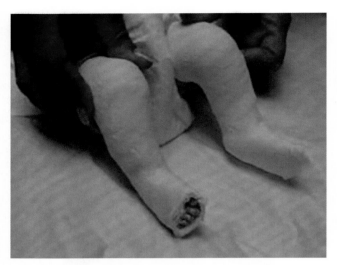

FIGURE 60.17 A child in bilateral above knee casts during Ponseti treatment.

Other Foot Problems

Congenital Vertical Talus

CVT is a similar but "opposite" deformity to CTEV, which is equally important to recognize because early treatment is indicated. As with CTEV, the hindfoot is in equinus, but in CVT, it is also in valgus (rather than varus). The midfoot is abducted and dorsiflexed. The talonavicular joint is subluxed, and the talar head is palpable plantarmedially in the sole of the foot. The overall appearance is of a "rockerbottom foot." Radiographs may be required to confirm the diagnosis. The Dobbs method of serial casting (a "reverse" Ponseti method) followed by limited surgery has gained popularity in recent years, but treatment is not as successful as for the CTEV. Treatment will not create a normal foot, but the outcome is better with early treatment as a neonate/infant.

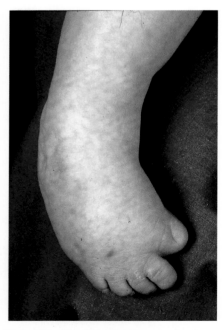

FIGURE 60.18 A child with a TEV deformity secondary to an amniotic band syndrome; note the short (part missing) big toe and the suggestion of a band around the distal lower leg.

Metatarsus Adductus

Metatarsus adductus may occur in isolation or as part of the molded baby syndrome; it should be distinguished from the more significant CTEV. The lateral border of the foot is curved, and there is often a medial crease on the sole of the foot. The foot appears "bean shaped." In most cases, the deformity is flexible, and the foot posture will improve over time. If the deformity is less flexible/more rigid, then stretching exercises may help and occasionally stretching casts may be required. The outcome is invariably good.

Talipes Calcaneovalgus

This is rarely a structural deformity, but rather a reflection of the foot's position *in utero*. The top of the foot lies against the anterior surface of the tibia, but the deformity is flexible and the foot usually corrects fully or to just past neutral with gentle manipulation. Treatment is gentle stretching exercises performed regularly during the day, for example, at nappy changes or when "playing" with the foot. More resistant deformities may require manipulation and serial casting. It is important that the positional talipes calcaneovalgus is not confused with a posteromedial bow of the tibia.

Upper Limb

As with the lower limb, failures of normal development make up the majority of the obvious abnormalities. Both longitudinal deficiencies of the forearm are often associated with abnormalities of the radial or ulnar sided digits, and overall long-term functional outcomes are influenced by form and function of the remaining fingers/thumb.

Sprengel Shoulder

A Sprengel deformity, although rare, is the most common significant congenital anomaly of the shoulder girdle. It represents a failure of embryologic descent of the scapula, and it is usually unilateral. The small scapula is too high, sited at the base of the neck, and rotated laterally (13). Due to its abnormal position and/or abnormal connections to the spinous processes of the cervical spine (an omovertebral bone), the neck may appear short and webbed on the affected side. Shoulder movements are often restricted, but this may be difficult to see in the neonate. It is often associated with a Klippel-Feil syndrome where fused vertebrae result in a short, stiff neck. No specific treatment is required in the neonatal period.

Congenital Pseudarthrosis of the Clavicle

This is an isolated anomaly, which is classically on the right side unless there is dextrocardia. It presents with painless angulation of the clavicle in association with a nontender mass in the midclavicular region. There is no loss of movement at the shoulder or neck. The importance of this condition lies in its differentiation from an acute traumatic or indeed nonaccidental injury. An x-ray confirms the pseudarthrosis, and usually both bone ends are bulbous. There is no healing of the "fracture" over time clinically or on radiographs.

Cleidocranial Dysostosis

The completely absent clavicle is usually associated with cranial dysostosis and/or a widened pubic symphysis due to a failure in intramembranous ossification. There are no symptoms in the neonate, and no treatment is required.

▌ ACQUIRED ABNORMALITIES

Birth-Related Brachial Plexus Injury

Damage to the brachial plexus is one of the more common birth injuries with an incidence of 0.9 to 2.6 per 1,000 live births (14). It creates a flaccid paralysis and thus an absent Moro reflex on the affected side. It is associated with high birth weight, shoulder dystocia, and is caused by the traction and lateral flexion applied to the neck when delivering the shoulder in a vertex delivery. The same injury can occur with breech deliveries when delivering the head. Bilateral lesions can occur but are very rare.

Injuries are classified according to involvement of the shoulder, elbow, wrist, and hand. There may also be associated damage to the phrenic nerve leading to tachypnea and a raised hemidiaphragm on chest x-ray or to the sympathetic chain resulting in the clinical picture of a Horner syndrome (Table 60.6).

Each of the many neurones in each of the nerve roots can be injured in a variety of ways including stretching, compression, and avulsion with or without injury to the tissues around them causing considerable complexity in assessment and determining the prognosis. Outcomes vary with the severity of the damage and although movement returns to the paralyzed muscles in around 90% of those affected, it is now recognized that at least 30% of children demonstrate long-term sequelae when assessed carefully over time.

The differential diagnosis includes those other conditions that present immediately after birth with a pseudoparalysis; thus, a radiograph to exclude a fracture of the clavicle or the humerus is required. Fractures frequently coexist with a birth-related brachial plexus injury (BRBPI). A pseudoparalysis secondary to sepsis usually presents a day or two after birth, and the arm is not flaccid but stiff as the infant uses their muscle to guard against movement of the joint.

The early treatment of BRBPI is conservative: careful repeated and documented assessment of the evolving neurologic picture is very helpful. The extent of neural damage can only be assessed by evaluating recovery over the course of time as nerve lesions of differing severity initially present with the same clinical features. Regular and frequent (with every diaper change) passive movement of all of the involved joints (shoulder and elbow +/– forearm, wrist, and hand) and sensory stimulation of the skin will ensure contractures do not occur. Information is also essential at this point with a clear explanation of the injury and the range of potential outcomes. Referral to an expert team is required if full recovery has not occurred by 6 to 8 weeks of age (15).

Fractures in the Neonate

The neonatal skeleton consists of a significant amount of cartilage as well as bone. The bones will fracture if or when a pathologic force is applied to them or if the bone is pathologically weak/brittle.

A fracture noted at or around birth is usually related to a difficult delivery, particularly of a large infant, those in a breech position or where fetal distress demands a rapid extraction, but it may be the first manifestation of a metabolic condition such as OGI. The fractures occur either in the mid shaft (the diaphysis) of the humerus or femur or through the growth plate (physis) most commonly at the proximal or distal humerus. With physeal injuries, the epiphysis is displaced from the metaphysis and may give the clinical appearance of a dislocated joint. The clavicle is also frequently fractured. Fractures below the elbow or below the knee are rare. In the neonate, as in any child, if there is no history of injury, then nonaccidental injury must be considered.

The fractures are characterized by reduced movement of the affected limb, pain and distress on handling, swelling, and possibly a change in shape of the limb. Pain and swelling may be minimal, but an acute fracture should be tender to palpation and is in the differential diagnosis of pseudoparalysis of a limb. The neurovascular status of the limb must be checked.

A plain radiograph will confirm a diaphyseal fracture; these are often spiral in nature due to the twisting force that was applied to the limb, often by the obstetrician, at delivery (**Fig. 60.19**). Physeal injuries, through cartilage, are not visible on x-ray, but the relationships between the visible bones will be abnormal (**Fig. 60.20**). Further detail can be seen with an USS. An MRI scan is rarely indicated.

Fractures in the neonatal period never require surgical management. Injuries to the clavicle and the humerus are treated by gentle immobilization of the upper limb, with the arm by the child's side under their clothes and some padding, if needed, between the arm and the chest.

Femoral shaft fractures may be splinted using a Pavlik harness with the leg resting in a "frog leg" position (as in Fig. 60.15).

For both upper and lower limb fractures, healing is rapid and the child will begin moving their arm and kicking their leg within 7 to 10 days of injury at which time the splint can be removed. The fractures always heal, no matter what position they are in and any deformity remodels with time. The family may become aware of a hard mass at the site of the fracture representing the mass of healing bone, but this too will improve with time.

Physeal injuries also heal rapidly, and again despite significant initial displacement, nonoperative management is invari-

TABLE 60.6			
Narakas Classification			
Narakas Classification	**Parts of the Arm Affected by the Flaccid Paralysis**	**Likely Nerve Root Involvement**	**Clinical Picture**
1	Shoulder and elbow	Upper trunk (C5, C6)	Shoulder flaccid and arm adducted and internally rotated Hand and wrist normal
2	Shoulder, elbow, and wrist	Upper and middle trunks (C5, C6, C7)	As above but also with flaccid wrist (wrist drop) Fingers flexed and held in fist
3	Whole arm • shoulder, elbow, wrist, and hand	Upper middle and lower trunks (C5, C6, C7, C8, T1)	No movement at any level of the affected arm Hand flaccid and open
4	Whole arm • shoulder, elbow, wrist, and hand • Horner syndrome	Upper middle and lower trunks (C4, C5, C6, C7, C8, T1) • Sympathetic chain	Flaccid paralysis of upper limb Raised hemidiaphragm Ptosis and constricted pupil

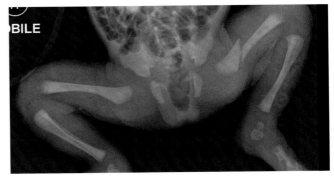

FIGURE 60.19 Left femoral fracture, which occurred during delivery of large breech position infant. This fracture is through normal bone.

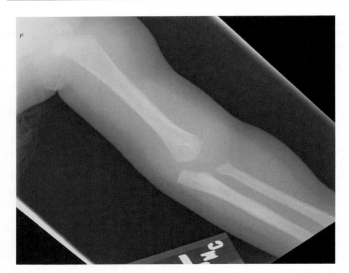

FIGURE 60.20 A neonatal elbow x-ray—there is not enough distance between the distal humerus and the proximal ulna meaning this is a transphyseal separation of the distal humerus. The distal epiphysis and the radius and ulna have been displaced posteriorly. An USS would confirm this.

ably the preferred treatment option. Remodeling results in normal or near-normal alignment and good function. Despite the injury affecting the growth center, significant growth disturbance is rare.

All fractures should be referred for an orthopedic opinion and followed up in clinic.

Bone and Joint Infections

Both osteomyelitis and septic arthritis occur in the neonate and may present with pseudoparalysis of the affected limb: the mode of presentation differs from that seen in older children. The neonatal immune system is immature, and, in contrast to older infants, there is a transphyseal blood supply that links the metaphysis with the epiphysis, increasing the likelihood of extension of an osteomyelitis into the joint itself. Infection is more common in preterm infants, and a high index of suspicion combined with regular, careful physical examination is essential for early diagnosis and treatment. Multiple foci are common, and bone or joint involvement should be considered wherever there are soft tissue abscesses. All neonates with a diagnosis of MSK infection will require long-term follow-up.

Acute septic arthritis is primarily hematogenous in origin but on occasion it may be secondary to inadvertent puncture of a joint (usually the hip joint) during venipuncture. Preterm infants with indwelling lines are at particular risk (16). The neonate is generally unwell, but there may be few localizing signs. The child may present with failure to thrive, pseudoparalysis, pain on passive motion, swelling and local warmth. The deep seated hip joint is the joint most frequently affected, but here visible swelling and palpable warmth are difficult to detect in the early case. Nevertheless, the leg will tend to lie flexed, abducted, and externally rotated. Routine observations and hematologic investigations are essential, but results may not show the expected abnormal levels if the sepsis is overwhelming.

Plain radiographs are requested to exclude a fracture and established osteomyelitis. They may show a widened joint space and/or joint subluxation due to fluid within the joint. USS will identify the joint effusion and may be able to comment on the nature of the fluid. The report should also comment on edema of the soft tissues, changes within the bone suggestive of a concomitant osteomyelitis, and thickening of the periosteum with/without a subperiosteal abscess. The shoulder joints and hip joints may be visible on chest and abdominal radiographs taken as part of the assessment of an unwell child, and the diagnosis of a septic arthritis must always be considered.

A septic arthritis is an orthopedic emergency, and drainage of the purulent fluid with irrigation of the joint is required. For some joints, repeated needle arthrocenteses and irrigation will suffice, but many surgeons believe for the hip joint an open surgical procedure (arthrotomy) is preferable and allows a full inspection of the joint while facilitating irrigation (17). Specimens should be inoculated into blood culture bottles, and, if available, a PCR assay performed in addition to routine culture and sensitivity.

A delay in diagnosis of septic arthritis of the hip joint and shoulder joint in particular has grave consequences on the vascular supply to the epiphysis. The blood supply is vulnerable to the increased intra-articular pressure associated with the joint effusion, and the purulent contents promote vascular occlusion and degeneration of the articular cartilage. Joint distension and the continued accumulation of purulent fluid may lead to joint subluxation and dislocation. In such situations, following surgical drainage, the joint may need to be splinted in the reduced position with, for example, a Pavlik harness.

Osteomyelitis is also invariably due to hematogenous spread. The pathology begins in the metaphyses of the long bones where the terminal sinusoids of the nutrient artery are associated with low flow, which encourages bacterial stasis and replication. The subsequent inflammatory process within the bone is followed by small vessel thrombosis and the formation of pus and an abscess with destruction of some bony trabeculae (18). The exudate spreads via Volkmann canals to the subperiosteal space. The periosteal elevation so caused provokes new bone formation (involucrum). In joints where the metaphysis is intra-articular when pus spreads through the periosteum, a secondary septic arthritis develops. In the neonate, due to the persistent transphyseal vessels, spread into the epiphysis is facilitated and destruction of the ossification centre here will be associated with significant shape abnormalities of the joint in later life. In preterm infants, infection may occur secondary to direct inoculation following a heel prick or a line insertion.

The neonate with hematogenous osteomyelitis presents in a similar manner to one with septic arthritis, and the two may coexist. The child may be hypothermic rather than pyrexial. There is a reluctance to move the affected limb. Soft tissue swelling occurs early and may be visible on a plain radiograph before any bony changes are seen, so osteomyelitis should be considered whenever significant limb swelling is present.

In any infant who is seriously ill or failing to thrive, careful examination of the extremities should be performed, with observation for any evidence of tenderness, pain, and swelling that may indicate the presence of osteomyelitis (or indeed a septic arthritis). The most common organisms are *Staphylococcus aureus* (and Staph epidermidis in the premature infants particularly), but group B beta-hemolytic streptococcus also occurs along with Gram-negative organisms. In some countries, community acquired strains of methicillin-resistant Staph aureus are also relevant.

Prompt treatment with appropriate antibiotics and other supportive measures is essential. Immobilization/splintage may rest the infected tissues and provide pain relief. Once abscess formation has occurred, surgical drainage will be required.

REFERENCES

1. Rubio AS, Griffet JR, Caci H, et al. The moulded baby syndrome: incidence and risk factors regarding 1,001 neonates. *Eur J Pediatr* 2009;168(5):605. doi: 10.1007/s00431-008-0806-y
2. National Organisation for Rare Diseases. Available from: https://rarediseases.org/rare-diseases/amniotic-band-syndrome
3. Bamshad M, Van Heest AE, Pleasure D. Arthrogryposis: a review and update. *J Bone Joint Surg Am* 2009;91:40.
4. Calder AD, Foley P. Skeletal dysplasias: an overview. *Paediatr Child Health* 2018;28:84.

5. Pauli RM. Achondroplasia: a comprehensive clinical review. *Orphanet J Rare Dis* 2019;14:1. doi: 10.1186/s13023-018-0972-6
6. Van Dijk FS, Sillence DO. Osteogenesis imperfecta: clinical diagnosis, nomenclature and severity assessment. *Am J Med Genet A* 2014;164(6):1470. Correction in: *Am J Med Genet A* 2015;167(5):117.
7. AIUM Practice parameter for the performance of an ultrasound examination of the neonatal and infant spine. *J Ultrasound Med* 2016;35:1. Available from: https://www.aium.org/resources/guidelines/neonatalSpine.pdf
8. Rampal V, Mehrafshan M, Ramanoudjame M, et al. Congenital dislocation of the knee at birth—Part 2: impact of a new classification on treatment strategies, results and prognostic factors. *Orthop Traumatol Surg Res* 2016;102(5):635.
9. Rhodes AML, Clarke NMP. A review of environmental factors implicated in human developmental dysplasia of the hip. *J Child Orthop* 2014;8(5):375.
10. Biedermann R, Eastwood DM. Universal or selective ultrasound screening for developmental dysplasia of the hip? A discussion of the issues. *J Child Orthop* 2018;12:296.
11. Barlow TG. Early diagnosis and treatment of congenital dislocation of the hip. *J Bone Joint Surg* 1962;44-B:292.
12. Ponseti IV, Campos J. The classic: observations on pathogenesis and treatment of congenital clubfoot. *Clin Orthop Relat Res* 2009;467(5):1124.
13. Matsuoka T, Ahlberg PE, Kessaris N, et al. Neural crest origins of the neck and shoulder. *Nature* 2005;436:347.
14. Coroneos CJ, Voineskos SH, Christakis MK, et al.; Canadian OBPI working group. Obstetrical brachial plexus injury (OBPI): Canada's national clinical practice guideline. *BMJ Open* 2017;7:e014141.
15. Smith BW, Daunter AK, Yang LJ, et al. An update on the management of neonatal brachial plexus palsy—replacing old paradigms: a review. *JAMA* 2018;172:585.
16. Paakkonen M. Septic arthritis in children: diagnosis and treatment. *Paediatric Health Med Ther* 2017:8;65.
17. Givon U, Liberman B, Schindler A, et al. Treatment of septic arthritis of the hip joint by repeated ultrasound-guided aspirations. *J Pediatr Orthop* 2004;24(3):266.
18. Ogden JA, Lister G. The pathology of neonatal osteomyelitis. *Pediatrics* 1975;55:474.

61 Dermatology

Kaiane A. Habeshian, Ha-young Choi, and Robert A. Silverman

INTRODUCTION

The skin is the largest and most readily visible organ in the human body. Its primary obvious function is to serve as a barrier between the internal body and the external world, protecting against infection and fluid losses. In addition, increasing evidence points to the critical role of the skin and skin microbiome in the development of a healthy immune system (1). Conversely, imbalances in neonatal skin likely play a role in the development of systemic inflammatory diseases such as atopic dermatitis and psoriasis. The skin can also serve as an indicator of internal disease that may not otherwise be readily apparent. The clinician caring for the newborn must be able to distinguish between worrisome and benign skin disorders.

SKIN DEVELOPMENT, STRUCTURE, AND FUNCTION

There are three anatomic layers (epidermis, dermis, and fat) and three adnexal structures (hair, nails, and glands) that create the structure of the skin. While the structural development of skin is completed at an early gestation, in early premature birth, the functional activity of the skin is underdeveloped (**Fig. 61.1**).

During development, skin and its structures are thought to migrate along the "lines of Blaschko," which were first described by Alfred Blaschko based on observations of the distribution of skin lesions (2). Blaschko lines are believed to represent pathways of epidermal keratinocyte and not mesodermal cell migration. They are not related to dermatomes or to cutaneous neural pathways. Skin disorders following these lines are manifestations of genetic mosaicism, thought to result from a single postzygotic mutation of a single clone of cells or from a mutation on an X chromosome that is exposed by X inactivation (3). Affected keratinocytes influence the development of underlying dermal structures, which may account for dermal pathology seen within a Blaschko linear pattern.

The epidermis is composed of four layers, from deep to superficial: stratum basale, stratum spinosum, stratum granulosum, and stratum corneum. Keratinocytes, the main cell type of the epidermis, are produced from stem cells in the basal layer and migrate upward, during which time they flatten and lose their nuclei, becoming more compact. The extracellular space becomes increasingly lipidized with ceramides, fatty acids, and cholesterol within the supper layers of the epidermis. This structure is referred to as the "brick (keratinocytes) and mortar (lipids)" of the epidermis (4,5).

The epidermis is critical for maintaining fluid homeostasis and a barrier between the internal organs and the outside environment. The stratum corneum is relatively waterproof and prevents transepidermal water loss (TEWL) due to its composition rich in hydrophobic lipids (4,5). In addition, the skin is a biologically active organ that helps prevent infection and modulates the immune system. In addition to the presence of lymphocytes, neutrophils, and histiocytes in the dermis, keratinocytes themselves directly produce cytokines and antimicrobial peptides and play a critical role in both innate and adaptive immunity (6,7). In addition, the cutaneous microbiome and the immune system interact in a dynamic fashion, an area of active research (7).

The appearance and texture of newborn skin differs based on the newborn's gestational age and postnatal age. Premature infants have skin that appears thin and transparent, with visible veins. Infants born after 40 weeks of EGA have thicker skin with wrinkles and peeling. Most term infants are also born with a pasty substance on the skin called the vernix caseosa, which is composed of lipids and waxes, sloughed corneocytes, and shed lanugo hair (8). It has an important role in moisturizing the skin, creating a hydrophobic barrier against maceration within the amniotic fluid, and providing lubrication during the birth process. The vernix also likely plays an important role in innate immune defense, as it contains antimicrobial agents that are active against fungal and bacterial pathogens (9). Most premature and postmature infants have little vernix.

Prematurity and a number of skin disorders disrupt epidermal permeability barrier function and may allow for massive TEWL (10). Premature infants can lose up to 30% of their total body weight in 24 hours. Their rate of TEWL may be 10 to 15 times greater than in a full-term infant, as they lack vernix caseosa and have an underdeveloped stratum corneum (11,12). The fluid management of premature infants must take into account the increased TEWL. By contrast, the skin of a full-term infant is well developed and likely as effective at preventing TEWL as an adult's skin (13).

Epidermal barrier development is accelerated by exposure to the dry, extrauterine environment (11). This barrier maturation typically takes 2 to 4 weeks and may be delayed for 8 weeks in extremely premature infants. Thus, premature infants are particularly vulnerable to infections and toxins, particularly during the first week of life when approximately two-thirds of all neonatal deaths worldwide occur. A proportion of late-onset sepsis may be linked to the colonization of the preterm infant's skin with pathogenic bacteria.

CARE IN THE NEONATAL INTENSIVE CARE UNIT

During an infant's care in the neonatal intensive care unit (NICU), many questions may arise regarding general skin care. While there are no universal protocols, each hospital should create guidelines that address general skin care and common iatrogenic skin injuries. These protocols might include guidance on incubator settings to decrease TEWL for premature infants and others at risk of TEWL, cleansing, and intravenous catheter care.

Incubator Care

Humidified incubators slow fluid losses from the underdeveloped epidermal skin barrier. Premature skin begins to mature upon birth, resembling that of full-term babies in about 2 to 4 weeks. Even during this period of maturation, it may be appropriate in hemodynamically stable infants to use skin-to-skin or "kangaroo mother care" (KMC), when the infant is placed directly in contact with the mother's skin, usually on her chest. Though it is unclear if the microenvironment created during skin-to-skin mitigates some of the loss of the humidified incubator, there are numerous benefits to KMC (12). See Chapters 25 and 26.

Likewise, collodion babies require incubator care even when born at term because they are at high risk of hypernatremic dehydration until the abnormal collodion membrane sheds, which takes on average 2 to 4 weeks (14). The degree of humidification and the length of time in the incubator have not been strictly studied. However, most published experiences describe anywhere from 40% to 100% humidity, with breaks for appropriate bonding as tolerated (14–17).

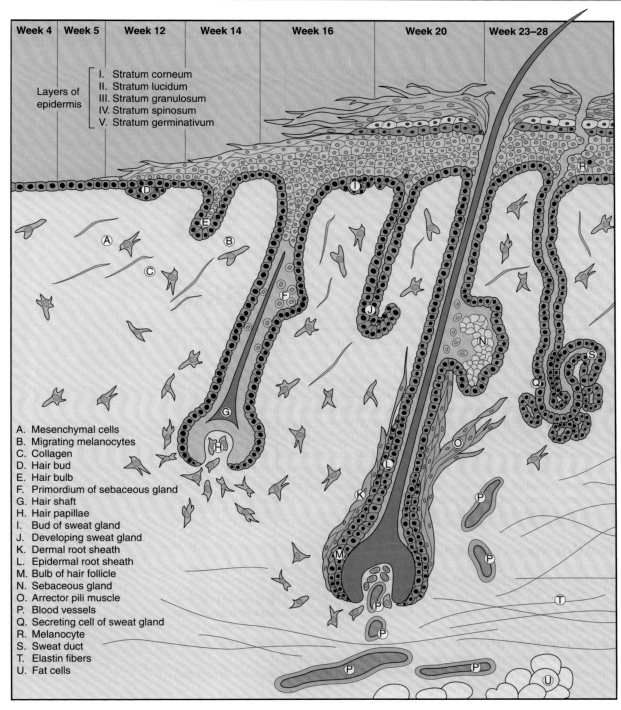

Week 4	Week 5	Week 12	Week 14	Week 16	Week 20	Week 23–28

Layers of epidermis
- I. Stratum corneum
- II. Stratum lucidum
- III. Stratum granulosum
- IV. Stratum spinosum
- V. Stratum germinativum

A. Mesenchymal cells
B. Migrating melanocytes
C. Collagen
D. Hair bud
E. Hair bulb
F. Primordium of sebaceous gland
G. Hair shaft
H. Hair papillae
I. Bud of sweat gland
J. Developing sweat gland
K. Dermal root sheath
L. Epidermal root sheath
M. Bulb of hair follicle
N. Sebaceous gland
O. Arrector pili muscle
P. Blood vessels
Q. Secreting cell of sweat gland
R. Melanocyte
S. Sweat duct
T. Elastin fibers
U. Fat cells

THE NEWBORN INFANT

FIGURE 61.1 Structure of the skin. (Reprinted with permission from Fletcher MA. *Physical diagnosis in neonatology.* Philadelphia, PA: Lippincott-Raven Publishers, 1998.)

Obstetrical Effects

Obstetric procedures that are commonly used in management of the fetus during pregnancy and delivery are associated with specific skin findings. Though wounds to a fetus were long thought to be inconsequential, fetal injuries as early as 16 weeks of gestation can heal with scarring (18). Amniocentesis has been associated with skin dimpling that is presumably due to needle puncture (19). Fetal scalp electrodes, which are frequently used during labor to measure fetal heart rate, may lead to transient superficial lacerations (20). Infrequently, the lacerations can become infected and form abscesses or serve as an inoculation point for herpes simplex (21). Halo scalp ring, a nonscarring alopecia of the scalp, is often

associated with primigravidas with prolonged labor (22). It is secondary to pressure necrosis on the vertex of the scalp from the cervix, leading to hair loss and sometimes permanent scarring alopecia in a classic annular pattern. Recognition of these common patterns of skin injury in neonates is important to prevent unnecessary workup and for monitoring of complications.

Intensive Care Effects

Anetoderma of prematurity appears as well-circumscribed wrinkly atrophic patches of skin with decreased elastic tissue, usually at the site of prior monitoring leads (23). These lesions are not present at birth and may be preceded by a bruise-like appearance or a

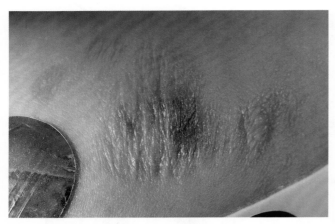

FIGURE 61.2 Anetoderma of prematurity follows the location of cardiopulmonary monitoring electrodes.

TABLE 61.1

Steps in a Newborn Skin Examination

1. Assess skin integrity.
   Skin breakdown
   Texture
   Hydration
   Swelling
2. Determine primary and secondary skin lesions (see **Table 61.2**).
3. Determine the location, configuration, and distribution of the skin lesions.
4. Evaluate mucous membranes, palms, soles, hair, and nails.
5. If there is a rash, determine whether it is fixed or evolving.
6. Develop a differential diagnosis.
7. Perform appropriate diagnostic tests.
8. Consider referral to a specialist.

Reprinted with permission from Dinulos JB. *Avery's neonatology*, 7th ed. Philadelphia, PA: Wolters Kluwer, 2016.

known history of lead placement at that site (**Fig. 61.2**). While an exact mechanism of anetoderma of prematurity is unknown, it is thought that pressure or traction during lead removal from immature skin lead to local hypoxia and tissue damage (24).

Hypothermia is extremely dangerous in preterm newborns, associated with increased risk of IVH, respiratory issues, hypoglycemia, and sepsis; thus, methods of heat regulation such as warming the delivery room, skin-to-skin, and plastic wrap are recommended for resuscitation and the care of newborns (25). When available, thermal heat pads and incubators may also be used. However, because neonatal skin can burn at low temperatures, application of warmers should occur according to strict manufacturer recommendations. The use of hot water bottles or other nonregulated, nonuniform heat sources pose a great risk of burn. Even the warmth from transilluminators, commonly used to visualize veins or pneumothorax, can cause thermal burns. The risk of transilluminator-related thermal burns may be decreased with the use of light-emitting diode (LED) lights, which do not create as much heat as do traditional incandescent fiber optic "cold" light lamps (26). Even pulse oximeters have been reported to cause burns, highlighting the importance of close diligence of even the most routine devices in the NICU (27).

Antiseptic agents, while essential to decrease infection risk, can lead to chemical burns of the skin. Even alcohol, commonly used for skin preparation in minor procedures, such as IV placement, can cause burns in premature infants (28). Other antiseptic solutions such as chlorhexidine and iodine are usually dissolved in alcohol and can cause burns, especially if allowed to pool under an infant during a procedure.

Peripheral intravenous (IV) lines, essential in neonatal care, can lead to infiltrates of fluid and chemicals into the surrounding subcutaneous tissue. Many of the infusions used in neonatal medicine can be caustic, including parenteral nutrition, calcium, potassium, sodium bicarbonate, vasopressors, antibiotics, and antivirals. Severe extravasation injuries cause tissue damage and require immediate attention. There are multiple antidotes used to decrease the severity of extravasation injuries, including saline flushout, hyaluronidase, topical nitroglycerine, and phentolamine, but these antidotes must be applied quickly for optimal effect (29–32). The type of antidote used depends on the extent of injury, the infant's stability, availability, and health providers' experience.

EXAMINATION OF NEWBORN SKIN

The general examination of the newborn should include a thorough skin exam with adequate exposure of the skin and lighting to allow for easy assessment. With exposure of the skin for assessment, care must be taken to ensure a neutral environment to minimize reactive vascular changes. A natural light source is best, as artificial lights can cast hues or mask hues to the skin; side lighting and dermatoscopes may be useful. The exam of the skin should include global assessment of skin integrity, texture, color, hydration, and edema and should include the often overlooked portions of the skin exam such as the mucous membranes, palms, soles, hair, and nails (**Table 61.1**). When a specific skin finding is noted, it should be assessed for primary and secondary skin lesions, location, configuration, and distribution (**Table 61.2**).

COMMON BENIGN SKIN FINDINGS IN THE NEONATE

Rashes are common in the first month of life, affecting 80% of newborns (33). During the first week of life, the vast majority of term and post-term infants will have superficial peeling or desquamation of skin; it rarely occurs in those under 35 weeks of gestation. Deeper skin peeling that results in denuded skin and continuous peeling for longer than 1 week are potential warning signs of an underlying systemic process.

Erythema Toxicum Neonatorum

Erythema toxicum neonatorum (ETN) is a common benign transient eruption seen most commonly in healthy full-term Caucasian babies. It is characterized by evanescent pink macules and papules and pustules on an erythematous base (**Fig. 61.3**), most prominent on the face, torso, and extremities, with sparing of the palms and soles. The pustules may coalesce to form large pustular plaques. Typically, lesions are not present at birth but develop within 24 to 72 hours of life and continue to appear for the first week of life. A smear of a pustule showing abundant eosinophils and no bacteria or yeast may confirm the diagnosis but is usually unnecessary. The cause of ETN is not fully understood but is postulated to occur as a healthy appropriate immune response to the novel extrauterine environment and colonization of skin organisms (34). It is more common in warm seasons and climates. ETN is self-resolving, and treatment is not necessary.

Cutis Marmorata

Cutis marmorata is a transient net-like erythema caused by constriction of capillaries and venules occurring in newborns exposed to cold. It usually disappears quickly with rewarming. Persistent and extensive cutis marmorata can be seen in association with trisomies 18 and 21 and Cornelia de Lange syndrome. Cutis marmorata should not be confused with a vascular malformation (VM) referred to as cutis marmorata telangiectatica congenita (CMTC).

TABLE 61.2

Primary and Secondary Skin Lesions, Configurations, and Locations

1. Primary lesions

    Macule (<0.5 cm) and patch (>0.5 cm)—well-circumscribed flat lesion

    Papule (<0.5 cm) and plaque (>0.5 cm)—well-circumscribed raised lesion

    Vesicle (<0.5 cm) and bullae (>0.5 cm)—fluid-filled raised lesion

    Pustule—well-circumscribed raised fluid-filled lesion containing leukocytes

    Nodule (>0.5 cm)—deep-seated raised lesion

    Tumor—a large nodule

    Wheal (hive)—raised transient (<24 h) lesion

    Cyst—fluid-filled nodule

    Telangiectasia—dilated dermal blood vessel

    Petechiae—areas of extravasated red blood cells resulting from broken capillaries

2. Secondary lesions

    Atrophy—depressed lesion

    Erosion—superficial break in the skin

    Ulceration—full thickness (i.e., break in the skin through the dermis)

    Scale—flakes of skin

    Crust—scale with serum

    Fissure—linear erosion

    Scar—fibrosis of the dermis

3. Configuration

    Blaschko—embryologic lines of skin cell migration (i.e., whorled)

    Linear—straight

    Annular—round with normal skin in central "ring"

    Iris—round with a dark center

    Nummular—round, "coin shaped"

    Clustered—numerous adjacent lesions

4. Location

    Symmetric—both sides of the body

    Localized—one area

    Widespread—generalized

    Intertriginous—skin folds

    Acral—ears, nose, hands, feet

Reprinted with permission from Dinulos JB. *Avery's neonatology,* 7th ed. Philadelphia, PA: Wolters Kluwer, 2016.

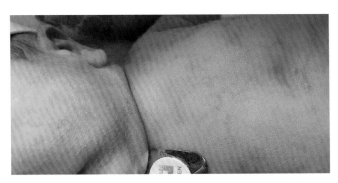

FIGURE 61.3 Erythema toxicum neonatorum is a common and benign skin eruption in the first few weeks of life.

Sebaceous Gland Hyperplasia

Sebaceous gland hyperplasia is seen in the vast majority of term infants and occasionally in preterm infants. Close examination of the nose, upper vermilion lip border, and malar areas at birth reveals numerous pinpoint yellow to white papules that are caused by enlargement of the pilosebaceous glands in response to maternal androgens. After the increased androgen exposure ceases shortly at birth, the condition self-resolves by 2 to 6 months of age.

Milia

Milia can resemble sebaceous gland hyperplasia, but these small discrete yellow-white papules are slightly larger than those seen at birth with sebaceous gland hyperplasia and usually occur on the forehead, nose, cheeks, chin, and forehead as well as on the body, including acral surfaces. Most milia arise spontaneously (primary milia) and can affect 40% to 50% of newborns (35). Milia can also result from other causes (secondary milia) such as trauma or genetic conditions (epidermolysis bullosa [EB], pachyonychia congenita). No treatment is required, and most will resolve within the first few months, though larger milia can persist. Persistent milia can be extracted.

Miliaria

Miliaria is caused by sweat retention in blocked eccrine ducts (Fig. 61.4). It is usually found in intertriginous areas due local humidity and occlusion, as well as the trunk, and commonly occurs in hot and humid environments. The condition will usually resolve with a cool environment, although it may require low-potency

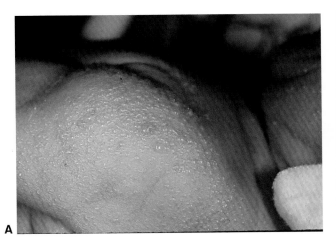
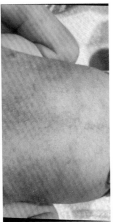

FIGURE 61.4 Miliaria crystallina (A) and miliaria rubra (B) can be present at birth but resolve quickly with a cool environment.

topical corticosteroids to calm the inflammatory response. There are four types of miliaria, depending on the depth of the blockage. Deeper blockages take longer to resolve. Miliaria crystallina occurs due to occlusion in the outermost layer of the skin, the stratum corneum, and appears as small superficial clear noninflammatory vesicles. This is commonly seen in neonates. Miliaria rubra, commonly called "prickly heat," occurs due to blockage at the dermoepidermal junction and appears as small pink papules and vesicles that may itch. Miliaria pustulosa is similar to miliaria rubra but occurs due to blockage at the mid-dermal level and appears as pustules on an erythematous base. Miliaria profunda occurs due to blockage at the deeper dermal layers and appears as firm pink nodules.

Sucking Blisters

Blisters and erosions present at birth on the thumb, index finger, wrist and lip, and occur at sites of *in utero* sucking (**Fig. 61.5**). Sucking blisters do not appear inflammatory and are transient and limited in extent. They should be differentiated from mechanobullous eruptions such as EB and bacterial and viral infections. Localized involvement in classic locations and lack of generalized skin fragility are helpful clues.

TRANSIENT PHENOMENON IN NEONATES

Purpuric Light Eruption

Purpuric light eruption is a transient generalized purpuric eruption occurring in newborns who have received blood transfusions or IVIG and also receive treatment with phototherapy. The purpura appears within 4 days of the light therapy and spontaneously clears within 1 week of stopping phototherapy. The area of purpura is limited to areas exposed to intensive phototherapy—and so will be notably absent under leads, eye patches, and the diaper area. The underlying cause of this eruption is unknown, but it may be related to a transient increase in porphyrins (36).

Harlequin Color Change

This is a rare transient vascular phenomenon presenting as sharply demarcated erythema that develops on the dependent half of an infant who is in the lateral decubitus position. It occurs in both healthy and ill newborns (especially low birth weight infants), lasts 1 to 30 minutes, and reverses if the infant is placed on the opposite side. The underlying mechanism for harlequin color change is unknown. This reaction may occur for up to 3 weeks and is not associated with long-term sequelae.

COMMON SKIN RASHES IN THE OLDER NEONATE AND INFANT

Neonatal Cephalic Pustulosis

Neonatal cephalic pustulosis (formerly neonatal acne) occurs in the first 2 weeks to 3 months of life. It manifests as monomorphic tiny papules and pustules on an erythematous base located on the face, especially the cheeks, and sometimes the scalp, chest, and arms, without comedones (**Fig. 61.6**). It may represent an inflammatory reaction to colonization by the *Malassezia* spp. fungal skin flora. Topical antifungal creams can be helpful for more severely affected newborns, but treatment is not necessary, as it generally self-resolves over weeks to months.

Seborrheic Dermatitis

Seborrheic dermatitis, commonly referred to as "cradle cap," is characterized by white-yellow waxy scale, sometimes with underlying erythema, on the scalp and the eyebrows. It also affects intertriginous areas in which typical scale is absent, leading to a characteristic shiny pink appearance in babies. Concurrent staph, strep, or yeast infections may occur. Unlike atopic dermatitis, it is not pruritic. The eruption typically begins at 2 to 3 weeks of age and in some infants becomes widespread over the next few months before improving significantly during the first year of life. Persistent and severe seborrheic dermatitis may be associated with human immunodeficiency virus (HIV) infection and other underlying systemic diseases. The cause of seborrheic dermatitis has not been established, but alterations in fatty acid metabolism, immunity, or infection with yeast such as *Malassezia* appear to be associated with seborrheic dermatitis.

No therapy is required as seborrheic dermatitis is generally asymptomatic and self-limited. For more adherent, thick scalp scale, warm mineral oil covered with a warm moist towel or gentle rubbing with a soft-bristled brush assists in removing scale. Olive oil may worsen seborrheic dermatitis as it may facilitate growth of *Plasmodium ovale* and promote inflammation (37). Parents should be instructed to comb gently if they wish to remove the scales in order to prevent alopecia. Topical antifungal or anti-inflammatory agents may be used judiciously.

Irritant Contact Dermatitis

Irritant contact dermatitis (ICD) or diaper dermatitis is common in newborns. It is easily recognized as an erythematous rash in the diaper area (**Fig. 61.7**) affecting the perianal skin and

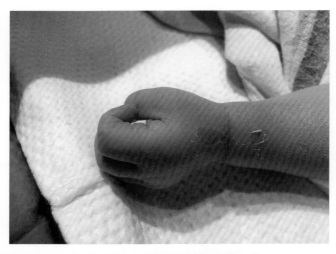

FIGURE 61.5 Sucking blister on the wrist of a well newborn.

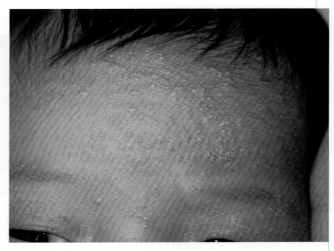

FIGURE 61.6 Neonatal cephalic pustulosis, previously termed neonatal acne, will self-resolve over time.

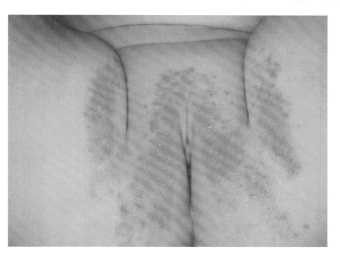

FIGURE 61.7 Diaper dermatitis is frequently due to contact with an irritant and spares creases.

convex surfaces with relative sparing of the inguinal creases due to decreased contact with irritants in those areas. ICD is caused by contact with moisture, sweat, urine, and stool exacerbated by occlusion and friction from the diaper.

Increased hydration of the stratum corneum makes the skin more susceptible to friction from the diaper material. Irritation from elevated pH caused by urinary ammonia disrupts the skin barrier (38–40). The potential for irritation is compounded in the presence of both urine and feces, as fecal proteases and lipases are activated in the alkaline urinary milieu. Breast-fed infants have been noted to have stools with lower pH, which may account for their decreased incidence of diaper dermatitis. Severe ICD can lead to Jacquet erosive dermatitis, which presents as painful erosions, often with heaped-up borders, and may resemble HSV infection (Fig. 61.8).

Though ICD is by far the most common culprit of diaper dermatitis, it should be distinguished from numerous other dermatologic conditions affecting the diaper area. ICD leaves the skin susceptible to secondary infection, especially with *Candida albicans*, *Staphylococcus aureus*, and *Streptococcus pyogenes*. Thus super-infection should be considered in recalcitrant diaper dermatitis or if other exam findings raise suspicion. *C. albicans* causes pustules on a "beefy" red base that, after rupture, form erosions surrounded

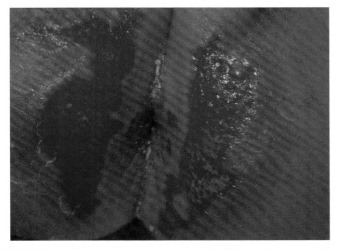

FIGURE 61.8 Ulcerations can occur as a result of irritant diaper dermatitis, especially in the more vulnerable skin of premature infants.

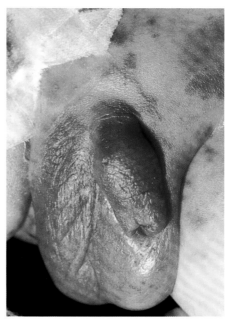

FIGURE 61.9 Bright "beefy" red diaper dermatitis that involves the inguinal and gluteal folds is suspicious for infection with *Candida albicans*. Often, there will be pustules that rupture and leave behind erosions with fine scale.

by fine superficial white scale and frequently involves the creases and folds of the skin (Fig. 61.9). *S. aureus* and *S. pyogenes* impetigo can present as pustules on a red base or by superficial erosions and crusting. The affected skin folds often have a shiny, wet, glossy appearance accompanied by malodor (Fig. 61.10A). Certain types of *S. aureus* produce an epidermolytic toxin, causing superficial bullae (bullous impetigo) (Fig. 61.10B).

The differential diagnosis of ICD includes psoriasis, seborrheic dermatitis, secondary syphilis, Langerhans cell histiocytosis, acrodermatitis enteropathica (AE), and cystic fibrosis (due in part to diarrhea and nutritional deficiency) (41). However, while the appearance of the rash in the diaper area can mimic diaper dermatitis, these conditions often affect the skin outside the diaper area or have additional exam findings.

The mainstay of ICD treatment is decreasing excessive moisture to the skin and decreasing contact with feces and the organisms it carries. Frequent diaper changes also help to minimize wetness and are a proven method to treat diaper dermatitis (42). Disposable diapers are superior to cloth diapers in decreasing skin wetness and maintaining an acidic skin pH because cloth diapers do not absorb and wick away moisture as well, though they are more economical and environmentally friendly (43,44). In developing countries, disposable diapers may help prevent spread of infectious diseases within nurseries (42). More evidence is needed for diaper-free time, which may be more cost-effective but impractical in certain situations.

Barrier ointments are used primarily to decrease contact time between the skin and urine or feces. Common over-the-counter zinc oxide containing products, while creating a strong barrier, are sticky and difficult to remove, so care should be taken not to cause more irritation to the skin during diaper changes, as complete removal of the barrier cream is unnecessary. Cholestyramine compounded in Aquaphor helps neutralize bile acids and is effective in erosive dermatitis (45).

There is no definitive evidence to suggest the superiority of water-moistened cloths, soap and water, or modern wet wipes. A mild alkaline gel cleanser is the preferred soap when needed, and irritating additions such as fragrances and dyes should be avoided.

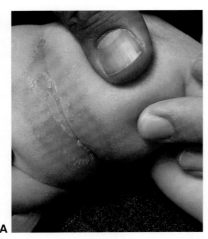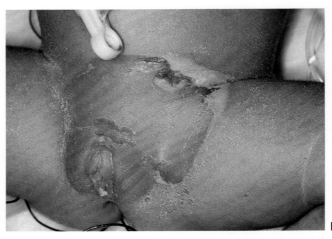

FIGURE 61.10 A: The wet, glossy appearance within the intertriginous folds of the upper thigh is secondary to *S. aureus* and *S. pyogenes* impetigo, similar to that also seen in diaper dermatitis. **B:** Bullous impetigo can be seen in exotoxin-producing strains of *S. aureus*.

Low- to mid-potency topical corticosteroids may be needed for short periods of time when inflammation is significant. However, higher-potency topical steroids should generally be avoided on thin perineal skin due to the occlusive nature of diapers, which increase the risk of systemic absorption and cutaneous atrophy, striae, cutaneous and systemic infection, adrenal suppression, and Cushing syndrome. Combination antifungal–steroid compounds such as Lotrisone and Mycolog II contain high- to mid-potency topical corticosteroid (betamethasone dipropionate and triamcinolone 0.1%, respectively). They have no use in treating neonatal skin conditions involving the diaper area; the FDA has issued a warning for the former medication in this context. As reflected in the literature, use of high-potency topical steroids for diaper dermatitis is likely more common in countries in which these medications are available without a prescription. Two cases of iatrogenic Cushing syndrome due to high-potency topical steroid use for diaper dermatitis were associated with disseminated CMV infection leading to death, presumably due to systemic immune suppression (46).

Fungal or bacterial superinfection can be managed with appropriate topical antimicrobial agents (47). Use of powders also should be avoided due to risk of inhalation. Topical antifungal agents such as nystatin, clotrimazole, miconazole, or ketoconazole can be safely applied to newborn skin. Bacterial infection generally responds to mupirocin. Over the counter, bacitracin and neomycin carry a high risk of allergic contact sensitization and should be avoided. For more severe bacterial and fungal infections, oral agents may be considered.

Atopic Dermatitis

Atopic dermatitis, frequently referred to as eczema, is a pruritic dermatitis occurring in up to 20% of children. Newborns with atopic dermatitis develop ill-defined red, itchy scaly patches, papules, and plaques (Fig. 61.11). The distribution may be focal, often with facial accentuation due to irritation from saliva and food, or more widespread, with relative sparing of the diaper area. The distribution in newborns is more commonly over extensor surfaces, whereas it is more commonly seen in older children in flexural areas. The occlusive nature of diapers provides hydration and can provide relative protection against atopic dermatitis in this area, although concomitant irritant dermatitis or seborrheic dermatitis may be present in this area. In the young infant, pruritus may not be evident because of lack of scratching but may manifest as wiggling of the body or rubbing of the scalp. There are diagnostic criteria for atopic dermatitis (48). Common patterns noted in atopic dermatitis that are not necessary for the diagnosis include a family

history of atopy, asthma, or atopic dermatitis, as well as concurrent food hypersensitivity in the child. The etiology of atopic dermatitis is complex and multifactorial, related to genetics, impaired skin barrier function, aberrant innate and adaptive immune system function, and decreased production of antimicrobial peptides by keratinocytes (48). Atopic dermatitis leaves the skin vulnerable to coinfection. Colonization with *S. aureus* is common and likely exacerbates the eczema. Coinfection with viruses is also common, including herpes simplex virus, coxsackie virus, molluscum contagiosum virus, and human papillomavirus. Mainstays of treatment include liberal emollient and moisturizer use, low- to mid-potency topical steroids, topical calcineurin inhibitors, topical crisaborole, diluted bleach baths, avoidance of irritants, and prevention and treatment of secondary infections.

COMMON BIRTHMARKS IN NEONATES AND INFANTS

Nevus Simplex

Nevus sebaceus (NS) is a type of capillary malformation that can appear as red midline patches on the nape ("stork bite"), eyelids ("angel kisses"), and glabella that are more noticeable with crying

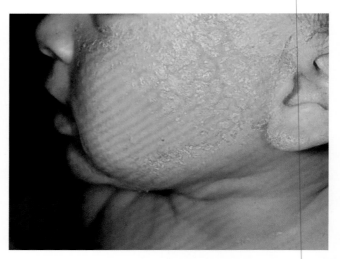

FIGURE 61.11 Atopic eczema is commonly found on the face due to irritation from saliva and food.

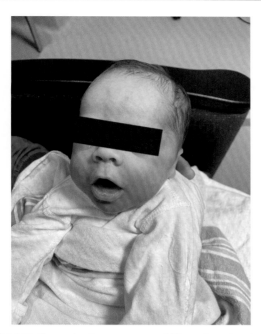

FIGURE 61.12 Nevus simplex appears as midline red patches that usually fade with time, though some glabellar patches will persist into adulthood.

(Fig. 61.12). They are found in at least 50% of newborns and fade with time, though most nuchal patches and some glabellar patches persist into adulthood. They may be prone to an intermittent dermatitis that can be managed with moisturizer and a low-potency topical steroid if needed. Extensive NS are rarely associated with syndromes (e.g., Beckwith-Wiedemann), which tend to have a presentation much more dramatic than the NS themselves. Parents of babies with NS should be reassured.

Dermal Melanocytosis

Dermal melanocytosis arises as a result of increased numbers of melanocytes within the dermis and appears most commonly as blue-gray patches on the mid dorsal aspect of the body (Fig. 61.13). The lower back and buttock are the most commonly affected areas. The posterior shoulders, upper arms and dorsal hands and feet may be affected as well. They are very common in

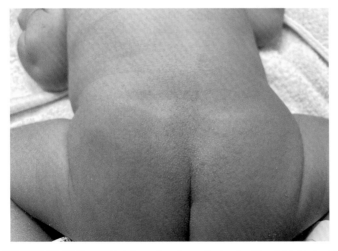

FIGURE 61.13 Congenital dermal melanocytosis should not be confused with bruising.

newborns of color and should not be confused with child abuse. Dermal melanocytosis tends to fade on the buttock and back over years but may be more persistent on the extremities. Extensive dermal melanocytosis has been described as an early sign of GM1 gangliosidosis. The historic term mongolian spot should be avoided.

Infantile Hemangioma

Hemangiomas of infancy are the most common vascular tumor of infancy, seen in 4% to 5% of the population, (49) and more commonly in premature, low birth weight, and firstborn babies. They consist of proliferating endothelial-like cells (50–53). They may be classified as superficial, deep, mixed (superficial and deep) based on depth, and localized (focal), indeterminate, segmental, and multifocal (>5) based on size and distribution. IHs arise as a precursor lesion seen as a patch of vasoconstricted pallor, bruise-like macule, or pink telangiectatic patch (Fig. 61.14A and B). They then undergo a proliferative phase, in which a bright "strawberry" red plaque develops in superficial IH, and involutional phases of development (Fig. 61.14C). The most rapid growth of an infantile hemangioma (IH) occurs between 5.5 and 7.5 weeks of age (54). This proliferative growth principally occurs in volume and not radial growth, and 80% of IHs irrespective of depth or subtype reach their maximal size by 3 months (55). Most IHs end the growth phase by 9 months, although deep, mixed, and segmental IHs may demonstrate a prolonged proliferative phase (56). Deep IHs tend to show a delayed onset of growth by about 1 month and may proliferate for a month longer than superficial IHs (55). Involution takes place over a period of years, but recent studies have shown that involution ends at a median age of 3 years and 92% by 4 years (57). Sometimes, infants are at risk for cosmetic and functional impairment from the IH, and it is important to distinguish these cases early in life and refer for intervention to minimize complications.

Large segmental IHs occurring in specific locations on the body, especially the head and neck, lumbosacral, perineal, and lower extremity regions have been associated with regional congenital anomalies (Fig. 61.15). Since Frieden et al. described PHACE syndrome in 1996, investigators have been examining the association of IHs with regional congenital anomalies (58). PHACE syndrome is a neurocutaneous syndrome characterized by the following features: posterior fossa abnormalities, hemangiomas, arterial malformations, cardiac defects, and eye anomalies. IHs in PHACE syndrome are large facial plaque segmental IHs. PHACE syndrome is seen mostly in girls and term infants. Cerebrovascular anomalies are the most common extracutaneous findings associated with PHACE syndrome, followed by structural cerebral anomalies and coarctation of the aorta (59). Because of these cerebrovascular anomalies, infants with PHACE syndrome are at increased risk of stroke. Infants with large facial segmental IHs should be evaluated with magnetic resonance imaging (MRI) and magnetic resonance angiogram (MRA) of the head and neck, echocardiogram, and an ophthalmologic examination (60).

Three acronyms are commonly used to describe congenital anomalies associated with lumbosacral, perineal, and lower extremity segmental IHs. These include the following: PELVIS syndrome (perineal hemangiomas, external genitalia malformations, lipomyelomeningocele, vesicorenal abnormalities, imperforate anus, and skin tags) (61), SACRAL syndrome (spinal dysraphism, anogenital anomalies, cutaneous anomalies, renal and urologic anomalies, and angioma of lumbosacral localization) (62), and LUMBAR (lower body infantile hemangiomas and other skin defects, urogenital anomalies and ulceration, myelopathy, bony deformities, anorectal malformations and arterial anomalies, and renal anomalies) (63). Infants with large sacral IHs should be screened for internal manifestations with a lumbosacral MRI (64).

THE NEWBORN INFANT

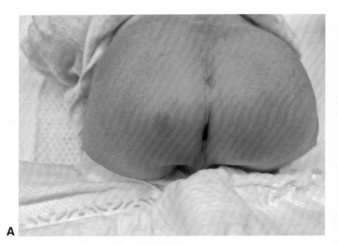

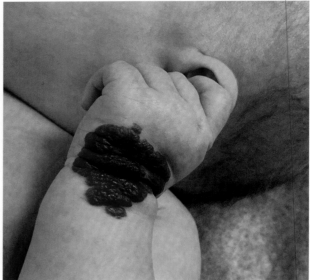

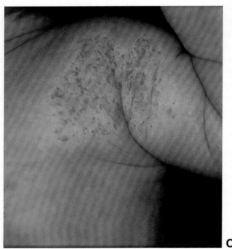

FIGURE 61.14 **A:** The precursory lesion to an infantile hemangioma is often a vasoconstricted area of pallor, or pink telangiectatic macule or patch. **B:** Rapid proliferation occurs, leading to a bright red papule or plaque. **C:** Finally, involution occurs.

Isolated IHs can require specialist care for treatment if they develop complications such as ulceration, gastrointestinal bleeding, or visceral involvement. The most common complication of IHs is

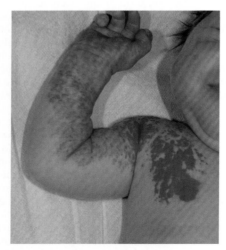

FIGURE 61.15 **Large segmental infantile hemangiomas can be associated with congenital anomalies, as with PHACE syndrome.** Posterior fossa malformations, Hemangioma, Arterial anomalies of the head and neck, Cardiac abnormalities, and Eye abnormalities.

ulceration, occurring in 15% to 25% of infants (65,66). Any infant with complications such as ulceration should be referred for specialist care for treatment. Large size, segmental distribution, and location on the neck, anogenital area, and lip are risk factors for ulceration (65,67). The greatest risk for cutaneous ulceration occurs during the proliferation phase in the first few months of life. Many IHs develop an ominous white color on the surface (in contrast to the normal graying and central fading), which is thought to be a predictor for ulceration (68) (Fig. 61.16A). Ulceration causes pain, bleeding, scarring, and sometimes infection (Fig. 61.16B). Gastrointestinal bleeding can also occur, though rarely, with isolated IHs and more commonly is seen in two clinical scenarios: multiple cutaneous IH and large segmental IH (69–71).

Only 30% of infants have more than one IH, and only 3% have more than five IHs. Infants under the age of 5 months with five or more IHs should be screened with an abdominal ultrasound, as 16% of these patients may have liver hemangiomas, which can lead to high output cardiac failure and consumptive hypothyroidism (69). The most common location for visceral hemangiomas is the liver, although the gastrointestinal tract, brain, mediastinum, and lung may also be involved (72).

The majority of IHs may be managed conservatively with watchful waiting, utilizing parental education and photographs. Complicated IHs at risk for ulceration and cosmetic and functional compromise should be treated early in life, ideally before or during the most rapid proliferative period to help reduce the risk of complications. Factors to consider include IH subtype, patient age,

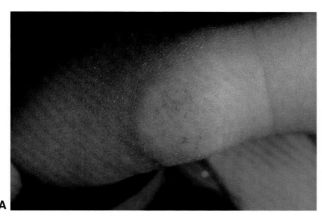 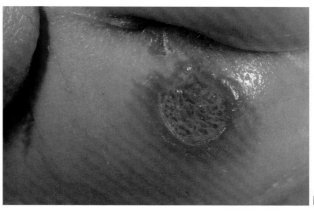

FIGURE 61.16 A: Ulceration is sometimes preceded by a black eschar or rapid white pallor to the surface. Ulceration is more likely to occur in hemangiomas with large size, segmental distribution, or location on the neck, anogenital area **(B)**, and lip. High-risk and ulcerated IH should be referred to a specialist due to risk of pain, bleeding, scarring, and infection.

anatomic location, and lesion size. Bulky IH on the upper eyelids can cause lid lag and those adjacent to the eyes can block the visual axis, leading to impaired development of the visual cortex. IH near the ear can have a similar effect by blocking hearing, and involvement of external ear and nasal cartilage can lead to disfigurement and lead to conductive hearing loss and respiratory difficulties, respectively. IH on the lip are prone to ulceration and can impair feeding in addition to leading to significant facial differences that are known to affect psychosocial wellbeing at a young age. Treatments include topical and systemic medical agents, laser, and surgery.

Systemic corticosteroids (prednisone or prednisolone) were the mainstay of treatment for complicated IH, but more recently, the use of propranolol has become more widespread. Propranolol is administered orally at a dose of 2 mg/kg/d divided two to three times per day. Although propranolol is generally safe, adverse effects such as bradycardia, hypotension, asymptomatic hypoglycemia, and bronchospasm have been described. Starting the medication at a lower dose with gradual upward titration and close monitoring for possible complications is recommended. Other delivery methods for propranolol such as intralesional injection have been employed with limited success for IHs (73). Other beta-blocking agents such as atenolol, nadolol, and acebutolol have been used off label (74–76). Topical timolol is used as well and is currently in clinical trials. Propranolol's mechanism of action in the treatment of IHs is unknown, but possible mechanisms include constriction of blood supply due to uninhibited alpha-receptor induced vasoconstriction, inhibition of angiogenesis, and induction of apoptosis (77,78).

Infants with high-risk IHs should be referred to specialty care no later than 4 weeks of age. IHs that have not adequately involuted by age 3 may be referred for a surgical consultation to prevent potential adverse psychological implications (57).

Pigmented Birthmarks

Pigmented birthmarks, including café au lait spots (CALs), congenital melanocytic nevi (CMN), and nevus depigmentosus, are very common and discussed below.

Nevus Sebaceus

NS is a common congenital hamartoma of the sebaceous glands. NS presents most commonly on the scalp as pink to yellow round, ovoid, or curvilinear rubbery alopecic plaques (Fig. 61.17). They become more raised, yellow, and cobblestoned over time under the influence of androgenetic hormones, though the alopecia is permanent due to lack of functional pilar adnexa. Some NS may present with a cerebriform or papillomatous morphology and may be mistaken for heterotopic brain tissue. Most NS occur on the head and neck and are isolated, benign findings. Rarely, extensive facial NS, especially those involving the midline, can be associated with underlying bony, neurologic, ocular, and palatal abnormalities (nevus sebaceus syndrome). In some instances, benign tumors (trichoblastoma, syringocystadenoma papilliferum) and malignant tumors (most commonly indolent basal cell carcinoma, rarely squamous cell carcinoma or adnexal carcinomas) arise within NS, prompting prophylactic surgical excision of these lesions before puberty. The incidence of malignant tumors arising within NS is subject to some controversy, as is the need for prophylactic

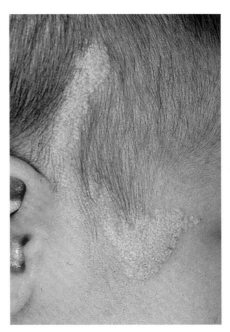

FIGURE 61.17 Nevus sebaceus is a common benign lesion usually seen in the scalp, though larger lesions may be associated with nevus sebaceus syndrome.

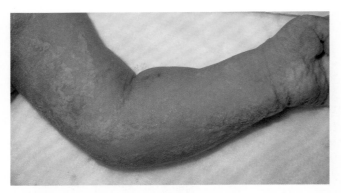

FIGURE 61.18 Epidermal nevus at birth presenting as blaschkoid bands of spongiform hyperkeratosis.

removal, which is often discouraged due to lack of evidence toward improved outcomes (79). Monitoring is usually reasonable, though management should be individualized to the patient. Large scalp lesions may be removed in infancy because the skin of the scalp is more elastic and the scalp is easier to close at a younger age.

Epidermal Nevi

Epidermal nevi are keratinocyte hamartomas that present as verrucous or hyperkeratotic pink, tan, or brown papules and plaques that develop within the lines of Blaschko in a curvilinear pattern (**Fig. 61.18**). They can become more raised and textured over time. Typically, the lesions are solitary and unilateral but may also be multifocal or bilateral and rarely associated with underlying neurologic deficits, ocular findings, skeletal dysplasia, and cardiac abnormalities (epidermal nevus syndrome). Epidermal nevi are thought to result from in utero somatic mutations in keratinocytes. Mutations occurring early in development lead to more extensive skin involvement. Systemic involvement is likely due to mutations in ectodermal progenitor cells. Mutations have been identified in the genes encoding RAS, fibroblast growth factor receptor 3 (FGFR3), phosphatidylinositol-4,5-bisphosphate 3-kinase catalytic subunit alpha (PIK3CA), and keratins. Genotype–phenotype correlations have not yet been deciphered. Epidermal nevi resulting from mutations in keratin 1 and/or keratin 10 demonstrate epidermolytic hyperkeratosis (EHK) on histopathology, and rarely, females with gonadal tissue involvement can give birth to infants with systemic EHK.

DEVELOPMENTAL ANOMALIES IN THE NEONATE

Cysts in neonates are generally benign and may be transient, as with milia, or persistent, as with cysts due to developmental anomalies, including dermoid cysts and branchial cleft anomalies.

Aplasia Cutis Congenita

Aplasia cutis congenita (ACC) is congenital absence of the skin. It is a descriptive term; there are multiple underlying etiologies. The morphology can range from small and round to large and jagged with irregular borders depending on the cause. Some authors categorize ACC into the following groups: (a) ACC of the scalp without multiple systemic anomalies; (b) ACC with associated limb abnormalities; (c) ACC with organoid and epidermal nevi; (d) ACC with overlying embryologic abnormalities; (e) ACC with associated fetus papyraceus or placental infarcts; (f) ACC associated with EB; (g) ACC localized to the extremities without blistering; (h) ACC caused by teratogens; and (i) ACC associated with malformation syndromes (80). Most infants have isolated benign scalp ACC (Group 1). Eighty percent of the lesions are near the parietal scalp whorl and 76% are solitary lesions. Up to one-third of cases of ACC have underlying defects in the bone, risk factors for which include midline vertex location, hair collar sign, and size greater than 5 cm (81). Further workup with MRI may be considered in some cases, especially in larger irregular ACC. Sometimes, ACC is partially healed at birth, giving variable morphologies from a small patch of alopecia to full-thickness ulceration with an underlying bony defect (**Fig. 61.19A and B**).

Dermoid Cysts and Sinuses

Dermoid cysts are common cysts composed of tissue of all three embryonic tissues along lines of fusion. They can occur in any cutaneous site but are most common on the head and neck, especially on the lateral eyebrow (82). Most are firm and fixed to the underlying bone. Dermoid cysts can be superficial, or they can have a deeper component that involves muscle and bone. They may remain unchanged or grow somewhat in size and occasionally become inflamed. Midline cysts should raise concern for a possible underlying connection with the central nervous system (CNS) or spinal dysraphism and prompt radiologic evaluation. An imaging study such as a CT scan or MRI is needed before operating on a midline lesion. Treatment is surgical excision.

Dermoid sinuses are far less common but are more likely to be associated with complications (83). They present along the nasal midline as a pit, classically with protruding hairs. The pit may

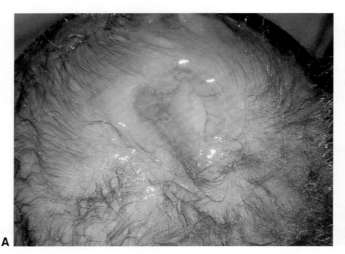
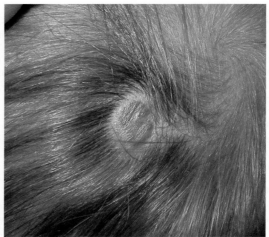

FIGURE 61.19 Cutis aplasia can show a full-thickness ulceration (A) or may be partially healed (B).

secrete keratinaceous debris or hairs, and bouts of inflammation or infection are not uncommon. There is a higher risk of intracranial connection than with dermoid cysts, and infection can lead to serious complications such as osteomyelitis and meningitis. Imaging studies are required with surgical management dependent on the findings.

Other Developmental Anomalies

Branchial cleft abnormalities can produce pits, nodules, and cysts along closure lines on the corresponding branchial arch of the face and neck and may have a deeper underlying component extending to bone. Therefore, excision should be left to an experienced surgeon. Others include accessory tragus (first branchial arch) in the preauricular region, midline clefts (first branchial arch), preauricular cysts (first branchial arch), lateral cervical cysts, sinuses, and fistulae (second branchial arch). Thyroglossal duct cysts occur in the midline neck and are as a result of failure of fusion of the thyroglossal duct. Bronchogenic cysts usually occur on the midline on the chest and develop as a result of abnormal development of the primitive foregut. They can drain mucous fluid. Median raphe cysts occur along the ventral surface of the penis and scrotum. They are thought to occur because of entrapped epidermal or urethral cells. If median raphe cysts enlarge or become infected, they can be surgically removed.

ERYTHEMATOUS SCALY RASHES

Psoriasis

Psoriasis presents as sharply demarcated thick salmon pink plaques with firmly adherent thick white (micaceous) scale. It can produce various cutaneous patterns such as guttate (teardrop) papules, pustules, and plaques. Psoriasis is often self-limited in infants and most often presents in the anogenital region in patients under the age of 2 years (84). In this region, the scale may be minimal. One can also see isolated nail and nailfold involvement. Rarely, newborns develop generalized pustular erythroderma with fever.

The cause of psoriasis is multifactorial with both genetic and environmental factors playing a role. Children with two psoriatic parents have an approximately 50% lifetime risk (85). Infection (*S. pyogenes*), cold weather, emotional stress, medications (beta-blockers, antimalarials), and withdrawal from systemic corticosteroids have all been shown to provoke psoriatic flares. Severe psoriasis in infancy should raise concern for a monogenic mutation.

A family history of psoriasis and "soft signs" of psoriasis (e.g., gluteal cleft fissures, nail pitting, geographic tongue, and rash in the umbilicus) are useful aids to diagnoses.

Medium-strength topical corticosteroids and topical calcineurin inhibitors are the mainstay of therapy for infantile psoriasis. Biologic treatments targeting T lymphocytes and associated cytokines have not been studied in infants.

Erythroderma

Erythroderma describes widespread erythema (>80% total body surface area) and can result from a number of inherited and acquired conditions. The differential diagnosis is broad and includes inflammatory conditions (atopic dermatitis, seborrheic dermatitis), neoplastic conditions (mastocytosis), infectious conditions (syphilis, herpes, *S. aureus*), metabolic conditions (methylmalonic aciduria, maple syrup urine disease, cobalamin deficiency), genetic skin diseases (ichthyoses, including Netherton syndrome), and immunodeficiency (severe combined immunodeficiency, common variable hypogammaglobulinemia). Erythroderma compromises skin barrier function with the risks of hypothermia, fluid imbalances, and sepsis. The diagnosis is guided by the history, exam,

and biopsy if needed. Supportive care is critical and involves intravenous fluids, liberal use of emollients, and incubators with warm humidified air. The caloric requirements of the infant are dramatically increased, and parenteral nutrition is sometimes required. Fissures may be treated with topical antibiotics such as mupirocin. Infants with signs of skin infection (e.g., crusting, oozing, malodor) and sepsis should have cultures and treated with appropriate systemic antibiotics.

Neonatal Lupus Erythematosus

Neonatal lupus erythematosus (NLE) may present as annular, red, scaly plaques resembling subacute cutaneous lupus erythematosus (SCLE), classically on the face in a periorbital distribution ("raccoon eyes") (Fig. 61.20). The rash can be purpuric and appear lacy. While the face, head, and neck are most commonly affected, photoprotected areas may also be involved. Systemic manifestations include hepatobiliary abnormalities (elevated aminotransferases, cholestasis, hepatomegaly, rarely splenomegaly), hematologic abnormalities (anemia, neutropenia, thrombocytopenia), and/or congenital heart block. Congenital complete atrioventricular heart block is the most life-threatening manifestation of NLE. It develops in the second trimester and requires a lifelong pacemaker in the majority of cases. Otherwise, most infants thrive and appear well, as the causative maternal autoantibodies are transient.

NLE occurs in newborns born to mothers with autoantibodies to Sjögren syndrome types A and B autoantigens (SS-A/anti-Ro and SS-B/anti-La antibodies, respectively) due to transplacental transfer (86). More recently, anti-U1RNP antibody has been implicated as well (87). The incidence of NLE in mothers with SS-A or SS-B antibodies, which can be found in systemic lupus erythematosus, Sjögren syndrome, rheumatoid arthritis, and undifferentiated connective tissue disorder or in asymptomatic patients, is approximately 2%. Recurrence rate is about 20% in subsequent pregnancies. Skin biopsy may assist in diagnosis. Histopathology shows vacuolar interface dermatitis with perivascular and perifollicular lymphocytes and increased mucin within the superficial and deep dermis. Newborns with NLE should receive special

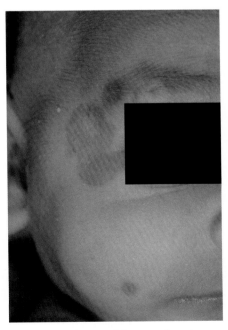

FIGURE 61.20 The rash of neonatal lupus erythematosus resembles that of subacute cutaneous lupus erythematosus (SCLE), as an annular, red, scaly plaque, usually on the face, head, and neck.

protection from ultraviolet radiation. Cutaneous NLE has an excellent prognosis with most symptoms resolving by 1 year of age, though telangiectasias, atrophy, and dyspigmentation may persist. Maternal hydroxychloroquine during pregnancy is thought to be cardioprotective for infants.

Inherited Conditions

Inherited causes of diffuse erythematous scaly rashes are discussed in the Genetics section below.

VESICULAR AND PUSTULAR ERUPTIONS

There are many common to uncommon benign inflammatory pustular eruptions in neonates. Infectious causes must be considered and investigated by history, physical examination, and laboratory tests. Langerhans cell histiocytosis and the genetic disorder incontinentia pigmenti must be considered as well.

Inflammatory Eruptions

Transient Neonatal Pustular Melanosis

Transient neonatal pustular melanosis is a less common, benign eruption occurring at birth in up to 0.2% to 0.6% of healthy newborns, and even more commonly in darker skin tones (88). The rash is characterized by superficial pustules on a nonerythematous base that easily rupture to form fine collarettes of scale that heal with residual hyperpigmented macules (Fig. 61.21). The pustules may rupture before birth, and the only finding may be small round scattered hyperpigmented macules. The most common sites are the head and neck folds. Pustules and scales resolve over 1 to 3 weeks; however, hyperpigmented macules can persist for several years. The fluid within the pustules is sterile and if examined would show neutrophils and rare eosinophils.

Infantile Acne

Infantile acne is far less common than neonatal cephalic pustulosis and is characterized by true open and closed comedones, papulopustules, and occasionally nodules and cysts on the cheeks, chin, and forehead, as seen in adolescent acne (Fig. 61.22). It develops most commonly in boys at 6 months of life, though onset may be much earlier, and resolves by 3 years of age (89). The etiology is attributed to transient increases in gonadal and adrenal hormone

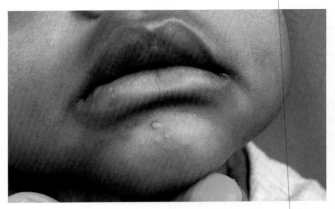

FIGURE 61.22 Infantile acne, as opposed to neonatal cephalic pustulosis, shows true comedones and often requires treatment to prevent scarring.

secretion. Treatment options include sodium sulfacetamide and/or low-strength benzoyl peroxide washes, topical antibiotics such as erythromycin or clindamycin, and topical retinoids. Babies with severe infantile acne may require oral antibiotics or oral isotretinoin to prevent scarring and should be referred to a dermatologist for management. Endocrine workup may be considered in severe persistent cases.

Acropustulosis of Infancy

Acropustulosis of infancy is an uncommon benign recurrent pustular eruption, occurring most commonly at 3 to 6 months of age. Infants develop pruritic pink papules on the palms and soles that quickly evolve into vesicles and pustules. Most infants are irritable and have pruritus. Pustules resolve in 7 to 14 days, leaving white scale, but tend to recur in crops in 2- to 4-week cycles. The cause of acropustulosis is unknown, though many infants with suspected acrodermatitis of infancy have scabies. It may represent a post-scabetic hypersensitivity reaction. Diagnostic evaluation should include a scabies preparation and bacterial and fungal cultures. Topical corticosteroids and oral antihistamines help to treat symptoms.

Eosinophilic Pustular Folliculitis

Eosinophilic pustular folliculitis is a rare condition in neonates and infants that leads to recurrent crops of very pruritic papules and pustules on the head and neck, especially the scalp, lasting approximately 1 week (90). The scalp can develop a yellow scale crust that resembles seborrheic dermatitis or impetigo. A smear of the pustule contents shows abundant eosinophils without bacteria or fungus. Due to the significant pruritus, infants should be treated with low- to mid-potency topical corticosteroids. Unlike that in adults, eosinophilic pustular folliculitis of infancy is not associated with HIV infection. The eruption typically resolves within the first year of life.

Infections

There are numerous viral, bacterial, and fungal infections that must be considered in neonates, who are particularly vulnerable to sepsis and do not always present with fevers, even when critically ill. Herpes simplex virus infection should always be on the differential diagnosis of skin vesicles in a newborn and will be discussed below. Infection with varicella-zoster virus must be considered in neonates with disseminated skin vesicles or dermatomal erosions or scarring with musculoskeletal hypoplasia. Congenital candidiasis can present with widespread erythema and pustules in addition to nail involvement with onychomycosis and paronychia, which can help distinguish Candida from other disseminated infec-

FIGURE 61.21 Transient neonatal pustular melanosis is a benign condition that starts as pustules on a nonerythematous base that easily rupture, leaving fine collarettes of scale that heal with small hyperpigmented macules. The various morphologies can be seen concurrently.

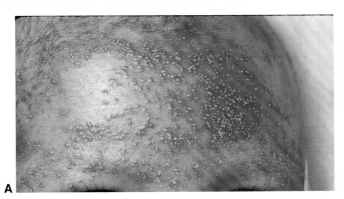 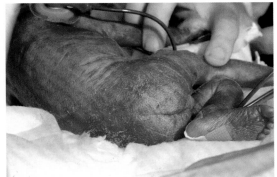

FIGURE 61.23 A: Congenital Candida can present as disseminated infection with widespread erythema and pustules. **B:** Candida can cause a burn-like dermatitis, especially in susceptible premature infants.

tions (Fig. 61.23A and B). In infants, scabies infestation must be considered with vesiculopapular eruptions, especially when the intertriginous areas, wrists, palms, ankles, and soles are heavily involved (Fig. 61.24A and B). The linear burrow is a pathognomonic sign of scabies but is not always visible. Other clues to scabies are intense pruritus and concomitant eczematous changes.

Herpes Simplex Infection

The primary cutaneous lesion of HSV is a vesicle on an erythematous base with a central dell. The vesicles are small, monomorphous, and clustered or grouped. Within 1 to 2 days, the vesicles develop into pustules and then form crusts (Fig. 61.25A and B). The border of a group of herpes vesicles appears scalloped. HSV in neonates can be acquired either congenitally or perinatally, leading to variable presentations and outcomes (21). It can occur to mothers both with and without a known history of HSV; primary infections acquired during pregnancy can be asymptomatic and cause more severe disease, as do active infections at the time of delivery. Congenital HSV acquired within the first two trimesters can result in intrauterine growth restriction, microcephaly, chorioretinitis, seizures, limb atrophy, and scars and ACC in additional to classic vesicles. Perinatal HSV acquired just before or at the time of delivery presents within the first week of life as infection localized to the skin, eyes, or mouth (SEM disease), disseminated disease, or CNS disease. Disseminated HSV presents as

septic shock and multiple organ failure. CNS disease presents as encephalitis. Localized disease can disseminate, and both disseminated and CNS disease can present without skin findings.

HSV infections are best diagnosed with a swab for HSV PCR obtained from the base of a vesicle, when possible, or viral culture. Direct immunofluorescence can be performed by unroofing a vesicle and scrapping the base of the vesicle. Skin biopsy can show signs of viral cytopathic effect in the epidermis. If HSV is suspected, swabs should be obtained immediately and empiric acyclovir started as soon as possible (see Chapter 46 Congenital Infections).

Staphylococcal Scalded Skin Syndrome

Staphylococcal scalded skin syndrome (SSSS) is a staphylococcal epidermolytic toxin (exfoliative toxins A and B)–mediated disease characterized by painful, diffuse redness of the skin with accentuation in flexural and periorificial areas (91). Common foci of staphylococcal infection or colonization include the nasopharynx, umbilicus, urinary tract, a cutaneous wound, and the conjunctivae. An obvious source is often lacking. These bacterial toxins cleave the cadherin protein desmoglein 1 within the granular layer located in the superficial epidermis, leading to a superficial split resembling a sunburn. Neonates are more susceptible to SSSS because of reduced renal clearance as well as lack of lifetime acquisition of antibodies to ET. Initial signs may include

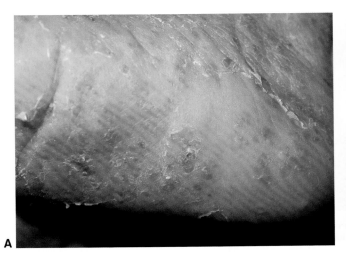 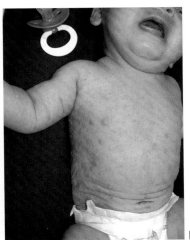

FIGURE 61.24 A: The serpiginous burrow pathognomonic of scabies infestation is found mostly on the palms, soles, wrists, and genitals. **B:** Generalized eruptions of scabies may include the scalp in neonates and can develop as early as 1 to 2 weeks of age.

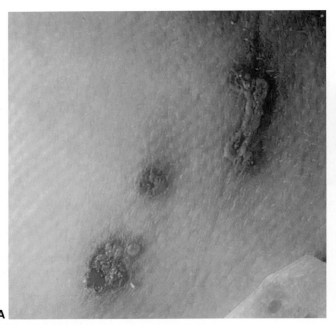
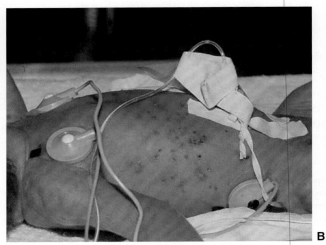

FIGURE 61.25 A and B: These classic HSV skin lesions show small, monomorphous clustered, and grouped vesicles on an erythematous base.

bright erythema of the face that then spreads to the body. In 2 to 5 days, the skin develops superficial peeling and fine flaky desquamation, especially in the flexural surfaces. Severely affected newborns can develop widespread sterile, flaccid blisters that easily rupture with gentle shear forces (Nikolsky sign), leaving large areas of open, weeping skin (Fig. 61.26). SSSS causes a distinctive crust and fissuring with a radial orientation around the eyes, mouth, and nose but without mucosal membrane involvement. Widespread skin breakdown puts newborns at risk for sepsis, fluid and electrolyte imbalance, and temperature instability. Prognosis is good with an overall mortality rate of 0.31% in hospitalized patients under 18 years of age, significantly less than the mortality in adults (92).

SSSS may be mistaken for a number of other disorders, including scarlet fever, bullous impetigo, EB, EHK, diffuse cutaneous mastocytosis, drug or viral eruption, and drug-induced toxic epidermal necrolysis (TEN). While both TEN and SSSS lead to skin pain and blistering, TEN results in full-thickness epidermal necrosis, with a blister cleavage plane at the dermal–epidermal junction. TEN is distinguished by its exuberant, hemorrhagic mucositis of two or more mucous membranes, deeper depth of blistering exposing the dermis, dusky appearance of the necrotic skin, distribution of skin findings with initiation of the rash on the face and trunk with spread toward the extremities, and a history of drug ingestion,. Distinguishing between these conditions is based on clinical exam and does not require a biopsy. Mortality rates are

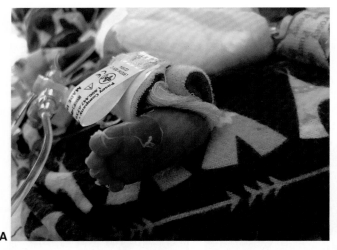
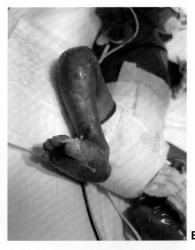

FIGURE 61.26 Staphylococcal scalded skin syndrome starts with diffuse erythroderma and positive Nikolsky sign with skin easily ruptured by gentle shear forces. A: The foot of a premature infant with SSSS shows diffuse erythema and superficial peeling of skin where physical contact was made for a routine capillary blood draw. **B:** Shows that same premature infant's foot 1 day later, with less erythema but continued superficial peeling and fine flaking. There is a transparent dressing over the knee of the infant.

much higher in TEN, and avoidance of the offending drug is crucial to prevent a recurrence. In SSSS, recovery usually is rapid once appropriate antibiotic therapy is begun. Parenteral therapy with nafcillin, oxacillin, vancomycin, or clindamycin should be administered promptly. In addition to treatment of the bacteria itself, clindamycin or linezolid are often added to aid in inhibition of toxin synthesis. Gentle skin care, emollients, pain control, IV fluids, and semiocclusive dressings to provide lubrication and minimize pain are also important. The use of Betadine and silver sulfadiazine should be avoided due to the risks of excessive absorption of these topic agents and their associated risks (thyroid dysfunction, kernicterus). Attention must also be turned to isolation procedures in the NICU to prevent an outbreak of SSSS. Healing occurs without scarring in 10 to 14 days although postinflammatory pigment alteration may be seen.

Purpura Fulminans

Purpura fulminans appears as widespread purpuric cutaneous lesions with disseminated intravascular coagulation (DIC) as a result of deficiencies of proteins C and S (93). The etiology of protein C and S deficiency can be either acquired on inherited. It can occur in the setting of overwhelming sepsis such as in Group B Streptococcal sepsis, so initiating investigation for sepsis and treatment with antibiotics is warranted while identifying the cause of purpura fulminans. However, it also occurs due to congenital deficiency of Protein C or Protein S, inherited as a homozygous recessive trait. The mainstay of acute treatment is correction of DIC, using blood products and protein C replacement therapy in combination with anticoagulation. Ongoing treatment is recommended for congenital Protein C deficiency.

Neoplastic

Langerhans Cell Histiocytosis

Langerhans cells are skin antigen-presenting cells derived from the bone marrow. LCH is a malignant condition that results from abnormal clones of Langerhans cells within the skin, internal organs, or both. Infants with LCH can develop a range of cutaneous findings, including a seborrheic dermatitis–like rash, crusted papules, shiny red to purple hemangioma-like papules, pustules, vesicles, bullae, petechiae, purpura, and nodules (Fig. 61.27A and B). The presence of multiple morphologies is a clue to the diagnosis. Lesions can occur in the "seborrheic areas" (scalp, face, and flexural areas) and extremities, including the palms and soles. Cutaneous features of LCH often precede systemic signs (e.g., fever, hepatosplenomegaly, lymphadenopathy, anemia), and longitudinal care of these patients is required.

A high index of suspicion is required for diagnosis, as LCH can mimic numerous benign conditions, including seborrheic dermatitis and IHs. A skin biopsy is mandatory if there is concern for LCH; classic histopathologic and immunohistochemical patterns are diagnostic. Acral vesicles and bullae must be differentiated from bullous impetigo, scabies, and syphilis. If scabies is suspected, a scrape and prep with mineral oil or KOH can be undertaken and may show adult scabies, eggs, or scybala (feces).

All infants with LCH should have an evaluation for systemic involvement (hematologic, pulmonary, hepatic, renal, and skeletal screening) (94), and they should be followed closely, because extracutaneous relapses may occur months to years after diagnosis. Infants with systemic involvement should be followed by pediatric hematology and oncology.

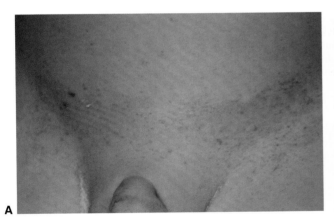

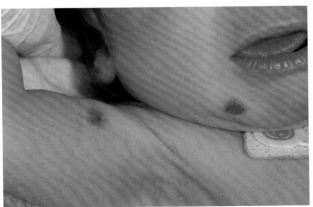

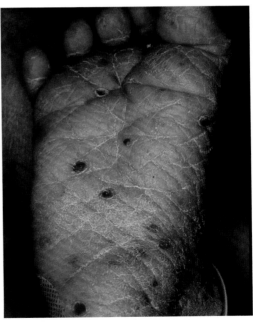

FIGURE 61.27 Skin findings in Langerhans cell histiocytosis (LCH) can be varied, including seborrheic dermatitis–like rash (**A**), crusted papules (**B**), as seen at birth on the sole of this neonate's foot and (**C**), regressing on this neonate's chin and arm, among many other presentations.

SUPERFICIAL PAPULES AND DERMAL TUMORS

Papules and superficial tumors in neonates and infants can result from a number of benign etiologies, though entities with potential systemic involvement and malignant behavior must be considered as well.

Juvenile Xanthogranuloma

Juvenile xanthogranuloma (JXG) is a common benign non–Langerhans cell histiocytosis seen in infants and children. Typically, JXG appears as single or multiple discrete firm pink to yellow papules on the head and trunk (**Fig. 61.28A and B**). Most JXG are congenital or appear within the first year of life, though some arise later (95,96). Solitary lesions are most common, but patients may have multiple lesions. Lesions resolve spontaneously over a period of months to several years, leaving few cutaneous sequelae. Hyperpigmentation and atrophic scars remain in some patients. Periocular JXG or multiple JXG should raise the suspicion of intraocular lesions, which can lead to hyphema and blindness, and these infants should be referred to an ophthalmologist. However, a 2018 meta-analysis suggests that the risk of intraocular involvement is extremely low (0.24%) and that most patients have ocular symptoms or known ocular disease at the time of presentation to dermatology (96). JXG in patients with neurofibromatosis type I can be associated with juvenile chronic myeloid leukemia and warrants a workup with blood counts and evaluation by hematology. Rarely, JXG can be systemic. Systemic JXG refers to involvement of two or more internal organs, including the liver, spleen, lungs, CNS, and eyes, usually with skin involvement (95,97). It may be indolent, self-resolving, or fatal and warrants management by hematology or oncology. Systemic JXG seems to be associated with multiple JXG, but the risk in patients with multiple JXG is not known, and formal screening guidelines do not exist. Some authors suggest that the presence of two or more cutaneous JXG is an indication for screening (97). However, a 2018 meta-analysis suggests an extremely low risk of systemic JXG (0.75%), though patients with multiple cutaneous JXG are overrepresented (96). Cutaneous findings usually precede systemic symptoms, so monitoring patients with multiple JXGs is prudent.

Mastocytosis

Mastocytosis is a heterogeneous condition that can present as solitary mastocytomas, urticaria pigmentosa (UP), systemic mastocytosis, and mast cell leukemia. In children, the former two presentations represent the majority of cases, and life-threatening systemic involvement is rare. Adult mastocytosis, by contrast, is far more aggressive and concerning. Solitary mastocytomas can present as large solitary orange-brown plaques or nodules. UP presents as hyperpigmented golden-brown macules, papules, and nodules on the face, scalp, trunk, and extremities, which can form wheals with rubbing (Darier sign). Although this sign is characteristic of mast cell disease, other conditions such as leukemia cutis can form wheals when rubbed. Thus, skin biopsy should be done if the diagnosis is in doubt. In some instances, frank bullae develop, especially on the palms and soles. Most cases of UP are congenital or develop in the first year of life, though onset can occur in childhood or adolescence (98). Cutaneous involvement gradually resolves by an average of 10 years of age, but many cases persist through adolescence. Systemic mastocytosis occurs in less than 2% of patients with cutaneous mastocytosis, most of whom present with diffuse cutaneous involvement with infiltration, thickening, and blistering (Fig. 61.29). However, systemic mastocytosis can also occur with minimal cutaneous involvement. Flushing, diarrhea, respiratory distress, tachycardia, hypotension, lymphadenopathy, and/or hepatosplenomegaly should prompt evaluation for systemic mastocytosis with serum tryptase levels (to assess overall mast cell burden), blood counts, and abdominal ultrasound. If abnormalities are present, patients should be referred to hematology, oncology, or mast cell disorder specialist, and bone scan and bone marrow biopsy should be considered.

The utility of EpiPens is debated. The risk of anaphylaxis appears to be very low in healthy children with UP (98). Parents should be educated regarding triggers of mast cell degranulation including opiates, radiocontrast dyes, citrus foods, and bee stings. Antihistamines such as hydroxyzine (Atarax) and diphenhydramine (Benadryl) can help control pruritus.

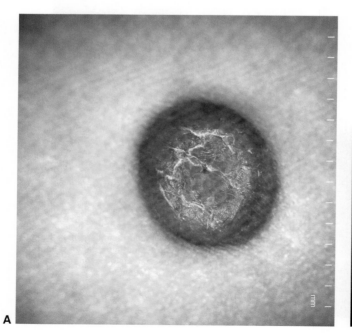

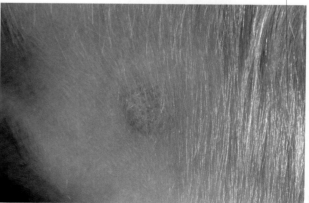

FIGURE 61.28 Juvenile xanthogranulomas (JXG) presents as a firm pink papule (A) that becomes *yellow* as histiocytes become lipidized (B).

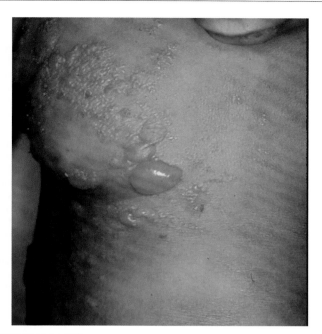

FIGURE 61.29 Diffuse cutaneous mastocytosis can be associated with systemic symptoms.

NODULES

Nodules refer to deeper palpable skin lesions and have a wide range of benign and malignant causes.

Malignant Causes of Nodules

Multiple Red-Blue Nodules ("Blueberry Muffin Baby")

The "blueberry muffin" presentation of multiple violaceous to red macule to nodules is caused by infiltrative conditions in the skin. The differential diagnosis includes leukemia cutis, extramedullary hematopoiesis, Langerhans cell histiocytosis, neuroblastoma, congenital syphilis, congenital toxoplasmosis, and erythroblastosis fetalis. Skin biopsy is necessary to help elucidate the cause and guide further workup and management.

Infantile Myofibromatosis

Infantile myofibromatosis, so called because the cells within the tumor exhibit characteristics of both smooth muscle cells and fibroblasts, is a mesenchymal disorder characterized by firm nodules palpated within the subcutaneous fat (Fig. 61.30A). The overlying skin can be either purplish or normal in color, and these nodules are usually located on the head, neck, and trunk (99). If the lesion is not palpated, the purple color can sometimes be confused for a deep/subcutaneous hemangioma. Often necrosis in the center of the nodule is visible, whether with the eye or with ultrasound (Fig. 61.30B). Bony involvement is often difficult to distinguish on radiograph from other osteolytic lesions, thus is best confirmed through pathology (100). While rare, infantile myofibromatosis is the most common fibrous tumor of infancy, accounting for 35% of soft tissue tumors in newborns (100). The tumor itself is benign; however, depth and visceral involvement can cause complications.

Infantile myofibromatosis exists in three classifications, solitary, multicentric without visceral involvement, and rarely multicentric with visceral involvement. When confined to the skin and bones, these nodules will mostly spontaneous regress in 1 to 2 years (101). Visceral involvement has very poor prognosis; thus, when multicentric infantile myofibromatosis is diagnosed, the patient may require further imaging to determine visceral involvement. When the viscera are involved, the tumors can lead to failure to thrive, infection, hemorrhage, or obstruction. Due to the high mortality associated with visceral involvement, surgical excision and chemotherapy have been proposed in treatment, and the successful use of methotrexate and vinblastine has been reported (101,102).

Neonatal Soft Tissue Sarcomas

Benign vascular tumors are common in infancy and at times difficult to distinguish from more malignant soft tissue tumors. Soft tissue sarcomas of the neonatal period are exceedingly rare, with incidence rising with age (103). Malignant lesions such as rhabdomyosarcoma, infantile fibrosarcoma, and malignant rhabdoid tumors are often very locally aggressive and, in the case of rhabdomyosarcoma, have the propensity to metastasize. Treatment depends largely on diagnosis and propensity to invasion of neurovascular structures and organs in addition to the presence of or propensity toward metastasis.

About half of soft tissue sarcomas are rhabdomyosarcomas, with only about 1% to 2% of cases congenital and another 5% to 10% diagnosed under a year (103). It most commonly presents in the head and neck, genitourinary tract, and extremities and is unfortunately very difficult to distinguish on exam or via imaging techniques from vascular lesions. Thus, atypical and rapidly growing masses should be biopsied for diagnosis. Treatment is generally a combination of chemotherapy and radiotherapy, with surgical resection when possible. Unfortunately, treatment is nuanced due

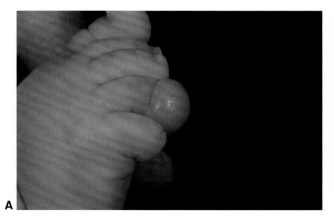
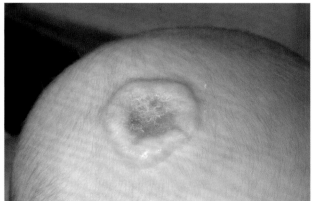

FIGURE 61.30 A: This digital fibroma is a benign tumor. **B:** This solitary giant infantile myofibroma displays central necrosis.

to the side effects of therapy and prognosis is rather poor, with 5-year survival about 38% to 44% (103).

Conversely, infantile fibrosarcomas have the best outcome, with 5-year survival of about 83% to 94% (104). Infantile fibrosarcomas present as rapidly growing noninflammatory, often vascular soft tissue masses, generally in the extremities (103). Chemotherapy is generally effective, with surgical excision only after treatment failure, due to the often disfiguring outcomes of primary surgical treatment.

Nonmalignant Nodules
Subcutaneous Fat Necrosis

Subcutaneous fat necrosis presents as red-purple, indurated subcutaneous nodules or plaques on the extremities, trunk, or buttocks during the first weeks of life (105) classically in pressure bearing areas, though the cheeks can be affected as well. It has been attributed to trauma, shock, cold, and asphyxia and can be seen in NICUs, especially in cases of infants who have undergone whole body cooling for hypoxic–ischemic encephalopathy. Infants appear healthy, although subcutaneous fat necrosis has been associated with hypercalcemia and laboratory monitoring is recommended periodically until 6 months of age. Lesions spontaneously resolve over a period of weeks to months. Rarely, sterile abscesses form with attendant atrophy and scarring. The sterile abscesses should not be drained.

Sclerema Neonatorum

Extensive subcutaneous fat necrosis is referred to as sclerema neonatorum and is more prone to happen in preterm or severely ill term infants, but is rarely seen with modern NICU care. The extremities may be involved at first, but generalized involvement occurs quickly within 3 to 4 days. When it affects the chest wall and torso, it can cause rigidity and difficulty with ventilation. If the infant survives, scleromatous skin changes resolve within about 3 weeks. The cause is unknown. Other than treating any associated illness, no specific therapy is indicated.

Vascular Anomalies

See section below.

DISORDERS OF PIGMENTATION (BROWN SPOTS/WHITE SPOTS)

Most irregularities in pigmentation are normal; however, pigment alterations can be the first indicator of an underlying inherited genetic skin condition. Hyperpigmentation or hypopigmentation occurring in whorls or in straight lines is thought to be a result of genetic mosaicism. Newborns with extensive alterations in skin pigment following the lines of Blaschko should be evaluated closely for associated extracutaneous defects.

Brown Spots
Café Au Lait Spots

CALs are round, ovoid, or geometric tan to brown macules or patches with crisp smooth or feathery borders. They can be quite large and involve a large surface area of the body (segmental CALs). They are more common in heavily pigmented children and in children with light skin and red or blond hair (106). CALs result from increased melanin content of the basal melanocytes and keratinocytes. The number and size of CALs increase during infancy and early childhood. Although 19% of normal children have CALs, they are seen in increased numbers in several genetic conditions. Six or more CALs larger than 0.5 cm in prepubescent children is one of the diagnostic criteria for neurofibromatosis type 1 (NF1) and should prompt additional workup. Crowe sign (axillary and inguinal freckling) is another diagnostic feature of NF1. Plexiform neurofibromas, which are pathognomonic of NF1, may be misdiagnosed as CALs but are a darker color and have underlying substance, ill-defined borders, and overlying hypertrichosis. Segmental CAL is associated with McCune-Albright syndrome. The differential diagnosis of a segmental CAL includes Becker nevus, which is found most commonly on the trunk or shoulder of males and may develop hypertrichosis under the influence of androgens.

Congenital Melanocytic Nevi

CMN appear at birth or within the first week of life and are thought to occur in 1% of infants (105,107) and represent benign clonal proliferations of melanocytes. CMN typically appear as small to large brown plaques with terminal hair growth though they may be lighter in color and flatter in some instances. CMN encompasses "birthmark moles" of all sizes including those formerly referred to as giant hairy nevus (108) (Fig. 61.31A). CMN are categorized by projected adult size: small less than 1.5 cm, medium 1.5 to 20 cm, and large/giant ≥20 cm.

Certain characteristics are associated with risk of melanoma in patients with CMN: (a) melanoma risk increases with the size of the nevus and may be as high as 5% to 15% in large/giant CMN (107); (b) the risk in small, single CMN is likely comparable to that of an acquired melanocytic nevus; (c) melanoma in large CMN may arise earlier; (d) satellite nevi are a marker for melanoma risk (108); (e) melanoma risk is greatest for infants with large CMN located on the trunk, large CMN greater than 40 cm, and multiple satellite nevi (109); and (f) melanoma may arise within CMN or within the brain. More recently, data have been published suggesting that the presence of CNS anomalies on MRI of the brain and spinal cord is associated with melanoma risk (107). Pathogenic NRAS mutations have been identified in melanomas arising within CMN, in contrast to BRAF (proto-oncogene B-Raf) mutations in other melanomas (107,110). Therefore, these melanomas may not be amenable to treatment with B-RAF inhibitors.

CMN may rarely develop associated nonmelanocytic tumors, including rhabdomyosarcoma and liposarcoma, and benign melanocytic tumors such as proliferative nodules and growths of undifferentiated spindle cells that can mimic melanoma (111,112). Proliferative nodules can show worrisome features, including rapid growth, hemorrhage, and ulceration and should be evaluated closely and biopsied to rule out melanoma (Fig. 61.31B). Histologic criteria have been developed to differentiate these nodules from malignant melanoma (112). An experienced pathologist should evaluate these specimens to avoid unnecessary worry and treatment. There is no evidence that prophylactic excision of CMN decreases melanoma risk or improves outcomes (107); cosmetic outcome of large CMN excision is generally poor.

Neurocutaneous melanosis (NCM) describes melanocytic proliferations within the leptomeninges and the brain parenchyma in patients with CMN that may be asymptomatic or associated with symptoms. Risk factors include large/giant size and multiple satellite nevi. Although formal screening criteria have not been established, experts recommend obtaining a baseline MRI of the leptomeninges, brain parenchyma, and spinal cord in high-risk patients (two or more CMN or large CMN), ideally before 6 to 8 months of age, when complete myelinization may obscure findings, with follow-up MRI based on the development of clinical signs or symptoms (113). Symptoms and signs of increased intracranial pressure, hydrocephalus, seizures, cranial nerve palsies, sensorimotor defects, bowel and bladder dysfunction, and developmental delay usually occur by age 2, but may be delayed until adulthood. The prognosis for symptomatic NCM is poor with over 50% mortality within the first 3 years of diagnosis (108). Other CNS abnormalities that have been described in patients with NCM include Dandy-Walker malformation, posterior fossa cysts, defects of the skull or vertebra, a tethered spinal cord, and corpus callosum agenesis (114).

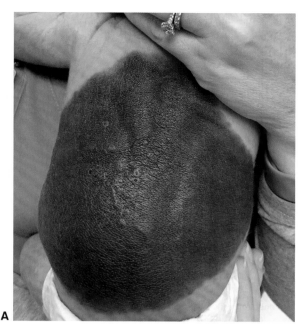
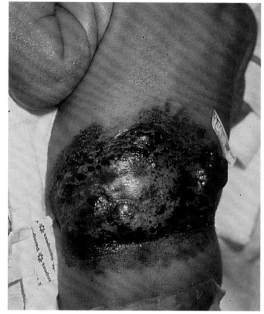

FIGURE 61.31 A: Congenital melanocytic nevi (CMN) are fairly homogeneous in color at birth but can develop variable focal nevi ranging in color from *pink* to *black*. Overlying hypertrichosis is common. Giant CMN are most commonly found on the trunk. **B:** They are benign but carry a risk of melanoma, rarely congenital melanoma seen in this giant CMN at birth. Rapid change, deep nodules, bleeding, and ulceration are considering signs that warrant evaluation.

White Spots

White birthmarks usually occur due to decreased number or function of melanocytes. The exception is nevus anemicus (NA), which is caused by constitutive blood vessel constriction. NA loses its border with diascopy (pressure), does not become erythematous when rubbed, and does not show a color change with Wood light examination and can be an early marker of neurofibromatosis type 1 (115). Hypopigmentation or decreased pigment should be distinguished from depigmentation or absence of pigment using fluorescent light (Wood light). Depigmentation displays a bright white color, while hypopigmentation does not accentuate significantly or leads to an off-white color.

Ash Leaf Macules

Ash leaf macules are small well-defined lancet-shaped patches of decreased pigmentation. They are seen in 3% to 5% of the normal population but can be an indicator of tuberous sclerosis, especially when three or more hypopigmented macules ≥5 mm in size are present. Other cutaneous signs of tuberous sclerosis include connective tissue nevus (shagreen patch), periungual fibromas, confetti hypopigmentation, gingival fibromas, and facial angiofibromas (adenoma sebaceum).

Hypomelanosis of Ito

Hypomelanosis of Ito consists of extensive whirls of hypopigmentation following Blaschko lines that can be seen in association with seizures, developmental delay, and ocular and/or skeletal anomalies. If limited to the skin, it is best called pigmentary mosaicism, which is a benign and often inherited skin finding.

Nevus Depigmentosus

Nevus depigmentosus (nevus achromicus) is a well-demarcated hypopigmented patch that generally presents as an isolated patch but can also present as linear streaks, in which case the term pigmentary mosaicism is preferred. Affected areas are usually unilateral and may be small, or they may be very broad affecting a large part of the body. The borders are often feathery, a clue to diagnosis (116). Nevus depigmentosus is not associated with extracutaneous organ involvement. It is a misnomer, as biopsy demonstrates the presence of melanocytes. They may produce an off-white color with a Wood lamp.

Diffuse Hypopigmentation/Depigmentation

Generalized hypopigmentation or pigment dilution can be seen in newborns with oculocutaneous albinism, Chédiak-Higashi syndrome, or phenylketonuria.

▌ VASCULAR ANOMALIES

Vascular anomalies are categorized as either tumors or malformations by the International Society for the Study of Vascular Anomalies (ISSVA), with tumors demonstrating proliferative capacity and malformation remaining relatively static. However, this is admittedly an oversimplification, as VMs can indeed grow over time, albeit more indolently compared with vascular tumors.

Vascular Tumors

Vascular tumors can range from benign to borderline or malignant. Fortunately, the vast majority are benign and are most often IHs as described above. The differential diagnosis for a deep IH includes the rare kaposiform hemangioendothelioma, which can be complicated by Kasabach-Merritt syndrome, in which a localized consumptive coagulopathy (decreased platelets and fibrinogen) within the borderline aggressive tumor can lead to a sudden increase in size, overlying petechiae, bleeding, spontaneous widespread bruising, and DIC (Fig. 61.32).

IH should be distinguished from the less common congenital hemangioma (CH), which are fully formed at birth and either involute rapidly (RICH) starting in the first several weeks of life with complete resolution by 6 to 14 months of age, do not involute (NICH), or involute partially (PICH) (Fig. 61.33). CH have a unique morphology, associated set of complications (potential for transient thrombocytopenia in CH, rarely severe), and natural history compared with IH (117).

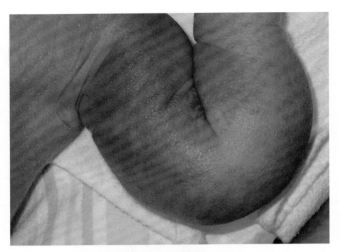

FIGURE 61.32 Kaposiform hemangioendothelioma are at risk for Kasabach-Merritt syndrome, which presents as *purple* or bruise-like nodules, plaques, or tumors.

Pyogenic Granuloma

Pyogenic granulomas or lobular capillary hemangiomas are small pink to red papules occurring on the head, neck, torso, and mucous membranes (Fig. 61.34). They are collections of endothelial cells that are thought to arise from trauma and have a propensity for prolonged bleeding with minor trauma. They are rare in the newborn period. Without treatment, they may persist for years and are a nuisance.

Vascular Malformations

Vascular malformations result from abnormal morphogenesis of blood vessels and lymphatics. As such, they are all congenital but can present later as they grow. In contrast to IHs, they do not involute but rather gradually progress through life to varying extents. VMs can undergo apparent rapid increase in size as they fill up with blood or lymph fluid. Localized intravascular thrombosis can lead to pain. VMs are classified by vessel type (capillary, venous, arterial, lymphatic, mixed, and arteriovenous) and the flow characteristics (high and low flow). New genes are being discovered in both spontaneous and

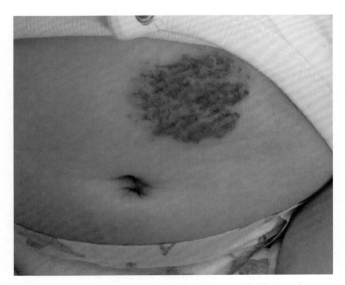

FIGURE 61.33 Unlike infantile hemangiomas, congenital hemangiomas are fully formed at birth. These lesions are rapidly involuting (RICH) or noninvoluting (NICH).

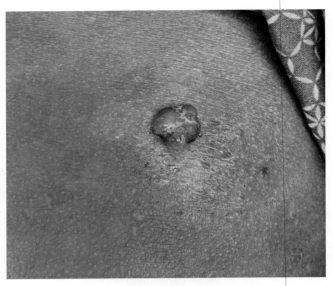

FIGURE 61.34 Pyogenic granulomas grow rapidly and bleed repeatedly and profusely.

familial cases. Doppler ultrasound with flow and MRI with angiography are helpful to assess the extent of an AVM.

Capillary Malformations
Port Wine Stain

Capillary malformations involving segments of skin, most often the face but also the limbs and trunk, are termed port wine stains (PWSs) or birthmarks (Fig. 61.35). Distinct patterns of PWS facial segments have been described, thought to reflect the embryonic development of the vasculature rather than dermatomal patterns. Approximately 10% of newborns with high-risk PWS (S1, S4) also have ocular and CNS involvement. This triad is referred to as Sturge-Weber syndrome (SWS). Patients with SWS can develop glaucoma, seizures, and facial asymmetry as a result of overgrowth of soft tissue and facial bones. Timing of screening for CNS anomalies with MRI of the brain varies among neurologists and institutions. Almost all capillary malformations occur as isolated defects. They have been described, however, in association with trisomy 13 and Rubinstein-Taybi, Beckwith-Wiedemann, and Klippel-Trenaunay-Weber syndromes. Some lesions lighten with age, but most darken. Vascular lasers are used to treat capillary malformations,

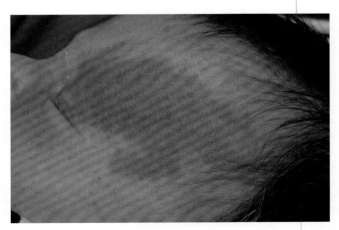

FIGURE 61.35 Infants with port wine stain patterns on the upper face (forehead and centrofacial placodes) are at risk for Sturge-Weber syndrome and should be evaluated for ocular and CNS involvement.

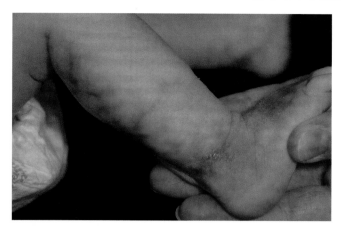

FIGURE 61.36 **Cutis marmorata telangiectatica congenita, seen here, is a vascular malformation distinct from the more common transient net-like erythema of cutis marmorata.**

though multiple treatments are required throughout life and they tend to regrow, necessitating touch-ups throughout life.

Cutis Marmorata Telangiectatica Congenita (Fig. 61.36)

Infants with CMTC are born with atrophic net-like red–blue patches in a segmental pattern, usually on the lower extremities but the trunk and upper extremities may be involved. Limb girth discrepancy is the most common associated complication followed by limb length discrepancy. Evaluation by orthopedics is indicated if the length discrepancy is greater than 2 cm, as this can interfere with gait. The atrophic areas may ulcerate and scar. Lesions have a tendency to become less noticeable by adulthood (118). Rarely, CMTC is associated with underlying CNS, glaucoma, or cardiac malformations, especially with generalized CMTC (119).

Venous Malformations

Malformations of the veins are slow-flow VMs, taking on a variety of clinical appearances: varicosities, isolated local spongy nodules, or large complex infiltrating channels, both on the skin and mucosa and in internal organs. The vast majority of venous malformations (VMs) are sporadic, although they can be inherited in autosomal dominant and recessive manners. Multiple lesions are more likely to be inherited. TEK2 gene mutations have been identified in sporadic and inherited forms. Blue rubber bleb nevus syndrome presents with numerous VMs on the acral and mucosal surfaces as well as GI involvement leading to GI bleeds and anemia and occasional CNS involvement. Patients with venous malformations often experience pain and swelling, especially in the morning with ambulation. Large combined type venous malformations can be debilitating and prohibit ambulation and workplace productivity. Venous stasis, intravascular thrombosis, and calcifications (phleboliths) are thought to be responsible for the pain. Extensive venous thrombosis can result in widespread coagulopathy. Treatment options include deep vascular lasers such as the Nd:YAG laser, embolization with interventional radiology, and surgical excision, as well as oral sirolimus in extensive cases with internal involvement.

Lymphatic Malformations

Lymphatic malformations (lymphangiomas) result from dilated, aberrant lymphatic channels. They can be classified broadly as microcystic (small channels), macrocystic (large channels), or mixed.

Microcystic lymphatic malformations have been referred to as lymphangioma circumscriptum, which appears as small clustered translucent pseudovesicles that resemble "frog spawn." Commonly, some of the vesicles are hemorrhagic, and there may be an underlying deep component giving a blue hue. Microcystic lymphatic malformations can occur on any site; however, axillary folds, neck, shoulders, proximal limbs, perineum, tongue, and buccal mucous membranes are more commonly involved. These malformations have been mistaken for warts and can be confused with sexual abuse (120). They may be small (<1 cm) or very large, covering an extensive surface area. Patients can develop cellulitis in the involved areas, and lymphatic malformations commonly recur around previously excised sites.

Macrocystic lymphatic malformations (cystic hygroma) are large single or multiple masses occurring on the neck, axillae, groin, and/or chest. Most commonly, these malformations are detected within the first 2 years of life and can cause significant morbidity and even death as a result of airway compromise and infection. They may be detected *in utero* by ultrasound and increased α-fetoprotein levels and may be associated with Down syndrome or Turner syndrome. The lesions are persistent and can expand, although spontaneous remission has been described, usually after infection. Treatment measures have included sclerotherapy and surgical excision, but the benefits are often palliative and temporary.

Arteriovenous Malformations

Arteriovenous malformations (AVM) are fast-flow malformations that are dangerous and can produce cardiovascular instability. Increased warmth, swelling, bruits, and thrills are signs of an AVM. Small AVMs can result from trauma. They are most common in the head and neck region but also occur on the extremities. A warm swollen extremity with an associated capillary malformation can be a sign of an underlying AVM. These malformations are difficult to manage and may require surgery and/or endovascular embolization.

Edema

Congenital lymphedema is rare and can be primary or secondary. Milroy disease describes primary congenital lymphedema that is primarily located distally on the lower legs and feet. Initially, the edema is pitting but later becomes firm and nonpitting. Turner syndrome and Noonan syndrome are two important conditions associated with congenital lymphedema.

GENETIC SKIN DISEASES

Collodion Baby

Collodion baby is the general term for infants that present at birth with a collodion membrane, resembling a thick "saran-wrap" covering of skin (**Fig. 61.37**). The collodion membrane is a temporary condition in the newborn period but can cause morbidity until resolution and can be indicative of other underlying dermatologic conditions. In the early newborn period, this covering can produce respiratory distress, painful cracks and fissures, temperature and fluid instability, and increase susceptibility to infection. Newborns frequently require respiratory support, a humidified air incubator, and liberal applications of emollients. The eyes should be liberally lubricated because desiccation may cause corneal scarring. Supportive care measures should be provided at least until the membrane is completely shed. No matter the underlying cause, the initial collodion membrane sloughs over a period of 2 to 4 weeks, and after this shedding, the causative skin disorder may be differentiated. Long-term complications include ectropion (eversion of the eyelids) and eclabium (eversion of the lips). The vast majority of infants who present with a collodion membrane have an autosomal recessive congenital ichthyosis (ARCI) including lamellar ichthyosis (LI), nonbullous congenital ichthyosiform erythroderma (NB-CIE), and rarely Harlequin ichthyosis (HI). Other causes of collodion membrane include trichothiodystrophy, Sjögren-Larsson syndrome,

THE NEWBORN INFANT

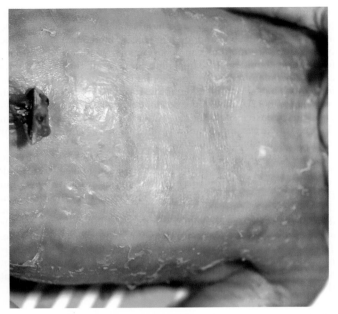

FIGURE 61.37 Collodion babies present at birth with the appearance of "Saran wrap"–like skin that gradually sloughs over 2 to 4 weeks. (This is thicker than postmature desquamation.)

Conradi-Hünermann syndrome, Gaucher disease (type IIB), and Refsum disease. Ten to fifteen percent of infants have no underlying disorder and will have normal skin when the collodion membrane resolves. Skin biopsy during the period of collodion membranes does not help to distinguish the various underlying causes.

Ichthyosis

Ichthyosis is a term utilized to describe inherited and acquired conditions that produce "fish-like" scales (**Fig. 61.38**). Ichthyosis vulgaris, the most common form, is inherited in an autosomal

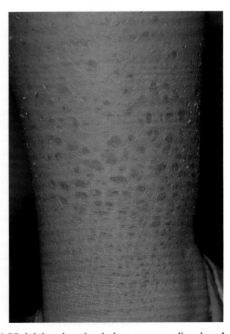

FIGURE 61.38 Ichthyosis vulgaris is a common disorder of cornification that produces fish-like scales, especially on the lower extremities, as seen in this older child.

dominant manner and can be associated with atopic dermatitis. There are numerous rare causes of ichthyosis, the most important of which are discussed below. Newborns with ichthyosis are primarily managed with petroleum-based emollients, such as Vaseline and Aquaphor. A thinner lotion may be preferable. Keratolytic emollients containing lactic and salicylic acid should be avoided in babies, because they can be systemically absorbed. Infants with severe forms of ichthyosis can benefit from topical and/or systemic retinoids, but these medications should be used in consultation with a dermatologist. Genetic testing should be done to confirm the diagnosis. Genetic counseling is essential for families of infants with ichthyosis. "F.I.R.S.T, the Foundation for Ichthyosis and Related Skin Types, (firstskinfoundation.org) has a tele-ichthyosis diagnostic and therapeutic consultative service for health care providers."

X-Linked Ichthyosis

X-linked ichthyosis is caused by a mutation in the steroid sulfatase gene, which results in retention of keratinocytes. These patients are frequently born after prolonged labor due to increased fetal production of DHEAS and decreased placental estrogen. In the first months of life, the skin develops thick brown firmly adherent scale with relative sparing of the flexural regions. Undescended testes, testicular cancer, and corneal opacities are classically associated with X-linked ichthyosis and are clues to diagnosis. Therefore, these patients should be evaluated by urology and ophthalmology. Moisturizers are recommended to help ameliorate the skin findings.

Autosomal Recessive Congenital Ichthyosis

ARCI is a rare subset of ichthyosis that includes LI, NB-CIE, and rarely HI. Most of these babies present with a collodion membrane and may have the ensuing complications. In NB-CIE, there is often underlying erythema that becomes more visible as the collodion membrane resolves. A fine white powdery scale develops over time. Most cases are caused by mutations in lipoxygenase genes. In LI, thick brown scales develop after the collodion membrane resolves. These scales are taut and lead to tension on the skin, which leads to worsening ectropion and eclabium, hypoplasia of the nasal and external ear cartilage, and painful fissures. Approximately half of the cases are due to mutations in transglutaminase-1 (121). Both NB-CIE and LI may be associated with hypohidrosis and overheating due to occlusion of the sweat ducts. Palmar keratodermas with painful fissures are common. Alopecia may be present. Infants with HI are born with an extremely thick and cracked, armor-like covering with pronounced eclabium and ectropion. HI is exceedingly rare, and these patients usually die during infancy; however, there are some long-term survivors (122). This condition is inherited in an autosomal recessive manner by mutations in the *ABCA12* gene, which is important for normal epidermal development. Treatment with a systemic retinoid may increase survival (122).

Netherton Syndrome

Netherton syndrome is an ichthyosis that can present as severe erythroderma and cause progressive and diffuse cutaneous findings. Newborns are frequently born prematurely and fail to thrive, in part due to high metabolic demands from the skin. They are at risk for hypernatremic dehydration and sepsis. Frequent systemic infections requiring hospitalization should raise suspicion for NS; an altered immune systemic is to blame in part. Infants develop sparse scalp hair as a result of hair fragility (123). The characteristic hair shaft abnormality referred to as trichorrhexis invaginata ("bamboo hair" or "ball-and-socket hair") develops after 3 months of age and can serve as a marker for NS. Only 30% of hairs may be involved, and the eyebrows are the most promising location to identify this finding. The characteristic ichthyosis linearis circumflexa ("double-edged scale") is generally not a prominent feature in the newborn. There are no specific laboratory abnormalities, except most infants have elevated levels of immunoglobulin E

(IgE). Patients with suspected NS should be referred to genetics, as mutations in the SPINK5 gene, which encodes a serine protease inhibitor (LEKTI), are well known to cause the syndrome (124). Patients are managed with cautious use of topical corticosteroids, emollients, and antihistamines. Tacrolimus and pimecrolimus should be used with caution in infants with Netherton syndrome, with consideration for checking serum tacrolimus levels, because high serum levels of tacrolimus have been detected in some infants due to increased absorption from the skin. The scaly rash can be quite pruritic and refractory to treatment. Food allergies are common as well, complicating the management of these patients.

Genetic Blistering Disease

Genetic skin conditions are rare but important causes of blisters and bullae in the newborn period. The differential includes autoimmune blistering disorders, which occur due to transplacental passage of maternal autoantibodies from mothers with known disease or rarely through a primary disease process, as well as infection.

Epidermolytic Hyperkeratosis (Epidermolytic Ichthyosis, Bullous Congenital Ichthyosiform Erythroderma)

EHK is a rare autosomal dominant condition that results from mutations in genes encoding keratin 1 (KRT1) and keratin10 (KRT10). It is named for its characteristic finding on histopathology, in which the keratinocytes of the spinous and granular layer demonstrate granular and vacuolar degeneration, a pathognomonic finding termed EHK (125). Keratins 1 and 10 are intermediate filament proteins found in the superficial layers of the epidermis; thus, alterations in these proteins weaken the epidermis. Affected newborns develop widespread areas of erythroderma, denuded skin, superficial blisters, and skin fragility. Newborns should be treated with topical emollients and be monitored closely for signs of infection and sepsis, as they are at risk for secondary cutaneous infections. Later in infancy and early childhood, blistering becomes less evident and the skin develops verrucous-appearing thick scale that is prominent in the flexures. Typically, involved areas are heavily colonized with bacteria, producing an odor. Diagnosis is established by genetic testing.

Epidermolysis Bullosa

EB represents a large group of inherited skin disorders characterized by blisters and breakdown of the epidermis deeper than that seen in EHK. This condition is caused by mutations in various genes responsible for structural proteins important in maintaining

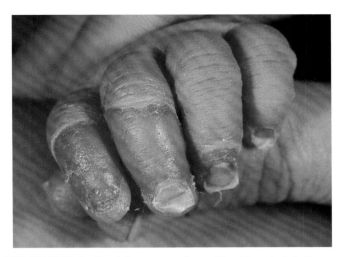

FIGURE 61.39 Sucking injury on a newborn with epidermolysis bullosa.

the skin integrity. EB should be suspected in newborns with blisters and erosions that result from minor friction (**Fig. 61.39**). Mucosal and extracutaneous involvement may occur depending on the EB subtype. Although classification schemes may change as new genes are identified, traditionally, EB has been classified as EB simplex, junctional EB, and dystrophic EB. EB simplex is due to alterations in proteins found in the basal layer of the epidermis (keratin 5/keratin 14) (**Fig. 61.40A**). Junctional EB is as a result of altered proteins at the dermoepidermal junction (laminin 5) (**Fig. 61.40B**). Dystrophic EB is as a result of altered proteins below the dermoepidermal junction (collagen type VII). As such, the blisters of EB simplex are more superficial than those of junctional EB, which are more superficial than those in dystrophic EB. The severity of disease is determined only in part by the layer of the split; the quantitative and qualitative degree of protein alteration is also critical. Genotype–phenotype correlations will become more apparent in the future. Mucosal involvement can be mild to severe, with some neonates requiring intubation, classically in junctional EB-Herlitz type. Laryngeal, urologic, and gastrointestinal involvement is seen in more severely affected infants. In the newborn period, distinguishing between EB subtypes on clinical appearance alone can be extremely difficult, because all forms of EB can present with widespread blisters. Diagnosis is best made

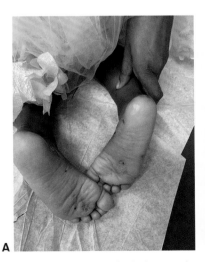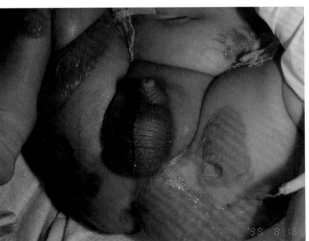

FIGURE 61.40 A: Mild EB simplex lesions are the most superficial. **B:** Junctional EB lesions on a neonate show blisters and erosions.

THE NEWBORN INFANT

by genetic testing via a panel of known causative genes done on serum rather than tissue.

Managing newborns with severe EB is difficult and should include multidisciplinary support with wound care or burn care specialists. Friction should be minimized as much as possible and wounds should be carefully dressed with a nonadherent dressing (Vaseline gauze, Mepitel, Exu-Dry) followed by gauze wrap. Tense blisters will easily spread in EB patients, so large blisters should be drained in a sterile manner with a sterile needle to the blister base, allowing the fluid to drain spontaneously with the roof left in place as a "natural" dressing. Cautious use of silver dressings and topical mupirocin can be helpful to prevent wound infection in open areas, though bacterial resistance (*S. aureus*) to mupirocin has occurred. Prophylactic oral or intravenous antibiotics should be avoided. Though dressing removal may be onerous, the skin must be assessed daily, especially for areas of possible infection. Dressings should be removed gently, similar to burn patients. Dressing removal can be facilitated by soaking the dressing in warm water; extra application of Vaseline prior to application of dressings can make them less adherent and more easily removed.

Newborns with EB have increased nutritional and fluid requirements. If intravenous catheters are required, they can be sutured in place, as tape should not be applied directly to the skin. Nasogastric tube feedings can be used sparingly to assist in the early newborn period with consideration to possible mucosal fragility. The use of special needs feeders, such as the Haberman feeder, may help feeding, as they are designed to allow the infant to feed without having to create negative pressure; instead, the parent may apply the pressure to the feeder to facilitate milk transfer into the infant's mouth, which compared to a regular bottle nipple decreases pressure on the infant's mucosal surfaces. Percutaneous gastrostomy tubes should be placed early if feeding and nutrition are problematic.

The diagnosis of EB is psychologically distressing for parents and families. Addressing these issues is an essential part of EB management. Advocacy groups such as Dystrophic Epidermolysis Bullosa Research Association of America (www.debra.org) are invaluable resources for families.

Incontinentia Pigmenti (Bloch-Sulzberger Syndrome)

IP is an X-linked dominant disease characterized by linear streaks and whorls of vesicles and bullae, which pass through stages and become verrucous or warty, then flatten forming hyperpigmented patches and finally hypopigmented and atrophic patches. Typically, these four stages occur in sequence, although patients can "skip" stages, and different stages can be seen together (**Fig. 61.41**). The vesicles that are seen in stage 1 develop within the first 2 to 3 weeks of life and can reoccur or flare with systemic infections, fevers, or vaccinations (126). They can be confused in the newborn period for infections such as herpes simplex, varicella, or impetigo.

IP is a result of X-linked dominant mutations in the NEMO gene on Xq28. This condition is usually lethal in males but can be seen in male patients with an XXY genotype and with postzygotic somatic NEMO mutations. Early on in the condition, a striking peripheral eosinophilia can be seen. Other extracutaneous findings include CNS abnormalities (seizures), ocular defects (retinal changes), immunologic abnormalities (elevated IgE), dental anomalies, and skeletal anomalies (spina bifida). Newborns suspected of having IP should have a skin biopsy and appropriate bacterial and viral cultures. Parents should be referred to a geneticist for diagnostic confirmation and genetic counseling. Care should be multidisciplinary.

Focal Dermal Hypoplasia of Goltz

Focal dermal hypoplasia (Goltz syndrome) is rare multisystem disorder that shows characteristic skin findings of thinned or absent dermis with fat herniation, and hyperpigmented and hypopigmented patches following the swirling lines of Blaschko. Other cutaneous signs include alopecia, brittle hair, nail dystrophy, atrophic scars, ACC, telangiectasias, dermatographism, and red raspberry-like papillomas (perioral, intraoral, perianal, vulvar) that are often not present at birth. It is an X-linked dominant disorder that is primarily seen in females, as males often have much more severe disease that can affect survival. Infants with Goltz syndrome are often small for gestation at birth and can have skeletal, ocular, dental, cardiac, renal, gastrointestinal, and neurologic defects, including microphthalmia, malformed ears, pointed chin, and ectrodactyly.

Metabolic and Nutritional Disorders

Various metabolic diseases and nutritional deficiencies can cause neonatal rashes (127). Examples include maple syrup urine disease, carbamoyl phosphate synthetase deficiency, argininosuccinic aciduria, propionic acidemia, methylmalonic aciduria, cystic fibrosis, biotinidase deficiency, multiple carboxylase deficiency, and essential fatty acid deficiency. AE (zinc deficiency) produces a unique rash and will be discussed in more detail.

Acrodermatitis Enteropathica

AE is caused by zinc deficiency (127). Infants develop a tetrad of diarrhea, periorificial and acral dermatitis, alopecia, and apathy. Zinc is an essential trace element that is used by the body in wound healing, neuron signaling, and gene regulation. Usually, the dermatitis is the first sign (**Fig. 61.42**) and has a classic well-demarcated shiny scaly brown–pink appearance or may appear vesiculobullous or eczematous. Symptoms often arise after weaning from breast milk but prior to introduction of solids, as

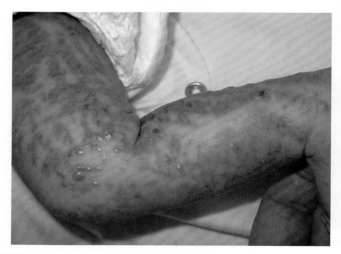

FIGURE 61.41 The lesions of incontinentia pigmenti, including the vesicles, verrucous papules, and hyperpigmented patches seen on this leg, travel in linear and whorling patterns along the lines of Blaschko.

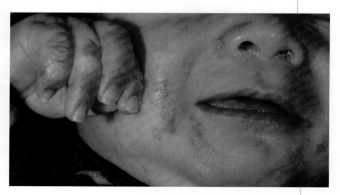

FIGURE 61.42 Acrodermatitis enteropathica skin findings typically include periorificial and acral dermatitis, plus diarrhea, alopecia, and apathy.

zinc is better absorbed from breast milk compared with formula. Autosomal recessive AE is as a result of an altered gastrointestinal zinc absorption due to mutations in the SLC39A gene, which encodes for the Zip4 intestinal zinc transporter. Clinical findings develop within the first several months of life (128). Acquired forms of AE are more common. Conditions that increase risk are intestinal malabsorption, diarrhea, liver disease, prematurity, prolonged TPN without adequate zinc, and HIV infection. However, it can also rarely result spontaneously from low or absent levels of zinc in the breast milk, because of altered transfer of zinc from maternal serum, levels of which are usually normal. Low levels of serum alkaline phosphatase, a zinc-dependent enzyme, may suggest the diagnosis, and a low plasma zinc level is strongly supportive, although AE can occur in the setting of normal zinc levels. Serum testing is unnecessary, as zinc supplementation of 3 mg/kg/d leads to rapid improvement in symptoms. Cystic fibrosis and biotinidase deficiency may also produce a similar rash (129).

DISORDERS OF HAIR AND NAILS

Hair

Newborns are sometimes born covered with very fine downy hair referred to as lanugo. The lanugo is normally shed and replaced with vellus hair within the first several months of life. Scalp hair undergoes repeated patterns of shedding with regrowth from front to back within the first year of life. Hair can be abundant (hypertrichosis) or absent (alopecia). Examples of genetic conditions associated with hypertrichosis include congenital hypertrichosis lanuginosa, Cornelia de Lange syndrome, and Rubinstein-Taybi syndrome. Congenital alopecia can be an isolated inherited condition, or it can be associated with a number of ectodermal dysplasia, as well as atrichia with papular lesions that presents as shedding of hair permanently in the first few months of birth.

Ectodermal Dysplasia

Ectodermal dysplasia is a term that refers to conditions resulting in abnormalities of the skin and adnexal structures (teeth, hair, and nails). There are many different forms of ectodermal dysplasia, many of which are associated with absent eccrine glands and subsequent risk of overheating. Hypohidrotic ectodermal dysplasia, hidrotic ectodermal dysplasia, and p63-related ectodermal dysplasias are examples. The diagnosis may be delayed because teeth are rarely present at birth, and most infants have sparse hair and thin nails, though unique features may be present as described below. Unexplained fevers may be the first clue to hypohidrotic ectodermal dysplasia, likely due to impaired temperature regulation due to lack of sweat glands. These patients also have characteristic facial features, including arched thin eyebrows, flattened nasal root, periocular hyperpigmentation, thick vermillion lips, and peg-shaped teeth. Female carriers, including mothers and sisters, may share similar attenuated morphologic features. Patients with p63-related ectodermal dysplasis may be born with ankyloblepharon, lacrimal duct defects, distal limb abnormalities including syndactyly and ectrodactyly, and cleft lip/palate. A constellation of these findings should raise suspicion for a genetic disorder and prompt workup with genetic testing.

There is no specific therapy for ectodermal dysplasia. Care is multidisciplinary with dermatology, dentistry, ophthalmology, surgery, and others. Patients with hypohidrosis should be counseled on methods for temperature regulation. Families should be referred to a dermatologist and geneticist to assist in diagnosis and genetic counseling. The National Foundation for Ectodermal Dysplasia (NFED.org) is an excellent resource for providers and families with newborns who have ED. Clinical trials for new therapeutic options for previously untreatable ED are available through NFED.

REFERENCES

1. Schoch JJ, Monir RL, Satcher KG, et al. The infantile cutaneous microbiome: a review. *Pediatr Dermatol* 2019;36(5):574.
2. Blaschko A. *Die Nervenverteilung in der Haut ihrer Beziehung zu den Erkrankungen der Haut.* Wiem: Wilhelm Braumuller, 1901.
3. Bolognia JL, Orlow SJ, Glick SA. Lines of Blaschko. *J Am Acad Dermatol* 1994;31(2 Pt 1):157; quiz 190.
4. Madison KC. Barrier function of the skin: "la raison d'etre" of the epidermis. *J Invest Dermatol* 2003;121(2):231.
5. Rassner U, Feingold KR, Crumrine DA, et al. Coordinate assembly of lipids and enzyme proteins into epidermal lamellar bodies. *Tissue Cell* 1999;31(5):489.
6. Gallo RL. The birth of innate immunity. *Exp Dermatol* 2013;22(8):517.
7. Sanford JA, Gallo RL. Functions of the skin microbiota in health and disease. *Semin Immunol* 2013;25(5):370.
8. Hoeger PH, Schreiner V, Klaassen IA, et al. Epidermal barrier lipids in human vernix caseosa: corresponding ceramide pattern in vernix and fetal skin. *Br J Dermatol* 2002;146(2):194.
9. Yoshio H, Tollin M, Gudmundsson GH, et al. Antimicrobial polypeptides of human vernix caseosa and amniotic fluid: implications for newborn innate defense. *Pediatr Res* 2003;53(2):211.
10. Grubauer G, Elias PM, Feingold KR. Transepidermal water loss: the signal for recovery of barrier structure and function. *J Lipid Res* 1989;30(3):323.
11. Rutter N. The immature skin. *Br Med Bull* 1988;44(4):957.
12. Abouelfettoh A, Ludington-Hoe SM, Burant CJ, et al. Effect of skin-to-skin contact on preterm infant skin barrier function and hospital-acquired infection. *J Clin Med Res* 2011;3(1):36.
13. Visscher MO, Adam R, Brink S, et al. Newborn infant skin: physiology, development, and care. *Clin Dermatol* 2015;33(3):271.
14. Johnson E, Hunt R. Infant skin care: updates and recommendations. *Curr Opin Pediatr* 2019;31(4):476.
15. Chi M, Han T, Chen C, et al. Clinical characteristics and prognosis of collodion babies. *Int J Clin Exp Med* 2018;11(10):10949.
16. Prado R, Ellis LZ, Gamble R, et al. Collodion baby: an update with a focus on practical management. *J Am Acad Dermatol* 2012;67(6):1362.
17. Nguyen MA, Gelman A, Norton SA. Practical events in the management of a collodion baby. *JAMA Dermatol* 2015;151(9):1031.
18. Morrison WA, Hurley JV, Ahmad TS, et al. Scar formation after skin injury to the human foetus in utero or the premature neonate. *Br J Plast Surg* 1999;52(1):6.
19. Seeds JW. Diagnostic mid trimester amniocentesis: how safe? *Am J Obstet Gynecol* 2004;191(2):607.
20. Ashkenazi S, Metzker A, Merlob P, et al. Scalp changes after fetal monitoring. *Arch Dis Child* 1985;60(3):267.
21. Anzivino E, Fioriti D, Mischitelli M, et al. Herpes simplex virus infection in pregnancy and in neonate: status of art of epidemiology, diagnosis, therapy and prevention. *Virol J* 2009;6:40.
22. Tanzi EL, Hornung RL, Silverberg NB. Halo scalp ring: a case series and review of the literature. *Arch Pediatr Adolesc Med* 2002;156(2):188.
23. Maffeis, L, Pugni L, Pietrasanta C, et al. Iatrogenic Anetoderma of Prematurity: a case report and review of the literature. *Case Rep Dermatol Med* 2014;2014:781493.
24. Goujon E, Beer F, Gay S, et al. Anetoderma of prematurity: an iatrogenic consequence of neonatal intensive care. *Arch Dermatol* 2010;146(5):565.
25. Wyckoff MH, Aziz K, Escobedo MB, et al. Part 13: neonatal resuscitation: 2015 American Heart Association Guidelines Update for Cardiopulmonary Resuscitation and Emergency Cardiovascular Care. *Circulation* 2015;132(suppl 2):S543.
26. Sümpelmann R, Osthaus W, Irmler H. Prevention of burns caused by transillumination for peripheral venous access in neonates. *Paediatr Anaesth* 2006;(16):1097.
27. Jung SN, Hwang DY, Kim J, et al. Pulse oximeter probe-induced electrical burn. *Burns* 2009;35(5):751.
28. Reynolds PR, Banerjee S, Meek JH. Alcohol burns in extremely low birthweight infants: still occurring. *Arch Dis Child Fetal Neonatal Ed* 2005;90(1):F10.
29. Gopalakrishnan PN, Goel N, Banerjee S. Saline irrigation for the management of skin extravasation injury in neonates. *Cochrane Database Syst Rev* 2017;7:CD008484.
30. Beaulieu MJ. Hyaluronidase for extravasation management. *Neonatal Netw* 2012;31(6):413.
31. Samiee-Zafarghandy S, van den Anker JN, Ben Fadel N. Topical nitroglycerin in neonates with tissue injury: a case report and review of the literature. *Paediatr Child Health* 2014;19(1):9.
32. Le A, Patel S. Extravasation of noncytotoxic drugs: a review of the literature. *Ann Pharmacother* 2015;48(7):870.
33. Cetta F, Lambert GH, Ros SP. Newborn chemical exposure from over-the-counter skin care products. *Clin Pediatr* 1991;30(5):286.

34. Monteagudo B, Labandeira J, Cabanillas M, et al. Prospective study of erythema toxicum neonatorum: epidemiology and predisposing factors. *Pediatr Dermatol* 2012;29(2):166.
35. Berk DR, Bayliss SJ. Milia: a review and classification. *J Am Acad Dermatol* 2008;59(6):1050.
36. LaRusso J, Wilson J, Ceilley R. Phototherapy-induced purpuric eruption in a neonate. *J Clin Aesthet Dermatol* 2015;8(3):46.
37. Siegfried E, Glenn E. Use of olive oil for the treatment of seborrheic dermatitis in children. *Arch Pediatr Adolesc Med* 2012;166(10):967.
38. Warner RR, Boissy YL, Lilly NA, et al. Water disrupts stratum corneum lipid lamellae: damage is similar to surfactants. *J Invest Dermatol* 1999;113(6):960.
39. Berg RW, Buckingham KW, Stewart RL. Etiologic factors in diaper dermatitis: the role of urine. *Pediatr Dermatol* 1986;3(2):102.
40. Buckingham KW, Berg RW. Etiologic factors in diaper dermatitis: the role of feces. *Pediatr Dermatol* 1986;3(2):107.
41. Bernstein ML, McCusker MM, Grant-Kels JM. Cutaneous manifestations of cystic fibrosis. *Pediatr Dermatol* 2008;25(2):150.
42. Burdall O, Willgress L, Goad N. Neonatal skin care: developments in care to maintain neonatal barrier function and prevention of diaper dermatitis. *Pediatr Dermatol* 2019;36(1):31.
43. Campbell RL. Clinical tests with improved disposable diapers. *Pediatrician* 1987;14(suppl 1):34.
44. Campbell RL, Seymour JL, Stone LC, et al. Clinical studies with disposable diapers containing absorbent gelling materials: evaluation of effects on infant skin condition. *J Am Acad Dermatol* 1987;17(6):978.
45. White CM, Gailey RA, Lippe S. Cholestyramine ointment to treat buttocks rash and anal excoriation in an infant. *Ann Pharmacother* 1996;30(9):954.
46. Tempark T, Phatarakijnirund V, Chatproedprai S, et al. Exogenous Cushing's syndrome due to topical corticosteroid application: case report and review literature. *Endocrine* 2010;38(3):328.
47. Darmstadt GL, Dinulos JG. Neonatal skin care. *Pediatr Clin North Am* 2000;47(4):757.
48. Eichenfield LF, Tom WL, Chamlin SL, et al. Guidelines of care for the management of atopic dermatitis: section 1. Diagnosis and assessment of atopic dermatitis. *J Am Acad Dermatol* 2014;70(2):338.
49. Kilcline C, Frieden IJ. Infantile hemangiomas: how common are they? A systematic review of the medical literature. *Pediatr Dermatol* 2008;25(2):168.
50. Drolet BA, Frommelt PC, Chamlin SL, et al. Initiation and use of propranolol for infantile hemangioma: report of a consensus conference. *Pediatrics* 2013;131(1):128.
51. Lee KC, Bercovitch L. Update on infantile hemangiomas. *Semin Perinatol* 2013;37(1):49.
52. Kwon EK, Seefeldt M, Drolet BA. Infantile hemangiomas: an update. *Am J Clin Dermatol* 2013;14(2):111.
53. Luu M, Frieden IJ. Haemangioma: clinical course, complications and management. *Br J Dermatol* 2013;169(1):20.
54. Tollefson MM, Frieden IJ. Early growth of infantile hemangiomas: what parents' photographs tell us. *Pediatrics* 2012;130(2):e314.
55. Chang LC, Haggstrom AN, Drolet BA, et al. Growth characteristics of infantile hemangiomas: implications for management. *Pediatrics* 2008;122(2):360.
56. Brandling-Bennett HA, Metry DW, Baselga E, et al. Infantile hemangiomas with unusually prolonged growth phase: a case series. *Arch Dermatol* 2008;144(12):1632.
57. Couto RA, Maclellan RA, Zurakowski D, et al. Infantile hemangioma: clinical assessment of the involuting phase and implications for management. *Plast Reconstr Surg* 2012;130(3):619.
58. Frieden IJ, Reese V, Cohen D. PHACE syndrome. The association of posterior fossa brain malformations, hemangiomas, arterial anomalies, coarctation of the aorta and cardiac defects, and eye abnormalities. *Arch Dermatol* 1996;132(3):307.
59. Metry DW, Haggstrom AN, Drolet BA, et al. A prospective study of PHACE syndrome in infantile hemangiomas: demographic features, clinical findings, and complications. *Am J Med Genet A* 2006;140(9):975.
60. Metry D, Heyer G, Hess C, et al. Consensus statement on diagnostic criteria for PHACE syndrome. *Pediatrics* 2009;124(5):1447.
61. Girard C, Bigorre M, Guillot B, et al. PELVIS syndrome. *Arch Dermatol* 2006;142(7):884.
62. Stockman A, Boralevi F, Taieb A, et al. SACRAL syndrome: spinal dysraphism, anogenital, cutaneous, renal and urologic anomalies, associated with an angioma of lumbosacral localization. *Dermatology* 2007;214(1):40.
63. Iacobas I, Burrows PE, Frieden IJ, et al. LUMBAR: association between cutaneous infantile hemangiomas of the lower body and regional congenital anomalies. *J Pediatr* 2010;157(5):795.
64. Drolet BA, Chamlin SL, Garzon MC, et al. Prospective study of spinal anomalies in children with infantile hemangiomas of the lumbosacral skin. *J Pediatr* 2010;157(5):789.
65. Chamlin SL, Haggstrom AN, Drolet BA, et al. Multicenter prospective study of ulcerated hemangiomas. *J Pediatr* 2007;151(6):684.
66. Hermans DJ, Boezeman JB, Van de Kerkhof PC, et al. Differences between ulcerated and non-ulcerated hemangiomas, a retrospective study of 465 cases. *Eur J Dermatol* 2009;19(2):152.
67. Shin HT, Orlow SJ, Chang MW. Ulcerated haemangioma of infancy: a retrospective review of 47 patients. *Br J Dermatol* 2007;156(5):1050.
68. Maguiness SM, Hoffman WY, McCalmont TH, et al. Early white discoloration of infantile hemangioma: a sign of impending ulceration. *Arch Dermatol* 2010;146(11):1235.
69. Horii KA, Drolet BA, Frieden IJ, et al. Prospective study of the frequency of hepatic hemangiomas in infants with multiple cutaneous infantile hemangiomas. *Pediatr Dermatol* 2011;28(3):245.
70. Vredenborg AD, Janmohamed SR, de Laat PC, et al. Multiple cutaneous infantile haemangiomas and the risk of internal haemangioma. *Br J Dermatol* 2013;169(1):188.
71. Drolet BA, Pope E, Juern AM, et al. Gastrointestinal bleeding in infantile hemangioma: a complication of segmental, rather than multifocal, infantile hemangiomas. *J Pediatr* 2012;160(6):1021.
72. Metry DW, Hawrot A, Altman C, et al. Association of solitary, segmental hemangiomas of the skin with visceral hemangiomatosis. *Arch Dermatol* 2004;140(5):591.
73. Torres-Pradilla M, Baselga E. Failure of intralesional propranolol in infantile hemangiomas. *Pediatr Dermatol* 2014;31(2):156.
74. Pope E, Chakkittakandiyil A, Lara-Corrales I, et al. Expanding the therapeutic repertoire of infantile haemangiomas: cohort-blinded study of oral nadolol compared with propranolol. *Br J Dermatol* 2013;168(1):222.
75. Raphael MF, de Graaf M, Breugem CC, et al. Atenolol: a promising alternative to propranolol for the treatment of hemangiomas. *J Am Acad Dermatol* 2011;65(2):420.
76. Bigorre M, Van Kien AK, Valette H. Beta-blocking agent for treatment of infantile hemangioma. *Plast Reconstr Surg* 2009;123(6):195e.
77. Storch CH, Hoeger PH. Propranolol for infantile haemangiomas: insights into the molecular mechanisms of action. *Br J Dermatol* 2010;163(2):269.
78. Tu JB, Ma RZ, Dong Q, et al. Induction of apoptosis in infantile hemangioma endothelial cells by propranolol. *Exp Ther Med* 2013;6(2):574.
79. Moody MN, Landau JM, Goldberg LH. Nevus sebaceus revisited. *Pediatr Dermatol* 2012;29(1):15.
80. Frieden IJ. Aplasia cutis congenita: a clinical review and proposal for classification. *J Am Acad Dermatol* 1986;14(4):646.
81. Patel DP, Castelo-Soccio L, Yan AC. Aplasia cutis congenita: evaluation of signs suggesting extracutaneous involvement. *Pediatr Dermatol* 2018;35(1):e59.
82. Orozco-Covarrubias L, Lara-Carpio R, Saez-De-Ocariz M, et al. Dermoid cysts: a report of 75 pediatric patients. *Pediatr Dermatol* 2013;30(6):706.
83. Cambiaghi S, Micheli S, Talamonti G, et al. Nasal dermoid sinus cyst. *Pediatr Dermatol* 2007;24(6):646.
84. Eichenfield LF, Paller AS, Tom WL, et al. Pediatric psoriasis: evolving perspectives. *Pediatr Dermatol* 2018;35(2):170.
85. Traupe H, van Gurp PJ, Happle R, et al. Psoriasis vulgaris, fetal growth, and genomic imprinting. *Am J Med Genet* 1992;42(5):649.
86. Vanoni F, Lava SAG, Fossali EF, et al. Neonatal systemic lupus erythematosus syndrome: a comprehensive review. *Clin Rev Allergy Immunol* 2017;53(3):469.
87. Izmirly PM, Halushka MK, Rosenberg AZ, et al. Clinical and pathologic implications of extending the spectrum of maternal autoantibodies reactive with ribonucleoproteins associated with cutaneous and now cardiac neonatal lupus from SSA/Ro and SSB/La to U1RNP. *Autoimmun Rev* 2017;16(9):980.
88. Brazzelli V, Grasso V, Croci G, et al. An unusual case of transient neonatal pustular melanosis: a diagnostic puzzle. *Eur J Pediatr* 2014;173(12):1655.
89. Miller IM, Echeverría B, Torrelo A, et al. Infantile acne treated with oral isotretinoin. *Pediatr Dermatol* 2013;30(5):513.
90. Darmstadt GL, Tunnessen WW Jr, Swerer RJ. Eosinophilic pustular folliculitis. *Pediatrics* 1992;89(6 Pt 1):1095.
91. Takahashi N, Nishida H, Kato H, et al. Exanthematous disease induced by toxic shock syndrome toxin 1 in the early neonatal period. *Lancet* 1998;351(9116):1614.
92. Arnold JD, Hoek SN, Kirkorian AY. Epidemiology of staphylococcal scalded skin syndrome in the United States: a cross-sectional study, 2010-2014. *J Am Acad Dermatol* 2018;78(2):404.
93. Price VE, et al. Diagnosis and management of neonatal purpura fulminans. *Semin Fetal Neonat Med.* 2001;16(3):318.
94. Haupt R, Minkov M, Astigarraga I, et al.; Euro Histio Network. Langerhans cell histiocytosis (LCH): guidelines for diagnosis, clinical work-up, and treatment for patients till the age of 18 years. *Pediatr Blood Cancer* 2013;60(2):175.
95. Janssen D, Harms D. Juvenile xanthogranuloma in childhood and adolescence: a clinicopathologic study of 129 patients from the Kiel Pediatric Tumor Registry. *Am J Surg Pathol* 2005;29(1):21.
96. Samuelov L, Kinori M, Chamlin SL, et al. Risk of intraocular and other extracutaneous involvement in patients with cutaneous juvenile xanthogranuloma. *Pediatr Dermatol* 2018;35(3):329.

97. Meyer M, Grimes A, Becker E, et al. Systemic juvenile xanthogranuloma: a case report and brief review. *Clin Exp Dermatol* 2018;43(5):642.

98. Heinze A, Kuemmet TJ, Chiu YE, et al. Longitudinal study of pediatric urticaria pigmentosa. *Pediatr Dermatol* 2017;34(2):144.

99. Zhao G, Zhu M, Qin C, et al. Infantile Myofibromatosis: 32 patients and review of the literatures. *J Pediatr Hematol Oncol* 2020;42(8):495.

100. Hausbrandt PA, Leithner A, Beham A, et al. A rare case of infantile myofibromatosis and review of literature. *J Pediatr Orthop B* 2010;19(1):122.

101. Larralde M, Ferrari B, Martinez JP, et al. Infantile myofibromatosis. *An Bras Dermatol* 2017;92(6):854.

102. Wu SY, McCavit TL, Cederberg K, et al. Chemotherapy for generalized infantile myofibromatosis with visceral involvement. *J Pediatr Hematol Oncol* 2015;37(5):402.

103. Ferrari A, Orbach D, Sultan I, et al. Neonatal soft tissue sarcomas. *Semin Fetal Neonatal Med* 2012;17(4):231.

104. Palumbo JS, Zwerdling T. Soft tissue sarcomas of infancy. *Semin Perinatol* 1999;23(4):299.

105. Pride HB, Tollefson M, Silverman R. What's new in pediatric dermatology?: part I. Diagnosis and pathogenesis. *J Am Acad Dermatol* 2013;68(6):885. e1; quiz 897.

106. St John J, Summe H, Csikesz C, et al. Multiple Café au Lait Spots in a Group of fair-skinned children without signs or symptoms of neurofibromatosis type 1. *Pediatr Dermatol* 2016;33(5):526.

107. Kinsler VA, O'Hare P, Bulstrode N, et al. Melanoma in congenital melanocytic naevi. *Br J Dermatol* 2017;176(5):1131.

108. Alikhan A, Ibrahimi OA, Eisen DB. Congenital melanocytic nevi: where are we now? Part I. Clinical presentation, epidemiology, pathogenesis, histology, malignant transformation, and neurocutaneous melanosis. *J Am Acad Dermatol* 2012;67(4):515.e1; quiz 528.

109. Vourc'h-Jourdain M, Martin L, Barbarot S. Large congenital melanocytic nevi: therapeutic management and melanoma risk: a systematic review. *J Am Acad Dermatol* 2013;68(3):493.e1.

110. Bauer J, Curtin JA, Pinkel D, et al. Congenital melanocytic nevi frequently harbor NRAS mutations but no BRAF mutations. *J Invest Dermatol* 2007;127(1):179.

111. Christou EM, Chen AC, Sugo E, et al. Proliferative nodules of undifferentiated spindle cells arising in a large congenital melanocytic naevus. *Australas J Dermatol* 2014;55(2):e24.

112. Nguyen TL, Theos A, Kelly DR, et al. Mitotically active proliferative nodule arising in a giant congenital melanocytic nevus: a diagnostic pitfall. *Am J Dermatopathol* 2013;35(1):e16.

113. Waelchli R, Aylett SE, Atherton D, et al. Classification of neurological abnormalities in children with congenital melanocytic naevus syndrome identifies magnetic resonance imaging as the best predictor of clinical outcome. *Br J Dermatol* 2015;173(3):739.

114. Price HN, Schaffer JV. Congenital melanocytic nevi—when to worry and how to treat: facts and controversies. *Clin Dermatol* 2010;28(3):293.

115. Vaassen P, Rosenbaum T. Nevus anemicus as an additional diagnostic marker of neurofibromatosis type 1 in Childhood. *Neuropediatrics* 2016;47(3):190.

116. Roh D, Shin K, Kim WI, et al. Clinical differences between segmental nevus depigmentosus and segmental vitiligo. *J Dermatol* 2019;46(9):777.

117. Baselga E, Cordisco MR, Garzon M, et al. Rapidly involuting congenital haemangioma associated with transient thrombocytopenia and coagulopathy: a case series. *Br J Dermatol* 2008;158(6):1363.

118. Fujita M, Darmstadt GL, Dinulos JG. Cutis marmorata telangiectatica congenita with hemangiomatous histopathologic features. *J Am Acad Dermatol* 2003;48(6):950.

119. Bui TNPT, Corap A, Bygum A. Cutis marmorata telangiectatica congenita: a literature review. *Orphanet J Rare Dis* 2019;14(1):283.

120. Darmstadt GL. Perianal lymphangioma circumscriptum mistaken for genital warts. *Pediatrics* 1996;98(3 Pt 1):461.

121. Richard G, Bale, SJ. Autosomal recessive congenital ichthyosis. In: Pagon R, Adam MP, Bird TD, et al., eds. *GeneReviews*. Seattle, WA: University of Washington, 2014.

122. Shibata A, Ogawa Y, Sugiura K, et al. High survival rate of harlequin ichthyosis in Japan. *J Am Acad Dermatol* 2014;70(2):387.

123. Sun JD, Linden KG. Netherton syndrome: a case report and review of the literature. *Int J Dermatol* 2006;45(6):693.

124. Chavanas S, Bodemer C, Rochat A, et al. Mutations in SPINK5, encoding a serine protease inhibitor, cause Netherton syndrome. *Nat Genet* 2000;25(2):141.

125. Rice AS, Crane JS. Epidermolytic hyperkeratosis (Bullous Ichthyosiform Erythroderma). In: *StatPearls* [Internet]. Treasure Island, FL: StatPearls Publishing, 2019.

126. Jefferson J, Grossberg A. Incontinentia Pigmenti Coxsackium. *Pediatr Dermatol* 2016;33(5):e280.

127. Gehrig KA, Dinulos JG. Acrodermatitis due to nutritional deficiency. *Curr Opin Pediatr* 2010;22(1):107.

128. Dinulos JG, Zembowicz A. Case records of the Massachusetts General Hospital. Case 32–2008. A 10-year-old girl with recurrent oral lesions and cutaneous bullae. *N Engl J Med* 2008;359(16):1718.

129. Darmstadt GL, McGuire J, Ziboh VA. Malnutrition-associated rash of cystic fibrosis. *Pediatr Dermatol* 2000;17(5):337.

THE NEWBORN INFANT

Index

ESRD. *See* End-stage renal disease (ESRD)
Essential Care for Every Baby (ECEB), 22–23
Estrogen, pulmonary maturation, 368
ETN. *See* Erythema toxicum neonatorum (ETN)
Every Newborn Action Plan (ENAP), 1, 3*t*, 22
Evidence-based Practice for Improving Quality (EPIQ), 23–24
Evolution of cerebral abnormalities, 809
Ex utero intrapartum therapy (EXIT), 211
Examination, 219–235
 abdomen, 227–228
 cardiac, 228–229, 229*t*–230*t*
 chest, 227–228, 227*t*
 color, 219, 220*f*
 conditions, 219
 ears, 224–225
 eyes, 224
 facies, 221–222, 222*f*
 general assessment, 219
 genitalia, 230, 230*t*
 genitourinary system, 229–230, 230*t*
 hair and scalp, 222
 head and neck, 222
 heart rate, 229*t*–230*t*
 inspection, 219
 lymph nodes, 225–227
 mouth and throat, 225, 226*f*, 227*f*
 musculoskeletal system, 230–231
 nervous system, 231–235
 nose, 225, 225*f*
 placenta and cord, 215–216, 216*f*
 posture, 217*f*, 221
 pulse, 229*t*–230*t*
 respiratory effort, 219–221
 skin, 225–227
 spontaneous activity, 221
 state, 219
 vital signs, 221
Excess intracranial mass, removal of, 846–847
Exogenous surfactant replacement therapy, 211
Expanded Ballard score, 217*f*
Extended-spectrum β-lactamase-producing (ESBL) gram negative organisms, 301–302
External genitalia, 664
Extracellular water (ECW)
Extracorporeal cardiopulmonary resuscitation (E-CPR), 498
Extracorporeal life support (ECLS), 61
Extracorporeal membrane oxygenation (ECMO), 64, 312, 487–488, 497
 for PPHN, 378
Extrauterine circulation, transition to, 195–197
Extreme hyperbilirubinemia (EHB), 731, 735*f*, 744*f*
 estimation of global Rh disease burden, 743
 global mortality, due to kernicterus, 743
 incidence of, 743, 743*f*
 National Guidelines and Impact on, 743, 744*f*

Extremely low birth weight infant (ELBW), 94, 216, 218, 300, 767, 772
Eye
 congenital anomalies, 892–896
 crusting, 224
 disorders, 891–904
 enlarged, 892–893, 893*f*
 examination, 224
 examination techniques, 891–892
 growth and development of, 891, 892*f*, 892*t*
 size and shape, anomalies, 892–893
 small, 893, 893*f*
Eyebrows, examination, 224
Eyelids
 abnormalities, 893–894, 894*f*
 tumors, 894

F

FA. *See* Fanconi anemia (FA)
Face masks, for breathing, 207
Face validity measures, 44–45
Facial palsy, 222*f*, 234
Facies, 221–222, 222*f*
Factitious hyperinsulinism, 686
Factor V Leiden (FVL) mutation, 724
FAIR principles for data (Findable, Accessible, Interoperable, and Reusable), 37
Familial focal segmental glomerulosclerosis (FSGS), 613–614
Familial hypocalciuric hypercalcemia, 612
Familial hypophosphatemic rickets. *See* X-linked hypophosphatemia
Familial isolated glucocorticoid insufficiency (FGD), 668
Familial juvenile hyperuricemic nephropathy, 596
Family care, early intervention in, 103
Family, definition, 80
Family-centered care, 7, 10, 58, 80–81, 87–88, 303
 definition, 80
 vs. family-integrated care (FICare), 81
 neonatologist's role in, 81
 recommendations for, 80–81, 81*t*
Family-Integrated Care (FIC), 90
Fanconi anemia (FA), 782, 905
Fanconi syndrome, 607–608
 causes of, 596–597, 608*t*
 disorders of energy metabolism, 607–608
 secondary causes of, 607
Fanconi-Bickel syndrome (FBS), 597, 608
FAS. *See* Fetal alcohol syndrome (FAS)
FASD. *See* Fetal alcohol spectrum disorder (FASD)
Fats
 absorption, 269
 cow's milk, 260
 digestion, 269
 in human milk, 260
 in infant formula, 270
 in preterm human milk, 270
 in preterm infant formulas, 271
 sources, 259–260
Fat-soluble vitamins, requirements, 264

Fatty acids, in preterm infant formulas, 271
FBS. *See* Fanconi-Bickel syndrome (FBS)
Feeding problems, 97–98
Female genital abnormalities, 652–655
Femoral shaft fractures, 927
Fentanyl, 308*t*, 309, 312
 chest-wall rigidity, 319
 dosage, 319*t*
 for pain, 317
Fentanyl–midazolam, for pain, 317
Fetal alcohol spectrum disorder (FASD)
 adverse effects, 171–172
 alcohol-related birth defects, 171–172
 definition, 172
 fetal alcohol syndrome (*see* Fetal alcohol syndrome (FAS))
 fetal and neonatal dysmorphogenesis features, 171–172, 171*t*
 prenatal alcohol exposure, 170
Fetal alcohol syndrome (FAS), 161, 169, 869
 diagnosis of, 171–172
 follow-up of infants with, 172
 hearing disorders, 172
 maternal risk factors for, 172
 prevalence, 172
 underdiagnosis of, 172
Fetal breathing, 190, 352
 during control and CO_2 rebreathing, 191*f*
 discovery of, 190
 in fetal lamb, 190, 190*f*
 oxygen, 190
Fetal breathing movements (FBMs), 187
Fetal cardiac assessment, indications, 471–472, 471*t*
Fetal chromosome anomalies
 biochemical serum screening, 118
 ultrasonographic screening, 118
Fetal circulation, 193, 194*f*
Fetal goiter, 131, 132*f*
Fetal growth restriction (FGR), 148, 150–151, 150*f*, 153, 218
Fetal hypoxia, 793
Fetal infections, in pregnancy, 160–161
 cytomegalovirus, 160
 parvovirus, 161
 rubella, 161
 toxoplasmosis, 160–161
 varicella–zoster virus, 161
 Zika virus, 161
Fetal inflammatory response syndrome (FIRS), 153
Fetal liver biopsy, 123
Fetal lung fluid, 187–188
 absorption, 189*f*
 clearance after birth, 189–190, 189*f*
 clearance at birth, 189
 clearance before birth, 188, 189*f*
 production of, 188
 secretion, 188*f*
 secretory activity, 187–188
Fetal Medicine Foundation (FMF), 118
Fetal metabolism, 678
Fetal pulmonary vascular resistance, regulation of, 193–195, 195*f*
Fetal reduction and selective termination, 130–131, 130*f*
Fetal shunts closure, 196–197